# Pediatrics and Perinatology

## THE SCIENTIFIC BASIS

### Second Edition

EDITED BY

## Peter D. Gluckman

*Professor of Perinatal and Pediatric Biology, and Director, Research Centre for Developmental
Medicine and Biology, University of Auckland, Auckland, New Zealand*

## Michael A. Heymann

*Professor of Pediatrics and Obstetrics, Gynecology and Reproductive Sciences, and Senior Staff
Member, Cardiovascular Research Institute, University of California, San Francisco, California, USA*

Assistant editors

Karen Goldstone and Paul D. Sagan

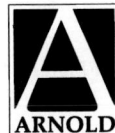

A member of the Hodder Headline Group
LONDON • SYDNEY • AUCKLAND
Co-published in the USA by Oxford University Press, Inc., New York

First published in Great Britain in 1993
as *Perinatal and Pediatric Pathophysiology*

Second edition published in 1996 by
Arnold, a member of the Hodder Headline Group,
338 Euston Road, London NW1 3BH

Co-published in the United States of America by
Oxford University Press, Inc.,
198 Madison Avenue, New York, NY10016
Oxford is a registered trademark of Oxford University Press

Whilst the advice and information in this book is believed to be true and
accurate at the date of going to press, neither the authors nor the publisher
can accept any legal responsibility or liability for any errors or omissions
that may be made. In particular (but without limiting the generality of the
preceding disclaimer) every effort has been made to check drug dosages;
however it is still possible that errors have been missed. Furthermore,
dosage schedules are constantly being revised and new side-effects
recognized. For these reasons the reader is strongly urged to consult the
drug companies' printed instructions before administering any of the drugs
recommended in this book.

*British Library Cataloguing in Publication Data*
A catalogue record for this book is available from the British Library

*Library of Congress Cataloging-in-Publication Data*
A catalog record for this book is available from the Library of Congress

ISBN 0 340 66190 9

Typeset in 9pt Sabon by Keyword Typesetting Services Ltd
Printed and bound in Great Britain by The Bath Press

# Contents

# List of Contributors

**Joel W. Adelson MD, PhD**
Professor of Pediatrics and Physiology and Director, Division of Pediatric Gastroenterology and Nutrition, Brown University, Rhode Island Hospital, Rhode Island, USA

**Thomas E. Adrian PhD, FRCPath**
Professor and Head, Department of Physiology, Department of Biomedical Sciences, Creighton University Medical School, Omaha, NE, USA

**Maureen Andrew MD**
Professor of Pediatrics, Children's Hospital at Chedoke-McMaster Hamilton Civic Hospitals Research Centre, Henderson General Division, Hamilton, Ontario, Canada

**Anita Aperia MD**
Professor of Pediatrics, Karolinska Institute, St Göran's Children's Hospital, Stockholm, Sweden

**Peter Århem PhD**
Associate Professor, University Lecturer in Neurophysiology, Nobel Institute for Neurophysiology, Karolinska Institute, Stockholm, Sweden

**Janette Atkinson PhD**
Professor, Department of Psychology, University College London, London, UK

**Michael Bauer PhD**
Senior Research Fellow, Research Centre for Developmental Medicine and Biology, School of Medicine, University of Auckland, Auckland, New Zealand

**David A. Belford BMedSc, BMBS, PhD**
Senior Research Scientist, CSIRO Division of Human Nutrition and The Child Health Research Institute, Women's and Children's Hospital, Adelaide, Australia

**Nicholas M. Birchall MBChB, FRACP**
Director of Dermatology Research, Genesis Research and Development Ltd, Auckland, New Zealand

**Einat Birk MD**
Department of Pediatric Cardiology, Children's Medical Center of Israel, Petah-Tiqva, Israel

**Stephen M. Black PhD**
Assistant Professor of Pediatrics, Division of Pediatric Critical Care, University of California, San Francisco, California, USA

**Werner F. Blum MD, PhD**
Clinical Research Physician, Lilly Deutschland GmbH, Homburg, Germany

**Robert A. Brace PhD**
Professor of Reproductive Medicine, Division of Perinatal Medicine, University of California, San Diego, La Jolla, California, USA

**James D. Bristow MD**
Associate Professor of Pediatrics, Department of Pediatrics, Division of Pediatric Cardiology, University of California, San Francisco, California, USA

**Robert T. Brouillette MD**
Professor of Pediatrics, McGill University; Division Head, Newborn Medicine Group, The Montreal Children's Hospital, Montreal, Quebec, Canada

**Georgette M. Buga PhD**
Department of Molecular and Medical Pharmacology, UCLA School of Medicine, Center for Health Sciences, Los Angeles, California, USA

**Barbara Cannon MD**
Professor and Chairman of Physiology, Wenner-Gren Institute, the Arrhenius Laboratories, Stockholm University, Stockholm, Sweden

**Anthony D. Care MA, BVMS, PhD, DSc, MRCVS**
Institute of Biological Sciences, University of Wales, Aberystwyth, UK

**Thomas Carlstedt MD, PhD**
Associate Professor, Department of Orthopaedics, Karolinska Institute, Stockholm, Sweden

**David P. Carlton MD**
Department of Pediatrics, Children's Research Center, Division of Lung Biology, University of Utah School of Medicine, Salt Lake City, Utah, USA

**Dale L. Chapman MD**
Granger Medical Clinic, West Valley City, Utah, USA

**Pierre G. Chatelain MD**
Professor of Pediatrics, Université Claude Bernard and INSERM, Hôpital Debrousse, Lyon, France

**Robert D. Christensen MD**
Professor of Pediatrics and Chief, Division of Neonatalogy, Department of Pediatrics, University of Florida College of Medicine, Health Science Center, Gainesville, Florida, USA

**Ronald I. Clyman MD**
Professor of Pediatrics, University of California, San Francisco, California, USA

**Mitchell B. Cohen MD**
Associate Professor of Pediatrics, University of Cincinnati, Children's Hospital Research Foundation, Cincinnati, Ohio, USA

**Garth Cooper MB ChB, DPhil, FRACP**
Professor of Biochemistry and Clinical Biochemistry, School of Biological Sciences and School of Medicine, University of Auckland, New Zealand

**Rodney D. Cooter MBBS, MD, FRACS**
Senior Lecturer, Plastic and Reconstructive Surgery, University of Adelaide, Adelaide, Australia

**Aurore Côté MD**
Assistant Professor of Pediatrics, McGill University, Division of Respiratory Medicine, The Montreal Children's Hospital, Montreal, Quebec, Canada

**Karen D. Crissinger MD, PhD**
Associate Professor of Pediatrics and Physiology, Division of Gastroenterology and Nutrition, Louisiana State University Medical Center, Shreveport, Louisiana, USA

**Staffan Cullheim MD, PhD**
Associate Professor, Department of Neuroscience, Karolinska Institute, Stockholm, Sweden

**Wayne S. Cutfield MB ChB, DCH, FRACP**
Senior Lecturer in Paediatrics, Department of Paediatrics, University of Auckland, Auckland, New Zealand

**Caroline H. Damsky PhD**
Professor of Stomatology and Anatomy, University of California, San Francisco, California, USA

**Suzanne L. Davis MB ChB, PhD**
Department of Paediatrics, University of Auckland, Auckland, New Zealand

**Michael Dragunow PhD**
Associate Professor, Department of Pharmacology and Clinical Pharmacology, University of Auckland, Auckland, New Zealand

**Lars Edström MD**
Department of Clinical Neuroscience, Division of Neurology, Karolinska Hospital, Stockholm, Sweden

**A. David Edwards MA, MB BS, FRCP**
Professor of Paediatrics and Neonatal Medicine, Hammersmith Hospital, London, UK

**Gilbert M. Eisner MD**
Adjunct Professor of Physiology and Biophysics; Clinical Professor of Medicine, Georgetown University Medical Center, Washington DC, USA

**Melissa E. Elder MD, PhD**
Associate Professor of Pediatrics, Department of Pediatrics, University of California, San Francisco, California, USA

**Miles L. Epstein PhD**
Professor, Department of Anatomy, University of Wisconsin Medical School, Madison, Wisconsin, USA

**Stefan Eriksson DDS, PhD**
Associate Professor of Physiology, Department of Physiology and Pharmacology, Karolinska Institute, Stockholm, Sweden

**Arthur R. Euler MD**
Senior Director, Clinical Nutrition, Wyeth Nutrition International, Philadelphia, Pennsylvania, USA

**Jeffrey R. Fineman MD**
Assistant Professor of Pediatrics, Division of Pediatric Critical Care, University of California, San Francisco, California, USA

**Susan J. Fisher PhD**
Professor of Stomatology, Anatomy, Obstetrics, Gynecology and Reproductive Sciences, Division of Oral Biology, University of California, San Francisco, California, USA

**Maria Fitzgerald BA, PhD**
Professor of Developmental Neurobiology, Department of Anatomy and Developmental Biology, University College London, London, UK

**Hans Forssberg MD, PhD**
Professor of Neuropediatrics, Department of Pediatrics, Karolinska Hospital, Stockholm, Sweden

**John T. France PhD, DSc, FAACB**
Associate Professor in Steroid Biochemistry, Department of Obstetrics and Gynecology, National Women's Hospital, University of Auckland School of Medicine, Auckland, New Zealand

**Stephen E. Gitelman MD**
Assistant Professor of Pediatrics, Department of Pediatrics, University of California, San Francisco, California, USA

**Michelle Glass PhD**
Department of Pharmacology and Clinical Pharmacology, University of Auckland, Auckland, New Zealand

**Peter D. Gluckman MB ChB, DSc, FRACP, FRSNZ**
Professor of Perinatal and Pediatric Biology and Director, Research Centre for Developmental Medicine and Biology, University of Auckland, Auckland, New Zealand

**Mitchell S. Golbus MD**
Professor of Obstetrics, Gynecology, and Reproductive Sciences and of Pediatrics, University of California, San Francisco, California, USA

**Anthony W. Goodwin PhD**
Associate Professor, Department of Anatomy and Cell Biology, University of Melbourne, Parkville, Victoria, Australia

**Glenn R. Gourley MD**
Professor of Pediatrics, University of Wisconsin School of Medicine, Madison, Wisconsin, USA

**Anne Green BSc, MSc, PhD, FRSC, FRCPath**
Consultant Biochemist, Department of Clinical Chemistry, Birmingham Children's Hospital, Birmingham, UK

**Dan Greitz MD, PhD**
Assistant Professor, Karolinska MR Research Center, Karolinska Institute, Stockholm, Sweden

**Alistair Gunn MB ChB, FRACP, PhD**
Research Fellow, Research Centre for
Developmental Medicine and Biology, University of
Auckland, New Zealand

**Tania R. Gunn, MBChB, MD, FRCPC**
Associate Professor, Department of Pediatrics,
National Women's Hospital, Epsom, New Zealand

**Victor K. M. Han MD, FRCPC(C), FRCP**
Associate Professor, Department of Paediatrics, The
Lawson Research Institute, St Joseph's Hospital,
University of Western Ontario, London, Ontario,
Canada

**Mark A. Hanson MD, PhD**
Professor of Fetal and Neonatal Physiology,
Department of Obstetrics and Gynaecology,
University College London Medical School, London,
UK

**Aviad Haramati PhD**
Professor of Physiology and Biophysics, Georgetown
University School of Medicine, Washington DC,
USA

**Terry O. Harville MD, PhD**
Assistant Professor of Pediatrics, Division of Allergy
and Immunology, Duke University Medical Center,
Durham, North Carolina, USA

**Samuel Hawgood MB BS**
Professor of Pediatrics, Department of Pediatrics and
Cardiovascular Research Institute, University of
California, San Francisco, California, USA

**William W. Hay, Jr MD**
Professor of Pediatrics, Division of Perinatal
Medicine, University of Colorado School of
Medicine, Denver, Colorado, USA

**Mikael Heimann PhD**
Associate Professor, Department of Psychology,
Göteborg University, Göteborg, Sweden

**David J. Henderson-Smart MB BS, PhD, FRACP**
Professor of Perinatal Medicine, King George V
Memorial Hospital, Camperdown, NSW, Australia

**James E. Heubi MD**
Professor of Pediatrics, University of Cincinnati
College of Medicine; Director, Clinical Research
Center, Children's Hospital Medical Center,
Cincinnati, Ohio, USA

**Michael A. Heymann MD**
Professor of Pediatrics and Obstetrics, Gynecology
and Reproductive Sciences, and Senior Staff
Member, Cardiovascular Research Instititue,
University of California, San Francisco, California,
USA

**David J. Hill PhD, DPhil**
MRC Group in Fetal & Neonatal Health &
Development, Lawson Professor & Diabetes
Research, Professor, Departments of Medicine,
Physiology & Paediatrics, The Lawson Research
Institute, St Joseph's Hospital, University of Western
Ontario, London, Ontario, Canada

**Julien I. E. Hoffman MD**
Professor of Pediatrics, University of California, San
Francisco, California, USA

**Barbara M. Holland MB, FRCP(Glas)**
Consultant Neonatologist, Queen Mother's
Hospital, University of Glasgow, Glasgow, UK

**Ieuan A. Hughes MB BS, FRCP**
Professor of Pediatrics, University of Cambridge
School of Clinical Medicine, Addenbrooke's
Hospital, Cambridge, UK

**Sir David Hull FRCP**
Professor, Department of Child Health, University
of Nottingham, Nottingham, UK

**Louis J. Ignarro PhD**
Professor of Molecular and Medical Pharmacology,
UCLA School of Medicine, Center for Health
Sciences, Los Angeles, California, USA

**Olle G. P. Isaksson MD**
Professor of Endocrinology; Chief Physician,
Department of Internal Medicine, Sahlgrenska
University Hospital, Göteborg, Sweden

**Jorgen Isgaard MD, PhD**
Department of Internal Medicine, Sahlgrenska
University Hospital, Göteborg, Sweden

**Harriet S. Iwamoto PhD**
Associate Professor of Pediatrics and Molecular and
Cellular Physiology, Children's Hospital Medical
Center, Cincinnati, Ohio, USA

**Alan A. Jackson MA, MD, FRCP**
Professor of Human Nutrition, Institute of Human
Nutrition, University of Southampton,
Southampton, UK

**Clinton H. Joiner MD, PhD**
Associate Professor of Pediatrics and Molecular and
Cellular Physiology; Director, Cincinnati
Comprehensive Sickle Cell Center, University of
Cincinnati College of Medicine, Children's Hospital
Medical Center, Cincinnati, Ohio, USA

**J. G. Jones BPharm, PhD**
Senior Lecturer in Biochemistry, University of Wales
College of Cardiff, Cardiff, UK

**Pedro A. Jose MD, PhD**
Professor of Pediatrics and Physiology and
Biophysics; Vice-Chair of Pediatrics, Georgetown
University Children's Medical Center, Washington,
DC, USA

**Nathalie Josso MD**
Unité de Recherches sur l'Endocrinologie du
Développement, Département de Biologie, Ecole
Normale Supérieure, Mont Rouge, France

**Stuart S. Kaufman MD**
Associate Professor, Department of Pediatrics, Joint
Section of Pediatric GI and Nutrition, Creighton
University School of Medicine, Children's Hospital,
Omaha, NE, USA

**Gideon Koren MD, ABMT, FRCP(C)**
Professor of Pediatrics, University of Toronto;
Director of the Motherisk Program, Division of
Clinical Pharmacology and Toxicology, The
Hospital for Sick Children, Toronto, Ontario,
Canada

**Krister Kristensson MD**
Professor of Neuropathology, Department of Neuroscience, Karolinska Institute, Stockholm, Sweden

**Jeffrey A. Kuller MD**
Director of Reproductive Genetics, Department of Obstetrics and Gynecology, Division of Maternal and Fetal Medicine, The University of North Carolina at Chapel Hill, Chapel Hill, North Carolina, USA

**Hugo Lagercrantz MD, PhD**
Professor of Pediatrics, Department of Pediatrics, Karolinska Hospital, Stockholm, Sweden

**Maggie Lai PhD**
Research Fellow, Research Centre for Developmental Medicine and Biology, University of Auckland, Auckland, New Zealand

**Urban Lendahl PhD**
University Lecturer, Department of Cell and Molecular Biology, Karolinska Institute, Stockholm, Sweden

**Gunnar Lennerstrand MD, PhD**
Professor of Ophthalmology, Department of Ophthalmology, Karolinska Institute, Huddinge University Hospital, Huddinge, Sweden

**Sir Graham C. Liggins MB, PhD, FRCS, FRCOG, FRS, FRSNZ**
Emeritus Professor of Obstetrics and Gynecology, University of Auckland, National Women's Hospital, Auckland, New Zealand

**Kee-Hak Lim MD**
Assistant Professor of Obstetrics, Gynecology and Reproductive Sciences, University of California, San Francisco, California, USA

**George Lister MD**
Professor of Pediatrics, Yale University School of Medicine, Section of Critical Care and Applied Physiology, New Haven, CT, USA

**Stephen J. Lye PhD**
Professor of Obstetrics and Gynecology and of Physiology, University of Toronto; Co-Head, Program in Development and Fetal Health, Samuel Lunefeld Research Institute of Mount Sinai Hospital, Toronto, Ontario, Canada

**Lynn K. McClean MD**
Department of Obstetrics, Gynecology and Reproductive Sciences, University of California, San Francisco, California, USA

**John McIntyre MRCP**
Research Fellow, Child development Centre, Addenbrooke's Hospital, Cambridge, UK

**I. C. McMillen MB BS, DPhil**
Professor and Chair, Department of Physiology, University of Adelaide, Adelaide, Australia

**Ronald R. Magness PhD**
Professor of Obstetrics, Gynecology and Meat/Animal Sciences, Perinatal Research Laboratories, University of Wisconsin, Madison, Wisconsin, USA

**M. Patricia Massicotte MD**
Research Fellow, Hamilton Civic Hospitals Research Center, Henderson General Division, Hamilton, Ontario, Canada

**Doreen Matsui MD, FRCP(C)**
Assistant Professor of Pediatrics, University of Western Ontario, Division of Pediatric Clinical Pharmacology, Children's Hospital of Western Ontario, London, Ontario, Canada

**R. David G. Milner DSc, MD, FRCP**
Research Professor, Department of Obstetrics and Gynecology, U Z Gasthuisberg, Leuven, Belgium

**Rebecca Eve Mischel MD**
Neonatology Fellow, Department of Pediatrics, University of California, San Francisco, California, USA

**Murray D. Mitchell DPhil, DSc**
Professor and Head, Department of Pharmacology and Clinical Pharmacology, University of Auckland, New Zealand

**William Mobley MD, PhD**
Professor of Neurology, Pediatrics and the Neuroscience Program, University of California, San Francisco, California, USA

**Kjeld Møllgård MD, PhD**
Professor of Anatomy and Rector of the University of Copenhagen, Institute of Medical Anatomy, The Panum Institute, University of Copenhagen, Copenhagen, Denmark

**Susan E. Mulroney PhD**
Assistant Professor, Department of Physiology and Biophysics, Georgetown University School of Medicine, Washington DC, USA

**Robert D. Murray MD**
Associate Professor of Pediatrics, Division of Gastroenterology and Nutrition, The Ohio State University, Children's Hospital, Columbus, Ohio, USA

**Leslie Myatt PhD**
Professor of Obstetrics and Gynecology, Pediatrics and Molecular and Cellular Physiology, The Perinatal Research Institute, University of Cincinnati, Cincinnati, Ohio, USA

**Jan Nedergaard MD, PhD**
Professor of Physiology, Wenner-Gren Institute, The Arrhenius Laboratories, Stockholm University, Stockholm, Sweden

**Jan G. Nijhuis MD, PhD**
Associate Professor of Perinatology, Department of Obstetrics and Gynecology, University Hospital Nijmegen, Nijmegen, The Netherlands

**Anders Nilsson MD, PhD**
RCEM, Department of Internal Medicine, Sahlgrenska University Hospital, Göteborg, Sweden

**Richard S. Nowakowski PhD**
Associate Professor, Department of Neuroscience and Cell Biology, UMDNJ-Robert Wood Johnson Medical School, Piscataway, New Jersey, USA

**Hans D. Ochs MD**
Professor of Pediatrics, Division of Immunology and
Rheumatology, Department of Pediatrics, University
of Washington School of Medicine, Seattle,
Washington, USA

**David M. Olson PhD**
The University of Alberta Perinatal Research Center,
Edmonton, Alberta, Canada

**Julie A. Owens BSc, PhD**
NHMRC Research Fellow, Department of
Obstetrics and Gynecology, University of Adelaide,
Adelaide, Australia

**James F. Padbury MD**
Professor and Vice Chair of Pediatrics, Brown
University School of Medicine, Department of
Pediatrics, Women and Infants' Hospital, Rhode
Island, Providence, RI 02905, USA

**R. Mark Payne MD**
Assistant Professor of Pediatrics, Division of
Pediatric Cardiology, Washington University School
of Medicine, St Louis, Missouri, USA

**William J. Pearce PhD**
Associate Professor of Physiology, Center for
Perinatal Biology, Department of Physiology, Loma
Linda University School of Medicine, Loma Linda,
California, USA

**J. Julio Pérez Fontán MD**
Associate Professor of Pediatrics and
Anesthesiology, Division of Critical Care Medicine,
Washington University School of Medicine, St Louis
Children's Hospital, St Louis, Missouri, USA

**Alan G. Pettigrew BSc, PhD**
Professor of Physiology, University of Queensland,
Australia and George Peabody College of Vanderbilt
University, Nashville, Tennessee, USA

**Anthony C. Poole, BSc (Hons), PhD**
Health Research Council Senior Research Fellow
Department of Anatomy, University of Auckland,
Auckland, New Zealand

**Richard H. Porter PhD**
Director de Recherche Centre National de la
Recherche Scientifique France, Laboratoire de
Comportement Animal, Nouzilly, France

**Martin Post PhD**
Professor of Pediatrics; Director of Research,
Division of Neonatology, University of Toronto,
The Hospital for Sick Children, Toronto, Ontario,
Canada

**Mary Anne Preece BSc, MSc, MCB**
Principal Biochemist, Department of Clinical
Chemistry, Birmingham Children's Hospital NHS
Trust, Birmingham, UK

**Bjørn Quistorff MD, DSc**
Professor of Biochemistry, NMR Centre, Institute of
Medical Biochemistry and Genetics, The Panum
Institute, University of Copenhagen & Blegalamsvej,
Copenhagen, Denmark 2200

**Francisco J. Ramos-Gomez DDS, MSc, MPH**
Assistant Professor, Department of Growth and
Development, Division of Pediatric Dentistry,
University of California, San Francisco, California,
USA

**Sandra Rees PhD**
Senior Lecturer, Department of Anatomy and Cell
Biology, University of Melbourne, Parkville,
Victoria, Australia

**Ian R. Reid MBChB, MD, FRACP**
Associate Professor of Medicine, Department of
Medicine, University of Auckland, Auckland, New
Zealand

**Edward O. Reiter MD**
Professor of Pediatrics, Tufts University; Chairman,
Department of Pediatrics, Baystate Medical Center
Children's Hospital, Springfield, Massachusetts,
USA

**Gail E. Richards MD**
Professor and Head, Department of Pediatrics,
University of Auckland, Auckland, New Zealand

**Bryan S. Richardson MD, FRCS(C)**
Professor of Obstetrics and Gynaecology and of
Physiology, University of Western Ontario, MRC
Group in Fetal and Neonatal Health and
Development, Lawson Research Institute, London,
Ontario, Canada

**R. Kirk Riemer PhD**
Assistant Professor of Surgery, Department of
Surgery, University of California, San Francisco,
California, USA

**Märten Risling MD, PhD**
Associate Professor, Department of Neuroscience,
Karolinska Institute, Stockholm, Sweden

**James M. Roberts MD**
Professor of Obstetrics, Gynecology and
Reproductive Sciences; Director of Research, Magee
Women's Research Institute, University of
Pittsburgh, Pittsburgh, Pennsylvania, USA

**Jean E. Robillard MD**
Professor and Chairman of Pediatrics, University of
Michigan, Ann Arbor, Michigan, USA

**Jeffrey S. Robinson MB ChB, BAO, FRACOG**
Professor and Chairman, Department of Obstetrics
and Gynaecology, University of Adelaide, Adelaide,
Australia

**Colin D. Rudolph MD, PhD**
Assistant Professor of Pediatrics, Division of
Pediatric Gastroenterology and Nutrition, University
of Cincinnati College of Medicine, Children's
Hospital Medical Center, Cincinnati, Ohio, USA

**M. Rundgren MD, PhD**
Associate Professor of Physiology, Department of
Physiology and Pharmacology, Karolinska Institute,
Stockholm, Sweden

**James P. Ryan PhD**
Professor and Deputy Chairman, Department of
Physiology, Temple University School of Medicine,
Philadelphia, Pennsylvania, USA

**Jossi Sack MD**
Professor in Pediatrics and Endocrinology, Tel-Aviv
University, Sackler School of Medicine, Tel-
Hashomer, Israel

**Yoel Sadovsky MD**
Assistant Professor of Obstetrics and Gynecology, Department of Obstetrics and Gynecology, Division of Maternal Fetal Medicine, Washington University School of Medicine, St Louis, Missouri, USA

**Lisa M. Satlin MD**
Associate Professor of Pediatrics, Rose F Kennedy Center, Division of Nephrology, Albert Einstein College of Medicine, Bronx, New York, USA

**Norman R. Saunders BSc, MB BS, PhD**
Professor and Head, Department of Physiology, University of Tasmania, Hobart, Tasmania, Australia

**Kurt R. Schibler MD**
Assistant Professor of Pediatrics, Divisions of Neonatology and Human Development and Aging, University of Utah School of Medicine, Salt Lake City, Utah, USA

**Arne Schousboe DSc**
Professor, PharmaBiotec Research Center, Department of Biological Sciences, Royal Danish School of Pharmacy, Copenhagen, Denmark

**Dennis Scolnik MB ChB, DCH, FRCP(C)**
Assistant Professor of Pediatrics, University of Toronto, Division of Emergency Services, The Hospital for Sick Children, Toronto, Ontario, Canada

**Thomas Sejersen MD, PhD**
Assistant Professor, Department of Cell and Molecular Biology, Karolinska Institute, Stockholm, Sweden

**Richard S. Shames MD**
Assistant Clinical Professor of Pediatrics, Director, Pediatric Allergy Section, University of California, San Francisco, USA

**Kevin Shannon MD**
Associate Professor of Pediatrics, University of California, San Francisco, California, USA

**Robert J. Shulman MD**
Associate Professor of Pediatrics, Section of Nutrition and Gastroenterology, Baylor College of Medicine; Director, Nutritional Support Team, Children's Nutrition Research Center, Texas Children's Hospital, Houston, Texas, USA

**Faye S. Silverstein MDCM**
Professor of Pediatrics and Neurology, Departments of Pediatrics and Neurology, University of Michigan, Ann Arbor, Michigan, USA

**Stephen J. M. Skinner PhD**
Head, Cell Biology, Research Centre for Developmental Medicine and Biology, University of Auckland, Auckland, New Zealand

**Stephen K. Smith MD, MRCOG**
Professor of Obstetrics and Gynecology, University of Cambridge, Cambridge, UK

**Scott J. Soifer MD**
Professor of Pediatrics; Director, Division of Pediatric Critical Care, University of San Francisco, San Francisco, USA

**Bonny L. Specker PhD**
Associate Professor, Department of Pediatrics, Division of Neonatology, University of Cincinnati Medical Center, Cincinnati, Ohio, USA

**Kurt R. Stenmark MD**
Professor of Pediatrics, Head, Division of Critical Care Medicine and Developmental Lung Biology, Department of Pediatrics, University of Colorado Health Sciences Center, Denver, Colorado, USA

**Lennart Stjärne MD**
Professor, Department of Physiology and Pharmacology, Karolinska Institute, Stockholm, Sweden

**N. Susan Stott MB, BCh, FRACS**
Senior Lecturer in Orthopaedic Surgery, Department of Surgery, School of Medicine, University of Auckland, Auckland, New Zealand

**Kathleen E. Sullivan MD, PhD**
Assistant Professor of Pediatrics, University of Pensylvania School of Medicine, Division of Allergy, Immunology and Infectious Diseases, Children's Hospital of Philadelphia, Pennsylvania, USA

**Toshiaki Tanaka MD**
Director, Department of Endocrinology and Metabolism, National Children's Medical Research Center, Tokyo, Japan

**David F. Teitel MD**
Professor of Pediatrics, University of California, San Francisco, San Francisco, California, USA

**Peter R. Thorne PhD**
Senior Lecturer, Department of Physiology, University of Auckland, Auckland, New Zealand

**Lars-Erik Thornell MD, PhD**
Professor of Anatomy, Department of Pediatrics, Karolinska Institute, Stockholm, Sweden

**Brun Ulfhake MD, PhD**
University Lecturer, Department of Neuroscience, Karolinska Institute, Stockholm, Sweden

**George F. Van Hare MD**
Associate Professor of Pediatrics and Medicine, Case Western Reserve University School of Medicine; Director, Pediatric Arrhythmia Service, Rainbow Babies' and Children's Hospital, Cleveland, Ohio, USA

**David L. Vaux MD, PhD**
Dunlop Cancer Research Fellow, The Walter and Eliza Hall Institute of Medical Research, Victoria, Australia

**David Walker PhD**
Senior Research Fellow, Department of Physiology, Monash University, Clayton, Victoria, Australia

**David Warburton BSc, MD, MRCP**
Professor of Surgery, Pediatrics and Craniofacial Molecular Biology, University of Southern California, Children's Hospital Los Angeles Research Institute, Los Angeles, California, USA

**Charles A. J. Wardrop MB, FRCPE, FRCPath**
Senior Lecturer in Hematology, University of Wales College of Medicine, University Hospital of Wales, Cardiff, UK

**James D. Watson PhD**
Scientific Director, Genesis Research and
Development Corporation Limited, Auckland, New
Zealand

**Mary C. Weiser PhD**
Instructor in Pediatrics, Division of Critical Care and
Developmental Lung Biology, Department of
Pediatrics, University of Colorado Health Sciences
Center, Denver, Colorado, USA

**Barry K. Wershil MD**
Assistant Professor of Pediatrics, The Combined
Program in Pediatric Gastroenterology and
Nutrition, Boston Children's Hospital and Harvard
Medical School, Boston, Massachusetts, USA

**Niels Westergaard PhD**
Department of Biological Sciences, Royal Danish
School of Pharmacy, Copenhagen, Denmark

**Jan Winberg MD, PhD**
Professor Emeritus of Pediatrics, Institution for
Women and Child Health, Karolinska Hospital,
Stockholm, Sweden

**Ingrid Winship MB ChB, MD**
Senior Lecturer in Clinical Genetics, Department of
Molecular Medicine, University of Auckland,
Auckland, New Zealand

**Christine C. Winterbourn PhD**
Professorial Research Fellow; Director, Free Radical
Research Group, Department of Pathology,
University of Otago, Christchurch School of
Medicine, Christchurch, New Zealand

**Jonathan R. Wispé MD**
Associate Professor of Pediatrics, Divisions of
Neonatology and Pulmonary Biology, University of
Cincinnati, Children's Hospital Medical Center,
Cincinnati, Ohio, USA

**Jan Ygge MD, PhD**
Associate Professor, Department of Ophthalmology,
Karolinska Institute, Huddinge Hospital, Huddinge,
Sweden

**Deborah Young MSc**
Department of Pharmacology and Clinical
Pharmacology, University of Auckland, Auckland,
New Zealand

**Francis de Zegher MD, PhD**
Department of Pediatrics, University Hospital
Gasthuisberg, University of Leuven, Leuven,
Belgium

**Eugen Zeisberger PhD**
Professor of Physiology, Physiological Institute,
Justus Liebig University, Giessen, Germany

**Jing Zheng PhD**
Postdoctoral Research Fellow, Perinatal Research
Laboratories, University of Wisconsin, Madison,
Wisconsin, USA

# Preface to Second Edition

This volume, *Pediatrics and Perinatology: The Scientific Basis*, is the second edition of our multi-author text, first published as *Perinatal and Pediatric Pathophysiology*. The change of name was suggested by many readers who felt that the original title was too narrow. We agreed: the new title far more accurately reflects the purpose of the book.

Clinical pediatrics and perinatology present many exciting challenges: first because of the interaction between the doctor, child, and family, and second because of the intellectual perspective. The latter reflects the remarkable changes in physiology consequent to passage from fetus to neonate to infant to child to adolescent. The major changes in normal body function apparent throughout this period are reflected in the patterns and processes of diseases observed. Furthermore, these disease processes themselves may alter the pattern of development. Consideration of normal and abnormal development, along with the range of pathophysiology and disease states encountered, requires that the pediatrician and perinatologist have a current and in-depth understanding of normal and abnormal biology from a developmental perspective. The rapid explosion of knowledge in cellular biology, molecular biology, biochemistry, and physiology increases this imperative: practicing pediatricians must understand developmental biology in order to fully advance clinical care. Conversely, experimentalists must look for clinical relevance in their studies to minimize the gap between clinical practice and contemporary biology.

This book arose from our concern that there were no easy avenues for pediatricians or perinatologists to attain a comprehensive understanding of the scientific basis relevant to their clinical disciplines. In our experience, this lack of access to essential information was compromising the ability to give pediatricians and perinatologists in training an understanding of the basic science essential to providing high-quality clinical care. This volume should also be of value to experimentalists who require an understanding of developmental and clinical perspectives.

The text has been revised extensively since the first edition. The chapters on membrane, cellular and molecular biology, and on immunology are totally rewritten. New chapters have been added on genetics and clinical genetics and on bone, connective tissue and skin development. The chapter on neurophysiology is greatly extended with reference to both basic physiology and developmental aspects. Many other contributions are totally rewritten, and all have been updated. While our intent has been to present only that information we consider essential for the modern practice of pediatrics and perinatology, in places we have asked authors to provide additional detail as exemplars of how new findings in medical biology will soon be applied to clinical practice.

Our approach has been to select contributors who are acknowledged leaders working at the cutting edge of their fields. We particularly sought contributions from active clinician-researchers or from experimentalists working in close collaboration with pediatricians or obstetricians to ensure the relevance of the data presented. We have demanded an emphasis on new knowledge and have been richly rewarded. At the same time, we have sought to be comprehensive so that pediatricians or obstetricians in training can find what is necessary in a single volume. While the text presents basic science, it does so from both a developmental and a clinical perspective. There are frequent italicized references to the disease states associated with disordered biology, and each chapter has a strong focus on developmental aspects. Separate chapters address the particular features of pediatrics: growth and important phases of development, including fetal life and puberty.

We thank all those who have contributed in a timely manner to this second edition. Our colleague, David Milner, who contributed much to both editions as chapter editor, died suddenly during the final phase of preparation of this volume. As a pediatric clinician-scientist he contributed much to our understanding of perinatal growth and development. We hope that the book will prove attractive to clinicians and experimentalists, and essential to pediatricians and perinatologists in training.

*Peter D Gluckman and Michael A Heymann*
*1996*

# PART ONE

# *Membrane and Cellular Biology*

**Editors: James D. Bristow, Stephen E. Gitelman and Stephen M. Black**

# 1

# Molecular Biology

Stephen M. Black and James D. Bristow

## STRUCTURE OF NUCLEIC ACIDS

When the term "gene" is used, most biologists will immediately think of deoxyribonucleic acid or DNA. DNA is known to be the molecule of heredity since it meets the following requirements necessary to qualify as the substance that transmits genetic information:

- it stores the information in a stable form
- it can be reproduced and transmitted intact to the next generation
- it can be expressed to produce other relevant biological macromolecules
- it is capable of variation.

However, genetic phenomena involve three types of biological macromolecules, DNA (as the genetic material), ribonucleic acid (RNA, the intermediary or messenger) and proteins (the functional entities of the cell). Each of these molecules will be considered.

## STRUCTURAL CONSIDERATIONS

Nucleic acids, both DNA and RNA, have three major components: pentose sugars, phosphoric acid and nitrogen-containing aromatic bases. The structural components of nucleic acids are shown in Fig. 1.1. The first two constituents can be considered as invariant, except for the presence (ribose) or absence (deoxyribose) of a hydroxyl group on the sugar residue at the 2'-position in RNA and DNA respectively (Fig. 1.1(b)). Thus only the aromatic bases differ. There are only five common nitrogenous bases which are found in all organisms from virus to man: the purines (adenine and guanine) and the pyrimidines (uracil, thymine and cytosine) (Fig. 1.1(c)). Each base is joined to the sugar moiety via a N-glycosyl bond resulting in the formation of a *nucleoside*. Furthermore, each nucleoside carries a phosphate group linked to the 5'-OH of the sugar moiety through a phosphoester bond, forming a *nucleotide* (Fig. 1.1(a)). One, two or three phosphate groups may be added through the formation of pyrophosphate linkages at the 5'-terminal phosphate resulting in the formation of nucleoside mono-, di-, or triphosphates. However, it is as a polynucleotide that nucleic acids function. In the polymerized form each nucleoside is linked via a 3',5'-phosphodiester bond formed when a single phosphate group connects adjacent sugar residues at the 3'- and 5'-hydroxyl positions (Fig. 1.2). This forms a regular sugar-phosphate repeating unit which is constant throughout the

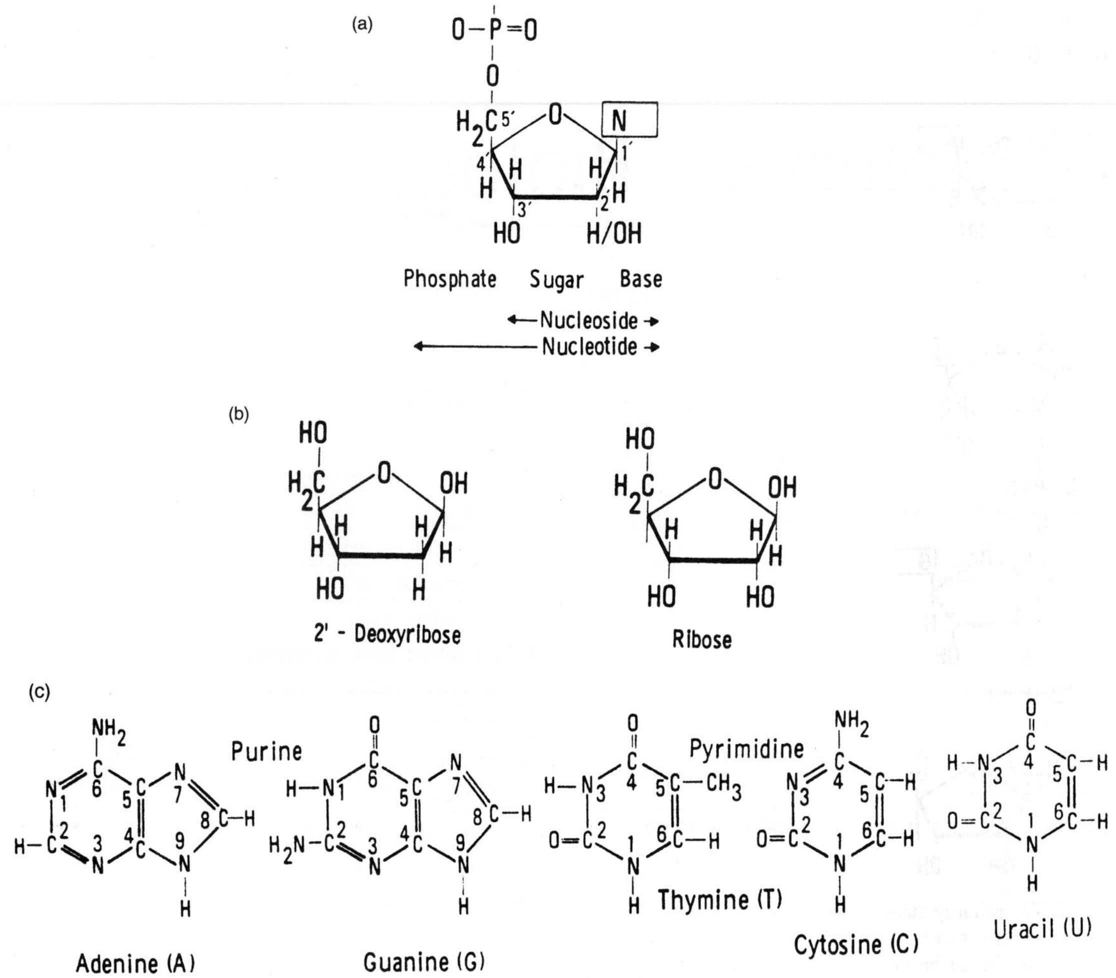

FIGURE 1.1 The three components of nucleic acids are shown in panel (a), where N refers to any nitrogenous base. Panel (b) shows the difference in the sugar components between DNA (2'-deoxyribose) and RNA (ribose). Panel (c) shows the structure of the five nitrogenous bases. It should be noted that uracil is only found in RNA molecules where it replaces thymine.

molecule. From this regular *backbone* extend the purine or pyrimidine bases. By definition the structure formed has polarity since the growing chain carries only a single 5'-terminal phosphate and a single 3'-hydroxyl group free of a sugar linkage.

## THE DOUBLE HELIX

Whereas the RNA chain is present in the single-stranded form shown in Fig. 1.2, DNA is more commonly found as a duplex. Thus two strands formed as in Fig. 1.2 become associated through weak non-ionic interactions known as *hydrogen bonds*. These interactions are limited such that the associations, known as *base-pairing*, can occur only between purines and pyrimidines (Fig. 1.3). Thus the 6-amino group of adenine pairs with the 4-keto group of thymine (A–T pairing), which along with interactions between the ring nitrogens form two hydrogen bonds. Similar interactions occur between the amino and keto groups of guanine and cytosine (G–C pairing) which in addition to the ring nitrogen interactions yields three hydrogen bonds and thus makes a G–C pairing more stable than an A–T pairing. Each strand thus becomes a complement of the other, with the sequence of one being dictated by the other, and produces two chains that are anti-parallel with respect to each other. Thus the 5'-terminus of one chain is attached to the 3'-end of its complement, and the internucleotide bonding is 3'→5' in one strand and 5'→3' in the other (Fig. 1.4). This phenomenon becomes more crucial when we examine the secondary structure of DNA.

In 1953, Watson and Crick correctly deduced that the two strands of the DNA molecule are coiled around a common axis with the purine and pyrimidine bases facing inwards and with the sugar and phosphate groups on the outside forming a *double helix* (Fig. 1.5). Each turn of the helix is separated by 10 nucleotide pairs (about 3.4 nm) and has a diameter of 2 nm. The base pair interactions form two grooves within the helix to produce the so-called minor and major grooves. The major groove appears to be involved in

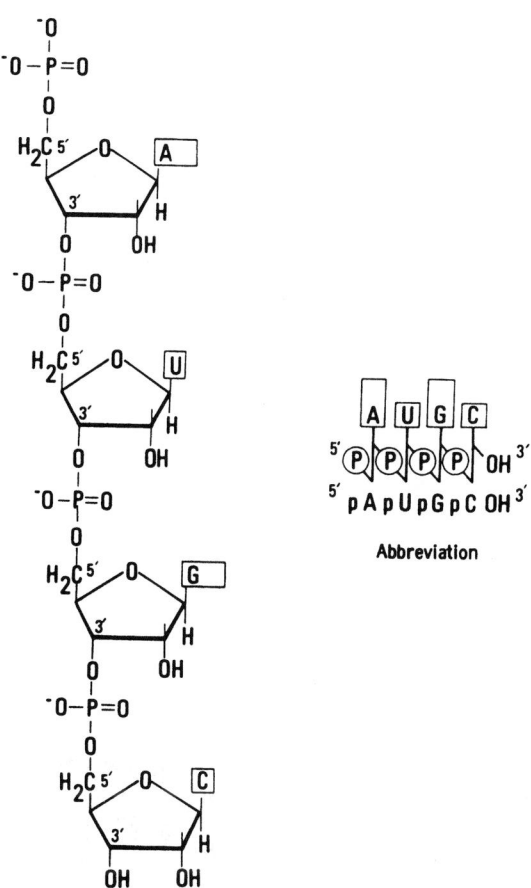

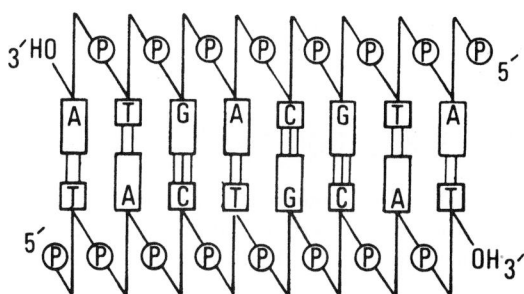

FIGURE 1.4 Formation of complementary sequences. An eight base-pair stretch of double-stranded DNA is shown according to the abbreviation depicted in Fig. 1.2. Note that each base-pair consists of a pyrimidine and a purine with either two (for the A–T pairing) or three (for the G–C pairing) hydrogen bonds. Note also the formation of the $5' \to 3'/3' \to 5'$ anti-parallel chains.

FIGURE 1.2 The primary structure of a polyribonucleotide. The full chemical structure is shown at left and the abbreviation on the right. It should be noted that no matter how long the linear sequence there is only a single $5'$- phosphoryl group and a single $3'$-hydroxyl group per molecule.

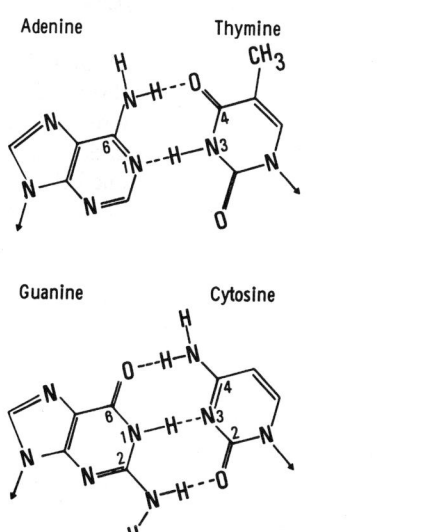

FIGURE 1.3 Nitrogenous bases allow hydrogen bonding. The dotted lines indicate the presence of hydrogen bonding. In each base pair there is pairing between a large purine and a small pyrimidine. Hydrogen bond formation is limited to adenine and thymine (forming two bonds) and guanine and cytosine (which form three bonds).

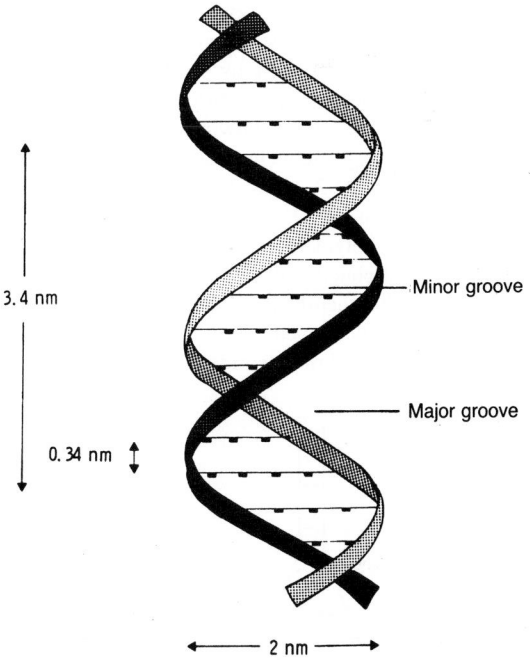

FIGURE 1.5 The double helix. The regular B-form of DNA has a pitch of 3.4 nm with an axial repeat distance of 0.34 nm corresponding to 10 base pairs per turn of the helix with both a major and minor groove. The width of the helix corresponds to 2 nm.

base-specific interactions with proteins which may ultimately serve to regulate the expression of specific genes.

## DNA REPLICATION

The DNA molecule must also be propagated from one generation to the next and thus there must be a mechanism to copy the DNA. This process of *DNA replication* involves opening up, and unwinding into single strands, the two strands of the double helix and the subsequent formation of new strands by insertion of new units as dictated by complementary base-pairing restrictions. The process occurs in both directions from a defined starting point. However, replication can only occur at the $3'$-hydroxyl end, and since the two strands are anti-parallel, it is not possible for synthesis to occur simply by the successive addition of single nucleotides. Instead, DNA replication occurs by the addition of short fragments (Okazaki fragments) which are then joined (Fig. 1.6). A specific enzyme, *DNA polymerase*, connects each nucleotide to the short fragment, and these are subsequently joined together by another enzyme, *DNA ligase*, to form the completed strand. The strand opposite that being newly synthesized acts as a *template* to ensure that the proper nucleotide is inserted onto the growing strand by the restrictions of complementary base-pairing. In addition, the growing strand itself can act as a primer, serving as a site for the addition of new nucleotides. DNA polymerase is thus incapable of synthesizing DNA *de novo* but can only copy a preexisting template. In most cases, the initial primer requirement for DNA replication is met by small DNA or RNA fragments associating with the origin(s) of replication. As the DNA double helix unwinds, at one or a few predetermined origin sequences, a *primase* synthesizes a short strand of DNA or RNA complementary to the unwound section of DNA. Once the priming has occurred DNA polymerase takes over with the addition of deoxyribonucleotides to the $3'$-end of the priming strand. Subsequently the primer is removed by a *nuclease* and the destroyed region is filled in with complementary deoxyribonucleotides. Finally the short fragments are joined together to complete the synthesis of the complete DNA strand.

## DNA TRANSCRIPTION AND TRANSLATION

Ribonucleic acid (RNA) plays a number of important roles in the expression of genetic information. To accomplish these roles RNA is found in three major forms: (1) messenger RNA (mRNA); (2) transfer RNA (tRNA); (3) ribosomal RNA (rRNA). There are three key chemical differences between RNA and DNA. First, RNA contains a *ribose* sugar rather than *deoxyribose*; second, RNA contains the base *uracil* instead of thymine; and third, except in certain viruses, RNA is not double-stranded.

### Messenger RNA (mRNA)

The existence of mRNA was first suspected because of the need for an intermediary in eukaryotic cells to carry information from the nucleus to the cytoplasm where proteins are synthesized. It was expected that an RNA intermediate would serve as a template on which amino acids were assembled to produce the required protein.

mRNA is now known to be synthesized from the DNA template by a process called *transcription*. In general, the DNA acting as the template is double-stranded, but only one of the two strands is transcribed, and this is known as the *sense* strand. Base-pairing rules are used to synthesize mRNA, and the mRNA is thus identical to the non-coding DNA strand. mRNA has only one known purpose: to be translated into protein. However, there are differences in both the synthesis and structure of mRNA in prokaryotes and eukaryotes. The most obvious difference is that in eukaryotes mRNA is synthesized as a large precursor molecule in the nucleus and undergoes a long and complex maturational process before being translated in the cytoplasm. In prokaryotes mRNA is transcribed in the same compartment in which it is translated with the processes occurring almost simultaneously.

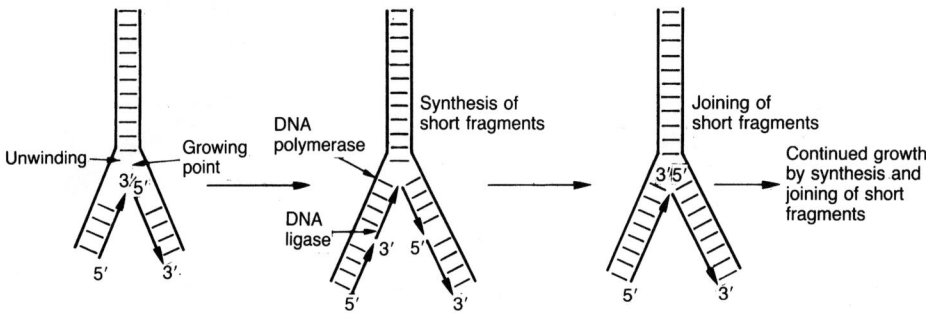

FIGURE 1.6 Replication of DNA. This process is limited to the $3'$-end of the two DNA strands. Thus, the direction of synthesis is invariably $5' \rightarrow 3'$. DNA polymerases add individual nucleotides to produce small DNA fragments (Okazaki fragments) which then are joined together by the action of DNA ligase to produce a single continuous strand of DNA.

Similarly, in prokaryotes a single mRNA can encode several different proteins whereas a eukaryotic mRNA is translated into only one polypeptide chain.

Transcription is carried out by *RNA polymerases* which catalyze the formation of phosphodiester bonds between ribonucleotides. RNA polymerases require the DNA template as well as the ribonucleotide triphosphates, ATP, CTP, GTP and UTP, which are polymerized with the release of two high-energy phosphate bonds. The sites at which RNA polymerases initiate mRNA synthesis are not random. For each gene there is a specific site called a *promoter region*, at which the RNA polymerase first binds. The sequences contained in these promoter regions and the control of transcription will be discussed later in the chapter.

## Transfer RNA (tRNA)

The translation of mRNA into the primary amino acid sequence of a protein is mediated by tRNA. The detailed structure of tRNA is now well understood. These molecules are short, single-stranded sequences with lengths varying from 73 to 93 nucleotides. Sequence comparisons have shown that there are certain structural aspects that are constant between different tRNA species and others which vary. tRNA molecules also contain some purine and pyrimidine bases that differ from the normal bases found in RNA owing to chemical modification, usually methylation. Although the molecular structure of tRNA is single-stranded, there are extensive double-stranded regions forming a so-called *cloverleaf structure*. The structure and function of this clover leaf will be discussed in greater detail in a later section on protein biosynthesis.

## Ribosomal RNA (rRNA)

Ribosomal RNA is the major component of the ribosomes that are required for protein synthesis although its exact role in the process is unclear. There are different sizes of rRNA which can be separated on the basis of their sedimentation characteristics. In *E. coli* there are three rRNA species, 5S, 16S and 23S, whereas in mammalian cells the 16S and 23S species are replaced with rRNA of 18S and 28S, respectively. rRNA is the most abundant of the three RNA species present in a cell, comprising up to 80 per cent of the total RNA.

## SELECTED READING

Goodfellow JM, Cruzeiro-Hansson L, Norberto de Souza O, *et al*. DNA structure, hydration and dynamics. *Int J Radiation Biol* 1994; 66: 471.

Lohman TM. *Escherichia coli* DNA helicases: mechanisms of DNA unwinding. *Molec Microbiol* 1992; 6: 5.

Ogasawara N, Moriya S, Yoshikawa H. Initiation of chromosome replication: structure and function of oriC and DnaA protein in eubacteria. *Res Microbiol* 1991; 142: 851.

Savic DJ, Jankovic M, Kostic T. Cellular role of DNA polymerase I. *J Basic Microbiol* 1990; 30: 769.

Zavitz KH, Marians KJ. Dissecting the functional role of PriA protein-catalysed primosome assembly in *Escherichia coli* DNA replication. *Molec Microbiol* 1991; 5: 2869.

# GENE REGULATION

## STRUCTURE OF BACTERIAL PROMOTERS

Attempts to identify the features within a gene that are necessary for the correct binding of RNA polymerase started by simply comparing the sequences of the known promoters. It was reasoned that any essential sequence should be found in all promoters. This allowed an idealized sequence to be formed, known as a *consensus sequence*, that represented the bases found most often at each position. From this analysis, the most striking feature is that within the ~60 bp of DNA with which the RNA polymerase is associated there is little conservation of sequences, indicating that most of this sequence is irrelevant to RNA polymerase binding. However, there are some short conserved sequences that are crucial for promoter function (Fig. 1.7).

The start of *transcription* is, in more than 90 per cent of instances, denoted by a purine residue which is preceded by a 6-bp region found in virtually all promoters. The center of this sequence is usually close to 10 bp upstream of the initiation site (–10) although the distance may vary from –9 to –18. The consensus sequence is TATAAT and often is called the *–10 sequence* or *Pribnow box region*. Similarities also occur at another sequence located ~35 bp upstream of the initiation site. This is called the –35 sequence and has a consensus of TTGACA. The distance separating the –10 and –35 regions is between 16 and 19 bp in more than 90 per cent of promoters and, although the actual sequence between the two sites appears to be irrelevant, the actual distance is crucial to hold the sites in the correct 3-dimensional alignment to allow RNA polymerase to bind efficiently.

## STRUCTURE OF PROKARYOTIC RNA POLYMERASE

In bacteria (prokaryotic organisms in which cells have no discrete nuclei) a single type of RNA polymerase is responsible for the synthesis of mRNA, tRNA and rRNA within the cell, with approximately 7000 molecules of enzyme present within each bacterial cell. In *E. coli* the *holoenzyme* has a molecular weight of ~480 kD with a subunit composition of $\alpha_2 \beta \beta' \sigma$

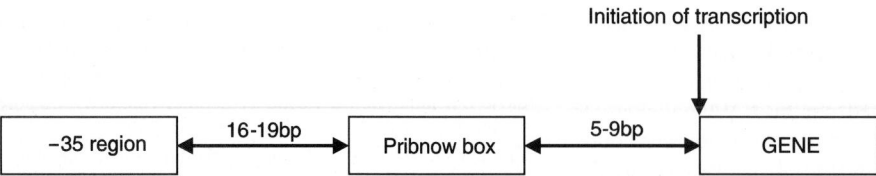

FIGURE 1.7 A consensus prokaryotic promoter. The promoter has three consensus components: the −35 region, the Pribnow box, and the transcriptional start point.

(Table 1.1). The core enzyme can be separated into two components consisting of the *core enzyme* ($\alpha_2 \beta \beta'$) and the *sigma factor* ($\sigma$). Only the holoenzyme can initiate transcription. The sigma factor is released from the complex after 8–9 bases of RNA are synthesized, with the core enzyme having the necessary components to complete RNA synthesis.

Once the sigma factor has been released, the core enzyme begins to move along the DNA template, producing an RNA copy of the DNA. As the template is extended, there is local unwinding of the DNA to free the template, with each of the DNA strands probably entering a separate site in the enzyme (Fig. 1.8(a)). The template strand of DNA is thus free just ahead of the area where the ribonucleotide is added to the growing chain, producing a region with a DNA/RNA hybrid (this region is of the order of ~12 bp). As the enzyme continues to migrate along the DNA, the duplex is reformed, thereby freeing the RNA chain.

## Role of sigma factor

Sigma factor functions to ensure that the RNA polymerase binds only to promoter sequences and not any other sequences. Sigma introduces a major change in the affinity of RNA polymerase for DNA by reducing the ability of the core enzyme to bind to any general DNA sequence (or *loose binding sites*) by a factor of ~$10^4$. At the same time sigma factor also confers the ability to recognize the specific binding sites found in bacterial promoter sequences. The holoenzyme binds very tightly to promoters, with, on average, $10^3$ times greater affinity than the core enzyme (Fig. 1.8(b)).

## CONTROL OF PROKARYOTIC GENES

In bacteria, gene activity is primarily regulated at the level of *transcription* rather than translation. The general principles are best exemplified by the genes

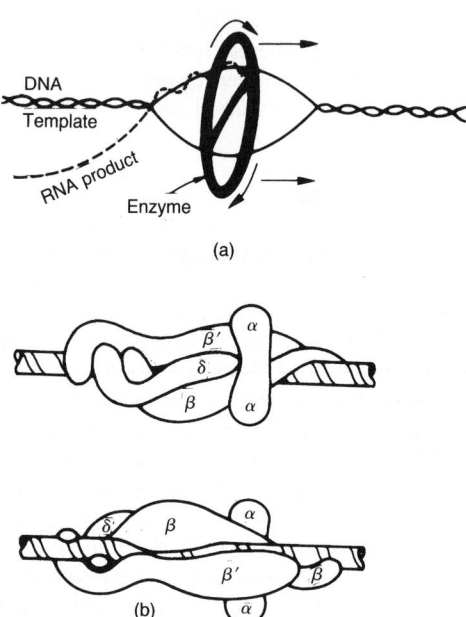

FIGURE 1.8 Schematic representation of *E. coli* RNA polymerase. Note that the enzyme has several active sites, including one for unwinding and one for rewinding the DNA duplex (panel (a)). Panel (b) represents the holoenzyme of RNA polymerase binding to the *lac* UV5 promoter, viewed from opposite sides.

involved in lactose and tryptophan metabolism and these will be discussed in detail.

## Lactose metabolism in *E. coli*

Lactose can be used by *E. coli* as a sole carbon source, being hydrolyzed to galactose and glucose by the enzyme β-galactosidase (Fig. 1.9). Under conditions in which the carbon source is not lactose there may

TABLE 1.1 The subunits of RNA polymerase in *E. coli*

| RNA POLYMERASE SUBUNIT | MASS (kD) | LOCATION | FUNCTION |
|---|---|---|---|
| α | 40 | Core | Binding to promoter |
| β | 155 | Core | Nucleotide binding |
| β' | 160 | Core | Template binding |
| σ | 85 | Holoenzyme | Initiation of transcription |

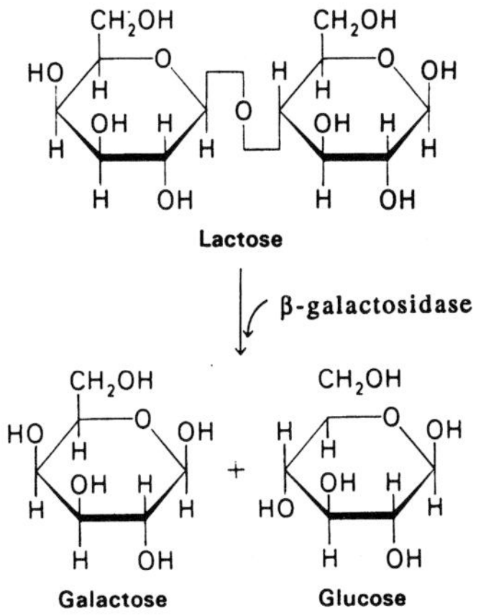

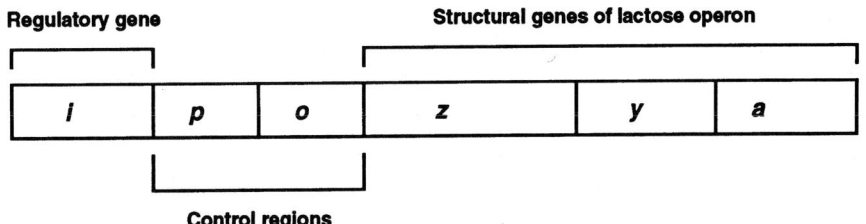

FIGURE 1.9 The activity of β-galactosidase

be fewer than 10 molecules of β-galactosidase present in the cell. However, in cells growing on lactose, β-galactosidase is induced to levels of several thousand molecules per cell. This induction occurs through *de novo* β-galactosidase synthesis rather than by the activation of a proenzyme. *In vivo*, the inducer of β-galactosidase is *allolactose*, which is formed from lactose by the transglycosylation of lactose by the action of the few molecules of β-galactosidase present in the cell.

Two other proteins are required for lactose metabolism, galactoside permease and thiogalactoside transacetylase, which are synthesized in concert with β-galactosidase. The permease transports lactose across the bacterial cell membrane, while the cellular function of the transacetylase remains unclear.

The β-galactosidase, permease and transacetylase enzymes are encoded by three contiguous genes called *lac z*, *lac y* and *lac a*, respectively. Jacob and Monod deduced that the rate of synthesis of these proteins was regulated by a common element separate from the structural genes, which they named *lac i*, and which encodes a cytoplasmic *repressor* protein. These results then led Jacob and Monod to propose the *operon model* for this type of regulation of protein synthesis (Fig. 1.10). The elements of this model are a *regulator gene*, an *operator site* and a set of *structural genes*. In the model, the regulator gene produces a repressor that can interact with the operator contained within the promoter of the operon. The promoter contains sequences to which the RNA polymerase binds to

begin transcribing the structural genes. The site for the initiation of transcription is located adjacent to the operator site, and in the presence of the repressor the RNA polymerase is prevented from binding, thus blocking the initiation of transcription. However, an inducer such as allolactose can bind to the repressor causing a conformational change which prevents the repressor from binding to the operator. The structural genes can then be transcribed to form a *polycistronic* mRNA molecule (Fig. 1.11).

There is another level of complexity in the regulation of the *lac* operon, and other catabolic operons, called *catabolite repression*. Obviously, it would be energetically undesirable to express catabolic enzymes when glucose is present as a carbon source. It was found that in an environment where glucose levels are high, the intracellular concentration of cyclic AMP (adenosine monophosphate) is low, while the opposite is true in a low-glucose environment. This led to the discovery that cAMP stimulates the initiation of transcription in the *lac* and other inducible operons.

The large amounts of cAMP produced in the absence of glucose are able to bind to a protein called CAP (Catabolite Activator Protein) to form a complex that stimulates transcription by binding to certain promoter sites. CAP activates the *lac* operon by binding just upstream of the site for the RNA polymerase. It is thought that the binding of CAP creates an extra interaction for the RNA polymerase, stabilizing its binding to the promoter and thereby increasing the frequency of transcriptional initiation. Conversely, the site for repressor binding is found within the binding region for RNA polymerase, and this prevents initiation by sterically inhibiting the binding of RNA polymerase to the promoter.

## The tryptophan operon

The *trp* mRNA is a 7-kb transcript in which there are five structural genes for tryptophan metabolism with translation of the mRNA occurring coincidentally with transcription (Fig. 1.12). *Trp* mRNA is synthesized within 4 minutes and is then subject to rapid degradation. This short half-life allows the bacteria to respond rapidly to the requirement for tryptophan, varying the production of tryptophan over a 700-fold range.

**Regulatory gene**

**Structural genes of lactose operon**

| *i* | *p* | *o* | *z* | *y* | *a* |
|-----|-----|-----|-----|-----|-----|

**Control regions**

FIGURE 1.10 The lactose operon of *E. coli*. The operon consists of the three structural genes (*z, y, a*) which are regulated by the action of the regulatory gene *lac i*, acting at the control site (*o*) to block transcription by RNA polymerase at the promoter (*p*).

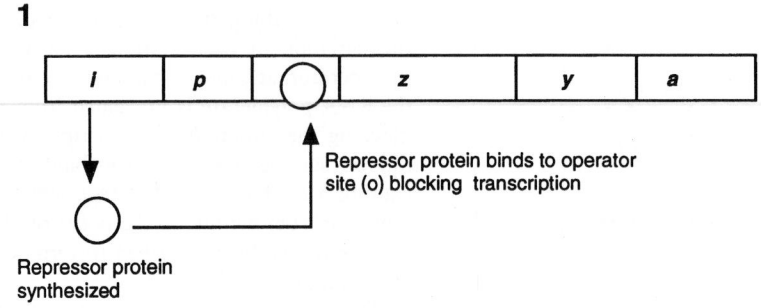

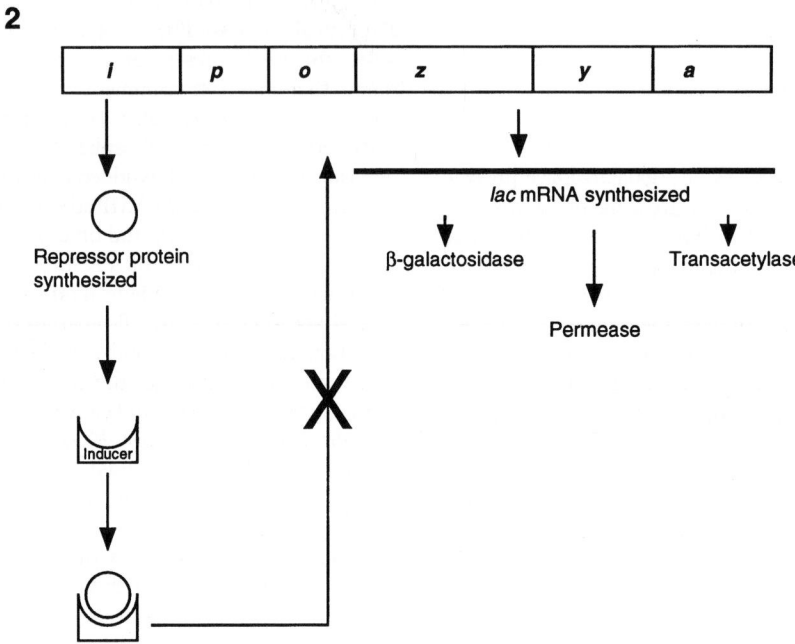

FIGURE 1.11 Regulation of the lactose operon. The operon can be either (1) repressed in the presence of glucose as a carbon source, or (2) induced in the presence of lactose.

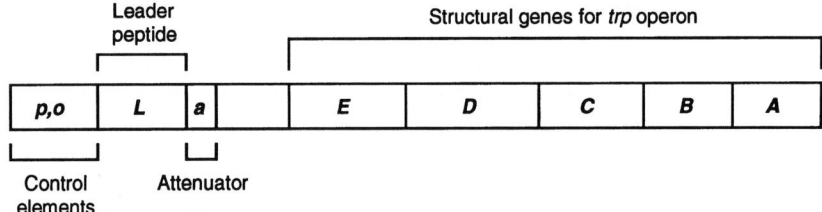

FIGURE 1.12 The tryptophan operon of *E. coli*. The operon consists of the five structural genes (*E, D, C, B, A*). Also shown are the promoter (*p*), operator (*o*), attenuator (*a*) and the leader sequence (*L*).

One level of control in this operon is achieved by the interaction of a specific repressor (encoded by *trp* R) with the *trp* operator site. This repression can only occur when tryptophan is complexed with the repressor, and thus tryptophan can be thought of as a *co-repressor*. Since the operator site overlaps the promoter site for transcriptional initiation, binding of the repressor prevents RNA polymerase binding and thus the *trp* genes are not transcribed. It was later found that certain deletion mutants between the operator and *trp* E

(the first gene in the operon) actually increased the production of *trp* mRNA. This led to the discovery that the *trp* mRNA has a 162-bp *leader sequence* prior to the *trp* E initiator codon within which the deletion mutants mapped. Furthermore, in the presence of high levels of tryptophan only the leader sequence was found to be transcribed, while the full-length 7-kb *trp* mRNA was expressed when tryptophan was scarce. This led Yanofsky to propose that the transcription of *trp* mRNA is regulated by a controllable termination sequence or *attenuator* located between the operator and the *trp* E gene. This sequence was found to have a two-fold axis of symmetry and to be composed of a GC-rich region followed by an AT-rich one.

## Attenuation of *trp* mRNA synthesis

An additional question about the tryptophan operon was how the attenuator sequence is regulated by the cellular levels of tryptophan. Key aspects of this regulation are, first, the close coupling of transcription and translation, with the ribosome following closely behind the RNA polymerase molecule transcribing the DNA template, and second, that the leader sequence contains two codons for tryptophan located in tandem. When tryptophan is abundant the complete leader is translated owing to the presence of sufficient tryptophanyl tRNAs, which results in termination of transcription (Fig. 1.13(a)). However, if tryptophan is in short supply then there is a lack of tryptophanyl tRNAs, which makes the ribosome that is translating the leader sequence stall at the tandem UGG *trp* codons. This stall ultimately leads to an alteration in the structure of the mRNA, allowing mRNA synthesis to continue beyond the attenuator sequence and into the structural genes (Fig. 1.13(b)).

## Transcriptional termination in prokaryotes

Once transcription has been initiated, RNA polymerase will continue to synthesize RNA until it meets a *terminator sequence*. As this point is reached no further nucleotides are added to the nascent RNA chain; the completed mRNA is then released both from the DNA template and the RNA polymerase, and the DNA duplex is re-formed.

Two types of terminator sequences have been defined in bacteria. The first type are known as *rho-independent* (or *simple*) *terminators*. In this case the core enzyme of RNA polymerase terminates in the absence of any other factors. Rho-independent terminators have two structural features (Fig. 1.14). These contain a *hairpin loop structure* formed from palindromic sequences formed within the RNA molecule, and a sequence of ~6 U residues at the very end of the RNA molecule. It is believed that the formation of the hairpin loop structure causes the RNA polymerase to either slow down or pause entirely. This pause lasts an average of 60 seconds. Since hairpins can be formed in other regions of the growing RNA molecule, this structure alone is insufficient for termination of transcription but only creates the opportunity for this to occur. Other sequences in the vicinity of the pause

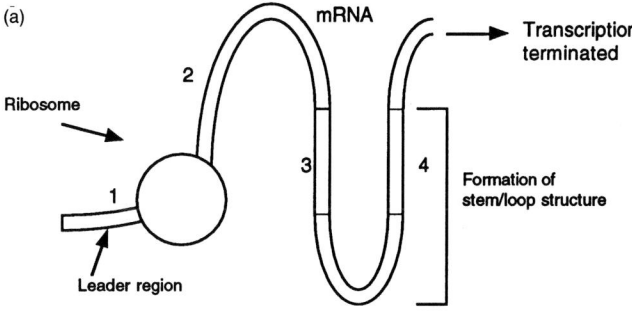

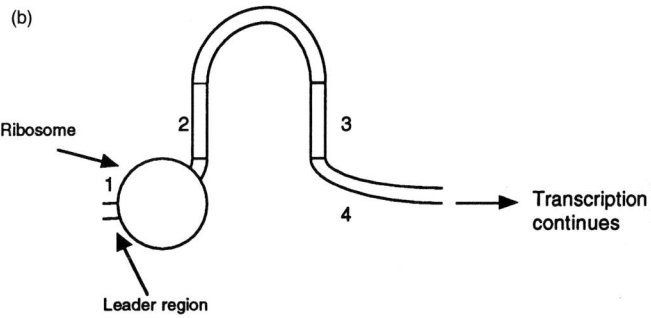

FIGURE 1.13 Attenuation in the *trp* operon of *E. coli*. When tryptophan levels are high the leader region (1) is fully translated, allowing region 2 to interact with the ribosome and leaving regions 3 and 4 free to form a stem–loop structure. This results in signaling to the RNA polymerase to abort transcription. When tryptophan is scarce the leader is not translated and regions 2 and 3 interact, rather than regions 3 and 4, and transcription continues.

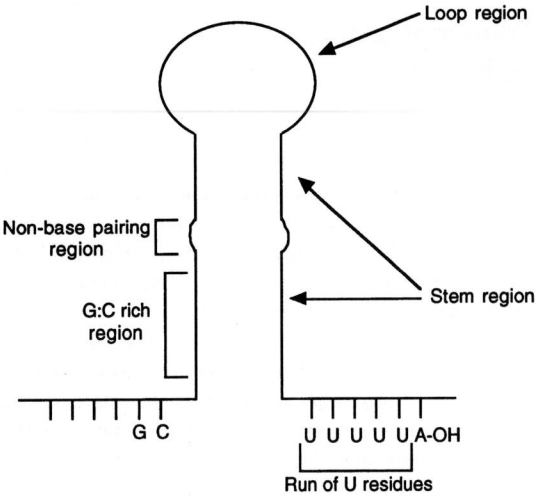

FIGURE 1.14 Structural features of rho-independent terminators. The hairpin loop structure can vary from 7 to 20 bp in length and is always followed by a string of U residues.

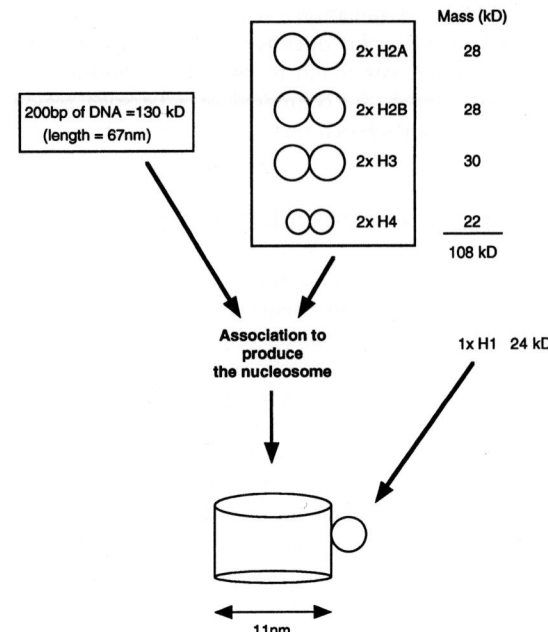

FIGURE 1.15 The nucleosome is the basic unit for DNA packaging and consists of ~50 per cent DNA and ~50 per cent protein. The proteins are the basic histones (H1, H2A and B, H3 and H4). The predicted mass of each nucleosome is 262 kD.

must play a role for termination actually to occur. The consecutive uridine residues are thought to be important in this regard. The DNA–RNA hybrid formed by dA–rU is a particularly weak one and requires the least amount of energy to break the association. Thus, as the RNA polymerase pauses at the hairpin loop structure, the DNA–RNA hybrid can be unraveled from the weak dA–rU region. The actual site of termination can take place at several sites following the string of U residues, possibly as the enzyme "stutters" during the termination event. The importance of the U-string is emphasized by deletional analysis experiments which remove this sequence. The result is transcriptional pause but *not* termination.

The second type of terminators found in prokaryotes are *rho-dependent*, which require the further presence of the *rho factor*. This factor allows RNA polymerase to terminate at certain sites to produce RNA molecules with unique 3′-ends. Rho factor is an essential protein in *E. coli*, but no features of sequence or structure have as yet been identified in rho-dependent terminators.

## EUKARYOTIC TRANSCRIPTION

## Chromatin structure

As an extended linear molecule, eukaryotic DNA would vastly exceed the size of the cell. Thus, in order to conform to the size constraints of the nucleus, the DNA is arranged in a tightly packed form called *chromatin*. Chromatin is a highly compact structure in which most DNA sequences are structurally inaccessible to RNA polymerases and are thus transcriptionally inactive (*heterochromatin*). Within this heterochromatin are the minority of transcriptionally active sequences (*euchromatin*). The fundamental subunit of

chromatin is the same in all eukaryotes (organisms in which cells have discrete nuclei), containing 200 bp of DNA organized by an octamer of proteins into a bead-like structure called a *nucleosome* (Fig. 1.15). The proteins within chromatin consist of two types: *histones* and *non-histones*. There are five classes of histones which are among the most conserved proteins found in all eukaryotes (Table 1.2).

The formation of the nucleosome is only the first step in the packaging of chromatin. The second is the coiling of the nucleosomes into a helical structure to form the *30-nm fiber*, and the final step is the packaging of the 30-nm fiber itself. The overall packaging by this hierarchical process is over 1000-fold in euchromatin.

Euchromatin is the only transcriptionally active chromatin and can be identified using DNase (deoxyribonuclease) I (an enzyme that hydrolyzes DNA). Most DNA in isolated nuclei is resistant to DNase I cleavage as it is surrounded by the protein components found in chromatin. However, euchroma-

TABLE 1.2 The histone proteins associated with the nucleosome

| HISTONE | MASS (kD) | RATIO OF BASIC/ ACIDIC AMINO ACIDS |
|---|---|---|
| H1 | 23 | 5.4 |
| H2A | 14 | 1.4 |
| H2B | 14 | 1.7 |
| H3 | 15 | 1.8 |
| H4 | 11 | 2.5 |

tin has a more open structure and is digested by DNase I. These *DNase I hypersensitive sites* frequently are found to map to the promoter regions of transcriptionally active genes. Presumably the open structure of euchromatin is required for the transcriptional machinery to gain access to the DNA and to initiate transcription.

# DNA methylation in eukaryotes

Between 2 and 7 per cent of mammalian cytosine residues are methylated, and it is believed that methylation at the 5′-end of a gene inhibits its expression. Genes that are not methylated (*hypomethylated*) are expressed. Hypomethylation appears to be associated with the ability to be transcribed rather than with the act of transcription itself.

Most methylation in eukaryotic DNA takes place in cytosine/guanosine rich areas (*CpG-rich islands)* in the 5′ regions of genes. This CpG sequence is statistically under-represented in the eukaryotic genome (~20 per cent of the expected frequency) and seems to be particularly prevalent in the promoters of constitutively expressed genes. In actively transcribed genes, the CpG islands are hypomethylated, and their presence has been used to delineate possible transcription units within eukaryotic genomes.

# RNA polymerases

As with prokaryotes, *transcription* is a major level at which gene expression is regulated in eukaryotes. However, the eukaryotic cell is more complicated, since there are three RNA polymerases (I, II, III) rather than the single one found in bacteria. Most research has focused on RNA polymerase II, which is responsible for transcribing protein-coding genes, and the control mechanisms for this polymerase will be discussed in greater detail than the control of polymerase I or III.

## RNA polymerase I

Eukaryotic ribosomal RNA (rRNA) genes are arranged in tandem arrays and are specifically transcribed by RNA polymerase I within the nucleolus, accounting for almost 50 per cent of the transcription that takes place within the cell. Each rRNA gene has an identical promoter region which is repeated about 200 times per haploid genome. The promoter consists of two domains. The first is obligate for transcriptional activity and is located in the 50 bp preceding the initiation site. The second domain has a variable effect on transcription and is located 50–150 bp upstream of the initiation site. Another property of Pol I transcription is that there is species specificity in its ability to recognize the promoters of rRNA genes. Thus the RNA

polymerase I transcription machinery of one species will not recognize the promoter of another.

## RNA polymerase III

This polymerase is responsible for transcription of genes that encode a variety of small, stable RNAs such as tRNA, 5S RNA and some small nuclear RNAs (snRNAs) required in RNA splicing. Most class III genes have intragenic promoter sequences, i.e. the promoters lie within the coding region of the gene. However, some have promoter domains located outside the coding sequence and they can either act in unison with the intragenic sequences or be independent. The external promoters have been found to have sequence characteristics of RNA polymerase II-dependent promoters containing TATA type motifs, which, when mutated, significantly reduce the level of transcription. It is likely that RNA polymerases II and III utilize the same *trans*-acting factors, as they are known to share subunits.

## RNA polymerase II

### General transcription factors of RNA polymerase II

RNA polymerase II cannot accurately initiate transcription unless it is supplemented with a wide variety of other proteins called *general transcription factors*. These factors permit RNA polymerase II to specifically recognize minimal promoter sequences. These sequences, by convention, consist of the TATA motif and the cap site only. Sequences that are found upstream, and that may be necessary for maximal transcriptional activity, are not considered part of the minimal promoter. The TATA motif is associated with many promoters, although a large percentage of RNA polymerase II-dependent genes, including many housekeeping genes, lack a TATA sequence.

In RNA polymerase II there are at least five general transcription factors (TFIIA, B, C, D and E) that have been identified as necessary cofactors to initiate transcription. Using reconstitution experiments, these factors have been shown to be required for the formation of the pre-initiation complex necessary to promote RNA polymerase-dependent transcription. While the action of these factors is still unclear, TFIID has been shown to be capable of specifically binding to the TATA box and its surrounding sequence (including the initiation site).

The proposed assembly of the pre-initiation complex is shown in Fig. 1.16. It is thought that the initial binding is by TFIIA, which alters the structure of the DNA around the TATA box and enhances TFIID binding. The formation of the promoter–TFIIA/TFIID complex facilitates the binding of RNA polymerase II and is followed by a complex of TFIIE/TFIIB, producing the pre-initiation complex. This complex, in the

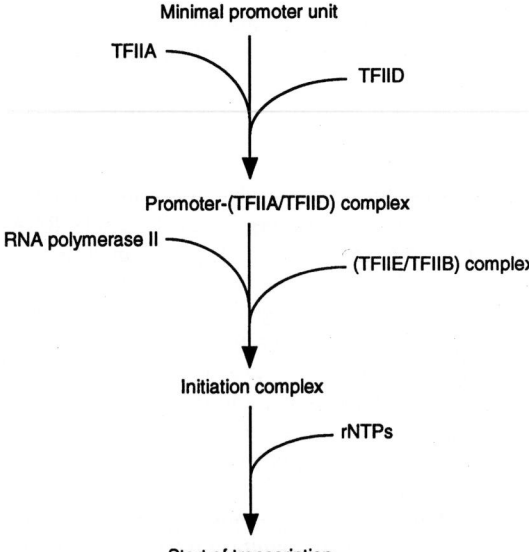

Minimal promoter unit

FIGURE 1.16 The assembly of the transcriptional initiation complex. This schematic representation details the proposed order of general transcription factor assembly to form a complex capable of transcription.

presence of ribonucleotide triphosphates (rNTPs), can begin transcription.

Promoter-specific transcription factors

In addition to *cis*-acting elements such as the TATA motif (that are shared by a variety of promoters), there are control elements that are found only in selective promoters. The main characteristics of these elements are distance dependence (i.e. will only function at a discrete distance from the transcriptional initiation site) and a location upstream of the cap site. It should be noted that promoter-specific elements can, in the correct location, function as enhancer elements, exhibiting distance and orientation independence. Some of the most common factors are discussed below.

*CCAAT box transcription factors (CTF)*

The sequence CCAAT is often found in eukaryotic promoters and usually is located 40–100 bp upstream of the cap site and is required for efficient transcription. This sequence, commonly called the CCAAT box, is orientation independent, i.e. functions in a sense or anti-sense orientation, and can act either alone or in tandem with other motifs to increase transcriptional activity. This motif is recognized by a family of transcription factors.

*SP1*

This binding motif was first identified in the SV40 viral genome. It has a core consensus sequence of GGGCGG and is recognized by the transcription factor SP1. This factor consists of two polypeptide chains of 105 and 95 kD, both of which can bind to the GGGCGG sequence. SP1 sequences are predominantly arrayed in tandem with the site closest to the initiation of tran-

scription mediating the strongest transcriptional activation.

*Octamer-binding factors*

These factors recognize the consensus sequence ATGCAAAT. This sequence is found in a wide variety of promoters and, in the appropriate setting, it also can act as an enhancer element. There are a variety of different members that make up this family, which can be either ubiquitous (found in all cells) or cell-specific (found only in a defined cell type).

*Heat-shock transcription factors (HSTF)*

All genes that are inducible by heat shock contain multiple copies of a consensus sequence CNNGAAANNTCCNNG, called a heat-shock element (HSE). This sequence is recognized by the 150-kD heat-shock transcription factor.

*Cyclic AMP-response-element binding factors (CREB)*

cAMP is one of the major second messenger systems found in eukaryotic cells. It acts through the activation of cAMP-dependent kinases which can in turn phosphorylate key regulatory proteins to either enhance or diminish their activity. CREBs are a family of *trans*-acting factors that bind to the cAMP response element (CRE), which has the consensus sequence TGACGTCA. The presence of a CRE within a promoter will confer cAMP inducibility on that gene.

Enhancers

As indicated previously, there is no clear distinction between enhancer and upstream *cis*-acting elements, rather there is an *enhancer effect*. This can be defined by the ability to cause transcriptional activation independent of both distance from the promoter and orientation to the promoter. For example, the octamer motif can either be part of an enhancer or be an integral part of the promoter.

The mRNA cap site

The 5′-ends of all eukaryotic mRNA species are further modified in the cytoplasm. In most cases transcription is initiated at a purine residue. However, the terminal base in the mature transcript is always a G residue. This is added by the enzyme guanyl transferase to all mRNA species in eukaryotes. This G residue is added in the reverse orientation to all the other nucleotides, producing a 5′–5′ triphosphate linkage between the first two nucleotides (Fig. 1.17). The subsequent structure is called a *cap*, which then can be methylated at several positions. The first methylation is identical in all eukaryotes and is at the 7-position of the terminal guanosine and yields *cap 0*. Further methylation can then occur at the 2′-O position (*cap 1*) of the penultimate base. Occasionally a methyl group also can be added to the $N^6$ position of the same base, but only if it is an adenine. Finally the third base also can be methylated at the 2′-O position, yielding *cap 2* (but only if the cap 1 already possesses two methyl groups).

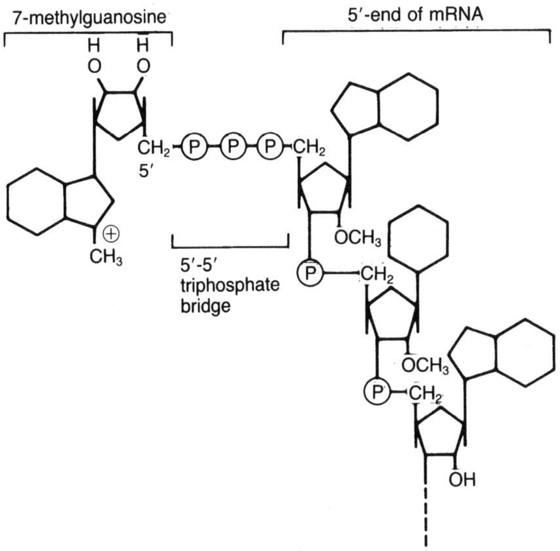

7-methylguanosine

5'-end of mRNA

5'-5'
triphosphate
bridge

**FIGURE 1.17** The formation of capped RNA in eukaryotes. Formation of the 5'–5'–base linkage blocks the end of the RNA, increasing its half-life.

## Transcriptional termination in eukaryotes

Each of the three RNA polymerases found in eukaryotes has evolved a different termination mechanism. Termination of RNA polymerase III transcripts appears to be relatively simple. The transcriptional termination signals are invariably short runs of T residues (at least four) surrounded by GC-rich regions. The 3' termini of RNA polymerase III genes are thus always poly U sequences. In contrast, RNA polymerase I termination events are much more complex, and the process is not fully understood. Nuclear runoff and *in vitro* transcription experiments have identified one termination site in the 28S rRNA gene. This sequence is located 500 bp past the 3'-end of the mature 28S

rRNA. The sequence contains a *Sal*I restriction site that is repeated eight times and binds to a protein that is proposed to be a termination factor. Since the termination of transcription occurs at least 500 bp downstream of the end of the mature 28S rRNA, there must be some processing of the RNA after termination, although the mechanism is largely unknown.

Little is known about the mechanisms of RNA polymerase II termination, and it is possible that this process may only be loosely specified. In some genes termination occurs more than 1 kb beyond the site of the mature 3'-end of the mRNA. Thus, instead of using specific termination signals, RNA synthesis may in fact be terminated at multiple sites located within *terminator regions*. The identity of the terminator sequences within these regions remains unclear. It is also thought that secondary structure formation within the mRNA species is an important factor for termination (as in rho-independent terminators in *E. coli*), although the exact sequence may be less important than the secondary structure formation.

It is known, however, that the mature 3'-ends of mRNA species are generated in a two-step process. The first step is cleavage of the transcript by a nuclease and the second is the addition of a poly A tract to the 3'-end (Fig. 1.18).

Comparisons of the 3'-ends of mRNA species has identified a consensus sequence, AAUAAA, found 20–30 bp upstream of the poly A tail. This sequence represents the most conserved sequence in RNA polymerase II transcribed genes and is necessary but not sufficient to determine the 3'-end of the transcript. Since the sequence AAUAAA occurs by chance in regions other than at the site of termination, searches were made to determine if other sequences were conserved. Results indicate that GT-rich or T-rich regions may be involved in the process and that the spacing of these regions from the AAUAAA sequence is also critical for correct 3'-end formation.

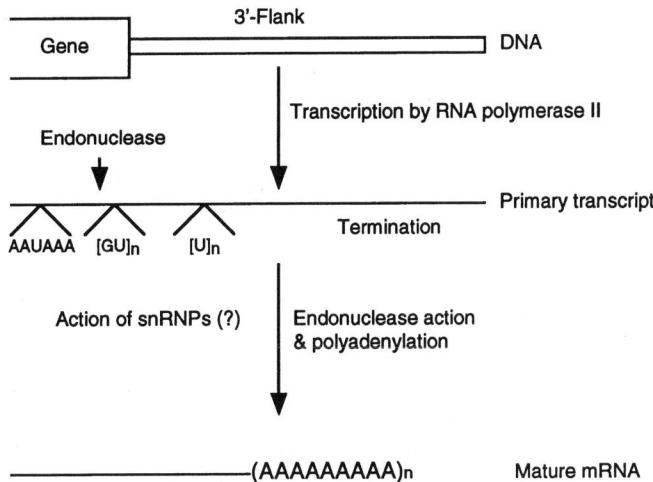

**FIGURE 1.18** The formation of the 3'-end of polyadenylated mRNA. See text for details.

After the 3'-end has been formed, the poly A tail is added by the action of poly A polymerase using ATP as a substrate. It was also found that if the analog 3'-deoxyadenosine was used in place of adenosine the appearance of mRNA in the cytoplasm was inhibited, indicating that polyadenylation is necessary for RNA maturation (although since only ~70 per cent of mRNA is polyadenylated in mammals, this is not a hard and fast rule).

Important factors in this process are *small nuclear ribonuclear particles* (snRNPs), which are now thought to act in all the processing events of the initial transcript. In this case the small nuclear RNA (snRNA) in the snRNP contains sequences that are complementary to sequences found around the polyadenylation site. This allows base-pairing between the nascent RNA species and the snRNA, leaving an extensive hairpin at the end of the snRNA. This hairpin structure may function either to initiate termination or possibly to assist in the cleavage reaction prior to polyadenylation.

## RNA splicing in eukaryotes

Another level of complexity in RNA synthesis unique to eukaryotes is *RNA splicing*. The majority of eukaryotic transcripts are composed not only of coding sequences (*exons*) but also of non-coding intervening sequences (*introns*). RNA splicing is the process whereby there is precise removal of the introns from the precursor RNA, leaving the adjacent exons, in the correct sequence, to produce the mature RNA species. Several theories have been suggested to explain the appearance of introns in eukaryotic RNA, but whatever the explanation it is clear that RNA splicing is essential for gene expression in eukaryotes. In some cases this process is actually used to regulate gene expression.

### Splicing mechanisms

Introns are found in many different RNA precursors including pre-mRNA, pre-tRNA and pre-rRNA. Examination of the intron structures and the mechanisms used for their removal have identified four classes of introns: nuclear pre-tRNA introns; group I introns; group II introns and nuclear pre-mRNA introns.

### Nuclear pre-tRNA splicing

This pathway was first elucidated in *S. cerevisiae* and was shown to be a two-step process (Fig. 1.19). In the first step there is endonucleolytic cleavage at the 5'- and 3'-splice sites to release a linear intron followed by ligation of the two exons. Other factors are required for proper splicing, including a 3'-cyclic phosphodiesterase which converts the terminus of the 5'-base from a 2',3'-cyclic phosphodiester to a 2'-phosphomonoester, and a kinase which phosphorylates

the 3' base to allow the formation of the required phosphodiester bond to ligate the two exons.

### Group I intron splicing

The mechanism for splicing of transcripts containing group I introns was elucidated in *Tetrahymena* 26S pre-rRNA. Introns in this class have two common features. First, the isolated RNA has the ability to splice itself (*autosplicing*). Second, the required sequence elements to define the splicing event are short sequences that can be organized into distinct secondary structures (Fig. 1.20).

The reaction requires only the pre-rRNA species, a monovalent and divalent cation and a guanine nucleotide (with a 3'-OH group). The guanine provides a free 3'-OH to which the 5'-end of the intron is transferred (Step I). This is followed by the newly created 3'-OH attacking the second exon (Step II). The intron is then released as a linear molecule but is then circularized by a third transfer reaction (Step III).

### Group II intron splicing

This class of introns is characterized by the following consensus 5'- and 3'-splice sites: /GUGCG and YUAYYNY(N)AY/. In addition, six internal hairpin loop structures have been postulated as necessary for correct splicing. As with group I introns, these introns can undergo self-splicing, although some do require additional nuclear encoded factors for splicing to occur efficiently.

### Nuclear pre-mRNA introns

Pre-mRNAs contain introns that can range in number up to 50 and can be up to 60 kb in length. Three conserved sequences have been identified in these introns: at the 5'- and 3'-splice sites, and within the intron itself near the 3'-splice site (the *branchpoint sequence*) (Fig. 1.21(a)).

The splicing of pre-mRNA introns requires the formation of a *spliceosome*. The formation of this large complex requires ATP, functional splice sites, small nuclear ribonuclear particles (snRNPs) and heterogeneous nuclear proteins (hnRNPs), as well as other as yet unidentified factors. Following assembly, the pre-mRNA is cleaved at the 5'-splice site, producing an exon I RNA fragment with a 3'-OH group (Fig. 1.21(b)). The phosphate group on the 5'-terminus of the intron is then esterified with the 2'-OH group of the conserved A residue within the branchpoint sequence, producing a branched circular RNA called a *lariat*. These steps generate two intermediates, an exon I species and a lariat–exon II species. These are held together as part of the spliceosome. The next step in the process is the cleavage of the lariat–exon II intermediate at the 3'-splice site, releasing a free lariat intron. This process appears to occur simultaneously with the final stage, which is the ligation of the two

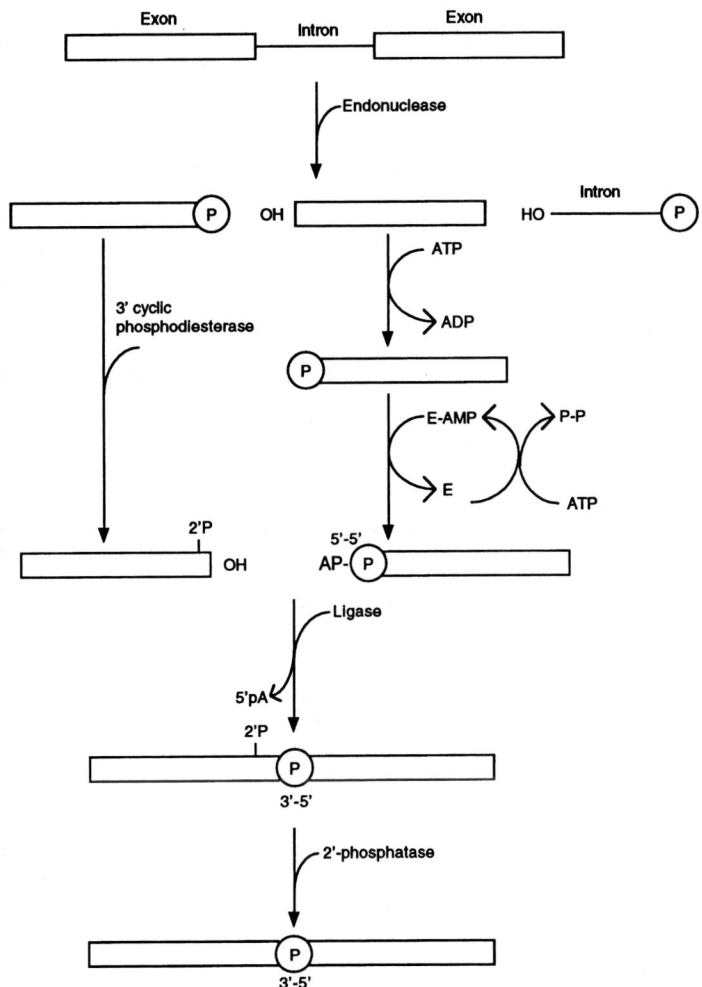

FIGURE 1.19 The mechanism of pre-tRNA splicing. The boxes represent the exons and the thin line the intron to be spliced out. E-AMP represents the adenylated enzyme complex. See text for details.

exons. The lariat itself is then *debranched* to produce a linear intron.

## mRNA stability

mRNA levels in eukaryotes can also be regulated post-transcriptionally as a means of regulating gene expression. This involves controlling the stability of the gene transcript. This process is especially prevalent in mRNA species that are required only transiently, such as various oncogenes growth factors. All these mRNAs have several tandem copies of the consensus sequence AUUU in their 3′ non-coding region. If these sequences are switched with the 3′ non-coding region of otherwise stable transcripts, they will yield a desta-bilized mRNA.

The poly A tail also affects mRNA stability, serving to increase mRNA stability. This effect has been demonstrated by removing the poly A tail of the α-globin mRNA, producing a transcript that had a trans-lational competency reduced from one week to a few hours in a *Xenopus* oocyte injection model.

## RNA EDITING

A central dogma in molecular biology is that the sequence of an mRNA molecule can only represent the sequence encoded in the DNA template. However, RNA editing is a newly discovered process in which information is changed at the level of the mRNA. It was first observed in situations where differ-ences were found between the DNA template and its transcribed RNA. The end result of this process is that the sequence of the protein produced cannot be deduced solely from examination of the gene sequence. This process is widely found in mitochondrial RNA species and occasionally in nuclear transcribed genes.

Editing appears to have at least two forms. In the first case, there is substitution of only a single base within the RNA producing a change in the encoded protein. A prominent example of this is editing of the

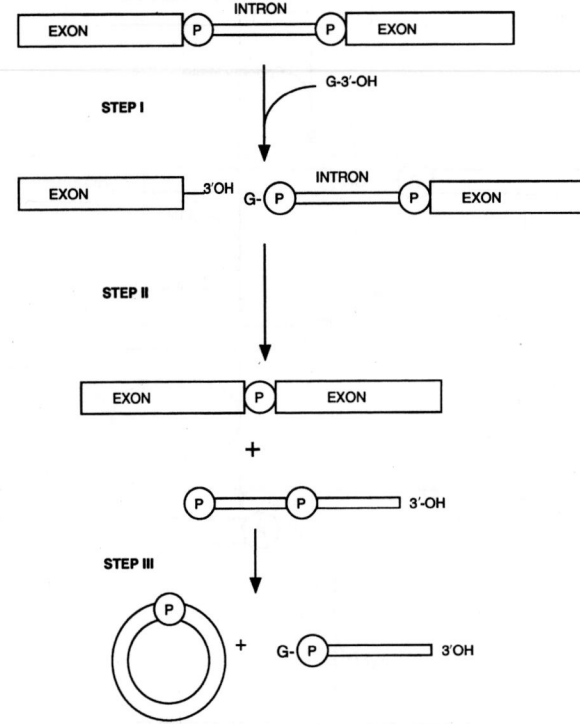

FIGURE 1.20 Group I introns are self-splicing. In some instances the excised linear exon covalently attached to the G cofactor is circularized, releasing a small 5′-terminal intron fragment.

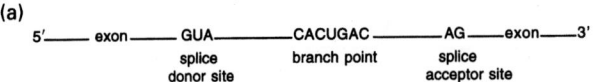

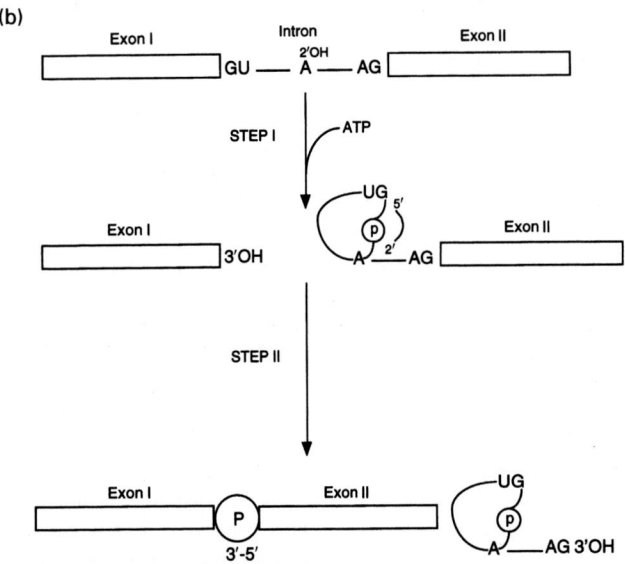

FIGURE 1.21 Mechanism of pre-mRNA splicing. Panel (a) shows the consensus sequences of the 5′- and 3′-splice donor and acceptor sites in vertebrates. Panel (b) represents a pathway that has been elucidated in metazoans and yeast for the splicing of pre-mRNA introns. This reaction requires multiple cofactors, including proteins and snRNPs.

apolipoprotein B gene in the liver. Normally, the mRNA encodes a 100-kD protein; however, mRNA editing in the liver introduces a stop codon resulting in the production of a 48-kD protein. It appears that the editing function is performed by a protein complex that is now being characterized.

The second type of editing is more complex, with both the addition and deletion of bases within the transcript. The factor(s) controlling this process is still not understood.

## SELECTED READING

Brown JD, Plumpton M, Beggs JD. The genetics of nuclear pre-mRNA splicing: a complex story. *Antonie Van Leeuwenhoek* 1992; **62**: 35.

Busch SJ, Sassone-Corsi P. Dimers, leucine zippers and DNA-binding domains. *Trends Genet* 1990; **6**: 36.

Cattaneo R. Messenger RNA editing and the genetic code. *Experientia* 1990; **46**: 1142.

Freundlich M, Ramani N, Mathew E, *et al*. The role of integration host factor in gene expression in Escherichia coli. *Molec Microbiol* 1992; **6**: 2557.

Haldenwang WG. The sigma factors of Bacillus subtilis. *Microbiol Rev* 1995; **59**: 1.

Kerppola TK, Kane CM. RNA polymerase: regulation of transcript elongation and termination. *Faseb J* 1991; **5**: 2833.

Krajewska WM. Regulation of transcription in eukaryotes by DNA-binding proteins. *Int J Biochem* 1992; **24**: 1885.

Krumm A, Meulia T, Groudine M. Common mechanisms for the control of eukaryotic transcriptional elongation. *Bioessays* 1993; **15**: 659.

Latchman DS. Cell-type-specific splicing factors and the regulation of alternative RNA splicing. *New Biologist* 1990; **2**: 297.

Mattaj IW, Tollervey D, Seraphin B. Small nuclear RNAs in messenger RNA and ribosomal RNA processing. *Faseb J* 1993; **7**: 47.

Morimoto RI. Transcription factors: positive and negative regulators of cell growth and disease. *Curr Opin Cell Biol* 1992; **4**: 480.

Owen-Hughes T, Workman JL. Experimental analysis of chromatin function in transcription control. *Crit Rev Eukaryotic Gene Expr* 1994; **4**: 403.

Svaren J, Chalkley R. The structure and assembly of active chromatin. *Trends Genet* 1990; **6**: 52.

Zlatanova J, Yaneva J. DNA sequence specific interactions of histone H1. *Molec Biol Rep* 1991; **15**: 53.

Zlatanova JS, van Holde KE. Chromatin loops and transcriptional regulation. *Crit Rev Eukaryotic Gene Expr* 1992; **2**: 211.

# PROTEIN SYNTHESIS, SORTING, MODIFICATION AND SECRETION

## PROTEIN SYNTHESIS

### Initiation

The initial event in protein synthesis is the binding of the small ribosomal subunit to the mRNA leader sequence (Fig. 1.22). This binding, in prokaryotes, is established by the Shine–Delgarno sequence (consensus: $5'$-AGGA-$3'$) present within the leader sequence. In eukaryotes, this binding involves the small ribosomal subunit, the $M^7G(5')$ cap at the beginning of the mRNA, and a factor known as *cap-binding protein*. Following binding, the small ribosomal subunit "scans" along the leader sequence until the *initiator codon* is reached. The initiator codon is overwhelmingly AUG (but can occasionally be GUG). In eukaryotes the requirements for an initiator codon are not particularly stringent with only a few flanking nucleotides required for recognition. The flanking sequences are important, because AUG sequences may occur in any or all of the three possible *reading frames* for translation of mRNA into protein. The requirement that AUG be flanked by certain nucleotides for recognition allows efficient translation of only the correct reading frame.

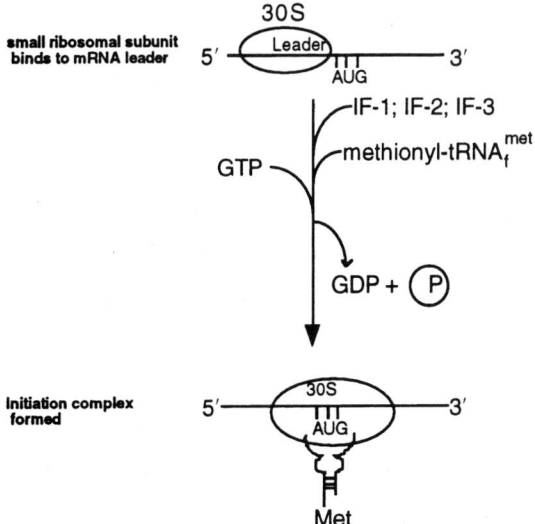

FIGURE 1.22 Initiation events in protein synthesis. The small ribosomal subunit (30S) binds to sequences at the $5'$ end of the mRNA molecule and scans to find the AUG initiator. Three protein initiation factors (IFs) are required to bind methionyl-tRNA charged with methionine to the initiator codon. The process requires energy supplied by the hydrolysis of guanosine triphosphate (GTP) to guanosine diphosphate (GDP).

The initiator codon is recognized by the initiator tRNA (tRNA$_f^{met}$). This tRNA is "charged" (or covalently linked) with methionine which, in prokaryotes, is then formylated. Thus in any polypeptide the first amino acid is invariably methionine (or N-formyl-methionine in prokaryotes) which may or may not be removed during post-translational processing. The interaction between the tRNA$_f^{met}$ anticodon loop, the initiator codon and the small ribosomal subunit requires at least three other components called *initiation factors* (IF-1, IF-2, IF-3) and energy liberated by the hydrolysis of a molecule of GTP (guanosine triphosphate). This results in the formation of an *initiation complex* which is then able to interact with the large ribosomal subunit to form an intact *ribosome*. This large subunit possesses two regions, a *peptidyl* site and an *aminoacyl* site. As the two subunits associate, the methionyl-tRNA$_f^{met}$ becomes bound to the peptidyl site, while the mRNA slots into a groove formed by the spatial orientation of the two subunits.

## Elongation

The alignment of the initiator codon with the methionyl-tRNA$_f^{met}$ within the peptidyl site serves to fix the

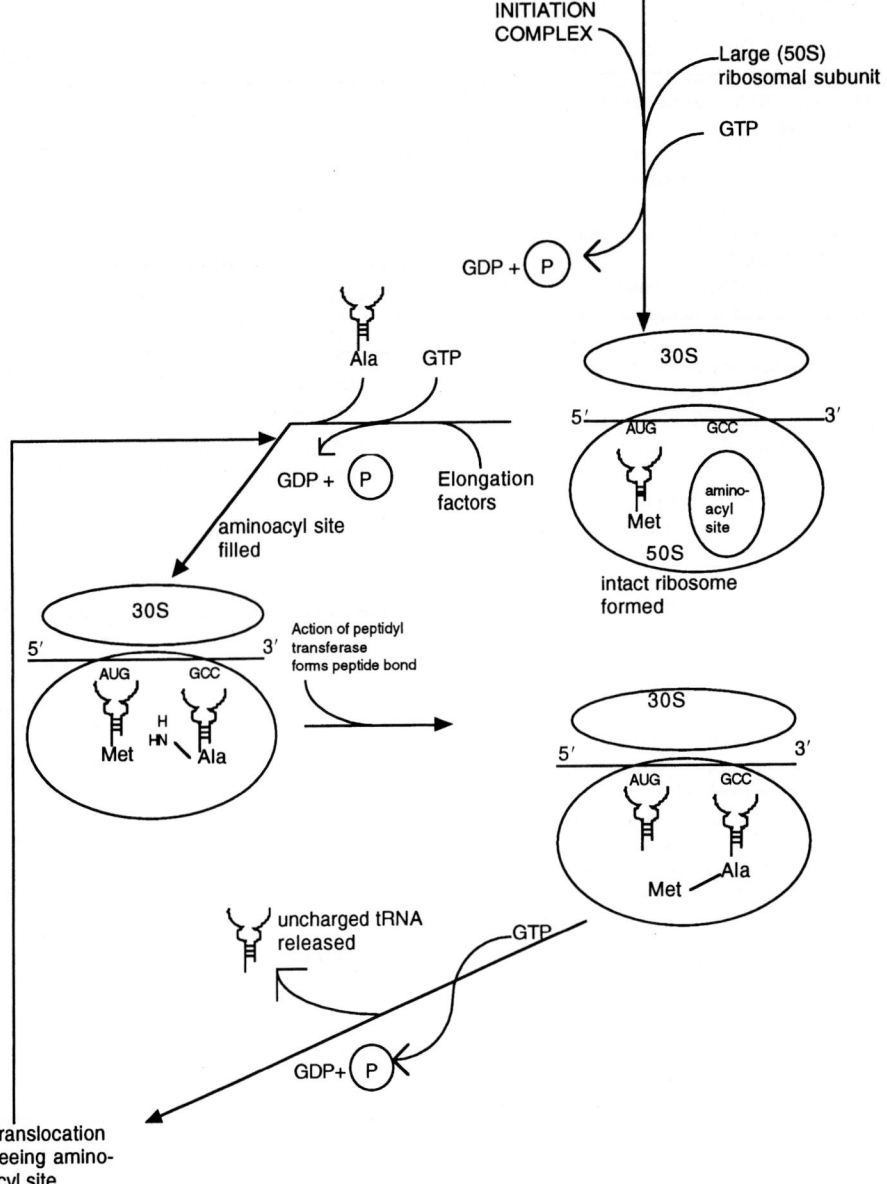

FIGURE 1.23 Elongation events in protein synthesis. In a process requiring GTP, the initiation complex binds the large ribosomal subunit which contains the aminoacyl site to be bound by the next amino acid. In a manner analogous to initiation, protein elongation factors, a charged tRNA, and energy are required for this process. The peptide bond is then synthesized by peptidyl transferase, and the uncharged tRNA is released as a third molecule of GTP is hydrolyzed.

alignment of the next codon and consequently the alignment of the aminoacyl site (Fig. 1.23). The next codon specifies alanine, thus an alanyl-tRNA$^{ala}$ occupies the aminoacyl site pairing with the mRNA codon. Again this association is GTP dependent and is mediated by a complex of *elongation factors*. At this stage the peptidyl site is still occupied by a methionyl group, covalently linked to its tRNA$_f^{met}$, and a displacement occurs to break the linkage to the tRNA$_f^{met}$ and form a *peptide bond* with the α-NH$_2$ group of the alanyl-tRNA$^{ala}$ present in the aminoacyl site. This process is mediated by the enzyme *peptidyl transferase* which is bound to the large ribosomal subunit and results in a tRNA$_f^{met}$ that lacks its methionine residue and a dipeptidyl-tRNA$^{ala}$.

The next two events occur simultaneously in a process called *translocation*, whereby the dipeptidyl-tRNA moves from the aminoacyl site to the peptidyl site, dislodging the empty tRNA$_f^{met}$. At the same time the complete ribosome shifts one codon along the mRNA. As a result, the alanine codon remains associated with the anticodon of the dipeptidyl-tRNA$^{ala}$ and a new codon appears in the aminoacyl site. These steps are then repeated with the incorporation of 8–15 amino acids per second in the growing protein. After about 25 codons have been translated, the 5' end of the mRNA molecule becomes free to form a second initiation complex and a second ribosome becomes attached and begins translation. Others can then follow, resulting in the formation of a *polyribosome* (or *polysome*).

## Termination

Protein synthesis is halted when a ribosome encounters a *terminator codon* within the mRNA sequence. These codons are not recognized by any of the anticodons present in normal aminoacyl-tRNAs. Thus no further amino acids can be added to the polypeptide chain. There are three codons that act as termination signals: UAA, UGA, and UAG.

When a termination codon moves into the aminoacyl site there is an initial interaction with one of two *release factors* (RF-1, which recognizes UAA and UAG, and RF-2, which recognizes UAA and UGA). This complex blocks further chain elongation (Fig. 1.24). The completed protein is then released from the final tRNA occupying the peptidyl site by a hydrolysis reaction mediated by another protein factor. The protein chain is then released along with the empty tRNA, and finally the ribosome dissociates into its two subunits which can then participate in another round of translation.

## PROPERTIES OF TRANSFER RNA

tRNA molecules play a key role in protein biosynthesis, by aligning amino acids within the ribosome in a manner dictated by the sequence of codons within the mRNA molecule. The structure of the mature tRNA is shown in Fig. 1.25. Every tRNA folds into a distinctive cloverleaf structure. Each tRNA molecule associates with a specific amino acid at its *3' acceptor end*; and since there are 20 amino acids present in proteins, there is a requirement for at least 20 different tRNA molecules. However, most amino acids are recognized by several different tRNA species called *isoacceptor tRNAs*. Once charged with the appropriate amino acid (Fig. 1.26) the tRNA is in a conformation that allows it to recognize a specific *codon* in the mRNA species owing to the presence of the *anticodon loop* (Fig. 1.25).

## THE GENETIC CODE

Unraveling of the genetic code was one of the major early problems in molecular biology. The basic problem was to decipher how a linear array of nucleic acids is translated by the protein synthetic machinery into a linear array of amino acids. In trying to deduce the nature of the genetic code it became immediately apparent that if a single nucleotide within the mRNA molecule specified a single amino acid, only four amino acids would be found in proteins, whereas in fact they contain 20. Similarly, a doublet code would generate only 16 combinations (4 × 4). Therefore, the simplest code that could specify the correct number of amino acids is a triplet code. When all triple combinations of the four nucleotides are made, 64 (4 × 4 × 4) combinations are possible. Because only 20 combinations are necessary, the code must be *degenerate*, meaning that an amino acid can be specified by more than one triplet.

The next step was to establish which nucleotide triplets specified which amino acids. Two complementary approaches were taken to solve this problem. The first was to synthesize polyribonucleotides of defined sequence and then incubate them in the presence of a *cell-free protein synthesis system*, containing all the necessary factors for protein synthesis to occur. Subsequent analysis of the protein products allowed assignment of amino acids to individual codons. A different approach involved synthesizing trinucleotides of known sequence, associating them with ribosomes, then testing the ability of the resulting complexes to stimulate the binding of specific aminoacyl-tRNAs. The combination of these approaches established the codon assignments for each of the amino acids as shown in Table 1.3.

Three generalizations emerged with the solving of the genetic code. First, when several codons specify the same amino acid, the first two bases of the triplet are constant whereas the third can vary. For example, all codons starting with GU specify valine (GUA, GUC, GUG, GUU). This flexibility in the third position of a codon may help to minimize the consequences of error. This led Francis Crick to propose the *wobble hypothesis* which postulated that once correct base-pairing has occurred between the first two bases of the

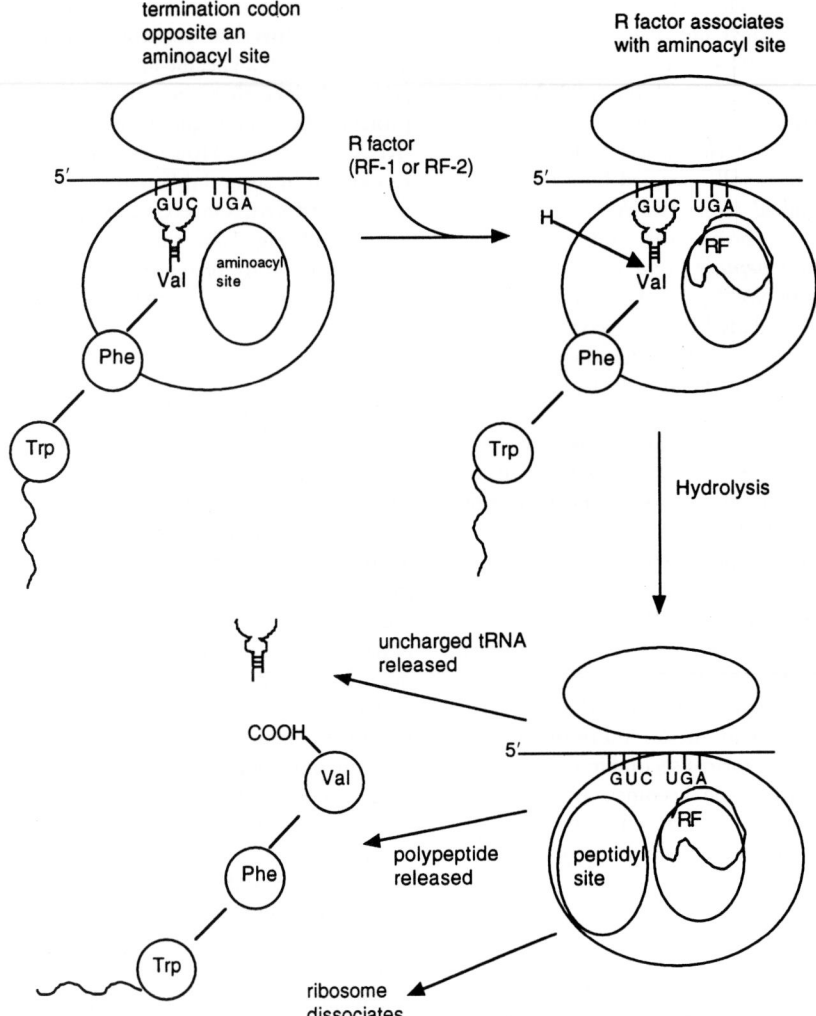

FIGURE 1.24 The termination of protein synthesis. The polypeptide chain is terminated when a termination codon (UGA) is reached. The aminoacyl site is then occupied by a release factor (RF) which pairs with the termination codon, stimulating release of polypeptide and uncharged tRNA, and dissociation of the ribosomal subunits.

mRNA codon and the tRNA anticodon, some wobble will be permissible at the third position. Thus certain tRNA species are able to recognize more than one codon for the same amino acid.

The second generalization was that amino acids with similar structural properties tend to have related codons. For example the aromatic amino acids phenylalanine (UUU, UUC), tyrosine (UAU, UAC), and tryptophan (UGG) all begin with uracil. Similarly, 13 of the 16 codons containing uracil in the middle position encode branched-chain amino acids (leucine, isoleucine, and valine). This feature of the code also serves to minimize the consequences of mistakes made during translation or of mutagenic base substitutions.

The final pattern that emerged was that the codons UAG, UAA, and UGA were not active as trinucleotides in promoting the binding of aminoacyl-tRNAs to ribosomes, and when they appeared in mRNA molecules they promoted the cessation of further synthesis. This led to the conclusion that these codons were chain termination codons. They are now known to be present in all mRNA species that code for polypeptides, and they cause the termination of further polypeptide chain elongation and promote the release of newly synthesized protein.

## PROTEIN TARGETING

Within eukaryotic cells there are two types of *ribosome* responsible for protein biosynthesis, those that are free in the cytosol and a second type which are bound to the *endoplasmic reticulum* (ER). Cytosolic proteins are synthesized by free ribosomes. If a protein is synthesized on the ER it has three fates. It can remain anchored to the ER, it can pass through the ER membrane and into the lumen to be directed to another subcellular organelle, or it can be transported to the

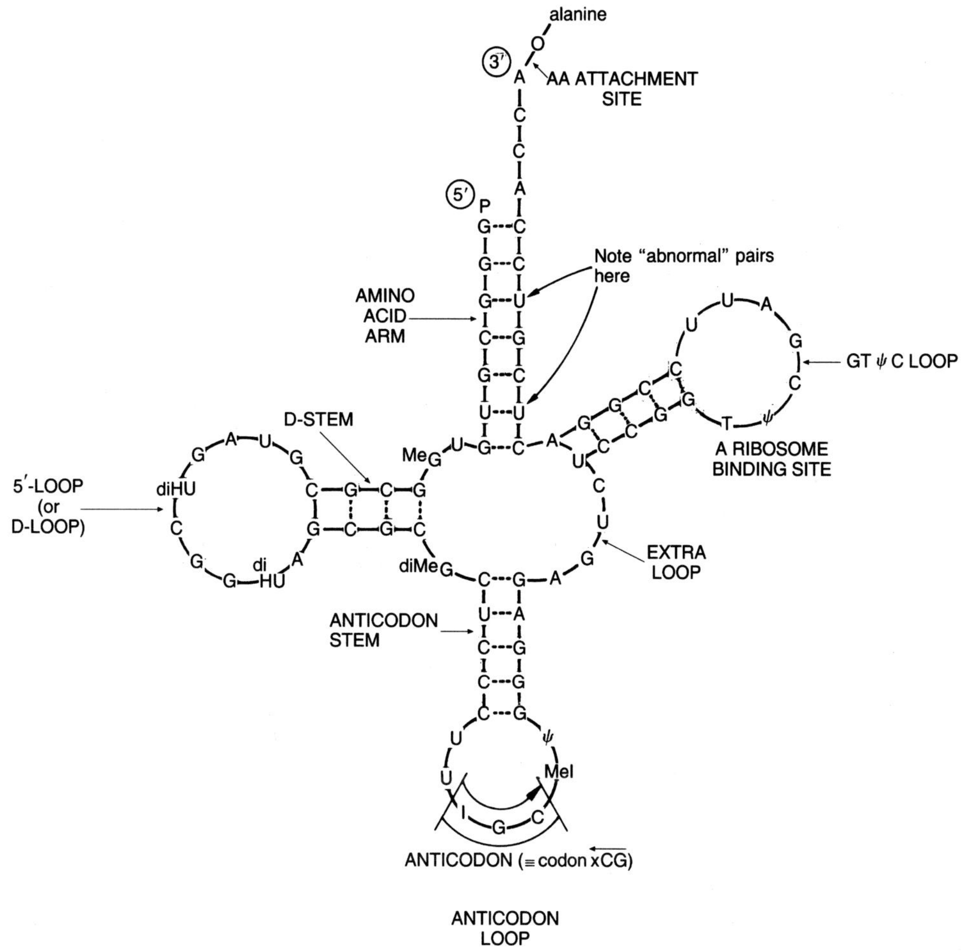

FIGURE 1.25 The structure of mature tRNA. The cloverleaf structure of a prototypical tRNA molecule is shown. Note especially the anticodon loop that recognizes the triplet codon in the mRNA corresponding to the amino acid with which the tRNA will be charged. The amino acid is covalently linked to the amino acid attachment site at the 3′ end of the tRNA. All tRNAs end with the sequence ACC at the aminoacyl (AA) attachment site.

TABLE 1.3 Genetic code and amino acid abbreviations

| FIRST POSITION (5′ end of mRNA) (read down) | SECOND POSITION (read across) | | | | THIRD POSITION (3′end) (read down) |
|---|---|---|---|---|---|
| | U | C | A | G | |
| U | phe | ser | tyr | cys | U |
| | phe | ser | tyr | cys | C |
| | leu | ser | Stop | Stop | A |
| | leu | ser | Stop | trp | G |
| C | leu | pro | his | arg | U |
| | leu | pro | his | arg | C |
| | leu | pro | gln | arg | A |
| | leu | pro | gln | arg | G |
| A | ile | thr | asn | ser | U |
| | ile | thr | asn | ser | C |
| | ile | thr | lys | arg | A |
| | met (start) | thr | lys | arg | G |
| G | val | ala | asp | gly | U |
| | val | ala | asp | gly | C |
| | val | ala | glu | gly | A |
| | val (start) | ala | glu | gly | G |

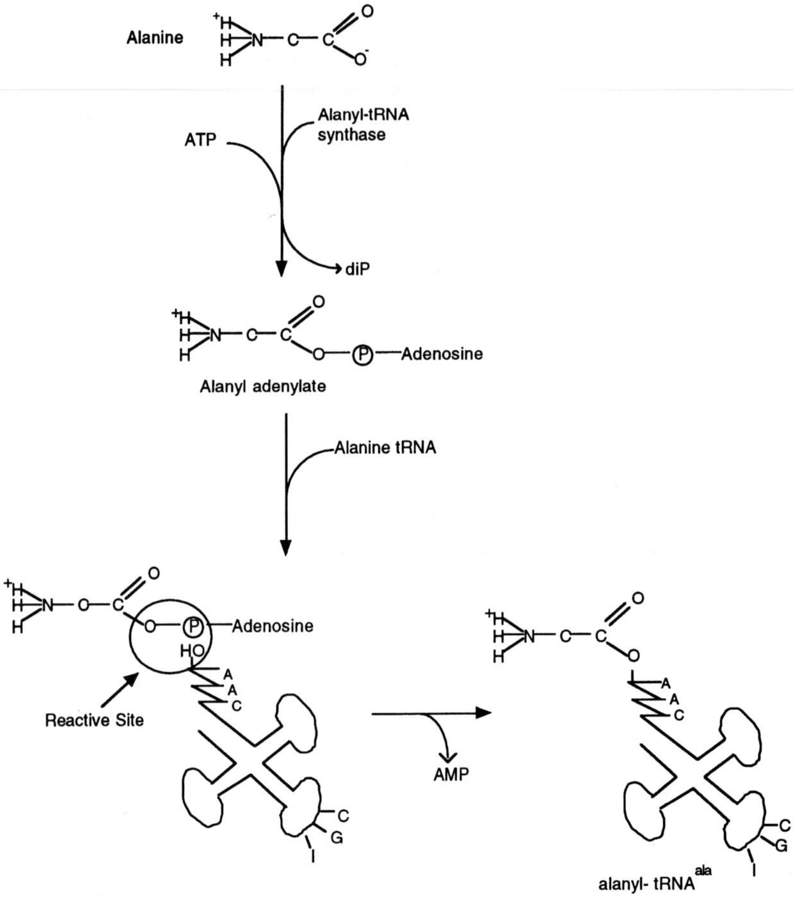

FIGURE 1.26 Charging of tRNA. Aminoacyl-tRNA synthase, in the presence of ATP, interacts with an amino acid (in this example alanine) to form an adenylated residue. This can then associate with the 3′-OH of the amino acid attachment site of an alanine tRNA. Finally there is hydrolysis of AMP to form an ester bond between the two to produce a tRNA$^{ala}$.

plasma membrane where it may reside or be released from the cell.

Studies completed over 20 years ago determined that there are *signal sequences* located within the amino terminus of the linear amino acid sequence of certain proteins that target these proteins (and the ribosome synthesizing the nascent protein) to the ER (Fig. 1.27). These sequences range from 15 to 30 amino acids in length and are distinguishable by a high concentration of hydrophobic residues. The signal sequence is recognized by the *signal recognition particle* (SRP) which guides the ribosome to a specific receptor on the ER. After insertion into the ER membrane, the signal sequence is thought to adopt conformations that either block further transfer of the protein (*stop-transfer sequences*) or are recognized by channel proteins to allow the passage through the membrane and into the lumen. As the protein passes through the membrane the signal peptide is usually cleaved by a peptidase found on the luminal side of the ER. Most often there is coupling between translation of the protein and transfer across the ER membrane (*co-translation*) although some proteins are transferred after translation is complete (*post-translation*). Post-translational insertion into membranes is most often associated

with proteins destined for the nucleus, mitochondrion or chloroplast (in plants). In these cases the proteins are synthesized on free ribosomes, released into the cytosol and then directed to the relevant organelle. These proteins also contain amino-terminal sequences that both direct the protein to the relevant organelle and are removed after transfer.

## GLYCOSYLATION AND PROTEIN TARGETING

Proteins moving along the biosynthetic/secretory pathway from the ER to their final destination (extracellular, plasma membrane, lysosome) are labeled, by glycosylation, to "tag" the protein to the correct pathway. There are two types of glycosylation. One involves N-linked glycosylation of the side chains of asparagine residues, and the second involves O-linked glycosylation of the side-chains of either serine or threonine. Even in heavily glycosylated proteins, not all asparagine or serine/threonine residues will be modified, because glycosylation is determined by flanking amino acids. The function of glycosylation has been demonstrated in yeast strains defective in

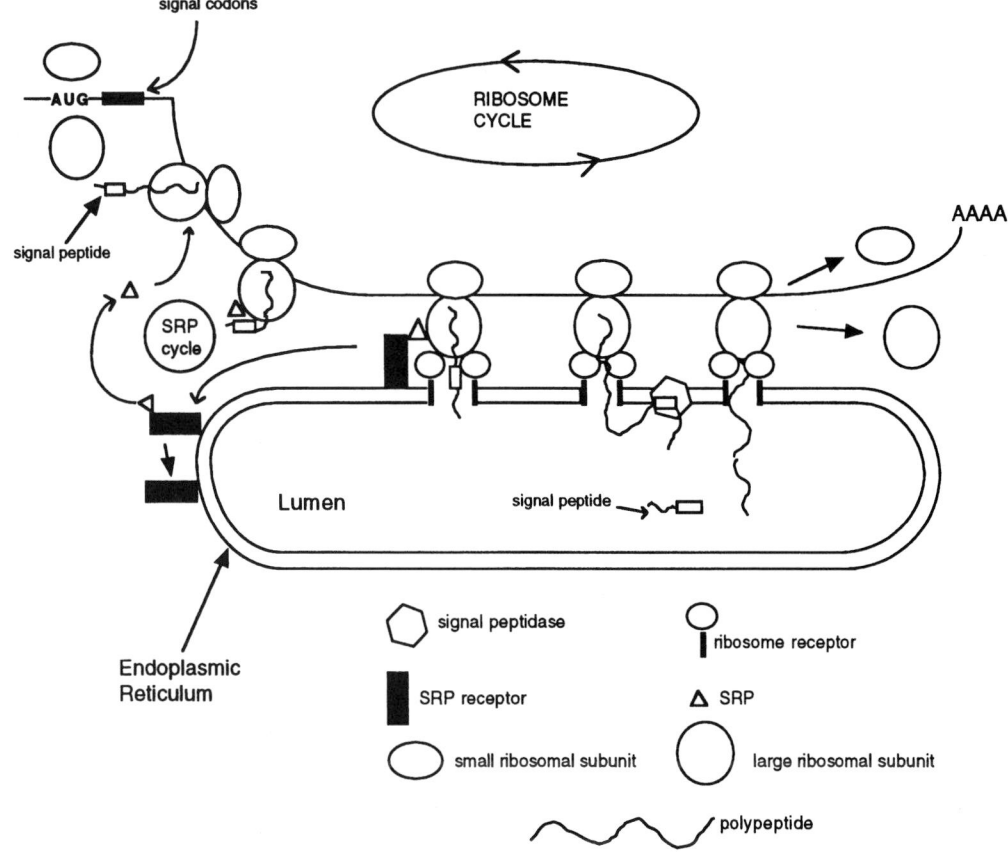

FIGURE 1.27 The signal hypothesis. In this model for the biosynthesis of secretory and membrane proteins, translation occurs in ribosomes associated with the membrane of the endoplasmic reticulum. The signal sequence is recognized by the signal recognition particle (SRP) and binds to a specific receptor on the ER. The signal sequence is then cleaved by the action of a signal peptidase as the protein passes through to the luminal side of the ER. The signal recognition particle and receptor then dissociate and are free to repeat the cycle.

this process; as a result these yeasts are unable to correctly route their proteins.

The process of glycosylation occurs in two stages. The first occurs in the ER itself where the primary oligosaccharides are added, and the second in the Golgi apparatus, where there is extensive modification of the oligosaccharide side-chains. The sugar residues to be transferred are first built on a carrier molecule, the lipid *dolichol phosphate*, by the action of a series of specific transferases which are located on the luminal side of the ER. The first sugars attached are N-acetyl glucosamines followed by mannose residues and finally glucose residues (Fig. 1.28). Finally the core oligosaccharide is transferred to a specific asparagine residue within the growing polypeptide chain. The consensus sequence for transfer appears to be Asn–X–Ser or Asn–X–Thr. Other conformational constraints seem to apply as only a few potential transfer sites are used in any given protein.

## THE GOLGI APPARATUS

Following glycosylation, proteins pass into the lumen of the ER and are ready for transport into the *Golgi*

*apparatus*, a stack of flattened membranous sacs in which the core oligosaccharides are trimmed and new sugar residues added. The Golgi apparatus is responsible for the sorting and packaging of glycoproteins and for their transport to a variety of cellular locations. The glycoproteins are delivered by vesicles coated in a polyhedral lattice formed by clustering of the protein *clathrin* on the outside of the vesicle. These *coated vesicles* bud from the ER and fuse with the Golgi stack. They also carry membrane proteins from the Golgi stack to other cellular locations such as lysosomes, and the plasma membrane, as well as transporting proteins and lipids from the plasma membrane to internal membrane locations.

Early electron microscopic studies showed that the Golgi has a polarized structure with secretory granules located on one side of the stack. These observations suggested that proteins are transported vectorially in a process involving the progressive movement of protein and membrane from the immature (*cis*) to the mature side (*trans*) of the Golgi structure. However, recent developments have considerably changed the picture of this secretory pathway. The series of compartments which participate in the vectorial transport of proteins are not static entities but rather are highly dynamic

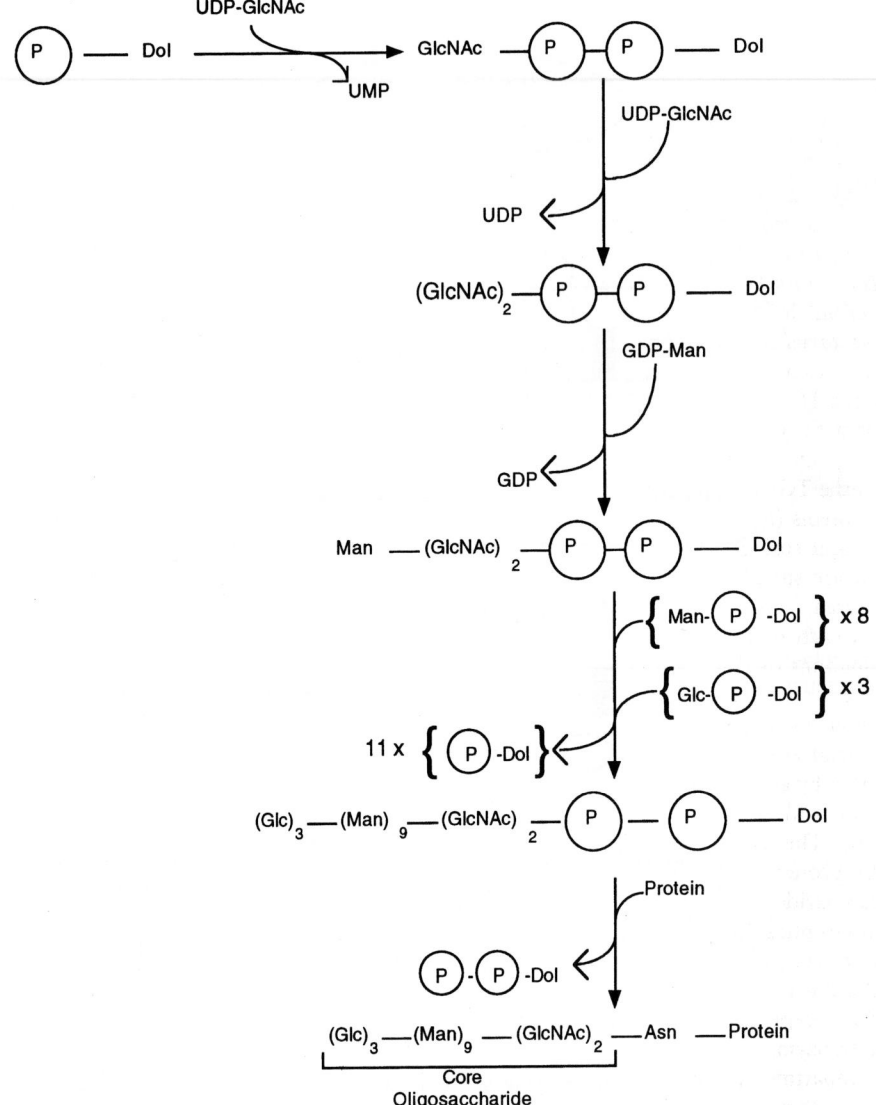

FIGURE 1.28 Glycosylation of eukaryotic secreted proteins. The sequential addition of single sugar units leads to the production of a core oligosaccharide that can then be transferred to the side-chain of an asparagine residue located on a protein in the lumen of the ER. Dolichol phosphate (Dol-P) is first charged with two N-acetyl glucosamine (GlcNAc) molecules and the first mannose molecule. Note that the initial sugars are transferred from UDP and GDP complexes. The last 11 sugars (8 mannose and 3 glucose) are transferred from dolichol phosphate complexes, producing 11 free dolichol phosphate molecules. In a final step, the core oligosaccharide is transferred to an asparagine residue.

membrane structures. Both the positioning and morphology of the ER and Golgi complex are in a constant state of movement. These two organelles also have been shown to be connected by a recycling pathway which can operate, for example, in the retention of a number of resident proteins within the lumen of the ER. Studies with the fungal inhibitor, brefeldin A, suggest that the integrity of the Golgi stack relies on the balance of the two-way traffic between the ER and Golgi and that this is tightly regulated by the interactions of the membrane and cytoskeletal components.

A new understanding of protein movement in the Golgi has arisen from the identification and analysis of temperature-sensitive yeast mutants. In these yeasts, protein trafficking within the Golgi is stopped by changing the growth conditions from the permissive to the sensitive temperature, with the result that proteins accumulate at sites proximal to the block. These changes can be seen by electron microscopy. Some mutations caused accumulation in the cis-Golgi while others caused accumulation in the trans-Golgi. Clearly the Golgi subcompartments, rather than being identical as the previous model supposed, are now known to have distinct functions in both protein sorting and membrane recycling. The Golgi can now be differentiated by morphological, genetic, and functional characteristics into the *cis*- and *trans*-Golgi networks (CGN and TGN).

## PROTEIN TARGETING AND SECRETION

Proteins that are destined for various targets within the cell, or are being secreted, are transported through the intermediate compartment and the Golgi complex to the *trans*-Golgi network (TGN). Transport appears to be in one direction (from *cis*- to *trans*-Golgi, and is referred to as *vectorial transport*. The transport of all these different classes of proteins is thought to occur by bulk flow until the TGN is reached where final protein sorting is thought to occur. In cells, with a regulated secretory pathway, there is a three-tiered sorting event which occurs in the TGN. In this process the constitutive secretory proteins (those that are secreted as they are synthesized and sorted), regulated secretory proteins (those that are stored within the cell until secretion is stimulated) and lysosomal enzymes are segregated from each other and are directed to their respective destinations by distinct mechanisms.

The constitutive secretory proteins are passively segregated by bulk flow into clathrin coated vesicles, while the lysosomal enzymes and regulated secretory proteins are sorted by active processes that direct them to pre-lysosomes and immature secretory granules (ISG) respectively. The mechanism by which the sorting of lysosomal proteins occurs involves modification of the oligosaccharide chain of these proteins to include mannose-6-phosphate. Mannose-6-phosphate is recognized by a specific mannose-6-phosphate receptor that is localized within the Golgi and also at the cell surface, and this receptor mediates both targeting of proteins to the lysozyme and their recapture from the extracellular compartment. In cells lacking the enzymatic machinery that adds mannose-6-phosphate, lysosomal proteins are secreted constitutively, and are not found in lysozymes or taken up from the external environment. This observation demonstrates both the importance of mannose-6-phosphate and its receptor in protein targeting and the passive nature of constitutive secretion.

Regulated secretory proteins leave the TGN as membrane-bound structures containing dilute solutions of the protein(s) to be secreted. This structure is known as a *condensing vacuole*. With time, the secreted protein combines with another glycoprotein of the condensing vacuole and a precipitate forms. The particle is then called a *secretory vesicle* and the precipitate within is called a *dense-cored aggregate* because of its appearance in the electron microscope. Because the precipitate is osmotically inactive, there is net movement of water out of the vesicle. This mechanism allows the maximum amount of protein to be delivered to the cell surface in the minimum volume, and hence with the minimum requirement for cellular membrane. Fig. 1.29 depicts a possible pathway for the

targeting and regulated secretion of proteins through the TGN.

## PROTEIN DEGRADATION

The proteins within a cell are in a constant state of synthesis and degradation. This allows the basic metabolic pathways present to be highly regulated in response to changing environmental signals. The process by which proteins are degraded is very specific and thus different proteins can be turned over at vastly different rates. Paradoxically this process has an absolute requirement for energy, which may endow the system with the aforementioned specificity.

In mammalian cells there are two separate degradation pathways which are either *lysosomal* or *non-lysosomal* associated. The lysosomal pathway is responsible for the degradation of proteins that enter the cell from without (for example by receptor-mediated endocytosis). This pathway can also degrade intracellular proteins, but this occurs mostly under conditions of extreme stress, such as starvation. The non-lysosomal pathways are responsible for the turnover of proteins that are required to keep the cellular machinery working smoothly under basic metabolic conditions.

One such pathway that has been extensively studied involves the polypeptide, *ubiquitin*. This protein is found in abundance in all eukaryotic cells. Ubiquitin modification of proteins within the cell is now known to play an important role in a variety of cellular processes. Amongst these are the regulation of gene expression, cell cycle, and division, cellular responses to stress, cell surface receptor activity, DNA repair, protein import into mitochondria, uptake of precursors into neurons and in the biogenesis of mitochondria, ribosomes, and peroxisomes. However, the best studied ubiquitin modification pathway is the one involving proteolysis.

### Ubiquitin-mediated proteolytic pathway

This is a non-lysosomal ATP-dependent proteolytic system that has been characterized and partially purified. The system consists of several essential constituents, one of which is ubiquitin, a 76-amino-acid polypeptide. The degradation of a polypeptide through this pathway can be separated into two steps (Fig. 1.30). The first involves the covalent attachment of multiple ubiquitin molecules to the targeted protein. The carboxy-terminal glycine of the ubiquitin is activated by ATP to produce a high-energy thiol-ester intermediate by the ubiquitin-activating enzyme (E1). Following this a ubiquitin-carrier protein (E2) transfers the ubiquitin from E1 to a ubiquitin protein ligase (E3). E3 then catalyzes the formation of an isopeptide bond between the activated glycine residue and $\varepsilon$-NH$_2$ groups of lysine residues within the target protein. This final step appears to involve the binding of the

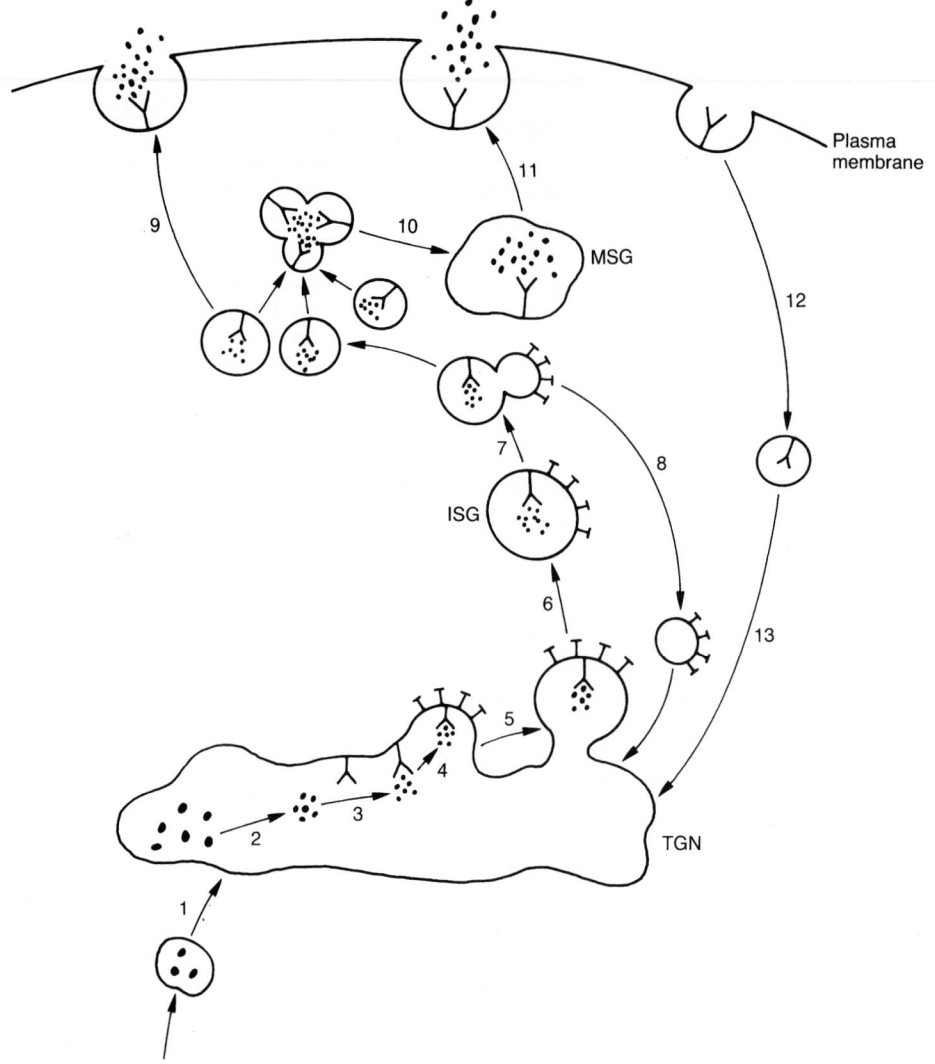

FIGURE 1.29 Transport through the *trans*-Golgi network (TGN). Secretory proteins are transported through the Golgi to the TGN (1) where there is the aggregation of proteins (2) and membrane association (3). Subsequently the aggregates are progressively engulfed in membrane (4 and 5) until there is budding of the immature secretory granule (ISG) which is partially clathrin-coated (6). This clathrin is then lost (7) and recycled back to the TGN (8). The ISG can then either fuse directly with the membrane to release its contents (9) or fuse with other ISGs to form the mature secretory granule (MSG) (10). MSGs are stored at the periphery of the cell until a signal is received which triggers their fusion with the membrane and their contents are released (11). The membrane components are then internalized (12) and returned to the TGN (13).

target protein to E3 prior to the interaction with ubiquitin. Thus E3 may play a very important role in determining which polypeptides are designated for degradation. In the second step the ubiquitin-protein substrate is degraded by a specific ATP-dependent protease to liberate free amino acids and reusable ubiquitin.

## SELECTED READING

Altmann M, Trachsel H. The yeast Saccharomyces cerevisiae system: a powerful tool to study the mechanism of protein synthesis initiation in eukaryotes. *Biochimie* 1994; **76**: 853.

Ciechanover A. The ubiquitin-mediated proteolytic pathway: mechanisms of action and cellular physiology. *Biolog Chem Hoppe-Seyler* 1994; **375**: 565.

Kozak M. A short leader sequence impairs the fidelity of initiation by eukaryotic ribosomes. *Gene Expr* 1991; **1**: 111.

Kozak M. Downstream secondary structure facilitates recognition of initiator codons by eukaryotic ribosomes. *PNAS* 1990; **87**: 8301.

Kozak M. Regulation of translation in eukaryotic systems. *Ann Rev Cell Biol* 1992; **8**: 197.

Lutcke H. Signal recognition particle (SRP), a ubiquitous initiator of protein translocation. *Eur J Biochem* 1995; **228**: 531.

Opdenakker G, Rudd PM, Ponting CP, Dwek RA. Concepts and principles of glycobiology. *Faseb J* 1993; **7**: 1330.

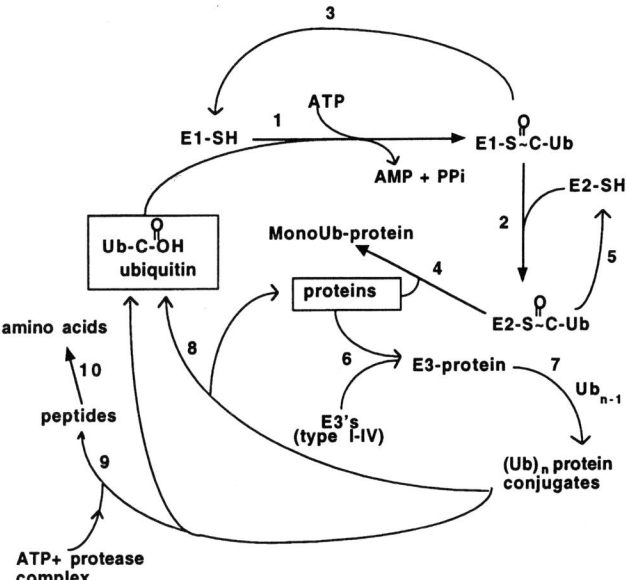

FIGURE 1.30 Proposed sequence of events in the ubiquitin-mediated protein degradation pathway. (1) Ubiquitin activation by ubiquitin activating enzyme (E1); (2) transfer of high-energy ubiquitin to ubiquitin-carrier protein E2; (3) E1 is recycled; (4) protein conjugation of ubiquitin; (5) E2 is recycled; (6) formation of a complex of ubiquitin protein ligase (E3) and protein; (7) protein molecule has multiple ubiquitins attached; (8) ubiquitin recycling; (9) energy-dependent degradation of the protein into peptide fragments; (10) release of amino acids from the peptides.

Rexach MF, Latterich M, Schekman RW. Characteristics of endoplasmic reticulum-derived transport vesicles. *J Cell Biol* 1994; **126**: 1133.

Rexach MF, Schekman RW. Use of sec mutants to define intermediates in protein transport from endoplasmic reticulum. *Meth Enzymol* 1992; **219**: 267.

Rucker RB, McGee C. Chemical modifications of proteins in vivo: selected examples important to cellular regulation. *J Nutrition* 1993; **123**: 977.

Wuestehube LJ, Schekman RW. Reconstitution of transport from endoplasmic reticulum to Golgi complex using endoplasmic reticulum-enriched membrane fraction from yeast. *Meth Enzymol* 1992; **219**: 124.

# RECOMBINANT DNA TECHNOLOGY

Once nucleic acids were identified as the genetic material, and it became possible to purify large quantities of DNA and RNA, a system for analysis of eukaryotic genes was needed. The fundamental problem was how to extract a single nucleic acid sequence of interest from a heterogeneous population of nucleic acid chains and then produce it in sufficient quantity and purity to allow subsequent analysis. Present techniques provide a variety of solutions to this fundamental problem, but all ultimately rely on the same basic principle; namely that the DNA of interest must be isolated from nearby sequences and *recombined* with DNA from one of several simpler microbial systems. When placed back in the original microbe or *host*, the DNA of interest will be replicated with very high fidelity by the host's genetic machinery. As the microbe divides over and over, a substantial quantity of the DNA of interest is produced. Because the DNA thus produced is identical, the process has been dubbed *cloning*.

The techniques for identification, cutting, pasting, and replication of DNA are outlined in the discussion that follows. Each section outlines a separate piece of the technology, but the techniques are unified by the principle that each relies on the utilization of genetic and enzymatic machinery normally occurring in nature. It is this fact more than any other that has allowed the molecular revolution to occur. Once the study of the genetics of microbial organisms revealed the power of these manipulable molecular factories, it was not long before they were being widely applied in the study of eukaryotic genes. Indeed, one of the truly remarkable things about modern molecular biology is the speed with which new biological mechanisms are translated into reagents for the next set of experiments.

## HOST RESTRICTION–MODIFICATION SYSTEMS

Many bacterial strains synthesize enzymes, called *restriction nucleases*, which protect them from invading foreign DNA. Each enzyme recognizes a specific DNA sequence of 4–8 nucleotides. The corresponding sequences in the genome of the bacterium are

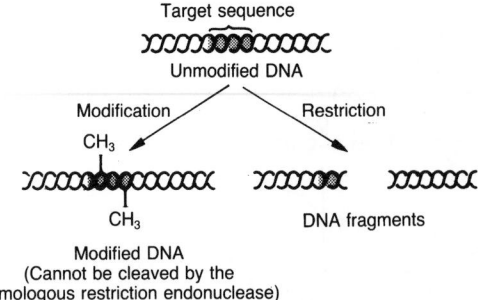

Target sequence
Unmodified DNA

Modification / Restriction

CH₃

CH₃ / DNA fragments

Modified DNA
(Cannot be cleaved by the
homologous restriction endonuclease)

FIGURE 1.31 Bacterial host restriction–modification systems. The methylation of A or C residues in the genome (represented by the CH₃) tags the DNA as host and protects it from digestion by restriction endonucleases.

"camouflaged" by methylation at certain A or C residues to prevent cleavage of the host DNA (Fig. 1.31). However, any DNA that enters the cell does not have this protection. Thus it is recognized as foreign and both strands of the DNA molecule are cleaved. Many of these restriction enzymes have been purified from various bacterial species. Most recognize unique nucleotide sequences, and are now commercially available.

Many restriction nucleases produce staggered, or *cohesive*, ends. These can form complementary base pairs with any other end produced by the action of the same enzyme. The cohesive ends generated by restriction enzymes have played a vital role in DNA technology because they allow any two DNA fragments to be joined, provided they are produced by the same enzyme and thus possess *complementary ends*. Once the two ends have been brought together they can be sealed by the action of the enzyme DNA ligase. These enzymes can form covalent phosphodiester bonds between the opposing ends of each DNA strand and thus seal the molecule. The combined use of restriction nucleases and DNA ligases has made it possible to clone fragments of DNA into self-replicating elements.

## VECTOR–HOST SYSTEMS

Fragments of DNA from any source can be amplified using one of the four main systems for cloning foreign DNA in *E. coli*. These cloning systems are plasmids, bacteriophage lambda (λ), cosmids and bacteriophage M13. These differ in their size and structure but share the following properties: they can replicate autonomously in *E. coli* even when linked to foreign DNA; they can easily be separated from bacterial nucleic acids and purified; and they contain regions of DNA not essential for propagation in bacteria, that can be replaced with foreign DNA, which then is treated as a normal component of the vector. Each system has its own particular advantages and disadvantages for molecular cloning purposes and a summary is detailed in Table 1.4.

## Plasmids

These are extra chromosomal genetic elements found in a variety of bacterial species. They are double-stranded, closed, circular DNA molecules which vary in size between 1 and 200kb. Plasmids often code for enzymes which are advantageous to the host under certain environmental conditions. Among the conferred phenotypes are resistance to antibiotics; production of antibiotics, colicins, and enterotoxins; and production of enzymes that can degrade complex organic molecules or are involved in host restriction–modification systems. Under natural conditions many plasmids are transmitted to new hosts by a process similar to bacterial conjugation. However, in the laboratory plasmids are transferred to new hosts by the process of *transformation*. This is accomplished by treating the bacterial cells in such a way, usually with $CaCl_2$, so as to make them permeable to small DNA molecules. The new phenotype conferred to the host allows for a simple selection of the transformed cells within the background population of non-transformed cells.

TABLE 1.4 Advantages and disadvantages of the various DNA cloning systems. The features that are required for different purposes are summarized in this table as either present (+) or absent (−) in the available systems.

|  | PLASMIDS | BACTERIOPHAGE λ | COSMIDS | SINGLE-STRANDED BACTERIOPHAGES |
|---|---|---|---|---|
| Cloning large DNA fragments | ±[a] | + | + | − |
| Constructing genomic libraries | − | + | + | − |
| Constructing cDNA libraries | + | − | − | − |
| Routine subcloning | + | − | − | − |
| Building new DNA constructs | + | − | − | − |
| Sequencing | + | − | − | + |
| Single-stranded probes | − | − | − | + |
| Expressing foreign genes in *E. coli* | + | − | − | − |

[a]Although there have been no defined limits to the size of DNA fragments that can be cloned into plasmids, the transformation efficiency and the yield of plasmid DNA containing more than ~10 kb of foreign DNA are extremely low.

Replication of plasmid DNA is usually carried out by the same set of enzymes that are responsible for the replication of the bacterial chromosome. The replication of some plasmids is defined as being under *stringent control*, meaning that their replication is coupled to that of the host so that only one, or at most a few, copies of the plasmid are present in any particular cell. Plasmids under *relaxed control* have copy numbers of 10–200 since their replication is relatively independent of the host. This number can be raised to several thousand per cell if host protein synthesis is stopped by the addition of chloramphenicol to the growth medium. In the absence of host protein synthesis, replication of relaxed plasmids continues, whereas the replication of host DNA ceases.

To be useful as a cloning vector, a plasmid should possess several properties: it should be relatively small and replicate in a relaxed way; carry one or more selectable markers to allow selection of transformants and to maintain the plasmid in the population; and contain a single recognition site for one or more restriction nucleases in regions of the plasmid not essential for replication.

The advantages of small size are that the plasmid DNA is easier to handle, as it is less susceptible to physical damage and possesses a simpler restriction map. Smaller plasmids generally have a higher copy number which increases the sensitivity with which bacteria carrying the foreign DNA sequences can be identified. However, smaller size can lead to the elimination of useful cloning sites. To extend this range, polylinkers are inserted. These are segments of DNA that contain closely spaced sites for several restriction enzymes.

## Cloning in plasmids

In principle, cloning foreign DNA into a plasmid is straightforward: plasmid DNA is cleaved with a restriction enzyme endonuclease and joined *in vitro* to the foreign DNA. The resulting recombinant plasmids are then placed back into *E. coli* by a simple process called *transformation*. However, in practice the plasmid vector must be carefully chosen to minimize the effort required to identify and characterize the recombinants. The major difficulty is to distinguish plasmids with foreign DNA inserts from recircularized plasmids with no insert. This recircularization can be minimized by adjusting the concentrations of foreign DNA and vector during ligation. There are other procedures that have been developed to further reduce recircularization, and to more readily identify recombinant molecules.

### Insertional inactivation

This procedure can be used if the plasmid carries two or more antibiotic resistance markers (Fig. 1.32). The

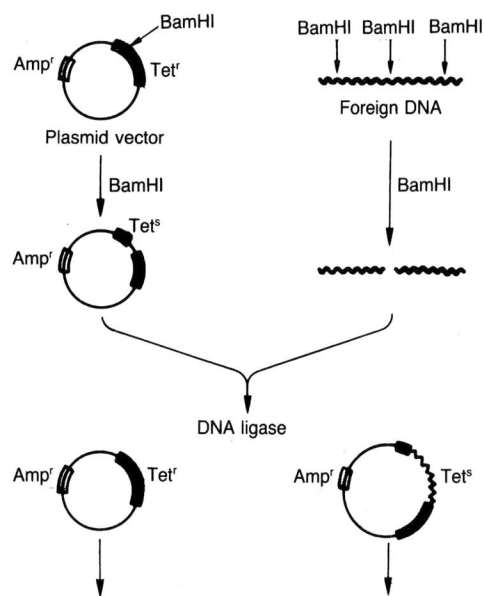

FIGURE 1.32 Insertional activation as a means to clone foreign DNA. The DNA and the plasmid in which it is to be cloned are cut with a restriction endonuclease that is present in one of the antibiotic (tetracycline) resistant genes (Tet$^r$) within the plasmid. The two are then ligated and transformed into *E coli*. The recombinants (b) will only grow in the presence of ampicillin, while the colonies formed from the religated vector (a) will grow in the presence of both tetracycline and ampicillin.

DNA to be inserted and the vector are digested with a restriction enzyme that recognizes a unique site in one of the resistance genes. After ligation the mixture is used to transform an *E. coli* strain sensitive to both antibiotics. These cells are then grown in the presence of the unrestricted antibiotic gene and the colonies which form contain a mixture of recombinant molecules and recircularized vectors. These colonies are then replica plated onto an agar plate containing the restricted antibiotic such that only the colonies containing the recircularized plasmid grow. Those that do not grow are likely to contain foreign DNA sequences.

A similar technique, now widely used in many commercially available cloning vectors, is the process of color selection. In these plasmids, the cloning site has been engineered to reside in the middle of a plasmid gene encoding a fragment of the enzyme β-galactosidase that is capable of joining with the non-functional β-galactosidase encoded on the bacterial chromosome to produce a functional enzyme. This process is called *complementation*. In the presence of an artificial substrate for β-galactosidase, a blue color is produced. When the plasmid gene is interrupted by foreign DNA, complementation cannot occur and the colonies are white rather than blue. This system has the advantage that replica plates need not be produced.

## Directional cloning

Most plasmids carry two or more unique restriction sites. For example the vector pBR322 has single *Hind* III and *Bam* HI sites. Thus, after cleavage with both enzymes the larger fragment can be obtained and ligated to foreign DNA containing compatible cohesive ends (Fig. 1.33). Since there is no complementarity between *Bam* HI and *Hind* III the vector cannot recirculate efficiently and thus only the vector should be able to successfully transform *E. coli*. Different combinations of enzymes can be used depending on the locations of restriction sites in the vector and the fragment of foreign DNA to be cloned.

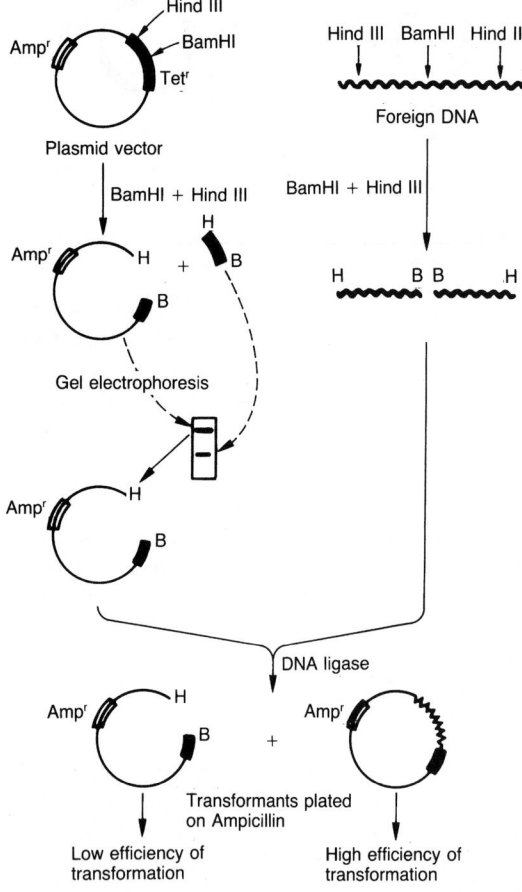

FIGURE 1.33 Directional cloning in plasmids. See text for details.

## Phosphatase treatment of linear plasmid vector DNA

During ligation, DNA ligase will catalyze the formation of a phosphodiester bond between adjacent nucleotides only if one contains a 5'-phosphate group and the other a 3'-OH group. Thus recirculation of the plasmid can be minimized by removing the 5'-phosphate from both ends of the linearized plasmid DNA (Fig. 1.34). This can be accomplished either by bacterial alkaline phosphatase or calf intestinal phosphatase. As a result neither strand of the duplex

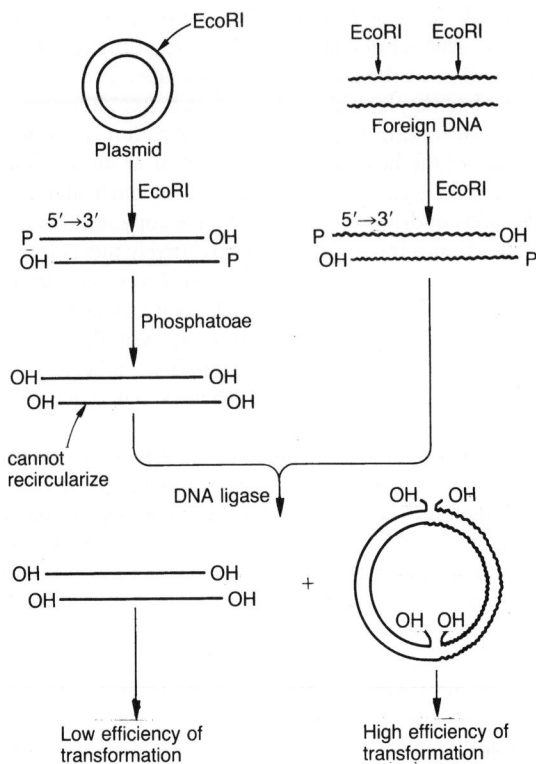

FIGURE 1.34 Phosphatase prevents the recircularization of plasmid DNA. See text for details.

can form a phosphodiester bond. However a foreign segment of DNA with terminal 5'-phosphate groups can be efficiently ligated to the dephosphorylated plasmid to produce an open circular molecule containing two nicks. Since open circular DNA transforms *E. coli* more efficiently than linear plasmid DNA, most of the transformants will contain recombinant plasmids.

## Bacteriophage lambda (λ)

Since the first demonstration that λ can be used as a cloning vehicle, a large number of related vectors have been constructed. λ is a double-stranded DNA virus of 50 kb in length. The DNA is found in a linear form within the viral particle containing single-stranded complementary ends, 12 bp in length. These ends are produced by the action of a viral enzyme which recognizes this 12 base sequence called the *cos* site. Upon entering the host, the DNA circularizes and one of two pathways is chosen (Fig. 1.35). The first is *lytic growth* where the circular DNA is replicated many-fold in the cell and many viral particles are formed prior to lysing the cell. The second pathway is *lysogenic growth*, where the viral genome is integrated into the host chromosome and is subsequently replicated and transmitted to progeny bacteria as any chromosomal gene.

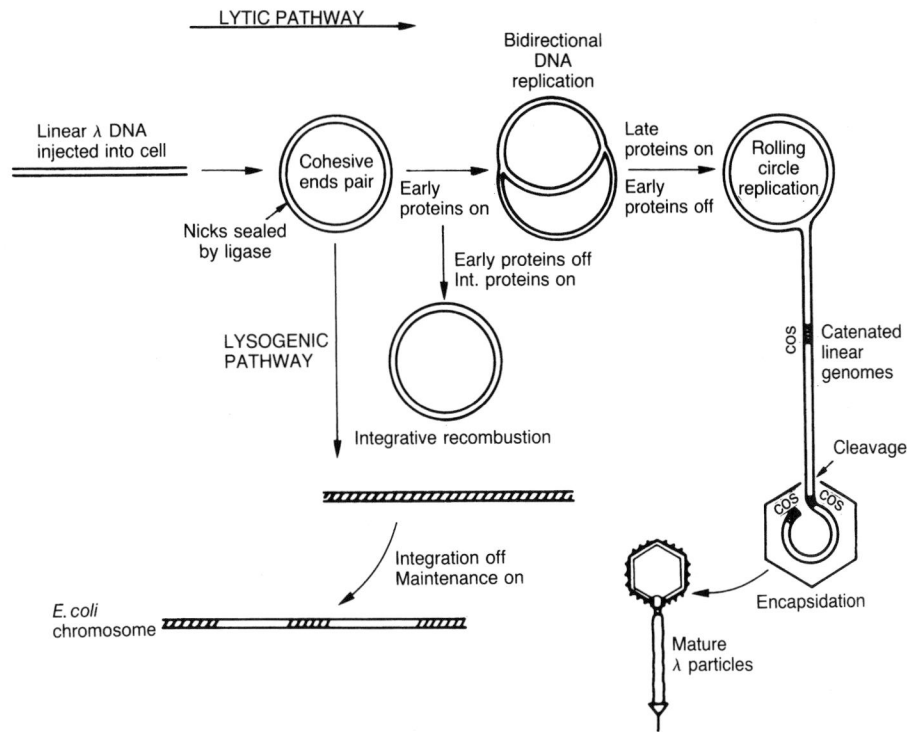

FIGURE 1.35 The bacteriophage λ life-cycle. Double-stranded λ DNA enters the cell as a linear duplex. The lytic pathway requires the activity of both early and late genes and leads to host cell lysis. The lysogenic pathway requires only the activity of early genes and allows the host cell to survive, although the rate of cell growth is usually slightly retarded.

## Construction of λ vectors

At first glance it would seem a bleak prospect to use λ, with its large and complex genome, as a vector. Its DNA contains several sites for many of the restriction enzymes that are most useful in cloning, and these sites are often in regions essential for lytic growth. Also, since the viral particle itself will only accommodate DNA molecules that are approximately the same size as the viral genome, it would appear that λ would only be useful to clone small pieces of DNA.

However, these problems are not as formidable as they appear. First, the central third of the genome, lying between the J and N genes, is non-essential for lytic growth. Second, knowledge of the genetics of restriction and modification systems provided the opportunity to select, *in vivo*, λ derivatives that are free of certain useful restriction enzymes. This has allowed the production of a large number of λ vectors which have a single target site at which foreign DNA can be inserted to produce what are known as *insertion vectors*. Similarly, λ vectors exist which have a pair of sites spanning a segment that can be replaced by foreign DNA, referred to as *replacement vectors*.

There is no single λ vector suitable for cloning all DNA fragments. It thus is necessary to choose one suitable for the task at hand. This choice is influenced by the restriction enzyme to be used and the size of foreign DNA fragment to be cloned. Although only 60 per cent of the viral genome is required for lytic

growth, bacteriophage viability decreases dramatically outside the size range of 78–105 per cent of the wild type genome size. Thus it is important to choose a combination of vector and DNA such that the recombinant phage falls within these size limits.

## Cosmids

The construction of libraries in λ vectors has proven to be an effective means of isolating specific segments of DNA from complex eukaryotic genomes. However, the limited size capacity (< 23 kb) of λ cloning vectors is a disadvantage in some situations, since some genes are too large to be cloned in a contiguous segment. For example, the chicken α-collagen I gene is 38 kb and had to be isolated as a series of overlapping genomic clones from a genomic λ library. Now, many genes are known that span more than 100 kb of genomic DNA. The laborious process of chromosome walking needed to characterize these large genes is facilitated by the ability to clone larger fragments of DNA.

*Cosmids* are vectors specifically designed for cloning large fragments of eukaryotic DNA (up to 45 kb in length). The essential components of cosmid cloning vectors are the presence of an antibiotic resistance marker, a plasmid origin of replication and one or more unique restriction sites. Cosmids also contain the λ *cos*

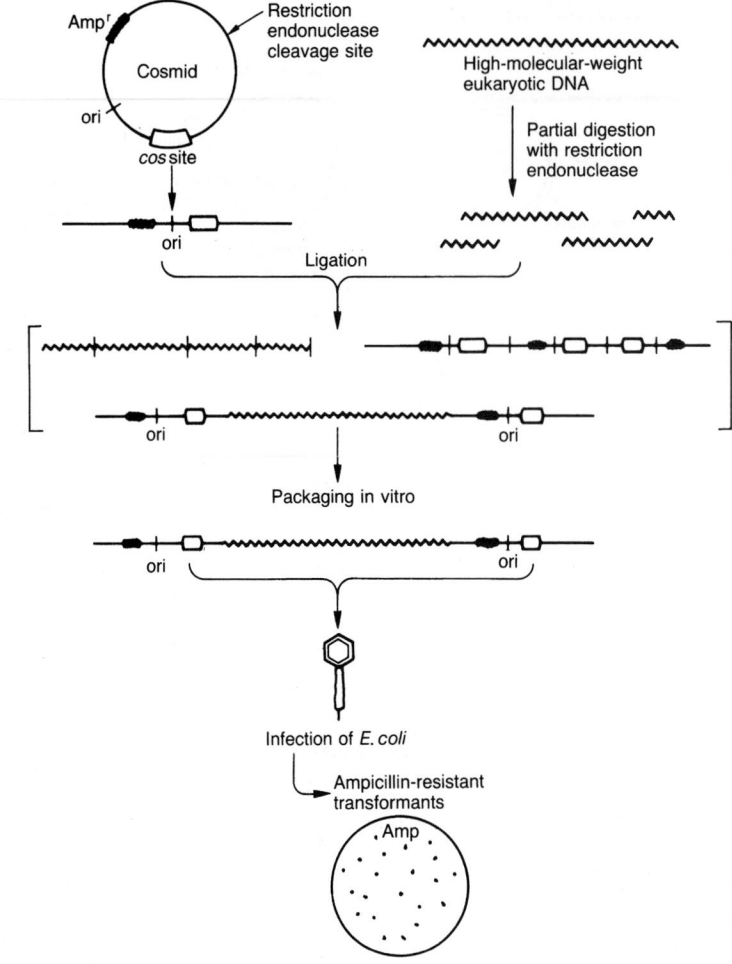

FIGURE 1.36 Cloning large fragments of DNA using cosmids. The details for the cloning procedure are related in the text.

site to allow the circularization of the recombinant molecules upon the infection of the bacterial host.

The basic principles of cloning in cosmids are detailed in Fig. 1.36. A ligation mixture is prepared containing high concentrations of cosmid and foreign DNA that have been digested with a restriction endonuclease. This results in the formation of *catenates* in which the foreign DNA is linked to the cosmid molecule. This is then incubated with a λ packaging extract, thereby allowing the recombinant cosmid molecules to produce mature λ particles. During the infection of *E. coli*, the recombinant DNA is injected by the bacteriophage into the host and then circularizes via the *cos* ends. Since the recombinant molecule contains essential plasmid elements, it can replicate as a plasmid and expresses the antibiotic resistance marker. Owing to the packaging limitations this process selects for bacteriophage particles with a total size of 40–50 kb, and owing to the small size of the cosmid genome up to 45 kb of contiguous foreign DNA can be cloned.

## Single-stranded bacteriophages

By far the best developed single-stranded DNA bacteriophage vectors are those derived from M13. This is a filamentous phage with a closed circular DNA genome of 6.5 kb. The phage attaches to the F-pili of *E. coli* and is thus only able to infect male cells (F′ or Hfr strains). After penetration, the single-stranded phage DNA is converted into the double-stranded replicative form. This can be isolated from cells and is used as a double-stranded cloning vector. After 1–200 copies have been produced M13 synthesis becomes asymmetric, producing large amounts of only one of the two DNA strands which is incorporated into mature phage particles. These particles are continually extruded from the cell, as M13 does not kill its host but only inhibits its growth.

The primary advantage of M13 as a cloning vector is that the phage particles released contain only single-stranded DNA, that is homologous to only one of the complementary strands of the cloned DNA, and can be used either as a template for sequencing using the

Sanger-dideoxy method (see below), to produce single-stranded DNA probes, or to serve as substrates for *in vitro* mutagenesis. The major problem in M13 cloning has been the instability of large DNA inserts. In general, cloned sequences >1 kb are unstable and give rise to deletions during propagation of the phage.

## LIBRARIES

One of the most frequent uses of λ phage and cosmids is the construction of libraries. A genomic library is a mixture of recombinant clones that together contain a complete representation of a particular genome. In practice, genomic DNA is digested with a restriction enzyme that cuts frequently, but under conditions that allow only a small subset of possible cleavage sites to be cut at random. This generates fragments of varying sizes, with the important property that fragments from different DNA molecules will have overlapping sequences. Fragments of approximately 20 kb are size-selected and cloned into a suitable vector. After packaging and infection, a large quantity of phage is produced. A λ clone containing a DNA sequence of interest then can be identified using hybridization techniques discussed below.

A second kind of library is frequently constructed in λ phage. These libraries represent all the mRNAs expressed in a given tissue or cell type in a given condition. Construction of these libraries (as well as study of mRNA sequences) was not possible until the discovery of a novel class of DNA polymerases, the *reverse transcriptases*. These polymerases will make a DNA copy that is complementary to the RNA template. The resulting single-stranded complementary DNA (cDNA) can be made double stranded by the usual DNA polymerases and then can be cloned in exactly analogous fashion to genomic DNA. The resulting library is termed a *cDNA library*. Because most mRNAs are less than 5 kb in length, they easily fit into the λ genome.

As noted above, cosmid vectors were developed to accommodate larger foreign DNA inserts than could be readily placed in phage λ. In the past several years, libraries have been constructed using three new cloning systems that were developed to accept even larger DNA inserts. The largest DNA inserts are found in *yeast artificial chromosomes* (YACs) that contain up to several million base pairs. Unfortunately, YACs frequently undergo recombination, so that the inserted DNA may contain substantial differences when compared with the genomic DNA from which it was derived. This difficulty has largely been overcome by the introduction of *bacterial artificial chromosomes* (BACs) which contain less DNA, but are more stable. Finally, *P1* clones containing 100 kb of DNA, and which can be handled very much like cosmid clones, are now available.

## DNA SEQUENCING

Much of what we know about the molecular machinery of cells has arisen from characterization of linear nucleic acid sequences. This is true for gene structure and the regulatory events that control gene transcription, mRNA translation and stability. Indeed, most of the known protein sequences were derived from nucleic acid sequences and not from the proteins themselves. This fundamental concept has led to complete sequencing of viral and bacterial genomes, and major projects are under way to sequence the *Drosophila*, mouse, and human genomes.

There are two main techniques that can be used to sequence DNA. The first involves the chemical cleavage method developed by Maxam and Gilbert. However, the more widely used technique, developed by Sanger, involves the controlled interruption of enzymatic replication of the DNA. The key to this method is the use of dideoxyribonucleoside triphosphates in which the 3′-OH moiety present in normal nucleotides is missing. When such a modified nucleotide is incorporated into a DNA chain, it blocks subsequent additions of nucleotides. Using a radiolabeled dNTP (usually $^{35}$S-dATP) and four different synthesis reactions, each with a different chain terminating nucleotide, DNA ladders can be produced that vary by a single base in length. These then can be separated by gel electrophoresis in four parallel lanes of a gel to derive the DNA sequence (Fig. 1.37).

## POLYMERASE CHAIN REACTION (PCR)

PCR is used to amplify a region of DNA that lies between two areas of known sequence. As shown in Fig. 1.38, two oligonucleotides, whose sequences match the DNA to be amplified, are used as primers for a series of reactions catalyzed by a DNA polymerase. The template DNA is first denatured by heating to temperatures over 90°C in the presence of excess oligonucleotides and the four dNTPs. The reaction mixture is then cooled to a temperature that allows each of the primers to anneal to their target sequences and to be extended by the action of the DNA polymerase. These cycles of denaturation, annealing and extension are then repeated many times over. Since the product synthesized in one round can act as a template for subsequent steps, each cycle essentially doubles the amount of the desired DNA sequence. The major product of these reactions is a segment of double-stranded DNA whose ends are defined by the sequence of the oligonucleotide primers used and whose length is the distance between the primers.

The original protocols for PCR used the Klenow fragment of *E. coli* DNA polymerase I to extend the primers. However, because this enzyme is inactivated by the temperature required to denature the strands of the DNA duplex, each round of synthesis required the addition of new enzyme. Similarly, these reactions

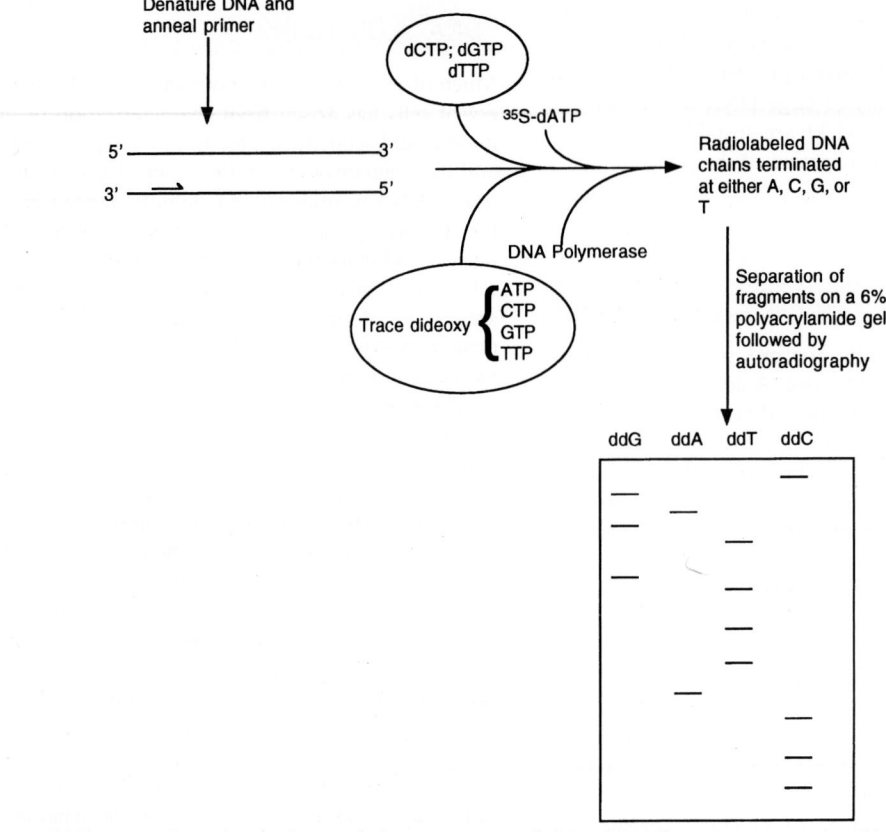

FIGURE 1.37 DNA sequencing using the Sanger chain-termination technique. DNA fragments are produced by mixing 2′,3′-dideoxy analogs for each of the four dNTPs in separate reaction mixtures. This blocks further growth of the chain when it is incorporated into the DNA sequence. The four sets of chain-terminated fragments are then separated by gel electrophoresis on polyacrylamide gels which have a resolution down to the single base-pair level. The sequence of the DNA is then read from an autoradiograph of the gel.

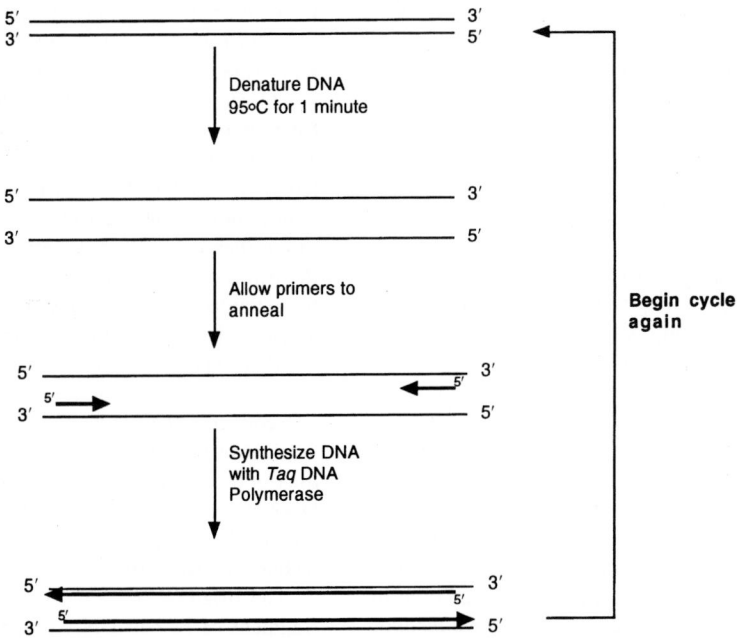

FIGURE 1.38 The steps involved in the polymerase chain reaction (PCR). The template is reduced to a single strand by heating to 95°C and then cooled to allow the primers to bind to their complementary sequences. The primer sequences are then extended with Taq polymerase, producing a copy of the sequence flanked by the two primers. This cycle can be repeated as often as required, with each cycle of the PCR reaction doubling the number of the copies of the target region.

were only applicable to the synthesis of small sequences of DNA (<200 bp). These problems were overcome with the introduction of a thermostable DNA polymerase purified from the thermophilic bacterium *Thermus aquaticus* (*Taq* DNA polymerase). This polymerase can survive extended incubation at 95°C and is thus not inactivated by the denaturation step in the procedure and does not need to be replaced after every cycle.

Although it is still a relatively new technique, PCR amplification is now used extensively in the diagnosis of genetic disease, in the genetic identification of forensic samples, as well as in a variety of tasks in molecular cloning. These include generation of specific sequences for use as probes, generation of probes specific for uncloned but related genes, generation of cDNA libraries from small amounts of mRNA (RT/PCR), and generation of large amounts of DNA for sequencing or mutational analysis. However, a limitation of PCR amplification is its relatively high error rate, with approximately a four-fold higher rate of base misincorporation than with other DNA polymerases. Thus any DNA product obtained using PCR amplification should be confirmed by sequencing the cloned DNA. This eliminates the possibility that misincorporation occurring in the early rounds of amplification might appear in every clone derived from a particular amplification reaction.

## NUCLEIC ACID HYBRIDIZATION

When DNA solutions are heated to temperatures of 100°C the complementary base pairs that hold the two strands together are disrupted, resulting in the dissociation of the double helix into two single strands. This process is called *DNA denaturation* and has been shown to be reversible. The process of *DNA renaturation*, or *hybridization*, is limited by the rate at which the two complementary nucleic acids collide. This process depends on the concentration of the complementary sequences within the solution. Similar hybridization reactions will also occur between any two single-stranded chains (RNA:DNA or RNA:RNA) provided that they have a complementary nucleotide sequence.

DNA fragments can also be produced in which radioactive nucleotides are incorporated into the DNA template. This DNA probe, when denatured, can be used to detect complementary nucleic acid sequences within a population. These hybridization reactions using radiolabeled DNA probes are sensitive enough to detect complementary sequences present at levels of only one copy per cell. Similarly this technique can be used to search for related but non-identical genes. For example, if a particular gene has been cloned from one species a DNA probe from part or all of the molecule can be used to identify the corresponding gene in other species. Alternatively, since hybridization reactions can occur between

DNA:RNA complementary sequences, DNA probes can be used to determine if a particular cell is expressing any given gene. In this case the DNA probe is hybridized with RNA prepared from the cell of interest to see whether the RNA species of interest is included in the RNA population. DNA probes are often used in conjunction with gel electrophoresis and nucleic acid transfer which separates the various nucleic acid species according to their size. This is followed by immobilization of the molecules on a membrane support before the hybridization reaction is carried out. There are two basic procedures, *blotting*, or *library screening*.

## Blotting

This technique has been one of the cornerstones of DNA analysis since its inception by Southern in 1975. Southern showed that it was possible to immobilize size-fractionated DNA fragments in a reliable and efficient manner (Fig. 1.39). DNA is first size-fractionated by gel electrophoresis and then denatured by treatment with alkali. Transfer from gel to membrane can be accomplished either by bulk fluid flow or electrophoretically. The DNA is immobilized onto the membrane either by baking under vacuum or crosslinking by irradiation of the membrane with high-energy UV light. The use of Southern transfer and the associated hybridization techniques makes it possible to obtain information about the physical organization of single and multicopy sequences in complex eukaryotic genomes. This technique also enables the study of restriction fragment length polymorphisms (RFLPs), which has opened up the science of genetic fingerprinting and the prenatal diagnosis of genetic disease.

The term *Southern blotting*, now used to describe any type of DNA transfer from gel to membrane, originally referred solely to capillary transfer onto nitrocellulose. However, the fragility of nitrocellulose membranes prompted the search for alternative types of support matrix, which resulted in the introduction of nylon membranes in the early 1980s. In comparison with nitrocellulose, nylon membranes have less stringent requirements regarding the composition of the transfer buffer.

Northern blotting is analogous to Southern transfer except that, rather than DNA, it is RNA that is separated electrophoretically and then transferred to a membrane support. In addition, because RNA is single-stranded and will be degraded in alkali, the denaturation step is skipped and transfer is accomplished at neutral pH.

## Library screening

A major use of DNA hybridization is the ability to identify a particular clone from a complex mixture of

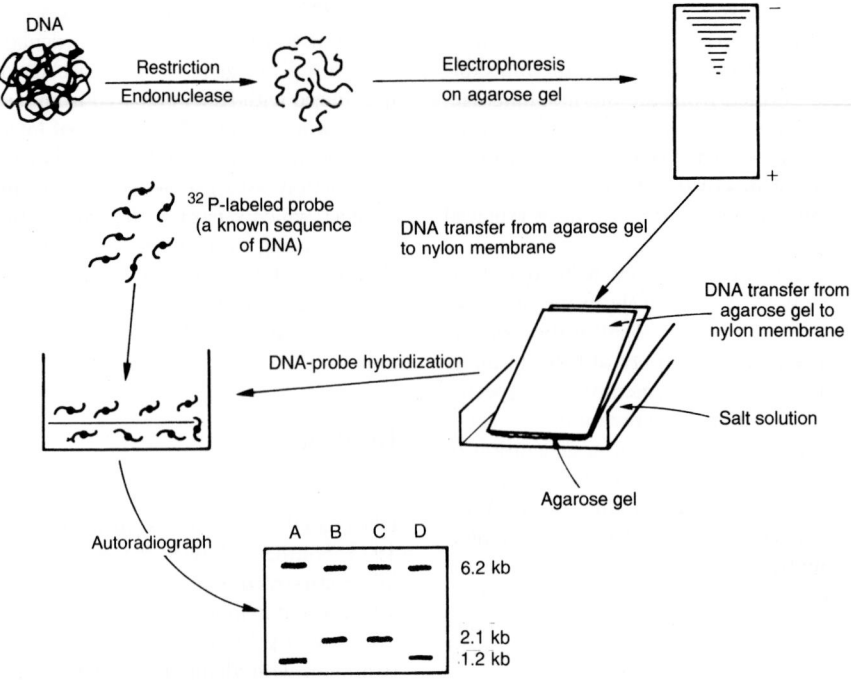

FIGURE 1.39 Southern blot analysis. The DNA of interest is cleaved using the desired restriction endonuclease, separated electrophoretically on an agarose gel and transferred to a support membrane. This is then hybridized with a radiolabeled probe produced from the target of interest. The signal is then seen by subjecting the filter to autoradiography.

clones (such as a genomic library) using a DNA fragment of known sequence. In practice, clones from the library must be plated out at sufficient density that the entire library is likely to be represented on the minimum number of bacterial plates. The bacterial, cosmid, or yeast colonies or λ plaques are then "lifted" directly onto a nitrocellulose membrane applied directly over the plate; the process usually is repeated so the experiment can be done in duplicate. The cells are lysed and DNA is immobilized onto the membrane as above. The stringency of subsequent hybridization can be adjusted depending upon the degree of identity that is anticipated. For example, if one is using a gene fragment to find the next upstream region of the gene in the same organism, high stringency will be used because only exact matches are desired. If, on the other hand, one is interested in cloning the human homologue of a gene found initially in mice, the stringency will have to be reduced substantially as the probe and target sequences are expect to have only about 70–80 per cent identity.

## SELECTED READING

Bickle TA, Kruger DH. Biology of DNA restriction. *Microbiol Rev* 1993; **57**: 434.

Kessler C, Manta V. Specificity of restriction endonucleases and DNA modification: methyltransferases – a review. *Gene* 1990; **92**: 1.

Maser RL, Calvet JP. Analysis of differential gene expression in the kidney by differential cDNA screening, subtractive cloning, and mRNA differential display. *Semin Nephrol* 1995; **15**: 29.

Murray NE. Special uses of lambda phage for molecular cloning. *Meth Enzymol* 1991; **204**: 280.

Murrell J, Trofatter J, Rutter M, *et al.* A 500-kilobase region containing the tuberous sclerosis locus (TSC1) in a 1.7-megabase YAC and cosmid contig. *Genomics* 1995; **25**: 59.

Palmer BR, Marinus MG. The dam and dcm strains of Escherichia coli – a review. *Gene* 1994; **143**: 1.

Pan LX, Diss TC, Isaacson PG. The polymerase chain reaction in histopathology. *Histopathology* 1995; **26**: 201.

Rashtchian A. Novel methods for cloning and engineering genes using the polymerase chain reaction. *Curr Opin Biotechnol* 1995; **6**: 30.

Sanger F, Nicklen S, Coulson AR. DNA sequencing with chain-terminating inhibitors. 1977 [classical article]. *Biotechnology*, 1992; **24**: 104.

2

# Membrane
# and Cellular Structure
# and Function

# MEMBRANE FUNCTION, ION TRANSPORT AND CELLULAR ION REGULATION

## MEMBRANE STRUCTURE AND FUNCTION

### Structure

The cell membrane is composed of lipids (predominantly phospholipids and cholesterol), proteins, and carbohydrates, which are highly ordered and interact in complex ways (Fig. 2.1). In general, lipids are arranged in a bilayer, with polar head groups oriented toward either the cytoplasmic or external surfaces. The fatty acid side-tail groups interact in the hydrophobic center of the bilayer, with each other and with sterol molecules. Acidic phospholipids (phosphatidyl serine, phosphatidyl ethanolamine, phosphatidyl inositol) are preferentially located at the cytoplasmic surface of the bilayer, while neutral phospholipids (phosphatidyl choline, sphingomyelin) are predominantly external. There is also evidence for ordered domains of phospholipid in the lateral plane of the membrane, and similar inhomogeneity of both lateral and transbilayer domains of cholesterol has been documented. The ratio of phospholipid to sterol and the composition of fatty acid side-chains affect various physicochemical properties of the membrane (e.g. fluidity, viscosity) which may affect protein function. In addition, specific

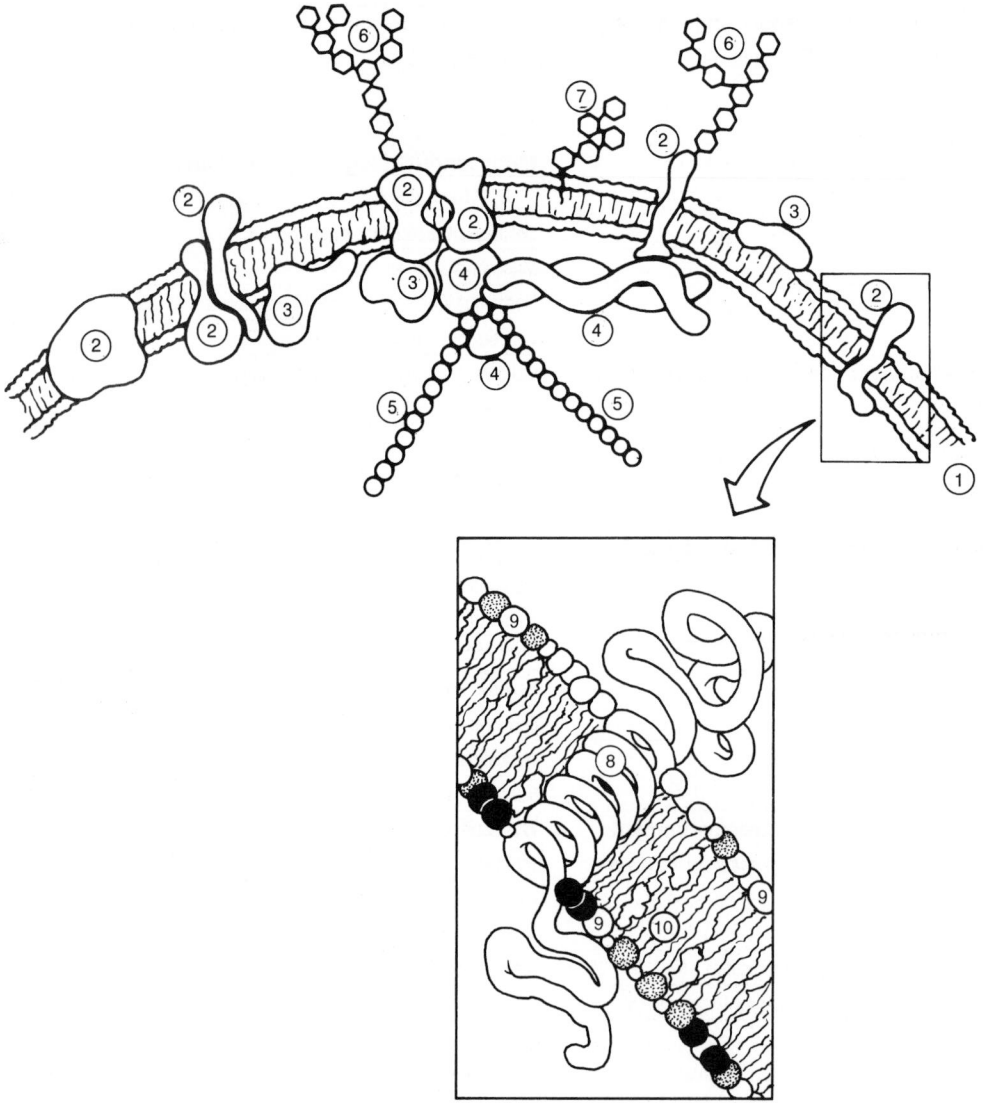

FIGURE 2.1 The plasma membrane. This schematic illustrates the major structural features of the plasma membrane of mammalian cells. Shown are the lipid bilayer (1), integral membrane proteins (2), peripheral membrane proteins (3), membrane skeleton proteins (4) attached to microfilaments (5), surface polysaccharides attached to proteins (6) or lipids (7). The insert shows higher-resolution detail depicting an integral membrane protein traversing the bilayer in an α-helical conformation (8); the inhomogeneous distribution of phospholipid (9) and cholesterol (10) is illustrated.

lipid–protein interactions may have important physiological effects. Hydrolysis of certain membrane phospholipids plays a central role in transmembrane signaling (*see* page 60).

Integral membrane proteins are embedded in the lipid bilayer or are covalently bound to lipids; they cannot be removed without disruptive treatment with detergents. Peripheral membrane proteins are associated with the membrane via weaker interactions and can be removed by changes in ionic strength or salt composition. Other proteins may be intermittently attached to the membrane in response to regulatory events; e.g. phosphorylation of protein kinase C leads to binding to the membrane. Interactions between integral membrane proteins and the membrane skeleton (composed of a number of peripheral membrane proteins which include the spectrins (fodrins), ankyrin, protein 4.1 and several other peripheral membrane proteins) provide structural support for the membrane and are major determinants of cell shape and mediators of cell mobility.

Simple and complex carbohydrates are covalently linked to lipids and proteins at the external surface of the membrane. These molecules modulate many cell–cell and receptor–ligand interactions and are important immunological determinants.

## Functions

Most membrane functions may be viewed as extensions of the fundamental role of the membrane as a barrier, separating the cellular interior from the extracellular milieu and compartmentalizing one region of the cell from another. Membranes organize the cell and its interior, control the size and shape of the cell, mediate the movements of substances into and out of the cell, send and receive biochemical and hormonal signals, and serve as the primary interface between the cell and its environment. This section of the chapter will focus on ion transport and its role in cell volume regulation, and subsequent sections will address additional membrane functions.

The movements across cell membranes of most materials (salts, water, and substrates) are mediated by specialized proteins and are intricately controlled by the cell's regulatory machinery. Transport processes may be divided into two major functional classes: those pertaining to the maintenance of cellular homeostasis and those mediating the bulk transfer of material across epithelia. Cellular ion homeostasis involves volume regulation, control of intracellular pH, maintenance of $Ca^{2+}$ ion concentration in the nanomolar range, and creation of monovalent cation gradients to support a variety of cellular functions, including electrical activity, secondary active transport processes, and the movement of metabolic substrates and waste products across the cell membrane. Epithelial transport is responsible for secretion and absorption of salt and water, and of the nutrients and waste products in the gut, kidneys, respiratory tract, and other tissues. Virtually all transport systems are subject to cellular regulatory control, and many exhibit physiologically important changes during development.

## TYPES OF TRANSPORT MECHANISMS

The mechanisms that mediate the movement of substances across cell membranes can be divided into *active* and *passive* transport processes on the basis of whether the substance in question moves up or down its electrochemical gradient.

## Active transport

Active transport of molecules against an electrochemical gradient requires energy, either from the hydrolysis of ATP (*primary active transport*) or from the downhill movement of another substance (*secondary active transport*). The $Na^+$-$K^+$-ATPase, $Ca^{2+}$-ATPase, and $H^+$-$K^+$-ATPase are members of a family of transport ATPases, which mediate active ion transport in many tissues and which have close structural homologies and functional similarities. A variety of secondary active transport processes are responsible for the transmembrane movement of many organic substances, as well as cations and anions. Most of these *transporters* utilize the energy stored in the transmembrane $Na^+$ gradient to drive the movement of another substance against its electrochemical gradient. Systems that move substances in the same direction as $Na^+$, i.e. into the cell, are called *symporters* and are exemplified by the $Na^+$-$K^+$-$Cl^-$-cotransporter and $Na^+$-coupled transporters for sugars and amino acids. *Antiporters* couple the downhill movement of $Na^+$ to the uphill transport of another ion in the opposite direction, i.e. out of the cell. Physiologically important antiport systems include $Na^+$-$H^+$ and $Na^+$-$Ca^{2+}$-exchangers. Such carriers may also function to regulate the movement of ions down their electrochemical gradients. Such is the case of the KCl cotransporter mediating $K^+$ loss to control cell volume, or the $Na^+$-$H^+$ exchanger catalyzing $H^+$ loss from an acidified cell. Likewise, the anion exchanger, another physiologically important antiporter, exchanges $HCO_3^-$ for $Cl^-$ to dissipate the transmembrane gradients of these ions.

## Passive transport

Passive movements of hydrophilic organic compounds are mediated by transporters that catalyze and regulate their passage through the hydrophobic lipid bilayer. The *facilitated diffusion* of certain sugars, amino acids, and other organic compounds is mediated by "carrier" molecules, which have binding sites with discrete affinities for transported substrates and maximal velocities of transport and which exhibit saturation kinetics. Diffusional movement of ions generally is mediated by *channels* that are specific for certain ions, exhibit characteristic, discrete electrical conductances, and exist in either an open or closed state, subject to cellular regulatory control. Ion movements through channels are always driven by the electrochemical gradient of the transported ion. Ion channel function and its appropriate regulation are central to the function of excitable cells and epithelial tissues. In most cells, the transmembrane movement of water is also controlled by specialized channels, the regulation of which is best exemplified by the modulation of water permeability of the collecting duct of the kidney by vasopressin. Transport via channels is very fast (typically one million molecules per second per channel), while transmembrane movement via facilitated diffusion carriers, symporters, antiporters, and ATPases is generally much slower (around 1000 molecules per second per carrier). A notable exception is the anion exchanger which can catalyze $Cl^-$-$HCO_3^-$ exchange at a rate of one million ions per second.

Lipid-soluble substances, such as gases ($O_2$, $CO_2$, and $N_2$), hydrocarbons, protonated organic acids, and anesthetic gases, pass through the lipid bilayer by simple diffusion, without mediation by protein carriers or channels.

## CELLULAR ION HOMEOSTASIS

## The $Na^+$-$K^+$-ATPase

### Transmembrane ionic gradients

Maintenance of the intracellular ionic milieu is one of the most basic cellular functions. Intracellular $Na^+$ and $K^+$, as well as water, behave as if in free solution in most cells, i.e. the amount of ion or water bound to cellular proteins and lipids is relatively small. In most animal cells, water is at osmotic equilibrium across the membrane, and there is no hydrostatic pressure gradient across the cell membrane. Cellular $K^+$ is maintained at 90–120 mmol/L cell water, while $Na^+$ varies from 5 to 50 mmol/L cell water, depending on cell type and functional mode. These concentrations are the result of the activity of the $Na^+$-$K^+$-ATPase, which couples the energy of ATP hydrolysis to the movement of ions across the membrane against their electrochemical gradient. The potential energy of these gradients is used by the cell to perform a variety of vital functions, including regulation of cellular volume and pH, electrical activity in excitable cells, modulation of cell $Ca^{2+}$, and membrane transport of organic compounds. Accordingly, the $Na^+$-$K^+$-ATPase is vital to cellular homeostasis and is found in virtually all cells. Its biochemistry, physiology, and molecular biology are better understood than any other transport protein and serve as a paradigm of this important class of membrane proteins.

## $Na^+$-$K^+$-ATPase structure

The $Na^+$-$K^+$-ATPase comprises two protein polypeptides (referred to as the $\alpha$ and $\beta$ chains), which are present in a heterodimer ($\alpha\beta$) in the membrane. A third polypeptide chain ($\gamma$) has been described, but its functional significance is not clear. The $\alpha$ chain mediates the catalytic/transport functions of the complex, although the $\beta$-subunit is necessary for activity and seems to be required for the proper insertion of the newly synthesized $\alpha$-subunit into the membrane. Although relative transcription rates for the $\alpha$ and $\beta$ chain mRNAs vary considerably among different cells and tissues, the two polypeptide chains are always found in a 1:1 ratio in the membrane.

Three isotypes of the $\alpha$ chain have been identified ($\alpha1$, $\alpha2$, and $\alpha3$) and possess characteristic tissue specificities and functional differences. The isotypes exhibit greater homology across species lines than they do with each other, i.e. rat $\alpha1$ is more like human $\alpha1$ than like rat $\alpha2$. The $\alpha1$ isoform predominates in kidney, lung, and stomach but is detectable in virtually all tissues and cells. Cardiac and skeletal muscle contain appreciable amounts of $\alpha2$ mRNA, and neuronal tissue contains all three isoforms. Currently, information about the physiological differences among the different isoforms is sketchy, but evidence indicates that the kinetic characteristics and responses to cellular regulatory processes differ among the isoforms. For example, the $Na^+$ affinity of the $\alpha2$ isoform found in muscle is considerably lower than that of $\alpha1$ and is altered by insulin stimulation (see below). Cell- and tissue-specific patterns of $Na^+$-$K^+$-ATPase isoform expression and developmental changes in those patterns are likely to have important physiological correlates in enzyme function and its regulation.

The $\alpha$ chain is approximately 1000 amino acids in length with a molecular weight of 100 kD, and contains the ATP hydrolysis site, cation, and cardiac glycoside-binding sites, as well as cytoplasmic domains that interact with the regulatory machinery of the cell to modulate $Na^+$-$K^+$-ATPase activity. The molecule (Fig. 2.2) has 6–10 membrane-spanning $\alpha$-helical domains (depending on isotype and species) and several small extracellular domains, one of which binds inhibitory cardiac glycosides. Isotype and species differences in primary sequence in a small segment of one of the extracellular domains are associated with differences in cardiac glycoside-binding affinity. Several of the transmembrane domains of the protein have clusters of anionic amino acids, which are thought to be involved in the binding and translocation of cations across the membrane. Located at the cytoplasmic surface is a binding domain for ATP, which is highly conserved across species and isotype lines and which is shared by other members of the P-type ATPase class of enzymes, including the ubiquitous $Ca^{2+}$-ATPases and the $H^+$-$K^+$-ATPase responsible for acid secretion in lysosomes and gastric parietal cells.

The $\beta$-subunit of the $Na^+$-$K^+$-ATPase is a 35-kD polypeptide that traverses the membrane once. The

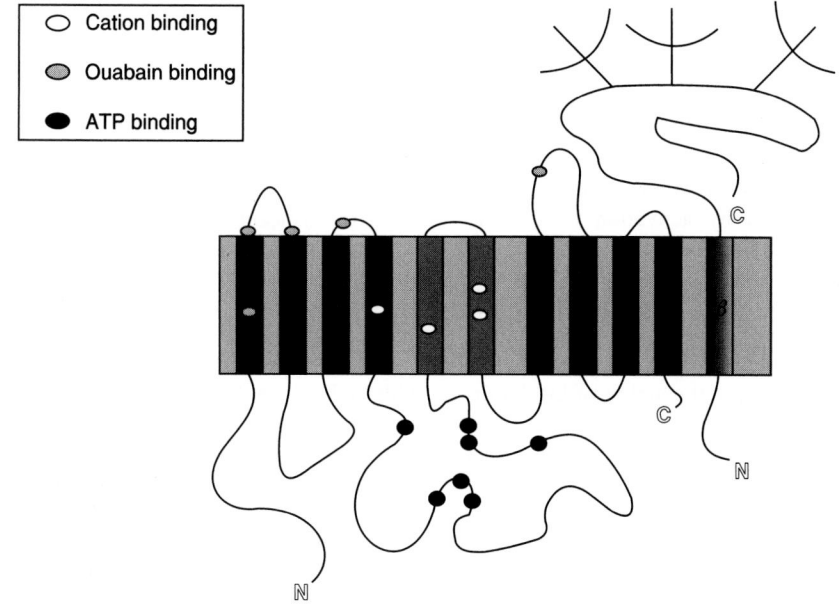

FIGURE 2.2 Structure of the Na⁺-K⁺-ATPase. Ten transmembrane segments are shown for the α-subunit, with a cytoplasmic –COOH terminus. Amino acids involved in function of the ATPase have been identified by chemical modification or site-directed mutagenesis. Residues associated with the ATP binding site are shown on the cytoplasmic face, one of which is phosphorylated during the catalytic cycle. Cation binding residues are located in the transmembrane segments, and the ouabain binding site is predominantly extracellular. The single transmembrane segment of the β-subunit is shown with an extensively glycosylated extracellular domain. (Figure courtesy of S. Lutsenko and J.H. Kaplan, Department of Biochemistry and Molecular Biology, Oregon Health Sciences and University.)

cytoplasmic domain is small, and the extracellular region has three sites bearing oligosaccharides, giving this glycoprotein a molecular weight of 53 kD. Glycosylation has no effect on enzyme activity. Although the β-subunit has no intrinsic catalytic or transport function, its presence is required for the α-subunit to function. Furthermore, the β-subunit appears to play an important role in the insertion of newly synthesized polypeptide into the endoplasmic reticulum membrane and its transfer to the plasma membrane.

## The catalytic cycle

The catalytic cycle of the Na⁺-K⁺-ATPase begins with the interaction of the cytoplasmic domain with Na⁺, which promotes the phosphorylation of the protein by ATP at a specific aspartyl residue on the α chain, producing ADP at the cytoplasmic surface. In association with the phosphorylated enzyme, three Na⁺ ions are then translocated across the membrane. Next, two external K⁺ ions bind to the enzyme and induce the hydrolysis of the phosphoprotein, releasing the inorganic phosphate at the cytoplasmic surface. Subsequently, the K⁺–enzyme complex reorients to the interior of the membrane, and the K⁺ ions are released when the complex binds Mg²⁺-ATP. The enzyme is then poised to interact with Na⁺ to begin the cycle again. These events are associated with discrete conformation changes in the protein, which are detectable by physicochemical techniques such as changes in its susceptibility to proteolysis, binding of certain ligands,

and spectrophotometric methods. Rather than gross movements of large segments of the protein across the membrane, these conformational changes are thought to represent small alterations in the relative positions of various domains in the protein, such as two adjacent α-helical transmembrane domains. Membrane lipids may play a role in modulating catalytic activity by facilitating or inhibiting these conformational changes.

## Na⁺-K⁺-ATPase regulation

The activity of Na⁺-K⁺-ATPase in the cell is subject to at least four types of physiological regulation: acute modulation of activity by changes in Na⁺ and K⁺ concentrations, modification by cellular regulatory processes, mobilization of enzyme from storage pools to the plasma membrane, and control of Na⁺-K⁺-ATPase gene expression. The first and last of these mechanisms are the most important.

Short-term control of Na⁺-K⁺-ATPase activity represents a kinetic response to demand. The affinity ($K_m$) of the ATPase for internal Na⁺ is around 20 mM in most cases, so that under steady-state conditions with intracellular Na⁺ of about 10 mM, the pump operates well below its maximal capacity. If cellular Na⁺ concentrations rise, Na⁺-K⁺-ATPase activity increases on the basis of substrate (Na⁺) availability. Because of the kinetic characteristics of the system, relatively small changes in cellular Na⁺ concentration can result in large increases in pump activity. Once the perturbation of membrane permeability has subsided and cellular Na$^+$ levels are brought back to normal by the Na$^+$-K$^+$-ATPase, its activity returns to normal. Most examples of acute stimulation of Na$^+$-K$^+$-ATPase activity by hormones or drugs involve this secondary reaction to increased intracellular Na$^+$, which results from the primary action of the stimulant to increased Na$^+$ influx into the cell by activation of Na$^+$-H$^+$ exchange or opening of Na$^+$ channels. The $K_m$ of the pump for external K$^+$ is 1 mM, so that alterations of K$^+$ within the physiological range (3–5 mM) have little effect on Na$^+$-K$^+$-ATPase function.

An important example of a direct regulatory effect on Na$^+$-K$^+$-ATPase activity is the action of insulin on skeletal muscle. In the resting state, the majority of Na$^+$-K$^+$-ATPase molecules (about 75 per cent) in this tissue are composed of $\alpha$2 isoform. This isoform has low affinity for internal Na$^+$ in the resting state, so that the turnover of these pumps is quite low. Insulin acts via a tissue-specific membrane receptor to increase the affinity of the Na$^+$-K$^+$ pump for internal Na$^+$, thereby increasing the pumping rate appreciably. Although the mechanistic details of this phenomenon are not entirely clear, it is known to the clinician because it manifests as a reduction in serum K$^+$ following insulin infusion.

Several factors influence the number of Na$^+$-K$^+$-ATPase molecules in the plasma membrane of a cell. A number of hormones, notably mineralocorticoids and thyroid hormone, increase Na$^+$-K$^+$-ATPase gene expression, thereby increasing the number of pump sites on cells containing their respective receptors. In addition, prolonged elevation of intracellular Na$^+$ enhances expression of both $\alpha$ and $\beta$ chains, which represents a response of the cell to added demand for Na$^+$ pumping. Experimentally, this is manifest as an increase in mRNA levels for the $\alpha$ and $\beta$ genes and an increase in Na$^+$-K$^+$-ATPase activity assayed immunochemically or by $^3$H-ouabain-binding sites within several hours of incubation of cells in the presence of low external K$^+$ or cardiac glycosides, both of which inhibit the pump and cause cellular Na$^+$ to rise. Biologically, this means that stimulation of Na$^+$ entry into the cell, e.g. by activation of Na$^+$ channels or Na$^+$-H$^+$ exchange or by damage to the cell membrane, results in a compensatory increase in Na$^+$ pumping capacity. This must be borne in mind when examining the physiological or developmental changes in Na$^+$-K$^+$-ATPase expression, because, as discussed above for acute modulation of Na$^+$-K$^+$-ATPase activity by physiological stimuli, some of the changes in gene expression may be secondary to an increase in cellular Na$^+$ induced by the primary event.

## Cell volume regulation

Water occupies 70–90 per cent of the volume of an animal cell, most of the remainder representing the volume of solutes, mostly protein. Because the membrane of most cells is highly permeable to water, no osmotic gradient exists between the intracellular and extracellular space in the steady state. This means that the water content of most cells is strictly a function of the osmotically active species of cell, and that the *control of cell volume hinges on the regulation of cation content*. The presence of negatively charged, membrane-impermeant proteins and organic phosphates in high concentrations in the cell creates electrical and colloid osmotic driving forces for cations and water to enter the cell (known as the Donnan effect). In the steady state, the cell uses the energy of the cation gradients established by the Na$^+$-K$^+$-ATPase, combined with tightly regulated passive permeabilities of the ions, to offset the tendency of the cell to gain cation and swell.

Note that the capacity of the Na$^+$-K$^+$-ATPase to carry out net extrusion of cations is not essential to this mechanism, only that it function to exchange Na$^+$ for K$^+$. The steady-state cation content and therefore cell volume is a function of Na$^+$-K$^+$ pump activity and its coupling ratio (Na$^+$ extruded:K$^+$ taken in) and the passive permeabilities of the membrane to Na$^+$ and K$^+$. This model, formulated for the mammalian red blood cell by Tosteson and Hoffman in 1960, also applies to nucleated cells, with the additional complexity that such cells are capable of rapidly altering passive cation permeabilities in response to changes in cell volume.

Cell volume regulation has been studied extensively in the nucleated red blood cells of fish, amphibians, and birds, as well as in the human reticulocyte, and there is evidence that other human somatic cells have similar mechanisms. Cell swelling (by reduction in medium osmolality) elicits a volume regulatory decrease in which cation and water are lost by the cell to return it to its original volume. In the human reticulocyte, a KCl cotransport system performs this function. A brief review of this system illustrates the principle of downward volume regulation (Fig. 2.3). Upon acute reduction of extracellular osmolarity, a transient osmotic gradient is created across the membrane, causing water to move into the cell with resultant increase in volume; in reticulocytes, such osmotically driven water movements are complete within seconds. This swelling of the cell activates the KCl transporter, which moves K$^+$ out of the cell down its electrochemical gradient, coupled with the movement of Cl$^-$ and carrying with it osmotically obliged water. The reticulocyte returns to its original volume within minutes. The mechanism of activation of the KCl cotransporter by cell swelling is not certain, but evidence suggests that sulfhydryl groups are involved in the volume-sensing mechanism and regulation of protein phosphorylation–dephosphorylation controls in the activity of the cotransporter.

Two distinct mechanisms have been described for volume regulatory increase in response to shrinkage in red cells. One system (Fig. 2.4), modeled in avian erythrocytes, involves a Na$^+$-K$^+$-Cl$^-$ cotransporter stimu-

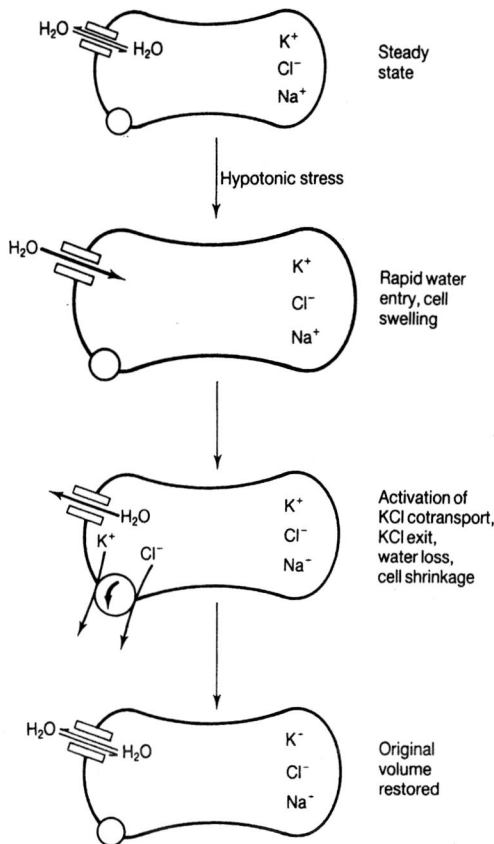

FIGURE 2.3 Volume regulatory decrease in the red cell

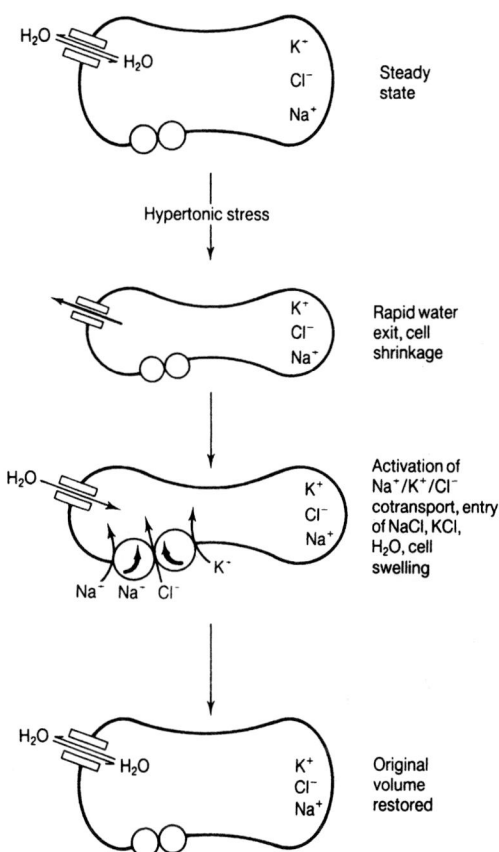

FIGURE 2.4 Volume regulatory increase via $Na^+$-$K^+$-$Cl^-$ cotransport

lated by catecholamines via a cAMP-dependent mechanism and inhibited by loop diuretics such as furosemide, which moves salt into the cell to restore volume. A different system is found in fish red cells, which respond to cell shrinkage by activating a $Na^+$-$H^+$-exchanger that moves $Na^+$ into the cell in exchange for $H^+$; the resultant alkalinization of the cell interior increases the concentration of $HCO_3^-$, which is exchanged for extracellular $Cl^-$ by the anion exchanger (Fig. 2.5). The net result is the uptake of NaCl and osmotically obliged water. $Na^+$-$H^+$ exchange is activated by a variety of tissue-specific receptors coupled to protein phosphorylation mechanisms. The response to changes in osmolality is demanded of cells in the gut and kidney, and volume control is also required of other epithelial cells in which the transcellular movement of large amounts of solute may perturb cell volume.

Both $Na^+$-$H^+$ exchange and $Na^+$-$K^+$-$Cl^-$ cotransport systems are known to exist in a variety of cell types in mammals and are likely to participate in volume regulation of these cells. In addition, certain $K^+$ and $Cl^-$ channels appear to be opened in some cells by swelling, permitting electrically coupled KCl efflux from the cell. In brain, and possibly other tissues, certain amino acids (glutamine, taurine), carbohydrates (myo-inositol) and organic cations (choline, betaine) may also play important roles in cell volume regulation. In response to osmotic perturbations, the intracellular content of these osmolytes may be regulated by transport into or out of the cell or by synthesis or degradation of the compound.

## Cellular pH regulation

Intracellular pH is normally slightly more acidic (by 0.1–0.3 pH units) than the extracellular compartment, reflecting the Donnan distribution of protons and the production by cellular metabolism of acidic compounds such as lactic acid and $CO_2$. Cellular pH is often perturbed by a number of physiological processes, including environmental pH changes, increased cellular metabolism, and *hypoxemia–ischemia*. Intracellular buffers, including $HCO_3^-$, phosphates, and proteins, absorb some of the protons produced by these processes, but the cell also has mechanisms to remove excess $H^+$, the two most important being $Na^+$-$H^+$ exchange and $Cl^-$-$HCO_3^-$ exchange.

$Na^+$-$H^+$ exchange functions as an antiporter to move $Na^+$ into the cell and $H^+$ outward, and is stimulated by increased intracellular $H^+$ concentration

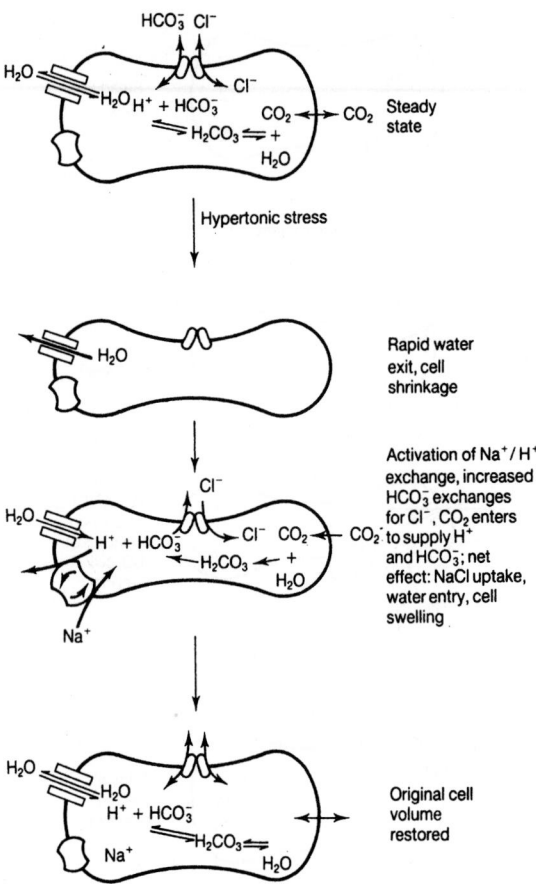

FIGURE 2.5 Volume regulatory increase via Na$^+$-H$^+$ exchange functionally coupled to Cl$^-$-HCO$_3$-exchange

(decreased pH) (Fig. 2.6). The excess cellular Na$^+$ must be removed from the cell by the Na$^+$-K$^+$-ATPase. Under hypoxic–ischemic stress, when the cell's ATP supply falls below the level that can sustain ATPase activity, cell Na$^+$ may rise, causing cell swelling and tissue edema. This mechanism may underlie the cere-

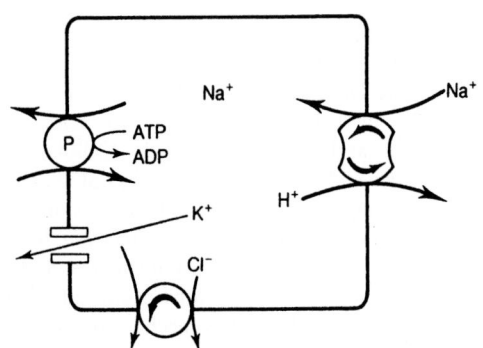

FIGURE 2.6 Recovery from acid load via Na$^+$-H$^+$ exchange. Cellular acidification activates Na$^+$/H$^+$ exchange, extruding H$^+$; increased Na$^+$ stimulates Na$^+$/K$^+$ pump. Excess K$^+$ is recycled via K$^+$ channel and/or KCl cotransporter.

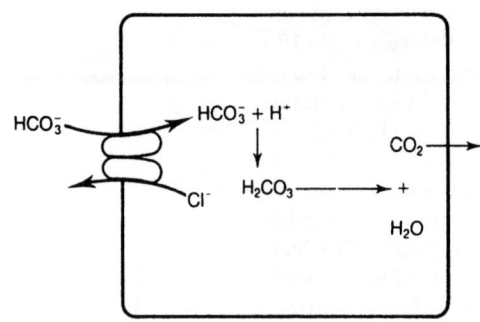

FIGURE 2.7 Recovery from acid load via Cl$^-$-HCO$_3^-$ exchange

bral edema associated with hypoxic–ischemic brain injury. In certain cells, neurohumoral stimuli activate Na$^+$-H$^+$ exchange via cAMP-mediated protein phosphorylation, and the resultant alkalinization may trigger other cellular responses.

Under steady-state conditions, Cl$^-$-HCO$_3^-$ exchange tends to remove HCO$_3^-$ from the cell as a consequence of the transmembrane gradients of the transport ions (Fig. 2.7). However, under conditions of acid stress, Cl$^-$-HCO$_3^-$ exchange can also function to maintain cellular pH. When cells experience intracellular acidification, H$^+$ reacts with HCO$_3^-$, and the resultant H$_2$CO$_3$ is converted to water and CO$_2$, which diffuses from the cell; the cell's HCO$_3^-$ supply is then replenished by exchange of internal Cl$^-$ for extracellular HCO$_3^-$, permitting ongoing H$^+$ buffering. The anion exchanger is therefore essential to the efficient functioning of the CO$_2$-HCO$_3^-$ buffer system.

Cl$^-$-HCO$_3^-$ exchange is also crucial to the respiratory function of the erythrocyte. As the red cell traverses the capillary, CO$_2$ diffuses into the cell, where it is converted into carbonic acid (H$_2$CO$_3$) by carbonic anhydrase. H$_2$CO$_3$ dissociates to form H$^+$, which is absorbed by intracellular buffers (mainly hemoglobin and phosphates), and HCO$_3^-$, which leaves the cell in exchange for Cl$^-$. This process, known as the Hamburger shift after the nineteenth-century physiologist who described it, is reversed in the lung and increases the blood's CO$_2$-carrying capacity by minimizing the perturbation of plasma and red cell pH.

## Ca$^{2+}$ homeostasis

The control of ionized Ca$^{2+}$ concentration is another vital cellular function that depends primarily on ion transport and regulated membrane permeability. The precise regulation of Ca$^{2+}$ is mandated in all cells by its universal role as a second messenger governing multiple cellular processes, and by its toxicity to the cell when concentrations rise above micromolar levels. In addition, in both smooth and striated muscle cells, Ca$^{2+}$ is the primary determinant of contractile protein function. In the steady state in most cells and the resting state in contractile cells, intracellular ionized $Ca^{2+}$ is maintained at 10–100 nM; with an extracellular concentration of 1–2 mM, a 10 000–100 000-fold transmembrane concentration gradient exists for $Ca^{2+}$, one of the largest of any physiologically relevant compound. This gradient is maintained by the $Ca^{2+}$-ATPase, which exists in several isoforms in different tissues and is a member of the common transport ATPase family. The high affinity of this enzyme for $Ca^{2+}$ and ATP, its rapid reaction rate, and relatively high abundance contribute to its ability to keep intracellular $Ca^{2+}$ concentrations low and to respond to the rapid changes in $Ca^{2+}$ levels associated with stimulus secretion or excitation–contraction coupling. In skeletal and cardiac muscle, large amounts of $Ca^{2+}$-ATPase are found in the endoplasmic reticulum into which $Ca^{2+}$ is pumped and sequestered after contraction occurs. In other cells, the enzyme is located in the plasma membrane and functions to extrude $Ca^{2+}$ from the cell.

In addition to the $Ca^{2+}$-ATPase, $Ca^{2+}$ is removed from some cells via a $Na^+$-$Ca^{2+}$ exchanger; the inward movement of three $Na^+$ ions energizes the outward movement of one $Ca^{2+}$ ion against its large electrochemical gradient. The mechanism of cardiac glycoside inotropy is thought to involve this transporter: glycoside inhibition of the $Na^+$-$K^+$-ATPase leads to increased cellular $Na^+$, which diminishes the driving force of the $Na^+$-$Ca^{2+}$ exchanger, an important regulator of $Ca^{2+}$ concentration in cardiac muscle. This raises steady-state cellular $Ca^{2+}$ levels, thereby augmenting the contractile function of the muscle.

$Ca^{2+}$ entry into the cytoplasmic space, from either the extracellular space or endoplasmic reticulum, is mediated by a variety of intricately regulated channels. In cardiac and skeletal muscle, voltage-gated $Ca^{2+}$ channels in the plasma membrane and sarcoplasmic reticulum are opened when an action potential depolarizes the membrane in which they reside. After a brief period in the open state, during which $Ca^{2+}$ flows into the cytoplasm, the channel closes; the duration of the open state may be modulated by regulatory processes, mediated by receptor-linked protein kinases. This family of channels is blocked by compounds such as verapamil, nifedipine, and diltiazem. In neurons, arrival of the action potential at the presynaptic membrane opens a voltage-dependent $Ca^{2+}$ channel, and the resultant $Ca^{2+}$ influx triggers neurotransmitter release. In some non-excitable cell types, the occupation of membrane receptors by a variety of hormones, growth factors, secretagogues, etc. increases cytoplasmic $Ca^{2+}$ by activation of $Ca^{2+}$ channels. In some cells, $Ca^{2+}$ channels in the plasma membrane are activated by receptor-linked protein kinases. In other cells, receptor-linked

activation of phospholipase C increases hydrolysis of inositol phospholipids to produce inositol-1,4,5-triphosphate (ITP), which activates an ITP-specific $Ca^{2+}$ channel in the endoplasmic reticulum membrane, releasing $Ca^{2+}$ into the cytoplasm. As a second messenger, $Ca^{2+}$ may affect many cellular functions, by activating or inhibiting channels for other ions, specific protein kinases, proteases, or other enzymes.

$Ca^{2+}$ movements across the apical membrane of certain epithelia in the gut, kidney and placenta associated with transepithelial $Ca^{2+}$ movement appear to be mediated by carrier proteins, rather than channels, based on the physiological characteristics of $Ca^{2+}$ transport in these tissues. The molecules associated with these functions have not yet been characterized.

## Electrical activity

The membrane potential ($E_m$) of all cells is a function of the transmembrane gradients of charged species and their respective permeabilities, expressed in the Goldman equation, shown below. In most cells, $Na^+$, $K^+$, and $Cl^-$ ($HCO_3^-$) are the ions which determine $E_m$.

In excitable cells, such as nerve and muscle, the action potential results from the coordinated opening and closing of $Na^+$ and $K^+$ channels. In the resting state, both $Na^+$ and $K^+$ channels are closed, and because the resting permeability of the membrane for $K^+$ is high relative to that of $Na^+$ and $Cl^-$, the membrane potential approximates the $K^+$ equilibrium potential, around 90 mV interior negative. As the action potential approaches an area of membrane, it begins to depolarize owing to current flowing across the membrane nearby; this depolarization activates the $Na^+$ channel. The rapid increase in $Na^+$ permeability causes the membrane potential in that area of the membrane to approach the $Na^+$ potential (+40 mV). This strong depolarization opens $K^+$ channels, which returns the membrane voltage toward the $K^+$ potential. After a discrete period of time, both $Na^+$ and $K^+$ channels close to return the membrane permeability of both ions to resting values, and the action potential has passed. The $Na^+$-$K^+$-ATPase plays a crucial secondary role in these cells to maintain the transmembrane gradients of $Na^+$ and $K^+$. Neurotransmitters interact with specific receptors on target neurons to activate or inhibit certain ion channels. Transmitters that activate $Na^+$ channels depolarize the membrane to initiate an action potential, and therefore are stimulatory. Transmitters that activate $K^+$ channels inhibit neuronal activity by hyperpolarizing the membrane.

In striated muscle cells, the acetylcholine receptor is itself a subunit of a non-specific $Na^+$ and $K^+$ channel at

$$E_m = -61 \log \frac{(P_{Na}[Na]_i + P_K[K]_i + P_{Cl}[Cl]_o + P_{HCO_3}[HCO_3]_o + P_{Ca}[Ca]_i^2 + P_{Mg}[Mg]_i^2)}{(P_{Na}[Na]_o + P_K[K]_o + P_{Cl}[Cl]_i + P_{HCO_3}[HCO_3]_i + P_{Ca}[Ca]_o^2 + P_{Mg}[Mg]_o^2)}$$

The Goldman Equation

the motor end plate. Binding of acetylcholine to the receptor opens these channels, depolarizing the plasma membrane and propagating an action potential in the muscle cell membrane. The arrival of this action potential via transverse tubules depolarizes the endoplasmic reticulum membrane, activating a voltage-dependent $Ca^{2+}$ channel and causing the release of $Ca^{2+}$ into the cytoplasm, which initiates muscle contraction. The tonic contraction of smooth muscle is a function of intracellular $Ca^{2+}$ levels, in turn a function of membrane potential determined by $Na^+$ and $K^+$ permeabilities of the plasma membrane, which can be modulated by neurohumoral influences.

Cells other than nerve or muscle may also exhibit physiologically important changes in membrane potential, either primarily or secondarily associated with cellular functions. Stimulus-secretion coupling involves changes in membrane potential or activation of specific

ion channels. For example, the coupling of insulin secretion to serum glucose concentrations involves the regulation of several ion channels in the β islet cell of the pancreas (Fig. 2.8): glucose availability modulates ATP levels in the β cell; high ATP levels associated with high glucose concentrations close a specific $K^+$ channel, which depolarizes the membrane; in response to this change in membrane potential, a voltage-dependent $Ca^{2+}$ channel is opened, permitting $Ca^{2+}$ influx and increasing cytoplasmic $Ca^{2+}$ concentration; this triggers $Ca^{2+}$-dependent protein phosphorylation responsible for exocytosis and insulin release; meanwhile, $Ca^{2+}$ activation of a second $K^+$ channel allows repolarization of the membrane, damping and controlling the response.

Even in cells that do not undergo large changes in membrane potential, activation of $Ca^{2+}$ channels by certain stimuli underlies the mechanism by which

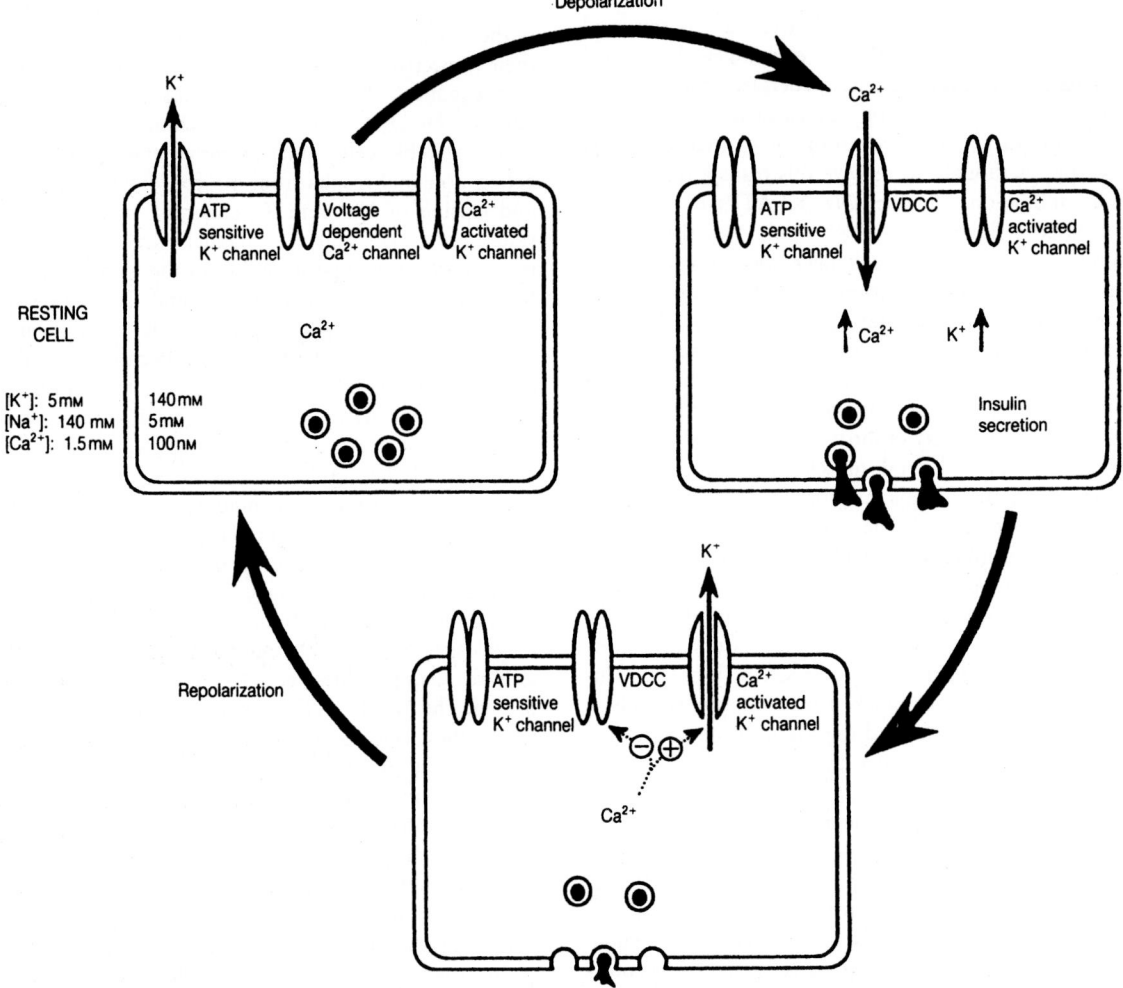

FIGURE 2.8 Ion-channel modulation of insulin secretion. Resting membrane potential in pancreatic β cells is governed by $K^+$ conductance through ATP-sensitive $K^+$ channels. Closure of these channels leads to cell depolarization and $Ca^{2+}$ influx through voltage-dependent $Ca^{2+}$ channels (VDCC). Rise in free cytosolic $Ca^{2+}$ triggers insulin secretion. In addition, rise in cytosolic $Ca^{2+}$ activates $Ca^{2+}$-activated $K^+$ channels to enhance $K^+$ efflux and inactivate $Ca^{2+}$ channels. This results in cell repolarization and reversion to resting state. (Reprinted with permission from Rajan AS *et al. Diabetes Care* 1990; **13**: 341. Copyright © 1990 by the American Diabetes Association, Inc.)

$Ca^{2+}$ acts as a second messenger of hormone action. In transporting epithelia, changes in the membrane potential caused by the opening of one ion channel may alter the properties of other channels or transport proteins to maintain the functional activity of the cell. Virtually all of the regulated ion channels are susceptible to protein phosphorylation, and there are many examples in which hormones that may not have a primary regulatory action on a cellular process can modulate that process by affecting the activity of an ion channel via kinase–phosphatase interactions, thereby fine-tuning the cell's response to its primary stimulus.

## EPITHELIAL TRANSPORT

Fluid movements into and out of the various luminal cavities of the body are controlled by transport of salt across epithelia. Epithelial cells of the kidney, of the respiratory, gastrointestinal, and genital tracts, of the exocrine, mucous, and sweat glands, and of the choroid plexus all perform important secretory and/or absorptive functions. Neurohumoral stimulation or inhibition of these processes modulates tissue functions to meet physiological needs.

Although tissue- or cell-specific mechanisms exist for movement of $H^+$, $K^+$, $Ca^{2+}$, and other substances, the regulation of water movements generally involves the active absorption of $Na^+$ (lumen to blood) and the secretion of $Cl^-$ (blood to lumen). The basic mechanisms underlying these processes will be detailed here, with specific examples of physiological regulation for individual tissues.

## Sodium absorption

The absorption of $Na^+$ is driven by the $Na^+$-$K^+$-ATPase located in the basolateral membrane of the epithelial cell. The energy derived from the hydrolysis of ATP is used to pump $Na^+$ against its electrochemical gradient out of the cell (where $Na^+$ concentration is low) into the interstitial space (where it is high). $Na^+$ enters the cell's apical (luminal) membrane through a specific mechanism, usually either a regulated $Na^+$ channel or a $Na^+$-$H^+$ exchanger. In some cells in the renal tubule, $Na^+$-$Cl^-$ or $Na^+$-$K^+$-$Cl^-$ cotransport is responsible for transepithelial NaCl absorption, and the inhibition of this type of transporter by furosemide (Lasix®) accounts for the powerful diuretic effect of this drug. Channel-mediated $Na^+$ absorption is pictured in Fig. 2.9 and will be considered first. The function of an apical $Na^+$-$H^+$ exchanger will be considered below.

Under quiescent conditions, the $Na^+$ channel remains closed and little $Na^+$ entry occurs. Upon stimulation, the channel opens and $Na^+$ enters the cell by diffusion down its electrochemical gradient. Intracellular $Na^+$ rises and stimulates the $Na^+$-$K^+$-ATPase to pump at a faster rate. A basolateral $K^+$ channel is also opened by the same initial stimulus or by the

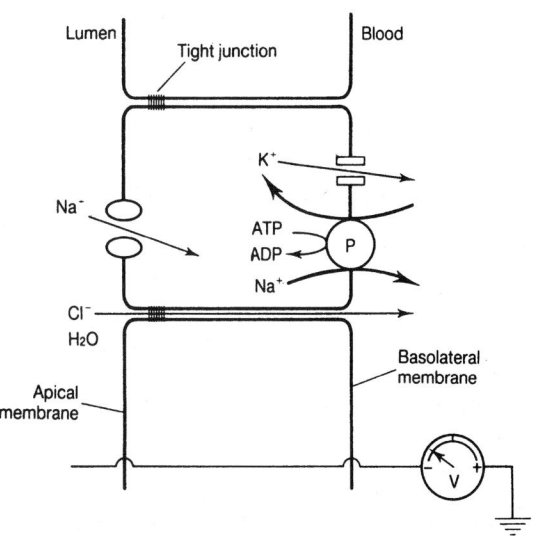

FIGURE 2.9 Epithelial $Na^+$ absorption via the apical $Na^+$ channel

depolarization of the membrane, which accompanies the opening of the $Na^+$ channel and functions to permit exit of $K^+$ brought into the cell by the pump in exchange for $Na^+$. The movement of $Na^+$ across the epithelium causes an electrical potential difference to develop across the cell layer (lumen negative relative to interstitial space), which drives the movement of $Cl^-$. Chloride enters the interstitium either transcellularly by means of $Cl^-$ channels in both apical and basolateral membranes, or via a paracellular route through the tight junctions that join the epithelial cells together. Water follows the movements of $Na^+$ and $Cl^-$, driven by osmotic forces and moving across the cell membrane and through the paracellular pathway. In certain regions of the kidney tubule where passage of water is restricted, luminal fluid becomes hypotonic upon absorption of NaCl; but in most epithelia, isotonic conditions prevail on both sides of the cell and water moves along with salt.

In some epithelia, notably in the kidney and intestine, the primary entry step for $Na^+$ at the apical membrane is not a $Na^+$ channel, but rather a $Na^+$-$H^+$ exchange system (Fig. 2.10), and in this case the epithelium functions to excrete $H^+$ and absorb $HCO_3^-$. The intracellular proton secreted in exchange for luminal $Na^+$ reacts with luminal $HCO_3^-$ to produce $H_2CO_3$. Luminal carbonic anhydrase catalyses the production of $H_2O$ and $CO_2$, which diffuses back into the cell and forms $H^+$ and $HCO_3^-$. The $H^+$ is available for exchange with $Na^+$, and the $HCO_3^-$ is extruded to the interstitium by a $Cl^-$-$HCO_3$-exchanger located on the basolateral membrane. The net result is $NaHCO_3$ absorption. This mechanism occurs in the intestine and is a predominant mode of $Na^+$ and $HCO_3^-$ absorption in the kidney proximal tubule. The diuretic actions of amiloride and acetazolamide result from inhibition of $Na^+$-$H^+$ exchange and carbonic anhydrase, respec-

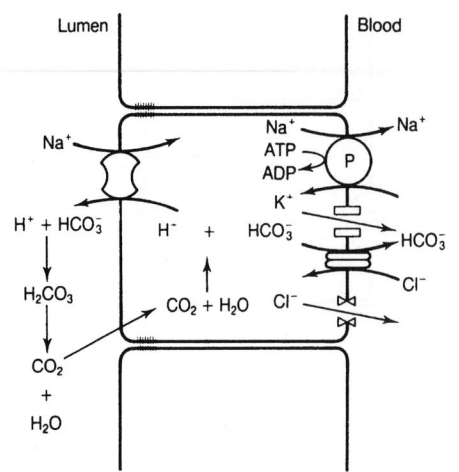

FIGURE 2.10 Absorption of $NaHCO_3$ via coupling of $Na^+$-$H^+$ exchange and $Cl^-$-$HCO_3^-$ exchange

tively. Amiloride also blocks the $Na^+$ channel. In addition, the dependence of $Na^+$ and water absorption on $Na^+$-$K^+$-ATPase activity renders the process susceptible to inhibition by hypokalemia, metabolic depletion and the cardiac glycoside, ouabain.

To stimulate salt and water absorption, a variety of neurohumoral agents activate the $Na^+$-$H^+$ exchanger or apical $Na^+$ channels in absorptive epithelia. Most responses are mediated by cAMP and activation of protein kinase A. Phosphorylation of the channel increases the time it spends in the open state, and activation of the exchanger changes its affinity for $Na^+$ and/or $H^+$.

$Na^+$ channel activity is also affected by aldosterone. Acutely, this hormone increases $Na^+$ channel activity by stimulating methylation of the channel or its regulating subunits. Aldosterone may also have a long-term effect of increasing the number of $Na^+$ channels in the membrane. Such mechanisms may play a role in regulating renal $Na^+$ absorption.

$Na^+$ channels have been purified or cloned from several tissues in various species and differ considerably in molecular weight and protein subunit type and number. Nevertheless, the membrane-spanning domains, which are thought to form the actual channel structures, exhibit considerable homology among proteins derived from different tissues and species. These domains conform to the general motif of membrane transport proteins, with multiple hydrophobic α-helical sequences. The cytoplasmic domains, which interact with cellular regulatory mechanisms to modulate channel activity, are often quite different among tissues and species. Some of the components of multi-subunit channels may have primarily regulatory functions. There are striking sequence and structural homologies among $Na^+$, $K^+$, and $Ca^{2+}$ channels within functional subclasses, such as voltage-gated channels, particularly in the membrane-spanning domains. This suggests that

some of these families of channel proteins diverged from a common ancestral membrane protein.

## Chloride secretion

Fluid secretion by epithelial tissues also depends on energy derived from ATP hydrolysis by the $Na^+$-$K^+$-ATPase, because $Cl^-$ movements are driven by the $Na^+$ gradient. This is accomplished by a $Na^+$-$K^+$-$Cl^-$ cotransport system (possibly a $Na^+$-$Cl^-$ cotransporter) located on the basolateral membrane (Fig. 2.11).

Although intracellular $Cl^-$ concentration may be lower than external $Cl^-$, the resting membrane potential is negative, so that the electrochemical driving force (the algebraic sum of electrical and chemical forces) favors $Cl^-$ exit in the steady state; thus, net movement of $Cl^-$ from the interstitial space into the cell is *uphill* and requires energy, which is supplied via the cotransporter as $Na^+$ moves into the cell down its electrochemical gradient. $Na^+$ is pumped out again by the $Na^+$-$K^+$-ATPase and cellular $K^+$ is *recycled* by specific channels located at the basolateral membrane, as in $Na^+$-absorbing epithelia. Secretion of $Cl^-$ is accomplished by opening of $Cl^-$-specific channels at the apical surface of the cell. Chloride then moves down its electrochemical gradient into the lumen, creating an electrical potential across the membrane (lumen negative) that causes $Na^+$ and osmotically obliged water to move via paracellular pathways. Because of the transport systems involved, $Cl^-$ secretion is susceptible to inhibition by ouabain and by the

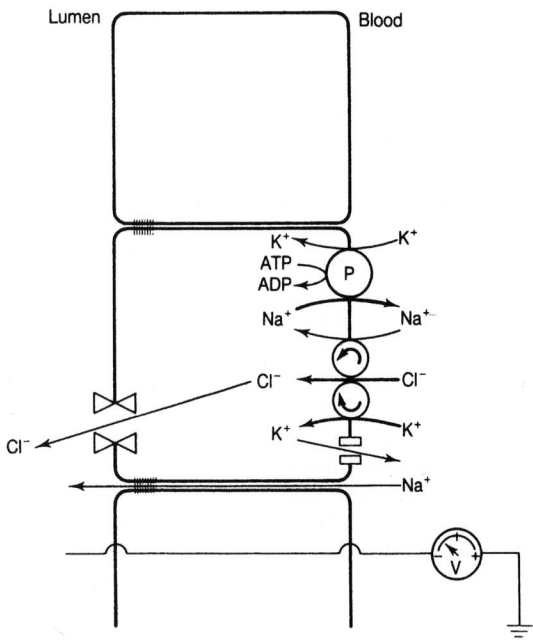

FIGURE 2.11 Epithelial $Cl^-$ secretion

loop diuretics (furosemide), which inhibit $Na^+$-$K^+$-$Cl^-$ cotransport.

As with $Na^+$ channels, $Cl^-$ channels exhibit tissue-specific regulation by a variety of neurohumoral agents coupled to various second messengers. For example, $Cl^-$ secretion in the trachea is stimulated by catecholamines and mediated by the cAMP-dependent protein kinase A, which apparently phosphorylates and activates the $Cl^-$ channel. In the intestine the $Cl^-$ channel associated with secretion is also activated by a cAMP-mediated kinase. *Cholera toxin* activates a G-protein leading to uncontrolled stimulation of adenylyl cyclase and producing high levels of cAMP. This results in maximal opening of this $Cl^-$ channel and produces the secretory diarrhea characteristic of cholera. Some $Cl^-$ channels are also activated by $Ca^{2+}$, and some are voltage-dependent.

Several different $Cl^-$ channels have been identified physiologically and characterized molecularly. These molecules exhibit the channel motif described above for $Na^+$ channels, with helical and hydrophobic transmembrane segments and cytoplasmic domains that interact with cellular regulatory machinery. Of considerable interest is the $Cl^-$ channel defect associated with cystic fibrosis. In this disorder, the response of $Cl^-$ channel function to β-adrenergic stimulation is abnormal in a number of tissues, although basal (i.e. unstimulated) $Cl^-$ channel function may be normal. The protein affected by the gene defect in *cystic fibrosis* (dubbed the Cystic Fibrosis Transport Regulatory [CFTR] protein) resembles the family of proteins known as multiple drug resistance proteins, associated with extrusion of xenobiotics from cells. Recent research indicates that the CFTR is in fact a $Cl^-$ channel that is either abnormally regulated by cellular protein kinases and consequently does not open under physiological conditions, or is improperly processed upon synthesis and is therefore degraded before reaching the plasma membrane. In either event, the result is a $Cl^-$ secretion abnormality, which manifests as dehydration of pulmonary secretions and abnormal exocrine and sweat gland function.

The asymmetric distribution of channels and transporters between the apical and basolateral membranes of the epithelial cell is a key determinant of the physiological capabilities of the epithelium. For example, in the case of the $Cl^-$-secreting cell described above, if the locations of the $Cl^-$ channel and NaCl cotransporter are reversed so that the channel is basolateral and the cotransporter apical, the epithelium can now function as an absorptive surface, carrying out the transcellular movement of $Cl^-$ again driven by the $Na^+$ gradient. This mechanism has in fact been verified in certain tissues. In the distal tubule of the kidney, which regulates $K^+$ secretion, $K^+$ channels are located in both apical and basolateral membranes and are independently regulated, so the cell can control whether $K^+$ is secreted into the lumen or cycled to the interstitial space for reabsorption. The specific function of an epithelial cell, therefore, depends on the types of ion channels and transporters present, their polarized location on the cell membrane, and the nature of the cytokine or hormone receptors and associated regulatory mechanisms present in the cell.

## DEVELOPMENTAL ASPECTS

## Placental transport

One fundamental purpose of the placenta is to mediate the transport of nutrients to the developing fetus. Unfortunately, this process has proved difficult to study, and knowledge of placental transport is incomplete. This is due in part to the remarkable differences in placental anatomy and physiology among different species. Nevertheless, several generalizations are possible about transport of certain substances across the hemochorial placenta of humans.

Water, gases, and lipophilic substances diffuse freely across the placenta. Permeability to ions and even large polar solutes and proteins is quite high and has prompted speculation that relatively large pores exist in the syncytiotrophoblast, although no such pores have been demonstrated anatomically. This suggests that many high-capacity mechanisms exist for the transport of non-lipophilic substances. Transport systems known to exist in syncytiotrophoblast membranes include $Na^+$-$K^+$-ATPase, $Ca^{2+}$-ATPase, $Cl^-$-$HCO_3^-$ and $Na^+$-$H^+$ exchange, $Na^+$-dependent and independent glucose carriers, a variety of amino acid transporters, and other transport proteins. Active, uphill transport of $Ca^{2+}$, $Mg^{2+}$, and possibly $K^+$ have been demonstrated across the placenta, but the details of these processes are not known. As suitable trophoblast culture systems are developed and molecular biological techniques are applied to the study of placental transport, new insights into this important area of fetal physiology are likely to emerge.

## Fetal life and perinatal changes in transport functions

The association between ion transport regulation and cell differentiation and development is illustrated by the fact that within minutes of fertilization, $Na^+$-$H^+$ exchange is activated in the zygote. The resulting alkalinization of the cell interior is thought to trigger increases in DNA synthesis and protein translation, formation of microtubules and microfilaments, and increased $K^+$ conductance. Similarly, activation of $Na^+$-$H^+$ exchange is one of the early events in receptor- or chemical-induced differentiation of some cultured cells. It is likely, though unproved, that many of the cellular differentiation processes that occur during fetal development involve changes in cellular ion homeostasis, and the function and regulation of specific ion channels and transporters. The differentiation of epithelial cells and establishment of transport function involve the translation and transcription of transport protein genes, modification of the protein and its insertion into the appropriate membrane, and the presence of appropriate regulatory mechanisms. Because epithelial transport involves multiple channels and transporters located at different membranes, any one component might be rate-limiting to the establishment of transport function. Very little is currently known about these processes in development, which constitute a fertile area for future research.

The development of ion transport capacity of the pulmonary epithelia involves changes in fluid secretion, which are important to the crucial transition from fluid-filled to air-filled lung (see also page 813). In fetal life, the lung secretes fluid, producing up to 500 ml per day in the late-gestation sheep fetus, in which most experimental work has been done. This fluid contributes to amniotic fluid volume, and the distention of the lung produced by the constant flow of fluid has an important effect on pulmonary development. Fluid is produced by proximal and distal airway epithelial cells by means of a $Cl^-$-secretion mechanism similar to that described above. This mechanism persists in the adult trachea and is stimulated by adrenergic agents. Late in gestation, however, an absorptive mechanism appears, which is also sensitive to adrenergic stimulation. This mechanism may be similar to the $Na^+$ absorption system found in adult bronchi, which features an apical $Na^+$ channel (see Fig. 2.9), or may involve the $Na^+$-$H^+$ exchange system known to be present in alveolar type II cells. Regardless of the mechanism involved, late in gestation adrenergic stimulation results in a reversal of tracheal fluid flow, so that net secretion changes to net absorption. This suggests that the absorption by the airway epithelium can override the secretion of fluid under the influence of catecholamine near term. An increase in $Na^+$-$K^+$-ATPase gene expression (mRNA levels) in mouse lung epithelium late in gestation also supports the notion that the capacity for ion transport increases in the perinatal period.

Studies in rabbit lung indicate that total lung water diminishes near term, and morphological studies demonstrate that a portion of the fluid filling the alveoli is absorbed before birth. Immediately after birth, fluid collects in the peribronchial space, presumably transported across the airway epithelium, before being removed by the pulmonary circulation and lymphatics. The maturation of the surfactant system also plays an important role in the ability of the newborn to maintain a "dry" airway. Once the alveoli are air-filled, surface tension represents a significant hydraulic driving force for water entry into the alveoli from the interstitial space, which must be offset by other mechanisms of fluid removal, including active $Na^+$ transport. Reduction of surface tension by surfactant diminishes this driving force, thereby hastening fluid removal and lessening the tendency for pulmonary edema.

As in lung, many of the epithelial transport functions of the gut, kidney, and other organs mature in late fetal or neonatal life to the level characteristic of the adult animal. For example, the fetal proximal tubule of the kidney exhibits less than one-half the rate of $Na^+$-$H^+$ exchange as the adult kidney; this changes rapidly over the neonatal period, and reaches adult levels by 6 weeks of age. This relative deficiency of $Na^+$-$H^+$ exchange accounts for the poor handling of $Na^+$ and $HCO_3^-$ by preterm kidney, which is often apparent clinically, and may relate to low levels of expression of the $Na^+$-$H^+$-exchanger in the tubular epithelial cells. $Na^+$-$K^+$-ATPase expression also increases in the kidney during the late fetal and neonatal period. A similar pattern of perinatal development of $Na^+$-$H^+$ exchange capacity is also observed in the small intestine.

## GENETIC DEFECTS

It has long been recognized that a number of human disease states reflect abnormalities in membrane function. Recently the origins of a number of hereditary disorders have been traced to gene mutations in specific membrane proteins. As noted above, a single amino acid deletion in the CFTR $Cl^-$ channel accounts for almost three-fourths of the cases of cystic fibrosis, and other mutations in the same protein account for most of the remainder. A defect in a different class of $Cl^-$ channels in skeletal muscle produces the phenotype of myotonia congenita. A point mutation in a P-type ATPase responsible for copper transport, results in Wilson disease, and a different mutation in the same protein causes Menkes disease. Cystinuria results from a defect in an amino acid transporter expressed in the renal proximal tubule. A mutation in the intestinal $Na^+$-glucose transporter produces a rare disorder marked by glucose/galactose malabsorption. The hemolytic red cell disorders, hereditary spherocytosis and hereditary elliptocytosis, result from a variety of mutations in the membrane skeleton proteins (spectrin, ankyrin, protein 4.1) or their attachment sites on the membrane (anion exchange protein, glycophorin). A kindred has been described with a recessive mutation in the erythrocyte spectrin gene which results in the absence of spectrin synthesis and produces a phenotype of severe erythroblastosis fetalis in the homozygous state. Duchenne muscular dystrophy is a consequence of a mutation in dystrophin, a member of the spectrin superfamily of proteins expressed in skeletal muscle. Neurofibromatosis type 2 results from a defect in another skeletal protein in the 4.1 superfamily. It is likely that the explosion of information on the molecular genetics of membrane and transport proteins currently underway will reveal that a great many pathological states have a direct origin in membrane dysfunction.

## CONCLUSION

Regulation of membrane permeability and ion transport is a vital cellular function, central to the maintenance of cell volume and pH; many cellular functions are primarily or secondarily affected by the intracellular ionic milieu. The transmembrane $Na^+$ gradient, maintained by the $Na^+$-$K^+$-ATPase, is important in many of these processes and also represents an energy source for the transport of other ions and substrates. Many pathological processes and pharmacological actions can be traced to effects of an injury or drug on a transport process.

Membrane transport of most ions and compounds is mediated by specific transport proteins. These ATPases, carriers, and channels share many common structural features, especially within functional classes. Species, tissue, and cell specificity often reside in the regulatory components of these membrane protein complexes. Intricate cellular regulation of transport protein activity is accomplished by a variety of acute and long-term mechanisms. These include substrate availability, phosphorylation–dephosphorylation mechanisms, sulfhydryl oxidation, $Ca^{2+}$ activation, voltage sensitivity, and regulation of transcription, translation, and membrane insertion of transport protein.

Changes in ion transport occur during development from the zygote to the postnatal period. Some of these changes affect differentiation of cells, while others reflect the development of specific transport capacities in tissue such as renal tubule and intestinal epithelia. Much more information about the molecular biology, biochemistry, and physiology of these processes is required to build a coherent picture of this important component of developmental physiology.

## SELECTED READING

Benos DJ, Sorcher EJ. Ion channels. In: Seldin DW, Geibish G, eds. *The Kidney: Physiology and Pathophysiology*, Vol I. New York: Raven Press, 1992: 587.

Bennet V, Gilligan DM. The spectrin-based skeleton and micron-scale organization of the plasma membrane. *Ann Rev Cell Biol* 1993; 9: 27.

Boron WF. Control of intracellular pH. In: Seldin DW, Geibish G, eds. *The Kidney: Physiology and Pathophysiology*, Vol I. New York: Raven Press, 1992: 219.

Demaurex N, Grinstein S. $Na^+/H^+$ antiport: modulation by ATP and role in cell volume regulation. *J Exp Biol* 1994; 196: 389.

Hay WW, Jr. Metabolic interrelationships of placenta and fetus. *Placenta* 1995; 16: 19.

Joiner CH. Cation transport and volume regulation in sickle red blood cells. *Am J Physiol* 1993; 264: C251.

Lauf PK, Bauer J, Adragna NC, et al. Erythrocyte KCl cotransport: properties and regulation. *Am J Physiol* 1992; 263: C917.

Law RO. Regulation of mammalian brain cell volume. *J Exp Zool* 1994; 268: 90.

Lingrell JB, Orlowski J, Shull MM, Price EM. Molecular genetics of Na,K-ATPase. *Nucleic Acid Res Mol Biol* 1990; 38: 37.

Poole RC, Halestrap AP. Transport of lactate and other monocarboxylates across mammalian plasma membranes. *Am J Physiol* 1993; 264: C761.

Spring KR, Hoffman EK. Cellular volume control. In: Seldin DW, Geibish G, eds. *The Kidney: Physiology and Pathophysiology*, Vol I. New York: Raven Press, 1992: 147.

Thorens B, Charron MJ, Lodish HF. Molecular physiology of glucose transporters. *Diabetes Care* 1990; 13: 209.

Welsh, MJ, Tsui L-C, Boat TF, Beaudet AL. Cystic Fibrosis. In: Scriver CR, Beaudet AL, Sly WS, Valee D, eds. *The Metabolic and Molecular Basis of Inherited Disease*. New York: McGraw-Hill, 1995: 3799.

# RECEPTORS

## CELL SIGNALING

Survival of unicellular organisms depends on their ability to respond to extracellular signals. Coordinated function of multicellular organisms requires not only response to environmental signals, but also communication with neighboring and remote cells. To allow transfer of information into the cell, a signal must gain access across the cell membrane. Although lipid-soluble ligands, such as steroids, may enter the cell directly, the hydrophobic nature of the cell membrane prohibits entry of many signaling ligands, such as amines and peptides, into cells, and they require the presence of a transmembrane communication system. Receptors are specialized structures, designed to transmit signals between ligands and target molecules. Membrane receptors allow transmission across the phospholipid cell membrane, while intracellular receptors initiate signal transduction by lipophilic agents. To allow coordinated function, intracellular enzymes detect the transmitted stimulus and generate signaling molecules called "second messengers," which lead to an orchestrated and reversible cell response (Fig. 2.12).

Recent progress in understanding cell signaling stems primarily from improved isolation and purification techniques, along with the ability to sequence, clone, and express the receptors in host cells. These techniques have allowed determination of the sequences that confer ligand and effector specificity, and insight into conformational changes that trigger transmembrane signaling. These approaches have also identified structural "families" of receptors, some even functionally unrelated, yet with a high degree of similarity (homology) in portions of the amino acid sequences. Important portions of these molecules are identified by the fact that their sequences are virtually unchanged (conserved) across a wide range of species.

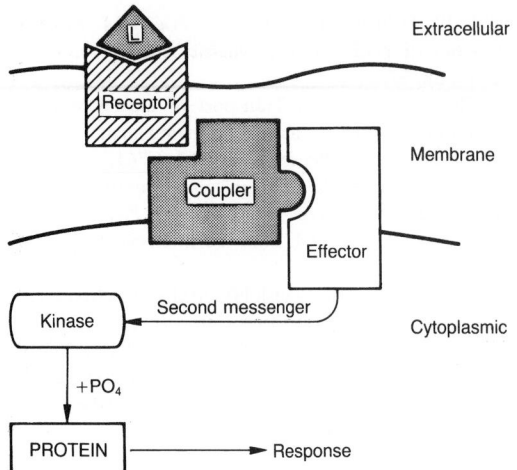

FIGURE 2.12 Diagrammatic overview of a ligand (e.g. β-adren-ergic agonist) stimulated response. Ligand (L) binding to the receptor activates a coupling protein (e.g. G-protein), which stimulates an effector (e.g. adenylyl cyclase) to generate a second messenger (e.g. cAMP). The second messenger acti-vates a protein kinase (e.g. kinase A) which phosphorylates a target protein leading to a cellular response (e.g. ion channel activation, muscle contraction, and DNA synthesis). For other receptors (e.g. tyrosine kinase receptors) this system is combined in one membrane-spanning protein which includes the ligand recognition site, coupler, and the kinase.

Receptors contain two functional domains: a ligand-binding domain, which determines initial inter-action with the ligand, and a catalytic domain, which interacts with effectors for further signal processing and response. Membrane receptors also contain a transmembrane anchoring domain. In addition, a regulatory domain is present in many receptors. This domain contains phosphorylation sites, which provide targets for homologous regulation, induced in a recep-tor by its own specific ligand (e.g. tachyphylaxis), or heterologous regulation by other effectors (e.g. kinase A induced desensitization of β-adrenergic receptors). This complex signal transmission machinery of sen-sors, modulators, and effectors determines the specifi-city of response, conferred by expression of different receptors among various cell types, and is capable of signal sorting and amplification of the message.

This section of the chapter describes receptor sys-tems that illustrate these principles (*see* Chapter 33 (page 459) for additional details on specific receptors). These systems (Fig. 2.13) include G-protein-coupled receptors, tyrosine kinase receptors, endocytosis-asso-ciated receptors, membrane-bound and cytosolic gua-nylyl cyclase, cell adhesion receptors, and the steroid receptor superfamily.

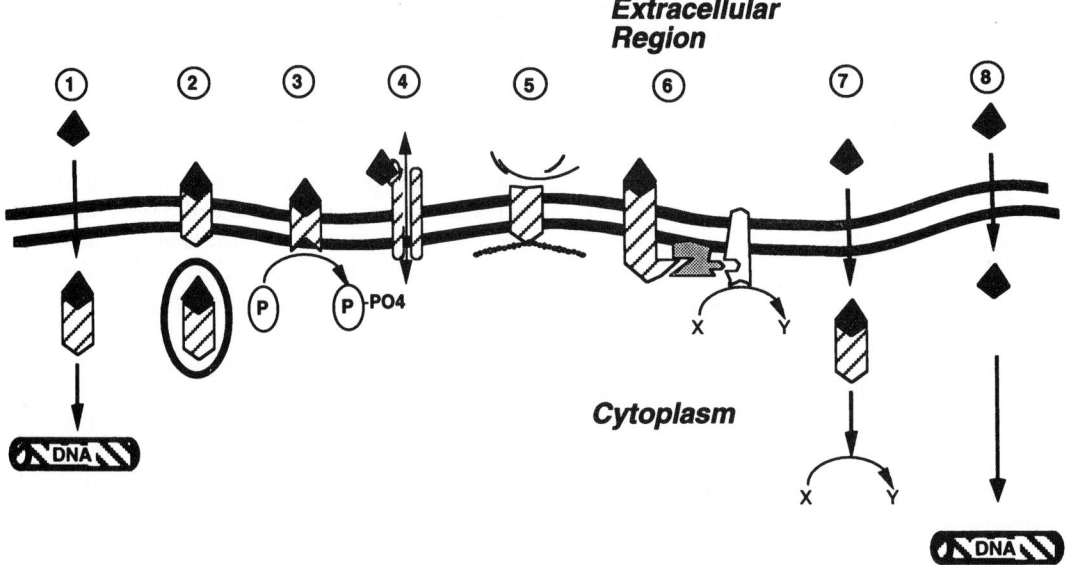

FIGURE 2.13 Diagrammatic representation of receptor-mediated transmembrane signaling. (1) Lipid-soluble ligands, capable of crossing the lipid bilayer, interact with intracellular receptors (e.g. steroids) and regulate gene expression. (2) Ligands are transported across the membrane via receptor-mediated endocytosis (e.g. low-density lipoproteins). (3) Ligands bind to the extracellular region of the receptor (e.g. epidermal growth factor), resulting in allosteric changes that activate a cytoplasmic catalytic domain, which phosphorylates ($PO_4$) cytoplasmic proteins (P). (4) Ligands (e.g. acetylcholine) bind to a receptor, which includes an ion channel, and open the channel to ion flux into the cells. (5) Ligands, which are a component of the extracellular matrix, bind to a receptor (e.g. integrin) that interacts with cytoskeleton. (6) Ligands bind to receptors (e.g. β-adrenergic receptors) that span the membrane, causing activation of G-protein on the cytoplasmic side of the membrane, which converts inactive enzyme (X) to an active effector (Y). (7) Ligands (e.g. nitric oxide, NO) cross the lipid bilayer, and bind to receptors that contain a catalytic domain. (8) Signaling by ligand/nuclear proteins (e.g. lactoferrin) that cross the cell membrane and directly effect gene transcription.

## CELL MEMBRANE RECEPTORS

Receptors in the cell membrane utilize several strategies to transfer information from hydrophilic ligands across the hydrophobic cell membrane. In some cases (e.g. G-protein-linked receptors) these receptors interact with proteins on the cytosolic face of the membrane to access intracellular targets, while in others (e.g. tyrosine kinase receptors) the receptor itself interacts with the effectors. Still others (e.g. low density lipoprotein (LDL) receptors) carry the ligand into the cell.

## G-protein-linked receptors

The activation of cellular signaling mechanisms by many ligands is mediated by receptors that interact with a special group of guanosine-5′-triphosphate (GTP)-binding "coupling" proteins termed *G-proteins*. G-protein-linked receptors represent the largest family of membrane receptors. Examples include receptors for adrenergic, muscarinic, and dopaminergic activators, somatostatin, opiates, serotonin, adenosine and rhodopsin. All transmembrane receptors linked to G-proteins have a similar structure (Fig. 2.14). Seven transmembrane domains (M-I to M-VII) span the bilayer, with an extracellular amino terminus and an intracellular carboxy terminus. The hydrophilic domains include the extracellular (E-I to E-III) and cytoplasmic (C-I to C-III) loops. Disulfide bonds within cysteine-rich residues in the ligand-binding domain stabilize ligand-binding pockets. The transmembrane region, which includes segments of 20–28 amino acids, contains conserved regions also crucial for ligand binding. The cytoplasmic domain is involved in coupling with G-proteins, and specificity of this interaction is determined by the C-III loop.

Adrenergic receptor coupling to G-proteins is the most completely elucidated model of receptor and G-protein interaction (*see* Fig. 2.19). There are several distinct types of adrenergic receptors, defined by physiological action, pharmacological specificity, and deduced amino acid sequence. β-Receptors activate the enzyme adenylyl cyclase to stimulate cyclic-3′,5′-adenosine monophosphate (cAMP) generation. This effect is mediated by $G_s$-protein. $α_2$-Receptors are coupled by $G_i$-protein to inhibit adenylyl cyclase. In recent years the subtypes were further divided (e.g. $α_{2a}$, $α_{2b}$, and $α_{2c}$), and selective expression of these subtypes may explain tissue specific responses. $α_1$-Receptors are coupled by G-proteins (e.g. $G_q$) to phospholipase C.

Characteristic of these receptors is their ability to undergo regulatory modifications. For the β-adrenergic receptors, for example, phosphorylation of the receptor protein results in alteration of interaction between the cytoplasmic domain and G-protein, sequestration of the receptor into membrane vesicles, internalization into the cytoplasm, and consequent receptor degradation.

Phosphorylation of specific serine and threonine residues in the C-III loop produces the pharmacological phenomenon of desensitization by several independently regulated processes. These regulatory steps may be affected by the native ligand (homologous desensi-

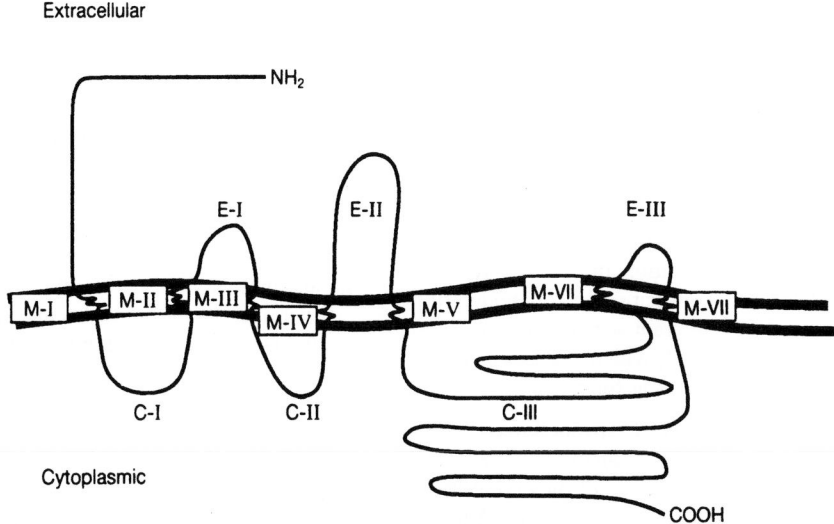

FIGURE 2.14 Diagrammatic representation of G-protein-linked receptors. The receptor is composed of seven α helices, which span the membrane bilayer. Stimulatory ligands interact with extracellular loops (E-I to E-III) and transmembrane helices (M-I to M-VII). G-protein interacts with cytoplasmic loops (C-I to C-III). The carboxy terminus and C-III contain multiple serine and threonine residues, targets for phosphorylation, which induces receptor desensitization.

tization). The β-adrenergic receptor kinase, which phosphorylates agonist-occupied receptors, reduces the ability of agonists to activate β-adrenergic receptors. The phosphorylated receptor also has increased affinity for another regulatory protein, β-arrestin, which binds to the receptor and prevents its interaction with $G_{s\alpha}$ thus impeding activation of the second messenger cascade. Ligands that stimulate cAMP generation through other receptors can also reduce receptor function (heterologous desensitization) by phosphorylation through cAMP-dependent protein kinase (kinase A). The precise mechanisms of receptor regulation are currently under investigation. Because G-proteins are activated by synthetic peptides composed of the receptor domain that interacts with G-proteins, agonist binding seems to result in an allosteric change of the receptor, allowing this portion to interact with G-protein. This disinhibition of the receptor by an agonist seems to be a common theme of activation.

## Tyrosine kinase receptors

This group of receptors binds growth factors, such as epidermal growth factor (EGF), platelet-derived growth factor (PDGF), fibroblast growth factor (FGF), insulin-like growth factors (IGFs), and insulin (*see also* page 463). The structure of tyrosine kinase receptors includes an extracellular ligand-binding domain, a transmembrane region, and a cytoplasmic catalytic domain that contains the tyrosine kinase active site. The composition of the extracellular and intracellular domains defines the several subclasses of tyrosine kinase receptors. The extracellular glycosylated ligand-binding domain consists of cysteine-rich repetitive sequences (Fig. 2.15), which in some cases (e.g. PDGF receptor) resemble the immunoglobulin structure. The hydrophobic transmembrane region anchors the receptor to the plasma membrane and plays a passive role in signal transduction. The cytoplasmic portion of the receptor is composed of three domains:

- the juxtamembrane domain, which is thought to be a target for modulation by heterologous stimuli;
- the highly conserved tyrosine kinase domain, required for phosphorylation of tyrosine residues in intracellular target proteins and for modulation of interactions with different second messengers;
- the carboxy terminal tail, which exerts a negative control on receptor signaling functions.

There are three subclasses of tyrosine kinase receptors. Receptor activation by a ligand such as EGF results in a conformational change of the extracellular domain and dimer formation (subclass I). Alternatively, type-1 IGF and insulin receptors (subclass II) exist as a dimer even prior to ligand binding, while PDGF receptors (subclass III) undergo dimerization after binding a dimeric ligand to the receptors. Activa-

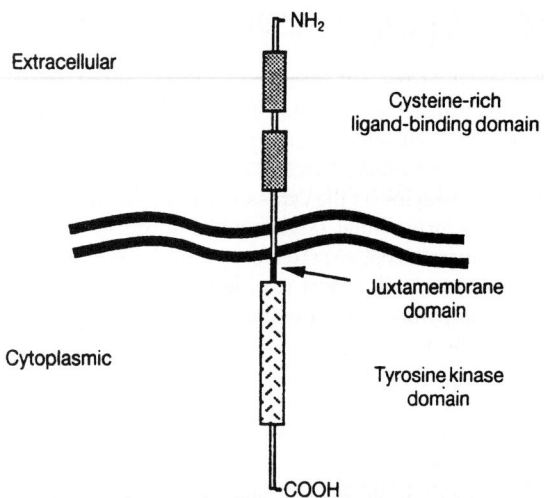

FIGURE 2.15 Illustration of the epidermal growth factor receptor as representative of the tyrosine kinase receptor family. The extracellular ligand-binding domain undergoes dimerization after ligand binding. The cytoplasmic region is composed of a regulatory juxtamembrane domain, a conserved catalytic tyrosine kinase domain, and a carboxy terminal tail (COOH), which modulates the action of the tyrosine kinase domain.

tion of the receptor leads to signal transduction by phosphorylating tyrosine residues of cytosolic targets. The tyrosine kinase receptor also phosphorylates its own tyrosine residues, leading to modification of the receptor conformation, which enhances the kinase activity. Activation is followed by aggregation at specialized membrane regions, which on electron microscopy appear as depressions coated with "fuzzy" material. These "coated pits" are characterized by constitutive invagination activity. Following aggregation, the receptor–ligand complex undergoes internalization and intracellular degradation, and provides a downregulation mechanism to decrease receptor concentration. The signal is terminated by hydrolytic action of specific phosphatases.

Cytokines bind specific membrane receptors, many of which (like the tumor necrosis factor family of cytokines) contain a tyrosine kinase-like domain in their cytoplasmic region. Interestingly, soluble forms of cytokine receptors, which retain their ability to bind ligands, may be modulators of cytokine action.

Several signaling pathways are modulated by tyrosine kinase receptors. Ligand binding and auto-phosphorylation lead to recruitment of Src homology 2 (SH2) domain-containing proteins to phosphorylated tyrosine residues on the receptors. SH2 domain-containing proteins (such as inositol phosphate 3-kinase, phospholipase C and Src family kinase) lead to activation of signaling molecules through several mechanisms, such as tyrosine phosphorylation, conformational changes and plasma membrane translocation. Other signaling systems such as $Ca^{2+}$ influx, $Na^+/H^+$ exchange, glucose, and amino acid transport are also enhanced by tyrosine kinase receptor activation. Thus these diverse pathways regulate growth as well as differentiated functions.

## Receptors mediating endocytosis

Many large macromolecules enter the cell via receptor-mediated endocytosis (Fig. 2.16). Examples include low-density lipoproteins (LDL), transferrin, transcobalamin, and immune complexes. LDL receptors, which regulate plasma clearance of these lipoproteins, serve as a model for the mechanism of action of this receptor.

The LDL receptor is a highly conserved membrane glycoprotein composed of five domains. The ligand-binding domain at the amino terminus mediates interaction of the receptor with the lipoproteins apo B and apo E. The transmembrane domain serves to anchor the receptor to the membrane. The cytoplasmic

domain contains an O-linked carbohydrate chain domain and an EGF-like domain, the function of which remains unclear. LDL receptor concentration is regulated by the availability of its ligand, with cholesterol intake down-regulating LDL receptor synthesis.

As described for tyrosine kinase receptors, LDL receptors also aggregate at coated pits. In general, the internalization of the receptor-ligand complex of receptors mediating endocytosis results in recycling or degradation of the two components (*see* Fig. 2.16). Following internalization and endosome formation, the LDL receptor dissociates and free LDL is delivered to lysosomes and is degraded, while the unliganded receptor recycles to the cell membrane. This outcome is different among receptors. As described for EGF, both the ligand and receptor may be degraded. Alternatively, when the internalized iron–transferrin receptor complex dissociates, both transferrin and its receptor recycle to the plasma membrane where free transferrin is available for iron binding.

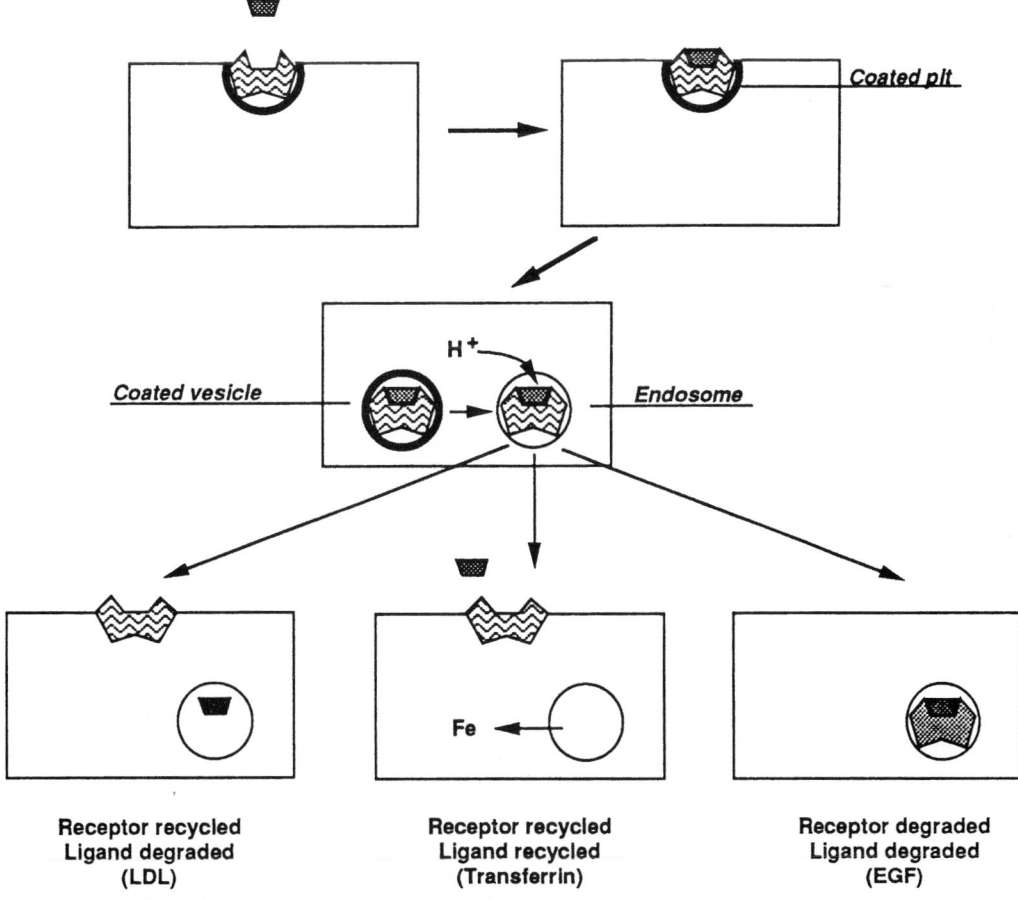

FIGURE 2.16 Diagrammatic representation of receptor-mediated endocytosis. Ligand binds to receptors clustered in coated pits. The coated pits undergo internalization and form coated vesicles, becoming endosomes following acidification ($H^+$). Low-density lipoprotein (LDL) receptors recycle to the cell membrane while the LDL is degraded in lysosomes. For transferrin, both receptor and ligand recycle after iron (Fe) release in the cell. Epidermal growth factor (EGF) and its receptors are both degraded in the lysosomes.

## IGF-II/mannose 6-phosphate receptors

Although the IGF-II/mannose 6-phosphate receptor shares many features with receptors for other growth factors, this receptor type is distinguished by the lack of tyrosine kinase activity in its cytoplasmic region. Similarly, nerve growth factor (NGF) receptors also lack intrinsic tyrosine kinase activity. The mechanism of signal transduction by growth factors that lack kinase activity is not yet identified. Possibly, the major role of these receptors, which bind IGF-II and lysosomal enzymes bearing the mannose 6-phosphate recognition marker, is transport of the ligand into the cell, as described above for LDL receptors, with subsequent mechanisms, such as G-protein$_{1\alpha}$ and Ca$^{2+}$-gated signaling, resulting in intracellular signal propagation.

## Membrane-bound guanylyl cyclases

Membrane-bound guanylyl cyclases are structurally similar to tyrosine kinase receptors. They consist of an extracellular ligand-binding domain at the amino terminus, a transmembrane domain, and a highly conserved cytosolic domain that includes the catalytic site. The catalytic domain contains sequences homologous to the catalytic domain of tyrosine kinase receptors.

There are several isoforms of membrane-bound guanylyl cyclase, each responsive to specific ligands. Not surprisingly, the major heterogeneity of these receptor subtypes is in the ligand-binding domain. At present a few endogenous ligands have been identified, all small peptides. Examples include atrial natriuretic peptide and heat-stable enterotoxin of *E. coli*. Interestingly, a truncated form of this receptor, lacking its intracellular domain, can be found in the serum, and may represent a degradation pathway of this receptor.

## Receptors that include ion channels

The most direct receptor–ion channel interaction is found in receptors such as the nicotinic acetylcholine receptor, which is included as an integral part of the channel structure (single element signaling). The receptor is a pentamer made up of five polypeptide subunits. These polypeptides, all of which cross the lipid bilayer more than once, form a cylindrical structure 8 nm in diameter. Other transmitter-gated ion channels can be divided into excitatory and inhibitory receptors. Among the excitatory receptors are cation channels gated by acetylcholine, serotonin or glutamate, and inhibitory channels gated by GABA (γ-aminobutyric acid) and glycine. Recently, special attention was given to glutamate receptors, which have been implicated in neuronal plasticity, in acute neuronal degeneration, and as an important component of memory

termed long-term potentiation, which involves a subgroup of glutamate receptors that can be activated by N-methyl-D-aspartate (NMDA) receptors. The function of NMDA receptors in synaptic plasticity and long-term potentiation depends on two unique features. First, current flows through these receptors only when glutamate is bound and the membrane is strongly depolarized. Second, Ca$^{2+}$, which is important for long-term potentiation, can pass through these channels along with Na$^{+}$ and K$^{+}$ ions.

## Cell adhesion receptors

Virtually all cells contain adhesion receptors, mediating cell–cell and cell–extracellular matrix interactions. These receptors are divided into two major types (Fig. 2.17): the immunoglobulin superfamily (e.g. cadherins), which bind to their identical molecules (homophi-

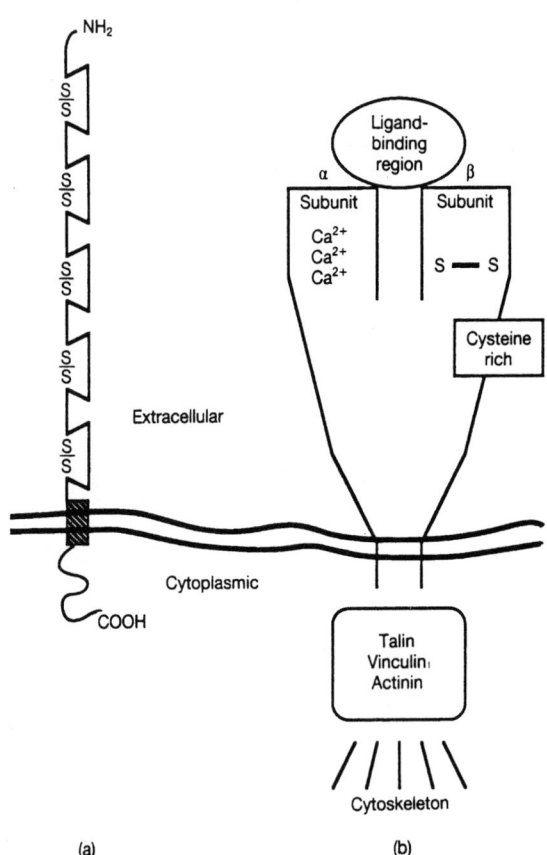

FIGURE 2.17 Diagrammatic representation of cell adhesion receptors. (a) Cadherin contains an extracellular domain folded into five immunoglobulin-like regions, with disulfide bonds (SS) connecting the ends of each loop. (b) Integrin, composed of two noncovalently associated subunits: α, which contains areas thought to bind Ca$^{2+}$, and β, which contains four cysteine-rich repeats, and is characterized by disulfide bonds (S-S). The small cytoplasmic domain binds cytoskeleton elements.

lic binding), and the integrin superfamily, which can bind to nonidentical adhesion receptors (heterophilic binding).

Cadherins are Ca²⁺-dependent adhesion molecules and have a structure characteristic of the immunoglobulin type of adhesion molecule. The extracellular amino terminus determines interaction specificity. The intracellular domain is a conserved region, and determines the adhesive properties of the receptor. This is associated with actin-binding cytoplasmic proteins called catenins. By contrast, the ligand-binding domain of the integrins contains two non-covalently associated subunits: the α-subunit, which has multiple Ca²⁺ binding residues, and a highly conserved β-subunit, folded into a loop stabilized by disulfide bonds. Several forms of both α- and β-subunits have been identified, and the specificity of ligand binding (e.g. fibronectin, laminin) is determined by the combination of these subunits. The interaction of the cytoplasmic domain with actin filaments is mediated by additional cytoskeleton molecules. This domain also contains a tyrosine phosphorylation site, a possible target for regulation.

Cell adhesion receptors also have a role in selective interactions among cells during morphogenesis. Cadherins are found on presumptive neural crest cells. When these cells convert from an ectoderm form to a migratory form they lose detectable cadherins. It has also been suggested that adhesion molecules have a role in cell signaling, mediated by the cytoplasmic domain.

## INTRACELLULAR RECEPTORS

## The nuclear receptor superfamily

This superfamily includes receptors for steroids and other lipid-soluble agonists, such as thyroid hormone, retinoic acid, and vitamin D. These hormones regulate development, cellular proliferation, and differentiation by crossing the hydrophobic cell membrane and binding to specific cytosolic (e.g. glucocorticoids) or nuclear (e.g. estrogen, thyroid) receptors. Cloning of these receptors and deducing their amino acid sequences reveals a high degree of similarity, leading to their classification as a "superfamily." In addition, many other proteins, which share a high degree of homology with steroid receptors, but for which there is as yet no known ligand, constitute the subset of "orphan receptors."

The modular structure of members in this family includes several independent domains. The conserved ligand-binding domain confers ligand specificity, and a region necessary for receptor dimerization. Binding of the receptor to DNA is at the cysteine-rich DNA-binding domain of the receptor, characterized by cysteine residues folded around a zinc ion to form "zinc fingers." Transcriptional activation function is located in both the carboxy- and amino-termini for most

receptors. Receptor activation induces allosteric alterations, which enable the receptor to dissociate from heat shock proteins. Many members of this family then dimerize and bind to specific receptor response elements in the promoter regions of target proteins. Dimerization may involve two identical proteins (homodimerization, e.g. estrogen receptor dimers), or two different members of this family (heterodimerization, e.g. thyroid hormone or retinoid X receptors) (Fig. 2.18). Other receptors (e.g. the orphan receptor, steroidogenic factor 1) bind the DNA as a monomer. DNA response elements can be composed of two repeats (half-sites) in several orientations, or a single "half-site." Receptor binding to its response element alters the expression of the target gene, causing stimulation or inhibition of protein synthesis through interaction with additional cellular coactivators and proteins which are part of the basal transcription machinery.

Several cellular proteins were recently shown to function as both extracellular ligands and DNA binding proteins. These proteins cross the cell membrane, and bind DNA without activation of signaling intermediates. Examples of such proteins include lactoferrin, and the viral proteins TAT and Tax-1. In addition, several homeodomain proteins traverse the cell membrane and bind DNA directly, indicating that these transcription factors can act in a paracrine fashion. The exact sequence used by such proteins for gaining entry into the cell remains obscure. It has been suggested that their intranuclear activity may be modulated by glycoseaminoglycans, which can modify the transcriptional activity of nuclear proteins.

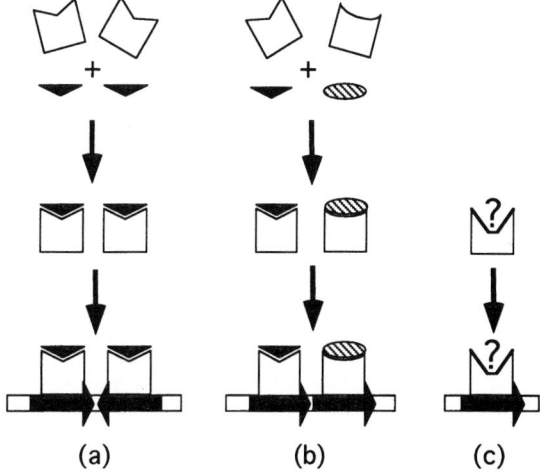

FIGURE 2.18 DNA binding by members of the steroid receptor superfamily. (a) Two identical proteins, bound by their ligands, homodimerize and bind two inverted DNA "half-sites" (palindrome). (b) Two non-identical members, bound by their respective ligands, heterodimerize and bind two "half-sites" arranged as a "direct repeat." (c) An orphan receptor binds a single "half-site" as a monomer

## Cytosolic guanylyl cyclase

In addition to a membrane-bound form, guanylyl cyclase also is present as a soluble intracellular enzyme. Unlike the former, the cytosolic form is a heterodimer, composed of two subunits, the assembly of which is determined by the specific tissue in which the enzyme is localized. The carboxy terminus is homologous to the cytosolic domain of the membrane-bound enzyme and also to the cytosolic portion of adenylyl cyclase.

The primary agonist for this receptor is nitric oxide (NO). This lipid-soluble agonist, which is synthesized from L-arginine by several forms of the enzyme nitric oxide synthase (NOS) (*see* Chapter 10 for further details), recently has been recognized as an important signaling molecule (involved, for example, in neuro-transmission, smooth muscle relaxation, and mediation of inflammatory responses). Another gas, carbon monoxide (CO), also can act as an intracellular signal. It is synthesized by heme oxygenase and utilizes the same guanylyl cyclase signaling system as NO. Like NO, CO also is a smooth muscle relaxant. These two gasses readily diffuse through the cell membrane and bind to, and stimulate, cellular guanylyl cyclase to produce cyclic-3′,5′-guanosine monophosphate (cGMP). cGMP has at least three broad cellular targets: cGMP-dependent kinases, which are most abundant in smooth muscle cells, platelets, and the cerebellum, cGMP-dependent ion channels, important for intact function of photoreceptors, olfactory and renal epithelium, and cGMP-binding phosphodiesterase, which is widely distributed in mammalian tissues.

## SELECTED READING

Albeda SM, Buck CA. Integrins and other cell adhesion molecules. *Faseb J* 1990; 4: 2868.
Hollenberg MD. Structure-activity relationship for transmembrane signaling: the receptor's turn. *Faseb J* 1991; 5: 178.
Lincoln TM, Cornwall TL. Intracellular cyclic GMP receptor protein. *Faseb J* 1993; 7: 328.
O'Malley B. The steroid receptor superfamily: more excitement predicted for the future. *Mol Endocrinol* 1990; 4: 363.
Prochiantz A, Theodore L. Nuclear/growth factors. *Bioassay* 1995; 17: 39.
Schneider WJ. The low density lipoprotein receptor. *Biochim Biophys Acta* 1989; 988: 303.
Ullrich A, Schlessinger J. Signal transduction by receptors with tyrosine kinase activity. *Cell* 1990; 61: 203.
Verma A, Hirsch DJ, Glatt CE, *et al.* Carbon monoxide: a putative neuronal messenger. *Science* 1993; 259: 381.

# POSTRECEPTOR MECHANISMS

Intracellular signaling molecules that couple membrane events to intracellular effector systems are called *second messengers*. To define a molecule as a second messenger, its concentration should be modified by a ligand-stimulated receptor system and lead to a parallel change in the cellular response. The second messenger should also elicit an appropriate response when applied, even in the absence of the receptor or its ligand. These molecules participate in the processing, sorting, amplification, and targeting of the initial signal. This section of the chapter describes the major postreceptor messengers and pathways mediating intracellular signal transduction and integrated response.

## G-PROTEINS

The G-proteins are a subset of a larger family of guanosine-5′-triphosphate (GTP)-binding proteins that also includes ribosomal protein synthesis components and $p21^{ras}$ protein. These proteins have GTPase activity, and their function is regulated by bound guanyl nucleotide (i.e. GTP or guanosine-5′-diphosphate [GDP]). G-proteins are located on the cytoplasmic surface of cell membranes. They sort, amplify, and relay signals from membrane receptors to proteins that generate intracellular second messengers (e.g. inositol phosphates, cAMP, and $Ca^{2+}$).

G-proteins mediate diverse effects, but share a common general structure and mechanism of activation (Fig. 2.19). G-proteins are heterotrimeric, consisting of α-, β-, and γ-subunits. There are at least 20 $G\alpha$-subunits, 5 β-subunits and 6 γ-subunits. Specificity is conferred by the interaction of specific types of $G\alpha$-proteins with the βγ-subunits. In the heterotrimeric form, GDP is bound to $G_\alpha$ and stabilizes the complex. Agonist binding facilitates interaction of the receptor with G-protein, causing allosteric alteration of $G_\alpha$ leading to the dissociation of GDP, which is replaced by GTP, present in excess intracellularly. GTP destabilizes the complex, and the βγ complex dissociates. The α-subunit is then free to bind and activate effector proteins. Effector molecule activation is terminated by GTPase-induced hydrolysis of GTP to GDP and subsequent reassociation of the heterotrimer complex. This cycle demonstrates one of the principles of signal amplification. A receptor's signal of a few milliseconds is converted by the G-protein into several seconds of effector activation, dictated by the timing of the "turn off" signal by GTPase. Thus one receptor can activate many cytoplasmic messengers. Although it was thought that βγ-subunits reverse the action of the α-subunit, it is clear that the βγ-subunit can directly interact with the effector, producing an effect which may be independent (such as $K^+$ channel regulation),

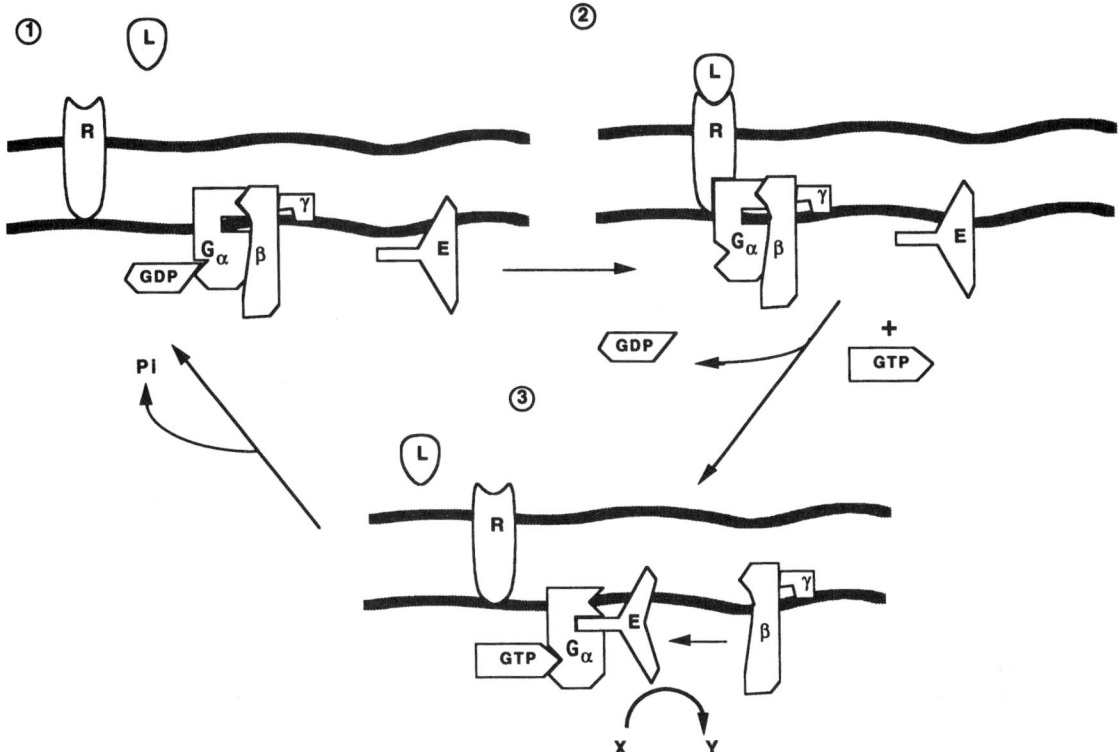

FIGURE 2.19 Diagrammatic representation of receptor-mediated activation of adenylyl cyclase as an example of G-protein function. (1) In the resting state, $G_{sa}$ is bound to $\beta\gamma$ complex, and this heterotrimer binds to GDP. (2) Ligand (L) activation of the receptor (R) facilitates GDP dissociation from $G_{sa}$, and replacement by GTP. (3) GTP binding reduces the affinity of $G_{sa}$ for $\beta\gamma$ complex, and the dissociation of this complex allows $G_{sa}$ stimulation of adenylyl cyclase (C) activity. GTP hydrolysis by intrinsic $G_{sa}$-GTPase action returns $G_{sa}$ to the GDP-bound state, which then recycles to form the heterotrimer with $\beta\gamma$ complex.

synergistic (such as adenylyl cyclase II activation) or antagonistic (such as adenylyl cyclase IV activation) to the effect of the $\alpha$-subunit. $G\beta\gamma$-subunits also may be regulated by cytoplasmic proteins, such as calmodulin. This interaction modulates heterotrimer association with target proteins.

The identity and mechanism of action of several G-proteins were determined originally by the effect of specific bacterial toxins, and more recently by using mutated G-proteins. The first G-protein identified, $G_s$, was found to be irreversibly activated by cholera toxin, which inhibits the GTPase "turn off" reaction. Several G-proteins are substrates for another bacterial toxin, pertussis toxin, which prevents receptor activation by interfering with the release of GDP. Using these approaches it was found that $G_s$ activates not only adenylyl cyclase but also cardiac $Ca^{2+}$ channels. Three inhibitory G-proteins ($G_i$) have been identified, and found to suppress adenylyl cyclase action in response to adrenergic, muscarinic, or opioid ligands. The mechanism of inhibition appears to be partially explained by liberation of $\beta\gamma$ complexes, which bind to $G_{sa}$ and inhibit adenylyl cyclase. Whether the dissociation is in fact the principal action of these heterotrimers or merely a minor effect is not clearly established. The unliganded $G_{ia}$ can, for example, activate phosphatidylinositol-phospholipase C, phosphati-

dylcholine-phospholipase C, phospholipase $A_2$ as well as $K^+$ channels (Fig. 2.20). Other forms of G-proteins have also been identified. $G_q$-protein activates the phosphatidylinositol-phospholipase C pathway (Fig. 2.21), and is neither a target for cholera nor pertussis toxin. $G_t$ links photoreceptors in the retina to cGMP phosphodiesterase, while $G_{olf}$ couples olfactory receptors to adenylyl cyclase activation in the olfactory epithelium. The function of further members of the G-protein family is yet to be determined.

The selective activation of a specific G-protein is determined by its cytoplasmic region. Within this region, specific recognition sequences interact with cell-specific receptors and effectors. Several receptors can interact with more than one G-protein. Subsequent activation of several effectors is regulated by the kinetics of the G-protein–effector interaction. For example, effectors may modulate the rate of GTP hydrolysis of one G-protein, and not the other, thereby affecting the lifetime of effector activation. Cell-specific response pathways also may be determined through G-protein modifications by phosphorylation, binding of lipid residues (e.g. prenylation), interaction with cellular proteins, or by compartmentation with unique signaling proteins. The application of each of these mechanisms to mammalian systems is yet to be determined.

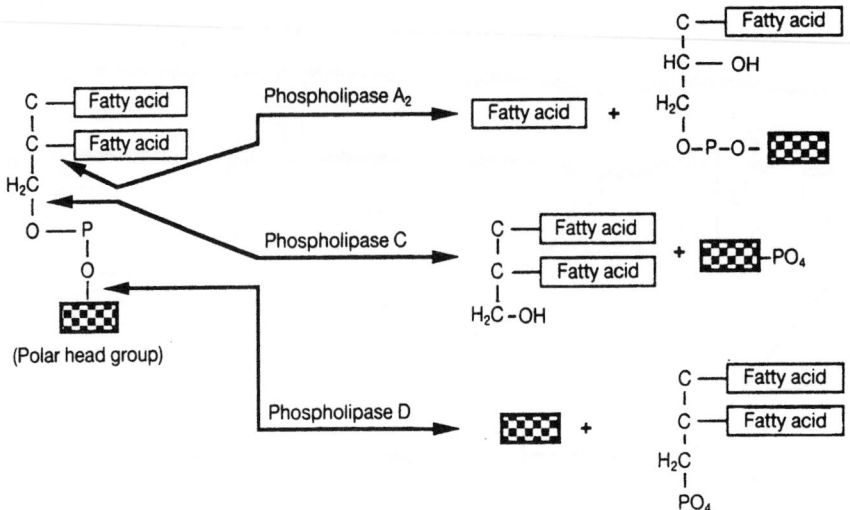

FIGURE 2.20 Diagrammatic representation of phospholipid hydrolysis by phospholipases. Two fatty acids and a polar head group (e.g. choline, inositol, ethanolamine) are bound to the glycerol backbone. Phospholipase $A_2$ hydrolyzes the fatty acid (e.g. arachidonic acid) at the second position, yielding fatty acid and a lysophosphatide. Phospholipase C generates DAG and a phosphorylated head group, such as inositol phosphate. Phospholipase D generates a free polar head group and phosphatidic acid. Not illustrated: phospholipase D also catalyzes the transphosphatidylation of phospholipids (see text).

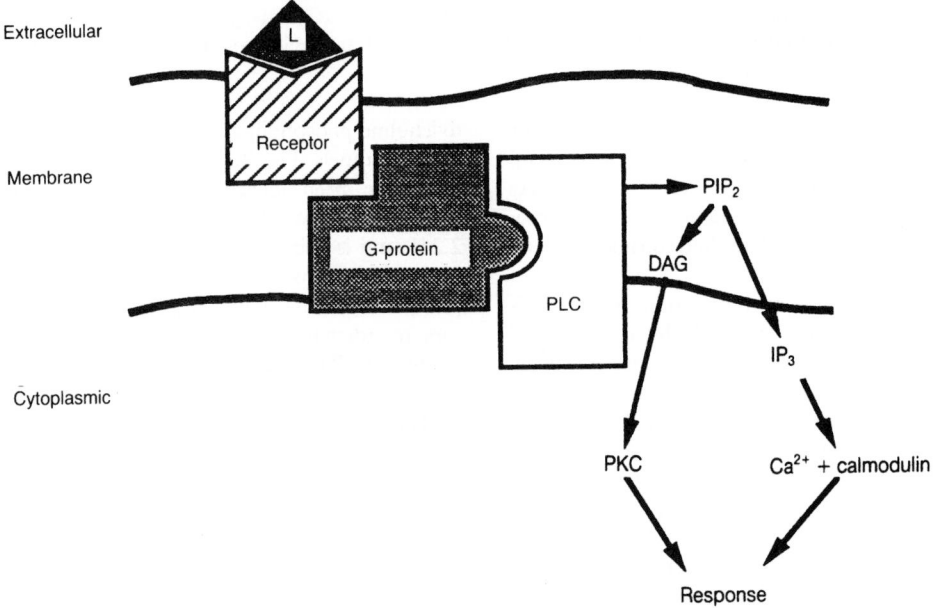

FIGURE 2.21 Schematic representation of phospholipase C (PLC) mediated response. Receptor activation (e.g. $\alpha_1$-receptor) by a ligand (L) activates a G-protein (e.g. $G_q$), which stimulates PLC hydrolysis of phosphatidylinositol-4,5-bisphosphate ($PIP_2$), releasing inositol-1,4,5-trisphosphate ($IP_3$) and 1,2 diacylglycerol (DAG). $IP_3$ enhances the release of $Ca^{2+}$, which binds to calmodulin and stimulates cellular response (e.g. smooth muscle contraction). Diacylglycerol activates intracellular protein kinase C (PKC), which stimulates response by phosphorylation of specific cytoplasmic proteins.

## EXTRACELLULAR SIGNAL-REGULATED PROTEIN KINASES

In complex signal trafficking, the requirement for phosphorylation of a target at multiple sites ensures specificity and fine-tuning, since only a unique combination of modifications will overcome the activation threshold while allowing a low degree of crosstalk between signaling cascades. An example of one such regulatory pathway is the mitogen-activated protein kinase (MAPK) pathway, part of the family of extracellular signal-regulated kinases (ERKs). The MAPK pathway consists of three protein kinases (Fig. 2.22): a serine/threonine protein kinase (MAPK kinase kinase, MAPKKK), which phosphorylates and activates a protein kinase (MAPK kinase, MAPKK), which in turn phosphorylates another kinase (MAPK). This phosphorylation cascade ultimately links a cell surface signal to a nuclear target. There are several families of MAPKs, and their regulation of transcription factors can occur in the cell membrane, cytoplasm or nucleus. Insulin action, for example, is mediated through this cascade (see page 463). The Jun N-terminal/stress-activated protein kinases (JNK/ SAPK) regulate intranuclear phosphorylation of Jun. Phosphorylation of a cytoplasmic target can be seen in the case of NF-κB, where several regulatory phosphorylation signals converge on cytoplasmic regulation of its inhibitor, I-κB.

In contrast, other pathways are capable of "short-circuiting" this multistep second messenger cascade. They include transcription factors which activate or repress gene transcription through direct DNA binding and interaction with basal transcription machinery. Transcription factors are regulated by postreceptor signaling mechanisms which exert their effect either by phosphorylation of the transcription factor, modifying its nuclear localization signal, or by directly effecting oligomerization of transcription factors and DNA binding. For example, the transcription factor p91, when activated by cytokine bound surface receptors (e.g. interferons), directly binds DNA and activates gene transcription. This rapid signaling mechanism is regulated by the Janus kinase/signal transducer and activator of transcription (Jak/STAT) pathway, which is involved in modulation of these rapid signaling cascades through phosphorylation of transcription factors.

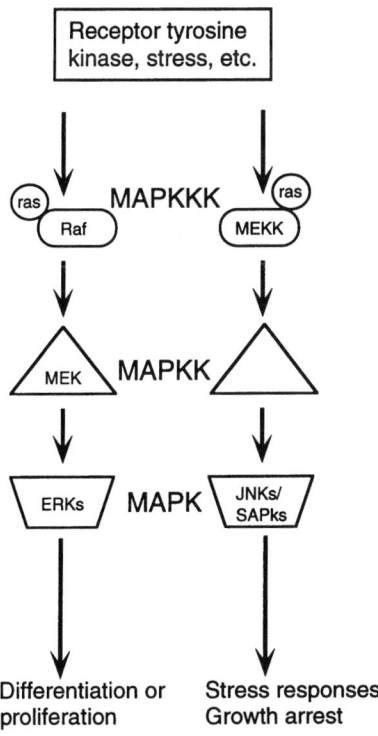

FIGURE 2.22 Mitogen-activated protein kinase (MAPK) pathway. Receptor tyrosine kinase, cytokines or other physical changes activate a kinase of MAPK kinase (MAPKKK) (e.g. Raf, MEK kinase [MEKK]). This activation is regulated by a specific G-protein signaling mechanism. Subsequent phosphorylation of a MAPK kinase (MAPKK) (e.g. MEK) leads to phosphorylation of a MAPK (e.g. ERK, JNK/SAPK), which regulates diverse cellular function.

## ION CHANNEL SIGNALING PATHWAYS

Ion channels play a vital role in the maintenance and modulation of the electrochemical gradient across the cell membrane. These structures allow the flux of channel-specific ions down a concentration gradient, and thus have lower energy requirements than ion pumps, which are responsible for maintenance of the concentration gradient. The dependence of enzymes involved in signal transduction on the cytoplasmic electrochemical milieu explains the ability of ion channels to effect signal transduction.

Ion channels are characterized by their ion specificity, the ligand that activates the channel (e.g. glycine, acetylcholine), and the tissue type. The ion channels are coupled to signaling pathways at several levels.

### Direct coupling at the cell membrane

While some ion channels contain a receptor within the channel structure (single-element signaling, described in the previous section), the regulation of ion channels found in the brain, peripheral neurons, skeletal muscle, smooth muscle, epithelial cells, and many other tissues is mediated through G-proteins (multielement signaling). In the cardiac muscle, for example, muscarinic $M_2$ acetylcholine receptors activate $G_i$-proteins, which are coupled to inward $K^+$ channels. G-proteins including $G_i$ and $G_z$ mediate $Ca^{2+}$ channel inhibition induced by several ligands, such as somatostatin, $GABA_B$, dopamine, enkephalins, adenosine and atrial natriuretic peptide. Although response time is slower in a multielement signaling system (500 ms for $M_2$ acetylcholine receptor vs 1 ms for single-element nicotinic end-plate receptor), more complex regulation is possible than in a single-element system.

### Indirect coupling via second messengers

These pathways utilize intracellular effectors, and commonly include at least four components. In ventricular myocytes, for example, norepinephrine binding to β-adrenergic receptors activates $G_s$, leading to adenylyl cyclase-mediated cAMP production, which permits protein kinase A phosphorylation of an intracellular regulatory site within the $Ca^{2+}$ channel. Interestingly, the same channels can be directly regulated by $G_s$, bypassing intracellular components. Other ion channels (e.g. $K^+$ channels) are activated through the phospholipase $A_2$ pathway or phospholipase C-mediated inositol phosphate generation. This pathway is the slowest, but also the most amenable to modulation.

## SECOND MESSENGERS

## Cyclic-3′,5′-adenosine monophosphate (cAMP)

The formation of cAMP is catalyzed by the enzyme adenylyl cyclase, which is regulated by $G_s$- and $G_i$-proteins. cAMP effects are extensive and include positive chronotropic and inotropic effects in the myocardium, mediation of β-adrenergic enhancement of glycogenolysis and lipolysis, vasopressin-induced renal water retention, and hormonal steroid production and secretion. cAMP acts primarily by activation of the specific cAMP-dependent kinase, kinase A. Kinase A is a tetramer with two regulatory and two catalytic subunits. The regulatory subunits inhibit the catalytic subunits. Binding of cAMP to the regulatory subunit causes tetramer dissociation, allowing the catalytic subunit to phosphorylate target proteins. The signal generated by this phosphorylation can be reversed only by a specific phosphatase. Covalent modification by phosphorylation amplifies the receptor stimulus because it confers "memory" to the system which persists long after the dissociation of the hormone-receptor complex. It also provides an additional site of regulation, determined by the "turn off" action of the phosphatases.

Kinase A is structurally similar to a family of intracellular enzymes (kinases) that catalyze protein phosphorylation. Although subunit structure and regulatory regions vary, the catalytic core is conserved among all of these proteins.

## Cyclic-3′,5′-guanosine monophosphate (cGMP)

Formation of cGMP is through the enzyme guanylyl cyclase. In many respects the actions of cGMP are mediated in a manner similar to cAMP, through activation of an intracellular kinase (G-kinase). Unlike the ubiquitous cAMP, cGMP action has been demonstrated in only a few cell types. For example, cGMP mediates vascular smooth muscle relaxation induced by nitric oxide (NO). In the intestinal mucosa, cGMP mediates water and electrolyte secretion by *E. coli* endotoxin. In contrast, high concentrations of cGMP in the retinal rods characterize the inactive dark state. Photons activate cGMP hydrolysis by cGMP phosphodiesterase, resulting in decreased cGMP levels and membrane hyperpolarization, which lead to visual signal transmission.

## Phospholipid hydrolysis products

Stimulation of surface receptors coupled to specific G-proteins leads to the activation of several phospholipases (*see* Fig. 2.20). The hydrolysis products can act directly as second messengers or serve as precursors for other second messengers.

Phospholipase C (PLC) hydrolysis results in the release of phosphorylated sugars and diacylglycerols (*see* Fig. 2.21). The most extensively characterized form of this enzyme is the phosphatidylinositol-4,5-bisphosphate ($PIP_2$)-specific PLC. The products of $PIP_2$ hydrolysis are inositol-1,4,5-trisphosphate ($IP_3$) and 1,2 diacylglycerol (DAG). Both of these products act as second messengers. $IP_3$ acts on intracellular organelles to stimulate $Ca^{2+}$ release, while DAG activates the intracellular enzyme kinase C. Several PLC isoenzymes have been characterized and cloned; most are membrane-bound, although a few are cytoplasmic. Proteolytic cleavage of the membrane-anchoring domain and cytosolic enzyme release appear to play a role in signal transduction.

$IP_3$ is subject to extensive further metabolism, resulting in the formation of a myriad of phosphorylated inositols, some of which may also be biologically active. $IP_3$ is inactivated primarily by phosphorylation to inositol-1,3,4,5-tetrakisphosphate, with subsequent sequential dephosphorylation to free inositol.

DAG allosterically activates the cytosolic enzyme protein kinase C, which catalyzes phosphorylation of many cellular proteins with diverse intracellular effects, such as smooth muscle contraction and gene transcription. In addition to stimulatory activities, it is a mediator of negative feedback systems. Thus kinase C-stimulated phosphorylation inhibits PLC activity, decreases $IP_3$ generation, enhances phosphatidylinositol degradation, and decreases the affinity of EGF for its receptor. Diacylglycerols formed from $PIP_2$ are a rich source of arachidonic acid. Over 60 per cent of DAGs from $PIP_2$ contain arachidonic acid, and their hydrolysis by diglyceride lipase results in the release of arachidonic acid, the precursor for the synthesis of prostaglandins and other eicosanoids (Fig. 2.23) (*see* Chapter 8).

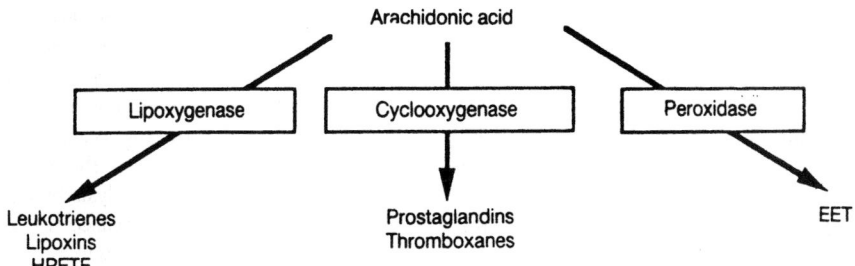

FIGURE 2.23 The major eicosanoid pathways. Arachidonic acid is converted by cyclooxygenase to prostaglandins and thromboxanes. Metabolism by lipoxygenase yields leukotrienes and lipoxins and stimulates hydroxy-peroxy-eicosatetraenoic acid (HPETE) production. Arachidonic acid can also undergo auto-oxidation to HPETE. Peroxidase (cytochrome $P_{450}$ enzyme) converts arachidonic acid to epoxy-eicosatetraenoic acid (EET).

Another species of PLC has phosphatidylcholine as a preferred substrate, resulting in the release of DAG and phosphorylated choline, which has yet to be established as a second messenger. The DAG formed from phosphatidylcholine is slowly metabolized to phosphatidic acid by diglyceride kinase. The reduced rate of recycling is apparently related to the low content of arachidonic acid of DAG in phosphatidylcholine, because DAGs that originate from $PIP_2$, which are rich in arachidonic acid, are rapidly degraded. Thus it appears that the important consequence of phosphatidylcholine hydrolysis by PLC is a sustained elevation of DAG concentration.

Phospholipase D (PLD) hydrolyzes the polar head group of phosphatidylcholine, phosphatidylinositol, and phosphatidylethanolamine (see Fig. 2.20), with preferred substrate determined by the cell type. The active products include phosphatidic acid or phosphatidylated compounds, which result from the exchange of the polar head group for hydroxyl groups of intracellular molecules (transphosphatidylation). Although the understanding of the regulation and consequences of PLD activity is still incomplete, G-proteins, $Ca^{2+}$, and kinase C appear to be involved. Phosphatidic acid and the transphosphatidylation product phosphatidylethanol can, for example, modify $Ca^{2+}$ channel activation. Phosphatidic acid has also been suggested to act as an intracellular signal. Transphosphatidylation of nucleotides also occurs, and may alter response by modifying the intracellular nucleotide concentration; alternatively, phosphatidylnucleotides themselves might serve as second messengers. Phosphatidic acid is also a source of DAGs through hydrolysis by phosphohydrolase. PLC and PLD are closely linked. In several systems PLC activation precedes PLD, yet this is not the case for all tissues, and this temporal relationship may be secondary to differential activation by the same stimulator (e.g. G-protein).

Phospholipase $A_2$ hydrolysis of phospholipids liberates arachidonic acid (5,8,11,14-cis-eicosatetraenoic acid), which serves as a precursor for biologically active eicosanoids (see Fig. 2.23). The specific eicosanoid produced is determined by three major enzymatic pathways: the cyclooxygenase pathway produces prostaglandins and leukotrienes; the lipoxygenase pathway forms leukotrienes, lipoxins, hydroxy-eicosatetraenoic acids (HETE), and hydroxyperoxy-eicosatetraenoic acids (HPETE); and the peroxidase pathway forms epoxy-eicosatrienoic acids (EET). These eicosanoids play an important modulatory role in tissue development and functions, e.g. chemotaxis, smooth muscle contraction, hormone release, and modulation of voltage-gated $K^+$ channels in the cardiac atrium. Unlike other second messengers, the eicosanoids also serve as primary ligands and affect neighboring cells either by binding to membrane receptors or, due to their lipid solubility, by direct intracellular actions.

Recent findings indicate the synthesis of inositide phosphate products within the nucleus, more likely bound to the nuclear skeleton than the nuclear membrane. The exact pathway and targets are yet to be determined, but they may relate to regulation of specific nuclear kinases which regulate the cell cycle.

## Calcium (see also Chapter 43)

The intracellular concentration of free $Ca^{2+}$ ion regulates a myriad of enzymes involved in vital cell function, such as contractile protein action, secretory mechanisms, and transcellular communication via gap junctions or synaptic transmission. Many signaling systems converge on the regulation of the cytoplasmic concentration of unbound $Ca^{2+}$ ion (approximately 100 nM), which is 10 000-fold lower than $Ca^{2+}$ concentrations in the extracellular or intracellular $Ca^{2+}$-sequestering compartments. Cytoplasmic free $Ca^{2+}$ concentration is determined by both transmembrane channel-mediated $Ca^{2+}$ influx and second messenger-induced $Ca^{2+}$ release from intracellular compartments, both leading to a transient 10-fold increase in cytoplasmic $Ca^{2+}$ ion concentration. The resting $Ca^{2+}$ concentration is restored by $Ca^{2+}$-ATPase pumps and $Ca^{2+}$-$Na^+$ exchangers, which couple $Ca^{2+}$ efflux with $Na^+$ influx. Using these pumps, $Ca^{2+}$ is actively sequestered into the endoplasmic reticulum (where it is bound to buffering molecules such as calsequestrin), into mitochondria, and into the Golgi network. The actions of intracellular $Ca^{2+}$, in many cases, are secondary to the kinase C-mediated phosphorylation previously described. At least as important are interactions with another ubiquitous intracellular signaling protein, calmodulin. Calmodulin is an intracellular $Ca^{2+}$-binding protein composed of a single polypeptide chain that contains four $Ca^{2+}$-binding sites. $Ca^{2+}$ binding to calmodulin activates the protein with subsequent calmodulin binding to target proteins or activation of $Ca^{2+}$-calmodulin-dependent kinases.

$Ca^{2+}$ entry into the cell across the plasma membrane is stimulated by depletion of intracellular $Ca^{2+}$ stores. The mechanism underlying this phenomenon is not entirely clear; however, it appears to involve a change in the cellular membrane potential, signaled by discrete factors, such as the recently isolated $Ca^{2+}$-influx factor. $Ca^{2+}$ release from intracellular stores is regulated by at least two receptors: the $IP_3$ receptors and the ryanodine receptors, whose internal ligand appears to be cyclic ADP ribose.

Recent studies suggest that $Ca^{2+}$ release from discrete intracellular stores may lead to an oscillating $Ca^{2+}$ signal. Direct measurements of intracellular $Ca^{2+}$ indicate that $Ca^{2+}$ concentration spikes periodically above a constant baseline, with spike frequency being cell-type-dependent. $Ca^{2+}$ spikes depend on the size of the intracellular pool, the rapidity of $Ca^{2+}$ sequestration to the pools, and its extrusion to the extracellular space. The oscillating $Ca^{2+}$ signal may be explained by $Ca^{2+}$-induced positive feedback on $IP_3$-mediated $Ca^{2+}$ release. $PIP_2$ hydrolysis is negatively regulated by DAG activation of kinase C. Thus either increase in DAG or depletion of $Ca^{2+}$ terminates the $IP_3$ signal.

Increased $Ca^{2+}$ concentration triggers $Ca^{2+}$ release from adjacent $Ca^{2+}$ pools, leading to intracellular signal propagation. The propagating signal originates at the location of stimulated receptors. For example, the receptors at the site of egg-sperm fusion dictate the origin of $Ca^{2+}$ signal propagation in the egg.

## SUMMARY

In a simplified model, a signal presented to a cell directly generates a response proportional to the original signal. However, the complex cellular communication system described allows processing, sorting, and amplification of the transmitted stimulus. This complexity is achieved by supplementing direct ligand–effector coupling with multijunctional pathways, capable of vertical and horizontal regulation. Temporal regulation is conferred via covalent modification of

target molecules by phosphorylation, allowing the signal to persist after dissociation of receptor and agonist. The signal is terminated by dephosphorylation of the target molecule by phosphatases, which themselves are subject to activation/inactivation by external signals. Integration of these converging and diverging signals forms the basis of coordinated cellular functions.

## SELECTED READING

Berridge MJ, Irvine RF. Inositol phosphates and cell signalling. *Nature* 1989; 341: 197.
Bourne HR, DeFranco AL. Signal transduction and intracellular messengers. In: Winberg RA, ed. *Oncogenes and Molecular Origins of Cancer*. Cold Spring Harbor: Cold Spring Harbor Laboratory Press, 1989: 97.
Clapham DE. Calcium signaling. *Cell* 1995; 80: 259.
Hill CS, Treisman R. Transcriptional regulation by extracellular signals: mechanism and specificity. *Cell* 1995; 80: 199.
Neubig RR. Membrane organization in G-protein mechanisms. *Faseb J* 1994; 8: 939.
Shimizu T, Wolfe LS. Arachidonic acid cascade and signal transduction. *J Neurochem* 1990; 55: 1.
Stahl N, Farruggella TJ, Boulton TG, et al. Choice of STATs and other substrates specified by modular tyrosine-based motifs in cytokine receptors. *Science* 1995; 267: 1349.

# CELLULAR INTERACTION WITH THE MICROENVIRONMENT

## INTRODUCTION

Cells interact with extracellular matrices (ECM) and neighboring cells through cell surface adhesion molecules which promote reorganization of the cytoskeleton and regulate adhesive strength, cell shape and motility. In addition, adhesion molecules are involved in transduction of signals from the external environment, which in turn can regulate intracellular signaling as well as their own affinity for various ligands. This dynamic interaction between a cell and its microenvironment is critical in cell migration, proliferation, differentiation and morphogenesis. Although these cell functions are fundamental to many biological processes, recent work in mammalian embryonic development highlights the complex and dramatic nature of cells' interactions with the surrounding microenvironment and their regulatory influences in cell function and morphogenesis.

Normal morphogenesis and differentiation depend heavily on the coordination of cell–cell and cell–ECM interactions. With regard to early development, cell–cell interactions play a predominant role during initial lineage decisions and in the initial stages of epithelial-mesenchymal transitions that take place throughout this period. Cell–ECM interactions probably dominate morphogenesis and differentiation of extraembryonic tissues, particularly the placenta. Furthermore, in conjunction with other proteoglycans in extracellular matrices, adhesion molecules can modulate local effects of growth factors: cell surface proteoglycans can function as adhesion receptors by recognizing glycosaminoglycan (GAG)-binding domains present on many ECM glycoproteins via their GAG side-chains and bind to various growth factors.

This section of the chapter first describes major families of cell adhesion molecules and major ECM components that are noted to be important in development. Recent work regarding mammalian placental and embryonic formation is reviewed. The role of cell–cell and cell–ECM interactions during early mammalian development is examined as an example of how these interactions can guide cell behavior, tissue organization and ultimately morphogenesis. The section begins with morphogenetic events within the pre- and peri-implantation embryo as well as early stages of implantation, emphasizing work with the mouse. The section concludes by summarizing adhesive interactions that are critical to formation of the placenta, emphasizing work in the human.

## ADHESION MOLECULES INVOLVED IN CELL–CELL INTERACTIONS

Cell–cell interactions are mediated largely by three classes of adhesion molecules (Fig. 2.24):

- cadherins (calcium-dependent adhesion molecules, CAMs)
- immunoglobulin superfamily adhesion receptors, and
- selectins.

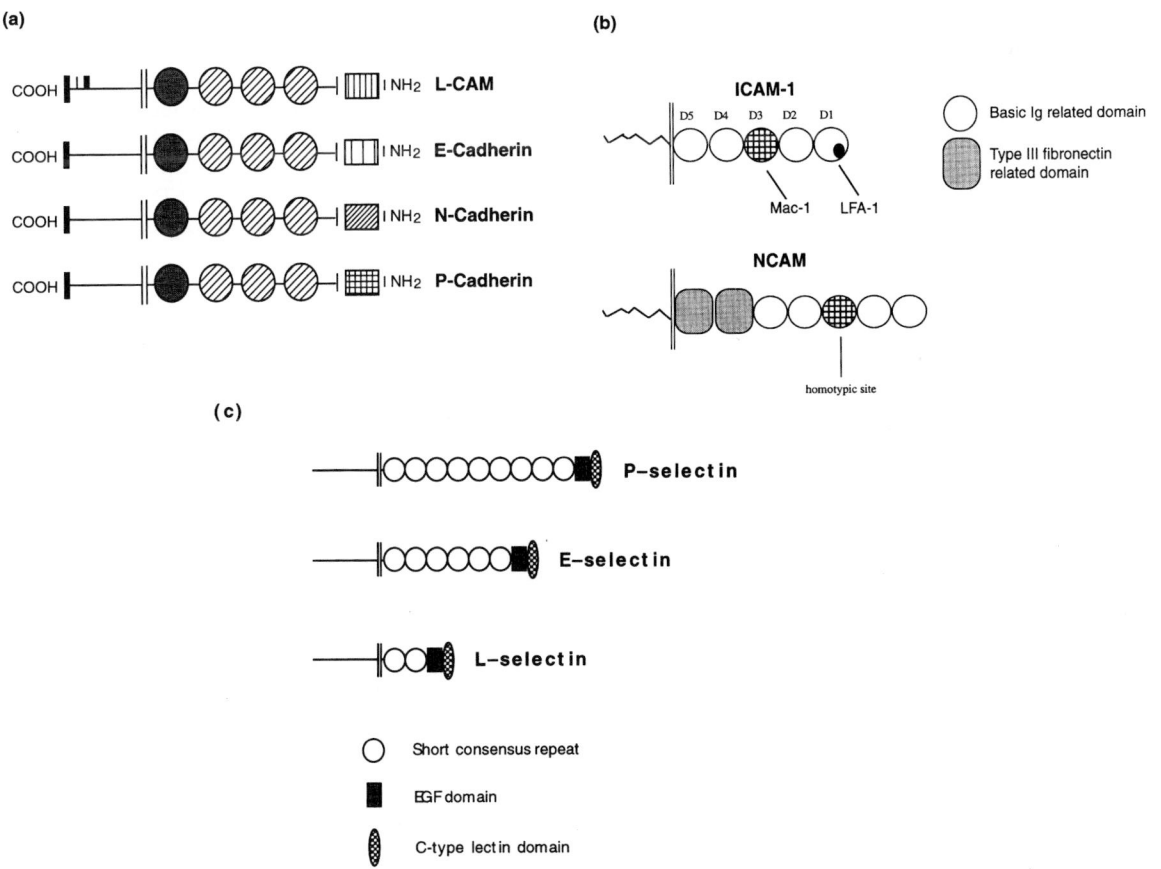

**(a)**

COOH — L-CAM — NH₂
COOH — E-Cadherin — NH₂
COOH — N-Cadherin — NH₂
COOH — P-Cadherin — NH₂

**(b)**

ICAM-1
D5 D4 D3 D2 D1
Mac-1  LFA-1

○ Basic Ig related domain
▨ Type III fibronectin related domain

NCAM
homotypic site

**(c)**

P–selectin
E–selectin
L–selectin

○ Short consensus repeat
■ EGF domain
C-type lectin domain

FIGURE 2.24 Schematic representations of molecules involved in cell–cell adhesion. (a) Cadherins are Ca²⁺-dependent adhesion molecules that mediate homotypic cell aggregation. Their ligand specificities are determined by the 110 amino acid residues at the NH₂ terminal. (b) Cell adhesion molecules belonging to the immunoglobulin superfamily contain the repeat immunoglobulin domains. As summarized in Table 2.1, these molecules perform a wide variety of functions. The molecules in this class mediate either heterotypic cell adhesion (ICAM) or homotypic adhesion (NCAM). The locations of their ligand binding sites are shown. (c) Selectins recognize carbohydrates as their ligands and are involved in leukocyte transmigration from the blood vessels during inflammation. Three members are represented schematically. P- and E-selectins are expressed, among others, by endothelial cells, and L-selectin is expressed by leukocytes.

## Cadherins

Of the cadherins, the four most widely studied subclasses are E- (epithelial or uvomorulin), N- (neural), P- (placental) and L-CAM (liver) cadherins. These molecules were named for tissues in which they were first studied, and despite their restrictive names, they are expressed by a wide variety of cells and tissues. It is now clear that the cadherin family of cell–cell adhesion molecules is very large and that cadherin switching accompanies virtually all events throughout development where one group of cells either aggregates or segregates from another. During early development, cell–cell interactions govern the initial lineage decisions as well as the initial stage of epithelial–mesenchymal transitions that take place during this period. This observation raises the possibility that cadherin molecules could play an important role in early development.

Structurally, the extracellular component of the cadherin molecule contains three repeated domains, and the 113-amino-acid region at the $NH_2$ terminus is responsible for the binding specificities of these molecules (Fig. 2.24(a)). Among the subclasses, about 50 per cent of the amino acids are conserved when compared within a single species. The extent of conservation varies with the region of the molecules. The highest percentage of conservation is found in the intracellular domain. The importance of highly conserved intracellular domains has been demonstrated in deletion experiments. Either partial or complete deletion of the COOH-terminal half of the intracellular domain disrupts its function as a cell–cell adhesion receptor, suggesting that the association of cadherin with the cytoskeleton may be crucial for the cell-binding function of the extracellular domain.

Expression of cadherins is developmentally regulated and correlates with a variety of morphogenetic events that involve cell aggregation or dispersion. Each of the subclasses displays a unique pattern of tissue distribution, and cadherin binding is subclass-specific: e.g. E-cadherin binds selectively with E-cadherin. In many types of cells, multiple cadherin subclasses are coexpressed in varying combinations. Each cell type thus can be characterized by the expression of a particular cadherin subclass or set of cadherin subclasses. Thus, expression of cadherin facilitates homotypic cell aggregation, and down-regulation is associated with segregation—two important processes in embryonic development. In addition to morphogenesis, cadherins are involved in *tumor invasion* and *metastasis*. Altered or decreased cadherin expression is observed in highly metastatic tumor cell lines, suggesting that invasiveness of tumor cells is associated with aberrant cadherin function.

## The immunoglobulin superfamily

The immunoglobulin superfamily is the most abundant family of cell surface molecules that contain one or more immunoglobulin domains. The immunoglobulin (Ig) domain, which is composed of approximately 100 amino acids arranged in two sheets of anti-parallel strands, has evolved to serve many different functions including receptors for growth factors (colony-stimulating factor-1 (CSF-1), platelet-derived growth factor (PDGF) and fibroblast growth factor (FGF) receptors), receptors for the Fc region of Ig, as well as adhesion molecule receptors (Fig. 2.24(b)). The molecules belonging to this family are involved in a wide variety of biological functions and include intercellular adhesion molecule-1 (ICAM-1), ICAM-2, ICAM-3, vascular cell adhesion molecule (VCAM-1), neural cell adhesion molecule-1 (NCAM-1), CD2, CD3 (T-cell receptor), CD4, CD8, major histocompatibility complex (MHC) classes I and II and carcinoembryonic antigen (Table 2.1).

ICAM-1 is the major ligand for a leukocyte integrin receptor LFA-1 ($\alpha_L\beta_2$) and Mac-1, a receptor found on neutrophils, monocytes and some lymphocytes. ICAM-1 can be found on endothelial, epithelial, and fibroblast cells as well as on leukocytes; and its expression, which can be induced by cytokines within 4 hours of stimulation, can serve as a rhinovirus receptor as well as a ligand for *Plasmodium falciparum*. In addition to functioning as an adhesion receptor, ICAM-1 has been implicated in antigen presentation, T-cell stimulation, and cytotoxicity of T cells.

ICAM-2 also binds to Mac-1 and is mostly expressed on non-neutrophil hematopoietic and endothelial cells. Unlike ICAM-1, ICAM-2 is not regulated by cytokines or phorbol esters and thus may be more important for adhesion in the basal state. ICAM-

TABLE 2.1 Partial list of immunoglobulin superfamily cell-surface receptors. Each molecule contains immunoglobulin homology units.

| BIOLOGICAL PROPERTIES | IMMUNOGLOBULIN SUPERFAMILY |
|---|---|
| Immune interactions | ICAM-1, ICAM-2, VCAM, PECAM-1, MHC I, MHC II, TCR, CD4, CD8, CD3γ, Thy-1 |
| Signal transduction | PDGF, CD3$_E$, PECAM, TCR, N-CAM, L1, CSF-1, CD4 |
| Neural development | N-CAM, Mag, Ng-CAM |
| Tumor associated | CEA, NCA, BGP, DCC |
| Proteoglycan interactions | N-CAM, PECAM |
| Viral receptors | ICAM-1, CD4 |

3 is only expressed by leukocytes and is thought to play a role in the initiation of the immune response as it mediates adhesion of resting T lymphocytes.

VCAM-1, another cell adhesion receptor in this family, is expressed on vascular endothelium as well as a variety of other tissues. It is one of the major ligands for VLA-4 ($\alpha_4\beta_1$ integrin), and its expression is stimulated by interleukin (IL)-4, IL-1, endotoxin, and TNFα. VCAM-1 can support the adhesion of lymphocytes, monocytes, and eosinophils. In addition, VCAM-1 has been shown to play a critical role in chorioallantoic fusion and placental formation in mice. In up to half of homozygous mouse embryos with targeted mutations in genes encoding either $\alpha_4$ integrin subunit or VCAM-1, the allantois does not fuse with the chorion. Embryonic death occurs in one to three days. In the subset of VCAM-1-deficient embryos in which chorioallantoic fusion occurs, allantoic mesoderm is abnormally distributed over the chorionic surface. In this context, VCAM-1 function appears to be mediated by interaction with VLA-4, as similar defects are found in $\alpha_4$ integrin–deficient mice.

## Selectins

Selectins are a three-member adhesion receptor family that regulate the first reversible interaction between leukocytes and endothelial cells in lymphocyte extravasation during inflammation. E-selectin (endothelial leukocyte adhesion molecule-1 [ELAM-1]) and P-selectin (platelet activation-dependent granule external membrane) are inducible endothelial cell surface antigens which bind myeloid cells and subsets of lymphocytes. L-selectin (lymphocyte homing receptor), on the other hand, is expressed by leukocytes and recognizes inducible surface antigens on endothelial cells. This family of adhesion molecules contain a $NH_2$-terminal lectin (carbohydrate-binding protein) domain, an epidermal growth factor domain, 2–9 complement regulatory repeats, a transmembrane domain, and a short cytoplasmic domain (Fig. 2.24(c)).

Vascular endothelial cells up-regulate E-selectins in response to a variety of stimuli including IL-1β, TNFα, endotoxin, and interferon-γ. P-selectin is constitutively synthesized and stored in granules of platelets and endothelial cells. It can be redistributed within minutes to the cell surface after a variety of stimuli, including thrombin, histamine, and terminal complement components. L-selectin is constitutively expressed by most leukocytes. It was originally described as a participant in lymphocyte homing to peripheral lymph nodes. L-selectin also participates in the recruitment of neutrophils and monocytes to sites of inflammation. Interaction between selectins and carbohydrate ligands appears to be essential for the initial contact of leukocytes with activated endothelium. Under conditions of fluid shear stress, this contact is evidenced by rolling of

leukocytes along the endothelial lining of the vessel wall – a prelude to more stable adhesion and transmigration into tissue. Up-regulation of selectin has been documented in sepsis and other inflammatory diseases. In baboons, E-selectin expression is increased in vascular beds of lung, kidney, liver, intestine, and skin in septic shock. Expression of E-selectin in the cutaneous microcirculation has been detected in patients during the early phases of *peritonitis*. In addition, serum of patients with *septic shock* contains elevated amounts of a soluble form of E-selectin. In animal models, antibodies against E-selectin, P-selectin, and ICAM-1 are protective, to varying degrees, against lung damage induced by several stimulants.

## ADHESION MOLECULES IN CELL–EXTRACELLULAR MATRIX INTERACTIONS

### Integrins

The major classes of cell surface receptors that mediate cell–ECM interactions are the integrins and the cell surface proteoglycans. The integrins are heterodimeric transmembrane adhesion receptors composed of αβ subunits that mediate mostly cell–ECM interactions (Fig. 2.25(a)). Recently some integrins have been shown to play a role in cell–cell interactions as well. The large number of known integrin αβ combinations (Fig. 2.25(c)), redundancies in their ligand preferences, alternative splicing of cytoplasmic domains and the existence of multiple affinity states for many integrins mean that cells have the potential to regulate integrin expression and function at many levels and to express a great variety of adhesion phenotypes. For example, fibronectin and laminin are each recognized by at least six different integrin heterodimers. Integrins seem to recognize arginine–glycine–aspartic acid (RGD) sequences in the ECM components they bind, and their cytoplasmic domain is bound to the cytoskeleton. Integrins, therefore, are excellent candidates for transducing signals from ECM into cytoplasm.

While the combined function of two subunits is important in their ligand specificity, the interaction with the intracellular component and an integrin is mediated mostly by the β subunit. The cytoplasmic domain of the integrin $\beta_1$ subunit can bind directly to at least two structural proteins of focal contacts, α-actinin and talin, and focal contact sites of fibroblasts can be disassembled following injection of α-actinin fragments. All the information necessary for $\alpha\beta_1$ integrins to translocate to focal contact sites resides in the cytoplasmic domain of the $\beta_1$ subunit. In addition to major structural components such as α-actinin, talin and vinculin, focal contact sites in spread fibroblasts also contain several additional non-enzy-

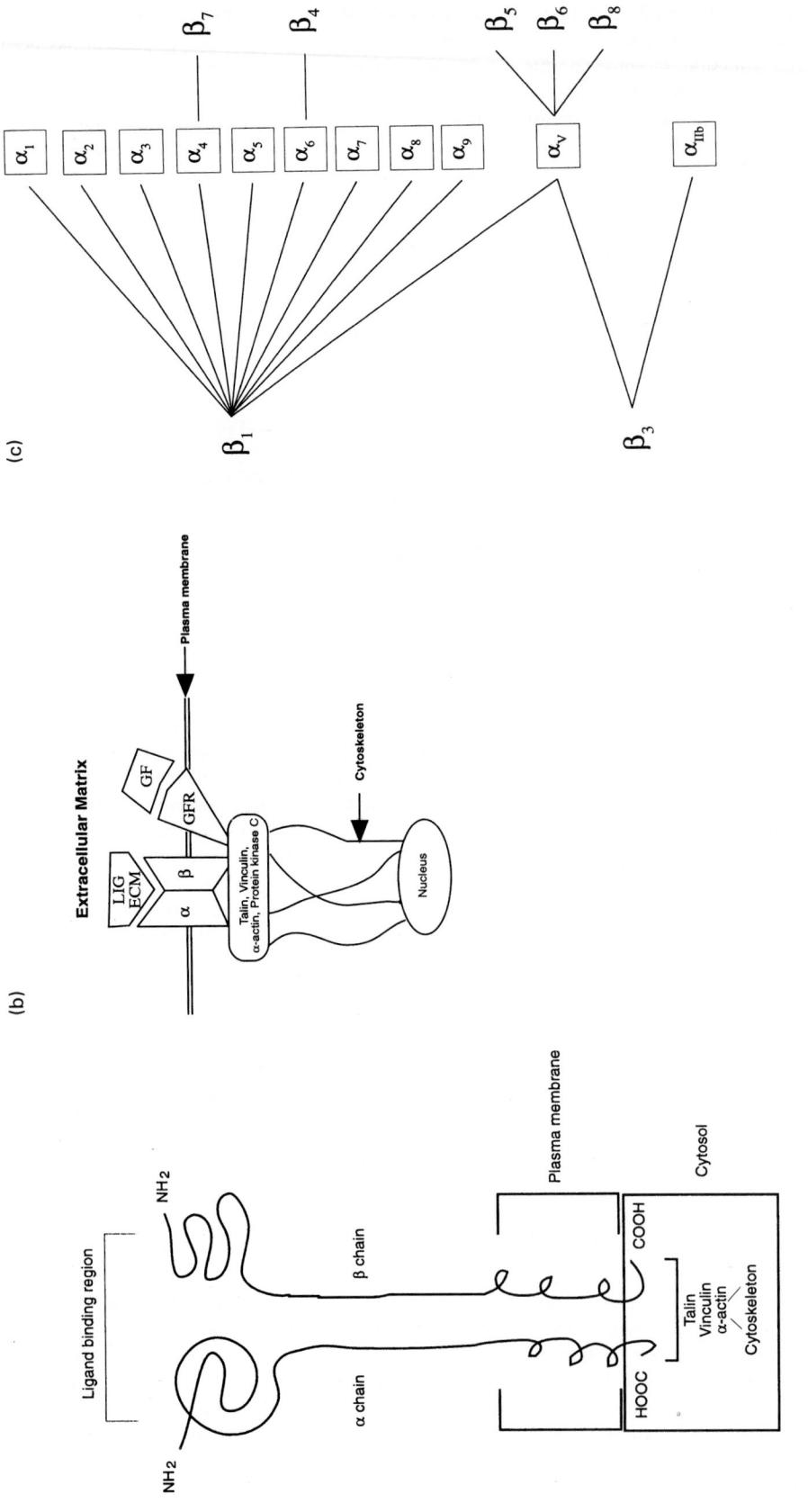

FIGURE 2.25 (a) Integrins are heterodimeric transmembrane adhesion receptors that mediate mostly cell–extracellular matrix inter-actions. Because the intracellular domain of this molecule is attached to the cytoskeletal network (b), integrins are ideal candidates for transmitting signals from extracellular matrices to the intracellular space (GF, growth factor; GFR, growth factor receptor). Owing to a wide array of α and β heterodimeric combinations (c), these molecules have a wide repertoire of ligands (Table 2.3). Furthermore, integrins can interact with various growth factor receptors, which could explain the close relationship between cell adhesion and cell differentiation and growth.

matic proteins that are present at low levels, suggesting that they may play a regulatory role. These include paxillin, which is a major substrate for tyrosine kinases, and tensin, which has an *SRC* homology 2 (SH2) domain. As SH2 domains recognize tyrosine phosphate sites on other proteins, they could potentially link regulatory molecules that become associated with the cytoskeleton as it is reorganized during fibroblast spreading.

Integrins can transduce signals cooperatively with other classes of adhesion receptors or with growth factor receptors (Fig. 2.25(b)). Furthermore, the ability of integrins to interact with the cytoskeleton appears to be fundamental to their mechanism for signal transduction.

Recent studies suggest that chemical signals from integrins and growth factor receptors are rapidly integrated after cell surface receptor binding. For example, stimulation of inositol lipid turnover and subsequent signaling events in fibroblasts requires both PDGF and adhesion to ECM. In suspended cells, PDGF binds its receptors and activates phospholipase C (PLC), yet there is minimal inositol lipid breakdown or release of $IP_3$. Instead, cellular levels of 4,5 phosphatidylinositol bisphosphate ($PIP_2$), the substrate for PLC, decline when cells are placed in suspension and recover following reattachment to fibronectin (FN). Thus binding to integrins stimulates synthesis of a critical regulatory substrate ($PIP_2$), whereas growth factor receptors activate the enzyme that is responsible for its breakdown. These findings provide one possible explanation for why both soluble mitogens and insoluble matrix components are required for growth.

There are multiple congenital disorders associated with integrin deficiencies. *Leukocyte adhesion deficiency* is an autosomal recessive disorder characterized by recurrent bacterial infection, impaired pus formation and wound healing as well as delayed umbilical cord separation. The genetic defect has been localized to chromosome 21q22.3 which is the location for integrin $\beta_2$ subunit. The neutrophils in these patients lack adhesion molecules that require integrin $\beta_2$ subunit (CD18) and demonstrate impaired mobility. In *Glanzmann thrombasthenia* (diminished clot retraction) platelet integrin $\alpha_{IIb}\beta_3$ is found to be deficient. These patients have bleeding diathesis with normal clotting time, platelet count and coagulation time, but with deficient clot retraction and abnormal platelet morphology.

Another major group of adhesion receptors is cell-surface proteoglycans. These can recognize the glycosaminoglycan (GAG)-binding domains present on many ECM glycoproteins via their GAG side-chains. In addition, cell-surface proteoglycans can bind factors critical for the regulation of growth and differentiation, either via the core protein or GAG side-chain. An example of this type of proteoglycan will be given later.

## EXTRACELLULAR MATRIX PROTEINS

ECM is composed of a variety of polysaccharides and proteins that are secreted locally and assemble into an organized meshwork. Expression of ECM molecules is tightly regulated; some are transiently expressed at particular times in development, whereas others are continually expressed into adulthood and have unique compositions in each organ of the body. The diverse forms of ECM are primarily a function of variations in the relative amounts of the different types of matrix macromolecules and the way they are organized in the ECM. The ECM is generally believed to have evolved as a response to the mechanical forces acting on organisms. From ground substances in simple systems to collagen fibers and cartilages in higher organisms, the complexity of the ECM seems to correlate with the increasing tensile and compressive forces present in various organisms. This view of the mechanical role of the matrix is now being supplanted by a growing awareness of the importance of the matrix in governing the behavior of cells.

Over the years it has become clear that ECM molecules are involved in promotion of cell adhesion, activation of intracellular signaling pathways, and modulation of activities of several growth factors and proteins. The major components of the ECM include cell adhesive molecules such as fibronectin, vitronectin, laminin and anti-adhesive tenascins; the structural components, such as collagens and elastin; and the proteoglycans, a complex array of proteins with glycosaminoglycan side-chains. In addition, SPARC (secreted protein acidic and rich in cysteine), which is a 43-kD collagen-binding glycoprotein, has been added to the list. ECM molecules interact with each other and with their specific receptors on the cell surface (Table 2.2). Although the biological importance of all these molecules cannot be overstated, detailed

TABLE 2.2 Partial list of receptors for various extracellular matrix (ECM) components. Integrins play a major role in cell interaction with ECM.

| ECM COMPONENTS | RECEPTORS |
|---|---|
| Collagens | Integrins ($\alpha_1\beta_1$, $\alpha_2\beta_1$, $\alpha_3\beta_1$), CD44, syndecan, proteoglycans |
| Laminins | Integrins ($\alpha_1\beta_1$, $\alpha_2\beta_1$, $\alpha_3\beta_1$, $\alpha_6\beta_1$ and $\alpha_7\beta_1$; $\alpha_v\beta_3$, $\alpha_6\beta_4$), lactose-binding lectins, proteoglycans |
| Fibronectin | Integrins ($\alpha_v\beta_3$, $\alpha_v\beta_6$, $\alpha_3\beta_1$, $\alpha_5\beta_1$), CD44, syndecan, proteoglycans |
| Proteoglycans | Integrins |

description of every molecule is beyond the scope of this chapter. Therefore, the discussion of these molecules will be limited to collagen, laminin, fibronectin and proteoglycans.

## Collagens

The collagens are a family of highly fibrous proteins found in all multicellular animals and are the major protein of the extracellular matrices. Collagens are composed of three polypeptide chains, called α chains (each about 1000 amino acids long), wound around in a regular superhelix format. The chains are rich in proline and glycine, both of which are important in the formation of the triple-stranded helix (Fig. 2.26(a)). Approximately 25 gene products are recognized as collagen types, and 14 major type members of this family are divided into groups based on shared characteristics. Types I, II, III, V and XI are fibril-forming collagens, types XII, IX, and XIV are fibril-associated collagens with interrupted triple helices (FACITs),

types IV, VIII and X are sheet-forming collagens, and types VI and VII are beaded filament-forming and anchoring fibril constituents. Sheet-forming collagens, which include type IV collagen, differ from the other groups in that the secreted "procollagen" molecules are not cleaved, and the secreted molecules interact via their uncleaved propeptide domains to assemble into a sheet-like multilayered network rather than into fibrils. Type IV collagen is the major form of collagen found in basement membranes, and identified integrins that interact with type IV collagens are $\alpha_1\beta_1$, $\alpha_2\beta_1$, and $\alpha_3\beta_1$. The role of collagen in embryonic development and placentation will be discussed later.

There are many examples of inherited collagen disorders including *Ehlers–Danlos syndrome*, *Marfan syndrome* and *osteogenesis imperfecta*. Ehlers–Danlos syndrome has been associated with abnormal types I and III collagens as a result of a defect in collagen-processing peptidase, and osteogenesis imperfecta type I has been associated with abnormalities in the type I procollagen gene, although this is not the only

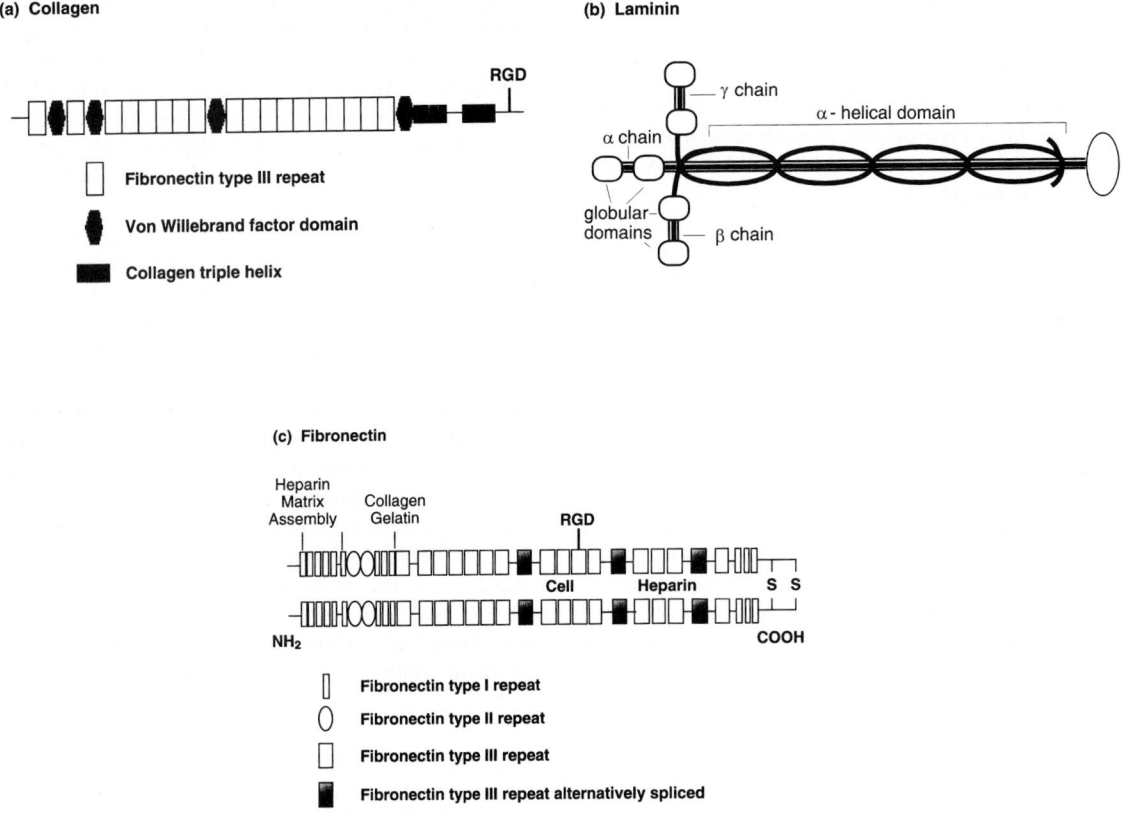

FIGURE 2.26 Three abundant extracellular matrix proteins are shown. In addition to mechanical support, these components of extracellular matrices play a critical role in mediating cell differentiation and migration. Collagen (a) is the most abundant protein in the ECM, and laminin (b) is the most abundant non-collagenous protein. Although fibronectin (c) is not one of the abundant proteins in ECM, it plays an important role in cell migration and differentiation.

mutation that has been associated with this disorder. Decreased levels of type III collagen are noted in *coarctation of the aorta*, which has been associated with an increased incidence of *berry aneurysm*. Marfan syndrome is associated with a gene mutation defect in fibrillin.

## Laminin

Laminin, the most abundant non-collagenous protein in basement membranes, is a multidomain protein (850 kD) composed of three distinct polypeptide chains connected by disulfide bonds (Fig. 2.26(b)). In 1994, a new nomenclature for laminin was adopted. The previous A, B1 and B2 chains are now referred to as $\alpha$, $\beta$ and $\gamma$ chains. The laminin isoforms are numbered with Arabic numerals in the order in which they were discovered. For example, the first laminin identified from Engelbreth–Holm–Swann (EHS) tumor was designated laminin-1 with the chain composition $\alpha$-1/$\beta$-1/$\gamma$-1. The genes for these three chains are *LAMA1*, *LAMB1* and *LAMC1*. Structurally, $\alpha$, $\beta$ and $\gamma$ polypeptide chains are arranged in the shape of an asymmetric cross with three short arms of 36 nm and a long arm of 77 nm. Laminin consists of a number of functional domains: one binds to type IV collagen, one to heparan sulfate, and one or more to laminin receptor proteins on the surface of cells. A single entactin molecule is thought to be tightly bound to each laminin molecule where the short arms meet the long one. Entactin is a sulfated glycoprotein (158 kD) that is expressed with laminin in normal tissues and is laid down in the basement membrane matrix as a noncovalent complex with laminin.

Along with collagen, laminin functions *in vitro* as a very potent modifier of cell behavior. This effect has been demonstrated in a number of culture models including cytotrophoblasts, mammary cells and neurons, to name a few. In a mouse mammary cell culture system, addition of laminin can increase $\beta$-casein production in a concentration-dependent manner. Laminin and different isoforms promote neurite outgrowth by ciliary ganglion neurons *in vitro*. In addition, tumor interaction with the P1 region of laminin has been reported to induce metalloproteinases, ECM-degrading enzymes that play a critical role in tumor metastasis. $\beta_1$ class integrins act as laminin receptors, and at least five different $\alpha$ subunits ($\alpha_1$, $\alpha_2$, $\alpha_3$, $\alpha_6$, and $\alpha_7$) can combine with the $\beta_1$ subunit to form heterodimers. In addition, $\alpha_V\beta_3$ and $\alpha_6\beta_4$ have been reported to function as laminin receptors.

Absence of laminin in the basement membranes of capillaries and the dermal–epithelial junction is associated with a congenital syndrome called *neonatal cutis laxa* with Marfanoid phenotype. Affected individuals can manifest cutis laxa, emphysema, cardiac abnormalities, diaphragmatic hernia, or mild contractures at the elbows, hips and knees. Chromosome studies show either a break or translocation involving 7q31, which is the location of the *LAMB1* gene. Immunostaining of tissues from affected individuals shows an absence of laminin in the basement membranes of capillaries and at the dermal–epidermal junction.

## Fibronectin

Fibronectin, a widely expressed ECM component, is one of the major adhesive glycoproteins. It binds to both cells and other matrix macromolecules. Fibronectin is a multifunctional molecule in which the various globular domains play different roles (Fig. 2.26(c)). For example, one domain binds to collagen, another to heparin, another to specific receptors on the surface of various types of cells. These multiple functions allow fibronectin to contribute to the organization of the matrix and help cells attach to it. Cells attach to fibronectin via integrins that recognize various domains, including the RGD-containing domain, which is near the middle of the molecule. There are at least four integrin heterodimers that recognize fibronectin (Table 2.2), and these receptor–ligand interactions are involved in cell migration and adhesion. Fibronectin is expressed in the developing brain as well as along the pathways of neural crest migration and peripheral nerve outgrowth. Fibronectin can also modulate tissue invasion. Hence exogenous fibronectin can block matrix invasion by cytotrophoblasts, while function-perturbing antibody to $\alpha_5\beta_1$ (one of the fibronectin receptors) can enhance cytotrophoblast invasion *in vitro*.

## Proteoglycans

Proteoglycans are macromolecules composed of glycosaminoglycan chains covalently bound to a protein core. Many distinct genes encode the protein cores present in proteoglycans. The number, size and composition of glycosaminoglycan chains attached to individual core proteins vary according to cell types. Important functional domains are present in both the protein and carbohydrate moieties. Their potential functions include roles as receptors, components of ECM, and modulators of growth factor actions. Multiple groups of glycosaminoglycan can be bound to a protein core of a proteoglycan. Four main groups of glycosaminoglycans have been noted: (1) hyaluronic acid, (2) chondroitin sulfate and dermatan sulfate, (3) heparan sulfate and heparin, and (4) keratan sulfate.

In addition to proteoglycans found in the ECM, there is a group of proteoglycans found on the cell surface such as syndecan and betaglycan. Both core protein and glycosaminoglycan moieties found in these cell-surface proteoglycans can interact with growth factors. In particular, heparan sulfate chains can bind different growth factors, including basic fibroblast growth factor (bFGF), acidic FGF, granulocyte colony-stimulating factor, IL-3, and interferon-γ. In addition, these proteoglycans can interact with the ECM through the glycosaminoglycan binding sites present on many ECM constituents. An example of a cell-surface proteoglycan that can interact with growth factors and ECM molecules is syndecan-1. Syndecan-1 can bind to collagen, fibronectin, thrombospondin, and tenascin. In addition, it forms a complex with bFGF via its heparan sulfate moiety, a step that is thought to be necessary for bFGF binding to its signal-transducing bFGF receptor. In fact, variant cells, selected for low expression of syndecan-1, show dramatically reduced responsiveness to FGF. Thus, syndecan-1 may function both as a cell adhesion-promoting receptor for ECM proteins and one type of low-affinity growth factor receptor that facilitates the interaction of bFGF binding to its signal-transducing bFGF receptor.

## ADHESIVE INTERACTIONS IN EARLY EMBRYOGENESIS, IMPLANTATION AND PLACENTATION

Cellular interactions with the microenvironment play a critical role in embryonic development and morphogenesis. As an example, we will examine the adhesive interactions starting within the pre- and peri-implantation mouse embryo. Preimplantation development is defined here as the period from fertilization to hatching of the blastocyst (embryonic day 0 [day E0]–E4.5 in the mouse). Peri-implantation period encompasses the further development of the hatched blastocyst through E7.5 in the mouse, by which time trophoblast invasion is well underway and gastrulation is in progress. During this period there is a strong emphasis on the segregation and differentiation of extraembryonic lineages (visceral and parietal endoderm and trophoblast). This is essential, as the mammalian egg has little endogenous nutrient supply for the growing embryo. The lineages for these tissues are set aside before implantation, and their subsequent morphogenesis and "organogenesis" occur before those of any embryonic tissues. The first polarization events, ECM deposition, cell migrations, invasion, epithelial–mesenchymal transitions and tissue-specific gene expression programs in mammalian development take place in the extraembryonic lineages. Therefore, understanding how such events are regulated in extraembryonic tissues and what contributions are made to such processes by cell-surface adhesion receptors is important in its own right, as well as being instructive for analogous events occurring later in the embryo.

## Cell–cell interactions mediating initial steps in lineage segregation during preimplantation development

Shortly after fertilization, the first two lineage decisions in the embryo set aside cells that go on to form trophectoderm and extraembryonic endoderm. The trophectoderm is the forerunner of the trophoblast and fetal portion of the placenta, whereas the initial extraembryonic endoderm layer goes on to form the visceral and parietal yolk sacs (Fig. 2.27). The Ca$^{2+}$-dependent

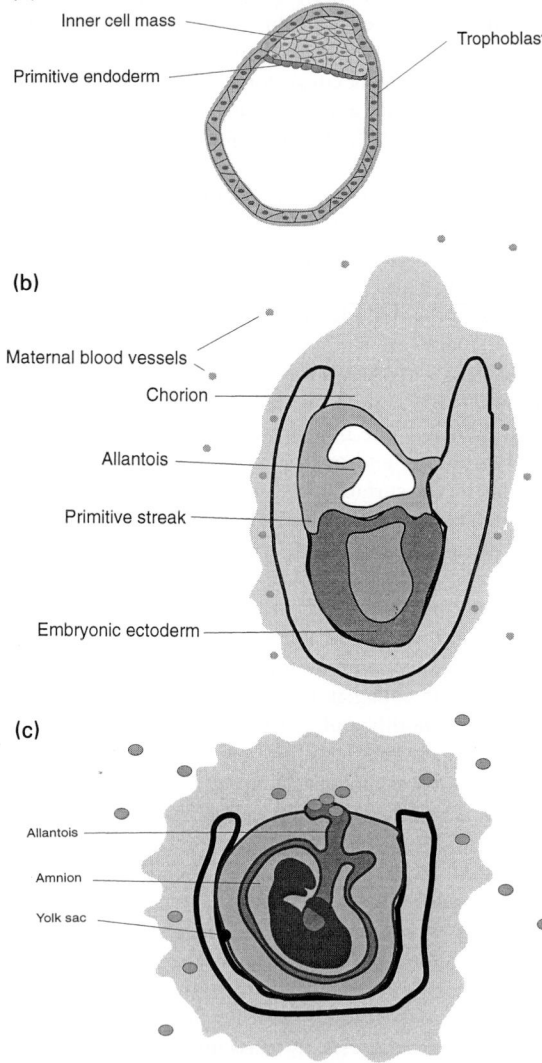

FIGURE 2.27 Mouse embryo development. (a) Peri-implantation blastocyst at day 4.5 has trophoblast, inner cell mass and primitive endoderm. Cell–cell interactions appear to guide the cell lineage decisions in inner cell mass formation (compaction) and differentiation of primitive endoderm. (b) Allantois formation starts during the early postimplantation period. (c) The allantois eventually will fuse with the chorion to form the chorioallantoic placenta, a process which is completed by day 9.5 of mouse development. Interactions between VCAM-1 and integrin $\alpha_4$ play a critical role during this process.

cell–cell adhesion molecule E-cadherin has been specifically implicated in these decisions. Other cell–cell adhesion mechanisms may also be very important. However, studies with E-cadherin best exemplify the general principle that cell–cell interactions play a particularly dominant role in morphogenesis in the pre- and early peri-implantation period.

The first step in setting aside the trophoblast lineage occurs at compaction when blastomeres of the eight-cell mouse embryo maximize their cell–cell contact and create a tight ball composed of "outside" cells, which will go on to form the trophectoderm of the blastocyst, surrounding a core of "inside" cells, the inner cell mass (ICM). E-cadherin, the only member of the $Ca^{2+}$-dependent cell adhesion molecule family expressed at this time, is required for compaction. Interestingly, E-cadherin is present from the outset of development and is uniformly distributed over the surface of all blastomeres until compaction, at which time it becomes enriched at areas of cell–cell contact. E-cadherin also becomes serine phosphorylated at this time. Furthermore, compaction can be triggered prematurely at the four-cell stage by treatment with compounds that activate protein kinase C. These data suggest strongly that compaction is triggered by a phosphorylation event that activates E-cadherin such that it has enhanced affinity for both the cytoskeleton (via its interaction with catenins) and homotypic binding to E-cadherin on neighboring blastomeres.

The first step in setting aside the extraembryonic endoderm lineages occurs at the late blastula stage by a process that may be similar to that just described. In this case, the layer of the ICM that faces the blastocele cavity forms a polarized epithelium that becomes separated from the remainder of the ICM by deposition of a basement membrane: the first organized ECM formed during development. E-cadherin, which is uniformly distributed around all cells of the ICM prior to endoderm segregation, becomes redistributed to the lateral surfaces of the polarizing endoderm. Furthermore, anti-E-cadherin blocks endoderm segregation. Therefore, activation of E-cadherin function may play as critical a role at least in the initial stages of endoderm segregation, as it does in initial segregation of trophectoderm.

## CELL–ECM INTERACTIONS IN PRE- AND PERI-IMPLANTATION DEVELOPMENT OF THE MAMMALIAN EMBRYO

Although preimplantation morphogenesis in the mouse appears to be regulated primarily by cell–cell interactions, cell–ECM interactions play an increasingly important role in peri-implantation development and implantation, as they are critical for promoting morphogenesis, motility, and differentiation of the extra-embryonic lineages following their initial segregation.

## Production of a broad repertoire of ECM constituents and receptors by the mouse embryo at the onset of development

The preimplantation mouse embryo also produces a surprisingly broad repertoire of integrins and ECM ligands. Several integrins ($\alpha_5\beta_1$, $\alpha_{6B}\beta_1$, $\alpha_V\beta_3$) are detected on the unfertilized egg and on the embryo from the outset of embryonic gene transcription (late two-cell stage) using either RT-PCR to detect mRNA, or immunoprecipitation to detect protein. The cell-surface proteoglycan syndecan-1, as well as several ECM constituents, are also produced during this period. Thus, by the time blastulation starts there is considerable diversity in the adhesion receptor and ECM ligand repertoire. However, there is no organized ECM evident during this period, and broadly reacting anti-integrin antibodies do not interfere with any aspect of preimplantation development. Furthermore, the ECM constituents and integrin subunits appear to be either sequestered intracellularly or distributed uniformly around all cells of the embryo. This suggests that their expression in the preimplantation period is a prelude to later events and that the functional interaction of ECM receptors and their ligands requires a process of activation and redistribution (see previous discussion of E-cadherin). Several integrins are known to exist in more than one state of activation. Therefore it is possible that integrins are expressed in an inactive form at these very early stages of development.

## ECM reorganization and a second wave of integrin and ECM expression accompany morphogenesis of the hatched blastocyst: acquisition of adhesiveness by trophoblast

Striking changes take place in adhesion receptor expression and in the spatial organization of ECM ligands and receptors subsequent to blastocyst hatching. Two important morphogenetic events take place at this time: the endoderm layer segregates from the ICM, and the embryo becomes attachment-competent. Deposition of the first organized basement membrane occurs both at the interface of the primitive endoderm and ICM (future embryonic ectoderm), and at the internal surface of the trophectoderm, along which the parietal endoderm cells will migrate as they disassociate from the periphery of the endoderm layer. Collagen IV and laminin, which are in large part sequestered intracellularly until this time, as well as fibronectin and syndecan-1, become enriched at these sites of matrix deposition, while the $\alpha_6\beta_1$ integrin laminin receptor becomes enriched on the newly segregated endoderm layer. The triggers for this intricate redistribution of cell–ECM adhesion-related molecules are unknown, although activation of integrin ECM receptors could be involved.

The embryo becomes attachment-competent about 12–16 h after hatching. The previously non-adhesive, quiescent apical (external) surface of the trophectoderm becomes adhesive and displays vigorous protrusive activity. Following this transition, the blastocyst is able to interact with a wide variety of cell layers and ECM ligands. This change also coincides with the ability to detect heparan sulfate proteoglycan and integrins, reactive with a pan-integrin antiserum, on the apical surface of the trophectoderm for the first time. This could arise from redistribution of existing integrins and/or the onset of expression of new integrins not expressed in the preimplantation period.

A broadening of the integrin repertoire accompanies the morphogenetic events described above (Table 2.3). At least three integrin α subunits ($\alpha_2$, $\alpha_{6A}$ (an alternatively spliced form of the $\alpha_6$ subunit), $\alpha_7$) are newly expressed at the late blastocyst stage: the time of endoderm segregation and acquisition of adhesiveness by trophoblast. Two other integrin subunits ($\alpha_3$ and $\alpha_1$) are not detected until trophoblast outgrowth is underway, suggesting that their expression is a response to contact with ECM. Interestingly, dissection of the 7.5-day embryo into extraembryonic ectoplacental cone (primarily trophoblast and its derivatives) and embryonic regions shows that the $\alpha_1\beta_1$, $\alpha_{6A}\beta_1$ and $\alpha_7\beta_1$ complexes are detected only in the extraembryonic ectoplacental cone region, suggesting that they are specific for trophoblast-derived tissues at this time. Thus, differentiation and outgrowth of the trophoblast, which is the forerunner of the placenta, is accompanied by the onset of expression of three integrins that appear to be trophoblast-specific ($\alpha_1\beta_1$, $\alpha_7\beta_1$ and $\alpha_{6A}\beta_1$), as well as other integrins that are more broadly distributed. This provides for an expanded ability of these cells to interact with laminin and collagen as they differentiate and invade the uterine wall.

# Embryo–uterine epithelial interactions: a great unsolved cell–cell recognition mystery

The mammalian embryo is free-living until shortly after it hatches from the zona pellucida at the late blastocyst stage (about E4.5 d). Considerable information is available about how the attachment-competent embryo interacts with ECM and uterine stroma. However, the molecular basis of the hormonally regulated blastocyst–uterine epithelial recognition and adherence continues to elude investigators. After it becomes attachment-competent, the blastocyst is able *in vitro* to attach to and invade virtually any cell monolayer or ECM. Yet *in vivo*, initial blastocyst–uterine epithelial attachment is tightly regulated, indicating that the uterine lining controls the time and the site of embryo implantation.

The coordinated expression of molecules that inhibit blastocyst–uterine interactions with those that promote this process is likely. Data on the mouse system suggest that heavily glycosylated, polylactosamine-bearing glycoproteins and mucin(s) expressed on the luminal surface of uterine epithelium act as a barrier to inappropriate blastocyst attachment, while other glycosylated epitopes may promote embryo–uterine epithelium interactions. The fact that carbohydrate-mediated interactions usually have lower affinities than those mediated by proteins could account, at least in part, for the relative difficulty in identifying the partner adhesion molecules that mediate implantation. Carson and colleagues suggest that heparan sulfate-binding sites on uterine epithelium promote embryo attachment by interacting with heparan sulfate proteoglycans, such as perlecan, which is present on the blastocyst surface at the time attachment-competence develops. In addition to recognizing heparin binding domains via its GAG chains, perlecan has also been shown to recognize the integrin $\alpha_V\beta_3$ via its core protein. Interestingly, the $\beta_3$ subunit has been shown by immunocytochemistry to be temporally regulated on human uterine epithelium, appearing

TABLE 2.3 Integrins detected in early mouse development and their ligand specificities (in temporal order of detection)

| INTEGRIN | LIGAND SPECIFICITY | PERI-IMPLANTATION DISTRIBUTION |
|---|---|---|
| *Constitutive* | | |
| $\alpha_V\beta_3$ | Vn, Fn, Tsp, Ln (P1) | Embryonic/extraembryonic |
| $\alpha_{6B}\beta_1$ | Ln (E8) | Primarily endoderm |
| $\alpha_5\beta_1$ | Fn | Embryonic/extraembryonic |
| *Regulated* | | |
| $\alpha_3\beta_1$ | Fn, Ln (E8), Col | Embryonic/extraembryonic |
| $\alpha_7\beta_1$ | Ln (E8) | Primarily trophoblast |
| $\alpha_{6A}\beta_1$ | Ln (E8) | Primarily trophoblast |
| $\alpha_2\beta_1$ | Ln, Col | Embryonic/extraembryonic |
| $\alpha_1\beta_1$ | Ln (P1, E1), Col | Primarily trophoblast |

Abbreviations: Vn, vitronectin; Fn, fibronectin; Tsp, thrombospondin; Ln, laminin; Col, collagen.

only during days 19–24 of the menstrual cycle, the period of optimum uterine receptivity. The relevance of this observation is supported by the fact that $\beta_3$ was not present on uterine epithelium on days 20–24 in infertile women with luteal phase biopsies that were three or more days out of phase. It is not known whether $\alpha_V\beta_3$ is temporally regulated on mouse uterine epithelium. Another potential blastocyst–uterine epithelial interaction could involve $\alpha_V\beta_3$ on the embryo surface and one of its many potential ligands, osteopontin, which is present on the apical surface of both uterine and fallopian tube epithelium. The functional significance of the regulated expression of specific adhesion molecules remains to be determined.

## Integrins are critical for trophoblast invasion

Trophoblast outgrowth on ECM in culture has been studied as a model for trophoblast interactions with decidualized stroma of the uterine wall. It is clear that integrins are critical for trophoblast–ECM interactions *in vitro*, as a pan-integrin antiserum blocks blastocyst outgrowth on many defined ligands and on reconstituted basement membrane. Although trophoblasts encounter many matrix components during their invasion of the uterine stroma, their interaction with laminin is likely to be particularly important. Migrating trophoblast expresses at least seven integrin complexes capable of recognizing laminin. Furthermore, laminin and collagen are both up-regulated by uterine stromal cells in response to the presence of the attaching embryo.

It is important to point out that some integrin–ligand interactions may transmit information to cells that does not primarily affect adhesive behavior. For example, tumor cell interaction with the P1 region of laminin has been shown to induce metalloproteinases, whereas the $\alpha_V\beta_3$ integrin has been shown to regulate proteinase expression in melanoma cells invading EHS tumor matrix. If a similar situation exists in invasive trophoblast, certain integrin-mediated interactions with ECM ligands or their fragments could contribute to an autocrine induction of higher levels of matrix-degrading enzymes, further facilitating invasion.

*In vitro* studies of blastocyst–ECM interactions in the mouse have showed that trophoblast differentiation is a stepwise process that is accompanied by temporally regulated changes in both adhesiveness and integrin expression. Functional studies have shown that trophoblast–ECM interactions are integrin-dependent and lead us to suggest that trophoblast interactions with laminin are particularly complex and critical. These kinds of studies cannot be carried out on early human embryos. However, the principal conclusions from the mouse studies summarized above have been reinforced by studies of later stages of trophoblast differentiation and establishment of the placenta in humans.

## TROPHOBLAST DIFFERENTIATION AND FORMATION OF THE HUMAN PLACENTA

*See also Chapter 13*

## Trophoblast differentiation along the invasive pathway is a complex process that requires the regulated expression of several classes of molecules

The process of placentation (establishment of a functional fetal–maternal interface) is highly variable among even closely related mammals. Many species, including mouse and human, form a hemochorial placenta in which the fetal trophoblasts from chorionic villi come in direct contact with maternal blood. In order to access the maternal circulation, the trophoblast must invade the uterine wall and its arterial network and promote the formation of sinusoidal spaces in which blood can come in direct contact with the trophoblast subpopulations engaged in nutrient and gas exchange. The morphology of the placental bed (area of trophoblast interaction with the uterine wall and vasculature) is distinct even among species that form a hemochorial placenta. For example, the depth of trophoblast invasion is relatively limited in mice when compared to humans.

By 6–12 weeks' gestation the fetal portion of the human placenta consists of both floating and anchoring chorionic villi (Fig. 2.28). In the floating chorionic villi mononuclear trophoblasts (cytotrophoblasts) remain as a monolayer of polarized epithelial cells attached to the chorionic villus basement membrane. These cells replicate and fuse to form the overlying syncytiotrophoblast layer that contacts maternal blood and carries out the exchange and transport functions of the placenta. However, at the tips of some of those villi the cytotrophoblasts detach from the basement membrane, and aggregate into multilayered columns of non-polarized cells that rapidly invade the uterus. This unusual behavior, which forms the anchoring villi, is confined spatially to the endometrium, the first third of the myometrium and the associated spiral arterioles, and temporally to early pregnancy (Fig. 2.28). Particularly striking is the precision with which cytotrophoblasts home to and invade the uterine arterial system and replace the endothelial lining of these vessels throughout their endometrial and inner third of their myometrial segments.

Although we will focus on the role of cell–ECM interactions in trophoblast invasion, other classes of molecules are also clearly important. For example, the regulation of cell–cell interactions is likely to be critical in the acquisition of an invasive phenotype. In both the mouse and human systems E-cadherin is down-regulated during trophoblast invasion. In addition, a specific metalloproteinase (the 92 kD type IV

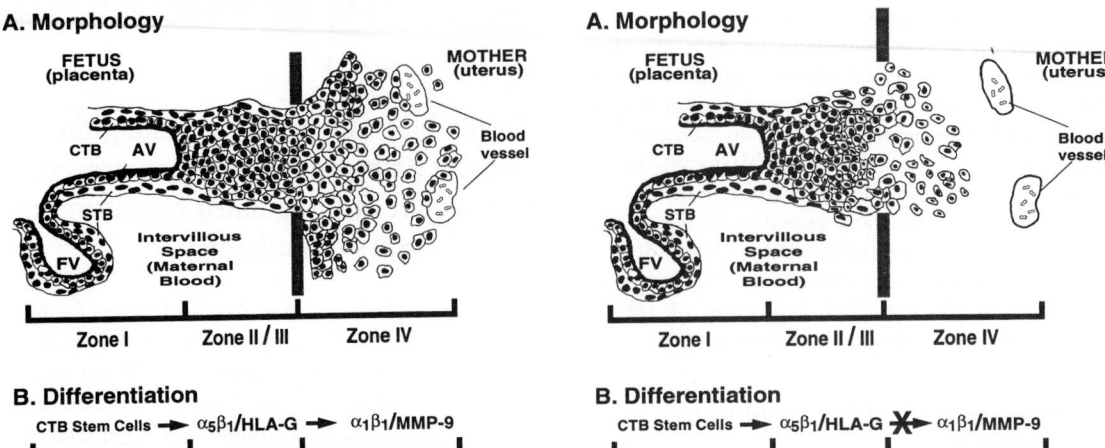

FIGURE 2.28 A schematic presentation of floating villi (FV) and anchoring villi (AV) and invading cytotrophoblasts (CTB). In normal pregnancy, the invading cytotrophoblasts undergo a dramatic alteration in their integrin profile as they migrate into maternal tissue. During this process, these cells also up-regulate metalloproteinases and express a novel MHC class I antigen, HLA-G. The invading cytotrophoblasts gain access to maternal blood vessels where they replace the muscular intima and endothelium, rendering these vessels incapable of vasoconstriction. This process is critical to establishing a low-resistance, high-flow placental circulation. In preeclampsia the invading cytotrophoblasts fail to undergo differentiation along the invasive pathway, as evidenced by their altered interactions with the extracellular matrix, and do not invade the maternal blood vessels. (STB = syncytiotrophoblast.)

collagenase: MMP-9 ) is rate-limiting for trophoblast invasion *in vitro* in both species. Finally, successful pregnancy requires that the embryo evade maternal immune rejection. Recent evidence suggests that human cytotrophoblasts express a novel class I HLA molecule, HLA G, for this purpose.

## Altered expression of integrins and their ECM ligands during trophoblast differentiation changes the invasive potential of the cells

The authors have used immunocytochemistry and tissue samples from the fetal–maternal interface at different gestational ages to study the expression of adhesion receptors and their ECM ligands during human trophoblast invasion *in vivo*. In the first trimester, undifferentiated villus cytophoblastic cells, attached to basement membrane, stain for $\alpha_6$ and $\beta_4$ integrin subunits and multiple forms of laminin. Cytotrophoblasts that leave their basement membrane and form aggregates (cell columns) undergo a striking modulation of their adhesion phenotype. Expression of $\alpha_6\beta_4$ is down-regulated, and the cells turn on expression of $\alpha_5$ and $\beta_1$ integrin subunits, as well as a fibronectin-rich matrix. Cytotrophoblasts within the uterine wall again change their repertoire of adhesion receptors. These cells stain for the $\alpha_1$ subunit for the first time and continue to stain for the $\alpha_5$ and $\beta_1$ integrins. They do not stain for most ECM ligands, suggesting that they interact primarily with surrounding maternal cells and matrices.

To investigate directly whether these tightly regulated integrins are critical for trophoblast invasive activity, we have used an *in vitro* Matrigel model for cytotrophoblast differentiation and invasion that has already demonstrated the importance of the 92-kD matrix metalloproteinase. The adhesion phenotype of the cytotrophoblasts invading Matrigel *in vitro* resembles that of cytotrophoblasts within the uterine wall *in vivo*. We have recently shown that antibodies against collagen IV and laminin, and against the $\alpha_1\beta_1$ integrin receptor for these ligands, block cytotrophoblast invasion in the Matrigel assay. In contrast, antibodies against the $\alpha_5\beta_1$ fibronectin receptor stimulate invasion, whereas addition of exogenous fibronectin to the Matrigel blocks invasion. This suggests that there is a balance between cytotrophoblast–ECM interactions that promote invasion (i.e. laminin and collagen interactions with the $\alpha_1\beta_1$ integrin) and those that restrict invasion (i.e. fibronectin interactions with the $\alpha_5\beta_1$ integrin). Altered regulation of this balance may profoundly influence the depth of trophoblast invasion.

## Regulation of expression of integrins and MMP-9 during cytotrophoblast differentiation is defective in preeclampsia

*Preeclampsia*, a serious disease of pregnancy, is characterized by abnormally shallow trophoblast invasion of the uterine wall and by an absence of blood vessel invasion (Fig. 2.28). Cytotrophoblasts in the superficial endometrium of preeclamptic patients fail to down-regulate the $\alpha_6\beta_4$ complex. At the same time expression of the $\alpha_1\beta_1$ complex is not up-regulated. In contrast, the $\alpha_5\beta_1$ complex is regulated normally. When cytotrophoblasts isolated from patients with preeclampsia are cultured on Matrigel, their expression of integrin $\alpha_1\beta_1$ complex and MMP-9 were markedly reduced compared with gestationally matched controls. The cytotrophoblasts from preeclamptic pregnancies, however, retained their ability to express $\alpha_5\beta_1$ complex, confirming the observation made in the placental bed biopsy samples.

The observations on integrin and MMP-9 disregulation in preeclampsia reveal an early defect in the differentiation program of trophoblasts which is likely to contribute significantly to the observed alteration in placental anatomy and function: insufficient invasion by trophoblasts of the maternal myometrium and blood vessels. In particular, these observations point to an important role for the regulated expression of the $\alpha_1\beta_1$ integrin in normal trophoblast invasion. It is likely that other regulatory events are proximal to the defective cytotrophoblast integrin expression seen in preeclamptic placentas. Understanding the mechanisms underlying the regulation of integrin and MMP-9 expression during placentation is therefore a high priority.

# Mechanisms of regulation of integrin-mediated cell–ECM interactions

Growth factors and cytokines released by maternal immune and decidual cells, or by the fetal trophoblasts themselves, are likely to play important roles in regulating integrin expression during trophoblast differentiation. Trophoblast cells produce a large number of growth/differentiation factors, many of which are known to regulate expression of integrins in other systems. For example, TNF$\alpha$, which promotes ECM remodeling, tumor cell invasion and angiogenesis, up-regulates $\alpha_1\beta_1$ and down-regulates $\alpha_6\beta_1$ expression in endothelial cells. TGF$\beta$ stimulates ECM and integrin expression and suppresses the invasive phenotype in some systems. Thus, if the net effects of growth factors and cytokines on the integrin repertoire of cytotrophoblasts is altered in preeclampsia, this could affect profoundly their invasiveness of the uterine wall and vasculature. These or other factors could also affect the net activity of matrix-degrading proteases at sites of trophoblast invasion by regulating expression or activation of these enzymes or their inhibitors. Some aspects of these hypotheses can be tested directly using our *in vitro* model and cytotrophoblasts isolated from normal and preeclamptic placentas.

## SUMMARY

This chapter has emphasized the role of cell–cell and cell–ECM interactions in early mammalian development. Along with other critical factors involved in this process, cell interaction with the microenvironment clearly guides cell recognition, lineage restriction, and the dynamic processes of epithelial–mesenchymal transformation, migration, and invasion. It is evident that genetic defects in ECM components or cellular receptors can have profound consequences in morphogenesis and cellular and organ function. ECM signaling for differentiation is likely to involve the pathways of other regulators of cellular function. Growth factors and tissue- and developmental stage-specific hormones act in concert with ECM. It is possible that ECM binding to specific transmembrane receptors could affect the dimerization or phosphorylation of some hormone receptors and activate those particular signal transduction pathways. Cell interaction with the microenvironment is a dynamic process that plays a critical role in a wide variety of biologic events ranging from embryonic development to tumor metastasis. Being able to understand and manipulate these intricate and powerful interactions will serve as effective tools in investigating fundamental issues in cell biology, pathophysiology and ultimately disease treatment.

## SELECTED READING

Buck C. Immunoglobulin superfamily: structure, function and relationship to other receptor molecules. *Curr Opin Cell Biol* 1992; 3: 179.

Cross JC, Werb Z, Fisher SJ. Implantation and the placenta: key pieces of the development puzzle. *Science* 1994; 266: 1508.

Damsky CH, Librach C, Lim KH, et al. Integrin switching regulates normal trophoblast invasion. *Development* 1994; 120: 3657.

Damsky CH, Sutherland A, Fisher S. Extracellular matrix 5: adhesive interactions in early mammalian embryogenesis, implantation, and placentation. *Faseb J* 1993; 7: 1320.

Damsky CH, Werb Z. Signal transduction by integrin receptors for extracellular matrix: cooperative processing of extracellular information. *Curr Opin Cell Biol* 1992; 4: 772.

Hynes RO. Integrins: versatility, modulation, and signaling in cell adhesion. *Cell* 1992; 69: 11.

Paulsson M. Basement membrane proteins: structure, assembly, and cellular interactions. *Crit Rev Biochem & Molec Biol* 1992; 27: 93.

Ranscht B. Cadherins and catenins: interactions and functions in embryonic development. *Curr Opin Cell Biol* 1994; 6: 740.

Rosen SD, Bertozzi CR. The selectins and their ligands. *Curr Opin Cell Biol* 1994; 6: 663.

Takeichi M. Cadherin cell adhesion receptors as a morphogenetic regulator. *Science* 1991; 251: 1451.

Venstrom KA, Reichardt L F. Extracellular matrix 2: role of extracellular matrix molecules and their receptors in the nervous system. *Faseb J* 1993; 7: 996.

# MITOCHONDRIAL BIOGENESIS AND FUNCTION

Energy demands for cellular functions are met largely through the process of oxidative phosphorylation. Cytosolic glycolysis can also produce energy (ATP) in the absence of $O_2$ (anaerobic metabolism); however, this process is inefficient and cannot meet the extraordinarily high energy needs of tissues such as brain, muscle, and heart. Thus energy for highly active cellular functions is generated within mitochondria, either through β-oxidation of fatty acids or via glycolysis and the citric acid cycle. With either pathway, efficient ATP production requires the enzyme complexes of the respiratory chain, the cytosolic components of an energy transduction system, and molecular $O_2$. The following discussion describes the biogenesis and unique genetics of mitochondria, their function in normal cellular metabolism, and the diseases that can follow from disordered mitochondrial function.

## EVOLUTION OF MITOCHONDRIA

The appearance of mitochondria in mammalian cells represents a bacterial endosymbiotic event over 1.5 billion years ago, probably of a particular type of purple photosynthetic bacterium that lost its photosynthetic capabilities but retained its respiratory chain. With the appearance of bacteria that could use water as the H+ source for the reduction of $CO_2$, $O_2$ began to appear in the atmosphere, allowing the development of bacteria and more complex life forms that utilized aerobic metabolism to make ATP. In turn, the greater energy released from the breakdown of complex organic molecules and carbohydrates to $H_2O$ and $CO_2$ rapidly advanced the growth and evolution of these organisms. Because this endosymbiotic event occurred so early in evolution, virtually all complex single and multicellular organisms contain mitochondria or their equivalent. For example, plants contain chloroplasts, which closely resemble mitochondria in structure, and have many of the same enzymes, genetic codes, and functions of eukaryotic mitochondria. Yeast and molds also contain mitochondria that are functionally and structurally very similar to mammalian mitochondria. The key point of this evolutionary history of mitochondria, aside from the selective advantages they offered to the host cell, is that it is the basis for the unique properties of mitochondrial biogenesis and has significant implications for mitochondrial disease processes.

## MITOCHONDRIAL BIOGENESIS

Mitochondria are double-membraned organelles, each membrane having very different characteristics and creating two internal compartments (Fig. 2.29). The inner compartment is called the *matrix* and is enclosed by the *inner mitochondrial membrane* (IM): this is the major working space of the mitochondrion. The matrix contains the mitochondrial genome and replication machinery as well as the enzymes for β-oxidation of fatty acids and for the citric acid cycle. The inner mitochondrial membrane contains most of the enzymes of the electron transport chain necessary for oxidative phosphorylation and is folded into extensive cristae to increase its surface area. Three different enzyme systems are located on, or within, the inner membrane:

- the enzymes of the electron transport chain, e.g. cytochrome *c*;
- the ATP synthase enzyme complex that produces ATP; and
- specific transport proteins that regulate and perform the movement of metabolites, ions, and ATP into and out of the matrix, e.g. the adenine nucleotide translocase (ANT), which is responsible for moving high-energy phosphates (ATP) out of, and ADP into, the mitochondria.

The space between the inner and outer mitochondrial membranes is called the *intermembranous space* (IMS), and generally contains enzymes the function of which is to phosphorylate other compounds, such as mitochondrial creatine kinase, which transfers a high-energy phosphate from ATP to creatine (creatine phosphate). The *outer mitochondrial membrane* (OM) contains multiple copies of a protein called porin, which allows free passage of small molecules less than 10 kD in molecular weight. It also contains receptors that recognize the precursor proteins specifically targeted to mitochondria and several enzymes that function to convert lipid substrates into forms that can be metabolized in the matrix. Approximately 67 per cent of the total mitochondrial protein is contained in the matrix, 21 per cent in the inner mitochondrial membrane, 6 per cent in the IMS, and 6 per cent in the outer membrane. Thus, whereas the OM is highly permeable to small metabolites and ions, the inner membrane is virtually impermeable to ions and proteins and creates a matrix space that is substantially different in composition from either the cytosol or the IMS, which is relatively "open" to the cytosol.

Mitochondria contain their own genome, and a single mitochondrion usually contains multiple copies (5–10) of this genome. It is double-stranded, and both strands are "read" from opposing directions during transcription (Fig. 2.30). Compared with the nuclear genome, the mitochondrial genome is very small, 16 569 nucleotide pairs (np) in length in humans, and extraordinarily compact with virtually no intronic sequences, or untranslated regions, between the coding genes. Because of the asymmetric distribution of guanines and cytosines between the two strands, one strand is heavier (more guanines) and designated the *H-strand*, and the opposing lighter strand (cytosine

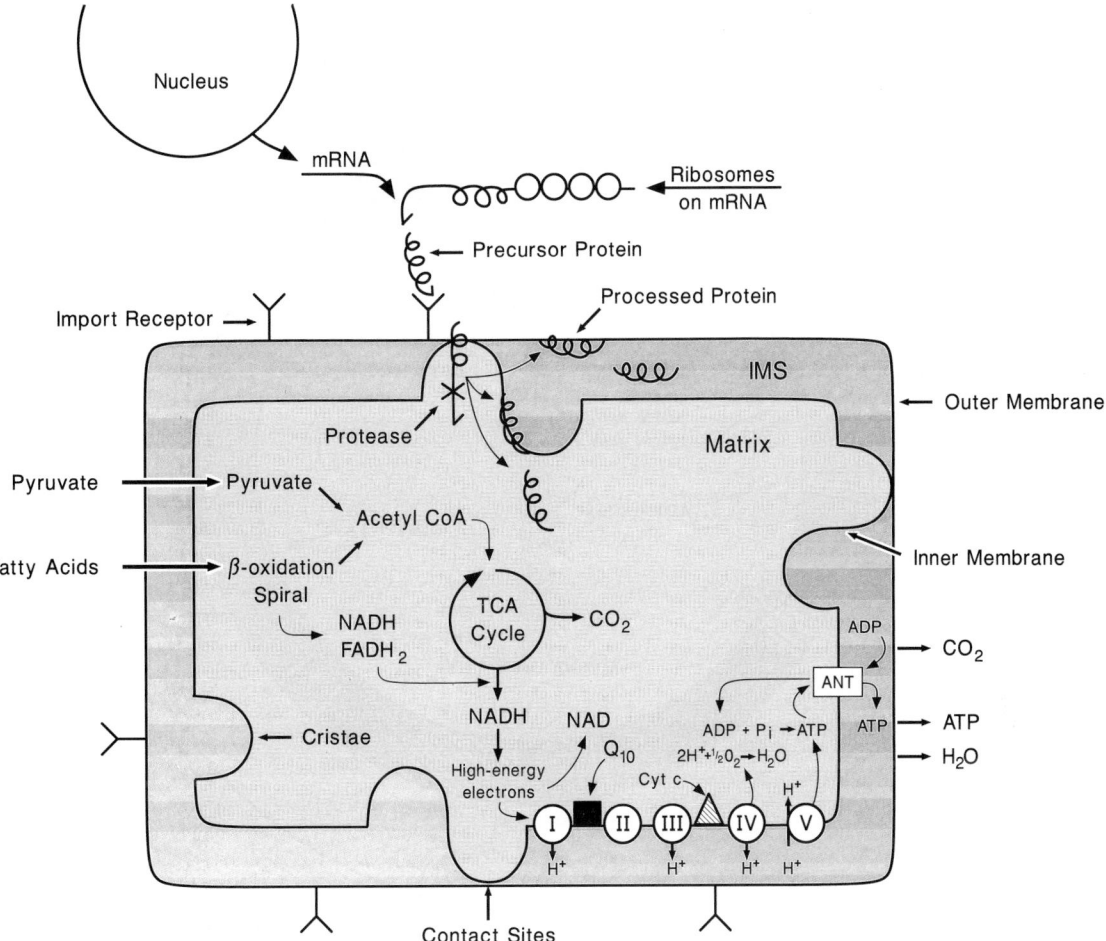

FIGURE 2.29 Mitochondrial organization and structure. Four basic processes in energy generation are depicted: (1) Import of nuclearly encoded, cytosolically translated proteins across the mitochondrial membranes at the contact sites. Precursor proteins are recognized by a receptor, translocated across the import apparatus at the contact site, the transit peptide is clipped off by specific proteases, and the mature peptide is localized to one of four locations: outer or inner membrane, matrix, or intermembranous space (IMS). (2) Fuels enter the matrix as pyruvate from glycolysis, or fatty acids which enter the β-oxidation spiral. Both are converted to acetyl CoA which enters the citric acid cycle producing high-energy electrons in the form of NADH and FADH$_2$, ATP, and CO$_2$. (3) High-energy electrons from both the TCA cycle and β-oxidation of fatty acids are passed down the electron transport chain, shown as complexes I to IV. The electrochemical gradient established by pumping three protons out of the matrix per electron is used by complex V to produce ATP from ADP. ATP is transported across the inner membrane by the adenine nucleotide translocase (ANT).

rich) is designated the *L-strand*. The L-strand encodes eight transfer RNA (tRNA) genes and one subunit gene (ND6 of complex I). The H-strand encodes the 12S and 16S ribosomal genes (rRNA), 14 tRNA genes, and 12 oxidative phosphorylation (OXPHOS) subunit genes. Because of simplified codon–anticodon pairing, mitochondrial translation is accomplished with only 22 tRNAs compared with a minimum of 32 tRNAs required to read the nuclear genetic code. The origin of the H-strand replication (O$_H$) is contained within the D-loop, a 1122-bp stretch of DNA containing the genetic information for replication and transcription of the mtDNA. Both the H-strand promoter (HSP) and L-strand promoter (LSP) are contained within the D-loop. Binding of these regions by the nuclearly encoded mitochondrial *trans*-acting factor, mtTF1, initiates

transcription of either H- or L-strands, depending on whether multiple (HSP activation) or single (LSP activation) mtTF1 molecules are bound. The mtTF1 molecule also represents an important control point of mitochondrial replication by the nuclear genome.

The majority of the hundreds of proteins in mitochondria are encoded by the nuclear genome, translated in the cytosol of the cell, then targeted and imported into the mitochondrion by special amino acid sequences contained in the imported protein itself (Fig. 2.29). Receptors on the outer membrane of the mitochondrion recognize and bind the targeting signal in the amino terminus of the precursor protein, and transport the protein to the *import apparatus* located at the contact sites. *Contact sites* are a unique feature of mitochondria where the inner and outer membranes

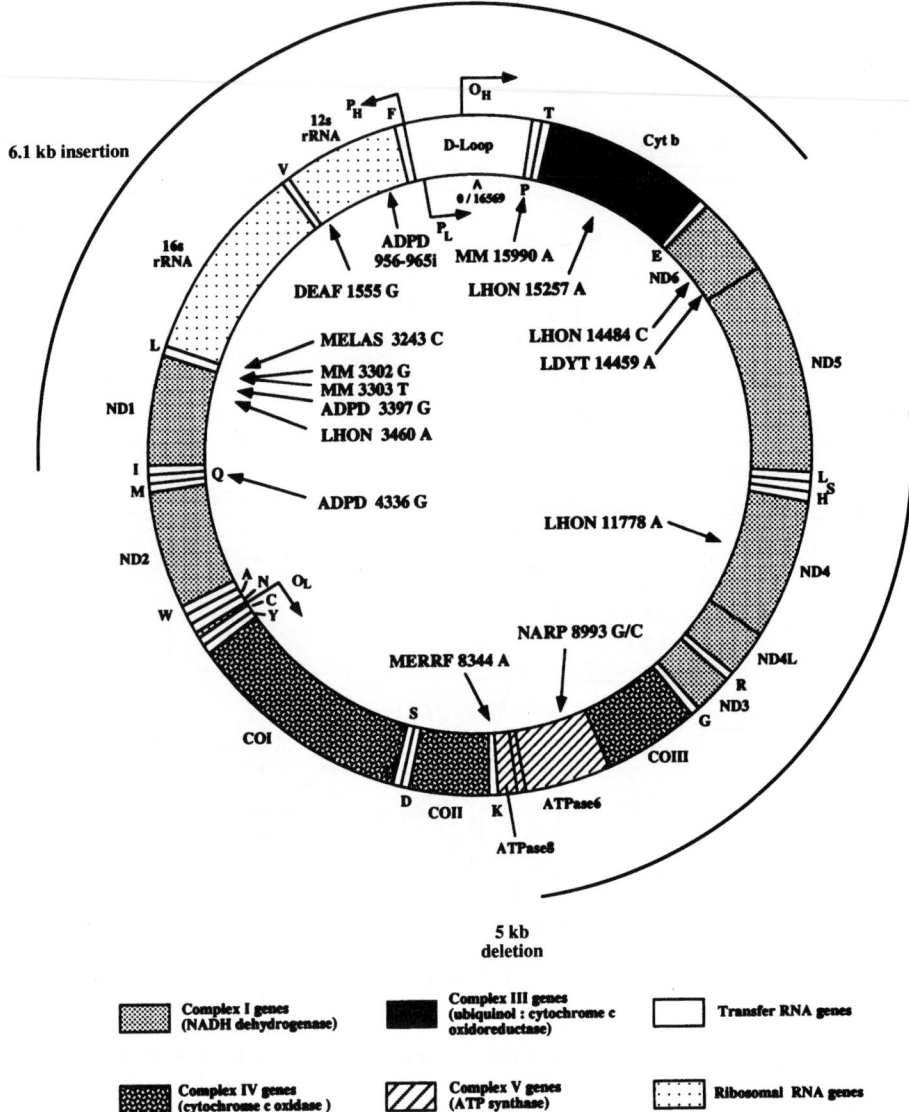

FIGURE 2.30 Human mtDNA structural and morbid map showing locations of genes and mutations. The tRNAs are indicated by their cognate amino acid single-letter code. The genes encoded by the G-rich heavy (H) strand are on the outside of the circle, while those for the C-rich light (L) strand are on the inside. The H- and L-strand origins ($O_H$ and $O_L$) and promoters ($P_H$ and $P_L$) are shown. The positions of representative base substitutions are shown on the inside of the circle. The disease acronyms are defined in the text, with the exception that ADPD stands for Alzheimer and Parkinson disease and DEAF for neurosensory hearing loss. Two representative rearrangements are shown outside the circle, the common 5-kb deletion associated with ocular myopathy and Pearson marrow/pancreas syndrome, and the 6.1-kb insertion observed in the maternally inherited diabetes and deafness family harboring the trimolecular heteroplasmy. (Reprinted with permission from the 1994 William Allan Award Address, *Am J Hum Genet* 1995; 57: 201. Copyright © 1995 by the University of Chicago Press.)

fuse; it is probably at these contact sites that import of nuclearly encoded proteins into mitochondria occurs via the import apparatus, which is a multi-subunit complex of proteins spanning the contact site, and which functions selectively to import proteins targeted to mitochondria. The precursor protein is pulled into the mitochondrial matrix in a linear form where enzymes called processing proteases clip off the targeting signal, and the imported protein is directed to its final location (OM, IMS, IM, or matrix) by signals and processes not yet fully understood. A relative few pro-

teins bypass this import process and integrate directly into the outer membrane without processing. Study of the targeting and translocation of nuclearly encoded, mitochondrial proteins has been informative in two simple eukaryotic organisms, yeast (*Saccharomyces cerevisiae*) and slime mold (*Neurospora crassa*). However, the corresponding mammalian genes encoding these proteins have not been isolated. This is important because this process is complex, and impaired targeting and import of mitochondrial proteins may result in diseases that are not yet defined for lack of the proper reagents. Thus, although the mitochondrial genome replicates independently of the nuclear genome, to control the complex process of energy production clearly requires an important level of interdependence and communication between the nuclear and mitochondrial genomes, which may represent a potential source of disordered mitochondrial function.

# BIOCHEMISTRY OF MITOCHONDRIAL ENERGY GENERATION

Oxidative energy generated from mitochondria derives primarily from two fuels, *pyruvate* from cytosolic glycolysis of glucose, and *fatty acids*, which enter the β-oxidative pathway (see also Chapter 7). Glycogen is the major intracellular storage form of glucose that is broken down via the glycolytic pathway to pyruvate in a nine-step reaction that is energetically favorable (the free energy change is less than zero). Glucose is the primary fuel of brain tissue, which cannot utilize fatty acids. However, the brain readily oxidizes the ketone bodies derived from the acetyl CoA and acetoacetyl CoA produced from β-oxidation of fatty acids in the liver. Fats are the intracellular storage form for fatty acid oxidation, a process that releases more than six times the energy of an equivalent mass of hydrated glycogen. Fatty acid oxidation is the major source of energy in tissues such as heart. Glycogen is a readily available, but rapidly consumed, source of fuel. After an overnight fast, most of the energy substrate for oxidative phosphorylation derives from fatty acids, whereas after a meal, most of the acetyl CoA entering the citric acid cycle comes from the breakdown of carbohydrates (foodstuffs) into glucose. In mammalian cells, sugars are readily converted to fats, but fats cannot be converted to sugars. It is also important to note that fuel substrates change dramatically around the time of birth in most mammals. Glucose is a major fuel for the fetus, but after birth, fats derived from milk become much more important in metabolism. Thus, the enzymes of mitochondria, and mitochondrial functions, are developmentally regulated to accommodate these changes in fuel source. Finally, both fatty acids and pyruvate are selectively transported into the mitochondrial matrix where they are converted to *acetyl CoA*, which then enters the *tricarboxylic acid cycle* (TCA) (Fig. 2.29).

Pyruvate is converted to acetyl CoA in the mitochondrial matrix by the *pyruvate dehydrogenase* (PDH) complex, located in the mitochondrial matrix. Pyruvate dehydrogenase is a large enzyme complex, composed of multiple copies of three different catalytic enzymes, five different coenzymes, and two regulatory enzymes, all encoded by the nuclear genome. The oxidation of pyruvate to acetyl CoA is a complicated process that is irreversible in mammalian tissues. It is summarized by the equation:

$$\text{Pyruvate} + NAD^+ + CoA \rightarrow \text{acetyl CoA} + NADH + H^+ + CO_2$$

and is an energetically favorable reaction by generating electrons ($\Delta G^\circ = -8.0$ kcal/mol). Defects in the PDH complex are associated with disease (*PDH complex-$E_1$ deficiency*) characterized by lactic acidosis, neurologic impairment, and early death. Pyruvate can also be converted to the amino acid alanine by alanine aminotransferase, to lactate by lactate dehydrogenase, or to oxaloacetate by pyruvate carboxylase.

Fatty acids must reach the mitochondrial matrix where they are converted to acetyl CoA by β-oxidation (Fig. 2.31). Long-chain fatty acids (>10 carbons) depend upon the four-step carnitine cycle for transport into the mitochondrial matrix, whereas fatty acids with fewer than 10 carbons traverse the inner mitochondrial membrane freely. The β-oxidation spiral is an enzymatic, stepwise removal of two carbons from the carboxyl end of fatty acid molecules producing one molecule of acetyl CoA, and one molecule each of $FADH_2$ and NADH, with each turn of the cycle (see also Chapter 7). This acetyl CoA then enters the TCA cycle for generation of ATP. Defects in both the carnitine transport cycle, and in the β-oxidation spiral, are associated with diseases presenting early in life (infancy).

The TCA cycle begins with the condensation of acetyl CoA with the four-carbon oxaloacetate to produce the six-carbon citric acid for which the cycle is named. Through seven enzymatic steps, two carbons are removed from citric acid regenerating oxaloacetate, and producing two $CO_2$ molecules, one ATP via a GTP intermediate, and two high-energy electrons. This reaction can be summarized as follows:

$$CH_3COOH \text{ (as acetyl CoA)} + 2H_2O + 3NAD^+ + FAD \rightarrow 2CO_2 + 3NADH + FADH_2$$

The TCA cycle (citric acid cycle) does not consume $O_2$ directly, but rather extracts high-energy electrons from the conversion of two carbon atoms from acetyl CoA into $CO_2$. These electrons, in the form of NADH and $FADH_2$, are fed into the *electron transport chain* located in the inner membrane, combined with molecular $O_2$, and used to convert ADP + $P_i$ to ATP. Hence, this process is termed *oxidative phosphorylation*. $H_2O$ is a byproduct of this process, whereas $CO_2$ is the byproduct of the TCA cycle.

The electron transport chain consumes the energy stored in the high-energy electrons (NADH and $FADH_2$) from the TCA cycle in a stepwise fashion to pump protons from the mitochondrial matrix across the inner membrane to the intermembranous space. This creates an *electrochemical proton gradient* across the impermeable inner membrane, which, in turn, drives the membrane-bound enzyme complex, *ATP synthase*, to catalyze the conversion of ADP + $P_i$ to

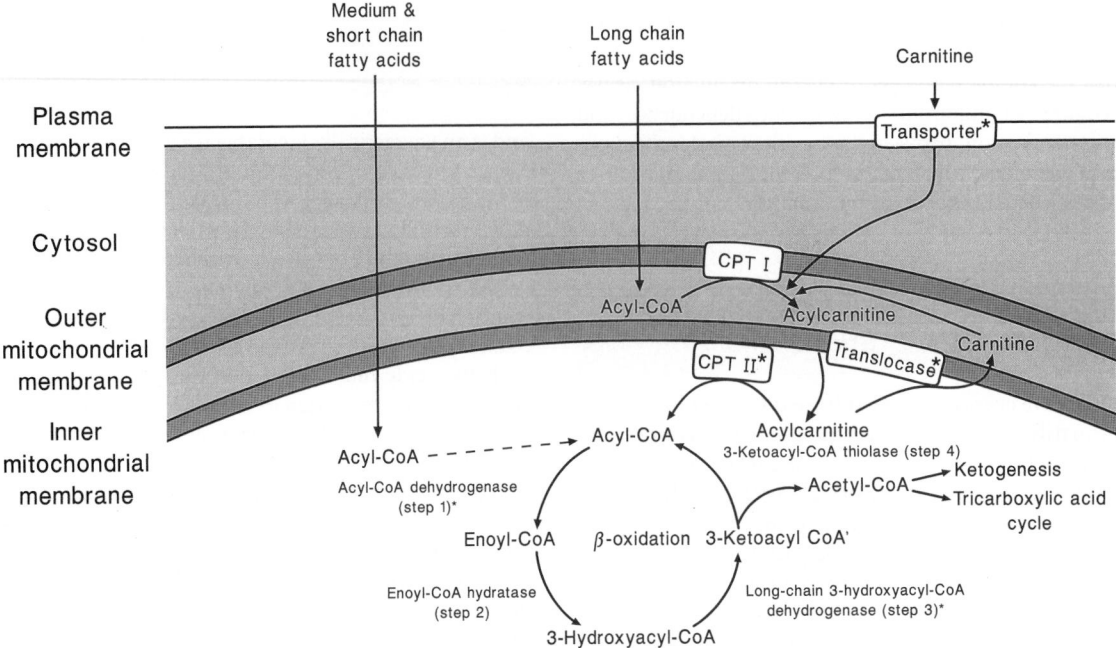

FIGURE 2.31 The β-oxidation pathway of fatty acids and specific defects causing cardiomyopathy. The pathways of fatty-acid oxidation and cellular carnitine metabolism are shown. Defects known to cause cardiomyopathy (indicated by the asterisks) include abnormalities in carnitine or acylcarnitine transport (carnitine transport defect, carnitine palmitoyltransferase II (CPT II) deficiency), and carnitine (acylcarnitine translocase (translocase) deficiency), and errors in steps 1 and 3 of mitochondrial β-oxidation (long-chain acyl-coenzyme A dehydrogenase deficiency and long-chain 3-hydroxyacyl-coenzyme A dehydrogenase deficiency, respectively). CPT I denotes carnitine palmitoyltransferase I; and AD short-chain, medium-chain, long-chain, and very-long-chain acyl-CoA dehydrogenase. (Copyright ©: reprinted with permission from Kelly DP, Strauss AW, *N Engl J Med* 1994; **330**: 913.)

ATP. The energy from the reversible flow of protons down this gradient, i.e. from the intermembranous space to the matrix, also transports various metabolites into the matrix, such as $Ca^{2+}$, which is used for intracellular signaling and which must be kept low in the cytosol.

The electron transport chain is composed of five complexes to which the mitochondrial genome contributes all of its 13 encoded proteins. Complex I (NADH:ubiquinone oxidoreductase, or NADH dehydrogenase) encompasses more than 40 proteins, including 7 from mitochondrial DNA (mtDNA) (MTND1, -2, -3, -4, -4L, -5, and -6), and functions to remove electrons from NADH for transfer to ubiquinone (coenzyme $Q_{10}$). This includes electrons generated by cytosolic processes, such as glycolysis, which are transported across the inner mitochondrial membrane by the malate–aspartate shuttle to form NADH. Complex II (succinate:ubiquinone oxidoreductase) is composed of four nuclear encoded proteins, and collects the electrons from the dehydrogenation of succinate to fumarate in the TCA cycle. It is located on the matrix side of the inner membrane and is the only OXPHOS enzyme complex entirely encoded by the nuclear DNA. Thus, both complex I and II collect electrons from various sources and transfer them to coenzyme $Q_{10}$. Coenzyme $Q_{10}$ is a fat-soluble quinone that transfers electrons to complex III; it is also a powerful

antioxidant found in the cell nucleus, microsomes, and cytosol. Complex III (ubiquinol:ferrocytochrome *c* oxidoreductase, or cytochrome $bc_1$ complex) is composed of 11 proteins, of which 1 (cytochrome *b*) is encoded by the mtDNA, and catalyzes the transfer of electrons between ubiquinol and cytochrome *c*. Cytochrome *c*, like ubiquinol, is a mobile electron carrier loosely attached to the matrix side of the inner membrane, and is a small, nuclear-encoded protein containing a covalently bound heme group. The final enzyme complex for electron transport is complex IV (ferrocytochrome $c$:$O_2$ oxidoreductase, or cytochrome *c* oxidase). It contains 13 protein subunits of which 3 (subunits I, II, and III) are encoded by the mitochondrial genome. Complex IV transfers electrons to $O_2$ to yield $H_2O$.

The entire process of transferring one electron to $O_2$ generates three protons, one each at complexes I, III, and IV, which are pumped across the inner mitochondrial membrane to create an *electrochemical proton gradient* (Fig. 2.29). This electrochemical gradient has two major components: (1) a pH gradient across the inner mitochondrial membrane with a lower $H^+$ concentration in the matrix compared with the cytosol, and (2) a voltage gradient across the inner mitochondrial membrane with a negative matrix and positive outside. This membrane potential is termed $\Delta\psi$, and is also a motive force for the movement of precursor proteins into mitochondria. Complex V (ATP synthase) uses the energy of this electrochemical gradient to condense ADP + P$_i$ to ATP in the mitochondrial matrix. Complex V is composed of 12 or 13 subunits of which two, ATPase 6 and 8, are encoded by the mitochondrial genome.

The ATP produced in this process is translocated across the inner membrane by the *adenine nucleotide translocase* (ANT translocase) to the intermembranous space. From the intermembranous space, ATP either can diffuse into the cytosol and be consumed directly in intracellular functions, or can be used by one of several kinases, such as mitochondrial creatine kinase, to phosphorylate high-energy intermediate metabolites. Diffusion of ATP into the cytosol is an inefficient means of energy transmission because it is slow, and multiple processes break down ATP. In fact, the cytosolic milieu is not homogeneous, as would be predicted by a diffusion model for energy distribution, but rather is very structured with regard to metabolic compartmentalization; *metabolite channelling* of high-energy substrates is crucial to the metabolic regulation of respiration.

Metabolite channeling results from the action of several systems that direct and regulate the flow of high-energy substrates within the cell. The best understood example is the family of creatine kinase enzymes. The purpose of this enzyme family is to phosphorylate creatine reversibly. *Creatine phosphate* then becomes the cytosolic storage and transport form of high-energy phosphate in the cell and forms part of a highly regulated shuttle of energy from the mitochondrion to the site of utilization. Mitochondrial creatine kinase phosphorylates creatine in the intermembranous space of the mitochondria, and the cytosolic creatine kinases, MCK and BCK, use creatine phosphate to rephosphorylate ADP to ATP, thus maintaining very high local concentrations of ATP at sites of high energy consumption. Creatine then shuttles back to the mitochondria for rephosphorylation. This cycle, termed the *creatine phosphate shuttle*, operates in tissues with repetitious, fluctuating high-energy demands, such as heart and skeletal muscle, and in static, high-energy tissues as well, such as brain, sperm, and the visual system.

The process of oxidative phosphorylation is remarkably efficient. About 12 molecules of ATP are produced from every molecule of acetyl CoA that enters the TCA cycle. Thus, each molecule of glucose (6 carbons) yields 24 molecules of ATP because it makes two molecules of acetyl CoA (3 carbons), and each molecule of a 16-carbon fatty acid, palmitate, yields about 96 molecules of ATP. Counting energy from processes prior to the formation of acetyl CoA, each molecule of glucose yields a total of 36 molecules of ATP, and each molecule of palmitate yields 129 molecules of ATP. Obviously, the energy density of fats is much higher than that of carbohydrates (glucose), but the generation of acetyl CoA from fatty acids is also more involved and slower than consuming intracellular glycogen. Overall, conversion of the energy stored in carbohydrates and fatty acids into the chemical bonds of high-energy phosphates exceeds 50 per cent and is a direct result of the *stepwise* release of small amounts of energy from the oxidation of fuels.

## GENETICS OF MITOCHONDRIAL DISEASES

In addition to the endosymbiotic origin of mitochondria, four unique features of these organelles are responsible for the unusual characteristics of mitochondrial diseases. First, mitochondria are inherited from the maternal germ line. Even though the sperm is tightly packed with mitochondria, they are stripped away in the process of fertilizing the egg, and virtually no male mitochondrial DNAs survive entry into the ovum. Each ovum contains 200 000 to 300 000 mitochondria, and each mitochondrion contains a single genome. Thus, mitochondrial diseases are inherited through the mother and do not follow mendelian laws of inheritance: affected males do not pass on their disease. Additionally, because mitochondria do not recombine to share genomes, the lineage of any person's mitochondrial DNA reflects the early evolutionary history of women with regard to migration and mutations: individual mutations can be tracked along radiating female lineages. Based on these characteristics, analysis of mtDNA migrations indicate that the human mtDNA tree originated in Africa approximately 150 000 years ago, and, as females migrated to colonize new lands, new mutations became established that created continent-specific mutations. An important point, then, about mitochondrial genetics is that the only manner in which the mitochondrial genome can change is through the sequential accumulation of mutations along radiating maternal lineages over time.

Second, the high copy number of mitochondria per cell (hundreds to thousands), their cytoplasmic location, and their semiautonomous replication contribute to the unusual genetics of mitochondria. The population dynamics of mitochondria most closely resemble intracellular microorganisms in that mutations arising in the mtDNA result in a mixed population of normal (wild type) and mutant mitochondria distributed randomly within the cytoplasm. This mixture of wild type and mutant mitochondria is termed *heteroplasmy*, and a pure population of either type of mitochondria is termed *homoplasmy*. Thus, with repeated divisions of a heteroplasmic cell, random chance incorporation of mitochondria into the daughter cells will change the proportion of mutant to wild type mitochondria and result in relatively pure populations of either type of mitochondria in the cells over time. This process is termed *replicative segregation* and is one reason why mitochondrial diseases can show up later in childhood or in adulthood; repeated division of somatic cells carrying a deleterious mtDNA mutation will result in a higher percentage of defective cells leading to the phenotypic expression of disease. Additionally, because *deletion* mutants have a smaller mitochondrial genome than wild type mtDNA, mutant mtDNA has a replicative advantage over the wild type mtDNA (see below). If replicative segregation occurs during the proliferation of female germ-line cells (meiosis) which become oocytes, the oocytes will contain differing amounts of wild type and mutant mtDNAs. If the mutation is deleterious, then the offspring resulting from an oocyte high in mutated mtDNA can have a very early appearance of severe disease in spite of a normal-appearing heteroplasmic mother.

Third, whether or not a mutation produces a disease state (a phenotype) is a product of the nature of

the mutation, the percentage of mutant mtDNAs in the cells, and the reliance of the tissue upon mitochondrial function; this is termed *threshold expression* (Fig. 2.32). As mitochondrial ATP production decreases over time, there will be a point where cellular function becomes impaired, and symptoms appear rapidly. Different tissues have differing bioenergetic thresholds reflecting their reliance upon oxidative phosphorylation. For example, heart and skeletal muscle (red muscle) are tightly packed with mitochondria and depend heavily upon oxidative phosphorylation for production of energy. White blood cells have few mitochondria, and red cells have none; their primary source of energy is cytosolic glycolysis. Aging is also important

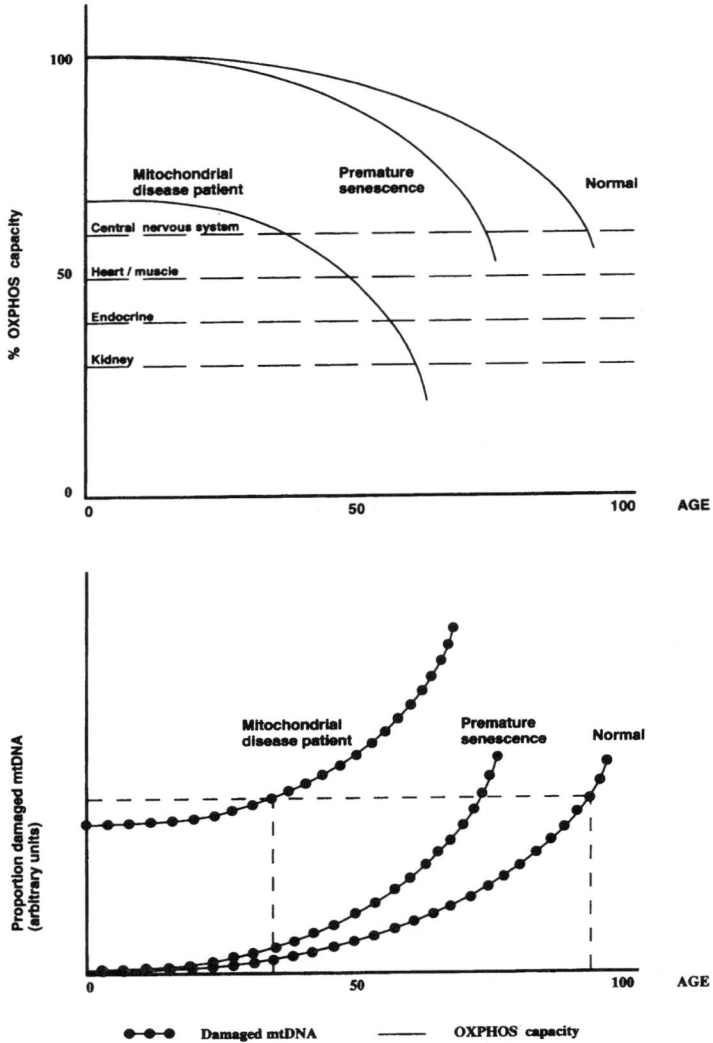

FIGURE 2.32 Hypothesis relating the acquisition of mtDNA mutations (inherited and somatic) to the age-related decline of oxidative phosphorylation (OXPHOS) and the progression of OXPHOS diseases and senescence. The dashed horizontal lines in both panels represent different tissue-specific expression thresholds. The top panel shows the age-related decline of OXPHOS in individuals born with a normal OXPHOS phenotype, a mutant OXPHOS gene, and an increased mtDNA somatic mutation rate. The bottom panel shows the relative levels of defective mtDNA with age for each of these individuals. (Reprinted with permission from the 1994 William Allan Award Address, *Am J Hum Genet* 1995; **57**: 201. Copyright © 1995 by the University of Chicago Press.)

to the expression of mitochondrial function because of accumulation of damage to the mtDNAs, and replication of this damaged mtDNA. Thus, the visual system and brain are affected earliest in mitochondrial disorders because they are most reliant on mitochondrial energy production, followed by heart and skeletal muscle, kidney, endocrine systems, and liver.

Finally, the spontaneous mutation rate of mtDNA is very high compared with nuclear DNA. Thus, the mitochondrial genome has a *sequence evolution rate* (mutation X mutation fixation) that is 10–20 times greater than nuclear genes of similar function, meaning that mtDNA is much more likely to acquire a deleterious mutation. The high mutation rate in mtDNA arises from three factors:

■ About 90 per cent of cellular $O_2$ is consumed by mitochondria in the process of oxidative phosphorylation, and generates free radicals in the matrix that can damage DNA and proteins (see Chapter 9). Defensive systems against oxidative damage consist of enzymes such as superoxide dismutase, glutathione peroxidase, and catalase. However, these mechanisms can be overwhelmed by conditions that generate free radicals, such as chronic infections, degradation of fatty acids by peroxisomes, environmental conditions (smoking), and drugs such as Adriamycin, which target cancer cells by producing reactive $O_2$ species.
■ Mitochondria lack histone proteins, which protect nuclear DNA.
■ Mitochondria lack the efficient enzyme systems for repair and proofreading of mtDNA that the nucleus has. Thus, over time and with repeated oxidative stress, extensive oxidative damage accumulates in mtDNA that is unrepaired.

Clearly, the impact of a mtDNA mutation depends both upon when the mutation occurred in the individual life-cycle and where it occurred in the mitochondrial genome. Mutations transmitted through the maternal germ-line can be either neutral (causing no disease) or deleterious. Obviously, mutations that are neutral or mildly deleterious will have a long female lineage, as high as tens of thousands of years, and can reach very high levels of mutated mtDNA (homoplasmy) before the appearance of a disease phenotype. Moderately severe, or very severe, mutations cause disease making their lineage recent and their mtDNA content heteroplasmic: progeny are eliminated by natural selection. The effect of somatic mutations in mtDNA depends upon multiple factors: type of mutations, tissue(s) in which they occur, and age at which they occur. For example, repeated ischemic or anoxic insults, such as in the coronary blood supply of smokers, generate free radicals that damage mtDNA. Over time, these mitochondria accumulate, cardiac function suffers, and the cycle is accelerated.

## DISEASES OF IMPAIRED MITOCHONDRIAL FUNCTION

From the foregoing discussions two points should be clear.

■ The process of energy production is detailed, involving hundreds of steps and proteins. Multiple processes must be coordinately regulated by two separate genomes, and disordered mitochondrial function can arise from defects in either the *mitochondrial* or the *nuclear DNAs*. Thus, the opportunity for biochemical misadventure is great; however, relatively few known diseases are the result of mitochondrial dysfunction.
■ Many components of mitochondrial biogenesis and function have not been well studied or characterized, and thus, the reagents necessary to define and determine the etiology of a disease at a basic level are lacking. An example would be the multistep process of targeting nuclearly encoded proteins to mitochondria, and their translocation across the mitochondrial membranes. Whereas many of the genes and steps for this process have been discovered in simple organisms, the homologous genes, proteins, and processes have yet to be isolated in humans and may well be associated with a disease phenotype if impaired.

## Defects of the mitochondrial genome

Defects in the mitochondrial genome fall into three classes (Table 2.4).

### Missense mutations

*Missense mutations* are point mutations in the mtDNA that alter polypeptide genes by creating amino acid substitutions, and can be associated with multiorgan dysfunction. Two of the best studied examples of this are *Leber hereditary optic neuropathy* (LHON), and *neurogenic muscle weakness, ataxia, and retinitis pigmentosa* (NARP) in association with *Leigh syndrome*. LHON is a syndrome of male predominance, maternally inherited, adult-onset blindness (central), and has cardiac conduction defects consisting of arrhythmias and heart block, and results from single base substitutions of the OXPHOS complex I, primarily in the mtDNA ND4 gene. Two missense mutations have been identified in the mtDNA ATP6 gene (complex V: proton-translocating ATP synthase) producing NARP and Leigh syndrome phenotypes, which present in childhood. Both mutations convert a highly conserved leucine to either arginine or proline. Both are highly pathogenic heteroplasmic mutations generating a broad spectrum of symptoms and reduced reproductive fitness.

TABLE 2.4 Summary of the phenotypes resulting from defects in oxidative phosphorylation (OXPHOS) (*see* Figure 2.30 for location of mutations in the mitochondrial DNA)

*Missense mutations*

Leber hereditary optic neuropathy (LHON): ND4 gene of Complex I affected
Neurogenic muscle weakness, ataxia, and retinitis pigmentosa (NARP): ATP6 gene of Complex V affected
Leigh disease: subacute necrotizing encephalomyelopathy; a severe expression of the ATP6 defect in Complex V

*Protein synthesis mutations*

Myoclonic epilepsy and ragged-red fibers (MERFF): primarily Complexes I and IV affected
Mitochondrial encephalomyopathy, lactic acidosis, and stroke-like symptoms (MELAS): Complex I enzymes affected
Maternally inherited myopathy and cardiomyopathy (MMC): combined Complex I and IV defects with both infantile, and adult patterns of onset
Lethal infantile mitochondrial myopathy (LIMM): preliminary evidence suggests the tRNA$^{ile}$ gene at bp 4317, and a second defect at tRNA$^{thr}$ may cause this fatal defect
Ocular myopathy associated with ptosis, ophthalmoplegia, and mitochondrial myopathy: occasional patients harbor mutations in tRNA$^{lys}$ (bp 8334), tRNA$^{leu}$ (bp 3242), tRNA$^{ser}$ (bp 12246), tRNA$^{leu}$ (bp 12308), and tRNA$^{gly}$ (bp 10006)

*Deletion/duplication mutations*

Kearns–Sayre syndrome (KSS): age at onset less than 20 years; mitochondrial genome duplications also described
Chronic progressive external ophthalmoplegia (CPEO): age of onset greater than 20 years; both KSS and CPEO involve loss of 9 per cent to 50 per cent of the mitochondrial genome; deletions usually 5 kb, or 7 kb, in size; CPEO PLUS when other organ systems involved
Pearson marrow/pancreas syndrome: deletions are sporadic within pedigrees
Diabetes mellitus (DM) and deafness: maternally inherited early deafness, and late-onset Type II DM with strokes; 10.4-kb deletion with defects in Complexes I, III, and IV
Malignant migraines and strokes: 5-kb mtDNA deletion with childhood onset of migraines; Complexes I, III, and IV affected

## Protein synthesis mutations

*Protein synthesis mutations* are point mutations in the mtDNA that create mutant tRNAs: mitochondria are unable to translate their own genes. These defects tend to have more systemic phenotypic consequences than do the missense mutations. Nearly 30 mutations have been described in the tRNA and rRNA genes, and 11 of these are in the tRNA$^{Leu(UUR)}$ gene. Their clinical phenotypes vary from severe to mild. However, because the moderate and severe protein synthesis mutations cause severe symptoms in childhood, they, like the NARP missense mutations, reduce reproductive fitness of the affected individuals, making most of these mutations heteroplasmic. The milder protein synthesis mutations frequently do not appear until after reproductive age; thus, these mutations are often homoplasmic and are maintained in the population for many generations.

*Cardiomyopathies* frequently are associated with oxidative phosphorylation defects, including protein synthesis mutations, and are most often hypertrophic with decreased function. A second clinical feature commonly associated with protein synthesis mutations is a delayed onset of symptoms and progression over time. *Myoclonic epilepsy and ragged-red fiber disease* (MERRF) produces epilepsy, hearing loss, dementia, renal failure, and a dilated cardiomyopathy, and presents in adults both during and after reproductive years, making for large pedigrees with a high (85–95 per cent) percentage of mutant mtDNA. In most pedigrees, the mutation is at bp 8344 altering tRNA$^{lys}$. This primarily affects complexes I and IV of the oxidative phosphorylation pathway, and the enzyme defect is directly proportional to the severity of the disease consistent with the threshold theory. *Maternally inherited myopathy and cardiomyopathy* (MMC) is associated with both dilated and hypertrophic cardiomyopathies, and is caused by a mutation at bp 3260 (tRNA$^{leu}$) of the mtDNA. This affects both complex I and IV of the oxidative phosphorylation pathway. Patients with *mitochondrial encephalomyopathy, lactic acidosis, and reversible stroke-like symptoms* (MELAS) primarily have a mutation at bp 3243 altering tRNA$^{leu}$. Complex I enzymes of the oxidative phosphorylation pathway are affected. Severely affected patients may have strokes, hypertrophic cardiomyopathy and renal failure; adults may present with milder symptoms (neurosensory hearing loss and adult-onset diabetes) if they have lower percentages of mutant mtDNA. Between 1 and 3 per cent of all *type II diabetes* is the result of the bp 3243 mutation. Finally, *lethal infantile mitochondrial myopathy* (LIMM) represents a heterogeneous group of tRNA mutations associated with severe lactic acidosis, hypotonia and neurological deficits, cardiomyopathy, ragged red fibers on histology, and death in the first year. One case was associated with a mutation in the tRNA$^{ile}$ gene at bp 4317, but other cases have not been well characterized.

Thus, all protein synthesis mutations have been associated with tRNA mutations, and have a characteristic phenotype that is associated with mitochondrial myopathies: ragged red fibers and abnormal mitochondria on histology. The age at presentation is generally somewhat older than early childhood, and the clinical symptoms involve many organ systems.

## Deletion/insertion defects

*Deletion/insertion defects* are mutations that rearrange the mitochondrial genome. Over 100 such defects in the mtDNA have been associated with degenerative diseases of mitochondria, of which the majority are deletions. Deletion defects are almost always spontaneous, with no family history, suggesting that most of these defects are new mutations occurring during development; thus, different tissues will have differing burdens of mutant mtDNA. Diseases associated with deletions usually progress with age, and symptoms are proportional to the accumulation of deleted mtDNAs. This is in distinct contrast to the point mutations where age and other undefined factors influence the expression of the mtDNA defects. Thus, the clinical phenotypes in deletion defects can be quite variable and reflect the chance distribution of the deleted mitochondrial genomes among various tissues through replicative segregation.

Mitochondrial genome rearrangements fall into three clinical phenotypes.

- *Pearson marrow/pancreas syndrome* is a generally fatal disease of childhood with the findings of pancytopenia, splenic atrophy, and pancreatic fibrosis. Accumulation of rearranged mtDNA in the bone-marrow cells results in loss of blood-forming elements and early death. The most common deletion defect removes about 5000 bp of the mitochondrial genome, although mtDNA duplications also occur. Some patients survive and progress to a mitochondrial myopathy (KSS) presumably because the marrow repopulates with stem cells containing normal mtDNA.

- The ocular phenotypes, which include *Kearns–Sayre syndrome* (KSS) and *chronic progressive external ophthalmoplegia* (CPEO), have the prominent features of ophthalmoplegia and ptosis, along with a mitochondrial myopathy that includes the ragged red fibers typical of mtDNA defects. Both tend to have multisystem involvement; however, the age at onset is different. Both are caused by mtDNA deletions probably occurring during embryogenesis: 80 per cent of KSS, 70 per cent of CPEO PLUS, and 40 per cent of CPEO patients have deletions of mtDNA, while the rest most likely represent point mutations of the mtDNA. These deletions can remove 9–50 per cent of the mitochondrial genome, and are heteroplasmic. Duplications of the mtDNA have also been described, and are clinically indistinguishable from the deletion defects.

- *Maternally inherited diabetes and deafness* presents with sensory neural hearing loss appearing as early as childhood to early twenties, and type II diabetes mellitus occurring between 20 and 40 years of age. Patients also may experience strokes. In contrast to type I diabetes mellitus, which usually appears in childhood, type II diabetes mellitus appears much later in life, is ketoacidosis-resistant, and often is associated with obesity. Evaluation of one large pedigree revealed a large, 10.4-kb heteroplasmic deletion from the mtDNA, and maternal relatives had a 6.1-kb tandem insertion (duplication) in their heteroplasmic mtDNA. Skeletal muscle biopsy showed no evidence of mitochondrial myopathy, but oxidative phosphorylation biochemistry of these mitochondria demonstrated severe defects in complexes I, III, and IV. Thus, this pedigree represented a heteroplasmic, trimolecular defect of mtDNA involving normal, deleted, and duplicated mtDNA. Epidemiology of type II diabetic patients older than 25 years indicates a three- to four-fold increase in maternal transmission of disease, suggesting the possibility that mitochondrial mutations may be an important cause of late-onset diabetes mellitus.

Finally, it should be noted that mitochondrial deletions (e.g. a heteroplasmic 5-kb mtDNA deletion) have been described in which the initial symptoms were neurological, i.e. migraine headaches and strokes, with no evidence of muscle weakness. Migraines and strokes are also features of the mitochondrial point mutations (see above), but the presence of the myopathy helps guide diagnosis towards a mitochondrial defect. Thus, patients with malignant migraines should be considered as possibly having oxidative phosphorylation defects, even if classical findings of myopathy associated with mitochondrial defects are absent. A family history of maternal transmission of migraine headaches would suggest including oxidative phosphorylation defects in the evaluation.

# Defects in nuclearly encoded mitochondrial proteins

As noted above, the mitochondrial genome encodes only a few of the hundreds of proteins found in mitochondria; the rest are encoded in the nuclear genome. Defects in nuclear genes have mendelian characteristics of inheritance, and many single-gene defects have been described for the multiple steps of energy generation. This includes the four major components of oxidative phosphorylation: (1) glycolysis, (2) β-oxidation of fatty acids, (3) the citric acid cycle, and (4) the electron transport chain (respiratory chain). Of these, components (2)–(4) occur within mitochondria, and all four have disease phenotypes associated with biochemical defects. Defects in glycolysis and the production of pyruvate are not discussed in this section because this is a cytosolic process. Obviously, many other defects in mitochondrial function have been described, and many other disease associations will be made as new understanding and reagents become available, e.g. targeting and translocations of proteins into mitochondria.

## β-Oxidation of fatty acids

Inborn errors of the enzymes and transport proteins involved in the β-oxidation of fatty acids are among the most common of the inherited metabolic diseases, with an estimated incidence from 1 in 10 000 to 1 in 15 000 live births. At least 15 proteins directly involved in this process have been identified as having defects producing disease in humans (Fig. 2.31). Fatty acids are the primary source of energy for the heart, and defects in the enzymes of the β-oxidation spiral have been associated with cardiomyopathy and sudden death in childhood, including *sudden infant death syndrome* (SIDS).

*Medium-chain acyl CoA dehydrogenase* (MCAD) deficiency is the most common defect in the β-oxidation pathway, and is associated with familial SIDS and cardiomyopathy (Fig. 2.31). MCAD acts on a broad range of acyl CoA compounds from 4 to 12 carbons in length, and about 80 per cent of patients are homozygous for a single point mutation in the nuclear gene (A985G). MCAD is a rate-limiting enzyme of the β-oxidation spiral with overlapping substrate specificities that catalyze the first step in the β-oxidation processing of fatty acids. If blocked, patients are unable to metabolize fats adequately for energy in the heart, or for production of ketones by the liver, which brain and muscle can utilize as fuel: glucose becomes the main fuel source in these patients. Liver is the only tissue that can channel the product of β-oxidation (acetyl CoA) into ketone body formation. This process provides an alternative fuel substrate for brain oxidative metabolism, preventing proteolysis and sparing glucose oxidation. The intermediary metabolites resulting from this block, such as long-chain acylcarnitines, may be toxic to myocardium (arrhythmogenic), resulting in death or cardiomyopathy. Thus, an episode of decreased caloric intake resulting in low serum glucose, such as vomiting from a viral gastroenteritis, can progress rapidly to liver failure, coma, and death. Clinically, MCAD deficiency typically presents in the child less than 2 years of age as *hypoketotic hypoglycemia*, and can be confused with Reye syndrome. Thus, both an inherited defect in fatty acid oxidation, and a triggering event, such as hypoglycemia, are necessary for expression of the disease.

Other inherited defects in the enzymes of fatty acid oxidation have been described. These include long-chain acyl CoA dehydrogenase (LCAD), short-chain acyl CoA dehydrogenase (SCAD), very-long-chain acyl CoA dehydrogenase (VLCAD), and long-chain 3-hydroxyacyl-CoA dehydrogenase (LCHAD). Manifestations of the acyl CoA dehydrogenase (AD) deficiencies include a Reye-like syndrome with hypoglycemia, fatty liver, coma, and death. Cardiomyopathies, either dilated or hypertrophic, and skeletal myopathies are also associated with the AD deficiencies. Unexplained sudden death following a viral illness is the presenting sign in as many as 25 per cent of cases of MCAD deficiency, usually in the first 2 years of life. A *family history* of sudden death, episodes of hypoglycemia and lethargy, and elevations of transaminases and prothrombin time all favor the diagnosis of fatty acid oxidation defects. The diagnosis can be determined biochemically by measuring plasma and urinary intermediary metabolites, such as dicarboxylic acids (a general indication of disordered β-oxidation), and specific metabolites that accumulate proximal to the block in the metabolic pathway. If an AD deficiency is suspected, other family members can be screened using the techniques of molecular biology to identify the mutation. The inheritance of the AD deficiencies is autosomal recessive. Avoidance of hypoglycemia can prevent the serious and fatal outcome of this disease.

## The carnitine cycle

The carnitine cycle (Fig. 2.31) (*see also* page 150) is required for the transport of long-chain fatty acids into the mitochondrial matrix, and has four components:

- a plasma membrane carnitine uptake transporter (CU) that functions to maintain a high intracellular level of carnitine;
- carnitine palmitoyltransferase I (CPT I) in the outer mitochondrial membrane, which converts acyl-CoA compounds to their acylcarnitine analogues;
- carnitine/acylcarnitine translocase (CT) in the inner mitochondrial membrane, which facilitates the exchange of carnitine and acylcarnitines across the inner membrane;
- carnitine palmitoyltransferase II (CPT II) located on the matrix side of the inner mitochondrial membrane, which functions in reesterification of acylcarnitines to acyl-CoA esters for the β-oxidation spiral.

Fatty acids less than 10 carbons in length traverse the mitochondrial membrane as free acids without the need for transport systems.

Defects in the *CU transporter* have two clinical scenarios: about half present early in life (3 mo to 2.5 yr) with episodes of hypoketotic hypoglycemia, hyperammonemia, elevated transaminases, and some with cardio- or skeletal myopathies. The other half present with isolated, progressive cardiomyopathies (dilated) and skeletal muscle weakness, with an onset later in childhood (1–7 years). They will have very low plasma carnitine concentration secondary to carnitine wasting by the kidneys, and no significant dicarboxylic aciduria. Treatment with oral L-carnitine is effective.

Defects in *CPT I* are associated with a fasting illness (diarrhea, viral gastroenteritis). Symptoms include coma, hepatomegaly, seizures, and hypoketotic hypoglycemia with normal plasma carnitine concentrations presenting during infancy to 2 years of age. Cardiomyopathies and skeletal muscle weakness are not part of the presentation. Because the patients cannot transport long-chain fatty acids into mitochondria, the treatment is based on a diet rich in medium-chain triglycerides (MCT oil), which readily traverse the mitochondrial membranes as free fatty acids.

Deficiency of *carnitine/acylcarnitine translocase* (CT) has been described once.

Deficiency of *CPT II* has two distinct clinical presentations. Classical CPT II deficiency presents in male adults with exercise or fasting-induced myoglobinuria and muscle weakness. A second form of CPT II deficiency occurs in infancy, is severe and usually fatal, presenting with hypoketotic hypoglycemia, coma, seizures, hepatomegaly, skeletal muscle myopathy, and cardiomegaly with arrhythmias. Urinary dicarboxylic acids are low, as are plasma and serum carnitine concentrations, of which the long-chain acylcarnitine fraction is elevated. Diagnosis is made by demonstration of decreased CPT II activity in fibroblasts. Because of the defect, long-chain acylcarnitines are translocated across the inner mitochondrial membrane, but cannot be efficiently converted to their acyl-CoA analogues. Accumulation of long-chain acylcarnitines in the matrix may produce cardiac arrhythmias.

## Defects of nuclear encoded OXPHOS genes

Very few defects of nuclear genes encoding the large number of proteins of the oxidative phosphorylation pathway, i.e. the TCA cycle and the respiratory chain, have been identified and characterized. This is most likely due to the extreme lethality that complete defects would present with subsequent fetal demise *in utero*. Consequently, most defects will probably be "leaky" and compatible with life, making them hard to detect.

*Glutaric acidemia type II*, or multiple acyl-CoA dehydrogenation deficiency, is an autosomal recessive deficiency of the oxidative phosphorylation pathway as a result of deficiency of either electron transfer flavoprotein (ETF), or electron transfer flavoprotein-ubiquinone oxidoreductase (ETF-QO). Both ETF and ETF-QO are encoded by separate nuclear genes, and function to transfer electrons from the flavin-containing acyl CoA dehydrogenases, such as LCAD, MCAD, SCAD, and VLCAD in β-oxidation of fatty acids, to the electron transport chain. Complete deficiencies of ETF or ETF-QO are associated with hypoketotic hypoglycemia, severe metabolic acidosis, and fatty degeneration of liver parenchymal cells, renal tubular epithelium, and myocardium. Biochemically, the metabolites of compounds oxidized by enzymes that transfer electrons to ETF/ETF-QO accumulate in tissues.

Glutaric acidemia type II has three classical presentations. Multiple acyl CoA dehydrogenase deficiencies presenting in the neonatal period are severe (MADD:S), and can be associated either with prematurity and multiple congenital anomalies, including renal cystic disease and a characteristic dysmorphology, or with the metabolic disorder but without the phenotypic appearance. Most patients presenting in the neonatal period die within the first few months, usually from a severe cardiomyopathy. *Later-onset glutaric acidemia type II* (MADD:M) has a milder course with a longer, adult life-span. Diagnosis is established by the presence of a characteristic organic acid pattern in urine associated with nonketotic hypoglycemia and metabolic acidosis, especially in the newborn period, and by enzyme assays of ETF/ETF-QO in fibroblasts. Treatment of severe phenotype has been unsuccessful, whereas MADD:M has responded to riboflavin, carnitine, and diets low in protein and fats.

## SUMMARY

Mitochondria have multiple functions as a result of their capacity for oxidative phosphorylation: generation of energy in the form of ATP, reoxidation of NADH and $FADH_2$, and regulation of temperature by heat generation. Impairment of these functions reduces both reproductive capacity and survival of the individual. Control of mitochondrial function is complex and involves multiple levels of communication and control between the nuclear and mitochondrial genomes. Defects in the mitochondrial genome can be either neutral or deleterious, and phenotypic expression of defects is heavily influenced by multiple factors: defect type, dosing of mutant mtDNAs, environment, age, and tissue type. Based on biochemical analysis, many of these defects can be diagnosed, and patients counseled and treated. However, many processes that are important to mitochondrial biogenesis are unknown and may represent points that are vital to normal function, yielding disease phenotypes when disturbed. Clearly, much investigative work remains in the elucidation of mitochondrial biogenesis and interaction with its cellular host.

## SELECTED READING

Alberts B, Bray D, Lewis J, Raff M, Roberts K, Watson JD, eds. *Molecular Biology of the Cell*. New York: Garland Publishing, Inc., 1983.

Luft R. The development of mitochondrial medicine *Proc Natl Acad Sci USA* 1994; **91**: 8731.

Scriver CR, Beaudet AL, Sly WS, Valle D, eds. *The Metabolic and Molecular Bases of Inherited Disease*, Vol I. St. Louis: McGraw-Hill, 1995.

Wallace DC. 1994 William Allan Award Address: Mitchondrial DNA variation in human evolution, degenerative disease, and aging. *Am J Hum Genet* 1995; **57**: 201.

# PROTO-ONCOGENES, TUMOR SUPPRESSOR GENES AND GROWTH CONTROL

## OVERVIEW

*Cancer* results from a set of discrete genetic alterations in a single immature cell, and repeated rounds of cell division ultimately lead to a detectable tumor. Human cells express a complex repertoire of genes during the process of cell division and differentiation. A fundamental aspect of cancer cells is that proliferation and differentiation become uncoupled, resulting in deregulated growth. Because the differentiation of muscle cells requires coordinated expression of a set of genes that is distinct from those that are used by a neutrophil, it is not surprising that *rhabdomyosarcomas* (an embryonal neoplasm of early muscle cells) show a molecular "signature" that is distinct from that seen in *myeloid leukemia*. At the same time, it has become increasingly apparent that a small group of genes that play a central role in either stimulating or restraining cell growth are altered in many different types of cancer. Members of this class of genes include the proto-oncogenes *MYC* and *Ras* and the tumor suppressor genes *p53* and *RB1*.

The term "clonal" refers to the fact that almost all cancers arise from a single cell. This initiating cell has a proliferative advantage that eventually results in clonal expansion and, in many cases, inhibition of normal cellular functions as a result of invasion and overgrowth (for example, in *acute leukemia*, replacement of the bone marrow by the malignant blast cells suppresses normal blood cell production). The clonality of cancer cells has been established by a variety of experimental techniques. Not all malignant cells divide rapidly; however, these cells are uniformly unable to respond to the extracellular signals that normally regulate growth and differentiation. Because all of the cancer cells in a given patient are derived from the same malignant precursor, they show similar morphologic, biochemical, and genetic characteristics.

The idea that a particular disorder is "genetic" in origin generally implies that it is transmitted within families. This is true of childhood disorders such as cystic fibrosis, Duchenne-type muscular dystrophy, and hereditary spherocytosis. While some human cancers are heritable genetic disorders, most patients have no known susceptibility to cancer, and malignant transformation results from a series of somatic mutations in a target cell. Cancer is therefore unique in that acquired (somatic) genetic alterations play a major role in its pathogenesis. In some families, the predisposition to develop cancer is transmitted from parent to child, and children with germline mutations of cancer susceptibility genes are at high risk of developing specific malignant tumors. Heritable cases of cancer have been extraordinarily informative in defining genetic mechanisms and in localizing and identifying the responsible genes. In addition, a number of the genes that confer a genetic predisposition to childhood cancer play a central role in normal cellular growth control.

## CLASSES OF CANCER GENES

The genes that are mutated in cancer cells fall within two functional classes: *oncogenes* and *tumor suppressor genes*. General characteristics that distinguish these types of genes are described and contrasted in this section of the chapter. The proto-oncogenes (normal cellular homologues of oncogenes) and tumor suppressors encode proteins that have opposite effects on cell growth.

Proto-oncogenes generally encode proteins that stimulate cell growth and division. Expression of many of these genes correlates with an undifferentiated phenotype. The types of proteins that are encoded by proto-oncogenes include molecules that act as soluble growth factors, growth factor receptors, proteins that transduce proliferative signals from the cell surface to the nucleus, and nuclear proteins that drive cell division by directing transcription of target genes.

Oncogenes are mutated versions of proto-oncogenes and are carried in the genomes of many rapidly-transforming viruses. Somatic mutations or amplification of endogenous cellular proto-oncogenes converts them to oncogenes in human cells. Oncogenic proteins are actively expressed in cancer cells. Oncogene mutations behave as dominant genetic traits in cancer cells (that is, mutation of only one allele is required to deregulate growth). An important feature of oncogenes that has facilitated isolating and characterizing them and their protein products is that they confer a pattern of abnormal growth (or transformation) when they are introduced into non-malignant primary cells or host cell lines. Proto-oncogenes are characteristically altered by cytogenetic translocation and/or amplification in tumor cells.

The adult type of *chronic myeloid leukemia* (CML) is a highly instructive example that illustrates some of the features of oncogenic transformation. A molecular hallmark of this disorder is a characteristic translocation that fuses a gene called *BCR* on chromosome 22 with the gene called *ABL* on chromosome 9. The 9;22 translocation was the first non-random cytogenetic alteration to be associated with a type of human cancer. The finding that the *ABL* gene was altered by the 9;22 translocation was an exciting discovery because a mutated homologue (*v-abl*) had previously been identified in a transforming virus. The translocation involving *BCR* and *ABL* invariably results in the production of a chimeric messenger RNA species which encodes a protein that combines upstream (5′) *BCR* sequences with downstream (3′) *ABL* sequences.

This chimeric Bcr-Abl protein has abnormal biochemical activity in two important respects: (1) it has an enhanced ability to phosphorylate target proteins on tyrosine residues (tyrosine kinase activity), and (2) it directly interacts with proteins that activate signaling through Ras. A plasmid encoding the Bcr-Abl fusion protein was transduced into murine hematopoietic cells to ask if this was capable of transforming cells as a single event. When these transduced cells were transplanted into lethally-irradiated recipient animals, the recipients developed leukemia at high frequency. These data establish that the Bcr-Abl fusion protein plays a primary role in malignant transformation. Ironically, recent evidence suggests that the wild-type Abl protein normally functions to suppress growth.

The genetics and function of tumor suppressor genes are opposite to those of the proto-oncogenes in many respects. Proteins encoded by tumor suppressor genes negatively regulate cell growth and stimulate differentiation. Tumor suppressor alterations behave as recessive genetic traits in cancer cells (that is, inactivation of both alleles is required to deregulate growth). The proteins encoded by these genes negatively regulate cell growth, and they therefore do not induce transformation when introduced into non-malignant cell lines. Furthermore, because loss of function is critical for the growth of cancer cells, inactivation of tumor suppressor genes eliminates RNA and protein expression in cancer cells. Chromosomal deletions are the cytogenetic hallmark of mutations that affect tumor suppressor genes in cancer cells.

Germline mutations of tumor suppressor genes account for almost all of the known inherited cancer predispositions. According to the Knudson model, these individuals are at markedly increased risk of cancer because all of their somatic cells have one inactive copy of the target gene ("first hit"). This model is summarized in Fig. 2.33. An acquired mutation of the remaining normal allele in any susceptible cell ("second hit") inactivates the tumor suppressor function and contributes to the development of cancer. Thus, the Knudson model postulates that both alleles of tumor suppressor genes must be inactivated by separate events during tumorigenesis. Because every somatic cell contains the first hit, patients with germline mutations of tumor suppressor genes develop cancer at a relatively young age and are prone to multiple independent tumors. Although loss of growth control is recessive at the cellular level, the cancer predisposition is transmitted as a dominant trait. Offspring have a 50 per cent chance of inheriting the predisposing mutant allele from an affected parent. Because every cell has already sustained one inactivating mutation, a "second hit" is likely to occur in one cell from this relatively large population of susceptible target cells. The Knudson model also correctly predicted that the same tumor suppressor genes would be involved in the pathogenesis of non-familial cases of cancer. In these patients, both copies of the tumor suppressor gene are affected by independent acquired mutational events.

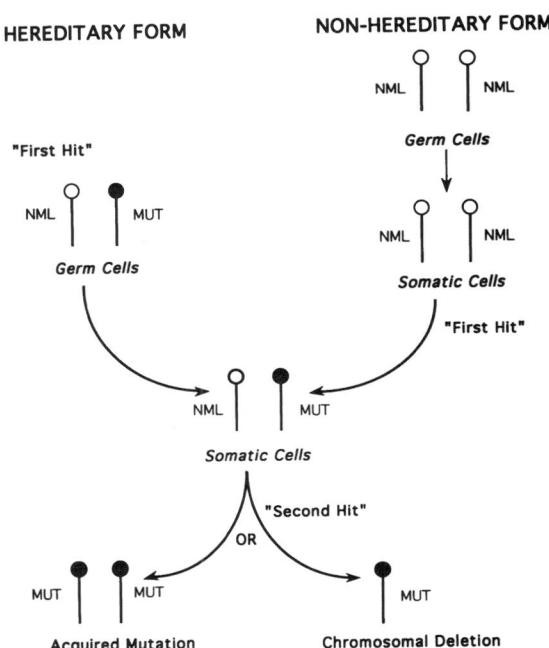

FIGURE 2.33 The Knudson hypothesis. Predisposition to cancer is conferred by a mutation in one allele of a tumor suppressor gene: a "first hit." In hereditary forms of cancer due to mutations in tumor suppressor genes, the "first hit" is present in the germline, and hence is passed to offspring in an autosomal dominant manner. In non-hereditary forms, the disabling mutation occurs in the tissue type responsible for the tumor and the germ line is unaffected. In either case, a subsequent mutation or "second hit" is required in the somatic cell to produce transformation. The second mutation can be either a nonsense mutation or a deletion of the tumor suppressor gene. (Reprinted with permission from Rudolph AM, ed. *Pediatrics*, 20th edn. Copyright © 1995 by Appleton & Lange.)

Inactivation of tumor suppressor genes occurs by a variety of genetic mechanisms including structural deletions, point mutations, or gene conversion.

The malignant eye tumor *retinoblastoma* is a landmark example of a genetic cancer predisposition that involves loss of function of a tumor suppressor gene. The predisposition to cancer is inherited in a dominant fashion in some kindreds; in an occasional family, the individuals at risk of developing retinoblastoma also carry a small interstitial deletion of chromosome 13. These data are provocative because cytogenetic analysis of both familial and non-familial retinoblastoma cells frequently demonstrate acquired deletions of the same region of chromosome 13. Molecular genetic analysis confirmed that many retinoblastomas without visible cytogenetic deletions nevertheless show allelic losses in the same area of chromosome 13. This region was narrowed down by mapping the extent of the genetic deletions present in multiple individuals and determining where these overlapped. A gene called *RB1* was ultimately isolated. Biochemical investigation of the Rb protein has shown that its phosphorylation status plays a central role in regulating the cell cycle—loss of this critical "checkpoint" allows cells to proceed through DNA synthesis and mitosis in an unregulated manner.

The identification of tumor suppressor genes has been problematic because of their biologic features. In particular, it is technically much more straightforward to characterize the dominant mutations that activate proto-oncogenes than it is to find genes that show loss of function during tumorigenesis. For this reason, most of the existing tumor suppressor genes were identified by "reverse genetics" (that is, their protein products were only known after the gene was cloned by ascertaining the position of the gene by linkage and microdeletion analysis). Long-range mapping technologies such as yeast artificial chromosomes and pulse-field gel electrophoresis have facilitated the search for tumor suppressor genes. Once in hand, the technique of targeted homologous recombination into murine embryonic stem (ES) cells has proven invaluable in characterizing how tumor suppressor genes function in both normal development and in tumorigenesis. Studies of these "knockout" mice have shown that a number of tumor suppressor genes are absolutely required for intrauterine development. For example, homozygous inactivation of the murine *Rb1* gene is an embryonic lethal because of erythropoietic failure while disruption of the neurofibromatosis type 1 (*NF1*) tumor suppressor gene causes complex cardiac anomalies. These defects were unanticipated inasmuch as children with *RB1* mutations are predisposed to eye tumors while those with neurofibromatosis develop neural crest neoplasia and myeloid leukemia.

## MULTISTEP MODELS OF HUMAN CANCER

Fortunately for all of us, the development of the common human cancers requires alterations of multiple genes. While inactivation of *RB1* may be both necessary and sufficient for the development of malignant eye tumors, this circumstance is atypical. Experimental data and clinical experience suggest that alterations of other genes cooperate with germline mutations of tumor suppressors to induce full malignant transformation. This paradigm has been most clearly established for colon cancer, where mutations of the tumor suppressors *APC*, *DCC*, and *p53* and of the proto-oncogene *RAS* all participate in tumorigenesis.

## Leukemia in children with *Neurofibromatosis type 1* (NF1): Clinical features, genetics, and biochemistry

The predisposition to *myeloid leukemia* among children with NF1 is an instructive example of some of the principles discussed above. Although fewer than 1 per cent of children with NF1 develop leukemia, this

incidence is 200–500 fold above that in the general population. When the *NF1* gene was cloned in 1990, a computer-assisted search of existing genomic databases showed that it shared DNA sequence homology with a GTPase-activating protein (GAP) for RAS. This was an extraordinary observation because proteins encoded by the p21$^{ras}$ (*RAS*) family of proto-oncogenes play a central role in the control of cellular growth by cycling between an active guanosine triphosphate (GTP)-bound state (Ras-GTP) and an inactive guanosine diphosphate (GDP)-bound state (Ras-GDP) (Fig. 2.34). *RAS* genes commonly acquire activating point mutations during the development of human cancer which perturb the biochemical activity of Ras proteins by elevating the level of Ras-GTP. This occurs, at least in part, because mutated RAS proteins no longer respond to negative regulation by GAPs. GAPs normally control the biologic activity of Ras proteins by accelerating GTP hydrolysis, thereby "switching" Ras to its inactive, GDP-bound conformation. Activating *RAS* mutations are very common in most types of myeloid leukemia. Because many hematopoietic growth factors stimulate cell growth by activating Ras proteins, it has been hypothesized that the effect of *RAS* mutations in hematopoieitc cells is to allow them to proliferate autonomously (in the absence of growth factor stimulation). All of the above suggested that *NF1* functioned as a tumor

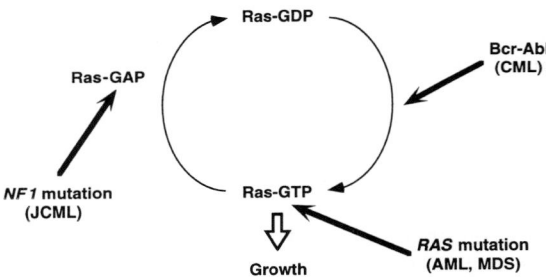

FIGURE 2.34 The role of *RAS* in myeloid leukemia. The Ras protein is cycled between a growth-promoting GTP-bound form and an inactive GDP-bound form. Three different kinds of mutations appear to produce myeloid leukemias by activation of Ras. First, acquired mutations of the *RAS* gene may activate the *RAS* protein directly, leading to uncontrolled growth. These somatic mutations must affect only one allele and thus exert a dominant effect. Second, the mutant Bcr-Abl fusion protein may stimulate conversion of Ras to its GTP-bound form. This mutation is also a dominant cellular mutant. Finally, mutations leading to inactivation of *NF1* will diminish cycling of Ras to its inactive GDP-bound form. This mechanism must involve inactivation of both *NF1* alleles, and hence its cellular effect is recessive. (GTP = guanosine triphosphate; GDP = guanosine diphosphate; GAP = GTPase-activating protein; NF1 = neurofibromatosis type 1; CML = chronic myeloid leukemia; AML = acute myeloid leukemia; MDS = myelodysplastic syndrome; JCML = juvenile chronic myelogenous leukemia.)

suppressor gene in myeloid cells and offered a testable experimental model. If *NF1* is acting as a tumor suppressor gene, careful genetic analysis should demonstrate loss of the normal copy of *NF1* in many leukemias. This proved to be true. In addition, if loss of *NF1* function were sufficient to deregulate the biochemical activity of Ras proteins, the leukemias of children with NF1 would not be expected to show activating *RAS* mutations. This has also been shown. Like children with NF1, mice that are heterozygous for a disrupted allele of *NF1* are predisposed to myeloid leukemia. It thus appears that the protein encoded by the *NF1* tumor suppressor gene negatively regulates the growth of immature myeloid cells through its biochemical effect on the protein encoded by the *RAS* proto-oncogene. It thus appears that the Ras signaling pathway can be deregulated by three independent genetic mechanisms during the development of myeloid leukemia: (1) production of the chimeric Bcr-Abl protein; (2) activating point mutations of the *RAS* proto-oncogenes; and, (3) loss of *NF1* function (summarized in Fig. 2.34). All result in elevated levels of Ras-GTP. These observations emphasize that the Ras deregulation plays a central (and perhaps essential) role in myeloid leukemogenesis.

## APOPTOSIS

While it has been clear for over a decade that the interplay between tumor suppressor and proto-oncogene products influence how cells "decide" to divide and differentiate, the important role of apoptosis in human cancer has emerged more recently (*see also* page 100).

Apoptosis, or programmed cell death, refers to an active process by which cells are eliminated from the body. This process is important in regulating both lymphoid development and the size of hematopoietic progenitor cell pools. Apoptosis may be activated by exposure to radiation or by other types of cellular injury. Recent data have shown that this response is mediated through the p53 protein in some cells. Inhibition of apoptosis in lymphoma cells results from activation of the *BCL-2* proto-oncogene by translocation in some lymphomas. This provides direct evidence that suppression of apoptosis may contribute to cancer development by providing the abnormal clone with a survival advantage.

## GENOMIC IMPRINTING AND GENE DOSAGE

If the simple genetic principles described by Mendel were applicable in all cases, various combinations of dominant oncogenic and recessive tumor suppressor mutations would act together to induce all human cancers. Most inherited predispositions are explained by the Knudson model (dominant inheritance) or by a simple recessive mechanism (e.g. in patients with *Fanconi anemia*). However, recent observations in children who are predisposed to some types of cancer show that these disorders sometimes do not follow Mendelian inheritance or conform to the Knudson model. It has become clear that the function of some genes depends on whether they were inherited from the mother or father. The term "genomic imprinting" refers to these differences in gene activities that are specific to the parent-of-origin.

*Wilms tumor* is the best example of how imprinting plays a role in the development of cancer. The dominant mode of inheritance, and the observation that the risk of Wilms tumor co-inherits with a small deletion of chromosome 11 in some families, suggested that a tumor suppressor gene was located in this region. Indeed, molecular investigation with probes from chromosome 11 demonstrated frequent loss of one copy of this region in tumors removed from children who had the common, non-familial form of Wilms tumor, and a tumor suppressor gene called *WT1* was cloned from this segment. However, when chromosome 11 losses occur in non-familial cases of Wilms tumor, the mother's chromosome is lost in about 90 per cent of tumors. This is unexpected as the Knudson model predicts no difference between the mother's and father's DNA with respect to the frequency of acquired mutations or deletions. The most likely reason that maternal alleles are lost preferentially from sporadic Wilms tumors is that the mother's chromosome is essential to regulate growth properly and that some critical gene (or genes) in this region of the father's chromosome is normally "turned off" (imprinted).

Additional evidence for the importance of genomic imprinting in this region of chromosome 11 comes from studies of children with *Beckwith–Wiedemann syndrome*, many of whom have a duplication of their father's genes and loss of the mother's DNA. Children with Beckwith–Wiedemann syndrome are at high risk of developing Wilms tumor, probably because they lack an active maternal copy of a tumor suppressor gene (or genes) located in the imprinted region of chromosome 11.

Children with *Down syndrome* are at increased risk of developing leukemia and also commonly show a transient leukemia-like disorder in infancy. In addition, acquired trisomies of various chromosomes occur nonrandomly in certain human cancers. These findings suggest that over-expression of certain genes is important in some cancers. There is no direct evidence that loss of a single copy of any autosomal gene deregulates growth in cancer cells. Proving the existence of dosage loss will be challenging because both inactivation due to imprinting or the presence of a new tumor suppressor gene in the same chromosomal region are plausible alternative explanations.

## RECESSIVE GENETIC DISEASES ASSOCIATED WITH CHILDHOOD CANCER

*Ataxia-telangiectasia, xeroderma pigmentosa, Bloom syndrome*, and *Fanconi anemia* are inherited disorders that are associated with a high risk of childhood cancer. Genetic instability is a cardinal feature of all of these syndromes and excessive rates of cellular death and/or cytogenetic rearrangements are observed either spontaneously or after exposure to agents that damage DNA. Although all of these conditions appear to result from loss of function of the gene in question, they are not generally classified as tumor suppressors because people with only one abnormal copy of these genes do not show an obvious cancer predisposition. Cancer susceptibility is inherited as a mendelian recessive trait.

## IMPLICATIONS BEYOND CANCER RESEARCH

Cancer cells embody how normal patterns of proliferation, differentiation, and death are subverted. As such, they provide a unique experimental system for characterizing the genes that are crucial for these functions in normal cells and for dissecting the relevant biochemical pathways. While studies of cancer initially called attention to genes such as *RB1, Ras*, and *p53*, perhaps the most interesting aspect is how the proteins they encode regulate the growth of normal cells. Inactivation of a number of tumor suppressor genes has unanticipated effects on murine fetal development. These data, in turn, implicate the encoded proteins as critical in a variety of developmental processes. Similarly, the burgeoning interest in the role of apoptosis in cancer (see later) raises novel questions about the normal physiologic role of this process. Apoptosis is likely to be particularly important during embryonic and fetal life when there are profound changes in developing tissues throughout the body.

## SELECTED READING

Aaronson SA. Growth factors and cancer. *Science* 1991; **254**: 1146.

Friend SH, Dryja TP, Weinberg RA. Oncogenes and tumor suppressing genes. *N Engl J Med* 1988; **318**: 618.

Knudson AG. All in the (cancer) family. *Nature Genet* 1993; **5**: 103.

Shannon K.M. The Ras signaling pathway and the molecular basis of myeloid leukemogenesis. *Curr Opin Hematol* 1995; **2**: 305.

Solomon E, Borrow J, Goddard A. Chromosome aberrations and cancer. *Science* 1991; **254**: 1153.

Weinberg RA. Tumor suppressor genes. *Science* 1991; **254**: 1138.

# THE CELL CYCLE

## THE CYCLE

### See also Chapter 18

The most basic of biological functions is reproduction. Eukaryotic somatic cells reproduce by division into two similar daughter cells in a process called *mitosis*. In a continuously dividing population of cells, the steps required for cell division, such as replication of the DNA, occur in a highly regulated, coordinated way. The cycling of cells from one round of division to the next is divided into four segments based on the content of DNA (Fig. 2.35). During *S (synthesis) phase*, DNA is being replicated. At *M phase (mitosis)* the cell splits in two so that the DNA content per cell halves from 4N to 2N (diploid). The S and M phases are separated by two G (gap) phases during which the content of DNA does not change. During $G_1$ the enzymes necessary for DNA replication must be synthesized, and during $G_2$ mitotic apparatus such as the spindle must be prepared.

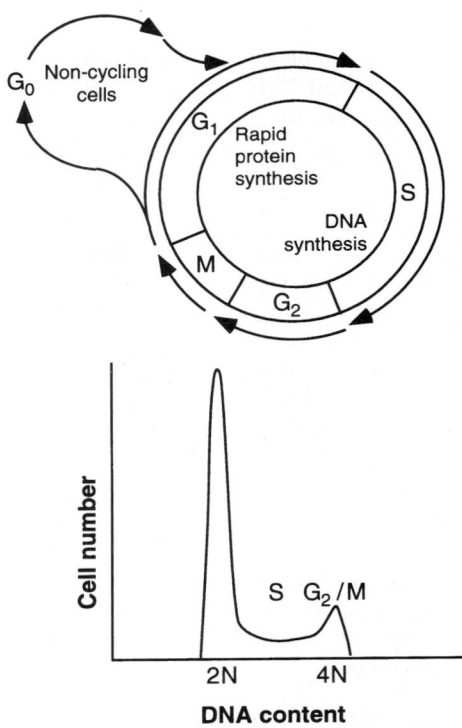

FIGURE 2.35 When cycling, cells pass through $G_1$, S, $G_2$ and M phases. Most cells in the body are not actively cycling, and are said to be in $G_0$. The DNA content of a resting, $G_0$ cell is diploid (2N). In $G_1$ phase the cell produces many of the enzymes needed for DNA synthesis. During S phase the DNA is being replicated, so the DNA content increases to 4N. During $G_2$ and M phase the DNA content is 4N, and is reduced to 2N again once mitosis has occurred.

Most of the cells in the body are not cycling, but exist in a quiescent, non-proliferating state termed $G_0$. In $G_0$ cells remain viable and metabolically active, performing the required tissue-specific functions for an extended period. Many $G_0$ cells retain the ability to re-enter the cell cycle if they receive extracellular signals to do so, such as when fibroblasts begin to proliferate during wound healing.

Damage to the genes that regulate the cell cycle can lead to uncontrolled cell proliferation or premature cell division, which in turn can cause further genetic abnormalities. While there are fail-safe mechanisms to guard against these genetic errors, alterations to genes involved in the cell cycle play a major part in most human cancers.

Control of the cell cycle is carried out by sets of proteins that, for this review, have been divided into five groups. Members from each family interact with each other in complex cross-regulatory and feedback loops. The first set of proteins are the *cyclins*, which were identified because the abundance of each varies during the cell cycle. The cyclins can pair in different combinations to a set of kinases called *cyclin-dependent kinases* (cdks) because their ability to phosphorylate requires a cyclin partner. Activity of the cyclin/cdk complex can be influenced by a third set of proteins that inhibit their function, acting as a brake on the cycle. The fourth family of proteins include the product of the *retinoblastoma gene* (pRb) and its relatives, p107 and p130. These proteins bind to and inhibit the cycle-dependent transcription factors that comprise the fifth protein family. These transcription factors promote production of messenger RNA from genes that encode proteins, such as DNA polymerase, needed at specific stages of the cycle.

Many of the genes necessary for normal functioning of the cell cycle were initially identified in yeast, and were termed *cell division cycle* (cdc) genes. As the specific role of these genes was determined, their names have been changed. Not surprisingly, many cdc genes turned out to be cdks, while others encoded ligase, thymidylate synthetase, etc. For these historical reasons the terminology can be confusing, with many genes having alternate names, such as *cdk1*, which is also frequently called *p34cdc2*.

## The cyclins

At least 10 cyclins (to date, cyclins A, B, C, D1–3, E, G and H) exist in mammalian cells, and all share a region of structural homology of 150 amino acids called the *cyclin box*. It is through this conserved region that cyclins interact with the cdks. Cyclins are newly synthesized at specific phases of the cell cycle (Fig. 2.36), but are rapidly degraded by specific proteases, releasing their cdk partner, soon after. The proteases that remove the cyclins may in turn be switched off by phosphorylation by another cyclin–cdk combination.

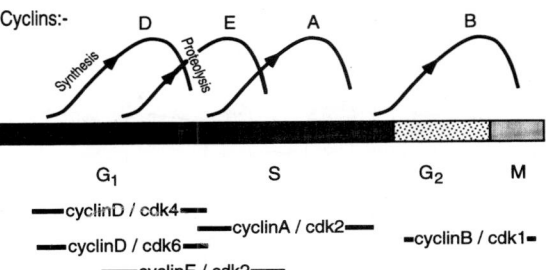

FIGURE 2.36 As the cell cycle progresses different cyclins are produced in sequence. They are then rapidly degraded by proteases that are themselves active at certain stages of the cycle. The cyclins pair with cyclin-dependent kinases (cdks) to form complexes capable of phosphorylating various substrates.

This is one of many ways by which cyclins and cdks can regulate each other.

## Cyclin-dependent kinases (cdks)

The cdks are serine/threonine protein kinases that can transfer phosphate groups to proteins only when they are bound to a cyclin. Their function is to phosphorylate serines or threonine residues of a range of different substrates, and by that means, regulate them. Different cyclins and cdks act at different stages of the cell cycle. More than six cdks have been identified in mammalian cells, and are proteins of about 34 kD. Their substrate specificity depends on both the cdk and the cyclin it is bound to, so that a given cdk may phosphorylate different substrates depending on its partner.

Although the cdks can add phosphates to other proteins, the cdks themselves can be regulated by being phosphorylated. Control of the activity of the cdk/cyclin complex is achieved by phosphorylation or dephosphorylation of the cdk on tyrosine and threonine residues. A few examples illustrate how phosphates are used to allow cyclins and cdks to be regulated and to regulate each other. Phosphorylation on one threonine residue of a cdk helps to activate its kinase activity, and this is carried out by an enzyme that itself resembles a cdk. cdk2 and 4–containing cyclin complexes are phosphorylated by a cyclin activating kinase (CAK) which complexes with another cyclin, cyclin H. Phosphorylation is also used to inactivate cdks, as phosphorylation of tyrosine or threonine residues in the ATP binding site of a cdk can prevent it from functioning (Fig. 2.37). Removal of these phosphates, leading to activation of the cdk, is achieved by a family of phosphatases (cdc25 A, B and C).

The cdks thus are regulated by cyclins and by the pattern of phosphate groups they carry. We now know that one of the first cell-cycle factors identified, mitosis

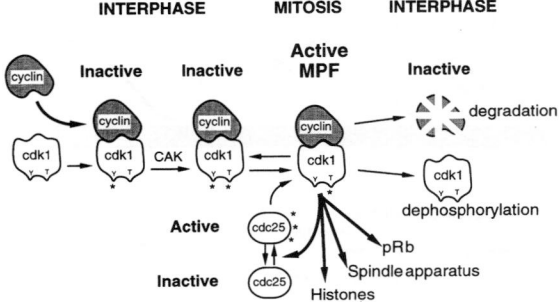

FIGURE 2.37 Cyclins pair with cdks, to form a complex. Phosphorylation (*) on some residues such as tyrosine (Y) by cyclin activating kinase (CAK) is required to activate the complex, whereas phosphorylation on other residues such as threonine (T) inhibits cyclin/cdk activity. MPF, or mitosis promoting factor, is the active form of the cyclin B/cdk1 complex that can phosphorylate a number of substrates, including cdc25, a phosphatase that can remove an inhibitory phosphate to activate the cyclin/cdk complex. cdc25 is itself activated by being phosphorylated by the cyclin/cdk complex. In this way a positive feedback loop is established. Negative regulation is carried out by other kinases and phosphatases that have not been shown, and by proteases that degrade the cyclin.

promoting factor (MPF), which can induce mitosis when injected into *Xenopus* oocytes, is a cyclin/cdk complex that has been activated by phosphorylation on the appropriate residues. cdk activity is not only controlled by the pattern of phosphorylation and cyclins, but can also be controlled by cell-cycle inhibitory proteins (see below).

The substrates regulated through phosphorylation by cdks include a variety of proteins, such as the product of the retinoblastoma gene (pRb) and structural components such as histones, which have essential functions in the cell cycle.

## Cycle inhibitory proteins

Precise control of the sequence and timing of the cell cycle is necessary to prevent mitosis before DNA replication has been successfully completed, and to prevent S phase before the required enzymes have been synthesized. Orderly sequential activation of the cdks usually allows smooth transition from one phase to the next, but control points, or "*checkpoints*" exist to halt the cycle if for some reason mitosis or DNA replication is delayed. For example, the cell is able to detect incompletely replicated DNA and activate the mitotic entry checkpoint, delaying the commencement of mitosis at the $G_2$ to M transition until the DNA is completely copied. Another checkpoint exists at the exit from mitosis that allows completion of mitosis only if a functional spindle has been formed. Less well understood checkpoints occur prior to S phase that allow

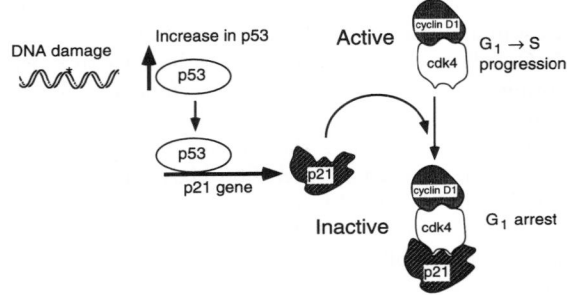

FIGURE 2.38 Damaged or abnormal DNA can be detected by the cell and leads to an increase in p53 protein. p53 acts as a transcription factor to induce transcription of the p21 gene. p21 is a cell-cycle inhibitory protein that binds to, and inactivates cyclin D/cdk4, causing arrest in $G_1$. The cell then will either repair the DNA damage or may undergo apoptosis. p53 acts as a tumor suppressor gene, as in its absence the cell copies damages DNA before it can be repaired, leading to the rapid accumulation of mutations.

entry dependent on integrity of the genome and growth factor and nutrient status.

$G_1$ phase arrest of cells with damaged DNA is achieved by the p53 tumor suppressor gene. Levels of p53 increase when the DNA is damaged by ionizing radiation. p53 is a DNA binding transcription factor that stimulates expression of a protein called p21. p21 and another inhibitor, p27, can bind to cyclins A or E complexed to cdk2, as well as to D cyclins bound to cdks 4 and 6, thereby inhibiting the function of these cyclin/cdk complexes. By inducing p21, p53 can arrest cells in $G_1$ and prevent entry into S phase, thus preventing mutations in the DNA being copied when the DNA is replicated (Fig. 2.38).

p27 can be activated by transforming growth factor-β (TGFβ), and thus TGFβ can prevent assembly and activation of cyclin E/cdk2 complexes. Growth arrest by contact inhibition, which is seen in normal cells but is frequently lost in tumor cells, is also mediated by p27.

A separate family of inhibitors known as p16 and p15 act on cdks 4 and 6. Deletion of these genes is often found in cancer cells. Presumably losing these genes allows the tumor cells to proliferate free from internal restraints, as well as those imposed by neighboring cells.

## Retinoblastoma gene family

Individuals who inherit one non-functional copy of the retinoblastoma gene have a greatly increased incidence of retinoblastoma. The product of this gene, pRb, and of related genes, p107 and p130, are collectively known as "pocket proteins" because they are able to repress the activity of transcription factors, such as E2F (see below) by binding them to a pocket in their sur-

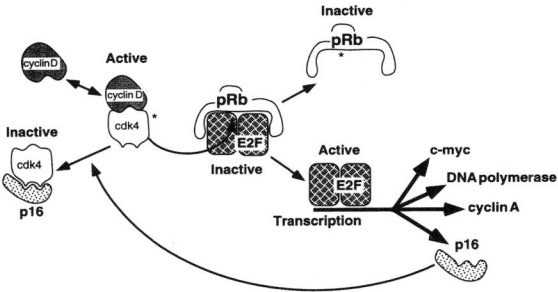

FIGURE 2.39 The pocket protein pRb can be phosphorylated (*) by a cyclin/cdk complex which causes it to free the transcription factor E2F, allowing it to stimulate transcription for genes needed in S phase. One of the many genes induced by E2F is the gene for the inhibitor protein p16, which can bind to and inactivate the cyclin/cdk complex. Retinoblastoma cells, which lack pRb, prematurely enter S phase.

face. However, when pRb is phosphorylated (by cyclin/cdks) at the $G_1$/S transition it releases E2F from this constraint, allowing it to stimulate transcription of genes needed for entry into S phase. If the cell is not ready to divide, p53 can prevent the phosphorylation of pRb by induction of p21, and thus stop transcriptional activity of E2Fs (Fig. 2.39). The other pocket proteins work in a similar way to pRb, but at different phases of the cell cycle. While pRb associates with E2F mainly during late $G_1$, p130 forms its complex during $G_0$ and p107 does so during $G_1$ and S.

## Transcription factors

*Transcription factors* are proteins that bind to DNA and regulate production of messenger RNA from the genes. Many of the proteins needed for the cell cycle are produced when required at specific stages of the cycle. Production of these proteins is dependent on transcription of the appropriate mRNA and this is regulated by transcription factors. In a cell-cycle dependent manner, cyclin/cdk complexes can turn on and off gene regulators such as the E2F family of transcription factors. For example, cyclin A/cdk2 binds to p107, a relative of the product of the retinoblastoma gene, and E2F, in a cell-cycle regulated manner. This allows cyclin A/cdk2 to regulate gene transcription during $G_1$ and S by controlling E2F activity via p107. When cyclin A/cdk2 phosphorylates *p107*, E2F is freed, allowing it to bind to DNA, which transcriptionally activates specific sets of genes. In a similar way cyclin E/cdk2, p107 and E2F form a quaternary complex, but this assembles at a different phase to the cyclin A complex.

Genes that contain binding sites for E2F, and thus can be regulated by cyclins in a cell-cycle dependent manner, include thymidine kinase and DNA polymerase, which are necessary for DNA synthesis, as well as

cycle-related proteins, such as cdk1, B-Myb, cyclin A, and c-myc (Fig. 2.39).

## THE CELL CYCLE AND DISEASE

## Cell-cycle genes as oncogenes and tumor suppressor genes

As cancer is essentially the pathological accumulation of cells, it is not surprising that disruption to the normal functioning of the cell cycle could be found in cancer cells, or be oncogenic. However, as major disturbances to the cell cycle could be expected to prevent cells from being able to divide, genetic changes to cell-cycle genes associated with cancer have largely been confined to proteins that act as checkpoints and controls. Mutations to *p53* are found in more than half of human tumors, and deletion of *p16* has often been found in immortalized cells *in vitro*. Loss of function of these proteins would increase the likelihood of cells dividing before they had the chance to repair damaged or mutated DNA. The *Rb* gene also acts as a tumor suppressor gene. Cells lacking pRb could prematurely transcribe from E2F dependent genes, and enter S phase too early.

Alterations to the *Cyclin D1* gene have been found in several types of cancer. It was found to be translocated in B cell malignancies, where it was originally designated the *BCL-1* oncogene. The *Cyclin D1* gene has also been rearranged in parathyroid adenomas, and amplified in some other tumor types. All these changes would be expected to increase the abundance or activity of cyclin D, and increase the likelihood of uncontrolled cell proliferation.

## Cell-cycle genes as targets for cancer chemotherapy

Most anticancer drugs are not specific for tumor cells, but rely on the fact that most tumors are a clone of dividing cells, whereas most of the other cells in the body are in $G_0$. The fact that this is an over-generalization is evidenced by the poor response of some malignancies to chemotherapy, and the damage that these drugs can do to dividing normal cells, such as those in the bone marrow or epithelia. Nevertheless, many cancer chemotherapies kill cells by interfering with different cell-cycle events. Radiation can mutate DNA, leading to death of cells mediated via induction of *p53*, $G_1$ arrest, and apoptosis. Even in tumor cells with mutated *p53*, radiation can kill cells by causing double-stranded DNA breaks that, when repaired, prevent separation of the chromosomes at metaphase. Topoisomerases are enzymes that allow the DNA to be broken and twisted for packaging and for replication. Topoisomerase I inhibitors, such as camptothecin, act to kill cells at $G_1$, whereas topoisomerase

II inhibitors, such as etoposide, act in S phase. Taxol acts in M phase, by preventing depolymerization of tubulin, and methotrexate inhibits production of thymidine, which is needed for synthesis of DNA.

At some stage in the future it may be possible for cancer chemotherapeutics to directly target abnormal cell-cycle proteins. For example, drugs might be made that could act as adapters to allow mutated p53 to function normally. Alternatively, small pharmaceutical agents might be made that could mimic the activity of cell-cycle inhibitors such as p21.

## SELECTED READING

Cobrinik D, Dowdy SF, Hinds PW, Mittnacht S, Weinberg RA. The retinoblastoma protein and the regulation of cell cycling. *Trends Biochem Sci* 1992; **17**: 312.

Hartwell LH, Kastan MB. Cell-cycle control and cancer. *Science* 1994; **266**: 1821.

Hunt T, Sherr CJ. Cell multiplication, checks and balances. *Curr Op Cell Biol* 1994; **6**: 833.

King RW, Jackson PK, Kirschner MW. Mitosis in transition. *Cell* 1994; **79**: 563.

Lam EW, La Thangue NB. DP and E2F proteins: coordinating transcription with cell-cycle progression. *Curr Op Cell Biol* 1994; **6**: 859.

Murray A. Cell-cycle checkpoints. *Curr Op Cell Biol* 1994; **6**: 872.

Nurse P. Ordering S phase and M phase in the cell-cycle. *Cell* 1994; **79**: 547.

Picksley SM, Lane DP. p53 and Rb: their cellular roles. *Curr Op Cell Biol* 1994; **6**: 853.

# APOPTOSIS

## INTRODUCTION

The death of cells as a normal, physiological occurrence is a fundamental process in all multicellular organisms. It most commonly occurs for two reasons: to remove unnecessary cells as a normal developmental or regulatory process, or as a defense mechanism, to get rid of cells that are potentially dangerous, such as those that bear mutations or are infected with viruses. The fate of most of the cells produced in a human is for them to kill themselves by a molecular mechanism that has changed little over the last billion years of evolution.

Physiological cell death is frequently referred to by other terms, such as *apoptosis* or *programmed cell death* (PCD). The term "apoptosis" was used by Kerr, Wyllie and Currie in 1972 to refer to dead or dying cells seen in histological sections in which there was no evidence of pathology, or reason to think that the cells were being injured or killed. Apoptosis is an ancient Greek word meaning "a dropping off," as of leaves from a tree, another situation in which death of cells is a normal occurrence. They suggested that apoptosis was how the body removed a cell, just as mitosis allowed production of a new cell by cell division.

A term that is now often used synonymously with apoptosis, programmed cell death, was used to refer to cell death that occurred to certain cells in a predictable way at a predetermined time, such as cell death seen during metamorphosis of insects and amphibia, or during embryonic development of chicks or nematodes. As the same molecular mechanism is usually used in both programmed and non-programmed cell death, this term now is less generally applied.

Apoptosis is a descriptive term for cells dying while displaying certain characteristic features such as cell shrinkage, condensation of the chromatin around the margins of the nucleus, and formation of "blebs" in the plasma membrane, but relatively few changes to the mitochondria. These cells then tend to divide into well-contained, membrane-bound fragments termed *apoptotic bodies*. These bodies, and cells undergoing apoptosis, are disposed of by being engulfed and degraded by neighboring cells, which may not be professional phagocytic cells (Fig. 2.40). Typically there is no associated inflammation, and no subsequent scarring or changes to the tissue architecture.

In contrast, cells dying in unphysiological circumstances, such as following arterial occlusion, typically exhibit a different appearance, termed *necrosis*. Cells undergoing necrosis swell, and changes to the mitochondria occur at an early stage. Loss of membrane integrity follows, and the cellular debris is removed by an inflammatory infiltrate of neutrophils and macrophages. Unfortunately, histological appearances are often mixed, and while they may give an indication of the mode of cell death, they are not always a reliable guide to the underlying molecular mechanisms.

## MECHANISMS

It is convenient to think of three phases of cell death; the *activator* phase, in which the signals for cell death are received and integrated; the *effector* phase where the killing machinery acts; and the *post mortem* phase in which the dead cell is removed and degraded (Fig. 2.41).

Many different signals and pathways can serve to activate a common effector mechanism. Some of these signals originate from outside the cell and are mediated via cell surface receptors for *growth factors* or *cytokines* such as *tumor necrosis factor* (TNF) or the ligand for the *Fas antigen*. Other cell death activation signals, such as damaged DNA, originate inside the cell. Several different signal transduction pathways, some involving gene transcription, have been implicated in passing the cell death signal. In many cases cell death can be blocked by RNA or protein synthesis inhibitors, which supports the notion that cells need to participate actively in their own demise. It is now clear, however,

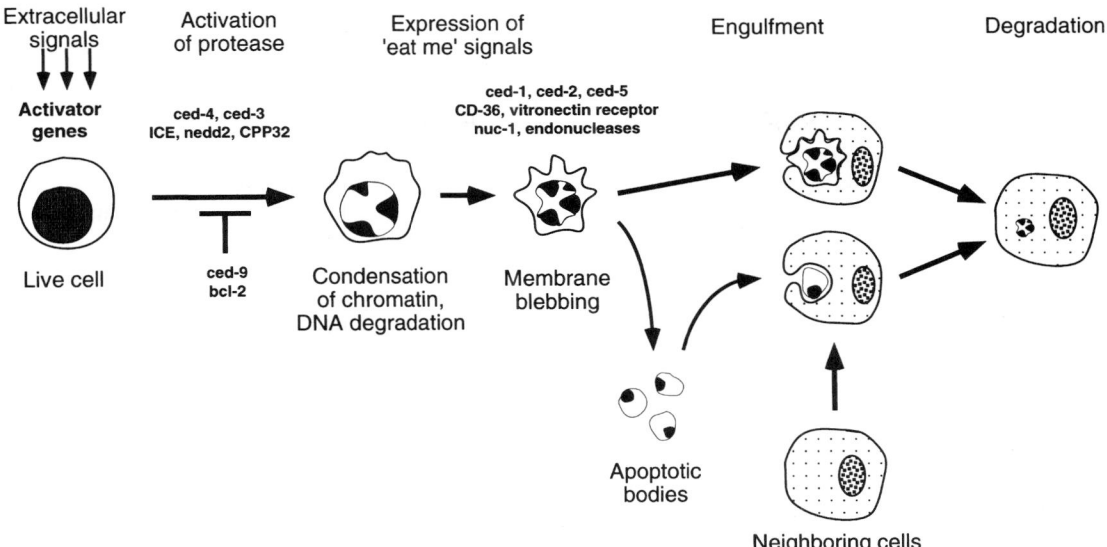

FIGURE 2.40 For apoptosis to occur, proteases such as ced-3 or ICE are required. They are activated by signals from inside or outside the cell, but cell death can be blocked by ced-9 or bcl-2. The earliest changes are seen in the nucleus. The dead cell tends to divide and is engulfed and fully degraded by another cell in a process that requires expression of specific molecules on the surface of both the dead and engulfing cells. The gene products listed are examples only, as new homologs are reported regularly.

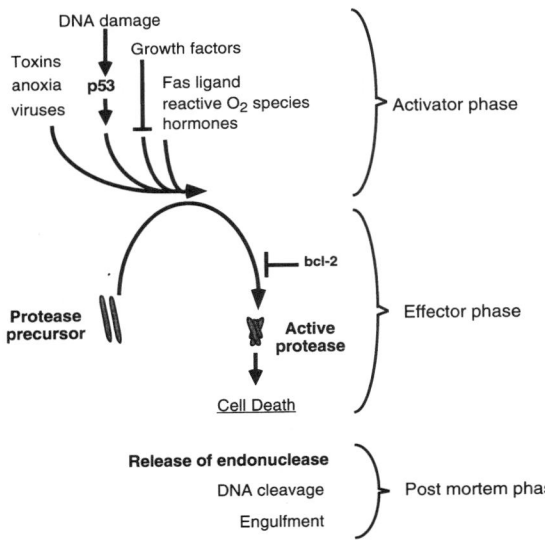

FIGURE 2.41 Cell death occurs in three phases. Multiple signals originating inside or outside the cell can converge to activate a common cell death effector mechanism in the cytoplasm. A cysteine protease resembling ced-3 is converted from an inactive precursor to the active tetramer. Bcl-2 is able to block cell death, either by preventing the activation of the protease or by preventing it reaching its substrate. The protease cleaves as yet unidentified substrates in the cell leading to the changes recognizable as apoptosis. Nucleases gain access to and degrade the DNA in the nucleus. The cell corpse, which may have contracted into membrane-bound apoptotic bodies, is recognized and engulfed by neighboring cells that then fully degrade it

that the effector mechanisms for apoptosis involve activation of preexisting proteases, but that the activation phase of cell death is sometimes transcriptionally regulated.

Much of our understanding of the molecular effector mechanisms that carry out cell suicide have come from genetic studies of cell death in the nematode *Caenorhabditis elegans*, in which over a dozen cell death genes have been identified. Of the 1090 cells formed during development of the hermaphrodite worm, 131 die as their normal cell fate. The dead cells are rapidly engulfed and degraded by neighboring cells. Most of the *cell death abnormal* (*ced*) genes are involved in removal of the cell corpses. Two genes, *ced-3* and *ced-4*, are required for cell death to occur. In the absence of either of these two genes the worm ends up with an extra 131 cells, and these have been shown to be able to function. Thus *ced-3* and *ced-4* are thought to encode "killer" proteins. *Ced-9* has the opposite effect to *ced-3* and *ced-4*, as worms with a mutation to *ced-9* that increases its activity also have the extra 131 cells. It seems likely that the ced-9 product either prevents activation of *ced-3* or *ced-4*, or prevents them from functioning (Fig. 2.41).

Identification of cell death genes in mammals has been much slower than in *C. elegans*. The first mammalian cell death gene identified was a human gene called *BCL-2* (B cell leukemia/lymphoma gene 2) that lies at the site of translocations typical of the common hemopoietic malignancy follicular lymphoma. Bcl-2 can block apoptosis, and is thought to cause follicular lymphoma indirectly by allowing the accumulation of B cells that are rendered unable to kill themselves. High levels of Bcl-2 can protect many cells from an enormous array of insults, including removal of growth factors, heat shock, cytotoxic drugs and irradiation. This showed that the same process of cell death, the one that Bcl-2 can block, can be activated in many different ways, but it did not reveal the nature of this mechanism. However, once it was shown that Bcl-2 could also inhibit cell death in *C. elegans* it became clear that the process of cell death is highly conserved, and homologues of the other nematode cell death genes are responsible for cell death in mammals (Fig. 2.41).

## The *BCL-2* gene family

A family of genes have now been identified that have sequence similarity with *BCL-2*. The products of some of these genes act like Bcl-2 to inhibit cell death, whereas others antagonize the protection offered by Bcl-2. Examination of the sequences has not provided any clues as to how *BCL-2* or its relatives function. Most of these molecules have a hydrophobic carboxy terminus and are located on the cytoplasmic side of internal membranes in the cell. From experiments in mammalian cells and *C. elegans* outlined below, Bcl-2 directly or indirectly appears to regulate the activity of a family of cysteine proteases, either by preventing their activation or by blocking access to their substrates.

## Cytoplasmic proteases

The "killer" gene from *C. elegans*, *ced-3*, encodes a protein that is similar to the mammalian cysteine protease, *interleukin-1β converting enzyme* (*ICE*), and another mammalian gene product called nedd2. All three genes are likely to encode proteases that, when activated, cleave as yet unidentified substrates, culminating in apoptosis. ICE is known to exist in many cells as an inactive p45 precursor molecule that is processed into active 2(p10/p20) tetramers during the process of apoptosis. *BCL-2*, which is similar to a cell death inhibitor gene from *C. elegans* called *ced-9*, is able to prevent death of cells in tissue culture mediated by overexpression of *ced-3*, *ICE* or *NEDD2*.

## Nucleases and DNA degradation

A frequent accompanying feature of apoptosis is cleavage of the DNA of the cell into about 180 base pair fragments that give a characteristic "ladder" appearance upon gel electrophoresis. The size of the fragments corresponds to the length of DNA wrapped around each nucleosome. The nucleases responsible for cleavage presumably cut the DNA preferentially at the inter-nucleosomal sites where it is more accessible. Debate exists over the identity of the nuclease(s)

responsible for cleaving the DNA in apoptosis, but many cells contain nucleases in an inactive state. While detection of DNA cleavage is often a convenient indicator of apoptosis, DNA cleavage is probably a post-mortem event that is not required for cell death, as apoptotic changes can be seen in enucleated cells, and mutation of the *C. elegans* endonuclease-encoding *nuc-1* gene prevents DNA degradation, but does not block cell death.

## Disposal of apoptotic cells

In both mammals and nematodes, cells that have died of apoptosis are quickly removed by being engulfed by neighboring cells. Genetic experiments in *C. elegans* have shown that engulfment is not required for cell death to occur, and several genes are needed for efficient disposal of the cell corpses. It is likely that these genes encode "eat me" signals on the surface of the dead cell, and receptor molecules on the engulfing cell that recognize these signals. In mammals, efficient recognition of apoptosing neutrophils and their engulfment by macrophages is mediated by several molecules, including the vitronectin receptor, phosphatidyl serine, CD36, and thrombospondin, but the molecular details of this process have not been fully elucidated.

## USES FOR PHYSIOLOGICAL CELL DEATH

How, when and why cell death evolved is not known, but in organisms as diverse as plants, bacteria and animals the most common uses for cell suicide are: (1) as a defense mechanism, to limit the spread of pathogens or remove mutated cells, and (2) for morphogenesis and homeostasis of cell number.

## Cell death during development

During development of the infant many more neurons are produced than are needed. Those that have made the correct connections receive a signal from their target cell that allow them to live. The remaining cells activate their suicide mechanisms by default.

Unnecessary cells are removed during organogenesis. For example, cell death is used to remove the webbing between the fingers, allowing them to separate. Tissues needed in only one sex may be removed by apoptosis in the other. For example, breast epithelia dies in males under the influence of testosterone.

## Cell death as part of homeostasis

In the adult, tissues which turn over rapidly – such as white blood cells or cells of the gut or skin – kill themselves by apoptosis at a predetermined age, rather than living until they are injured or degenerate. In some cases instructions to live or die are sent through receptors on the cell surface, but in other cases the survival period may be linked to the number of cell divisions or by an internal clock. Growth factors can give combinations of signals for survival, proliferation or differentiation. Adhesion molecules can also pass survival signals. On the other hand, engagement of receptors such as the Fas antigen or the TNF receptors may give a death signal.

## Cell death as a defense mechanism

Many cells undergo apoptosis when they are infected with intracellular pathogens such as viruses. This can prevent the pathogen from replicating and spreading to other cells, eventually threatening the organism as a whole. The nature of the molecular change caused by the infectious particle that alerts the cell to its presence is not known, but the tendency of cells to apoptose in response to a great variety of drugs and toxins may be due to the cell interpreting metabolic changes caused by these drugs as evidence of a viral infection. Many types of cells respond to inappropriate activation of their DNA synthetic machinery by apoptosis. It makes sense for cells to keep a close watch on their cell-cycle machinery as viruses may try to use it to replicate, and loss of regulation can lead to unrestrained growth and cancer. The product of the tumor suppressor gene p53 can activate apoptosis, and may be part of the mechanism that monitors the DNA and the cell-cycle machinery.

It seems that viruses have come up with their own strategies to disable this defensive host response. These viruses carry anti-apoptosis genes that inactivate the cell-death mechanisms. Several viruses encode proteins that can inactivate p53. Adenovirus, for example, uses E1B 55K protein to bind to, and inactivate, p53 while Human Papilloma Virus (HPV) specifically targets p53 for proteolytic degradation. Other viruses, such as Epstein Barr Virus, have proteins that resemble Bcl-2, and some, such as Cowpox Virus, have products that can block ICE. These viruses can block cell autonomous, defensive apoptosis.

Cell death may also help in the defense against cancer. DNA mutations can cause stabilization of p53, which can activate cell death mechanisms. Blocking cell death by over-expression of BCL-2 predisposes towards cancer in humans and mice.

## Cytotoxic T cell killing

Our main defense against viruses comes from *cytotoxic T cells* (CTL). These can specifically recognize and cause apoptosis of infected cells. CTL can efficiently kill cells expressing high levels of Bcl-2, so they may activate the effector mechanisms downstream of the step where Bcl-2 acts. As some viruses carry *BCL-2* like genes, it makes sense for CTL to be able to kill in a way that is not sensitive to viral anti-apoptosis genes.

CTL have granules in their cytoplasm that contain *perforin* and proteases called *granzymes*. After binding to a target cell, the contents of these granules are emptied into the intercellular space. Perforin forms pores in the plasma membrane of the target cell, through which the granzymes can enter. Directly adding perforin and granzyme B can cause the rapid apoptosis of cells. Added alone, perforin can cause the plasma membrane to leak slowly, but kills ineffectively. Rapid cell death, with early DNA degradation and apoptotic morphology, requires both perforin and granzymes.

## CELL DEATH AND DISEASE

Because the process of cell death is ubiquitous, and irreversible, yet required for normal functions, it needs to be carefully regulated. Failure of cells to die, or inappropriate cell death is a significant cause of human disease.

## Cancer

Failure of cell death can lead to the persistence of damaged or mutated cells that can become malignant. This occurs in follicular lymphoma, where cell death is blocked by constitutive BCL-2 expression from the t14:18 translocation. Part of the antitumor effect of p53 is due to its ability to send cells with damaged DNA to their deaths. Some of the greater than 50 per cent of human cancers that have mutant p53 alleles thus can be attributed to failure of cell death mechanisms. As human genes similar to the nematode cell death genes ced-3 and ced-4 are likely to be necessary for apoptosis of cancer cells in humans, these homologues of ced-3 or ced-4, such as ICE or NEDD2, may be tumor suppressor genes. Individuals inheriting mutated copies of these genes may run an increased risk of cancer.

Many cancer cells show signs of apoptosis when treated with anticancer drugs, while others do not. Killing of cancer cells by radiotherapy often occurs by apoptosis. It may be that a significant proportion of cells in a tumor die not by the direct action of a chemotherapeutic drug, but commit suicide even when exposed to otherwise sublethal levels of the drug; in other words the cells commit suicide in response to a drug before they are killed by it. Increasing the proportion of tumor cells liable to undergo apoptosis may help increase the effectiveness of cancer therapies, by decreasing the total tumor burden. Blocking genes like BCL-2 could increase the response of cancers to chemotherapy or radiation.

## Autoimmune disease

Autoimmune diseases may result from loss of tolerance due to failure of self-reactive T or B cell clones to die. In support of this idea, transgenic mice expressing *BCL-2* in their B cells, and mice with non-functioning *Fas* genes, develop an autoimmune disease that resembles SLE. However it is unlikely that any autoimmune disease can be attributed purely to loss of tolerance through inhibition of cell death, as the development of autoimmune disease in animal models such as these is strongly influenced by the genetic background.

## Ischemic disease

In certain model systems it has been shown that cells exposed to anoxia, or tissues deprived of blood supply, die showing signs of apoptosis. Furthermore, in some cases expression of *BCL-2* can prevent or delay anoxia-induced cell death. This suggests that some cells may respond to sub-lethal levels of anoxia by activating cell suicide mechanisms. Drugs that could block this response may limit cell death post-stroke or post-infarct. They may be able to protect fetal neurons from transient periods of anoxia during childbirth, for example (*see* page 445).

## SELECTED READING

Ellis RE, Yuan JY, Horvitz HR. Mechanisms and functions of cell death. *Ann Rev Cell Biol* 1991; 7: 663.

Nagata S, Golstein P. The Fas death factor. *Science* 1995; 267: 1449.

Raff MC. Social controls on cell survival and cell death. *Nature* 1992; 356: 397.

Stellar H. Mechanisms and genes of cellular suicide. *Science* 1995; 267: 1445.

Stewart BW. Mechanisms of apoptosis: integration of genetic, biochemical, and cellular indicators. *J Natl Cancer Inst* 1994; 86: 1286.

Thompson CB. Apoptosis in the pathogenesis and treatment of disease. *Science* 1995; 267: 1456.

Vaux DL, Haecker G, Strasser A. An evolutionary perspective on apoptosis. *Cell* 1994; 76: 777.

Wyllie AH. The biology of cell death in tumours. *Anticancer Res* 1985; 5: 131.

# PART TWO

# *Genetics*

**Editor: Ingrid Winship**

# 3

# Genetics

Ingrid Winship

## CHROMOSOME STRUCTURE AND FUNCTION

Chromosomes are present in all nucleated cells and contain DNA with associated acidic and basic proteins. The basic structure of the chromosome, 11 nm in diameter comprises nucleosomes which are octomeric histones around which the DNA wraps approximately twice. The length of DNA joining two nucleosomes is associated with a linker molecule of histone. The elementary fiber composed of linked nucleosomes is in turn coiled into a fiber of 36 nm diameter which is the chromatin fiber. A central scaffold of the metaphase chromosome formed of acidic proteins to which the chromosome fiber is attached at repeated sequences. Loops of fiber emanate from the scaffold to form the body of the chromatin, about 0.6 μm in diameter. This compaction allows 3 m of double-stranded DNA to be packaged for cell division into metaphase chromosomes. These range in size from 10 μm, comprising 200 Mb of DNA (chromosome 1), to 2 μm comprising 40 Mb of DNA (chromosome 21) (Fig. 3.1).

The chromosome complement of each species is specific in number and form and this is known as the karyotype of the species. The normal human karyotype comprises 46 chromosomes. These are arranged as 23 matching or homologous pairs (Fig. 3.2). The autosomes are arranged in decreasing size, numbered 1 to 22. The 23rd pair are the sex chromosomes, of which there are two X chromosomes in the normal female and an X and a Y in a normal male. One of each pair of autosomes and the X chromosome are maternally derived, while the father would contribute a second X to a female, the Y to a male and the other 22 autosomes. Each chromosome has a short arm (p) and a long arm (q) divided by a narrow waistline, the centromere. The tip of each arm is the telomere. The centromere, which is the site of attachment of the spindle fibers in mitosis, is constant in position for each chromosome. By convention, the subgroups of chromosomes are identified by the position of the centromere:

- metacentric – the centromere is in the middle (chromosomes 1, 3, 16, 19, 20);
- acrocentric – the centromere is placed at one end (chromosomes 13, 14, 15, 21, 22, Y);
- submetacentric or subacrocentric – the centromere has an intermediate position.

Detailed DNA measurements by flow cytometry demonstrate that chromosomes show variations in DNA content between individuals which are inherited. The X chromosome shows least variation, while the Y chromosome is most variable. These differences are called heteromorphisms which are genetic polymorphisms, e.g. fragile sites. Size polymorphisms usually involve repetitive DNA; the degree of variation shows a Gaussian distribution. These are not usually associated with clinical anomalies.

Cytoplasmic DNA exists in addition to nuclear chromosomes. Human mitochondria have their own chromosomes which comprise approximately 10 single, circular, double helices (16 kb) of DNA which are self-replicating. Human mitochondrial DNA differs from nuclear DNA in its codon recognition for several amino acids. It has no introns and both strands are transcribed and translated. Its significance is discussed further on pages 80 and 119.

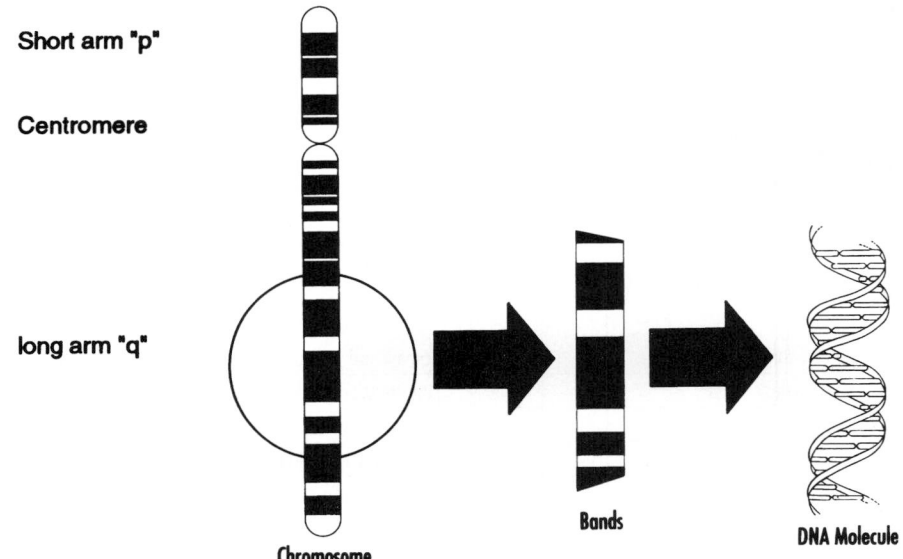

FIGURE 3.1 Normal chromosome structure, with an area magnified to demonstrate the DNA double helix.

## THE CELL CYCLE AND GAMETOGENESIS

The cell cycle depends on an orderly sequence of events in which synthesis of enzymes and other gene products occurs at specific times, so maintaining a smooth progression of cellular events (*see also* Chapter 2). Each event depends on preceding events and in turn determines successive events. Proteins, such as $H_1$ kinase and cyclins, appear to control the cycle by mechanisms as yet unknown. Mitosis occupies up to one hour of the total cycle; DNA synthesis for replication takes up to eight hours (Fig. 3.3).

## Mitosis

Mitosis is the division of somatic cells whereby the cell produces two identical daughter cells. Five arbitrary

stages exist in mitosis: interphase, which includes $G_1$, S, and $G_2$ phases, prophase, metaphase, anaphase and telophase (Fig. 3.4).

### Interphase

A cell that is not actively dividing is in interphase. This phase comprises Gap 1 ($G_1$), S (DNA synthesis) and Gap 2 ($G_2$). Replication of DNA occurs during the S phase so that the nucleus in $G_2$ has twice the diploid amount of DNA present in $G_1$. Cells may withdraw to the resting phase $G_0$.

Each chromosome has its own pattern of DNA synthesis, and some segments replicate earlier than

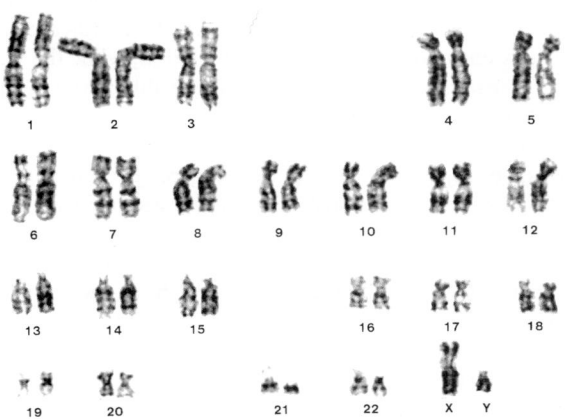

FIGURE 3.2 A normal male karyotype: 46 XY. The chromosomes are arranged, by convention, according to their size and centromere position.

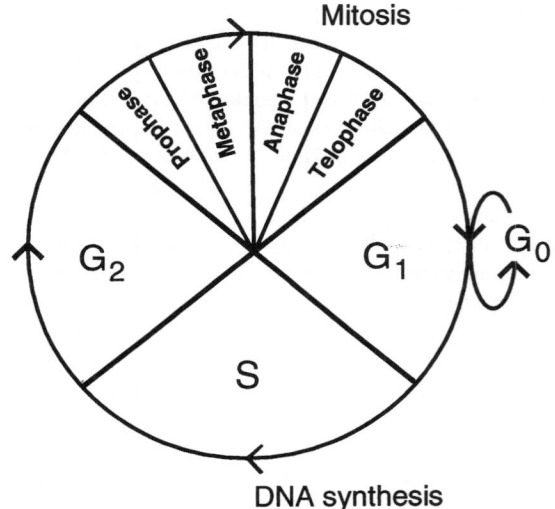

FIGURE 3.3 The cell cycle depends on an orderly sequence of events, including mitosis and DNA synthesis, each with intervening rest periods.

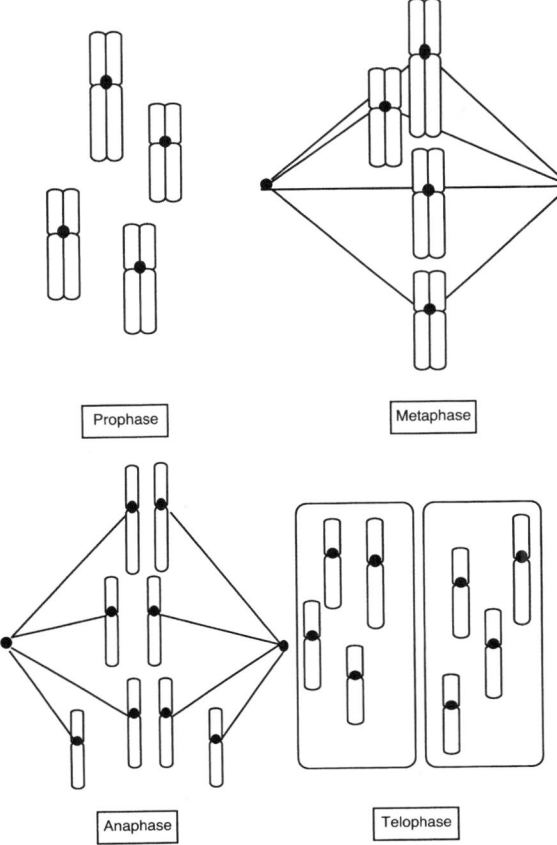

Prophase

Metaphase

Anaphase

Telophase

FIGURE 3.4 Mitosis comprises five stages and results in two daughter cells with an identical genetic constitution. The active phases of two chromosome pairs are shown.

others. The inactive X is always the last chromosome to replicate. In replication, exact copies of parent DNA are produced with resultant transfer of identical genetic information to daughter cells. Each strand of the DNA helix serves as a template on which a complementary strand is formed by base-pairing with free nucleotides (*see* Chapter 1). These nucleotides are joined together by the action of the enzyme DNA polymerase III and are hydrogen-bonded to the template strand. DNA replication takes place at "replication forks" with the synthesis being continuous on the strand moving away from the fork, and discontinuous on the strand moving towards the fork. Resultant duplex DNA consists of one parent strand and one newly replicated strand. This is known as semiconservative replication.

## Prophase

Chromosomes become visible during prophase; they are seen as a pair of long parallel strands which are sister chromatids, held together at the centromeres. At this time crossovers between sister chromatids with exchange of material may occur. The nuclear mem-

brane disappears, the centriole divides, and its products migrate towards opposite poles of the cell.

## Metaphase

During metaphase, chromosomes have reached their maximal contraction. Once this occurs they move to the equatorial plate of the cell. The mitotic spindle forms, and chromosomes attach at the centromere in an orderly fashion.

## Anaphase

Anaphase is the point at which the centromeres divide. The paired chromatids separate to produce two identical daughter chromosomes. The spindle fibers contract and draw the daughter chromosomes, centromere first, to the poles of the cells.

## Telophase

At the final stage of division the daughter chromosomes reach the poles of the cells. The cytoplasm divides along with nuclear material, and the cell plates form to produce two daughter cells. The chromosomes start to unwind, and at the same time the nuclear membrane reforms. Active cell division is now complete, and interphase follows. Mitosis results in two daughter cells with an identical genetic constitution.

# Gametogenesis

Gametogenesis occurs in the gonad, where the somatic diploid (2N) chromosome complement is halved to the haploid number (N), to provide a single copy of the chromosome. Each mature gamete therefore contains one member of each pair of chromosomes. This is achieved by a specialized cell division, *meiosis*. Fusion of the egg and sperm restores the diploid chromosome content in the fertilized ovum.

Meiosis (Fig. 3.5) consists of two successive processes: first meiotic division (reduction division) halves the chromosome number; and second meiotic division follows reduction division. DNA replicates once only during meiosis.

## Meiosis I

The first meiotic division comprises three stages: prophase, metaphase and anaphase.

### Prophase

Prophase is complex; five stages are identifiable. During leptotene, the chromosomes are visible as threadlike structures. In zygotene, pairing of homologous chromosomes occurs. Thickening of the chromosomes is evident in pachytene. Chiasmata mark the location of crossing over. Chromatids of homologous chromosomes approximate and exchange material in

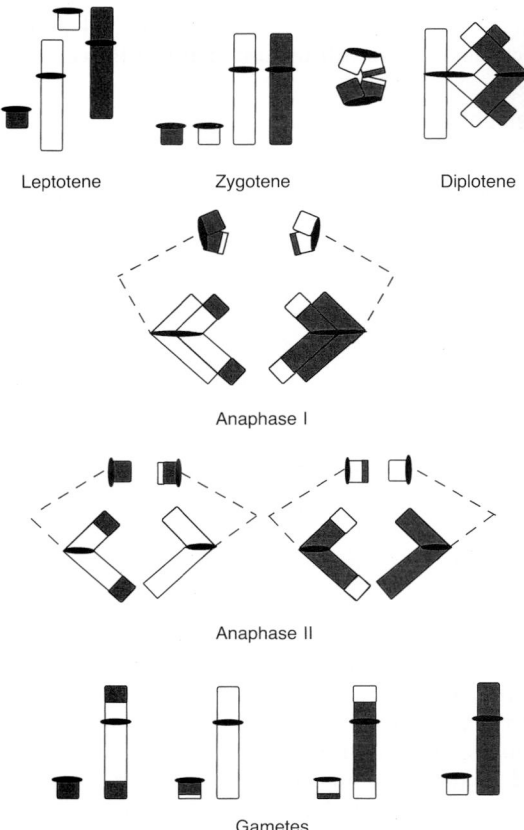

Leptotene    Zygotene    Diplotene

Anaphase I

Anaphase II

Gametes

FIGURE 3.5 This cartoon shows two chromosome pairs in some of the stages of meiosis. Chromosomes from one parent are shaded. In leptotene the chromosomes become threadlike. In zygotene, homologous chromosomes pair. During diplotene, chiasmata at the points of contact between chromosomes mark the location of crossovers, where chromatids of homologous chromosomes have exchanged material in late pachytene. At anaphase the two members of each bivalent disjoin, one going to each pole.

later pachytene. The chromatids that have exchanged material are called recombinants (Fig. 3.6). The fourth phase is diplotene, during which time chromosomes appear double. Finally, diakinesis occurs where the homologous chromosomes move apart.

### Metaphase

During metaphase the nuclear membrane disappears and the chromosomes move to the equatorial plate.

### Anaphase

In anaphase the two chromosome members separate or disjoin, one going to each pole of the cell, assorted independently. At this time the cytoplasm divides to form two cells. Each of these cells has 23 single chromosomes, each of which is a pair of chromatids which differ from one another only as a result of crossing over during prophase.

### Meiosis II

This follows meiosis I without an interphase. It is similar to mitosis where centromeres divide and sister chromatids move to opposite poles.

The significance of meiosis is to produce gametes that contain only one member of a homologous pair of chromosomes. The disjunction of chromosome pairs results in random assortment of maternal and paternal chromosomes. Crossing over between homologous chromosomes with resultant exchange of material ensures genetic variation.

## Spermatogenesis (*see also* Chapter 38)

Spermatogenesis occurs from sexual maturity onwards in the seminiferous tubules of males. The primary spermatocyte is derived from a committed spermatogonium, which then undergoes the first meiotic division to produce two secondary spermatocytes which contain the haploid number of chromosomes. The second stage of meiosis follows, and two spermatids are formed. The spermatids mature into sperm without further division. The entire process takes approximately 64 days, and the semen produced contains between 50 and 100 million sperm/mL. Numerous replications, with increasing age, increase the chance for mutation to occur; a number of single gene mutations are more common in the offspring of older fathers, e.g. *achondroplasia, neurofibromatosis.*

## Oogenesis (*see also* Chapter 38)

The process of oogenesis begins at the end of the first trimester prenatally and is almost complete at birth. The *oogonia* are derived from primordial germ cells, which are the central cells of the developing follicles. During the prenatal period the oogonia become *oocytes* and may enter the first meiotic division. These primary oocytes remain in suspended prophase until the girl reaches sexual maturity. As follicles mature, oocytes are released into the fallopian tubes. It is at this time that the first meiotic division is completed, so that the completion of meiosis I in a female may take as long as 45 years. The extended time period between the start and finish of meiosis I explains the high incidence of meiotic errors associated with advanced maternal age.

Meiosis I results in uneven division of the cytoplasm whereby the secondary oocyte receives the majority, with a lesser quantity going to the polar body. Meiosis II is not completed until after fertilization. This results in a mature ovum and a second polar body.

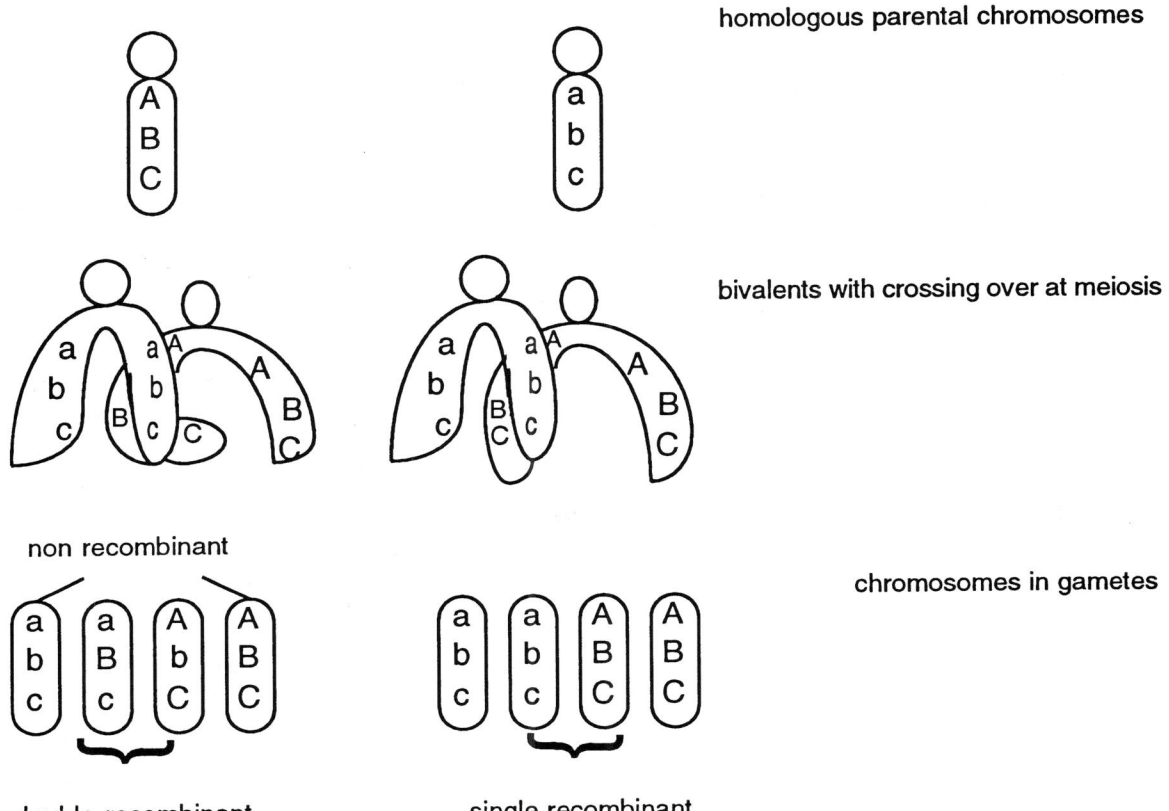

homologous parental chromosomes

bivalents with crossing over at meiosis

chromosomes in gametes

non recombinant

double recombinant

single recombinant

FIGURE 3.6 Crossing over occurs in late pachytene, where there is exchange of material between the chromatids of homologous chromosomes.

Genetic disorders can be divided into the following groups: chromosome disorders, single gene disorders, multifactorial or polygenic inheritance, somatic cell disorders, non-traditional inheritance and sporadic cases.

## CHROMOSOMAL ANOMALIES

Chromosomal disorders result from microscopically identifiable changes in the chromosomes. Up to 20 per cent of all conceptions have a chromosome disorder. Most of these are spontaneously aborted and the frequency of chromosomal disorders in live-born infants is approximately 0.6 per cent. Chromosome disorders occur in about 60 per cent of early spontaneous abortions, whereas in late spontaneous abortions and stillbirths the frequency is 5 per cent.

Abnormalities of the chromosomes may involve autosomes or sex chromosomes and are classified as follows: numerical abnormalities, structural abnormalities and other abnormalities.

## Numerical aberration

Somatic cells contain the diploid (2N) number of chromosomes, 46; mature gametes have the haploid (N) number, 23. Polyploidy is a chromosome number which is an exact multiple of the haploid number greater than two: aneuploidy is an abnormal chromosome number which is not a multiple of the haploid number.

### Polyploidy

Triploidy implies a complete extra set of chromosomes (3N or 69). This usually results from dispermy or the formation of a diploid gamete due to failure of one of the maturation divisions of either the sperm or the egg.

### Aneuploidy

Aneuploidy usually results from non-disjunction which is the failure of paired chromosomes or sister chromatids to disjoin during anaphase in meiosis (Fig. 3.7). Aneuploidy may also be caused by anaphase lag, delayed movement of a chromosome at anaphase.

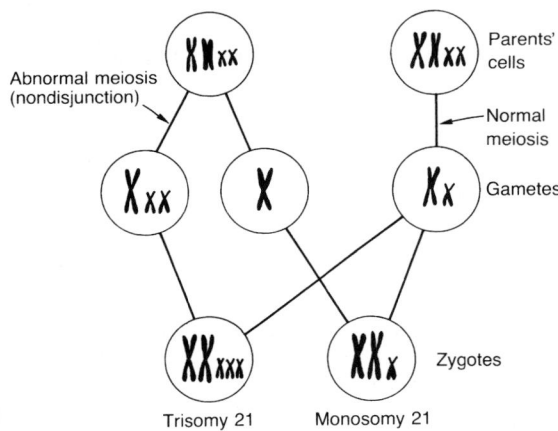

FIGURE 3.7 Non-disjunction occurs when chromosomes fail to disjoin during meiotic division. This results in gametes with an uneven distribution of chromosomes; such a gamete, if fertilized, would result in a zygote with either a trisomy or a monosomy.

Failure to cross over or form chiasmata may also play a role. The oocytes wait suspended in the first meiotic division for longer periods with advancing maternal age; it is believed that aneuploidy may be due to problems with maternal spindle function. However, a recent postulate is that aneuploidy associated with increased maternal age is the result of failure to spontaneously abort an aneuploid fetus rather than an increased frequency of ova with damaged chromosomes. There may be genetic factors which predispose to non-disjunction since a familial tendency to chromosomal abnormalities exists. In addition, the incidence is raised with consanguineous unions. Maternal hypothyroidism, irradiation, viral infection and teratogenic agents may play a role in causing aneuploidy. Paternal non-disjunction contributes approximately 5–10 per cent of aneuploidy.

## Structural abnormalities

Chromosomal breakages cause structural aberrations. Chromosomes break, resulting in two unstable sticky ends, which are rejoined immediately by repair mechanisms. If multiple breaks occur, one sticky end cannot be distinguished from another and the wrong ends may be rejoined. The rate of chromosomal breakage may be raised by exposure to ionizing radiation or mutagens.

Seven types of structural abnormalities exist: translocation, deletion, ring chromosome, duplication, inversion, isochromosome and centric fragments.

### Translocation

A translocation is defined as the transfer of chromosomal material between chromosomes. The process either involves breakage of the chromosomes involved, with repair in an abnormal rearrangement, or accidental meiotic recombination between non-homologous chromosomes. This "balanced translocation" usually results in no loss of DNA and the individual may be clinically normal. However, a balanced translocation carrier is at risk of producing offspring with chromosomal imbalance. Translocations may be: reciprocal, Robertsonian or insertional.

### Reciprocal translocation

In reciprocal translocation, chromosomal material distal to breaks in two chromosomes is exchanged. Any pair of chromosomes may be involved, whether homologous or non-homologous, and this breakage may involve the short or long arms of the chromosome. Six possibilities exist for the gametes of a couple of whom one is a translocation carrier. Of these six possibilities one gamete has normal chromosomes and one has a balanced translocation. The other four result in various imbalances of the two chromosomes involved; large numbers of genes may be gained or lost and affected offspring have multiple congenital abnormalities, or the fetus may abort spontaneously.

### Robertsonian translocation

Breaks at or near the centromere in two acrocentric chromosomes and cross-fusion of the products cause Centric fusion or Robertsonian translocations. The breaks are usually just above the centromeres and result in a single dicentric chromosome with two centromeres, and an acentric fragment bearing both satellites. The acentric fragment cannot undergo mitosis and is usually lost at a subsequent division.

It is possible that centric fusion is due to accidental crossover between homologous sequences on non-homologous chromosomes during the first meiotic division. The most frequent translocation in humans is centric fusion of chromosomes 13 and 14, and of 14 and 21. A carrier of a Robertsonian translocation is usually clinically unaffected; however uneven transmission of chromosomal material to gametes may result in abnormalities in their offspring. Translocations involving chromosome 21 account for some 4 per cent of individuals with *Down syndrome*. Fig. 3.8 illustrates the segregation of a 14/21 translocation.

### Insertional translocation

Three breaks are required in one or two chromosomes to produce an insertional translocation. Insertional translocation carriers are clinically normal but may produce children with either a duplication or a deletion.

### Deletion

A deletion is a loss of any region of a chromosome. Three mechanisms for deletion exist. Interstitial deletions occur when there is loss of a part of the chromosome between two breaks. Secondly, there may be unequal crossing over in meiosis. Finally, in parental translocation, the deleted segment will be lost at subsequent cell division because it has no centromere.

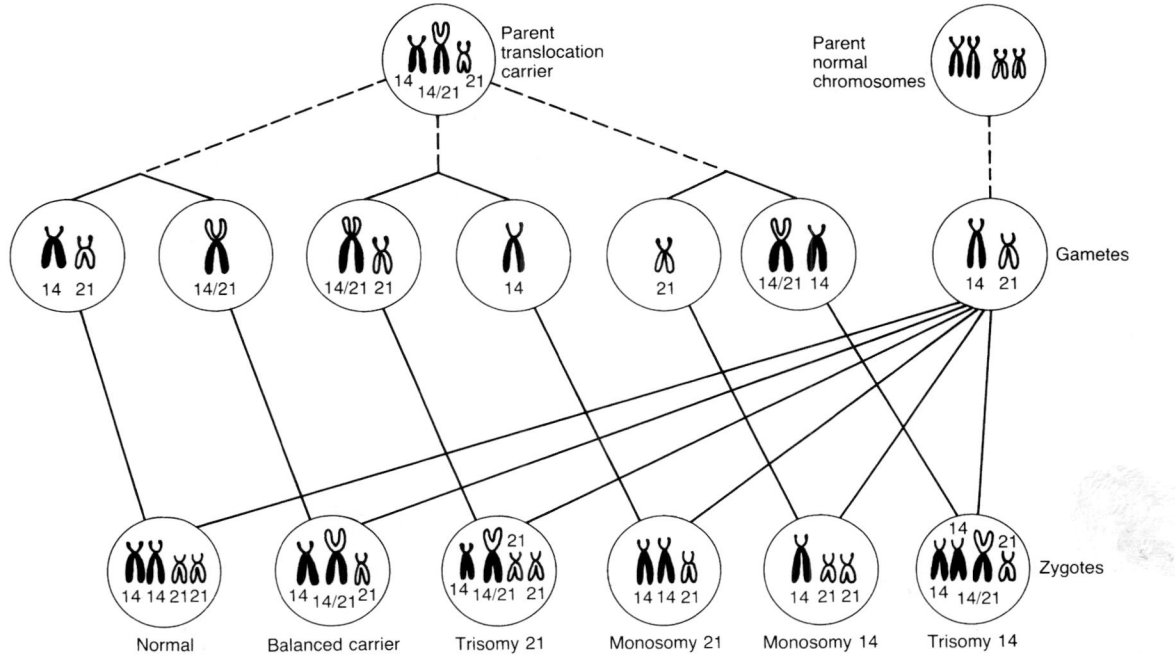

FIGURE 3.8 The possible gametes produced as a result of a parent who is a balanced carrier of a Robertsonian translocation (14/21) are shown. The resultant zygotes, assuming normal chromosomes in the other parent, are demonstrated.

The smallest visible loss from a chromosome is about 4000 kb; individuals with such deletions are monosomic for variable numbers of contiguous genes and may have corresponding clinical disability.

## Ring chromosome

A ring chromosome arises from breaks at both ends of a chromosome. The terminal ends of each are lost and the two proximal "sticky ends" join to form a ring. A ring chromosome that has a centromere is able to undergo cell division.

## Duplication

Duplication is where two copies of a segment of a chromosome derive from an unequal crossing over during meiosis; the reciprocal product is a deletion. Duplication may occur in meiosis in parents who carry a translocation, inversion or isochromosome. Duplications occur more frequently than deletions, but cause fewer clinical abnormalities.

## Inversion

Inversions result from two chromosomal breaks with rotation through 180° of the fragment between the breaks. Paracentric inversion results from breaks in a single arm and the centromere is not included; pericentric inversion involves breaks on either side and inclusion of the centromere. Inversions are rarely responsible for clinical pathology but may cause unbalanced gametes.

## Isochromosome

An isochromosome has a deletion of one arm with a duplication of the other. These result from transverse division of the centromere during cell division or from an isochromatid break which fuses above the centromere. Isochromosomes of the long arm of the X chromosomes may result in *Turner syndrome* due to short-arm monosomy and long-arm trisomy. Isochromosomes of the Y chromosome are also seen in live births, but most autosomal isochromosomes induce spontaneous early abortion.

## Centric fragments

Small, metacentric additional fragments may be detected during routine karyotyping. Some are familial as the result of a Robertsonian translocation in a parent. If the centric fragment contains only repetitive and ribosomal DNA there are usually no clinical abnormalities. Unusually, transcribed genes are also included, with consequent anomalies.

# Other chromosomal anomalies

## Mosaicism

A mosaic is an individual with more than one cell line derived from a single zygote. This implies the concurrent presence of normal cells and cells carrying a mutation. Mosaicism accounts for about 1 per cent of patients with *trisomy 21*, and karyotyping confirms normal and trisomic cell lines. Mosaicism is usually a post-zygotic event; the zygote has *trisomy 21*, and a normal cell line is produced at a subsequent mitosis by anaphase lag. Alternatively, the original zygote may be normal and a trisomic cell line results from non-disjunction at a later mitosis.

Somatic mosaicism results from a chromosomal anomaly or a gene mutation arising in somatic cells which then divide to produce daughter cells carrying the same mutation. Such mutations are not inherited, nor are they transmitted to the carrier's children. Somatic mutation may occur at any time where there is cell division.

Germ line (germinal) mosaicism occurs when an individual develops both normal and mutation-carrying germ line cells. This mutation may be passed to offspring. It will not be detected in the parents unless it is also carried in the somatic cells and will only manifest when expressed in the offspring. The presence of unexpressed germ-line mutations has important implications in "new" mutations in autosomal dominant and X-linked conditions, where recurrence of a phenotype within a family would not be expected.

## Chimeras

A chimera is an individual with two cell lines which have been derived from two separate zygotes. This could result from the exchange of hemopoietic stem cells *in utero* by dizygotic twins, by early fusion of dizygotic twin zygotes, or by double fertilization of the egg and a polar body.

## Uniparental disomy and isodisomy

Inheritance of both paternal and maternal copies of each autosome are required for normal development. This is illustrated by *hydatidiform moles* and by certain syndromes, e.g. the *Prader-Willi* and *Angelman syndromes*.

Uniparental disomy (UPD) is the inheritance of both chromosomes of a pair from only one parent. Two identical copies of the chromosome constitute uniparental isodisomy, while two different copies of that chromosome from one parent constitute uniparental heterodisomy.

The most likely explanation for UPD is that the zygote begins as a trisomy because of a meiotic error. Most trisomic conceptions are lethal and the embryo is aborted unless a cell line with only two copies of the chromosome, i.e. a disomic cell, arises and survives. If one of the copies is lost during cell division to produce a disomic cell line, the result will be uniparental disomy. In one-third of cases, both chromosomes in the pair will come from one parent. Depending on the chromosome involved, the extra copy may be lost as early as the four-cell stage or as late as two to three weeks after the beginning of embryogenesis. There are

several chromosomes which are more likely to exhibit this phenomenon: chromosome 15 as well as chromosomes 4, 6, 7, 11, 14, 16 and 21.

If the two copies of the chromosome coming from one parent are identical (isodisomy) and each carries an abnormal recessive gene, then uniparental disomy can lead to the expression of a recessive disorder in the child. There have been reports of *cystic fibrosis*, an autosomal recessive disease, in which both chromosomes 7 have come from the mother while the father of the affected individuals is not a carrier for CF. Uniparental disomy is one of the mechanisms for genomic imprinting.

## SINGLE GENE DISORDERS

The principles of inheritance were first determined in 1865 by an Austrian monk, Gregor Mendel. He observed that there were discrete units of heredity and that these were transmitted in a predictable pattern from parent to offspring, with one copy of each gene coming from each parent and both copies being expressed equally. He introduced the concepts of *dominant* and *recessive* inheritance.

Single gene disorders are caused by mutations on one or both of a pair of autosomal genes, or the X or Y chromosome. More than 4000 disorders have been identified that are inherited according to mendelian patterns. The following patterns of inheritance have been described:

■ autosomal inheritance: dominant, recessive, or codominant;
■ sex-linked inheritance: X-linked recessive, X-linked dominant, or Y-linked (holandric).

## Autosomal inheritance

Twenty-two pairs of autosomes exist. Each gene occupies a specific locus on a chromosome. Autosomal genes present in pairs: one paternal, one maternal. Alternate forms of a gene are called alleles. If both members of a gene pair are identical, the person is homozygous for that locus. If the alleles differ, the person is heterozygous.

### Autosomal dominant (AD) inheritance

Autosomal dominant disorders are transmitted from generation to generation, irrespective of gender, and these manifest in the heterozygous form. An affected individual has one normal allele and one mutant. This individual will pass either the normal gene or the mutant to his or her offspring, with a 50 per cent chance. Many AD disorders when present in the homozygous form have a very severe phenotype, e.g. *familial hypercholesterolemia*. *Huntington chorea*, by contrast, is a true AD condition where heterozygotes and homo-

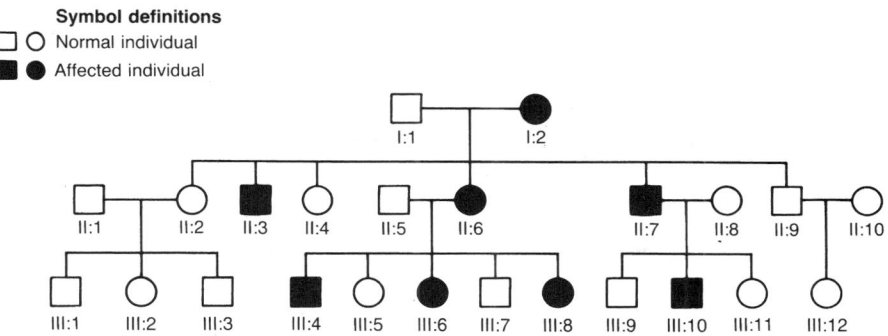

FIGURE 3.9 An autosomal dominant pedigree shows a vertical pattern of inheritance. Male-to-male, female-to-female, male-to-female and female-to-male transmission all occur.

zygotes are equivalent in phenotype. An example of an autosomal dominant pedigree with its vertical pattern of transmission is shown in Fig. 3.9.

## Penetrance

This is the frequency of expression of a genotype. Full penetrance implies that all individuals who have the mutant gene are phenotypically affected. Non-penetrance may occur, leading to a skipped generation in an AD pedigree, e.g. *ectodactyly*. Late-onset disorders may mimic non-penetrance.

## Expressivity

This is the variation in the severity of a phenotype, e.g. *neurofibromatosis* where even intrafamilial variation is evident.

## Epistasis

This is the influence on a gene by an allele at another locus. It may explain variable severity of clinical manifestations of a syndrome within a family.

## Domains

Mutations may occur in different domains of a protein product and therefore affect different functions of the same protein. Two different mutations in the same gene can produce different phenotypes.

## New mutations

These occur on a regular though unpredictable basis. Mutation frequency ranges from 1 in 30 000 to 1 in 100 000 live-born infants.

## Pleiotropism

A single abnormal gene may produce multiple, unrelated abnormalities. The understanding of the pathogenic mechanisms for such disorders will elucidate their common cause.

## Germinal mosaicism

This explains the recurrence of an AD trait or XLR in siblings with overtly normal parents. A mutation in gonadal cells only will not express in the parent, but may be passed to the next generation.

## Paternal age effect

Advanced paternal age accounts for an increase in "new mutation" of several autosomal dominant disorders, including *achondroplasia* and *Apert syndrome*.

## Autosomal recessive (AR) inheritance

If an AR gene exists in the heterozygous form, the individual will be a carrier of that disorder. Affected individuals inherit the homozygous form, with identical mutant alleles at a locus. Thus, a 25 per cent chance exists that the offspring of two carriers will be affected. A 50 per cent chance exists of their children being gene carriers. A pedigree illustrating autosomal recessive inheritance in a consanguineous union (horizontal pattern) is shown in Fig. 3.10.

## Consanguinity

The common ancestry of a couple increases the proportion of shared genes, and therefore increases the risks of AR conditions.

## Carrier detection

This is the confirmation of carrier status in relatives of individuals with AR conditions.

## Compound heterozygotic

This is an individual who inherits two differently abnormal alleles of the same gene. This may affect the phenotype.

## Complementation

Two different alleles of the same gene may compensate for each other, resulting in a normal phenotype.

## Autosomal codominant inheritance

The pattern of codominance resembles autosomal dominant, where two alleles can be followed together through a family. The ABO blood groups are inherited codominantly.

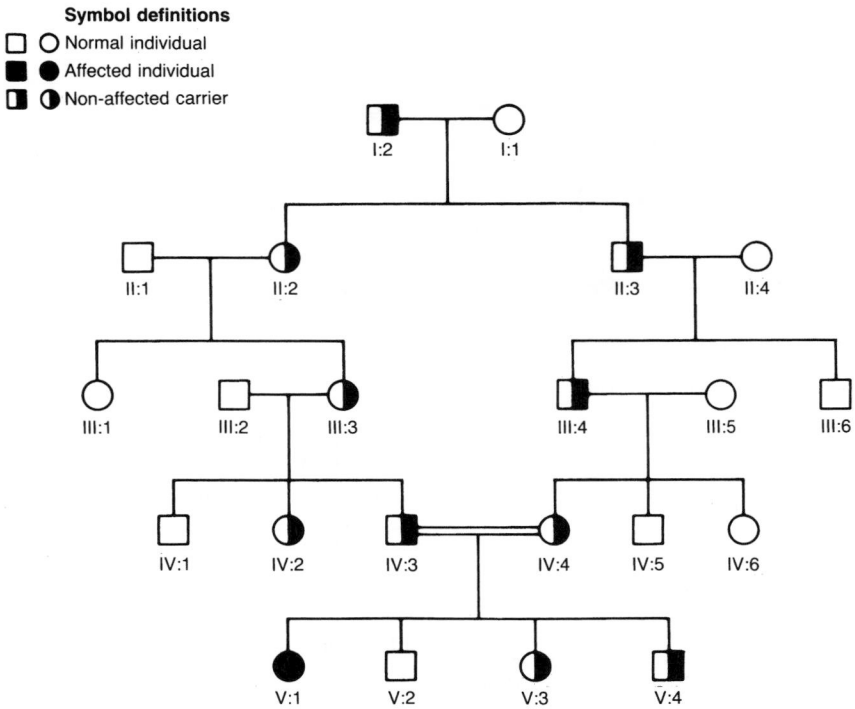

**Symbol definitions**
☐ ○ Normal individual
■ ● Affected individual
◧ ◑ Non-affected carrier

FIGURE 3.10 A pedigree illustrating autosomal recessive inheritance (horizontal pattern). The double line between IV:3 and IV:4 denotes the consanguineous union.

# Sex-linked inheritance

The female has two X chromosomes. One of the X chromosomes may be inactivated in each somatic cell, by a process known as lyonization. Lyonization is the inactivation of one X chromosome in somatic cells except for a few XY homologous genes. It occurs at approximately 16 days' gestation by a process of methylation. This ensures that the amount of X-linked gene products in somatic cells of females is equivalent to male cells.

The male (XY) is hemizygous for each X chromosome gene; he has only one copy for each locus on the X chromosomes.

## X-linked recessive (XLR) inheritance

Heterozygous females are clinically unaffected (carriers) but may transmit the disorder to their hemizygous sons. Thus, a female carrier has a 50 per cent chance of affected sons and a 50 per cent chance of carrier daughters. All daughters of affected males are obligate carriers. An example of a pedigree of X-linked recessive transmission within a family is shown in Fig. 3.11.

Normally, lyonization is random such that different cells do not inactivate the same X chromosome. However, all daughter cells from a given cell will continue to inactivate the same X chromosome. In certain situations (e.g. some immunodeficiency disorders such

as X-linked *severe combined immunodeficiency syndrome* and *Wiskott–Aldrich syndrome*, or in the presence of a structural abnormality of the chromosome) X inactivation is non-random. Female carriers of some X-linked disorders (e.g. *Duchenne muscular dystrophy* and *hemophilia A*) may manifest symptoms if a greater portion of cells have the mutation on the active X chromosome; they are known as *manifesting heterozygotes*.

## X-linked dominant (XLD) inheritance

Males are usually severely affected by X-linked dominant disorders whereas manifestations in females are variable because of lyonization. The pedigree resembles AD, but no male-to-male transmission is possible and all daughters of affected males are affected. Examples of these disorders are *incontinentia pigmenti* and *focal dermal hypoplasia*.

## Male lethality

XLD conditions exist in females where the phenotype is so severe in males that spontaneous abortions occur. It is thought that the cells in which the abnormal gene has been inactivated due to lyonization survive, and cells that express only the abnormal gene die, producing a "patchy" phenotype, e.g. *incontinentia pigmenti*. Males carrying only the abnormal gene are not viable. An explanation for the small number of males who do survive with manifestations of these XLD disorders is *somatic mosaicism*.

**Symbol definitions**

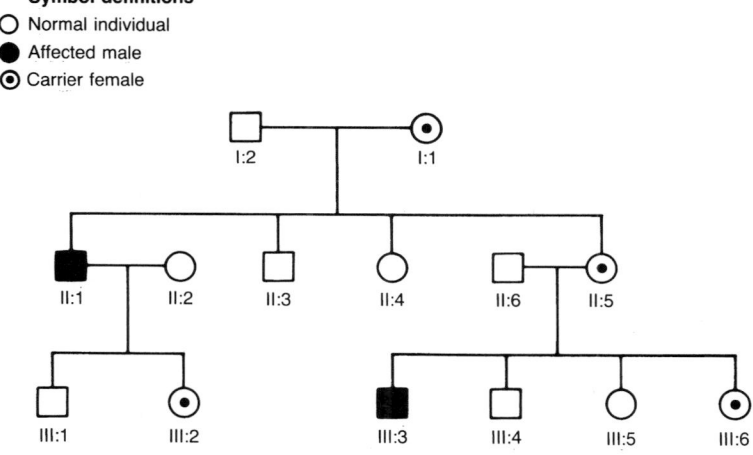

FIGURE 3.11 A pedigree showing X-linked recessive inheritance, with carrier females transmitting a disorder which affects sons. Daughters of affected males are obligate carriers.

## Y-linked inheritance

The Y chromosome is passed from father to son. No human disorders transmitted by the Y chromosome have as yet been identified.

# Mutations

The molecular lesion in a single gene disorder may occur at any point in the pathway from DNA to protein product. Genetic heterogeneity results from diverse molecular pathology. The defect therefore may be a gene mutation, defective regulation of transcription to mRNA or mRNA processing, an error in translation to the initial protein, or a post-translational processing anomaly. A mutation is a change in the DNA sequence of the gene.

If a mutation occurs in the coding region of a gene the protein product is changed and may result in defective function. If the mutation occurs in the regulatory region of a gene it may affect the protein quantitatively, or it may completely block its synthesis. Despite the fact that DNA polymerase has a sensitive "proofreading" mechanism to detect and repair errors in replication, mutations still occur at the frequency of about $10^{-6}$ per gene per cell.

For practical purposes, mutations of DNA are divided into point mutations (alteration of the genetic code with no gain or loss of genetic material) and length mutations (gain or loss of genetic material).

## Point mutation

A point mutation is the replacement of a single nucleotide base with another. Purine to purine, or pyrimidine to pyrimidine is a transition; transversions are purine to pyrimidine change, or vice versa. This may result in no change to the amino acid coded for, e.g. CAA and

CAG both code for Glutamine. Alternatively, substitution of another amino acid causes a missense mutation, while alteration to a chain terminator or stop codon causes a nonsense mutation. These are designated by standard nomenclature dependent upon the mutation type, the genetic code and the position of the amino acid within the protein.

Point mutations are largely spontaneous, with a mutation rate of approximately 1 base pair substituted for every $10^9$ base pairs replicated. A variety of mutagens, including ionizing radiation and chemical agents, alter the rate of mutation by a number of different mechanisms. Mutagens generally cause point mutations. The mutation rate alters dependent upon the time and dose of exposure to irradiation or the other mutagens. These mutagens are largely somatic.

X-rays cause chromosome breakage but uncommonly lead to point mutations. In contrast, a range of mutations are attributed to the effects of ultraviolet light. Pyrimidine bases adjacent to each other are linked by carbon–carbon bonding resulting in thymidine dimers. This bonding distorts the DNA region. The resultant crosslinks interfere with the synthesis of DNA and the transcription of RNA.

Temperature changes cause the loss of approximately 5000 purine bases from every cell on a daily basis as a natural phenomenon. In parallel, the deamination of at least a hundred cytosines to uracil occurs on this basis. DNA would soon lose normal function without the existence of repair mechanisms for these changes. A large range of specific enzymes, DNA glycosylases, and nucleases play a role in the repair of depurination and deamination. An example of a defect in certain nucleases is xeroderma pigmentosa, where an inability to perform excision repair results in skin cancer.

Not all deamination is identifiable and the mechanisms for repair are not as clear. Certain transitions appear not to be repaired, e.g. the deamination of methylated cytosine to thymidine, with a parallel adenine to guanine change on the complementary DNA strand. Up to half of all point mutations may be caused by C to T translations.

## Length mutations

Length mutation may be duplications, deletions, or insertions. The length of the mutation may be one base pair to thousands of kilobases. There are a number of mechanisms for deletion including chromosomal breakage *de novo* or via parental translocation. Unequal meiotic crossing over may occur, particularly where genes are duplicated within a region. Slipped mispairing may result in the loss of a single stranded loop, and consequent gene loss. Large deletions cause the loss of a number of contiguous genes which may manifest as a single gene disorder phenotype with additional unexplained anomalies. Transcription will be prevented if an entire gene is lost. Deletion may alter the reading frame of the mRNA if they are smaller or greater than three base pairs long. This alteration may result in premature termination of translocation if there is a stop codon in the out-of-frame message. These are frameshift mutations. In the same way, the reading frame may be changed by duplication mutations.

Either point or length mutations may result from nonreciprocal recombination, which may occur during mitosis or meiosis. In this gene conversion, one allele is replaced by another. The effect of this is unbalanced and a segment of DNA is lost.

## Trinucleotide repeats

A number of human neurological disorders have been identified as having a different type of mutation as their cause, the expansion of trinucleotide repeats. These triplet repeats are normally polymorphic and exonic although they do not always have a coding function. In the disorder states they become unstable and may expand by thousands of repeats in a single generation. The consequent changes occur in gene expression, message stability and protein structure. These disorders all show a marked variation in clinical symptoms as well as the phenomenon of genetic *anticipation*, which is the progressive worsening of the severity of the phenotype in successive generations. Table 3.1 illustrates the features of *fragile X syndrome*, *Huntington chorea*, *spinocerebellar ataxia*, *Kennedy disease*, *myotonic dystrophy* and *FraXE*, all of which result from triplet repeat mutations.

*Fragile X* syndrome is a common cause of mental retardation that is inherited as an X-linked dominant disorder with reduced penetrance. Fragile X syndrome has been shown to be caused by an unstable trinucleotide repeat, CGG, within the fragile X mental retarda-

tion type 1 (*FMR-1*) gene at Xq27. The CGG repeat lies within the 5′ untranslated region of the first exon. This CGG repeat is polymorphic in normal individuals and ranges from 6 to 52 repeats, with an average size of 29 repeats. Individuals with fragile X mental retardation have an increase or expanded region of CGG repeats which makes the gene unstable. Affected individuals have expansion resulting in 200–1000 repeats and this is known as a full mutation. When the trinucleotide repeat is this size, the DNA of the entire 5′ region becomes abnormally methylated. This methylation extends upstream into and beyond the promoter region and results in transcriptional suppression of the *FMR-1* gene. Affected males generally have no detectable *FMR-1* mRNA, and the absence of the encoded protein Fmr-p is thought to cause the phenotype. The premutation allele is of intermediate length, between 50 and 200 repeats, and occurs in female carriers, non-penetrant males and normal transmitting males. The premutations are unmethylated and transcriptionally active, and these alleles produce normal levels of Fmr-p. Males who carry the mutation but are intellectually normal are carriers, but account for the reduced penetrance of the transmission of this disorder. The premutation is extremely unstable when transmitted, and the offspring have alleles distinct from the parental premutation. When transmitted from the mother, the premutation can change and lengthen, but may also undergo expansion to a full mutation. Transmission of a premutation allele through the male line may cause some slight lengthening but does not result in the full mutation. The mechanism limiting the expansion of premutation to full mutation to maternal transmission is unknown, but may be associated with lethality of the full mutation in sperm and/or an influence of X-inactivation on the expansion process.

## MULTIFACTORIAL INHERITANCE

Multifactorial or polygenic traits result from an interaction of a number of genes at different loci together with environmental factors. Multifactorial traits may be continuous, i.e. lacking a distinct phenotype (e.g. height), or discontinuous with distinct phenotypes (e.g. *spina bifida*). In discontinuous disorders the risk of recurrence to members of an affected family is raised above the general population risk, but it is lower than the risk in mendelian traits. The study of twin concordance in monozygotic twins, as well as correlation of data within a family, may help to discern the proportion of heritability in the causation of such a disorder. Twins are concordant if both are positive for a discontinuous trait and discordant if only one manifests that trait. Monozygotic twins are genetically identical as they are derived from a single zygote which divides into two embryos during the first two weeks of gestation. By contrast dizygotic twins result from two fertilized ova by two spermatozoa and are therefore genetically equivalent to two siblings.

The environment, both intrauterine and postnatal in twins, tends to be similar and it is difficult to distinguish the proportion of genes or the environment to that multifactorial trait. Studies of twins who have been adopted in infancy and raised apart may yield important information.

## SOMATIC-CELL GENETIC DISORDERS

Somatic cell disorders arise only in specific somatic cells; mutations can occur at any time when there is cell division. Cancer syndromes, which may involve an interaction between a genetic predisposition and environmental factors, represent a paradigm for somatic cell disease. The accumulation of multiple genetic changes underpins the process of tumorigenesis. Both dominantly acting oncogenes and inactivated tumor-suppressor genes may simulaneously exist in the same tumor. Individual mutations are thought to contribute independently to the phenotype. Several examples have been found of mutations in genes that act on contact points via a number of mechanisms, either to ensure genome stability or to regulate common pathways that signal cell proliferation, survival and differentiation. Mutations at these loci may have multiple and apparently unrelated phenotypic consequences.

*Bilateral retinoblastoma* is inherited as an autosomal dominant trait. A deletion in the *Rb* gene on chromosome 13q14 is inherited, i.e. the "first hit." A second somatic mutation at the same locus of the homologous chromosome in the tumor causes functional homozygosity at this locus, i.e. the "second hit." This loss of heterozygosity at a critical locus results in the phenotype.

Retinoblastoma cells of both familial or spontaneous tumors have altered function of the *Rb* protein. The major role of this protein is to sequester cell-cycle specific transcription factors; the *Rb* protein bonds to these factors, inhibiting their action for most of the cycle. During the G1–S stages, *Rb* is phosphorylated by a protein kinase and loses the ability to bind these transcription factors, which are then free to bind to their DNA target sequences and modify the expression of numerous genes. At a specific point in the cell cycle, the inhibitory phosphates are removed and *Rb* re-sequesters the transcription factors. It appears that tumor formation is due to abrogation of the transcription binding capacity of the *Rb* protein and deregulation of transcription.

## NON-TRADITIONAL INHERITANCE

The mendelian laws of inheritance have been the basis for our understanding of genetics. However, recent studies have demonstrated that not all inherited traits follow these laws and that the genes from both parents do not always make an equal contribution to offspring, nor are they always equally expressed. These phenomena include cytoplasmic inheritance, uniparental dis-

omy (see chromosome disorders) and genomic imprinting.

## Cytoplasmic inheritance (*see also* page 85)

The cytoplasmic route of inheritance occurs as a result of mitochondrial inheritance with some influence from the mitotic spindles and endoplasmic reticulum. The nucleus does not carry all of our genetic material; the mitochondria contain a separate genome comprising more than 16 kb of DNA and each somatic cell contains $10^3$–$10^4$ copies of the mitochondrial genome. The inheritance of these genes follows a strictly maternal line of transmission and these genetic traits or susceptibility to a trait are passed only through women to offspring of both sexes. This differs from X-linked recessive traits whereby only male offspring are affected. Transmission of mitochondrial genes ends with sons, since they do not pass mitochondrial material on to their offspring. Spermatozoa introduce a small number of mitochondria into the egg at fertilization, but these are digested soon after penetration.

Mammalian mitochondrial DNA codes for 13 enzymes used in the mitochondrial energy generating pathway of oxidative phosphorylation, 22 tRNAs and two rRNAs. Although all transcripts of mitochondrial DNA remain in the mitochondria, most proteins used in the mitochondria are derived from nuclear DNA and are imported after synthesis on cytoplasmic ribosomes.

Mitochondria play a critical role in cellular energy metabolism, and deletions or point mutations of the mitochondrial DNA produce a variety of disorders in organ syndromes. The clinical expression of mitochondrial diseases is variable and depends on the nature of the mutation as well as the proportion of mitochondria in the body tissues and the proportion of mitochondria carrying mutant versus wild-type DNA. *Heteroplasmy* is the term used to describe the presence of both wild-type and mutant mitochondrial genomes in an individual. *Homoplasmy* may result if the mutant DNA has a replicative advantage (e.g. smaller size due to the presence of a deletion).

Multiple deletions of mitochondrial DNA have recently been described in a number of patients with neurological disorders. Point mutations, deletions and depletion of the mitochrondrial genome are associated with disorders including LHON (*Lebers hereditary optic neuropathy*), MERRF (*myoclonus epilipsia with ragged red fibers*), and MELAS (*mitochondrial myopathy, encephalopathy, lactic acidosis* and *stroke-like episodes*). Onset may be late, with central or peripheral nervous system involvement, short stature, deafness and myoglobinuria. Mitochondrial DNA-encoded enzyme activity is reduced in skeletal muscle. Deletions in mitochondrial DNA occur at multiple sites between the replication initiation sites, and most deletions seem to be flanked by direct sequence repeats shown to be "hot-spots" in the case of single large deletions. A defect in a nuclear gene may result in multiple deletions of mitochondrial DNA. Both the clinical and molecular observations indicate genetic heterogeneity based on a disturbance in the crosstalk between nuclear and mitochondrial genomes.

## Genomic imprinting

Genomic imprinting refers to the process whereby specific genes are differentially marked during parental gametogenesis with the result that there is differential expression of these genes in the embryo and the adult. It is the understanding of genomic imprinting which explains the uneven inheritance of several autosomal disorders depending on maternal or paternal transmission. Early studies in the 1980s using pronuclear experiments in mouse models demonstrated that paternal and maternal inheritance was unequal in mammals. The first gene which was found to be imprinted was the *IGF-II* gene; this gene was expressed as mRNA only from the paternal allele. By contrast, genes encoding for the IGF-II receptor (*IGF-IIR*) and a differentiation-related fetal RNA (*H19*) were expressed only from the maternal allele. The process of genomic imprinting in the human is complex, involving an interplay of gene-specific and chromosomal domain events, including DNA methylation, chromatin compaction and DNA replication.

Any biochemical modification of DNA and/or chromatin which may account for imprinting would have to satisfy four requirements: the modification should be made prior to fertilization; the modification should confer transcriptional silencing and must be transmitted in a stable form via mitosis in somatic cells; and this modification must be reversible on passage through the opposite parental germ line.

Methylation of DNA in mammalian cells occurs exclusively at cytosine residues in the context of CpG dinucleotides. CpG methylation of genes, especially in promoter regions, can render them transcriptionally silent and CpG is faithfully transmitted through cell divisions by the maintenance action of DNA methyltransferase.

A model for genomic imprinting in human disorders is the comparison of the *Prader-Willi syndrome* (PWS) and the *Angelman syndrome* (AS) which have two distinct phenotypes. In PWS the deletions of chromosome 15 are exclusively paternal, while the deletions in AS are maternal. PWS patients who do not have an obvious deletion of chromosome 15 show uniparental disomy (UPD) as a result of non-disjunction during parental gametogenesis and/or early embryonic development. This non-disjunction leads to absence of the paternal chromosome 15. Similar events occur in AS to cause uniparental disomy, but in AS there is an absence of maternal chromosome 15. The net effect of either a deletion or uniparental disomy is a functional

loss of paternal genes in PWS and a functional loss of maternal genes in AS. The uniparental disomy class of patient suggests that the corresponding maternal genes in PWS and paternal genes in AS are normally silent and it appears that a contribution at this locus from both parents is necessary.

Two DNA methylation imprints are known to exist at the 15q11-q13 locus; *PW71* is associated with an endogenous retroviral solo LTR sequence and *snRPN* in the 5th intron of the small nuclear ribonuclear protein peptide N. These imprints are recognizable as epigenetic differences in DNA between the two parental alleles, and this type of modification satisfies all the requirements necessary for specifically marking parental alleles in the germ line and for subsequent maintenance during embryonic and adult development. Individuals with the PWS with either deletion or UPD, therefore, have only a maternal DNA methylation imprint, while the AS patients have only a paternal methylation imprint. These DNA methylation imprints can be used for molecular diagnostic purposes in PWS and AS.

A number of AS patients exist with neither a deletion nor UPD. This group do not have a DNA methylation imprint characteristic of AS but have a normal biparental pattern. Included among these patients are a number of familial cases in which the etiologic imprinted gene is linked to chromosome 15q11-q13. It is thought that this is likely to be due to a point mutation or a small rearrangement in a single imprinted *AS* gene producing the AS phenotype. These mutations may not affect the determinants of the imprint such as chromatin structure or DNA methylation. This is probably not the case in PWS; there is no significant group of patients with PWS with inheritance consistent with a single segregated gene, and this would suggest that multiple genes may play roles in the classic PWS phenotype. The *snRPN* gene in the *Prader-Willi* region is found to be functionally imprinted since it is expressed only from the paternal chromosome. However, evidence suggests that the regulation of imprinted genes may involve domain structures and it is possible that genes outside the critical regions may have an effect on the phenotype. For example, studies of small deletions in critical regions of *PW71* and *snRPN* in human chromosome arrangements in 15q11-q13 suggest that DNA methylation imprints are altered at distant loci including a zinc finger gene, *ZNF127*. Therefore, the regulation of imprinted genes may involve domain structures and it is possible that genes outside the critical regions may have an effect on the phenotype.

In addition to deletions and UPD, specific mutations which affect the imprinting mechanism may cause silencing of the normal, active parental allele. A model has been postulated whereby a *cis* mutation in the germ line of one grandparent results in failure to restore the imprinting signal in the parental germ line, which results in the phenotype and familial occurrence of PWS or AS. A new concept of *imprinting control elements* (ICE) has been suggested where mutations cause *cis*-active elements to be defective in PWS and AS. These ICE differ in each syndrome so that the imprinting mutation would affect each syndrome specifically.

Timing of the DNA replication of imprinting genes and their flanking loci is important. Most genes replicate synchronously during the S phase of the cell cycle. However, all known imprinted genes in human and mice replicate asynchronously, with the paternal allele usually replicating before the maternal allele. The loci in PWS and AS critical regions all show early paternal replication. This phenomenon has also been observed in imprinted *H19* and *IGF-II* genes in the mouse and in the Philadelphia chromosome in *chronic myeloid leukemia*. It is possible that the distal 15q11-13 region contains an ICE regulating an imprinted locus in this region. It is unknown how differential DNA replication of a chromosomal domain and differential DNA methylation at individual loci are coordinated, although DNA methyltransferase may localize to sites of DNA replication. It is likely that specific proteins expressed during male or female gametogenesis are involved in the specification of the epigenetic imprint in addition to DNA methylation.

There is a second group of imprinted genes, known as the triplet repeat disorders (*see* Table 3.1). In the fragile X syndrome, for example, when a tract of CGG repeats in the gene *FMR-1* becomes longer than a critical length, the repeat region becomes unstable and can undergo massive length expansions during cellular DNA replication. Expansions occur as a multistep process over several generations. Premutations are smaller expansions which do not result in clinical manifestations, whereas the much larger full mutation causes functional inactivation of the *FMR-1* gene and results in the fragile X phenotype. Imprinting in the repeat

area may provide an explanation for the observation that a premutation in a female may go on to a full mutation in her offspring, whereas a premutation in a male is transmitted to the next generation as a premutation. Other evidence for imprinting in these triplet repeat disorders are the earlier onset of *Huntington chorea* when transmitted paternally, and the earlier onset and congenital phenotype of myotonic dystrophy. The explanation for this association between imprinting and expansion is not apparent. The fragile X triplet repeat and nearby region contains CpG sites which are highly methylated only in the expanded allele. Maternal-specific hypermethylation associated with X-inactivation could play a role in marking the premutation for subsequent expansion.

The third area of evidence for imprinting is in tumorigenesis. This is initially observed in the *inherited paraganglioma syndrome* which usually presents with bilateral carotid body tumors and is inherited as a maternally imprinted/paternally expressed dominant oncogene. The locus responsible is 11q23-qter and this rare syndrome only manifests after transmission from fathers. The *Beckwith–Wiedemann syndrome* (BWS) is characterized by overgrowth and tumorigenesis. There is good evidence for genomic imprinting in BWS; chromosomal inversion or translocation in the 11p15.4 or 11p15.5 region may only be expressed after passage of these structurally abnormal chromosomes through the maternal germ line. A number of patients with BWS without cytogenetic anomalies have shown genetic linkage to the region, again only via the maternal line. There is evidence of paternal duplication, or isodisomy, for the 11p15.5 region. Tumors seen in patients with BWS show frequent loss of heterozygosity for DNA markers at the 11p15.5 locus with 95 per cent maternal allele loss. Human *IGF-II* and *H19* genes display methylation imprinting, and the

TABLE 3.1 Summary of expansion mutations

| DISORDER | FRAGILE X SYNDROME | MYOTONIC DYSTROPHY | HUNTINGTON CHOREA | SPINOCEREBELLAR ATAXIA TYPE 1 | SPINOBULBAR MUSCULAR ATROPHY (KENNEDY'S DISEASE) | FRAXE |
|---|---|---|---|---|---|---|
| Inheritance | X-linked dominant with incomplete penetrance | Autosomal dominant | Autosomal dominant | Autosomal dominant | X-linked recessive | X-linked recessive |
| Anticipation | Anticipation | Anticipation | Anticipation | Anticipation | Unknown | Unknown |
| Sex bias for transmission of severe form | Maternal (full mutation) | Maternal (congenital DM) | Paternal (early onset) | Paternal | Unknown | ?Maternal |
| Repeated trinucleotide | CGG | CTG | CAG | CAG | CAG | CGG |
| Size of repeat (normal) | 6–52 | 5–35 | 9–34 | 19–36 | 11–33 | 6–25 |
| Disease alleles | 52–230 (premutation) 230–2000 (full mutation) | 50–80 (protomutation) 80–2000 (affected) | 30–100 | 43–81 | 40–62 | ? ›25 ›200 premutation ? ›200 full mutation |
| Gene locus | Xq27.3 | 19 | 4p16.3 | 6p22 | Xq28 | ?Xq27.3 |
| Gene | *FMR-1* gene (5′ untranslated) | Mytonin protein kinase (3′ untranslated) | *IT1-5* (coding sequence) | *SCA-1* Unknown | Androgen receptor (coding region) | Unknown |

relationship between imprinting and the *IGF-II* gene have been implicated in *Wilms tumor* and BWS.

## SPORADIC CASES OF GENETIC DISORDER

All single gene disorders have arisen by mutation at some time; the proportion of individuals with each genetic disorder is held in genetic equilibrium. The loss of genes, for example due to reduced ability to survive or reproduce, is balanced by the gain of these genes by mutation. In sporadic cases of hereditable disorders the following possibilities exist.

- New mutation may occur in AD or XLR disorders. Approximately one-third of boys with XLR disorders have new mutations. Advanced paternal age increases the possibility of new mutations in AD disorders, e.g. *Apert syndrome* and *achondroplasia*.
- The affected person may have a recessive gene in the homozygous state. The possibility is strengthened by parental consanguinity.
- Variable expression with a very subtle phenotype, missed clinically in the parent, may result in apparent non-penetrance.
- Germ line (germinal) mosaicism may occur in the parent. A phenotypically unaffected parent has the mutation in his/her germ cells which is transmitted to the offspring.
- Somatic mutation may occur.
- Uniparental disomy may occur.
- Contiguous gene deletions may occur, resulting in a chromosomal anomaly.
- Phenocopy may occur. This results from an environmental factor producing the same phenotype as a single gene disorder, e.g. *warfarin embryopathy* and *chondrodysplasia punctatum*.

## TECHNIQUES TO EVALUATE GENETIC DISORDERS

## Cytogenetics

### Karyotyping

Human chromosomes are most easily studied using peripheral blood, but almost any dividing cells can be used including bone marrow, skin fibroblasts or cells from amniotic fluid or chorionic villi. After 48–72 hours of incubation, cell division is arrested at metaphase by the addition of colchicine. The chromosomes (chromos = colored, soma = body) have the ability to take up stains, which produce approximately 500 alternating light and dark bands. These are characteristic for each chromosome pair. Special Banding allows more accurate identification of each chromosome. Deletions or duplications of 4000 kb or more can be visualized on routine chromosomal analysis. Higher resolution of smaller defects is possible by arrest of cell division in prometaphase (long chromosomes).

### Flow cytometry

Flow cytometry measures the DNA content of chromosomes. This demonstrates inherited variations in this content between individual chromosomes. The X chromosome shows least variability, the Y chromosome most. These differences are known as heteromorphisms and are genetic polymorphisms, e.g. fragile sites. Size polymorphisms generally encompass repetitive DNA, varying in this size within a normal distribution. Chromosome heteromorphisms are rarely implicated in disorders, other than *Fragile X syndrome*.

### High-resolution imaging

These techniques, which include fluorescent *in situ* hybridization (FISH), electron microscope *in situ* hybridization (EMISH), primed *in situ* labeling (PRINS) and comparative genomic hybridization, form a natural bridge between cytogenetic and molecular genetic studies and allow for the physical mapping of sequences of DNA within a chromosome.

## Biochemical analysis

A variety of biochemical markers are used in the study of genetic disorders, ranging from measurement of α-fetoprotein concentrations in maternal screening tests, to specific enzyme studies in the inborn errors of metabolism.

## Techniques for DNA analysis

### Source of material

Genomic DNA can be extracted from any tissue containing nucleated cells. Peripheral blood lymphocytes are the usual source of DNA, but amniotic fluid cells and chorionic villi are an important source of DNA in prenatal diagnosis.

### Family linkage studies

Two genes are linked if their loci are close together on a chromosome, so that they tend to be inherited together and meiotic recombination is unlikely. Polymorphic markers, which can be used in this way in family linkage studies include blood groups and enzymes, as well as restriction fragment length polymorphisms (RFLPs) and variable number of tandem repeats (VNTRs – minisatellites and microsatellites).

## DNA cloning (*see also* Chapter 1)

The term "recombinant DNA" refers to the ability to join genes from different species and have them functionally expressed; i.e. transcribed into mRNA then translated into protein. All cells from bacteria to humans have the enzymes and factors needed to read the DNA. A fragment of DNA with a particular sequence can base-pair or hybridize with any other DNA molecules which have a complimentary sequence. This enables a fragment of DNA with a known sequence to be used as a "molecular probe" to search for a particular gene. Restriction endonucleases are enzymes derived from bacteria which cut or "digest" DNA at specific sequences. Genomic DNA thus can be cut into smaller fragments at predictable sites, which allows the construction of recombinant vectors.

Cloning is the production of multiple identical copies of a DNA fragment. The DNA fragment, termed the insert, is inserted into a range of autonomously replicating DNA molecules, termed vectors. These vectors carry restriction enzyme sites which permit the cloning of insert DNAs. If the insert and the cloning vector site have been cut with the same enzyme, the base sequence of their free ends will be identical and a new recombinant DNA will be formed by the action of DNA ligase. These recombinant DNA molecules then are introduced into a host cell to produce multiple copies. Thereafter, vector and insert can be separated by restriction enzyme digestion of the purified recombinants, with the subsequent isolation of multiple identical copies of the insert DNA. DNA then can be sequenced to determine the exact order of the bases on the length of a single strand.

If a probe is known for a particular gene, the gene can be cloned by constructing a genomic library. This is created by digesting genomic DNA with restriction enzymes and inserting the resulting fragments into viral DNA vectors. Alternatively a complementary DNA (cDNA) library may be used; mRNA from tissue culture is used with the enzyme reverse transcriptase to generate cDNA.

## Southern blotting

Mutations may be analyzed using Southern blots. A specific probe and restriction enzyme can be used in combination to identify differences in the DNA sequence between a pair of chromosomes. A probe is a radioactively labeled sequence of DNA which is used to identify complementary sequences in the genomic DNA.

## Polymerase chain reaction (PCR)

PCR can rapidly amplify amounts of DNA of less than 1 μg for DNA analysis. A PCR requires two specific primers complementary to the flanking sequences of the DNA of interest. Single-stranded primers anneal to denatured DNA; thereafter DNA synthesis using added deoxyribonucleotide triphosphates proceeds 5' to 3' under the control of a heat-stable Taq-DNA polymerase. A cycle of heating and cooling in this way results in the production of larger amounts of double-stranded DNA, the ends of which are precisely bound by the primers and their complementary sequences. The amplified DNA then can be digested with a restriction endonuclease and the resulting fragments separated by gel electrophoresis. Following ethidium bromide staining, these DNA fragments can be visualized with ultraviolet light.

## Mutational analysis

Initially RFLP studies depended upon linkage analysis, i.e. the use of markers close to the gene of interest. This type of analysis necessitated family studies with comparison of affected and unaffected individuals. Recent advances in the identification and sequencing of genes have enabled intragenic investigation of disorders, no longer requiring family studies.

A number of PCR-based techniques are available for the detection of mutations at known DNA sites. These include RFLP analysis and allele-specific oligonucleotide hybridization. In addition, many techniques allow for the detection of mutations at unknown sites in PCR-amplified DNA; denaturing gradient gel electrophoresis, RNase A mismatch cleavage of either RNA:DNA or RNA:RNA heteroplexes, hydroxylamine/osmium tetroxide (HOT) mismatch cleavage (also known as chemical cleavage of mismatch method), electrophoresis of heteroduplex DNA, and single-strand conformation polymorphism analysis of PCR products.

Exon amplification, a technique useful in the search for gene defects, has been used successfully in the analysis of *Duchenne muscular dystrophy*. Exon amplification facilitates the analysis of expressed sequences from large regions of genomic DNA. This method of isolation is efficient, rapid and sensitive and has, to a large extent, streamlined diagnostic procedures that have in the past relied on restriction enzyme digestion and Southern blotting analysis.

Once a gene has been isolated, the exact sequence of that gene can be determined. The information gained from this sequence can be utilized in the understanding of the genotype/phenotype correlations, and for the development of specific gene therapy.

## SELECTED READING

Connor JM, Ferguson Smith MA. *Essential Medical Genetics* 4th Ed. Oxford: Blackwell, 1993.

Davies KE. *Human Genetic Disease Analysis*, 2nd edn. New York: IRL Press, 1993.

Demetrick BJ. Molecular biology primer for the paediatric pathologist. *Paed Pathol* 1994; **14**: 339.

Koshland D. Mitosis: back to the basics. *Cell* 1994; **77**: 951.

Langlois S. Genomic imprinting: a new mechanism for disease. *Paed Pathol* 1994; **14**: 161.

Monckton DG, Caskey CT. Unstable triplet repeat diseases. *Circulation* 1995; **91**: 513.

Nichols RD. New insights reveal complex mechanisms involved in genomic imprinting. *Am J Hum Genet* 1995; **54**: 733.

Orr HT. Unstable trinucleotide repeats and the diagnosis of neuro-degenerative disease. *Hum Pathol* 1994; **25**: 598.

Spagnolo DV, Turbett GR, Dix B, Iacopetta B. Polymerase chain reaction and single-strand polymorphism analysis (PCR-SSCP): a novel means of detecting DNA mutations. *Adv Anatomic Path* 1994; **1**: 61.

Sutherland GR, Richards RI. DNA repeats – a treasury of human variation. *N Engl J Med* 1994; **331**: 191.

Trask BJ. Fluorescent in situ hybridisation. *Trends Genet* 1991; **7**: 149.

Trent RJ. *Molecular Medicine*. London: Churchill Livingstone, 1994.

Warburton D. De novo balanced chromosome rearrangements and extra marker chromosomes identified at prenatal diagnosis: clinical significance and distribution of breakpoints. *Am J Hum Genet* 1991; **49**: 995.

Warren ST, Nelson DL. Advances in molecular analyses of fragile X syndrome. *JAMA* 1994; **271**: 536.

# PART THREE

# Biochemistry and Metabolism

## Editors: R. David G. Milner[†] and Garth Cooper

† Deceased

# 4

# Protein and Amino Acid Metabolism

Garth Cooper and R. David G. Milner

All forms of life arose from a common ancestor, and all are subject to the laws of physics and chemistry. Proteins exemplify this underlying unity of life. They constitute the primary substance or fundamental material of the bodies of animals and plants. They play central roles in almost all biological processes, acting as crucial structural and functional components of all living organisms. Indeed, the name "protein" embodies the importance of their contribution to the existence of life itself, being derived from the Greek word *proteios*, which means literally "primary" or "of the first rank."

Examples demonstrating the significance and scope of their contributions to life processes are legion. They include the mediation by proteins of the following structures and processes: enzymatic catalysis; coordination and execution of metabolic pathways; transport and storage systems; formation of the cytoskeleton and enablement of cellular movement systems; generation of the extracellular matrix and provision of mechanical support; immune function; regulation of growth and development; execution of the processes of DNA replication, transcription and translation; and communication within and between cells.

## DIETARY PROTEIN REQUIREMENTS

Dietary protein contributes all of the amino acids and fixed nitrogen necessary for the biosynthesis of tissue proteins and non-protein nitrogenous compounds such as purines and pyrimidines. Each day more amino acids are degraded and resynthesized in the body than are ordinarily consumed in the diet. The balance of protein degradation and resynthesis is called *protein turnover*. Dietary amino acids are required for the synthesis of new tissue constituents at all ages but particularly during growth. Amino acids consumed in excess of these needs are not stored but are degraded, the nitrogen being excreted and the carbon skeleton recycled.

All 20 fundamental amino acids must be present for protein synthesis to occur. Indeed, all proteins in all species, from bacteria to humans, are constructed from the same set of 20 amino acids, a fundamental alphabet of proteins which is at least two billion years old. The remarkable range of functions mediated by proteins results from the diversity and versatility of these 20 distinct building blocks. Nine amino acids, histidine, isoleucine, leucine, lysine, methionine, phenylalanine, threonine, tryptophan and valine, are not synthesized in the human body and are therefore "essential" for well-being. In addition, arginine is essential in infancy, and in the preterm infant there is a transient need for dietary tyrosine and cysteine as well.

The nutritional quality of dietary protein is influenced by its essential amino acid content. This implies that the protein intake contains sufficient "non-essential" amino acids to minimize metabolic diversion of essential amino acids to cover non-specific nitrogen requirements. The interrelationship between efficiency of utilization of amino acids and total dietary intake of energy also must be considered. In particular, the protein-sparing effect of an adequate energy intake is important, in that it can significantly decrease the total dietary requirement for protein.

An adequate protein intake contains all of the essential amino acids in sufficient quantities to satisfy maintenance needs and to provide a surplus sufficient for the processes of normal growth and development. Serum concentrations of albumin and total protein serve as clinical indicators of the sufficiency of dietary protein intake in the absence of systemic disease. From a practical standpoint, the protein foods of animal origin commonly consumed in western countries (milk, meat, fish and eggs) supply all of the essential amino acids; some foods of vegetable origin supply most of them in adequate amounts.

It is important to maintain a balanced intake of amino acids in the diet, and to understand the relationships between different groups of amino acids, and other nutrients such as vitamins. For example, when the most limiting amino acid in a diet generally poor in protein is increased, a deficiency of the next most limiting amino acid may occur. Excessive intakes of certain amino acids, which may or may not be limiting, when added to a diet that is marginal in certain of the B vitamins, may result in an increased severity of the vitamin deficiency. In other cases, an excess of an amino acid may reduce the utilization of another amino acid, that is provided in normally adequate amounts, to such an extent that a deficiency occurs.

Dietary protein requirements to maintain health are modest when judged by western intakes: an adult needs no more than 1 g protein/kg bodyweight and a baby no more than 3 g/kg each day, but dietary protein deficiency remains the most serious nutritional problem in the world and causes *kwashiorkor* in toddlers. A balanced shortage of all nutrients due to starvation results in *marasmus*.

## Women in normal pregnancy

The recommended daily allowance (RDA) of protein during pregnancy includes an additional 30 g/day beyond the 44 g/day recommended for non-pregnant women. Protein is relatively abundant in the diet of most western countries, and inadequate intake during pregnancy is relatively uncommon. Studies have associated diets containing 20 per cent of total calories from protein (as compared with the 12–14 per cent usually recommended) with a higher risk of premature deliveries and neonatal mortality and suggest that protein intakes significantly higher than those recommended may be harmful (*see also* page 300).

## The fetus

A fetus near term requires about 6–8 g of protein/day. Most of this comes as small amounts of essential and non-essential amino acids received continuously from the mother via the placental circulation. Free amino acid concentrations in the umbilical artery and vein are higher than those in the mother's blood, indicating active metabolic transport across the placenta. A second source of protein is the amniotic fluid swallowed by the fetus, which is estimated to yield up to 0.75 g/day.

## The newborn and infant

Protein requirements are proportionally greater in infants and children than in adults. Dietary protein intake in infancy must be sufficient to support increases in body protein ranging from an average of 3.7 g/day for the first month of life in males and 3.3 g/day in females down to 1.8 and 1.7 g/day, respectively, for months 9–12. These needs are generally met by protein intakes of about 1.8 g/100 kcal for infants during the first month of life, decreasing to 1.2 g/100 kcal for infants 4–6 months of age. The US Infant Formula Act of 1980 established a minimum standard for the protein equivalent content of infant formulas in that country, 1.8 g/100 kcal. The RDA of 2.2 g/kg for the first 6 months and 2.0 g/kg for months 7–12 also considers protein quality.

## Infants of low birthweight

Before 26 weeks' gestation, the fetal gastrointestinal system is too immature to digest proteins or other macronutrients; fully competent digestive processes do not develop until about 32–36 weeks' gestation. Feeding of such infants necessitates the provision of adequate calories and nutrients in a form that the immature digestive system and excretory systems can handle and that does not cause complications. Providing 95–160 kcal and about 3 g of protein/kg per day (maintained at about 10 per cent of calories ingested as the infant grows) in the context of a balanced intake of other nutrients helps achieve adequate nutrition for low-birthweight infants.

Parenteral nutrition is often used in the first days to weeks of life to support anabolism in infants who cannot tolerate full enteral feeding. Solutions of amino acids are usually used as the protein source, and amounts administered are limited to those that do not cause elevated plasma amino acid concentrations or the accumulation of ammonia in the blood.

## The normal child

The energy requirements of children are determined by their individual basal metabolic and growth rates, and activity patterns. Therefore, appropriate intakes for children of the same age, sex, and size vary. Higher than normally recommended levels of energy intake are required to compensate for inadequate bodyweight due to low birthweight, growth retardation or other factors.

Children need protein for the maintenance of body tissues, changes in body composition, and the synthesis of new tissues. During growth, the protein content of the body increases from about 15 per cent at 1 year to 18–19 per cent by 4 years, which is also the value for adults. Estimates of protein needs for growth range from 1 to 4 g/(kg.day). The RDA decreases from 1.8 g/(kg.day) at 1 year to 0.8 g/(kg.day) at 18 years.

## PROTEIN-ENERGY MALNUTRITION IN INFANCY AND CHILDHOOD

### See also Chapter 22

Animal and human studies have shown that severe malnutrition during fetal growth and early infancy can result in altered development of the brain, but the cognitive and behavioral effects of less severe nutritional deprivation cannot easily be distinguished from other environmental defects. Data from populations in which malnutrition is endemic indicate a relationship between growth retardation of infants and young children and low performance in tests of mental function. Children with protein-energy malnutrition in infancy who were tested at ages 5–11 years, had poorer academic performance than children who were well nourished in infancy, but the effects of socioeconomic disadvantage frequently complicate such studies. Children subjected to prenatal malnutrition have been shown to overcome cognitive defects and exhibit cognitive function levels that correlate most strongly with those of their parents. Other recent studies suggest that prenatal undernutrition could play a role in the appearance of adult diseases such as *hypertension* and *non-insulin-dependent diabetes mellitus*.

The relationship between protein-energy malnutrition and general indices of growth is more firmly established. Growth status during childhood is accepted almost universally as the best indicator, in field studies, of nutritional status at the levels of both individuals and communities. The response of the previously malnourished infant and pre-school age child to nutritional supplementation and therapy is still unclear, however. The potential for catch-up growth has been striking in some studies, with no permanent physical deficit after nutritional rehabilitation. On the other hand, some workers have suggested that the effects of early infant malnutrition are long-term.

## PROTEIN DIGESTION AND ABSORPTION

### See also Chapter 60

Dietary protein is digested by proteolytic enzymes and peptidases in the gut. Many of the proteolytic enzymes are produced in the exocrine pancreas, from which they are secreted as inactive precursors, called zymogens. Pepsinogen (a 40.4-kD peptide) is secreted from the chief cells in the wall of the stomach in response to gastrin, which simultaneously stimulates the release of HCl from the parietal cells causing the pH of the stomach contents to drop and pepsinogen to be autocatalytically activated to pepsin (32.7 kD). Pepsin itself then causes the further conversion of pepsinogen as well as cleaving dietary proteins into large peptides. Gastric protein hydrolysis is important but not essential in protein digestion. Passage of the stomach contents into the duodenum stimulates the release of the hormones, secretin and pancreozymin from the duodenal mucosa, which in turn cause the secretion of pancreatic juice that is both alkaline and rich in digestive enzymes. Secretin alone causes the secretion of an alkaline, protein-poor pancreatic juice, whereas pancreozymin causes the secretion of an enzyme-rich juice. There is a family of pancreatic proteolytic enzymes. Some, such as trypsin, chymotrypsin and elastase, split proteins and polypeptides at specific internal sites, in contrast to carboxypeptidases that cleave individual amino acids from the carboxyl ends of polypeptide chains. The end products of pancreatic digestion are free amino acids, dipeptides and small peptides. Further amino acid hydrolysis takes place in intestinal mucosal cells by aminopeptidases and dipeptidases.

Both amino acids and small peptides are absorbed by stereospecific transport systems located in the membrane of the intestinal mucosal cell. There are at least five specific transport systems: one each for small neutral amino acids, large neutral and aromatic amino acids, basic amino acids, proline and glycine, and acidic amino acids (Table 4.1). Most of the transport mechanisms are coupled to Na$^+$ transport. Many if not all the transport mechanisms participate in the γ-glutamyl cycle immediately after the stereospecific uptake

TABLE 4.1 Specific intestinal transport systems for amino acids and diseases associated with transport defects

| AMINO ACID TRANSPORTER GROUP | EXAMPLES OF TRANSPORTED AMINO ACIDS | DEFICIENCY DISEASE |
| --- | --- | --- |
| Acidic | Aspartic and glutamic acids | |
| Basic | Arginine, lysine, ornithine, cysteine | Cystinuria |
| Small neutral | Alanine, serine, threonine | |
| Large neutral and aromatic | Isoleucine, leucine, valine, tyrosine, tryptophan, phenylalanine | Hartnup disease |
| Glycine, proline | | Glycinuria |

step. This involves the tripeptide, glutathione serving as a donor of a γ-glutamyl group to form a dipeptide with the absorbed α-amino acid. Once in the cell the dipeptide is cleaved and the glutamyl group resynthesized in a five-step cycle. One turn of the cycle costs three ATP molecules. Proline is not transported via this cycle. Any absorbed peptides are hydrolyzed in the mucosal cell and only amino acids are released into the portal blood. Inherited defects of an amino acid transport system in both the gut and the kidney may result in conditions such as *cystinuria*, *glycinuria*, or *Hartnup disease* (Table 4.1). Despite the inability of the intestine to transport large neutral and aromatic amino acids in *Hartnup disease*, the patient faces few problems because essential amino acids bypass the block by being absorbed as peptides.

## AMINO ACID CATABOLISM

## Deamination

Following absorption, amino acids pass via the portal circulation to the liver to enter the metabolic pool of the body where they can undergo *transamination* (Fig. 4.1) or oxidative deamination. Both processes produce keto acids, but oxidative deamination produces ammonium ions directly whereas the amino group passes to another keto acid (e.g. α-ketoglutarate) via transamination. The coupling of the glutamate dehydrogenase reaction, in which the amino group is split from glutamate to produce α-ketoglutarate and ammonium, to a glutamate-requiring transaminase reaction produces a system capable of making ammonium from almost all amino acids. *Aspartate aminotransferase* is of particular significance because it contributes an amino group to oxaloacetate to make aspartate, which is the donor of one of the two nitrogen atoms in urea synthesis. The deamination of amino acids by the L-amino acid oxidases of the liver and kidney is of lesser importance. These enzymes have a broad specificity but a slow rate of oxidation. The fate of amino acid nitrogen is described in Chapter 5.

## Fate of the carbon skeleton

The fate of the amino acid carbon skeleton is particularly important during fasting when gluconeogenesis is essential for maintaining substrate delivery. Most of the amino acids utilized come from skeletal muscle. A certain amount of amino acid catabolism takes place *in situ* to cater to the energy needs of muscle, but a potential problem arises because the nitrogen generated from transamination and deamination can only be converted to urea in the liver. This is resolved by the synthesis, from pyruvate, of *alanine*, which then acts to transport nitrogen to the liver where transamination yields glucose for the return journey; this process is referred to as the "glucose–alanine cycle" (Fig. 4.2). Another important pathway for exporting nitrogen from muscle is via the synthesis of glutamine from glutamate. Glutamine can release its amine group in either the intestine or kidney. The latter organ also uses serine to transport excess nitrogen to the liver.

Carbon skeletons derived from amino acids provide energy via conversion into ketones (ketogenic), glucose (glucogenic), or both. Most amino acids are glucogenic, with only leucine being solely ketogenic. Isoleucine, lysine, phenylalanine, tyrosine and tryptophan are both ketogenic and glucogenic. The entry points of the amino acid skeletons into the metabolic pool and citric acid cycle are summarized in Fig. 4.3. More important than learning details of the cycle is the appreciation that both types of precursor are energy sources and that certain enzyme deficiencies in amino acid catabolism result in inborn metabolic errors which are clinically important. One example, *maple syrup urine disease*, will be given here. The reader should consult a reference text on inborn metabolic errors for information on other specific disorders.

The three-branched chain amino acids leucine, isoleucine and valine are essential components of the

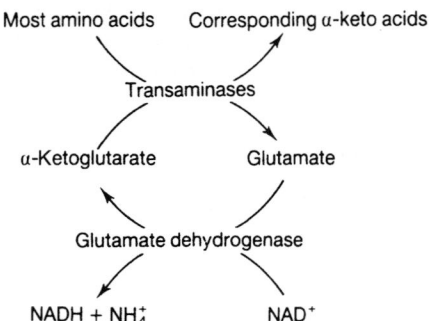

FIGURE 4.1 Schematic representation of transamination

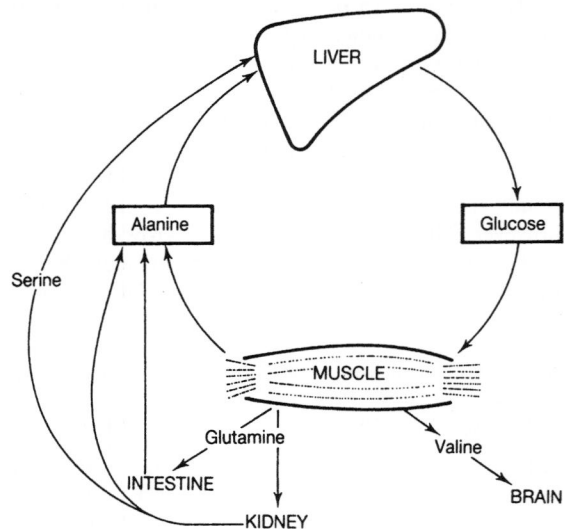

FIGURE 4.2 The glucose–alanine cycle and other pathways of nitrogen transport

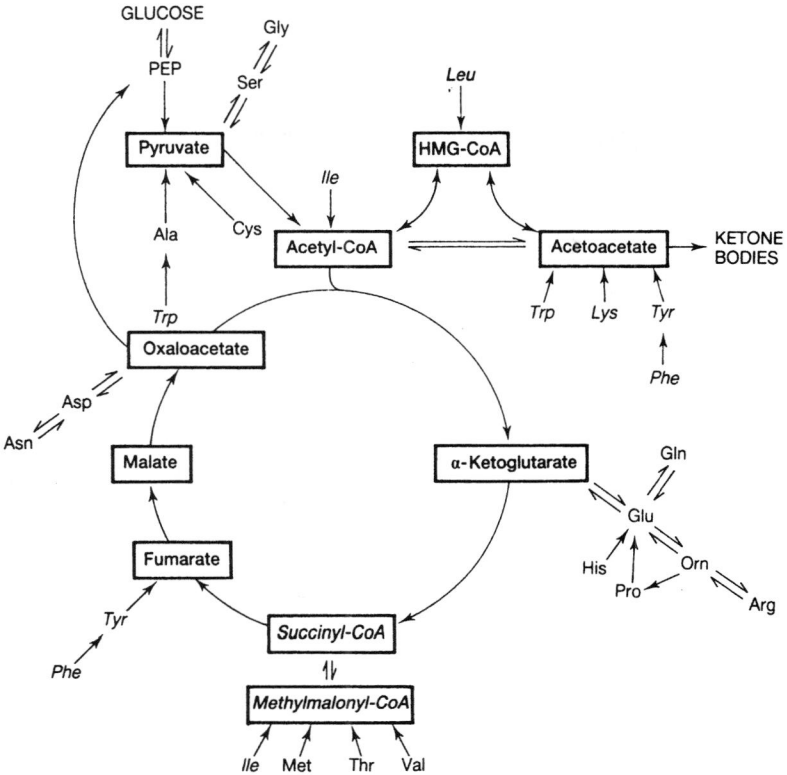

FIGURE 4.3 The metabolic fates of the amino acid carbon skeletons. Amino acids shown in italics may be ketogenic. Only leucine and lysine must be ketogenic.

human diet, since enzymes for their *de novo* synthesis are not present in human cells. Following uptake by the cell, they are either incorporated into proteins or broken down for energy. In patients with maple syrup urine disease, accumulation of branched-chain amino acids results from impaired oxidative decarboxylation of the branched-chain α-ketoacids. The disorder may result from one of several different inherited defects in the mitochondrial multi-enzyme complex, branched-chain α-keto acid dehydrogenase, and results in increased concentrations of the branched-chain amino and α-ketoacids in body cells and fluids. If the disorder is not diagnosed in the neonatal period and treated with diets restricted in the branched-chain amino acids, permanent mental and physical retardation results.

## AMINO ACID SYNTHESIS

### General principles

The ratio of amino acids present in the diet is not in the proportions required by the body and must therefore be modified. Changes take place in the gut mucosa and the amino acid spectrum in the portal blood differs from that of the food ingested, with alanine levels being higher and glutamate and aspartate being lower. Alanine is the principal vector for transport of

fixed nitrogen to the liver both from ingested food and from skeletal muscle during fasting.

Non-essential amino acids can be synthesized by transamination of intermediates from the glycolytic pathway and the citric acid cycle. Glutamate is the commonest amino donor in all transamination reactions. Within the citric acid cycle, glutamate and aspartate act as reciprocal amino donors in the transamination couplings, glutamate/α-ketoglutarate and aspartate/oxaloacetate (*see* Fig. 4.1). Glutamate provides the amino acid for the transamination pairs, pyruvate/alanine and 3-phosphoglycerate/serine which occur in the glycolytic pathway. Serine is the precursor of glycine which is formed by transfer of the serine hydroxymethyl group to tetrahydrofolate.

Both aspartate and glutamate can be converted into their respective amides, asparagine and glutamine. Glutamine is formed by the direct linking of glutamate and ammonium in a reaction catalyzed by glutamine synthetase, and asparagine is formed by the donation of an amino group from glutamine to aspartate in a reaction catalyzed by asparagine synthetase; one molecule of ATP is consumed in each case.

Methyl group transfer is an important biological process that can be illustrated conveniently by the biosynthesis of cysteine from methionine. Hepatic methionine adenosyl transferase catalyzes the formation of *S*-adenosylmethionine (SAM) from methionine and

ATP. SAM is the principal methyl donor in the body and examples of the end products include: creatine, phosphatidylcholine, methylated RNA, methylated DNA and epinephrine. In yielding up the methyl group SAM becomes *S*-adenosylhomocysteine which is then split by a hydrolase to homocysteine and adenosine. Homocysteine can be metabolically reconverted to methionine by two routes. In one transmethylation reaction, betaine, derived from the oxidation of choline, acts as donor. The other mechanism is important in folate and vitamin $B_{12}$ metabolism and involves donation of a methyl group by 5-methyl tetrahydrofolate.

## Specific amino acids

The anabolic pathways in humans through which selected amino acids are synthesized will now be presented in summary form. These have been chosen to illustrate general principles, or because defective enzyme function in selected pathways can cause inherited disease in humans.

### Cysteine

Cysteine is synthesized from a sulfhydryl group derived from homocysteine and a carbon skeleton from serine.

The two amino acids condense under the influence of cystathionine synthetase to form cystathionine which is then split by cystathionase to give homoserine and cysteine. *Homocystinuria* is due to a mutation of the cystathionine synthetase gene and *cystathioninuria* to a defective cystathionase molecule with decreased affinity for its coenzyme, pyridoxal phosphate. In addition to being required for protein synthesis, cysteine is also used to make the tripeptide glutathione and the non-essential amino acid taurine.

### Tyrosine

If sufficient dietary phenylalanine is available, adequate amounts of tyrosine can be synthesized by humans. The enzyme catalyzing this process is phenylalanine hydroxylase, which requires the electron carrier, tetrahydrobiopterin (THB), as a coenzyme. Deficiency of the enzyme, or more rarely of the THB cofactor, results in *phenylketonuria*, an autosomal recessive condition characterized by mental retardation, under-pigmentation and hyperphenylalaninemia.

Tyrosine has a number of biosynthetic roles; it acts as a precursor for biosynthesis of triiodothyronine and thyroxine, melanin pigments and catecholamines (Fig. 4.4). Elevated blood concentrations of tyrosine may be found in all forms of *liver failure*, but are also characteristic of *hepatorenal tyrosinemia (tyrosinemia type I)*,

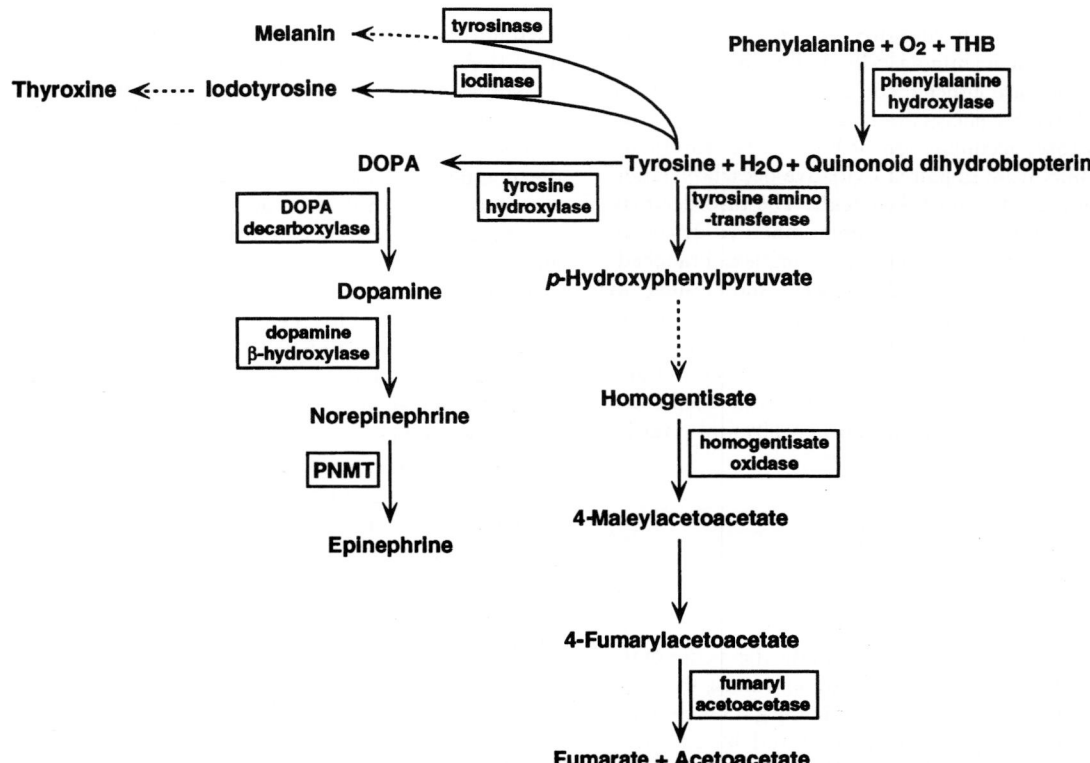

FIGURE 4.4 The metabolic fate of tyrosine, showing both the degradation pathway and the synthetic pathway for thyroxine, melanin and catecholamines. (PNMT = para-*N*-methyl transferase; THB = tetrahydrobiopterin.)

a genetically transmitted disorder due to fumaryl acet-oacetase deficiency which presents as *infantile cirrhosis* and *renal Fanconi syndrome*. Tyrosine aminotransfer-ase (TAT) deficiency (*Richner–Hanhart syndrome or tyrosinemia type 2*) also causes high tyrosine concen-trations and is characterized by keratosis and corneal dystrophy. *Alcaptonuria* is due to deficiency of homo-gentisate oxidase and was the original condition from which Garrod recognized the link between enzymes and genes.

## Proline

Proline is synthesized from arginine via a series of reac-tions. In the first, arginase splits arginine to ornithine and urea. The ornithine is then transaminated to yield glutamate-γ-semialdehyde which, by closure of the Schiff base to form a ring and by subsequent reduction, is converted to proline.

## Arginine and histidine

While both arginine and histidine are non-essential in adults, they may be needed in the diet of infants who cannot synthesize adequate amounts for growth. Arginine is synthesized from ornithine in the urea cycle. The status of histidine as an essential/non-essential amino acid is not clear as deprivation experi-ments in man have been short-term and under these conditions histidine shortage can be made good by conversion of the related molecule, carnosine.

## ALTERNATIVE ROLES OF AMINO ACIDS

Several amino acids have physiological functions in addition to their principal roles as building blocks of peptides and proteins. For example, glycine is an inhi-bitory neurotransmitter in the CNS, acting via the opening of glycine-gated $Cl^-$ channels to suppress neu-ronal firing by maintaining the polarization of post-synaptic membranes. By contrast, glutamate acts as an excitatory neurotransmitter, opening glutamate-gated cation channels and causing an influx of $Na^+$ that depolarizes the postsynaptic membrane toward the threshold potential for firing an action potential. Two further amino acids, aspartate and taurine, are also thought to act as neurotransmitters in the CNS.

## Amino acids as precursors of biologically active metabolites

Some of the most important biologically active com-pounds derived from amino acids are neurotransmit-ters. Acetylcholine is formed from choline, in turn derived from serine via ethanolamine (Fig. 4.5). Catecholamines are derived from dopamine, in turn derived from tyrosine via L-dopa (Fig. 4.4).

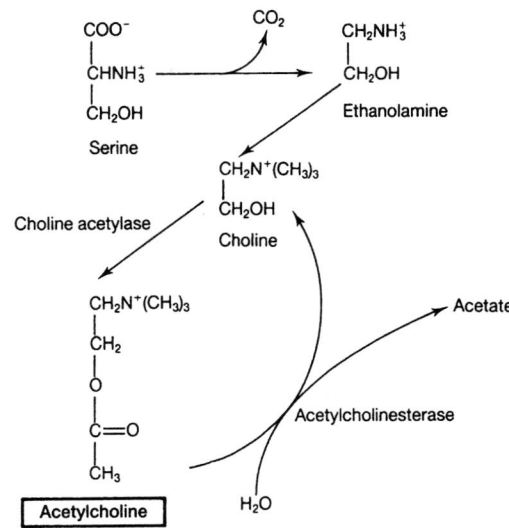

FIGURE 4.5 The synthesis and hydrolysis of acetylcholine

5-Hydroxytryptamine, or serotonin, a neurotransmit-ter found in the central nervous system and gut mucosa, is synthesized by the hydroxylation and dec-arboxylation of tryptophan. The decarboxylation of glutamate catalyzed in neurons by glutamic acid dec-arboxylase produces γ-aminobutyrate (GABA), an inhibitory transmitter in the central nervous system. The potent vasodilator histamine is formed from histi-dine by decarboxylation.

Glycine and arginine are both used in the synthesis of creatine, an important muscle metabolite. The amount of ATP in muscle serves to sustain contractile activity for less than a second. Vertebrate muscle con-tains a reservoir of high-energy phosphoryl groups in the form of creatine phosphate, which can readily transfer its phosphoryl group to ATP in a reaction catalyzed by creatine kinase. This high-energy com-pound serves to maintain a high concentration of mus-cle ATP during exercise, acting as the major source of energy during the first few seconds of extreme muscu-lar exertion. Hydrolysis of creatine phosphate gener-ates creatinine which is commonly measured in the blood and urine as an index of both renal function and muscle turnover.

Carnitine is a small nitrogen-containing molecule involved in the transport of fatty acids across mito-chondrial membranes. It is synthesized from protein-bound lysine. *Inborn metabolic errors of fatty acid β-oxidation* result in a fall in circulating carnitine due to an accumulation of esterified carnitine, and dietary carnitine therapy is beneficial in such cases.

Arginine generates nitric oxide (NO), an important cellular signal molecule (see Chapter 10). NO has recently been shown to play an important role as a signal molecule in a number of signal transduction processes. This free-radical gas is synthesized endogen-ously from arginine in a complex reaction catalyzed by nitric oxide synthase (NOS), an enzyme group structurally and functionally similar to the cytochrome P$_{450}$ oxygenases. NO readily diffuses across membranes, but has a half-life less than a few seconds, a property that makes it well suited to serve as a transient signal molecule within and between adjacent cells.

## BIOSYNTHESIS AND STRUCTURE OF PROTEINS

### See also Chapter 1

The following is an outline designed to illustrate the principles involved. Natural proteins are linear and unbranched polymers of the 20 naturally occurring amino acids, linked together through *peptide bonds*. Proteins of molecular weight less than several kilodaltons are sometimes called *polypeptides*, although the distinction is somewhat arbitrary. Proteins have precise lengths and amino acid sequences, usually with a free amino group at one end (the N or amino-terminus) and a free carboxylic acid group at the other (the C- or carboxyl-terminus). Every protein has a unique sequence of amino acid residues which determines both its biological and physicochemical properties. Differences in length and sequence distinguish one protein from another and make possible the great diversity of structures and functions. The linear chains of most naturally occurring proteins share the basic property of being able to assume specific three-dimensional structures, called *conformations*, which in turn subserve their specific functions. Indeed, the key to the functional diversity of proteins lies largely in the formation of such specific structures.

When amino acids are joined together to form proteins, their potential for flexible movement is variably restrained by the backbone of peptide bonds acting in combination with covalent cross-linkages such as those produced by disulfide bonds, as well as by non-covalent forces generated by electrostatic repulsion, hydrogen bonding and ionic, van der Waals and hydrophobic interactions. The amino acid sequence of a protein is referred to as the *primary structure*, and the overall three-dimensional shape it adopts as the *tertiary structure*. Protein chains are often folded locally into α-helices or β-sheets, which generate the local conformation of the polypeptide backbone, known as the *secondary structure*. Both of these localized conformations are stabilized by hydrogen bonds, and may coexist within the same polypeptide chain. Many proteins exist naturally as non-covalently bound aggregates of two or more polypeptide chains, which may be either identical or different. These polypeptide chains are referred to as *subunits* or *monomers*, and the overall aggregate as the *quaternary structure*. The tertiary and quaternary structures of proteins are vital to their roles as binding molecules in which specificity is all-important. Examples include the binding of O$_2$ to hemoglobin, hormones to receptors, and enzymes to substrates.

The mechanism of protein synthesis is a complex process, called "translation" because the four-letter code of nucleic acids is translated into the entirely separate code of amino acids (*see also* Chapter 1). Ultimate direction of protein synthesis resides in the nucleotide sequences of DNA transcribed into specific mRNAs, each separate protein being encoded by a specific gene. Translation requires the coordinated interaction of more than a hundred different macromolecules, including aminoacyl-transfer RNAs, mRNA and many proteins. The process is coordinated on ribosomes, which act as template-directed catalysts of peptide bond formation, and takes place in the amino-to-carboxyl direction. Following the assembly of an entire polypeptide chain and its release from a ribosome, the structure and function of the nascent protein can be changed through post-translational modification, whereby structural alterations such as covalent addition of sugars (glycosylation) or other substituent groups, coordination with metal atoms or other protein molecules, removal or modification of individual amino acid residues, and the formation of intra- or inter-chain disulfide bonds can occur. Consequently, the amino acid sequence of the final protein is not necessarily the same as that specified by the gene sequence.

Proteins are generally detected by physical processes such as ultraviolet light absorption or protein mass spectrometry, or by various procedures employing reagents that measure either peptide bonds or the side-chains of component amino acids. Proteins have been classified in various ways, such as by their solubility, size, mobility in electrical or centrifugal fields, or their ability to combine with antibodies of known specificity using techniques such as immunoassays or protein blotting (Western blot). Methods for determination of the covalent structures of proteins include the determination of amino acid composition, of amino acid sequence (which identifies a protein unambiguously), and of disulfide bonding pattern. The study of protein structure and function has also been greatly aided by the development of methods for chemical peptide synthesis.

The characterization and properties of proteins will now be illustrated by reference to the proteins commonly found in the blood. The normal protein concentration of plasma is 60–80 g/L, of which 30–50 g/L is albumin and 15–30 g/L a mixture of globulins. In the clinical laboratory, plasma protein concentrations are usually measured by colorimetry, and individual proteins separated by electrophoresis, which permits their classification into albumin, α$_1$-globulins, α$_2$-globulins, β-globulins and γ-globulins. The γ-globulins are primarily synthesized by plasma cells whereas most of the other plasma proteins are synthesized by hepatocytes.

Albumin is the most abundant protein in plasma. It is a globular protein of 66.3 kD which consists of a single polypeptide chain that is strongly negatively charged at physiological pH. The main functions of albumin are to generate osmotic pressure within the vascular compartment and to transport small molecules. Albumin is the primary transporter of poorly soluble molecules, such as free fatty acids and bilirubin, that must be moved from one compartment to another to be metabolized. It also binds sparingly soluble drugs such as aspirin, digoxin and barbiturates, all of which can displace natural metabolites. In addition, albumin is the principal transporter of small cations and anions; for example, roughly half of the $Ca^{2+}$ present in plasma is bound to albumin.

$\alpha_1$-Globulins are mainly glycoproteins and high-density lipoproteins (HDL). $\alpha_2$-Globulins include the following: haptoglobin, the transport protein for free hemoglobin; ceruloplasmin, the main copper transport protein; prothrombin, a proenzyme involved in blood clotting; glycoproteins; and very-low-density lipoproteins (VLDL). The major $\beta$-globulins are transferrin, the iron transport protein, and low-density lipoproteins (LDL). The $\gamma$-globulins are the immunoglobulins, which are grouped into five subclasses, each of which is heterogenous and contains many thousands of structurally distinct molecules. Five subclasses of immunoglobulins are recognized, IgG, IgA, IgD, IgE and IgM, each of which mediate distinct effector functions. All of these molecules share a similar general quaternary structure of two light and two heavy polypeptide chains.

## DEVELOPMENTAL ASPECTS

## Before birth (see also Chapters 13 and 22)

Prenatal growth involves much protein synthesis, the bulk of which is added in the second and third trimesters. The normal human newborn contains about 500 g of protein, most of which is accumulated in a linear manner from gestational week 22 to term as the fetus grows from 250 g to 3500 g. The rate of protein synthesis slows as pregnancy advances but it is always greater than in the adult. Increased synthetic rates are accompanied by increased breakdown, rates of fetal protein turnover being much greater than occurs postnatally. There is also marked variation between organs in the rate of protein synthesis. Studies in fetal lambs towards term indicate that the half-life of protein synthesized in the liver and heart is approximately 1 day, whereas that in skeletal muscle is about 1 week. The rate of placental protein turnover is similar to that in the fetal liver and heart. Although protein turnover in all fetal tissues slows with advancing gestation, it remains 4–6 fold faster than in the adult. Substrate delivery is the main controlling influence on fetal protein synthesis. Insulin stimulates protein synthesis in muscle only and then only in the presence of hyperaminoacidemia. Insulin-like growth factor I (IGF-I) may also play a role in regulating fetal protein synthesis. In addition to being used for protein synthesis, amino acids are important sources of metabolic fuel for the fetus in which they account for up to 25 per cent of consumption. This implies an early ontogeny for transamination pathways and nitrogen metabolism.

A consequence of the dynamism of fetal amino acid metabolism is that plasma circulating concentrations are higher than after birth. In contrast, maternal circulating amino acid concentrations are low throughout pregnancy and the fetal/maternal ratio is greater than 1, being greatest in the second trimester (approximately 3) and falling towards term (approximately 1.6). The pattern of amino acids in the maternal circulation differs from that of the non-pregnant woman, with glycine, leucine, ornithine, lysine, arginine, serine and $\alpha$-amino butyrate concentrations all being significantly reduced. In contrast, concentrations of alanine, the amino acid metabolic shuttle between muscle and liver, are increased. *Toxemia of pregnancy* impairs placental transport of nutrients to the fetus and amino acids in particular: both maternal and fetal plasma amino acid concentrations rise, but the maternal proportionately more, with a consequent fall in the fetal/maternal amino acid ratio. Prolonged pregnancy associated with *intrauterine growth retardation* is also characterized by a drop in the fetal/maternal amino acid ratio due largely to a rise in maternal circulating concentrations. Overt *maternal malnutrition* during pregnancy results in changes in both the mother and newborn infant resembling those seen in *kwashiorkor*. The plasma aminogram of the pregnant woman shows significant increases in ornithine and glycine and a high glycine/valine ratio. In the first hours after birth, the aminogram of the infant shows increased concentrations of alanine, proline, glycine and taurine and a slower-than-normal postnatal fall in branched-chain amino acid concentrations. In contrast, women from low socioeconomic groups, who subsequently gave birth to light-for-dates babies, had aminograms that were reduced 20 per cent overall but which showed both increases and falls in different groups of amino acids. Ornithine, arginine and aspartic acid were all reduced more than 30 per cent, while isoleucine, methionine, valine and cysteine were all higher than found in normal pregnancy. The changes again suggest selective alterations in different placental transport groups and/or fetoplacental amino acid metabolism.

Despite fetal plasma concentrations of amino acids being higher than maternal, placental cytosolic levels are higher still. The transport of amino acids across the placenta involves both the direct active transfer of essential amino acids from maternal to fetal plasma and placental cytosolic synthesis of non-essential amino acids. The placental concentrations of the metabolically labile straight-chain and acidic amino acids are particularly high partly as a consequence of *de novo* synthesis. There are considerable inter-species differences in placental amino acid transport but in humans amino acid transport occurs both by passive diffusion and Na⁺-independent and Na⁺-dependent carrier-mediated systems (*see* page 224).

The concept of an essential amino acid acquires a new dimension when one considers the fetus (*see also* page 301). Both fetal and placental tissues possess a wide variety of transaminases and deaminases by which fetal tissues can readjust the mixture of amino acids taken up by the placenta. However, rapid protein synthesis, coupled with an uneven pattern of enzyme maturation, means that certain amino acids which are non-essential postnatally are essential to the fetus and preterm infant. For example, cystathionase, the enzyme responsible for metabolism of methionine to cysteine, is completely absent from the fetal human liver, so the fetus is entirely dependent upon the mother for cysteine, which is considered essential in the preterm infant. Phenylalanine and tyrosine are also poorly metabolized in premature infants. Furthermore, the *trans*-sulfuration pathway that converts methionine to cysteine only develops postnatally, so it is prudent to regard cysteine as remaining essential for some time after birth. Histidine also appears to be essential for the fetus since infants fed a low-histidine diet show impaired nitrogen retention and poor weight gain.

## Neonatal changes

Large changes in plasma amino acid concentrations occur rapidly after birth. Overall there is a fall in most amino acids which is significant at 4 hours and progresses to become maximal by 24 hours. The fall is greatest in the essential amino acids, with the non-essential amino acids, and in particular glycine, showing a modest rise. The ratio of non-essential amino acids to essential amino acids is 1.3 in cord blood, rises to a maximum of 2.8 at 24 hours and then remains about 2.0 for several days. Preterm infants show exaggerated changes, and in those suffering *intrauterine growth retardation* the glycine/valine ratio correlates directly with the degree of weight deficit.

The fate of the different amino acids remains less clear. Protein synthesis continues at a rapid pace immediately after birth. Fat is the principal source of energy in the newborn, and it is unlikely that amino acids normally provide a significant source of calories to milk-fed infants. However, metabolic balance studies on parenterally fed preterm infants show that fat can be replaced as a caloric source by carbohydrate and amino acids.

## SELECTED READING

Alberts B, Bray D, Lewis J, Raff M, Roberts K, Watson JD. *Molecular biology of the cell*, 3rd edn. New York: Garland Publishing, 1994.

Creighton TE. *Proteins: structures and molecular properties*, 2nd edn. New York: W.H. Freeman, 1993.

Falkner F, Tanner JM. *Human growth: a comprehensive treatise*. New York: Plenum Press, 1986.

Felig P. Amino acid metabolism in man. *Ann Rev Biochem* 1975; **44**: 933.

Harper AE, Elvehjem CA. Importance of amino acid balance in nutrition. *JAMA* 1955; **158**: 655.

Lowrey GH. *Growth and development of children*, 8th edn. Chicago: Year Book Medical Publishers, 1986.

Montgomery R, Conway TW, Spector AA. *Biochemistry: a case oriented approach*. St Louis: C.V. Mosby, 1990.

Scriver CR, Beaudet AL, Sly WS, Valle D. *The metabolic basis of inherited disease*, 6th edn. New York: McGraw-Hill, 1989.

Stryer L. *Biochemistry*, 4th edn. New York: W.H. Freeman, 1995.

Suskind RM, Lewinter-Susking L (eds). *Textbook of pediatric nutrition*, 2nd edn. New York: Raven Press, 1993.

US Department of Health and Human Services. *The Surgeon General's report on nutrition and health*. Washington, DC: DHHS (PHS) publication No 88-50210, 1988.

# 5

# Ammonia Metabolism: the Urea Cycle

### Anne Green and Mary Anne Preece

## AMMONIA AND AMMONIUM

Ammonia is generated during metabolism by all organs. It is produced from the catabolism of amino acids and as a product of purine and pyrimidine metabolism. It exists predominantly (95 per cent) as the ammonium ion ($NH_4^+$) at physiological pH. Large quantities are produced during exercise by the skeletal muscle (purine nucleotide cycle), and from the gastro-intestinal tract by bacterial metabolism of amino acids.

Ammonia is toxic – the non-ionized form ($NH_3$) is more diffusible and hence more toxic than ammonium. Most of the ammonium generated is detoxified by amination of glutamate to glutamine (Fig. 5.1). Glutamine acts as a short-term buffer and is transported in the blood and taken up by the intestinal epithelial cells. Ammonium is then transported by the portal vein for subsequent metabolism in the liver by the urea cycle. Approximately 30 per cent of $NH_4^+$ arises from protein digested in the gut, with the majority from circulating glutamine. Effective detoxification results in tight control of blood ammonium concentrations, i.e. <40 µmol/L in normal circumstances.

## THE UREA CYCLE

Detoxification of ammonia occurs by synthesis of urea (the urea cycle – see Fig. 5.2). The complete pathway is confined to the liver, although the steps from citrulline to ornithine are present in a variety of other tissues. In man approximately 80 per cent of excreted nitrogen is urea. Some urea may be recycled to amino acids, par-

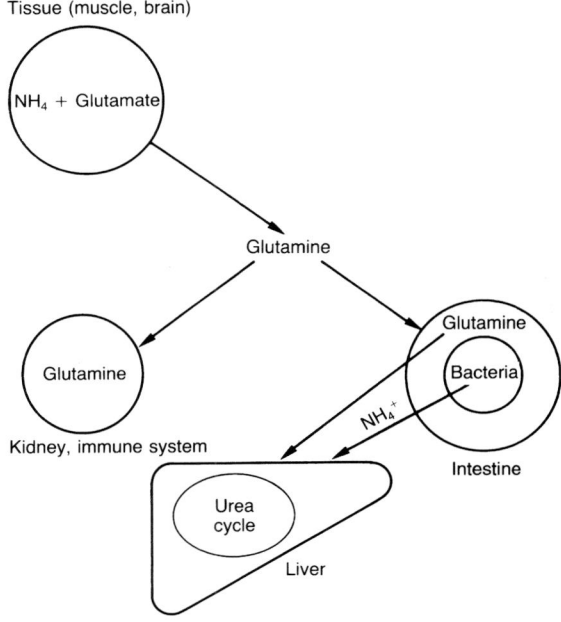

FIGURE 5.1 Ammonia production and the central role of glutamine

ticularly in early infancy, by metabolism (hydrolysis) by colonic bacteria.

Synthesis of urea starts in the mitochondria with the formation of carbamyl phosphate from ammonium and bicarbonate, and then condensation of ornithine with carbamyl phosphate to form citrulline. Citrulline

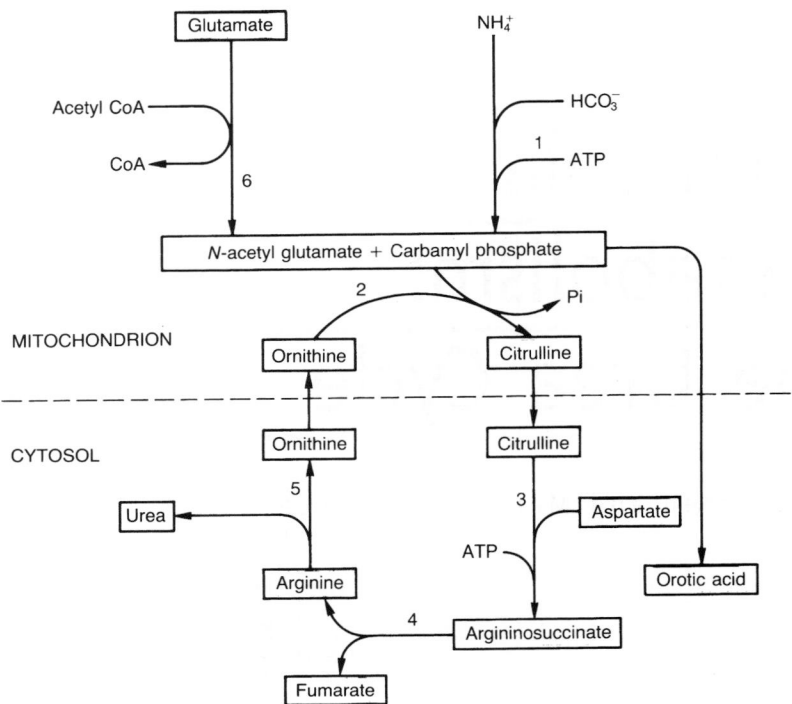

Numbers represent enzymes in the urea cycle

1 Carbamyl phosphate synthetase
2 Ornithine carbamyl transferase
3 Argininosuccinate synthetase
4 Argininosuccinate lyase
5 Arginase
6 N-acetylglutamate synthetase

FIGURE 5.2  The urea cycle and inherited defects

crosses the mitochondrial membrane into the cytoplasm where the cycle is completed. In the human fetus, urea cycle enzyme activity is found at 10–13 weeks' gestation. At 20 weeks' gestation the enzyme activity is 50–90 per cent of that found in adults.

Impairment in the synthesis of urea, either as a primary enzyme defect or as a secondary effect, leads to accumulation of the ammonium ion and potential toxicity and arginine becomes an essential amino acid. The mitochondrial enzyme N-acetylglutamate synthetase is susceptible to toxins and results in secondary hyperammonemia in *inherited defects of organic acid and fatty acid oxidation.*

## HYPERAMMONEMIA

Ammonia is toxic and prolonged or recurrent *hyperammonemia* causes irreversible brain damage. The precise biochemical mechanisms are not known, although interference with neurotransmitter metabolism and mitochondrial energy production is likely. Symptoms may occur if blood levels exceed 80 μmol/L. Hyperammonemia is a possible contributor to encephalopathy arising from *liver failure,* although asso-

ciated metabolic disturbances make it impossible to distinguish the specific effects of ammonium toxicity.

The clinical features associated with hyperammonemia are seizures, and drowsiness with progression to coma, cerebral edema and death. Postmortem findings show an edematous brain with swollen astrocytes. Astrocytes are rich in glutamine synthetase and the pathology is attributed to accumulation of glutamine, resulting in osmotic shifts of water into the cell and swelling.

In the urea cycle disorders, with the exception of *arginase deficiency,* arginine can no longer be produced and thus becomes an essential amino acid. Chronic deficiency of this amino acid is characterized by dermatological features.

## Causes of hyperammonemia

Poor sampling is unfortunately a common problem which may result in an artefactually elevated blood ammonium concentration. Asphyxia, shock and septicemia may cause hyperammonemia. Increased production may occur in *urinary tract infections, leukemia* and intravenous amino acid loads, i.e. as part of parenteral nutrition. Defective functioning of the urea cycle, either as one of the primary enzyme defects or secondary deficiencies such as inhibition by drugs/toxins/metabolites, may cause increased ammonium levels. Other inherited disorders which are associated with hyperammonemia include *methylmalonic acidemia* and *propionic acidemia*. Sodium valproate therapy may cause/exacerbate hyperammonemia by inhibiting the urea cycle at the carbamyl phosphate synthetase step, as well as having a direct effect on the CNS to enhance the encephalopathic effect of ammonium. Ammonium concentrations may be very high (in excess of 1000 μmol/L), particularly in the severe forms of *ornithine carbamyl transferase (OTC) deficiency*.

## INBORN ERRORS OF THE UREA CYCLE

Inherited defects of all five enzymes of the urea cycle can occur (Table 5.1). In addition, *N-acetylglutamate synthetase deficiency* has been reported. With the exception of *OTC deficiency*, which is X-linked, the inheritance pattern of the *urea cycle defects* (UCDs) is autosomal recessive.

The disorders share a similar spectrum of clinical presentation, the severity dependent on the extent of the reduced activity of the deficient enzyme. The most severe types present in the neonatal period with a rapidly developing encephalopathy. The less severe types present later in infancy/childhood with vomiting, lethargy, behavior disturbance, often as an episodic illness precipitated by intercurrent illness or high protein intake. In OTC deficiency the males are usually severely affected, although partial deficiency can occur with a less severe clinical picture. Female carriers of OTC deficiency are usually asymptomatic unless there is disproportionate representation of the mutant allele in the liver.

Defects of the urea cycle have specific plasma and urine amino acid abnormalities which enable diagnosis in some cases, e.g. citrullinemia (Table 5.1). Distinction between carbamyl phosphate synthetase (CPS) and OTC deficiencies can be made by urinary orotic acid measurement, although tissue enzyme measurements are required for definitive diagnosis.

## MOLECULAR BIOLOGY OF UREA CYCLE ENZYMES

The genes for all the enzymes involved in the urea cycle have been located. To date, no common mutations have been found. Despite this fact, many families with *urea cycle defects* are informative by linkage analysis or by the presence of polymorphisms. The *OTC* gene has been mapped to the short arm of the X chromosome and approximately 30 per cent of cases are thought to arise as a result of new mutations. Both gene deletions and point mutations have been found. Because of the high rate of new mutations in cases of *OTC deficiency*, it is important to establish carrier status in female relatives (i.e. siblings and aunts) of a male index case. These individuals may be clinically and biochemically normal because of favorable lyonization.

## SELECTED READING

Brusilow SW. Inborn errors of urea synthesis. In: Lloyd, Scriver CR, eds, *Genetic and metabolic disease in paediatrics*. London: Butterworth, 1985: 140.

Brusilow SW, Horwich AL. Urea cycle enzymes. In: Scriver CR, Beaudet AL, Sly WS, Valle D, eds, *The metabolic and molecular basis of inherited disease*, Vol. 1, 7th edn. New York: McGraw-Hill, 1995: 1187.

Bachmann C. Urea cycle disorders. In: Fernandes J, Saudubray J-M, Tada K, eds, *Inborn metabolic diseases:*

TABLE 5.1 Biochemical findings in inherited disorders of the urea cycle

| DISORDER | AMINO ACIDS | | URINE OROTIC ACID SECRETION | TISSUES IN WHICH THE ENZYME DEFECT IS EXPRESSED |
|---|---|---|---|---|
| | PLASMA[a] | URINE | | |
| Carbamyl phosphate synthetase deficiency | Glutamate + Alanine ↑ Citrulline ↓ | Glutamine + Alanine ↑ | Normal | Liver |
| Ornithine carbamyl transferase deficiency | Glutamine + Alanine ↑ Citrulline ↓ | Glutamine + Alanine ↑ | ↑↑↑ | Liver |
| Citrullinemia (argininosuccinate synthetase deficiency) | Citrulline ↑ | Citrulline ↑ | ↑ | Liver Skin fibroblasts |
| Argininosuccinic aciduria (argininosuccinate lyase deficiency) | Argininosuccinate ↑ Citrulline ↑ | Argininosuccinic acid ↑ | ↑ (during acute attacks) | Liver Red blood cells Skin fibroblasts |
| Arginase deficiency | Arginine ↑ | Arginine, Ornithine, Cystine, Lysine ↑ | ↑/normal | Liver Red blood cells |
| *N*-acetylglutamate synthetase deficiency | Glutamine + Alanine ↑ | Glutamine + Alanine ↑ | Normal | Liver |

[a]Plasma arginine concentrations are low/low normal in all the disorders except arginase deficiency.

*diagnosis and treatment*, Part V. Berlin: Springer-Verlag, 1990: 211.

Pollitt RJ. Amino acid disorders. In: Holton JB, ed. *The inherited metabolic diseases*, 2nd edn. Edinburgh: Churchill Livingstone, 1994: 67.

Tuchman M. The clinical, biochemical, and molecular spectrum of ornithine transcarbamylase deficiency. *J Lab Clin Med* 1992; **120**: 836.

# 6

# Purine and Pyrimidine Metabolism

Mary Anne Preece and Anne Green

## INTRODUCTION

Purines and pyrimidines are heterocyclic aromatic bases which are important constituents of many biochemical molecules. The parent compounds are shown in Fig. 6.1. The best known bases are the purines, adenine and guanine, and the pyrimidines, cytosine, thymine and uracil which form the base-pairs in the nucleic acids DNA and RNA (see Chapter 1). There are also a number of other purine and pyrimidine derivatives found in small amounts in DNA and RNA. Purine and pyrimidine bases also form part of a number of other biologically important molecules including adenosine triphosphate (ATP), nicotinamide adenine dinucleotide (NAD), and its phosphate NADP, coenzyme A, cyclic adenosine monophosphate (AMP) and uridine diphosphate glucose (UDPG). Many of these compounds have an important function in the formation of coenzymes and active intermediates in carbohydrate and phospholipid metabolism.

Nucleic acids consist of chains of nucleotides – in DNA they are deoxyribonucleotides, in RNA they are ribonucleotides (see also Chapter 1). Nucleotides are made up of three components, a base (purine or pyrimidine), a pentose sugar (deoxyribose or ribose) and one molecule of phosphoric acid. Nucleosides are formed from nucleotides by hydrolysis and loss of the phosphate moiety of the molecule and consist of a base and a pentose (Fig. 6.2). Nucleosides can exist in monophosphate, diphosphate and triphosphate forms (e.g. for adenosine these are AMP, ADP and ATP). These phosphorylated nucleosides play an important role in metabolism in three ways. First, they are energy carriers. ATP for example is a carrier of phosphate and

**Nucleoside (e.g. adenosine)**

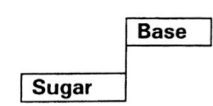

**Nucleotide (e.g. adenosine monophosphate)**

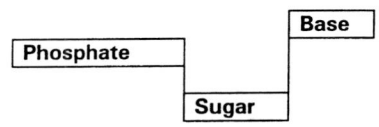

FIGURE 6.2 Diagrammatic representation of the structure of nucleosides and nucleotides

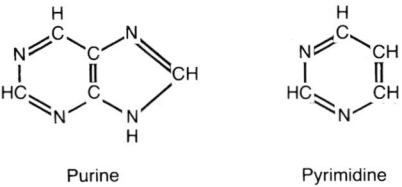

Purine          Pyrimidine

FIGURE 6.1 The chemical structures of purine and pyrimidine

pyrophosphate in reactions involving transfer of chemical energy. Some other triphosphates can also channel energy into specific biosynthetic pathways. Second, they function as specific carriers of building-block molecules; for example, UDP glucose is a specific donor of glucose for synthesis of glycogen, and CDP choline is a specific donor of phosphocholine for synthesis of choline-containing phosphoglycerides. Third, they are energy-rich precursors of mononucleotides for the synthesis of the nucleic acids RNA and DNA.

## METABOLIC PATHWAYS

### See Figs. 6.3 and 6.4

Purine and pyrimidine nucleotides can be synthesized *de novo* from simple molecules (purines from ribose-5-phosphate and pyrimidines from bicarbonate and glutamine). There are also alternative "salvage" pathways which recycle the bases to their corresponding nucleotides. These salvage pathways are simpler and require less energy than the *de novo* pathways and are responsible for the majority of nucleotide production.

Catabolism takes place by initial conversion to the base which, after further breakdown, results in uric acid as the end product of the purine pathway and β-alanine and β-aminoisobutyric acid as the end products of the pyrimidine pathway. The main contributor to nucleotide catabolism is RNA which has a relatively

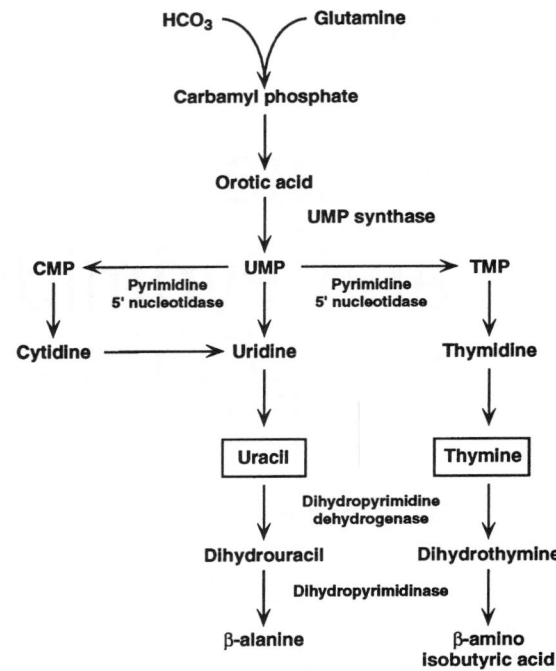

FIGURE 6.4 Synthesis and catabolism of pyrimidines. The pyrimidine bases are shown in boxes.

short half-life. DNA is only catabolized upon cell death. DNA, however, is ingested in the diet and may be broken down. Cancer chemotherapy results in massive cell death and therefore greatly increased

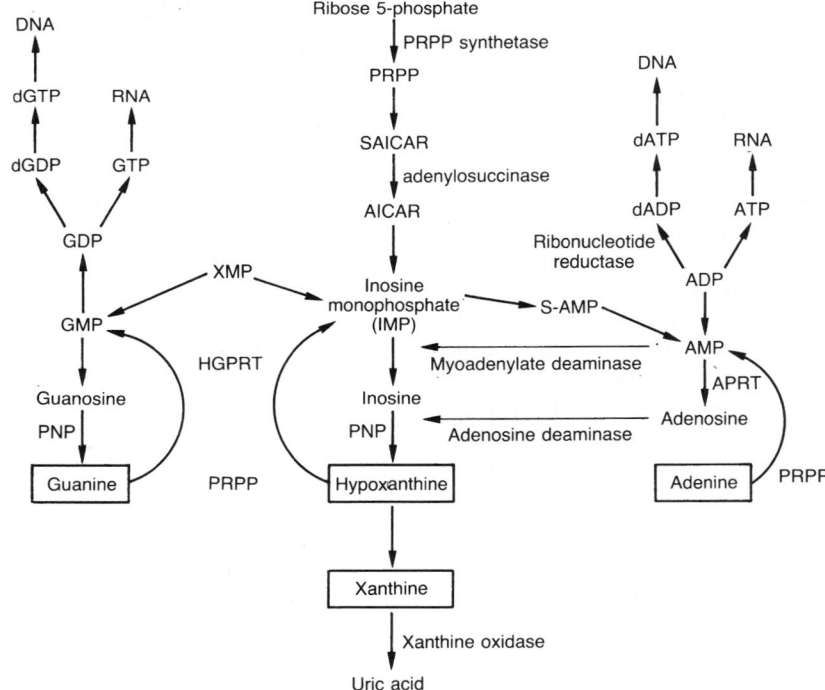

FIGURE 6.3 Synthesis and catabolism of purines. The purine bases are shown in boxes. AICAR = 5-aminoimidazole-4-carboxamide ribonucleotide; XMP = xanthylate; S-AMP = adenylo-succinate; SAICAR = 5-aminoimidazole-4-*N*-succinocarboxamide ribonucleotide. For further abbreviations see Table 6.1.

flux through the catabolic pathways, which may result in *uric acid nephropathy*.

## INHERITED METABOLIC DISORDERS

There are several inherited disorders of purine/pyrimidine metabolism. All of these disorders are individually rare, but the wide range of presentations serves to illustrate the importance and wide-reaching effect of purines and pyrimidines in the body. The clinical features range from benign (some cases of *xanthine oxidase deficiency*) to severe life-threatening symptoms in the neonatal period (*immunodeficiency* or *neurological problems*) – *see* Table 6.1. There is considerable heterogeneity of presentation for a particular biochemical defect, and some disorders can present at any age. The inheritance is mainly autosomal recessive with the exception of *hypoxanthine–guanine phosphoribosyl transferase* (HGPRT) *deficiency* and *phosphoribosyl pyrophosphate* (PRPP) *synthetase superactivity* which are X-linked. PRPP synthetase superactivity is due to structural defects of the enzyme causing it to become insensitive to regulatory mechanisms and therefore resulting in continuous *de novo* purine synthesis, which ultimately ends up as uric acid.

## MOLECULAR BIOLOGY

The structural genes for the inborn errors of purine metabolism with a known enzyme defect have all been located. The extent of knowledge about a particular molecular defect varies for different disorders, but in none of the disorders has a common mutation been described. Probably the most work has been carried out on the *HGPRT* gene which causes *Lesch–Nyhan syndrome*, in which over 50 different defects as point mutations, substitutions, deletions and duplications have been described.

## BIOCHEMICAL ASSESSMENT OF PURINE AND PYRIMIDINE METABOLISM

The only widely available biochemical test of purine or pyrimidine metabolism is measurement of uric acid, the end-point of purine metabolism. Further investigation of purine and pyrimidine metabolism requires specialized assays. Orotic acid is a test primarily used to aid in the diagnosis of *urea cycle defects*. Some disorders of pyrimidine metabolism may be detectable by urinary organic acid analysis.

TABLE 6.1  Inborn errors of purine and pyrimidine metabolism and their main presenting clinical signs

| DISORDERS | CLINICAL SIGN |
| --- | --- |
| *Purine disorders* | |
| Phosphoribosyl pyrophosphate (PRPP) synthetase superactivity | Arthritis<br>Kidney stones (urate) |
| Adenylosuccinase deficiency | Psychomotor retardation<br>Epilepsy<br>Autistic features |
| Myoadenylate deaminase deficiency | Muscle cramps |
| Adenosine deaminase deficiency | Recurrent life-threatening infections (severe combined immunodeficiency disease) |
| Purine nucleoside phosphorylase (PNP) deficiency | Recurrent infections |
| Xanthine oxidase deficiency | Kidney stones (xanthine) in 50% of cases |
| Molybdenum cofactor deficiency (xanthine oxidase and sulfite oxidase) | Neonatal fits<br>Lens dislocation<br>Mental retardation |
| Hypoxanthine–guanine phosphoribosyl transferase deficiency (HGPRT) | Delayed motor development<br>Choreoathetosis, self-mutilation<br>Kidney stones (urate) |
| Adenosine phosphoribosyl transferase (APRT) deficiency | Kidney stones (2,8-dihydroxy adenine) |
| *Pyrimidine disorders* | |
| Hereditary orotic aciduria (UMP synthase deficiency) | Megaloblastic anemia<br>Orotic acid crystalluria |
| Pyrimidine 5'-nucleotidase deficiency | Hemolytic anemia |
| Dihydropyrimidine dehydrogenase deficiency | ? Neurological problems |
| Dihydropyrimidinase deficiency | ? Neurological problems |

# Uric acid

Approximately two-thirds of uric acid is excreted via the kidney and one-third via the gut where it is broken down by bacteria. Plasma urate concentrations are dependent upon age, sex, ethnic origin and diet, and are also affected by renal function and some drugs, including ethanol and thiazide diuretics.

Hyperuricemia can cause *gout* by inducing the deposition of urate crystals, resulting in recurrent attacks of inflammatory arthritis, tophaceous deposits in joints, and renal stones. *Primary gout* predominantly affects middle-aged males: a specific genetic defect has been identified in less than 1 per cent of patients. The basic problem appears to be due to a reduced ability to excrete urate via the kidney.

*Familial juvenile gout* is a recently described disorder which generally presents around puberty in both males and females. The fractional excretion of urate is grossly decreased and is even lower than in primary gout. If untreated this disorder often results in a rapid decline to renal failure and death. It appears to be inherited in autosomal dominant manner with high penetrance. Inherited disorders of purine metabolism can also result in hyperuricemia and gout. *HGPRT deficiency* and *PRPP synthetase superactivity* both lead to hyperuricemia because of purine nucleotide and uric acid overproduction, secondary to an increased availability of PRPP. *Glycogen storage disease type I* (*glucose-6-phosphatase deficiency*) causes hyperuricemia due to increased production and decreased excretion of urate, thought to be due to competing mechanisms for renal transport of lactate. Exercise-induced hyperuricemia is found in *glycogen storage diseases types I, V, VII* and also in *myoadenylate deaminase deficiency*. In these disorders the cause is thought to be due to rapid utilization of ATP greater than the regenerative ability.

Secondary hyperuricemia can result from rapid tissue breakdown or accelerated cell turnover, e.g. in *leukemia* or in the *tumor lysis syndrome* secondary to chemotherapy. Decreased clearance of urate, as in volume depletion, starvation or ketoacidosis and secondary to drugs (e.g. thiazide diuretics), can lead to hyperuricemia.

Hyperuricemia can be treated by uricosuric drugs which inhibit the post-secretory reabsorption of uric acid and thereby promote the excretion of uric acid by the kidney. Alternatively, uric acid production can be decreased by the use of allopurinol which inhibits xanthine oxidase.

Hypouricemia is observed in *xanthine oxidase deficiency* and *molybdenum cofactor deficiency*.

# Orotic acid

Orotic acid is an early intermediate in the biosynthetic pathway of pyrimidines. It is increased in hereditary *orotic aciduria (UMP synthase deficiency)*. Orotic acid also is increased in some of the *urea cycle defects* (*see* Chapter 5) as well as secondarily to some pharmacological agents.

## SELECTED READING

Van der Berghe G. Disorders of purine and pyrimidine metabolism. In: Fernandes J, Saudubray J-M, Tada K, eds, *Inborn metabolic diseases: diagnosis and treatment*, Part IX. Berlin: Springer-Verlag, 1990: 455.

Simmonds HA. Purine and pyrimidine disorders. In: Holton JB, ed. *The inherited metabolic diseases*, 2nd edn. Edinburgh: Churchill Livingstone, 1994: 297.

Scriver CR, Beaudet AL, Sly WS, Valle D, eds, *The metabolic and molecular basis of inherited disease*, Vol. II, 7th edn. New York: McGraw-Hill, 1995: 1655.

# 7

# Fat and Carbohydrate Metabolism

R. David G. Milner

The decision to consider carbohydrates and lipids together stems from their great importance as energy sources and the central role of pancreatic hormones in controlling energy delivery. Carbohydrates and lipids also form part of large structural molecules (e.g. myelin and glycoproteins) and other molecules of particular pediatric relevance (e.g. surfactant).

The largest energy requirement of the fetus is for anabolism, but after birth thermogenesis and the skeletal and visceral metabolism associated with homeothermic independence must be added to the total caloric requirement of the infant and child. Glucose plays a special role in energy homeostasis because some tissues, notably the brain, are partially or wholly glucose-dependent.

## CELLULAR ENERGY BALANCE AND THE KREBS CYCLE

The ultimate source of free energy in living organisms comes from oxidative reactions. In biological oxidation, hydrogen is removed from the substrate being oxidized and then reacts with molecular oxygen to form water. Part of the energy released by the oxidation is conserved in the form of "high-energy compounds" with large negative free energies of hydrolysis. Most high-energy compounds are phosphorylated (e.g. adenosine triphosphate (ATP)), creatine phosphate and phosphoenol pyruvate), but some, such as acetyl coenzyme A (acetyl-CoA), are not. The production of such compounds is termed "oxidative phosphorylation," in which the oxidative and phos-

phorylative processes are simultaneous and tightly coupled. This takes place in the respiratory chain located on the inner mitochondrial membrane (see page 83). Oxidative phosphorylation can be blocked by uncouplers which cause increased oxidation, decreased phosphorylation and the production of extra heat which if excessive may result in fever. Natural uncouplers include bilirubin and some bacterial toxins. The physiological uncoupler uniquely present in brown fat mitochondria is a protein, thermogenin (see Chapter 48). Synthetic uncouplers include dicoumarol and 2,4-dinitrophenol.

Sugars, fat and amino acids enter a final common energy-generating pathway as molecules containing two to six carbon atoms that are mainly organic acids or acid derivatives. This pathway is the tricarboxylic acid cycle, or Krebs cycle (Fig. 7.1), which is the source of most of the $CO_2$ made in the body, and provides much of the reduced coenzyme pool that enables the respiratory chain to produce ATP. It is also the means whereby excess energy is converted into fatty acid, prior to triglyceride formation, and thus to fat deposition. In the Krebs cycle, carbohydrates can be converted to fatty acids or amino acids, and amino acids to glucose or fatty acids, but fatty acids cannot be metabolized to glucose. All the enzymes of the Krebs cycle are found on the matrix side of the inner mitochondrial membrane or in the matrix space, close by those of the respiratory chain.

A major entry point to the cycle is the 2-carbon molecule acetyl-CoA. This is formed either from pyruvate under the influence of the pyruvate dehydrogen-

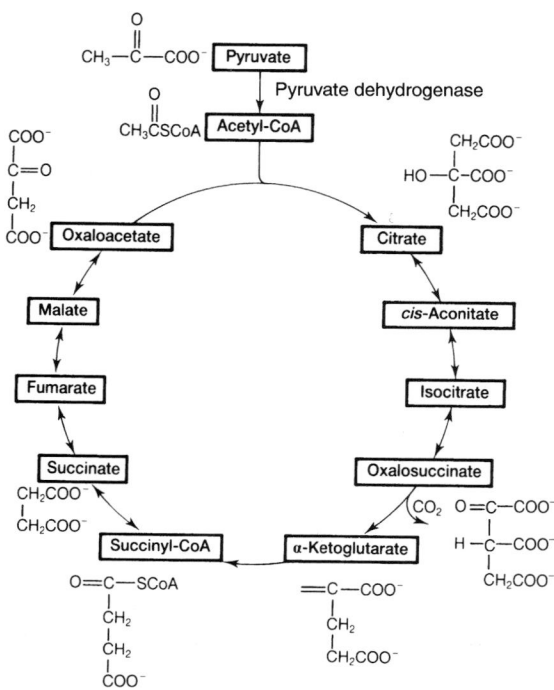

FIGURE 7.1 A simplified diagram of the Krebs (citric acid) cycle showing the formulae of only the more clinically important intermediates

ase complex or by β-oxidation of fatty acids. Both reactions take place within the mitochondria. The pyruvate dehydrogenase complex is subject to several control mechanisms. It is activated by dephosphorylation (pyruvate dehydrogenase kinase). The kinase is activated by cyclic AMP and ATP. The phosphatase is inhibited by ketosis or high concentrations of fatty acids.

The first step in the Krebs cycle using acetyl-CoA as the starting point is condensation with oxaloacetate to form citrate under the unidirectional control of citrate synthetase, which is found only in mitochondria. Citrate is then converted to isocitrate in two steps, both catalyzed by the unidirectional and highly specific aconitase. Isocitrate is next transiently dehydrogenated to oxalosuccinate which remains bound to isocitrate dehydrogenase before being decarboxylated to α-ketoglutarate. This molecule is then decarboxylated by an enzyme complex, α-ketoglutarate dehydrogenase, which closely resembles the pyruvate dehydrogenase complex except in its specificity for substrate. The product is succinyl-CoA, which is converted to succinate and CoA-SH by succinate thiokinase with the production of GTP from GDP. This is an example of phosphorylation not involving the respiratory chain and one of the few instances when GDP and not ADP is involved. Succinate passes through the intermediates, malate and fumarate, en route to becoming oxaloacetate in a manner similar to the conversion of citrate to isocitrate. The enzymes involved are succinate dehy-

drogenase, fumarase and malate dehydrogenase. The net effect of one turn of the wheel is the formation of $CO_2$ and water from acetic acid, yielding the precursors of 12 mol ATP with an efficiency of approximately 40 per cent. The Krebs cycle is the largest single source of ATP.

Acetyl-CoA, as the universal carrier of acyl groups, is the principal building block in long-chain fatty acid construction which takes place in the cytoplasm. Under adequate nutrition, it is formed from carbohydrate by glycolysis to yield pyruvate, which is converted to acetyl-CoA under the control of pyruvate dehydrogenase, or from protein by the transamination of amino acids which enter the Krebs cycle at various points. Certain amino acids are homologues of Krebs cycle intermediaries, e.g. pyruvate/alanine and α-ketoglutarate/glutamate, and these can be converted in either direction as required under the control of transaminases (see page 130). When amino acid supply exceeds the need for protein biosynthesis the acids are made available to the Krebs cycle in a variety of ways. A homologue is deaminated by an aminotransferase and the carbon skeleton processed through the cycle to yield acetyl-CoA. Direct transamination is possible for only a minority of amino acids such as alanine, aspartate and glutamine. Others, such as serine, threonine, glycine and cysteine, are transaminated, converted to pyruvate and processed by that route. A third mechanism is oxidative deamination involving amino acid oxidase to produce ammonium ions or amide groups and carbon skeletons that enter the Krebs cycle.

There is no net synthesis of glucose from fatty acids because each acetyl-CoA entering the cycle generates two molecules of $CO_2$. Therefore all the fuel entering the cycle is converted into high-energy phosphate bonds or heat, leaving no carbon available for glucose synthesis.

While the above pathways provide the major route for the generation of ATP, some high-potential electrons must be conserved for biosynthetic purposes. This is done via the synthesis of NADPH as a hydride ion (electron) donor for reductive biosynthesis. The synthesis of NADPH occurs via the pentose phosphate pathway (hexose monophosphate pathway).

$$\text{Glucose 6-PO}_4 + 2\text{NADP}^+ + \text{H}_2\text{O} \rightarrow \text{ribose 5-PO}_4 + 2\text{NADPH} + 2\text{H}^+ + \text{CO}_2$$

This pathway is more active in adipose tissue than muscle because large amounts of NADPH are needed for fatty acid synthesis from acetyl-CoA. Because many cells need more NADPH for reductive biosynthesis compared with the requirement for ribose 5-phosphate incorporation into nucleotides (see page 141), the ribose 5-phosphate can be converted into glyceraldehyde 3-phosphate (and thence to pyruvate), and fructose-6-phosphate by transketotolase and transaldolase, thus creating a reversible link between the pentose phosphate pathway and glycolysis.

## LIPID METABOLISM

Lipids are poorly soluble in water and are found in the body as cell membranes, metabolic fuel, storage forms of energy and emulsifying agents. Lipids can be classified chemically into five groups:

- fatty acids, which are a major source of energy and also building blocks for more complicated lipids;
- glycerol esters, which include the triglycerides, the storage form of fatty acids, and phosphoglycerides, the main lipid component of cell membranes;
- sphingolipids, which are also membrane components;
- sterols, which include cholesterol, bile acids, steroid hormones and vitamin D;
- and terpenes, which include the other fat-soluble vitamins (A, E, K).

Attention will be focused on fatty acids and the glycerol esters.

## Fatty acids and glycerol esters

*Fatty acids* may be represented by the formula R-COOH, where R is an alkyl chain composed of carbon and hydrogen atoms. They are commonly classified according to chain length and degree of saturation. Long-chain fatty acids contain 12–26 carbon atoms, medium-chain 6–10, and short-chain 2–4. Almost all naturally derived fatty acids contain an even number of carbon atoms. Fatty acids with one unsaturated bond are *monoenoic* and polyunsaturated fatty acids are *polyenoic*. Dietary fat is made up of a mixture of fatty acids mainly present as triglycerides. The fatty acids in animal fat (e.g. butter and lard) are generally more saturated than those in vegetable oils (e.g. olive oil). The unsaturated fatty acid composition of vegetable oils varies, resulting in the need to mix them judiciously in the preparation of commercial infant formulas.

Not all polyenoic fatty acids can be synthesized and those that must be obtained from the diet are termed *essential fatty acids*. In man the linoleic and linolenic classes are essential. Linoleic acid derivatives are precursors of certain prostaglandins (*see* page 162) and linolenic acid metabolites are found in retinal photoreceptor membranes. Essential fatty acid deficiency may occur clinically, especially during prolonged parenteral nutrition, and is characterized by dermatitis and poor wound healing.

*Glycerides* are the fatty acid esters of glycerol and may be mono-, di- or tri- depending on the number of glycerol hydroxyl groups esterified. Triglycerides are the most prevalent, being the major storage and transport form of fatty acids. Phosphoglycerides are acyl-glycerols containing phosphoric acid esterified at the C3-hydroxyl group. They form bilayers when dispersed in an aqueous solution and in this form are the main structural components of cell membranes. *Lecithin* is the common name for phosphatidylcholine.

## Digestion and absorption of fat (*see also* Chapter 56)

Most dietary lipid is triglyceride which makes up 20–40 per cent of the caloric intake. Fat must be emulsified and hydrolyzed in the intestinal lumen before being absorbed. Emulsification takes place in the aqueous chyme of the duodenum under the influence of bile salts, to produce micelles. *Micelles* are aggregates of molecules made up of both polar (hydrophilic) and non-polar (hydrophobic) groups. These are known as amphipathic molecules when the molecule is long enough for each end to demonstrate its own solubility characteristics. Phosphatidylcholine is an example of a substance that forms micelles, the non-polar fatty acid chains being aggregated inwardly while the polar phosphorylcholine groups orient outwards to interact with the surrounding water molecules. Triglyceride and cholesterol esters are not amphipathic, but are able to reside within the non-polar interior of the micelles where they are digested.

Pancreatic lipase cleaves the fatty acids from positions 1 and 3 of a triglyceride. The resulting fatty acids and 2-monoglyceride are then absorbed by diffusion into the mucosal cells of the upper small intestine. Pancreatic lipase is activated by a cofactor, co-lipase, also secreted by the pancreas. Co-lipase binds to the mixed micelle containing triglycerides and facilitates adsorption of lipase to the complex. Once inside the mucosal cell the fatty acids and monoglycerides are resynthesized into triglyceride before passing into the circulation. These reactions consume energy but permit remodeling of the triglyceride entering the circulation. Triglycerides are released into the lymph in the form of a lipoprotein, the chylomicron.

After birth, fat quickly replaces glucose as the major energy source, but the mechanisms for lipid digestion and absorption are not fully developed. In the newborn infant, and especially the premature, both pancreatic lipase and bile salt concentrations are low. Lipid digestion therefore is mainly intragastric and is under the control of lingual and gastric lipases which have a broad pH optimum (2.5–7.0) and, unlike pancreatic lipase, are not dependent on bile salts. The products of lipolysis, monoglyceride and free fatty acids (FFAs), compensate for the reduced bile salts by acting as emulsifiers.

*Medium-chain triglycerides* (MCT) do not appear in the food we eat but have an important role in therapeutic diets. They are synthetic triglycerides with fatty acid chains of 8–10 carbon atoms. MCTs are absorbed intact by the intestinal mucosal cells where they are hydrolyzed by an intracellular lipase to fatty acid and glycerol. These are not re-esterified but pass directly into the portal vein bound to albumin to be taken up and further metabolized by the liver. MCTs are a useful caloric supplement in diseases where one or more of the steps in normal lipid digestion are either not fully developed as in prematurity, or are defective such as in *pancreatic insufficiency* where there is inadequate lipase secreted, or *abetalipoproteinemia* in which chylomicrons cannot be synthesized.

## Lipid transport

There are three important routes for lipid movement in the body:

- dietary triglyceride is transported from the intestine to the tissues;
- triglyceride synthesized by the liver is secreted and transported for storage in adipose tissue;
- adipose tissue triglyceride is taken to other tissues in the form of free fatty acids (FFAs).

A small amount of free fatty acid comes from the hydrolysis of triglyceride in chylomicrons and very-low-density lipoproteins (VLDL) by lipoprotein lipase at the point of delivery. Cholesterol absorbed from the gut, or synthesized in the liver, must be transported to other tissues as substrate for steroid and membrane synthesis.

Although free fatty acids are only about 3 per cent of the total fatty acids in the circulation, they are metabolically important. FFAs are transported tightly bound to albumin. On average each molecule of albumin binds 1–2 free fatty acid molecules with a dissociation constant in the order of 1 $\mu$M. The small amount of unbound FFA is readily taken up by tissue for oxidation or tissue lipid synthesis and the half-life of plasma FFA is only 1–2 minutes.

The remainder of the fatty acids and cholesterol are carried by lipoproteins which have a micellar structure with triglycerides and cholesterol esters in the core surrounded by amphipathic lipids and proteins. There are five main classes of plasma lipoprotein (Table 7.1).

Chylomicrons are very large molecules, but have the lowest density because they are approximately 98 per cent lipid. VLDLs contain about 90 per cent lipid of which more than half is triglyceride. They are synthesized in the liver and are primarily responsible for the transport of triglyceride from the liver to other tissues, notably adipose tissue. Triglycerides are transported mainly by chylomicrons and very-low-density lipoproteins, whereas cholesterol esters are carried by low-density lipoproteins and phospholipids by high-density lipoproteins.

Lipoproteins can also be separated by electrophoresis. The band remaining at the origin contains the chylomicrons. The next, called the $\beta$-lipoproteins, migrates with the $\beta$-globulins and contains the LDL. The band migrating in front of the $\beta$ region contains the VLDL and is called the pre-$\beta$-lipoproteins. The final band, the $\alpha$-lipoproteins, migrates with the $\alpha$-globulins and contains the HDL.

Lipoproteins contain a wide variety of apoproteins (Apo-) which are synthesized in various organs and have other functions as well as lipid transport. For example, Apo-AI which is the main structural protein of HDLs is also an activator of lecithin cholesterol acyltransferase, and Apo-CII which is found in VLDL and HDL activates lipoprotein lipase. *Abetalipoproteinemia* is a rare autosomal recessive condition in which there is deficient synthesis of lipoproteins containing Apo-B. The formation of chylomicrons, VLDL and LDL are all deficient with resulting fat malabsorption, ataxic neuropathy, acanthocytosis and ataxic neuropathy.

## Lipolysis

The hydrolysis of triglyceride in the circulation is governed by lipoprotein lipase. This is present in most tissues including the heart, mammary gland and adipose tissue where its activity is increased by insulin. Lipoprotein lipase is secreted and passes through the capillary endothelium where it binds to the surface membrane of the endothelial cells. The enzyme is activated by apoprotein CII, one of the low-molecular-weight proteins present in VLDL and HDL. It hydrolyzes triglyceride at positions 1 and 3; the resulting fatty acids are taken up locally and the monoglyceride is transported to the liver where it is metabolized. Intravenous heparin liberates lipoprotein lipase into the circulation from both the capillary endothelium

TABLE 7.1 Classes of lipoproteins separable by density ultracentrifugation and electrophoresis

| LIPOPROTEIN | MAJOR LIPIDS | ELECTROPHORETIC MOBILITY |
|---|---|---|
| Chylomicron | Triglyceride | None |
| Very-low-density (VLDL) | Triglyceride | Pre-$\beta$ |
| Intermediate-density (IDL) | Triglyceride and cholesterol esters | $\beta$ |
| Low-density (LDL) | Cholesterol esters | $\beta$ |
| High-density (HDL) | Phospholipids and cholesterol | $\alpha$ |

and the liver. The capillary lipase is inactivated by protamine, but the hepatic lipase is not.

Lipoprotein lipase activity can vary between tissues and this may be important in the growth and maturation of individual organs. There is low activity in fetal muscle and heart, but more in the lung possibly related to surfactant biosynthesis. Lipoprotein lipase is present in fetal adipocyte precursors which can hydrolyze exogenous triglyceride and are hormone- and heparin-sensitive. Lipoprotein lipase activity increases in all tissues immediately after birth irrespective of whether this occurs at term or prematurely. There is impaired clearance of circulating triglyceride in premature infants owing to low lipoprotein lipase activity, which is directly proportional to the degree of prematurity. When babies are fed parenterally using Intralipid, a 10 per cent soybean oil emulsion, as a rich caloric source they may develop marked lipemia. Intralipid particles are similar in size to chylomicrons and are also cleared by lipoprotein lipase.

Stored triglyceride, needed as fuel elsewhere in the body, is mobilized from adipocytes by hormone-sensitive lipase which is activated, via the adenylyl cyclase mechanism, by hormones such as glucagon and catecholamines or by sympathetic stimulation. Thyroxine and growth hormone also stimulate lipolysis but do so more slowly, probably by increasing the synthesis of an intracellular regulatory protein rather than by activating adenylyl cyclase.

Triglyceride destined for intracellular catabolism is hydrolyzed by lysosomal acid lipase which has a pH optimum of 5.

# Lipid storage

Fat differs from protein and carbohydrate, neither of which has specialized storage arrangements in the body. The only quantitatively important energy reservoir is adipose tissue. There are two kinds of adipose tissue, brown and white.

Brown adipose tissue is important for thermogenesis, white for energy homeostasis. Brown adipose tissue is composed of large multilocular cells packed with mitochondria and has a rich blood supply and sympathetic innervation. Lipolysis is controlled by hormone-sensitive lipase which is stimulated by catecholamines of both sympathetic and adrenal origin. The resulting FFAs are oxidized locally in the mitochondria and peroxisomes to produce heat by uncoupled oxidation due to the presence of thermogenin (see Chapter 48). Mitochondria preferentially oxidize saturated medium-chain FFAs and peroxisomes oxidize long-chain polyunsaturated FFAs. Mitochondrial FFA oxidation requires high concentrations of carnitine for transmembrane FFA transport. When endogenous substrate stores are exhausted, brown adipose tissue can take up FFAs from the circulation.

White adipose tissue exists as subcutaneous fat and deep body fat. Adipose tissue stores develop late in gestation, the concentration of fetal lipids before 32 weeks being low and constant. In the last 8 weeks of pregnancy subcutaneous fat increases exponentially from 20 to 350 g, and deep body fat from 10 to 80 g. Conditions characterized by fetal hyperinsulinemia, such as *infant of a diabetic mother* (IDM) and *Beckwith–Wiedemann syndrome*, are associated with increased adipose tissue development. *Obesity* is associated with an increase in both adipocyte size and number. The extent to which feeding in the first months of life can influence growth of white adipocytes and thereby produce a liability to obesity in later life remains unresolved.

In adipocytes, triglyceride synthesis occurs from FFAs, which may be synthesized from glucose metabolism or more likely are delivered to the cell as triglyceride in chylomicrons or VLDL. Insulin stimulates the production of lipoprotein lipase and glucose uptake, thereby enhancing the delivery of both FFAs and the glycerol moiety of triglyceride. Lipolysis in adipocytes results in both FFAs and glycerol being released into the circulation because adipocytes lack glycerol kinase. Most of the glycerol is metabolized by the liver, but the FFAs are taken up by nearly all tissues and may be recycled within the adipose tissue.

# Fat oxidation

Fatty acids are a major fuel. When catabolized completely to $CO_2$ and $H_2O$, 60 per cent of the energy is released as heat and 40 per cent is conserved to form ATP. Fatty acid catabolism occurs in the mitochondria by "β-oxidation" in which two carbon fragments are progressively removed in the form of acetyl-CoA which is then catabolized to $CO_2$ and water in the Krebs cycle.

The first step in β-oxidation is formation of the acyl-CoA thioester by combination with CoA-SH under the control of acyl-CoA synthetase. There are at least three acyl-CoA synthetases for short-, medium- and long-chain fatty acids, respectively. The long-chain activating enzyme is located in the outer mitochondrial membrane and endoplasmic reticulum, but the other two are purely mitochondrial. The acyl-CoA formed in the outer mitochondrial membrane must then be transesterified from CoA-SH to carnitine in order to traverse the inner mitochondrial membrane and arrive at the site of the β-oxidation enzyme system (Fig. 7.2). This is controlled by carnitine acyltransferase (CAT) located on the inner mitochondrial membrane and is a reversible reaction. Further oxidation takes place within the mitochondrial matrix. Deficiency of an acyl-CoA synthetase results in one of the inborn errors of fatty acid oxidation, such as *glutaric aciduria types 1 and 2*, which have diverse clinical presentations including hypoglycemia, neurological dysfunction and

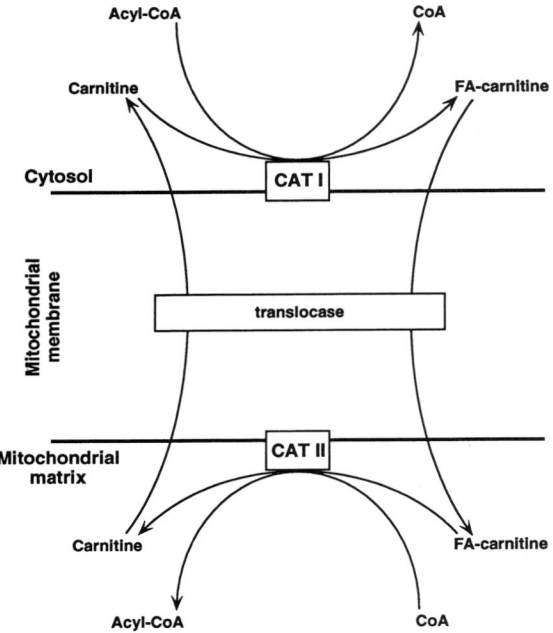

FIGURE 7.2 Translocation of long-chain fatty acid acyl groups across the mitochondrial membrane. CAT = carnitine acyl-transferase

failure to thrive. A β-oxidation loop involves sequentially, oxidation of the acyl-CoA thioester, hydration, oxidation and thiolysis to produce an oxyl-CoA shortened by two carbon atoms plus $FADH_2$, NADH and acetyl-CoA. A single β-oxidation cycle yielding 1 mol of acetyl-CoA produces 5 mol of ATP (2 from each $FADH_2$ and 3 from NADH) and the resulting oxidation of the acetyl-CoA a further 12 mol of ATP (Fig. 7.3).

The energy of cardiac contraction comes mainly from fatty acid oxidation and there are important quantitative changes in the perinatal period. Fatty acid oxidation in the fetus is limited by a low concentration of carnitine in the heart and a relative paucity of mitochondria, both of which increase rapidly after birth. Prior to birth, cardiac energetics depend primarily on glucose and to a lesser extent lactate as a source of energy. Other fetal tissues, such as liver, brain, placenta and lung, also have a limited capacity to oxidize fatty acids, probably owing to limited production of palmitoyl carnitine by palmitoyl carnitine transferase A. After birth, fatty acid oxidation increases markedly and remains high until the time of weaning. Carnitine is potentially rate-limiting and its inclusion in infant formulae or parenteral nutrients may have an important subsidiary role in the development of fatty acid oxidation. *Carnitine deficiency* may also arise as an inborn metabolic defect in carnitine synthesis, from the trapping and excretion of carnitine esters in *metabolic errors of fatty acid oxidation*, and also from

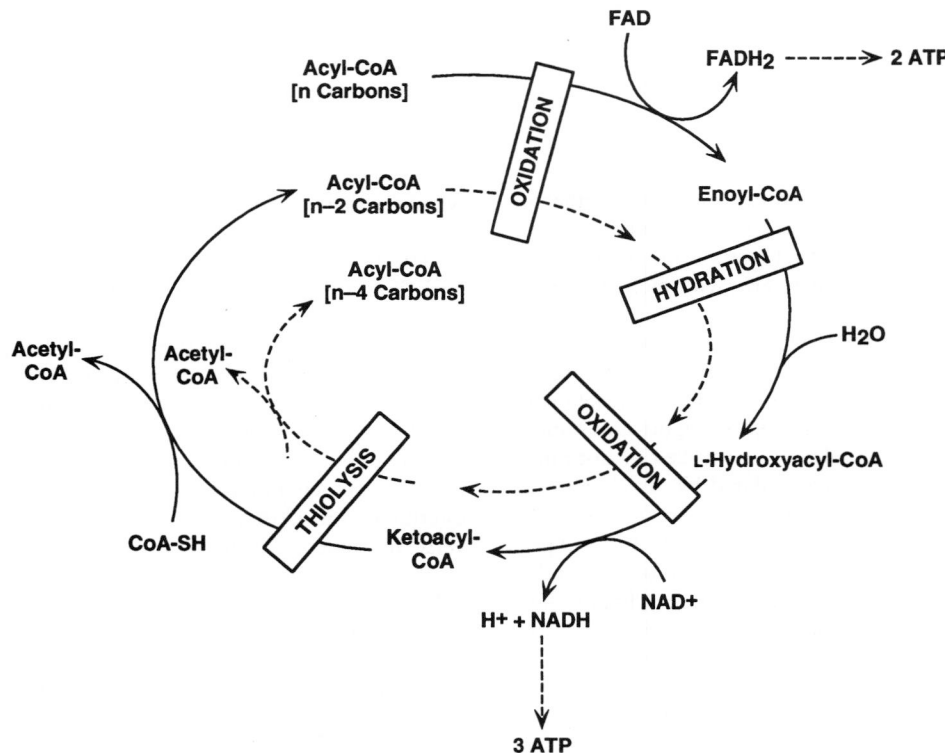

FIGURE 7.3 A loop of the β oxidation cycle in which acyl-CoA is shortened by two carbons which are released as acetyl-CoA

excessive losses in renal conditions such as the *Fanconi syndrome, cystinosis* and *chronic dialysis*.

## Ketones

The efficiency with which two carbon residues can be oxidized in the Krebs cycle depends on glucose availability. If imbalance occurs, as in *starvation* or *diabetes mellitus*, there is an accumulation of acetyl-CoA which is then condensed to form the ketone bodies, acetoacetate, β-hydroxybutyrate and acetone. Ketone body synthesis is blocked by malonyl-CoA, which is the link molecule between glucose and fatty acid metabolism, inhibiting carnitine acyltransferase I. Ketone bodies pass from the liver into the circulation to be used by brain, muscle and heart as an energy source. When the body's capacity to oxidize ketones is saturated, they spill into the urine and are exhaled, producing a sickly sweet smell.

Ketone bodies in the fetal circulation can arise from the partial oxidation of fatty acids, but they also may be of maternal origin. Fasting during pregnancy causes a rapid rise in maternal ketone levels and maternal–fetal ketone body transfer during labor may be appreciable. During the latter part of pregnancy the capacity to oxidize hydroxybutyrate has been demonstrated *in vitro* in fetal liver, brain and placenta. On balance, ketones in the fetal circulation are used more for lipid synthesis than as a source of immediate energy.

## Lipogenesis

Fatty acids may be synthesized in three ways. The most important quantitatively is *de novo* synthesis from glucose in the cell cytosol. Pyruvate derived from glucose enters the mitochondrion and is converted to acetyl-CoA by the pyruvate dehydrogenase enzyme complex. The acetyl-CoA thus formed cannot traverse the inner mitochondrial membrane and must leave the mitochondrion as citrate to be cleaved by citrate lyase in the cell cytoplasm to produce acetyl-CoA and oxaloacetate (Fig. 7.4). All but one of the acetyl-CoA units that will end up as two carbon blocks in a FFA molecule must first be carboxylated to malonyl-CoA by the enzyme complex acetyl-CoA carboxylase. This is the rate-limiting step in fatty acid synthesis. The assembly of the fatty acid then proceeds under the control of the fatty acid synthetase complex, which consists of six enzymes and a carrier protein. *De novo* fatty acid synthesis always results in an even-numbered carbon product because the acetate primer contains two carbons and each malonate unit condensing with it donates two more.

*De novo* fatty acid synthesis is under short- and long-term control. Short-term control involves modulation of acetyl-CoA carboxylase which is aggregated and activated by citrate and disaggregated by palmi-

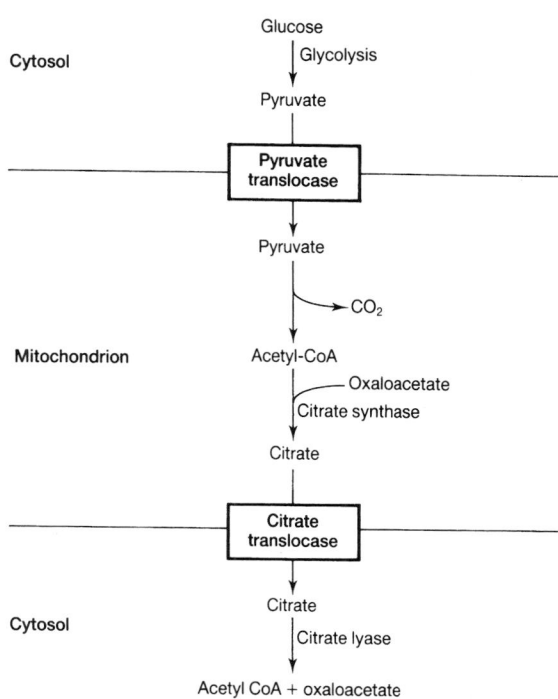

FIGURE 7.4 Conversion of glucose to acetyl-CoA

toyl-CoA. Long-term control involves the synthesis of new fatty acid biosynthetic enzymes which have a short half-life. This is stimulated in the liver by glucose and insulin and inhibited during *starvation* or *insulin-deficient diabetes*.

Fatty acid synthesis is active in hepatic cytosol in late fetal life, declines after birth when the diet becomes fat-rich milk, and then increases again at weaning when dietary fat intake falls. Human fetal tissue of 12–20 weeks' gestation is capable of incorporating glucose, fructose, acetate, citrate and amino acids into lipids *in vitro*. The liver also takes up maternal fatty acids which cross the placenta easily. Long-chain unsaturated fatty acids must be provided by the mother. Fetal fatty acid synthesis is stimulated by insulin and inhibited by glucagon or cAMP. Triglyceride synthesis from palmitate has been demonstrated in slices of liver, lung and brain from abortions of 12–16 weeks' gestation.

## Phosphoglycerides

Phosphoglycerides are derived from glycerol by two pathways. In the main pathway the phosphoglyceride is produced from glycerol 3-phosphate derived from glucose (Fig. 7.5). This is first converted to a diacylglycerol and then phosphate is removed under the influence of phosphatidic acid phosphatase. This is also the pathway for triglyceride synthesis. The final step is a reaction with a cytidine diphosphate derivative of

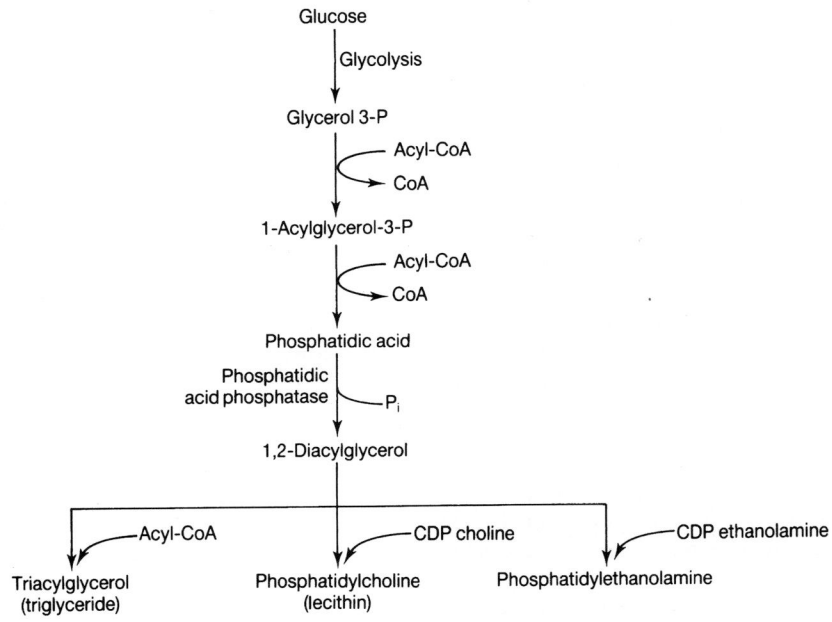

FIGURE 7.5 The synthesis of triacylglycerol, phosphatidylethanolamine and phosphatidylcholine from glucose

either ethanol or choline (CDP ethanolamine or CDP choline). Phosphatidylcholine (lecithin) and phosphatidylethanolamine take up about 75 per cent of the phosphoglycerides in most tissues and body fluids. All the enzymes involved in phosphoglyceride and triglyceride synthesis are associated with the endoplasmic reticulum. The second pathway bypasses the formation of 1,2-diacylglycerol and involves the reaction between phosphatidic acid and cytidine diphosphate diacylglycerol yielding, in the main, cardiolipin and phosphatidylinositol. Phosphoglycerides are metabolized by phospholipases which remove the acyl residues from the glycerol backbone.

*Surfactant* is a lipoprotein secreted by pulmonary type II epithelial cells and is essential in lowering the surface tension of the alveoli and permitting normal gas exchange. Surfactant contains a characteristic lecithin, dipalmitoyl phosphatidylcholine, which makes up about half the surfactant lipid. This is an unusual phosphatidylcholine in being saturated; most cell membrane phosphatidylcholine is unsaturated. Another important component of surfactant is phosphatidyl glycerol. The surfactant complex contains two specific proteins, one of 38 kD and the other 10 kD. The larger protein molecule is thought to be involved in the secretion of surfactant and the smaller in its recycling. A deficiency of surfactant results in the *respiratory distress syndrome* (RDS) (*see* Chapter 77).

## Sphingolipids

Sphingosine is an 18-carbon dihydric alcohol containing an amino group at C17. It is synthesized from palmitoyl-CoA and serine. Ceramide which is formed by the N-acylation of sphingosine is the key intermediate in sphingolipid synthesis. Ceramide reacts with CDP choline to form choline P-ceramide (sphingomyelin), UDP galactose to form galactosylceramide and UDP glucose to form glucosylceramide, both examples of cerebrosides. Gangliosides are formed by the addition of hexose residues to glucosylceramide. Sphingomyelin is degraded by sphingomyelinase which removes the phosphorylcholine residue. Cerebrosides and gangliosides are hydrolyzed by hexosidases which are lysosomal enzymes. Inherited deficiencies of these catabolic enzymes results in the *lipid storage diseases* or *lipidoses* in which there is intracellular accumulation of sphingolipid leading to visceromegally and neurological degeneration.

## CARBOHYDRATE METABOLISM

The term "carbohydrate" was used originally to describe naturally occurring compounds such as glucose, sucrose, glycogen, cellulose and starch which can be represented by the formula $C_x(H_2O)_y$, but now also includes more complex molecules which have a sugar in them. Carbohydrates represent about half of the total caloric intake and come mainly from plant sources. The physiologically important monosaccharides are glucose, galactose and fructose. The physiologically important disaccharides are lactose (glucose, galactose), sucrose (glucose, fructose) and to a lesser extent maltose (glucose, glucose). Starch is the most important polysaccharide ingested and glycogen the most important in the body.

## Carbohydrate digestion and absorption (*see also* Chapter 56)

The glycoside bonds of saccharides are hydrolyzed by glycosidases to give reducing sugars. Mastication stimulates the secretion of salivary amylase which acts on starch in a random manner to produce glucose, maltose and smaller starch fragments called dextrins. Thorough chewing will reduce starch to an average chain length of less than eight glucose units. Amylase action is stopped by the acidity of the stomach, but as the food enters the small intestine and is rendered alkaline by pancreatic juice, digestion of the starch dextrins is continued by pancreatic amylase. The resulting carbohydrate mix from a typical meal is glucose, maltose, isomaltose, lactose and sucrose. Ingested cellulose is non-digestible but contributes to stool bulk.

The important monosaccharides, glucose, fructose and galactose, can be absorbed across the intestinal mucosa against a concentration gradient, but under normal conditions the intraluminal concentration is greater and the pump functions mainly to prevent sugars leaking back into the intestinal lumen. Disaccharide digestion occurs in the brush border of the upper jejunum where the resulting monosaccharides are absorbed. The postprandial rate of sugar absorption is approximately 1 g/kg bodyweight per hour. The products of digestion are then delivered to the liver. Apart from a contribution to complex glycoproteins and glycolipids, most galactose and fructose enters the glucose metabolic pool.

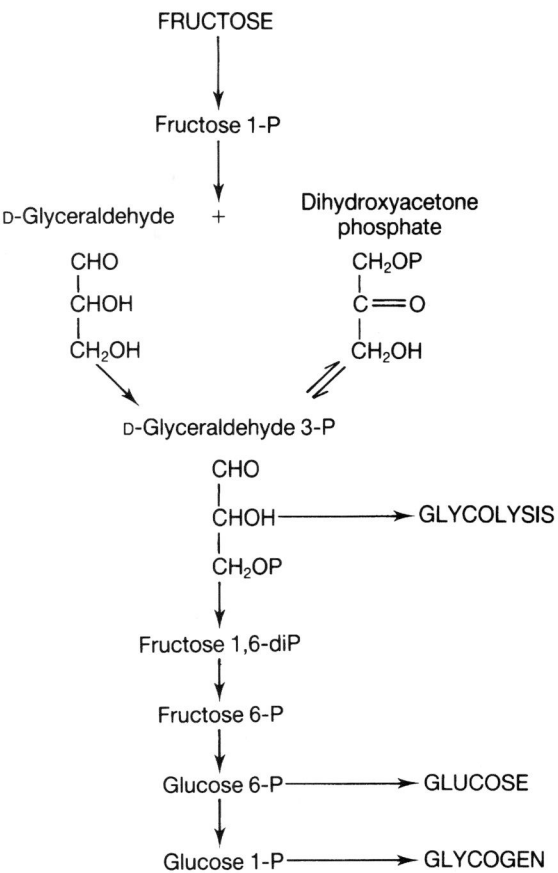

FIGURE 7.6 Hepatic metabolism of fructose

## Monosaccharide metabolism

There are specific kinases for the initial phosphorylation of the monosaccharides. Cells also contain less specific hexokinases at a relatively constant concentration which convert monosaccharides to the relevant 6-P ester and which are subject to product inhibition. Glucokinase is found only in the liver where its concentration is determined by the circulating insulin level. Skeletal and visceral cellular uptake of glucose occur as a function of the blood glucose and insulin concentrations. Hepatic glucose uptake differs from that in the rest of the body in being dependent on glucokinase which is deficient in insulinopenic conditions such as *diabetes mellitus* or *starvation*. Because glucokinase is not subject to feedback inhibition, glucose uptake is enhanced postprandially when glycogenesis is promoted. In contrast the tissue hexokinase, which has a much lower $K_m$, becomes more important during fasting.

Fructose metabolism involves splitting fructose 1-phosphate to two triose fragments by an aldolase (Fig. 7.6). These trioses are glyceraldehyde and dihydroxyacetone phosphate which may then be catabolized by glycolysis or condensed to produce fructose

1,6-diphosphate which is available for glycogenesis via glucose 6-phosphate. Deficiency of the aldolase causes *hereditary fructose intolerance*, a potentially life-threatening condition characterized by vomiting, hypoglycemia, metabolic acidosis and mental retardation.

Galactose is rapidly taken up by the liver, where after phosphorylation by galactokinase, it is converted to glucose 1-phosphate by galactose 1-phosphate uridyl transferase. Deficiency of galactokinase results in *galactosemia*, which is characterized by galactosuria and the development of cataracts. Deficiency of galactose 1-phosphate uridyl transferase results in the accumulation of intracellular galactose 1-phosphate and is the cause of classical *galactosemia*, a serious disease characterized by vomiting, hypoglycemia, cataracts, mental retardation and hepatosplenomegaly.

## Glycogen

Glycogen metabolism is at the heart of glucose homeostasis. Glucose 6-phosphatase is the key enzyme in the liver and kidney which permits glucose 6-phosphate, derived from glycogen breakdown, to be converted to glucose and thus access the circulation. Other tissues, such as muscle, may have glycogen synthetic capacity but are obliged to metabolize glucose stores locally by entering glucose 6-phosphate into the glycolytic pathway. Glycogen, mainly hepatic in origin, is the immediate glucose reservoir in times of need. Conversely, when glucose is plentiful there is a finite capacity for glycogen synthesis and any excess glucose is converted to fat. Glycogenesis is controlled by glycogen synthetase and branching enzyme (D-glucosyl-4,6-transferase) which causes irreversible sequential addition of glucosyl residues to a branched glucose polymer (Fig. 7.7). Glycogenolysis is under the control of phosphorylase and debranching enzymes (oligo-1,4 → 1,4-glucantransferase and amylo 1,6-glucosidase) which split the terminal glucose residues to yield glucose 1-phosphate (Fig. 7.8). This then must be transferred by phosphoglucomutase to glucose 6-phosphate to allow glucose release. During *starvation* glycogen stores are rarely completely depleted. A nucleus remains for future glycogen synthesis when refeeding occurs.

Nearly every cell is capable of glycogen metabolism and the flow of glucosyl units to or from storage is under the hormonal and substrate control of the relevant enzymes. Both glycogen synthetase and phosphorylase exist in two forms, which differ in being phosphorylated or not. The phosphorylation of each pair of enzymes is under the control of ATP and the protein kinase/cAMP/adenylyl cyclase cascade. Adenylyl cyclase is stimulated by glucagon and catecholamines to result in the production of the active form of phosphorylase (A) and the inactive form of glycogen synthetase (I). Glycogen synthetase (I) requires the presence of glucose 6-phosphate to work. Glycogen synthesis is activated by insulin, stimulating glucokinase to produce glucose 6-phosphate and inhibiting phosphorylation of the glycogenolytic enzymes. In adults the balance between glycogen synthesis or breakdown depends largely on the phosphorylation state of the enzymes, but in the fetus the concentration of enzyme, especially that of synthetase, is more important. Towards term there is a rapid accu-

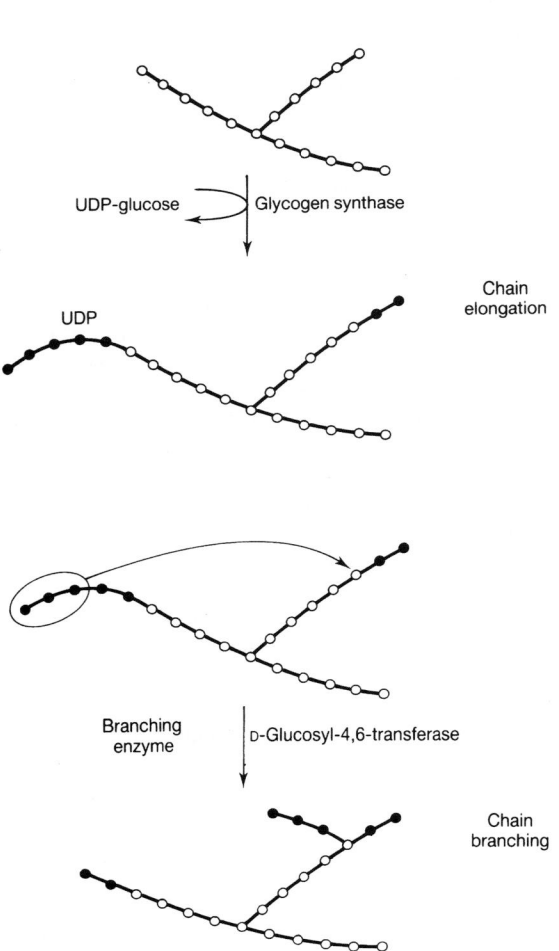

FIGURE 7.7 Glycogen synthesis by chain elongation and branching. UDP = uridine diphosphate.

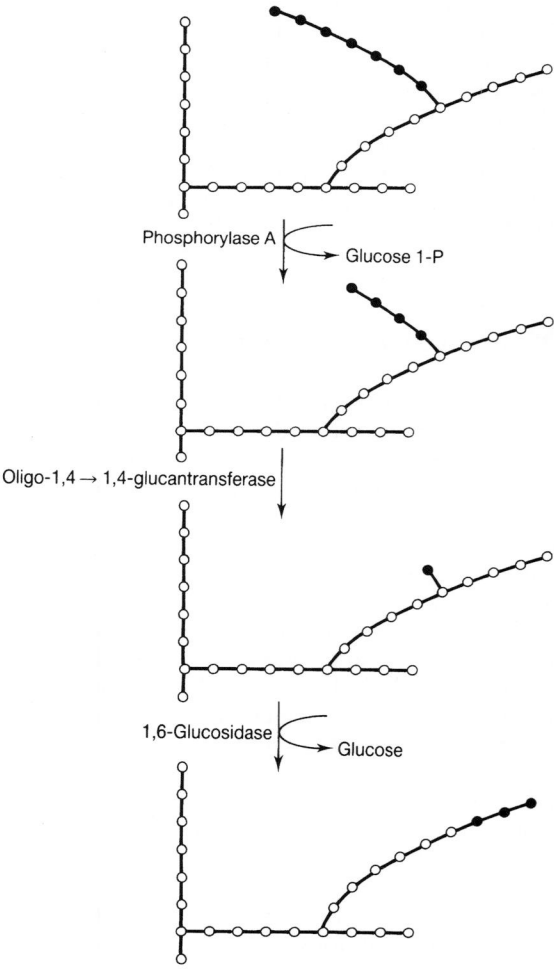

FIGURE 7.8 Glycogen breakdown by chain shortening, rearrangement and debranching

mulation of hepatic glycogen under the control of adrenal glucocorticoids. Both enzymes for glycogenolysis are present in the fetus, but they do not become active until after birth when complete depletion of liver glycogen can occur within 12 hours.

Deficiency of any of the enzymes involved in glycogen metabolism in any tissue results in one of the *glycogen storage diseases* which are variously characterized by hypoglycemia, visceromegally, muscle weakness and metabolic acidosis.

## Glycolysis

*Anaerobic glycolysis* of one glucose molecule generates lactate and two ATP, whereas *aerobic glycolysis* to $CO_2$ and $H_2O$ yields 38 ATP (Fig. 7.9). The three carbon compounds of glycolysis link it to other metabolic pathways; for example, pyruvate is a precursor of alanine synthesis, glycerol 3-phosphate is a precursor of triglyceride and phospholipid synthesis, and 2,3-diphosphoglycerate is an important erythrocyte metabolite.

In anoxic or hypoxic conditions, pyruvate acts as a temporary hydrogen acceptor and lactate is formed, but in normal circumstances hydrogen generated in glycolysis is taken up by $NAD^+$. This buffering action of pyruvate is an important homeostatic mechanism. Vigorous exercise by a healthy individual produces an $O_2$ debt and a transient rise of blood lactate, whereas normal exercise by a catabolic, feverish patient may be associated with a sustained rise in blood lactate. *Deficiency of lactic dehydrogenase*, the enzyme converting lactic acid to pyruvate, or of any of the enzymes involved in the synthesis of glucose 6-phosphate from pyruvate or the entry of pyruvate to the citric acid cycle, all cause clinically important *lactic acidosis* which may be associated with hypoglycemia, hyperventilation and neurological abnormalities.

## Gluconeogenesis

Gluconeogenesis is the synthesis of glucose from non-carbohydrate precursors (*see* Fig. 4.3). The main sites of gluconeogenesis are the liver and kidney which, having glucose 6-phosphatase, are able to release glucose into the circulation. Most other cells have the capacity for gluconeogenesis, which is important in the nervous system and erythrocytes but not in muscle. Amino acids are the principal carbon sources for gluconeogenesis. Transamination occurs between amino/keto acid homologues (e.g. pyruvate/alanine) and also between non-homologous pairs such as pyruvate/glutamine and oxaloacetate/glutamine. The blood concentrations of the enzymes controlling these reactions (SGPT and SGOT) are useful clinical markers of disease.

The molecule through which all carbon skeletons must pass in gluconeogenesis is 2-phosphoenol pyruvate (PEP). The enzymes linking PEP and glucose are cytosolic and reversible. In contrast the deaminated keto skeletons, pyruvate, α-ketoglutarate and succinate, all traverse part of the Krebs cycle before exiting at oxaloacetate which is converted to PEP under the control of PEP carboxykinase. These reactions are intramitochondrial and irreversible. The key regulatory enzymes in gluconeogenesis are pyruvate carboxylase, PEP-carboxykinase, fructose 1,6-diphosphate 1-phosphatase and glucose 6-phosphatase. Pyruvate carboxylase controls the reaction between pyruvate and acetyl-CoA to produce intramitochondrial oxaloacetate and is a crucial meeting point of carbohydrate and lipid metabolism. The 1-phosphatase is inhibited by AMP and ADP whereas the glucose 6-phosphatase is inhibited by glucose and inorganic phosphate. Cortisol stimulates, and insulin inhibits, the synthesis of all four enzymes.

## PANCREATIC CONTROL OF ENERGY HOMEOSTASIS

Insulin and glucagon are the two islet hormones most intimately concerned with energy homeostasis, but they should not be thought of in isolation because they are members of a larger family of peptide signals found in the gut and central nervous system.

## The endocrine pancreas

The mature islets of Langerhans are compact, round or ovoid groups of polygonal epithelial cells irregularly distributed throughout the exocrine pancreas. Each islet is surrounded by an incomplete pseudocapsule which is continuous with the connective tissue interstitial septa of the exocrine gland. The islet has a rich blood supply of wide, thin-walled, anastomosing sinusoids that form a glomerulus with one afferent arteriole and several efferent capillaries. The islets have both

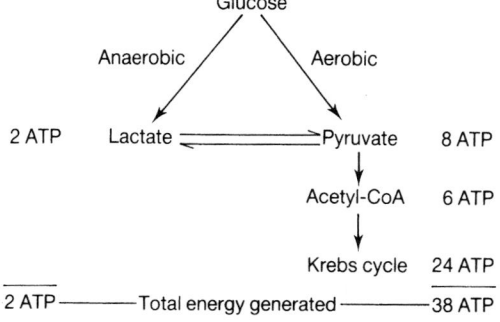

FIGURE 7.9 Glycolysis: the pathway for the generation of energy by the anaerobic or aerobic oxidation of glucose

sympathetic and parasympathetic innervation but the physiological importance of this remains unclear.

The islets originate from the primitive ducts of the embryonic pancreas whose cells are pluripotential for development to mature islet cells. There are four undisputed islet cell types: the β-cell contains insulin, the α-cell contains glucagon, the δ-cell contains somatostatin, and the PP cell contains pancreatic polypeptide. The biosynthesis and secretion of each of the four hormones occurs by the same general mechanism. First there is ribosomal synthesis of a preprohormone, from which the leader sequence is removed during passage of the newly formed polypeptide through the endoplasmic reticulum membrane to leave the prohormone in the intracisternal space, from which it passes to the Golgi vesicles where it is stored as granules. The granule contents are secreted by exocytosis in which the granule membrane and cell membrane fuse and break down, allowing release of the granule contents to the circulation.

The proportions of different islet cell types vary depending on the embryological origin of the pancreas, which grows as two outpouches of the duodenum that fuse together by the eighth week of gestation to form a ventral and dorsal lobe. The ventral lobe matures to become the uncinate process and posterior part of the head of the pancreas, whereas the dorsal lobe becomes the anterior part of the head, the body and tail of the gland. Islets rich in pancreatic polypeptide (PP) cells are found only in pancreas derived from the ventral lobe. α cells develop before β cells and islets remain α-cell-rich throughout fetal life. β-cell density (the product of cell size and number) increases with development to reach a peak 2 months after birth, after which it falls. This phenomenon is clinically important in the histopathological evaluation of pancreas when a diagnosis of *nesidioblastosis* is being considered, because comparison with normal pancreas from older infants may give a misleading impression of pathological β-cell overdevelopment.

Abnormal islet development occurs in the *infant of the diabetic mother* (IDM) where there is β-cell and islet hyperplasia together with an increase in the PP-cell fraction in the ventral lobe. In *erythroblastosis fetalis* there is hyperplasia of all four islet cell types but only in the islets of the ventral lobe. *Nesidioblastosis* represents a persistent hyperplasia of β-cells and the islet may be disorganized with a loss of normal paracrine relationships between different cell types.

# Insulin

## Structure, storage and secretion

The molecules insulin, relaxin and the insulin-like growth factors (IGF) -I and -II are a structurally related family. The insulin gene is on chromosome 11 as a single copy. There is a TATA box 30 base-pairs from the start site for transcription and three exons. Insulin is first synthesized as preproinsulin which contains a leader sequence of 24 amino acids. Proinsulin contains 84 amino acids in a single chain and is cleaved by proteolysis of a 33-amino-acid segment to produce insulin which has A and B chains of 21 and 30 amino acids linked by two disulfide bonds. The residue of the cleaved segment is called the connecting or C-peptide and this is retained in the granule and secreted in equimolar amounts with insulin. Insulin, proinsulin and C-peptide can all be measured by radioimmunoassay. The half-life of circulating insulin is 10 minutes whereas that of C-peptide is appreciably longer, 30 minutes. In some circumstances the measurement of the circulating C-peptide or proinsulin concentration is a more accurate reflection of insulin secretion than the plasma insulin concentration.

## Stimulation of secretion

The important nutritional stimuli to insulin secretion are glucose and amino acids. Other monosaccharides also cause insulin release, but glucose is the most important quantitatively. Oral glucose is more potent than intravenous glucose causing the same blood glucose rise. This is due to the enteroinsular axis through which the digestion and absorption of food stimulates the release of messengers from the gut that affect endocrine pancreatic secretion. Messengers with this action have been named *incretins*. Gastric inhibitory polypeptide (GIP) is a 42-amino-acid straight-chain peptide arising from the epithelium of the duodenum and upper jejunum. GIP release is stimulated by glucose and galactose transport across the gut. Besides inhibiting gastric activity, GIP is also insulinotropic, but only in the presence of hyperglycemia. It thus fulfills the definition of an incretin. Pancreatic glucagon and the post-translational fragments GLP (1–37) and GLP (7–37) generated by cleavage of proglucagon in the intestine are also insulin secretagogues and potential incretins.

Insulin release is stimulated by amino acids, and the mechanism of action of leucine differs from that of other amino acids. Arginine stimulation of insulin secretion is glucose-dependent and diazoxide insensitive whereas the opposite is true for leucine. *Leucine-sensitive hypoglycemia* is probably the result of a normal physiological stimulus acting on an increased β-cell mass – this is part of the spectrum of disorders extending to *nesidioblastosis*. The mixture of amino acids resulting from a protein-rich meal is a more powerful insulin secretagogue than any individual amino acid.

Lipids have no consistent effect on insulin secretion. Medium-chain triglycerides (MCT) stimulate insulin release either directly or via a metabolite and their action is synergistic with that of oral glucose. This may be clinically important in patients fed artificial therapeutic diets.

The islets are innervated by the autonomic nervous system and the catecholamines: epinephrine and norepinephrine are powerful inhibitors of insulin secretion. β-adrenergic mimetics stimulate insulin release but their use therapeutically, as in asthma therapy, is not thought to be clinically important in glucose homeostasis. The methylxanthines inhibit cyclic 3,5-AMP phosphodiesterase and thereby stimulate insulin secretion. The stimulatory effects of sulfonylureas are pertinent to pediatric practice only in the context of poisoning. Diazoxide blocks insulin secretion by interfering with $Ca^{2+}$ uptake and is useful in the management of some *hyperinsulinemic states* of infancy and childhood.

*Insulin-dependent diabetes mellitus* results from a relative or absolute insulin deficiency in infancy or childhood. *Transient neonatal diabetes* is a self-limiting insulin-dependent diabetes whose pathophysiology is poorly understood. Excessive spontaneous insulin release occurs transiently in the *infant of the diabetic mother* and in the *erythroblastotic newborn*. Sustained or reactive hyperinsulinemia may occur in *nesidioblastosis* and in *Beckwith–Wiedemann syndrome*.

## Mechanism of action

Insulin binds to specific receptors on the cell surface. The insulin receptor is closely related to the IGF-I receptor and is a glycoprotein of about 350 kD made up of two pairs of subunits. The α pair of 135 kD is entirely extracellular and has binding specificity. The β-subunits have a small extracellular domain connecting them to the α-subunits, a transmembrane domain of about 20 amino acids, and a large intracellular domain that contains tyrosine kinase sites.

Insulin binding results in autophosphorylation. Following autophosphorylation a cascade of intracellular protein phosphorylation events occurs. The major substrate IRS-1 is first phosphorylated and in turn this leads to phosphorylation of several different proteins (*see* page 463). One protein phosphorylated is phosphatidylinositol-3-kinase which initiates activation of phosphatidylinositol-3 phosphate. In turn this leads to transcriptional activation. Another protein phosphorylated is Grb2, which in turn activates SOS which activates Ras, then Raf and then the MAP-kinases leading to transcriptional activation (*see also* Chapters 2 and 18). Phospholipase C is also activated, offering a further signal transition pathway. The insulin receptor may be deactivated by phosphorylation of serine groups by other kinases, e.g. protein kinase C. Insulin receptors are also found in the cytosol and on the nuclear membrane, possibly as part of a receptor recycling control mechanism. Insulin-sensitive cells such as adipocytes and hepatocytes have higher receptor densities than other cells.

All the actions of insulin are directed towards anabolism and the lowering of blood glucose. Some actions are seen at fasting plasma insulin concentrations, others only in the presence of postprandial raised insulin concentrations. Some actions of insulin are rapid, others slower. Among the slow and longer lasting actions are the induction of enzymes whose gene transcription is under partial insulin control. Enzymes stimulated in this way include glucokinase, pyruvate kinase and glyceraldehyde 3-phosphate dehydrogenase which result in glycogenesis and increased glycolysis. Pancreatic amylase is also stimulated, thereby enhancing starch digestion and saccharide uptake.

Muscle protein is in a state of dynamic flux and its turnover increases with immaturity. Muscle protein turnover of an infant is in the order of 6 g/kg bodyweight per day, whereas that of a middle-aged man is only about 1.5 g/kg bodyweight per day. Protein synthesis and breakdown in muscle are subject to a number of influences; for example, muscle activity causes anabolism and excess glucocorticoids induce catabolism. High plasma insulin concentrations that occur postprandially stimulate protein synthesis by increasing the cellular uptake of amino acids and peptide synthesis independently, with the consequence that the intracellular concentration of amino acids falls and tissue nitrogen increases. Low plasma insulin concentrations as seen in fasting inhibit but do not abolish proteolysis. Under these conditions muscle produces amino acids, particularly alanine and glutamate which are substrates for hepatic and renal gluconeogenesis. A slight increase of circulating insulin during fasting can depress plasma amino acids and urea nitrogen excretion without influencing circulating lipid metabolites.

Glucose crosses cell membranes by interaction with specific cell membrane proteins, the glucose transporters. These are a superfamily of at least five proteins, some of which are primarily located on the cell membrane for constitutive glucose entry. The five well-characterized isoforms have been designated GLUT 1 to GLUT 5. They are primarily expressed in different tissues and have different physiological functions. They have a high degree of structural homology with 12 transmembrane domains and are 492–524 amino acids in length. Both the N and C terminals are internally orientated. The characteristics of GLUT 1–5 are described in Table 7.2. In addition to the facilitative glucose transporter superfamily, glucose transport in the kidney and intestine also involves the $Na^+$ dependent glucose transporter (SGLT) which is an entirely separate class of molecule. SGLT is involved in the active uptake of dietary glucose from the small intestine and reabsorption of filtered glucose in the proximal intake of the kidney. GLUT 1 and GLUT 3 have high affinity for glucose whereas GLUT 2 has low affinity for glucose. This latter characteristic, together with the high capacity of GLUT 2, means that the rate of flux through this

TABLE 7.2 Mammalian glucose transporters: major site of expression and physiological functions

| ISOFORM | SIZE (AMINO ACIDS) | PRIMARY TISSUE DISTRIBUTION | FUNCTION |
|---|---|---|---|
| GLUT 1 | 492 | Brain endothelial cells, erythrocytes, placenta, kidney, colon | Blood/tissue barrier transport basal transport |
| GLUT 2 | 524 | Pancreatic β cell, small intestine, kidney, liver | β-cell glucose sensor, uptake and release of glucose by hepatocytes, release of absorbed glucose from basal surface of small intestine and kidney epithelium to blood stream |
| GLUT 3 | 496 | Neurones, placenta, many other tissues | High affinity transporter, basal uptake of glucose to all cells, including brain, placental transport |
| GLUT 4 | 501 | Heart and skeletal muscle, brown fat, white adipose tissue | Insulin-stimulated glucose transport |
| GLUT 5 | 501 | Small intestine, sperm, brain endothelial cells, skeletal muscle | Fructose transport |

transporter is directly proportional to the glucose concentration. GLUT 2 is the primary sensor molecule for glucose in the islet cell. Whereas the other GLUTs are located primarily in the cell membrane, GLUT 4, the insulin-sensitive transporter which is found only in fat and muscle, is primarily located in the Golgi apparatus and is translocated to the cell surface in response to insulin. Insulin promotes glucose uptake by increasing the amount of glucose transporter synthesized and by increasing the movement of transporter to the plasma membrane in both muscle cells and adipocytes, but not in hepatocytes which are freely permeable to glucose.

Insulin stimulates both glycolysis and glycogenesis. Glycolysis is activated by direct stimulation of phosphofructokinase and unblocking the inhibitory action of fructose 2,6-biphosphate. Glycogen synthesis is promoted by a sequence of events started by the tyrosine kinase of the insulin receptor, leading eventually to the dephosphorylation of both the glycogen phosphorylase and synthetase which are reciprocally inactivated and activated. At low fasting concentrations insulin inhibits hormone-sensitive lipase and thus adipocyte lipolysis. Lipogenesis is promoted by insulin at postprandial concentrations.

# Glucagon

Glucagon is a member of a multigene family which also includes secretin, vasoactive intestinal peptide (VIP), gastric inhibitory peptide (GIP) and glicentin. The glucagon gene is on chromosome 2q36–2q37 and comprises six exons and five introns. Preproglucagon is a 180 residue protein that contains the sequences of glucagon, glicentin and two glucagon-like peptides (GLP), GLP-1 and GLP-2. Glucagon is a 29-amino-acid single chain which is synthesized and secreted from the α-cells of the islet in a manner analogous to insulin.

## Stimulation of secretion

The stimuli to glucagon secretion and its actions are largely the opposite of those of insulin. Glucagon release is stimulated by hypoglycemia and inhibited by glucose. Fasting increases plasma glucagon concentrations. Both glucagon and insulin release are stimulated by amino acids and arginine is a potent glucagon secretagogue. The simultaneous rise of both hormones after a protein-rich meal ensures the proper conversion of excess glucogenic amino acids to glucose and utilization of the glucose. The α-cell is more sensitive to the inhibitory effect of glucose and stimulatory effect of arginine than the β-cell. A rise in plasma free fatty acids or ketones inhibits glucagon release and a fall is stimulatory. Other members of the gut peptide family may stimulate glucagon secretion. Catecholamines and sympathetic nervous stimulation result in glucagon release.

## Mechanism of action

Glucagon binds to a specific cell-surface receptor which is coupled to adenylyl cyclase by a $G_s$-protein. Activation of adenylyl cyclase results in the synthesis of cAMP from ATP in the presence of magnesium. This acts on a cAMP-dependent kinase which then adds phosphate groups to the serine and threonine groups of other proteins. cAMP is hydrolyzed by a specific phosphodiesterase that can be inhibited by methylxanthines. Glucagon causes hyperglycemia by promoting glycogenolysis and inhibiting glycogen synthesis via cAMP-induced phosphorylation. At the same time hepatic gluconeogenesis is stimulated by reduction of fructose 2,6-biphosphate concentration, leading to activation of gluconeogenesis and inhibition of glycolysis. Glycolysis raises the blood glucose faster than gluconeogenesis. Adipocyte lipolysis is stimulated via activation of hormone-sensitive lipase. Hepatic lipogenesis is inhibited because acetyl-CoA production from glucose falls with the block of glycolysis. Ketogenesis is stimulated by glucagon induction of carnitine acyltransferase I, which is the rate-limiting enzyme for the transfer of fatty acids from the cytosol to the mitochondria.

*Glucagon deficiency* is extremely rare but has been reported and results clinically in a presentation characterized by hypoglycemia which is responsive to glucagon therapy.

## Other islet hormones

Somatostatin is widely distributed throughout the body in a variety of endocrine cells as well as in the central nervous system. It is a 1.63-kD peptide containing 14 amino acids synthesized and secreted in a manner analogous to insulin. The stimuli to somatostatin secretion are unknown, but local innervation may be important. The physiological role of somatostatin released from the δ cells of the islets remains unclear; it seems more likely to be a paracrine inhibitor of other islet hormone secreting cells than a true endocrine messenger. Synthetic somatostatin analogs have been used experimentally in the treatment of refractory hyperinsulinemic hypoglycemia.

Amylin is a 37-amino-acid polypeptide, first isolated from amyloid deposits in pancreatic islet cells from type II diabetics. It shows a close structural homology to calcitonin gene-related peptide (CGRP), an alternate splice product of the calcitonin gene. Amylin is a β-cell hormone which colocalizes with and probably is cosecreted with insulin. It appears to inhibit both insulin secretion and the sensitivity of peripheral tissues to insulin and has been implicated as an etiological factor in *type II diabetes*.

Pancreatic polypeptide (PP) contains 36 amino acids and is 4.24 kD. In man both neural and nutritive stimuli are important secretagogues, vagal activity in the anticipatory preprandial phase and protein ingestion both being effective. The actions of pancreatic polypeptide are mainly on the stomach and duodenum where it has actions on muscle tone, pancreatic fluid production, bicarbonate and enzyme release, and bile secretion.

## DEVELOPMENTAL ASPECTS

## Before birth (*see also* Chapter 13)

Carbohydrate, predominantly glucose, provides about 60 per cent of fetal energy needs. The normal fetus does not produce glucose but receives it by facilitated placental diffusion at a rate of 4–6 mg/kg per minute. In late gestation, fetal gluconeogenesis may contribute to fetal and placental glucose utilization if fetal glucose supply is reduced by, for example, maternal fasting or intrauterine growth retardation. A proportion of the glucose taken up by the placenta is metabolized there to produce lactate which then passes to the fetal and maternal circulations. Fetal $O_2$ consumption is directly related to the sum of the fetal glucose and lactate uptake. Only 50 per cent of the glucose taken up by the fetus in late gestation is oxidized, the remainder being converted to glycogen in the liver and muscle, and to fat in the liver and adipose tissue. In the last trimester, glucose storage is controlled primarily by insulin but glucocorticoids are also involved in the early ontogeny of glycogen synthetic pathways. Most fetal tissues oxidize glucose preferentially, and some – the brain, adrenal medulla, renal cortex and erythrocytes – are obligatory glucose consumers.

The molar transport of lipid molecules may be small in comparison with carbohydrate, but their carbon-rich skeleton may make a significant contribution to fetal metabolism. Net transplacental flux of FFA can occur by (1) direct carrier-mediated transport, (2) placental synthesis and release into the umbilical circulation especially of essential fatty acids produced by chain elongation and desaturation, or (3) lipolysis of complex triglycerides, lipoproteins or phospholipids derived from either the maternal or fetal circulations. Since fetal fatty acid composition varies with maternal diet, placental selectivity in fatty acid transport is probably not of major importance.

Fetal metabolic rate determined by net fetal $O_2$ consumption is linked directly, but not tightly, to fetal energy supply. The extent to which the placenta determines net glucose and lactate delivery to the fetus influences fetal metabolic rate slightly, but the fact that fetal $O_2$ consumption remains constant while glucose oxidation varies two-fold indicates that a reciprocal relationship exists between glucose oxidation and that of other energy-producing substrates. Amino acids are taken up by the fetus in excess of protein synthetic rates and fetal urea production is high, both indicating a contribution to fetal energy supply. Fetal protein catabolism is regulated by non-protein energy supply and when necessary the amino acids released are transaminated to glucose or oxidized to maintain fetal and placental metabolic rate, potentially to the detriment of fetal growth.

The placenta is impermeable to both insulin and glucagon, both of which are found in fetal blood from week 10 of gestation. Insulin acts cooperatively with circulating metabolites and paracrine growth factors to maintain an anabolic effect throughout pregnancy. In the first two trimesters the most important insulin secretagogue may be amino acids. Glucose stimulates insulin release in the third trimester only and at this stage of development insulin is both strongly glycogenic and lipogenic. In addition to promoting glucose storage, insulin also stimulates glucose oxidation with a consequent sparing of amino acids. Glucagon secretion is unaffected by acute changes in blood glucose concentration, but increases during chronic fetal hypoglycemia.

During prolonged maternal fasting or subnutrition there is a fall in both maternal and fetal blood glucose, and after several days fetal glucose utilization also declines together with plasma insulin. Fetal glucose delivery is augmented by gluconeogenesis from lactate of placental origin and to a lesser extent from fetal amino acids. This is reflected by fetal glucose utilization remaining higher than umbilical glucose delivery. Hepatic glycogen is not mobilized and is protected for the neonatal transition, even in the face of marked intrauterine growth retardation. Fetal and maternal ketones also contribute to fetal energy demands and have a glucose sparing effect. Fetal hypoxia is associated with hyperglycemia and a reduced fetal glucose clearance probably due to fetal catecholamine release and inhibition of insulin secretion. There is also increased fetal glucose production possibly arising from catecholamine stimulated hepatic glycogenolysis.

## After birth

Following birth, blood glucose is derived from hepatic glycogen for a few hours only, after which gluconeogenesis from lipid is necessary for glucose homeostasis. Tissue fat is mobilized for this purpose until milk intake is adequate. In the normal term infant, plasma glycerol concentrations rise sharply in the first minutes after birth and FFAs in the early hours, while glucose concentrations fall gently. Part of this is associated with the initiation of brown fat thermogenesis. By 12 hours after birth, FFA concentrations have stabilized at three to four times the umbilical cord blood concentration, whereas glucose has fallen by approximately one-third. The respiratory quotient of the infant falls over the same interval, from 1.0 to 0.7, signifying a transfer to fat as the principal source of energy. The newborn brain uses both glucose and ketone bodies as fuel. Ketones may provide 10 per cent of the energy requirement in normal circumstances and more during starvation.

The rate of FFA mobilization in the newborn depends not only on neuronal and hormonal stimulation and inhibition of lipolysis, but also on changes in the uptake, re-esterification and oxidation of FFAs within adipose tissue. Early postnatal lipolysis occurs in a thermoneutral environment due to increased sympathetic activity, but cold exposure can exaggerate the rise in plasma glycerol and FFAs. Acidosis has little or no acute effect on lipolysis, but if prolonged is inhibitory. Heparin stimulates lipolysis and when added in low dose to neonatal infusion fluids may have desirable metabolic effects.

Fasting is characterized by low but detectable plasma insulin concentrations and modestly raised plasma glucagon concentrations. There is hepatic gluconeogenesis and ketogenesis but no glycolysis or lipogenesis. Similarly there is adipocyte lipolysis and no lipogenesis or glucose uptake. In muscle there is slight proteolysis and no glucose uptake.

The hormonal and metabolic responses to feeding vary depending on the nutrient mix. A protein-rich meal causes both insulin and glucagon secretion and stimulates both lipogenesis and gluconeogenesis in the liver, while glycolysis and ketogenesis are suppressed. Glucose uptake is promoted in both muscles and adipose tissue where protein synthesis and lipogenesis, respectively, are stimulated. In contrast, a carbohydrate-rich meal stimulates insulin but not glucagon secretion and causes hepatic lipogenesis and glycolysis but no gluconeogenesis. Glucose uptake is strongly stimulated in both muscle and fat with a consequential promotion of lipogenesis and an equivocal stimulation of protein synthesis. A mixed meal rich in both protein and carbohydrate is the strongest stimulus of insulin secretion and causes marginal glucagon release. This is strongly stimulatory to hepatic lipogenesis, glucose uptake by muscle and adipose tissue and the subsequent protein synthesis and lipogenesis.

## HYPOGLYCEMIA

*Hypoglycemia* is a common clinical manifestation of disordered energy metabolism and is important because the obligatory consumption of glucose by the brain means that sustained hypoglycemia may cause neuronal damage. The pathophysiology of hypoglycemia divides neatly into those examples resulting from increased glucose consumption, usually as a consequence of insulin excess, and those due to inadequate glucose production. There are important differences in the etiology of the two mechanisms in the neonate, the toddler and the older child and it is convenient to consider each separately.

The physiological blood glucose range is lower in the newborn, but the absolute glucose concentration is less important than the overall clinical assessment of the baby. Neonatal hypoglycemia associated with abnormal physical signs is called *symptomatic hypoglycemia* and is potentially lethal. Conventional teaching states that "asymptomatic hypoglycemia" is benign, but recent evidence suggests otherwise and it is prudent to keep a baby's blood glucose above 2.6 mmol/L; there is electrophysiological evidence for neurological dysfunction at concentrations lower than this. The preterm infant, especially the very low birthweight infant, lacks both hepatic carbohydrate and subcutaneous adipose stores, with the result that circulating fuel concentrations are low and may run out, leading to exhaustion of cardiac and respiratory muscle and cerebral damage. Small-for-dates infants also are characterized by a tendency to hypoglycemia. Hypoxia and acidemia in the newborn are associated with an inefficient oxidative metabolism and a tendency to hypoglycemia. Cold exposure is detrimental for babies because an increased metabolic rate is necessary to maintain a constant body temperature.

The typical *infant of a diabetic mother* (IDM) has an exaggerated fall in blood glucose and an attenuated rise of FFA because of hyperinsulinemia, but the hypoglycemia is not prolonged past the first few days after birth. Persistent hypoglycemia in an infant clinically resembling an IDM should arouse suspicion of abnormal β-cell development as in *nesidioblastosis* or *pancreatic adenoma*. *Beckwith–Wiedemann syndrome* is also characterized by hyperinsulinemic hypoglycemia. Prenatal exposure to drugs such as sulfonylureas which cross the placenta, also may have profound effects on glucose concentrations.

A toddler may have an inborn metabolic error causing inadequate glucose production. In such cases the presence of acidosis and/or hepatomegaly are important clinical clues to which specific biochemical investigations are pertinent (Table 7.3). The *inborn errors of fatty acid metabolism* are unusual because they are the only metabolic defects resulting in non-ketotic hypoglycemia. Other uncommon but important conditions that may present as non-ketotic hypoglycemia at this age are endocrine deficiencies, in particular *congenital hypopituitarism* and *adrenocortical insufficiency*.

In toddlers and later childhood the principles governing metabolic balance associated with feeding and fasting are no different from those applying to the adult, but the younger the child, the shorter the time during fasting that euglycemia can be sustained. It is important to appreciate that among children of the

TABLE 7.3 Examples of inborn metabolic errors characterized by hypoglycemia associated with acidosis and/or hepatomegaly

| INBORN METABOLIC ERROR | ACIDOSIS | HEPATOMEGALY |
| --- | --- | --- |
| Glucose 6-phosphatase (GSD I) | + | + |
| Amylo 1,6-glucosidase (GSD III) | − | + |
| Phosphorylase | + | + |
| Fructose 1,6-diphosphatase | + | + |
| Fructose intolerance | + | + |
| Galactosemia | − | + |
| Pyruvate carboxylase | + | − |

same age or weight there is a biological spectrum of tolerance of fasting. Some children labeled as having *ketotic hypoglycemia* may have a subtle or partial metabolic defect or they may be examples of one end of the physiological spectrum.

## SELECTED READING

Montgomery R, Conway TW, Spector AA. *Biochemistry: a case oriented approach*, 5th edn. St Louis: C.V. Mosby, 1990.

Senior B, Sadeghi-Nejad A. Hypoglycemia: a pathophysiological approach. *Acta Paediatr Scand Suppl* 1989: 352:1.

Pessin JE, Bell GI. Mammalian facilitative glucose transporter family: structure and molecular regulation. *Ann Rev Physiol* 1992; **54**: 911.

# 8

# Biochemical Regulation of Arachidonic Acid Metabolism

Murray D. Mitchell

## PATHWAYS OF ARACHIDONIC ACID METABOLISM

*Eicosanoids* are derivatives of 20-carbon polyunsaturated fatty acids, one of which, arachidonic acid (all *cis*-5,8,11,14-eicosatetraenoic acid), is the precursor of the most important group of eicosanoids, the *prostaglandins*. Formation of these eicosanoids via fatty acid cyclooxygenase requires that arachidonic acid be in the non-esterified form.

## Arachidonic acid release

Fatty acids such as arachidonic acid do not exist in the free form in cells to any significant extent. Rather they are esterified in triacylglycerols (triglycerides), glycolipids (sugar-containing lipids) or phospholipids (the major class of membrane lipids).

Glycerophospholipids (phosphoglycerides) are a key subset of phospholipids. They have a glycerol backbone, with the hydroxyl groups of C-1 and C-2 esterified to the carboxyl groups of two fatty acids and the hydroxyl group of C-3 esterified to phosphoric acid (Fig. 8.1). Polyunsaturated fatty acids tend to be esterified at C-2 (at the *sn-2* site) while saturated fatty acids tend to be esterified at C-1 (at the *sn-1* site). The phosphate group is generally esterified to an alcohol, with the most common ones being choline, glycerol, inositol and ethanolamine.

Arachidonic acid is a typical polyunsaturated fatty acid, present in cells predominantly in an esterified

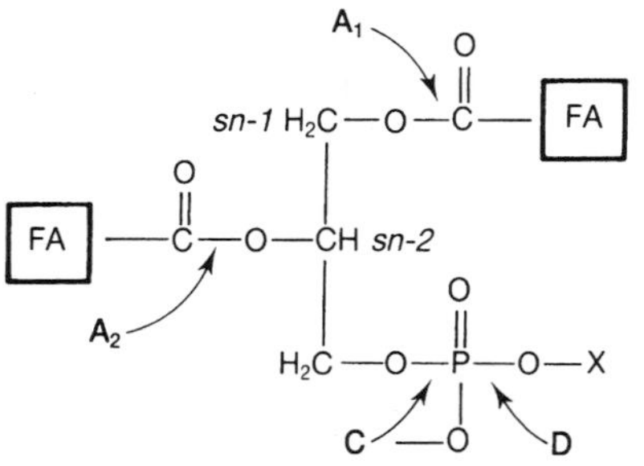

FIGURE 8.1 The structure of a generalized glycerophospholipid. Alcohols found in phosphomonoester linkage are depicted as X. Sites of phospholipase hydrolysis are shown by $A_1$, $A_2$, C and D. A saturated fatty acid is typically esterified at the *sn-1* position and a polyunsaturated fatty acid at the *sn-2* position. Fatty acids are represented by FA. (Adapted from Hillier K, ed. *Eicosanoids and reproduction*. Dordrecht, Holland: MTP Press, 1987: 109, with permission.)

form, usually in the *sn-2* position of a glycerophospholipid (Fig. 8.1). The liberation of arachidonic acid from glycerophospholipids, by hydrolysis at the *sn-2* position, is a rate-limiting step in the biosynthesis of eicosanoids that is accomplished either directly (e.g. from phosphatidylcholine or phosphatidylethanolamine) by the action of phospholipase $A_2$ (PLA$_2$) or indirectly (e.g. from phosphatidylinositol) by action of phospholipase C followed by the action of diacylglycerol and monoacylglycerol lipases (Fig. 8.2).

Phospholipases $A_2$ may be divided into two major categories, extracellular and cellular (or cytosolic). The extracellular forms have relatively low molecular

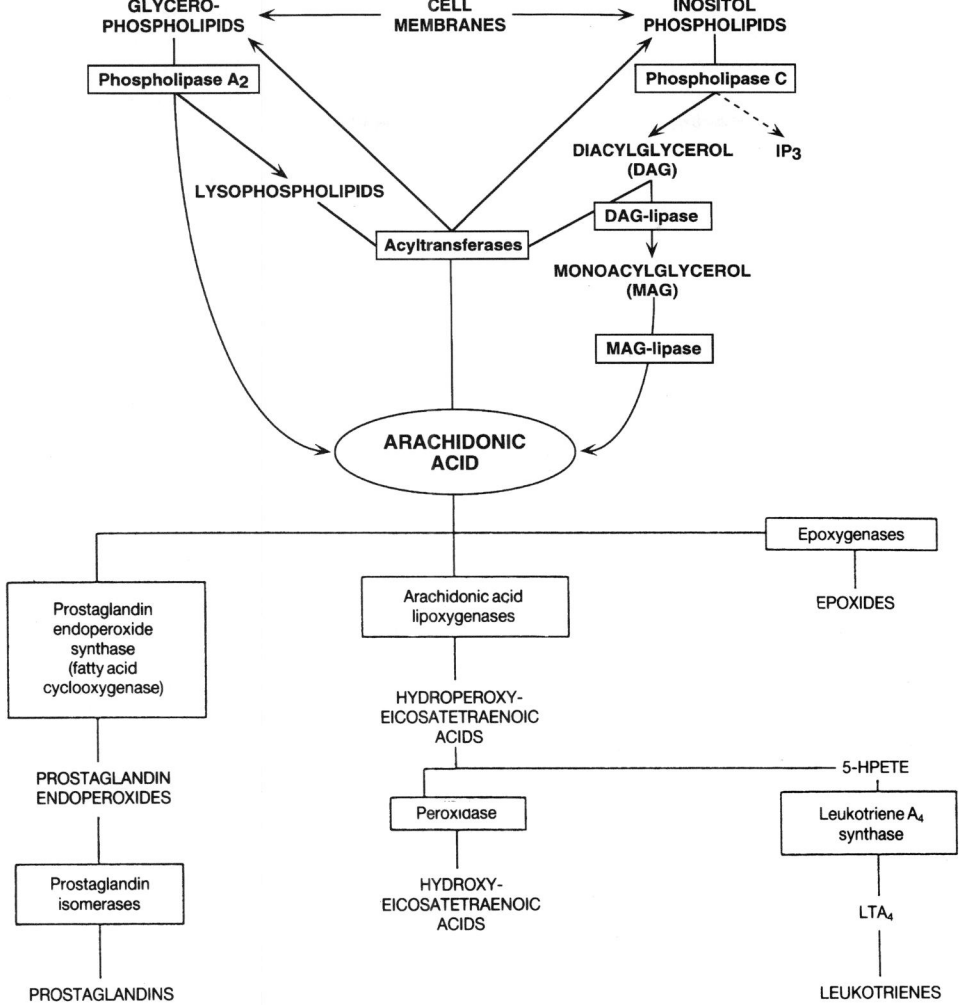

FIGURE 8.2 The enzymatic pathways of arachidonic acid metabolism. Inositol triphosphate = $IP_3$. (Reprinted with permission from Mitchell MD. *Semin Perinatol* 1986; **10**(4): 243.)

weights (14 kD), virtually identical catalytic mechanisms, similar geometry of the active site residues and an absolute requirement for $Ca^{2+}$. Mammals, including humans, have both type I and type II phospholipases. The type I enzyme is a digestive enzyme produced in the pancreas, whereas the type II enzyme is found in many other tissues, although its specific functions are not fully defined. These two enzymes differ structurally mainly in the location of their seven disulfide bonds. Recent studies have shown the presence in gestational tissues of a type II secreted 14-kD form of phospholipase $A_2$. It is important to note that this secreted form can be taken up by other tissues and show activity.

Another species of phospholipase $A_2$ recently purified and cloned is larger (85–110 kD, dependent upon glycosylation), cytosolic and not secreted. This cytosolic phospholipase $A_2$ preferentially hydrolyzes phospholipids containing arachidonic acid in the *sn-2* position. It is responsive to intracellular concentrations of $Ca^{2+}$ (1 μM) which differentiates it from extracellular phospholipases $A_2$, which require millimolar concentrations of $Ca^{2+}$ for activation. These phospholipases have been found in cytosols from several tissues and cells including monoblast and macrophage cell lines, macrophages, platelets, renal mesangial cells and kidney. It is thought that these cytosolic enzymes play an important role in cellular signal transduction pathways.

The regulation of phospholipase C and its isoforms is extremely complex. These enzymes are initially assigned into one of three categories (β, γ and δ), each of which is further subdivided by number (1, 2, 3 etc.). Each phospholipase C isoform has different selectivity in terms of the hydrolysis of inositol-containing phospholipids, and thus produces differing ratios of cyclic to non-cyclic products. In general, phospholipases $C_β$ are activated by G-protein-linked receptors including that for thromboxane $A_2$.

Phospholipases $C_γ$ are activated by growth factors via tyrosine kinase activation, and are G-protein-independent. In both cases, activation of protein kinases A and C can offset receptor-coupled increases in phospholipase C activity. Little information is available on phospholipases $C_\delta$ in general, or any of the isoforms in reproductive tissues. The major phosphoinositide-specific phospholipase C in amnion has been characterized and no change in total phospholipase C activity has been found in amnion, chorion and decidua with labor, although more subtle changes as within or between isoforms have not been ruled out.

Arachidonic acid liberated by these reactions is metabolized in three major pathways (Fig. 8.2): cyclooxygenase, lipoxygenase and cytochrome $P_{450}$ (epoxygenase). Each pathway results in the formation of a variety of biologically active products (Fig. 8.3).

## FATTY ACID CYCLOOXYGENASE (COX)

This enzyme is also known as *prostaglandin endoperoxide synthase*. At least two forms of this enzyme exist: PGHS-1 (cyclooxygenase 1, COX1) and PGHS-2 (cyclooxygenase 2, COX2). PGHS-1 is known as the constitutive enzyme whereas PGHS-2 is known as the inducible enzyme. The latter is induced by serum, phorbol esters, growth factors and many other substances. Arachidonic acid metabolism via this pathway involves the *bis*-dioxygenation reaction to form the unstable prostaglandin (PG) endoperoxide $PGG_2$ which is subsequently reduced by a hydroperoxidase to $PGH_2$. All subsequent PGs are derived from this intermediate.

- $PGH_2$ is converted to thromboxane (Tx) $A_2$ by thromboxane synthase which is present in platelets and a number of other cells. $TxA_2$ is a potent constrictor not only of vascular beds but also of airway smooth muscle.
- $PGH_2$ is converted to prostacyclin ($PGI_2$) by prostacyclin synthase which is in endothelial cells, the uterus and a number of other cells. $PGI_2$ is a potent vasodilator, particularly of the perinatal pulmonary circulation (*see* Chapter 73), and also inhibits platelet adhesion (*see* pages 887 and 888).
- $PGH_2$ is converted to $PGD_2$ by serum albumin and PGD isomerase. $PGD_2$ is found in highest concentrations in the central nervous system. When administered systemically it has multiple effects, one of which is pulmonary vasodilatation in the immediate newborn period. $PGD_2$ is the principal cyclooxygenase product of mast cells.
- $PGH_2$ is converted to $PGE_2$ by isomerization. $PGE_2$ is the major arachidonate product of a number of cells and is produced by the placenta. PGs of the E series inhibit gastric secretion and relax bronchial

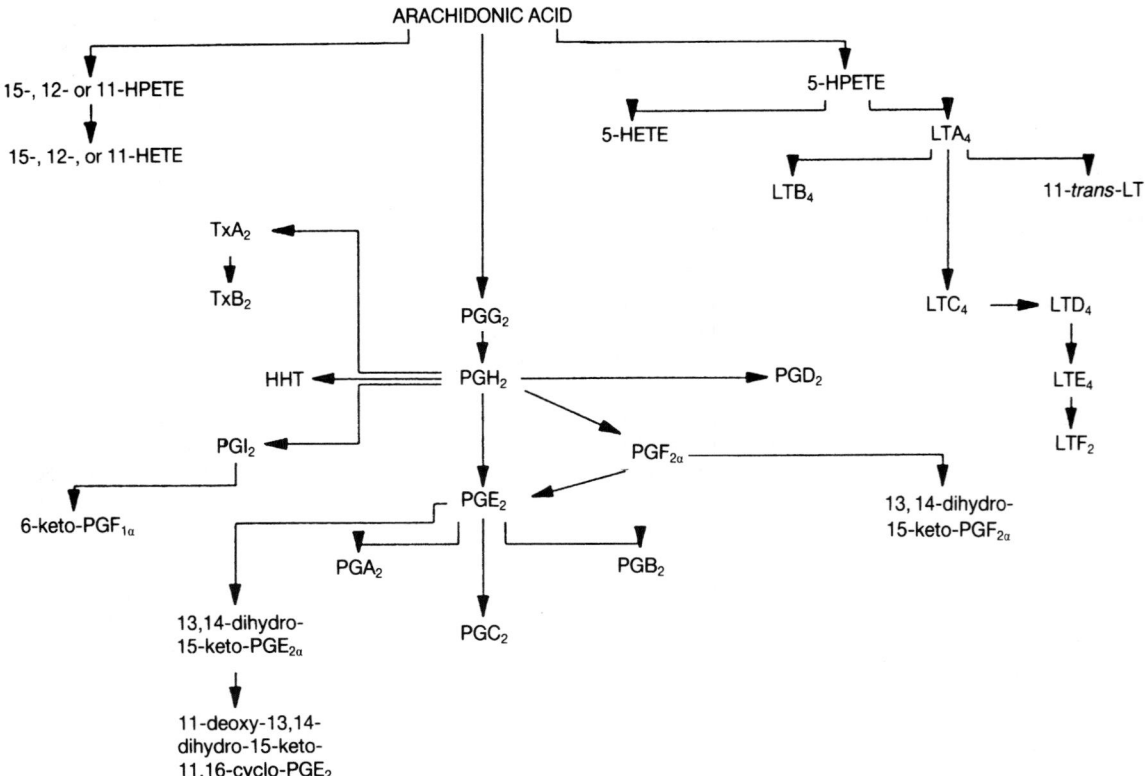

FIGURE 8.3 A simplified outline of the pathways of arachidonic acid metabolism. (Reprinted with permission from Mitchell MD. *Semin Perinatol* 1986; **10**(4): 243.)

smooth muscle directly by inhibition of acetylcholine release. $PGE_2$ also dilates the ductus arteriosus (*see* page 755 and below). $PGE_1$, derived from dihomo-γ-linolenic acid, inhibits neutrophil adherence and neutrophil-mediated injury to endothelial cells.

▪ $PGH_2$ is converted to $PGF_{2\alpha}$ usually by non-specific reduction. $PGF_{2\alpha}$ acts as a potent bronchoconstrictor and elevated $PGF_{2\alpha}$ concentrations in acute asthma have been reported.

## 15-Hydroxyprostaglandin dehydrogenase

The first step in the catabolism of PGs is effected by the cytosolic enzyme 15-hydroxyprostaglandin dehydrogenase (PGDH). The 15-keto derivatives formed are rapidly converted to the 13,14-dihydro-15-keto derivatives which are the major but biologically inactive circulating forms. The lung is a major metabolic venue: almost all biologically active PGs are metabolized during one passage through the lungs. Metabolism occurs by uptake into pulmonary cells and then by the action of PGDH. Biologically active PGs are further eliminated by a series of β- and ω-oxidations that result in the formation of products that are excreted in the urine. There are exceptions to this general pattern: $PGD_2$ is an extremely poor substrate for PGDH and $PGI_2$ may not be completely metabolized by the lungs since it is a poor substrate for the pulmonary cellular uptake mechanism.

## Inhibitors of prostaglandin biosynthesis

The most common endogenous inhibitors of PG biosynthesis are the antiphospholipase proteins known as *lipocortins*, which are related to *calpactins* and thus fall under the broad umbrella of *annexins*. The mechanisms by which these substances inhibit phospholipase activity remain controversial. Both a direct action on phospholipase enzymes and binding of substrate have been suggested. Annexins have been found in gestational tissues, and also an antiphospholipase protein termed *gravidin* is produced by chorion; gravidin is identical to the secretory component of IgA.

The most commonly used inhibitors of PG biosynthesis are the non-steroidal anti-inflammatory drugs (NSAIDs) such as indomethacin, naproxen, mefenamic acid and ibuprofen. These drugs act at the level of fatty acid cyclooxygenase and block the biosynthesis of all PGs. Glucocorticoids also inhibit PG biosynthesis, either by an action on the phospholipases via stimulation of antiphospholipase proteins such as macrocortin, lipomodulin, lipocortins and annexins, or via inhibition of PGHS-2.

## Lipoxygenases

Lipoxygenases are a group of iron-containing dioxygenases which catalyze the insertion of oxygen into polyunsaturated fatty acids including arachidonic acid. Three distinct enzymes insert oxygen at carbons 5, 12, and 15 of arachidonic acid. Additionally, others exist which also insert oxygen at the 8 and 11 positions.

12-Hydroperoxy-eicosatetraenoic acid (12-HPETE) formed by 12-lipoxygenase reduces secretion of neutrophil specific granules and augments immunoglobulin (Ig)-E-mediated mast cell release. Biological effects of 12-lipoxygenase products are found only at high concentrations.

15-HPETE and its secondary derivatives are the principal products of arachidonic acid metabolism by the 15-lipoxygenases in the lung and eosinophils.

5-HPETE formed by 5-lipoxygenase is the precursor of leukotrienes (LTs) which are important in many inflammatory processes. The key step is the conversion of 5-HPETE to $LTA_4$ which is then metabolized in a number of ways. Water may be added at C-12 opening the epoxide at C-6 and creating $LTB_4$, or the epoxide at C-6 may be opened by the sulfhydryl group of glutathione with the formation of $LTC_4$. $LTC_4$ may be metabolized further by the sequential elimination of glutamic acid and glycine to form $LTD_4$ and $LTE_4$. Conversion of $LTE_4$ to $LTF_4$ occurs by addition of a g-glutamyl residue to the amino group. The further metabolism of LTs is complex.

$LTB_4$ is a chemoattractant for neutrophils and eosinophils. $LTC_4$, $D_4$ and $E_4$ constrict smooth muscle in airways and vascular and intestinal beds. It should be noted that 15-HPETE can be metabolized by other routes to yield lipoxins that have many important biological properties.

## Cytochrome $P_{450}$ (epoxygenase)

Metabolism of arachidonic acid by cytochrome $P_{450}$ leads to various oxygenated products. The epoxy acids exhibit significant biological activity *in vitro*: stimulation of peptide hormone release, mobilization of intracellular $Ca^{2+}$, and alteration of net $K^+$ and $Na^+$ fluxes.

## Eicosanoid receptors

Prostaglandin receptors are classified as FP, EP, DP, IP and TP, with subsets of EP-1, EP-2, EP-3. The first letter corresponds to the type of prostaglandin that is a major ligand: PG(F), PG(E) and PG(D) with PG(I) for prostacyclin and T for thromboxane. The subset definitions are based on responsiveness to drugs; for example EP1 and EP3 mediate contractile activity of PGE whereas EP-2 mediates relaxant activity. The full range of prostanoid receptors has been found in non-pregnant and term pregnant human myometrium.

Receptors have been described for leukotrienes $B_4$, $C_4$, $D_4$ and $E_4$ as have one or more binding protein for 12-HETE. A classification for leukotriene receptors has been proposed based on actions of agonist and antagonists. These membrane receptors are found in various tissues and cells including trachea, bronchial smooth muscle, ileum and polymorphonuclear leukocytes. Signal transduction processes have been elucidated particularly in relation to leukotriene $D_4$ receptor action. When activated by leukotriene $D_4$ these receptors interact with at least two G-proteins resulting in the mobilization of $Ca^{2+}$.

## FUNCTION OF PROSTAGLANDINS IN DEVELOPMENT

The relative abundance of arachidonic acid in uterine tissues is higher than in many other tissues; it accounts for 7–20 per cent of the non-esterified fatty acids. Concentrations of non-esterified arachidonic acid in amniotic fluid increase several-fold during labor. This increase exceeds those of other fatty acids and indicates a degree of specificity in the mobilization of arachidonic acid. There also is a significantly lower arachidonic acid content in fetal membranes (amnion and chorion) from women in labor compared with women not in labor. Separation of the total glycerophospholipids of amnion into individual classes has revealed a significant reduction in the arachidonic acid content of (diacyl) phosphatidylethanolamine and phosphatidylinositol with early labor. Similar changes have been observed in chorion.

In amnion there is a phospholipase $A_2$ that is $Ca^{2+}$-dependent and has a substrate preference for phosphatidylethanolamine that contains arachidonic acid. This is consistent with the release of arachidonic acid from phosphatidylethanolamine in amnion during labor. There also is a phosphatidylinositol-specific phospholipase C in amnion that is $Ca^{2+}$-dependent. Moreover, diacylglycerol and monoacylglycerol lipase activities have been detected in amnion. This is consistent with the release of arachidonic acid from phosphatidylinositol during early labor.

Limited available information on the products of the lipoxygenase and monooxygenase enzymes focuses attention on the cyclooxygenase products.

## Before birth

### Preterm

$PGE_2$ and $PGF_{2\alpha}$ play a key part in the mechanisms controlling labor (see page 252) since both contract uterine smooth muscle and soften the cervix at all stages of gestation. They are used as abortifacients.

$PGE_2$ is ten times more potent than $PGF_{2\alpha}$. Inhibitors of PG synthesis such as the non-steroidal anti-inflammatory drugs have been used to treat preterm labor. They should be used with extreme caution or even avoided since results from controlled studies are not available and severe side-effects may occur, such as reduction in cerebral blood flow or constriction of the ductus arteriosus. $PGI_2$ relaxes vascular smooth muscle and inhibits platelet aggregation whereas thromboxane has the opposite actions. Low-dose aspirin is used to prevent pre-eclampsia and intrauterine growth retardation because it alters the $PGI_2$/thromboxane balance in favor of $PGI_2$.

### At term

Labor at term is initiated in part by increased intrauterine synthesis of PGs. There are substantial increases of both intra-amniotic and plasma $PGE_2$ and $PGF_{2\alpha}$ concentrations, leading to uterine contractions. Stimuli of fatty acid cyclooxygenase often fail to elicit a release of arachidonate and it is possible that an endogenous activator of phospholipase $A_2$ or C is likely to be involved to increase PG synthesis during parturition.

### After birth

The ductus arteriosus (DA) (see Chapter 73) is maintained patent by $PGE_2$ and is relatively unresponsive to other PGs both in vivo and in vitro. A major source of fetal circulating $PGE_2$ is the placenta, and since only 10 per cent of the fetal cardiac output goes to the lungs where $PGE_2$ mainly is metabolized, the systemic circulating concentration is high. Blocking PG synthesis by cyclooxygenase inhibition causes constriction of the fetal ductus arteriosus and the effect of indomethacin in this respect is greater in immature than mature fetuses. Maturation of ductal PG insensitivity can be triggered by corticosteroids. The fetal ductus arteriosus is open, not because of passive dilatation, but due to a balance between constricting and relaxing stimuli. After birth, circulating $PGE_2$ concentrations fall due to increased pulmonary blood flow and removal of the placenta. This permits the ductus arteriosus to become more sensitive to constricting stimuli such as rising oxygen tension.

Knowledge of the physiological control of the ductal diameter can be applied clinically in congenital heart defects. For example: in aortic arch anomalies or left ventricular outflow tract obstruction the patent ductus supplies most or all of the systemic blood; in transposition of the great arteries ductus arteriosus patency allows pulmonary/systemic mixing via bidirectional shunting; and in right ventricular outflow obstruction the patent ductus supplies the pulmonary blood flow. $PGE_2$ has been used to maintain ductus arteriosus patency at infusion rates of 0.02–0.05

μg/kg bodyweight per minute. PGs influence many systems and their pharmacological use or inhibition of their synthesis will always have multiple effects that must be monitored.

## SELECTED READING

Challis JRG, Patrick JE. The production of prostaglandins and thromboxanes in the feto-placental unit and their effects on the developing fetus. *Semin Perinatol* 1980; 4: 23.

Clyman RI. Eicosanoids and the ductus arteriosus. In: Mitchell MD, ed. *Eicosanoids in reproduction*. Florida: CRC Press, 1990: 273.

Heymann MA. The role of eicosanoids in the fetal and perinatal circulations. In: Mitchell MD, ed. *Eicosanoids in reproduction*. Florida: CRC Press, 1990: 285.

Holtzman MJ. Arachidonic acid metabolism. *Am Rev Respir Dis* 1991; **143**: 188.

Mitchell MD. Prostaglandin synthesis, metabolism and function in the fetus. In: Jones CT ed. *Biochemical development of the fetus*. Amsterdam: Elsevier, 1982: 425.

Myatt L. Placental biosynthesis, metabolism and transport of eicosanoids. In: Mitchell MD, ed. *Eicosanoids in reproduction*. Florida: CRC Press, 1990: 169.

# 9

# Free Radicals, Oxidants and Antioxidants

Christine C. Winterbourn

The discovery of superoxide dismutase (SOD) in 1968 led to the realization that free radicals are produced physiologically, and opened up the field of free radical biology. It is now clear that not only are free radicals formed during normal metabolism but they are also involved in a number of pathological and toxicological processes. In some cases they are a prime cause of injury, in others they are a consequence. These may amplify the injury, such that protection by radical scavengers would be beneficial. Alternatively they may be an epiphenomenon with no pathophysiological importance.

## DEFINITIONS

A *free radical* is any chemical species containing one or more unpaired electrons. Most free radicals have a lifetime of less than a second and react with a wide range of biological molecules. Some cause oxidation, some reduction, and others, like superoxide, are capable of both. Oxidative reactions are most likely to be injurious.

Molecular oxygen ($O_2$) is a terminal electron ($e^-$) acceptor and has a high affinity for electrons. Complete reduction of $O_2$ via the cytochrome oxidase pathway adds four electrons and produces two molecules of $H_2O$ without releasing any partially reduced intermediates, which remain bound to the cytochrome oxidase complex throughout the process. The partial reduction of $O_2$ by sequential single electron steps pro-

duces three intermediates, the *superoxide radical* (superoxide anion) ($O_2^{\bullet-}$), *hydrogen peroxide* ($H_2O_2$), or the *hydroxyl radical* ($OH^\bullet$), each more reactive than $O_2$ itself.

$$O_2 \xrightarrow{e^-} O_2^{\bullet-} \xrightarrow{e^-/2H^+} H_2O_2 \xrightarrow{e^-/H^+} OH^\bullet + H_2O \xrightarrow{e^-/H^+} H_2O$$

Superoxide is in equilibrium with its protonated form, the hydroperoxyl radical ($HO_2^\bullet$), with a pKa of 4.8. Superoxide breaks down by spontaneous dismutation to $H_2O_2$.

$$O_2^{\bullet-} + HO_2^\bullet + H^+ \longrightarrow O_2 + H_2O_2$$

Together these intermediates of $O_2$ reduction are referred to as either *activated oxygen* or *reactive oxygen species*. *Oxidative stress* in cells refers to the increased generation of superoxide and $H_2O_2$. *Oxidative damage* is the tissue injury caused by free radicals or other strong oxidants.

A free radical scavenger is any compound that intercepts radicals. To be an effective antioxidant, it must do this without propagating further radical reactions. Some scavengers may be relatively specific, such as for hydroxyl or lipid peroxyl radicals; others are more general. *Antioxidant defense* encompasses both free radical scavengers and enzymatic mechanisms that remove radicals and reactive oxidants.

## SOURCES OF FREE RADICALS AND REACTIVE OXIDANTS

### Radiation

Ionizing (nuclear) radiation is harmful because of free radical reactions. Its prime target is tissue water and, in the presence of $O_2$ the main radical species produced are superoxide and hydroxyl radicals. These water-derived radicals cause damage by reacting with DNA and other macromolecules. Ultraviolet radiation is sufficiently energetic to generate free radicals and also produces electronically excited species that decay by initiating radical reactions. Injury by these mechanisms is seen in *sunburn, porphyria* and *hyperbilirubinemia* treated by phototherapy.

### Metabolic generation of radicals

#### Mitochondria

Free radicals are produced during normal metabolism from several sources, the major one being mitochondrial respiration. Aerobic life depends on the energy released in the conversion of $O_2$ to $H_2O$ without forming radical intermediates. This is achieved in the mitochondria by cytochrome oxidase in the respiratory chain. However, about 1 per cent of the $O_2$ consumed is released as superoxide.

#### Xanthine oxidase

Another significant source of free radicals is the oxidation of xanthine and hypoxanthine to uric acid under the control of xanthine oxidase with the concomitant reduction of $O_2$ to superoxide and $H_2O_2$. This reaction proceeds normally under the control of xanthine dehydrogenase using NAD+ (nicotinamide adenine dinucleotide) as a hydrogen acceptor, but switches to the oxidase in the presence of raised intracellular $Ca^{2+}$ or ischemia. Ischemia also results in breakdown of adenine nucleotides to hypoxanthine, so that if $O_2$ is reintroduced, there is a sudden burst of production of superoxide and $H_2O_2$ (Fig. 9.1). This process is blocked by the xanthine oxidase inhibitor, allopurinol.

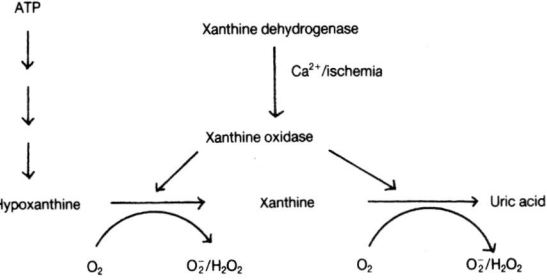

FIGURE 9.1 Mechanism of activation of xanthine oxidase and the production of superoxide and hydrogen peroxide from xanthine and hypoxanthine

### Heme proteins

Oxidation of oxyhemoglobin and oxymyoglobin to their met forms is accompanied by the release of heme-bound $O_2$ as superoxide. Since the ferric proteins recycle, there is continuous net generation of superoxide corresponding to the oxidation of about 3 per cent of red cell hemoglobin per day.

### Free radical production through chemical autoxidation and metabolism

A number of compounds autoxidize (are oxidized by molecular oxygen) to give free radicals. These include physiological compounds, such as catecholamines, flavins and sugars, as well as many drugs and environmental chemicals (xenobiotics). Autoxidation is catalyzed by transition metals, particularly iron and copper, and is an important factor in metal toxicity. Other toxic chemicals (xenobiotics) are metabolized to free radicals, by reduction by NADH or NADPH-dependent reductases (e.g. menadione) or by oxidation by cytochrome $P_{450}$, hemoglobin or heme peroxidases (e.g. acetaminophen). Radicals such as menadione semiquinone react with oxygen to give superoxide and allow continued reduction of the parent compound. This process is known as *redox cycling* (Fig.

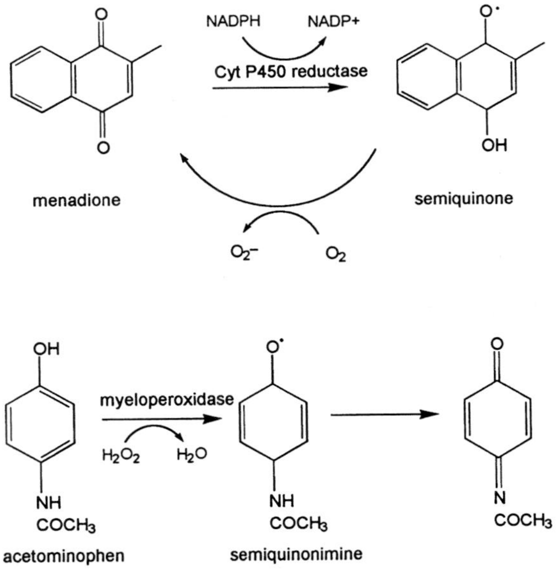

FIGURE 9.2 Redox cycling

9.2).

### Phagocytes

Granulocytes and mononuclear phagocytes produce large amounts of reactive oxygen species to kill microorganisms. Phagocytic stimuli and a wide variety of inflammatory mediators activate an NADPH oxidase located in the cell membrane, causing a burst of $O_2$ uptake and conversion to superoxide (Fig. 9.3).

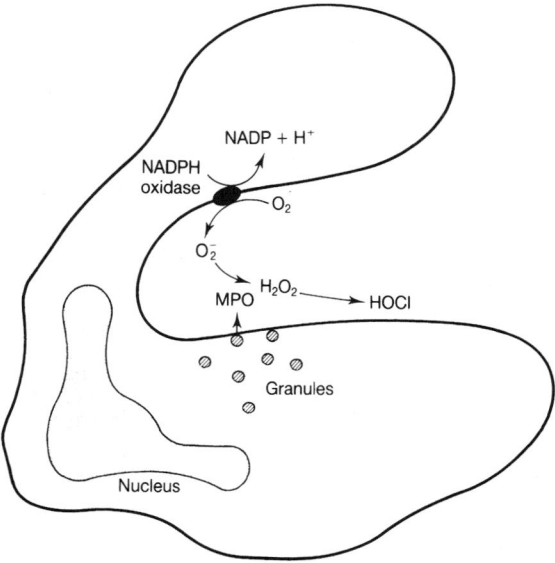

FIGURE 9.3 Oxidant release by a neutrophil, following phagocytosis of microorganisms or stimulation by inflammatory mediators. Degranulation releases myeloperoxidase (MPO) as well as proteinases, hydrolyases and other antibacterial peptides (see text for abbreviations).

Superoxide is generated on the external surface of the membrane and released either into the extracellular medium or into the phagocytic vacuole. In *chronic granulomatous disease* superoxide production is absent and recurrent bacterial and fungal infections occur. Superoxide production by phagocytes can be detrimental when host rather than invading cells are the target. Such tissue injury is important in *chronic inflammation*, and plays an amplifying role in conditions such as *ischemia/reperfusion* when neutrophils are attracted to the site of initial injury.

Although superoxide is the primary product of the oxidative burst, its principal effect in microbicidal activity or host cell killing is via $H_2O_2$ and other reactive oxygen species. Hypochlorous acid (HOCl) is the most powerful oxidant produced by neutrophils and monocytes. It is generated from $Cl^-$ and $H_2O_2$ under the control of myeloperoxidase when the cells are stimulated. Eosinophils contain a related peroxidase that converts bromide to hypobromous acid by an analogous mechanism. HOCl reacts rapidly with many biological molecules and is very effective at killing both bacterial and mammalian cells. Thiols and methionine residues are particularly susceptible to HOCl. Amines react to give chloramines, which have more limited oxidizing properties. Neutrophils employ oxidative and non-oxidative mechanisms for killing microorganisms. While oxidative killing is predominantly myeloperoxidase-dependent, alternative mechanisms provide adequate defense in myeloperoxidase deficiency. There is little evidence that neutrophils produce significant amounts of hydroxyl radicals, although they may arise through the interaction of neutrophil $H_2O_2$ with iron complexes in target tissue.

# Nitric oxide

Nitric oxide (NO; see Chapter 10) is a free radical gas that functions both as a signaling molecule in endothelial cells and the brain and as a killer molecule in activated immune cells. It is produced from L-arginine by oxidative deamination by nitric oxide synthase. This enzyme is constitutively expressed in endothelial and brain cells where it is activated by increases in intracellular $Ca^{2+}$. In macrophage-like cells it is induced by cytokines and its activity is not $Ca^{2+}$-dependent. In macrophages, NO production is associated with antimicrobial and antitumor activity. In the vasculature, NO has been identified as endothelial derived relaxing factor and acts on smooth muscle cells. Its signaling role in the brain has not been fully elucidated, but it appears to be related to glutamate receptors and may be involved in synaptic plasticity. Conditions such as *endotoxic shock* and *cerebral ischemia* lead to excessive NO production with consequent pathological effects. NO acts as a messenger by binding to the heme of guanylyl cyclase, and is inactivated primarily by binding to hemoglobin. Reactions with intracellular iron proteins and with thiols probably contribute to its cytotoxic effects. Most of its cytotoxicity, however, it is likely to be mediated by peroxynitrite ($ONOO^-$), a strong hydroxyl radical-like oxidant. Peroxynitrite is formed in an extremely rapid reaction between NO and superoxide. Nitration of proteins attributed to peroxynitrite has been detected in the brain and at sites of inflammatory tissue injury, including the lungs of infants with *bronchopulmonary dysplasia*.

Inhalation of low concentrations of NO is now being used experimentally as one form of therapy in conditions where there is pulmonary hypertension (*see* page 754). However, a full assessment of potential toxicity and the significance of any reaction with superoxide from inflammatory cells in the lungs is yet to be made.

## ANTIOXIDANTS AND FREE RADICAL SCAVENGERS

A complex system of antioxidant defenses preserves the balance between oxidant production and removal. When the balance is upset, by either excess radical production or a defective defense mechanism, oxidative stress and tissue injury can occur. A general scheme for oxidant production and defenses is depicted in Fig. 9.4.

# Enzymatic defenses

Antioxidant enzymatic systems are present for removal of superoxide and hydrogen peroxide. Superoxide dismutase (SOD) catalyzes the breakdown of superoxide to $O_2$ and $H_2O_2$ 1000 times faster than occurs spontaneously.

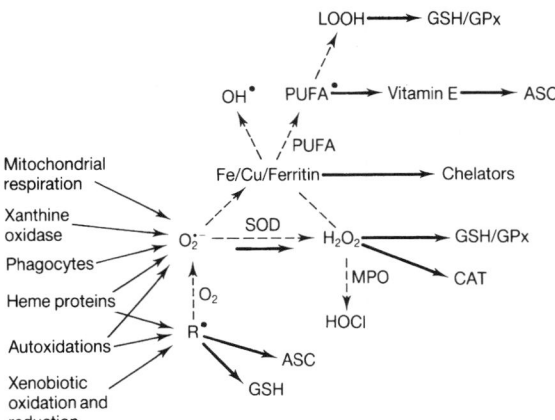

FIGURE 9.4 Scheme showing mechanisms of radical production and metabolism. Route of radical production (prooxidants) is shown by normal arrows, the interconversion of radicals or reactive oxidants by the broken arrows and radical or oxidant removal by the heavy arrows. $R^{\bullet}$ = unspecified radical; SOD = superoxide dismutase; CAT = catalase; GSH = glutathione; ASC = ascorbate; GPx = glutathione peroxidase; MPO = myeloperoxidase; PUFA = polyunsaturated lipid; PUFA- = lipid radical; LOOH = lipid hydroperoxide (for remainder see text).

---

**Superoxide dismutase**
$$2O_2^{\bullet-} + 2H^+ \longrightarrow H_2O_2 + O_2$$

---

SOD is present in all mammalian cells, both as copper/zinc SOD in the cytoplasm and as manganese SOD in the mitochondria. Low concentrations of another copper/zinc SOD are also found extracellularly. The gene for copper/zinc SOD is encoded on chromosome 21 and the concentration of the enzyme is raised in *Down syndrome.*

Hydrogen peroxide is broken down to $H_2O$ and $O_2$ by catalase.

---

**Catalase**
$$2H_2O_2 \longrightarrow 2H_2O + O_2$$

---

Glutathione peroxidase removes both hydrogen peroxide and lipid hydroperoxides (LOOH) by catalyzing their reaction with reduced glutathione (GSH).

---

**Glutathione peroxidase**
$$H_2O_2 \text{ (or LOOH)} + 2GSH \longrightarrow 2H_2O \text{ (or LOH} + H_2O) + GSSG$$

---

GSH is regenerated by NADPH from the hexose monophosphate pathway and this pathway is therefore necessary for the glutathione cycle. Catalase also requires NADPH for maximal activity.

In genetic disorders of the hexose monophosphate pathway, such as *glucose 6-phosphate dehydrogenase (G6PD) deficiency,* since both systems for peroxide removal may be compromised, there is a susceptibility to drug-induced hemolytic anemia. Glutathione peroxidase contains the trace element selenium and its activity is reduced when selenium intake is restricted due to low soil selenium or special diets such as *total parenteral nutrition* or diets for *phenylketonuria* or *cystic fibrosis.* Very low selenium in parts of China causes a *cardiomyopathy (Keshan disease).*

## Low-molecular-weight scavengers

The most abundant physiological free radical scavengers are vitamin E (α-tocopherol), vitamin C (ascorbic acid) and glutathione. Vitamin E is lipid soluble and found in cell membranes where it intercepts lipid peroxyl radicals and breaks the chain reaction of polyunsaturated fatty acid peroxidation. Ascorbate and glutathione are found in the cytoplasm and other aqueous environments where they intercept primary radicals and repair radical damage to macromolecules. Since the reaction between a radical and a scavenger generates another radical, the scavenger is an effective antioxidant only if its radical breaks down benignly. Ascorbate is particularly good because its radical decays mainly by reacting with itself. α-Tocopherol radicals can do likewise or they may react with ascorbate. The latter reaction permits ascorbate to spare α-tocopherol and provides a link between the aqueous and the lipid phase antioxidants. The glutathione radical probably reacts mainly with $O_2$ to give superoxide which can be eliminated by SOD. Vitamin A, β-carotene and ubiquinol (coenzyme Q10) can all act as lipid antioxidants in experimental circumstances, and other dietary constituents have antioxidant properties.

As illustrated by the examples given above, there is a close interrelationship between the different antioxidants, both enzymatic and non-enzymatic, such that oxidant–antioxidant balance is regulated by the whole integrated system. In view of the accumulating experimental and epidemiological evidence that antioxidants protect against various diseases, there is considerable interest in pharmacological use of antioxidants. A number of compounds show promise experimentally. An important factor is the property of radical scavengers to act as an antioxidant in some situations and prooxidant in others, and any pharmacological agent must act synergistically with the natural antioxidant system to boost its effect.

## Metal binding

Iron, copper and other transition metals promote the formation of free radicals. Iron is more significant physiologically, and important facets of antioxidant defense are the storage and transport of iron in an inert form and the maintenance of very low free iron concentrations. The transport proteins, transferrin and lactoferrin, are inactive as free radical catalysts and ferritin stores iron within a protein shell. However, superoxide and other radicals can release iron from ferritin and this may contribute to their toxicity. Iron overload enhances free radical damage when iron-binding capacity is exceeded. Frequent transfusions of premature infants can saturate their transferrin.

## REACTIVE OXYGEN SPECIES AND OXIDATIVE DAMAGE

Superoxide and $H_2O_2$ are formed in many free radical reactions. Both oxidatively stress the cell by depleting reducing equivalents and energy supplies. The associated alteration in cell redox state (ratio of oxidizing to reducing species), as discussed below, can have major effects on cell function, including gene expression, differentiation and programmed cell death. Alternatively, free radical reactions may damage tissue constituents in ways that are directly toxic. Superoxide and $H_2O_2$ on their own are not particularly damaging, although they can inactivate iron–sulfur and heme proteins. They do, however, act as precursors of much more reactive species, particularly peroxynitrite and hypochlorite (see above) and hydroxyl radicals.

## Hydroxyl radical production

Hydroxyl radicals (or an oxidant with similar high reactivity) are formed when certain ferrous or cuprous complexes react with hydrogen peroxide (Fenton reaction).

$$Fe^{2+} + H_2O_2 \longrightarrow Fe^{3+} + OH^- + OH^\bullet$$

Reduction of the iron is necessary for it to act catalytically. This can be brought about by superoxide (via the Haber–Weiss reaction) and other reducing radicals, and by physiological concentrations of ascorbate and glutathione. Iron (and copper) concentrations are normally extremely low and limit hydroxyl radical production. Superoxide and other radicals can enhance the reaction by releasing iron from ferritin and iron–sulfur proteins.

Hydroxyl radicals react rapidly with most biological molecules. They react close to their site of generation, and this, rather than relative reactivity with different compounds, determines their specificity. Thus hydroxyl radicals generated close to DNA react mainly with DNA, and those generated extracellularly do not penetrate the cell. If the metal involved in the Fenton reaction is bound to a target such as a protein molecule, the hydroxyl radical can react specifically with that molecule. The most abundant compounds, such as albumin in extracellular fluid, are likely to be major targets for hydroxyl radicals, although not necessarily critical ones. As hydroxyl radicals are so reactive and non-specific, any one compound is unlikely to prevent reactions with other tissue constituents. Specific hydroxyl radical scavengers are seldom able to reach high enough concentrations to be effective *in vivo*.

## Lipid peroxidation

Peroxidation of polyunsaturated fatty acids is a classical free radical reaction that occurs in biological membranes and lipoproteins. It is a chain reaction (Fig. 9.5) involving lipid radicals and $O_2$ that produces unstable

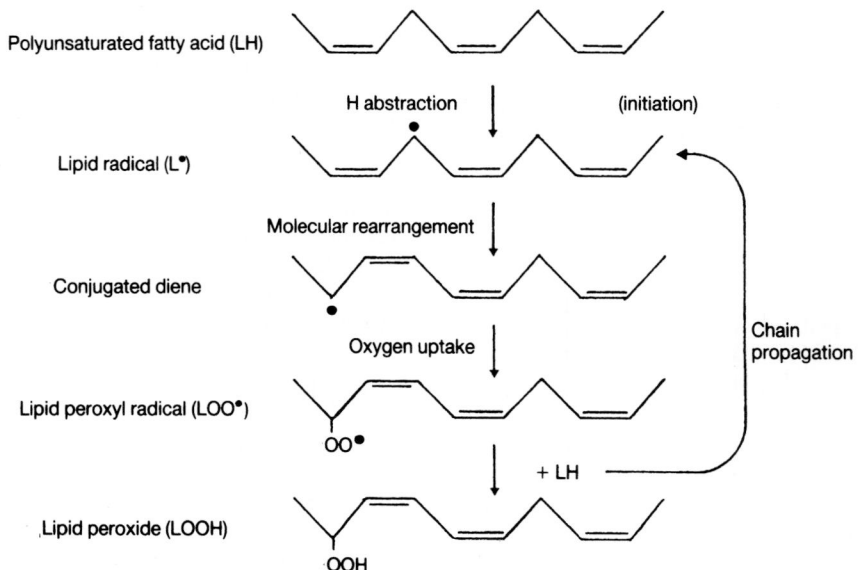

FIGURE 9.5 Initiation and propagation of lipid peroxidation. Minor breakdown products and relatively unstable lipid hydroperoxides include malondialdehyde, 4-hydroxynonenal and ethane. Various assay methods measure these products.

and structurally disruptive fatty acyl hydroperoxide groups in the membrane plus a variety of reactive side products. Peroxidation can be initiated by hydroxyl radicals, but mechanisms involving an iron catalyst and a reducing agent such as superoxide or ascorbate, or a heme protein plus peroxide, are more significant. Lipid peroxidation is a widely measured index of free radical injury. With the specific assays now available this can be a definitive and sensitive measure. However, some of the simpler techniques are not necessarily specific and have limitations when used for basal tissue concentrations. In some conditions lipid peroxidation is an important cause of tissue injury. It also occurs as a consequence of gross tissue disorganization, so in other situations it just may be a non-specific marker of such pathology.

## CONSEQUENCES OF OXIDATIVE STRESS

Investigation of free radical pathology has until recently focused mainly on gross damage to tissue constituents and on direct cytotoxicity. It is now realized that more subtle changes to the redox state of the cell, as a result of oxidative stress, can have equally profound effects. These changes involve oxidation of protein thiol groups and effects include reversible inactivation of enzymes and activation of binding proteins or transcription factors. These can translate into alterations in metabolic pathways, elevation of cell $Ca^{2+}$, activation of gene expression or programmed cell death (apoptosis – see Chapter 2). Direct cytotoxicity also occurs as a result of more extreme oxidative stress and irreversible damage to biomolecules.

## Oxidative damage

Proteins, lipids and nucleic acids are susceptible to oxidative damage. Oxidation of DNA results in single- or double-strand breaks and modification of the bases. Much of the damage is repaired, but persisting modifications at key sites are mutagenic. Radical reactions can cross link proteins or oxidize amino acids, resulting in enzyme inactivation or structural alterations to the cytoskeleton or connective tissue. Lipid peroxidation mainly affects cell membrane structure and permeability, and some of the minor peroxidation products damage DNA and proteins.

## Detection of *in vivo* oxidative damage

Although there are strong implications for free radical involvement in a number of diseases, direct evidence has been difficult to obtain. Free radicals are so short-lived that they can rarely be detected directly *in vivo* and products of oxidative injury are frequently unstable or metabolized. Radical scavengers and transition metal chelators are useful supportive evidence but not necessarily specific. Recent developments that have been applied successfully to *ex vivo* samples

include assays for oxidized DNA bases; e.g. 8-hydroxydeoxyguanosine, protein carbonyl groups, specific lipid peroxides and peroxidation products such as 8-isoprostane. For most diseases where radicals are implicated in the pathology, rigorous use of such techniques is still needed before this is proven.

## Oxidants, gene regulation and apoptosis

An increasing number of genes are being shown to be under redox control. The best characterized are those regulated by the transcription factors NF-$\kappa$/$\beta$ and AP1. NF-$\kappa$/$\beta$ controls expression of a range of cytokines, adhesion molecules and other proteins involved in the inflammatory response. While some oxidants cause direct activation, other receptor binding inducers such as TNF$\alpha$ act by switching on endogenous oxidative events. Gene activation is suppressed by a wide range of antioxidants.

Endogenous oxidant production is involved in lymphocyte differentiation, and at least one of the mechanisms leading to programmed cell death (apoptosis). Apoptosis, characterized by chromatin condensation, membrane blebbing and DNA fragmentation, is important in tissue differentiation during development and as a control mechanism for destroying damaged cells that could otherwise lead to cancer. Oxidants such as menadione, which at high concentrations cause necrosis, at lower doses produce apoptotic cell death.

## FREE RADICAL PATHOLOGY

Free radicals and oxidative stress have been implicated, but not proven, in many pathological conditions. The evidence is strong in diseases of aging such as *atherosclerosis* and *cataract*, in inflammatory diseases such as *rheumatoid arthritis, inflammatory bowel disease, emphysema, adult respiratory distress syndrome* and *toxic shock*, and in conditions involving *ischemia and reperfusion*. Inflammation and ischemia are common neonatal pathologies. Furthermore, free radical injury is strongly implicated in the major diseases of the premature infant.

## Inflammation

Neutrophils and other inflammatory cells are attracted to sites of injury by activated complement, immune complexes and inflammatory cytokines. Such stimulants cause the cells to release large amounts of reactive oxygen species. In experimental systems, neutrophil oxidants kill cells in culture, increase capillary permeability, denature basement membrane and cartilage components, inactivate $\alpha$1-proteinase inhibitor so that it does not inhibit neutrophil elastase, and decrease the activity of pulmonary surfactant. Nitric oxide production by macrophages, particularly in combination with superoxide, is also potentially injurious.

## Ischemia and reperfusion injury

When a tissue is deprived of $O_2$ owing to impaired blood flow, cells are injured and may die. Although restoration of blood flow is essential for recovery, it is now appreciated that providing the ischemia does not do irreversible damage, reperfusion may be responsible for much of the total injury. Inhibitors such as SOD and radical scavengers provide dramatic protection in a number of experimental studies, but despite this, the extent to which oxygen radicals are involved in ischemia/reperfusion injury remains controversial. Results vary depending on the system and index of tissue injury used. Much of the controversy is centered on the heart and *myocardial infarction*. Evidence is stronger for free radicals contributing to *ischemia/reperfusion injury* in the gut, kidney, muscle and particularly brain, arising from trauma, crush or pressure injury and in *perinatal asphyxial encephalopathies*.

One way in which free radicals can be produced in ischemia/reperfusion is by disruption of mitochondrial integrity during ischemia, so that when $O_2$ is reintroduced there is less control and more superoxide release. A second mechanism involves conversion of xanthine dehydrogenase to xanthine oxidase and the accumulation of xanthine and hypoxanthine during ischemia (*see* Fig. 9.1). This is not a problem until reintroduction of $O_2$ allows the enzyme to act, producing superoxide and $H_2O_2$. Support for this mechanism comes from studies using the xanthine oxidase inhibitor, allopurinol. Neutrophils recruited in response to the initial injury amplify the damage by releasing reactive oxygen species.

## Oxidative injury and the common diseases of prematurity

*Bronchopulmonary dysplasia* and *chronic lung disease* are common conditions that develop in very-low-birthweight infants who have required mechanical ventilation. Causes include a combination of elevated inspired $O_2$ concentrations, barotrauma, the secondary recruitment of neutrophils due to mechanical injury, and lung immaturity. The toxicity of high $O_2$ concentrations has been shown experimentally to be due to oxygen radical generation, and circumstantial evidence points to radical involvement in neonatal lung injury where some evidence for oxidative injury has been found. While in animals antioxidant enzyme levels in the lung rise steeply just before term, apart from catalase and GSH, markedly lower levels are not found in the lungs of preterm infants. However, they are low in GSH and antioxidant vitamins, and it is possible that antioxidant therapy would be beneficial.

*Retinopathy of prematurity* is an oxidative injury caused primarily by high inspired $O_2$ concentrations. It may be compounded by light-induced radical generation, iron overload and immature antioxidant defenses. Vitamin E has been found in some, but not other, studies to ameliorate the condition, and, since it may be harmful, controversy remains about whether or not it should be given prophylactically.

Current evidence suggests that oxidative injury resulting from ischemic insults followed by reperfusion contributes to *intraventricular hemorrhage* in the newborn. Vitamin E administration has in some studies been shown to improve outcome.

*Hemolytic anemia* in the newborn is another oxidative injury that is seen when vitamin E levels are low. It is exacerbated by high iron status.

*Perinatal asphyxia* and *cerebral trauma* have many characteristics in common with other brain injuries where oxygen radicals are known to be involved, and there is suggestive evidence for reperfusion injury in these conditions. Observed increases in uric acid concentrations could indicate xanthine oxidase activity, and the rise observed in extracellular glutamate could be due to inactivation of glutamine synthetase which is very susceptible to oxidative inactivation.

## ANTIOXIDANT THERAPY

The therapeutic use of oxygen radical scavengers is under active investigation, particularly in relation to *inflammatory and ischemic diseases*. One approach has been to use the enzymes SOD and catalase. In some cases protective effects have been dramatic, in others not. Both enzymes suffer from short plasma half-lives, inaccessibility to intracellular sites of radical production, and inability to cross the blood–brain barrier. Liposomal encapsulation and intratracheal infusion have been used with some success, but overall the initial hopes for enzyme therapy have not been realized. Low-molecular-weight scavengers have better accessibility and are receiving considerable attention. Scavengers of hydroxyl radicals or HOCl have major limitations because of the high concentrations required. However, inhibitors of lipid peroxidation are effective at achievable concentrations and both natural and synthetic lipid antioxidants are being studied. Thiol compounds such as *N*-acetylcysteine increase antioxidant activity, either directly or via glutathione.

An alternative approach is to prevent oxidant production. Allopurinol is effective when xanthine oxidase is involved and is proving beneficial in some ischemic conditions. Inhibitors of the neutrophil oxidative burst or myeloperoxidase have so far received little attention, but monoclonal antibodies against cell adhesion molecules that prevent neutrophils attaching to the endothelium have shown impressive protection in several animal models of inflammation and ischemia. Since transition metals play an important role in radical reactions, another approach is the administration of chelators such as desferrioxamine. In all these approaches a balance must be preserved between therapeutic effect and preservation of essential physiological functions. Diet is an important factor, particularly in the neonatal period when intakes of micronutrients may be suboptimal. Low intakes of antioxidant vitamins are reflected in tissue levels and low dietary selenium and sulfur amino acids result in decreased glutathione and glutathione peroxidase activities.

## SELECTED READING

Ängård E. Nitric oxide: mediator, murderer, and medicine. *Lancet* 1994; 343: 1199.

Frank L. Developmental aspects of experimental pulmonary oxygen toxicity. *Free Radical Biol Med* 1991; 11: 463.

Halliwell B, Gutteridge JMC. *Free radicals in biology and medicine*, 2nd edn. Oxford: Clarendon Press, 1989.

Heffner JE, Repine JE. Pulmonary strategies of antioxidant defense. *Am Rev Respir Dis* 1989; 140: 531.

Holley AE, Cheeseman KH. Measurement of free radical reactions in vivo. *Brit Med Bull* 1993; 49: 494.

Kelly FJ. Free radical disorders of preterm infants. *Brit Med Bull* 1993; 49: 668.

Saugstad OD. Oxygen toxicity in the neonatal period. *Acta Paediatr Scand* 1990; 79: 881.

Vannucci RC. Current and potentially new management strategies for perinatal hypoxic–ischemic encephalopathy. *Pediatrics* 1990; 85: 961.

Weiss SJ. Tissue destruction by neutrophils. *N Engl J Med* 1989; 320: 365.

# 10

# Nitric Oxide: Molecular Basis for Production and Biologic Action

R. Kirk Riemer

## INTRODUCTION

Nitric oxide (NO), a reactive gas, has long been recognized as an environmental pollutant, a byproduct of the internal combustion engine, and a key member of the industrial pollutant gases that contribute to the destruction of the Earth's ozone layer. The discovery of NO as an important biological messenger, however, came about through classical scientific detective work which exemplifies basic research: the convergence of separate lines of inquiry linked arginine-dependent nitrate production by endotoxin-exposed macrophages, endothelium-dependent vascular relaxation in response to acetylcholine, and neuronal glutamate receptor stimulated cyclic-3′,5′-guanosine monophosphate (cGMP) production, to the common element, nitric oxide. Since the seminal observations in the 1980s, research on the biologic effects of NO has expanded in epic proportions on a global basis, and continues to gain momentum. We are finding that NO is the link in an enormous number of previous gaps in our understanding of virtually every aspect of physiology, most notably the vascular, nervous and immunologic systems, but including a variety of pathophysiologic states as well. Another significant breakthrough arising from the discovery of NO is the realization that a class of life-saving drugs – the nitrovasodilators such as nitroglycerin and nitroprusside –

which have been used for decades, act by releasing NO.

Much is still being learned about this novel chemical messenger, NO, and along the way, nearly every attempt at general classification of the NO synthases (NOSs) and their regulatory properties has fallen victim to exceptions save for one: cellular production of NO either is *continuous* at maximal levels (as exemplified by the macrophage form of the enzyme), or production is controlled by the intracellular ionized calcium concentration (as in the neuronal and endothelial forms of the enzyme).

## THE DISCOVERY OF NO AS A BIOLOGIC MESSENGER

Production of NO by a biologic system was first realized as a result of studies in the field of immunology, conducted to understand why nitrate production was increased in animals exposed to endotoxins. Subsequent observations revealed that macrophages were the source of the increased nitrate production, that arginine was the source of the nitrate, and that authentic NO gas killed tumor cells in a manner indistinguishable from that caused by cytokine-activated macrophages.

Discovery of NO synthesized by vascular tissue arose from studies of the vasodilatory action of acetylcholine. Dr Robert Furschgott observed that a new technician was unable to obtain the relaxant responses of arterial segments to acetylcholine which he had been studying. He observed that when the delicate endothelium was rubbed away, this caused the vessels to contract instead of relax. The pursuit of this fundamental observation gave birth to the monumental discovery of the endothelium-dependent relaxing factor (EDRF) which we now believe to be NO. Separate studies underway at the same time by Ignarro and others showed that vasodilator drugs such as nitroglycerine act by releasing NO, and led them to reach the conclusion that EDRF is NO.

Although the vascular activity of NO spurred its discovery as a signaling molecule, the molecular basis for its biologic synthesis, the molecular cloning of the first NO synthase enzyme, was the fruit of a search for the protein which produced the activator of brain guanylyl cyclase. The activator was reasoned to be EDRF/NO on the basis of studies demonstrating that glutamate-stimulated neuron cultures produced a substance which could dilate blood vessels. Bredt *et al.* used standard molecular cloning strategies based on peptide sequences of purified brain NO synthase to isolate the first cDNA for NO synthase in 1991.

## CHEMISTRY OF NO: BIOLOGIC MESSENGER AND CYTOTOXIN

As shown in Fig. 10.1, NO is chemically similar to the anesthetic gas nitrous oxide ($N_2O$). However, the presence of its unpaired electron renders NO (correctly written NO$^\bullet$, but generally abbreviated as NO) an extremely reactive substance – whether released as an atmospheric pollutant or produced as a biologic signal. The uncharged NO radical undergoes rapid reaction with molecular oxygen ($O_2$), superoxide ($O_2^{\bullet -}$), organic thiols such as cysteine residues of proteins, and transition metal ions such as the Fe(II) heme centers of hemoglobin and the Fe(III) centers of porphyrin-containing proteins such as the soluble form of guanylyl cyclase. The products of these reactions (e.g. peroxynitrite [OONO$^-$], RS-NO) may undergo further reactions with other nucleophiles. In biologic systems, heme centers and thiols such as cysteine residues of proteins are particularly abundant, so thiol- and metal-containing proteins are prevalent targets of NO reactivity. The high reactivity of the NO molecule has prevented rigorous proof that EDRF is actually NO rather than NO$^+$ or NO$^-$ or some other NO-adduct such as a nitrosyl thiol. It is most likely that NO exists

as different molecular species – each with different activities and reactivity potential – under different cellular and metabolic conditions.

In the signaling cascade of NO, the best characterized downstream effector of NO is the soluble form of guanylyl cyclase, which contains a heme-porphyrin center. Reaction of NO with the heme center brings about a conformational change as formation of the Fe-NO adduct shifts the charge distribution within the protein, resulting in the activation of the catalytic domain of the cyclase to convert guanosine-5'-triphosphate (GTP) to cGMP and PPi (pyrophosphate). A similar interaction of NO with the heme centers of hemoglobin produces methemoglobin. Interestingly, the deep red coloration of meats preserved with nitrate salts is the result of NO interaction with myoglobin heme centers. Other reactions of NO which constitute signaling paths are discussed below. The reaction of NO with a metalloprotein is reversed slowly if at all, a reflection of the stability of the adduct formed. The formation of NO-adducts may result in the activation or inactivation of the protein's function, and such changes are the basis for the cytotoxic action of NO. The formation of complexes with heme centers of respiratory enzymes results in the cessation of respiration and death of biologic systems – whether an invading bacterium or a brain neuron. One of the major questions left to be understood is how a cell such as a macrophage can produce enough NO to kill adjacent tumor or bacterial cells without killing itself. A mechanism to protect against the essentially irreversible toxic effect of NO must exist, and the ability to harness such an effect may enable broader therapeutic use of NO as a selective cell-killing agent in, for example cancer, or in protecting us from the harm of air pollutants.

## Drugs that release NO

Perhaps the greatest benefit to the field of pharmacology arising through the discovery of NO is the realization that we have been using NO as a drug for decades, without knowing it. We now know that the class of drugs known as nitro-vasodilators, and typified by agents such as glyceryl trinitrate, isosorbide dinitrate and sodium nitroprusside, exert their effects via the release of NO. NO gas is currently being evaluated as an inhalant therapy for different *respiratory distress* conditions. Newer classes of NO-releasing agents are being developed to provide spontaneous or sustained controlled release of NO for uses as disparate as the production of penile erection and the suppression of premature labor contractions.

An important new class of drugs currently being developed are the NOS inhibitors which are truly selective for the different isoforms. These drugs will enable the more selective treatment of conditions where an excess of NO is being produced, such as *septic shock*

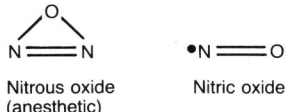

Nitrous oxide (anesthetic)          Nitric oxide

FIGURE 10.1 Shown are the chemical structures of the anesthetic gas nitrous oxide ($N_2O$) and the signaling molecule NO, which is also a gas

or *reperfusion following ischemia*, without negatively affecting other NO-dependent systems.

## MOLECULAR BASIS FOR NO PRODUCTION: NO SYNTHASES

## NO synthase genes

Following rapidly after the molecular cloning of the rat neuronal form of NO synthase (*ncNOS*, nNOS, NOS I, see below for current designations), the cloning of the NOS forms expressed by murine macrophage cells induced by interferon-γ and endotoxin (*iNOS*, NOS II) and by human vascular endothelium (*ecNOS*, eNOS, NOS III, endothelial NOS) were reported. All three gene products were found to code for a single polypeptide chain which contained amino acid sequence motifs recognized as binding domains for the known cofactors of the isolated enzymes: flavins, NADPH, tetrahydrobiopterin (THB) and calmodulin (CM) (Fig. 10.2). A comparison of these three gene products reveals sufficient structural homology to consider them distinct isoforms within a family of homologous proteins. Among the three isoforms, ncNOS is structurally distinguished by the presence of an extra 200 amino acids at its amino terminus, iNOS is distinguished by the deletion of a region proximal to the putative calmodulin binding site, and ecNOS is distinguished by the presence of a consensus site for N-terminal myristoylation. ecNOS is known to be present as a myristoylated (covalently modified by addition of a 14 carbon saturated fatty acid chain), membrane-anchored form in endothelial cells. All three isoforms can undergo phosphorylation at certain serine residues, although it is still unclear how such modification affects *in vivo* NOS function since the effects of phosphorylation *in vitro* are quite variable. A common feature of the NOS gene family members is the near identity of the C-terminal half of the peptide chain with that of cytochrome $P_{450}$ reductase. Subsequent studies have led to the realization that the single-chain NOS molecule actually functions analogously to the two-chain cytochrome $P_{450}$ reductase–cytochrome $P_{450}$ complexes in catalyzing the oxidation of arginine (see below). Other unique enzymatic features of the NO synthases include their representing the only known examples of calmodulin-requiring oxidative enzymes and the only soluble form of $P_{450}$ reductase known to be expressed in eukaryotic organisms.

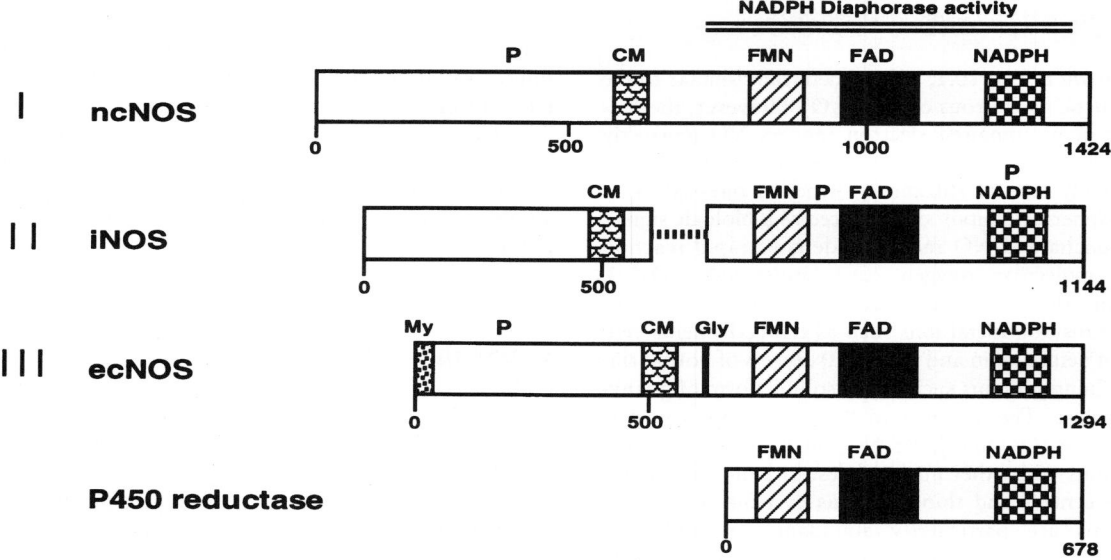

FIGURE 10.2 The relative positions of protein structural features of known NOS gene products are depicted, along with those for $P_{450}$ reductase. The numbering refers to amino acid residues in the translated protein. Abbreviations: ncNOS = "constitutive," $Ca^{2+}$ plus calmodulin stimulated neuronal form; iNOS = calcium-insensitive macrophage form; ecNOS = "constitutive," $Ca^{2+}$ plus calmodulin stimulated vascular endothelial form; FMN = flavin mononucleotide binding site; FAD = binding site for flavin adenine dinucleotide; NADPH = site for NADPH nucleotide binding. The portion of the ncNOS molecule that confers NADPH diaphorase activity is indicated by the double bar. Consensus motifs for calmodulin binding (CM) are present in the neuronal and endothelial forms, but may be different in the macrophage form. Similarly, consensus phosphorylation sites (P) for cAMP-dependent kinases, calcium plus CM-dependent kinases and protein kinase C (i.e. a serine/threonine kinase phosphorylation motif), are present only in neuronal and endothelial enzyme sequences. A myristoylation motif (My, a potential membrane anchoring site) and an N-glycosylation motif (Gly) are found only in the endothelial form, which also is the only NOS activity found primarily in membranous fractions. In terms of sequence alignment, the ncNOS is 220 AA longer than the other forms at the $NH_2$ terminus, iNOS has an internal mid-sequence deletion (40 AA) relative to ncNOS and is 15 AA shorter at the C terminal, while ecNOS is an additional 20 AA shorter than iNOS at the N terminus, but does have the middle and C-terminal sequences which are missing from iNOS.

TABLE 10.1 Molecular properties of the NOS gene products

| TYPE | NAME | ORIGINAL SOURCE | $Ca^{2+}$ STIM. | Mr (kD) | cDNA (kb) | mRNA (kb) | UNIQUE FEATURES |
|------|------|-----------------|----------------|---------|-----------|-----------|-----------------|
| I | ncNOS[a] | Cerebellum | Yes | 155 | 4.6 | 10.5 | Extra 220 AA @ $NH_2$ |
| II | iNOS[b] | Macrophage | No | 131 | 3.8 | 4.4 | Altered CM site |
| III | ecNOS[a] | Endothelium | Yes | 135 | 4.1 | 4.8 | Myristoylation site |

[a]$Ca^{2+}$ plus calmodulin stimulated (formerly designated "constitutive" NOS)
[b]$Ca^{2+}$ insensitive (formerly designated "inducible" NOS)

The physical properties of the NOS gene products are listed in Table 10.1. The NOS enzymes are homodimers containing per subunit (e.g. 130 000 Mr iNOS monomer) an average of 1 FAD, 1 FMN, 1 heme, 0.1 to 1 THB, and variable amounts of calmodulin.

## Enzymatic NO production

The enzymatic reaction of the NO synthases is the stoichiometric conversion of L-arginine and molecular oxygen to NO and L-citrulline via an hydroxyarginine (NOH-Arg intermediate). This catalysis is one of the most complex reactions known to be carried out by a single enzyme. In addition to $O_2$, NO synthases require the cofactors NADPH, THB, FAD, FMN, magnesium ion and $Ca^{2+}$-ligated calmodulin (Fig. 10.3). The catalytic conversion of arginine involves its transitional hydroxylation by $O_2$, facilitated by a tightly bound heme (iron protoporphrin IX) and this reaction probably is assisted by the tightly-bound THB prosthetic group. Although NO synthases are $P_{450}$ cytochromes by definition, and bind heme in a similar manner, they differ in the sequence of the heme binding domains and the novel use of the biopterin prosthetic group in the NOS.

Biological production of NO in neuronal and endothelial cells is regulated acutely (i.e. the activation is brief) by changes in the intracellular concentration of ionized calcium, which activates NOS via interaction with the $Ca^{2+}$ binding protein calmodulin. In these cells, the influx or release of $Ca^{2+}$ consequent to receptor activation by hormones (such as acetylcholine, aspartate, endothelins) increases NO production, which is subsequently attenuated by the reversal of $Ca^{2+}$ mobilization through the homeostatic mechanisms which enable the cell to recover from hormonal stimulation. In macrophages and other cells expressing the so-called "inducible" form of NOS (iNOS), NO production is independent of ambient levels of intracellular $Ca^{2+}$, and is sustained at a high level which is regulated only by the availability of the substrate L-arginine, the cofactor THB, and the stability of the enzyme protein. The explanation for the apparent $Ca^{2+}$ insensitivity of the iNOS isoform, despite its ability to bind $Ca^{2+}$-ligated calmodulin, lies in the essentially irreversible binding of calmodulin by this isoform; without the reversible association of calmodulin, the response to changes in ambient $Ca^{2+}$ levels is lost.

The production of NO in the presence of molecular oxygen is dependent on an adequate supply of two key molecules: the amino acid L-arginine and the nutrient cofactor THB. L-Arginine is synthesized by the kidney and liver, and is usually transported into other cells via the $y^+$ transporter. L-Arginine can also be produced from L-citrulline via a salvage pathway consisting of the urea cycle enzymes, arginosuccinate synthase and arginosuccinate lyase. In endothelial cells and vascular smooth muscle, these enzymes are co-induced by cytokines which induce iNOS expression. Therefore, the L-arginine substrate required for high sustained levels of NO production (characteristic of iNOS), can apparently be maintained without an increase in supply of exogenous L-arginine. When L-arginine availability is low, but NADPH is abundant, NOS actually produces superoxide or hydrogen peroxide.

THB is an allosteric activator of NO synthases which also may function in catalysis. Cellular levels

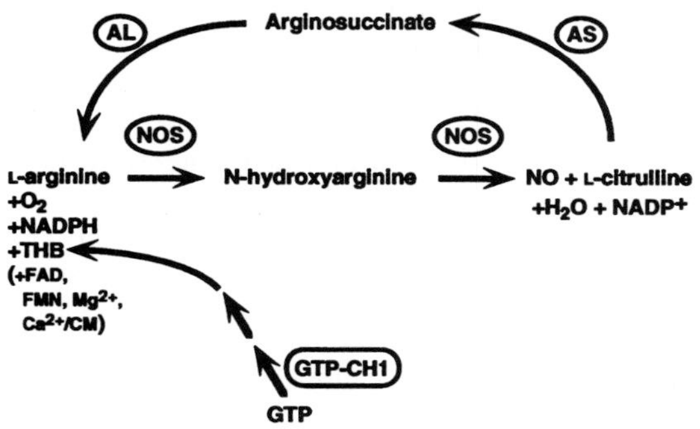

FIGURE 10.3 The NO synthase catalytic reaction. The reaction sequence for the conversion of L-arginine to nitric oxide (NO) is shown. L-arginine is converted to NO via an hydroxyarginine intermediate. Although only the cofactors NADPH and tetrahydrobiopterin (THB) are thought to function in catalysis, NOS also requires the binding of FAD, FMN, $Mg^{2+}$ and $Ca^{2+}$-ligated calmodulin ($Ca^{2+}$/CM) to be functional. Also depicted are the pathways for THB synthesis and for the recycling of L-citrulline back to L-arginine, both of which can occur in a variety of cells. The rate-limiting enzyme for THB synthesis is GTP cyclohydrolase-1 (GTP-CH1). The salvage pathway for L-arginine synthesis uses the urea cycle enzymes arginosuccintate synthase (AS) and arginosuccinate lyase (AL) to convert L-citrulline to arginosuccinate and then to L-arginine.

of THB are also regulated, and may serve as a mechanism for the control of NO production within endothelial cells and vascular smooth muscle cells. The rate-limiting step in THB synthesis is the enzyme GTP-cyclohydrolase-1(GTP-CH1) which converts GTP to dihydroneopterin triphosphate. This enzyme is up-regulated in concert with stimuli which induce iNOS expression in several cell types including endothelium and smooth muscle. Endothelial cells in long-term culture have a diminished capacity for NO production despite the presence of ecNOS; THB levels were decreased in this setting, and NO production could be restored either by supplying this cofactor or by augmenting its production. Consistent with this, inhibitors of THB synthesis (e.g. 2,4 diamino-6-hydroxy-pyrimidine, a GTP-CH1 inhibitor) have a protective effect against experimental endotoxin-induced shock in a mouse model.

## Cell and tissue distribution of the NO synthases

To identify forms of NOS, earlier studies relied on the localization to a cellular compartment (membranes vs cytosol) and dependency upon $Ca^{2+}$ in addition to cell or tissue type. Although as many as six isoforms of NOS were thought to exist on the basis of protein purification studies, molecular identification has reduced the apparent complexity of NOS isoforms. Adding to the confusion over the identity of NOS isoforms, has been the use of antibodies that ultimately were revealed to react with more than one NOS isoform. At present, only three distinct NOS gene products have been isolated and their gene structure and chromosomal locations determined to be different (i.e. chromosomes 12, 7 and 17 for ncNOS, ecNOS and iNOS, respectively). Structural studies have revealed the basis for several sequence variations based on alternate-splicing of the gene products. At least three forms of ncNOS are now known and variants of ecNOS which are not myristoylated are thought to exist under certain physiologic conditions. The current picture of NOS isoforms and their subcellular distribution is that all three isoforms can be isolated from both soluble and membrane fractions of cells.

The relative ability of different arginine analogs to inhibit NO production (i.e. rank order of potency) has not proven to be a foolproof means for identification of an NOS isoform, although newer, potentially isoform-selective compounds are being developed. The use of nucleic acid probes representing sequences unique to an isoform is the most reliable means for molecular identification of previously uncharacterized sources of NOS activity. The clearest delimiter for NOS isoforms on the basis of activity is the sensitivity to $Ca^{2+}$; only iNOS activity is insensitive to $Ca^{2+}$ and calmodulin inhibitors (e.g. calmodizolium). The functional classification of NO synthases thus should be based on $Ca^{2+}$-dependency. Since they are all gene products, they are all "inducible," so the label "iNOS" is best interpreted as the $Ca^{2+}$-insensitive NOS form and "ncNOS" and "ecNOS" as the $Ca^{2+}$ plus calmodulin-stimulated neuronal and endothelial NOS forms, respectively.

Neuronal NOS has been found in both the central (e.g. cerebellar cells) and peripheral nervous system (e.g. myenteric plexus of the intestine). This form has also been isolated from human skeletal muscle and rat skeletal muscle. Endothelial NOS may be membrane anchored via myristoyl modification, but it has been shown that such modification is necessary but insufficient for localization of this isoform to the membrane. Further post-translational modification of ecNOS, by addition of palmitic acid, is now thought to control membrane anchoring of this form. The iNOS form has been demonstrated in many diverse cell types (macrophages, vascular, uterine and fallopian tube smooth muscle cells, hepatocytes, chondrocytes, several epithelia), and can be induced in a cell-type specific manner by an increasing list of diverse stimuli including a variety of cytokines (bacterial endotoxin plus interferon-γ, IL-1β, TNFα). The putative promoter region of the *iNOS* gene contains binding sites for transcription factors which are known to be activated by these cytokines (NF-1, IRE, TNF, NF-IL6, and AP1) and by endotoxin (NF-κB). In vascular smooth muscle cells, agents which elevate cellular levels of cyclic-3′,5′-adenosine monophosphate (cAMP) also induce iNOS.

## ROLE OF NO IN INTERCELLULAR SIGNALING

The signaling functions of NO are mediated by several different mechanisms, and generally serve to signal between cells, rather than within a cell. The most distinctive feature of the NO signaling system is that it uses a distinctively non-classical receptor mechanism: the "receptors" for NO serve both a molecular recognition and signal transduction function and are themselves targets for chemical reaction with NO. This is quite different from the reversible association between signaling molecules, characteristic of classical hormone receptors. For example, NO reacts with the heme moiety of soluble guanylyl cyclase to activate its catalysis of cGMP synthesis. While none of the signaling pathways which involve NO are completely understood, patterns of NO responses have emerged, and so some generalizations can be made. The reader should be aware, however, that little is known about this signaling system, and that as our knowledge increases, some of what is known today will have to be revised.

NO is a gas which has a high aqueous solubility and freely permeates cellular membranes. However, because NO is also highly reactive, it is thought to exert its physiologic actions within closely adjacent cell layers rather than by diffusion across great distances; it serves a paracrine or intracrine signaling function. NO concentrations decline by 50 per cent at a distance of $100\,\mu m$ from the point of production in aortic endothelium, where NO apparently is released in a manner which directs it towards the smooth muscle of the medial layer rather than towards the vessel lumen. The local availability of superoxide dismutase, which prolongs the stability of NO, also governs the potential for NO to react distant from its point of generation. The potential for diffusion and the permeability of NO is further complicated by the observation that nitrosylthiol adducts (RS-NO) of NO do not readily cross cell membranes. Therefore, limited or directional permeation of NO may be a function of the presence of reactive groups within adjacent cells or of extracellular matrix composition.

At present, most of the acute signaling effects of NO production are thought to be mediated via cGMP produced by the activation of soluble guanylyl cyclase. cGMP effects changes in cellular function by increasing the level of phosphorylation of key cellular proteins (Fig. 10.4). The phosphorylation function is performed by the catalytic component of cGMP-dependent protein kinase, which is activated upon its release from its complex with a regulatory subunit which bears specific binding sites for cGMP. The cGMP signaling cascade is terminated as a result of the metabolism of cGMP by a specific phosphodiesterase to yield GMP. Dephosphorylation of cellular protein effectors is a continuous process which maintains homeostasis, so all that is needed to cease a signaling process is to cease the generation of the second messenger (cGMP), and the reversal will normally ensue.

The area of greatest ignorance in the cGMP signaling pathway, as it is in most signaling pathways, is the nature and function of the proteins which become phosphorylated as a result of the signal. Phosphorylation acts as a molecular switch, causing changes in the conformation and charge distribution throughout molecules. The resultant effect is to alter a substrate's access to an enzyme's active site, alter ion gating via membrane channels, or, either directly or allosterically, alter the ability of molecules to associate with others. In most situations, the signaling cascade seems to lead to several changes, including amplification/attenuation steps as other kinases and phosphatases are activated. Although many of the proteins which undergo changes in their phosphorylation status in response to some signals have been identified, the system is enormously complex, and we still have little insight into the manner in which the events convey a discrete cellular signal to modify cellular function. For example, two types of targets of cGMP-dependent protein kinase are proteins which inhibit phosphatases when phosphorylated and phosphodiesterases which metabolize either cAMP, cGMP, or both.

Perhaps the best understood NO signaling pathway is that of the vascular response, where the role of the endothelial cell is to control the extent of smooth muscle contraction in the adjacent media as a means of regulating blood pressure. Humoral mediators such as acetylcholine and bradykinin mobilize endothelial cell $Ca^{2+}$ via specific receptor ($M_1$ and $B_1$, respectively) coupled $G_q$ activation of a phospholipase C, to increase inositol trisphosphate production ($IP_3$). $IP_3$ triggers the release of intracellular $Ca^{2+}$ stores and transmembrane $Ca^{2+}$ influx, raising intracellular $Ca^{2+}$. Elevation of free $Ca^{2+}$ levels increases $Ca^{2+}$ binding to calmodulin which then binds to, and activates, ecNOS to produce NO (see also Chapter 67). Even in this extensively studied system we still have incomplete proof that cGMP mediates the effect of NO to limit $Ca^{2+}$ influx in the smooth muscle cells, although cGMP is provisionally presumed to be the mediator. At issue is whether cGMP production is causal rather than coincident with the final effect on $Ca^{2+}$ mobilization. NO can activate a $Ca^{2+}$-gated $K^+$ channel on the aortic smooth muscle cell, thereby causing hyperpolarization and reduced $Ca^{2+}$ influx, suggesting that cGMP may not be critical to the relaxation mechanism. These issues can be resolved only through further studies which provide finer detail of the signaling cascade elicited by NO.

In the neuronal cell, NO mediates neurotransmitter release in response to ncNOS activation through depolarization-associated $Ca^{2+}$ influx. An example of this is the release of vasoactive intestinal peptide (VIP) in gastrointestinal neurons. $Ca^{2+}$ influx may be mediated via activation of voltage-dependent $Ca^{2+}$ channels (by depolarization) or receptor-operated channels (by a neurotransmitter). In the central nervous system, the NMDA-sensitive subtype of glutamate receptors contain an integral $Ca^{2+}$ channel which activates influx upon agonist occupancy. The ncNOS-containing neurons are designated nitrergic or NANC (non-adrenergic, non-cholinergic) to distinguish them. However, the coexistence of other transmitters (e.g. peptides) will probably prove to be a common feature of the nitrergic neurons, at least in the periphery. NO produced within the neuron is thought to freely diffuse to adjacent neurons where it stimulates cGMP production and subsequent phosphorylation of neuronal proteins. In this manner NO transmits signals to adjacent neuronal, glial, and probably vascular cells. Tests of ncNOS function have been attempted by intron deletion ("knock out") in transgenic mice. The resulting mice were quite normal at birth, showing only enlarged stomachs, but with no obvious CNS deficits. Subsequently, it has been found that these mice may have been protected by the expression of an alternate form of ncNOS during fetal life.

As discussed above, NO production by macrophage cell iNOS occurs in a $Ca^{2+}$-independent manner and in a constant, high level of output, which has the apparent purpose of exerting a cytotoxic action against nearby bacteria or determinedly non-host cell types (e.g. tumor cells or rejected allografts). Much less clear is the functional role of iNOS in non-macrophage cell types such as smooth muscle, epithelial and hepatic cells. That iNOS can be induced in these cells is proven, but the physiologic effect of iNOS expression and

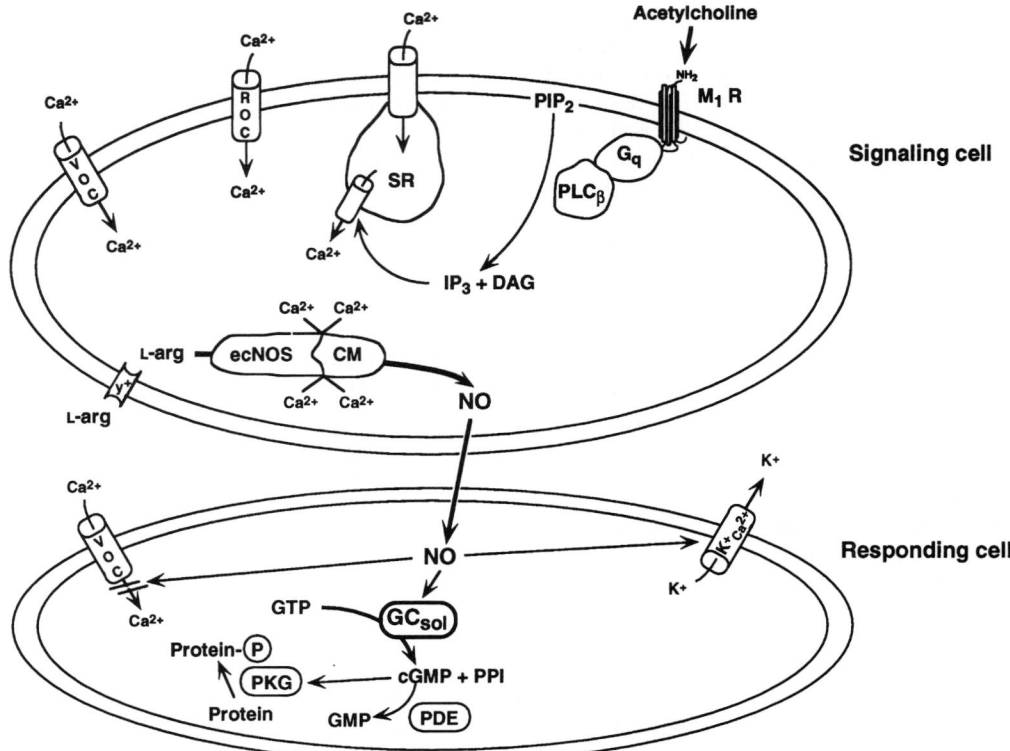

FIGURE 10.4 Intercellular signaling by nitric oxide. This scheme depicts a representative cascade through which NO signals from one cell to another. The signal is initiated when a calcium ($Ca^{2+}$) mobilizing agonist (e.g. acetylcholine) activates its receptor ($M_1$ R [muscarinic cholinergic receptor]). The $M_1$ receptor is coupled via a G-protein ($G_q$) to activate phospholipase $C_\beta$ ($PLC_\beta$), which catalyzes the conversion of phosphatidylinositol-4,5 bisphosphate ($PIP_2$) to inositol-1,4,5-trisphosphate ($IP_3$) and 1,2 diacylglycerol (DAG). $IP_3$ triggers a $Ca^{2+}$ mobilization cascade by interacting with its receptor/channels on the surface of the sarcoplasmic reticulum (SR). The resulting elevation in free intracellular $Ca^{2+}$ ion concentration triggers $Ca^{2+}$ entry via sarcolemmal channels of both the voltage (VOC) and voltage-independent, receptor-operated (ROC) types. The phosphorylation events triggered by the activation of protein kinase C by DAG support the calcium mobilization event triggered by $IP_3$ action. L-Arginine, transported into the cell via the $y^+$ carrier, is converted to NO by NOS which is activated upon the binding of $Ca^{2+}$-ligated calmodulin (CM). The NO so generated is free to diffuse across the cell membrane to signal adjacent responding cells. The relaxation signal received by the responding smooth muscle cell is mediated by both cGMP-dependent and -independent events. Activation of soluble guanylyl cyclase ($GC_{sol}$) causes cGMP levels to rise and to activate cGMP-dependent protein kinase (PKG). PKG then catalyzes the phosphorylation of a variety of proteins which serve to complete the signaling process and terminate the signaling event (by activation of phosphodiesterases (PDE)). NO can directly inactivate calcium channels (VOCs) and directly activate calcium-gated potassium channels ($K^+_{Ca^{2+}}$), thereby blocking $Ca^{2+}$ influx and promoting membrane hyperpolarization via $K^+$ efflux. For clarity, certain events are shown to occur in separate cells, such as is thought to occur in signaling between the vascular endothelium and vascular smooth muscle. The reader should be aware that any or all of these signals could emanate from the same cell, constituting an intracellular signaling cascade. PPI = pyrophosphate.

NO production is incompletely understood. NO production within a smooth muscle cell would be expected to elicit the same signaling cascade as if NO came from outside the cell: cGMP production and the inhibition/reversal of $Ca^{2+}$ influx. Thus, the iNOS-expressing smooth muscle cell should be constantly in a relaxed or inhibited state. Some insight into the physiologic implications of this situation arise from studies of the atherogenic response, where, as a result of endothelial injury and cytokine release from recruited macrophages, iNOS is induced in the smooth muscle cells and the endothelium. One conceivable scenario is that increased NO production inhibits contraction and, in a positive feedback loop, results in a spreading pattern of chronic vascular relaxation; this results in compensatory medial hyperplasia to attempt to restore wall tension, ultimately resulting in the pathology of atherosclerosis. Consistent with this putative pathophysiologic response mechanism, in septic shock patients where severe hypotension is unresponsive to vasoconstrictors, NOS inhibitors can elevate blood pressure, suggesting that endotoxin-induced iNOS activity is mediating the vascular hypo-responsiveness.

A variety of other receptors (more accurately viewed as targets) for NO besides soluble guanylyl cyclase are being recognized and their mechanisms elucidated (Fig. 10.5). The two major classes of NO targets are distinguished on the basis of the reacting

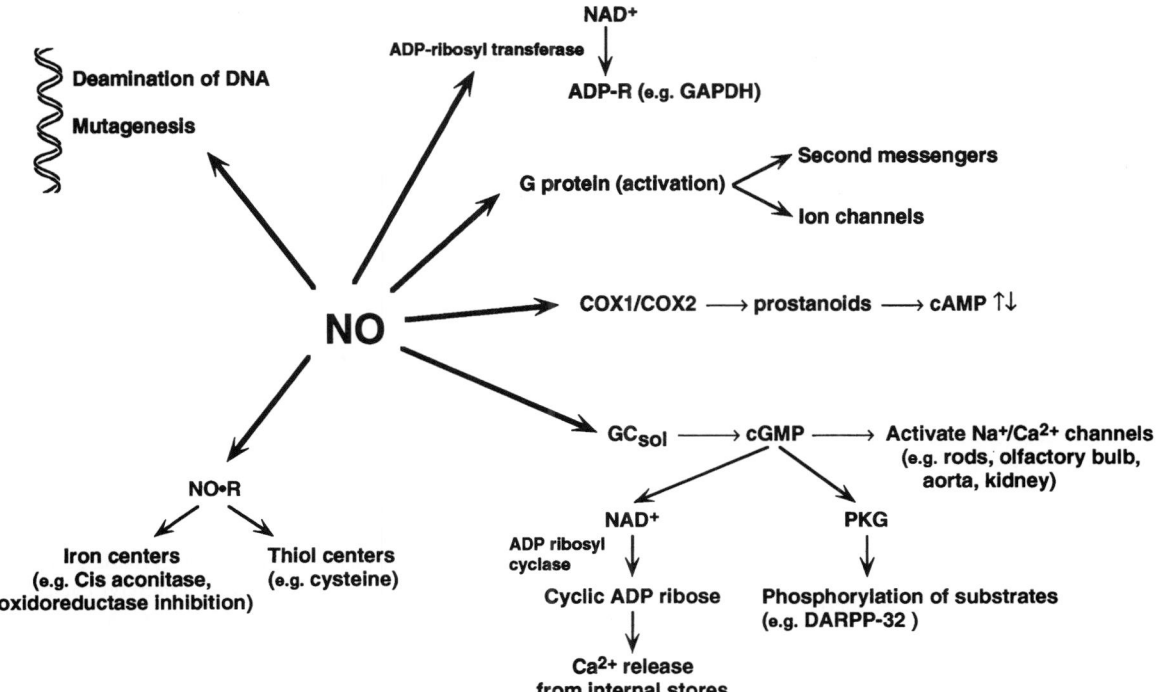

FIGURE 10.5 Molecular targets of NO. This scheme depicts some of the variety of signaling events which are initiated by NO. The interaction of NO, or an NO adduct (NO•R), with iron (hemes) or thiol (cysteines) centers of proteins often inhibits their function, but may also activate them through direct or allosteric mechanisms. Interaction with DNA leads to deamination of cytosine residues, C→T transitions and the induction of inheritable mutations. Several signaling enzymes are known to be activated by NO, e.g. ADP-ribosyl transferase which catalyzes the transfer of ADP-ribose from NAD to proteins such as GAPDH. G-proteins are activated by thiol interaction, leading to many potential signals, including ion channel modulation and second messenger production. The cyclooxygenase (COX) enzymes, COX1 and COX2, are activated by NO, leading to prostanoid production and the elevation of cAMP levels in some cells. The best-characterized target for NO action, the soluble form of guanylyl cyclase ($GC_{sol}$), is activated by reaction of NO with the heme-containing subunit of $GC_{sol}$. The general understanding is that all effects of cGMP are mediated via the activation of cGMP-dependent protein kinase (PKG), which catalyzes the serine phosphorylation of a variety of proteins. For example, the neuronal protein DARPP-32 is an inhibitor of the general protein phosphatase type 1. Phosphorylation of DARPP-32 by PKG inactivates it, and thus maintains other proteins (enzymes, receptors, channels) in a phosphorylated state. There are two reportedly direct effects of cGMP, although no mechanism for this action has been demonstrated. Cyclic GMP apparently activates ADP ribosyl cyclase, which catalyzes the cyclization of $NAD^+$ to cyclic ADP ribose which acts to release $Ca^{2+}$ from internal stores (ryanodine- and caffeine-sensitive), and which are distinct from the $IP_3$-sensitive $Ca^{2+}$ stores. It also has been reported that cGMP can directly activate the $Na^+/Ca^{2+}$ channels of visual rods, olfactory, aortic and kidney cells.

nucleophile: thiol or transition metal. Another important target of NO is the DNA molecule, where NO can bring about the deamination of cytosine residues, effecting a heritable mutation via a C→T transition. This genotoxic reaction of NO may involve the formation of a peroxynitrite radical which carries out the nucleophilic attack upon the cytosine ring $NH_2$.

Biologically important metal-NO adducts are typified by guanylyl cyclase and hemoglobin, but include a variety of cytosolic enzymes including cyclooxygenases, catalase, peroxidase, mitochondrial oxidoreductases I (NADH) and II (ubiquinone), and cytochrome c aconitase, as well as NOS and $P_{450}$ cytochromes. The result of NO reaction with these enzymes is, in most cases, inhibition of their activity, since the heme group can no longer undergo the switching mechanism via a conformational change in the *trans*-

imidazole ligand. Cyclooxygenase enzymes are activated by NO, and this exception to the pattern is still incompletely understood. The nuclear transcription factor Sox, which is involved in sensing changes in the oxidative states of cells, may be NO responsive as well.

A large number of nitrosyl-thiol adducts of NO are known and continue to be found. These adducts include membranous and cytosolic proteins as well as nuclear and extracellular proteins. The membrane proteins targets of NO comprise components of trans-membrane signaling systems: ion channels such as the NMDA receptor and a $Ca^{2+}$-gated $K^+$ channel; pertussis toxin-sensitive G proteins and $p21^{ras}$; adenylyl cyclase and protein kinase C. Cytoplasmic targets of NO include the Krebs-cycle enzyme GAPDH (glyceraldehyde-3-phosphate dehydrogenase), actin, glutathione, aldehyde and alcohol dehydrogenases, and tissue plasminogen activator. The transcription factors AP1 and NF-κB, and the extracellular proteins glutathione and albumin also undergo thio-nitrosylation reaction with NO. The molecular basis for the alteration of protein function by thio-nitrosylation involves the role of the critical cysteine residue(s) which undergo reaction with NO. Consequent alterations in trans-molecular $H^+$ bonding or electrostatic interactions likely lead to conformational changes at allosteric or catalytic sites. Either activation or inhibition of function may result from reaction with NO by thiol adduct formation, depending upon the protein targeted. For example, GDP release from $p21^{ras}$ is accelerated, G proteins, ion channels, AP1 and NF-κB are activated while GAPDH and alcohol dehydrogenase activities are decreased by NO. Of note, NO activation of NF-κB completes a positive feedback loop to augment NOS expression. Nitrosothiol activation of G proteins may modulate ion channels or any of the various signaling functions which are known to be mediated by these proteins, thereby widening the signaling capacity/complexity of NO. The interaction of NO with growth factor signaling has recently been reported, where the mitogenic response to fibroblast growth factor (FGF), but not platelet-derived growth factor (PDGF) or serum, was augmented by exogenous NO. Other reactions of NO which might constitute signaling paths include the stimulation of the adenosine-5′-diphosphate (ADP)-ribosylation of cellular proteins, and the reaction with superoxide to produce toxic peroxynitrites. Conceivably, these alternate signaling pathways could function in place of or in concert with the cGMP cascade, perhaps to provide a subtle difference in the spatial or temporal aspects of an NO-initiated signal.

## PHYSIOLOGIC ROLES FOR NO: WHERE DOES NO NOT HAVE A ROLE?

A role for NO in the neuronal, vascular and immunologic systems is not surprising since these are rich sources of the NO synthases. We have come to find that NO is to some extent involved in the function of virtually every organ system of animals, and roles for it in the biology of plants and bacteria and fungi are reported on a continual basis. Following discovery of cerebellar ncNOS, other studies have revealed important roles throughout the central and peripheral nervous systems in both physiologic function and pathologic responses. Vascular-derived NO has been found to mediate penile and clitoral erection as well as renal tubular function and to play a key role in the pathogenesis of septic shock, atherosclerosis, and myocardial failure. Macrophage-derived NO forms the cytotoxic basis of immunosurveillance, yet apparently all cells have the capacity for inductive expression if iNOS under physiologic as well as pathophysiologic

conditions. Hypoxic/reperfusion injury of tissues also involves NO production, and the normal quiescence of the pregnant uterus may depend upon sustained NO production.

## Conclusions/Perspective

The NO signaling system comprises an array of unique synthetic enzymes, a versatile signaling molecule and a diverse system of intercellular signal transduction systems. For several decades, drugs which release NO have been used and a variety of subcellular phenomena have been observed with an incomplete understanding of their mechanisms. An understanding of the NO system holds the promise of illuminating the major missing link in physiologic signaling in virtually all of biology. Much more is still unknown than is known about the NO signaling system, although considerable progress in our understanding has been made in a relatively short time. It is evident that guanylyl cyclase is only one of many targets of NO action. As we learn about the other target molecules, we will see the role of NO in biologic signaling continue to broaden. Two areas of inquiry which are critical to our harnessing of this system for use in therapy can be identified. First, the basis for the discreet signaling ability of NO must be understood so that the implications of therapeutic modification of NO levels can be known. Second, the potential for virtually every cell in the body to elevate its expression of iNOS in non-pathologic conditions must be better understood to provide insight to the relevance of this mechanism.

## SELECTED READING

Bredt DS, Hwang PM, Glatt CL, *et al.* Cloned and expressed nitric oxide synthase structurally resembles cytochrome $P_{450}$ reductase. *Nature* 1991; **351**: 714.

Garthwaite J, Boulton CL. Nitric oxide signaling in the central nervous system. *Ann Rev Physiol* 1995; **57**: 683.

Griffith OW, Stuehr DJ. Nitric oxide synthases: properties and catalytic mechanism. *Ann Rev Physiol* 1995; **57**: 707.

Gross SS, Wolin MS. Nitric oxide: pathophysiological mechanisms. *Ann Rev Physiol* 1995; **57**: 737.

Janssens SP, Shimouchi A, Quertermous T, *et al.* Cloning and expression of a cDNA encoding human endothelium-derived relaxing factor nitric oxide synthase. *J Biol Chem* 1992; **267**: 14519.

Lyons CR, Orloff GJ, Cunningham JM. Molecular cloning and functional expression of an inducible nitric oxide synthase from a murine macrophage cell line. *J Biol Chem* 1992; **267**: 6370.

Moncada S, Higgs A. The L-arginine-nitric oxide pathway. *N Engl J Med* 1993; **329**: 2002.

Nathan C, Xie QW. Regulation of biosynthesis of nitric oxide. *J Biol Chem* 1994; **269**: 13725.

Stamler JS. Redox signaling: nitrosylation and related target interactions of nitric oxide. *Cell* 1994; **78**: 931.

# PART FOUR

# *Phases of Development*

**Editors: Peter D. Gluckman and Michael A. Heymann**

# 11

# Morphogenesis and Teratogenesis

Jeffrey A. Kuller, Lynn K. McClean and
Mitchell S. Golbus

## EMBRYOGENESIS

Human embryogenesis can be divided into several stages: fertilization and implantation, the embryonic period, and finally, the fetal period.

Mitosis and cleavage of the zygote (formed by fusion of the egg and sperm) result in a ball of cells, the *morula*. As the morula grows, an inner and outer cell mass and a cell-lined fluid space develop. This structure, called the *blastocyst*, enters the uterus and implants in the endometrium toward the end of the first post-conception week. At the conclusion of the second week, the blastocyst is completely embedded in the endometrium. The outer cell mass or *trophoblast* then differentiates into an external layer, the syncytio-trophoblast, and an internal layer, the cytotrophoblast. The inner cell mass or embryoblast develops into a two-layered structure composed of the ectodermal and endodermal *germ layers*.

During the third week the primitive streak becomes evident with a primitive knot at the cephalic end. The primitive streak is a midline thickening of rapidly multiplying ectodermal cells. The embryo becomes polarized with discernible cranial and caudal, and right and left orientations. The invaginating cells of the primitive streak develop a third germ layer, the mesoderm, which forms between the ectodermal and endodermal layers. The chorionic villi also proliferate during this third post-conception week, invade maternal vessels, and acquire adequate nutrition and oxygen from the maternal circulation.

Post-conception weeks 4–8 constitute the *embryonic period*. This is the time of early embryogenesis and therefore represents the peak vulnerability to the occurrence of major congenital anomalies. As each germ layer differentiates, specific organ systems develop. The *ectoderm* is the source of the nervous system, the sensory organs (eye, ear, nose), as well as the integument. *Mesoderm* develops into the musculos-keletal system, connective tissue, the cardiovascular system, most of the urogenital system, and the adrenal glands. *Endoderm* provides the epithelium of the respiratory and gastrointestinal tracts and the urinary bladder. Endoderm also develops into a variety of glandular organs, including the thyroid and parathyroid glands, the pancreas, thymus, tonsils, and liver.

Week 9 begins the *fetal period*, which continues to term. Embryonic growth and early fetal growth occur by cell hyperplasia (increase in cell number). Later, both the size and number of cells increase. The combined cellular hyperplasia and hypertrophy continue throughout the fetal period into the postnatal period. The gross malformations that may result from an insult in the embryonic period rarely occur in the fetal period.

Each organ system develops at slightly different times. The first evidence of *cardiac development* occurs on day 18 or 19 when mesenchymal cells begin to differentiate into angiogenic clusters. These cells proliferate and form a primitive vascular plexus called the *cardiogenic area*. The cardiogenic area canalizes to become the first cardiac structures. These are called the endocardial heart tubes, which fuse to form the single primary heart tube. As the primary heart tube grows, it begins to undergo looping and segmentation. The four cardiac chambers develop between weeks 4 and 7. Peristaltic contractions of the heart begin on day 22.

*Lung development* occurs in four progressive phases: the embryonic, pseudoglandular, canalicular, and alveolar periods. Days 22–26 are the embryonic period, during which a ventral endodermal diverticulum evaginates from the embryonic foregut. The epithelial lining of the respiratory tract results from this anlage. The pseudoglandular period begins at 4 weeks, and branching and division of airways and blood vessels occur during this time. At 16 weeks, the canalicular period begins, during which time there is vascular proliferation as well as further development of the bronchial tree. The terminal sac or alveolar period commences with the 25th gestational week. During this interval, the respiratory tree develops an increased number of respiratory bronchioles and saccules. The surface area for gas exchange becomes sufficient to accommodate extrauterine breathing. Although the fetal lung has no ventilatory function, it is metabolically active.

*The gastrointestinal tract* develops from the primitive gut, which is an elongated tube extending nearly the entire length of the embryo. It is composed of the foregut, midgut, and hindgut. The foregut develops into the pharynx, lower respiratory tract, esophagus, stomach, proximal duodenum, liver, biliary system, and the pancreas. The midgut evolves into the small intestine, cecum, appendix, ascending colon, and proximal transverse colon. The midgut rapidly elongates and soon outgrows available space in the abdominal cavity. After counterclockwise rotation, the herniated intestine returns to the abdominal space at 10 weeks' gestation. The hindgut derivatives are the distal transverse colon, descending colon, sigmoid, rectum, and superior portion of the anus.

*The urinary system* is complex, and "three generations" of kidneys evolve. The first generation is called the pronephros; this rudimentary structure disappears by the fourth week. Most of the pronephric ducts are incorporated into the next renal generation, termed the mesonephros. The mesonephric ducts persist in the male to function as genital ducts. In the female they degenerate, becoming only vestigial organs. The third generation, or metanephros, becomes the permanent kidney. Appearing in the fifth post-conception week, it begins to function in the 11th or 12th week, and the fetus excretes urine into the amniotic fluid. True renal function does not begin until birth because the placenta eliminates metabolic end-products from the fetus. The urinary bladder and urethra are derived from the urogenital sinus. The fetal uterus is formed by 18 weeks, at which time vaginal canalization commences. The testes begin to descend at 20 weeks; this is completed at term.

*Hematopoiesis* progresses through a mesoblastic period, a hepatic period, and a myeloid period. These three maturational stages overlap in time. The mesoblastic period is characterized by the release of cells from blood islands in the yolk sac into the blood stream. This stage begins at 16–19 days and ends at approximately 12 weeks. The second phase of hematopoiesis, the hepatic period, begins at approximately 5 weeks. During this time hematopoiesis occurs primarily in the liver. During the third and fourth months, the spleen also contributes to hematopoiesis. The hepatic period is almost exclusively erythropoietic in nature and ends in

the sixth month. Finally, the myeloid period begins between the fourth and fifth months. Hematopoiesis moves to the bone marrow, where it continues throughout postnatal life. During the third trimester of pregnancy the bone marrow becomes the main hematopoietic organ. Erythropoiesis begins when the hemocytoblasts are committed to an erythrocytic line of maturation. This is indicated by the appearance of hemoglobin in the cytoplasm. Erythropoietin probably begins controlling erythropoiesis in the third trimester. Until 36 weeks' of gestation, approximately 90 per cent of hemoglobin in the fetus is hemoglobin F. Hemoglobin A (adult hemoglobin) is increasingly produced after 36 weeks. Lymphopoiesis is initiated in the third month in lymph nodes and thymus. Mature lymphocytes are first identified in the fetal circulation at this time.

*The central nervous system* develops from ectoderm. The neural tube is formed from the folding and fusion of the neural plate. The cranial neuropore closes on day 25 and the caudal neuropore on day 27. Three primary brain vesicles develop at the expanded cephalic end of the neural tube. These are the forebrain, the midbrain, and the hindbrain. The forebrain eventually forms the cerebral hemispheres and the third ventricle. The midbrain develops into the cerebral aqueduct, the red nuclei, nuclei of the third and fourth cranial nerves, and the substantia nigra. The hindbrain differentiates into the pons, cerebellum and the fourth ventricle. The spinal cord develops from the caudal portion of the neural tube. After the embryonic period, the fetal brain undergoes significant growth of the cerebral hemispheres. The vascular bed of the germinal matrix is the most critical locus of the blood supply to the fetal brain. The vast majority of intraventricular hemorrhages in premature neonates occur in this area.

*External fetal characteristics* and proportions change throughout gestation. At the onset of the fetal period, the head constitutes one-half of the total fetal length. The relative size of the fetal head then begins to diminish, and at term occupies only one-fourth of the length of the body. The face becomes more infantile during gestation, and the eyes migrate from the lateral aspect of the face medially. At 26 weeks, the eyes are partly open and eyelashes are visible. The ears are low-set at an early age, then later occupy their ultimate position. The limbs lengthen and the external genitalia begin to be discernible at 12 weeks. Intestinal loops, forced from the peritoneal cavity by the enlarging liver, migrate back into the abdomen at 10–11 weeks' gestation.

## TERATOGENESIS

## Principles

Teratology, the study of abnormal development, is directed at understanding the causes and mechanisms of maldevelopment. A teratogen is a substance, organism, or physical agent that produces abnormal embryonic structural or functional development. To be considered a teratogen, the agent must act during the embryonic period (Fig. 11.1). An exposure occurring during the fetal period that causes a structural or functional abnormality is called *fetotoxic*. Fetotoxic effects may mimic defects caused by teratogens, and some teratogens are also fetotoxic (e.g. alcohol).

Approximately 1 in 400 liveborn infants has a malformation due to a teratogenic exposure. Teratogens are implicated in approximately 10 per cent of all *birth defects*. Most human teratogens have been discovered by astute clinicians (e.g. *thalidomide syndrome*). Basic science and epidemiological studies have primarily played a confirmatory role in teratogen identification, usually verifying clinical findings after numbers of children with anomalies have been reported. There is approximately a 55 per cent correlation between teratogenicity in animals and teratogenicity in humans.

## Wilson's principles of teratology

Wilson's six principles of teratology provide a framework of how structural or functional teratogens may act. The first principle is that susceptibility to a teratogen depends on the genotype of the conception and the interaction between the genotype and environmental factors. Teratogenic differences based on genetic susceptibility could be the result of either polygenic inheritance or monogenic inheritance. An example of genetic variability to potential teratogenic agents is that exposed fetuses with low levels of the

enzyme epoxide hydrolase are much more likely to manifest the fetal hydantoin syndrome than those with higher levels.

The second of Wilson's principles is that susceptibility of the conceptus to teratogen varies with the developmental state at the time of exposure. During the first 2 weeks of life, the embryo is relatively resistant to teratogenic insults. A large insult may kill the embryo; surviving embryos usually manifest no organ-specific anomalies. During the second to eighth week of development, while organogenesis is occurring, susceptibility to teratogens is maximal. After organogenesis, a teratogen generally only affects the overall growth of the embryo or the size of a specific organ.

Wilson's third principle is that teratogenic agents act by specific mechanisms on developing cells and tissues. A teratogen may act by causing a gene mutation, by chromosome breakage or non-disjunction, by depletion or inhibition of precursors, energy sources, or enzymes, or by causing changes in membrane integrity. These events may result in cell death, decreased cell division, abnormal intracellular interactivity, disruption of cell migration, or mechanical disruption.

Wilson's fourth principle is that the final manifestations of abnormal development are death, malformation, growth retardation, and functional disorders. The teratogenic manifestation may depend on the developmental stage at which exposure occurs.

Wilson's fifth principle is that access of adverse environmental influences to developing tissues depends on the nature of the agent. Some agents are more ter-

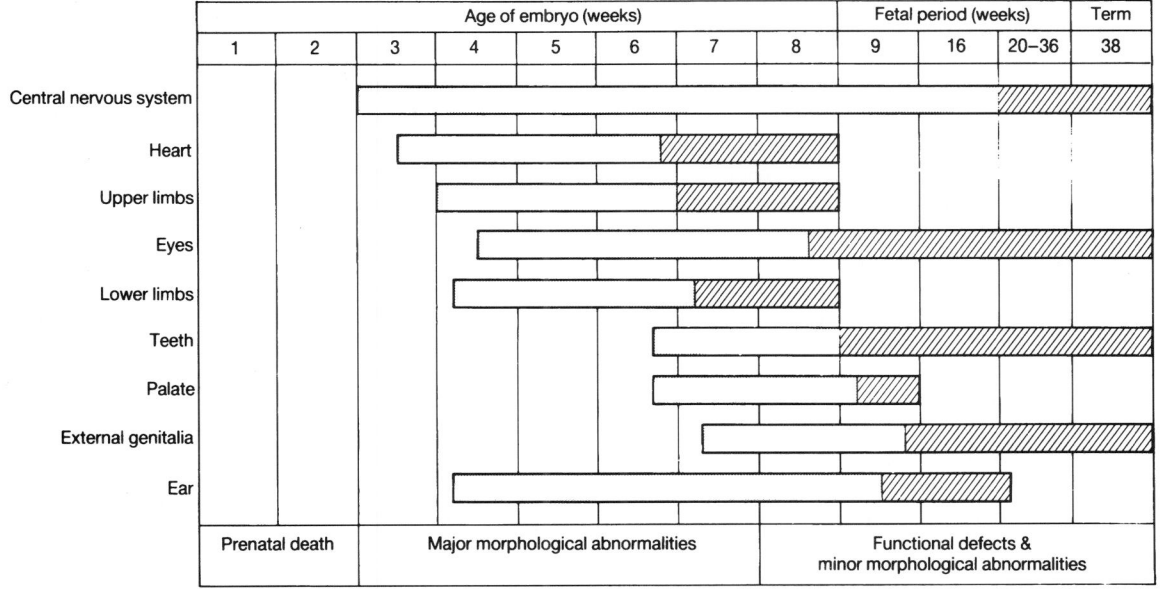

FIGURE 11.1 Vulnerable periods in embryonic and fetal development. During the first 2 weeks (predifferentiation stages) of development, the embryo generally is not susceptible to teratogens and a substance either damages all or most of the cells, resulting in death, or damages only a few cells, allowing the embryo to develop without defects. Periods of greatest sensitivity to teratogens are indicated by the non-hatched portion of the bar; later stages (hatched bar) are less sensitive. (Modified from Moore KL, *The developing human: clinically oriented embryology*. Philadelphia: WB Saunders, 1988: 143, with permission.)

atogenic than others. Moreover, an agent may be teratogenic only in a certain species. A perfect example is thalidomide, which produces *phocomelia* in primates but not in rodents.

Wilson's sixth and final principle is that the degree of abnormal development increases as dosage increases. An embryo may respond to a teratogen in one of three ways. At a low dose, there may be negligible effects or none. At intermediate dosages, organ-specific malformations can result. Finally, at high doses, the effect may be lethal. Route of administration and chronicity of exposure certainly may influence the dosage effect.

Proof of teratogenicity is difficult, but a number of observations may at least implicate a particular agent. First, subjects exposed to the agent should have a particular malformation more often than non-exposed controls. A specific anomaly or pattern of anomalies is consistently associated with the suspected agent. The agent must have been present during the stage of organogenesis when the anomaly should have occurred. The anomaly should be less common prior to the presence of the potential teratogen. Finally, the anomaly can be reproduced in experimental animals.

Human teratogens can be divided into several categories: radiation, illicit drugs, medications, infectious diseases, chemicals, and maternal disease. Each of these will be described in brief.

## Radiation as a teratogen

Ionizing radiation is a wave or particle with energy sufficient to break bonds and create ions (*see* page 169) capable of causing tissue damage (and therefore teratogenesis). Microwaves, because of their lower energy, cannot produce ionization. Neither can magnetic resonance imaging (MRI) because it utilizes radiofrequency waves. Ultrasound, a mechanical wave, is also incapable of producing ionization. Likewise, video display terminals have not been shown to cause increased risk of congenital anomalies.

Ionizing radiation, the first known environmental human teratogen, was identified around 1920. Both the radiation dose and the gestational age at exposure are critical in determining fetal risk. Moreover, there is virtually no fetal risk associated with a diagnostic study that does not include the maternal pelvis (e.g. chest X-ray, head CT scan). For larger maternal exposures, the embryonic exposure may need to be calculated in conjunction with a radiation physicist.

An exposure of 5 rad or less ("rad" is an acronym for *radiation absorbed dose*) causes no measurable risk to the embryo. The threshold for most radiation effects is in the range of 15–20 rad (0.15–0.20 Gy). Exposures to diagnostic radiation of even 20–50 rad represent an extremely low risk to the embryo. However, more than 50 rad of exposure poses a significant fetal risk regardless of the gestational age at exposure.

It is generally felt that significant radiation exposure earlier than 2 weeks after conception causes an "all or none" effect, i.e. abortion or a normal fetus. Exposure from 2 to 18 weeks can cause *intrauterine growth retardation* and *mental retardation*. In addition, exposure during the embryonic period may result in *microcephaly*, *microphthalmia*, and *cataracts*. Beyond 18 weeks' gestation, the fetus may have effects similar to adult *radiation sickness*, i.e. hair loss, bone marrow hypoplasia, and skin lesions. Whether *in utero* exposure to radiation increases the incidence of childhood as well as adult cancers is unclear at this time.

In counseling a pregnant patient after radiation exposure, there is considered to be no medical justification for terminating pregnancy in women exposed to 5 rad or less of ionizing radiation.

## Illicit drugs as teratogens

Unfortunately, abuse of alcohol and drugs (prescribed and illegal) continues to increase, and a significant proportion of the people abusing drugs are reproductive age women. It is estimated that on average a woman ingests between three and four medications during a pregnancy. Many women stop taking medications, drinking alcohol and/or abusing drugs when they realize they are pregnant, but the fetus may have already been exposed at its most critical time.

The prototypic agent is alcohol; it has been estimated that 1–2 per cent of women of childbearing age in north America are alcoholics. The *fetal alcohol syndrome (FAS)* is the most common known non-genetic cause of mental retardation. It affects 1/300 to 1/2000 live births and is present in 30–40 per cent of children of alcoholic mothers. The minimum quantity of alcohol that will result in the FAS is unknown, but the consumption of less than two drinks per day appears to be associated with a lower risk. The effects on the human fetus from episodic or 'binge' drinking are still unclear.

FAS is characterized by pre- and postnatal growth retardation and cardiovascular, limb, and craniofacial defects. The notable craniofacial features are microcephaly, short palpebral fissures, short upturned nose, midface hypoplasia, thin vermilion border, and smooth philtrum. Children have impaired fine and gross motor functions, impaired speech, and significant developmental delay.

*Cocaine* use leads to an increased incidence of major and minor congenital anomalies. These are probably secondary to vascular disruption related to the vasoconstrictive and hypertensive action of the drug. Reported malformations include genitourinary tract anomalies, limb reduction defects, disruptive brain anomalies, and segmental intestinal atresia. In addition, there is an increased risk of placental vascular anomalies, particularly abruptio placentae.

While *tobacco* use is clearly associated with an increase in low-birthweight infants, it has not been shown to be a teratogen. *Marijuana* use has not been associated with any specific congenital malformations. Moreover, the incidence of congenital anomalies does not appear to be increased in women who take methamphetamines during pregnancy. *Heroin* has been shown to cause an increased incidence of intra-uterine growth retardation, neonatal withdrawal, and prenatal death. However, the frequency of anatomical malformations has not been found to be significantly increased in several cohort series. Likewise, methadone does not appear to lead to an increase in congenital malformation. Benzodiazepine, barbiturates, and LSD have not been implicated as obvious teratogens. However, making definitive statements regarding teratogenicity is often difficult, as multiple agents may be used simultaneously, especially with alcohol.

## Medications as teratogens

To detail the fetal risks of widely prescribed medications is beyond the scope of this chapter. Selected agents will be briefly described. The Food and Drug Administration classifies medications into several categories (Table 11.1). This system has some limitations because pharmaceutical manufacturers rate the drugs, not the FDA.

Thalidomide was a sedative/hypnotic used in the early 1960s. The *fetal thalidomide syndrome* was characterized by phocomelia, facial hemangioma, esophageal or duodenal atresia, external ear anomalies, cardiac and renal anomalies.

*Diethylstilbestrol (DES)* is an estrogenic hormone that was used in approximately six million mothers between 1940 and 1971 to prevent reproductive problems such as miscarriage and premature delivery. The drug later was found to be ineffective in preventing these outcomes. Females exposed *in utero* before the 12th week of gestation were first noted to have an increased incidence of rare malignancy, adenocarcinoma of the vagina. Other female genital tract anomalies were also increased, including uterine anomalies, hypoplastic cervix, vaginal septum, and vaginal adenosis. Males exposed to DES *in utero* are also thought to have an increased incidence of genital tract abnormalities including epididymal cysts, hypo-

trophic testis, varicocele, microphallus, and abnormal semen.

*Isotretinoin*, a vitamin A isomer, has proved very useful in the treatment of severe, recalcitrant cystic acne. It has been estimated that 38 per cent of isotretinoin users are women of reproductive age. The teratogenicity of this agent in animals was well documented before its approval for human use. The recently described *retinoic acid embryopathy* consists of multiple craniofacial anomalies including microtia/anotia, cleft palate, micrognathia, and ocular abnormalities. In addition, heart and central nervous system defects as well as spontaneous abortions are increased. The risk of major congenital malformation in exposed pregnancies that do not spontaneously abort is approximately 20 per cent. The critical time of exposure appears to be 2–5 weeks post-conception. By taking the usual daily dose of isotretinoin, a woman is consuming the equivalent of thousands of times the recommended daily allowance of vitamin A. The presumed teratogenic mechanism of isotretinoin and its main metabolite, 4-oxo-isotretinoin, is thought to be from an adverse effect on the initial differentiation and migration of cephalic neural crest cells. There does not appear to be an increased incidence of spontaneous abortions or fetal structural malformations in women who discontinue isotretinoin prior to conception.

Seizure medications are associated with a 2- to 3-fold increased risk of fetal malformations. Notably, however, pregnant women with epilepsy who are not receiving anticonvulsant agents have a risk that is above the baseline 2–3 per cent risk of having a child with a congenital malformation. The prototypic agent is phenytoin, a hydantoin anticonvulsant. The teratogenic effects of phenytoin were recognized in 1964. The *fetal hydantoin syndrome* comprises craniofacial abnormalities, including cleft lip and palate, limb defects, including hypoplasia of distal phalanges and nails, and growth and mental deficiency. Recently, carbamazepine has been found to cause a similar spectrum of anomalies. Both anticonvulsants are metabolized using the epoxide hydrolase enzyme to degrade the active metabolite. Studies have shown that decreased epoxide hydrolase enzyme activity below 30 per cent is associated with a significantly increased incidence of fetal hydantoin syndrome. Decreased enzyme activity is inherited as an autosomal recessive trait and may be measured in fibroblasts or amniocytes. Preconception determination of the parents' epoxide hydrolase enzyme activity levels may allow high-risk couples to be identified. In this situation the woman may be switched to another anticonvulsant or prenatal diagnosis may be offered.

*Valproic acid* and its salt form, sodium valproate, are associated with a 1–2 per cent incidence of neural tube defects if used between 17 and 30 days after fertilization. No cases of anencephaly, however, have been associated with its use. Various other anomalies have been reported, including craniofacial, urogenital, cardiac, and skeletal abnormalities.

TABLE 11.1 Food and Drug Administration drug classifications

| Category A: | Controlled studies in humans have demonstrated no fetal risk |
|---|---|
| Category B: | Either animal studies indicate there are no fetal risks and there are no human studies, OR adverse effects have been demonstrated in animals, but not in well-controlled human studies |
| Category C: | No adequate studies are available |
| Category D: | Evidence of fetal risk, but benefits outweigh risk |
| Category X: | Proven fetal risk and contraindicated during pregnancy |

*Coumadin* derivatives are oral anticoagulants used for treatment and prophylaxis of thromboembolism. First-trimester use of coumadin derivatives may result in an embryopathy (*fetal warfarin syndrome*) in 15–25 per cent of exposed fetuses. The common characteristics are nasal hypoplasia and stippled vertebral and femoral epiphyses. Other features that may be present include ocular defects, limb hypoplasia, and mental retardation. The critical period of exposure seems to be 6–9 weeks of gestation. Interestingly, coumadin agents are both teratogenic and fetotoxic.

After years of debate, it is generally felt that first-trimester oral contraceptive exposure does not cause an increased incidence of cardiovascular, central nervous system, or limb defects. In contrast, some synthetic progestogens may cause masculinization of the female infant.

## Infections as teratogens

The fetus is protected from many infections by the maternal immune system and placenta. However, it is possible for some agents to infect the fetus, including viruses, bacteria, spirochetes and parasites. Intrauterine infection may have devastating effects on the developing fetus. The effects of fetal infection, which usually occurs by hematogenous transplacental spread, are diverse and may result in a spectrum of problems, including resorption and death of the embryo, intrauterine growth retardation, and congenital anomalies.

*Rubella* virus is transmitted *in utero* during the course of primary maternal infection. Approximately 10 per cent of reproductive age women do not have antibody to rubella and are therefore at risk for infection. The risk of fetal damage following a rubella infection depends on the timing of the infection: almost 50 per cent of children with a history of maternal rubella infection in the first month of pregnancy have significant and permanent damage. The incidence decreases to 22 per cent with rubella infection in the second month of pregnancy, 10 per cent in the third month, and 6 per cent in the fourth and fifth months. Classic congenital rubella is diagnosed by the presence of cataracts, congenital glaucoma, congenital heart disease, radiolucent bone lesions, hepatosplenomegaly, petechiae, and thrombocytopenia. The most frequent abnormalities are deafness and heart disease.

*Cytomegalovirus (CMV)*, a herpes virus, occurs as a primary infection in approximately 1–2 per cent of pregnant women. Higher CMV infection rates are reported among child daycare workers. The risk of fetal infection is approximately equal for primary and recurrent maternal infections. However, almost all fetal damage is related to a primary maternal infection. Approximately 40 per cent of women who have documented primary infection transmit the infection to their fetuses. However, only 10–15 per cent of these infected infants have clinically apparent disease. The

most frequently seen permanent damage includes deafness and mental retardation. More severe disease is quite rare and includes microphthalmia, microcephaly, hydrocephaly, chorioretinitis, and hepatosplenomegaly.

*Varicella*, or chicken pox, an acute, highly contagious disease, most commonly occurs in childhood. Approximately 95 per cent of adult women are immune to varicella because of infection in childhood. The risk of congenital varicella infection is thought to be approximately 1–2 per cent following maternal varicella infection during the first or second trimester. A child with congenital damage due to maternal infection during the first 5 months of pregnancy may have a variety of abnormalities, including low birthweight, skin lesions, eye abnormalities, limb hypoplasia, cortical atrophy, mental retardation, and early childhood death. The mechanism of these anomalies appears to be the development of *in utero* herpes zoster with an associated encephalitis.

There has been an epidemic of *syphilis* in the United States since 1985, with a significant proportion of the cases being in reproductive age women. The number of cases of congenital syphilis reported to the Centers for Disease Control has also risen dramatically, in part due to changes in the reporting criteria but also because of a true rise in the incidence. Risk of damage to the fetus depends on the gestational age when the infection occurs and the time elapsed before maternal treatment. The formation of immune complexes is thought to play a role in the teratogenic effects of the infection, so infection that is treated before 18 weeks' gestation is unlikely to be associated with any fetal malformations. Early congenital syphilis is characterized by prematurity, hydrops, and an enlarged placenta. The newborn may have hepatosplenomegaly, lymphadenopathy, hematological abnormalities, mucocutaneous manifestations, bony lesions, and chorioretinitis. Late congenital syphilis, diagnosed in children over 2 years old, may present with craniofacial anomalies including Hutchinson teeth, mulberry molars, saddle nose, eighth nerve deafness, skin lesions called rhagades, and central nervous system abnormalities including mental retardation, hydrocephalus, convulsions, and paresis.

*Toxoplasmosis* is caused by a protozoan parasite. Maternal toxoplasmosis may be asymptomatic or present as a mild mononucleosis-like illness. If the pregnant woman acquires the infection in the first trimester, the infection is transmitted to the fetus approximately 15 per cent of the time. This rate increases to 25 per cent in the second trimester, and 60 per cent in the third trimester. Manifestations of congenital toxoplasmosis are likely to be more severe when maternal infection is acquired early. The clinical spectrum of toxoplasmosis in the newborn is characteristic but not specific, and may include chorioretinitis, convulsions, jaundice, hydrocephaly or microcephaly, fever, hepatomegaly, lymphadenopathy, optic abnormalities, rash and pneumonia. Chorioretinitis is the most common single manifestation.

*Herpes simplex virus (HSV)* infection in the neonate is usually devastating. Most newborn infections are acquired intrapartum by direct fetal contact with the infected maternal genital secretions. Although extremely rare, more than a dozen cases have been reported in which maternal herpes infections early in pregnancy resulted in severe fetal consequences. These included skin lesions, chorioretinitis, microcephaly, hydrocephaly, and microphthalmia. Data suggesting a higher rate of spontaneous abortions in women with genital HSV provide indirect evidence that intrauterine infection from HSV may occur. Because the risk of *in utero* transmission is so small, therapeutic abortion or maternal treatment is not recommended or indicated at present.

## Chemicals as teratogens

Exposure to *organic mercury compounds* is uncommon but is still possible, primarily through the consumption of contaminated fish. Methyl mercury easily crosses the placenta and accumulates in embryonic and fetal tissues, particularly the brain. While obvious structural anomalies are not caused by antenatal exposure to mercury, significant neurological abnormalities may result.

The relationship between antenatal exposure to *anesthetic gases* and reproductive risk has been debated. Chronic first-trimester exposure (e.g. occupational) may increase the risk of spontaneous abortion. Although no recognizable pattern of malformation has been found following maternal exposure to anesthetic gases, some investigations have found an increased rate of all birth defects in infants born to exposed parents. General anesthesia during early pregnancy does not appear to be teratogenic; several large studies have found no increase in the risk of congenital malformations.

## Maternal disease as a teratogen

*Infants of insulin-dependent diabetic mothers (IDM)* have a 2 to 4-fold increased incidence of major malformations. A derangement in maternal metabolism, primarily maternal hyperglycemia, is the proposed teratogenic mechanism. The congenital defect thought to be most characteristic of diabetic embryopathy is sacral agenesis or caudal dysplasia. This anomaly is found 200–400 times more often in offspring of women with diabetes than in offspring of women without diabetes. Central nervous system abnormalities including neural tube defects and holoprosencephaly are increased 10-fold. In addition, cardiac anomalies, especially ventricular septal defects and complex lesions such as transposition of the great arteries, are increased 5-fold. Moreover, women whose diabetes is less well controlled are at higher risk for spontaneous abortion and infants with malformations.

Pregnancy in an untreated mother with *phenylketonuria (PKU)* exposes the fetus to a very high level of phenylalanine and its derivatives. A high percentage of offspring from women with high phenylalanine levels have mental retardation, growth retardation, and congenital anomalies including microcephaly, congenital heart defects, vertebral anomalies, and craniofacial features resembling the fetal alcohol syndrome. Importantly, infants whose mothers follow a strict low-phenylalanine diet beginning before conception and whose mothers maintain blood phenylalanine levels less than 10 mg/dL appear to exhibit no increased incidence of congenital malformations.

An association between neural tube defects (NTD) and dietary deficiencies was supported by an increased incidence of NTD following the famine in Holland in 1944–45 and food shortages in Germany after World War II, as well as animal studies. Recent studies have demonstrated a significant decrease in the incidence of NTD in women on folic acid supplementation. In the future there will need to be studies examining the relationship between the incidence of congenital malformations and the nutritional status of the mother.

## SELECTED READING

Beckman DA, Brent RL. Mechanisms of teratogenesis. *Ann Rev Pharmacol Toxicol* 1984; 24: 483.

Briggs GG, Freeman RK, Yaffe SJ. *Drugs in pregnancy and lactation*, 3rd edn. Baltimore: William & Wilkins, 1990.

Grose C, Itani O, Weiner CP. Prenatal diagnosis of fetal infection: advances from amniocentesis to cordocentesis – congenital toxoplasmosis, rubella, cytomegalovirus, varicella virus, parvovirus and human immunodeficiency virus. *Pediatr Infect Dis J* 1989; 8: 459.

Jones KL. *Smith's recognizable patterns of human malformation*, 4th edn. Philadelphia: WB Saunders, 1988.

Moore KL. *The developing human*, 4th edn. Philadelphia: WB Saunders, 1988.

Remington JS, Klein JO. *Infectious diseases of the fetus and newborn infant*, 3rd edn. Philadelphia: WB Saunders, 1990.

# 12

# Physiology and Pathophysiology of Fetal Sexual Differentiation

Nathalie Josso

Sex differentiation can be defined as the series of events which leads to the development of male or female characteristics in various organs. The gonads, internal genital tract and external genital organs successively become sex-oriented during fetal life; gender identity, brain sex and secondary sex attributes differentiate after birth.

Sex differentiation is a complex physiological process, governed by coordinated genetic and hormonal factors operating in an asymmetrical manner. In mammals, the testis imposes masculinity on structures which are programmed to become female. In the absence of testicular hormones, Müllerian ducts persist and develop into uterus and tubes, Wolffian derivatives degenerate and do not masculinize. Thus, the binary switch that determines the subsequent steps is the commitment of the primitive gonads to develop either as testes or ovaries: the development of the full sexual phenotype being merely a consequence of that initial decision.

## THE HUMAN TESTIS-DETERMINING GENE (*TDF*)

In most vertebrate species, sex differentiation is determined by genetic material present in the heterogametic sex. Sex determination in humans is governed by gene(s) lying on the Y chromosome; the number of accompanying X chromosomes is irrelevant, as shown by the male phenotype of XXY individuals with *Klinefelter syndrome*. Embryos lacking a Y chromosome, whether 46,XX or 45,X, develop ovaries at least initially, unless DNA endowed with testis-determining activity has been transferred to another chromosome, thus giving rise to XX male progeny, as discussed below.

The Y chromosome contains a pseudoautosomal region of approximately 2600 kb, which participates in homologous recombination with the X chromosome at meiosis (Fig. 12.1), ensuring that correct segregation

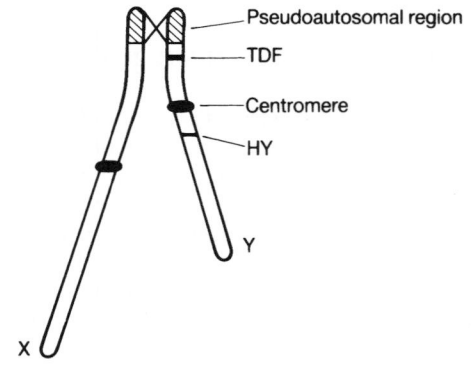

FIGURE 12.1 Diagram of sex chromosomes, showing the pseudoautosomal pairing region and the location of the testis-determining gene (TDF). The minor transplantation antigen HY, a former candidate for the title, now has been mapped to the Y chromosome long arm.

of sex chromosomes will occur. Loci proximal to the pseudoautosomal boundary normally abstain from exchange with the X chromosome and exhibit patrilineal inheritance. The location of the testis-determining gene (*TDF*) in the non-recombining, Y-specific, region is essential for the chromosomal basis of sex determination. Claims of several Y-located genes to the TDF title have been examined by analyzing the DNA of sex-reversed patients. By definition, the *TDF* gene can be located only in those Y-specific sequences which are invariably present in XX males and invariably absent in XY women. It has been mapped to the most distal part of the Y chromosome short arm, only 5 kb from the pseudoautosomal boundary, and has been named SRY for Sex-determining Region Y. Earlier, a more proximally located gene, *ZFY* (Fig. 12.2), was excluded as the candidate *TDF* because it was shown to be absent in several XX males whose DNA did contain material originating from the Y pseudoautosomal boundary. The *SRY* gene is Y-specific among a wide range of mammals and encodes a testis-specific transcript. SRY-mediated testicular development is blocked if a locus on the short arm of the X chromosome, named DSS for Dosage-Sensitive Sex reversal, is duplicated or if *SOX9*, a gene on chromosome 17, is defective.

## GONADAL SEX DIFFERENTIATION

### Testis differentiation

In the mammalian fetus, the gonadal primordium is represented by the gonadal ridge, a thickening of the celomic epithelium covering the anterior surface of the mesonephros, which is progressively colonized by primordial germ cells traveling from the stalk of the allantois through the mesentery and the wall of the fetal gut. The first recognizable event of testicular differentiation, which occurs at 6 weeks in the human fetus, is the development of a new cell type, the primordial Sertoli cell. Sertoli cells soon aggregate to form seminiferous tubules in which germ cells become enclosed. Germ cells in extragonadal locations, such as the adre-

nal, may survive and differentiate into oocytes. XY oocytes have also been observed in XX/XY female mice, suggesting that the differentiation potential of the mammalian germ cells is predominantly female, and is lost only in a testicular environment, for reasons which remain to be identified. In contrast, sexual differentiation of the gonad is not dependent upon the presence or karyotype of germ cells.

Fetal Sertoli cells are large, clear cells, with abundant cytoplasm containing vesicles of rough endoplasmic reticulum. In these is stored, prior to secretion, a glycoprotein, anti-Müllerian hormone (AMH) (also called Müllerian inhibiting substance, MIS), which, as shown by the classical experiments of Alfred Jost, is responsible for inhibition of the development of the Müllerian ducts in male fetuses. AMH is the first cognate protein produced by the fetal testis and is expressed immediately after testicular differentiation. Leydig cells differentiate somewhat later, at 8 weeks' gestation in the human fetus. Their number increases dramatically until 12–14 weeks, at which time they begin to degenerate. At birth, very few remain in the interstitial tissue. Fetal Leydig cells produce testosterone, the hormone responsible for the virilization of Wolffian derivatives, urogenital sinus and external genital organs. Initiation of testosterone secretion is constitutive but stimulation by luteinizing gonadotrophin (either chorionic gonadotrophin or fetal pituitary LH) is necessary for sustained production.

### Ovarian differentiation

Slower than the testis to differentiate initially, the fetal ovary eventually reaches a more advanced stage of maturation. Up to the second month of gestation, ovogonia mix freely with somatic cells in the gonadal blastema. Later, growth of connective tissue sheets from the medulla outwards delineates ovigerous cords, containing actively dividing ovogonia, which tend to accumulate near the ovarian surface. At 12–13 weeks, some oogonia, located in the deepest layer of the cortex, have entered meiotic prophase. Maturation progresses

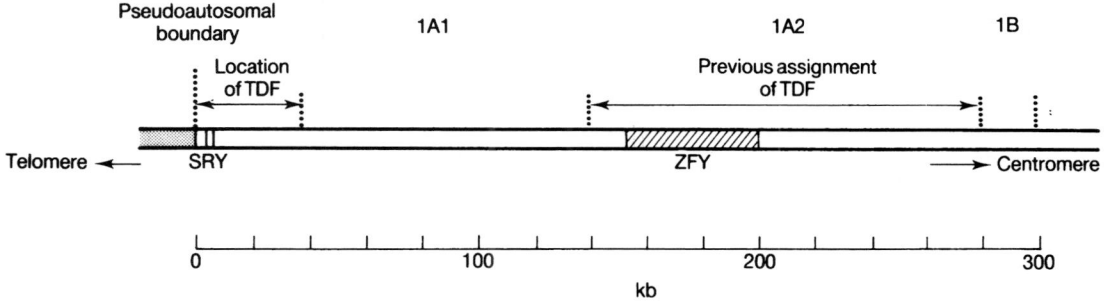

FIGURE 12.2 Mapping of TDF: respective localization of SRY and ZFY on the short arm of the Y chromosome. 1A1, 1A2 and 1B represent sections of the Y chromosome identified by probe hybridization. (Reproduced with permission from Hawkins JR, Sinclair AH. *Semin Dev Biol* 1991; 2: 251.)

from the center of the gonad towards the periphery, until, at approximately 7 months' gestation, all germ cells have entered or completed the meiotic prophase, and mitotic divisions are no longer seen. In parallel, the germ cell pool is severely depleted by waves of degeneration, which preferentially affect cells undergoing mitotic divisions or in the meiotic prophase. Germ cells enclosed in follicles are relatively protected from degeneration.

Primordial follicles can be recognized by 17 weeks, Graafian follicles by 26 weeks. Fetal granulosa cells produce estrogen at the same developmental stage at which fetal testes produce testosterone, suggesting that the acquisition of the enzymatic activities that allow specific endocrine function by these two tissues may be regulated by similar factors during embryonic development. In contrast, ovarian production of AMH can be demonstrated only after birth.

Normal ovarian development requires the presence of two X chromosomes. Thus, in both classical 45,X and in variant forms of *Turner syndrome* such as XXpi or XXqi, germ cells degenerate, leading to fibrous degeneration of the ovaries. The somatic abnormalities of Turner syndrome are thought to be the result of monosomy for a gene(s) common to the X and Y chromosome, residing on Yp and perhaps on Xq, with the reservation that efforts to map the Turner phenotype on the X chromosome have failed to yield a consistent localization.

## SOMATIC MASCULINIZATION

In contrast to the recent controversies concerning gonadal sex determination, the concepts regarding sex differentiation of the genital tract have undergone no major change since the now classic contribution of Alfred Jost, who showed that masculinization must be actively imposed upon the genital tract by the hormonal secretions of the fetal testis (Fig. 12.3). Genital primordia can be masculinized only during a short, discrete developmental period, the "critical stage," which differs for each element of the genital tract.

## Müllerian regression: anti-Müllerian hormone (AMH)

Shortly after gonadal differentiation, the genital tract of male or female fetuses consists of unipotential Wolffian and Müllerian ducts, and bipotential urogenital sinus and external genital primordia. Müllerian regression is the first sign of male differentiation of the genital tract. In the human fetus, the first signs of regression appear in embryos at 8 weeks and regression is more or less complete at 10–12 weeks. Female Müllerian ducts cease to respond to AMH by 8 weeks.

Müllerian regression is mediated by AMH, a 145 000-kD glycoprotein dimer synthesized by imma-

ture Sertoli cells under the influence of steroidogenic factor 1, very soon after testicular differentiation. Serum concentrations remain high until approximately 2 years of age, and then progressively decrease to become more or less undetectable after puberty. AMH, also called Müllerian-inhibiting substance (MIS) or factor (MIF), is also produced by postnatal granulosa cells, although the function of ovarian AMH has not yet been identified. The 2.8-kb gene has been cloned and mapped to chromosome 19. It consists of five exons, the last one exhibiting a 30 per cent homology with members of a superfamily of dimeric proteins involved in growth and differentiation, the TGFβ family. The receptor for AMH, like those of other members of the TGFβ family, is a serine/threonine kinase with a single transmembrane domain: it has been mapped to chromosome 12 and is expressed around the Müllerian duct and in gonads of both sexes.

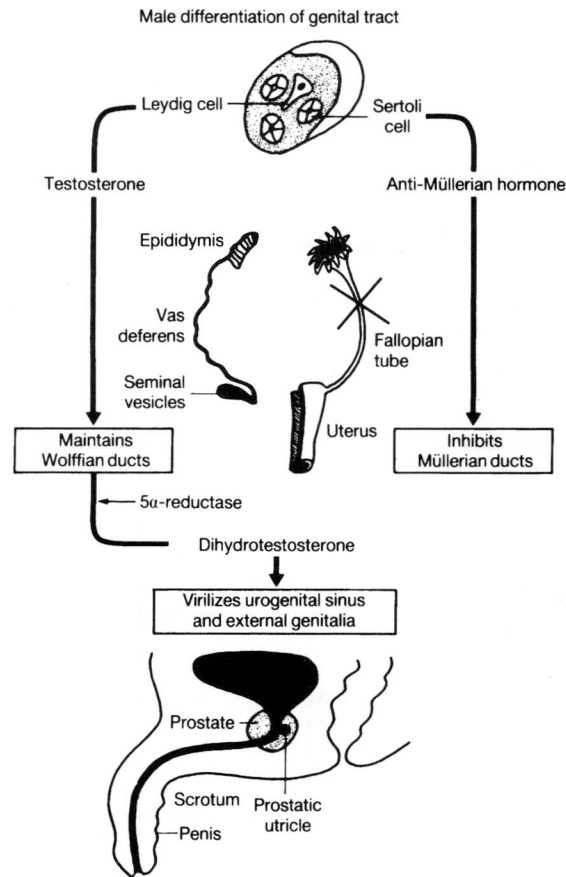

FIGURE 12.3 Cartoon of male sex differentiation. Testosterone, produced by fetal Leydig cells, maintains Wolffian ducts and, after reduction to dihydrotestosterone, virilizes the urogenital sinus and the external genital organs. Anti-Müllerian hormone inhibits the development of Müllerian ducts. (Reproduced with permission from Josso N, ed. *The intersex child*. Basel: Karger, 1981: 6.)

AMH can now be measured in human serum and has clinical usefulness as a marker of immature testicular function. Prior stimulation by gonadotrophins is not necessary. In XY babies in whom the gonads cannot be palpated, AMH measurement can discriminate between *anorchia* and *bilateral cryptorchidism*. In sexually ambiguous XX children, detection of circulating AMH rules out the diagnosis of *female pseudohermaphroditism* in favor of true *hermaphroditism*. The reverse, however, is not true, because dysgenetic testicular tissue may produce little or no AMH. Serum AMH concentrations usually correlate relatively well with Müllerian anatomical status but exceptions are possible, since presence or absence of Müllerian derivatives reflect the biological activity of AMH at 8 weeks' gestation, while serum AMH is a marker of Sertoli cell function at the time of investigation. Production of AMH is maintained throughout childhood and is curtailed by testosterone at the time of puberty, except in androgen-insensitive patients, whose serum AMH concentrations may rise to very high levels after puberty and also during the first semester of life.

## Development of Wolffian derivatives, masculinization of external genitalia and testicular descent

Wolffian ducts, originally the excretory canals of the primitive kidney, become incorporated into the genital tract, developing into the vasa deferentia, epididymes and seminal vesicles. Prostatic buds develop around the opening of the ducts at approximately 10–11 weeks of age while fusion of outgrowths of the urogenital sinus forms the prostatic utricle, the male equivalent of the vagina. Testosterone, not AMH, prevents the downgrowth of the vaginal rudiment and the acquisition of a separate perineal opening. In severely masculinized *female pseudohermaphrodites*, a short vaginal canal communicating with the uterus and tubes contacts the wall of the urethra just beneath the bladder neck and may be difficult to opacify radiologically. In contrast, the blind vaginal pouch of *androgen-insensitive male pseudohermaphrodites* has a separate perineal opening (Fig. 12.4). Only the upper part of the vagina is of Müllerian origin and responds to AMH and not testosterone.

At approximately 10 weeks' gestation, the genital tubercle elongates and urethral folds fuse over the urethral groove, leading to formation of the scrotum and penile urethra. Male anatomical development is completed at approximately 90 days of gestation, but at that time no appreciable size difference exists between the penis and clitoris. Penile growth occurs between 20 weeks and term, at a time when paradoxically, serum testosterone concentration is declining.

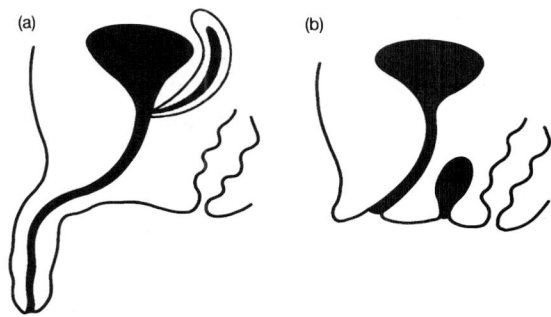

FIGURE 12.4 Dissociation between uterine (Müllerian) and vaginal development in intersexuality. (a) Female pseudohermaphroditism with complete virilization of the external genitalia and urogenital sinus for example in severe 21-hydroxylase deficiency: vaginal development has been repressed and the uterus contacts the posterior urethra just beneath the bladder neck. (b) Male pseudohermaphroditism due to complete androgen insensitivity: Müllerian ducts have regressed, but the vagina has developed normally and acquired a perineal opening. It may be short, due to the fact that the upper part of the vagina is of Müllerian origin.

Testicular descent takes place in two phases: transabdominal, which brings the testis to the internal inguinal ring by 12 weeks, and passage through the inguinal canal, which occurs between 7 months and term. The hormonal control of testicular descent is not well understood; androgens and gonadotrophins are apparently implicated only in the transinguinal phase. Testicular insufficiency is often associated with *cryptorchidism*, particularly in cases where Müllerian regression has not occurred. This could be partly due to mechanical causes, since Müllerian derivatives are tightly attached to the testis and may prevent it from reaching the scrotum.

## Testosterone: biosynthesis, 5α-reduction and binding to the androgen receptor

Except for Müllerian regression, male sex differentiation is mediated by androgens produced by fetal Leydig cells from 8 weeks onwards. Serum testosterone peaks at approximately 12–14 weeks, and then progressively falls, so that in late pregnancy, testosterone concentration is not significantly different in males and females (Fig. 12.5). Androgen production by the fetal Leydig cell is controlled initially by placental hCG (*see* page 207), but fetal pituitary gonadotrophins take over during late fetal life, explaining why micropenis and cryptorchidism are frequently observed in *congenital hypopituitarism*. A protein involved in cholesterol transport and five steroidogenic enzymes are needed for the biosynthesis of testosterone from cholesterol (Fig. 12.6). Because the same enzymes operate also in the adrenal, male pseudohermaphroditism due to steroidogenesis defects is often associated with *congenital adrenal hyperplasia* (*see* page 508).

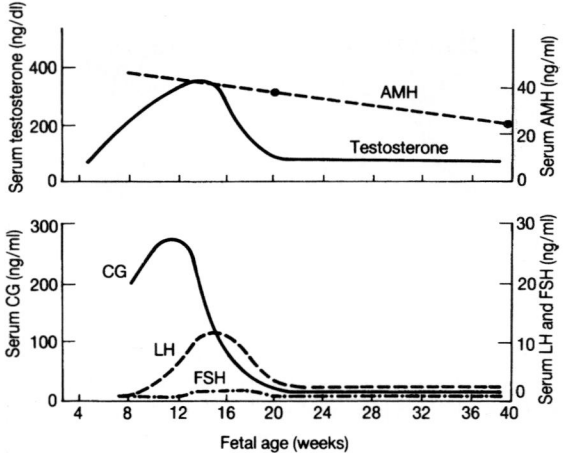

FIGURE 12.5 Ontogeny of AMH, testosterone and gonadotrophins in human fetal serum. Data for AMH before 20 weeks are extrapolated from measurements performed in fetal bovine serum, which have shown high values. (Values at 20 and 40 weeks are taken from Josso N, Lamarre I, Picard JY, *et al.*, Anti-Müllerian hormone in early human development. *Early Hum Dev* 1993; 33: 91. Values for other hormones are taken from Reyes FI, Winter JSD, Faiman C. In: *Diabetes and other endocrine disorders during pregnancy and in the newborn*. New York: Alan Liss, 1976: 83.)

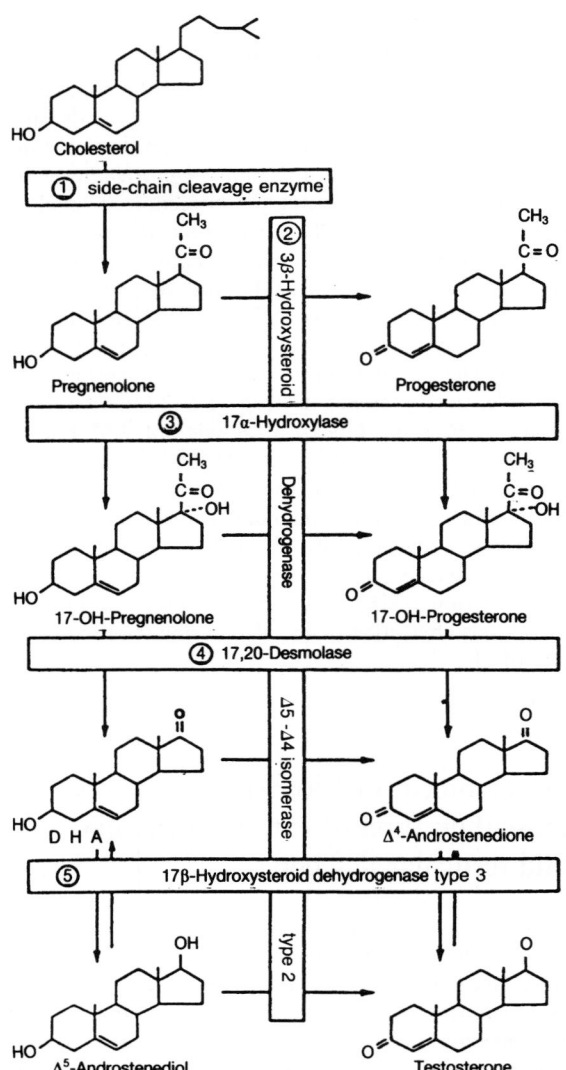

FIGURE 12.6 Enzymes necessary for testosterone biosynthesis. (Modified from Forest MG. In: Josso N, ed. *The intersex child*. Basel: Karger, 1981: 133, with permission.)

Testosterone exerts its biological activity by binding to an X-linked receptor molecule. The receptor has much greater affinity for the reduced derivative of testosterone, dihydrotestosterone, than for testosterone itself. Therefore, in tissues such as the urogenital sinus and external genitalia, containing 5α-reductase activity which enables them to generate dihydrotestosterone, the latter is the active androgen. Wolffian ducts, at the time of sex differentiation, do not yet express 5α-reductase activity, and consequently are the only fetal organs controlled by testosterone itself. This is perhaps the reason why they respond only to the high testosterone concentrations achieved by local uptake in the vicinity of the testis, but cannot be maintained by circulating androgen.

The gene coding for the androgen receptor is located on the X chromosome between the centromere and q13; it belongs to the superfamily of steroid receptors (Fig. 12.7). The human androgen receptor gene,

which spans a minimum of 54 kb, is divided into eight exons. Exons 2 and 3 code for the DNA-binding domain which consists of two zinc finger domains that are important for recognition and binding of promoter elements of androgen-responsive genes.

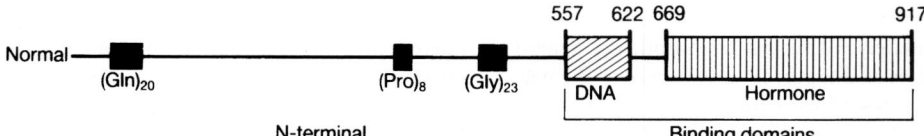

FIGURE 12.7 Structure of the androgen receptor protein. Note the stretches of repeated glutamines, prolines and glycines in the first exon and the separate hormone and DNA-binding domains. (Modified from Marcelli M, Tilley WD, Wilson CM, *et al.*, Definition of the human androgen receptor gene structure permits the identification of mutations that cause androgen resistance: premature termination of the receptor protein at amino acid residue 588 causes complete androgen resistance. *Mol Endocrinol* 1990; 4: 105, with permission.)

Mutations in this region have been found in patients with the so-called "receptor-positive" form of *androgen insensitivity syndrome*, because binding of dihydrotestosterone is not affected. Most mutations, however, have been described in exons 4–8, which code for the steroid hormone-binding domain. Deletions and point mutations in this region have been recognized in patients suffering from "receptor-negative" androgen insensitivity syndrome. The N-terminal part of the androgen receptor, encoded by the first exon, is important for transcriptional activation. In contrast to estrogen and progesterone receptors, which reside in the nucleus even in the absence of ligand-binding, nuclear translocation of the androgen receptor is promoted by androgen. The nuclear targeting signal is located within the hinge region between the DNA and steroid-binding domains.

## Female development

Female sex differentiation appears to lag behind male organogenesis, although sex determination – defined by the "critical period" of sensitivity of genital primordia to testicular hormones – occurs at the same time in males and females. In the female, Müllerian ducts persist to form Fallopian tubes, uterus and upper part of the vagina, Wolffian ducts degenerate, and the vagina differentiates at the level of the Müllerian tubercle, between the openings of the Wolffian ducts where the prostatic utricle forms in males. The main difference between male and female organogenesis of the urogenital sinus lies in the downgrowth of the vagina. Whereas in males, the prostatic utricle opens just beneath the neck of the bladder, in females, the lower end of the vagina slides down the posterior wall of the urethra to acquire a separate opening on the body surface.

Feminization of the external genitalia begins by the formation of the dorsal commissure, between the labio-scrotal swellings, which give rise to the labia majora. The urethral folds do not fuse and become the labia minora; the stunted phallus develops into the clitoris.

All these steps are constitutive and occur in the absence of hormonal stimulation of any kind. Although the fetal ovary does produce estrogens, female hormones do not promote female development. A female karyotype does not protect against masculinization by testicular hormones. Female fetuses with *congenital adrenal hyperplasia* may undergo total masculinization of the external genital organs, including formation of a penile urethra. However, in the absence of locally secreted testosterone, no Wolffian ducts differentiate, for reasons discussed above. Under normal conditions, human females are never exposed to AMH during fetal life. However, AMH-induced Müllerian regression has been described in bovine freemartins united by placental anastomoses to a male co-twin.

## Brain sex

The brain controls the endocrine system through the hypothalamus and pituitary gland. Anatomical differences between male and female brains have been detected in the anterior hypothalamus, thought to control sexual orientation, the anterior commissure, and the corpus callosum, which could be involved in cognition and patterns of lateralization. From an endocrine perspective, sexual dimorphism lies essentially in the control of gonadotrophin secretion. Already in the perinatal period, gonadotrophin levels differ between males and females, FSH levels being higher in the latter. At puberty, a cyclic LH preovulatory surge characterizes female reproductive function. In rodents, the ability of the female hypothalamus to release LHRH cyclically can be definitively destroyed by exposure to androgens during a critical period, which ends 5 days after birth; conversely, males castrated during the critical period, but not later, do exhibit a cyclic pattern of LH release at puberty. However, in contrast to rodents, androgen sex imprinting of the fetal hypothalamus cannot be demonstrated in either humans or subhuman primates: females exposed to androgens during fetal life because of *congenital adrenal hyperplasia* can ovulate at puberty if treated properly.

## Gender identity

Establishment of sexual identity occurs in several stages. The awareness of being either male or female may be evident as early as 13 months of age. Sex-typed behavior is clearly present at 3 years of age or earlier while the orientation of erotic interest emerges with pubertal maturation.

The question of the relative influence of hormonal and environmental factors in the determination of gender identity has been heavily debated. It was initially proposed that gender identity was ruled by the sex of rearing and irreversibly established after 3 years of age; however, recent evidence supports the conclusion that in *male pseudohermaphrodites* unambiguously raised as girls, pubertal masculinization may override social pressure and induce the individual to adopt a male gender role. Examples of successful "sex-reversal" are rare, however, and every effort should be made to ensure that, in sexually ambiguous children, the sex of rearing chosen in the neonatal period will fit anatomical and endocrine status in adulthood.

The unraveling, albeit incomplete, of the genetic and hormonal mechanisms of normal sex differentiation allows considerable insight into the nature of clinical disorders of sex differentiation. The demonstration that the fetal testis produces two discrete hormones, testosterone and AMH, is central to our understanding of sexual ambiguity and gonadal dysgenesis. Normally, genetic, gonadal and somatic sex are coherent, either all male or all female. Inadequate sex differentiation at any level, or discrepancy between its various elements, results in sex ambiguity.

## Testes without a Y chromosome: XX males and true hermaphrodites

As discussed above, *SRY*, the candidate testis-determining gene, not the Y chromosome *per se*, is responsible for testicular differentiation. Transfer of *SRY* to an X chromosome during paternal meiosis is facilitated by the closeness of *SRY* to the pseudoautosomal boundary (Fig. 12.8) and results in testicular development in XX individuals. Moreover, XX maleness cannot always be explained by transfer of Y-related DNA. Approximately 30 per cent of XX males type Y-negative when their DNA is probed with Y-specific probes. These patients are often incompletely masculinized and other *XX males* or *true hermaphrodites* can be traced in the family. Males developing in the absence of *SRY*, could harbor activating mutations in "downstream" autosomal gene(s) regulated by the *SRY* gene product. It also has been suggested that *SRY* could act by repressing the function of a negative regulator of testicular development and that testicular development in the absence of *SRY* could be due to "loss of function" mutations of this putative negative regulator.

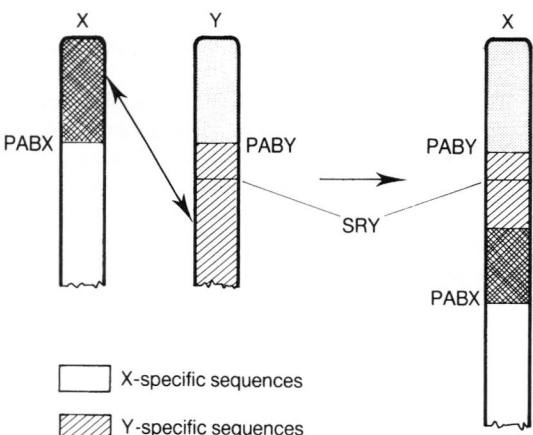

□ X-specific sequences
▨ Y-specific sequences

FIGURE 12.8 Abnormal X/Y interchange, leading to the generation of XX maleness. Y-specific sequences close to the pseudoautosomal boundary and containing *SRY* have been involved in crossing over between the X and Y chromosomes during paternal meiosis. The resulting X chromosome carries the *SRY* gene and will yield male offspring. PABX and PABY: pseudoautosomal boundary from X and Y chromosomes, respectively. (Modified from Weissenbach J, Petit C. *Médecine Sciences* 1990; 6: 785, with permission.)

## Masculinization without testes: anorchia and female pseudohermaphroditism

Masculinization of XY individuals with no testicular tissue is due to testicular degeneration during fetal life. The clinical picture in *anorchia* depends upon the timing of gonadal demise. If testes degenerate before 8 fetal weeks, the phenotype is usually female except for the absence of Müllerian derivatives. XY individuals with a female phenotype including a uterus and tubes are classified under the term *pure gonadal dysgenesis* because there is no evidence that testicular tissue developed at any time. If testicular degeneration occurs between 9 and 14 weeks' gestation, the clinical picture is that of *male pseudohermaphroditism*, with variable degrees of scrotal fusion and vaginal development. After 14 weeks, the masculine phenotype is complete, but micropenis is usually present (*congenital anorchia*).

*Female XX pseudohermaphrodites*, with sex ambiguity in the presence of normal ovaries, always possess a normal uterus and tubes, since in the fetus, AMH is made exclusively by testicular tissue, which they lack by definition. Masculinization is due to aggression by exogenous androgens, usually of adrenal origin, as in the various forms of *congenital adrenal hyperplasia*. Deficiency of 21-hydroxylase or other steroidogenic enzymes leads to enhanced androgen secretion, which can produce complete masculinization of the external genitalia. Bilateral cryptorchidism, even without hypospadias, should always be considered with suspicion. Testosterone-dependent masculinization is also reflected in the inhibition of lower vaginal development: the deeper the masculinization, the higher the opening of the vagina in the urogenital sinus. However, not all cases of *female pseudohermaphroditism* are due to testosterone overproduction: malformations, which usually also involve neighboring organs such as the kidney, uterus and terminal gut, may lead to clitoral hypertrophy and labial fusion which mimics the effect of androgens.

## Incompetent testes: male pseudohermaphroditism

Failure of testicular tissue to achieve complete masculinization, *male pseudohermaphroditism*, results from many different causes, most associated with an XY karyotype or mosaic cell line. When both AMH and testosterone-dependent steps of sex differentiation are impaired, in other words when persistence of Müllerian derivatives is associated with incomplete masculinization of the external genitalia and urogenital sinus, testicular dysgenesis is necessarily involved, since no biochemical cause can explain combined defects in the production or action of a steroid such as testosterone and a glycoprotein such as AMH. The frequent occurrence of testicular degeneration in so-called "*dysgenetic male pseudohermaphroditism*," characterized by the presence of Müllerian ducts, is therefore not surprising. *True hermaphrodites* have a similar phenotype; their lack of masculinization is due to an insufficient amount of testicular tissue, and also to severe testicular dysgenesis.

When Müllerian regression has occurred normally, biochemical defects affecting testosterone synthesis or peripheral effect should be sought (Table 12.1). Mutations of enzymes necessary for testosterone production are rare, often affect adrenal steroidogenesis, and can be recognized through measurement of hormone precursors. Decreased testosterone production, even in the absence of Müllerian derivatives, can also be due to the late occurrence of *testicular dysgenesis*; in this case, circulating AMH concentrations are also low. Since testosterone action requires transformation into dihydrotestosterone and its binding to an androgen receptor, biochemical defects of androgen target organs can also lead to sex ambiguity limited to testosterone-dependent steps. In *5α-reductase deficiency*, target organs are unable to produce dihydrotestosterone, and only testosterone is available for binding to the androgen receptor. Paradoxically, although the external genitalia are very poorly masculinized at birth, virilization occurs at puberty with the marked rise in sex steroid production that ensues. Many different mutations in the gene coding for 5α-reductase type 2, the major isoenzyme expressed in genital tissues, have been detected in affected subjects, approximately half of which are compound heterozygotes. *Androgen insensitivity*, an X-linked disorder due to lesions of the androgen receptor gene, is a much more common disorder, and displays a variety of phenotypes. From a clinical standpoint, androgen insensitivity may be complete or partial, with either female or ambiguous genitalia. Biologically, the capacity of the androgen receptor to bind dihydrotestosterone is either impaired ("receptor-negative form") or normal ("receptor-positive form"), suggesting abnormalities in distinct domains of the androgen receptor gene (*see above*).

Finally, in rare instances, the external genitalia and urogenital sinus are normally masculinized, but Müllerian ducts do not regress. This condition, the *persistent Müllerian duct syndrome*, is heterogeneous. A dozen different mutations of the *AMH* gene have been described in patients with low or undetectable serum concentrations of the hormone. Target organ insensitivity to *AMH* is involved in patients with normal levels of serum *AMH*. A splicing mutation in the *AMH* receptor has recently been described in such a case.

## SELECTED READING

Bardoni B, Zanaria E, Guioli S, *et al.* A dosage sensitive locus at chromosome Xp21 is involved in male to female sex reversal. *Nat Genet* 1994; 7: 497.

Ferguson-Smith MA, Lovell-Badge R, McLaren A. eds *Mechanisms in vertebrate sex determination.* Philosophical Transactions of the Royal Society of London, Series B, Vol. 350. London: The Royal Society, 1995.

Gorski RA. Sexual differentiation of the endocrine brain and its control. In: Motta M, ed. *Brain endocrinology.* New York: Raven Press, 1991: 71.

Hawkins JR. Genetics of XY Sex reversal. *J Endocrinol* 1995; 147: 183.

Quigley CA, De Bellis A, Marschkle KB, *et al.* Androgen receptor defects. Historical, clinical and molecular perspectives. *Endocrine Rev* 1995; 16: 271.

Rey R, Mebarki F, Forest MG, *et al.* Anti-Müllerian hormone in children with androgen insensitivity. *J Clin Endocrinol Metab* 1994; 79: 960.

Shen WH, Moore CCD, Ikeda Y, *et al.* Nuclear receptor steroidogenic factor 1 regulates the mullerian inhibiting substance gene: a link to the sex determination cascade. *Cell* 1994; 77: 651.

Thigpen AE, Davis DL, Milatovich A, *et al.* Molecular genetics of steroid 5α-reductase 2 deficiency. *J Clin Invest* 1992; 90: 799.

Wilson JD. Syndromes of androgen resistance. *Biol Reprod* 1992; 46: 168.

Wilson JD, Griffin JE, Russell DW. Steroid 5α-reductase-2 deficiency. *Endocrine Rev* 1993; 14: 577.

TABLE 12.1 Molecular basis of male pseudohermaphroditism

| AFFECTED STEP | DEFECTIVE PROTEIN | TRANSMISSION |
| --- | --- | --- |
| Testosterone biosynthesis | Steroidogenic acute regulatory protein | Recessive autosomal |
| | 17,20 desmolase | Recessive autosomal |
| | 17α-hydroxylase | Recessive autosomal |
| | 3β-HSD type 2 | Recessive autosomal |
| | 17β-HSD type 3 | Recessive autosomal |
| Testosterone responsiveness | 5α-reductase type 2 | Recessive autosomal |
| | Androgen receptor | X-linked |
| AMH biosynthesis | AMH | Recessive autosomal |
| AMH responsiveness | AMH receptor | Recessive autosomal |

Defects in both testosterone and AMH-dependent steps are usually sporadic and result from testicular dysgenesis, often due to chromosomal abnormalities.

# 13

# The Placenta

## DEVELOPMENT OF THE HUMAN PLACENTA

The suggestion that the intrauterine environment may have long-term consequences for postnatal and adult health of the fetus has stimulated interest in the growth and development of the placenta. In the past, studies focused on the latter stages of pregnancy when classical complications such as *pre-eclampsia, intrauterine growth retardation (IUGR)* and *antepartum hemorrhage* occurred. Recently realization of the key importance of the earliest days of human development, particularly implantation and other events that precede placentation, has arisen. Considerable effort is now being used to understand this crucial part of development. It is no longer thought that abnormal implantation is of no clinical significance, as it will lead to miscarriage.

The development of the human placenta is dependent not only on the genetic information retained within the conceptus but also on the maternal adaptation that provides a receptive endometrium and the subsequent vascular alterations in the mother that facilitate the development of the placental bed (*see also* page 77).

## THE RECEPTIVE MATERIAL ENVIRONMENT

For implantation to occur the endometrium must undergo adaptive changes. In rodents, these changes are closely regulated by ovarian steroids, and the receptive window can be measured in hours. In primates, endometrium also undergoes developmental changes influenced by steroids but it is not clear how tight the implantation window is. Several key features of these changes are recognized.

■ Epithelial cells on the endometrial surface express glycoproteins which are required for successful apposition of the embryo with the endometrium.
■ Most strikingly, the spiral arterioles of the uterus undergo profound growth. These vessels supply about 10 mm$^2$ of the endometrial surface. They grow during the follicular phase of the cycle and continue to do so in the luteal phase. Their rate of growth exceeds the increase in thickness of the endometrium and they become coiled. These spiral arterioles subsequently become invaded by the trophoblast and provide the maternal blood supply to the placenta.
■ Decidualization of the endometrium occurs at the end of the luteal phase of the menstrual cycle and *after* implantation has occurred. In this sense it is not

obligatory for implantation but represents part of the adaptive response of the maternal environment.

## IMPLANTATION

Fertilization occurs at the ampullary–isthmic junction, and development of the embryo proceeds with the extrusion of the first polar body. Mitosis continues as the embryo travels down the fallopian tube and has reached the morula stage by the time it reaches the cornua of the uterus. Blastulation has usually occurred by the time the embryo enters the uterine cavity approximately 6 days post-ovulation. At this stage the outer wall of the trophoblast is distinguishable from the inner cell mass, a small group of cells which will become the embryo, cord and amnion. These cells also provide mesenchyme and blood vessels to the placenta.

In humans, implantation is of the intrusive type in which trophoblast cells intrude between the uterine epithelial cells and migrate into the stroma of the endometrium. Shortly after this stage of development, the trophoblast cells proliferate to form a double cell layered structure, the outer layer being the syncytiotrophoblast facing the maternal tissue and the cytotrophoblast being the remaining cells on the inside of this structure. Syncytium forms by fusion of cytotrophoblast cells which are not able to undergo further differentiation. The remaining cytotrophoblasts retain the capacity to proliferate, differentiate and migrate.

At around day 8 or 9 post-ovulation, vacuoles appear in the syncytium, grow and fuse into a system of lacunae. This occurs most obviously at the implantation pole and is thicker than over the rest of the trophoblast. It is this structure which becomes the placenta. At this stage three depths of the primitive placenta can be identified:

- The *primary chorionic plate* is a layer consisting of cytotrophoblasts.
- The *lacunar system*. Below the primary chorionic plate are situated lacunae which arise in the syncytium, itself formed by the fusion of cytotrophoblasts. During the course of the next few days, cytotrophoblasts from the chorionic plate invade the syncytium around the lacunae. When they reach the limit of the lacunar system, they form the trophoblastic shell.
- The *trophoblastic shell*. This previously consisted of syncytiotrophoblasts only but now contains cytotrophoblasts as well (Fig. 13.1).

## TROPHOBLAST–VASCULAR INTERACTIONS

Central to understanding placentation has been the requirement of the invading placenta to establish a blood supply with the mother. Initial studies suggested that cytotrophoblasts proliferate and migrate into the decidua and invade the maternal blood vessels. However, there is considerable doubt as to whether this simple explanation is true. In rodents, vascular casts of implantation sites reveal a circle of occluded blood vessels in the placental bed at the earliest stages of implantation. In humans, cytotrophoblasts can be seen in the spiral arterioles but they occlude the vasculature. Finally, recent Doppler flow studies have failed to find a blood flow signal in the placenta before 10 weeks of gestation.

It now seems likely that in the early stages of pregnancy the invading trophoblast serves to protect the embryo by blocking blood vessels. At 10–12 weeks of pregnancy, remodeling of the vessels occurs in which the vascular smooth muscle undergoes atrophy and the intravascular trophoblast "takes over" from the original endothelium. The consequence of these changes is the development of low-resistance blood vessels which supply the intervillous space.

## VILLOUS DEVELOPMENT

The initial invasion of the syncytium by trophoblasts marks the beginning of the villous development of the placenta. Further proliferation and invasion by extraembryonic mesenchyme forms the secondary villi which, if they reach the trophoblastic plate, become the anchoring villi. Around 3 weeks after ovulation, fetal capillaries arise in the mesenchyme in the villi, and this marks the development of the tertiary villi. The villous tree undergoes further complication during the course of the pregnancy. *Stem villi* contain fibrous stroma and well-defined arteries and veins. The stem villi that constitute the anchoring villi are connected to the basal plate by a cell column. Distal to the stem villi are the *intermediate villi*. The final ramification is the terminal villi which contain large numbers of capillaries and dilated sinusoids; this is the main site of feto-maternal exchange (Fig. 13.2).

## FETAL BLOOD SUPPLY OF THE PLACENTA

Around the sixth week of pregnancy fetal endothelial cells are found in the villi. These fuse with fetal vessels that invade the villous tree via the connective stalk which becomes the umbilical cord. It is only later that these primitive vessels become distinguishable as arterioles and venules, probably as a consequence of pressure differences within the vessels. Stem villi contain a clearly defined artery with media and adventitia. In addition a paravascular network of capillaries exists just below the trophoblast. As would be expected, the terminal villi contain a rich network of capillaries, which in addition form loops or sinusoids resulting in significant reduction in blood flow, facilitating feto-maternal exchange.

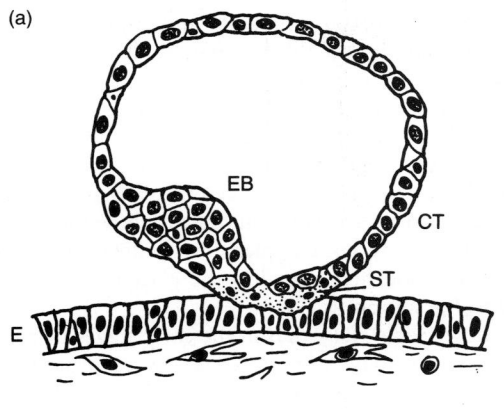

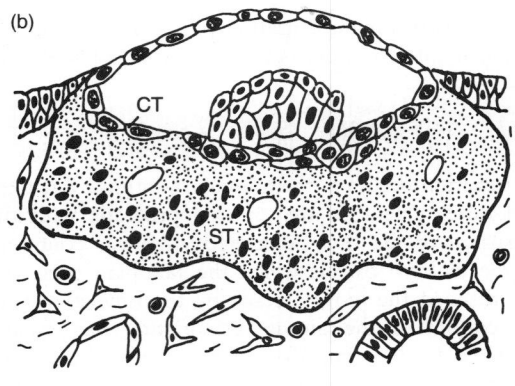

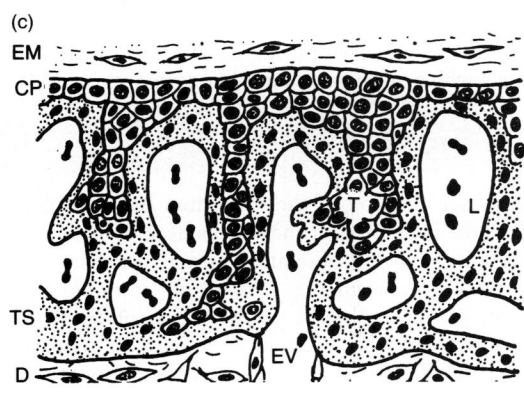

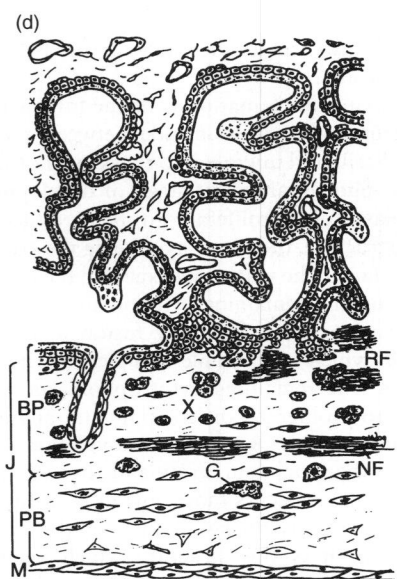

FIGURE 13.1 (a) Days 6–7: The early human embryo opposes to the endometrium (E) with the embryoblast (EB) closest to the surface epithelium. The trophectoderm has differentiated to cytotrophoblast (CT) which begins to form syncytiotrophoblast (ST) near the epithelium. (b) Days 7–8: The syncytiotrophoblast fuses and lacunae (L) appear. (c) Days 12–15: Cytotrophoblast migrates into the trabeculae (T) and primary villi form the primary chorionic plate (CP). EV = endometrial vessel; TS = trophoblastic shell; EM = extraembryonic mesoderm; D = decidua. (d) Day 18 to term: These cells reach the outermost part of the placenta at the basal plate (BP) and line the better defined tertiary villi. At the tips of the villi, cytotrophoblast pans between the syncytiotrophoblasts. They continue to divide and invade the decidua, becoming the extravillous trophoblast. RF = Rohr fibrinoid; NF = Nitabuch or uteroplacental fibrinoid; X = X cells or extravillus cytotrophoblast; G = trophoblastic giant cell; J = junctional zone; PB = placental bed; M = myometrium. (Adapted from Benirschke K, Kaufmann P, *Pathology of the human placenta*, 2nd edn. New York: Springer-Verlag, 1990, with permission.)

It is not known what initiates the developmental differentiation path which defines the blood vessels. The first identifiable marker of endothelial origin is the receptor (KDR) for the angiogenic growth factor, vascular endothelial growth factor (VEGF). Fetal macrophages or Hofbauer cells express the ligand VEGF, and it is possible that macrophages play a key role in regulating vascular development. As the placenta grows, angiogenesis results in sprouting from the original vessels (*see* page 77). Growth of the capil-laries exceeds that of the terminal villi, resulting in coiling of the capillaries.

## TROPHOBLAST INVASION

An important aspect of placental development is inva-sion of the decidua by the trophoblast. This invasion is regulated by locally released cytokines, and maternal–embryonic interactions are needed for this to be

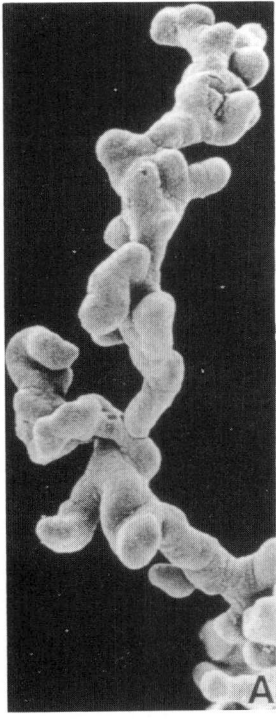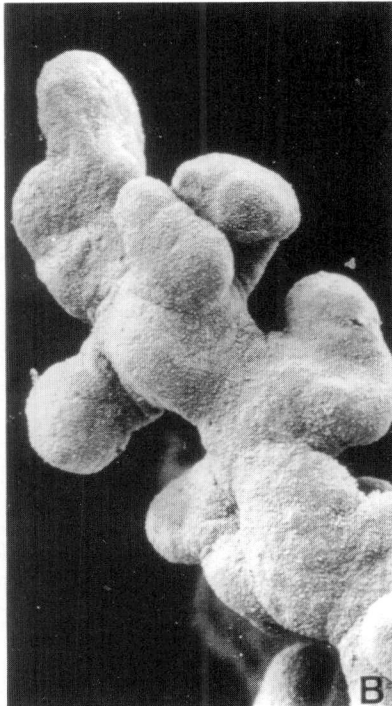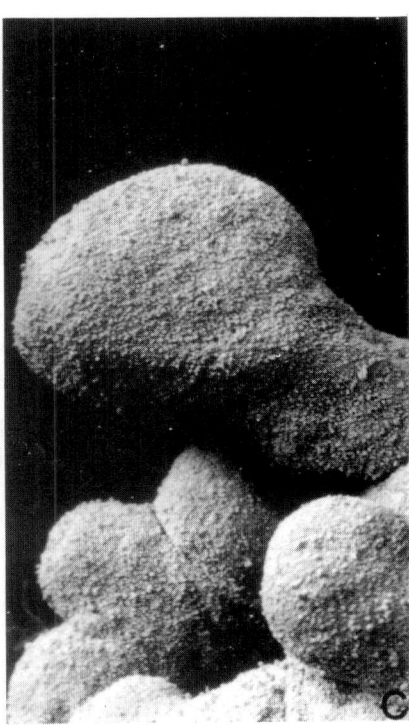

FIGURE 13.2 Scanning electron micrographs of terminal villi. Terminal villi contain extensive fetal capillaries, and it is possible that their structure reflects the response of trophoblast to capillary growth and branching. (Reproduced with permission from Benirschke K, Kaufmann P, *Pathology of the human placenta* 2nd edn. New York: Springer-Verlag, 1990.)

successful. Mice deleted for leukemia inhibitory factor (LIF) are able to ovulate and their oocytes will develop into embryos. These embryos can implant into wild type dames but *cannot* implant into the host mother. Thus maternal LIF but not fetal LIF is obligatory for murine implantation. A range of cytokines including CSF-1, GM-CSF, IFN γ, TNFα, TGFβ, IL-1, IL-2, IL-3, IL-6, IL-8 are expressed at the feto-maternal interface. Cells of the lympho-hematopoietic lineage at the implantation site express these cytokines, as does the trophoblast, and corresponding receptors are found on the same or other cells. For example, trophoblast expresses stem cell factor (SCF) and its receptor, *c-kit*, is found on macrophages close to the invasion site. It is likely that there exists a highly redundant but closely regulated cytokine network that regulates trophoblast invasion by permitting communication between the maternal and fetal environments.

A key feature of this process is the expression by trophoblast of integrins which bind to extracellular matrix, facilitating proliferation, differentiation and migration. As part of the invasive process, both trophoblast and decidua express metalloproteinases and tissue inhibitors of metalloproteinases which regulate the degradation of the extracellular matrix, permitting trophoblast invasion.

Other growth factors also may be critical to the process of implantation. Epidermal growth factor (EGF) is expressed by endometrium, and its receptor appears to be an important determinant of trophoblast differentiation, defining the intermediate trophoblast that can invade. Similarly, the insulin-like growth factors (IGFs) and their binding proteins appear to be involved in placental development. VEGF, assumed to be an angiogenic growth factor, is expressed by maternal macrophages at the implantation site and can influence trophoblast growth as well. It is not yet clear which are the key players in this complex interplay of cytokines and growth factors, in which redundancy probably plays an important role. In view of the importance of reproduction to the survival of the species, it is not surprising that the system incorporates so many fail-safe mechanisms. Despite this, human implantation remains an imperfect system, with 30–40 per cent of pregnancies resulting in miscarriage.

## ABNORMAL PLACENTATION

In view of the explosion of knowledge concerning human placental development, many groups have sought a cause and effect relationship between observed changes and common disorders of pregnancy. No effective means has been found to prevent *recurrent abortion* nor to correlate placental changes with this condition. *IUGR* on the other hand is associated with reduced capillary development in the terminal villi which are themselves inhibited in their development. What causes this change is not known, though if terminal villi development is dependent on capillary growth, then factors regulating angiogenesis must be important. There is confusion as to whether this is a primary event or follows defective early implantation resulting in fetal and placental hypoxia. Evidence for placental hypoxia is scanty. In *pre-eclampsia*, reports of impaired invasion of trophoblast into myometrium are not always consistent with the reduced capillary growth found in IUGR, which would be expected to be the case if there exists a simple relationship. In any case it does not explain why the trophoblast failed to invade in the first place!

Growth retardation is associated clinically with increased vascular resistance as determined by Doppler flow studies. Histologically this is reflected in *IUGR* by impaired capillary development, but this is not the case in about 50 per cent of *pre-eclamptic* patients. Here the role of vasoactive agents such as endothelins, prostaglandins and nitric oxide may be relevant. All of these can influence angiogenesis and their role on placental development remains to be elucidated. All in all, understanding of placental physiology has not yet permitted clinicians to in any way modulate placental function. In which case the common complications of human pregnancy, *IUGR*, *pre-eclampsia* and *antepartum hemorrhage*, remain beyond the reach of conventional medicine.

## SELECTED READING

Benirschke K, Kaufmann P. *Pathology of the human placenta*, 2nd edn. New York: Springer-Verlag, 1990.
Ward RHT, Smith SK, Donnai D, eds, *Early fetal growth and development*. RCOG Press, 1994.

TABLE 13.1 Hormonal and protein products of the human placenta

*Steroidal hormones*
Estradiol
Estrone
Estriol
Progesterone

*Miscellaneous proteins*
Corticotrophin-releasing hormone-binding protein (CRH-BP)
Free α-subunit of hCG
Free β-subunit of hCG
Free α-subunit of inhibin
Pregnancy associated plasma protein A (PAPP-A)
Pregnancy specific β1-glycoproteins

*Enzymes*
Oxytocinase
Placental alkaline phosphatase

*Peptide and protein hormones*
Corticotrophin-releasing hormone (CRH)
Gonadotrophin-releasing hormone (GnRH)
Growth hormone-releasing hormone (GHRH)
Thyrotrophin-releasing hormone (TRH)
Somatostatin
Human chorionic gonadotrophin (hCG)
Human placental lactogen
Human placental growth hormone (hGH-V)
Activin A and B
Inhibin A and B
Follistatin
Neuropeptide Y
Proopiomelanocortin derived peptides
– placental corticotrophin (ACTH)
– β-endorphin
– β-lipoprotein

# PLACENTAL ENDOCRINE FUNCTION

## INTRODUCTION

As an endocrine organ, the placenta is remarkable for the large variety of peptide, protein and steroid hormones it produces (Table 13.1). Through these hormones it effects marked changes in the homeostasis of the mother, which are important for the maintenance and successful outcome of the pregnancy.

The trophoblastic cells, particularly the syncytiotrophoblasts, are the source of placental hormones. Anatomically, the syncytiotrophoblast cells, which line the maternal side of the chorionic villi, come into direct contact with the mother's blood. The fetal blood supply, in contrast, is separated from the trophoblastic cells by several barriers, a basement membrane, the mesenchymal stroma of the villous core and the endothelium of the fetal capillaries. These structural relationships ensure that the hormones produced by the placenta are largely secreted into the maternal circulation.

Factors recognized as important to placental hormonogenesis are the mass of the trophoblasts and the uteroplacental and fetoplacental blood flows, which govern the rates at which precursor substrates, $O_2$ and nutrients are supplied to the placenta and at which hormones and other products are removed. Hormone production in the placenta, nevertheless, does not occur in an autonomous uncontrolled manner. Recent *in vitro* studies have revealed that many placental hormones themselves act endogenously as local paracrine and autocrine regulators of hormone biosynthesis.

This section of the chapter will focus on a selection of the hormones which especially contribute to the unique endocrine aspects of human pregnancy or which currently are attracting research interest as newly identified placental products.

# HUMAN CHORIONIC GONADOTROPHIN

Human chorionic gonadotrophin (hCG), a glycoprotein with a molecular weight of 36–40 kD, is a product of the syncytiotrophoblast. Structurally, hCG is composed of an α-subunit of 92 amino acids non-covalently linked to a distinctive β-subunit of 145 amino acids, and resembles the pituitary glycoproteins, luteinizing hormone (LH), follicle stimulating hormone (FSH) and thyroid stimulating hormone (TSH). The α-subunit of these hormones all share a common peptide structure coded for by a single gene on chromosome 6. The β-subunit of hCG is coded for by six genes clustered with the gene for the β-subunit of LH on chromosome 19. Variation in the expression of these genes, together with variation in the amount of glycosylation of the peptide core, explains placental production of different isoforms of hCG.

The β-subunit of hCG has greater than 80 per cent sequence homology with the 121–amino acid β-subunit of LH but differs in having a 24–amino acid extension at the carboxy terminus. The extension of the β-subunit with its associated carbohydrate markedly increases the *in vivo* half-life of hCG. The disappearance of hCG from the circulation occurs in two phases, the first with a half-life of 7 hours and the second with a half-life of 39 hours. In comparison, LH disappears with an initial phase half-life of 40 minutes and a second phase half-life of 2 hours.

hCG has similar luteotrophic actions to LH and plays a vital role during early gestation to ensure the continuance of the pregnancy. Immediately following implantation of the blastocyst, the primitive trophoblast begins secreting hCG into the maternal circulation. The hCG acts on the ovary to maintain the corpus luteum, preventing its degeneration and stimulating its further development to the corpus luteum of pregnancy. Under the stimulus of hCG the ovarian secretion of progesterone and estradiol rises. These two hormones are necessary for the maintenance of pregnancy. Progesterone is particularly important through its action in inhibiting myometrial contractility (*see* page 252). By 6–8 weeks of pregnancy, however, the ovary has been replaced by the placenta as the main source of these hormones and pregnancy is no longer dependent on an active corpus luteum.

hCG becomes detectable in maternal blood between 7 and 12 days after conception and in urine about 15 days after conception. Placental hCG production increases exponentially and reaches a peak at between 8 and 10 weeks gestation, when serum concentrations range between 40 000 and 200 000 IU/L. Thereafter, production rapidly declines, yielding serum concentrations of 8 000 to 20 000 IU/L throughout the remainder of gestation (Fig. 13.3). Urinary excretion closely reflects circulating concentrations.

In the fetus, hCG plays a role in male sexual differentiation by promoting a supply of the vital hormone testosterone (*see* page 197). At a critical time in the

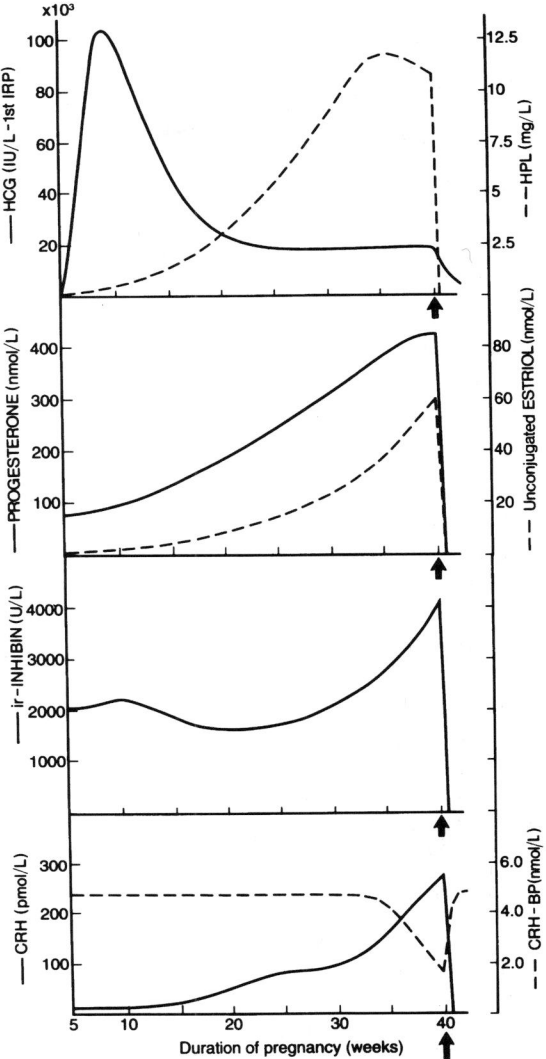

FIGURE 13.3 Diagrammatic representation of the changes in maternal serum concentrations of human chorionic gonadotrophin (hCG), human placental lactogen (hPL), progesterone, unconjugated estriol, immunoreactive (ir) inhibin, corticotrophin-releasing hormone (CRH), and corticotrophin-releasing hormone-binding protein (CRH-BP) during normal pregnancy and following delivery

differentiation process, at between 10–14 weeks' gestation, the trophoblast derived hCG circulating in the fetus serves in the male as a surrogate for LH and stimulates the testes to produce testosterone. Testosterone production is sustained later in pregnancy by fetal pituitary LH. The testosterone acts directly on the Wolffian ducts to effect the development of the epididymis, vas deferens and seminal vesicles. In the genital tubercle and urogenital sinus, testosterone is converted to the more potent androgen 5α-dihydrotestosterone, which effects development of the male external genitalia.

*In vitro* studies indicate hCG plays a regulatory role in the placenta itself, stimulating the synthesis of progesterone and inhibin.

The abrupt decline in hCG production around the tenth week of pregnancy is at variance with the ongoing increase in the mass of syncytiotrophoblastic tissue which continues until near term. This decline may result from limited availability of the β-subunit, for while production of the α-subunit continues to rise during pregnancy, production of the β-subunit mirrors that of hCG. Progesterone *in vitro* decreases placental hCG secretion and it is possible that the progesterone rise in pregnancy inhibits biosynthesis of the β-hCG subunit.

Immunoassay of serum or urinary hCG (or its β-subunit) is the most common laboratory test of pregnancy. Elevated serum and urinary hCG concentrations are common in women with trophoblast disease (*hydatidiform mole* and *choriocarcinoma*) and in men with certain *testicular cancers*. Measurements of the hormone are important in the diagnosis and follow-up of these conditions. Depressed concentrations occur in *ectopic pregnancy*. Measurements of serum hCG or of its free subunits combined with the assays of serum unconjugated estriol and α-fetoprotein form the basis of a prenatal second trimester screening test for *trisomy 21*.

## HUMAN PLACENTAL LACTOGEN

Human placental lactogen (hPL), sometimes referred to as human chorionic somatomammotrophin (hCS), is a 191–amino acid single-chain protein of molecular weight 22 kD. The amino acid sequence is 96 per cent homologous to that of human growth hormone (hGH) (*see* page 471). A family of five closely related genes grouped together on chromosome 17 encode for these hormones and their variant proteins. With their close structural similarity it is not surprising that hPL and hGH have similar biological properties though hPL is less potent.

The mechanisms that regulate hPL production are unclear. The protein also is synthesized by syncytiotrophoblasts, and the amount produced is related to the mass of syncytiotrophoblast tissue. Growth hormone-releasing hormone (GHRH), somatostatin and insulin-like growth factor-I (IGF-I), produced by trophoblast cells, may regulate hPL secretion much as they regulate GH secretion in the pituitary. Neurotransmitters such as dopamine which directly or indirectly control pituitary secretion of prolactin and GH have been found to have no effect on placental secretion of hPL. Short-term variations in maternal glucose, amino acid and lipid concentrations have little effect on hPL production, though prolonged fasting in early pregnancy raises hPL concentrations.

hPL first becomes detectable in the maternal circulation at around five weeks' gestation. Thereafter concentrations steadily increase to plateau (between 5 and 15 mg/L) at 35 weeks reflecting production in late pregnancy of more than 1 g per day (Fig. 13.3). hPL is rapidly cleared from the maternal serum with a half-life of 10–15 minutes.

hPL has a wide range of biological activities, and a number of the major metabolic changes that occur in pregnant women may be attributable to this hormone. The hormonal activities of hPL include actions that elevate maternal blood free fatty acid, glucose and insulin concentrations. hPL increases the degree of lipolysis and increases insulin resistance. The latter effect impairs glucose uptake and gluconeogenesis. These actions on nutrient repartitioning in the maternal compartment have the net effect of enhancing glucose and amino acid availability to the fetus. Only a small fraction of placental hPL production enters the fetal circulation. It is uncertain if this is sufficient to influence fetal growth.

hPL also shares structural similarity with human prolactin (*see* page 475). However, while hPL has been shown to be lactogenic in animals, there is little persuasive evidence of a similar role in the human. *In vitro* experiments have shown that hPL stimulates proliferation of epithelial cells in breast tissue, and its effect on the human breast may be confined to this action.

Though the actions of hPL are of significance in pregnancy, they are not essential. Normal pregnancies, leading to birth of a normal baby, have been reported in gene deletions which lead to an absolute deficiency in hPL production. The placenta also produces a variant form of growth hormone (hGH-V) which is 96 per cent homologous to pituitary hGH. Production of hGH-V in late gestation suppresses maternal pituitary hGH production. It is presumed that there is a redundancy in function between hPL and hGH-V.

## INHIBIN AND ACTIVIN

Inhibin and activin are members of a family of glycoproteins which includes transforming growth factor β and anti-Müllerian hormone (AMH) (formerly called Müllerian inhibiting factor, MIF). Inhibin structurally consists of two dissimilar α and β subunits linked by disulfide bonds and has a molecular weight of 32 kD. The α subunit consists of 133 amino acids. There are two distinctive β subunits, βA of 116 amino acids and βB of 115 amino acids, leading to two possible forms of inhibin, inhibin A (αβA) and inhibin B (αβB). Activin, a dimer of the inhibin β-subunit, can exist in three forms, A, B and AB, with a molecular weight of 26–28 kD.

Recently the placenta has been found to be a source of both inhibin and activin. Synthesis of the inhibin subunits apparently takes place in both cytotrophoblast and syncytiotrophoblast cells with a predominance of α- and βA-subunits being produced. Formation of the inhibin and activin dimers presumably is dependent on the relative predominance of subunits at the site of synthesis.

Placental secretion of inhibin and activin is mainly into the maternal circulation. Serum concentrations of both bioactive and immunoreactive inhibin (native hormone and free α-subunit) increase during pregnancy particularly during the third trimester (Fig. 13.3).

Following delivery, inhibin concentrations fall abruptly in parallel with progesterone and estradiol concentrations. Maternal serum activin concentrations rise significantly from 20 weeks' gestation. A further marked increase occurs with the onset of labor, both preterm and term. The significance of this increase in the mechanism of parturition is at present uncertain.

The elevated concentrations of inhibin in pregnancy act, with estradiol and progesterone, to suppress secretion of FSH by the maternal pituitary, accounting for the depressed serum concentration of this hormone and the consequential absence of maternal follicular activity. The main function of inhibin and activin in pregnancy, however, may be as local regulators of placental function. *In vitro* evidence implicates activin and inhibin as modulators of placental synthesis of gonadotrophin-releasing hormone (GnRH), hCG, progesterone and possibly other hormones. In a different role, activin has been proposed as a signaling protein and growth factor in embryogenesis.

## NEUROHORMONES

The human placenta produces most of the peptide neurohormones that normally are associated with the hypothalamus. They include GnRH, thyrotrophin-releasing hormone (TRH), somatostatin, GHRH, corticotrophin-releasing hormone (CRH), and the opioid peptides. They are produced predominantly by the cytotrophoblast cells and express activity in the neighboring syncytiotrophoblasts in regulating the synthesis of protein hormones such as hCG, hPL and chorionic ACTH. This interplay between cytotrophoblasts and syncytiotrophoblasts resembles the interplay between hypothalamic neurosecretory cells and anterior pituitary cells but without a portal blood supply as an intermediary.

## Gonadotrophin-releasing hormone (GnRH)

Placental GnRH is a decapeptide identical to the hypothalamic derived hormone. GnRH secretion by the placenta is regulated by changes in intracellular $Ca^{2+}$ levels in a manner similar to its release from the hypothalamus. Epinephrine promotes GnRH production, suggesting that cAMP is also a modulator of GnRH release.

Syncytiotrophoblast cells contain a specific GnRH receptor in the plasma membrane and respond to the receptor–ligand interaction by increasing intracellular

$Ca^{2+}$ concentration. The influx in $Ca^{2+}$ ions promotes the synthesis of both α- and β-subunits of hCG and secretion of the native hormone. Maternal serum concentrations of GnRH are elevated in pregnancy with the highest levels observed between 7 and 17 weeks' gestation, declining thereafter. Though the pregnancy profiles of serum GnRH and hCG levels are not synchronous, they are consistent with an involvement of GnRH in the regulation of placental production of hCG.

## Corticotrophin-releasing hormone (CRH)

Hypothalamic CRH was initially defined by its regulation of the hypothalamic–pituitary–adrenal axis. This 41–amino acid peptide controls ACTH secretion by stimulating synthesis of the precursor protein proopiomelanocortin in the anterior pituitary. The placenta is an additional site of CRH production and is the source of the high maternal circulating concentrations during pregnancy. Placental CRH synthesis occurs in the syncytiotrophoblasts. The amnion, chorion and maternal decidua are other intrauterine tissues of pregnancy that also produce CRH.

Serum CRH concentrations are barely detectable in non-pregnant women, but in pregnancy they begin to rise during the second trimester, increasing steeply between 36 weeks and term (Fig. 13.3). After delivery, CRH concentrations fall precipitously and are undetectable within 24 hours. Higher concentrations occur in patients with a twin pregnancy, in patients with pregnancy-induced hypertension, and in patients with a growth-restricted fetus. Raised serum CRH concentrations also are observed in patients prior to, but destined for, preterm labor, suggesting that measurement of the serum CRH concentration might be a useful test for predicting patients at risk of preterm labor.

For much of pregnancy CRH circulates in the blood bound to CRH-binding protein (CRH-BP). In this bound state it is unlikely that CRH can function biologically, and thus the possible action of placental CRH on the pituitary to stimulate ACTH release is blocked. CRH-BP is produced by the placenta and the liver. The serum concentrations of CRH-BP remain relatively constant close to non-pregnancy levels until the last three weeks of pregnancy when they fall markedly (Fig. 13.3). There is recovery to non-pregnant values within 48 hours postpartum.

The decrease in CRH-BP in the last weeks of pregnancy, at a time when placental production of CRH is increasing, enhances the availability of free bioactive CRH in the maternal and fetal compartments. The rise in CRH to concentrations that exceed the binding capacity of CRH-BP, indeed, may cause the fall in circulating concentrations of CRH-BP as bioavailable CRH promotes the metabolic clearance of the binding protein. The influence of the increased levels of free CRH on the anterior pituitary of the mother is uncertain for at the same time levels of free cortisol also are raised, and there may be a balance in the effects of the two hormones. The small increase in maternal serum concentrations of ACTH seen in late pregnancy is more likely a result of enhanced placental secretion of ACTH stimulated by the paracrine action of CRH.

The most important function of placental CRH, however, may be in processes involved in the onset of labor. As well as promoting placental synthesis of proopiomelanotonin and, derived from this protein, ACTH and β-endorphin, CRH has pronounced effects on the uterine myometrium and fetoplacental vasculature. A receptor for CRH has been characterized in the myometrium of pregnant and non-pregnant women. Presumably working via this receptor, CRH has been shown *in vitro* to potentiate the action of oxytocin on myometrial contractions markedly. CRH may further affect uterine contractility by stimulating production of prostaglandins $PGF_{2\alpha}$ and $PGE_2$ by the amnion, chorion, decidua and placenta. These two prostaglandins have long been implicated in the process of labor by stimulating contractility of the pregnant myometrium. Interestingly, in *in vitro* experiments $PGF_{2\alpha}$ and $PGE_2$ have been found to stimulate CRH production by placental cells, the fetal membranes and decidua. Hence, in late pregnancy, CRH and these prostaglandins may enter into a positive feedback interaction enhancing their availability to the myometrium to drive uterine contractions. Recent *in vitro* studies have found CRH to be 50 times more potent than prostacyclin ($PGI_2$) in causing vasodilatation of the placental vasculature. This action is likely to be of importance in maintaining a low vascular resistance in late pregnancy and during labor.

The evidence of a link between placental CRH and the timing of parturition has recently been interpreted as reflecting the activity of a "placental clock." This hypothesis proposes that early in human pregnancy a longitudinal process is established in the placenta which determines the subsequent timing of labor and delivery. The culmination of this process, regulated by the setting of the clock, is an increase in placental secretion of CRH and an exponential rise in the concentration of the hormone in the circulation. The rising concentrations of CRH prepare the fetus for extrauterine life by stimulating, via the pituitary–adrenal axis, cortisol-induced maturational changes. On reaching critical levels in the placenta, fetal membranes, decidua, and myometrium, CRH initiates prostaglandin synthesis and the other processes outlined above which bring about the onset of labor. Preterm labor, it is proposed, would result from an advanced setting of the clock. Proof of the hypothesis rests with future research, but clearly, even if true, other factors can override the clock. Intrauterine infection, for example, is well recognized as a cause of premature labor; cytokines produced by the membranes in response to infection induce prostaglandin production.

## STEROID HORMONES

As well as peptide and protein hormones, the human placenta produces considerable progesterone and estrogenic steroids. Unlike other endocrine glands that produce steroids, the placenta is extremely limited in ability to synthesize *de novo* from acetate the steroid nucleus in the form of cholesterol. Further, the placenta lacks expression of 17α-hydroxylase/17,20 lyase activity ($P_{450c17}$) and is thus unable to convert the $C_{21}$-steroids pregnenolone and progesterone to C19-products, the precursors of the estrogens. Consequently, biosynthesis of progesterone and estrogen in the human placenta requires a supply of appropriate steroidal precursors provided from other sources.

## Progesterone

Progesterone is synthesized by syncytiotrophoblast predominantly from low-density lipoprotein cholesterol present in the maternal circulation. This process occurs largely independent of the fetus. The progesterone is secreted both to the mother (90 per cent) and to the fetus (10 per cent) where it undergoes further metabolism. Production of progesterone steadily increases during pregnancy until a few weeks before term, when it levels off at a rate of approximately 300 mg/day. Maternal serum concentrations of progesterone in late pregnancy are commonly between 400 and 500 nmol/L (Fig. 13.3). The main urinary metabolite of progesterone is pregnanediol glucuronide. Its excretion over 24 hours accounts for about 15 per cent of the daily production of progesterone.

Several products of progesterone metabolism are themselves hormonally active. Progesterone is actively converted by 21-hydroxylation to deoxycorticosterone (DOC), a potent mineralocorticoid, principally at extra-adrenal sites including the kidneys and blood vessels. Dramatically high concentrations of DOC are observed in the mother and the fetus in late pregnancy. Intriguingly, the pregnant woman successfully adapts to the elevated production of DOC, and it is doubtful in normal pregnancy if DOC has any significant influence on maternal blood pressure. An involvement of DOC in the pathophysiology of *pregnancy induced hypertension* is uncertain since levels of DOC do not differ between affected and normal pregnancies.

Other metabolites of progesterone are known to function as neurosteroids (*see* page 465). The 3α- and 5α-derivatives of progesterone, e.g. allopregnanolone (3α-hydroxy-5α-pregnan-20-one), act in the brain independent of the steroid hormone receptor to modulate function of the γ-aminobutyric acid (GABA) type A receptor. They bind to the $GABA_A$ receptor where they act as allosteric agonists to enhance GABA binding and hence exhibit $GABA_A$-ergic effects. Anesthetic, sedative, anxiolytic and memory impairment effects have been attributed to the interaction of the progesterone-derived (and similar DOC-derived) neurosteroids with brain GABA$_A$ receptors. To what degree these neurosteroid-induced effects contribute to behavioral changes during human pregnancy and in the postpartum period remains to be clarified.

Maternal serum progesterone concentrations can readily be determined by radioimmunoassay. However, though progesterone production is related to placental mass and function, studies of high-risk pregnancies have found that serial serum progesterone estimations are not reliable for assessing fetal well-being.

## Estrogens

Estrogen production increases almost 1000-fold during human pregnancy, exceeding 80 mg/day near term and resulting in a highly estrogenic state for both mother and fetus. In the non-pregnant woman the weak estrogen, estriol, arises as an end-product of hepatic metabolism of estradiol. However in pregnancy estriol is a secretory product in its own right and is the major product of placental estrogen synthesis.

Estrogen production in pregnancy intimately involves both the fetus and placenta (*see also* page 244) and is dependent on:

- a live fetus
- functioning fetal adrenal glands
- an unimpeded fetoplacental circulation
- a functioning placenta

The cooperative relationship between the fetus and placenta (the fetoplacental unit) seen in the production of estrogens arises because of placental lack of the P$_{450C17}$ enzyme which has both 17α-hydroxylase and 17,20 lyase activity. The fetus, on the other hand, has an abundance of this enzyme in its adrenal cortex where it produces considerable quantities of the C$_{19}$ steroid dehydroepiandrosterone sulfate (DHEAS), a substrate suited to the placenta, which is rich in the other enzymes required for its conversion to estrogen.

Estrogen biosynthesis in the fetoplacental unit of human pregnancy involves the following steps. The fetal adrenal, stimulated by ACTH, converts LDL cholesterol to pregnenolone. While some of the pregnenolone enters the biosynthetic pathway to cortisol, the majority is converted to DHEAS which is secreted into the fetal circulation where it passes to the placenta and is converted into estrone and estradiol. This conversion involves as a first and compulsory step, the removal of the sulfate moiety through action of the enzyme steroid sulfatase. The DHEA then interacts in turn with 3β-OH-dehydrogenase/Δ$^4$ isomerase to produce androstenedione, some of which is converted to testosterone. Both serve as substrates for the aromatase enzyme system to yield estrone and estradiol, respectively. While these two estrogens are secreted mainly into the maternal compartment, some is shunted back to the fetus where a part is converted to estriol. The major pathway to estriol in the fetoplacental unit, however, involves the precursor 16α-hydroxydehydroepiandrosterone sulfate (16OH-DHEAS). The fetal adrenal produces 16OH-DHEAS, but by far the larger proportion comes from 16-hydroxylation by the fetal liver of circulating DHEAS. The placenta converts 16OH-DHEAS to estriol through the same sequence of enzyme reactions used in converting DHEAS to estrone/estradiol. The pathway is shown in Fig. 13.4.

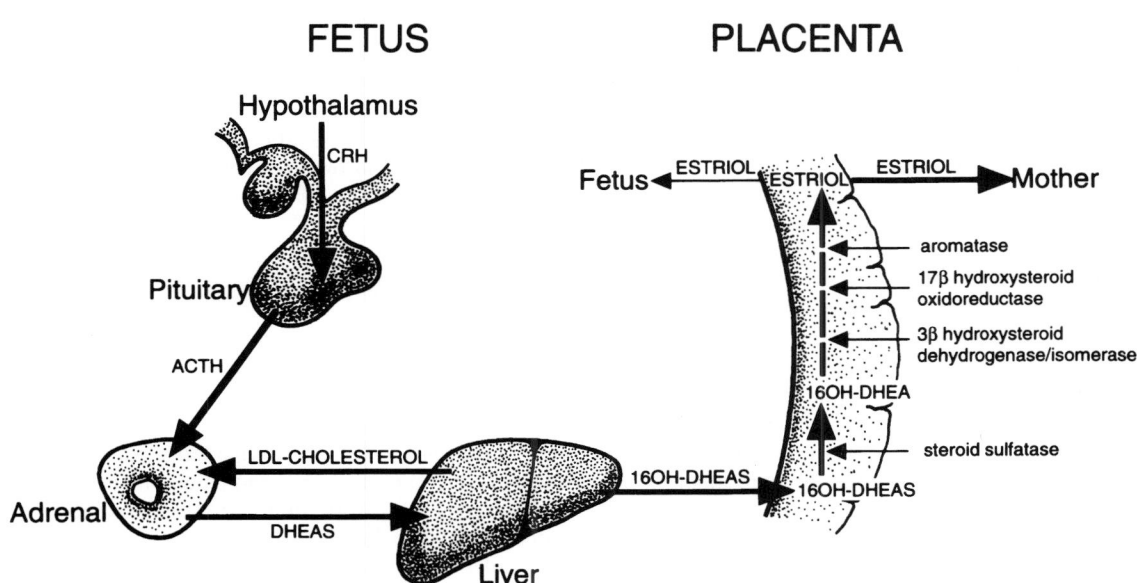

FIGURE 13.4 Diagrammatic representation of the pathway of estriol biosynthesis in the fetoplacental unit of human pregnancy

The DHEAS secreted by the maternal adrenal can be utilized by the placenta for estrogen biosynthesis. In the last 10 weeks of pregnancy about 50 per cent of estrone and estradiol produced arises from this source, but only about 10 per cent of the estriol.

In the past, the measurement of maternal urinary or serum concentrations of estriol was commonly used during the third trimester of pregnancy as a laboratory test for assessing fetal well-being, but it is infrequently used nowadays, being replaced by more direct clinical methods.

## Hormonal action of progesterone and estrogens in pregnancy

The reason why such large quantities of steroidal hormones are produced in human pregnancy is not known. The mother and fetus protect themselves from the high concentrations of these hormones through highly active hydroxylation enzyme systems and the formation of steroid conjugates. Nevertheless, in late pregnancy maternal serum concentrations of progesterone and estradiol, the most potent of the estrogens, average around 400 nmol/L and 100 nmol/L, respectively. In comparison, the highest concentrations reached by these hormones in the menstrual cycle average 60 nmol/L and 1000 pmol/L respectively.

The initial actions of estrogen and progesterone in pregnancy are to produce a uterine environment favorable for implantation of the conceptus and for subsequent nourishment of the developing embryo.

Progesterone is necessary throughout the gestation period for maintenance of the pregnancy by its action in maintaining the uterus in a quiescent state. Estrogen and progesterone acting synergistically stimulate growth of the uterus. The uterus also has a growth response to the mechanical stimulation of tension arising from the growing conceptus within it. The latter stimulus may be the more important as uterine growth continues normally in pregnancies associated with impaired estrogen production.

Estrogens promote growth and softening of the tissues of the birth canal to allow passage of the fetus without trauma. Other actions of estrogen in the process of human birth are unclear. In certain species, such as the sheep, a fall in progesterone concentrations and a rise in estradiol concentrations precedes, and is involved in, parturition through the enhancement of intrauterine prostaglandin synthesis. In human pregnancy, however, placental production and maternal serum concentrations of progesterone and the estrogens do not show these changes prior to labor.

The high estrogen concentrations have an effect on the maternal liver, stimulating the production of proteins which bind cortisol, testosterone and thyroxine in the serum. The hepatic effects also include increasing the hepatic production of LDL and HDL cholesterol.

In the breast, estrogens cause proliferation of the duct system, while progesterone acting synergistically with estrogen promotes development of the glandular tissue. These two hormones also act on the breast to inhibit milk secretion, blocking the stimulus from rising blood concentrations of prolactin, a consequence itself of estrogen action at the hypothalamus/pituitary. Following delivery, with the loss of placental production of estrogen and progesterone, their inhibitory influence is withdrawn and lactation can be established.

## Inborn errors of steroid metabolism affecting placental endocrine function

### Steroid sulfatase deficiency

This enzyme defect is inherited as an X-linked recessive trait so only males are affected. It occurs with an incidence of about 1 in 5000 male births. The gene encoding the steroid sulfatase enzyme is located on the distal portion of the short arm of the X chromosome (Xp22.3). In the large majority of instances the deficiency is the result of complete deletion of the gene.

During fetal life the disorder reveals itself as *placental sulfatase deficiency*, causing a marked decrease in placental estrogen production, particularly that of estriol, through failure of the necessary hydrolysis of the estrogen precursors DHEAS and 16OH-DHEAS. The pregnancies otherwise appear clinically normal, though at term a significant minority may show failure of cervical ripening and may not progress into spontaneous labor. In postnatal life, affected individuals develop the hyperkeratosis skin condition of *X-linked ichthyosis*, usually within three months of birth. Evidence strongly suggests steroid sulfatase deficiency as the cause of the ichthyosis.

In a small percentage of individuals affected with steroid sulfatase deficiency other abnormalities may also occur, such as *hypogonadotrophic hypogonadism with anosmia (Kallmann syndrome)* and *chondrodysplasia punctata*. These abnormalities probably arise through codeletion of genes contiguous with the steroid sulfatase gene.

### Aromatase deficiency

This is a rare abnormality inherited as an autosomal recessive trait. The enzyme deficiency appears to arise from mutation of the aromatase gene rather than deletion of the gene.

In pregnancy with an affected fetus, placental estrogen production is impaired and maternal and fetal concentrations of estriol and the other estrogens are depressed. The lack of aromatase activity results in considerable placental secretion of testosterone and androstenedione, which may, but not always, result in late pregnancy in virilization changes in the mother.

If the fetus is a female, virilization of the external genitalia occurs.

In later life after birth, affected females will be of short stature and will not experience puberty. They will exhibit signs of virilization and of estrogen deficiency. Affected males, following puberty, will be of tall stature with delayed bone maturation and epiphyses which remain unclosed until exposed to administered estrogen.

## SELECTED READING

Albrecht ED, Pepe GJ. Placental steroid hormone biosynthesis in primate pregnancy. *Endocrine Rev* 1990; **11**: 124.

Casey ML, MacDonald PC. Placental endocrinology. In: Redman CWG, Sargent IL, Starkey PM, eds. *The human placenta*. Oxford: Blackwell Scientific Publications, 1193: 237.

Cole LA, Kardana A, Park S-Y, Braunstein GD. The deactivation of hCG by nicking and dissociation. *J Clin Endocr Metab* 1994; **79**: 502.

Conte FA, Grumbach MM, Ito Y, *et al.* A syndrome of female pseudohermaphrodism, hypergonadotrophic hypogonadism, and multicystic ovaries associated with missense mutations in the gene encoding aromatase (P450 arom). *J Clin Endocr Metab* 1994; **78**: 1287.

de Kretser DCM, Foulds LM, Hancock M, Robertson DM. Partial characterization of inhibin, activin and follistatin in the term human placenta. *J Clin Endocr Metab* 1994; **79**: 504.

Jameson JL, Hollenberg AN. Regulation of chorionic gonadotropin gene expression. *Endocrine Rev* 1993; **14**: 203.

McLean M, Bisits A, Davies J, *et al.* A placental clock controlling the length of human pregnancy. *Nature Med* 1995; **2**: 460.

Petraglia F, Vaughan J, Vale W. Inhibin and activin modulate the release of gonadotropin-releasing hormone, human chorionic gonadotropin and progesterone from cultured human placental cells. *Proc Natl Acad Sci USA* 1989; **86**: 5114.

Petraglia F, De Vita D, Gallinelli A, *et al.* Abnormal concentration of maternal serum activin-A in gestational diseases. *J Clin Endocr Metab* 1995; **80**: 558.

Riley SC, Challis JRG. Corticotrophin-releasing hormone production by the placenta and fetal membranes. *Placenta* 1991; **12**: 105.

Shapiro LJ. Steroid sulfatase deficiency and X-linked ichthyosis. In: Scriver CR, Beaudet AL, Sly WS, *et al.*, eds. *The metabolic basis of inherited disease*, Vol. 2, 6th edn. New York: McGraw-Hill Information Services, 1989: 1945.

Strauss, III JF, Gåfvels M, King BF. Placental hormones. In: De Groot L, Besser M, Burger HG, *et al.*, eds. *Endocrinology*, Vol. 3, 3rd edn. Philadelphia: WB Saunders, 1995: 2171.

# PLACENTAL FUNCTION

The placenta is a specialized organ of exchange, interposed between the fetal (umbilical) and maternal (uterine) circulations to provide nutrients and $O_2$ to the fetus and to excrete fetal waste products. The placenta also has considerable metabolic activity, with $O_2$ and glucose consumption rates approaching or exceeding those of brain and tumor tissue, and an impressive array of metabolic activities including glycolysis, gluconeogenesis, glycogenesis, carbon substrate oxidation, protein synthesis (especially of hormones necessary to maintain pregnancy and to prepare lactation), amino acid interconversion, triglyceride synthesis, and chain lengthening and shortening of individual fatty acids. Evaluation of placental function, therefore, involves consideration of placental transfer and exchange of nutrient substances and waste products between the maternal and fetal circulations, as well as metabolic processes in the placenta.

## PLACENTAL MORPHOLOGY AND PLACENTAL FUNCTION

Although earlier investigators suggested that placental function was directly related to the degree of chorionic invasion of the uterine mucosa (Fig. 13.5), current understanding is quite different. Many other factors contribute to placental function, including total placental blood flow, intraplacental blood flow patterns, thickness of the various placental membranes, genetically determined transport properties (e.g. transport proteins and ion channels), the surface area and structure of the membranes, the physical–chemical properties of the membranes, the metabolic activity of the placenta, and various mechanisms of transfer (for example, simple diffusion, carrier mediated transfer, and active transfer).

Nevertheless, there are wide variations among placental morphological types with respect to placental transport processes. To some extent these variations depend on the structural complexity of the trophoblast, including the supporting tissues and blood flow patterns. For example, IgG is transported by the yolk sac in rabbits, by pinocytosis in the human placenta, but is not transported in sheep; iron is transported in red blood cells in sheep and cats, but by transferrin in humans. Diffusional and transporter-mediated placental transport mechanisms also differ among placental structural types. Complex lipid, lipoprotein, and polypeptide molecules cross hemochorial placentas (human, rat, guinea pig) easily, by direct mechanisms as well as by transporters and metabolic pathways, whereas there is little direct transport in the epitheliochorial placentas of sheep and pigs. There are probably differences among species and placental morphological types for placental metabolism as well, but these have been more difficult to characterize.

Therefore, no single structural characteristic is sufficient to classify placental type, especially regarding functional characteristics of transport and metabolism. Comparative studies have demonstrated important quantitative roles for the histology of the placental barrier (hemochorial, endotheliochorial, epitheliochor-

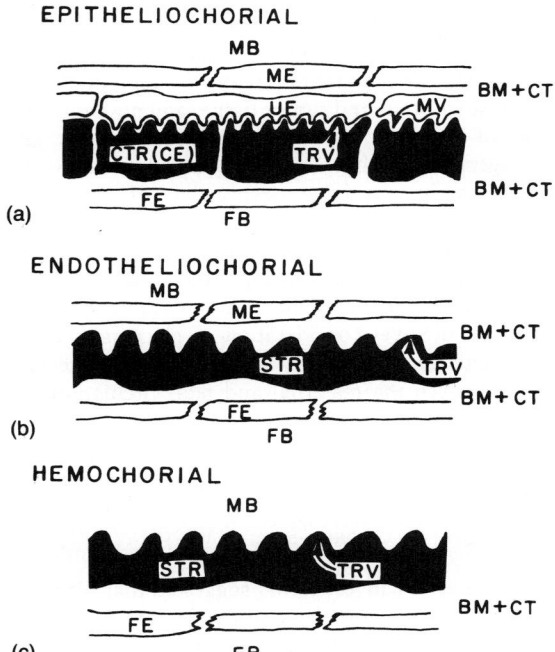

(a)

(b)

(c)

FIGURE 13.5 Diagrammatic representation of the three main anatomical types of placenta, classified according to histological structure. (a) Epitheliochorial, which has both fetal and maternal endothelial and epithelial structures, the latter apposing an intervening cytotrophoblast or chorionic epithelium. This type of placenta is found in sheep, swine, and cattle. (b) Endotheliochorial, which has both fetal and maternal endothelia that appose a syncytiotrophoblast. This type of placenta is common among the carnivores. (c) Hemochorial, which has a fetal endothelium and a syncytiotrophoblast but no uterine epithelium or endothelium. The trophoblast has eroded through the maternal (uterine) epithelium and endothelium, allowing maternal blood to circulate through the intervillous space, bathing directly the maternal-facing microvillous membrane of the syncytiotrophoblast. This type of placenta is found in humans. MB = basement membrane; CT = connective tissue; UE = uterine epithelium; MV = maternal epithelial microvilli; TRV = trophoblast microvilli; CTR = cytotrophoblast; CE = chorionic epithelium; FE = fetal endothelium. (Reproduced with permission from Hay WW Jr, Wilkening RB, Metabolic activity of the placenta. In: Thorburn G, Harding R, eds, *Textbook of fetal physiology*. Oxford: Oxford University Press, 1994: 31.)

ial), surface area (compact or diffuse), and perfusion pattern (concurrent or countercurrent). Each of these properties is important with respect to some aspect of placental function and does not co-vary with the other properties.

## PLACENTAL GROWTH AND PLACENTAL FUNCTION

### Placental growth

Fig. 13.6 shows human placental growth curves, derived from cross-sectional measurements of placen-

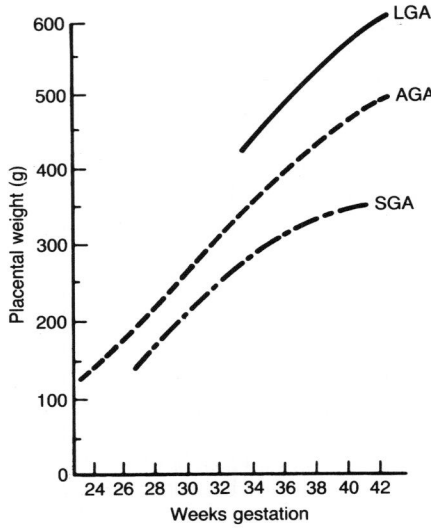

FIGURE 13.6 Human placental weights are shown to increase with gestational age and to fit three categories, AGA (average or appropriate for gestational age), SGA (small for gestational age), and LGA (large for gestational age), which also correspond to fetal weight/gestational age categories. (Reproduced with permission from Molteni RA, *et al.*, *Repro Med* 1978; **21**: 327.)

tal weights at delivery at advancing gestational ages. These data demonstrate two important characteristics of placental growth and function. First, fetal weight in late gestation is directly related to placental weight. Evidence from several models in which placental growth is experimentally restricted demonstrates that fetal growth in fact is dependent on placental growth. Second, small, average and large fetuses are directly related to small, average and large placentas, indicating that ordinarily the fetus does not outgrow the placenta. In studies in sheep, using carunculectomy to reduce placentation, however, among the growth-restricted fetuses the fetal : placental weight ratio was increased, indicating the possibility that an increase in placental functional capacity may partially compensate for the reduction in size.

### Placental transfer function

The placental capacity for functional adaptation has been documented in most detail in sheep, in which placental weight is maximal at 50 per cent of gestation and declines slightly toward term. Fetal growth continues progressively until term, however, demonstrating a marked change in placental functional capacity to meet the increasing nutrient needs imposed by fetal growth (Fig. 13.7). Functional maturation of the placenta has been quantified by estimates of transfer capacity. Placental urea permeability (or diffusing capacity) increases dramatically over the second half of gestation commensurate with the increase in fetal growth. More recent studies have focused on the change in placental

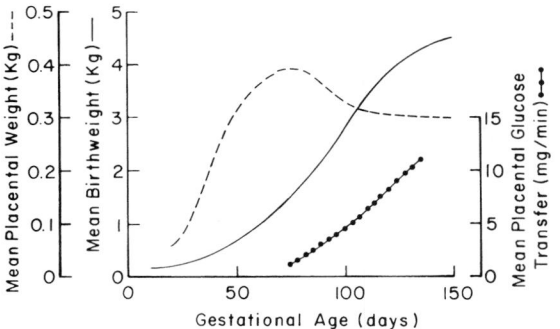

FIGURE 13.7 In sheep, placental weight (- - - -) peaks at midgestation and may decrease by 15–20 per cent by term. In contrast, placental glucose transfer (-●-●-●-) increases over the second half of gestation, reflecting the increased glucose needs of the growing fetus (——). (Reproduced with permission from Hay WW Jr, Placental nutrient metabolism and transport. In: Herrera E, Knopp R, eds, *Perinatal biochemistry*. Boca Raton: CRC Press, 1992: 100.)

glucose transport capacity (PGT) during the second half of gestation. PGT increases approximately 10-fold from mid to late gestation, a small part of which is due to increased fetal glucose consumption, and another small part to the increase in maternal-to-fetal glucose concentration gradient produced by an increase in the rate of placental glucose consumption; this even though the proportion of uterine glucose uptake consumed by the placenta relative to that of the fetus actually declines. As shown in Fig. 13.8, however, approximately 60 per cent of the late-gestational increase in placental glucose transport is accounted for by the increase in transport capacity *per se*. Thus, late gestation is marked by a progressive increase in functional transport capacity of the placenta that is quite separate from placental weight. In this regard, when

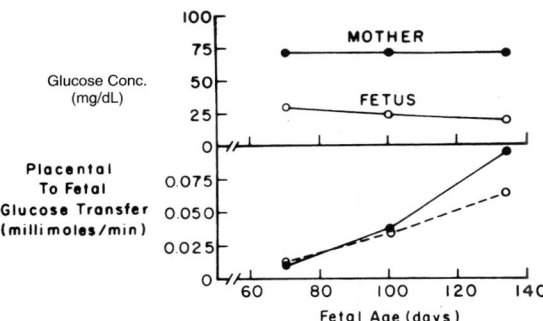

FIGURE 13.8 Upper panel: Basal glucose concentrations tend to decrease in fetal sheep over the second half of gestation; maternal concentrations were fixed for study purposes at 70 mg/dL plasma. Lower panel: Glucose transfer to the fetus from the mother via the placenta increases about 8-fold over this same period (-●-); this increase in transport primarily reflects an increase in transport capacity, as 60–70 per cent is not accounted for by the increase in transplacental glucose concentration gradient (-- ○ --). (Adapted from Molina RA *et al.*, *Am J Physiol* 1991; **261**: R697.)

the placenta is of normal size and function, any slowing of fetal growth in apparently normal fetuses in late gestation is unlikely to be due to placental limitation of nutrient supply. Thus, placental size and functional capacity are two important characteristics of placental development during gestation that directly determine the rate of fetal growth.

## MECHANISMS OF PLACENTAL TRANSFER

Placental transfer occurs by a large variety of mechanisms, each unique for a specific substance or a small set of substances with similar physical–chemical properties. General examples are illustrated in Fig. 13.9.

### Membrane transfer (flux)

Any inert substance that can cross the placental membranes will do so according to *Fick's law* (not to be confused with the Fick principle). Thus

$$\text{Flux}_{net} = D \left(\frac{A}{T}\right) (C_M - C_F) \text{ mol/(s·g)}$$

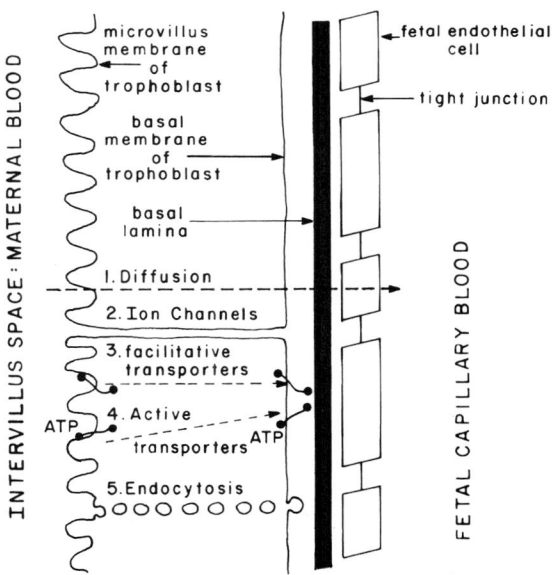

FIGURE 13.9 Schema of different transport mechanisms for the placenta illustrated for a hemochorial placenta as in humans. (1) Simple diffusion of gases (molecularly lipophilic); (2) paracellular or transcellular molecular ion channels (e.g. for $Na^+$, $Cl^-$, bicarbonate, etc.); (3) facilitative transporters, as for glucose, that mediate transport but have a specific binding affinity and maximum transport capacity; (4) active or energy-dependent transporters, as for amino acids; (5) endocytosis, which is receptor mediated, moves many large molecules such as lipoproteins, transferrin-iron complexes, and immunoglobulin G. (Reproduced with permission from Hay WW Jr, Placental nutrient metabolism and transport. In: Herrera E, Knopp R, eds, *Perinatal biochemistry*. Boca Raton: CRC Press, 1992: 102.)

where $D$ is a proportionality constant for the capacity of a substance to diffuse across the placenta; it includes the reflection coefficient ($\sigma$) unique for each substance ($\sigma$ is the fractional permeability of the membrane to each solute: 1.0 = completely permeable; 0 = completely impermeable) and the lipid solubility unique for each substance (1.0 = completely lipid soluble and highly diffusable; 0 = completely lipid insoluble and poorly diffusable), and reflects the combination of different structural components of the tissues between maternal and fetal plasma (M and F). $A$ is the surface area of the placental exchange area, and $T$ is the thickness of the placental tissues. $C_M$ and $C_F$ are the mean substance concentrations in maternal and fetal plasma, respectively, as they flow past the exchange area. The combined expression $D(A/T)$ is a constant known as $P$ or the "permeability" of the placenta for a particular substance. Thus, for any substance transferred across the placenta

$$\text{Flux}_{net} = P \text{ (concentration difference)}$$

$P$, therefore, is the proportionality coefficient between transfer rate and the concentration difference of a given substance across the placenta.

## Net membrane transfer (flux) rates

On each side of the placenta, net transfer rate or flux of a substance across the placental membrane is expressed by the Fick principle:

$$\text{Flux}_{net} \text{ across the uterine (maternal) side of the placenta} = F (C_{MA} - C_{MV})$$

where $C_{MA}$ and $C_{MV}$ are the concentrations of the substance in the uterine artery and vein, respectively, and $F$ is the rate of uterine blood flow. $C_{MA}$ is greater than $C_{MV}$ for substances that are transported in net into the uterus and placenta from the maternal circulation.

$$\text{Flux}_{net} \text{ across the umbilical (fetal) side of the placenta} = f(C_{Fv} - C_{Fa})$$

where $C_{Fv}$ and $C_{Fa}$ are concentrations of the substance in the umbilical vein and artery, respectively, and $f$ is the rate of umbilical blood flow. $C_{Fv}$ is greater than $C_{Fa}$ for substances that are transported in net into the fetal circulation from the placenta.

## Placental blood flow patterns and transport

In a placenta with concurrent (same direction or parallel) flow of the umbilical and uterine circulations, $C_M$

and $C_F$ will be most closely approximated by $C_{MV}$ and $C_{Fv}$. Thus

$$\text{Flux}_{net} = P(C_{MV} - C_{Fv})$$

Since $C_{MV} = C_{MA} - (\text{Flux}_{net}/F)$ and $C_{Fv} = C_{Fa} + (\text{Flux}_{net}/f)$, then

$$\text{Flux}_{net} = \frac{C_{MA} - C_{Fa}}{[1/P + 1/F + 1/f]}$$

which shows how the transplacental diffusion rate of a substance is related to the arterial concentrations of the substance in the uterine (maternal) and umbilical (fetal) circulations, the permeability of the placenta to the substance, and the actual uterine and umbilical blood flow rates. Similar calculations can be made for a concurrent (opposite direction) flow pattern.

## Placental clearance

It is essential to understand that the direction and magnitude of the transfer rate of a substance across the placenta depend on the maternal and fetal arterial concentrations of the substance. These are not exclusive properties of the placenta; they may depend, for example, on maternal diet, hormonal status, or metabolic rate for any given substance. Thus, placental transfer rate ($\text{Flux}_{net}$) is not a completely or even sufficiently satisfactory index of placental transfer function. As with renal physiology in which renal clearance is a better measure of renal function than is urinary excretion rate, it is better to define the placental transfer rate of a substance in relation to the arterial concentrations of the substance on both sides of the placenta and express placental transfer as a clearance.

$$\text{Placental clearance} = \frac{\text{Flux}_{net}}{C_{MA} - C_{Fa}}$$

Therefore, in the model shown above

$$\text{Placental clearance} = \frac{1}{[1/P + 1/F + 1/f]}$$

Clearance would be zero if either permeability or one or both of the flows were zero, because transport across the placenta requires the placenta to be permeable and perfused. Clearance of different inert substances varies between two limits: (a) permeability (or diffusion) limited clearance, and (b) flow-limited clearance. If permeability has a far more effective role relative to uterine and umbilical blood flows in controlling transfer of a given substance across the placenta (a very low permeability coefficient), then placental clearance of that substance is virtually equal to, and limited by, membrane permeability. Permeability-limited substances include most ions such as $Na^+$, and most nutrients such as the amino acids, glucose, lactate, and fatty acids.

Conversely, if permeability has a far less effective role relative to uterine and umbilical blood flows in controlling transfer of a given substance across the placenta, then placental clearance of that substance is virtually equal to, and limited by, the absolute values of uterine and umbilical blood flow. This condition is known as flow-limited clearance and indicates that blood flow, and thus the rate of "delivery" of a given substance to the placenta, will determine the rate of transfer of the substance across the placenta. $O_2$ is a good example of a flow-limited substance with respect to placental clearance and transfer.

## Diffusion-limited placental transfer

Diffusional transport will be passive (due only to permeability, maternal–fetal concentration differences, and blood flow rates and relationships) or transporter-mediated (Table 13.2). Transporter-mediated transport depends on the interaction of the transported substance with molecules or molecular structures that contribute to the overall placental permeability. Transporters can be facilitative, in which case they are saturable but at less than saturation assist transport according to concentration gradients, or active, in which case they are saturable but their activity depends on energy-consuming processes that can move the transported substance against a concentration gradient (e.g. certain amino acid transporters which transport amino acids to higher concentrations in the trophoblast).

## Ion transfer

$Na^+$ transfer is membrane-limited and thus is greater in the hemochorial human and rat placentas than in the epitheliochorial placenta of the sheep. $Na^+$ transfer is linked to neutral amino acid transfer (co-transport), $Cl^-$, $SO_4$, and succinate ion co-transport, and $H^+$ exchange ($Na^+$ in, $H^+$ out at the microvillous membrane). At the fetal membrane, $Na^+$ ion exchanges actively with $K^+$ ion, using energy generated by $Na^+$-$K^+$-ATPase. $Cl^-$ ion also passes through membrane-spanning $Cl^-$ channels. $SO_4$ exchanges at the fetal membrane in the fetal direction although the mechanism is not known. $Ca^{2+}$ appears to enter the trophoblast cytosol across the microvillous membrane by co-transport inward with $Na^+$ and exchange with $H^+$ according to electrochemical gradients established by inward $Na^+$ pumping and $H^+$ outward exchange at the base of pits in the microvillous membrane known as caveolae. $Ca^{2+}$ ions are actively transported across the fetal membrane into the fetal plasma by a putative $Ca^{2+}$ pump.

Thus, transporter-mediated transfer in the placenta can depend primarily on extraplacental concentration gradients established by non-placental mechanisms (facilitative transfer, as for glucose) or may be linked to energy supplied by metabolism within the placenta and at the placental membranes (as for amino acids and $Ca^{2+}$). The distinction between active and passive transfer mechanisms is not always so clear, as co-transport and exchange mechanisms may include passive partners such as $Cl^-$, $PO_4$, and certain amino acids. Also, transport can be active at one membrane and not the other. For example, the amino acid taurine is actively concentrated across the microvillous membrane into the trophoblast cytosol but may then diffuse more passively down a concentration gradient into the fetal plasma. In contrast, $Ca^{2+}$ appears to enter the

TABLE 13.2 Factors affecting placental substrate transfer

1. Uterine/umbilical blood flows: absolute rates (substrate delivery), the ratio of their flows (substrate delivery versus uptake and transport capacity), and the role of vasoactive substances (local or circulating) that alter uterine and/or umbilical blood flow (e.g. reduction in flow with epinephrine, enhancement of flow with nitric oxide)
2. Circulating hormone concentrations, placental receptors, and second messengers (e.g. hormone stimulation of cAMP-responsive increase in $Ca^{2+}$ channel and intracellular $Ca^{2+}$ release, activating substrate metabolism and transporter activity)
3. Transporter proteins in the trophoblast membranes: ontogeny, location (maternal-facing microvillus, or fetal-facing basal, or both), regulation by local or circulating factors
4. Transport capacity, measured by $V_{max}$ (maximum transport rate, affected by number of active transporters, number of transporters per unit membrane area, and total membrane surface area)
5. Transporter-substrate binding affinity, measured by $K_m$ (plasma substrate concentration at half $V_{max}$)
6. Competition for transporters among similar substrates
7. Turnover of transporters (rates of synthesis, degradation, or both)
8. Diffusional leaks: (a) into or out of cells; (b) via paracellular pathways
9. Intracellular, maternal, fetal, and maternal–fetal substrate concentration gradients
10. Metabolism of substrates by the trophoblast (e.g. oxidation of glutamate, conversion to other amino acids or substrates such as serine to glycine and leucine to ketoisocaproic acid (KIC), protein synthesis, deamination producing $NH_3$)
11. Inhibitory effects of drugs (e.g. alcohol, nicotine, cocaine)
12. Energy supply (glucose plus $O_2$)
13. Ion channel activity, ion gradients: $Na^+$-$K^+$-ATPase; $Na^+$, $H^+$, $Cl^-$ gradients (e.g. inward $Na^+$ gradient with System A co-transport)

trophoblast cytosol somewhat passively according to H⁺ exchange and Na⁺ co-transport at the microvillous membrane but then be actively pumped into the fetal plasma (the same may be true for $SO_4$ and $PO_4$ ions as well).

## Flow-limited placental transfer

Substances that are highly lipid-soluble diffuse passively through the placental membranes and cells very rapidly; thus, they have a permeability coefficient of nearly 1 and their transfer across the placenta depends almost completely on their transplacental concentration gradients and the directional relationships and flow rates of the umbilical and uterine circulations.

There are two types of umbilical and uterine blood flow relationships: concurrent and countercurrent. In the *concurrent* pattern, most characteristically found in sheep, umbilical and uterine blood pass through the placenta in parallel so that the umbilical venous blood is last equilibrated with and most closely resembles the composition of uterine venous blood. In this case, placental metabolism has strong influences on the composition of umbilical venous blood. In the *countercurrent* pattern, most characteristically found in rats, rabbits, and cats, umbilical blood flows through the placenta in the opposite direction to the uterine circulation so that umbilical venous blood last equilibrates with and more closely resembles the composition of uterine arterial blood. This produces a more efficient transfer capability. Placental metabolism still can affect the composition of umbilical venous blood. Quantitative comparisons of the effects of countercurrent and concurrent flow patterns on the flow-limited effectiveness of placental transfer (defined as clearance/flow) are shown in Fig. 13.10 for "effectiveness" versus the permeability/flow ratio and in Fig. 13.11 for "effectiveness" versus the uterine/umbilical flow ratio, based on data from rabbit and sheep.

The human hemochorial placenta has an *intermediate* pattern with respect to the anatomical arrangement of uterine and umbilical blood flows and transfer efficiency. Both concurrent and countercurrent flow patterns are present as the maternal blood circulates around the fetal villi. On balance, the human placenta functions more like a concurrent exchange system in that both cordocentesis blood samples obtained prior to delivery and cord blood samples obtained at cesarean section have failed to show an umbilical $Po_2$ above that in a simultaneously sampled uterine vein. Although micropuncture data from *in vitro* perfused human placentas show slightly higher umbilical venous $Po_2$ values than those measured in samples obtained simultaneously from the intervillous space, the relationship between such *in vitro* data and the normal *in vivo* condition is highly uncertain.

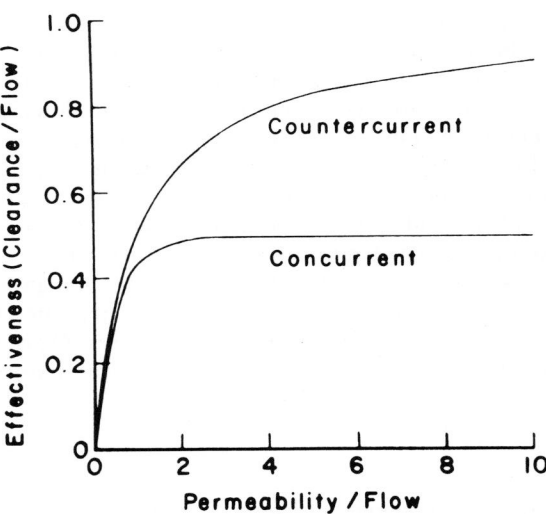

FIGURE 13.10 Relation of effectiveness of placental transfer to the permeability–flow with a ratio of 1.0 for two types of blood flow patterns. In both the countercurrent and concurrent models of placental exchange, effectiveness tends toward a flow-limited maximum as permeability increases in relationship to blood flow rate. (Reproduced with permission from Battaglia FC, Meschia G, *An introduction to fetal physiology.* Orlando: Academic Press, 1986: 34.)

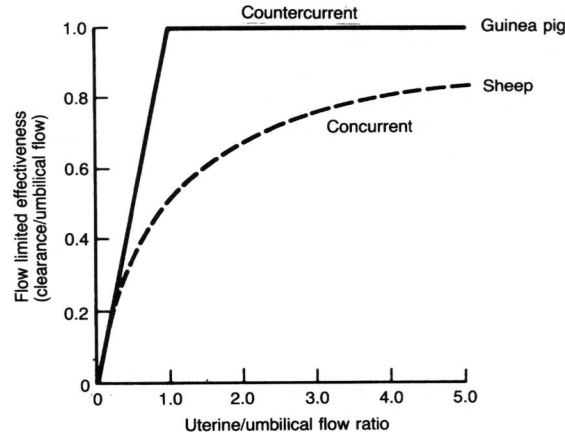

FIGURE 13.11 Comparison of experimental data testing the flow-limited effectiveness of the guinea pig and sheep placenta for tritated water. Guinea pig data from Moll and Kastendieck; sheep data from Wilkening, *et al.* (Adapted from Battaglia FC, Meschia G, *An introduction to fetal physiology.* Orlando: Academic Press, 1986: 46, with permission.)

## Endocytosis and exocytosis and placental transfer

Endocytosis and exocytosis involve transfer by fusion of membrane vesicles around a solute or transported substance, either into the cell (endocytosis) or out of the cell (exocytosis). The first phase is called *pinocyto-*

*sis* and involves extended invagination of pits in the membrane surface which capture and pull into the cytosol the substances to be transferred. Presumably, ligand-receptor mechanisms unique to the substances to be transferred initiate the invagination, vesiculation, and transfer processes, although such processes are not well understood. As with $Ca^{2+}$ entry into the trophoblast cells by caveolae, passive and active co-, anti-, and exchange-type transport processes may be involved at the base of the invaginations, as well as actual extrusion of the membrane-bound substance into the cytosol with subsequent release by lysozomal degradation of the endocytosed vesicle membrane. Examples of endocytotic uptake by the human placenta include low-density lipoproteins, transferrin/iron complex, and immunoglobulin G. IgG is transported intact but for transferrin/iron and LDL, and many other substances as well, intra-trophoblast metabolism alters what is subsequently transferred to the fetal plasma. In other cases, there is trans-syncytial migration of the vesicle containing the transferred substance (by unknown mechanisms), followed by fusion of the vesicle membrane with fetal-facing trophoblast membrane and exocytosis.

## Water transfer across the placenta (*see also* Chapter 14)

Based on measurements with radioactively labeled water (e.g. $^3H_2O$), unidirectional transfer rates of water across the sheep placenta are extremely rapid, many-fold greater than net transfer. Beyond that, the regulation of water transfer across the placenta is not well understood. Clearly, there is no reason to think that osmotic, oncotic, and hydrostatic mechanisms are not the essential regulating factors, but it has not been possible to identify and quantify their contributions. At best, it is clear from all species that water acquisition by the growing fetus is proportional to body weight, with some diminution of water content as fetal cellularity increases in the later part of gestation. Thus, the principal driving force for water transport is the growth of fetal cells and their components, all of which are governed by cell division and cell hypertrophy processes that require many solutes of many kinds, all of which drag water with them.

## METABOLIC ACTIVITY OF THE PLACENTA

## Oxygen

### Placental $O_2$ transfer

$O_2$ transfer across the placenta is flow-limited; thus, the net driving force across the placenta for $O_2$ is the partial pressure difference between maternal and fetal blood. In an ideal concurrent system, the umbilical venous blood $Po_2$ should be equal to that in the uterine vein. This is not the case, however, because of shunting (some maternal and fetal blood does not pass close to the site of exchange) and/or uneven perfusion (maternal–fetal blood flow ratios are different between different segments of the placenta). The largest cause of a lower umbilical venous $Po_2$ compared with that in the uterine vein, however, is placental $O_2$ consumption.

These relationships are illustrated in Fig. 13.12, which shows how placental $O_2$ uptake by the uterus and transfer of $O_2$ to the fetus are curvilinearly related to uterine blood flow. A significant reduction in placental $O_2$ transfer does not occur until uterine blood flow is reduced to less than 50 per cent of normal. Thus, in spite of major decreases in $O_2$ delivery, the transplacental driving force for $O_2$ transfer (the transplacental $Po_2$ gradient) and placental $O_2$ permeability are sufficiently large enough that transfer is maintained unless the uterine circulation is severely compromised.

Another factor involved in $O_2$ transfer across the placenta is the difference in $O_2$ affinity between maternal and fetal hemoglobin (*see* page 871) (Fig. 13.13).

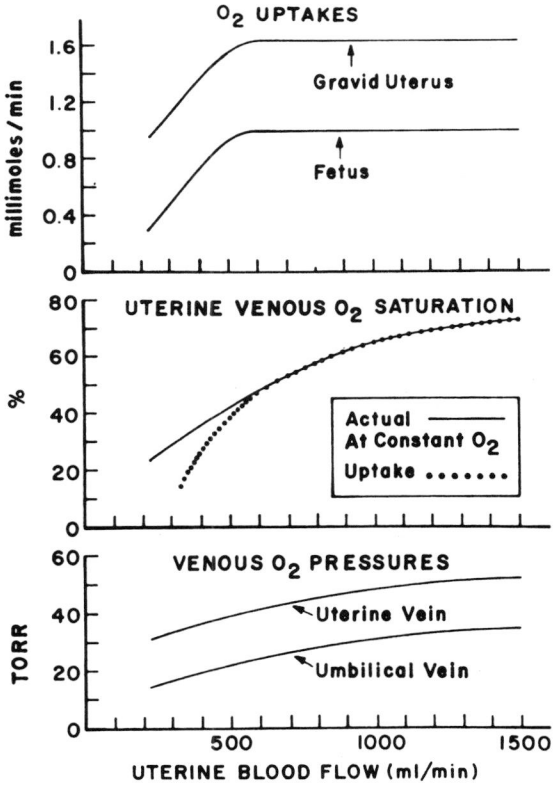

FIGURE 13.12 Effect of decreasing blood flow on uterine and fetal $O_2$ uptakes, uterine venous $O_2$ saturation, and the $Po_2$ in uterine venous and umbilical venous blood. (Reproduced with permission from Battaglia FC, Meschia G, *An introduction to fetal physiology*. Orlando: Academic Press, 1986: 170.)

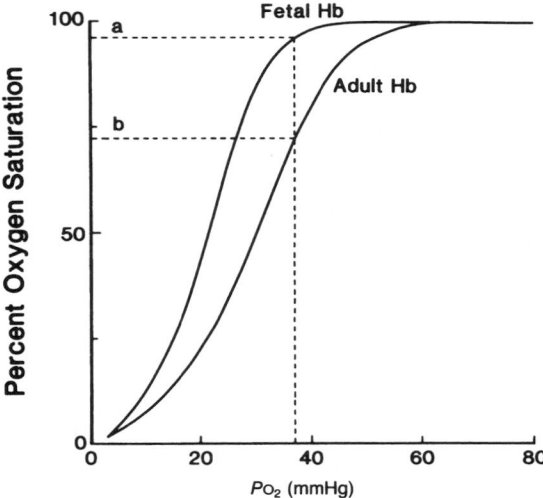

FIGURE 13.13 Fetal hemoglobin has a higher affinity for $O_2$ than does adult hemoglobin. This allows the blood $O_2$ saturation to be higher in the fetus (dotted line "a") compared with the mother (dotted line "b") at the relatively low $P_{O_2}$ values characteristic of the maternal blood bathing the fetal villi and last equilibrating with the uterine venous blood $P_{O_2}$ (intersection of vertical dotted line with x-axis).

Fetal hemoglobin has a higher affinity for $O_2$, which helps to guarantee sufficient $O_2$ supply for the high metabolic demands of the growing fetus. For example, replacement of fetal blood with maternal blood produces an umbilical venous saturation only half that of normal fetal blood and a marked decrease in net transfer rate of $O_2$ from maternal to fetal blood. This may be important clinically if maternal blood is used to directly transfuse the fetus who is markedly anemic from *hemolytic disease*. A decrease in fetal blood $O_2$ saturation under these circumstances is only a partial complication, however, as the principal benefit of the transfusion is the correction of the deficit in $O_2$ transport capacity by supplying red blood cells. Because of the higher affinity of fetal blood compared with maternal blood, fetal blood also will have a lower $P_{O_2}$ for any given saturation.

## Placental $O_2$ consumption

The placenta has one of the highest rates for $O_2$ consumption ($\dot{V}O_2$) of all tissues in the body. For example, in sheep the uteroplacental tissues consume approximately half of the uterine $O_2$ uptake; the balance is transported to and consumed by the fetus. On a weight-specific basis, however, $O_2$ consumption by the uteroplacental tissues is 4 to 5-fold greater than that of the fetus which itself has a metabolic rate approximately twice that of the adult. While these average values for uteroplacental $O_2$ consumption are quite high, they probably considerably underestimate $O_2$ utilization by placental cellular tissue alone. Placental cellular tissue has been calculated to have a metabolic rate as high as that in brain, liver, kidney and many tumor cells ($O_2$ consumption of about 1.5 to 2 μmol/(min·g)).

It is assumed that the high placental $O_2$ consumption is essential to maintain active processes such as ATP production, ATP-dependent concentration of amino acids in the trophoblast cytosol, active transplacental ion transfer, and protein synthesis (particularly of glycoproteins such as chorionic gonadotrophin). Limitation of $O_2$ supply, in fact, has been shown to decrease placental transfer of at least some amino acids. *In vivo* data also show a respiratory quotient (RQ) of about 1.0. *In vivo*, uteroplacental $O_2$ consumption increases over the second half of gestation both in absolute terms and on a weight-specific basis. Many synthetic and transport activities of the uteroplacenta increase markedly over the same gestational period. Presumably such activities and the increase in metabolic rate of the uteroplacental tissues are directly linked. Thus, although the proportion of uterine $O_2$ uptake consumed by the fetus also increases considerably over the second half of gestation, this by no means indicates a senescence of uteroplacental metabolic activity.

The quantities of $O_2$ taken up and consumed by the uteroplacental tissues (about 0.1–0.4 mmol/(kg·min) at term in humans and 0.5–2.0 mmol/(kg·min) in animals) are quite variable, reflecting the different species studied and particularly the different *in vivo* and *in vitro* technics and conditions applied. Stressful perturbations such as anesthesia, interference with either maternal or fetal perfusion, cold, and physical handling all affect the measurements. Much of the information obtained from *in vitro* studies of placental metabolism demonstrate a marginally functioning placenta limited by, and thus dependent upon, the supply of $O_2$ and metabolic substrates.

## Glucose

### Placental glucose transfer and metabolism

The uptake of glucose by the placenta and its transfer to the fetus occur by *facilitated diffusion* in which the glucose concentration gradient across the placenta is the principal regulator while perfusion has a much lesser role. This process is mediated by specific transporter proteins that have specificity for hexose molecules and differentiation among hexose molecules that favors glucose molecules. Glucose transporters are found on both the maternal-facing microvillus membrane of the trophoblast and on the fetal-facing basal membrane. The activity of placental glucose transporters on either the maternal or fetal surface appears dependent on glucose concentration alone; changes in insulin concentration in either the maternal or fetal circulation in all species studied to date, *in vivo* and *in vitro*, appear to have no effect on placental glucose transport or placental glucose consumption. Molecular studies have found only GLUT 1 and GLUT 3 glucose transporters in placental tissue, neither of which is insulin-sensitive in other tissues.

According to the transporter-mediated, facilitated diffusion model of placental glucose uptake and transfer, the glucose transfer rate approaches a maximum as maternal and fetal glucose concentrations are increased beyond physiological limits.

$$PGT = V_{max} [(G_A/G_A + K_m) - (G_a/G_a + K_m)] - \dot{q}p$$

where $V_{max}$ is the maximum rate of net glucose transport across the placenta; $G_A$ and $G_a$ are maternal and fetal arterial plasma glucose concentrations, respectively; $K_m$ is the maternal arterial plasma glucose at $V_{max}/2$; and $\dot{q}p$ is the net rate of placental glucose consumption from fetal-to-placental glucose transfer when maternal and fetal arterial plasma glucose concentrations are equal. The net placental glucose consumption contributes significantly to the physiological hypoglycemia of the fetus and helps to establish the glucose concentration gradient by which both placenta and fetus compete for glucose molecules.

The equation for glucose transport by the placenta indicates that changes in the maternal or fetal concentration of glucose will affect transport and, thus, affect uterine glucose uptake and placental glucose consumption. The effect of maternal glucose concentration is

shown in Fig. 13.14(a), which demonstrates a saturable increase in glucose uptake by the uterus at increasing maternal arterial plasma glucose concentrations. Uptake and net consumption of glucose by the uteroplacenta in relation to maternal arterial plasma glucose concentration also show saturation kinetics with a $V_{max}$ of about 41 mg/min. $K_m$ and $K_s$ ($K_s$ = maternal arterial glucose concentration at which $V_{max}$ is reached) were 19 mg/dL and 145 mg/dL, respectively, not significantly different from the same variables for uterine glucose uptake. Fetal glucose uptake (net transfer rate of glucose from the placenta to the fetus) also increases according to saturation kinetics as maternal glucose concentration increases (Fig. 13.14(b)).

In contrast to these studies in which both maternal and fetal glucose concentrations co-varied, other *in vivo* studies have demonstrated that at a constant maternal glucose concentration, net fetal glucose uptake increases as fetal glucose concentration decreases (Fig. 13.14(b)). At the same time, placental glucose consumption is directly related to fetal glucose concentration and is relatively independent of maternal glucose concentration (Fig. 13.14(c)). In fact, when the transplacental glucose concentration gradient is abolished, approximately 75–80 per cent of the glucose consumed by the uteroplacenta is supplied by the fetal circulation. This observation implies that the fetal side of the uteroplacenta is markedly more permeable to glucose than the maternal side (approximately

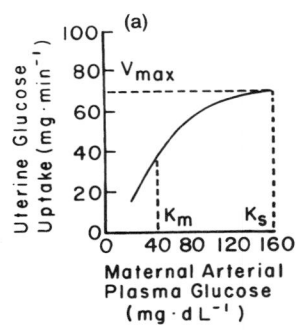
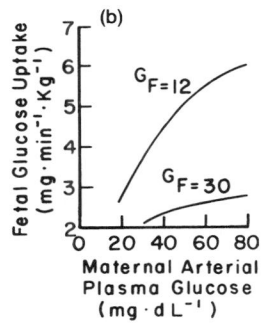
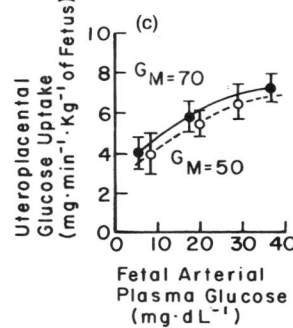

FIGURE 13.14 (a) Schematic representation of effect of maternal glucose concentration on uterine glucose uptake, based on experiments in which glucose was infused into pregnant sheep after an overnight fast to produce a large variety of maternal arterial blood glucose concentrations. Fick principle measurements were then made of net uterine glucose uptake rates versus the maternal arterial plasma glucose concentration which shows saturation kinetics with an approximate $K_m$ value in the physiological range of maternal glucose concentration (about 50–60 mg/dL). (Adapted with permission from data in Hay WW Jr, *et al.*, *Proc Soc Exp Biol Med* 1989; **190**: 63.) (b) Fetal glucose uptake (net transfer rate of glucose from placenta to fetal circulation) plotted against maternal arterial glucose concentration showing a saturable dependence of fetal glucose uptake on maternal glucose concentration. In addition, this relationship is left-shifted as fetal glucose concentration is decreased, showing that as fetal glucose concentration is decreased relative to that of the mother, which increases the maternal–fetal glucose concentration gradient, placental-to-fetal glucose transfer increases. (Adapted from data in Hay WW Jr *et al.*, *Am J Physiol* 1990; **258**: R569, with permission of the American Physiological Society.) (c) Net rate of uteroplacental glucose consumption in sheep, expressed per kilogram of fetus, plotted against fetal arterial plasma glucose. Solid line: values measured while maternal arterial plasma glucose was clamped at about 70 mg/dL. Dotted line: values measured while maternal arterial plasma glucose was clamped at about 50 mg/dL. These data show that although maternal glucose concentration determines glucose entry into the uteroplacenta and fetus, actual uteroplacental glucose consumption is regulated largely by the fetal glucose concentration. (Adapted from data in Hay WW Jr *et al.*, *Am J Physiol* 1990; **258**: R569, with permission of the American Physiological Society.)

8-fold) and indicates that changes in fetal glucose concentration should have strong influence on placental glucose flux and metabolism. This point is illustrated in Fig. 13.15. An increase in fetal glucose concentration, that is independent of the maternal glucose concentration, separately and significantly regulates uteroplacental glucose consumption, in contrast to the total entry of glucose into the uterus, uteroplacenta, and fetus that is regulated by maternal glucose concentration.

## Gestational maturation of placental glucose transfer

Approximately 60 per cent of the increase of placental glucose transport is accounted for by the increase in placental transport capacity, explained primarily by an increase in the number of glucose transporters. Fig. 13.16 presents a schema of how the increase in placental glucose transfer capacity over the second half of gestation in sheep interacts with fetal metabolism to guarantee an increase in placental transfer of glucose to meet the increasing glucose needs of the growing fetus. The fetal metabolic adjustments include increased insulin production and concentration, increased insulin action, and an increase in the fraction of fetal bodyweight accounted for by insulin-sensitive tissues (primarily skeletal muscle), all combining to produce increased fetal glucose utilization, increased fetal plasma glucose clearance, a relatively lower fetal

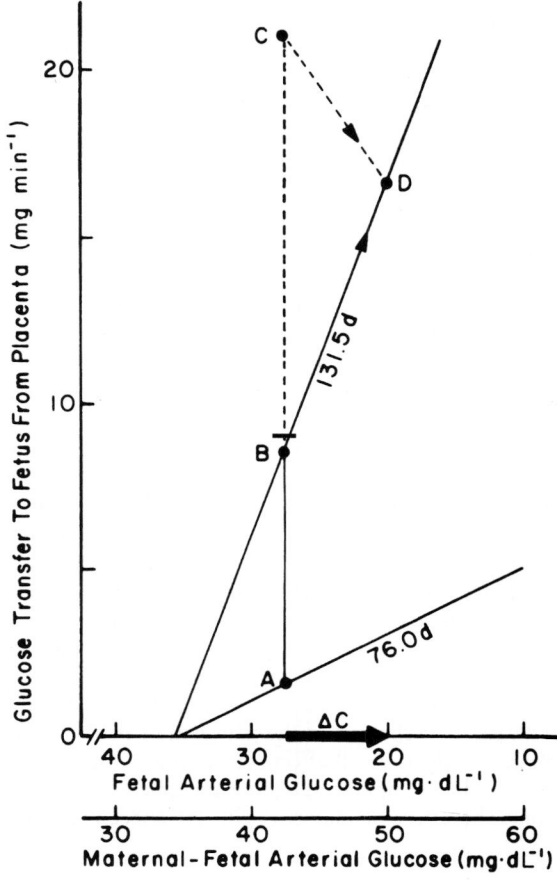

FIGURE 13.16 Graphic illustration of interrelationships among developmental changes in placental glucose transport capacity, fetal glucose demand, and fetal glucose concentration from mid- to late-gestation in the sheep model. Placental glucose transfer capacity increases over gestation, shown by the increased slope of the 131.5-day gestational age line versus the slope of the mid-gestation, 76-day line, supplying more glucose to the fetus (A→B). Fetal growth demands more glucose, however, represented by point C. Additional glucose is provided by the simultaneous decrease in fetal glucose concentration relative to that of the mother which increases the transplacental glucose concentration gradient (x-axis segment ΔC), producing the actual glucose supply to the fetus at point D (which is less than point C because the lower fetal glucose concentration also decreases the mass action transfer of glucose into fetal cells). (Reproduced from data in Molina RD, *et al.*, *Am J Physiol* 1991; **261**: R697, with permission of the American Physiological Society.)

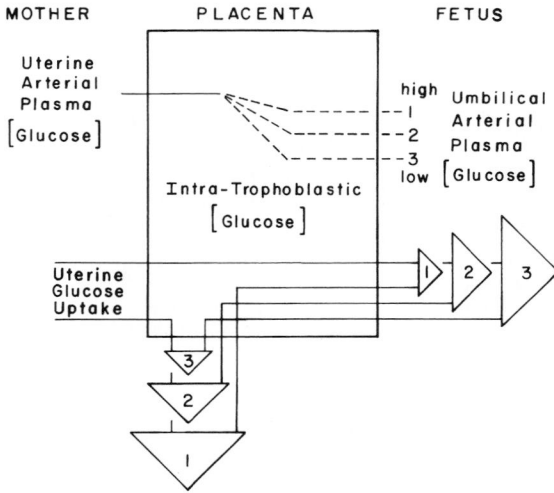

FIGURE 13.15 Schema of effects of fetal glucose concentration on placental glucose transfer to the fetus and uteroplacental glucose consumption, adapted from data in sheep. A decrease in fetal glucose concentration relative to maternal glucose concentration promotes maternal-to-fetal glucose transfer at the expense of uteroplacental glucose consumption. These findings demonstrate a reciprocal relationship between placental glucose transfer and uteroplacental glucose consumption that is determined by the fetal glucose concentration. (Reproduced with permission from Hay WW Jr, *Proc Nutr Soc* 1991; **50**: 321.)

plasma glucose concentration, and ultimately an increase in the maternal–fetal plasma glucose concentration gradient leading to increased glucose transfer across the placenta to the fetus.

## Placental glucose oxidative metabolism

Glucose carbon consumed by the placenta produces $CO_2$ and $H_2O$ by oxidation. If all of the glucose consumed were oxidized it could account for as much as 45 per cent of placental $O_2$ consumption. This value assumes that all of the lactate production by the placenta is derived from net placental glucose metabolism, although certain amino acids such as alanine are likely alternative sources of placental lactate production. In fact, however, only 50 per cent or less of glucose is oxidized *in vivo* in the sheep placenta and even less (as little as 5 per cent) *in vitro* in human and rat placentas.

The placenta also produces glycogen from glucose. Rates of production and regulation of this process are not known, although placentas from pregnancies complicated by *hyperglycemia* (e.g. *diabetes*) may have increased glycogen content. *In vitro* studies demonstrate that placental glycogen is synthesized rapidly in the placenta early in pregnancy and that this synthetic rate decreases toward term.

## Placental lactate metabolism

Lactate is produced by the placenta in all species and in large amounts (averaging approximately 28 μmol/(kg placental weight·min) in sheep) and enters in net into the maternal and fetal circulations (at approximately equal rates in sheep). *In vivo* human studies have not consistently demonstrated placental lactate production although accurate measurements during normal conditions have not been made yet. Placental lactate production is a normal process that occurs during aerobic metabolism and is unaffected by small to moderate changes in maternal or fetal blood $Po_2$, blood $O_2$ content, or uterine and/or umbilical blood flows. In sheep the amount of lactate taken up by the fetus is about half of net fetal glucose uptake at normal glucose concentrations and about one-third of fetal lactate utilization. Thus, the majority of fetal lactate is produced by the fetus although it is clear that lactate produced in the placenta is a relatively large net source of carbon for fetal utilization. Lactate metabolism thus appears to be responsible for at least as much of the oxidative activity in the placenta as glucose. The ability to metabolize lactate to meet placental energy requirements may permit other potential oxidative substrates to be spared for transport to the fetus. Lactate may be one of the substrates essential to the hypothesis that a reciprocal relationship exists between placental glucose oxidation and the oxidation of other substrates.

## Placental fructose metabolism

Placental production of fructose is unique to ruminants and does not occur to any appreciable extent in humans. Fructose can be oxidized in the placenta but at a very low rate; it also produces a small amount of lactate in the placenta although there is no measurable net conversion to glucose nor to placental glycogen.

# Amino acids

## Placental amino acid uptake and transfer

Most amino acids are concentrated in the trophoblast cytosol by so-called "active" or energy-dependent transporter proteins found at the maternal-facing microvillous membrane. Acute changes in maternal amino acid concentrations probably have little influence on this process of active concentration in that acute maternal hypoaminoacidemia or hyperaminoacidemia produce little or no change in fetal amino acid concentrations, at least over brief periods of an hour or so. Energy deficiency and $O_2$ deficiency do, however, reduce placental uptake and transfer of selected amino acids. Thus, for those amino acids directly transported from the maternal to the fetal plasma, the quantity and activity of their transporters in the placenta help to determine how much and what relative proportions of these amino acids get to the fetus, providing unique quantitative and qualitative control over fetal amino acid supply and plasma concentrations.

Table 13.3 lists the currently known placental amino acid transporters, the individual or group of amino acids that they transport, regulatory influences, and location on maternal or fetal membranes. Net transport of most of the amino acids into the fetus produces fetal plasma concentrations greater than maternal. Some amino acids simply may be concentrated in the trophoblast cytosol and then move more by facilitative transport down a concentration gradient into the fetal plasma whereas others are actively transported into the fetal plasma.

## Placental amino acid metabolism

In addition to amino acid uptake and transport to the fetus, the placenta has a large variety of metabolic processes that significantly alter amino acid supply to the fetus. Examples of these processes are shown in Fig. 13.17.

At term the placenta contains a large variety of enzymes capable of metabolizing amino acids through a diverse number of metabolic pathways including gluconeogenesis, glycogen synthesis, protein synthesis, amino acid oxidation, and ammoniagenesis. Amino acid flux through these pathways has been demonstrated *in vitro*. Other protein requirements include an undetermined amount for synthesis of secreted protein products. Quantitative aspects of placental amino acid requirements are not certain because the net uptake of amino acids by the placenta provides an extraction ratio equal to or less than the accuracy of their plasma concentration measurements. Based on placental nitrogen content at term in the human placenta, however, it has been estimated that placental growth over gestation would require about 10.6 g of nitrogen or 66 g of protein, which is a minimum estimate of nitrogen and protein requirements for

TABLE 13.3 Placental amino acid transport mechanisms in human placental fragments

| SYSTEM | SUBSTRATES | CONDITIONS | MEMBRANE |
|---|---|---|---|
| *Na⁺-dependent* | | | |
| A | Neutral amino acids: alanine, glycine, serine, proline, threonine, glutamine, MeAIB | $Na^+$-dependent, slowed by extracellular $H^+$. Excludes anionic and cationic amino acids, BCH, and leucine | M,F |
| ASC | Alanine, serine, cysteine, anionic (acidic) amino acids | $NA^+$-dependent, slowed by extracellular $H^+$. Excludes MeAIB, cationic amino acids and proline | F |
| N | Glutamine, histidine, asparagine | $NA^+$-dependent. Excludes cysteine, MeAIB, trans-stimulated | M |
| $X^-_{AG}$ | Anionic (acidic) amino acids, glutamate, aspartate | $NA^+$-dependent. Uptake from fetal blood. Non-competitive with other amino acids. Excludes non-anionic amino acids | M,F |
| β | Taurine | $Na^+$, $Cl^-$-dependent. Highest intracellular concentration of all amino acids. Excludes α-amino acids | M |
| *Na⁺-independent* | | | |
| l | Branched-chain amino acids: (leucine, isoleucine, valine), tryptophan, BCH, phenylalanine, tyrosine, alanine, serine, threonine, glutamine | $Na^+$-independent, enhanced by extracellular $H^+$. Excludes anionic amino acids, proline, MeAIB | M,F |
| $y^+$ | Lysine, arginine | Major cationic amino acid transporter. Excludes anionic amino acids. Inhibited by neutral amino acids (fetal side > maternal side) | M,F |
| $b^{o,+}$ | Lysine, arginine | Excludes anionic amino acids | F |
| $y^+L$ | Lysine, arginine | Excludes anionic amino acids | M |
| *Other not well-defined transporters specific for:* | | | |
| | Methionine | $Na^+$-dependent | M |
| | Proline | $Na^+$-dependent | F |
| | Cysteine | $Na^+$-independent | M |
| | Alanine, serine | $Na^+$-independent | M |
| | Tyrosine | $Na^+$-independent | F |

F = fetal; M = maternal. (Adapted from Yudilevich *et al.* Transport of amino acids in the placenta. *Biochim Biophys Acta* 1985; 822: 169; Smith *et al.* Nutrient transport pathways across the epithelium of the placenta. *Ann Rev Nutr* 1992; 12: 183.)

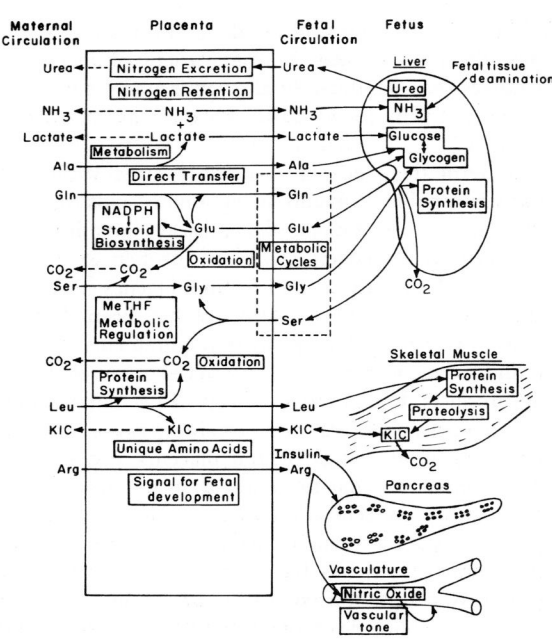

FIGURE 13.17 Schema of placental amino acid uptake, metabolism, and transfer, based on data in the pregnant sheep. Top: Ammonia ($NH_3$) is the end-product of placental amino acid deamination; it is taken up by the umbilical vein and can be used for urea formation in the fetal liver. Some amino acids also are metabolized to lactate while many are directly transported to the fetus after concentration in the trophoblast cytosol. Middle: Although serine and glycine may not be taken up appreciably by the placenta from the uterine circulation, placental production of glycine, fetal hepatic uptake of glycine and production of serine, and serine uptake by the placenta indicate active fetal–placental metabolic cycles, as well as placental oxidative metabolism and the formation of methyltetrahydrofolate which may be important for metabolic regulation. Similarly, glutamine is directly transported to the fetus (some may be used to produce glutamate in the placenta) where it is used in fetal tissues but in the liver produces glutamate, much of which is then taken up by the placenta and oxidized. Bottom: Leucine can be used for placental protein synthesis and oxidation, but continued deamination of leucine in the placenta produces α-ketoisocaproic acid which then is taken up by the umbilical circulation. Other amino acids may serve as important signals or substrates for unique fetal development, such as the role of arginine in pancreatic insulin secretion and nitric oxide formation. (Adapted with permission from Hay WW Jr, *Proc Nutr Soc* 1991; 50: 321.)

placental growth. In fact, placental amino acid consumption for other metabolic purposes may be much higher in order to provide carbon for oxidation, ammonia production, lactate production, conversion to other amino acids or to proteins that are excreted into the umbilical or uterine circulations, and incorporation into placental proteins.

The placenta has several unique metabolic processes for amino acid metabolism. For example, the placenta actively produces ammonia which is delivered in net into both the uterine and umbilical circulations. This appears to be a normal process in mammalian placental metabolism and in fetal sheep, occurs over a large part of gestation, with an absolute rate of uteroplacental ammonia production of about 25 µmol/min. This process is consistent with *in vitro* evidence of negligible urea cycle activity in placental tissue over the entire length of gestation. Such a relatively high placental ammonia production in mid-gestation probably contributes to the higher concentration of ammonia (approximately two-fold) found in fetal blood in mid-gestation at which point the fetus is much smaller and its ammonia clearing capacity is markedly reduced relative to term.

Another example of unique placental–fetal interaction involving amino acid metabolism is demonstrated by placental–fetal hepatic relationships between certain amino acids (examples from sheep). For example, glutamine and glycine are taken up in net by the fetus from the placenta and by the liver from the umbilical vein, whereas their metabolic products, glutamate and serine, respectively, are produced in net by the fetal liver and taken up in net by the placenta. The interorgan cycling of glycine and serine between the placenta and the fetal liver is quantitatively significant, contributing importantly to energy and protein balance in the fetal–placental unit. Furthermore, fetal serine production and uptake by the placenta from the umbilical circulation appears to be much larger at mid-gestation than near term, suggesting an active developmental process regulating this interorgan cycling. The serine–glycine cycle may be important for methyl group supply to and conservation in the fetus, and thus may be important for control of fetal growth. Placental uptake of glutamate may be important not only to produce glutamine for supply to the fetus where it can promote growth, but also to provide another substrate for placental oxidation (70–80 per cent of placental glutamate uptake from the fetus in sheep is oxidized to $CO_2$). This process also may help control fetal plasma glutamate concentration and modulate its potential neurotoxicity as an excitatory amino acid.

A further example of placental–fetal amino acid cycling involves the metabolic function of relatively high concentrations and activities of branch-chain amino acid aminotransferases found in the placenta (at least in the sheep and human). Studies in sheep suggest that net placental uptake and transamination to the corresponding ketoacid can occur for leucine (to ketoisocaproic acid). The importance of this process to placental and fetal amino acid metabolism and fetal growth remains to be determined. It is clear, therefore, that the placental free amino acid pool, derived from a variety of sources including the maternal and fetal circulations, and intraplacental interconversions, cannot be treated as a single homogeneous pool.

# Lipids

## Placental lipid transfer and metabolism

The amount and type of fatty acid or lipid moiety transported by the placenta varies among species, being greatest in the hemochorial placenta of the human, guinea pig, and rabbit, and least in the epitheliochorial placenta of ruminants and the endotheliochorial placenta of carnivores. Furthermore, the fat content of the fetus at term among species varies directly with the lipid transport capacity of the placenta.

A schema of lipid uptake, metabolism, and transport in the human placenta is shown in Fig. 13.18. After entering into the placenta, fatty acids may be used for triglyceride synthesis, cholesterol esterification, membrane biosynthesis, direct transfer to the fetus, or for oxidation. A variety of factors regulate the flux of lipid carbon into these various pathways of transport and metabolism. The most important factor appears to be the maternal plasma free fatty acid (FFA) concentration. For example, placental triglyceride content increases in women who are fasting, who deliver preterm infants, or who have *diabetes mellitus*, conditions in which maternal plasma FFA concentrations are increased. Fatty acids may be transferred directly to the fetus by specific transporter proteins or after modification by processes such as desaturation, elongation, or partial oxidation. Although most fatty acids appear to be transported by direct transporter-mediated mechanisms, some studies suggest that chain-altering metabolism in intra-trophoblast peroxisomes may lead to a greater transfer of medium chain fatty acids into the fetal circulation. This would be advantageous to fetal lipid metabolism which is limited in its capacity for oxidation of long-chain fatty acids by low carnitine concentrations. Fatty acids, as well as mono- and diglycerides carried in the maternal plasma or released from circulatory lipoproteins by placental lipoprotein lipase, also can be esterified to di- and triglycerides and to phospholipids in the trophoblast cells. These may be stored transiently or long-term as well as being hydrolyzed by phospholipases and acylglycerol lipases to release fatty acids to the fetal circulation. Fatty acids may also be synthesized in the placenta in free form or as lipoprotein particles and then transported to the fetal plasma. As a result of all of these processes, both maternal diet and metabo-

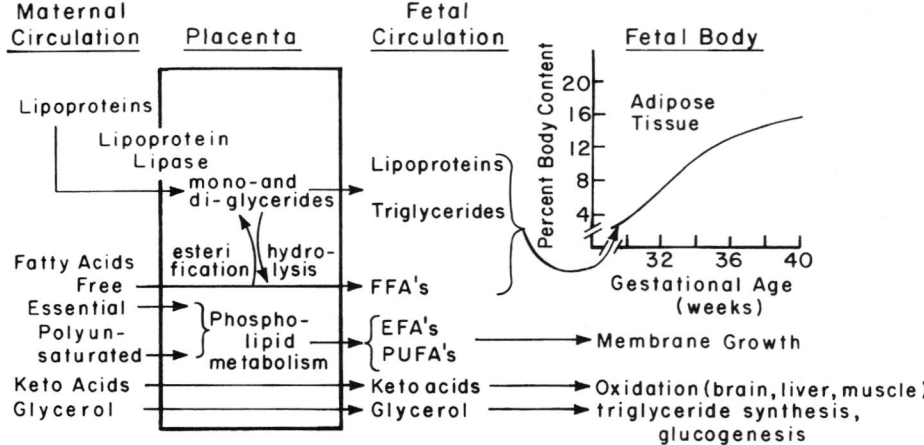

FIGURE 13.18 Possible pathways of placental lipid metabolism and transport to the fetus. Lipoprotein-carried triglycerides, phospholipids and cholesterol esters, and partial glycerides that have been released by placental lipase may be taken up and undergo esterification or further hydrolysis within placental cells. Maternal serum free fatty acids and the fatty acids that have been released by placental lipoprotein lipase may enter the placenta using specific transporters. Within placental cells, the free fatty acids taken up directly and those released by intracellular hydrolysis may be transported to the fetal circulation. Alternatively, these fatty acids may be re-esterified to form triglycerides which are transiently stored. The endogenously synthesized triglycerides may then be hydrolyzed and the released fatty acids may be transported to the fetus. Lipids that enter the fetus can then be used for a variety of metabolic pathways although oxidation is limited and tissue synthesis is primary. (Adapted with permission from Hay WW Jr, Metabolic interrelationships of placenta and fetus. *Placenta* 1995; **16**: 19.)

lism, which determine maternal lipid concentrations, and placental lipid transport and metabolic capacities, interact to produce a unique supply of lipids to the fetal circulation.

The placenta also is vitally important for metabolizing cholesterol. LDL cholesterol is taken up by endocytosis into trophoblast cells and degraded by lysozymes. It appears to be the major precursor for placental production of progesterone and estrogen. HDL cholesterol also contributes to placental progesterone production in cultured human trophoblast cells. Some of this cholesterol is transferred directly to the fetus, although the role of this transport is uncertain, given the large capacity and rate of cholesterol synthesis in the fetal liver.

In spite of major differences in placental lipid transport among species, all fetuses require essential fatty acids and their derivatives to produce structural components of membranes, particularly in the central nervous system. Thus, even the sheep placenta is an important source of essential fatty acids, such as linoleic and arachidonic acids, which are incorporated into phospholipids in the placenta and transferred into the fetal circulation. The same is true for the human placenta which transfers arachidonic acid directly from maternal to fetal plasma. Thus, the placenta has an important role in producing, modifying, and transporting to the fetus essential fatty acids and long-chain polyunsaturated fatty acids via phospholipid metabolism, thereby contributing to the quality as well as the quantity of fetal membrane phospholipids.

## CONCLUSIONS

Clearly the placenta is more than a passive membrane. While it serves the vital role of transporting substances between the uterine and umbilical circulations, it is also an extremely active metabolic organ, accounting for more than half of the uptake of $O_2$ and glucose by the conceptus (uterus, placenta, and fetus). In fact, a large portion of the gradients that passively and facilitatively drive $O_2$ and glucose from the uterine to the fetal circulations is accounted for by placental $O_2$ and glucose consumption. The energy produced by such oxidative metabolism is also used for the concentration of amino acids in placental cells to very high levels from which the amino acids then diffuse facilitatively into the fetal plasma. Other metabolic pathways in the placenta for $O_2$, carbohydrates, amino acids, and lipids are diverse and complex. They serve not only unique metabolic requirements in the placenta but they also modify the delivery to and concentration in the umbilical circulation of nearly all essential nutrients. Placental transport mechanisms and placental metabolism thus play major roles, independently and together, in providing for the nutritional requirements of fetal growth and metabolism.

## SELECTED READING

Battaglia FC. New concepts in fetal and placental amino acid metabolism. *J Anim Sci* 1992; **70**: 3258.

Battaglia FC, Meschia G. Fetal nutrition. *Ann Rev Nutr* 1988; **8**: 43.

Carter BS, Moores RR, Battaglia FC. Placental transport and fetal and placental metabolism of amino acids. *J Nutr Biochem* 1991; **2**: 4.

Coleman RA. Placental metabolism and transport of lipid. *Fed Proc* 1986; **45**: 2519.

Desoye G, Shafrir E. Placental metabolism and its regulation in health and diabetes. *Mol Aspects Med* 1994; **15**: 505.

Hay WW Jr. Metabolic interrelationships of placenta and fetus. *Placenta* 1995; **16**: 19.

Hay WW Jr. Placental metabolism of glucose in relation to fetal nutrition. In: Nathanielsz PW, ed. *Fetal and neonatal development. Research in perinatal medicine*, Vol. 7. Ithaca, NY: Perinatology Press, 1988: 58.

Hay WW Jr. Placental supply of energy and protein substrates to the fetus. *Acta Paediatr* 1995; **83** (Suppl. 405): 13.

Hay WW Jr. Placental transport of nutrients to the fetus. *Hormone Res* 1994; **42**: 215.

Hay WW Jr, Molina RA, DiGiacomo JE, Meschia G. Model of placental glucose consumption and glucose transfer. *Am J Physiol* 1990; **258**: R569.

Lemons JA. Fetal–placental nitrogen metabolism. *Semin Perinatol* 1979; **3**: 177.

# 14

# Fetal Physiology

## FETAL ADAPTIVE RESPONSES TO HYPOXEMIA

The fetus lives and grows in a relatively "hypoxic" environment and yet normally exists with a surplus of $O_2$ for metabolic needs. When oxygenation is compromised, the fetus is capable of a number of adaptive responses, both protective and potentially pathologic. These adaptive responses in turn provide a physiologic basis for the monitoring techniques used in the clinical assessment of fetal health.

### FETAL METABOLISM AND OXYGEN TRANSPORT

The fetal consumption of $O_2$ and of substrate, primarily glucose, serves two basic requirements (Fig. 14.1): (1) provision of fuel for energy production through maintenance of oxidative metabolism, and (2) provision of building materials for tissue growth. Although oxidative metabolism is the major component of total substrate needs, tissue growth requirements may not be insignificant depending on the rate of growth relative to ongoing energy requirements. For the ovine fetus near term, tissue growth requirements in fact account for approximately one-third of total substrate needs when expressed in terms of caloric equivalents. Furthermore, an unknown fraction of the energy produced from oxidative metabolism must fuel tissue growth. A variable "savings" in both ATP energy requirements and substrate building needs might therefore be realized with a falloff in tissue growth when $O_2$ and substrate availability to the fetus becomes limited.

The transport of $O_2$ from the atmosphere to the fetal tissues requires a series of steps alternating bulk

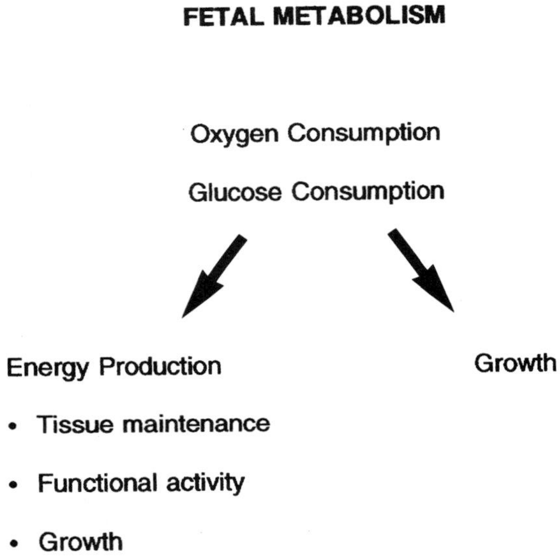

### FETAL METABOLISM

Oxygen Consumption

Glucose Consumption

Energy Production                    Growth

• **Tissue maintenance**

• **Functional activity**

• **Growth**

FIGURE 14.1 Outcomes of fetal metabolic processes

transport with transport by diffusion (Fig. 14.2). The normally low fetal arterial blood partial pressure of $O_2$ ($Pa_{O_2}$) of approximately 20 mmHg (2.66 kPa) can be attributed largely to two aspects of this transport process: (1) the venous equilibration of placental gas exchange whereby functionally both maternal and fetal vascular streams run in the same direction, and (2) the admixture of umbilical venous and inferior vena caval blood within the fetus. Nevertheless, the transport of $O_2$ to fetal tissues appears more than adequate, with no evidence for anaerobic glycolysis as a terminal source for energy production. This is due in part to the increased $O_2$-carrying capacity of fetal blood, in turn due to the higher hemoglobin concentration which increases throughout gestation, and to the higher $O_2$ affinity, which permits the saturation

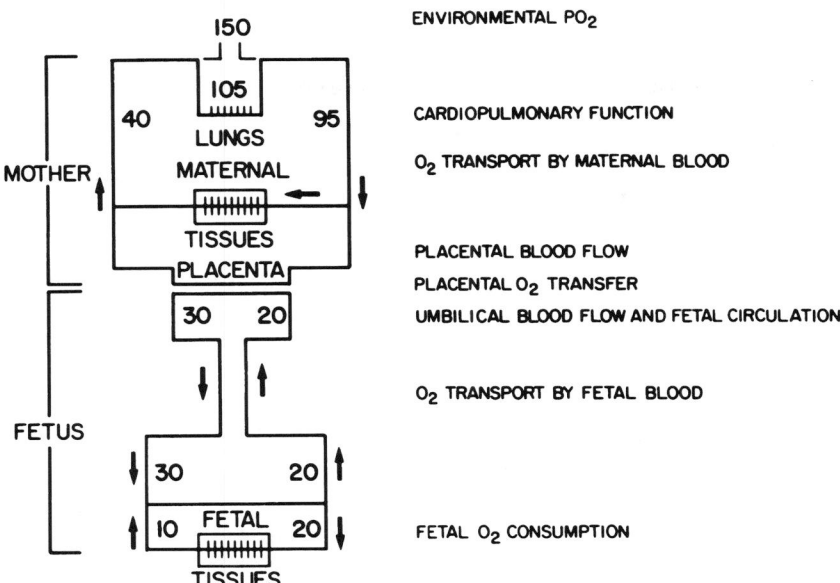

FIGURE 14.2 Maternal and fetal circulations. Numbers refer to $P_{O_2}$ of each compartment (i.e., inspired air, alveolar air, maternal arterial and venous blood, umbilical venous and arterial blood, and fetal venous blood). (Modified from Towel M. Fetal respiratory physiology. In: Goodwin JW, Godden JO, Chance GW, eds, *Perinatal medicine*. Toronto: Longman-Canada Ltd, 1976: 171, with permission.)

of fetal blood with $O_2$ at a lower $P_{O_2}$ (*see* Chapter 81). A second means whereby the oxygenation of fetal tissues is maintained is the relative overperfusion of fetal organs in comparison with their $O_2$ requirements. The result is an $O_2$ concentration in fetal blood only slightly less than that in maternal blood and $O_2$ delivery to some organs actually in access of their adult counterparts.

## FETAL RESPONSES TO HYPOXEMIA

Interference with the transport of $O_2$ (and possibly of $CO_2$) to (and from) the fetus can occur at any one of the transport steps indicated in Table 14.1. However, the extent to which gas exchange is impaired covers a spectrum and may lead to mild hypoxemia alone, or to severe hypoxemia with attendant hypercapnia and progressive metabolic acidemia. Likewise, the time course over which the impairment in gas exchange occurs may operate acutely over minutes or hours, subacutely over days, or chronically over weeks. Both the extent and the duration of the impairment of gas exchange will bear on fetal adaptive responses (outlined in Table 14.2) which can be categorized as those affecting fetal metabolism or those affecting fetal $O_2$ transport.

## Oxygen margin of safety

Fetal $O_2$ consumption ($\dot{V}O_2$) equals the product of umbilical blood flow ($\dot{Q}umb$) and veno-arterial $O_2$ content difference across the umbilical circulation (Fick equation):

$$\text{Fetal } \dot{V}O_2 = \dot{Q}umb \times (C\bar{u}vo_2 - Cuao_2)$$

TABLE 14.1 Factors decreasing $O_2$ transfer to the fetus, and examples of causes

| |
|---|
| Reduced environmental $P_{O_2}$ |
|   High altitude |
| Altered maternal cardiopulmonary function |
|   Cyanotic heart disease |
| Decreased $O_2$ transport by maternal blood |
|   Anemia |
|   Cigarette smoking |
| Decreased placental blood flow |
|   Hypertension |
|   Diabetes |
|   Uterine contractions |
| Decreased placental $O_2$ transfer |
|   Abruptio placentae |
|   Placental infarcts |
| Decreased umbilical blood flow and fetal circulation disturbances |
|   Umbilical cord occlusion |
|   Heart disease |
| Decreased $O_2$ transport by fetal blood |
|   Anemia |
|   Hemorrhage |

TABLE 14.2 Fetal responses to hypoxemia

> Fetal metabolism
>   "Oxygen margin of safety"
>   Substrate alterations
>   Decreased growth
>   Behavioral state alterations
>   Decreased fetal movements
> Fetal $O_2$ transport
>   Increased blood $O_2$ capacity
>   Blood flow redistribution

TABLE 14.3 The $O_2$ margin of safety

> Increased fractional oxygen extraction
> Maintenance of oxygen consumption

$O_2$ consumption = $O_2$ delivery × $O_2$ fractional extraction

where $\overline{Cuv}o_2$ is mixed umbilical venous blood $O_2$ content and $Cua o_2$ is umbilical arterial blood $O_2$ content. On rearrangement of this equation, fetal $O_2$ consumption is related to the product of umbilical $O_2$ delivery and fractional $O_2$ extraction (i.e. the $O_2$ consumed as a fraction of that delivered) (Table 14.3). Factors leading to impairment of fetal blood gas exchange ultimately give rise to either a lowered umbilical venous $O_2$ concentration or a lowered umbilical blood flow with a corresponding reduction in $O_2$ delivery to the fetus. With a decrease in $O_2$ delivery, however, the fetus is capable of a compensatory increase in fractional $O_2$ extraction, thus maintaining $O_2$ consumption. As $O_2$ extraction is a function of diffusion, any increase must involve an increase in the $Po_2$ gradient across the umbilical circulation, ultimately resulting in a drop in the $Pao_2$ and thus fetal hypoxemia. The degree to which fractional $O_2$ extraction can increase and fetal $Pao_2$ can fall before tissue $O_2$ supplies are inadequate and become rate-limiting for $O_2$ consumption, is the "$O_2$ margin of safety," which is an indicator of the $O_2$ reserve available for the fetus when $O_2$ delivery is decreased.

With acute reduction in $O_2$ delivery, the ovine fetus is capable of increasing $O_2$ extraction from approximately 33 per cent to approximately 66 per cent, thus maintaining $O_2$ consumption until $O_2$ delivery is reduced by half. That fetal $O_2$ consumption is maintained despite such a decrease in $O_2$ delivery, and thus a moderate degree of hypoxemia, is somewhat surprising since the metabolic costs of fetal movement activity and growth should diminish quickly (see below). This suggests that other aspects of fetal metabolism are increased in response to acute hypoxia; these may relate to the cardiovascular and hormonal changes that occur. The human fetus undoubtedly also is capable of this adaptive response, and this likely gives rise to an increased tolerance of obstetrical emergencies such as *umbilical cord prolapse* with the fetus at birth being hypoxemic, but usually without metabolic

acidemia. However, the $O_2$ reserve available to the human fetus may be less than that of the ovine fetus, as the $O_2$ extraction with uneventful vaginal or cesarean delivery normally measures somewhat higher than that of the ovine fetus *in utero*.

With prolonged reduction in fetal $O_2$ delivery over several days, the ovine fetus shows little change in $O_2$ extraction with $O_2$ consumption a linear function of $O_2$ delivery; thus there is no evidence for an "$O_2$ margin of safety." This indicates that the fetus responds differently to long-term reduction in oxygenation (and/or other substrate deficiencies) with the ability to "turn off" oxygen-consuming processes, such as growth and perhaps certain aspects of behavioral activity, contributing to a reduction in $O_2$ needs over time.

## Substrate alterations (Table 14.4)

Although oxidative metabolism has been studied extensively during induced hypoxemia in the ovine fetus, there is less information on the metabolic fate of other substrates. With acute short-term reduction in oxygenation, the exogenous uptake of glucose

TABLE 14.4 Substrate alterations

> Decreased glucose uptake
> Decreased lactate uptake
> Decreased amino acid uptake

across the umbilical circulation is variably decreased and, coupled with increased glycogen metabolism, serves to ensure placental glucose supply. Fetal lactate uptake also decreases and may give way to net lactate production. As fetal lactate concentrations rise this may also become an important source of substrate to sustain the placenta. In addition, the exogenous uptake of amino acids decreases such that fetal protein accretion, and therefore growth, must be curtailed.

During prolonged, but mild, hypoxemia such as occurs with induced *intrauterine growth restriction (IUGR)*, the ovine fetus again shows a variable decrease in umbilical glucose uptake while lactate uptake is variably increased, on both an absolute and per kilogram fetal weight basis. These metabolic changes are associated with fetal blood substrate changes whereby glucose concentrations are lower and lactate concentrations are higher. There also is a sustained rise in alanine concentrations in keeping with a decrease in amino-nitrogen utilization for growth and perhaps in oxidative metabolism. Cordocentesis data from *human growth restricted fetuses* indicate variable degrees of hypoglycemia, hyperlacticemia, and increases in alanine concentrations suggesting metabolic changes similar to those seen in the ovine fetus with experimental IUGR.

TABLE 14.5 Intrauterine growth restriction

| |
| --- |
| Decreased growth rate |
| Decreased substrate requirements |
| Metabolic normalization |

## Intrauterine growth restriction (Table 14.5)

In the ovine fetus with acutely induced hypoxemia of several hours' duration, protein synthesis is decreased with a corresponding decrease in the energy requirements for growth equivalent to approximately 10 per cent of total $O_2$ consumption. With both prolonged reduction in fetal $O_2$ delivery over several days and induced IUGR, total $O_2$ consumption is reduced approximately 20 per cent. This decrease in fetal oxidative metabolism again represents the energy "savings" from decreased tissue growth but also may reflect, in part, changes in behavioral activity and in associated energy requirements. The ovine fetus thus demonstrates a rapid adaptation to a limitation in substrate delivery with a decrease in growth rate (and activity) and thereby substrate needs, resulting in remarkable metabolic normality with a variable degree of hypoxemia and usually little evidence of metabolic acidosis or anaerobic metabolism. Of note, if decreased fetal growth is sufficient, the falloff in $O_2$ consumption may balance that for $O_2$ delivery such that fetal $Pao_2$ is in fact normalized.

The human fetus also undergoes intrauterine growth restriction, determined clinically by serial ultrasound assessment. Cordocentesis data indicate variable degrees of hypoxemia, although in many instances blood gas values are within the normal range, suggesting a degree of normalization with the falloff in growth. However, the extent to which this mechanism is protective by decreasing substrate requirements for energy and growth, or gives rise to pathologic development of certain organ systems with time, is not known. It is possible that abnormalities in brain growth and development may contribute to the minimal cerebral dysfunction noted in follow-up studies of growth-restricted infants.

## Behavioral state alterations

Behavioral states are evident in both the human and ovine fetus near term and are similar to those in human infants in which metabolic rate differences also are found ($O_2$ consumption approximately 5 per cent higher during the active or rapid eye movement (REM) sleep state when compared with the quiet or non-rapid eye movement (NREM) sleep state). A similar increase in overall $O_2$ consumption also is noted in the human adult during REM sleep when compared with NREM sleep; this is attributed largely to the cor-

responding increase in cerebral $O_2$ consumption. While behavioral state appears to have little effect on the overall metabolic rate of the ovine fetus, there is an increase in cerebral metabolic rate during the low-voltage electrocortical or REM state. Doppler flow velocity studies in the human fetus suggest a similar relationship given the tight flow-metabolism coupling within the brain.

In the ovine fetus REM state activity is variably decreased during hypoxemia, which would indicate a change to a metabolic state with lower oxidative needs, at least for the brain. However, a marked and significant decrease is only evident with moderate to severe hypoxemia. As such this adaptive process is more likely to be of benefit with acute rather than chronic reductions in fetal oxygenation. In the *growth restricted human fetus* there is a developmental delay in the appearance of well-defined behavioral states and periods of increased activity indicative of the awake state are less evident than in the appropriately grown fetus. Although possibly reflecting a metabolic compensatory response to a decrease in oxygenation, these alterations in behavioral state activity may instead reflect underlying neurologic dysfunction.

## Decreased fetal movements (Table 14.6)

Although the overall effect of behavioral state on fetal metabolic rate is minimal, at least for the ovine fetus, that of state-related biophysical parameters appears considerably greater. Neuromuscular blockade in the ovine fetus results in an approximate 20 per cent decrease in $O_2$ consumption, presumably due in part to a decrease in breathing activity and other gross body movements. Conversely, fetal $O_2$ consumption is increased to a similar extent during periods of fetal breathing activity when compared to apneic periods. As such, a decrease in fetal movements in response to a compromise in oxygenation should reduce energy expenditure and thus $O_2$ requirements depending on the extent to which muscular activity is decreased.

In the near-term ovine fetus, moderate hypoxemia of short-term duration results in a marked decrease in movement activity, including forelimb, eye and breathing movements. However, if this degree of hypoxemia is maintained in the absence of metabolic acidemia, movement activity returns toward normal after several hours. With prolonged and graded reductions in fetal oxygenation over several days, a marked decrease in fetal movement activity is only seen as the degree of hypoxemia approaches the level at which acidemia becomes apparent. As such, fetal movement assessment

TABLE 14.6 Decreased fetal movements

| |
| --- |
| Decreased body movements |
| Decreased breathing movements |
| Decreased energy expenditure |

should be seen as a marker for moderate to severe hypoxemic change. Of note, the biophysical response of the preterm ovine fetus is less pronounced than that of the older gestational-aged fetus, which may affect survival and have implications for the success of antenatal assessment protocols. With induced intrauterine growth restriction in the ovine fetus and with chronic hypoxemia, breathing movements are marginally decreased, occurring approximately 20 per cent of the time. While of probable biologic importance and providing for a decrease in oxidative needs, this would not be a useful clinical marker given the effects of other influencing factors, including the diurnal and cyclic nature of breathing activity.

In the human fetus, movement activity has been extensively studied in the "high risk" obstetrical patient as a component part of biophysical profile assessment. For the dynamic fetal variables as presently scored, a decrease in body movements would appear to improve the positive predictive value for adverse perinatal outcome more than a decrease in breathing movements or a non-reactive non-stress fetal heart rate test. Conversely, blood gas data from the umbilical cord obtained immediately after biophysical assessment indicate that a non-reactive non-stress test and loss of fetal breathing are earlier signs of fetal acidosis and worsening hypoxemia than a loss of fetal movement and tone. This would imply a hierarchy within the fetal brain for the control of these activities in response to hypoxemia and/or acidemia. Although this may be true, as suggested by studies in the ovine fetus, the clinical evidence to date is based on arbitrary standards without relation to normal values for a given population. Of note, a small number of patients with adverse perinatal outcome are not predicted on the basis of dynamic fetal monitoring. This serves to emphasize that the monitoring of fetal movement activity only allows for an assessment of fetal health at the time of testing, and from which only a probability of continued health may be formulated. However, the time course over which these variables become abnormal prior to fetal death is not known and may well change with assorted disease processes and their severity.

In patients with *intrauterine growth restriction* and presumed chronic fetal hypoxemia, fetal movement activity is variably decreased and appears dependent on the severity of growth restriction. Although again of probable biologic importance with an associated decrease in energy expenditure, there is considerable overlap with population norms which would limit the usefulness of activity variables as markers for intrauterine growth restriction.

## Increased blood oxygen capacity

In the ovine fetus, acutely induced hypoxemia results in an increase in hematocrit and thus blood $O_2$ capacity with an associated increase in serum protein concentration, indicating a shift of water from the vascular to the extravascular space. The hematocrit of human fetal blood obtained from the fetal scalp during labor and from the umbilical cord at delivery is also increased in the presence of fetal hypoxemia and acidosis. Fetal hematocrit is likewise increased in both the ovine and human *growth-restricted fetus*, with stimulated erythropoiesis and increased red blood cell production presumably in response to chronic hypoxemia.

## Blood flow redistribution

Hypoxemia results in well-described changes within the fetal circulation, both centrally and peripherally (Table 14.7), thus enhancing the delivery of $O_2$ to so-called "vital organs." Acute hypoxic stress in the ovine fetus increases umbilical venous return through the ductus venosus, facilitating the delivery of the most highly oxygenated blood directly to the heart, without prior passage through the hepatic circulation. An increase in the preferential streaming of this blood through the foramen ovale into the left atrium and ventricle further enhances the delivery of available $O_2$ to the ascending aorta and thus to the heart and brain.

Peripherally, acutely induced hypoxemia results in a redistribution of cardiac output such that umbilical–placental flow is maintained, and the proportion to the heart, brain, and adrenals is increased, and that to other fetal tissues variously maintained or decreased depending on the means by which hypoxemia is induced and the severity of the insult. In the ovine fetus this redistribution of cardiac output results in a hyperbolic increase in blood flow directed to the heart and brain in inverse relation to arterial $O_2$ content, such that $O_2$ delivery to these tissues is maintained. This protective redistribution of cardiac output is maintained when acutely induced hypoxemia is sustained for up to 48 hours; studies with induced *intrauterine growth restriction* indicate a similar blood flow redistribution in response to chronic hypoxemia. While there has been limited study to date, the redistribution of blood flow to vital organs in response to hypoxic insults may be less effective for the preterm ovine fetus.

The introduction of combined real-time and pulsed Doppler ultrasound has provided a noninvasive means of monitoring the human fetal circulation. Doppler-

TABLE 14.7 Blood flow redistribution

| |
|---|
| *Central* |
| Increased umbilical blood flow through ductus venosus |
| Increased umbilical blood flow through foramen ovale |
| *Peripheral* |
| Increased flow to vital organs |
| Maintained flow to placenta |
| Maintained or decreased flow to other ("non-vital") organs |

measured indices derived from velocity waveforms are assumed to be a reflection of downstream vascular resistance, and as such may be important as an indirect measure of fetal circulatory change in certain high-risk pregnancies. In patients with *intrauterine growth restriction* and presumed chronic fetal hypoxemia, these waveform indices are variably altered with a decrease in the cerebral circulation and an increase in the descending aorta and lower extremity in keeping with a centralization of blood flow to vital organs as in the ovine fetus. However, there is considerable overlap with population norms as Doppler-measured waveform indices are also affected by other biologic and hemodynamic factors, thus limiting the clinical usefulness of these measurements.

## SUMMARY

The fetal environment is thus well suited for normal growth and development with $O_2$ availability exceeding oxidative needs. With impairments in blood gas exchange this excess $O_2$ acts as a "margin of safety," providing for the maintenance of oxidative metabolism through increases in fractional $O_2$ extraction, although with resultant fetal hypoxemia. Increases in blood $O_2$ capacity and redistribution of cardiac output in response to this hypoxemia further protect fetal oxygenation. Additional adaptive mechanisms involve a decrease in energy-consuming processes, including growth restriction, decreasing fetal movements, and behavioral state alterations. Although protective insofar as essential metabolic functions are maintained, pathologic change may occur as the "$O_2$ margin of safety" becomes limited or energy-conserving measures give rise to abnormal growth and development.

## SELECTED READING

Bocking AD. Fetal behavioural states: pathological alteration with hypoxia. *Semin Perinatol* 1992; 16: 252.

Edelstone DI. Fetal compensatory responses to reduced oxygen delivery. *Semin Perinatol* 1984; 8: 184.

Jensen A, Berger R. Fetal circulatory responses to oxygen lack. *J Dev Physiol* 1991; 16: 181.

Milley JR. Uptake of exogenous substrates during hypoxia in fetal lambs. *Am J Physiol* 1988; 254: E572.

Richardson BS. Fetal adaptive responses to asphyxia. *Clin Perinatol* 1989; 16: 595.

Richardson BS, Gagnon R. Fetal breathing and body movements. In: Creasy RK, Resnik R. eds, *Maternal–fetal medicine: principles and practice*. Philadelphia: W.B. Saunders, 1993: 258.

Rurak DW, Richardson BS, Patrick JE, Carmichael L, Homan J. Oxygen consumption in the fetal lamb during sustained hypoxemia with progressive acidemia. *Am J Physiol* 1990; 258: R1108.

Rurak DW, Richardson BS, Patrick JE, Carmichael L, Homan J. Blood flow and oxygen delivery to fetal organs and tissues during sustained hypoxemia. *Am J Physiol* 1990; 258: R1116.

Soothill PW, Ajayi RA, Nicolaides KN. Fetal biochemistry in growth retardation. *Early Hum Dev* 1992; 29: 91.

# FETAL AND AMNIOTIC FLUID BALANCE

Fluid balance in the fetus is dramatically different from that in the adult. This occurs for multiple reasons:

- The fetus has a much higher water content than the adult.
- The fetus interacts extensively with its surrounding amniotic fluid.
- The rates at which fluids move in the fetus are approximately one order of magnitude greater than in the adult relative to bodyweight.

This section integrates these concepts together with an overview of current knowledge regarding fetal and amniotic fluid balance. The primary message is that fluid movements of the fetus are highly dynamic with extensive interactions among fetal fluids, amniotic fluid and the maternal compartment.

## FETAL FLUIDS

Two fundamental concepts aid in understanding regulation of fetal and amniotic fluid balance. First, the chorion and placenta are the outer limits of fetal tissue, and hence any fluid within these limits is fetal fluid. Thus, amniotic fluid as well as the fluid within the fetal body is fetal fluid. However, when discussing fetal fluid balance, it is convenient to consider fluid within the fetal body separately from amniotic fluid. Second, all fetal fluid volumes and flows depend either directly or indirectly on fetal blood volume. In other words, fetal urinary output, swallowing, transcapillary filtration, lymph flow, etc. are regulated, at least in part, to maintain fetal blood volume within a normal range. This is accomplished largely through neural, endocrine and passive physical mechanisms.

A third and equally important fact is that most physiological information regarding regulation of fetal and amniotic fluid balance derives from animal studies, particularly in fetal sheep. Thus, the following is a synthesis from multiple sources using animal data when needed.

### Fluid distribution within the fetal body

The amount of fluid within the fetus is dramatically different from that in later life. In the normal adult, 50–60 per cent of bodyweight is water. In contrast, at term, the fetus is approximately 75 per cent water, and fetal water content is as high as 90–95 per cent at the beginning of the fetal period. Thus, the normal state of hydration during the fetal period is somewhat analogous to gross whole-body edema in the adult.

In addition to having more total body water, the fetus has a different distribution of fluid within its body when compared with the adult; the fetus has more extracellular fluid and less intracellular fluid relative to bodyweight. Further, the relationship between intracellular, extracellular and total body water changes throughout the fetal period (Fig. 14.3), with total body water and extracellular fluid decreasing as intracellular fluid increases.

## Blood and plasma volumes

Although some older literature has indicated that blood volume/unit fetal weight was higher in younger than older fetuses, more recent data indicate that blood volume/unit fetal weight is constant across gestation. The higher volumes determined in the earlier studies arose as an artifact because the labels used to determine blood volume escaped from the circulation into the tissues and thereby overestimated true blood volume.

Normal blood volume in the human fetus averages 105–115 mL/kg fetal bodyweight, which is essentially the same as in the ovine fetus. Further, both human and animal data indicate that fetal blood volume/kg fetal bodyweight does not vary over a range of fetal hematocrit from approximately 15 to 50 per cent.

Thus, the moderately anemic human fetus would be expected to have the same blood volume as the non-anemic fetus at the same gestational age.

Although the average fetal blood volume does not vary with hematocrit, in individual fetuses there can be a wide range of weight-normalized blood volumes. Fetuses with high blood volumes have high plasma and high red-cell volumes, whereas fetuses with low blood volumes have low red-cell and plasma volumes (Fig. 14.4). Although the responsible mechanisms have yet to be determined, change in fetal vascular compliance is a major factor.

In the human fetus, the hematocrit of circulating blood gradually increases throughout gestation. At 20 weeks, fetal hematocrit averages approximately 30–32 per cent. This increases linearly to 43 per cent at term, prior to the onset of labor, with further increases during labor and delivery. In view of the constancy of blood volume as discussed above, the gradual increase in fetal hematocrit prior to labor implies that, relative to bodyweight, fetal red-cell volume increases with advancing gestation and plasma volume/unit weight decreases simultaneously by the same amount.

The average fetal blood volume of 110 mL/kg noted above is approximately 50 per cent greater than the adult blood volume, which averages approximately 75 mL/kg (*see also* page 522), a value which depends on the amount of body fat. Approximately 30 per cent of circulating fetal blood resides in the umbilical cord and placenta. Thus, after excluding this

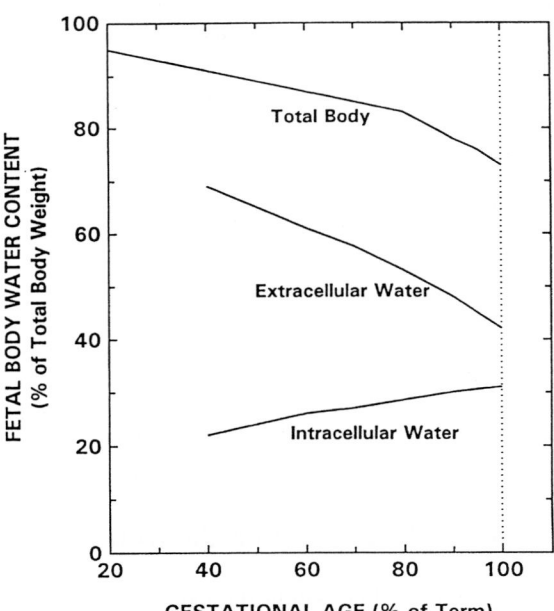

FIGURE 14.3 Human fetal body water content and water distribution as a function of gestational age

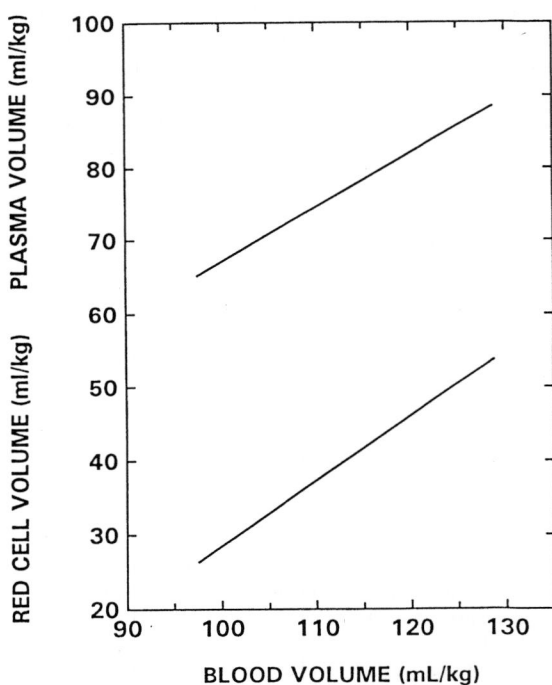

FIGURE 14.4 Interrelationships among red cell volume, plasma volume and blood volume in late-gestation ovine fetuses. Volumes are normalized per kg of fetal bodyweight. Solid lines are regression lines.

blood, the fetus has a net blood volume of approximately 80 mL/kg, similar to the weight- normalized blood volume in lean adult humans.

Just as total circulating blood volume/kg is higher in the fetus than in the adult, fetal plasma volume/kg is higher than in the adult, especially early in gestation when fetal hematocrit is low. Once again, after correction for plasma within the umbilical cord and placenta, plasma volume within the fetal body is only slightly larger than that which is normal for the adult. This similarity of fetal blood and plasma volumes/kg with those of the adult suggests that the blood volume and plasma volume regulatory mechanisms are established very early during the fetal period.

## Extrafetal fluids

The developing embryo and fetus are surrounded by amniotic fluid which, in turn, is surrounded by the amniotic membrane. The chorionic membrane extends outward from the edge of the placenta to form a closed sac which encompasses the amnion. In addition to the protruding yolk sac, fluid fills the space between the amnion and chorion early in gestation. This is variously referred to as coelomic fluid, extraembryonic coelomic fluid, and exocoelomic fluid. The coelomic fluid is straw-colored and viscous, in contrast to clear, low-viscosity amniotic fluid. Using ultrasound guidance, the coelomic fluid can be sampled by needle aspiration as early as 6 weeks' gestation until 10–12 weeks' gestation when the coelomic fluid disappears. The physical relationships among the fetus, coelomic and amniotic fluid are shown in Fig. 14.5.

In contrast to the transient existence of coelomic fluid, amniotic fluid volume increases progressively throughout the first half of gestation (Fig. 14.6). As shown by the 95 per cent confidence interval, there is a very wide range of amniotic fluid volume, particularly during the latter half of gestation. At any given gestational age, there is a skewing of amniotic volumes toward high values. During the second half of gestation, amniotic fluid volume increases gradually from approximately 340 mL at 20 weeks to a maximum of approximately 780 mL at 33 weeks. In prolonged pregnancies, amniotic fluid volume decreases and the average volume is approximately 400 mL at 43 weeks of gestation. In addition to recognizing that amniotic fluid volume varies widely among patients at any given gestational age, it is also important to recognize that within the same subject there may be relatively large day-to-day variations in amniotic volume.

## PHYSIOLOGICAL REGULATION OF FLUID VOLUMES

To understand the regulation of fetal and amniotic fluids, it is necessary to know the routes by which fluids move as well as the rate at which fluids flow by each route. Because of the influences of the mother, the regulation of fluid balance in the fetal compartment is much more complex than that in the adult (Fig. 14.7). This is further complicated because fluids are moving over multiple routes simultaneously. These include fluxes across the placenta, large volumes secreted by the fetal lungs which exit the trachea (tracheal flow), and large volumes of amniotic fluid which are absorbed across the fetal surface of the placenta into fetal blood (intramembranous flow). In addition, large volumes of fetal urine enter the amniotic sac each day, the fetus swallows very large volumes of fluid, and small amounts of amniotic fluid may cross

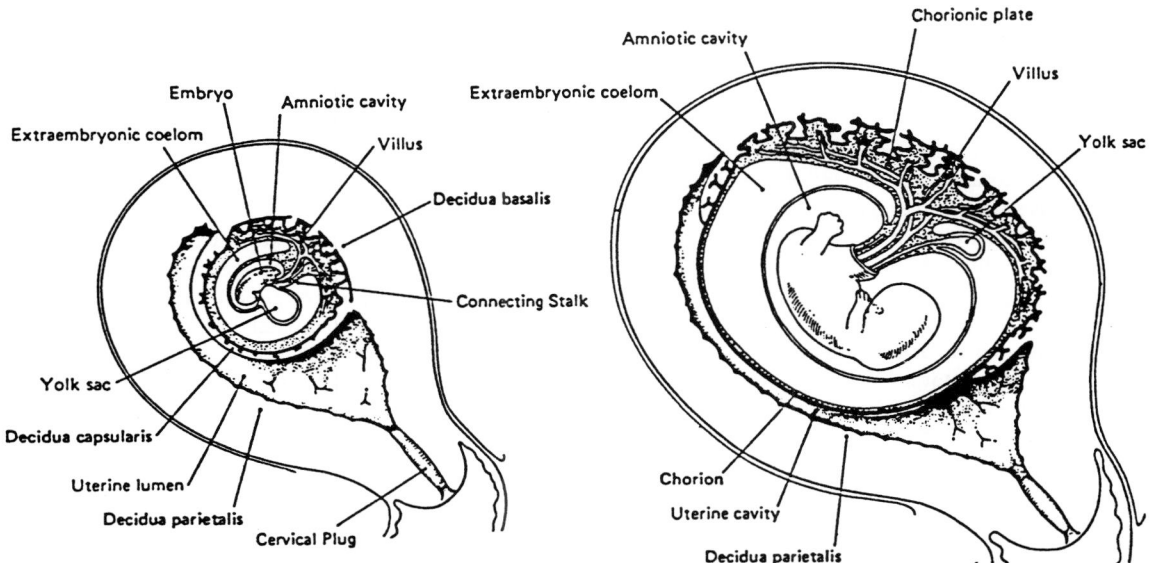

FIGURE 14.5 Schematic showing relationships among coelomic fluid, amniotic fluid, embryo and fetus early in gestation

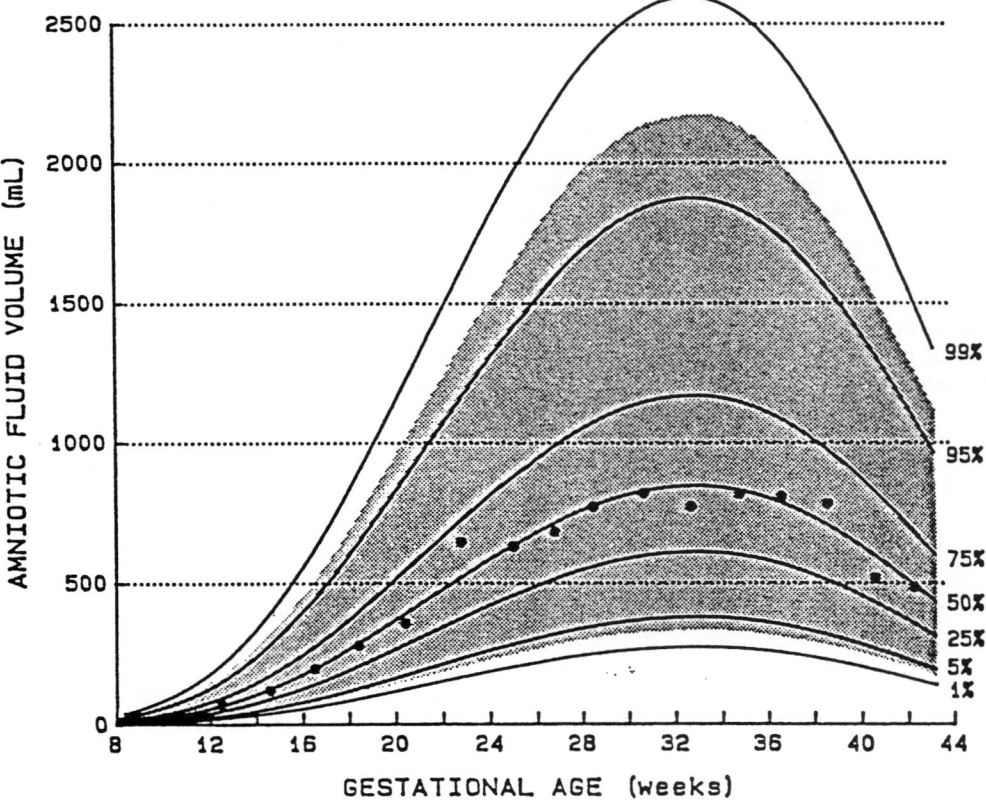

FIGURE 14.6 Distribution of amniotic fluid volume in 705 pregnancies as a function of fetal gestational age. Shaded area represents 95 per cent confidence interval above mean.

the amnion and chorion to be absorbed into the maternal blood perfusing the maternal uterine wall (transmembranous flow). Finally, there are undoubtedly secretions from the fetal oral and nasal cavities which enter the amniotic space.

## Flows within the fetus

By adding amniotic fluid volume plus fetal weight corrected for fractional water content, it can be calculated that the fetus gains an average of 20 mL of water a day over the last half of gestation. If 30 per cent is generated as a byproduct of metabolism, the late-gestation fetus needs to gain only approximately 15 mL/day of water from its mother. This flow is tiny compared with others which enter the fetal circulation (Fig. 14.8). For example, the late-gestation fetus may swallow as much as 25–50 per cent of bodyweight a day (i.e. 250–500 mL/(kg·day)). This fluid is absorbed through the digestive tract into the fetal circulation. In late-gestation fetal sheep, left thoracic duct lymph flow rate averages 0.5 mL/minute. Since this duct may carry only 70–80 per cent of the total, whole-body lymph flow rates may be as much as 1000 mL/day. The rate of transcapillary filtration within the fetal

body would be almost 1000 mL/day since only approximately 15 mL/day is needed to support fetal cellular and interstitial expansion with fetal growth.

Ultrasound studies in the 1970s showed that the human fetus has a high urinary output throughout the last half of gestation. However, more recent studies have demonstrated that true fetal urinary output is perhaps 1.5–2.0 times previous values. This underestimation of urinary output was due to frequent micturition (every 20–30 min) causing underestimation of dynamic changes in bladder volume with time. Thus, the human fetus produces approximately 120 mL of urine per day at 24 weeks of gestation, and this increases to 1000 mL/day at 40 weeks, the latter consistent with data from late-gestation ovine fetuses where urinary output averages 0.2 mL/(kg fetal bodyweight·min) or approximately 250 mL/(kg·day) over the last third of gestation.

In all mammalian fetuses studied to date, ligation or obstruction of the trachea in the latter half of gestation causes an overdistension of the fetal lungs. Thus it appears that lungs secrete fluid, and this is due to an active transport of chloride into the future airway spaces. Although no human data exist, ovine fetal lungs secrete a volume of fluid equal to 10 per cent of bodyweight per day over the last third of gestation. Because only about 1 per cent of this

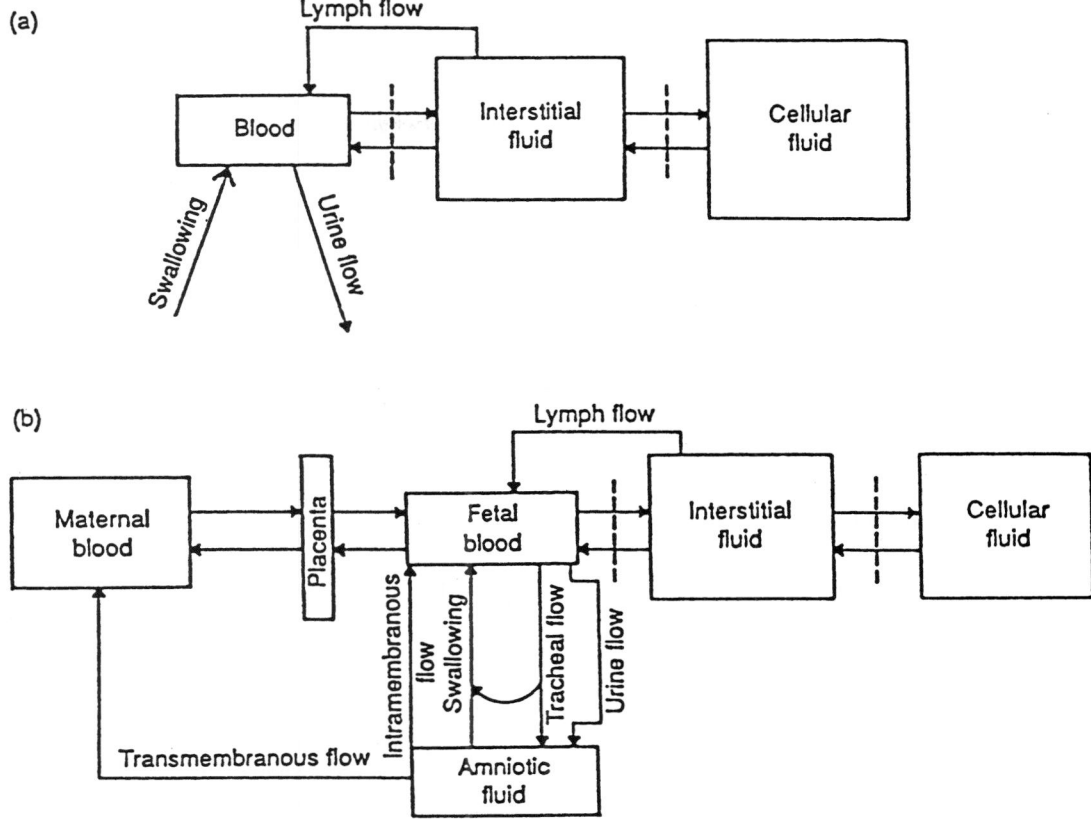

FIGURE 14.7 Schematics comparing major routes of fluid movement in (a) the adult and (b) late-gestation fetus. Note the much greater complexity in the fetus.

volume is needed for lung expansion with growth, a large volume of fluid must leave the lungs via the

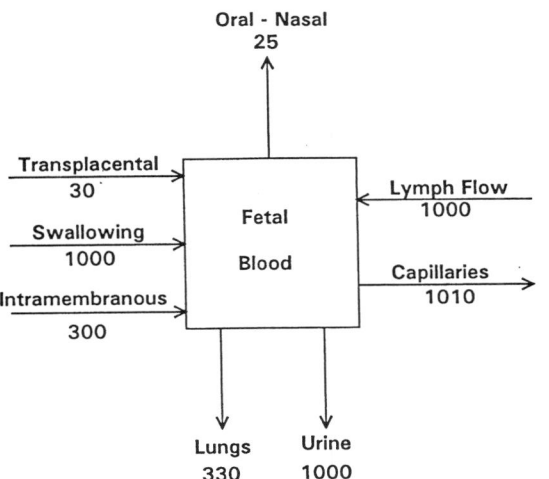

FIGURE 14.8 Estimated flows into and out of the blood stream of the late-gestation fetus. Flows have units of mL/day. Transplacental flow is sum of fluid needed by fetus for growth plus recovery of transmembranous losses. Swallowing is sum of amniotic fluid plus secreted liquid which is fluid swallowed.

trachea each day. This fluid enters the oral pharynx and from there either can be swallowed or passively enter the amniotic sac (a recent study under physio-logic conditions found that half entered the amniotic compartment and the other half was swallowed). This is of major importance for amniotic fluid volume with a near-term fetus secreting 300 mL/day from its lungs, a volume of 150 mL/day over many weeks would impact amniotic fluid volume.

The other flows which enter or exit the fetal blood stream or the amniotic compartment have been much more difficult to estimate. Although transmembranous flow may be as much as 80 mL/day, recent studies suggest that this might be at most in the order of 10 mL/day. Similarly, animal studies have suggested that the fetal oral and nasal cavities may secrete fluid at a rate of approximately 8 mL/(kg fetal bodyweight·day), with perhaps half of this entering the amniotic sac. In contrast to these low flows, both human and animal data suggest that solutes and water may move at a rapid rate across the fetal surface of the placenta and thereby provide a direct exchange between fetal blood and the amniotic fluid. Net volume flow rates have been estimated only in the ovine fetus and aver-age 250 mL of fluid per day absorbed from the amniotic compartment through the intramembranous pathway directly into the fetal circulation. This is a surprisingly large volume which would be a major determinant of amniotic fluid volume.

## Regulation of fetal blood volume

Fetal blood volume can change because of alterations in either red-cell volume or plasma volume. Fluid moves rapidly across fetal capillaries due to a capillary filtration coefficient which is about five times that in the adult, relative to bodyweight. Thus, any increase or decrease in fetal body capillary pressure can lead to rapid alterations in circulating fetal blood volume due to changes in plasma volume. Unlike plasma volume, red-cell volume changes slowly since the fetus does not have a store of releasable red cells as is present in the adult spleen. Thus, rapid changes in fetal red-cell volume only occur due to loss of blood via hemorrhage or blood sampling or due to transfusion. Fetal capillary pressure can be increased by at least three mechanisms: (1) fetal vasoconstriction with a subsequent rise in arterial and/or venous pressure, (2) vasodilatation as occurs to increase blood flow in several tissues during hypoxia, and (3) an increase in vascular volume. Fetal blood volume changes rapidly under several conditions. For example, acute hypoxia produces a rapid and sustained fall in blood volume of approximately 1 per cent per mmHg decrease in fetal arterial blood $O_2$ tension ($Pa_{O_2}$), due to a decrease in plasma volume. On return to normoxia, blood volume returns to normal in approximately one-half hour. Thus, even small changes in fetal capillary pressure have rapid and large effects on circulating blood volume.

More insight about blood volume regulation has been gained by exploring fetal responses to fluid volume loading. Following intravascular infusions of packed adult red cells, fetal plasma volume rapidly decreased so that within one hour blood volume was elevated by only 50 per cent of the transfused volume. In addition, when 20 mL/kg of physiologic saline was infused, only 6–7 per cent of the infused volume was retained within the circulation after one-half hour. This contrasts with 30–40 per cent retention in the adult under similar circumstances. The important point is that there are rapid and extensive movements of fluid across the fetal capillary walls into the fetal body tissues. If a colloidal solution such as 6 per cent Dextran 70 is infused into the fetus, blood volume increases by only about 50 per cent of the infused volume. In contrast, because 6 per cent Dextran 70 is hyperoncotic, the normal adult response is for blood volume to increase by 200 per cent of the infused volume. The failure of blood volume to expand by the same amount in the fetus is due to the fact that high-molecular-weight proteins and Dextran rapidly cross the fetal capillary wall. Thus, the fetal body capillaries are not only highly permeable to water and small-molecular-weight solutes, but also have a fairly large pore size and readily allow proteins to cross.

These studies demonstrate that the fetus can readily regulate its blood volume toward normal following volume expansion. If the opposite occurs, and the fetus has a mild to moderate hemorrhage over 5 minutes to 2 hours, fetal blood volume returns fully to normal within 2–5 hours after the hemorrhage. In contrast, in a number of species including humans, following hemorrhage of the adult, this takes 24–48 hours. An important observation is that blood volume in the fetus returns to normal only as plasma protein mass returns to normal. Because plasma proteins do not cross the placenta to any significant extent, both the proteins and fluid responsible for fetal blood volume restoration are likely to be derived from the fetal interstitial space with perhaps a small contribution from new protein synthesis.

## Regulation of fetal lymph flow

Basal lymph flow rates per kg in the late-gestation fetus are higher than in the adult, averaging about 20 per cent of bodyweight per day. Lymph flow rate is regulated by a number of factors, primarily venous pressure and interstitial fluid volume. Central venous pressure is the normal outflow pressure for the lymphatic system and in both adults and fetuses, increases in venous pressure decrease lymph flow rate (Fig. 14.9). Normal venous pressure in both the fetus and adult is approximately 3 mmHg. In adults, venous pressure can increase substantially before thoracic duct lymph flow decreases and pressure must increase to 26 mmHg before flow ceases. In contrast, in the

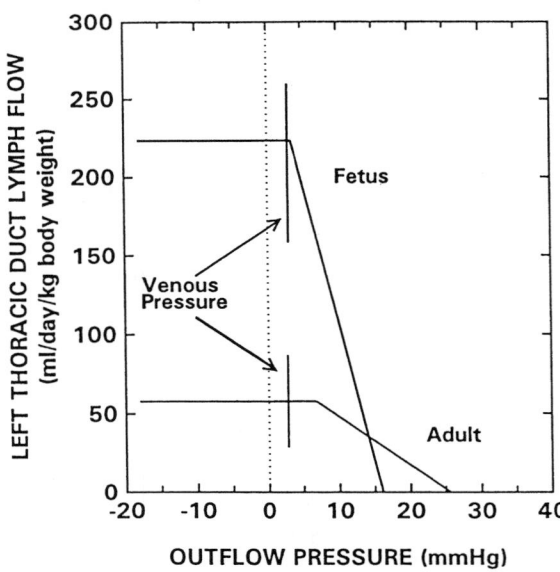

FIGURE 14.9 Lymph flow function curves in fetus and adult. Normal lymphatic outflow pressure is venous pressure.

fetus, only slight elevations in venous pressure cause lymph flow to decrease, and lymph flow ceases entirely at a venous pressure of 16 mmHg. Thus, there are major differences in the lymph flow function curves in the fetus compared with the adult.

Changes in interstitial fluid volume also affect fetal lymph flow rates. With an intravenous infusion of 20 mL/kg fetal bodyweight of physiologic saline, much of the infused fluid enters the interstitium and thoracic duct lymph flow rate increases by 5 per cent of the infused volume over 30 minutes, similar to the increase in flow in adults following a 20 mL/kg saline infusion. Larger volume infusions in the fetus can increase fetal thoracic duct lymph flow rates to a maximum of 3–4 times normal. Interstitial volume also can be altered by varying fetal hematocrit. When the ovine fetus is made progressively anemic over a period of many days, there is an inverse relationship between fetal lymph flow rate and hematocrit (Fig. 14.10). This curve is important because it shows that as fetal anemia becomes severe lymph flow rate does not yet become maximal. Thus, hydrops fetalis in association with fetal anemia does not appear to be due solely to a limitation of the fetal lymphatic system.

## Regulation of fetal urinary output

This discussion focuses on a few unique aspects of fetal urinary output, including the relationship to regulation of fetal blood volume (*see also* page 238). In the fetus, a rapid intravenous infusion of physiologic saline produces a short-term diuresis which is of the same relative volume as occurs in the adult. However, slow

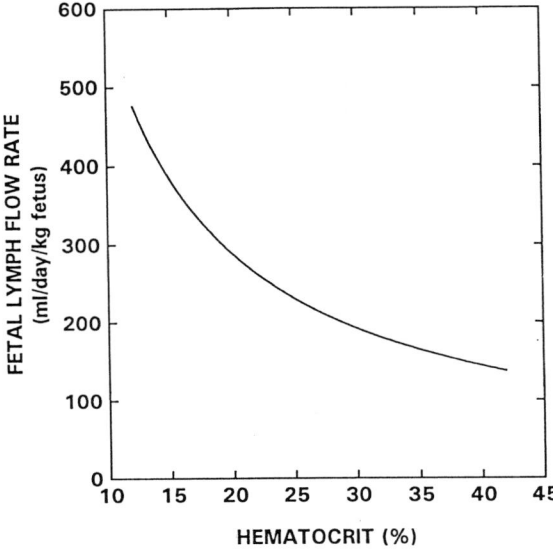

FIGURE 14.10 Steady-state left thoracic duct lymph flow rates in the ovine fetus under basal as well as chronically anemic conditions. The line is the regression line.

intravascular infusions of fluid in the fetus do not always produce a diuresis. As discussed above, fetal capillaries are highly permeable to fluid. In addition, the interstitial space within the fetal tissues is an order of magnitude more compliant than in adults. That is, for each mmHg increase in interstitial fluid pressure, the fetal interstitial space can hold about 15 times as much fluid as the adult interstitial space, relative to bodyweight. Thus, with a slow intravascular infusion to the fetus, the majority of the infused fluid is transferred to the fetal interstitial space, fetal vascular pressures are not elevated and there are no secondary changes in circulating hormones (e.g. atrial natriuretic peptide) which produce a fetal diuresis. Without changes in vascular pressures or in the endocrine environment, there is no driving force for a change in urinary output. However, if the slow intravascular infusions are maintained over a period of 24 hours or more, fetal urinary output increases to equal or slightly exceed the rate of intravenous infusion. Thus, the fetal kidneys have a tremendously powerful ability to diurese on a long-term basis in order to maintain blood volume close to normal.

## Regulation of fetal swallowing

Swallowing in the human fetus has been studied infrequently due to methodological limitations. Although difficult to interpret, these studies suggest that the near-term human fetus swallows 300–500 mL/day of amniotic fluid. However, this may be an underestimate as animal studies have shown that swallowing is reduced beginning a few days before the onset of labor. Nonetheless, earlier in gestation, the fetus swallows considerably less fluid. At 17 weeks the human fetus swallows about 2 mL/day, and this increases to 13 mL/day at 20 weeks' gestation. These numbers correspond to approximately 13 mL/(kg fetal bodyweight·day) at 17 weeks and 43 mL/(kg·day) at 20 weeks. In contrast the term fetus swallows approximately 150 mL/(kg·day). Thus not only does the absolute volume swallowed increase with advancing gestation but also the volume swallowed/kg of fetal weight. Although not extensively explored, data from the ovine fetus support this (Fig. 14.11).

## Regulation of pulmonary secretions

During the last third of gestation, the volume of liquid in the fetal lungs increases in proportion to fetal weight and averages 50 mL/kg fetal bodyweight. The normal rate of secretion of liquid into the fetal lungs is 100 mL/(kg fetal bodyweight·day). Net fluid secretion mostly is due to active $Cl^-$ secretion with $Na^+$ and water following passively. A reabsorptive process becomes active shortly before term. A variety of hormones modulate secretory processes while

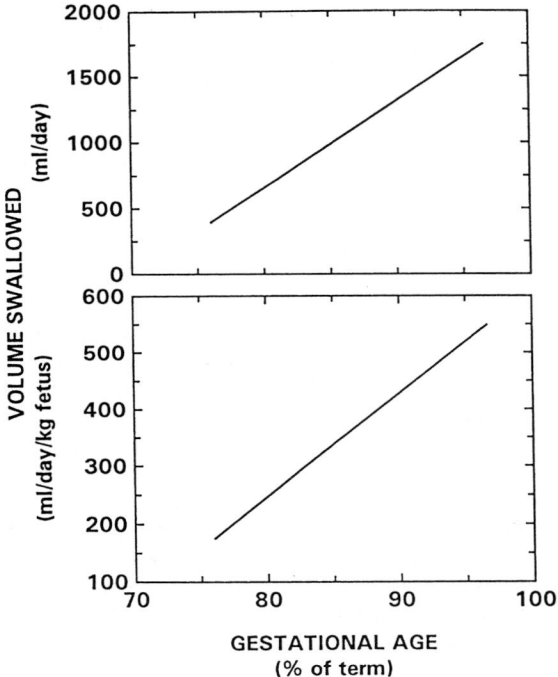

FIGURE 14.11 Volume of amniotic fluid swallowed by the late-gestation ovine fetus. Data are expressed as an absolute value as well as per kg of fetal weight. Lines are regression lines.

others stimulate reabsorptive processes; the influence of these on lung liquid secretion and reabsorption increases markedly as gestation progresses, particularly near term. β-adrenergic agonists, including epinephrine, inhibit secretion and reduce the fluid volume. Arginine vasopressin (AVP) has only a slight inhibitory effect until 1–2 weeks before delivery when it becomes increasingly effective at reducing the net secretory rate and producing a net reabsorption. Under basal conditions the net secretory process is dependent upon an active transport of $Cl^-$ in the lumen of the airways. In contrast, there may be little net reabsorption under basal conditions except near term. When reabsorption is stimulated, it is due to activation of a $Na^+$ channel, which promotes both water and $Na^+Cl^-$ movement from the airways back into the fetal circulation. Both adrenocortical and thyroid hormones regulate the maturation of these secretory and reabsorptive processes, but their exact role has yet to be defined. Nonetheless, the combination of endocrine changes over the last several days of pregnancy and the large increases in circulating vasoactive hormones during labor and delivery all act synergistically to inhibit secretion of fluid by the fetal lungs at the same time as stimulating reabsorption. Thus, the fetal lungs are prepared for air ventilation following delivery. It is also interesting to note that the very hormones that assist the lungs in this preparation are also those most importantly involved in regulating blood volume within the fetus.

## Regulation of intramembranous, transmembranous and transplacental flows

Little is known about what functionally regulates net flows across the intramembranous, transmembranous and transplacental pathways. From theory, hydrostatic and osmotic pressure gradients as well as concentration gradients provide the physical forces necessary for these fluxes; also changes in the effective pore size can have dramatic effects on net flux rate. However, studies to date have not evaluated the physiologic regulation of pore size or filtration coefficients.

Changes in either maternal or fetal osmolality are effective at moving large fluid volumes across the placenta, and this can occur over fairly short periods of time. Thus over a period of many minutes to a few hours, fetal osmolality readjusts to equilibrate with maternal osmolality whenever an osmotic disturbance is introduced. However, this provides little insight into the mechanisms by which the fetus normally gains water from its mother since the osmotic forces needed to provide the water necessary for fetal growth are immeasurably small. Thus, we are unable to explain the mechanisms by which the fetus accumulates the water needed for growth.

It is well established that amniotic fluid osmolality decreases progressively below maternal and fetal blood osmolality to average 250–260 mmol/kg at term in contrast to about 280 mmol/kg in fetal and adult blood. Since each mmol/kg of osmotic gradient produces an osmotic force of 19.3 mmHg at human body temperature, normally there are several hundred mmHg osmotic force to move water out of the amniotic compartment. However, there are few insights into the effectiveness of this driving force. One exception is a recent study which found that, if fetal urine was diverted to the exterior while fetal swallowing and tracheal outflow were simultaneously inhibited, there was a gradual increase in amniotic osmolality so that half the gradient between amniotic fluid and fetal blood dissipated over a period of 8 hours. This corresponded to a volume loss of approximately 250 mL/day. Thus the existing amniotic-to-fetal or amniotic-to-maternal osmotic force is responsible for large volumes of water leaving the amniotic compartment each day. This fluid enters the fetal circulation presumably by crossing the amniotic–fetal surface of the placenta. However, we know nothing of the regulatory processes.

# Regulation of amniotic fluid volume

In order for amniotic fluid volume to be regulated, there should be a sensor which detects volume changes and then activates mechanisms to return amniotic volume toward normal. However, we do not know whether such a sensor is present or if amniotic fluid volume is actively regulated.

In fact, we currently understand the factors which determine amniotic volume only under the most extreme conditions. For example, with fetal *anuria*, there is almost invariably severe *oligohydramnios* during the second half of gestation. Further, with *esophageal atresia* or *esophageal obstruction*, *polyhydramnios* frequently develops. However, there are many reported cases in which the fetus cannot swallow but amniotic fluid volume is normal. This occurs despite normal fetal urinary output. In view of studies which found little if any transmembranous flow, this suggests that intramembranous flow increases dramatically with esophageal obstruction so that a volume of fluid equal to the sum of fetal urinary output plus fetal lung secretions can be absorbed each day by the intramembranous pathway.

Much less is known about the maternal contribution to the regulation of amniotic fluid volume under physiologic conditions. Recent studies have suggested that if pregnant women with oligohydramnios drink 2 liters of water, there is a modest increase in amniotic fluid volume. However, the mechanisms involved are far from clear. Further, animals studies have shown that if the mother is water-deprived, amniotic fluid disappears over a few days. Thus, the mother appears to have access to fetal amniotic fluid. Again the mechanisms are unclear.

From Fig. 14.8 it is clear that fetal urine is a primary source of fluid which enters the amniotic sac and swallowing is the primary route by which amniotic fluid leaves the amniotic compartment. Thus it would be expected that physiologic regulation of fetal urinary output and/or swallowing should lead to changes in amniotic volume. However, there are no human data which support this concept, and only one study in pregnant sheep found large day-to-day variations in amniotic fluid volume which correlated positively with fetal urinary output and negatively with fetal swallowing. Thus, physiologic variations in fetal urinary output and/or swallowing will affect amniotic fluid volume. It is obvious that a great deal more needs to be learned in this area. This is particularly true of early gestation. For example, amniotic fluid is present long before the fetus begins to urinate or swallow at approximately 9–11 weeks' gestation, but virtually nothing is known about early amniotic fluid volume regulatory mechanisms.

## SUMMARY

Fluid moves very rapidly in the fetus. In the last third of gestation, fetal swallowing, urinary output, transcapillary filtration and lymphatic flow all average an order of magnitude greater in the fetus than in the adult relative to bodyweight. Further, following intravascular infusion or hemorrhage to the fetus, fetal blood volume returns to normal in approximately one-tenth the time required in the adult. These rapid and extensive fluid movements in the fetus are largely attributable to the fact that (1) fetal capillaries have a much higher filtration coefficient so water can rapidly move, and (2) the fetal interstitium has a much higher compliance so that fluid movements can be much more extensive. Each day large volumes of fetal fluid enter and leave the amniotic sac. Presumably, the fetus can use the amniotic space as a fluid reservoir so that fluid can be removed when needed or excess fluid can be deposited within the amniotic compartment when the fetus receives more than it needs from its mother. Finally, it also appears that in time of need, the mother can access amniotic fluid, presumably through the fetus after reabsorption across the placenta. It might also be speculated that, if the mother forces too much fluid to be transferred across the placenta, polyhydramnios would be the result as the fetal kidneys are usually very effective on a long-term basis at eliminating excess fluid within the fetal body.

## SELECTED READING

Brace RA, Ross MG, Robillard JE. *Fetal and neonatal body fluids: the scientific basis for clinical practice*. Ithaca, New York: Perinatology Press, 1989.

Gilbert WM, Brace RA. Amniotic fluid volume and normal flows to and from the amniotic cavity. *Semin Perinatol* 1993; **17**:150.

Hanson MA, Spencer JAD, Rodek CH. *Fetus and neonate: physiology and clinical applications. Vol. 1: The Circulation*. Cambridge: Cambridge University Press, 1993.

# 15

# Uterine Function

## REGULATION OF UTERINE ACTIVITY AND OF LABOR

### INTRODUCTION

The control of myometrial contractile activity during pregnancy represents an extraordinary example of physiologic regulation in reproductive biology. Throughout most of pregnancy this smooth muscle must be maintained in a quiescent and unresponsive state in order to allow the safe development of the embryo and fetus. Then, over a relatively short period, at the time of labor, the myometrium undergoes a remarkable transformation enabling it to develop the synchronous, intense contractions necessary for the effective expulsion of the fetus from the uterine cavity.

For the most part these events are subject to an exacting temporal control which allows this transformation of the myometrium to occur at a time when the fetus is relatively mature. Unfortunately, in human pregnancy these regulatory mechanisms can fail and lead to the premature birth of a baby whose physiologic organ systems have not matured to a degree where they are capable of sustaining life outside of the uterus. Preterm birth occurs in 5–10 per cent of all pregnancies but is associated with 70 per cent of all neonatal deaths and up to 75 per cent of neonatal morbidity. In the neonatal period, preterm infants are 40 times more likely to die than are term infants. They are also at significantly increased risk of major complications such as chronic lung disease, cerebral palsy and long-term neurobehavioral and learning disabilities.

Unfortunately, despite the myriad treatments that have been used in an attempt to prevent preterm labor, there have been no changes in the incidence of preterm birth over the past 40 years. Clinical and scientific data demonstrate that even β-adrenergic agonists, such as ritodrine, which are used extensively as tocolytics, do not prevent preterm birth nor significantly improve neonatal outcome. However, it is fair to say that such drugs do delay birth for a short period (about 72 hours) during which time the maternal administration of glucocorticoids may have a positive impact on fetal lung maturity. Why then have we been so unsuccessful at blocking myometrial contractions in women in preterm labor? There is no clear answer to this question, but our poor understanding of the mechanisms that maintain uterine quiescence during pregnancy and then induce a high level of contractility at the appropriate time at term is certainly a major factor.

### REGULATION OF UTERINE (MYOMETRIAL) CONTRACTILE ACTIVITY

During pregnancy, in virtually all species, the uterus is essentially quiescent: the muscle layer (myometrium) is relatively unexcitable and has little spontaneous activity. Those contractions that do occur are of low frequency and only capable of developing small increases in uterine pressure ("contractures"). In addition, the myometrium is relatively unresponsive to stimulants (e.g. oxytocin (OT), prostaglandins (PGs)) and the myometrial cells are not well coordinated. This significantly reduces the ability of the uterus to develop propagated contractions. In contrast, during labor the myometrium is highly excitable and spontaneously active. High-frequency, high-amplitude contractions are generated and spread rapidly across the surface of the uterus with a high degree of coordination. The myometrium also is very responsive to stimulation from endogenous agents at this time. This transformation in phenotype of the myometrium is termed *activation* (Fig. 15.1). Once activated the myometrium can respond effectively to endogenous stimulants (e.g. oxytocin, PGs) to produce labor contractions that aid in the expulsion of the fetus. This latter process is termed *stimulation* (Fig. 15.2).

The process of activation is believed to be due to marked changes in the synthesis of specific myometrial

## ONSET OF LABOR

### *PREGNANCY*

- Myometrium virtually quiescent
- Inexcitable
- Relatively unresponsive to uterotonic agonists
- Poorly coordinated

ACTIVATION

### *LABOR*

- High level of spontaneous activity
- Increased excitability
- Very responsive to uterotonic agonists
- Displays enhanced cell-to-cell coupling allowing generation of high frequency, intense, synchronous contractions of labor

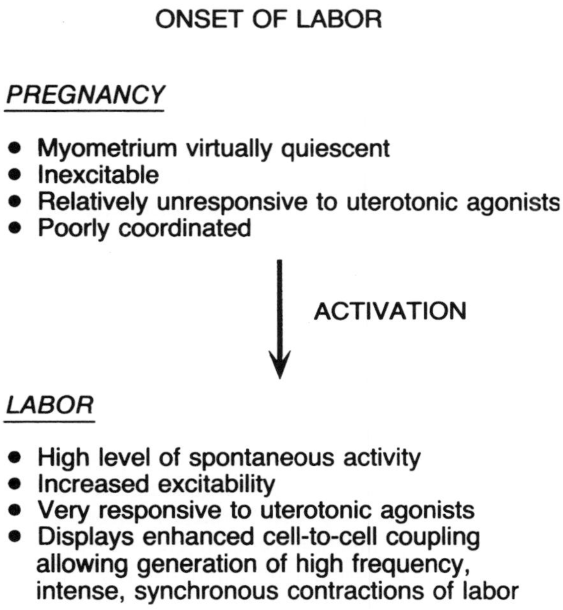

FIGURE 15.1 Myometrial activation: switch in the contractile characteristics of the myometrium with the onset of labor

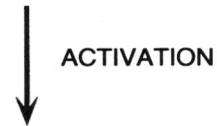

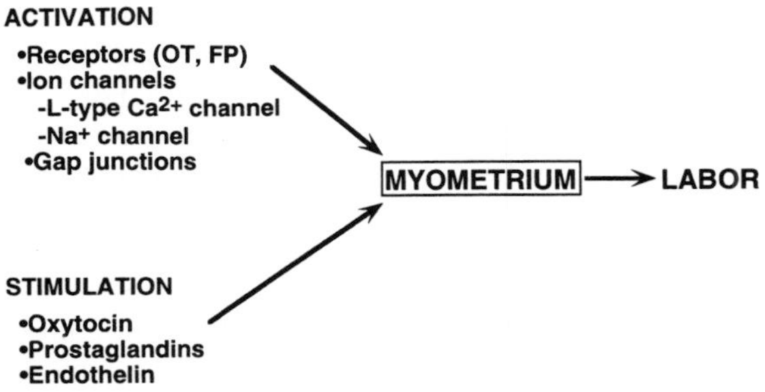

**ACTIVATION**
- Receptors (OT, FP)
- Ion channels
  - L-type $Ca^{2+}$ channel
  - $Na^+$ channel
- Gap junctions

MYOMETRIUM → LABOR

**STIMULATION**
- Oxytocin
- Prostaglandins
- Endothelin

FIGURE 15.2 Onset of labor. Myometrial ACTIVATION can be described biochemically by the activation of a cassette of "contraction-associated" genes encoding for proteins such as uterotonic receptors, ion channels and gap junctions; these enable the myometrium to more effectively respond to the increased STIMULATION afforded by the increased production of uterotonic stimulants such as oxytocin, stimulatory PGs and endothelin.

proteins ("contraction-associated proteins" (CAPs)) involved in regulating contractile activity. For example, excitability of the muscle is probably regulated by changes in the ion channel composition of the cell membrane, increased responsiveness is due to an increase in receptors for the stimulants, and increased coordination is associated with the appearance of gap junctions in myometrial cell membranes (Fig. 15.2).

Much of our knowledge of the regulation of activation comes from animals. In many (though not all) species progesterone and estrogen are believed to play critical roles in this process. In the sheep, progesterone reduces conductivity in the myometrium and blocks the response to oxytocin and PGs, probably by reducing synthesis of uterotonic receptors and gap junctions. However, spontaneous activity of the myometrium does not appear to be significantly affected by progesterone. In contrast, two other hormones present during pregnancy (relaxin, and prostacyclin ($PGI_2$, an inhibitory PG)) inhibit spontaneous contractions, thus contributing to uterine quiescence, but do not affect the response of the myometrium to stimulants. It is possible, therefore, that the pregnant myometrium is maintained quiescent by the combined effects of progesterone and other factors. In contrast, estrogen has opposite effects to progesterone and when administered to sheep, increases responsiveness to stimulants, increases spontaneous activity and increases conductivity.

In primates there is essentially no evidence to indicate that changes in systemic progesterone concentrations are responsible for the control of uterine activity. In rhesus monkeys, plasma progesterone concentrations remain at mid-luteal phase levels during the second half of gestation, with either no change or a small increase at the onset of parturition. Ovariectomy can be performed during early pregnancy without inducing abortion, and after fetectomy, the placenta is retained and the pregnancy continued without the development of normal uterine activity, even though basal systemic progesterone concentrations drop significantly. In humans maternal peripheral plasma progesterone concentrations increase progressively toward term.

Other mechanisms of progesterone withdrawal have been proposed to have a role in activation. A local or paracrine loss of progesterone within the fetal membranes is supported by data indicating the potential for 17β,20α-hydroxysteroid dehydrogenase to increase the estrogen/progesterone ratio in human amnion and chorion with the onset of labor. However, direct measurements of the absolute levels of estrone, estradiol and progesterone in amnion, chorion and decidua reveal no changes in these in relation to the onset of labor. Although there are fewer progesterone receptors in human myometrium at term than in nonpregnant women, there is no difference in the expression of progesterone receptor mRNA. A role for transforming growth factor β (TGFβ) as a natural inhibitor of progesterone-responsive genes, effectively resulting in progesterone withdrawal, has been proposed but is not confirmed.

Administration of the progesterone receptor blocker, RU486 (mifepristone), to rhesus monkeys in the mid-third trimester results in intense uterine contractions. However, the orderly sequence of contractile events that occurs during normal birth is not observed. The contraction pattern is quantitatively different both at night and during the day, as is the profile of increase in PGs. Moreover the cervix does not dilate, necessitating cesarean section 72 hours after beginning the administration of RU486. Thus, in the primate, it is unclear whether there is a functional withdrawal of progesterone at term. Even if this does occur it is doubtful that such a withdrawal in and of itself would lead to labor onset.

The major endocrine input to myometrial activation in the human is likely to involve estrogen. In humans and non-human primates, maternal plasma concentrations of estrogens increase progressively during gestation, reaching peak levels at term. This is not due to de novo placental synthesis from acetate or progesterone because the primate placenta lacks the 17α-hydroxylase/17,20 lyase ($P_{450c17}$) enzymatic system responsible for this pathway in sheep and some other species (see Fig. 15.7). Rather, the placenta converts fetal adrenal dehydroepiandrosterone sulfate (DHEAS) to estrogens (Figs. 15.3 and 15.7). During mid-gestation there is negative feedback control by placental estrogen on the secretion of fetal adrenal DHEAS, possibly by attenuating the tissue's responsiveness to trophic peptides. At late gestation this effect is lost, resulting in an elevated fetal DHEAS and the maternal estrogen increase observed at term. Spontaneous delivery in the rhesus monkey is preceded by increasing fetal levels of DHEAS, and rapid fetal adrenal maturation occurs before birth. Fetectomy in rhesus monkeys or baboons, and fetal decapitation, fetal death, or suppression of the fetal

adrenocortical axis with glucocorticoids in rhesus monkeys, cause peripheral maternal estrogen concentrations to decrease and significantly increase the length of gestation. Conversely, an increase in the production of fetal adrenal androgens and consequent increase in maternal estrogens, similar to that observed at term (184 days' gestation), has been reported in pregnant baboons (155–165 days' gestation) subjected to fetal hypoxic stress leading to preterm birth. As well, treatment of the fetus with ACTH or DHEAS results in elevated maternal estrogens, and androstenedione (an androgen) administration to fetal rhesus monkeys results in elevated maternal estrogens, labor-like uterine contractile activity and delivery. These data suggest an important role for maternal estrogens, derived from fetal androgens, in the activation of the human myometrium. Nevertheless, it is unlikely that estrogen alone is responsible for birth since primate parturition is not delayed indefinitely in situations, such as fetectomy, where maternal estrogens are low.

Another process which may facilitate uterine contractile activity, or the onset of parturition, is an increased availability of contractile hormones. During gestation, the uterine levels of enzymes which degrade endothelin, PGs and oxytocin are elevated, thus controlling the levels of these hormones. In labor, the levels of some of the degradatory enzymes decline. A reduced rate of degradation could increase hormone concentrations and consequently increase their effect on contractility.

The mechanisms that regulate myometrial activation remain to be fully determined. It is likely, however, that the process involves regulating the activity of genes encoding the CAPs. mRNA encoding the myometrial gap junction protein, connexin43 (Cx-43) is increased during labor, and the level of Cx-43 mRNA in rat myometrium is regulated positively by estrogen and negatively by progesterone. Possibly steroids regulate the expression of all the CAPs during labor, allowing their coordinated expression, leading to myometrial activation and an efficient labor process. There is substantial evidence, for example, that myometrial oxytocin receptors increase during late gestation, just before the onset of labor. PG receptors, on the other hand, were thought to remain constant in numbers during late gestation. Recent evidence in pregnant rats has suggested that this may not be true. Removal of the endogenous source of PGs by indomethacin treatment or by fetectomy increases the number of myometrial PGE and PGF receptors, whereas administration of PG decreases the number of receptors. Fetectomy of one horn increases PG receptors, coincident with the onset of labor, while in the intact contralateral horn no change in receptors occurs. It is probable that the number of PG receptors could increase at term, but the number is kept constant due to a comparable down-regulation by increasing PG production by the myometrium and other uterine tissues.

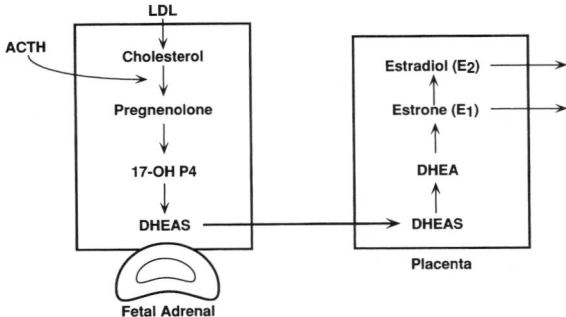

FIGURE 15.3 Synthesis of estrogens in primates. Estrogen synthesis by the primate placenta requires the provision of fetal adrenal androgen precursors (DHEAS, dehydroepiandrosterone sulfate). The production of adrenal DHEAS is increased in late pregnancy following ACTH-induced stimulation of this steroid synthetic pathway.

## MOLECULAR MECHANISMS OF MYOMETRIAL CONTRACTION

The biochemical pathways that result in the interaction of actin and myosin and lead to a contraction are shown in Fig. 15.4. The myosin molecule is a hexamer, approximately 160 nm in length, composed of two heavy chains (200 kD each) and two pairs of light chains (one pair around 17 kD and one around 20 kD). The heavy chain components form α-helices (130 nm in length). Towards the $NH_2$ terminal these chains unfold to form two globular heads. Each globular head contains: (1) ATPase activity (localized only on the heavy chain component); (2) an actin-binding site; (3) one light chain (20 kD) that can bind $Ca^{2+}$ and $Mg^{2+}$ and can be phosphorylated, and another light chain (17 kD), the functional role of which is unknown. The α-helical tail of the myosin molecule acts to transmit tension during shortening. The globular actin molecules (45 kD) polymerize into long filaments, 6–9 nm in diameter. In smooth muscles there are 11–15 thin filaments per myosin (thick) filament.

Interaction of actin and myosin occurs following the development of ATPase activity on the myosin head (Fig. 15.4). This then allows the formation of cross-links with the actin molecules. The myosin

head then rotates as a result of conformational changes in the protein structure, leading to a pulling on the actin filament to create tension and produce a relative spatial displacement. The energy required for these changes is believed to result from the phosphorylation (P) of the 20-kD myosin light chains (MLC20) by the enzyme myosin light chain kinase (MLCK). Other contractile proteins such as caldesmon, which interacts with myosin to increase the efficiency of actin–myosin coupling, may also play a role in regulating myometrial contraction.

MLCK can be considered a pivotal point in the regulation of smooth muscle contraction. MLCK has an absolute requirement for calcium–calmodulin ($Ca^{2+}$-CAM). In the presence of activating levels of $Ca^{2+}$ ($>10^{-6}$) the $Ca^{2+}$-CAM complex binds to a site on MLCK which in turn (presumably by some conformational change in MLCK) opens up the kinase site to enable the enzyme to phosphorylate MLC20 and hence initiate contraction (Fig. 15.5).

Relaxation of smooth muscle as a result of reduction in the phosphorylation of MLC20 occurs due to a decrease in MLCK activity with subsequent dephosphorylation of the light chains by MLC phosphatase. The reduction in MLCK activity can either be a result of a fall in intracellular $Ca^{2+}$ concentrations, leading to a decrease in $Ca^{2+}$-CAM levels, or possibly be due to phosphorylation of MLCK itself by a cAMP-dependent protein kinase (A-kinase). In this phosphorylated state the affinity of this regulatory protein for $Ca^{2+}$-CAM is reduced. Thus the contractile state of the cell can, in large part, be represented as a balance between the actions of $Ca^{2+}$ through CAM, and cAMP through A-kinase on the activity of the enzyme MLCK. cAMP also can affect contractility by reducing intracellular $Ca^{2+}$ levels either by increasing intracellular uptake of free $Ca^{2+}$ or by increasing $Ca^{2+}$ efflux from the myocyte.

The resting intracellular $Ca^{2+}$ concentration is $10^{-7}$–$10^{-8}$; this must increase to at least $10^{-6}$ for MLCK to be activated and for contraction to occur. Under normal resting conditions the extracellular $Ca^{2+}$ concentration is around $10^{-3}$, and in order to maintain this electrical imbalance active, ATP-dependent ($Ca^{2+}$-$Mg^{2+}$-ATPase) and ATP-independent ($Na^{+}$-exchange) cell-membrane $Ca^{2+}$ pumps have been developed.

An increase in intracellular $Ca^{2+}$ sufficient to initiate contraction within the myometrial cell can occur through several mechanisms (Fig. 15.5): (1) release of $Ca^{2+}$ from intracellular (sarcoplasmic reticulum, mitochondria, inner cell membrane bound) stores; (2) inhibition of $Ca^{2+}$ efflux; (3) increase in $Ca^{2+}$ influx from extracellular sources. Depending on the stimulus, one or more of these events may occur during contraction. The entry of $Ca^{2+}$ from extracellular sources may occur via potential-sensitive (during discharge of action potentials) or receptor-operated mechanisms. Mechanisms may also operate to link cell-membrane receptors to the intracellular $Ca^{2+}$ stores. Thus agonist–receptor activation of phospholipase C can

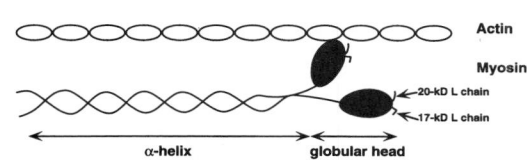

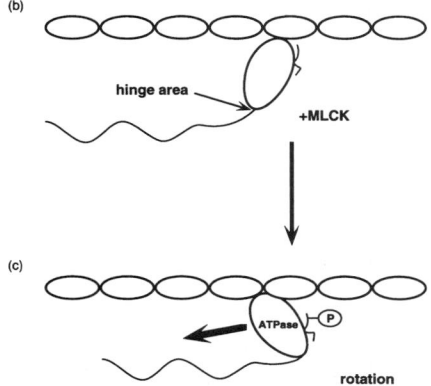

FIGURE 15.4 Molecular basis for myometrial contraction. (a) The globular actin molecules polymerize to form the long filaments of F–Actin to which the globular myosin head of the myosin filament attaches. (b) Myometrial contraction involves interactions between actin and myosin myofilaments. Phosphorylation (P) of the 20-kD myosin light chain on the myosin head by MLCK induces (c) an ATPase activity that supports a rotation in the myosin head relative to actin and consequently the sliding of the actin and myosin filaments in apposition to each other.

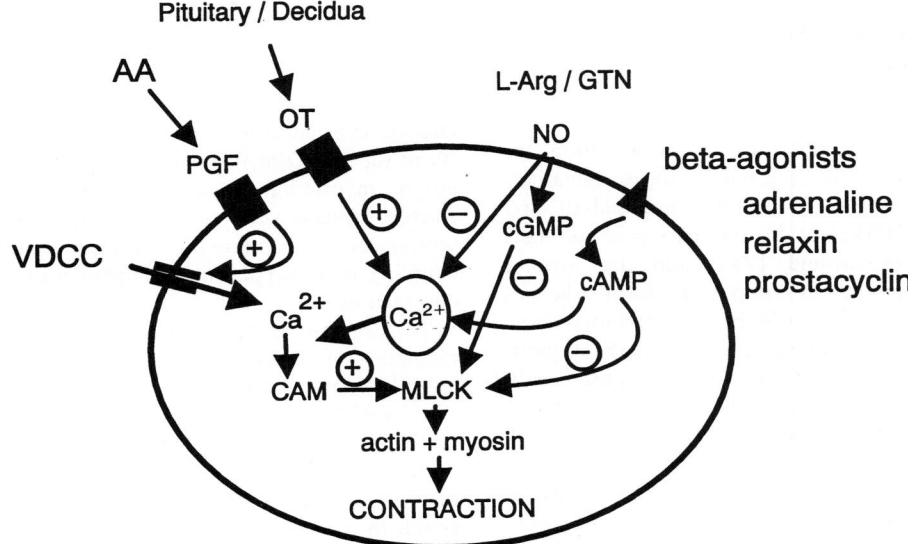

FIGURE 15.5 Intracellular biochemical pathways regulating myometrial contractions. The regulation of MLCK activity is central to the contraction of the myometrial cell. MLCK is activated by calcium–calmodulin (Ca$^{2+}$-CAM) following an increase in intracellular Ca$^{2+}$ levels. This increase is generated by uterotonic stimulants that activate signaling pathways resulting in an influx of extracellular Ca$^{2+}$ and/or release of Ca$^{2+}$ from intracellular stores. Intracellular signaling pathways involving cAMP (e.g. β-adrenergic agonists, prostacyclin, relaxin) or cGMP (nitric oxide, NO) act to inhibit contractile activity either by reducing intracellular Ca$^{2+}$ levels or by inactivating MLCK (see text for abbreviations).

lead to the hydrolysis of inositol phosphates leading to the release of inositol-1,4,5, trisphosphate (IP$_3$). IP$_3$ in turn can cause the release of Ca$^{2+}$ from intracellular stores. Diacylglycerol generated during inositol hydrolysis can interact with intracellular signaling pathways as well as be a substrate for PG synthesis. α-Adrenergic agonists and oxytocin operate through the inositol phosphate pathway. Stimulatory PGs act to increase the influx of Ca$^{2+}$ through voltage-dependent cell membrane Ca$^{2+}$ channels (VDCC), while oxytocin and PGs also have been reported to inhibit Ca$^{2+}$ efflux. A recent report also indicates that PGF$_{2\alpha}$ stimulates the hydrolysis of arachidonic acid from phospholipids and that this arachidonic acid can act, in turn, as a mediator of the release of intracellular Ca$^{2+}$. Hence PGs can have multiple actions to cause an elevation of intracellular Ca$^{2+}$. Agents which inhibit myometrial activity (progesterone, β-adrenergic agonists, relaxin) may operate to increase intracellular uptake or efflux of Ca$^{2+}$ which, by reducing the affinity of calmodulin for Ca$^{2+}$, would effectively reduce the activity of MLCK and hence inhibit contractile activity.

cAMP levels are regulated by adenylyl cyclase (cAMP synthesis) and phosphodiesterase (cAMP degradation). Inhibitors of myometrial activity, such as by β-adrenergic agonists, relaxin and prostacyclin, are known to increase cAMP probably through an increase in adenylyl cyclase activity. Recently it has been suggested that nitric oxide (NO) may also act as an endogenous inhibitor of myometrial contractile activity. The mechanism by which NO might inhibit myometrial contractions is unclear, but in other

smooth muscles it has been shown to increase intracellular cGMP levels, which in turn reduces intracellular Ca$^{2+}$ levels and hence contractile activity.

## CONTROL OF LABOR ONSET (PARTURITION)

## Role of the fetus in the initiation of labor

A central question regarding mechanisms that regulate the onset of labor is, does the signal originate within the mother or the fetus? It is a question that has been asked for centuries. The concept that the fetus initiates its own delivery dates back to 460 BC when Hippocrates suggested that, at the appointed hour, the fetus puts its feet on the fundus of the uterus and pushes. It was not until the 16th century that an Italian anatomist, Fabricius ab Aquapendente, proposed, against great opposition, that the chief agent of parturition was the muscular action of the uterus. By the 19th century, the importance of the link between fetal maturation and the initiation of labor was appreciated. In 1882, Spiegelberg wrote in a textbook of midwifery "...the reason why labor occurs at a definite time must be sought for, not in the uterus and its changes, but in the fetus. It is the maturity of the latter that gives the signal."

Across all species the role of the fetus in the initiation of labor varies. For example, in birds oviposition is a maternally regulated event initiated at the time of ovulation. In mammals, however, there is a wide spectrum of controls. In non-primates, there is convincing evidence that the fetus plays a major role in determining the timing of its own birth. Early experiments with cross-breeding of animals with different gestational lengths demonstrated that the fetal genotype plays a major role in determining the length of gestation. For example, while the length of gestation in the horse is 340 days and that of the donkey is 365 days, cross-breeding of these species leads to a pregnancy of intermediate length. This clear demonstration of the influence of fetal genotype led to the hypothesis that the conceptus has the means to trigger labor. Unfortunately, while it appears that in many species, such as the sheep, the fetus plays a significant role in the initiation of labor, the evidence in primates, humans in particular, is questionable.

## Initiation of labor in sheep

Because our greatest understanding of the role of the fetus in the initiation of labor is derived from studies in sheep, these mechanisms will be described in some detail. In 1963 the ingestion of the skunk cabbage (*Veratrum californicum*) by ewes during pregnancy was observed to be associated with prolonged pregnancy. The fetuses had cyclopean-type malformations with an absence, or abnormality, of neural connections to the pituitary, and the adrenal glands, which normally are comparatively large at birth, were atrophied. In 1965 Liggins developed experimental techniques for ablating the fetal sheep pituitary gland *in utero*, and in now classic experiments, investigated the role of the fetal brain in the initiation of labor (Fig. 15.6). The data from these and other studies over the past 25 years can be summarized as follows:

- Ablation of the ovine fetal pituitary or hypothalamus, or sectioning of the pituitary stalk, lead to a failure both of fetal adrenal growth and of the initiation of labor.
- Fetal blood concentrations of cortisol derived from the fetal adrenal in late pregnancy are high prior to the onset of labor. In contrast, fetuses in which the fetal pituitary stalk has been sectioned or fetuses which have been hypophysectomized (HPX) fail to show any increase in cortisol.

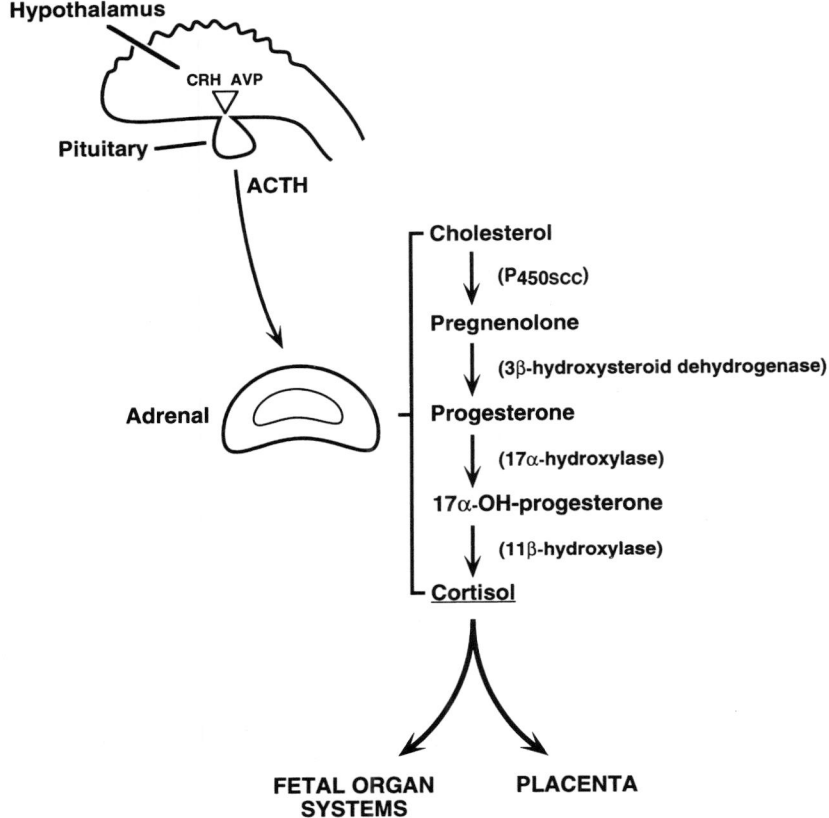

FIGURE 15.6 The fetal hypothalamic–pituitary–adrenal axis. Release of CRH/AVP from nuclei within the hypothalamus stimulates release of ACTH from the pituitary. The ACTH acts to increase 17α-hydroxylase activity within the adrenal cortex allowing progesterone to be metabolized to cortisol. The cortisol subsequently acts to regulate placental steroidogenesis (see text for abbreviations).

- Cortisol infusion into normal preterm fetuses results in the premature onset of labor, furthermore labor also can be induced by cortisol in HPX fetuses.
- Removal of the fetal adrenal glands prevents the onset of labor, and this can be reversed by cortisol administration.
- Administration of adrenocorticotrophin (ACTH) to normal preterm fetuses leads to an increase in fetal adrenal size and plasma cortisol concentrations and the premature onset of labor.
- Infusion of either corticotrophin-releasing hormone (CRH) or arginine vasopressin (AVP) into preterm fetuses can increase ACTH secretion and cortisol production.
- Ablation of the paraventricular nucleus (through which CRH and AVP neurons pass) prevents the onset of labor.

Thus in sheep, the fetal brain plays a critical role in triggering the onset of labor via activation of the adrenocorticotrophic axis. However, several questions remain to be answered.

1. Why is it that in adults and preterm fetuses, administration of cortisol acts in a negative feedback loop to inhibit ACTH release, whereas in fetuses at term, ACTH and cortisol rise in parallel?
2. Administration of $PGE_2$ to the fetus increases ACTH and cortisol through actions both at the pituitary and adrenal levels. $PGE_2$ is produced by the placenta during pregnancy, and fetal plasma concentrations increase around the same time as cortisol. What role might the placenta play in the onset of labor?

The above data strongly point to the pivotal role of cortisol in the events leading up to labor. The question is, how does cortisol bring about the changes in uterine activity? The first evidence came from measurements of maternal plasma hormone concentrations prior to labor. Plasma progesterone concentrations fall a day or two before labor starts while estrogen concentrations increase sharply in the 36 hours leading up to labor. The increase in estrogen is followed by an increase in maternal plasma $PGF_{2\alpha}$ concentrations, which acts to stimulate contractions. Both progesterone and estrogen are produced in the sheep placenta and are linked through the pathway shown in Fig. 15.7. During pregnancy placental 17α-hydroxylase activity is low; however, this activity increases prior to labor. Cortisol derived from the fetal adrenal increases activity of this enzyme and levels can be increased *in vitro* by incubation of placental tissue with glucocorticoids or *in vivo* by infusion of exogenous cortisol. The increase in 17α-hydroxylase provides increased substrate (17α-hydroxyprogesterone) and allows progesterone to be metabolized to estradiol-17β with the consequent switch from a progesterone to an estrogen-dominated state.

The mechanisms by which these steroid changes increase $PGF_{2\alpha}$ synthesis are not well understood. Extrapolation from knowledge of endometrial production in non-pregnant sheep suggests that estrogen promotes, while progesterone inhibits, $PGF_{2\alpha}$ synthesis. However, estrogen administration to late pregnant ewes does not elicit labor on its own.

Interestingly, cortisol not only induces placental enzyme synthesis but also induces systems in the fetal lung that bring about lung maturation, as well as affecting other organs including the kidney, thyroid, vascular system and GI tract. In this way, in the sheep, cortisol can be seen as acting to coordinate fetal organ maturation with the timing of birth.

## Initiation of labor in the human

Evidence for a role of the fetus in the initiation of parturition in the human is more circumspect. Unlike the sheep, absence of the pituitary (as occurs in *anencephalic fetuses*) does not prevent the onset of labor, although there is more scatter around the expected date of delivery and in some cases pregnancy can be prolonged. In the human there is no indication of a fall in progesterone or an acute rise in estrogen, either in plasma or within intrauterine tissues. However, recent data indicate that, while the concentrations of estrogen or progesterone may not change, there is an increase in estrogen receptor expression within intrauterine tissues. Thus the differences between sheep and the humans may be more superficial than originally thought, with the mechanisms regulating the onset of labor in the human occurring at a paracrine rather than endocrine level.

As with the sheep, it is believed by most investigators that concentrations of PGs, particularly $PGF_{2\alpha}$, and their stable metabolites increase prior to the onset of human labor and are responsible for stimulating the myometrium to contract (*see* page 252). Small amounts of exogenous $PGF_{2\alpha}$ or $PGE_2$ induce labor and reproduce the events of spontaneous labor. The importance of these uterotonic agonists is further demonstrated by the ability of inhibitors of PG synthesis to inhibit labor contractions. Prostaglandins are synthesized through a pathway involving release of arachidonic acid from membrane phospholipids (by the enzyme, phospholipase $A_2$), the formation of endoperoxides ($PGG_2$ and $PGH_2$) from arachidonic acid and the subsequent synthesis of primary PGs (by the enzyme, cyclooxygenase (COX)) (*see* Chapter 8 for further details). Indomethacin blocks the synthesis of PGs at this latter step. Within intrauterine tissues at least two COX enzymes are encoded by two separate genes, *COX1* and *COX2*. COX1 is active constitutively in most tissues while COX2 is an inducible form of the enzyme. Recent data suggest that only *COX2* expression is increased in intrauterine tissues

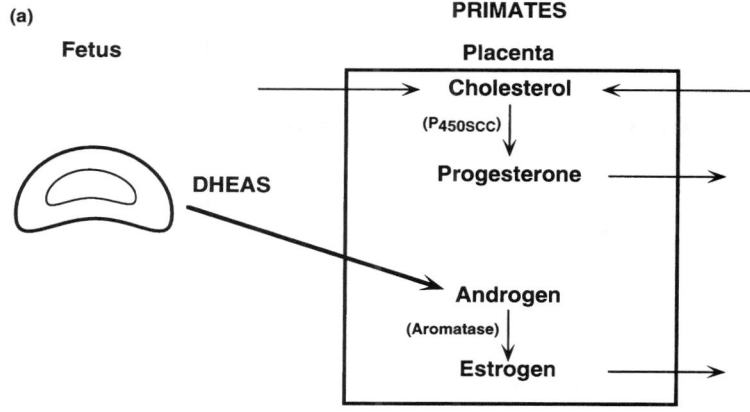

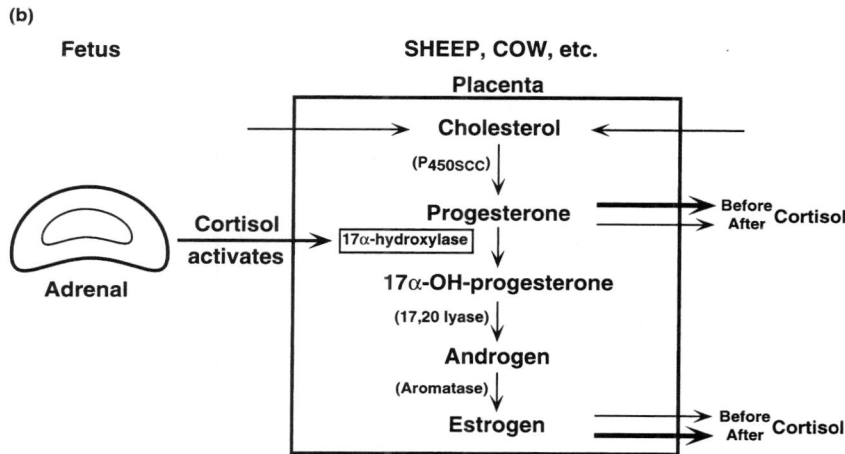

FIGURE 15.7 Pathways of steroid synthesis in the placenta in various species, demonstrating the fundamental difference depending on the presence or absence of 17α-hydroxylase. The primate (including human) placenta lacks the enzyme and depends on the fetal adrenal for substrate for estrogen synthesis. In sheep, cortisol derived from the fetal adrenal increases the activity of the rate-limiting enzyme, 17α-hydroxylase in the placenta. This allows progesterone to be metabolized through to estradiol-17β with the consequent switch from a progesterone to an estrogen dominated state. DHEAS = dehydroepiandrosterone sulfate.

during labor, leading to the observed increase in enzyme activity.

The source of the PGs postulated to stimulate myometrial contractions is controversial. Some investigators believe that PGs produced by the amnion diffuse through the chorion (which does not produce large amounts of PGs, but does metabolize them) and the decidua to reach the myometrium. Others believe that PGs produced within the decidua or placenta itself are important for stimulation of the myometrium and that these PGs can reach the myometrium either through a local paracrine route or through the systemic circulation. The mechanisms that stimulate PG production at term are equally controversial. PG production by amnion cells in culture is stimulated by glucocorticoids, though this steroid inhibits PG synthesis by fresh tissue. One hypothesis suggests that during pregnancy factors from the fetus or intrauterine tissues suppress decidual PGF production and that at term this paracrine support is lost or is inactivated leading to increased PGF production and stimulation of the myometrium. While several pieces of circumstantial evidence are consistent with such a hypothesis, there is no definitive information either way. Numerous cytokines and peptides stimulate PG synthesis *in vitro*, and the former have been suggested as mediators of infection-induced preterm labor (see below). Whether or not these factors operate as physiologic regulators of PG synthesis *in vivo* is not certain.

Humans are subject to several pregnancy complications that are associated with an increased risk of preterm birth. Perhaps most important of these is the association between intrauterine infection and premature labor. Several mechanisms have been postulated by which infection might lead to preterm labor. Direct stimulation of PG synthesis by release of bacterial phospholipase $A_2$ or an indirect pathway involving a maternal inflammatory response (as a result of exposure to bacterial wall products, e.g. lipopolysaccharides) leading to cytokine stimulation of PG synthesis are likely mechanisms. In the latter, the first step would involve infection of the intrauterine tissues by the invading bacteria. It is suggested that this infection induces an activation of decidual macrophages, production of cytokines by decidual and chorion cells, the recruitment of neutrophils and the consequent stimulation of intrauterine PG production. These PGs then would act on the myometrium to increase contractile activity. It also has been suggested that proteolytic enzymes, released either from bacteria or from maternal inflammatory cells, digest matrix proteins within the fetal membranes, weakening them and predisposing to premature rupture.

Of the other complications of pregnancy associated with preterm labor, those due to multiple fetuses and polyhydramnios are notable. Both conditions lead to an increase in uterine wall tension (stretch). Recent preliminary data suggest that stretch is a potent stimulus for increased expression of Cx-43, possibly mediated by c-fos, raising the possibility of a common mechanism by which hormonal and mechanical inputs might increase myometrial contractility and the onset of labor.

## CLINICAL APPLICATIONS OF REGULATION OF MYOMETRIAL CONTRACTILE ACTIVITY

## Induction of labor

A number of agents have been used clinically to induce labor at various times during pregnancy. The physiological stimulatory effects of oxytocin and stimulatory PGs (PGE, PGF) described above have led to their extensive use in this respect. However, while these agents will undoubtedly stimulate contractions, their effectiveness is determined by the prior level of activation of the myometrium. Thus unless the process of activation has already taken place, the myometrial response to the stimulation will not be optimal. Furthermore, in many cases the cervix has not undergone maturational changes that allow it to dilate rapidly and to efface. These problems may contribute to a relatively high incidence of cesarean section during induction (due to a failure of labor to progress effectively).

## Treatment of dysmenorrhea

*Dysmenorrhea* (pathologic menstrual cramps) is associated with an abnormal pattern of uterine contractile activity with either overproduction of stimulatory PGs, an imbalance of stimulatory versus inhibitory PGs or a hyper-response of the myometrium to normal PG levels. PG synthesis inhibitors are widely used to ameliorate the symptoms.

## Prevention of preterm labor

Preterm birth occurs in 5–10 per cent of all pregnancies and accounts for 75 per cent of neonatal deaths and for considerable neonatal morbidity. Because of the magnitude of the problem and the serious consequences to the neonate, the list of agents used as tocolytics is substantial. Unfortunately, none have proven effective. In large part this is due to our fragmentary knowledge of the mechanisms that affect myometrial inhibition as well as the multifactorial process of labor. The following is only a sample of some of the more recent treatment approaches.

### Progestins

Considering the mechanisms of action of progesterone described above one might think that progesterone would be an excellent choice as a tocolytic agent. To date, however, there is little evidence that progesterone, even in high doses, prevents or prolongs labor once initiated. This suggests that in the human, progesterone does not inhibit myometrial activity although at least one other possibility exists. Most of the effects of this steroid are mediated through protein synthetic events. Since these would take a number of hours to produce their effects, it could be that delivery might occur prior to the maximal effects of the steroid being apparent.

### Prostaglandin synthesis inhibitors

The critical role suggested for PGs in stimulation of the myometrium during labor has led to the use of PG synthesis inhibitors as a means of preventing preterm labor. The results of a number of clinical trials suggests that these compounds are effective in inhibiting uterine contractions in women in preterm labor. The slow acceptance of this form of therapy, however, is due to data concerning fetal side-effects connected with their usage. Indomethacin blocks the activity of both COX1 and COX2, the latter more effectively. Since COX1 may be important in generating PGs which act in a number of fetal physiologic processes including GI motility, regulation of vascular reactivity (particularly cerebral), maintenance of ductus arteriosus patency, urine output, etc., it is not surprising that blockade of both enzymes is often associated with generalized side-effects. While there are drugs that appear to be specific inhibitors of COX2, these have yet to be tested with respect to inhibition of labor contractions. Furthermore, new evidence shows that most fetal tissues express increasing amounts of COX2 in late gestation, suggesting that a COX2- specific blockade may not be without some fetal side-effects.

## Calcium antagonists

As described above $Ca^{2+}$ is central to the contractile events within the smooth muscle cell. Drugs which "block" the $Ca^{2+}$ channels, thereby preventing $Ca^{2+}$ influx, have been used to inhibit myometrial contractions. Although these drugs are effective in vascular smooth muscle, sufficient data are not yet available as to their effectiveness in the myometrium. As with many of these treatments, however, these drugs effect all types of smooth muscle, hence their use is associated with a number of side-effects.

## β-Adrenergic agonists

This group of compounds, probably the most commonly used agents for tocolysis, act by increasing cAMP within the smooth muscle cell. Unfortunately clinical trials suggest that while these drugs initially inhibit labor contractions, their effect is lost by 72 hours and there is no significant improvement in neonatal outcome associated with their use. Clinical and basic research studies suggest that this is due to an agonist-induced down-regulation of β-adrenergic receptors ultimately leaving insufficient receptors to maintain inhibition.

## Oxytocin antagonists

These agents bind to oxytocin receptors but do not induce any intracellular signaling. Since they compete with oxytocin for receptors they would act to inhibit the uterotonic effects of endogenous oxytocin. As yet there are limited data suggesting that such agents will be any more successful as tocolytics than any of the other pharmacologic treatments. Since, as described above, there are numerous ways (other than through oxytocin receptors) by which intracellular $Ca^{2+}$ can be increased, it would not be surprisingly if these drugs were only partially effective.

## Glyceryl trinitrate (nitroglycerin)

Glyceryl trinitrate acts as a nitric oxide (NO) donor (see also Chapter 10). In vitro studies have provided evidence that NO inhibits uterine smooth muscle contractile activity. There are also very limited data, mostly in humans, that NO has similar inhibitory effects in vivo. To date there is considerable debate as to the mechanisms of action of NO in the myometrium or indeed whether the effects of NO are direct or indirect. It has been suggested that NO is synthesized in the myometrium during pregnancy and that it acts

as an endogenous inhibitor of contractile activity. This has yet to be clearly demonstrated. At present, while it is likely that NO can act as a contractile inhibitor in the myometrium, there is little reason to believe that it will be any more effective as a tocolytic than other physiologic inhibitors.

## CONCLUSIONS

The mechanisms responsible for the onset of labor are complex and remain poorly understood. While common themes persist across mammalian species, significant species–species differences exist. This is especially problematic in understanding preterm labor, which has many etiologies and is rarely found in experimental animals. Currently there are no effective therapies that can prevent preterm birth in women in preterm labor. This may not be too surprising since while these therapies generally concentrate on one particular regulatory pathway (inhibition of PG synthesis, blockade of oxytocin receptors or $Ca^{2+}$ channels), the regulation of myometrial contractile activity involves multiple intracellular biochemical pathways. Future investigation in this area most probably will focus on the common elements between all species that are responsible for the both the *activation* of the myometrium, enabling it to develop the ability to produce effective contractile activity, and the production of uterotonic agonists that provide the *stimulus* to the activated myometrium.

## SELECTED READING

Challis JRG, Lye SJ. Parturition. In: Knobil E, Neill JD, eds, *The physiology of reproduction*, Vol. 2. New York: Raven Press, 1994: 985.

Lye SJ. The initiation and inhibition of labor – toward a molecular understanding. *Semin Reproductive Endocrinol* 1994;**12** : 284.

Word RA. Myosin phosphorylation and the control of myometrial contraction/relaxation. *Semin Perinatol* 1995; **19**: 3.

Olson DM, Mijovic JE, Sadowsky DW. Control of human parturition. *Semin Perinatol* 1995; **19**: 52.

Monga M, Creasy RK. Pharmacologic management of preterm labor. *Semin Perinatol* 1995; **19**: 84.

# HORMONES AND PROSTAGLANDINS: THEIR ROLE IN PARTURITION

The mechanism initiating parturition seems to result from the release of prostaglandin $F_{2\alpha}$ ($PGF_{2\alpha}$) from the uterine epithelium.

## PROSTAGLANDINS AND THEIR REGULATION

In some animal species the release of PGF$_{2\alpha}$ is stimulated at term by a rapid fall in progesterone and a sharp rise in estrogen levels. The changes in steroid synthesis result from rising concentrations of cortisol in the fetal circulation which induce the activity of 17α-hydroxylase, a placental enzyme necessary for the conversion of progesterone to estrogen (see Fig. 15.7). The placenta of primates, including man, lacks the enzyme, and parturition is not preceded by an alteration in the ratio of progesterone:estrogen. Nevertheless, PGF$_{2\alpha}$ and prostaglandin E$_2$ (PGE$_2$) are released in substantial quantities in human labor and are almost certainly responsible for the changes in uterine smooth muscle and connective tissue that lead to labor and delivery. The factors responsible for the control of uterine PG synthesis in human pregnancy remain uncertain. However, most investigators agree that human parturition is the outcome of paracrine rather than endocrine events, involving a maternal tissue (decidua) and fetal tissues (amnion and chorion).

•

## Actions of prostaglandins on the uterus

Administration of prostaglandins (PGs) to women at any stage of pregnancy leads to abortion or delivery provided that 8–12 hours is allowed for uterine responses involving protein synthesis to evolve. The changes involve both the smooth muscle and the connective tissue of the cervix and fetal membranes. The smooth muscle cells exposed to PGF$_{2\alpha}$ or PGE$_2$ develop gap junctions that transmit spike potentials, thereby propagating an electrical wave from a single pacemaker site. The resulting coordinated contraction of the whole uterus is effective in expelling the fetus, whereas the local, uncoordinated contractions that occur throughout pregnancy are ineffective. PGF$_{2\alpha}$ and PGE$_2$ are oxytocic (i.e. stimulate contractions) and, in addition, enhance the sensitivity of smooth muscle cells to oxytocin. Both PGF$_{2\alpha}$ and PGE$_2$, particularly the latter, cause changes in the uterine and amniotic connective tissues akin to those occurring in inflammation or tissue remodeling. Specifically, enhanced activity of collagenolytic enzymes causes mature, "tough" collagen to be degraded and partly replaced by young, more fragile collagen with fewer crosslinks. The concentration of strongly charged, sulfated glycosaminoglycans in the proteoglycan matrix is halved, leading to loosening of the tight packing of the collagen bundles. The overall effect of these biochemical changes is a 12-fold decrease in the mechanical strength of the intrapartum cervix compared with the non-pregnant cervix. Similar biochemical events in the amnion weaken this tough membrane sufficiently to allow labor contractions to burst it. Relaxin as well as PGE$_2$ and PGF$_{2\alpha}$ increase the compliance of the pregnant human cervix when applied topically, but whether relaxin has a physiological role in cervical ripening in women as it has in many animals is uncertain.

## Synthesis of uterine PGs (see page 248 and Chapter 8)

The various uterine tissues have different spectra of PG synthesis. The predominant PG released by the myometrium is PGI$_2$, whereas the decidua forms mainly PGF$_{2\alpha}$ and the amnion and cervix PGE$_2$. It is likely that PGF$_{2\alpha}$ of decidual origin is the major PG initiating labor. As in other tissues, uterine PGs require arachidonic acid as the mandatory substrate. Arachidonic acid is present in abundance in the phospholipids of uterine tissues, which are specifically enriched with this fatty acid, probably as a response to high levels of progesterone. The availability of free arachidonic acid determines the rate of synthesis, cyclooxygenase (COX) imposes a maximal production rate and the relative activities of the specific synthases determine the spectrum of end products (see Fig. 8.3, on page 164).

## Control of PG synthesis

Arachidonic acid is liberated by hydrolysis of glycerophospholipids either by phospholipase A$_2$ (PLA$_2$), present intracellularly in an inactive, membrane-bound form capable of almost instantaneous activation, or by phospholipase C and the subsequent action of di- and monoacylglycerol lipases. This pathway also liberates inositol triphosphate (IP$_3$) which mobilizes free Ca$^{2+}$ and enhances the activity of the Ca$^{2+}$-dependent PLA$_2$. A wide variety of physical, chemical, and bacteriological factors stimulate activity; many of them, such as stripping placental membranes, or intrauterine placement of hypertonic solutions, irritant solutions or foreign bodies, have been used clinically to induce labor or abortion. However, the physiological stimulus of PLA$_2$ in the human uterus remains uncertain.

## INTERACTION OF HORMONES REGULATING PARTURITION WITH PROSTAGLANDINS

### Progesterone

Progesterone has multiple actions on the uterus, including stimulation of smooth muscle cell hypertrophy, inhibition of gap junction formation, inhibition of oxytocin receptor synthesis and other effects that promote uterine quiescence. In addition, progesterone inhibits the activity of PLA$_2$ and the synthesis of PGs. A fall in the concentration of progesterone, by reversing these inhibitory effects, leads to increased uterine action and labor in some species. The weakness of the "progesterone withdrawal" hypothesis in human pregnancy is the absence of a prepartum fall in progesterone concentrations in plasma, myometrium or myometrial nuclear receptors. Progesterone concentrations may fall locally in target tissues despite maintained concentrations elsewhere, or alternately, tissue or receptor sensitivity to the same concentrations may be altered.

## Estrogen

Estradiol-17β is a potent stimulus of myometrial hyperplasia, gap junction formation, oxytocin receptor synthesis, $PLA_2$ activity and PG synthesis. However, like progesterone, estrogen shows no prepartum trends in concentration. Furthermore, administration of large amounts of estrogen to women at term is ineffective in inducing labor. Local concentrations of estrogen could be raised by conversion of the high concentration of estrogen sulfates in amniotic fluid to unconjugated estrogen. However, steroid sulfatase present in fetal membranes is no more active in tissues obtained at delivery than in tissues obtained before labor.

## Oxytocin

Oxytocin is the most powerful oxytocic agent known, yet its administration is ineffective in inducing labor, despite producing powerful contractions, unless the pregnancy is near term. The reason for this failure is that the various changes in the muscle and connective tissue induced by PGs are absent; the contractions are incompletely propagated and the cervix remains non-compliant. Recently, oxytocin has been found to stimulate decidual synthesis of $PGF_{2\alpha}$. The concentration of oxytocin in plasma remains low throughout pregnancy and rises only in the second stage of labor; the concentration of receptors increases with the onset of labor. Thus it is possible that oxytocin plays a part in initiating parturition by stimulating both contractions and decidual synthesis of $PGF_{2\alpha}$. The stimulus to oxytocin receptor synthesis is unknown, although estrogen stimulates receptors in experimental animals: the absence of an increase in estrogen concentrations before parturition in women excludes this as a cause. Uterine sensitivity to oxytocin increases during treatment with $PGF_{2\alpha}$ or $PGE_2$, suggesting an increase in oxytocin receptors but a postreceptor change cannot be excluded.

## Secretory component (gravidin)

Amniotic fluid contains secretory component of IgA, a 78-kD protein that binds tightly to IgA and facilitates passage of IgA through epithelial membranes. The protein is a potent inhibitor of PG synthesis by blocking the activity of $PLA_2$. Cultures of chorionic cells generate this secretory component in greater quantities when the cells are harvested before than when harvested during or after labor. These observations suggest that secretory component contributes to the maintenance of uterine quiesence to term and that a fall in the rate of synthesis may be one of the factors responsible for the liberation of $PGF_{2\alpha}$ associated with the onset of labor.

## Platelet activating factor

Platelet activating factor (PAF) is a potent stimulus of smooth muscle contractility by raising the intracellular concentrations of $Ca^{2+}$ as in its action on platelets. It is absent from amniotic fluid of women before labor starts but is usually present during labor. A PAF antagonist administered to rats prolongs labor but not the duration of pregnancy, suggesting that PAF is not an important component of the mechanism initiating labor. The production of PAF, a phospholipid-derived factor, may be a byproduct of $PLA_2$ activity during PG synthesis.

## Corticotrophin-releasing hormone (CRH)

The possible role of placental CRH as a biological clock determining the time of birth is described in Chapter 13.

## ROLE OF PGs IN PRETERM LABOR

Preterm labor is of two types involving primarily the connective tissue. In the first type, the connective tissue of the cervix undergoes the biochemical changes normally seen at term and dilates prematurely, painlessly and without uterine contractions; the membranes bulge through the cervix and rupture and the fetus is delivered after a brief second stage of labor. This so-called *incompetent cervix syndrome* presumably reflects the premature release of $PGE_2$ in cervical tissue, but the stimulus is unknown.

The second type of preterm labor results from premature activation of myometrial contractions; it mimics term labor and is probably dependent on release of $PGF_{2\alpha}$. In some instances, the cause is clearly related to an obstetric complication such as hemorrhage, uterine malformation, trauma or infection. In most instances, no cause is apparent and there is a tendency to recurrence in successive pregnancies.

The extent to which infection contributes to preterm labor is controversial. Some investigators claim that subclinical amnionitis is the cause of most cases of idiopathic preterm labor. Others consider that the common occurrence of low-grade amnionitis in preterm labor is a result rather than a cause. However, there is agreement that a variety of organisms have the ability to stimulate PG synthesis. The endotoxin lipo-polysaccharide, which is usually present in amniotic fluid in association with gram-negative amnionitis, is a potent stimulus of $PLA_2$ activity and PG synthesis. Cytokines such as interleukin-1α, interleukin-1β and tumor necrosis factor that mediate the inflammatory response stimulate PG synthesis. Controlled clinical trials of antibiotics in women at high risk of preterm labor so far have been unsuccessful in consistently reducing the incidence.

## SELECTED READING

Bleasdale JE, Johnston JM. Prostaglandins and human parturition: regulation of arachidonic acid mobilization. *Perinat Med* 1985; 5: 151.

Casey ML, MacDonald PC. The role of prostaglandins in labor. In: McNellis D, Challis J, MacDonald P, *et al.*, eds. *The onset of labor: cellular and integrative mechanisms*. Ithaca: Perinatology Press, 1988: 141.

Challis JRG, Lye SJ. Parturition. In: Clarke JR, ed. *Oxford reviews of reproductive biology*, Vol. 8. *Oxford: Clarendon Press, 1986: 61.*

Liggins GC. The paracrine system controlling human parturition. In: Jaffe RD, Dell'Acqua S, eds. *The endocrine physiology of parturition and the peripartal period*. New York: Raven Press, 1985: 205.

McClean M, Bisits A, Davies J, *et al.* A placental clock controlling the length of human pregnancy. *Nature Med* 1995; 1: 460.

# 16

# Puberty

Edward O. Reiter

Puberty is the period of transition between childhood and adulthood, during which individuals undergo a striking growth spurt, develop secondary sexual characteristics, achieve fertility and experience substantive psychological changes. The endocrine events of pubertal maturation are but a part of a developmental continuum extending from initial sexual differentiation through senescence. The key endocrine events are orchestrated by maturational changes in the gonadotrophic axis.

## REPRODUCTIVE ENDOCRINE SYSTEM

### See also Part 7

### Suprahypothalamic sites

Higher cortical centers and the limbic system influence synthesis and secretion of the decapeptide gonadotrophin releasing hormone (GnRH) by the arcuate nucleus of the hypothalamus. In addition, it is quite clear that many neurotransmitters, as well as sex steroids and varied gonadal peptides, affect the production of GnRH.

### Hypothalamus

The arcuate nucleus of the medial basal hypothalamus and its transducer neurosecretory neurons release GnRH in a periodic oscillatory fashion. This decapeptide is then transported from the median eminence to the anterior pituitary gland via the primary plexus of the hypothalamic pituitary portal circulation.

### Anterior pituitary gland

Upon reaching the anterior pituitary gland, molecules of GnRH bind to surface receptors on specialized cells, called pituitary gonadotropes, which synthesize and store the glycoprotein hormones, luteinizing hormone (LH) and follicle stimulating hormone (FSH). In response to this intermittent GnRH stimulation, LH and FSH are secreted in a pulsatile fashion, to enhance gonadal steroidogenesis and maturation of the germinal epithelium. The concept that LH secretory bursts are temporally related to a central episodic process such as GnRH release is supported by the finding that volleys of electrical activity have been recorded from the medial basal hypothalamus coincident with LH pulses.

## Gonads

In the female, ovaries are the site of sex steroid production in follicles and thecal tissue; ova are the germinal products. In the male, sex steroid production occurs in testicular Leydig cells, while spermatogenesis occurs in the germinal epithelium of the seminiferous tubules. Multiple peptides, including the insulin-like growth factors, the inhibin family, and diverse cytokines are also produced by the gonads and act in concert to produce functional maturation.

## PATTERNS OF GONADOTROPHIN RELEASE

The availability of sensitive and specific immunoassays and bioassays for the gonadotrophins has permitted their quantitation, both at the extremely low concentrations present through mid-childhood years and then at the rising concentrations which characterize pubertal change. Presumably because of the molecular heterogeneity of circulating LH and FSH, qualitative as well as quantitative changes in circulating gonadotrophins affect gonadal steroidogenesis and maturation of germinal tissues. The highly sensitive immunofluorometric assays (IFMA) appear to measure the circulating molecular forms responsible for the gonadotrophin bioactivity traditionally quantified by *in vitro* bioassays.

# Changes in levels of gonadotrophins

Production of gonadotrophins by the human fetal pituitary is demonstrable by 10 weeks' gestation, with hormonal secretion occurring by 11–12 weeks. In pituitary glands and serum of fetuses, gonadotrophin levels reach adult castrate levels by mid-gestation, with a decline thereafter to reach typical childhood values by term. Following the decrease in sex steroids during the first several days after birth, concentrations of FSH and LH increase again and exhibit wide fluctuations during the first months. These intermittent high gonadotrophin concentrations are associated with pubertal concentrations of testosterone in male infants and, to a less striking extent, increased estradiol concentrations in females. By 6 months of age in males and 1–2 years in females, concentrations of LH and FSH decrease to low levels, which then persist until the onset of puberty (Fig. 16.1).

In the immediate peripubertal period, basal gonadotrophin concentrations again begin to increase. In girls, FSH concentrations rise during the early stages of puberty and then plateau, whereas LH concentrations tend to rise during later stages. In boys, FSH concentrations rise progressively throughout puberty, and LH concentrations increase sharply during early pubertal development and then gradually rise throughout the remainder of the pubertal years.

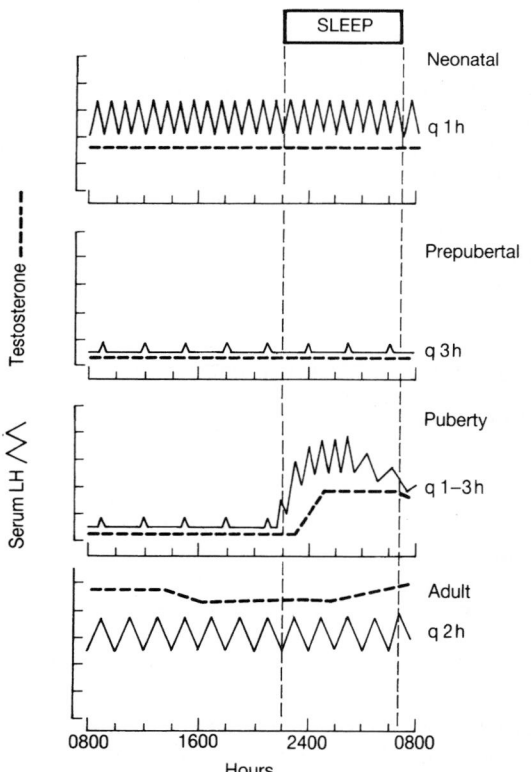

FIGURE 16.1 Luteinizing hormone (LH) and testosterone secretory patterns throughout sexual maturation in males

In addition to these changes in immunoreactive gonadotrophins, changes in the levels of biologically active LH have been quantitated throughout fetal life and in all stages of extrauterine life. In human studies, bioactive LH concentrations are generally undetectable during prepubertal years, then rise dramatically during pubertal maturation. The increment in mean LH concentrations from prepuberty to puberty is substantially greater when determined by bioassay than with standard immunoassay techniques. The utilization of IFMA measurements of LH confirm the striking increase of LH from prepuberty to adulthood, ranging to as high as 100-fold. This strong correlation between LH concentrations determined by bioassay and IFMA, in contrast to immunoassay, stresses the importance of using highly specific and sensitive measuring systems when assessing the very low gonadotrophin concentrations of early prepubertal children.

## Episodic circadian secretion

LH is secreted in a pulsatile (episodic) manner even in prepubertal children, but with a frequency and an amplitude lower than that in pubertal children or adults. The increment of mean LH concentrations during puberty corresponds to a rise in both the magnitude and frequency of LH pulses. A generally similar pattern occurs in FSH pulsatile release. In addition to these episodic bursts of LH and FSH secretion, a circadian rhythm exists which is augmented in late childhood and adolescent years. In prepubertal children, a small but detectable nocturnal enhancement of LH release is present.

During puberty, sleep-enhanced LH secretion increases progressively until the late pubertal years when the pattern of LH secretion appears to stabilize throughout the 24-hour period and is comparable to that seen in the adult. It appears, thus, that the increased concentrations of LH found during pubertal years are amplifications of pre-existing patterns of episodic and circadian gonadotrophin release that have been demonstrable even during the period of mid-childhood gonadotrophin secretory quiescence.

## REGULATION OF GONADOTROPHIN SECRETION

The generous secretion of LH and FSH by the fetal and neonatal pituitary diminishes by the third year, after which the entire reproductive endocrine system becomes relatively quiescent until the onset of puberty. Two different processes (i.e. a "dual mechanism of restraint") have been postulated to explain these developmental changes in gonadotrophin secretion: one is a sex steroid-dependent mechanism, i.e. a highly sensitive hypothalamic–pituitary–gonadal negative feedback system; the other is an apparently sex steroid-independent mechanism by which the central nervous system modulates gonadotrophin secretion, presumably by altering GnRH synthesis and release.

## Developmental changes in sex steroid-dependent control

It has been postulated that the hypothalamic–pituitary–gonadotrope system is highly sensitive, and rapidly responsive, to suppressive effects of tiny quantities of circulating sex steroids during the middle childhood years. With the onset of puberty, the hypothalamic arcuate nucleus and the pituitary gonadotropes appear to become progressively less sensitive to inhibitory effects of sex steroids on GnRH release, resulting in increased pulsatile GnRH release (altered frequency and heightened amplitude) with consequent increased secretion of gonadotrophins. The site of steroid action may involve both hypothalamic and pituitary cells. The sensing mechanism for this set point regulation of negative feedback control has been referred to as the "gonadostat." Though the concept of the gonadostat has proved useful in explaining many aspects of the normal physiological changes in gonadotrophin levels, it seems unlikely that a gonadostat change is the sole initiator of the fall of gonadotrophin concentrations during the midpubertal quiescent period. Nonetheless, in adult females, acquisition of an appropriate set point for negative feedback may be a prerequisite for appropriate gonadotrophin fluctuations during the early follicular phase of the menstrual cycle to allow appropriate ripening of a mature ovum.

## Sex steroid-independent control

The diphasic pattern of gonadotrophin secretion from infancy through adulthood (i.e. higher in the first 1–3 years of life than in the next 8–10 years with a subsequent secondary rise in adolescence into adulthood) is qualitatively similar in normal individuals and in patients with functional agonadism. The fall in gonadotrophin synthesis and secretion in children with agonadism (best studied in children with gonadal dysgenesis) has suggested the presence of intrinsic inhibitory CNS influences, largely independent of gonadal sex steroid production, that also act to diminish gonadotrophin production and release during middle childhood years and thus restrain the onset of puberty. The mechanism of this central nervous system inhibitory action remains unknown; endogenous opiates and the pineal gland, though well studied, seem not to be involved.

## Suprahypothalamic control

Recent studies in both primates and rodents demonstrate that GnRH or at least GnRH mRNA is present in abundant quantities in the hypothalami of immature monkeys and in rodents, suggesting adequate synthetic capacity for GnRH. Further, GnRH and consequent gonadotrophin release are quickly evoked by administration of excitatory neuroamines, such as N-methyl-D-aspartate (NMDA), to juvenile animals. Direct measurements of portal GnRH levels after electrical stimulation of the basal hypothalamus indicate that the capacity for GnRH release is similar to that for prepubertal and pubertal monkeys. Such data confirm an early potential for GnRH synthesis and secretion, supporting the notion that suprahypothalamic neuroregulatory factors may have major importance in the timing of puberty and in the regulation of function of the hypothalamic arcuate nucleus. A "desynchronization" of neurosecretory activity within the family of GnRH neurons may be associated with uncoordinated continuous low-grade GnRH release that must be "re-synchronized" to escape the prepubertal quiescent period. A role for the abundant glial cells which ensheath GnRH neurons is becoming apparent in this process.

LH and FSH appear always to be secreted in a pulsatile or episodic fashion with discrete bursts of hormone release from the gonadotropes, separated by intervals of quiescence. Modulation of frequency and amplitude of such secretory bursts occurs through an interaction of GnRH in its oscillatory rhythm, with sex steroids and gonadal inhibins/activins at the pituitary gonadotrope. This generates a pulsatile ultradian gonadotrophin concentration profile in the peripheral circulation. The frequency of GnRH pulses and the intermittent nature of its activating signal upon the gonadotropes appear critical in maintaining the responsiveness of the gonadotropes and also normal LH and FSH secretion. In the absence of exposure to pulsatile GnRH, the gonadotrope is unresponsive. Paradoxically, continuous infusion of GnRH will also inhibit gonadotrophin secretion through a process of "desensitization," or "down-regulation" of the GnRH receptors on the gonadotrope cell membranes.

## Interaction of synthetic gonadotrophin releasing hormone with pituitary gonadotrophin secretion

Since the augmented secretion of LH and FSH at the onset of puberty apparently results from decreased neurohormonal restraints on synthesis and pulsatile secretion of GnRH, the disinhibition of the arcuate GnRH oscillator should lead to increased GnRH pulses (frequency and amplitude) initially, followed by increased gonadotrophin secretion by the pituitary gonadotropes and, finally, enhanced sex steroidogenesis by the gonads. GnRH secretion cannot be measured readily in humans; nonetheless, endogenous GnRH release may be assessed indirectly and qualitatively by the gonadotrophin response to exogenous synthetic GnRH. With the availability of this synthetic decapeptide, pituitary sensitivity to GnRH and the dynamic reserve or readily releasable pool of pituitary LH and FSH have been carefully examined throughout the life cycle, as well as in many disorders of the hypothalamic–pituitary–gonadal system.

Results of such studies support the concept that the prepubertal stage is characterized by functional GnRH insufficiency. It must be noted that such studies do not clarify the issue of the primary or secondary nature of this functional GnRH insufficiency, but merely reflect a state of low exposure of pituitary gonadotropes to endogenous GnRH. The release of LH following administration of GnRH is minimal in prepubertal children beyond infancy, increases strikingly at the peripubertal period and throughout puberty, and increases further in adult males and females. The change in the maturity-related patterns of FSH release after administration of GnRH is quite different from that of LH and results in a striking reversal of the FSH:LH ratio of gonadotrophin release. Differing pulse frequency of endogenous GnRH and a significant role of ovarian steroid/peptid regulators account for the discordance of FSH and LH that evolves during sexual maturation. Prepubertal and pubertal females release much more FSH than males at all stages of sexual maturation. Prepubertal girls, indeed, appear to have a larger releasable pool of pituitary FSH than either pubertal girls or prepubertal or pubertal males. Circulating serum concentrations of FSH and LH (a summation of basal secretion) are similar in prepubertal children, a dramatic qualitative contrast to the amount of gonadotrophin release evoked by GnRH administration (the immediately available stores). The heightened LH release by pituitary gonadotropes in response to exogenous GnRH in peripubertal children, who do not yet exhibit physical signs of sexual maturation, provides evidence of slowly increasing levels of endogenous GnRH which augment pituitary responsiveness to exogenous GnRH. It should be noted that an enhanced nocturnal release of LH is also seen in this peripubertal period. The degree of previous exposure of gonadotropes to endogenous GnRH appears to affect both the magnitude and quality of LH responses to a single dose of GnRH.

Before puberty, the low set point of the hypothalamic–gonadostat to inhibitory feedback effects of low concentrations of plasma sex steroids and intrinsic CNS factors suppress secretion of GnRH. As a result, the prepubertal pituitary gonadotropes have small pools of releasable LH and, thus, diminished responsivity to an exogenous bolus of synthetic GnRH. With the onset of puberty, increased pulsatile release of endogenous GnRH increases the number of LH receptors on the gonadotrope, enhances pituitary sensitivity to exogenous GnRH, and enlarges the reserve of LH within the gonadotrope. In contrast, chronic continuous GnRH exposure desensitizes the gonadotrope. In clinical trials in patients with *hypogonadotrophic hypogonadism*, the administration of GnRH in a pulsatile manner results in the appearance of a pubertal pattern of gonadotrophin secretion and a maturation of pituitary–gonadal function.

## Positive feedback and ovulation

In normal adult women, the midcycle gonadotrophin secretory surge is attributed to a positive feedback effect of an increased, critical concentration of estradiol for a sufficient length of time during the latter part of the follicular phase. Estrogen is presumed to exert a positive feedback effect at both the pituitary gonadotropes and the hypothalamic GnRH neurons. This stimulatory effect of estradiol is a late maturational event, not occurring before midpuberty, and is absent in prepubertal and early pubertal girls. The development of positive feedback of estradiol requires:

- ovarian follicles primed by FSH to secrete adequate estradiol and maintain critical levels in the circulation;
- pituitary gonadotropes sensitized by estradiol to amplify and augment the GnRH effect and containing enough readily releasable LH to provide an LH surge;
- adequate GnRH stores for the hypothalamic GnRH neurosecretory neurons to increase GnRH acutely in response to estradiol stimulation;
- a sufficiently insensitive negative feedback system to allow estradiol concentrations to rise sufficiently to elicit an LH surge without blunting GnRH and gonadotrophin release.

Estrogen-induced positive feedback occurs directly upon pituitary gonadotropes which are simultaneously exposed to GnRH. It does not appear that frequency or amplitude modulation of the GnRH pulse is a prerequisite of the midcycle LH surge; nonetheless, changes in GnRH release at this period probably also occur.

## Control of the time of onset of puberty

The complexity of the specific mechanisms involved in the timing of pubertal onset have defied elucidation. The average age at menarche has followed a secular trend toward earlier occurrence over the past century. This decrease in the age of puberty has been explained by improvements in socioeconomic conditions, nutrition, and general health. That trend appears to have slowed or ceased during the past several decades in developed nations. Nonetheless, influences other than socioeconomic ones affect the age of puberty. An important role for nutritional factors and body composition upon the time of pubertal onset has been suggested by the earlier age of menarche in moderately obese girls, by delayed sexual maturation in the presence of *malnourishment* and *chronic illness*, and by the relationship of *amenorrhea* to states of diminished body fat such as *anorexia nervosa* and *voluntary weight loss*. Conditions of excessive energy expenditure, such as *vigorous physical conditioning*, may independently affect the onset and progression of the pubertal process. Metabolic signals potentially may affect pubertal maturation. Evidence of differences in utilization of energy stores by younger than older primates, perhaps relating to rates of energy consumption or availability of energy substrate, suggests some association between metabolic alterations during growth and the timing of pubertal onset.

The pineal gland–melatonin system and the opioidergic network do not appear important in the pubertal process; however, the activity of the noradrenergic system parallels GnRH release. Excitatory neuroamines, additionally, may fully activate the hypothalamic–pituitary–gonadal axis in primates, demonstrating their role as potential suprahypothalamic regulators of GnRH release. The temporal regulation of these processes remains undefined.

## ABNORMALITIES OF PUBERTAL MATURATION

### Delayed sexual maturation

The first sign of pubertal development in boys is testicular enlargement, largely based upon increased volume of the seminiferous tubules; this should occur by age 14. Breast budding is the initial physical manifestation of puberty in girls and should occur by 13 years of age. A higher incidence of *delayed sexual maturation* appears to be present in boys than in girls. The causes of delayed pubertal maturation are shown in Table 16.1 and demonstrate that there may be disorders of general health, of the central nervous system, as well as of gonadal function. The most common cause, however, is the syndrome of so-called "*constitutional delay of adolescence*" (or the

"syndrome of slow growth and delayed maturation"). This syndrome is characterized by: (1) familial late maturation; (2) delayed skeletal maturation; (3) an attenuated progression through the pubertal process; (4) an ultimate height that is generally within normal range for family. Differentiation between constitutionally delayed pubertal maturation and the syndrome of *hypogonadotrophic hypogonadism*, especially in early adolescence, is quite difficult. The diagnosis will surely become apparent by late adolescent years, but simply waiting until then is not generally an acceptable clinical option. Administration of exogenous GnRH has been used in an attempt to separate these two syndromes, but remarkable degrees of overlap occur in the readily releasable pools of LH and FSH, so that a definitive diagnosis is not possible based on the GnRH test results.

When considered in the light of the dual mechanism of restraint of puberty during normal mid-childhood, the *syndrome of delayed adolescence* is characterized by a more prolonged and intense degree of inhibition of hypothalamic GnRH synthesis and secretion. This results in a more profound and exaggerated period of GnRH insufficiency. In true *hypogonadotrophic hypogonadism*, either the central nervous inhibition does not disappear or there is an intrinsic abnormality of the synthesis in secretion of GnRH.

### Isosexual precocious puberty

A child is considered to have *precocious puberty* in North America when there is an appearance of testicular enlargement or pubic hair growth in the male prior to age 9 or breast budding or pubic hair growth in the female prior to age 8. This is based upon ages of mean pubertal onset 2.5 SD below the mean. Those children in whom evidence of sexual development occurs between ages 6 and 8 may have a syndrome variant that should be referred to as "*constitutional precocious puberty*"; this is simply an earlier onset of puberty without the accelerated pubertal maturation seen in those children with an even earlier onset of precocity. The differential diagnosis of true isosexual precocious puberty is shown in Table 16.2.

TABLE 16.1 Causes of delayed pubertal maturation

| GENERALIZED DISEASE | CENTRAL NERVOUS SYSTEM | GONADAL |
| --- | --- | --- |
| Malnutrition | Constitutional delay | Gonadal dysgenesis |
| Gastrointestinal | Congenital anomalies, e.g. craniopharyngioma | Noonan syndrome |
| Endocrine | Neoplasms | Orchitis |
| Renal | Post-inflammation states | Testicular regression syndrome |
| Cardiorespiratory | Trauma | Trauma |
| Hematology/Oncology | Hypogonadotrophic states, | Neoplasms |
| Collagen–vascular | e.g. Kallmann, Prader–Willi | Errors of testosterone biosynthesis |

TABLE 16.2 Causes of isosexual precocious puberty

*Gonadotrophin- (and GnRH)-dependent*
    Idiopathic
    Structural CNS abnormalities
    Neoplasms
    Congenital anomalies (e.g. septo-optic dysplasia, midline defects)
    Post-infection, trauma, irradiation

*Gonadotrophin- (and GnRH)-independent*
    HCG-producing neoplasm
    Sex steroid producing neoplasms of the gonads or adrenal
    Extragonadal androgen (males) – congenital adrenal hyperplasia
    Abnormalities of intragonadal regulation e.g. McCune–Albright syndrome, ovarian cysts, Leydig cell hyperfunction (testotoxicosis)

*Normal variants of development*
    Precocious thelarche
    Precocious adrenarche

"Complete" or "true" precocious puberty is dependent upon early initiation of gonadotrophin secretion consequent to premature attainment of a pubertal pattern of GnRH production by the arcuate nucleus of the hypothalamus. In this condition, the above-noted dual mechanism of restraint of puberty becomes attenuated at an early age so that the inhibitory controls of hypothalamic arcuate nucleus pulsatile GnRH secretion are diminished and gonadotrophin secretion increases. Activation of the hypothalamic–pituitary–gonadal axis is similar, then, to that seen in normal children but occurs at an earlier age. There are pubertal levels of sex steroid production, gonadotrophin concentrations in the pubertal range with the expected frequency of episodic secretion and circadian variability, and a mature level of GnRH-induced LH release.

The fact that continuous administration of GnRH leads to diminished release of pituitary gonadotrophins through a process of down-regulation of pituitary GnRH receptors has led to a major therapeutic advance in this area. Potent long-acting GnRH agonists, behaving like a continuous infusion, are now the standard of care for children with gonadotrophin-dependent sexual precocity. The hypothalamic–pituitary–gonadal axis is suppressed with concomitant slowing of sexual maturation and growth and an increase in final adult height outcome.

# Variants of pubertal maturation

## Precocious thelarche

Premature breast development without any other evidence of progressive sexual maturation is referred to as *premature thelarche*. This syndrome does not appear to be dependent upon prolonged activation of the hypothalamic–pituitary unit, but rather is due either to transient secretory burst of GnRH and the gonadotrophins or to a period of primary ovarian dysregulation of estrogen synthesis and secretion. The differential diagnosis of premature thelarche includes *true sexual precocity* and *ovarian cysts* or *tumors*. There do not appear to be any long-term developmental consequences of this variant of normal development.

## Precocious adrenarche (pubarche)

The appearance of sex hair prior to age 8 in girls or 9 in boys without any other evidence of progression of sexual development defines the syndrome of *precocious adrenarche (pubarche)*. It is more common in girls, especially those who are taller, heavier and having slightly advanced skeletal maturation. The regulation of adrenal androgenesis remains poorly understood. There is a significant increase in adrenal androgen secretion by age 8 in both boys and girls, antedating the pubertal increases of gonadotrophin and gonadal steroid production. The increasing levels of adrenal androgens correlate with development of the zona reticularis of the adrenal cortex. In general, maturation of this process of adrenal androgenesis and of the hypothalamic–pituitary–gonadal axis appear independent. The enhanced adrenal androgenesis seems to be, in part, an ACTH-dependent process, though other portions of the pro-opiomelanocortin (POMC) molecule have been implicated in the activation; changes of intra-adrenal enzyme action favoring synthesis and secretion of androgens have also been demonstrated. The differential diagnosis of precocious pubarche includes unusual cases of late-onset *congenital adrenal hyperplasia* and *adrenal or gonadal androgen-producing neoplasms*. Most commonly, however, this syndrome of early adrenal androgenesis is a variant of the normal. Onset of other pubertal events, the age of menarche and final adult height appear to be normal. The long-term risk of development of *polycystic ovarian disease* in association with this syndrome remains to be quantified.

## SELECTED READING

Apter D, Butzow TL, Laughlin BA, Yen SSC. Gonadotropin releasing hormone pulse generator activity during pubertal transition in girls: pulsatile and diurnal patterns of circulating gonadotropins. *J Clin Endocrinol Metab* 1993; 76: 940.

Grumbach MM, Styne DM. Puberty: ontogeny, neuroendocrinology, physiology, and disorders. In: Wilson JD, Foster DW, eds. *Williams' textbook of endocrinology*, 8th edn. Philadelphia: WB Saunders, 1992: 1139.

Kletter GB, Padmanabhan V, Brown MB, *et al*. Serum bioactive gonadotropins during male puberty: a longitudinal study. *J Clin Endocrinol Metab* 1993; 76: 432.

Ojeda SR. The neurobiology of mammalian puberty: has the contribution of glial cells been underestimated? *J NIH Research* 1994; **6**: 51.

Plant TM. Puberty in primates. In: Knobil E, Neill JD, eds. *The physiology of reproduction.* New York: Raven Press, 1988: 1763.

Reiter EO, Grumbach MM. Neuroendocrine control mechanism and the onset of puberty. *Ann Rev Physiol* 1982; **44**: 595.

Rosenfield RL. The diagnosis and management of delayed puberty. *J Clin Endocrinol Metab* 1990; **70**: 559.

Styne DM. Puberty and its disorders. *Curr Opin Endocrinol Diab* 1994; **1**: 46.

# PART FIVE

# *Growth*

**Editors: Peter D. Gluckman and Michael A. Heymann**

# 17

# Tissue and Organ Growth

Stephen J. M. Skinner and David Warburton

## INTRODUCTION

The regulation of tissue and organ growth in the embryo and through gestation to the newborn child is poorly understood. Yet these processes critically determine the development of healthy individuals. Morphogenetic processes are determined by genes, but whether or not the full genomic potential is achieved depends on fetal environmental conditions. Information gained from the new techniques of gene deletion and insertion are now being integrated with earlier observations from experimental embryology and this field is advancing with great speed.

Organs and tissues do not grow and differentiate in synchrony. The lung and heart are functional at birth while the immune system, digestive system, bones and gonads mature later. Organ and tissue development is controlled by intrinsic systems which consist of cascades of specific regulatory agents produced in spatially defined cellular zones of the embryo or fetus sequentially during development. The different peptide and protein signaling factors generated within, and secreted from, the cells of developing structures act at close range within the tissue, organ, or organ compartment and are themselves potent regulators of tissue growth and differentiation. The actions of diffusible and circulating signals on target organs will be determined by systems within the tissues which regulate specific receptor expression and function (*see also* page 459). External conditions and factors can impinge on the normal patterns of gene expression that determine organ development. Poor maternal nutrition and other environmental factors cause growth retardation where muscle, bone and many internal organs are poorly grown but the heart and brain are relatively spared. Under these conditions the lungs may be hypoplastic but are fully differentiated in terms of a functional surfactant system. On the other hand, in *diabetic mothers* the newborn infant can be very large (macrosomic) but often has a poorly developed lung surfactant system.

In order to understand the mechanisms which govern tissue and organ growth, and how pathologies may develop, it is necessary to consider some of the essential elements of the process of development.

## CELLULAR GROWTH, DIVISION, DEATH AND DIFFERENTIATION

Groups of cells are committed in the embryo to become specific structures and organs. These are generated and defined, by pattern-forming processes in the embryo, as progenitor fields or "anlage." For an organ to be generated, the cells in the field must divide and grow through many generations in a predetermined manner, with structural folding and always, to a greater or lesser extent, interacting with cells in adjacent anlage committed from other lineages, and with extracellular matrix. These events lead through progressive stages of cell commitment to different phenotypes and to the accumulation of tissue mass. The structure is "invaded" by hematopoietic cells and neural growth cones. Blood vessels are formed by the differentiation of mesenchymal cells into endothelial cells during the process of angiogenesis. These events are dependent on intercellular signaling between different cells and tissue structures within the organ.

At times in development many cells die or self-destruct in a completely normal process termed *apoptosis* (*see* page 100), apparently to cull or weed out the non-functional or detrimental members of the group. In the immune system and brain, the regressing Müllerian duct in the male fetus or the amphibian tadpole tail, apoptosis is a prominent part of development, allowing selection of the cells with correct function and death of the remaining majority of redundant cells.

The events leading to the final functioning phenotype are included in the general term *differentiation*. In many tissues the differentiation is terminal, the cell reaching a final committed task or phenotype and losing the capacity for further division. In some tissues, such as the brain and heart, the full complement of terminally differentiated cells is determined shortly after birth with a limited capacity for subsequent replacement.

## HOMEOBOX GENES AND INTERCELLULAR SIGNALING

Many of the concepts derived from research on developing embryos of such species as Xenopus, sea urchin, Drosophila, zebrafish and the nematode, *C. elegans*, have yielded major benefits to vertebrate biology. A variety of early and late structures are determined by protein products of homeobox (*Hox*) genes expressed at defined anatomical loci and with very precise timing. The characteristic anatomy and timing of *Hox* gene expression occurs in defined patterns where zones of expression can have sharply defined borders. The resultant proteins were classically considered nuclear proteins but now it is accepted that pattern forming genes can give rise to diffusible proteins that interact with receptors and with transcription sites on the DNA in neighboring cells. Receptor stimulation activates second messenger systems such as cyclic nucleotides, inositol phosphates, $Ca^{2+}$ mobilization and an ever-increasing array of phosphorylated signal proteins. These ligand and receptor mediated processes generate specific transcription factors, including the conversion of latent to active forms. Interaction of one or more transcription factors with specific, and often distant, binding sites on DNA to form looped complexes with RNA polymerase (Fig. 17.1), initiates or accelerates specific mRNA synthesis for generating a new wave of proteins for structural purposes and for intra- and extracellular signaling.

The diffusion of factors from one developing region across another may determine cellular commitment to a new phenotype or structure. In the early stages of development in some species, much of the cell–cell communication is via gap junctions which connect the cytoplasm of the cells in a syncitial arrangement. Here the changes in intracellular proteins and signaling factors can rapidly diffuse to all cells in the syncitium. Usually the signaling molecules (morphogens) diffuse in the extracellular spaces, interact with receptors on

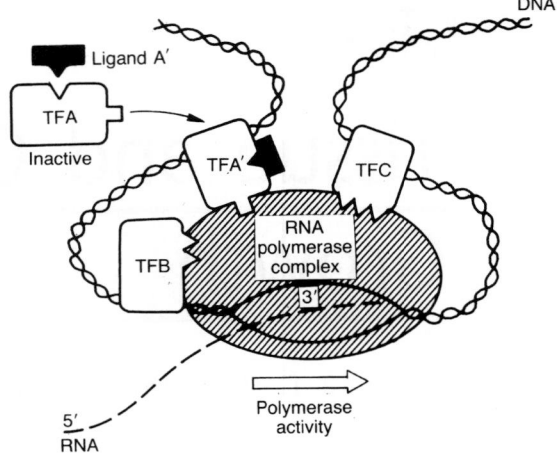

FIGURE 17.1 Control of gene expression by transcription factors. Transcription factors (TFA′, TFB and TFC) coordinate the binding and activity of the RNA polymerase complex to specific start sites on the DNA. The activation of TFA to TFA′ requires the binding of Ligand A′.

the cells and disappear as development progresses. Recent studies suggest that these morphogens, e.g. retinoids, molecules of the transforming growth factor β (TGFβ) or basic fibroblast growth factor (bFGF) families of proteins, form extracellular gradients across distances of about 300 µm (approximately 10 cell diameters) in mammalian tissues and control gene expression in cells with a functional receptor. A series of three-dimensional arrays of several morphogens, inducing or suppressing subsequent waves of morphogens, transcription factors and receptors, are envisaged as a sequential process (Fig. 17.2). Complex gradients of two or more morphogens in a three-dimensional system can control expression of many genes, determining such activities as cell proliferation, matrix adhesion and differentiation. Thus, zonal differences in the rates of cell proliferation in tubal structures such as the heart or kidney would induce folding (*see* page 929), as would transient adhesion to adjacent structures mediated by extracellular matrix and matrix receptor gene expression.

A common finding in *Hox* genes is their structural resemblance and often similar function in divergent species, from man and the higher vertebrates down to fruit flies, slime molds and yeast. The Drosophila gene *wg* was first found in wing mutants and later was shown to determine segmentation and dorsal–ventral orientation of certain structures. The vertebrate *Wnt* genes, equivalent to Drosophila *wg*, are an example of pattern forming *Hox* genes used repeatedly during development. *Wnt* genes have now been implicated in early mammalian processes such as gastrulation and the later events of somite, brain and kidney formation. Other pattern-forming genes are specific for the development of single organs – e.g. *Hox11*, which on deletion causes loss of the spleen in otherwise normal mice.

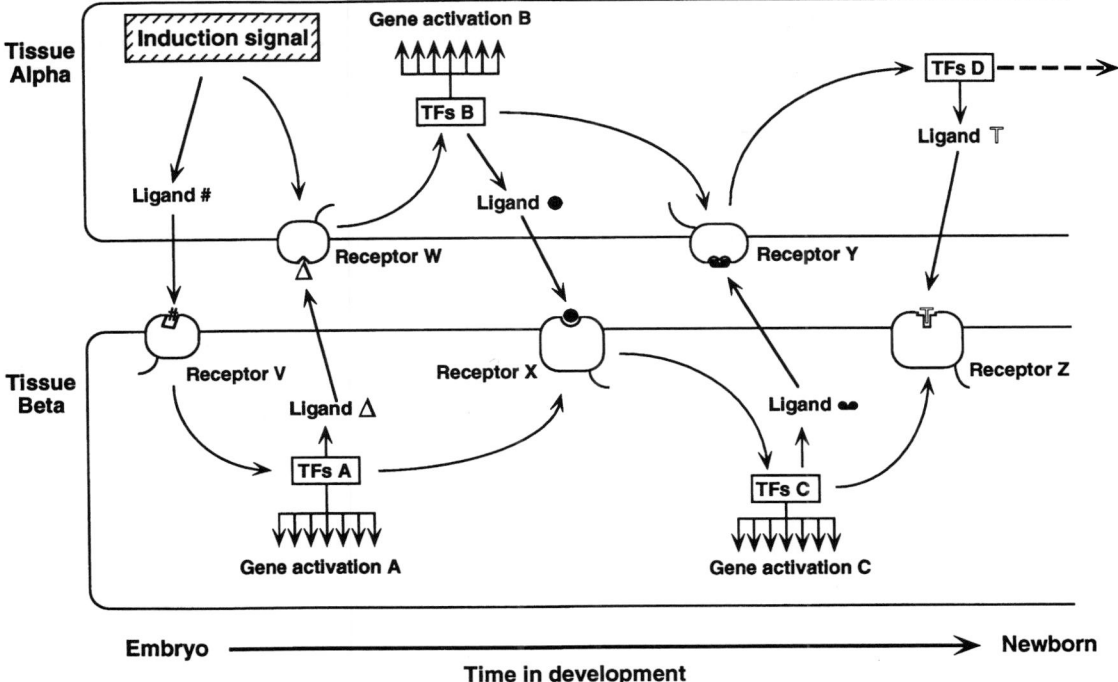

FIGURE 17.2 Activation of gene expression in interacting tissues during development. In this model a sequence of interactions are dependent on the INDUCER causing the production or activation of a ligand (#) and a receptor (Receptor W) in Tissue Alpha. Ligand # is secreted by Tissue Alpha and activates an existing receptor (Receptor V) in Tissue Beta. Active Receptor V causes specific transcription factor(s) (TFs A) to promote a battery of gene expression (Gene activation A) producing a number of proteins including at least one ligand (Δ) and one receptor (Receptor X). Ligand Δ stimulates the preexisting Receptor W, causing different transcription factor(s) (TFs B) to activate a battery of gene expression (Gene activation B) in Tissue Alpha, one of which is for ligand ● and one for Receptor Y. Ligand ● activates Receptor X on Tissue Beta, causing another set of genes to be expressed (Gene activation C), including Ligand ●● and Receptor Z. Ligand ●● activates Receptor Y in Tissue Alpha. The sequence can continue with inputs from other ligands diffusing from adjacent tissues or from direct interaction with migrating cells.

The poetically named *tinman* gene, if deleted, produces a heart-less Drosophila. In mice, deletion of a *tinman* analog (*Csx*) causes incorrect development of the heart, and in zebrafish similar deletions have been induced where valves or other cardiac structures are missing or poorly formed. These few examples demonstrate that the structures of the different *Hox* genes are largely homologous between species, indicating evolutionary conservation and great utility for survival.

## GROWTH FACTORS AND THEIR RECEPTORS

During development a number of protein and peptide factors are produced in tissues undergoing growth and differentiation (*see also* pages 273 and 280). These ligands interact with cell surface receptors and direct the cells in their progress through the cell cycle or into a new phenotype. Some are necessary for general cell growth and others are essential for growth and development of certain organs, depending on when and where the specific receptor is expressed; some examples follow.

The insulin-like growth factors (IGF-I and IGF-II) are about 60 per cent homologous with insulin and are general growth stimulators (*see* page 314). Deletion of IGF-I and its receptor system in mouse embryos causes severe *intrauterine growth retardation* with very poor muscle development and frequent neonatal death due to respiratory failure. Thus, IGFs are very important in fetal development and have a great impact on lung growth. However, the severe effects in these deletion models makes it difficult to determine whether death is due to a direct effect causing dysplastic pulmonary cell structures or simply inadequate respiratory muscle development.

A more selective experimental approach than general deletion has been devised using tissue-specific promoters linked to synthetic RNA generating systems. A lung epithelium-specific promoter (SP-C) was linked to a gene construct which blocks the activity of one of the FGF receptors (FGF receptor-3), and then transfected into mice. Newborn mice expressing this transgene were normal except for the lung where the epithelium, after initial budding from the fore-gut in the early embryo, failed to branch and grew only as two epithelial tubes extending from the trachea to the diaphragm.

This elegant experiment confirmed that FGF receptor expression is essential in the lung for epithelial branching morphogenesis. It is well established from fetal tissue microdissection and recombination experiments carried out in the 1960s that branching morphogenesis will not occur in lung epithelium without the associated mesenchyme. One explanation for this observation is that lung mesenchyme secretes bFGF, the ligand necessary to stimulate the epithelial receptor. These are examples, among many, which show that control systems for cell–cell signaling can determine not only when and where growth factors are produced but also specify where they may act by controlling the activity or expression of their receptors (*see* Fig. 17.2).

Another mechanism for controlling growth factor activity which has begun to command serious attention is the presence of growth factor binding proteins found in serum and extracellular matrix. Some growth factors, such as IGFs, are present in serum and tissues almost exclusively in the bound form (*see* page 314), whereas the closely related insulin is virtually always unbound. Most commonly these IGF binding proteins (IGFBPs) are present in serum but large quantities of certain IGFBPs sequester IGFs in the matrix (see below). Steroid hormones are another class of potent developmental regulators which have specific binding proteins in blood and tissue fluids.

## CELLS IN THREE DIMENSIONS

### Intra- and extracellular matrix

The importance of cellular position and anchorage in a defined matrix has been described and emphasized in recent years. Indeed the argument that the insoluble structures of higher organisms are of equal or greater importance to tissue and organ development than the liquid systems is difficult to deny. Many cells fail to grow and divide, remaining in the $G_1$ stage of the cell cycle, unless anchored and allowed to spread on an extracellular matrix. Loss of anchorage dependence may be a primary event in the development of tumors and the spread of malignant cells. Normal epithelial and endothelial cells spontaneously enter apoptosis and die if released from their matrix niche (anoikis).

### Tensegrity

It is now apparent that the nuclear matrix, the cytoskeleton and the extracellular matrix are linked in an integrated series. The engineering term that describes these interconnections is "tensegrity." The shape of cells is determined to a great extent by a network of cytoskeletal elements such as the polymers of tubulin and actin. These can be imagined as the poles, pillars and struts of a building, except that they constantly are

being remodeled by dissociation and reattachment. The cytoskeletal elements are attached to the internal cell surface at focal adhesion sites which comprise a number of proteins including vinculin and talin linked to actin polymers. A protein kinase termed "focal adhesion kinase" (FAK) is also located within this complex. FAK is activated when the complex is attached via a cell-surface integrin molecule to a substrate, such as fibronectin, which contains an RGD (arginine–glycine–aspartate) integrin recognition domain. The internal ends of the cytoskeleton are attached to cellular organelles, most importantly the nuclear membrane (Fig. 17.3). The nuclear membrane is attached to a nuclear matrix in which the chromosomes are embedded. Changes in cell shape can lead directly to changes in nuclear membrane permeability, allowing transcription factors and cyclin-dependent protein kinase complexes to enter the nucleus and activate transcription for differentiation or cell proliferation.

Thus, external mechanical stimuli such as breathing, muscle tension on bone, and shear stresses occurring when tissues move against each other (Fig. 17.4), are transmitted directly into the tissues not only at the level of the extracellular matrix but also to the cell membrane, cytoskeleton and the nuclear environment. Experiments suggest that without muscle activity before birth many tissues can be adversely affected.

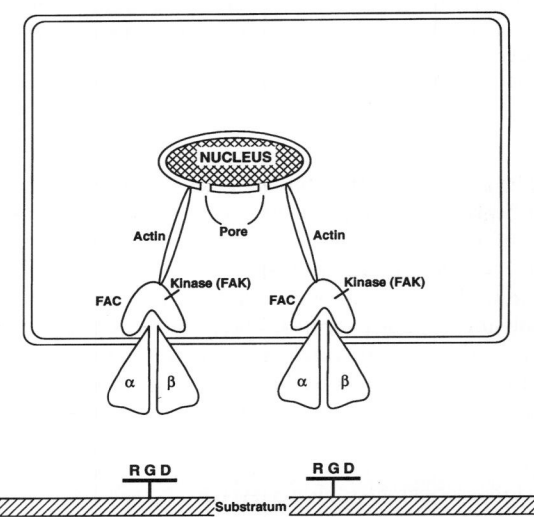

FIGURE 17.3 Connections between extracellular matrix, cell membrane, cytoskeleton and nucleus. The association of integrin receptor (α,β) with its ligand (RGD sequences in the primary structure of fibronectin and other proteins in the extracellular substratum) causes the formation of Focal Adhesion Complexes (FAC) which contain a number of proteins (vinculin, talin, α-actinin, paxillin) including a kinase. The kinase (Focal Adhesion Kinase, FAK), in association with other signaling proteins, has downstream effects on the MAP kinase system (*see* page 63). The FAC binds to actin which is tethered to a number of cell organelles including the nuclear membrane and the intranuclear matrix.

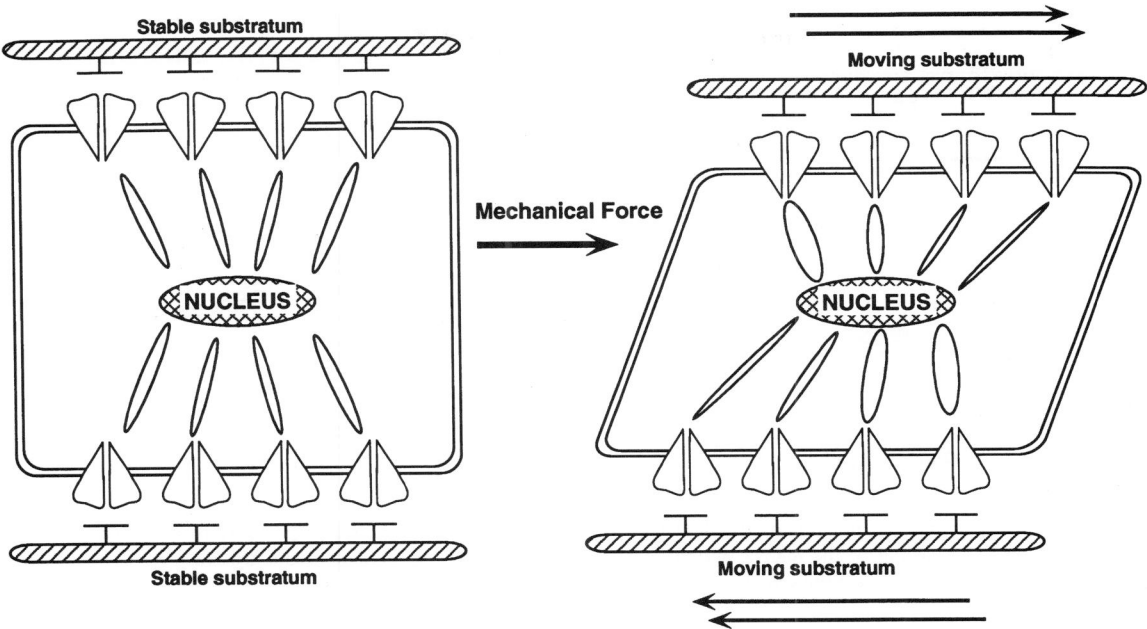

FIGURE 17.4 Tensegrity. Mechanical forces transmitted through the substratum act upon the cell components via integrin receptors, FACs and actin filaments and their connections to the cell membrane, nucleus and other organelles (*see* Figure 17.3). The cell tethered between the substrata is under tension. With changes in shape, distorting the cytoskeleton, the tensile forces become unequally distributed. The forces are transmitted throughout the cell, including the cell membrane and nuclear matrix. The cell responds by specific gene expression and by rapid remodeling of the cytoskeleton.

*Fetal akinesia* can cause facial and limb dysmorphology. A lack of regular diaphragmatic movements and intrapulmonary pressure changes *in utero* may cause *lung hypoplasia*.

## EXTRACELLULAR MATRIX AND GROWTH FACTORS

*See also* pages 66 and 282

While it is clear that cellular attachment to matrix via integrin and other receptors is extremely important, there are many growth regulating peptides and proteins which are intimately embedded in the matrix. These are attached by two main classes of amino-acid motifs within their structures: the RGD sequences and basic amino acid clusters, where groups of two or three of the basic amino acids arginine (R) and lysine (K) are separated only by one or two other amino acids. The RGD sequence, and flanking amino acids which confer specificity, bind to integrin receptors. These RGDs are present in a variety of growth regulators including some IGFBPs and the TGFβ family. The basic amino acid clusters within certain peptides were first exploited for peptide purification by binding to the acidic groups of heparin immobilized on chromatography columns. There are many examples of such basic amino acid clusters; in the coagulation proteins, some cytokines (GM-CSF), growth factors (bFGF) and

growth factor binding proteins (IGFBPs). Replacement of key basic amino acids in bFGF, by site-directed mutagenesis, destroys its activity. These basic clusters cause the molecule to bind to certain of the negatively charged proteoglycans and glycosaminoglycans in the extracellular matrix (Fig. 17.5). For example, TGFβ and bFGF are found sequestered in the basement membrane attached to heparin and chondroitin sulfates. Some IGFBPs, with associated IGFs, are found at high concentrations attached to the chondroitin sulfates of bone matrix.

The function of these extracellular depots of growth factors are not understood but it is likely that as tissues are remodeled during development, or during inflammatory events, the extracellular matrix will be broken down and resynthesized to accommodate repair or to allow the formation of bigger structures. As this occurs, the sequestered agents will be released in sufficient concentration to stimulate growth, differentiation or act as chemoattractants to cells in the immediate and perhaps wider environment. Some scientists in this field have suggested that the growth factors embedded in matrix may act as an environmental "memory." Where a matrix is established, but the cells are lost due to trauma, the cells which colonize, remodel and repopulate that microenvironment will be influenced by the composition of the matrix and the embedded growth factors they release.

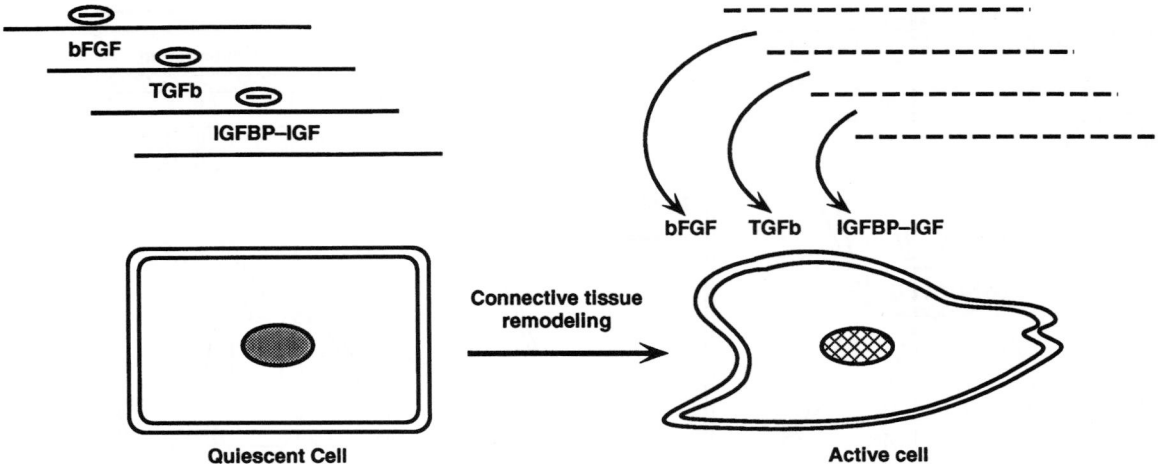

FIGURE 17.5 Mobilization of matrix bound growth factors. Negatively charged groups on the glycosaminoglycan chains of proteoglycans in extracellular matrix bind certain growth factors (or their binding proteins) containing positively charged basic amino acid clusters. With remodeling of the matrix during development, disease or inflammation, the growth factors are released, interact with receptors and activate the cell. The matrix thus acts as a depot for some growth factors.

## CHEMOTROPHIC AGENTS

The ability of developing organs to determine whether invading cells are guided in or are discouraged is often determined by the peptides or proteins they secrete (chemotrophic agents). Nerve cell processes and hematopoietic cells are invaders of the tissues and organs. They are guided by moving up the concentration gradients of chemoattractants secreted by the cells in a tissue. The first chemoattractant of interest in neural growth was designated "nerve growth factor" (NGF). Subsequently the netrins, which have equivalents in *C. elegans* (unc-6), have been characterized as products of the developing floor plate and lower spinal cord. These are positive signals to neural processes, probably guiding commissural axons to the floor plate. Negative signals have also been found, the collapsins, which diffuse through the matrix and, when in contact with neural growth cones, make them collapse. Thus growth cones can be guided, probably by a number of different positive and negative signals, to precise locations. Another example of a chemoattractant is platelet-derived growth factor (PDGF), also made in endothelial or epithelial cells and attracting vascular or subepithelial smooth muscle respectively. Basic FGF is an attractant for cells during angiogenesis, and airway epithelial cells migrate in response to calcitonin gene-related peptide (CGRP). Many chemoattractants, such as interleukins, have been described in the inflammatory response of the hematopoietic system. Another class of chemotrophic agents which stimulate random movement of cells are the motogens, such as hepatocyte growth factor (HGF), which stimulates the random migration of epithelial cells in a number of different tissues.

## DIFFERENTIATION

Differentiation is for most cell lineages a progressive activity which occurs during a series of commitments, generating a variety of phenotypes. Many cells attain a terminal differentiated state which is incapable of regeneration. Neurons and cardiac myocytes are examples cited above. In the lung, the mature alveolar epithelial cells are the Type I and Type II cells. The differentiation of primitive pulmonary "stem cell" epithelial cells into Type II surfactant-producing cells in late gestation is strongly influenced by glucocorticoids. This property is exploited in prenatal glucocorticoid therapy during premature labor to promote fetal lung maturation. If the alveolar surface is injured and subsequently denuded of Type I epithelium, the adjacent Type II cells can regain their progenitor status and proliferate to repopulate the gas exchange surfaces with Type I and Type II cells. Glucocorticoids are also potent differentiation agents for the gut and for hematopoietic cells in the thymus. The sex steroids, estrogen and testosterone, induce many aspects of differentiation such as Müllerian duct regression in the fetus (see above), and maturation of brain and bone at puberty (Fig. 17.6). It has been known for many years that brain differentiation requires estrogen, and that in the male testosterone is converted to estrogen in the brain. It has only recently been discovered from observations in a phenotypic male with a mutation in the estrogen receptor gene, that fusion of the epiphyses in bone at puberty depends on estrogen receptor activation in the growth plate, relying on testosterone conversion to estrogen within the male growth plate.

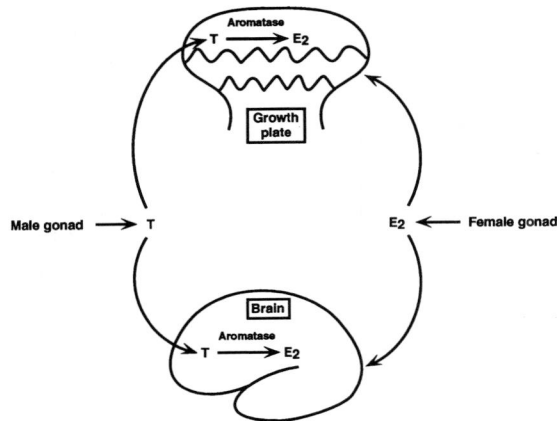

FIGURE 17.6 Steroid hormone synthesis in target organs. Brain and bone maturation depend upon sex steroids. In females, estradiol (E₂) is responsible for these changes. Previously it was believed that in males the key hormone was testosterone (T) or dihydrotestosterone. It is now known that in males the maturation requires the conversion of T to E₂ by the enzyme complex aromatase present within the developing brain and bone.

## SUMMARY

The complexity of tissue and organ growth makes it appear difficult to understand. Yet it is a rewarding and fascinating challenge. New information about gene regulation in development is likely to have increasing application in neonatal and pediatric disease. There are also many examples where tissue repair in the adult is substantially a recapitulation of what happened in the embryo. Disturbed development in the otherwise normal fetus or newborn can leave subtle but indelible flaws which may surface in adult organs and cause disease in later life.

## SELECTED READING

Barinaga M. Looking to development's future. *Science* 1994; **266**: 561.

Bernfield M. Developmental biology: preventive medicine for neonatology. *Pediatr Res* 1990; **27** (Suppl): S21.

Buckingham M. Molecular biology of muscle development. *Cell* 1994; **78**: 15.

Davidson E. Later embryogenesis: regulatory circuitry in morphogenetic fields. *Development* 1993; **118**: 665.

Ingber DE. The riddle of morphogenesis: a question of solution chemistry or molecular engineering. *Cell* 1994; **75**: 1249.

Nathan C, Sporn M. Cytokines in context. *J Cell Biol* 1991; **113**: 981.

Ruoslahti E, Reed JC. Anchorage dependence, integrins and apoptosis. *Cell* 1994; **77**: 477.

Smith EP, Boyd J, Frank GR, *et al.* Estrogen resistance caused by a mutation in the estrogen-receptor gene in a man. *N Engl J Med* 1994; **331**: 1056.

# 18

# Cellular Replication and Implications for Development

David Warburton and Stephen J. M. Skinner

Understanding the processes of cell proliferation and differentiation, which determine the eventual structure and function of the developing organism, are key to understanding both the pathobiologic processes of pediatric disease and possible future molecular approaches to pediatric therapeutics.

## REGULATION OF CELL REPLICATION

*See also Chapter 2, page 96*

The *cell cycle* is a term used to describe the orderly progression of cell replication through a *resting phase* ($G_0$ phase), through an *activation or gap phase* ($G_1$ phase) during which protein synthesis is initiated, through the phase of *DNA synthesis* (S phase), through a second gap phase ($G_2$ phase) and *mitosis* (M phase) (Fig. 18.1). The cell cycle is governed by two "checkpoints" during $G_1$/S phase and $G_2$/M phase. These checkpoints respectively prevent the cell from entering S phase from $G_0$/$G_1$ phase unless suitable growth-promoting conditions are present (this is analogous to START in yeast) and prevent the transition from $G_2$ to M phase unless DNA replication is complete. The cell cycle is particularly sensitive to the growth promoting or inhibiting actions of peptide growth factors in $G_1$ phase (Fig. 18.2), and is relatively insensitive to these factors after S phase. Thus, much interest has surrounded elucidating the mechanisms of positive and negative regulation of $G_1$ phase activation because of the clear therapeutic advantages of being able to manipulate this phase of the cell cycle.

## The role of cyclins and cyclin-dependent protein kinases

Cyclic accumulation and destruction of a class of molecules termed cyclins regulates progression through the cell cycle. The term "cyclin" was coined to describe proteins whose level of activity cycles up and down during the cell division cycle of Xenopus oocytes (*see* Fig. 2.36). By convention cyclins are named alphabetically in order of discovery. Another common nomenclature in the cell cycle field is to label proteins by their apparent molecular weight on SDS polyacrylamide gel electrophoresis, using the prefix p, e.g. $p36^{cyclinA}$. Cyclins function as regulatory subunits of the cyclin-dependent protein kinases (cdks), which in turn phosphorylate and regulate key cell cycle protein substrates such as the retinoblastoma protein, pRb. The ability of cyclins to activate the cdk complexes is in turn regulated positively by a family of cyclin-activating kinases (CAKs) and negatively by several classes of cdk inhibitors (Figs. 18.1–18.3). Dysregulation both of the cyclins, particularly cyclins A and D, and of the cdk inhibitors provides key targets for oncogenic transformation in certain types of cancer such as *hepatomas* and *parathyroid adenomas* respectively. Several cdk inhibitors, such as *p21*, may either function as, or are regulated by, tumor suppressor genes such as *p53*, providing a mechanism whereby dysfunction of the tumor suppressor can abrogate the function of the cdk inhibitor, resulting in unregulated cdk activation and therefore loss of tumor suppressor function.

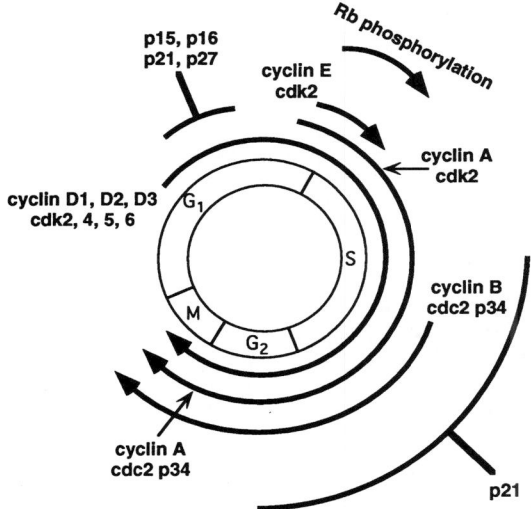

FIGURE 18.1 Expression of cell cycle proteins. Cyclins D1, D2 and D3 are expressed from mid $G_1$ through M phase. These proteins associate with cdk2, 4, 5 and 6. The kinase activity of the cyclin D/cdk complexes is negatively regulated by the cdk inhibitors p15, p16, p21 and p27. Cyclin E is transiently expressed in late $G_1$ and associates with cdk2. Cyclin A is expressed from late $G_1$ through S, $G_2$ and M phases. It associates with cdk2 in S phase and also with cdc2 p34 in M phase. Cyclin B is expressed from mid S phase through M phase. Cyclin B associates with cdc2 p34. The kinase activity of cyclin A and cyclin B/cdk complexes is negatively regulated by the cdk inhibitor p21. The Rb protein is phosphorylated during the $G_1$ to S transition and is a substrate for cyclin D, E and A/cdk complexes. The E2F family (see Figure 2.39) of transcriptional activators are displaced from Rb by phosphorylation of Rb binding pockets. These transcription factors are therefore activated in S phase.

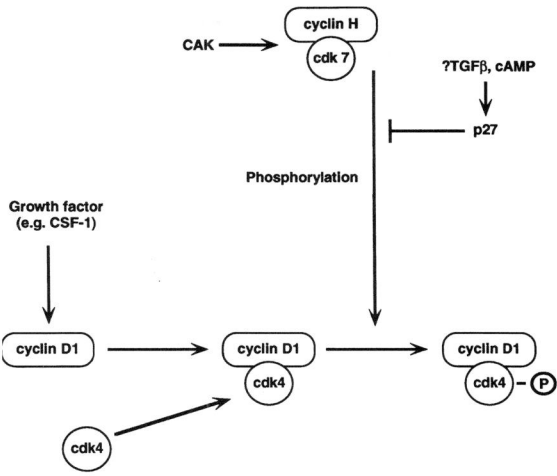

FIGURE 18.2 Regulation of $G_1$ to S phase progression. Cyclin H is a recently discovered early $G_1$ cyclin. It associates with cdk 7, and this complex is activated by cyclin activating kinase (CAK). The activation of cyclin H/cdk 7 complexes is in turn negatively regulated by the cdk inhibitor p27, which is probably activated by TGFβ and cAMP. Thus, growth factor stimulation (e.g. CSF-1) elevates cyclin D levels, cyclin D associates with cdk4, and this complex is then phosphorylated (P) and activated by association with CAK-activated cyclin H/cdk7 complexes.

The association and activation of cyclin–cdk complexes occurs sequentially during the cell cycle and regulates orderly progression from one phase to the next (Fig. 18.1). Association of cyclins D1, 2 and 3 with cdk4, and in some cells cdk6, is one of the earliest events in $G_1$ phase, that appears to transduce the growth-promoting activity of peptide growth factors and drives cells through the $G_1$ (START) checkpoint (Fig. 18.1). The Rb protein is hypophosphorylated through $G_1$ and is phosphorylated at the onset of S phase. The cyclin D/cdk4 complex is the best known candidate for the function of *in vivo* Rb kinase during $G_1$ phase (Fig. 18.2). Expression of the E-type cyclin peaks in $G_1$ after the onset of expression of the D-type cyclins. E-type cyclins are thought to play a role in the $G_1$/S phase transition, and may play a role in preparing the cell for DNA synthesis in S phase. Cyclin A/cdk2 complexes are in turn essential for progression through S phase and are again required in $G_2$/M phase (Fig. 18.1). Cyclin B/cdc2 forms the mitotic kinase complex that signals entry into M phase. The cyclin B/cdc2 complex accumulates and is maintained in an inactive form during S and $G_2$ phases by the Wee1/Mik1 protein kinase. Activation of the cyclin B/cdc2 complex

also requires the activation of the bifunctional threonine/tyrosine phosphatase cdc25 that dephosphorylates threonine 14 and tyrosine 15 to activate cdc2 kinase activity.

## The role of growth factors in cell replication

The growth promoting activity of serum is now known to comprise a number of peptide growth factors including platelet-derived growth factor (PDGF), insulin-like growth factors (IGFs), fibroblast growth factor (FGF), epidermal growth factor (EGF), colony-stimulating factor-1 (CSF-1), etc. Classical studies in Balb/c3T3 fibroblasts showed that PDGF and basic FGF act predominantly at the $G_0$/$G_1$ boundary to render cells "competent" to divide, while EGF acts early in $G_1$ and IGFs act later in $G_1$ to promote "progression" to S phase. Hence the classification of peptide growth factors into "competence" and "progression" factors.

Both positive and negative peptide growth factor signals are transduced by the activation of cognate receptors on the cell surface. Peptide growth factor receptors comprise two broad classes containing either tyrosine kinase (EGF, PDGF, IGF) or serine/threonine kinase (transforming growth factor β [TGFβ]) motifs on their intracellular domains (Fig. 18.3).

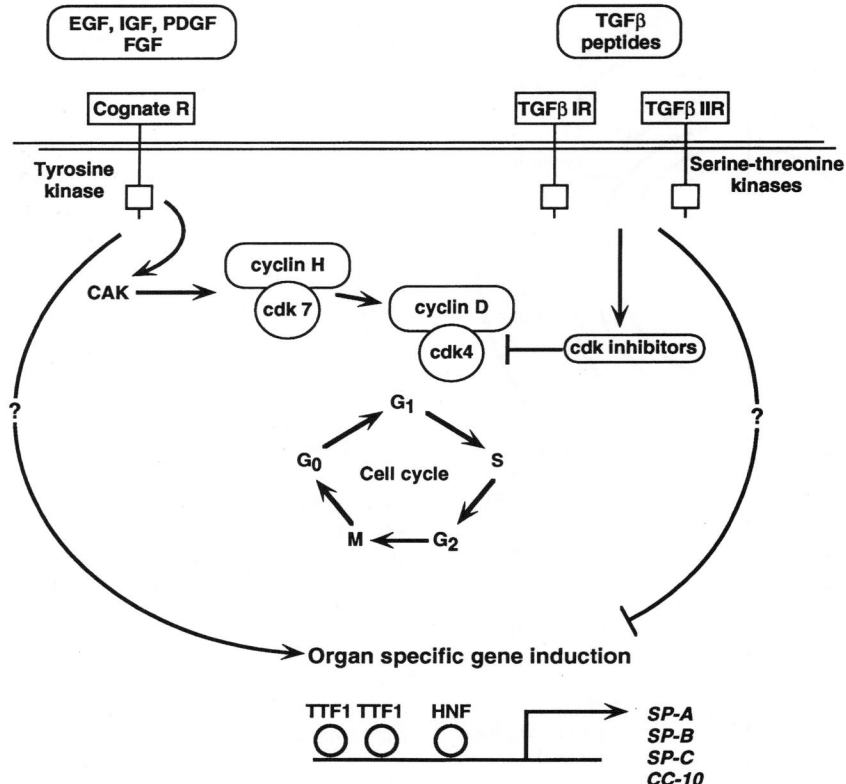

FIGURE 18.3 Specification of lung development by transcription factors and peptide growth factor signaling. Activation of cognate tyrosine kinase growth factor receptors such as EGFR, IGFR, PDGFR and FGFR stimulate lung epithelial cell proliferation and morphogenesis. Activation of cognate serine–threonine kinase receptors such as TGFβ IR and IIR negatively regulates lung epithelial cell proliferation and morphogenesis. It is speculated that these peptide growth factor–dependent mechanisms of organogenesis not only regulate the expression and activation of cell cycle genes during $G_1$ phase of the lung epithelial cell cycle, including CAK, cyclin H/cdk7 and cyclin D/cdk complexes, but also positively regulate the expression of lung cell lineage specific transcriptional factors such as TTF1 or HNF that induce the expression of lung cell lineage specific genes including *SP-A*, *SP-B*, *SP-C* and *CC-10*. On the other hand, TGFβ peptide signaling negatively regulates the $G_1$ to S phase transition of lung epithelial cells by negative regulation of cyclinD/cdk complexes and possibly also of cyclin H/cdk7 complexes by signal transduction mechanisms including the induction or activation of cdk inhibitors. TGFβ signaling is also speculated to play a role, perhaps in negatively regulating lung-specific gene expression.

## Tyrosine kinase associated growth factor receptors
(*see also* pages 56 and 463)

Positive growth signals are transduced by the cognate receptors of peptide growth factors that contain tyrosine kinase motifs in their C-terminal, internal domain. These receptors usually dimerize immediately following ligand binding, and activation of the intracellular tyrosine kinase domain results in autophosphorylation of several tyrosine residues in the C-terminal tail of the receptor. These phosphotyrosines are then recognized as docking sites for binding of downstream signaling molecules containing src-homology (SH-) domains. Effector signaling molecules may thus either bind directly to the receptor, or indirectly through binding of linking molecules such as Grb2 and Shc. Downstream signaling pathways activated in this manner include phospholipase c and phosphatidylinositol 3 kinase which activate phosphatidylinositol hydrolysis and diacylglycerol formation in the cell membrane, the Ras pathway, and the MEK/MAP kinase (MAPK) cascade leading to activation of ribosomal S6 kinase (S6K) and ribosomal protein synthesis. Direct activation both of tyrosine phosphorylated protein kinases such as the Janus (Jak) kinases and of transcription factors including p120, provide a direct link between positive growth factor signaling and the nucleus.

## Serine/threonine kinase receptors

The *TGFβ receptors* (TGFβR) (Fig. 18.3) constitute the best characterized and largest known family of serine/threonine kinase growth factor receptors. TGFβ signaling is capable of mediating many processes, including inhibition of the cell cycle in epithelial cells, stimulation of the expression of tyrosine kinase growth factor receptors in mesenchymal cells, and stimulation of extracellular matrix production through transcriptional activation of genes such as *PAI-1* that regulate the stability of extracellular matrix proteins.

The TGFβ receptors transduce signals instructed by members of the TGFβ peptide superfamily. In the best studied example, TGFβR I, II and III comprise a heterotrimeric signaling complex. TGFβ IIIR is a large proteoglycan that serves to present TGFβ peptide ligand to the TGFβ IIR and is devoid of intracellular signaling sequences. Ligand binding to TGFβ IIR then facilitates dimerization between the ligand occupied TGFβ IIR and TGFβ IR.

The constitutively active serine/threonine kinase of the TGFβ IIR is then able to cross-phosphorylate and activate the TGFβ IR. Downstream signaling from the TGFβ IR is currently much less well characterized than are tyrosine kinase receptors. However, immunophilins are the recently discovered first example of putative signaling molecules that bind to the internal domain of the TGFβ IR and appear to mediate intracellular signaling. In lymphoid cells, activation of immunophilins by drugs such as Rapamycin both blocks the cell cycle in $G_1$ phase and interferes with immunocompetence. Presumably other proteins that undergo protein–protein interactions with the TGFβR will emerge. It is likely that some will play a role, for example, in activation of the cdk inhibitor proteins, both at the transcriptional and post-transcriptional level.

## Cross-talk between growth factor signaling pathways

Cross-talk between growth factor signaling pathways can occur at all levels from the receptor to the nucleus. However, the integration of similar signals to yield different effects during such processes as differentiation and wound healing is a puzzle that has yet to be solved definitively. Clearly, the number of signaling receptors entering the signaling complex, the degree of phosphorylation of intracellular tyrosine, the relative numbers of SH-molecules bound to those tyrosines, and the relative levels of activation of such signaling molecules as Ras and the tyrosine phosphorylated transcription factors, are but a few concrete examples.

The Ras pathway is one of the best studied components of a cell membrane to nucleus signaling pathway. It is activated by growth factor receptor kinase addition of phosphates to tyrosines on Grb2, followed by the association and phosphorylation of the "son-of-seven-less" (SOS) protein with the complex, and activation of Ras at the cell membrane. Interestingly, the Ras pathway can tell the same types of cells to do different things, depending on its level of activation. For example, a Ras-mediated signal may tell a cell to divide, not to divide, to differentiate or to resist differentiation. Over-expression of Ras may also overwhelm the regulatory capacities of a cell, leading to transformation and uncontrolled proliferation. These developmental decisions depend partly on the previous developmental history of a cell. Thus, Ras activation may have one effect in a cell expressing a particular set of developmental genes, and an entirely different effect in another cell expressing a different set of signaling genes. A now classical example of this effect is shown in the abnormal development of the fruit fly eye, in developmental mutants lacking SOS function in which the seventh component of the omatidial complex fails to develop (hence the terminology "sevenless" and "son-of-sevenless").

## CELLULAR TRANSFORMATION, TUMOR SUPPRESSOR GENES AND APOPTOSIS

*See also* Chapter 2, page 92

Transformation of cells to form cancerous phenotypes may also be viewed as a developmental aberration. All proto-oncogenes described to date also have key functions in both normal development and normal cell physiology, as discussed above for the *Ras* proto-oncogene. Conversely, transformation can be accelerated by mutation or deletion of so-called tumor suppressor genes. Now classical examples of these mutations or deletions are the tumor suppressor genes for the retinoblastoma protein (pRb) and *p53*.

*Retinoblastoma* is a rare but fascinating eye cancer of childhood, which, in familial cases, has two deletions or mutations in the *Rb* gene product, pRb. pRb is a key component of the cell cycle machinery that becomes phosphorylated during late $G_1$ and S phase, in response to cyclin-dependent kinase activity. Several of these specific phosphorylations block binding domains in the Rb protein, known as the Rb binding pockets. This prevents so-called pocket-binding proteins from binding to pRb. The pocket-binding proteins have essential functions in promoting S phase of the cell cycle. Thus, deletion or mutation of key amino acid residues in the pRb protein prevent it from binding these proteins and overcomes the ability of this protein to maintain cells in $G_0$ or $G_1$.

*p53* is another important tumor suppressor gene, which is deleted or mutated in a high proportion of solid tumors including *carcinoma of the colon, breast and lung*. Among its many functions, *p53* serves as a positive transcription factor to regulate the expression of the potent cdk inhibitor *p21*. Thus, functional mutations in the *p53* gene prevent activation of *p21* and allow unopposed activation of cdks, leading to shortening of the cell cycle and a greater tendency to a malignant phenotype.

Over-expression of *p53* induces apoptosis in several cell lines (*see also* page 98). Apoptosis is a process characterized by dissolution of the chromatin and non-necrotic cell death without extracellular release of lysosomal contents. This suggests that *p53* also plays a role in developmental processes in which embryonic tissue is resorbed by apoptosis. *p53* also plays a role in DNA repair and has a key function in genome surveillance to determine where DNA repair is necessary. Thus, *p53* has been termed the "guardian of the genome." The reaction of skin keratinocytes to *sunburn* forms an intriguing and common example of how a common injury to the genome from ultraviolet light induced mutations induces abnormal *p53* function. Excessive ultraviolet light induces *p53*, presumably to perform the function of genome surveillance and DNA repair. However, in some keratinocytes excess *p53* induction leads to transient $G_1$ cell cycle arrest through the induction of *p21*, while in others, excess *p53* induction is associated with apoptosis. Of course, chronic over-exposure to sunlight is associated with a high incidence of *p53* functional mutations resulting in abrogation of the tumor suppressor functions of *p53*, and these are associated with *carcinoma in situ* and eventual metastasizing skin cancer such as *malignant melanoma*.

Because of the striking nuclear involution that occurs in apoptosis, it was assumed that nuclear events drove this process. However, apoptosis also is under the control of cytosolic factors, since cytoplasts prepared by removing the nuclei from fibroblasts can undergo apoptosis without the nucleus. Tumor necrosis factor α is capable of activating apoptosis in hematopoietic cells through a pathway that does not involve the nucleus. Thus, cells do not need a nucleus to undergo programmed cell death. In fact, cytoplasmic cell death proteins could be likened to "ninjas" waiting in the cytoplasm to execute the cell death program.

## SPATIOTEMPORAL INFORMATION, CELL REPLICATION AND DIFFERENTIATION IN ORGANOGENESIS

In addition to decisions to divide, remain quiescent, or to undergo apoptosis alluded to above, for the human organism to grow and develop normally, cells must also undergo decisions of when and where to exist and into which lineage to differentiate. We will consider the lung as an illustrative example of the current level of understanding of how these processes are accomplished in human organ development.

The lung develops as a bud which grows out from the epithelium lining the floor of the primitive pharynx into the surrounding mesenchyme. The placement of the primitive lung bud in a progenitor field along the axis of the gut epithelium is likely to be determined by a "bar-code" of transcription factors and morphogens including peptide growth factors and perhaps retinoic acid. The transcription factors involved in specifying the site and cell lineages of the primitive lung anlage include the hepatocyte nuclear factor family (HNF), and the thyroid transcription factor family (TTF) of transcription factors (Figs. 18.3 and 18.4). The HNF also are expressed in several structures along the gut axis and play a role in specifying the progenitor fields of a number of endoderm-derived structures including the thyroid, lung and liver. On the other hand, the TTF are expressed only in the thyroid and the lung, and preliminary results suggest that there may be lung-specific isoforms of the TTF. The

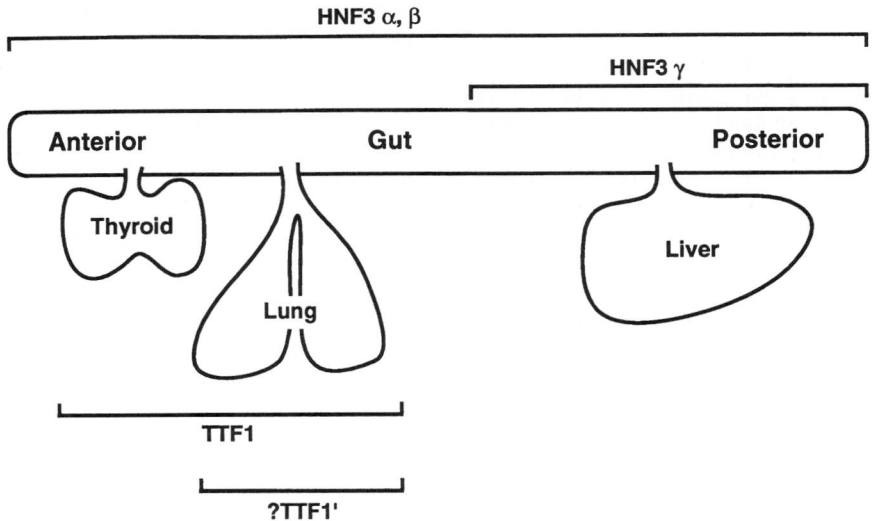

FIGURE 18.4 Specification of lung development by transcription factors and peptide growth factor signaling. The location of the lung bud along the axis of the embryonic gut is specified by at least two families of transcription factors: Hepatocyte nuclear factor family (HNF), the human homologue of the Drosophila Forkhead gene and the Thyroid transcription factor family (TTF). Co-expression of HNF and TTF1 appear to specify the location of the thyroid and lung in the floor of the primitive pharynx. TTF1 response elements are found in the 5′ promoters of several lung specific genes including *SP-A*, *SP-C* and *CC-10*.

TTF1 and HNF3 transcription factors bind to and activate the promoters of lung-specific genes including the *SP-A*, *SP-B* and *CC-10* gene promoters that are specifically expressed in certain pulmonary epithelial cell lineages. In addition, induction of the lung anlage is determined by epithelial–mesenchymal signaling mediated by peptide growth factors and their cognate receptors as well as by interactions between cells and the extracellular matrix, such as integrins binding fibronectin, and cell–cell interactions. Over-expression of a dominant negative FGF receptor (FGFR) coupled to the SP-C promoter completely abrogates lung morphogenesis and cell lineage differentiation distal to the major bronchi, suggesting that FGFR signaling is an important inductive signal for distal lung branching morphogenesis and for the emergence of distal epithelial cell lineages including Clara cells, pulmonary neuroendocrine cells and alveolar type I and II cells. Abrogation of EGF receptor (EGFR) signaling in embryonic mouse lung in culture likewise significantly inhibits embryonic lung branching and cytodifferentiation. On the other hand, PDGF signaling appears principally to play a role in lung cell proliferation. Evidence from gene knockouts of the IGFR further suggest that IGFs play a key role in the later stages of lung development and size increase.

Cell cycle genes also are important in determining the proliferative versus non-proliferative and differentiated phenotypes of cells during development. In the developing alveolar epithelium, for example, proliferative fetal rat epithelial cells express both cyclin D1 and D2 and the cyclin-dependent kinase cdc2 as well as the other key cell cycle regulators. However, in the non-proliferative, adult type II alveolar epithelial cell, cyclin D2 and cdc2 expression are significantly down-regulated, while cyclin D1 and many of the other cell cycle regulators continue to be expressed, suggesting that cyclin D2 expression may play a role in maintaining the proliferative fetal phenotype. This concept is further supported by the finding that abrogation of cyclin D2 expression in proliferating fetal rat alveolar epithelial cells using antisense cyclin D2 oligodeoxynucleotides arrests the cells in $G_0/G_1$ of the cell cycle. Differential expression of D-type cyclins also occurs in a number of other differentiating tissues including some immune cell lines that can be induced to differentiate and switch off specific cyclin D subtypes. Conversely, during the proliferative repair phase following acute hyperoxic lung injury, adult alveolar epithelial cells re-express cyclin D2 and cdc2 kinase; this expression then is suppressed again following return to quiescence later in the process of repair. It is interesting to note that cyclin D was discovered as a gene that is over-expressed in certain forms of cancer, particularly *parathyroid adenomas*. Thus, when over-expressed and uncontrolled, cyclin D also can function as a transforming oncogene.

## THE FUTURE: ORGAN REGENERATION AND ANTICANCER THERAPY IN PEDIATRICS

Developmental cues are now known to be initiated in a complex pattern of signaling networks that result in organ-specific gene activation, and specific sequential patterns of epithelial–mesenchymal and cell-cell interaction. Since nature recapitulates these complex developmental events based on information contained in the genome, it is now within our technical capacity to determine the precise temporospatial sequence of expression of these developmental genes. Thus, the morphogenesis of each individual organ system is instructed by a matrix of signaling pathways comprising transcription factors, including homeodomain proteins, morphogen receptors including the retinoic acid receptor superfamily, and peptide growth factors and their cognate receptors in addition to positional cues arising from cell–cell and cell–substratum interactions.

This new molecular information is informing novel rational therapeutic approaches to pediatric disease on many levels. For example, skin and bone regeneration using growth factor impregnated collagen substrates as "scaffolding" and which attracts stem cells to the site of wound healing, are now in preclinical development. Current efforts also are under way to devise inductive gene therapies, which, together with novel therapeutics, including rationally designed peptidomimetic molecules and monoclonal antibodies, may eventually facilitate repair of more complex developmental defects such as pulmonary and gastrointestinal hypoplasia. In this regard, the re-induction of a stem cell phenotype in damaged or so-called terminally differentiated tissues such as lung epithelium would be a major therapeutic goal. Gene therapies utilizing inducible antisense oligodeoxynucleotide vectors directed to down-regulate the expression of specific cell cycle genes also provide promise for the rational treatment of intractable pediatric cancers, particularly solid tumors and pulmonary metastases, by inducing cell cycle arrest.

## SELECTED READING

Bui KC, Buckley S, Wu F, Uhal B, Joshi I, Liu J, Hussain M, Makhoul I, Warburton D. Induction of A and D-type cyclins and cdc2 kinase activity during activity during recovery from short term hyperoxic lung injury. *Amer J Physiol* 1995; **12**: L625–L635.

Cohen GB, Ren R, Baltimore D. Modular binding domains in signal transduction proteins. *Cell* 1995; **80**: 237.

Heldin C-H. Dimerization of cell surface receptors in signal transduction. *Cell* 1995; **80**: 213.

Hill CS, Treisman R. Transcriptional regulation by extracellular signals: mechanisms and specificity. *Cell* 1995; **80**: 199.

Hunter T. Protein kinases and phosphatases: the yin and yang of protein phosphorylation and signalling. *Cell* 1995; **80**: 225.

Kaartinen V, Voncken JW, Shuler CA, Warburton D, Heisterkamp N, Groffen J. Abnormal lung development and cleft palate: defects of mesenchymal-epithelial interaction in mice lacking TGF-$\beta$3. *Nature Genetics* 1995; **11**:415–21.

Lewin B. Driving the cell cycle: M phase kinase, its partners and substrates. *Cell* 1990; **61**: 743.

Marshall CJ. Specificity of receptor tyrosine kinase signalling: transient versus sustained extracellular signal-regulated kinase activation. *Cell* 1995; **80**: 179.

Minoo P, Hamden H, Bu D, Warburton D, Stepanik P, deLemos R. TTF-1 regulates lung epithelial morphogenesis. *Developmental Biology* 1995; **172**: 694–8.

Murray A, Kirschner M. Dominoes and clocks: the union of two views of the cell cycle. *Science* 1989; **246**: 614.

Nurse P. Universal control mechanism regulating onset of M phase. *Nature* 1990; **344**: 503.

Ohtsubo M, Roberts JM. Cyclin-dependent regulation of $G_1$ in mammalian fibroblasts. *Science* 1993; **259**: 1908.

Pardee A. $G_1$ events and the regulation of cell proliferation. *Science* 1989; **246**: 603.

Pines J, Hunter T. p34$^{cdc2}$: the S and M kinase? *New Biologist* 1990; **2**: 389.

Reed SI. $G_1$ specific cyclins: in search of an S-phase promoting factor. *Trends in Genetics* 1992; **7**: 95.

Sherr CJ. Mammalian $G_1$ cyclins. *Cell* 1993; **73**: 1059.

Warburton D, Seth R, Shum L, Horcher P, Hall FL, Werb Z, Slarkin HC. Epigenetic role of epidermal growth factor expression and signalling in the regulation of embryonic lung morphogenesis. *Developmental Biology* 1992; **149**: 123–33.

Wu F, Buckley S, Bui KC, Warburton D. Differential expression of Cyclin D2 and cdc2 genes in proliferating and nonproliferating aveolar epithelial cells. *Amer J Resp Cell Mol Biol* 1995; **12**: 95–103.

# 19

# Role of Growth Factors in Tissue Development

David J. Hill and Victor K. M. Han

## INTRODUCTION

Growth of the embryo, fetus and child is a multifaceted process involving not only cell replication, hypertrophy and differentiation, but also the ordered migration of cells to defined anatomical sites, their condensation into organs, profound morphological events such as the formation of three germ layers, and programmed cell death. The integrated process of growth and development requires precise intercellular communication. The communication routes used are often not centrally controlled by the nervous system or circulating endocrine hormones, but depend on local cell–cell interactions via peptide growth factors and membrane-associated recognition molecules. Knowledge of how growth factors interrelate with each other and in the context of extracellular matrix and intercellular recognition molecules is central to understanding tissue development.

Peptide growth factors are peptide or glycoprotein hormones which are widely expressed in body tissues, and regulate aspects of tissue hyperplasia, differentiation, morphogenesis and cell migration. As a class of messengers, they typically act close to their sites of synthesis as paracrine or autocrine hormones, rather than as endocrine hormones transmitted via the circulation. This distinction is not mutually exclusive. For instance, the insulin-like growth factors (IGFs), also known as somatomedins, are widely expressed during development, yet are also present in blood (*see* page 314). In addition to IGFs, the other major types of growth factors that are involved in cellular growth and differentiation are epidermal growth factor (EGF), and its analog transforming growth factor $\alpha$ (TGF$\alpha$), platelet-derived growth factor (PDGF), fibroblast growth factors (FGFs), transforming growth factor $\beta$ (TGF$\beta$) and nerve growth factor (NGF). Several of these terms are generic and cover a family of related molecules.

## GROWTH FACTOR FAMILIES

There are two types of IGF, IGF-I and IGF-II, and two classes of receptor, type I and type II. The IGFs are mitogenic for isolated cell types derived from all three primitive germ layers. IGF-I typically has an $ED_{50}$ of 1–3 nM while IGF-II is an order of magnitude less active. IGFs are almost never found in free form but are complexed in tissues and biological fluids to a family of specific binding proteins (IGFBPs). In addition to extending the biological half-life of IGFs, IGFBPs are capable of modulating IGF bioactivity in either an augmentative or an antagonistic manner. For further discussion of the IGF and IGFBP system, *see* page 314.

EGF is a single-chain polypeptide with molecular weight 6 kD. Mouse EGF was first isolated from the submaxillary glands of male mice and the equivalent human peptide from urine. A structural analog of EGF is TGF$\alpha$ which shows a 30–40 per cent amino acid homology. TGF$\alpha$ is more abundantly expressed than EGF prior to birth. Both peptides share a high-affinity cell receptor. PDGF was first identified in the $\alpha$ storage granules of platelets. It exists as either homodimers or heterodimers of two separate peptide units, A and B, which are products of separate human chromosomes. In platelets, PDGF is always found as A–B heterodimers. The PDGF B chain is analogous to the product of the v-*sis* oncogene. The high-affinity PDGF receptor also has two subunit components, α and β, and can exist in homo- or heterodimer forms. Both EGF and PDGF act as mitogens for isolated mesenchymal cells with $ED_{50}$ values of 0.5–2.0 nM. EGF additionally has proliferative effects on epithelia.

The FGF family contains at least nine members, the best characterized of which are acidic and basic FGF, also now called FGF1 and 2, respectively. Various molecular sizes of FGF exist between 18 kD and 26 kD. Both acidic and basic FGF bind avidly to acidic sulfated glycosaminoglycans such as heparan sulfate and syndecans. Neither FGF has a signal peptide and they cannot be exteriorized by cells via the endoplasmic reticulum. However, abundant basic FGF is found in association with cell membranes and extracellular matrix, suggesting that it may be released complexed to glycosaminoglycans. Although basic FGF is an extremely potent mitogen for isolated connective tissue cell types with an $ED_{50}$ of 10–100 pM, its most dramatic effects are as an angiogenic agent. Proliferating endothelial cells express abundant basic FGF mRNA.

Transforming growth factor β also exists as multiple isomers of which TGFβ1, β2 and β3 are expressed in mammalian development. TGFβ is a homodimer of 25 kD, originally identified in platelets and as a tumor cell product. It is a potent inhibitor of epithelial cell proliferation and a bifunctional regulator of mesenchymal cell growth. Its growth inhibitory effects have been linked to an altered phosphorylation state of the retinoblastoma gene product, while its limited ability to promote cell growth may be mediated by an upregulation of PDGF B-chain expression. TGFβ binds avidly to extracellular matrix molecules such as decorin and is stored in large amounts in bone matrix. When released by cells it exists as a precursor form which is biologically inactive. The active TGFβ molecule can be released from the "latent" form experimentally by heat or acidic pH, while this may result from proteolytic activation by target tissues *in vivo*. An ability of TGFβ to greatly increase fibronectin and type I collagen production by fibroblasts underlies its ability to induce a fibrotic response and hasten wound healing *in vivo*.

Nerve growth factor (NGF) is a basic peptide of 13 kD and shares 25 per cent homology with the A and B chains of insulin. The storage form of NGF comprises three subunits, α, β and λ existing in a dimeric structure (so-called 7SNGF). The β-subunit is the biologically active component (NGF). Other neurotrophins, some with structural analogy to NGF are present in the mammalian brain; such as brain-derived neurotrophic factor (BDNF), ciliary neurotrophic factor (CNTF) and neurotrophins 3–6 (NT-3–6) (*see* page 368). NGF interacts with two types of receptors in neural tissues: the high-affinity, low-capacity receptor and the low-affinity, high-capacity receptor. The high-affinity receptor is a heterodimer comprising a member of the trk peptide family and the low-affinity NGF receptor. BDNF and NT-3 interact with related receptors involving trk-B and trk-C peptides in heterodimers with the low-affinity NGF receptor. Each of the neurotrophins has a different ontogeny and spatial distribution in the brain and different trophic activities on various neuronal phenotypes. The predominant effect of NGF is to promote the survival, differentiation and axonal outgrowth of sensory and sympathetic ganglia. It also has a weak mitogenic action for lymphoid tissues, which have the low-affinity, high-capacity receptors. NGF is selectively produced by peripheral tissues to which the neurites of the developing sensory and sympathetic neurons are attracted by chemotaxis. NGF is then transported retrogradely to the neuronal cell bodies, where it provides the crucial function of survival. Targeted disruption of either the NGF or *trk*A receptor genes causes neonatal lethality associated with poor development of sympathetic ganglia. Disruption of the *trk*B or *trk*C receptors causes behavioral and motor deficiencies associated with a failure of various CNS structures to adequately develop. For further discussion of NGF, *see* page 368.

## EXPRESSION AND DISTRIBUTION OF GROWTH FACTORS IN EARLY DEVELOPMENT

Messenger RNA encoding basic FGF is present at low levels in the oocyte but is absent following fertilization, to reappear as a product of the embryonic genome at the time of neurulation. Messenger RNAs for two other members of the FGF family, kFGF (FGF4) and *int*-2 (FGF3), are present in as early as the four-cell stage in mouse embryo and predominate prior to organogenesis. TGFβ mRNA and peptide is found in the four-cell mouse embryo and blastula, respectively, as is mRNA for the related peptide, activin.

During later embryonic development, basic FGF mRNA steadily increases in abundance until day 16 of gestation in mouse. Expression is greatest in the tail, face and developing limbs.

Conversely, the FGF-related oncogene *int*-2 is expressed in parietal endoderm, primitive mesoderm, the pharyngeal pouches and neuroepithelium of the hind-brain between 7.5 and 9.5 days of gestation. Different members of the FGF family appear to have distinct anatomical and ontological patterns of expression, which together cover almost every embryonic and fetal tissue. Similarly, TGFβ1, β2 and β3 have distinct patterns of expression in the rat fetus but are collectively expressed in every tissue. TGFβ mRNA is predominantly found in epithelial cells, but the peptides are predominantly found on mesenchyme following immunocytochemistry. This is likely to reflect the ability of TGFβ to bind to matrix elements in mesenchyme such as decorin. Animals lacking a functional TGFβ1 gene have severe cardiac abnormalities. However, this can be prevented *in utero* if the mother has a functioning TGFβ1 gene, since TGFβ1 can cross the placenta from mother to fetus. Specific deletions of FGF genes, or the expression of dominant negative mutant FGF receptors, cause severe anatomical abnormalities. For instance, a non-functional FGF receptor-3 is associated with a complete failure of branching within the respiratory tree. Mice exhibiting a naturally-occurring deletion of a PDGF receptor have severe craniofacial malformations, and other cellular deficiencies related to a failure of neural tube closure, and the migration of neural crest cells.

From studies with isolated embryonal carcinoma cells, it would appear that IGFs appear later in development than FGF or TGFβ. Undifferentiated cell lines do not express IGFs, but will produce IGF-II consequent to differentiation into either mesoderm or endoderm following exposure to retinoic acid. Similarly, IGF-II mRNA could not be detected in human embryos fertilized and cultured *in vitro* to the formation of blastocysts, but was detected in differentiated trophoblast from abortus tissue as early as 35 days post-conception. IGF-I mRNA does not appear in the rat embryo until around day 11 of gestation. In the late embryonic and fetal rat, abundant IGF-II mRNA was localized by *in situ* hybridization to the yolk sac, liver, skeletal muscle, precartilaginous mesenchymal condensations, chondrocytes, periosteum and centers of intramembranous ossification. The importance of IGF-II to fetal growth was demonstrated by studies in which one allele of the IGFBP gene was disrupted in the mouse embryo by homologous recombination. Animals which failed to express one IGF-II gene were smaller than wild type mice at birth, but postnatally grew at the same rate. However, mice lacking a functional IGF-I gene were also small at birth, showing that both IGF-I and -II are necessary for optimal fetal growth. Postnatally, IGF-II mRNA levels decline to negligible levels by weaning in most tissues except for brain, which continues to express IGF-II mRNA in the choroid plexus and leptomeninges. Conversely, IGF-I mRNA levels increase during neonatal life and achieve adult levels in rat liver, and other tissues, by 50 days after birth. One rat tissue which expresses abundant IGF-I mRNA postnatally is the epiphyseal cartilage of the growth plates within long bones. It therefore seems likely that the ability of IGF-I to potentiate longitudinal skeletal growth depends at least partly on a local synthesis within the growth plate.

In the human fetus of late first or early second trimester, IGF-II mRNA is present in every body tissue, but is most abundant in stromal tissues around and within organs. Conversely, immunocytochemistry has shown that IGF peptides are concentrated on epithelia in the gut, kidney and lung and in differentiated muscle. Since several IGFBPs show a similar immunocytochemical distribution it seems likely that the IGFBPs may direct the cellular distribution of IGFs.

Both IGF-I and II are detectable in human fetal plasma from at least 15 weeks of gestation. From 32 weeks until term, concentrations of both peptides increase 2-fold, but still remain lower than in the adult. Conversely, in the rat fetus, circulating IGF-II concentrations are 20- to 100-fold greater than in maternal serum. Despite an abundance of IGF-II in blood, correlations between circulating concentrations and weight or length of the fetus or newborn are poor. A positive correlation exists between these parameters and circulating IGF-I in the fetus. In infants who are small for gestational age, IGFBP-3 concentrations are low and IGFBP-I concentrations are increased. For further discussion, *see* page 288.

## BIOLOGICAL ACTIONS OF GROWTH FACTORS DURING DEVELOPMENT

An early embryonic expression of several peptide growth factors is logical with regard to the known synergistic interactions of growth factors during the cycle of cell replication (*see also* page 273). Studies with mouse Balb/c-3T3 fibroblasts showed that PDGF and basic FGF predominantly acted at the $G_0$/$G_1$ boundary and render cells "competent" to enter the cell cycle. In the same model, EGF acts in early $G_1$, and IGFs in late $G_1$, to allow the cells to progress to S phase and initiate DNA synthesis; they have therefore been termed "progression factors." Thus the controlled expression of a variety of growth factors may provide a fine control of cell proliferation rate in discrete tissues. During tissue remodeling, the release of proteolytic enzymes such as plasminogen activator will lead to local extracellular matrix degradation, which will in turn liberate additional stored growth factors such as TGFβ. This may serve to limit the proliferative events.

Such interactions between growth factors are well demonstrated in *in vitro* models of cell differentiation. The differentiation of the L6 rat myoblast cell line into postmitotic myotubes is prevented by basic FGF and EGF, but potentiated by IGF-I or II. TGFβ1 has little effect on myoblast proliferation rate but has an inhibitory effect on cell differentiation. Thus, altered local expression of particular growth factors can trigger specific events of cellular differentiation. These signals are, in part, supplied by the muscle cells themselves. FGF expression is high in proliferative myoblasts while IGF-II expression is low. As differentiation is initiated the expression of FGF declines while that of IGF-II rises. IGF-II increases the expression of differentiation-controlling genes such as myogenin and MYO-D.

Both basic FGF and TGFβ2 are able to mimic the actions of an endogenous morphogen and induce the development of mesoderm from primitive animal pole ectoderm removed from the Xenopus embryo. Messenger RNA encoding basic FGF is present in the Xenopus embryo at this time, and mesoderm-inducing activity can be partly neutralized with anti-basic FGF antiserum. Proof that the endogenous members of the FGF family were responsible for mesoderm formation was provided by expression of a dominant negative mutant of the FGF receptor in Xenopus embryo. Serious defects in gastrulation and in ventral mesoderm formation resulted, with no development of the somites of the tail. Bone morphogenetic protein-4 (BMP4) also induces ventral mesoderm. The β form of activin mRNA appears in Xenopus embryo coincident with mesoderm formation, and activin may be responsible for the development of dorsal mesoderm. A Xenopus ectodermal cell line releases a mesoderm-inducing activity which can be mimicked with activin or TGFβ2, and blocked by antiserum against TGFβ2. Thus, basic FGF, BMP4 and activin may jointly regulate the formation of the trilaminar embryo. FGF4 is expressed within the apical ectodermal ridge at the tip of the developing embryonic limb buds. FGF4 maintains limb outgrowth and also determines the pattern formation of skeletal elements within the limb.

TGFα and FGF are angiogenic and may contribute to the high density of uterine capillary formation around the site of embryonic uterine implantation. TGFα is expressed by the embryo in negligible amounts at this time compared with a massive expression in the maternal decidua adjacent to the embryo. TGFα mRNA levels were greatest at the time of implantation of the rodent embryo and subsequently showed a slow decline in parallel with decidual resorption. A surge of estrogen at the time of implantation may greatly increase the uterine expression of EGF/TGFα receptors. *In situ* hybridization of mRNA for PDGF B chain showed localization in trophoblasts as early as 21 days postconception in man, suggesting that PDGF may contribute to the invasive growth of placental implantation.

TGFβ1 and β2 are analogous to bone-derived factors previously known as cartilage-inducing factors A and B with the ability to induce chondrocyte formation from embryonic mesenchymal explants. Exposure of undifferentiated mesenchyme from primitive limb buds to TGFβ1 or β2 induced the appearance of chondrocytes. It is likely that TGFβ is responsible for specific events of differentiation in developing connective tissues, since TGFβ1–β3 mRNAs have been localized to chondrogenic areas in both the rat and human embryo.

## ONCOGENES

Oncogenes are normal components of the genome, which through an inappropriate degree of expression, translocation, or point mutation, are no longer under precise developmental control. This can lead to the expression of structurally or quantitatively aberrant oncogene-encoded proteins which can either be markers of neoplasia, or may contribute to the growth and metastasis of tumors. A pivotal finding was that viral oncogenes introduced into cells by retroviruses were homologous to normal cellular genes involved in the control of growth and differentiation. The virally inserted RNA is converted to DNA by host cells which express the aberrant oncogenic protein. The first published example of this was the finding that

the v-*sis* oncogene encoded a peptide related to the B-chain form of PDGF. Other oncogenes encode proteins which represent normal or altered growth factor receptors (v-*erb* is related to the EGF receptor, c-*met* is the hepatocyte growth factor receptor); intracellular second messenger components (c-*src* and c-*ros* encode tyrosine-specific protein kinases, c-*ras* encodes a GTP-binding protein); or DNA-binding proteins (c-*fos* and c-*myc*). The normal cellular equivalents of these oncogenes are expressed as part of the controlled pattern of embryogenesis and fetal development, often under the control of peptide growth factors. During the replicative cycle of fibroblasts, basic FGF will induce a transient elevation of c-*myc* and c-*fos* expression at the beginning of $G_1$. Later in $G_1$ a transient elevation of c-*ras* will occur in response to EGF. Within whole tissues a high expression of c-*myc* was found in the trophoblast during uterine invasion which declined as placental invasive growth ceased. The *src* gene appears to be preferentially active in embryonic neural tissues such as eye and brain of the embryo, while c-*ras* is expressed at high levels, compared with adult, in the human fetal brain and lung. The intracellular signaling pathways controlling mitogenesis in response to FGF, PDGF, EGF and IGFs all involve activation of c-*ras*, and of transcription factors such as c-*myc* and c-*fos*.

## MATRIX INTERACTIONS WITH GROWTH FACTORS

Extracellular matrix consists of two major classes of molecules: proteins such as collagens, fibronectin and laminin; and mucopolysaccharides such as hyaluronic acid, heparan sulfate, and chondroitin and keratin sulfate. Most epithelia are tightly attached to a basal lamina, or basement membrane, which is rich in type IV collagen and forms a connection with the fibrillar forms of collagen within the connective tissue stroma. The formation of the basal membrane and type IV collagen is stimulated by TGFβ, which is expressed by many developing epithelia.

The extracellular matrix of connective tissues contains fibronectin. Fibronectins form a bridge between cells such as fibroblasts and other matrix components such as type I collagen. Cellular attachment is via a family of integrin receptors with an arginine–glycine–aspartate (RGD) amino acid recognition sequence in the binding domain. Integrins are linked to actin within the intracellular cytoskeleton by the connecting peptides vinculin and talin. By their attachments fibronectin molecules are able to regulate cell shape during development, which is important during cell migration and differentiation. Migration routes are defined by tracts of fibronectin-rich mesenchymal matrix. These tracts are also rich in hyaluronic acid, a hydrophilic molecule which creates a loose gel through which migrating cells can pass easily. Hyaluronic acid is bound to the membrane of migrating cells, and appears to inhibit intercellular adhesion. When undifferentiated muscle cell precursors migrate into the embryonic limb buds from the somites they have pericellular hyaluronic acid coats. This phenotype is maintained by the presence of FGF molecules derived from the surrounding mesenchyme. When migration ceases, a reduction in hyaluronic acid presence allows muscle cell adhesion, and fusion following terminal differentiation. An important feature of tissue remodeling and cell migration is the ability of the tissue to produce neutral proteases such as plasminogen activator. The subsequent activation of plasminogen to plasmin results in the destruction of extracellular matrix at the site of remodeling. The ability of cells to release plasminogen activator is potentiated by basic FGF, and inhibited by TGFβ.

## ROLE OF GROWTH FACTORS IN REGULATING ORGAN GROWTH

The growth and functional maturation of several organs has been linked to the local expression of peptide growth factors and their interactions with endocrine hormones. Three examples will be given: the adrenal gland, placenta and brain. The adrenal gland is an extremely active steroidogenic organ *in utero* producing cortisol and $\Delta^5$ steroids such as dehydroepiandrosterone (DHA) and its sulfated derivative, DHAS. The latter are further metabolized by placenta to estrogens. The human fetal adrenal expresses large amounts of mRNA for IGF-II in early second trimester, and this was increased *in vitro* by exposure of adrenal tissue to adrenocorticotrophic hormone (ACTH) or dibutyryl cAMP, the second messenger activated by ACTH. Human fetal adrenal also contains mRNA for basic FGF, which is also up-regulated by ACTH. Proliferation of fetal adrenal cells is enhanced by IGFs, suggesting that they may partly mediate the trophic actions of ACTH on fetal adrenal hyperplasia, which is largely limited to the cortex. Extrapolation from studies with postnatal adrenal tissue suggests that growth factors may also contribute to adrenal function. When bovine fasciculata cells were maintained *in vitro* in the presence of IGF-I, receptors for angiotensin II were increased and ACTH-induced corticosterone and pregnenolone output elevated three- to sixfold. IGF-I most likely increased the availability of cholesterol and/or its transport to the mitochondria. FGF also plays an important role in the determination of neural crest cell differentiation into either sympathetic ganglia or adrenal medulla.

The finding of abundant IGF-II mRNA expression in the human cytotrophoblast and a high density of both type I and II IGF receptors on placental tissues suggests a role for IGFs in placental growth and perhaps function. IGFs promote the replication of isolated placental fibroblasts. Both IGF-I and insulin stimulate 3β-hydroxysteroid dehydrogenase activity, the rate-limiting enzyme in the conversion of pregnenolone to progesterone in isolated trophoblasts. In the same model IGF-I inhibited the activity of trophoblast aromatase necessary for estrogen production. While IGFs may regulate trophoblast function, this may be aided by a local expression of EGF or TGFα which will increase the differentiation of cytotrophoblastic cells into a functional syncytium *in vitro*. A high expression of basic FGF in placenta may contribute to endothelial cell proliferation, angiogenesis being a major feature of placental growth.

Multiple transcripts of IGF-I and II mRNA are found in the fetal and neonatal rat brain, as are IGF type I and II receptors. Cultured fetal rat neuronal and astroglial cells also release both IGF-I and II. Glial cells proliferate in response to exogenous IGF-I, and other growth factors such as EGF and basic FGF. The mitogenic actions of EGF are mediated in part by increased endogenous synthesis of IGFs. IGF-II will also promote the embryonic neurons and neurite formation in isolated rat sensory and sympathetic ganglia, and in human neuroblastoma cells. In these models IGF-II was synergistic with nerve growth factor. IGF-I was shown to increase the commitment of mixed glial cell cultures from the newborn rat cerebrum to form oligodendrocytes. The IGFs may also serve as neurotransmitters within brain since IGF-I was shown to stimulate acetylcholine release from rat cortical brain slices, and to cause the differentiation of catecholaminergic precursors in cultures of dorsal rat ganglia.

## SELECTED READING

Han VKM, Hill DJ. The involvement of insulin-like growth factors in embryonic and fetal development. In: Schofield P, ed. *The insulin-like growth factors, structures and biologic functions.* Oxford: Oxford University Press, 1990: 178.

Han VKM, Hill DJ. Growth factors in fetal growth. In: Thorburn GD, Harding R, eds. *Textbook of fetal physiology.* Oxford: Oxford Medical Publications, 1994: 48.

Lee DC, Han VKM. Expression of growth factors and their receptors in development. In: Sporn MB, Roberts AB, eds. *Peptide growth factors and their receptors,* Vol. 2. New York: Springer-Verlag, 1990: 611.

Sharpe PM, Ferguson MWJ. Mesenchymal influences on epithelial differentiation in developing systems. *J Cell Sci* 1988; Suppl 10: 195.

Sporn MB, Roberts AB, eds. *Peptide growth factors and their receptors.* Berlin: Springer-Verlag, 1990.

# 20

# Regulation of Intrauterine Growth

R. David G. Milner and Peter D. Gluckman

## INTRODUCTION

Growth can be defined as an increase in size and complexity, usually achieved by increases in cell size and cell number. In addition, an increased deposition of extracellular material contributes to growth. Growth early in life is accompanied by differentiation or the transformation of cells from a relatively unspecialized phenotype to specialized cells with specific functions. The human fetus undergoes the equivalent of some 42 successive mitotic divisions in progressing from a fertilized ovum to a term infant, with only five more divisions being necessary to achieve adult size. Growth occurs by changes in cell number and size: in the first trimester growth is by increase in cell number, in the second there is a stable rate of cellular division accompanied by an increase in cell size, while in the third trimester the rate of mitosis slows while growth by cellular hypertrophy continues. In the second or third trimesters *intrauterine growth retardation* (IUGR) can be caused by slowing of the mitotic rate or prevention of cellular hypertrophy. The earlier IUGR occurs, the more likely it is to be irreversible and lead to persistent postnatal growth failure (*see* Chapter 21).

Growth velocity expressed as fractional change per unit time is greatest for length at approximately 20 weeks and for weight at 34 weeks. The slowing of the rate of weight gain thereafter is due to "maternal constraint." In the last trimester the fetus doubles its bodyweight, from approximately 1.5 to 3 kg, due mainly to rapid acquisition of protein and fat. While of the first 1.5 kg bodyweight acquired over 28 weeks, only about 5 g is fat, of the second 1.5 kg accumulated after 28 weeks, 500 g is fat. At term the male fetus is heavier and has a greater lean body mass and less body fat than the female, possibly due to the effect of fetal testosterone production. Lipid accumulation by the fetus in the third trimester is an important determinant of birthweight and is primarily determined by nutrient availability and fetal insulin secretion.

Prenatal growth is a reflection of an interaction between maternal, placental and the fetal factors. Growth control is a mix of immutable genetic effects and the systems through which the genetic mechanisms are modulated. These are best considered as nutritional, endocrine and paracrine. Fetal survival and growth are absolutely dependent on delivery of nutrients to the fetus from the materno-placental unit, whereas after birth nutritional constraints are no longer all-powerful and genetic factors become the most important determinants of normal development to final adult size.

Mathematical models have been developed that partition the contribution of genetic and environmental factors in determining birthweight. Variation in birthweight can be partitioned roughly: one-third to genetic factors, one-third to recognizable environmental factors, particularly the maternal phenotype, and one-third unknown (Table 20.1).

## GENETIC FACTORS

Multiple gene loci contribute to birthweight of the normal fetus. Of the genetic component, maternal genotype is more important than fetal genotype. The paternal contribution is solely via the fetal genotype. Although the paternal contribution to birthweight is modest, the paternal genome is essential for trophoblast development, and in the presence of two copies of the paternal genome (*see* page 120) *trophoblast tumors* may occur. Gene targeting experiments in mice using insulin-like growth factor (IGF)-II and

TABLE 20.1 Factors determining variance in birthweight

| | PERCENTAGE OF VARIANCE | TOTAL |
|---|---|---|
| *Fetal* | | |
| Genotype | 16 | |
| Sex | 2 | |
| | | 18 |
| *Maternal* | | |
| Genotype | 20 | |
| Maternal environment | 24 | |
| Maternal age | 1 | |
| Parity | 7 | |
| | | 52 |
| *Unknown* | | 30 |

Derived from Penrose LS. *Proc 9th Int Congr Genetics* Part 1. 1954: 520.

IGF-II receptor genes have clearly shown the important effect genomic imprinting may have on development of the conceptus; for normal fetal and placental growth the IGF-II gene must be paternal and the IGF-II receptor gene maternal. In mice, over-expression of the IGF-II gene (paternal disomy) results in fetal overgrowth and under-expression (maternal disomy) results in dwarfism. In humans, isopaternal inheritance of IGF-II alleles is associated with the *Beckwith–Wiedemann syndrome* (*see* page 120).

## NON-GENETIC MATERNAL FACTORS

There is a high correlation between birthweight of siblings (Table 20.2). When birthweights between half siblings with a common mother are examined, the correlation remains high but is lost when half siblings with a common father are compared. Evidence of a maternal factor is seen even when the comparison is extended to first cousins. Such a maternal effect could be either genetic or environmental. The classic cross-breeding experiments between horses or pigs of different sized breeds first performed by Walton and Hammond together with subsequent embryo transplant experiments confirm that this effect is non-genetic in nature. For example, a small-breed embryo

TABLE 20.2 Correlations for birthweight

| BETWEEN | *r* |
|---|---|
| Monozygotic twins | 0.54 |
| Dizygotic twins | 0.67 |
| Full siblings | 0.52 |
| Half siblings | |
| common mother | 0.58 |
| common father | 0.10 |
| First cousins | |
| common maternal grandparents | 0.135 |
| common paternal grandparents | 0.015 |

Data from Robson ER, in Falkner F and Tanner JM, eds, *Human growth. Vol 1: Principles and prenatal growth.* New York: Plenum Press, 1978.

transplanted to a large-breed uterus will grow larger than a small-breed embryo remaining in a small-breed uterus: evidence that growth of the fetus is normally constrained. Conversely a large-breed embryo transplanted to a small-breed uterus will be smaller than in its natural environment.

Such studies demonstrate that the maternal environment normally determines and limits fetal growth. A fetus transplanted to a different uterus will grow at a rate appropriate to the genotype of the recipient mother. The phenomenon by which the maternal environment non-genomically influences fetal growth is physiological and is known as maternal constraint. The factors contributing to maternal constraint are poorly defined but include the limited capacity of the uterine circulation, uterus and placental bed to support placental function. Thus individual triplets on average weigh less than individual twins who weigh less than singletons. These non-genomic maternal factors are the most important single determinants of normal prenatal growth.

## Maternal nutrition

Fetal caloric requirements are 95 kcal/(kg·day) of which 40 are committed to growth and 55 are oxidized. To this minimum caloric cost of the fetus must be added the maternal metabolic burden of carrying the conceptus and preparing for lactation. Direct measurement has shown the extra caloric requirement for pregnancy to be in the order of 20 000 kcal (less than 100 kcal/day) but with marked individual and ethnic differences between women. The basal metabolic rate (BMR) of pregnant women in Europe rises slightly in the first trimester and then progressively thereafter. In contrast, Gambian women show a fall in BMR in the first trimester with a gradual rise just above prepregnancy reference values at term.

Despite the relatively high optimal plane of maternal nutrition, underfeeding has generally been considered to have a relatively small effect on fetal growth. Starvation, as experienced in Holland in 1944–45, led to a small fall in birthweight only when maternal intake fell below 1500 kcal/day in the third trimester. However, as discussed on page 302, more subtle degrees of undernutrition may have long-term consequences for postnatal growth and development. Such studies also demonstrate multigenerational effects. Women who starved during the first trimester gave birth to daughters of normal birthweight, but when the daughters reproduced, their babies were of lower than expected birthweight suggesting that grandmaternal undernutrition had influenced uterine growth in the mother.

## The placenta

Since the placenta is the conduit via which nutrients and O$_2$ are delivered to the fetus and waste products removed, consideration of placental structure and perfusion is pertinent in the context of nutritional control as each may profoundly influence delivery. The maternal–placental–fetal relationship is complicated and, since fetal survival depends on placental integrity, it is important to appreciate that at times fetal growth is sacrificed for placental well-being (see page 295).

The placenta grows faster than the fetus and reaches maximum weight at about 33 weeks' gestation, though surface area and vascularity continue to develop thereafter (see page 214). It is apparent that alterations in placental development of structure, or in either fetal or maternal arterial flow to the placenta, or of diffusion/transport properties of the placenta, can affect its capacity to deliver nutrients to the fetus.

Placental gas exchange is by passive diffusion (see page 219). The major physiological determinants of $O_2$ delivery to the fetus are maternal uterine and fetal umbilical flows and the relative affinities of fetal and maternal hemoglobin for $O_2$. If placental surface area is reduced or the diffusion distance increased (e.g. intervillous fibrin deposition), reduction in the overall $O_2$ diffusion capacity may restrict fetal growth.

The placenta influences fetal metabolism principally by regulating the transport of metabolites to the fetus. There are transporters or carriers for most substrates, some of which (e.g. glucose and fatty acids) diffuse passively whereas others (e.g. amino acids) move actively and largely uphill (see page 224). The amount of nutrients that pass to the fetus is influenced by the high metabolic rate of the placenta. The placenta may consume 30–50 per cent of glucose and $O_2$ taken from the maternal component. The extent of placental utilization is dependent on the status of the fetus and is discussed in detail in Chapter 13. However, given the relative magnitude of placental metabolism, alterations can have major effects on the supply of nutrients to the fetus. Little is known of the factors that regulate placental metabolism. Developmental changes in placental metabolism and transport capacity result in a changing fetal diet throughout gestation.

Near term the placenta contains a large variety of enzymes capable of metabolizing amino acids through pathways such as amino acid oxidation, protein synthesis, gluconeogenesis and glycogen synthesis. The net umbilical uptake of amino acids provides more than half the fetal carbon and more than one and a half times the nitrogen required for normal growth and development. This is reflected in a high fetal urea production rate. Not all amino acids contribute equally to the nitrogen excess; glycine, lysine, histidine, asparagine/aspartate and glutamine/glutamate are all taken up in similar amounts to net carcass accretion and any deficiency in maternal supply would be harmful to fetal growth. The capacity of the fetus to oxidize excess fetal amino acids appears to develop early in gestation. The placenta and fetus cycle amino acids and produce ammonia: ammonia from the placenta passes into both the maternal and the umbilical circulations. Glutamine and glycine are taken up by the fetus from the placenta and by the fetal liver from

the umbilical circulation, whereas the metabolically related products glutamate and serine are produced by the liver and taken up by the placenta. Lipid transport from mother to fetus is quantitatively slight, but the high carbon content of lipid molecules makes their contribution to fetal metabolism disproportionately great. Since fetal fatty acid composition varies with the maternal diet, it seems unlikely that the placenta exerts a significant selectivity in lipid delivery.

The fetal metabolic rate as reflected by net fetal $O_2$ consumption is only slightly associated with energy delivery to the fetus. The relative constancy of fetal metabolic rate at widely differing glucose concentrations indicates that there are important alternative substrates. In view of the limited availability and/or oxidation of other non-protein energy sources, a reciprocal relationship between glucose and amino acids in fulfilling fetal energy requirements is likely. The net uptake of amino acids is more than is needed for fetal protein synthesis and what is left over is oxidized or transaminated and stored as lipid. The fetus is commonly perceived as being both the gross and the net recipient of metabolic fuels but under some circumstances the fetus contributes to placental metabolic needs when these are not fulfilled from the maternal side. Fetal protein catabolism permits the release of amino acids for gluconeogenesis or direct oxidation by the placenta. When this happens fetal growth is compromised to ensure fetal survival by ensuring adequate nutrients for the placenta. If the fetus becomes catabolic in the last trimester the losses of fetal protein exceed those of lipids, and fetal wasting (detectable by ultrasound) may occur (see page 295).

## ENDOCRINE CONTROL OF FETAL GROWTH

## Maternal endocrine influences

The changes in maternal circulating growth hormone (GH) and GH-like peptides such as placental lactogen (hPL) which occur during pregnancy all combine to have a diabetogenic or anti-insulin effect on the mother so that metabolites such as glucose and free fatty acids (FFA) oscillate to higher levels and more wildly during feeding and fasting than in the non-pregnant state. This has important implications for fetal substrate delivery. The insulin resistance induced by these hormones is postulated to lead to increased maternal glucose and free fatty acid availability; the glucose being preferentially utilized by the feto-placental unit and free fatty acids used as a nutritional substrate by the mother. If maternal β islet cell function is disturbed as in *gestational diabetes mellitus*, and overt maternal hyperglycemia arises, then fetal hyperglycemia ensues. This in turn leads to fetal hyperinsulinemia and this leads to the classical adiposity and overgrowth of the *infant of the diabetic mother*.

# Placental endocrine influences

The placenta synthesizes and secretes into the maternal circulation a growth hormone variant (hGH-V or placental GH) which differs from pituitary GH in only 13 amino acids. First detected in midpregnancy, placental GH concentrations increase to term, but the biological significance of this peptide remains unclear. Its secretion is largely constant and it suppresses the pulsatile pattern of pituitary GH release. It may play a part in controlling maternal IGF-I production and in inducing maternal metabolic changes. What role, if any, is played by placental GH in the fetus is not known. Placental GH does not appear to be essential for successful pregnancy because normal fetal development has occurred in a woman who had a deletion of both the hGH-V and placental lactogen (hPL) genes; however, under these circumstances maternal pituitary GH secretion may be maintained.

The placenta makes large amounts of hPL (also known as chorionic somatomammotrophin), a molecule with close biological and chemical similarities to pituitary GH. More than 99 per cent of hPL is secreted into the maternal circulation where it is lipolytic and diabetogenic. It also may play a role in mammary gland development. Despite plasma concentrations in the fetus being 100-fold less, the hormone may play a part in fetal anabolism. Many fetal cells have hPL receptors, and hPL stimulates protein synthesis and cell division both directly and via an action on insulin release. Thus hPL may have an important role in normal fetal growth and in regulating maternal metabolism, but this action is permissive or redundant, as are the actions of other lactogenic hormones such as hGH-V, since there are case records of successful pregnancies in which the gene for hPL is missing.

# Fetal endocrine influences

The major hormones involved in the regulation of fetal growth in late gestation appear to be those which are under tight nutritional regulation. There is now overwhelming evidence that the IGF system plays a major role in regulating fetal growth. Insulin plays an essential but permissive role in fetal growth regulation and may also serve as the intermediate in the regulation of fetal IGF secretion by nutrient availability. Other hormones classically involved in postnatal growth such as GH play only a minor role in the regulation of fetal growth.

Peptide hormones do not cross the placenta, with the possible exception of limited permeability to thyroxine which may be of physiological significance. In contrast, steroid hormones are secreted and metabolized by the maternal–placental–fetal unit in its entirety (see page 206). Both peptide and steroid hormones play a part in fetal growth and organ maturation.

# Insulin-like growth factors

There is clear evidence that IGFs acting in both endocrine and paracrine fashions (see page 314) regulate fetal growth. IGF-I, IGF-II and their binding proteins (IGFBPs) are expressed in all fetal tissues. The patterns of expression of the IGFBPs suggest a role in focusing the actions of IGFs (see page 320). Both IGF-I and IGF-II can be extracted from human tissues from week 12 and are found in the circulation from week 15 of gestation. The expression of concentration of IGF-II mRNA in the tissues and the concentration of IGF-II in both tissues and plasma is consistently higher than that of IGF-I. The circulating concentrations of both IGF-I and IGF-II increase with gestation but remain lower than in maternal plasma at term. This is in contrast to some experimental species in which the concentration of IGF-I rises to adult levels during gestation and that of IGF-II is many times the maternal concentration at term.

IGF-I acting in both an endocrine and paracrine manner is probably the dominant fetal hormonal influence on fetal growth in late gestation, IGF-II may play a greater role earlier in gestation; IGF-I levels in fetal and umbilical cord blood correlate with birth size. The balance of evidence indicates that GH plays a minor role in controlling fetal IGF-I production and that fetal glucose levels and fetal insulin secretion are the primary determinants of fetal IGF-I levels in both the tissues and circulation.

The development of gene "knockout" models has provided additional evidence for the roles played by IGFs in fetal growth. Mice lacking the IGF-I gene have marked intrauterine and postnatal growth failure. Growth retardation does not become apparent until embryonic day 13.5 (E13.5), suggesting that IGF-I influences development only late in pregnancy. Most IGF-I null mutant mice die at birth because of diaphragmatic muscle hypoplasia. Other organs also are hypoplastic, ossification is retarded and neural development is affected. IGF-II knockout mice show fetal and placental growth-retardation from day E11 but resume a growth rate parallel to controls after day E18, suggesting a role for IGF-II in early fetal growth that is taken over by IGF-I later. IGF-I receptor knockouts are more growth-retarded than IGF-I or IGF-II knockouts. IGF-I and IGF-II double null mutants are similarly extremely growth-retarded, suggesting that both IGF-I and IGF-II act via the IGF-I receptor to regulate fetal growth (see page 322).

Whether IGF-I has separate actions in its paracrine and endocrine modes will be difficult to resolve for methodological reasons, but evidence from IGF-I infusions in fetal sheep suggests that the peptide affects fetal and placental metabolism in a manner conducive to promoting fetal growth. Placental lactate production and uptake of amino acids from the fetus were inhibited, whereas placental amino acid uptake from the mother was increased. There was greater fetal glucose uptake and a reduction in fetal urea production.

This is opposite to what occurs in fetal growth retardation and suggests that circulating fetal IGF-I may be both anticatabolic and anabolic.

The IGFBPs play a particular role in determining the biological role of IGF-I and IGF-II. In the fetus, circulating concentrations of the circulating IGF-II receptor, which acts as a specific IGF-II binding protein, are very high. This may reduce the biological effects of IGF-II. IGFBP-1 and IGFBP-2 levels are relatively high and IGFBP-3 levels relatively low. The latter is the consequence of relative GH resistance *in utero*. IGFBP-1 levels are particularly high in cord blood in IUGR, perhaps as a result of lower fetal insulin levels. In turn the higher IGFBP-1 levels may affect IGF-I availability and further impede fetal growth.

IGFs are presumed to play a significant role in placental growth; the placenta is a source of IGF-I, IGF-II and several of their binding proteins (IGFBPs). In IGF gene deletion mice, IGF-II deficiency is associated with a small placenta.

IGFs do not cross the placenta but recent evidence suggests that the maternal IGF-I system may influence fetal growth indirectly. In pregnant women IGF-I concentrations correlate with birthweight, and in IUGR, maternal IGF-I concentrations are lower than normal. The administration of IGF-I to pregnant rats or mice overcomes maternal constraint on fetal growth and may, in some instances, lead to enhanced fetal and placental growth and to an alteration in the placental expression of the glucose transporter GLUT 1. Short-term IGF-I administration to pregnant ewes causes a rise in maternal and fetal blood glucose concentrations, increased placental amino acid uptake and lactate production. This has led to speculation that a high circulating maternal IGF-I could lead to increased glucose availability to the fetus, a secondary rise of fetal IGF-I and improved fetal growth. Coordinated increases in fetal and maternal IGF-I levels would optimize placental metabolism and placental amino acid transfer for fetal growth.

## Insulin

Insulin was for many years considered the dominant hormone in the regulation of fetal growth. Its presence is clearly essential for normal fetal development. In the few reported cases of *pancreatic agenesis*, birthweight is about 2000 g. This demonstrates the essential role of insulin in allowing cellular uptake of glucose and amino acids. Pathological excess of insulin may lead to fetal overgrowth as observed in the *infant of the diabetic mother*, *nesidioblastosis* and the *Beckwith–Wiedemann syndrome*. However in general this increase in weight is largely due to an increase in fat cell mass and there is only a minor effect on muscular–skeletal mass. This small anabolic effect of insulin might be due either to its ability to enhance fetal IGF-I secretion or to its weak ability to bind at high concentrations to IGF-I receptors. Within the normal physiological range of fetal substrates and insulin concentrations, it is more likely that insulin is one factor determining the influence of nutrition on IGF-I and IGFBP production rather than having a direct regulating effect on fetal growth.

## Other hormones

Pituitary GH is found in the fetal circulation from week 12 of gestation, and by midpregnancy plasma concentrations are in the 100 ng/mL range and greater than at any other time before or after birth. The fall in GH which occurs in late gestation is thought to be related to the development of tonic inhibitory tone in the hypothalamic–hypophyseal axis. Despite the abundance of GH, the hormone was not thought to be the major endocrine determinant of fetal growth because *anencephalic fetuses* characteristically have a relatively normal bodyweight. *Laron dwarfism* is a heterogenous group of autosomal recessive conditions due to a lack or dysfunction of GH receptors. The normal birthweight of such infants and those with *congenital GH deficiency* was used as an argument for the unimportance of GH in growth in prenatal life, but recent studies have shown a reduced birth length and relative obesity in such babies. In experimental models also, fetal GH deficiency is associated with reduced long bone length and lowered IGF-I levels. GH receptors have been demonstrated on a variety of fetal cells in the second trimester and experimental studies have shown that the pituitary axis is important in producing the correct number and size of cells in different organs. GH receptors develop on fetal hepatocytes at about week 30 and may be responsible for the initiation of IGFBP-3 synthesis.

The pituitary–thyroid axis operates from week 10 of gestation and fetal thyroid function is characterized by reverse triiodothyronine ($rT_3$) being secreted in excess of triiodothyronine ($T_3$), but $rT_3$ is not thought to have significance for fetal development (*see* page 483). Late in gestation $T_3$ production rises due to an effect of cortisol on hepatic deiodinase. This is important for fetal lung maturation and explains the increased incidence of *respiratory distress syndrome* in *congenital hypothyroidism*. Fetal *hypothyroidism* which may arise from a structural anomaly or inborn error of metabolism results in delayed osseous and neuronal maturation but has no significant effect on overall body length.

The fetal pituitary–adrenal axis secretes more high-molecular-weight precursors and low-molecular-weight fragments of ACTH than after birth. They may play a part in the development and function of the fetal zone of the adrenal cortex which secretes large quantities of dehydroepiandrosterone (DHA) and DHA sulfate. Glucocorticoids in the fetal circulation originate in the mother and placenta as much as from the fetal adrenal.

Cortisol is involved in the maturation of a number of important enzymes involved in tissue and organ preparation for extrauterine life. From 32 weeks the choline phosphotransferase pathway becomes increasingly important in the manufacture of pulmonary surfactant and this is under the control of cortisol in association with thyroxine, prolactin and estrogens. Cortisol is involved in the maturation of glycogen synthetase upon which the accumulation of hepatic glycogen stores depends in the last trimester. Norepinephrine is converted to epinephrine in the adrenal medulla by phenylethanolamine-N-methyl-transferase which is induced by cortisol.

The possible role of other growth factors acting in a paracrine manner in organ and tissue development is discussed in detail in Chapter 17 and on page 279.

## SELECTED READING

Gluckman, PD. Insulin-like growth factors and their binding proteins. In: Hanson MA, Spencer JAD, Rodeck CH, eds. *The fetus and neonate. Vol. 3: Growth*. Cambridge: Cambridge University Press, 1994.

Han VKM, Hill DJ. Growth factors in fetal growth. In: Thorburn GD, Harding R, eds. *Textbook of fetal physiology*. Oxford: Oxford University Press, 1994: 48.

Robinson JS, Owens JA, Owens PC. Fetal growth and fetal growth retardation. In: Thorburn GD, Harding R, eds. *Textbook of fetal physiology*. Oxford: Oxford University Press, 1994: 83.

# 21

# Pathophysiology of Intrauterine Growth Failure

Jeffrey S. Robinson and Julie A. Owens

Variations in fetal growth and development, as indicated by birthweight, are associated with altered rates of perinatal morbidity and mortality. In particular, restricted fetal growth, or a low birthweight for a given gestational age, is associated with a high rate of perinatal morbidity and mortality. Individuals of low birthweight are also more likely to develop noncommunicable adult onset diseases, such as *hypertension* and *type II diabetes*. Fetal growth restriction, traditionally described as fetal or *intrauterine growth retardation* (IUGR), is therefore a major clinical problem.

## DEFINITION AND DIAGNOSIS OF FETAL GROWTH RESTRICTION

## Indicators

Fetal growth is characterized in terms of a range of anthropometric measures of size, including birthweight, length, head width (biparietal diameter) or circumference, femur length, abdominal circumference and body proportions. Indicators of body shape are ponderal index (weight [g] × 100/length [cm]$^3$) and birthweight to length ratio. These variables are most commonly measured at birth and give cross-sectional information on individual and population growth, but some can be measured serially by ultrasound, providing indices of growth velocity for the individual before birth.

These variables reflect growth of different systems within the individual which vary in their sensitivity to factors restricting or associated with slow growth *in utero*. Length reflects growth of both axial and appendicular skeletons, and femur length that of the appendicular skeleton. Birthweight is determined by growth of skeletal muscle and fat, and to a lesser extent by growth of visceral tissues. Head width or circumference is an indicator of brain growth. Abdominal circumference reflects growth of liver and gut. Indicators of body shape mainly reflect growth of soft tissues relative to that of skeletal tissues. Skinfold thickness and mid-arm or mid-thigh circumference reflecting fat deposition and growth of muscle can usefully add to the description of birth phenotype.

## Diagnosis and definition

*Fetal growth restriction* is defined and diagnosed as a fetus or neonate falling below a defined reference range of size or weight for a particular gestational age. In functional terms, growth-restricted fetuses are defined as individuals who have been restrained from achieving their genetic potential for growth, usually by factors extrinsic to themselves. However, this definition is difficult to use since it may be difficult or impossible to determine the genetic potential for growth. Such difficulties will be compounded by the phenomenon of imprinting (*see* page 120), which recent studies have shown ascribes special significance or influence to genes derived from a particular parent in the regulation of pre- and postnatal growth.

Diagnosis of *fetal growth restriction* is made difficult also by inaccurate knowledge or assessment of gestational age, as well as variations in fetal genotype and hence intrinsic growth potential. Thus an infant of low birthweight may be inappropriately diagnosed as growth-restricted, if gestational age has been overestimated or if the infant has a genotype leading to a low drive to growth.

## ORIGINS OF GROWTH RESTRICTION

The rate and pattern of fetal growth and development are largely determined by the interaction between the fetal genome and the availability of substrates essential for growth (*see* page 284). Fetal growth restriction or the failure of an individual to achieve its genetic potential for growth often results from inadequate supply or utilization of essential substrates. The major substrates for fetal growth are $O_2$, glucose, lactate and amino acids. Other substances which are required but in lesser amounts are lipids, ketone bodies and a range of micronutrients. The mother and her environment and the placenta are the major determinants of substrate supply to the fetus.

The mother must acquire sufficient essential substrates from the environment for the needs of the developing conceptus and for her own anabolic adaptations to pregnancy. In addition, through a variety of mechanisms she must ensure adequate delivery of these substrates to the conceptus. In turn, the placenta is a major determinant of substrate availability in the fetus because of

- its role as the organ responsible for transfer of substrates between mother and fetus;
- a high metabolic rate which makes it a significant competitor for substrates with the fetus;
- placental modification of substrates;
- exchange of substrates with the fetus (*see* page 215).

In addition, the placenta produces various hormones and factors which are secreted into the mother and fetus to coordinate and influence their metabolic and physiological activities during pregnancy (*see* page 206).

Many conditions are associated with human fetal growth restriction (Table 21.1). Some are extrinsic to the developing individual and include the maternal environment, the state of the mother herself or of the placenta. Others are intrinsic – that is, originate or act from within the fetus itself. In a significant proportion of cases of fetal growth restriction there is no obvious cause.

Most extrinsic conditions restrict fetal growth by a final common pathway: that of reduced delivery of essential substrates to the fetus. These factors are characterized by physiological or pathophysiological changes resulting in reduced availability of substrates within the maternal compartment, a reduced maternal capacity to deliver substrates to the placenta or impaired placental growth and development. Such

TABLE 21.1 Factors associated with intrauterine growth failure of the fetus

*Environmental problems*
  High altitude
  Toxic substances

*Maternal behavioral conditions*
  Malnutrition
  Delivery at age <16 years
  Low pre-pregnancy weight for height
  Low maternal weight gain
  Drug use, smoking, alcohol, hard drugs
  Low socioeconomic status

*Maternal factors*
  Maternal environment/maternal constraint
  Acute or chronic hypertension
  Severe chronic disease or infection
  Anemia
  Cyanotic heart disease
  Disseminated lupus erythematosus
  Malignancy
  Uterine abnormalities
  Uterine fibroids

*Pregnancy diseases*
  Pre-eclampsia
  Antepartum hemorrhage
  Lupus obstetric syndrome

*Abnormalities of the placenta*
Reduced blood flow
  Reduced area for exchange
  Infarcts
  Hematomas
  Placenta previa
  Placenta membranacea
  Extrachorial placenta
  Circumvallate placenta

changes will reduce delivery of substrates to the fetus and potentially restrict growth. Alternatively the passage of infectious agents or toxins to the fetus may interfere with cell replication.

High altitude reduces birthweight, as does restricted nutrition, although the impact of the latter depends on the timing and duration of undernutrition as well as the specific nutrients, which are limiting (*see* pages 285 and 298). Severe undernutrition in previously well-fed women, as occurred during the famine in Holland at the end of World War II, reduces birthweight to a modest extent, but only if experienced during the third trimester. In communities where nutrition is chronically restricted, supplementation of the maternal diet, sometimes but not always, increases birthweight, indicating that maternal undernutrition is contributing to fetal growth restriction. Globally, chronic maternal undernutrition probably accounts for much fetal growth restriction. Migration to a more developed community increases birthweight in the second generation. The role of specific macronutrients has been little examined in women: high protein density in dietary supplements actually decreases birthweight, indicating that further study is a priority.

The ability of a woman to sustain normal fetal growth is inversely related to the number of fetuses present. While multiple births were once a spontaneous biological phenomenon, more recently the incidence of higher-order multiple pregnancies owes much to ovulation induction and advanced reproductive technologies.

Maternal *substance abuse* is a factor frequently associated with slow fetal growth. *Maternal drug abuse* may retard fetal growth directly as in the toxic effects of acetaldehyde on placental hormone synthesis and fetal cellular mitosis, or indirectly by reducing maternal food intake or affecting placental function. *Smoking* has a dose-related effect on fetal growth; 20 cigarettes a day reduces birthweight by 200 g. Both nicotine and carbon monoxide (CO) are toxic. Nicotine increases uterine vascular resistance and decreases blood flow leading to fetal hypoxia and hypercapnia. CO leads to tissue hypoxia in both mother and fetus by the formation of carboxyhemoglobin. CO may also bind to cytochrome and impair placental nutrient transport. Smoking interacts with others factors associated with intrauterine fetal growth failure, particularly poor socioeconomic status. In some communities it may be the major factor associated with failure of fetal growth due to poor socioeconomic circumstances. Other adverse maternal factors include underlying maternal diseases (Table 21.1), young age, maternal nutrition or specific disorders of pregnancy (e.g. *pre-eclampsia* and *antepartum hemorrhage*).

The development of a normal placenta is crucial for normal fetal growth (*see* page 202). The spiral arterioles are converted to wide-bore low-resistance vessels by an intravascular invasion of trophoblasts, that replace the media and muscular wall. Initially the vessels are plugged, which protects the embryo from adverse effects of high $O_2$ tensions. Later the plug disappears, permitting increased flow. Failure of this invasion allows the persistence of thick-walled narrow vessels. Later in gestation, unconverted vessels may suffer a third wave of trophoblast invasion, which further compromises flow. Acute atherosis or loss of the endothelium with or without thrombosis may further compromise flow. Idiopathic *fetal growth restriction* is often accompanied by failure of such changes in the development of the placenta, which closely resemble those associated with *pre-eclampsia*. Fewer maternal spiral arterioles contribute to the maternal blood supply to the placenta and most of these have failed to undergo the normal physiological changes that increase vessel diameter and reduce vascular resistance to flow. The area for exchange within the placenta is reduced. On the fetal side of the placenta, the number of tertiary stem villi and their accompanying vessels may be greatly reduced and increase resistance to blood flow, which is evident

from Doppler flow velocity waveforms recorded from the umbilical artery. Infarction or other focal lesions may further reduce the functioning mass of the placenta.

Intrinsic factors may restrict fetal growth by limiting the ability of fetal cells and tissues to utilize essential substrates, even when provided in sufficient abundance. The genetic drive to growth may be reduced by chromosomal anomalies, which are usually associated with an intrinsically slower growth of the fetus due to a reduced rate of cell division. Aneuploidy (e.g. *Turner syndrome*) may be first suspected, when early onset of disproportionate fetal growth is noted on ultrasound examination. Triploidy and trisomies (e.g. *trisomy 21*) are accompanied by slow and often abnormal growth. Confined placental mosaicism may sustain the continued survival of the trisomic fetus, when the placental chromosomal constitution is normal. When the placenta contains the abnormal mosaic cells, fetal growth restriction correlates with the proportion of mosaic cells within the placenta and is subsequently followed by catch-up growth postnatally. Other intrinsic fetal factors, which slow growth, include malformation, single gene disorders and infection. Two of the more common fetal infections restricting fetal growth are *cytomegalovirus* and *toxoplasmosis*. However, occasionally, fetal infections (e.g. parvovirus and cytomegalovirus) are accompanied by apparent fetal overgrowth, due to fetal hydrops.

## PHENOTYPE OF GROWTH RESTRICTION

## Growth velocity

Fetal growth in terms of mass or size occurs largely in the second half of gestation in mammalian species (Fig. 21.1). Placental growth in terms of mass takes place substantially in the first half of pregnancy, although extensive structural remodeling of the placenta occurs in the second half of gestation to increase functional capacity and so meet the rapidly increasing fetal demand for substrates (*see* page 285).

Fetal weight, as calculated from variables measured longitudinally by ultrasound or measured cross-sectionally, increases continuously throughout the second and third trimesters, with little change in daily weight gain near term. Ultrasound monitoring of growth shows that infants born at term, with birthweights more than 2 standard deviations below the mean, grow more slowly in late gestation and may cease growth near term. Reductions in growth velocity have also been observed in some fetuses previously growing normally, indicating the onset of growth restriction, as well as "wasting" or reduction in abdominal circumference in others. This suggests that fetal growth restriction can vary in its time of onset and severity and that slower, or even reversal of, growth is possible in the human fetus.

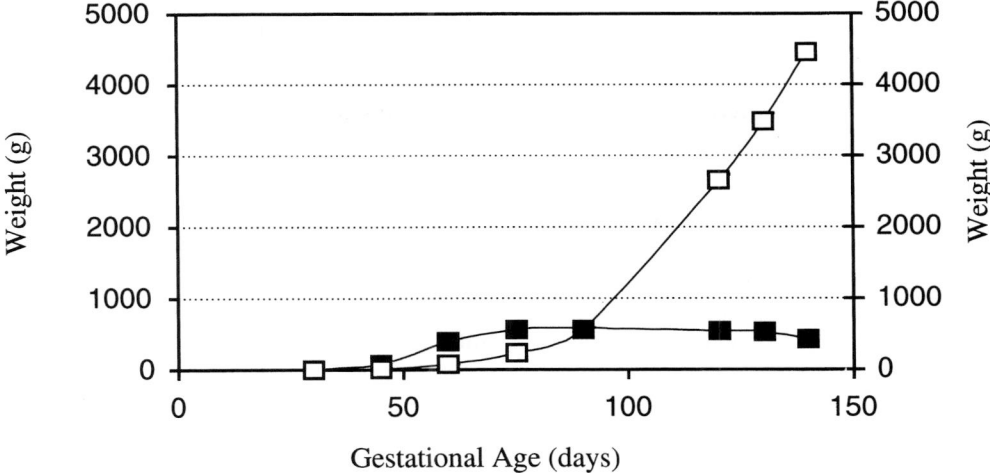

FIGURE 21.1 Ontogeny of placental and fetal growth in sheep: placental (■) and fetal (□) weight measured between days 30 and 140 of gestation (term ~150 days)

## Physical phenotype

Traditionally, two distinct patterns or phenotypes of human fetal growth restriction have been described: (a) primary growth restriction or low birthweight for gestational age with a normal ponderal index, reflecting a "symmetrical" reduction in growth, and considered to originate early in gestation; and (b) secondary fetal growth restriction, characterized by reduced birthweight and low ponderal index or "asymmetric" fetal growth restriction, considered to be of late onset. However, recent studies have found that when gestational age is accurately and independently determined, fetal growth restriction is generally disproportionate with increased length and head circumference for weight and increased variability in body proportions. Furthermore, disproportionality was just as evident at earlier gestational ages as near term and increased with the severity of the reduction in birthweight. Disproportionately or asymmetrically growth-restricted fetuses examined at autopsy have relative sparing of brain growth, while liver and lymphoid tissues are disproportionately reduced in size. They appear thin and wasted, reflecting their being relatively long for weight. Because of their malnourished appearance, the primary cause of fetal growth restriction is presumed to be restriction of the supply of essential substrates, $O_2$ and nutrients. The question as to whether human fetal growth restriction is largely disproportionate, regardless of the timing of onset, needs to be resolved, to improve diagnosis and our understanding of the causes and consequences of fetal growth restriction.

## Metabolic and endocrine phenotype

The metabolic state of the growth-restricted human fetus has been characterized directly using blood sam-

ples obtained at delivery by caesarean section and more recently, by ultrasound guided cord blood sampling (cordocentesis) before birth. Such procedures and the conditions under which they are carried out inevitably perturb the parameters under study to varying extents. In addition, many studies utilizing cordocentesis have characterized the pattern of growth of their subjects to a limited extent, relying on abdominal circumference or birthweight only, rather than body proportions. Thus some small but normally grown subjects may have been considered as growth-restricted in such studies. Cord blood sampling at delivery shows that disproportionate fetal growth restriction is characterized by perinatal hypoxemia and hypoglycemia. Cordocentesis throughout the second half of pregnancy shows that in some but not all fetuses with evidence of growth restriction, the circulating concentrations of the major substrates essential for maintenance and growth of fetal tissues, particularly $O_2$, glucose and essential amino acids, are reduced. Thus fetal hypoxia and acidosis (often a mixed acidosis with hypercapnia and lactic acidosis), hypoglycemia and reduced concentrations of essential and some non-essential amino acids are present in many growth-restricted fetuses. However, increased concentrations of triglycerides and of other non-essential amino acids, such as glycine and alanine, can also occur in growth-restricted fetuses, possibly reflecting an inability to utilize these substrates. In general, reductions in substrate abundance in the growth-restricted fetus also correlate with decreased placental perfusion or increased resistance in umbilical and uterine arteries, suggesting impaired placental function and substrate delivery is responsible.

These metabolic disturbances in the growth-restricted fetus are accompanied by various endocrine changes. The abundance of anabolic hormones and growth factors are reduced and that of inhibitory or catabolic factors increased in human fetal growth restriction. Fetal hypoinsulinemia occurs, and to a greater extent than expected from the degree of hypoglycemia present. Insulin is essential for fetal growth as it is needed to sustain cellular nutrition and by itself is capable of promoting fat deposition (*see* page 288). Reduced concentrations of insulin-like growth factor-I (IGF-I) and unchanged or decreased concentrations of IGF-II (near term) are also found in the growth-restricted fetus. The concentrations of IGF-binding proteins 1 and 2 in fetal cord blood plasma are increased in the growth-restricted fetus, while that of IGFBP-3 is decreased. The abundance of circulating IGFBP-1 can change rapidly and production is increased in response to a variety of stressful stimuli including hypoglycemia and hypoxia. This may alter the bioavailability of IGF-I.

Cortisol and noradrenaline are also increased in the small hypoxic fetus. Plasma concentrations of thyroid hormones decreased in some small fetuses and are related to the extent of fetal hypoxemia and acidemia (*see* page 484).

## OUTCOMES OF GROWTH RESTRICTION

Outcome for the growth-restricted fetus appears to vary according to phenotype, but more detailed studies are needed. Infants described as being symmetrically growth-restricted appear well-nourished and rarely show evidence of asphyxia. These infants have normal rates of perinatal morbidity and mortality, unless chromosomal abnormalities are present, but have lower than normal scores on parameters of mental development, and commonly fail to show catch-up growth. Some of these infants may be normally grown with a low genetic drive to growth.

Disproportionately growth-restricted infants have a high incidence of perinatal morbidity and mortality, including asphyxia during labor and acidosis, hypoglycemia and hypothermia after birth. The metabolic deficits noted earlier indicate that the growth-restricted fetus has little reserve in terms of substrate supply. This may be manifest on cardiotocography as decelerations in heart rate with either uterine or fetal activity, when demand for substrates such as $O_2$ exceeds their supply. Fetal distress in labor is common. Restriction of growth associated with substrate deficits, particularly of $O_2$, can cause fetal death and the risk of morbidity increases with the severity of the restriction. At autopsy, ischemic lesions have been observed in a number of organs including the brain and the heart. Fetal organs may show immaturity, in addition to restricted growth. Late in gestation, growth restriction can be associated with accelerated maturation of some organ systems and this may be reflected by a lesser need for support of the growth-restricted preterm baby in terms of lung function. However, metabolic disturbances are common and include severe hypoglycemia. After the immediate neonatal period, the growth-restricted baby frequently shows catch-up growth for the first few months and then it settles on a new growth centile. Long-term sequelae of severe fetal growth restriction include mental retardation, poor motor skills and cerebral palsy.

Recently an association between intrauterine fetal growth failure and common adult diseases, including *hypertension, coronary heart disease* and *mature onset diabetes mellitus*, has been increasingly recognized in various communities around the world. The risk for *hypertension* as an adult is increased by low birthweight and by having a large placenta relative to birthweight. Catch-up growth after birth does not alleviate this risk. In contrast, the incidences of both *coronary arterial disease* and *mature onset diabetes mellitus* are reduced by catch-up growth in the first year. These associations have been attributed to poor maternal nutrition altering fetal growth and development and there is some evidence experimentally that altering maternal nutrition restricts fetal growth and induces high blood pressure in offspring (*see also* page 302).

## MECHANISMS OF GROWTH RESTRICTION

The influence of various extrinsic and intrinsic factors on fetal growth and the mechanisms by which they can restrict fetal growth and alter outcome for the individual have been investigated experimentally in animals and help to delineate the pathways and the consequences involved in human intrauterine growth failure.

### Environmental and maternal factors

Reductions in the availability of substrates in the maternal environment restrict fetal growth. Experimental studies show clearly that either chronic maternal hypoglycemia or hypoxemia can restrict fetal growth and that the fetus and placenta appear to be most susceptible during periods of rapid growth: the first half of pregnancy for the placenta and the second half of pregnancy for the fetus.

Alterations in the capacity of the mother to adapt appropriately to pregnancy or to deliver substrates to the placenta for subsequent transfer to the fetus can restrict fetal growth. Chronic maternal hypertension, produced experimentally or occurring spontaneously in rats, restricts fetal growth, possibly in part by early restriction of placental growth.

Perturbation of the embryonic environment has substantial and long-term consequences for fetal growth and outcome. Variations in progesterone abundance during the peri-implantation period alter fetal growth and outcome: reduced progesterone abundance in mice restricts fetal growth, while progesterone supplementation in sheep increases fetal and placental growth. *In vitro* culture of sheep and cattle embryos (for longer periods than commonly used in human reproductive technology) increases fetal weight, birthweight and gestation length. In pregnancies generated through human advanced reproduction technology (*in vitro* fertilization, IVF, and gamete intrafallopian transfer, GIFT), fetal growth restriction is more common especially when the preexisting infertility is unexplained. The mechanisms involved are as yet unknown, but embryonic experience clearly influences later development.

## Placental factors

Environmental and maternal factors can restrict fetal growth in part by impairment of placental growth and development. Experimental restriction of implantation in sheep restricts placental and ultimately fetal growth. Experimental restriction of placental growth reduces placental weight and various functional characteristics, including the rates of uterine and umbilical blood flow, placental clearance of $O_2$, glucose and urea and the surface area of the exchange epithelia in late gestation (Fig. 21.2). Reduced delivery of $O_2$ and glucose to the conceptus and fetus occurs, producing chronic fetal hypoxemia and hypoglycemia (Fig. 21.3). Late in gestation, the concentrations of lactate in fetal blood increases with increasing fetal hypoxemia in the experimentally growth-restricted fetus.

Increased extraction of substrates occurs to help maintain consumption by the conceptus and fetus, but this compensatory response reduces the margin of safety between delivery and consumption (Fig. 21.3). Any increase in demand for substrates, such as occurs with increased fetal activity, or reduction in substrate delivery due for example to uterine contractures, may cause the reduced margin of safety between supply and demand to be exceeded. Continuous monitoring of $O_2$ saturation in placentally restricted fetal sheep shows evidence of such crises with transient reductions in $O_2$ saturation during fetal activity and uterine contractures. The consequences may be further altered development or damage to fetal organs and may contribute to the increased morbidity or even death *in utero* of the growth-restricted fetus. Other compensatory mechanisms are invoked when placental growth is restricted in this way, including redistribution of substrates such as $O_2$ and glucose from utilization by the placenta to the fetus (Fig. 21.4). Concomitantly, net loss of amino acids from fetus to placenta occurs, which may help sustain the placenta at further cost to fetal growth and may lead to fetal wasting (Fig. 21.4).

Experimental reduction of uteroplacental blood flow in the second half of pregnancy by a variety of methods restricts fetal growth, usually in association with fetal hypoxemia and hypoglycemia. Similarly,

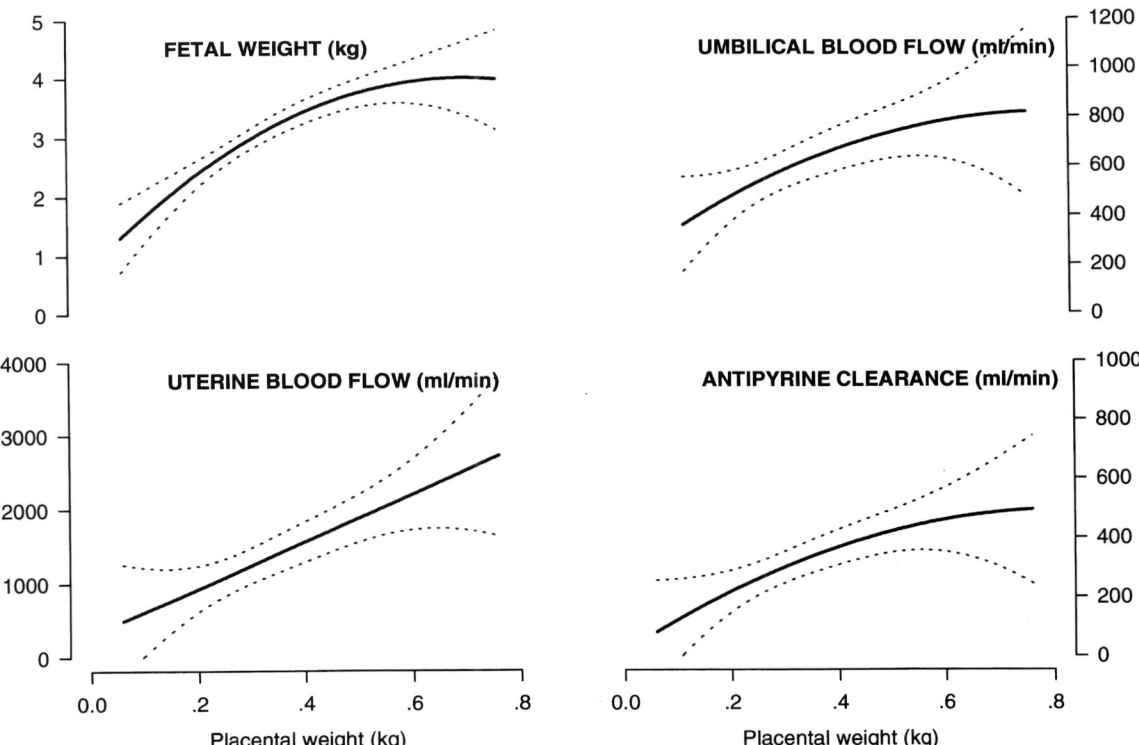

FIGURE 21.2 Relationship between function and growth in the ovine placenta in late gestation. Placental growth was restricted by surgical removal of most uterine implantation sites (carunclectomy) prior to pregnancy in some sheep. Uterine and umbilical blood flows and antipyrine clearance (an indicator of flow-determined transfer) were measured *in vivo* in sheep with indwelling vascular catheters.

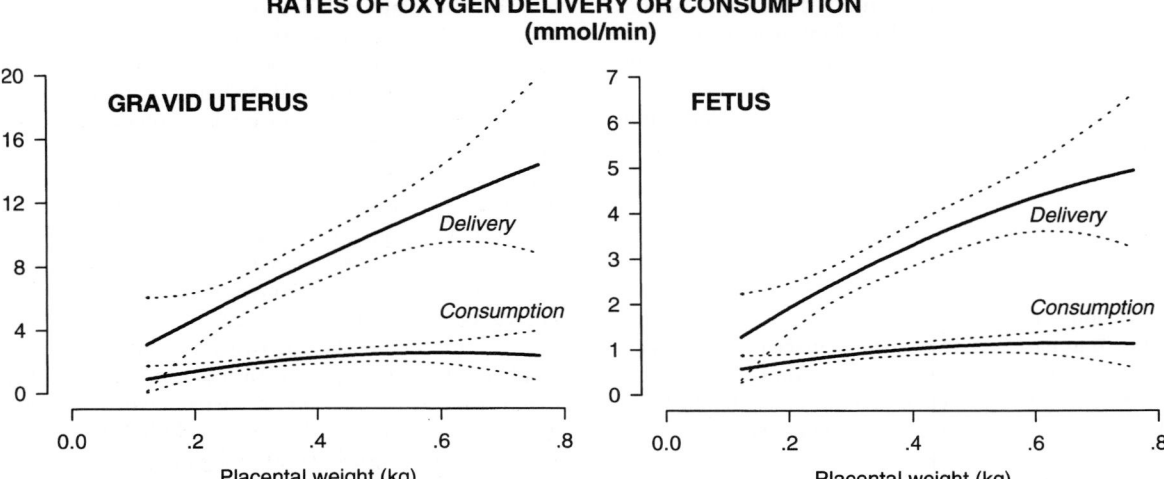

FIGURE 21.3 Effect of restricting placental growth on $O_2$ delivery to and consumption by the gravid uterus and fetus in sheep in late gestation. Placental growth was restricted as described in Figure 21.2.

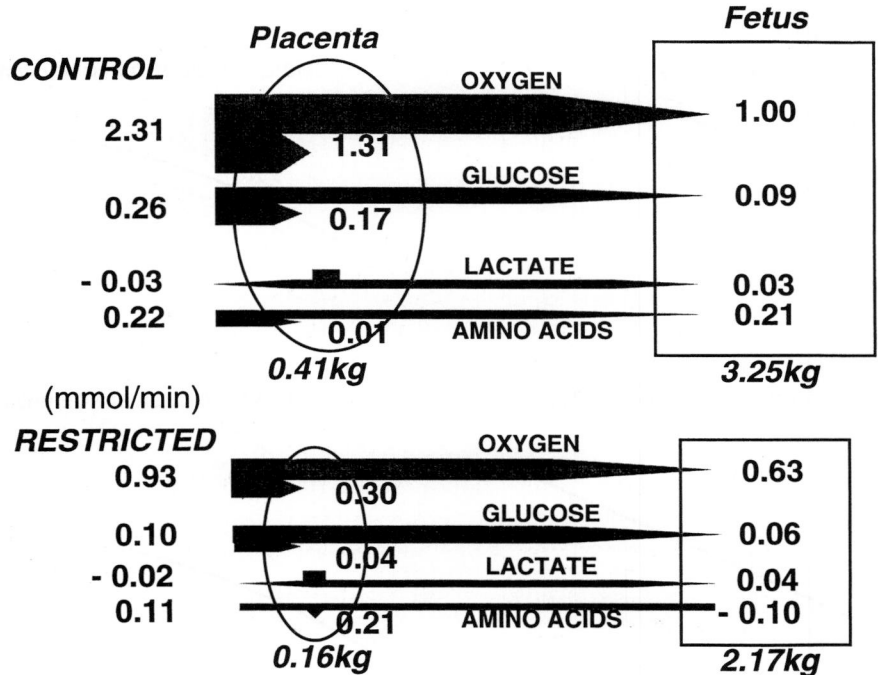

FIGURE 21.4 Partitioning of substrates between placenta and fetus: effect of restricting placental and fetal growth. Mean rates of flux of substrates in mmol/min between mother, placenta and fetus in control sheep and in sheep with restricted placental and fetal growth in late gestation are shown. Placental growth was restricted as described in Figure 21.2. Mean placental and fetal weights are shown in italics.

reduction in umbilical blood flow also reduces fetal growth, with fetal hypoxemia and hypoglycemia.

## Fetal factors

Ablation of various fetal endocrine glands has established that insulin, thyroid hormones and cortisol are essential for normal fetal growth and maturation, while gene disruption studies have established that IGF-I and -II are essential for fetal growth and IGF-II for placental growth (see page 287).

## CONSEQUENCES OF GROWTH RESTRICTION

## Metabolic and endocrine

A wide range of endocrine changes occur in the experimentally growth-restricted fetus, which substantially reflect the fetal response to perturbation of its environment, particularly changes in the supply of the essential substrates, $O_2$ and glucose. Fetal hypoxemia and hypoglycemia in the experimentally growth-restricted fetus are accompanied by reduced concentrations of the anabolic hormones, insulin, thyroid hormones and the growth factors, IGF-I and IGF-II (late in gestation). This is due to reduced production of these hormones and growth factors by fetal endocrine glands and various fetal tissues respectively and will reduce growth of a range of fetal tissues. An accelerated rise in the concentration of cortisol in fetal blood also occurs in the growth-restricted fetus in late gestation, which may enhance maturation of cortisol sensitive systems within the fetus, but induce premature delivery. Increased concentrations of catecholamines, but a delay in the ontogenic fall in the ratio of noradrenaline to adrenaline concentrations, are also observed in the growth-restricted fetus, which may contribute to redistribution of cardiac output and further inhibit insulin secretion.

## Functional

The consequences of most extrinsic experimental interventions are disproportionate fetal growth restriction, with bodyweight being reduced to a greater extent than crown–rump length. Brain weight is reduced but the ratio of brain weight relative to bodyweight is maintained or increased, while that of the liver, small intestine and lymphoid tissues are disproportionately reduced. Other organs are generally reduced in proportion to bodyweight. These changes in organ development are a consequence of alterations in the distribution of fetal cardiac output and in paracrine growth factor production. Cardiac output is redistributed preferentially to the heart, adrenals and brain; blood flow to other viscera and the carcass is reduced.

However, all organ systems studied to date show evidence of altered development, regardless of the impact of restriction on their size. For most, delayed maturation or immaturity is found. In the small intestine, wall thickness, surface area and epithelial regenerative capacity are reduced, and epithelial maturation is retarded. Development of the mucosal and submucosal layers of the fetal airways and reductions in the folding and ciliated border of the epithelial cells in the airways occurs. Neural function in the growth-retarded fetus is affected with structural evidence of altered connectivity. Neurological and neurophysiological examination in the neonate may show apparent transient precocial development (see page 390). Such changes in these and other tissues, which are essential for adaptation to postnatal life, indicate that altered functional capacity in experimental fetal growth restriction partly underlies the associated increase in morbidity and mortality observed in the perinatal period.

## SELECTED READING

Barker DJP. *Mothers, babies and diseases in later life.* London: BMJ Publishing Group, 1994.

Jones JI, Clemmons DR. Insulin-like growth factors and their binding proteins: biological actions. *Endocr Rev* 1995; 16: 3.

Owens JA, Owens PC, Robinson JS. Experimental restriction of fetal growth. In: Hanson MH, ed. *Growth.* Cambridge: University Press, 1995: 139.

Redman CWC, Sargent IL, Starkey PM, eds. *The human placenta.* Oxford, England: Blackwell Scientific Publishing.

Sharp F, Fraser RB, Milner RDG, eds. *Fetal growth. Proceedings of the Twentieth Study Group of the Royal College of Obstetricians and Gynaecologists.* London: Springer-Verlag, 1989.

Thorburn GD, Harding R, eds. *Textbook of fetal physiology.* Oxford: Oxford University Press, 1994.

Ward RHT, Smith SK, Donnai D, eds. *Early fetal growth and development.* London: RCOG Press, 1994.

# 22

# Perinatal Nutrition: the Impact on Postnatal Growth and Development

Alan A. Jackson

## INTRODUCTION

Growth is a complex process in which an increase in cell number and size leads to progressive differentiation of tissues and organs, an increase in the sophistication of their function and greater complexity of the interactions amongst systems. Because growth builds on previous experience and achievement, at any given age the shape, size and metabolic competence of an individual represents past experience and is the basis for the next phase. Normal growth is an ordered pattern of change in time at every level of organization, from the molecular to the whole organism. This blueprint, maintained as an intrinsic feature of the genome, can only be converted into reality if the nutrients which provide the energy, substrate and cofactors are available in the correct proportions and in adequate amounts, and the cell signaling mechanisms are intact. Intrauterine growth and development should enable the maturation of functions to a point where the infant can cope with the metabolic and physiological demands presented by the postnatal environment, while allowing for continued maturation, growth and development.

A metabolic demand must be met for cells and tissues to maintain function, to grow and to develop. This needs to be met by the provision of adequate amounts of energy and nutrients, in the fetus either through endogenous formation or via the placenta, at other stages in life through endogenous synthesis or from the diet. The cost of a metabolic shortfall is limitation of growth and constraint on function, which may have longer term "knock-on" effects for development.

## NUTRITIONAL RESTRICTION

The availability of energy is absolutely necessary, but not sufficient, for growth. Newborn size and body composition are determined by the energy available for intrauterine growth, and in turn determine the energy and nutrient requirements for maintenance and hence the potential ability of the infant to grow and develop in response to dietary intake and hormonal influences.

If at any stage demand for energy and nutrients exceeds supply, either because demand increases or supply is constrained, changes take place to facilitate survival, with essential functions taking priority. Brain growth and cardiovascular function have a higher priority than visceral or somatic growth. One cost of nutritional constraint is a limitation in net deposition of new tissue, which if sufficiently extensive is identifiable as growth failure. More subtle effects constrain the function of the systems which integrate metabolism. If these constraints act during critical periods of development, when a function is particularly sensitive to an adverse insult, the consequence might be a lasting effect on metabolic integration. As part of a continuous process of maturational change a constraint may, in turn, dictate both the metabolic demand for, and the handling of, energy and nutrients. Even a modest limitation of nutrient availability may influence the achieved mass and body composition, thereby compromising the maximum functional capacity for that individual (Figs. 22.1 and 22.2).

## REGULATION OF GROWTH

The fetus demonstrates a cranio-caudal gradient for development, and the brain is afforded a measure of protection from all but the most severe insults. The

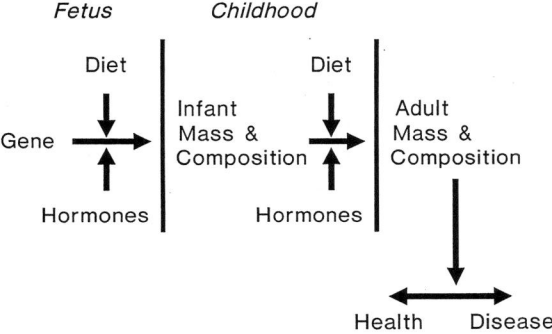

FIGURE 22.1 The interaction of body composition, hormonal profile and nutrient intake determines the growth and development in the fetus, which in turn sets the basis upon which infant and childhood growth takes place, themselves the consequence of an interaction of the same factors. In turn, adult mass and composition are dependent on fetal and childhood growth and are an important determinant of susceptibility to disease.

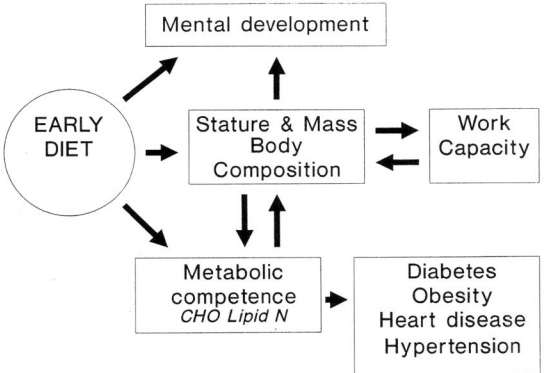

FIGURE 22.2 Achieved growth as influenced by early diet relates to the metabolic capacity of the individual (stature, mass, composition), and is an important determinant of functional competence (e.g. work capacity, mental development, metabolic competence) and susceptibility to disease

brain constitutes about 10 per cent of bodyweight, and demands a large proportion of the energy requirements throughout the first year of life. Brain size is a major determinant of head circumference. As brain growth is virtually complete by 2 years of age, the final adult head circumference is thus determined very early in life. Neuronal and glial proliferation, neuronal arborization and myelination take place in the perinatal period and are sensitive to nutrient availability. The ability to utilize long-chain polyunsaturated fatty acids for the formation of phospholipids, which comprise the membranes of cerebral neurones and supporting cells, is dependent upon maternal fatty acid profiles, the maturation of enzymes associated with fatty acid metabolism in the fetus and, postnatally, the pattern of fatty acids in the milk. The fatty acid profile of human milk has been associated with a specific pattern of phospholipids in the cerebral cortex, and improved cortical function, as measured by visually evoked responses for example. In preterm infants fed human milk there is improved developmental status at 18 months and a higher intelligence quotient later in childhood.

Linear growth failure, or stunting, is the most widely prevalent form of undernourishment in the world and has strong correlates with many indices of functional impairment, including intellectual development. The factors which affect the timing and extent of linear growth failure are major determinants of final adult stature. Although childhood stunting is very common in developing countries and amongst the poor, the differences in length are remarkably small at birth and during the first few months of life across a range of environments and cultures. Faltering in the rate of linear growth starts at about 2–3 months of age and is evident as a restriction in achieved length by 4–6 months of age. In normal Swedish infants and children, three distinct phases of postnatal linear growth have been identified: infant, childhood and pubertal, the so-called ICP model (see page 304). The overall growth curve from birth to maturity comprises these three additive and superimposed components, each of which is regulated by different growth-promoting systems. Although there is an interplay of nutrients, hormones and body composition, for each phase of growth the primary driver is different.

The infant phase of linear growth is a continuation of fetal growth, with progressive slowing to about 2 years. Whilst the size of the uterus and the supply of $O_2$ are clearly important for fetal growth, the primary driver is thought to be nutritional: the supply of substrates and cofactors act in conjunction with the two major hormonal systems, insulin and IGFs (see page 287). Growth hormone (GH) only has a limited role at this stage, but is the major driver for childhood growth in conjunction with thyroid hormone (see page 308). The exact age at which GH begins to exert a major influence upon linear growth is probably at around 6 months although the start of the childhood growth phase may not begin until 2 years. The timing of the start of the childhood phase is thought to be one of the most important determinants of the widely observed "nutritional stunting" commonly seen in children who are materially or emotionally deprived. Pubertal growth commences at around 10 or 11 years of age until adulthood with the major hormonal drive coming from sex hormones.

Any delay in the transition from infant to childhood growth will have profound effects on the attained height in subsequent years. The importance of maintaining an optimal rate of fetal–infant growth is clearly important. Timing of the initiation of the childhood growth period is related to the rate of fetal growth; as the rate of growth during infancy prior to the onset of the childhood phase is negatively related to the age of onset of the childhood phase. The rate of infant growth must result either from a lower capacity to grow in terms of attained size (small babies grow more slowly), an inadequate energy and/or nutrient intake or availability in relation to the demand, altered endocrine regulation, or a combination of all three factors. The effect of constraints on growth during each of the three phases tends to be additive: limited fetal–infant growth exerts a limitation on childhood growth, which in turn will tend to impair pubertal growth. Supplementation of energy and nutrient intake in children during infancy and early life shows clear benefits on size, work performance and psychological development during adulthood.

Weight, both absolute and relative to stature, is determined by the amounts and proportions of lean and adipose tissue, which in turn characterize metabolic and functional capacity. The rate of linear growth in the fetus is maximal at 16–22 weeks' gestation, whereas the rate of net protein deposition tends to be maximal at around 32 weeks with fat deposition in adipose tissue as a feature of the final weeks of pregnancy. Both lean and adipose tissue deposition may be sensitive to maternal nutritional status, but the details are not clear.

The extent to which catch-up growth can occur postnatally in those infants in whom there has been an intrauterine limitation of growth is important. The potential for catch-up growth is variable from infant to infant, but probably is determined by the nature of the insult which caused the limitation, its timing and duration. It is easier to replete deficits in adipose than in lean tissue, in weight than in length, and in length than in head circumference. The ability to catch-up will be limited by any lost potential for cellular hyperplasia and will require a pattern of energy and nutrient delivery appropriate for the metabolic needs of the infant at that time, taking into account the relative pattern and hierarchy of functional demands. Our knowledge of the pattern of specific nutrients needed to enable different patterns of growth, against the hormonal milieu which drives net tissue deposition, and the maturation of pathways for the endogenous formation of key nutrients, is not sufficient to know the extent to which it is potentially possible to completely reverse *intrauterine growth retardation* by enabling postnatal catch-up growth.

## MATERNAL NUTRITIONAL EFFECTS

Much of the evidence which relates fetal growth directly to aspects of maternal nutrition comes from animal studies, and it has been difficult to obtain unequivocal human data. The effects of severe specific nutrient deficiencies may be dramatic and obvious, e.g. *cretinism, vitamin A* or *folate deficiency*. It has been more difficult to identify the metabolic and dietary requirements for individual nutrients at each stage of pregnancy. Small changes over long periods of time are difficult to discern against the buffering effect of maternal nutritional status. Animal studies reinforce the idea that the maternal organism "prepares" by laying down a reserve of energy and nutrients in anticipation of a later demand. The reserve might be laid down before conception or during the early part of pregnancy itself. The nutritional state, and body composition, of a woman at the time she enters pregnancy are at least as important as her nutrient intake during the course of pregnancy itself for the growth of the fetus. The early plane of fetal nutrition and growth are in large part determined by the nutritional state of the mother around the time of conception. Thus the mother provides a buffer, or nutrient reserve, which may also play an important role in the endogenous formation of those nutrients for which the demand might be particularly high. Taller, heavier women have larger babies.

Natural experiments of extreme deprivation, such as the Dutch hunger winter (1944–45) and chronic or seasonal limitations in food availability in developing countries, have provided much of our understanding of the effects of nutrition on the outcome of pregnancy (*see also* page 285). These experiences emphasize the remarkable buffering ability of maternal tissues. In general, severe maternal food deprivation around the time of conception has the most marked influence upon linear growth, morbidity and mortality, whereas nutritional constraints later in gestation tend to be associated with relative wasting of adipose and lean tissues which is more easily reversed during postnatal catch-up weight gain. The effects of food deprivation can be ameliorated or reversed by maternal supplementation during pregnancy, leading to increases in birthweight. However, the balance of nutrient availability is critical: supplements which contain a high density of protein (more than 20 per cent of energy derived from protein, compared with 12–15 per cent in most normal diets) have a detrimental effect on the infant.

In primiparous women, who tend to be lighter at the start of pregnancy, an increase in maternal intake and weight gain is more obvious and an important determinant of fetal growth. Multiparous women tend to be heavier at the start of pregnancy and are better able to support fetal growth from their endogenous reserves.

During embryogenesis, quantitative requirements are relatively small. However, the embryo may be exquisitely sensitive to the provision of certain metabolites, as shown by the sensitivity of closure of the neural tube to maternal folate status, indicative of a high demand for methyl group metabolism during growth and development. The fetal pattern of nutrient demand varies in detail at each stage of gestation. The factors established as contributing to *intrauterine growth retardation* and amenable to modification in developed countries are prepregnancy weight, gestational weight gain, caloric intake, along with young maternal age, maternal education and cigarette smoking. In developing countries, *malaria* is added to the list. A number of studies carried out under very different conditions show that, for women in a marginal or deficient nutritional state, supplementation during pregnancy confers definite long-term benefits, both for physical growth and psychomotor function in the offspring.

## NUTRITION AND PERINATAL GROWTH

As the fetal and infant phases of growth are continuous aspects of the same process, birth acts as a temporary interruption. For term infants the transition from nutrition through the placenta to an established oral intake of breast milk requires a period of catch-up weight gain which returns the growth trajectory of the infant to that established during late fetal life. Postnatal constraints operate against this established pattern of growth.

All nutrients reach the fetus through the placenta (*see* Chapter 13). Placental size is indicative of placental capacity and in general relates directly to fetal growth. The placenta operates as a highly selective barrier between the maternal circulation and the fetus for transfer in both directions. In addition the placenta is metabolically active, modulating the pattern of nutrients available to fetal metabolism. There are situations where the placenta appears inappropriately large relative to the fetus, such as in women living at altitude or women with anemia. These examples suggest that the capacity of the placenta, either for transport or metabolic activity, is not always adequate for the demands of the fetus.

## Glucose and amino acids

Even though the embryo and fetus utilize glucose as the preferred source of energy, oxidation of amino acids provides a significant proportion of fetal energy requirements. The availability of glucose to the fetus is determined by maternal glucose concentration and the efficiency of placental glucose transport (*see* Chapter 13). Under normal circumstances the availability of glucose appears limiting, as over one-third of fetal energy requirements are satisfied by the oxidation of amino acids. When glucose availability is

obviously constrained, although protein synthesis appears to be protected, amino acids derived from protein degradation are oxidized at increased rates; hence, net protein deposition is decreased and the rate of fetal growth slowed. Increased amino acid oxidation is associated with an increased rate of urea formation, which passes readily across the placenta for excretion by the mother. After birth, amino acid oxidation and urea formation continue at a similar rate and the need to handle large amounts of urea persists (see below).

Based upon supplementation studies and estimates of the net accretion of amino acids and protein by the fetus, there is no evidence that the relative availability of essential amino acids from the mother is likely to constrain fetal or newborn growth. Indeed, any constraint is more likely to be within the endogenous formation of non-essential amino acids (especially for non-protein metabolic pathways), either through maternal, placental or fetal synthesis.

There are at least two quantitatively large amino acid cycles of functional importance between the placenta and fetus: glutamate/glutamine and glycine/serine, the details of which remain to be elucidated (*see also* page 286). Glutamine is of interest because of its importance for replicating cells, with a role in nucleotide formation and polyamine metabolism. Serine and glycine, also involved in nucleotide formation, are critical as the major source of 1-carbon groups for methylation reactions. In the close-to-term fetus, the metabolic demands for cysteine are relatively low and the pathways for cysteine formation have not yet matured. This ensures preferential re-methylation of homocysteine to methionine, utilizing a methyl group derived from serine, brought into metabolism by folate and vitamin $B_{12}$. As the carbon skeleton of serine is used for the formation of cysteine, a reduction in competitive demand through the pathway for cysteine formation increases the availability of serine either for methyl group generation, for glycine synthesis, or the formation of phosphatidyl serine. The availability of methyl groups from serine potentially conserves methyl groups from choline for the formation of phosphatidyl choline. Cell membrane formation, neural development and surfactant formation in the lungs are critically dependent upon adequate endogenous formation of phospholipids. At the same time, the generation of glycine makes a contribution to the competitive metabolic demands for increased formation of heme and collagen towards term.

Important metabolic functions of cysteine include being an integral component of cellular glutathione, thereby playing a central role in cellular antioxidant defenses, and participating in the excretion of xenobiotics as conjugates in the form of mercaptans. Both of these functions are limited during intrauterine life, but take on a more important role after birth once respiration and a dietary intake have been established.

The sequence and timing of the maturation of metabolic pathways related to amino acid metabolism around birth reflects shifting metabolic demands and exerts an important influence upon the dietary needs – reflected in the composition of human milk.

## The transition to postnatal nutrition

The pattern and nature of functional demand changes substantially at birth. Homeostasis has to be maintained and brain function is protected, while there is a shift from "intravenous" to oral food intake, and the presentation of $O_2$ through the lungs introduces new demands related to respiratory, gastrointestinal and liver function. The lungs and gastrointestinal tract, along with the skin, have to become effective physical barriers, which increases the nutrient demand for cell turnover, and immune and inflammatory function. Increased oxidizable substrate requires the maturation of the systems which protect against oxidative and free radical induced damage. The nutrient requirements for these functions are potentially competitive with the demands for growth. During the last weeks of pregnancy, the fetus lays down stores of nutrients, such as copper, iron, zinc and vitamin A, to be called on in the postnatal period. Subcutaneous adipose tissue acts as an insulation to conserve energy as well as providing energy directly, as the pattern of oxidizable substrate shifts from total dependence on glucose and amino acids. These functions are compromised in the preterm infant, and therefore preterm infants demand a different pattern of nutrients. Providing a more appropriate pattern of nutrients benefits growth, motor and psychological development at later ages.

The postnatal diet is high in fat as triacylglycerol, and contains many complex molecules which have to be digested before the nutrients can be presented for metabolic refinement through the liver to the rest of the body. The development of a metabolically active colonic flora participates in this metabolic interchange. For example, a high rate of amino acid oxidation continues for some time after birth, until fatty acid oxidation becomes established. If the urea produced were to be excreted by the kidney, the water requirements for urine formation would increase three- to four-fold. The alternative fate is for the urea to pass to the colon where it is hydrolysed by the micro flora, with the synthesis of amino acids (both non-essential and essential) which are of direct use to the host (see page 137). Bacterial synthesis of both fat- and water-soluble vitamins, e.g. vitamin K, play a critical role in the overall development of postnatal metabolic competence.

## FUNCTIONAL CONSEQUENCES OF IMPAIRED PERINATAL GROWTH

The timing of the physical development of tissues, and the maturation of processes in and around birth, is critical if functional development is to be integrated effectively. Although there is a reserve capacity for most functions, any compromise can be a constraint on function under conditions of stress. Cognitive function and psychomotor development can be impaired by nutrient limitation at any time during pregnancy until 5 years of age. Altered patterns of brain development give rise to functional changes in the CNS which result in a poorer quality of environmental interaction and exploration. Limitations of stature and muscularity directly impair work capacity, through a reduction in strength and work output over time. Muscle composition is modified with an increase in fast glycolytic fibers (Type IIa), in preference to slow oxidative fibers (Type I). Both the amount and composition of the fibers influences the functional and metabolic capacity. Through an effect upon type and amount of habitual physical activity, muscle composition modulates body composition and metabolic competence in terms of energy and substrate metabolism. The metabolic handling of dietary substrate in later life can be explained through differences in mass and composition, especially in terms of organ size and relative proportions of muscle to viscera. For example, whether an oral load of carbohydrate is either oxidized or stored (leanness compared with *obesity* and *diabetes mellitus*), is probably dependent on the relative proportions of lean body mass to adipose tissue, skeletal muscle to viscera and the relative proportions of slow to fast skeletal muscle fibers. The differing patterns of body composition are directly related to different patterns of energy expenditure and food choice. Small children become small adults with limited physical and intellectual competence and enhanced susceptibility to infections and chronic disease.

Since 1986, Barker and colleagues, using epidemiological evidence, have defined a close association between growth of the fetus and infant with the risk of developing *coronary heart disease*, *maturity onset diabetes mellitus*, *hypertension* and *chronic lung disease* during adult life. Birthweight and growth during the first year were shown to be significantly related to *coronary vascular disease*, with a two- to three-fold increased risk of death in adult men who at birth weighed 2.3 kg and by 1 year of age were 7.4 kg, compared with those with a birthweight of 4.6 kg who were 12.9 kg at 1 year. Later studies have emphasized that disproportionate growth carries a much higher risk, whether the disproportion is between the fetus and the placenta, or for the relative proportions of fetal head circumference, length and weight. Thus compromised nutrient delivery to the fetus, during critical periods of growth of individual tissues and organs, affects the size of individual tissues and also the maturation of metabolic competence, thereby permanently changing, or "programming," the metabolic function of the tissues. Small size at birth, or disproportion between head size, length and weight, represent differential effects on tissues related to the timing at which the insult occurred. Hence, although the prevalence of *non-insulin dependent diabetes mellitus* and impaired glucose tolerance in men aged 59–70 years increases from 14 per cent in those born weighing more than 4 kg to 40 per cent in those born weighing less than 2.5 kg, the risk of insulin resistance is greatly increased in those born thin. Thin neonates lack fat and muscle, the main site of the peripheral action of insulin. Relative insulin resistance can be demonstrated as early as 4 years of age in children who were thin as newborns. At 10 years of age the children of mothers who have limited fat reserves are more likely to have raised blood pressure. Thus metabolic competence and function in the child can be related to maternal nutritional status, fetal growth, and proportionate fetal growth. The human findings can be replicated in animal studies which show that manipulations of maternal nutritional state can have widespread, but specific, effects on the offspring. There is a close interrelationship between maternal body composition, nutrient intake and endocrine function which together influence placental function and the hormonal/metabolic programming of the developing fetus.

The observed changes fit in with a general model of development in which the ability of a tissue or organ to achieve maximum functional capacity is a central consideration (Fig. 22.3). The functional capacity of any metabolic step, process, tissue or organ is the maximum ability to carry out a function which defines the upper limit of metabolic capability. Growth represents an increase in functional capacity. On a normal day-to-day basis, the extent to which the maximum capacity is called upon varies, but for most functions the operating demand is well within the maximum capacity and there is a significant reserve capacity. In individuals who achieve a reduced maximum capacity because of earlier constraints on growth, the reserve capacity is proportionately smaller and the individual is less able to accommodate an increased demand, or stress for that function: i.e. with respect to that function,

"programming" represents a reduced maximum capacity. With normal aging there is a reduction in the functional capacity of all cells, and hence all functions, tissues and organs. At a critical threshold, the falling metabolic capacity is no longer able to maintain normal function (e.g. glucose disposal) and an identified pathology or disease condition becomes evident (e.g. *diabetes mellitus*). Those with a limitation in the maximal capacity, through a constraint during early growth, are more likely to reach the critical threshold at an earlier age. Therefore an appropriate nutrient intake relates not only to the demand set by the genomic potential for growth, but also to the metabolic capacity to handle the energy and nutrients taken in to drive that growth. Early constraints on growth lead to a reduced metabolic capacity, which in turn limits the ability to handle the generous availability of food at all later stages. An intake of energy and nutrients which consistently exceeds the metabolic capacity generates a metabolic stress, and disease supervenes.

## SELECTED READING

Barker DJP. *Mothers, babies, and disease in later life*. London: BMJ Publishing Group, 1994.

Institute of Medicine (US). Subcommittee on Nutritional Status and Weight Gain During Pregnancy. *Nutrition during pregnancy*. Washington, DC: National Academy Press, 1990.

Jackson AA, Wootton SA. The energy requirements of growth and catch-up growth. In: Scrimshaw NS, Schurch B, eds. *Activity, energy expenditure and energy requirements of infants and children*. Lausanne, Switzerland: IDECG, 1990: 185.

Kramer MS. Determinants of low birth weight: methodological assessment and meta-analysis. *Bulletin WHO* 1987; 65: 663.

Martorell R, Scrimshaw NS. The effects of improved nutrition in early childhood: the Institute of Nutrition of Central America and Panama (INCAP) follow-up study. *J Nutr* 1995; Suppl 4S: 125.

Rush D. Effects of changes in maternal energy and protein intake during pregnancy, with special reference to fetal growth. In: Sharp F, Fraser RB, Milner RDG, eds. *Fetal growth*. London: Springer-Verlag, 1989: 203.

Uauy R, Alvear J. Effects of protein–energy interactions on growth. In: Scrimshaw NS, Schurch B, eds. *Protein–energy interactions*. Lausanne, Switzerland: IDECG, 1992: 151.

Waterlow JC, Schurch B. Causes and mechanisms of linear growth retardation. Proceedings of an IDECG workshop. *Euro J Clin Nutr* 1994; 48: Suppl 1:S1.

Wootton SA, Jackson AA. Influence of under-nutrition in early life on growth, body composition and metabolic competence. In: Henry CJ, ed. *Early environment and later outcomes*. Society for the Study of Human Biology, Symposium. Cambridge: Cambridge University Press, 1995.

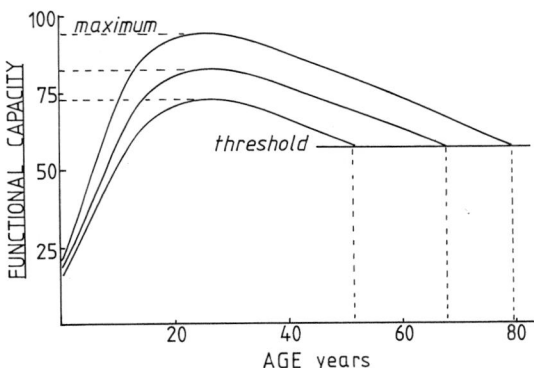

FIGURE 22.3 The maximum functional capacity achieved in adulthood, and the rate of its decline with aging towards a critical threshold below which disease supervenes, is determined by the extent to which the potential for functional capacity is set by tissue and organ growth during early life

# Postnatal Growth

# AN OVERVIEW

Postnatal growth is influenced by complex interactions between genetic, environmental and hormonal factors. The exact mechanisms of the interaction of these factors on growth are not yet fully understood.

## NORMAL GROWTH PATTERNS

Mean birth length at term is approximately $48 \pm 2$ cm, and adult height approximately $176 \pm 6$ cm for men and $164 \pm 6$ cm for women, generally achieved by the ages of 18 and 16 years, respectively. During this growth period, the linear growth rate is uneven. Postnatal linear growth is most rapid immediately after birth, falls rapidly until around 4 years, and gradually declines toward a nadir just before the onset of the pubertal growth spurt. At puberty, a rapid increase in growth rate occurs with a mean peak height velocity of approximately 10 cm/year in boys and 8 cm/year in girls.

Karlberg proposed the Infancy–Childhood–Pubertal (ICP) growth model to analyze postnatal human growth into three components: the rapid but rapidly decelerating growth of infancy, the more steady growth rate of the childhood period, and the growth spurt associated with puberty (Fig. 23.1). One extreme simplification is that growth in the infancy phase primarily depends on nutrition, growth hormone and thyroid hormone, growth in the childhood phase on growth hormone, and growth in the puberty phase on sex hormones.

Weight gain velocity almost parallels linear growth velocity. However, the proportions of the head, trunk, and legs differ with age. The head, which is big in infancy, becomes proportionately smaller, and the legs, which are small in infancy, become proportionately larger with age. The upper to lower body segment ratio falls from approximately 1.7 at birth to 1.0 in the female and 0.9 in the male adult.

There is no difference in average adult height among early-, normal- and late-maturing children. However, the timing of puberty influences the peak height velocity. Although height at onset of puberty is less in early-maturing children than in late-maturing children, the height difference at the onset of puberty is compensated for by the difference in the pubertal height gain. Thus early-maturing children show a higher peak height velocity than late-maturing children and the pubertal height gain is greater in early-maturing children than in late-maturing children. Therefore, early-, normal- and late-maturing children attain the same adult height on average (Fig. 23.2). However, prepubertal height at 6 years of age is greater in early-maturing children than late-maturing children. When the difference in height at 6 years is adjusted by selecting the children with the same height at 6 years, there is a significant positive correlation between age at peak height velocity and adult height. Therefore, when prepubertal height is the same, the later pubertal maturation occurs, the taller the adult height achieved (Fig. 23.3).

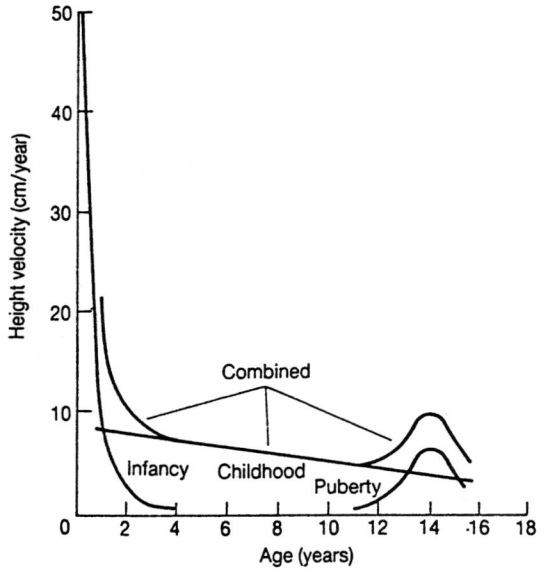

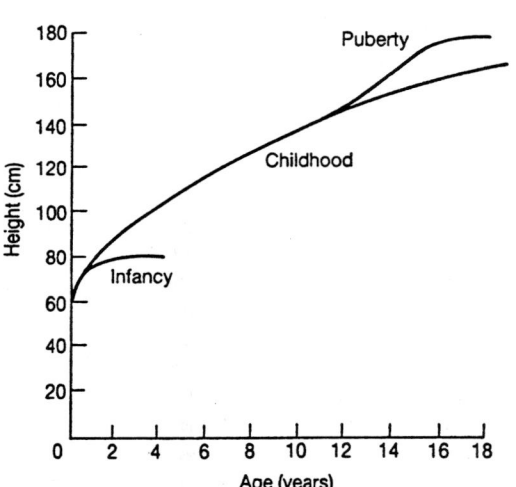

FIGURE 23.1 The Infancy–Childhood–Pubertal growth model of Karlberg, shown here for boys. Upper: the mean values for height velocity for each component (infancy, childhood, puberty) and their sum (combined velocity). Lower: the model for attained height (50th centile shown). (Reproduced with permission. © 1987 J. Karlberg.)

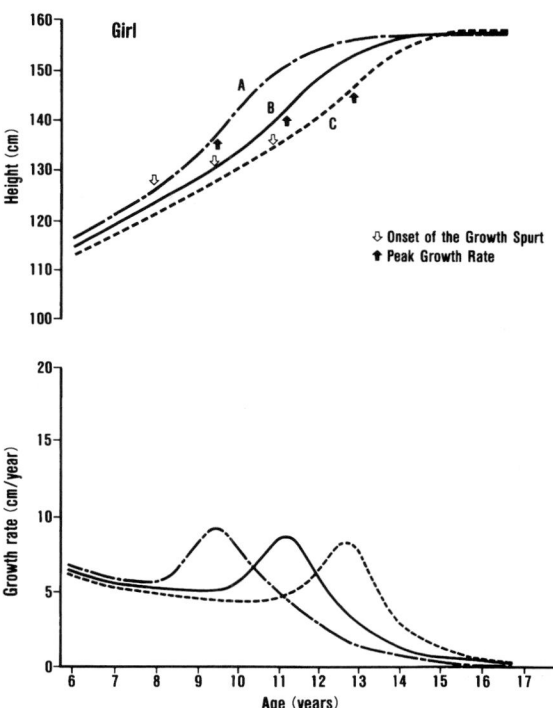

FIGURE 23.2 Upper: the mean growth curves, shown here for girls, of early-maturing children (A), average maturing children (B), and late-maturing children (C). There is no difference in mean final height. Lower: the mean growth curves of early-, average- and late-maturing children.

Organ and tissue growth in general parallel skeletal growth, with some notable exceptions. The eyes and brain are highly developed at birth and attain most of their adult size within the first few years of life. Lymphoid tissue mass increases throughout childhood, reaching a maximum just before puberty, and then declines throughout adult life. Reproductive tissues are relatively undeveloped until the onset of puberty when they grow rapidly and attain mature size within a few years.

## FACTORS INFLUENCING GROWTH

### Ethnic and genetic influences

There is a significant difference in size, body proportions, and timing of puberty among different races. Thus growth standards used should be appropriate for the population. Europeans are taller than Asians. Among Americans, African-Americans are taller than Americans of European ancestry. Even in *Turner syndrome*, the average adult height is shorter in Japanese Turner women than in European Turner women. Body proportions differ between racial groups; for example, Africans have longer legs than Caucasians. It has become apparent that bone maturation and pubertal development occur earlier in Japanese children than in British children. It is assumed that these racial differences in growth and pubertal onset are polygenic traits and that the timing of puberty influences the adult height.

Sexual differences in growth are well known. Male fetuses have a slightly higher average birthweight than female fetuses. Growth during infancy and childhood is not significantly different between the sexes, although boys are slightly taller than girls on average. The timing of puberty is 2 years earlier in girls than in

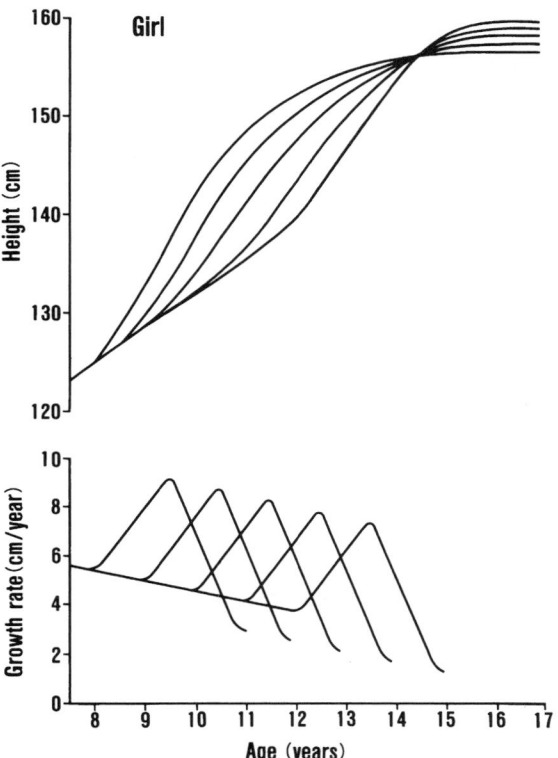

FIGURE 23.3 Schematic growth curves at peak velocity of groups of different ages at peak height velocity who had the same height before puberty. The later pubertal maturation occurs, the taller the final height achieved.

boys, and the peak height velocity is greater in boys than in girls. Therefore, both the height difference at onset of puberty (8–10 cm) and the difference in pubertal growth (3–5 cm) contribute to the adult height difference of approximately 13 cm between males and females.

There is a tendency for children of tall parents to become tall adults and children of short parents to become short adults. Quantitative characteristics such as height and weight are assumed to be polygenic traits. The correlation coefficient of height between parents and child has been reported to be 0.33, between siblings 0.38, between mid-parent height and child 0.65, between monozygotic twins 0.61 and between dizygotic twins 0.51. If height is determined only by genetic influences, the correlation coefficient between one of the parents and their child should be 0.5. Similarly there is a significant genetic component to the timing of pubertal maturation. Monozygotic twins have a higher correlation of age at menarche ($r=0.93$) than dizygotic twins ($r=0.62$). Thus genetic factors are the dominant determinant of adult height. Non-genetic factors such as intrauterine conditions, postnatal nutrition, and the endocrine milieu have a lesser effect.

Sex chromosome aberrations have significant effects on structural changes. It is well known that girls with *Turner syndrome* tend to be born small for dates and achieve short adult height. Average adult height in *XX males* is lower and in *Klinefelter syndrome* (47 XXY) is greater than the male standard; *47 XYY* syndrome individuals are even taller (Fig. 23.4). A pseudoautosomal growth gene, an X-specific growth gene, and a Y-specific growth gene are postulated to exist. Autosomal aberrations, such as *Down syndrome, 13 trisomy, 18 trisomy, 4p-syndrome*, and *cri du chat syndrome*, also manifest growth failure as well as mental retardation and multiple anomalies.

Specific genetic defects also affect skeletal growth and stature, directly and indirectly. Point mutation and deletions of the human growth hormone (hGH) gene are found in *isolated GH deficiency type 1A*, which manifests severe growth failure. *Laron syndrome*, also showing severe growth failure, is due to GH receptor gene abnormalities. A point mutation of the fibroblast growth factor receptor type-3 gene recently has been recognized in *achondroplasia*, which shows a short-limb-type growth failure. Many inborn errors of metabolism and organ system diseases may also affect growth indirectly, for example *cystic fibrosis*.

There are many syndromes, such as *Dubowitz syndrome, Seckel syndrome, Bloom syndrome, Smith–Lemli–Opitz syndrome, Cornelia de Lange syndrome*, and *Rubinstein–Taybi syndrome*, which show growth failure. Some are autosomal traits, but most are of unknown etiology. The mechanism of growth failure is not understood in these syndromes.

## Environment and nutrition

The most important environmental factor that influences growth is nutrition. Undernutrition during infancy and childhood leads not only to growth failure but also to retardation of brain development and decreased immunological response to infection. Because of malnutrition, underdeveloped countries with food shortages show an increased rate of low-birthweight children and an increased death rate of infants by infection. Malnourished children show a decreased growth rate, delayed bone age, delayed puberty and short adult height. Children who have been malnourished *in utero* or in infancy may subsequently show catch-up growth with adequate nutrition; however only 60 per cent of them do, and the occurrence of catch-up growth relates to the duration, severity, and timing of malnutrition. The mechanism of catch-up growth is not yet clarified. Most short children without GH deficiency are already short at 2 or 3 years of age. Since these children often show poor appetite, growth during infancy seems in part to depend on nutrition.

Nutritional status interacts with the endocrine regulation of growth. Indeed, the somatotropic axis can be viewed as the mediator of the interaction between

Height (cm)

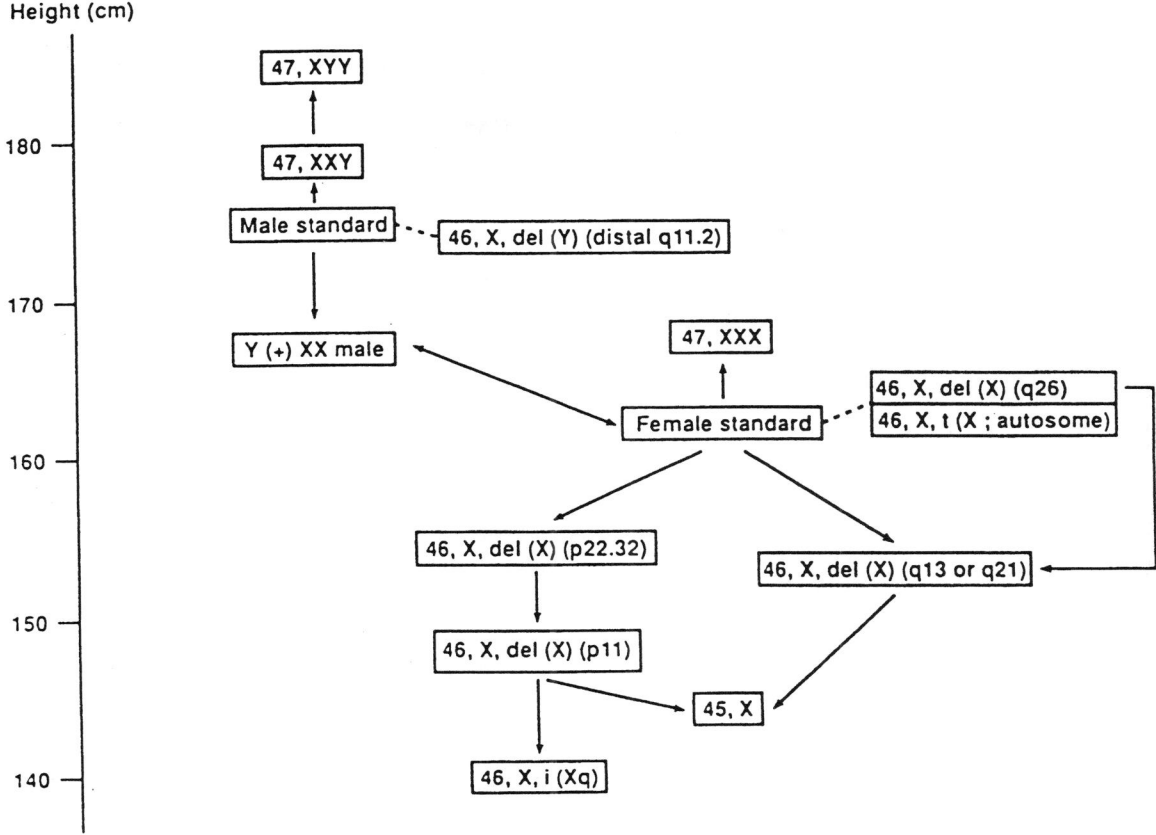

FIGURE 23.4 The distribution of mean adult heights in Caucasian patients with sex chromosome aberrations. The height differences designated by arrows are statistically significant by the two-tailed *t*-test, whereas no significant difference is found for the height differences indicated by dotted lines. (Derived from Ogata and Matsuo, *Hum Genet* 1993; **91**: 551.)

the genetic drive to grow and environmental factors such as nutrition. Severe undernutrition is associated with increased mean serum GH concentrations and increased GH pulse amplitude. Serum IGF-I concentrations, however, are decreased by undernutrition, and experimentally this has been demonstrated to be associated with down-regulation of the number of tissue GH receptors and with post-receptor resistance. Since IGF-I has been implicated as an anticatabolic hormone, this may be an adaptive response allowing preferential utilization of mobilized substrates to maintain homeostasis rather than for cell growth or proliferation.

A secular trend typically seen in Japan after World War II reveals an increased average male adult height from approximately 165 cm to 170 cm and average female adult height from approximately 153 cm to 158 cm in the space of 20 years. Average menarcheal age was 14.2 years in 1945 and 12.5 years in 1977. The age at peak height velocity in boys and girls was at 14.61 years and 12.70 years in 1949, and at 13.06 years and 10.98 years in 1969. This secular trend in Japan is believed to be influenced mainly by nutrition.

With overnutrition, children become obese and show an increased growth rate, slightly earlier pubertal

development, and slightly shorter adult height on average.

Other environmental factors, such as disease prevalence, socioeconomic class, physical activity, and emotional well-being, also influence growth. The *deprivation syndrome* associated with severe growth failure is accompanied by low spontaneous GH secretion. In general the endocrine abnormalities and growth are normalized by return to a healthy environment.

## HORMONAL REGULATION OF GROWTH

The essential event in growth is the proliferation of chondrocytes in the growth plate (*see* page 312), which is finally regulated by growth factors and hormones. Many hormones and growth factors, such as GH, IGF-I, thyroxine, sex steroids, and corticosteroids, are known to influence growth. Many other growth factors, such as epidermal growth factor and fibroblast growth factor, seem to act as local growth factors through autocrine and paracrine mechanisms, but the exact mechanisms are poorly understood.

## Growth hormone and IGF-I

It is well known that GH is an essential hormone for growth (*see* pages 309 and 471). GH secretion increases during puberty. Urinary GH and IGF-I concentrations change in parallel with the pubertal change in growth velocity in both males and females. *Isolated GH deficiency type 1A* and *Laron syndrome* show severe growth failure. Infants with *GH deficiency* diagnosed before the age of two years show a subtly reduced birth length and dramatic early postnatal growth failure. Therefore, growth hormone is necessary for normal growth, not only in childhood and puberty, but also from early infancy.

## Thyroid hormone

Patients with untreated *congenital hypothyroidism* manifest severe postnatal growth failure with epiphyseal dysgenesis and severe mental retardation. Thyroid hormone plays a major role in postnatal growth through influencing cartilage growth and ossification and in neurological development. Growth failure in hypothyroidism is in part mediated by secondary failure of growth hormone secretion. *Acquired hypothyroidism* manifests itself by growth retardation, bone age retardation, and sexual abnormality, such as delayed puberty or more rarely to precocious puberty. The latter may be due to hormonal overlap and increased hypothalamic TRH release acting with a degree of overlap on the gonadotrope.

Hyperthyroidism usually induces a mild acceleration of growth.

## Insulin

Insulin is an important factor in fetal life since *infants of diabetic mothers* are large (macrosomic) and patients with *leprechaunism* (insulin resistance) are small at birth. The fact that patients with *leprechaunism* and with inadequately treated *insulin-dependent diabetes mellitus* manifest growth retardation postnatally (*Mauriac syndrome*) also indicates the importance of insulin for postnatal growth. Some of the postnatal effects of insulin on growth appear to be mediated by insulin regulating GH receptor levels, sensitivity to GH and thus IGF-I release.

## Glucocorticoids

Glucocorticoids are essential to maintain homeostasis. Untreated *congenital adrenal hyperplasia* causes failure to thrive and leads to shock in severe cases. Overproduction of glucocorticoids, such as *Cushing syndrome*, shows deceleration of linear growth and obesity. *Nephrotic syndrome* and *chronic inflammatory disease* treated with high doses of glucocorticoids also show growth failure. Increased secretion or overdose of glucocorticoids seems to inhibit the action and expression of growth factors at the growth plate.

## Sex steroids

The main gonadal steroids in the male are testosterone and dihydrotestosterone and in the female, estrogens. Although gonadal steroids show high concentrations in serum in early infancy in both male and female, it seems that these steroids do not have any effects on infant growth, because boys with *anorchia* and patients with *testicular feminization syndrome* (an androgen receptor defect) do not show any growth failure during infancy. However, sex steroids are the most important factor for pubertal growth, since patients with *hypogonadism* (such as *Turner syndrome* or *Kallman syndrome*, etc.) and children treated with an LHRH analog do not show a pubertal spurt. Administration of HCG or testosterone to patients with *hypogonadism* induces a growth spurt. However, in addition to the acceleration of linear growth, sex steroids accelerate epiphyseal closure. Therefore, linear growth stops after the pubertal spurt. Bone age maturation in patients with *hypogonadism* or treated with an LHRH analog decelerates at around 14 years for boys and 12 years for girls with unclosed epiphyseal ends. Pubertal growth is mainly attributed to sex steroids but is in part mediated by increased pulsatile secretion of GH and thus IGF-I, induced by sex steroids. In mid-puberty, circulating IGF-I concentrations are within the acromegalic range. *Precocious puberty* characterized by increased secretion of sex steroids before pubertal age manifests itself by accelerated growth and accelerated bone age maturation as well as pubertal signs and thus early epiphyseal closure and loss of final height. Estrogen administration increases the growth rate at low doses but decelerates at high doses.

## Adrenal androgen

The progressive increased secretion of adrenal androgens such as DHEA, androstenedione, etc., at around seven years in both males and females is known as adrenarche. Although some children show a midgrowth spurt around adrenarche, the effect of adrenal androgen on growth is unclear. The onset of *premature adrenarche* associated with the early appearance of pubic hair may be associated with a mild advancement of height and bone age.

## Parathyroid hormone and calcium

Since patients with *rickets* and *pseudohypoparathy-roidism* (parathyroid hormone resistance) manifest growth failure, normal parathyroid hormone and $Ca^{2+}$ are also required for normal growth.

### SELECTED READING

Falkner F, Tanner JM, eds. *Human growth: A comprehensive treatise*, Vol. 2, 2nd edn. New York: Plenum Press, 1986: Chapters 1–12.

Hintz R, Rosenfeld RG, eds. *Growth abnormalities: Contemporary issues in endocrinology and metabolism*, Vol. 4. New York: Churchill Livingstone, 1987.

Laron Z, Perzelan A, Karp M, Keret R, Eshet R, Silbergeld A. Laron syndrome – a unique model of IGF-I deficiency. In: Laron Z, Parks JS eds, *Lessons from Laron syndrome (LS) 1966–1992*. Basel: Karger, 1993.

Ogata T, Matsuo N. Sex chromosome aberrations and stature: deduction of the principal factors involved in the determination of adult height. *Hum Genet* 1993; **91**: 551.

Pombo M, Rosenfeld RG, eds. *Two decades of experience in growth*. New York: Raven Press, 1993.

# ROLE OF GROWTH HORMONE IN POSTNATAL GROWTH AND METABOLISM

## PATTERNS OF GROWTH HORMONE (GH) SECRETION

The hypothalamus controls and regulates GH secretion through two peptides (with opposite effects) which are secreted into the portal vessel and affect the GH-producing somatotropes of the pituitary. Growth hormone releasing factor (GRF), which stimulates GH production and secretion, is produced in both the ventromedial and the arcuate nuclei of the hypothalamus. Somatostatin (SRIF), which originates from the anterior periventricular region and arcuate nucleus, is released in an episodic manner and blocks spontaneous and GRF-induced GH release. The biochemistry, ontogeny and control of GH secretion is discussed in detail in Chapter 35. However, certain aspects are specifically relevant to understanding the actions of GH. The interaction between the two hypothalamic peptides generates a pulsatile release of GH with regular GH peaks at 3–4 hour intervals separated by periods of low or undetectable GH plasma concentrations (Fig. 23.5).

The pattern of GH release is different in male and female rats and this sexual dimorphism has functional consequences. The male pattern consists of regular large multicomponent GH peaks separated by intervals

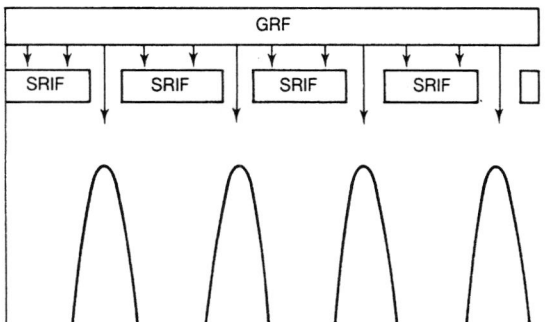

FIGURE 23.5 Schematic presentation of GH secretion through actions of growth hormone releasing factor (GRF) and somatostatin (SRIF)

of very low or undetectable levels of GH. In females, the plasma pattern is more irregular with more frequent pulses of lower amplitude and a constant elevated baseline secretion (Fig. 23.6). The intermittent responses to GRF in male rats could be explained by cyclic variations in SRIF tone whereas the uniform GH responses to GRF in the female rat may reflect a more continuous release of SRIF. In humans the differences between the sexes in the GH secretory pattern are less pronounced.

The sex differences in GH secretion are due to differential exposure to sex steroids. There are indications that testicular androgen secretion during a critical period of neural development (e.g. neonatal rat) influences the mature GH secretory pattern. This process appears analogous to the critical period in neural development when androgens determine other sexually dimorphic characteristics (*see* page 199).

Pulsatile GH secretion is more favorable for body growth than continuous GH release; this explains why

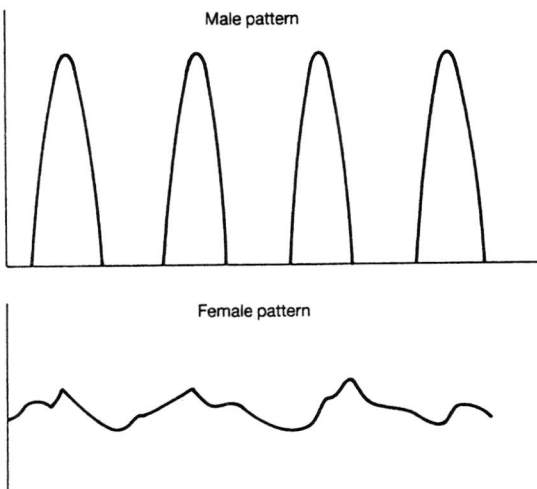

FIGURE 23.6 Illustration of the male and female GH secretory pattern.

male rats grow faster than females. A pulsatile infusion of GH stimulates increased weight gain and longitudinal bone growth more effectively than continuous infusion of GH. The GH secretory pattern also influences carbohydrate, lipid and protein metabolism. The effect on carbohydrate metabolism is mainly diabetogenic (anti-insulin-like) but GH also exerts a transient insulin-like effect under certain experimental conditions. The diabetogenic effect of GH is exemplified by the fact that 40–60 per cent of *acromegalic* patients have impaired glucose tolerance with elevated serum insulin concentrations. GH administration to experimental animals or man results in increased protein accretion, decreased lipid deposition, improved food efficiency and increased galactopoiesis.

The importance of the pattern of GH secretion for the metabolic effects of the hormone is not fully understood. The total plasma phospholipid concentration, which is higher in females than in males, appears to be regulated by the GH secretory pattern since continuous, but not intermittent, GH treatment increases phospholipid concentrations in hypophysectomized rats. Finally, the pattern of GH release explains the sex differences in serum apolipoprotein E and cholesterol concentrations in the rat.

The activity of several metabolic enzymes in the liver, including 5α-reductase, 5β-hydrolase, 16α-hydroxylase, carbonic anhydrase and serum cholinesterase, also is regulated by the pattern of GH secretion. The most dramatic effect is on the 16α-hydroxylase activity which is markedly elevated by the pattern of GH secretion. By intermittent GH administration the activity is increased and during continuous exposure the levels in hypophysectomized rats are decreased.

GH secretion also influences the concentrations of other peptide hormone receptors. The prolactin receptor concentration in the liver is higher in female rats than in male rats: this has been shown to be due to the continuous GH release in the female rat. In contrast, the episodic secretion of GH in male rats increases the number of hepatic epidermal growth factor receptors.

The physiological significance of GH in adults has only recently been studied. Adults with hypopituitarism have so far received replacement therapy with thyroid hormones, adrenal and sex steroids, but not GH. However, the recent availability of recombinant GH has made it possible to study the effect of GH replacement therapy. *GH-deficient adults* exhibit excess adipose tissue stored in the abdomen, in visceral and subcutaneous depots. Moreover, they show reduced lean body mass, low bone mineral content, decreased extracellular water, depressed renal function, impaired cardiac function, poor physical performance and finally signs of impaired psychological well-being such as reduced vitality, impaired emotional reactions and increased social isolation. Replacement therapy with GH decreases adipose tissue and increases lean body mass with no marked change in overall bodyweight. Recent studies also show an increase of extracellular fluid volume, total body nitrogen, bone mineral content, muscle volume, cardiac muscle mass, stroke volume and physical strength as well as vigor, ambition, sense of well-being and quality of life. By conventional replacement therapy with thyroid hormones, adrenal and sex steroids to hypopituitary patients, changes like decreased basal metabolic rate, glomerular filtration rate and blood volume have not been restored. This may indicate yet other important physiological functions of GH extending into adult life.

## THE GH RECEPTOR AND THE GH-BINDING PROTEIN

The biological actions of GH are initiated when GH binds to specific GH receptors (GHR) on the plasma membrane of the target tissue (Fig. 23.7). GH receptors have been detected in several tissues including the liver, kidney, heart, muscle, ovary and the epiphyseal growth plate. The human GH receptor was recently cloned and shown to be a protein consisting of 620 amino acids (aa) with a single transmembrane domain. The extracellular domain contains 246 aa, the

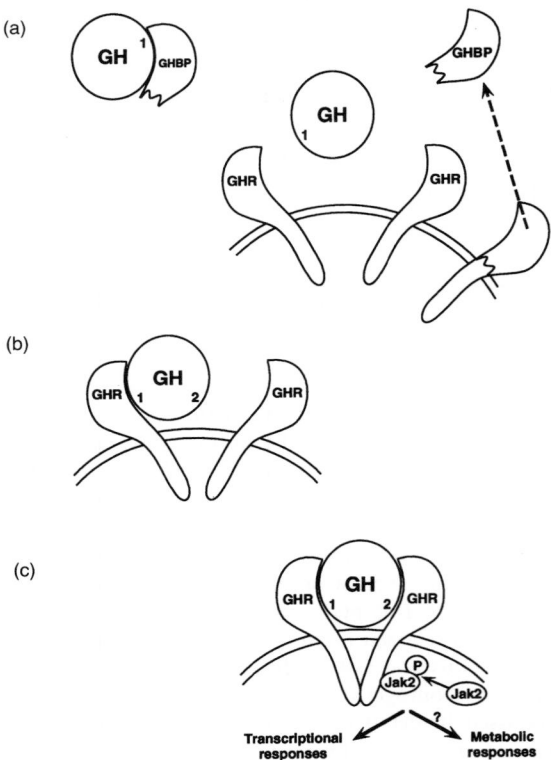

FIGURE 23.7 Hypothetical model of GH binding. (a) GH in the circulation may be free or complexed to GH binding protein (GHBP). (b) GH binds first via site 1 to membrane bound GH receptors (GHR) in monomeric form which activates site 2. (c) Following activation of site 2, dimerization of the receptor occurs. Jak2 becomes associated with the receptor and is phosphorylated thus initiating an intracellular cascade leading to transcriptional activation and interactions with other signaling systems.

transmembrane and the intracellular domain 24 and 350 aa, respectively. The extracellular domain has five potential N-linked glycosylation sites and seven cysteine residues forming three disulfide bonds. The function of the unpaired cysteine, located close to the plasma membrane, is not yet fully understood but it could be involved in the receptor dimerization which may be essential to activation of the receptor or interaction with membrane-associated proteins.

The human GH receptor gene contains at least 10 exons, spanning more than 85 kb. The extracellular domain of the receptor is encoded by exons 3–7, the transmembrane domain by exon 8, and exons 9 and 10 encode the intracellular domain. The GH receptor is closely related to a superfamily of hormone peptide receptors including the prolactin receptor, receptors of interleukins 2, 3, 4, 5, 6, 7 and the granulocyte–macrophage colony-stimulating factor receptor as well as the erythropoietin receptor. Subpopulations of slightly modified GH receptors may exist with different structures, binding characteristics or functions. These receptors are generated by alternative splicing of the GH receptor mRNA.

Studies in several species support the concept that the GH receptor is expressed at low levels at the time of birth with increased expression with advancing age. GH receptors are present in some areas of the fetal brain, although their function remains suppositional.

A specific binding protein for GH (GHBP) has been found in serum in man, rabbit, rat and mice. In rabbits the binding protein has an amino acid sequence identical to the extracellular portion of the GH receptor, and consequently could originate from proteolytic cleavage from the GH receptor. On the other hand, in rodents a specific mRNA encoding the BP has been cloned. This transcript is homologous to the extracellular domain of the GH receptor but the transmembrane and intracellular domains have been substituted by a short hydrophilic sequence. Circulating GHBP in rat is derived from an alternative spliced transcript of the GH receptor gene. It remains to be established by which mechanism the GHBP is generated *in vivo* in humans.

The function of the BP is not fully understood. In rats the GHBP transcripts are coexpressed with the GH receptor in all tissues analyzed. Circulating GHBPs have been shown to attenuate GH plasma peaks, diminish the troughs of the GH secretion, and inhibit GH elimination from the blood. This implies that the physiological function of the BP may be to modulate the half-life of GH in serum or modulate the amount of free GH at the receptor of the target cell.

*Laron syndrome* or *GH resistance syndrome* is an autosomally recessive inherited disease which is characterized by growth failure, low serum IGF-I, increased GH secretion and resistance to GH therapy. Many of these patients lack serum GHBP and preparations of hepatic membranes have low GH-binding activity. Such patients have mutations or deletions in the extracellular domain of the GH receptor. A mutation or deletion on the internal part of the GH receptor, which is important to the signaling mechanism, should also result in GH resistance and this may explain the recent observation that some children with *Laron syndrome* have normal concentrations of GHBP in their plasma. Another mutant has been described in which mutation in a single amino acid in the extracellular domain, close to the membrane, prevents dimerization of the receptor and thus signal transduction.

The GH receptor is regulated by a number of factors. GH itself increases the number of GH receptors in liver, muscle, adipose tissue and in chondrocytes. Sex steroids enhance hepatic GH receptor number and thus may be one mechanism operative in the pubertal growth spurt. Thyroid hormone may also affect the GH receptor. Undernutrition is associated with a reduction in GH receptor number at least in the liver and this effect may be mediated by insulin.

## SIGNALING MECHANISM OF THE GH RECEPTOR

The GH receptor sequence provided no evidence for earlier described signaling mechanisms (*see* page 53) such as ATP/GTP-binding sites or the presence of tyrosine kinase in the intracellular domain of the receptor. Recently, the crystal structure of the extracellular domain of the human GH receptor with bound GH was identified and has been used to infer the mechanism of GH–GH receptor interaction. The complex consists of one GH molecule and two molecules of the GH receptor (Fig. 23.7). GH has two binding sites for the GH receptor. Site 1 is utilized first and the conformational change in GH on binding to the first GH receptor molecule activates the second binding site which then binds to a second GH receptor molecule. Moreover, there is also a substantial contact surface between the carboxyl-terminal domains of the receptors, providing a mechanism for receptor dimerization. Receptor dimerization appears to be the first step in GH action. Multiple cascades are apparently initiated by GH binding and receptor dimerization (*see* page 462). These include activation of non-receptor tyrosine kinases, in particular Janus kinase 2 (Jak2). Other members of the cytokine receptor superfamily also activate Jak2. In turn a number of transcriptional responses are initiated (*see* page 463). In addition protein kinase C pathways and phospholipase C appear to be involved in the metabolic responses to GH. These various pathways may explain the diverse actions of GH in different tissues.

It may be that GHBP could be involved in the signaling mechanism by complexing with GH bound to the membrane-anchored GH receptor. Cytosolic GHBP also has been shown to be present in many cells and is identical in structure to the circulating GHBP. Immunoreactive GH receptors or GHBP have been found in the nuclei of several cell types, suggesting that GHBP could be involved in GH regulation of nuclear events.

## GH REGULATION OF TISSUE GROWTH

The absence of *in vitro* effects of GH resulted in the hypothesis that GH acts primarily on the liver and that the liver, in response to GH action, produces somatomedins (later renamed the insulin-like growth factors or IGFs) which are released into the blood stream. Although many of the *in vivo* effects of GH can be mimicked by IGF-I, there are several points of discrepancy between their actions. It is now recognized, however, that GH has receptors in many tissues where it could stimulate local IGF-I production. It is assumed that both the endocrine and paracrine somatotrophic axes play a role in growth regulation.

By studying the growth, differentiation and proliferation of preadipose cells, Green and coworkers made the important observation that GH has a specific stimulatory effect on preadipocyte cell conversion to adipocytes, which forms the basis of the "dual effector theory." According to this theory GH stimulates the differentiation of progenitor cells which subsequently become responsive to growth factors like IGF-I (Fig. 23.8). The role of the IGFs is discussed in detail on page 314.

## The epiphyseal growth plate and longitudinal bone growth (*see also* Chapter 44)

Many hormones and nutritional factors affect mammalian growth, but only GH has been shown to stimulate postnatal longitudinal bone growth in a specific and dose-dependent manner. In humans complete lack of GH, such as in *GH deficiency type Ia* due to a gene deletion, results in a final height of 120–130 cm while overproduction of GH before puberty leads to *gigantism*, or in adults to *acromegaly*.

Longitudinal bone growth is the result of cell proliferation in the epiphyseal growth plates which are located in the proximal and distal part of the long bones (*see* Fig. 44.2). The growth plate has a strict cellular organization with the germinative, proliferative, hypertrophic and degenerative cell layers. The germinative cell layer consists of rarely dividing cells, i.e. stem cells or progenitor cells. During the process of growth, stem cells initiate their program of differentiation and enter the proliferative cell layer, where frequent cellular divisions occur, forming continual cell columns. Subsequently, these cells stop dividing, mature and hypertrophy in the hypertrophic cell layer. Finally the chondrocytes degenerate and the matrix becomes a site for $Ca^{2+}$ deposition. As new progenitor cells continuously start their program of differentiation, the growth plate could be regarded as a constantly renewing tissue pushing the bony epiphysis further away from the center of the long bone.

Bone growth is the result of the recruitment of new cells from the stem cell layer and the number of cell divisions in the proliferative cell layer together with increasing size of cells within the hypertrophic cell layer. Under normal conditions the rate of stem cell recruitment, the cell proliferation and the mineralization are in balance, retaining the same thickness of the growth plate.

GH action on longitudinal bone has mostly been studied in hypophysectomized rats. In this animal model it has been shown that locally injected, or

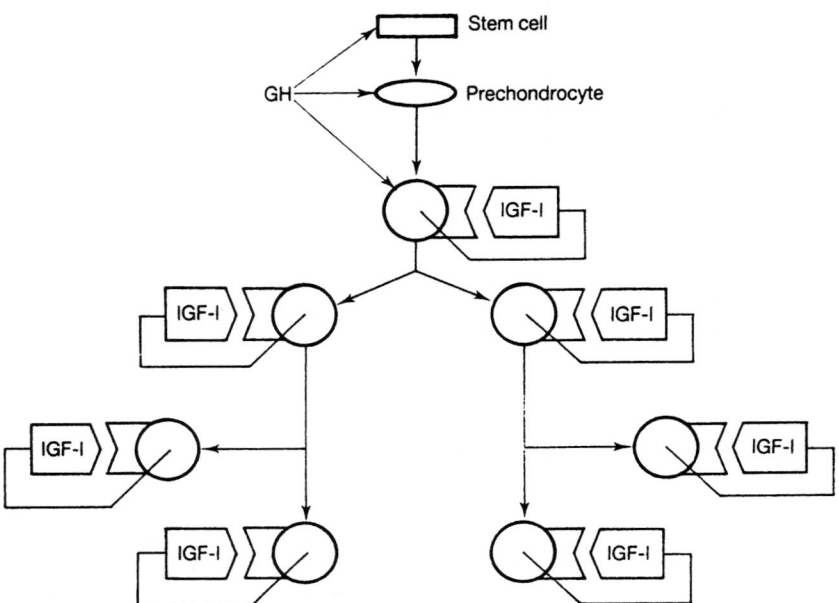

FIGURE 23.8 A hypothetical model of GH action on the longitudinal bone growth, based on the dual effector theory

locally infused, GH results in unilateral bone growth without a concomitant rise in serum IGF-I concentrations. Local GH treatment also resulted in local expression of IGF-I mRNA as well as increased presence of IGF-I protein. By co-infusing IGF-I antibodies with GH locally, the growth stimulation of GH was abolished. *In vitro*, culture of epiphyseal growth plate chondrocytes derived from GH-treated hypophysectomized rats showed increased response to IGF-I in subsequent culture. The application of the dual effector theory to these findings forms the basis for the proposed mechanism of action for GH on the epiphyseal growth plate. GH preferentially acts on the prechondrocytes, or young differentiating chondrocytes, in the germinative cell layer that have a high potential to divide. During the process of differentiation the cells become responsive to IGF-I and the gene encoding IGF-I is expressed, resulting in local IGF-I production. As a result IGF-I stimulates the differentiating cells by an autocrine or paracrine mechanism.

## Skeletal muscle

In skeletal muscle GH stimulates growth by increasing cell number rather than cell size. Thus, GH stimulates DNA replication in skeletal muscle. In analogy with GH effects on prechondrocytes, according to the dual effector theory it is possible that GH interacts with skeletal muscle progenitor cells. The proposed progenitor cells for myoblasts are the satellite cells. However, it remains to be determined whether GH can interact directly with these cells. *In vitro*, the differentiation of a cell line of myoblasts and the expression of myotubes is GH-dependent.

The role of IGF-I in muscle growth is not yet clarified. Several *in vitro* studies have demonstrated effects of IGF-I on a number of anabolic processes related to increased muscle mass or function. These include stimulatory effects on proliferation and promotion of differentiation of myoblasts to myotubes following cell division. *In vivo*, IGF-I has been shown to stimulate skeletal muscle protein synthesis and inhibit protein breakdown.

Studies regarding muscle regeneration in rats following ischemic injury have revealed increased expression of GH receptor mRNA and also increased expression of IGF-I, at both mRNA and protein levels, indicating a role for both GH and IGF-I during muscle regeneration. However, in regenerating muscle of hypophysectomized rats, IGF-I expression was also seen, suggesting that production of IGF-I may in part be independent of GH during certain conditions.

## Adipose tissue

Apart from its effects on somatic growth, GH is also an important regulator of intermediary metabolism.

*GH deficiency* results in an increase of body fat, whereas excessive GH, as in *acromegaly*, results in a decrease in body fat. When GH-deficient patients are treated with GH, total adipose tissue decreases. Moreover, the distribution of adipose tissue is affected since subcutaneous adipose tissue decreases less than visceral adipose tissue. The mechanism of this lipolytic effect is not certain; it may be independent of IGF-I. Recent data suggest that GH enhances the responsiveness of fat cells to other lipolytic agents. This may involve the action of GH inhibiting Gi protein.

GH also is diabetogenic. It inhibits the actions of insulin perhaps by interrupting G-protein-mediated signal transmission from the insulin receptor to phospholipase C.

GH also regulates the number of fat cells. Patients with short stature secondary to GH deficiency, despite large total fat cell mass, exhibit a low number of fat cells. This also is found in hypophysectomized rats where GH administration reduces total fat cell mass and increases fat cell number. Mature adipocytes are regarded as terminally differentiated cells unable to proliferate. Thus, increased fat cell number is the result of recruitment of cells from a preadipocyte population. During the process of adipose conversion a marked change in the cellular phenotype occurs. Synthesis of structural and membrane proteins is reduced, enzymes responsible for triglyceride synthesis are induced and hormonal sensitivity is modified. This process of fat cell differentiation has been extensively studied during experimental conditions and the velocity of the process has been found to be GH-dependent. Pretreatment of preadipose cells with GH increases the responsiveness of the cells to subsequently added IGF-I in terms of thymidine incorporation and the rate of adipose conversion, thus demonstrating that IGF-I was more effective at a later stage of differentiation.

## SELECTED READING

Bengtsson B-Å. *An introduction to growth hormone deficiency in adults.* Oxford: Oxford Clinical Communications, 1993.

Cunningham BC, Ultsch M, De Vos AM, *et al.* Dimerization of the extracellular domain of the human growth hormone receptor by a single hormone molecule. *Science* 1991; **254**: 821.

Daughaday WH, Rotwein P. Insulin-like growth factors I and II. Peptide, messenger ribonucleic acid and gene structures, serum and tissue concentrations. *Endocr Rev* 1989; **10**: 68.

Green H, Morikawa M, Nixon T. A dual effector theory of growth hormone action. *Differentiation* 1985; **29**: 195.

Isaksson OGP, Lindahl A, Nilsson A, Isgaard J. Mechanism of the stimulatory effect of growth hormone on longitudinal bone growth. *Endocr Rev* 1987; **8**: 426.

Roupas P, Herington AC. Postreceptor signalling mechanisms for growth hormone. *Trends Endocr Metab* 1994; **5**: 154.

# INSULIN-LIKE GROWTH FACTORS

## INTRODUCTION

The discovery of insulin-like growth factors (IGFs) is based on an observation in 1957 that the stimulatory effect of growth hormone (GH) on sulfate incorporation into cartilage matrix is mediated by a soluble substance termed "sulfation factor." During the following years multiple GH-dependent factors were identified which were designated "somatomedins" and subsequently were renamed insulin-like growth factors in view of their evolutionary relationship to insulin. The isolation of pure peptides revealed the existence of two major peptides, IGF-I and IGF-II. Somatomedins A and C were shown to be identical with IGF-I and multiplication stimulating activity (MSA) was recognized as the rat homologue of IGF-II. IGFs play pivotal roles in the regulation of proliferation, differentiation and specific functions of many cell types and in regulating body growth and metabolism. The IGFs are found in the circulation and are presumed to exert endocrine actions. The major source of circulating IGF-I is the liver. However, essentially all tissues express IGF-I and IGF-II and the IGFs have major paracrine and autocrine actions in the tissues of production.

In contrast to many other peptide hormones, especially those with short-term metabolic effects, IGFs are non-covalently bound to specific binding proteins (IGFBP). Only about 1 per cent of circulating IGFs exist in their free form.

## BIOCHEMISTRY

### IGF-I and IGF-II

IGF-I and IGF-II are single-chain polypeptides with 62 per cent sequence homology. IGF-I is a basic peptide of 70 amino acids (mol. wt = 7649). IGF-II is a slightly acidic peptide of 67 amino acids (mol. wt = 7471). Both are about 30 per cent homologous to proinsulin. By analogy to proinsulin their amino acid sequences can be divided into domains B, C, A and a short extension D at the C-terminus. The major sequence differ-

ences are in the C-peptide region. Several variant forms are described which may arise from alternative splicing of the primary gene transcript, incomplete processing of the prohormone, or proteolytic cleavage of the mature peptide. A truncated IGF-I form, lacking the first three amino acids (des 1-3N IGF-I), is a potent stimulator of IGF-I specific effects through high-affinity binding to the IGF type I receptor and has been identified in neural extracts and in colostrum. However, it does only weakly bind to some IGFBPs. Recently the specific protease required for generation of des 1-3N IGF-I has been identified in the circulation, raising the possibility that generation of des 1-3N IGF-I may be one mechanism for delivery of IGF-I from the circulation to tissues.

Different regions of the molecules are involved in the binding to the IGF type I and type II receptors and also to IGFBPs. Both IGFs are synthesized as prepropeptides with a molecular size of approximately 20–22 kD. Processing of the propeptide includes cleavage of the so-called E-domain which extends the length of the mature IGF peptides at the C-terminus. Pro-IGF forms are present in the circulation in certain clinical situations, e.g. *chronic renal failure* or in *non-islet cell tumor-induced hypoglycemia* (NICTH) which is caused by large tumors that produce excessive amounts of IGF-II.

## IGF-binding proteins

Six classes of IGFBPs (IGFBP-1–6) have been identified (Table 23.1). They show a high degree of sequence homology (about 40 per cent) especially within the N- and C-terminal regions where a relatively large number of cysteines is conserved. Biochemical characteristics of the various IGFBPs are listed in Table 23.1. IGFBP-1 and IGFBP-2 contain an Arg-Gly-Asp (single letter code: RGD) sequence near the C-terminal which is thought to facilitate binding to integrin receptors on the cell surface. Cell-surface adherent IGFBPs may modulate IGF-receptor interactions. IGFBP-4 and IGFBP-5 can exist in forms that bind to extracellular matrix or in soluble forms. IGFBP-4, IGFBP-5 and IGFBP-6 contain glycosylation sites. The carbohydrate moieties do not affect IGF binding to IGFBP-3, although they may influence interactions with the cell

TABLE 23.1  Biochemical characteristics of the human IGF-binding proteins

| IGFBP SEQUENCE | AMINO ACIDS | MOL. WT (kD) | CYSTEINE | GLYCOSYLATION | RGD |
|---|---|---|---|---|---|
| IGFBP-1 | 259 | 28.1 | 18 | − | + |
| IGFBP-2 | 289 | 31.3 | 18 | − | + |
| IGFBP-3 | 264 | 28.7* | 18 | + | − |
| IGFBP-4 | 237 | 26.3 | 20 | + | − |
| IGFBP-5 | 252 | 28.6 | 18 | − | − |
| IGFBP-6 | 216 | 22.8 | 16 | + | − |

*Glycosylated molecular weight 42–45 kD.

surface or the metabolic clearance. A further mechanism of post-translational modification of IGFBPs is phosphorylation which may modulate the affinity of the IGFBPs for IGFs.

IGFBP-2 and IGFBP-6 preferentially bind IGF-II whilst the other IGFBPs have a similar affinity for either IGF peptide. The affinity constants compare with the affinity constants of the IGF I and IGF II receptor. The association of IGFBP-3, the major circulating IGFBP postnatally, with either IGF is rapid. In contrast, the dissociation reaction is extremely slow with a half-time in the range of 17 hours.

Despite this very slow dissociation rate, physiological concentrations of free IGF would be restored within 10–30 minutes due to the high levels of the IGF/IGFBP-3 complex in the circulation. Although the mass action law could explain the release of IGF from the complex, it may be facilitated by specific proteases or by binding of glycosaminoglycans.

IGFBP-3 is unique among the IGF-binding proteins in that after association with either IGF-I or IGF-II it is then able to bind a so-called acid-labile subunit (ALS) thus constituting a large-molecular-weight ternary complex of 125–150 kD. ALS is a single-chain protein with a molecular size of 70 kD and is glycosylated, resulting in a total molecular weight of 84–86 kD. Although its affinity for the IGF/IGFBP-3 complex is clearly lower than the affinity of IGF for IGFBP-3, most of the IGF in the circulation is found in the large-molecular-weight range. This is caused by an excess of ALS which promotes the rapid formation of the ternary complex as soon as IGFs have bound to IGFBP-3. ALS itself is growth-hormone dependent.

Recently it has been recognized that there are specific proteases for several of the IGFBPs including IGFBP-3, IGFBP-4 and IGFBP-5. These proteases are serine proteases. Generally these proteases alter, but do not abolish, the affinity of the IGF for the binding protein. In the case of IGFBP-5, the affinity of the IGFBP for association with extracellular matrix is reduced by protease activity.

In addition, the extramembranous portion of the type II receptor is found in the circulation. This binds only IGF-II and is particularly high in fetal blood. Whether it acts as a further form of binding protein is unclear.

## MOLECULAR BIOLOGY

The IGF-I gene is located on the long arm of chromosome 12 and the gene for IGF-II at the end of the short arm of chromosome 11 contiguous to the insulin gene. Both genes are remarkably long and complex compared with other peptide hormones. The IGF-I gene spans about 95 kb and contains six exons. Multiple mRNAs are found due to the alternative use of different exons, alternative splicing of the primary transcript and to variable polyadenylation at the 3′ end of the mRNAs. The mature IGF-I peptide is encoded by

exons 3 and 4: exons 1 and 2 are used alternatively leading to class 1 or class 2 mRNAs. Most of the E-domain is encoded by exons 5 and 6. By alternative splicing of the primary transcript either of these two exons is used, resulting in two propeptides with different E-domains, Eb and Ea, respectively. The human IGF-II gene spans 35 kb and contains nine exons and four promoters adjacent to exons 1, 4, 5 and 6 at their 5′ ends. The mature IGF-II peptide is encoded by exons 7 and 8 and part of exon 9. Various mRNAs differing in length are found due to the alternative use of the various promoters and their adjacent exons.

The physiological meaning of the heterogeneity of IGF mRNAs is not fully understood but it may be relevant for the post-transcriptional regulation of IGFs. Large IGF-I mRNAs have a shorter half-life than smaller variants and the use of alternative 5′ sequences leads to different leader peptides which may be important for alternative targeting of the translation products. The concept that the heterogeneity of IGF mRNAs is physiologically relevant is supported by findings which show that the mRNA patterns are tissue and development specific.

## REGULATION

The regulation of IGFs is very complex owing to (1) the involvement of multiple regulatory factors, (2) their endocrine and paracrine modes of action, and (3) the importance of IGFBPs and their proteases in the regulation of physiological concentrations. While the regulation of circulating IGFs and IGFBPs may differ from local regulation, the major regulators of IGF-I (GH and nutrition) elicit a similar influence at both levels.

The regulation of circulating IGF-I and IGF-II cannot be regarded independently from IGFBPs. The most abundant IGFBP in blood is IGFBP-3, which represents 90 per cent of total circulating IGFBP in children and adults. A molar 1:1 ratio between total IGF (IGF-I plus IGF-II) and IGFBP-3 is found in the circulation in all situations except *chronic renal failure*. The reason why this 1:1 ratio is observed is that the metabolic half-life of free IGF-I and IGF-II is very short (4–15 minutes). Therefore only IGFBP-bound IGFs remain in the circulation. Consequently, total IGF-I and IGF-II serum concentrations are primarily determined by the IGFBP-3 concentrations. As IGF-I and IGF-II may displace each other from IGFBP-3, the ratio of IGF-I and IGF-II may be quite variable.

While the kidneys are not a primary site of IGF clearance, renal function plays a major role in the removal of IGFBPs from the circulation. In chronic renal failure IGF-I and IGF-II concentrations are normal and IGFBPs are markedly elevated owing to the accumulation of small-molecular-weight forms.

The plasma levels of both IGFs and the IGFBPs show age dependence but the patterns are quite different for each peptide (Fig. 23.9).

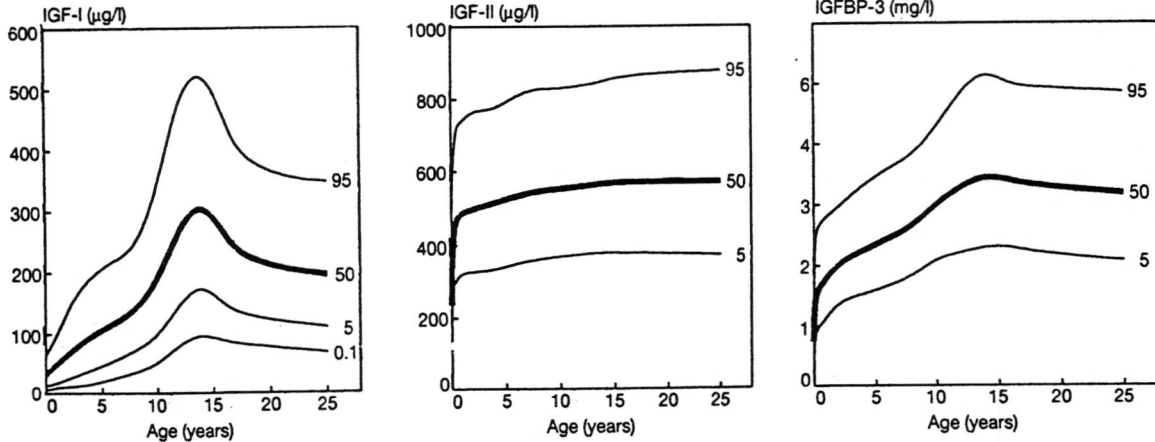

FIGURE 23.9  Age-dependent normal ranges of IGF-I, IGF-II and IGFBP-3 serum levels. The 5th, 50th and 95th centiles are shown.

# IGF-I

## Growth hormone

The major hormonal regulator of IGF-I, both in the circulation and in peripheral tissues, is GH. IGF-I serum concentrations are decreased in *GH deficiency* (GHD) and are increased in *acromegaly*. Administration of GH in patients with GHD, or in GH-deficient animals, produces a marked increase of IGF-I in the blood maximal after 12–24 hours due to induction of hepatic IGF-I synthesis. In addition, IGF-I expression is stimulated in multiple tissues including epiphyseal cartilage, which may be of particular importance for longitudinal growth (*see* page 312). As in many other hormonal regulatory systems there is a negative feedback loop mediated by IGFs on GH secretion at both the hypophyseal and hypothalamic levels. Thus in *undernutrition* or in *Laron syndrome* where there is GH resistance, IGF-I levels are low and circulating GH is high.

In patients with *hyperprolactinemia* normal IGF-I levels may be found despite obvious insufficient GH secretion. This can be explained by the weak affinity of PRL to the GH receptor.

## Other adenohypophyseal hormones

Other pituitary hormones besides GH or PRL have no direct influence on serum levels of IGF-I. They are, however, involved in the regulation of paracrine IGF-I synthesis in their specific target cells. TSH stimulates IGF-I production by thyroid follicular cells; LH (or hCG) stimulates IGF-I expression in granulosa and Leydig cells; FSH stimulates IGF-I in granulosa and Sertoli cells. This effect is mediated by cAMP and is modulated by the presence of other peptide growth factors.

Patients with *hypothyroidism* have impaired IGF-I serum concentrations that increase upon thyroxine substitution. The thyroxine effect is thought to act via the stimulation of GH secretion. In *hyperthyroidism* IGF-I concentrations are unchanged.

## Steroidal influences

Low-dose estrogen replacement therapy in *hypogonadal* patients increases serum IGF-I, possibly through the stimulation of the GH secretion. On the other hand, pharmacological doses of estrogens suppress IGF-I concentrations in normal individuals or in patients with *acromegaly*. This effect may be due to a direct inhibition of IGF-I expression in the liver as shown experimentally. From a clinical point of view it may also be relevant with respect to treatment of girls with *tall stature* with high doses of estrogens in order to reduce final height. In contrast to the liver, IGF-I expression is stimulated by estrogens in the uterus, underlining the divergent regulation of circulating IGF-I and local IGF-I production. In humans no direct effect of androgens upon IGF-I serum concentrations has been demonstrated. The increase observed in hypogonadal patients after androgen treatment is thought to be secondary to an increase of GH secretion. Also, the stimulatory effect of oxandrolone, an anabolic drug which is widely used in patients with *constitutional delay of growth and adolescence* to improve height velocity, may be explained by its weak androgenic activity.

In patients with *Cushing syndrome* or during *chronic high dose corticosteroid therapy*, IGF-I concentrations are normal or slightly elevated, contrasting with impaired growth, and suggesting glucocorticoids inhibit the effects of IGF-I. In addition there may be local effects as suggested by suppression of IGF-I production in osteoblast cell cultures.

## Other hormonal influences

PTH induces IGF-I synthesis in osteoblasts or bone tissue culture. However, it does not influence IGF-I serum concentrations.

IGF-I serum concentrations are decreased in untreated diabetes mellitus and normalize upon insulin treatment. It appears that insulin has a permissive effect on GH-stimulated IGF-I production in the liver and other tissues, perhaps by affecting the GH receptor.

There are a variety of paracrine peptide growth factors that stimulate local IGF-I production alone or in combination with trophic hormones (see page 279). These include platelet-derived growth factor (PDGF), epidermal growth factor (EGF), transforming growth factor α (TGFα), and basic fibroblast growth factor (bFGF). TGFβ has both inhibitory and stimulatory effects.

## Nutritional factors

The second most potent regulator of IGF-I serum concentrations besides GH is the nutritional status. IGF-I declines exponentially during fasting within a few days and is restored upon refeeding. This decrease is caused by a reduction of hepatic IGF-I gene expression which is also seen in non-hepatic tissues. Both protein and calorie intake play a role. If in human adults the daily caloric intake falls below a threshold of 12 kcal/kg, insensitivity to GH develops secondary to a decrease of GH receptor number and impairment of post-GH receptor events. IGF-I measurements can therefore be used to monitor nutritional status.

## Other influences on IGF-I secretion

In patients with sepsis IGF-I serum concentrations and IGF-I production in the liver decline and cannot be restored by GH administration. This may be due to a decrease in hepatic GH receptor density in the liver due to tumor necrosis factor (TNF). In patients with large solid tumors or with leukemia, IGF-I levels are significantly decreased and normalize during chemotherapy despite severe nutritional problems and cytotoxicity due to the treatment. This finding again indicates possible regulation of IGF-I by so-far unknown immunological factors.

From experimental studies it is known that lesions of various tissues – including muscles, tendons, nerves, brain, blood vessel endothelium, kidney, and subcutaneous or epidermal cells – cause a local transient increase of IGF-I production lasting about 3–5 weeks. Moreover, IGF-I may be released at the site of the lesion by platelets or macrophages. These findings suggest an important role of IGF-I in wound healing. Despite the local stimulation of IGF-I synthesis at the site of tissue lesions, IGF-I serum levels decline in severely traumatized patients, or after severe abdominal surgery, within a few days and are slowly restored within 2–3 weeks. This decline occurs even under calorically adequate parenteral nutrition. The mechanisms that are involved in this down-regulation are unclear.

As the liver is the main source of circulating IGFs and also IGFBPs, it is therefore not surprising that IGF-I serum concentrations decline in liver disease. A significant correlation is found with conventional indicators of liver function.

## IGF-II

Less is known about the regulation of IGF-II. This may in part be due to the divergent developmental patterns of IGF-II in different species. Whereas in the rat, for example, IGF-II serum concentrations decline postpartum to almost unmeasurable concentrations, they rapidly increase in humans during the first few weeks of life (Fig. 23.9). This makes the extrapolation of experimental findings in animal studies to the human situation difficult. A second problem arises from the fact that IGF concentrations in blood are largely determined by the IGFBP-3 levels. This is especially true for IGF-II which follows closely the IGFBP-3 concentration in many situations. It is therefore difficult to recognize whether IGF-II levels are directly controlled by a certain factor or whether any changes are secondary to variations of the binding proteins.

While GH is a firmly established regulator of IGF-I and IGFBP-3, it is doubtful that it also directly regulates IGF-II serum concentrations. In growth hormone deficiency, IGF-II serum concentrations are decreased and they increase during GH or IGF-I treatment following the increase of IGFBP-3. In contrast, in normal individuals a transient decrease of IGF-II concentrations is observed upon high-dose GH treatment, probably due to the displacement of IGF-II from IGFBP-3 by the increase in circulating IGF-I. Moreover, in patients with acromegaly, IGF-II concentrations are normal. In various other conditions IGF-II serum concentrations are diminished, closely paralleling the pattern of the decrease of IGFBP-3 rather than IGF-I: fasting or malnutrition, malignancies, trauma, severe surgical trauma, and hepatic insufficiency.

An increase of IGF-II mRNA following GH administration was found in rat brain, skeletal and cardiac muscle, whereas hepatic mRNA remained unchanged. Cortisol suppressed IGF-II mRNA in the liver. In human fetal adrenals and human granulosa cells, ACTH and FSH respectively stimulated IGF-II expression. These findings and others suggest that at least locally produced IGF-II may indeed be subject to the regulation of various hormonal factors.

## IGF-binding proteins

A most striking feature of IGFBP-1, IGFBP-2 and IGFBP-3 is that their control is quite independent, suggesting different and specific biological functions. Knowledge on the regulation of IGFBP-4, IGFBP-5, IGFBP-6 is still sparse. The regulation of the proteolysis may be the critical step in the regulation of IGFBP-4 and IGFBP-5 rather than regulation of their secretion.

## IGFBP-1

Basal circulating IGFBP-1 concentrations are high at birth (in humans, mean 0.070 mg/L), decline until adolescence (mean 0.016 mg/L) and increase again with aging. In contrast to IGFBP-2 and IGFBP-3, IGFBP-1 concentrations exhibit a marked circadian fluctuation with high concentrations at night which depend on food intake. Fasting causes a rapid rise of IGFBP-1 whilst refeeding suppresses IGFBP-1 concentrations. An increase of IGFBP-1 can also be induced by extreme physical exercise. These changes are related to the secretion of insulin which strongly impairs IGFBP-1 gene expression. Experimental evidence suggests that this effect is mediated by the availability of intracellular glucose. As a consequence, IGFBP-1 concentrations are significantly increased in *diabetes mellitus* and *undernutrition* and decline upon successful treatment.

IGF-I has a similar suppressive effect to insulin. There is an inverse relationship between IGFBP-1 and GH secretion. Local production of IGFBP-1 may be controlled by other factors such as progesterone and relaxin, e.g. in the decidualized cells of the endometrium.

## IGFBP-2

The age-dependent pattern of IGFBP-2 serum concentrations resembles that of IGFBP-1, although absolute concentrations are higher by an order of magnitude. There are relatively high concentrations in fetal and neonatal blood. There is, however, no circadian variation and insulin does not appear to have a major effect on IGFBP-2 concentrations. However, like IGFBP-1, IGFBP-2 shows an inverse relationship with the GH status. Interestingly, IGF-I administration to humans has an opposite effect, resulting in a moderate increase. A major regulator appears to be IGF-II which strongly binds to IGFBP-2. In patients with *non-islet cell tumor-induced hypoglycemia* secreting large amounts of IGF-II or its prohormone forms, IGFBP-2 concentrations are excessively elevated and can be used as a diagnostic marker.

## IGFBP-3

In contrast to IGFBP-1 and IGFBP-2, IGFBP-3 serum concentrations are low at birth. They rise rapidly during the first few weeks of life and show a peak at the time of puberty (*see* Fig. 23.9). There is no circadian rhythm. The regulation of IGFBP-3 serum concentrations resembles in many aspects the regulation of IGF-I.

The major regulator is GH. Levels are decreased in *growth hormone deficiency* and normalize upon treatment with GH within several days. On the other hand, IGFBP-3 concentrations are markedly elevated in *acromegaly* and normalize after successful therapy. Although *in vitro* studies suggest that IGF-I may directly stimulate IGFBP-3 production, IGF-I administration to normal humans, patients with *growth hormone deficiency* or patients with GH receptor deficiency (*Laron syndrome*) does not affect IGFBP-3 serum concentrations, indicating that the GH effect on circulating IGFBP-3 is not mediated by IGF-I.

Minor influences upon IGFBP-3 concentrations are exerted by thyroid hormones which may act via GH. The absence of sex steroids has no influence whereas in *precocious puberty* IGFBP-3 concentrations are markedly increased. Whether this effect is due to increased GH secretion remains unclear. In *Cushing syndrome*, IGFBP-3 concentrations are slightly increased, suggesting some regulatory influence of corticosteroids. IGFBP-3 concentrations are decreased by a number of non-hormonal factors, although the kinetics of the changes are slower and not as pronounced as with IGF-I: the conditions include fasting, polytrauma, severe surgical trauma, large tumors, leukemia, and impaired hepatic function.

In pregnancy, circulating concentrations of intact IGFBP-3 fall and lower-molecular-weight fragments appear due to the presence of a protease in pregnancy serum. Proteolytically cleaved IGFBP-3 has lower affinity for IGFs and this may be a mechanism for elevating free IGF-I and enhancing delivery of IGF-I to target tissues including the placenta. IGFBP-3 protease is also induced by surgery and trauma.

## IGFBP-4

Concentrations of IGFBP-4 in the circulation are low compared with those of IGFBP-3. It is generally considered an inhibitory binding protein for IGF action. In pregnancy IGFBP-4 concentrations fall, suggesting the presence of a protease; similar to the mechanism observed for IGFBP-3. IGFBP-4 is primarily expressed in connective tissue including bone. Vitamin D increases IGFBP-4 concentrations in osteoblasts. In granulosa cells, FSH induces the IGFBP-4 protease thus reducing IGFBP-4 activity and enhancing IGF-I action on follicular development. IGFBP-4 also is strongly expressed in myoblasts.

## IGFBP-5

IGFBP-5 concentrations are low in the circulation. It is expressed mainly in connective tissue where it binds to matrix via heparin-like sequences. A specific protease exists which reduces its binding to glucosaminoglycans. In the matrix bound form it potentiates the actions of IGF-I. This acts as a regulator of connective tissue proliferation. It is believed that tissue injury may affect the secretion of the protease and IGFBP-5. In bone, agents which increase osteoblast proliferation such as IGFs stimulate IGFBP-5 production, which in turn may enhance the action of IGF-I and IGF-II.

## IGFBP-6

IGFBP-6 was first identified in cerebrospinal fluid. It is also found in follicular fluid. IGFBP-6 values are low relative to IGFBP-3 in serum and similar to those of IGFBP-1 and IGFBP-2. The concentrations are higher in men than women and lower in pregnancy. Concentrations in amniotic fluid are similar to adult serum concentrations.

# ACTIONS OF THE IGFS

## IGF receptors

Both IGF-I and IGF-II act through membrane-bound receptors on the cell surface. Two classes of IGF receptors can be distinguished. The type I IGF receptor (or IGF-I receptor) consists of a heterotetramer and is highly homologous to the insulin receptor, being a member of the tyrosine kinase receptor family (*see* page 463). The type II IGF receptor (or IGF-II receptor) consists of a single-chain peptide which is identical to the cation-independent mannose-6-phosphate receptor. Both receptors are substantially glycosylated in the extracellular domains. Both IGF-I and IGF-II cross-react with the insulin receptor. Their affinities, however, are about 100-fold lower than the affinity of insulin which makes possible interactions unlikely under physiological conditions.

### IGF-I receptor

The gene is located on chromosome 15. The receptor is synthesized as a precursor protein consisting of 1337 amino acids with the α-domain at the amino terminus. Processing of the proreceptor involves proteolytic cleavage leaving two subunits, α and β (mol. wt 100–135 kD and 90–95 kD, respectively), that are linked by disulfide bridges. While the α-subunit is localized extracellularly, the β-subunit spans the cell membrane carrying a tyrosine kinase domain at the cytoplasmic portion. For full receptor activity the dimerization of two αβ-hemireceptor molecules is required. The affinity for IGFs and insulin decreases in the order IGF-I > IGF-II ≫ insulin. There is some receptor heterogeneity in various tissues, possibly due to different post-translational processing, which causes variability in the binding affinities for IGF-I and IGF-II.

The understanding of the events that take place after receptor activation by IGF is still developing. By analogy to the insulin receptor, tyrosine kinase seems to play a pivotal role. On binding of the ligand the β-subunit is auto-phosphorylated by an intramolecular reaction activating tyrosine kinase and thus to cascades involving phosphorylation of cytosolic protein leading ultimately to transcriptional activation. There is evidence that further signal transmission involves stimulation of phospholipase C generating 1,2-diacylglycerol and inositol 1,4,5-triphosphate as second messengers. After binding of IGFs to the type I receptor, phosphorylation of various intracellular proteins including IRS-1 is observed (*see* page 463).

It has been suggested that in some tissues insulin/IGF-I "hybrid receptors" are formed. These consist of an αβ component from the insulin receptor linked to the αβ component of the IGF-I receptor ($\alpha_{ins}\ \beta_{ins} - \alpha_{IGF}\ \beta_{IGF}$). Such receptors bind IGF-I with higher affinity than insulin and may mediate some of the metabolic actions of IGF-I.

### IGF-II receptor

The gene is located on chromosome 19 and the receptor protein is expressed in virtually every cell type. The single-chain polypeptide has a calculated molecular mass of 270 kD. There is a short hydrophobic membrane-spanning domain and an unusually short cytoplasmic portion. Ninety-two per cent of the receptor is extracellular, consisting of 15 conserved repeats. Confusingly, the receptor bears two binding sites for two totally unrelated ligands: one for mannose 6-phosphate (Man 6-P), which serves as a recognition marker for lysosomal enzymes, and one for IGF-II. Its affinity for IGF-I is lower by two orders of magnitude and is virtually absent for insulin. The role of this receptor in targeting acidic hydrolases from the trans-Golgi network, or from the cell surface to lysosomes, is well established. Less clear is the significance of IGF-II binding to the same protein. Since IGF-II impaired binding of Man 6-P labeled peptides, it has been speculated that IGF-II may be involved in the control of lysosomal enzymes that are secreted into the extracellular compartment during tissue remodeling. The type II receptor is also found in the circulation, particularly in the fetus, where it may act as an IGF-II specific binding protein.

Most IGF-II if not all effects appear to be mediated via the IGF-I receptor. Scattered evidence, however, suggests that at least in some cell types activation of the IGF-II receptor might be involved in IGF-II-stimulated DNA synthesis or specific cellular functions. More generally IGF-II is considered as a clearance receptor.

## Physiological role of IGFs

IGF-I and IGF-II influence a multitude of cell types of ectodermal, mesodermal and entodermal origin by stimulating (1) proliferation, (2) differentiation, (3) specific cell functions and (4) insulin-like metabolic effects. Examples where IGFs promote differentiation are myoblasts, chondroblasts, osteoblasts, neuroblasts, preadipocytes, lens cells and hematopoietic cells. Examples where IGFs stimulate specific functions of differentiated cells include the synthesis of proteoglycans and collagens by chondrocytes, steroidogenesis in gonadal cells, synthesis of thyroid hormones in thyroidal cells, or seemingly remote actions such as potentiation of natural killer cell activity. Many of these effects are of utmost importance in the growing organism. *In vivo* administration of IGF-I in animal models or in patients with *Laron syndrome* resulted in a clear promotion of linear growth.

The diversity of cells that respond to IGFs and of the responses that are promoted by these peptides raises the question of the physiological significance of such apparently non-specific signals. In particular, what is the information transmitted to the cells by IGFs? An answer cannot be given without considering the bimodal nature of IGF action: "autocrine/paracrine" versus "endocrine." An autocrine/paracrine mode of action means that IGFs elicit their effects at or in the near vicinity of their site of production. This view is supported by a number of findings:

- IGF-I and IGF-II are synthesized in many tissues and by many cell types, especially in cells of mesodermal origin.
- Their local expression is developmentally regulated.
- The regulation of local IGF synthesis is subject to tissue-specific hormonal or to non-hormonal factors.
- Local application of IGF-I promotes tissue repair or hypertrophy.

An endocrine mode of action means that IGFs are transported by the blood stream to a distant site of action. Evidence in favor of this view includes:

- While the main source of circulating IGFs is the hepatocyte, these cells are poor in IGF-I receptors, suggesting that they are not a target for locally produced IGF-I.
- Blood has the highest concentrations of IGF-I and, in humans, of IGF-II.
- Systemic application of IGF-I has metabolic effects, e.g. nitrogen retention, and promotes growth in the absence of GH, e.g. in *Laron syndrome*.
- Blood-borne IGF-I is rapidly transferred to peripheral tissues, where it is unevenly distributed mainly to functionally active cells.

Obviously, both modes of IGF action, autocrine/paracrine and endocrine, are of importance and the question is, how both perspectives can be reconciled to obtain a comprehensive understanding. A general feature of IGFs is that they primarily act on cells which are ready to proliferate or to perform a specific function. This particular status of a cell may be triggered by specific signals such as other peptide growth factors or tissue-specific trophic hormones. This view may be exemplified by the proliferation of fibroblasts.

Quiescent fibroblasts are rather unresponsive to IGF-I. If these quiescent fibroblasts are exposed to so-called "competence factors" like platelet-derived growth factor (PDGF) or basic fibroblast growth factor (bFGF), they become competent for proliferation. That is, the cells enter into the phase G of the cell cycle. To further traverse through G1 into the S-phase, where DNA replication takes place, requires the presence of so-called "progression factors," particularly IGF-I. The overall observable effect of IGF-I on the proliferation of quiescent fibroblasts would then be a synergistic potentiation of the mitogenic effect of PDGF or bFGF.

Similarly, IGF-I is synergistic with FSH, LH and hCG to promote steroidogenesis in granulosa cells, ovarian theca-interstitial cells, Leydig cells and Sertoli cells; with TSH to stimulate thyroid hormone synthesis in thyroid derived cells; with erythropoietin to stimulate erythropoiesis; with granulocyte–monocyte colony stimulating factor to stimulate granulopoiesis; with interleukin-2 to stimulate natural killer cells; and also with several other systems. It is thus evident that the IGFs are part of a complex interplay of diverse regulatory factors. A number of trophic hormones stimulate IGF expression in their target tissues (see above), thereby generating an auxiliary mechanism to potentiate their local effects (Fig. 23.10).

How do circulating IGFs fit into this scenario? Blood-borne IGFs may further increase local concentrations in the interstitial compartments. The major regulators of IGF-I in the blood are food intake and GH. IGF-I therefore provides information on the nutritional status of the organism at the cellular level. For cells which have become competent for proliferation it would be inappropriate to proliferate at a maximal rate if nutrient supply is insufficient due to chronic malnutrition. Decreases in IGF-I may thus decelerate mitosis or other cellular functions and adapt cellular activity to the nutritional situation. GH, on the other hand, integrates signals from the central nervous system (CNS) and the GH-IGF axis may therefore serve as a line of communication from the CNS down to the peripheral tissues. This may be exemplified by *psychosocial growth retardation*. If a child is raised in an unfavorable social environment, GH secretion becomes insufficient and consequently, IGF-I serum concentrations decline, resulting in poor growth. In summary, circulating IGFs and in particular IGF-I may provide information at the cellular level about the nutritional and environmental status of the organism and coordinate the whole body metabolic state (Fig. 23.10).

## Physiological role of IGFBPs

Direct evidence for one or the other physiological role of the IGFBPs is still scarce, but it appears that the various proteins have distinct functions. This is suggested by (1) their largely divergent patterns in different compartments, (2) their different developmental

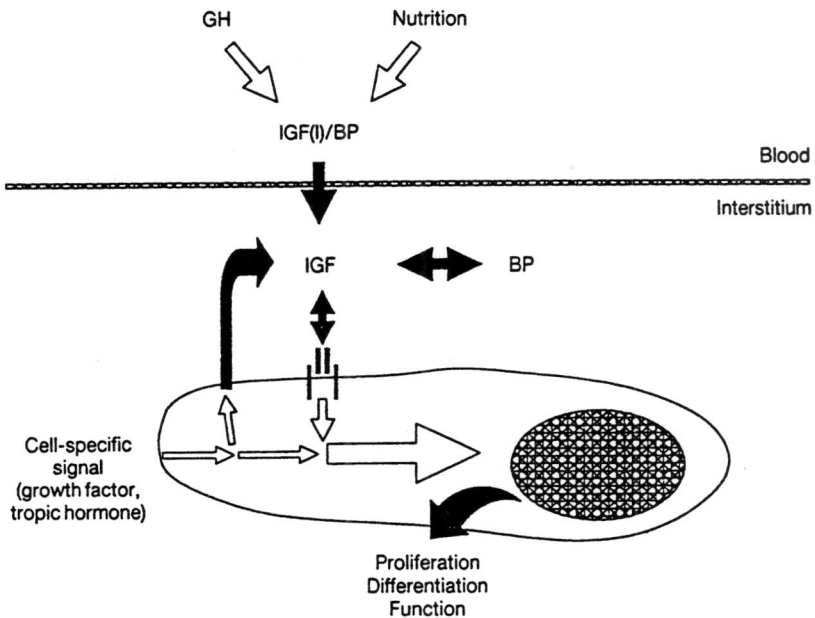

FIGURE 23.10 Schematic representation of the biological action of IGF. IGF synthesis is stimulated by cell-specific signals such as other peptide growth factors or trophic hormones. In addition IGFs are transferred from the circulation to the interstitium. They reversibly interact with their binding proteins (BP) and receptors on the cell surface. Activation of the receptor will then potentiate the response triggered by the cell-specific signal.

patterns, and (3) their different regulation by hormonal or non-hormonal factors. While IGFBP-3 is by far the most abundant IGFBP in the circulation after the first few weeks after birth, it is very low in cerebrospinal fluid, where IGFBP-2 and IGFBP-6 predominate. Similarly in human milk and in seminal plasma IGFBP-2 is present at very high concentrations. The pattern in the lymph varies considerably between different tissues.

The role of circulating IGFBP-3 as a reservoir for IGFs is widely accepted: it serves as a buffer preventing large fluctuations of free IGF. Formation of the ternary complex by binding of the ALS subunit may be of particular importance as the large complex is no longer subject to glomerular filtration. It may also prevent the transfer of IGFBP-3 to other extravascular compartments. Why is such a reservoir and buffer for IGFs necessary? First, there is no intracellular storage pool of IGFs. These peptides are secreted as they are synthesized. Secondly, large fluctuations would be unfavorable with respect to the physiological role of IGF-I in transmitting information on the nutritional and GH secretory status of the organism to the cells. Teleologically, acute food intake or a single GH pulse would be irrelevant for a competent cell to decide whether or not proliferation should take place at a maximal rate. Rather, the long-term nutritional or GH secretory status is important. The presence of a large pool of circulating IGFs releasing the peptides slowly provides a mechanism for integration of these factors over days.

Because of the very slow dissociation rate of the IGF/IGFBP-3 complex, the metabolic half-life of complexed IGF is markedly prolonged in comparison with free IGF. Owing to the very high affinity of IGFBP-3 for IGFs, free IGF is kept in a concentration range that would allow binding to the IGF receptors, but not to the insulin receptor, preventing acute insulin-like effects despite the very high total concentrations of IGFs.

IGFBP-1 and IGFBP-2 may be involved in the fine tuning of free IGF-I and IGF-II. IGFBP-1 is acutely suppressed by glucose ingestion. Such suppression could make free IGFs available, thereby complementing the effect of insulin. IGFBP-2 is consistently found to increase in situations where free IGF-II must be expected to be elevated. IGFBP-2 may therefore function as a buffer for free IGF-II, preventing acute insulin-like effects. In addition to these possible roles of IGFBP-1 and IGFBP-2 in the regulation of free IGFs, there is some evidence that they may also be involved in the transfer of IGFs to the extravascular space and in their specific targeting to cell types.

The influence of IGFBPs on IGF activity at a cellular level is complex. Both inhibitory and stimulatory effects are found which are not necessarily mutually exclusive. In the case of IGFBP-2 it has been demonstrated *in vitro* that the membrane-bound form enhances IGF-I action at low concentrations, and if the IGFBP-2 is modified so that it cannot bind to cell membranes or if it is in excess amounts it is inhibitory. This suggests that enhancing actions occur when the IGFBP fixes the IGF close to the receptor and inhibitory actions occur when excess soluble IGFBP exists. Similar observations have been made with respect to matrix-bound IGFBP-5. In all cases an excess of IGFBP inhibits IGF activity by competing for IGFs against the IGF-I receptor. At lower concentrations stimulatory effects on IGF-I activity can also be observed, especially when IGF-I and IGFBP are applied at an equimolar ratio. Although the exact molecular mechanisms are yet unclear, a constant supply of IGFs by release from the IGF/IGFBP complex may be causative. Modifications of the IGFBP molecules such as phosphorylation may be involved in determining an inhibitory or stimulatory function.

## SPECIFIC DEVELOPMENTAL ASPECTS

### Embryogenesis and fetal life

IGF-I and especially IGF-II have been assumed to play a role in fetal development. The evidence was, however, vague and circumstantial until recently, when direct evidence for the importance of both IGF-I and IGF-II for embryonic growth was demonstrated. In mice, who bear a disrupted IGF-II allele, IGF-II expression is markedly reduced and embryonic growth, but not late fetal or postnatal growth, is impaired. This is compatible with the absence of IGF-II expression in the postnatal rodent. IGF-I null mutants were also growth-retarded at birth but their growth retardation was more marked as it continued into late gestation and postnatally. Most IGF-I null mutants were not viable because of muscle hyperplasia. Double null mutants with both IGF-I and IGF-II deleted were more growth-retarded, suggesting both IGF-I and IGF-II play a role in fetal growth. IGF type I receptor mutants were similarly growth-retarded, suggesting that the action of both IGF-I and IGF-II on fetal growth are mediated via the IGF-I receptor (*see also* page 287).

In mouse embryos IGF-II is expressed along with the IGF-II receptor by the two-cell stage. In preimplantation 64-cell blastocytes IGF-II expression is found in every cell. During organogenesis, and later in mid-gestation fetuses of various species including man, there is abundant IGF-II mRNA in every organ, mainly in cells of mesodermal origin. The IGF-II receptor is abundant and ubiquitous until late gestation when it significantly declines. IGF-I expression commences later but not before embryo implantation, although type I IGF receptor mRNA could be demonstrated in mouse embryos as early as in the eight-cell stage. IGF-I and type I IGF receptor expression are widespread in every organ. Many cells express both IGF peptides, but this is not uniform.

With the appearance of IGF receptors, cells become responsive to IGF-I or IGF-II. Exogenous administration of either peptide stimulates embryogenesis. In early gestation, when no functional circulation has yet developed, their mode of action must necessarily be autocrine/paracrine. Later, circulating IGFs may also become important. From animal experiments it appears that GH has indeed some influence on fetal IGF-I concentrations. This is supported by the clinical observation that newborns with *Laron's syndrome* or *congenital GH deficiency* have a somewhat reduced birth length. Nutritional deprivation has also a suppressive effect on fetal serum IGF-I.

IGFBP-1 and IGFBP-2 are expressed in a variety of fetal tissues with the highest abundance in liver. Their serum concentrations in human fetuses are several-fold increased as compared with young children, whereas the concentrations of IGFBP-3 are several-fold decreased. Although the expression and the concentrations of the various IGFBPs are different in the fetus, their control is qualitatively similar to that described postnatally.

## Pregnancy

During pregnancy maternal IGF-I and IGF-II serum concentrations rise until late gestation and decline rapidly after delivery. IGF-I, but not IGF-II, was shown to positively correlate with birthweight and length, suggesting that maternal IGF-I may be important for fetoplacental development. The rise of IGFs may in part be due to a rise in IGFBP-3 which is high normal or slightly augmented in the second and even more in the third trimester. However, the IGFBP-3 circulates mainly in pregnancy as a 30-kD fragment which is generated from the complete protein by a specific protease. Although this protease is also present in other situations (e.g. in severely ill patients), its activity is particularly high after 7 weeks' gestation in humans. The 30-kD form still binds IGFs and is able to constitute the ternary complex, but its affinity for IGFs is somewhat reduced. The protease therefore may provide a mechanism to facilitate IGF release from the complex. IGFBP-1 concentrations clearly increase by mid-gestation whereas IGFBP-2 concentrations decline during pregnancy and both normalize after delivery.

Interestingly, IGF-I, IGF-II and IGFBP-3 concentrations normalize in pregnant women with *GH deficiency*. This strongly suggests that placental factors such as placental lactogen (hPL) or placental GH (variant GH) regulate IGF-I and IGFBP-3 during pregnancy and substitute for GH of hypophyseal origin.

## Postnatal life

Circulating IGFs and IGFBPs exhibit characteristic age-dependent patterns (*see* Fig. 23.9) which differ within various species. While IGF-II and IGFBP-3 rise rapidly after birth in humans, IGF-I increases slowly in early childhood with a most prominent peak at the time of puberty. IGF-I concentrations fall continuously in adult life whereas IGF-II and IGFBP-3 decrease only slowly between the third and sixth decade and decline more rapidly thereafter. In contrast, the IGFBP-1 and

IGFBP-2 serum concentrations are high at birth, decline until adolescence and increase again with aging. The physiological significance of these patterns remains unclear. There is good evidence that the pubertal peak of IGF-I and IGFBP-3 is caused by an increase of GH secretion at that time and it may be involved in the control of the pubertal growth spurt.

# CLINICAL APPLICATIONS

## Diagnostic use

The importance of IGFs for growth and development makes them interesting parameters for evaluation of growth disorders. Special care must, however, be taken to avoid interference of the IGFBPs in the IGF measurements which can cause grossly erroneous results.

IGF-I and IGFBP-3 and, with limitations, also IGF-II are shown to be of great interest in the evaluation of growth retardation. Subnormal concentrations indicate insufficient production due to one of the causes listed in Table 23.2. The combination of IGF-I and IGFBP-3 concentrations is particularly useful in identifying GH-responsive children with borderline GH secretion.

In tall young patients, or adult patients with clinical signs of acromegaly, elevated serum concentrations of IGF-I and IGFBP-3, but normal concentrations of IGF-II, are suggestive of pathologically increased GH secretion and further GH testing is required.

## Therapeutic use

The availability of recombinant IGFs and IGFBPs makes their use as therapeutic agents conceivable. Although this wide field is still at a very preliminary stage, first results of experimental studies and of clinical trials are promising. IGF-I may be beneficial for such diverse indications as: growth in patients with *Laron syndrome*, changing the catabolic to an anabolic state post-surgery, improving wound healing in polytraumatized or severely burned patients. With respect to wound healing, experimental results suggest that the administration of IGF-I complexed to IGFBP-3 may be effective.

# SELECTED READING

Baxter RC, Gluckman PD, Rosenfeld RG, eds. *The insulin-like growth factors and their regulatory proteins*. Amsterdam: Excerpta Medica, 1994.

Blum WF. Insulin-like growth factors and their binding proteins. In: Ranke MB, ed. *Functional endocrinologic diagnostics in children and adolescents*. Mannheim: J & J Verlag, 1992: 102.

Daughaday WH, Rotwein P. Insulin-like growth factors I and II. Peptide, messenger ribonucleic acid and gene structures, serum, and tissue concentrations. *Endocr Rev* 1989; **10**: 68.

Lowe WL. Once is not enough – promiscuity begets diversity among the insulin-like growth factor binding proteins. *Endocrinology* 1994; **135**: 1719.

Rechler MM, Nissley P. Insulin-like growth factors. In: Sporn MB, Roberts AB, eds. *Handbook of experimental pharmacology*. Vol. 95/I: *Peptide growth factors and their receptors I*. Berlin: Springer-Verlag, 1990: 263.

Spencer EM, ed. *Modern concepts of insulin-like growth factors*. New York: Elsevier, 1991.

TABLE 23.2 Clinical situations with abnormal serum concentrations of IGF-I, IGF-II and IGFBP-3

| DIAGNOSIS | IGF-I | IGF-II | IGFBP-3 |
|---|---|---|---|
| GH deficiency | -(-) | -(-) | -(-) |
| Laron syndrome | — | — | — |
| Diabetes mellitus | - | - | - |
| Hypothyroidism | - | - | - |
| Malnutrition/malabsorption | — | - | - |
| Liver insufficiency | -(-) | -(-) | -(-) |
| Malignancy | -(-) | -(-) | -(-) |
| Acromegaly | +(++) | n | +(++) |
| Precocious puberty | + | n | + |
| Chronic renal failure | n | n(+) | +(++) |

n = normal levels; - low levels; + increased levels.

# PART SIX

# *The Nervous and Muscle Systems*

**Editors: Suzanne L. Davis and Hugo Lagercrantz**

# Overview

Hugo Lagercrantz

The brain of the newborn is not a "tabula chaotica" as proposed by the behaviorists nor a "tabula rasa." The infant is born with a central pattern generator for locomotion (*see* page 407) and reacts to tastes, smells and pain with typical facial expressions, well recognized by the adult. The infant rapidly develops oral communication and is able to sort sound categories on the distribution of sounds in the parent's voice. The innate locomotion and sensory patterns must be genetically determined. The wiring of the $10^{12}$ neurons and $10^{14}$ synapses are contained in the human genome. There are probably only 30 000 genes within the human genome which govern the development of the central nervous system, and epigenetic processes are clearly involved.

During early embryonic life diffusible factors and surface molecules and then later sensory input activate specific subsets of genes at specific times. Homeobox and other phylogenetically conserved genes are involved in the organization of segmentation in the primitive neural tube (*see* page 357). There are basic genetic mechanisms for proliferation, migration and localization of neurons in the cerebral cortex (*see* page 360) which has a basic framework of columns of neurons within six layers. There are also cascades of expression of various neurotransmitters which have important functions during development (*see* page 341).

The developing brain is to a large extent a self-organizing learning system, once the general scaffolding has been built. Neuronal circuits which are active proliferate, while those which are not degenerate (*see* page 365). Edelman has coined the expression "neuronal Darwinism" for this selection process. Sensory and social environment thus reinforce the consolidation of connections formed early in development.

The neurobiology underlying developmental processes is presented in Chapter 24, followed by discussions of the developmental processes in Chapter 25. Subsequent sections detail basic neurobiology and developmental aspects of the sensory (Chapter 26) and motor (Chapter 27) systems, behavior (Chapter 28) and vegetative functions (Chapter 29). Chapter 30 discusses the cerebrovascular system. Chapter 31 discusses the pathophysiology of seizures, brain and peripheral nerve injury as relevant to perinatal and pediatric medicine. Chapter 32 discusses muscle physiology.

Many studies of the developing brain by their very nature must refer to experimental work. It is important to note that the degree of neural maturation at birth varies greatly between species. In altricial species, such as the rat, much neural maturation occurs after birth, relative to that observed in the human. Conversely in precocial species such as subhuman primates, guinea pig, and the sheep, neural maturation at birth is considerably advanced to allow for immediate locomotion.

## SELECTED READING

Changeux JP. *Neuronal man*. Oxford: Oxford University Press, 1985.

Edelman GM. *Bright air. Bright fire. On the matter of mind*. New York: Basic Books, 1992.

Mehler J, Dupoux E. *Naitre humaine*. Paris: Editions Odile Jacob, 1990.

# 24

# Basic Neurophysiology

# INTRANEURONAL BIOLOGY

Neurons show some similarities to other epithelial cells, but also present distinct structural and biological characteristics. These relate to the neuron's specialized ability to receive nerve impulses at the somato-dendritic junction and to transmit signals through the axon to another neuron or to an effector target. Synthesis of macromolecules, including those specific for neurotransmission, occurs in the cell body, the perikaryon, which contains the necessary organelles for this purpose. Neurons have an extensive dendritic tree and long axon of constant diameter. In order to generate this asymmetric structure, neurons have developed precise mechanisms for the sorting and intraneuronal transport of molecules to the different target areas. Non-neuronal epithelial cells (e.g. renal epithelium) also deliver materials asymmetrically to their functionally distinct apical and basolateral plasma membrane domains. The apical surface may be equivalent to axons and the basolateral domain to somato-dendrites, since similar molecules are transferred to these surfaces. For instance, molecules that are attached to the cell membrane by a glycolipid anchor are transported to apical and axonal surfaces, whereas the transferrin receptor travels to basolateral and somato-dendritic membranes (Fig. 24.1).

Neurons are unique for the striking spatial separation between the two cell membrane domains and by the requirement for long distance transportation of molecules in axons and dendrites. In addition, neurons, unlike other epithelial cells, have an asymmetric distribution of cytoskeletal elements in the cytosol. For example, the microtubule-associated protein, MAP2, is strictly localized to somata and dendrites, whereas another microtubule-associated protein, tau, is concentrated in axons.

## TARGETING IN THE PERIKARYON

Proteins synthesized at clusters of free ribosomes may remain in the cytosol, e.g. cytoskeletal proteins, or become specifically targeted to intracellular structures, e.g. the nucleus, mitochondria or peroxisomes. Signal amino acid sequences in the proteins for these transfers have been defined. Membrane associated protein synthesis commences with specific recognition between a nascent polypeptide–large ribosome subunit complex and the membrane of rough endoplasmic reticulum. A number of proteins are then translocated across the membrane to become content of cisterns or vesicles in the cell. Other proteins will become partly integrated in the membrane when stop transfer sequences inhibit their total translocation. A few proteins which express a specific recognition amino acid sequence remain in the endoplasmic reticulum. Such retained proteins may function as chaperons that play an important role in

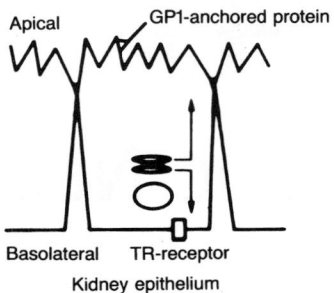

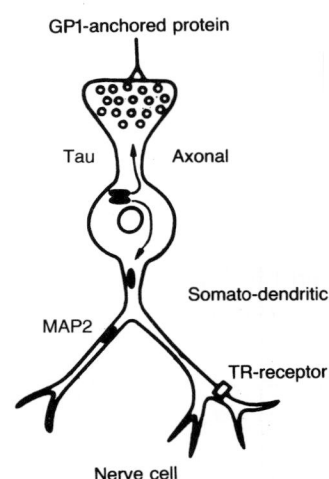

FIGURE 24.1 Comparison of cell asymmetry between a kidney epithelial cell and a neuron. Several molecules that are sorted to the apical surface of the kidney epithelial cell are transferred to the axon in the neuron. The basolateral and somato-dendritic domains are equivalent in a number of, but not all, aspects. In neurons, the microtubule-associated proteins, tau and MAP2, are asymmetrically distributed. GP1 glycolipid anchored protein; TR transferrin.

securing correct folding of other newly formed proteins. Interference with protein folding in neurons may be of pathophysiological importance, e.g. an altered protein configuration is a feature of *prion diseases* such as *Creutzfeld–Jakob disease*. After transfer through the smooth endoplasmic reticulum, which lacks attached ribosomes, transport vesicles shuttle the proteins to the Golgi apparatus for glycosylation. After passage through the Golgi apparatus further sorting occurs. Proteins destined to lysosomes are recognized by the presence of mannose-6-phosphate residues in their sugar component; lack of the residues causes *inclusion-cell disease*, in which hydrolases, by default sorting, are secreted from the cell instead of being targeted to lysosomes.

The majority of proteins made in the perikarya are transferred to dendrites or axons. Signals for this sorting may act either by retaining the material in the soma or by directing it to the processes. The axon hillock provides a functional barrier by which ribosomes and the Golgi apparatus are excluded from axons either by retention signals present in the perikaryon or by hindrance of cross-linked neurofilaments in the axons (see below). Transmembrane proteins in the vesicles may contain signals for directed transport. These can be located in their cytoplasmic tails and a deletion of the tails can inhibit asymmetric sorting. Recent data have indicated that a member of the family of Rab proteins in the cytosol, Rab8, may direct transport of vesicles specifically into dendrites, but the mechanism behind the vectorial movement of this cytosolic protein is not known. Although transport to only one plasma domain may be directed by sorting signals (the other being the result of default sorting), current research indicates that targeting of molecules to axons and dendrites depends on a number of different signals within the neuron and that the final position of a molecule on the cell surface is influenced by factors in the surrounding tissue.

## AXONAL TRANSPORT

### Fast anterograde transport

When entering axons or dendrites, vesicles are transported at a relatively rapid rate, about 400 mm/day, towards the periphery. Most experimental observations concern transport in axons. The vesicles destined for transport associate with kinesin, which is an ATPase that attaches one arm to the vesicle and the other to a microtubule. Thus, kinesin acts as the driv-

ing force for axonal transport of vesicles and microtubules serve as a track (Fig. 24.2). Axons also contain a system of continuous cisterns, the so-called axonal smooth endoplasmic reticulum. The relation of axonal smooth endoplasmic reticulum to that in the cell body is unclear, but evidence exists that some membrane proteins of the latter can bypass the Golgi apparatus to enter axons. The function of axonal endoplasmic reticulum was originally thought to be formation of synaptic vesicles at the axon terminals; other roles may include lipid synthesis or the storage of intra-axonal $Ca^{2+}$.

## Retrograde Transport

Vesicles that reach axon terminals can enter the pool of synaptic vesicles. Through a specific molecular interaction, the vesicles are docked to the membranes of the axon terminal (Fig. 24.2). After interaction, which involves two integral proteins of the synaptic vesicles (vesicle-associated membrane protein (VAMP)) and synaptotagmin) and two in the axon plasma membrane (syntaxin and synaptosome-associated protein 25 KDal (SNAP-25)), the membranes fuse and the vesicle releases its contents into the synaptic cleft. A compensatory incorporation of membranes from the surface of the axon terminals follows: the membrane is invaginated, coated with clathrin and encircled at its neck by a recently recognized protein, dynamin. The latter belongs to the guanosine triphosphat-(GTP)ase super-

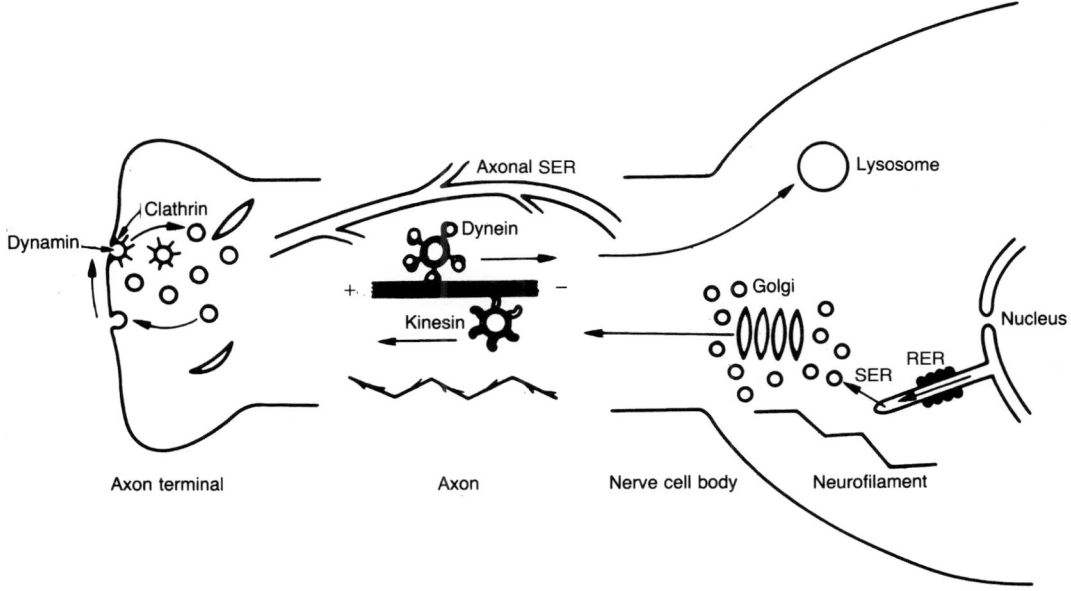

FIGURE 24.2 Intraneuronal traffic of membrane-associated molecules. They are synthesized in the rough endoplasmic reticulum (RER), pass through the smooth endoplasmic reticulum (SER) and are shuttled through transport vesicles to the Golgi apparatus. They are then transferred by fast anterograde axonal transport to the axon terminal. In axons kinesin serves as a motor and microtubules as tracks for the transport. After exocytosis, endocytic vesicles return via retrograde axonal transport to the cell body where their contents are broken down in lysosomes. Clathrin and dynamin are involved in formation of endocytic vesicles, and dynein serves as a motor for transport in the retrograde direction. In axons, the hinged heavy chain of the neurofilament triplets can cross-link organelles and thereby prevent free movement and give strength to the process.

family and pinches off the invaginated plasma membrane to form an endocytic vesicle. The vesicles may then return to the pool of synaptic vesicles or travel in retrograde direction to the cell body to fuse with lysosomes for protein degradation. The retrograde transport of endocytic vesicles in axons also uses microtubules as tracks, but the motor for the driving force is dynein instead of kinesin. The mechanism by which a vesicle is tagged to attach to the anterograde or to the retrograde transport machinery is not clear.

## Slow transport

A number of cytosolic proteins form the so-called cytoskeleton. They are synthesized in the perikaryon and transported slowly, 1–2 mm/day, out into the axons. The cytoskeleton is composed of microtubules and the microtubule-associated proteins, neurofilaments and microfilaments (actin). Although microtubules are present in all cells, some of the microtubule-associated proteins are specific for neurons. The latter may be asymmetrically distributed, e.g. microtubule-associated protein 2 (MAP2) localizes to somato-dendrites and does not, except for a period during development, extend into axons. The tau protein, on the other hand, is concentrated in axons. The functions of these microtubule-associated proteins include promotion of microtubule assembly and the spatial arrangement of the microtubules that contributes to the shape of axon or dendrites. Microtubules are polarized with their growing positive end directed to the periphery in axons. In dendrites, however, both positive and negative ends are oriented to the periphery. It is not clear if this difference in microtubule-polarity also contributes to the asymmetric delivery of proteins in neurons. Neurofilaments, which are neuron-specific members of the intermediate filament family, are transferred as triplets of different chain weights into the axons. Here they become phosphorylated, whereby the heavy outer chain is hinged providing arms to cross-link organelles. The function of intermediate filaments is in general not known, but may involve transport of RNA in the perikaryon. In axons, neurofilaments may increase the resistance of axons to stretching forces. The exact role played by actin in axons is not clear, but with its subsurface localization it may serve a skeletal function in maintaining the shape of the axon.

## PATHOPHYSIOLOGY OF AXONAL TRANSPORT

## Membrane flow

Vesicle cycling at axon terminals and their retrograde transport have a number pathophysiological implications.

- Botulinus toxin acts as an enzyme that specifically cleaves the docking proteins involved in synaptic vesicle release: botulinus toxin A cleaves SNAP-25. Consequently, one molecule of this potent toxin can block the function of a whole synapse.
- A number of neurotrophic viruses, e.g. *rabies*, *poliomyelitis* and *herpes simplex* can be taken up by endocytic vesicles at axon terminals and transported retrogradely to the nerve cell body for multiplication. Herpes simplex virus often remains latent in sensory ganglia. Upon activation it selects the peripheral branch of the axon to travel to the skin and not the central branch.
- Toxins, like tetanus toxin and certain lectins, can be transported retrogradely to exert their actions. The former, after reaching motorneuron cell bodies, can pass to inhibitory synaptic terminals, block their action by proteolytic cleavage of a synaptic vesicle docking protein and cause *tetanus*.
- The prion protein is glycolipid-anchored at axon terminals. Its endocytic incorporation may provide a means for axonal spread of infectious prions in *Creutzfeld–Jakob disease*.

## Cytoskeleton

The cytoskeleton is involved in a number of nervous system diseases ranging from abnormal phosphorylation of the tau protein in *Alzheimer disease* to large accumulations of neurofilaments at axon terminals in *neuroaxonal dystrophy* and during aging. The cytoskeleton is also the target for a number of toxic agents, like microtubule disassembly caused by vinblastine and neurofilament accumulations by hexacarbon solvents. Certain viruses can also cause selective cytoskeletal derangements.

## SELECTED READING

Holtzman E, Schacher S, Evans J, Teichberg S. Origin and fate of the membranes of secretion granules and synaptic vesicles: membrane circulation in neurons, gland cells and retinal photoreceptors. In Poste G, Nicolson L eds. *The synthesis, assembly and turnover of cell surface components*. Amsterdam: Elsevier, 1977.

Matus M. Microtubule-associated proteins: their potential role in determining neuronal morphology. *Ann Rev Neurosci* 1988; **11**: 29.

Pevsner J, Hsu S-C, Braun JEA, Calakos N, Ting AE, Bennett MK, Scheller RH. Specificity and regulation of a synaptic vesicle docking complex. *Neuron* 1994; **13**: 353.

Rodriguez-Boulan E, Powell SK. Polarity of epithelial and neuronal cells. *Ann Rev Cell Biol* 1992; **8**: 395.

Simons K, Zerial M. Rab proteins and the road maps for intracellular transport. *Neuron* 1993; **11**: 789.

Vallee RB, Shpetner HS, Paschal BM. The role of dynein in retrograde axonal transport. *TINS* 1989; **12**: 66.

# AXONAL CONDUCTION

The fundamental role of neurons in the nervous system is to process and transmit information in terms of electrical and chemical signals. The processing steps involve different regions of the neuron. A neuron comprises four essential components:

- an input component, consisting of the dendrites and soma, transforming chemical (synaptic) signals to localized potential changes.
- an integrative component, comprising trigger zones (mainly localized to the initial segment of the axon) transforming converging localized potentials to all-or-nothing action potentials.
- a conductile or long-range signaling component consisting of the axon which transmits the action potential from the integrative region to the output region.
- an output component, consisting of the branched axon (synaptic) terminal which transforms the transmitted action potentials to chemical signals.

The focus in this chapter will be on the conductile component of the neuron, i.e. the axon. The different functional roles for the dendrites and the axon are reflected in morphological and chemical differences, the most striking being the myelinization of vertebrate axons (see page 346). A myelinated axon is organized in long stretches (1–2 mm) of electrically passive myelinated segments, interrupted by short electrically active segments, the nodes of Ranvier.

The two principal types of electrical signals used by neurons are localized potentials and action potentials. A localized potential spreads only short distances (typically 1–2 mm) and is graded, i.e. its amplitude depends on the stimulus strength. An action potential is a regenerative all-or-nothing phenomenon, i.e. it is independent of stimulus strength and propagates along the axon without decrement in amplitude. The propagation speed depends on size and myelination of the axon and may vary between 0.5 and 100 ms. The change in membrane potential is caused by currents passing through specific proteins in the membrane bilayer, ion channels. Depending on whether the channels are regulated by the membrane potential or by ligands they are referred to as voltage- or ligand-gated. The ion channels involved in generation of the action potential belong to the voltage-gated group.

## THE RESTING POTENTIAL

A fundamental requisite for all cellular electrical signaling is a charged cell membrane at rest. The intact neuron has a resting membrane potential of –60 to –80 mV (intracellular relative to extracellular). The detailed mechanism for the resting potential at a molecular level is not fully understood. It is clear that the

unequal distribution of the $K^+$ ions across the cell membrane is essential for maintaining the resting potential in eukaryotic cells. This unequal distribution is maintained by ATP-dependent ion pumps. The intracellular $K^+$ concentration ($[K^+]$) in mammalian cells is about 140 mM; extracellular $[K^+]$, about 5 mM. If the nerve membrane was exclusively permeable to $K^+$ ions it can be inferred that such a $[K^+]$ difference would cause a resting potential of about –90 mV. The equation used is the Nernst equation:

$$E_K = \frac{RT}{z} F \ln \frac{[K^+]_o}{[K^+]_i}$$

where $E_K$ is the equilibrium potential for $K^+$; $R$, the gas constant; $T$, the absolute temperature; $z$, the valence of $K^+$; $F$, the Faraday constant; $[K^+]_o$, the extracellular and $[K^+]_i$, the intracellular $K^+$ concentration.

However, measured resting potentials are as a rule less negative than predicted for a pure $K^+$ permeable membrane, suggesting that the membrane is also permeable to other ions. Such a situation is described quantitatively by the constant field or Goldman–Hodgkin–Katz (GHK) equation, given below for the case of a membrane exclusively permeable for both $K^+$ and $Na^+$ ions:

$$V_r = \frac{RT}{F} \ln \frac{P_K [K^+]_o + P_{Na} [Na^+]_o}{P_K [K^+]_i + P_{Na} [Na^+]_i}$$

where $V_r$ is the resting potential; $P_K$, the permeability for $K^+$ and $P_{Na}$, the permeability for $Na^+$.

The molecular mechanism for the resting potential varies with cell type. Non-gated leak channels are suggested to be major determinants in many cells and non-protein ion pathways may play a role.

## THE ACTION POTENTIAL

The action potential is a transient membrane potential change (typically about 100 mV) that persists for 1–2 ms. In most axons the action potential is caused by transient changes in membrane permeability to $Na^+$ and $K^+$ associated with $Na^+$ and $K^+$ currents across the membrane (Fig. 24.3). The inward movement of $Na^+$, depolarization, is associated with the fast upstroke of the action potential. In some invertebrate axons this inward current is carried by $Ca^{2+}$. Repolarization is caused by an outward current of $K^+$. The action potential is a regenerative and cyclic process: depolarization increases $Na^+$ permeability,

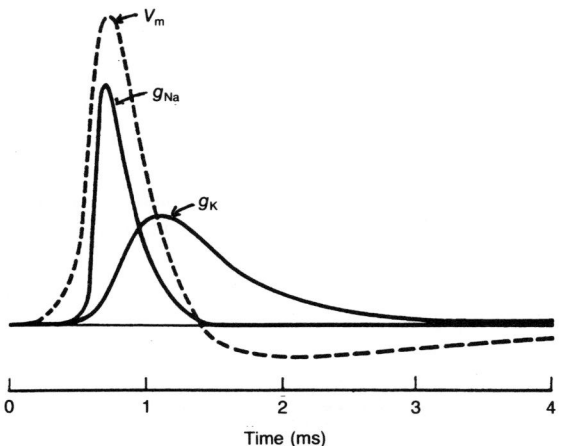

FIGURE 24.3 Computed action potential and underlying changes in sodium ($g_{Na}$) and potassium ($g_K$) conductances, defined as $g_{Na} = I_{Na}/(V_m - E_{Na})$ and $g_K = I_K/(V_m - E_K)$. $I_{Na}$ is sodium current and $I_K$ potassium current. $V_m$ is membrane potential. The computations are based on experimental data. (After Hodgkin AL. *The conduction of the nerve impulse.* Liverpool: Liverpool University Press, 1964.)

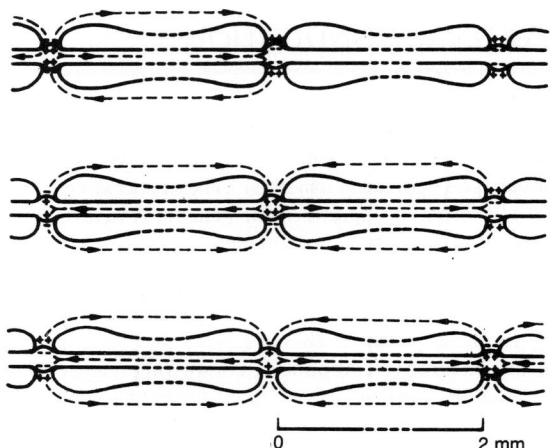

FIGURE 24.4 Schematic diagram of the current flow during action potential propagation in a myelinated axon. Saltatory conduction leads to action potentials only being generated at the nodes of Ranvier.

promotes Na⁺ flux and causes further depolarization. This regenerative process is the basis of the all-or-nothing principle which implies that signal intensity in axons is coded in frequency patterns rather than in the amplitude of action potentials. However, stimulus-dependent graded action potentials have been observed in certain central neurons, suggesting that some information processing in the brain may depend on amplitude modulation.

The propagation of the action potential along the axon depends on local current circuits. As a region of membrane generates an action potential, it causes depolarization and excitation of adjacent regions. Thus, the rate of propagation of action potentials along an axon depends not only on transient permeability changes but on static passive membrane properties such as membrane resistance, membrane capacitance and axoplasmic resistance, quantitatively described by the membrane time constant and the axon length constant. The higher the membrane resistance, the less attenuation of longitudinal current and the less membrane capacitance, the faster response to a change in longitudinal current. Myelinated axons are covered by segments of high-resistance and low-capacitance myelin layers resulting in faster propagation of action potentials by saltatory conduction compared to unmyelinated axons of similar size. Saltatory conduction is the propagation process in which action potentials are generated only at the nodes of Ranvier (Fig. 24.4).

## MOLECULAR MECHANISMS

The ion channels associated with the propagated action potential belong to the superfamily of voltage-gated

channels. The Na⁺ and Ca²⁺ channel families are relatively homogeneous with respect to molecular structure, suggesting a close evolutionary relationship. The pore-forming proteins of these channels consist of about 2000 amino acids organized in four conservative repeats or domains, each consisting of six transmembrane segments (S1–S6). One of these segments, S4, contains regularly repeated charged residues at every third position, and probably constitutes the voltage sensitive element of the channel. The linker between the S5 and S6 segments forms an essential part of the channel pore wall (Fig. 24.5). The voltage-gated K⁺ channel family is more diverse with respect to both kinetics and molecular structure. The pore-forming protein of voltage-gated K⁺ channels is smaller than corresponding Na⁺ and Ca²⁺ channel proteins and consists of about five hundred amino acids. It also consists of six transmembrane segments, the fourth (S4) being regularly charged. The channel is formed as a tetramer of these proteins (Fig. 24.5). The K⁺ channel family is probably more primitive than the Na⁺ and Ca²⁺ channels.

Most voltage-gated ion channels can exist in three main states; closed, open and inactivated. During an action potential the Na⁺ channel goes through all the states; from closed via open to the inactivated state. The existence of an inactivated state implies that the Na⁺ channel is refractory, i.e. has an interval of reduced membrane excitability, following the action potential.

## PHARMACOLOGICAL IMPLICATIONS

The molecular structure of ion channels may explain many of the observed effects of pharmacological agents on axons. Agents that are active at the axon belong to two main classes; blockers, such as the

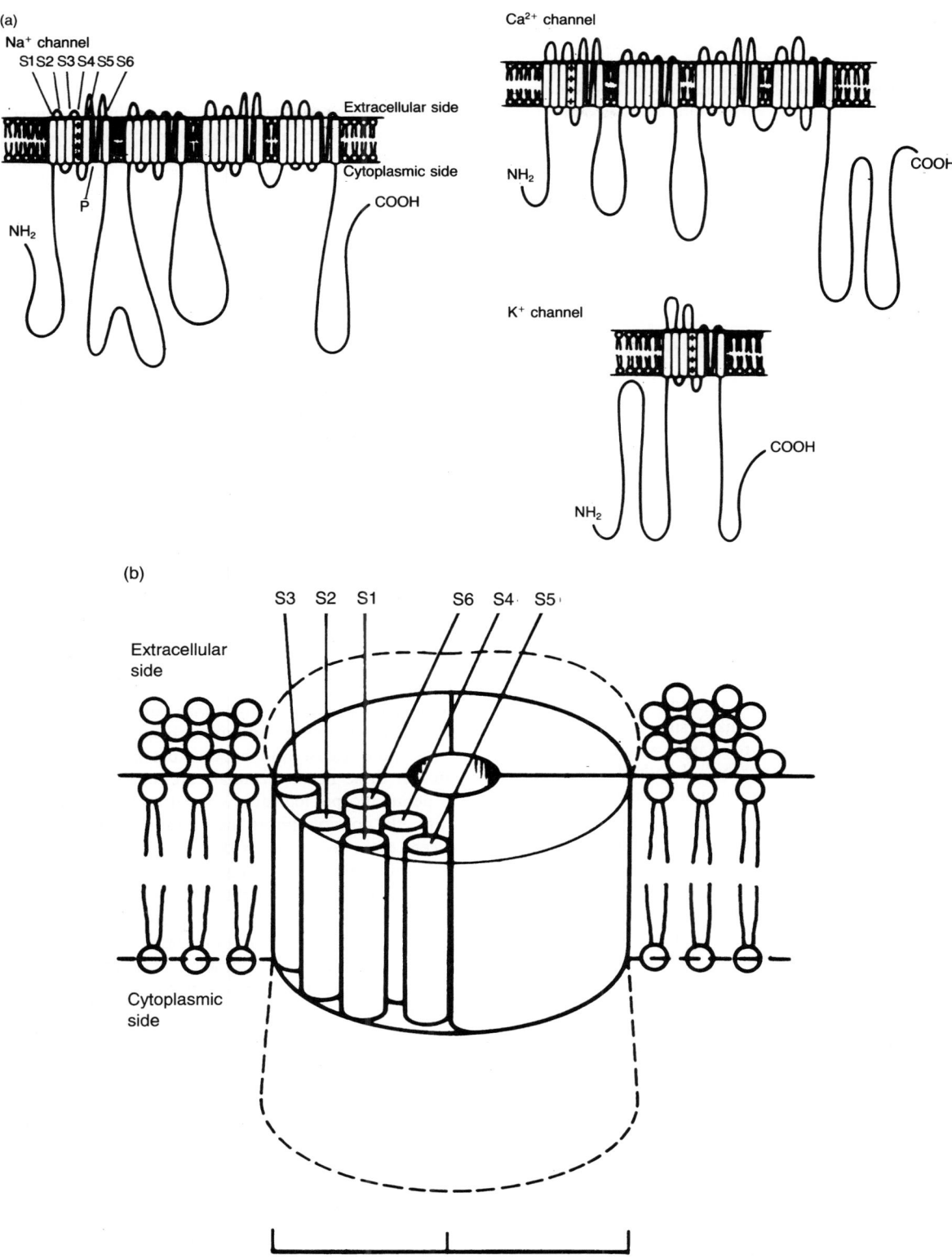

FIGURE 24.5 Proposed topology of voltage-gated ion channels. (a) The four domains of the $Na^+$ and $Ca^{2+}$ channels and the single domain of the $K^+$ channel are shown, as well as the six transmembrane helices (S1–S6) in each domain. The charged nature of the S4 segment is indicated. The linker between S5 and S6, assumed to form the pore wall, is marked by P. (b) The postulated three-dimensional structure of a channel is schematically illustrated. The six transmembrane helices are indicated in one domain. The $K^+$ channel is assumed to be formed by four single-domain subunits.

local anesthetics, and gating modifiers, such as $Ca^{2+}$ and $Mg^{2+}$. Local anesthetics probably block $Na^+$ and $K^+$ channels by binding to a hydrophobic site at an inner vestibule of the channel pore. The binding is use-dependent, i.e. it varies with channel state. Open and inactivated channels show higher affinity for the local anesthetic molecule than closed channels. Both $Ca^{2+}$ and $Mg^{2+}$ increase the threshold for elicitation of an action potential by modifying the potential dependence of the gating. This is largely explained by a neutralization of fixed surface charges on the external portion of the channel protein.

## SELECTED READING

Armstrong CM. Voltage-dependent ion channels and their gating. *Physiol Rev* 1992; 72: S5.

Hille B. *Ionic channels of excitable membranes*. 2nd edn. Sunderland: Sinauer, 1992.

Hodgkin AL. *The conduction of the nerve impulse*. Liverpool: Liverpool University Press, 1964.

Johnston D, Miao-Sin Wu S. *Foundations of cellular neurophysiology*. Cambridge MA: MIT Press, 1995.

# SYNAPTIC FUNCTION

The extremely complex interaction of the $10^{12}$ neurons in the human brain is traditionally assumed to be restricted to a specialized site, the synapse. The term synapse (Greek: to clasp) was coined by Sir Charles Sherrington nearly a hundred years ago to refer to the site of transmission between "neuron and neuron." The definition has been widened to include sites where a neuron interacts with non-neuronal target cells (e.g. neuromuscular endplate). Strict synaptic transmission is only a special case; the site of communication of some neurons with target cells is peri- or non-synaptic or even para- or neuroendocrine. Information flow across a "synapse" may be bidirectional. Some substances released from the nerve (transmitters) induce rapid changes in the target cells leading to distinct electrical, mechanical or secretory effects. Other substances released either from the nerve terminals or from target cells (modulators or trophins) have long-term effects, e.g. on synaptic strength, on the distribution of postsynaptic receptors, on the growth and differentiation of a neuron or on transmitter choice.

## NEUROTRANSMISSION VIA IONOPHORE RECEPTORS

Research concerning synaptic function has been focused mainly on synapses in which the released transmitter opens fast ionic channels. Rapid changes in the membrane potential or current may be used to monitor transmitter release on a pulse by pulse basis. Such synapses are often morphologically well defined. There is aggregation of synaptic vesicles at the active zone (or presynaptic grid), a region of the presynaptic membrane which is visibly thickened due to concentration of ion channels and possibly other protein components of the fusion machine. The synaptic cleft is characteristically narrow and there is thickening of the postsynaptic membrane due to clustering of neurotransmitter receptors. At the skeletal neuromuscular junction (Fig. 24.6) binding of two molecules of the released transmitter, acetylcholine, to the nicotinic receptor causes it to open a central pore and allow rapid influx of cations. Similar ionotrophic synapses occur in the central and peripheral nervous systems (Fig. 24.7, point A) where they may be either excitatory or inhibitory. The receptor channels opened by acetylcholine, glutamate or ATP are cation-selective; the effect is to depolarize the target cell, i.e. they are excitatory. The receptor channels opened by glycine or γ-aminobutyric acid (GABA) are anion-selective; the effect is to hyperpolarize the target cell, i.e. they are inhibitory.

## NEUROTRANSMISSION VIA G-PROTEIN-COUPLED RECEPTORS

Much more common are "synapses" in which the released transmitter acts via non-ionophore receptors. These synapses have been difficult to characterize both because of lack of methods with sufficient sensitivity and spatio-temporal resolution to measure per pulse transmitter release and because the preferred release sites in these nerve terminals are small and difficult to define morphologically with current staining methods. All non-ionophore neurotransmitter receptors, except those for nitric oxide (NO), have seven transmembrane-spanning domains (Fig. 24.7B–G). Transmitter actions via these receptors are mediated via G-proteins coupled to ion channels or to enzymes producing cAMP, cGMP, diacylglycerol or inositol 1,4,5 triphosphate ($IP_3$) (*see* page 341). These intracellular second messengers may act directly on ion channels or on protein kinases which in turn phosphorylate ion channels or other protein components that regulate the cell machinery.

Neurotransmitters which activate ionotrophic receptors may also be ligands of one or several G-protein-coupled receptors. The most extreme example is 5-hydroxytryptamine (serotonin; 5HT) for which 14 different G-protein-coupled receptor subtypes and one ionotrophic receptor have been cloned. Glutamate binds to three ionotrophic receptors (N-methyl-D-aspartate (NMDA), kainate and α-amino-3-hydroxy-5-methyl-4-isoxazole propionic acid (AMPA) receptors) and at least eight G-protein receptor subtypes (the so-called metabotrophic receptors). In general, the affinity of a receptor to its ligand transmitter increases with distance from the transmitter release site (Fig. 24.7).

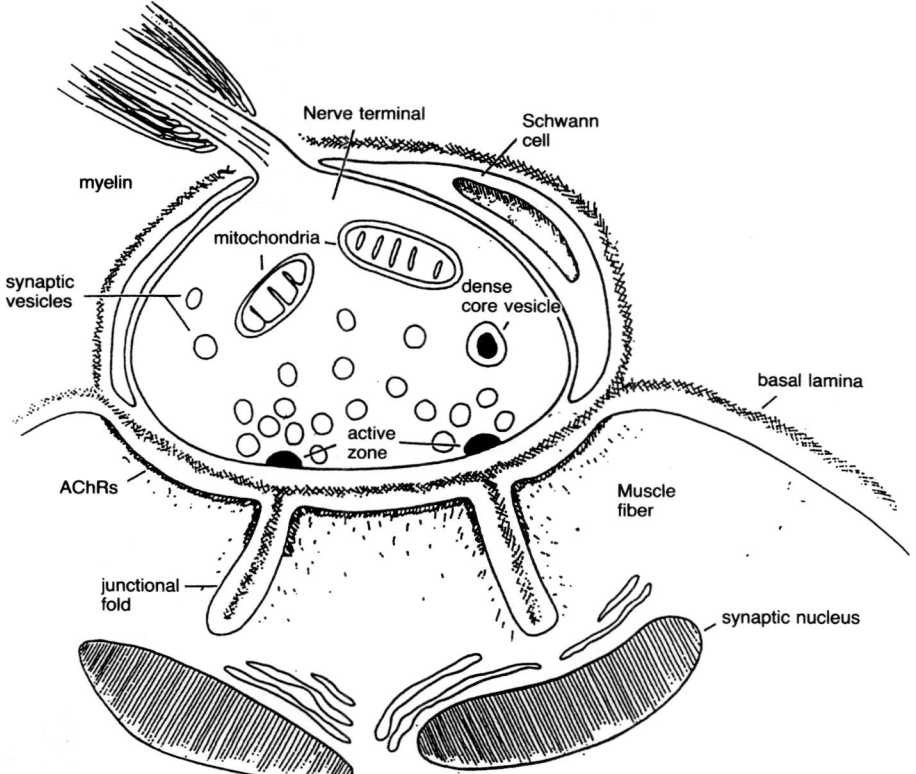

FIGURE 24.6 Essential elements of a morphologically well defined, classical peripheral synapse, in this case between a cholinergic motor nerve terminal and a skeletal muscle cell. Note (1) the pre- and postsynaptic elements separated by a narrow synaptic cleft and the unmyelinated Schwann cell sheath which encloses extrasynaptic regions of the nerve terminal, (2) the numerous small synaptic vesicles, the more sparse large dense core vesicles and mitochondria in the nerve terminal, (3) the clustering of small synaptic vesicles at active zones, (4) fusion of the basal laminae of nerve, muscle and Schwann cell, and (5) restriction of acetylcholine receptors (AChRs) to the intrasynaptic region of the muscle membrane.

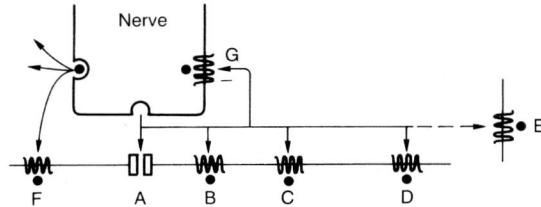

FIGURE 24.7 Small synaptic vesicles release transmitters by exocytosis from active zones. Exocytosis of large dense core vesicles occurs from other sites. Seven types of synaptic neurotransmission are illustrated. (A) Classical fast transmission via ionophore receptors located on the postsynaptic membrane opposite to the release site. (B) Slow transmission via seven transmembrane-spanning, G-protein-coupled receptors at the edge of the synapse. (C) Slower transmission via perisynaptic G-protein-coupled receptors. (D) Even slower transmission via nonsynaptic G-protein-coupled receptors. (E) Neuroendocrine transmission: the transmitter is carried by the blood stream to distant G-protein-coupled receptors (e.g. vasopressin). (F) Slow transmission mediated by three co-transmitters released from a large dense core vesicle, via G-protein-coupled receptors. (G) Autoinhibition of release mediated by released transmitter via G-protein-coupled receptors on the nerve terminal.

## DIFFERENT TYPES OF SYNAPTIC COMMUNICATION

In a chemical synapse, the signaling which induces short term electrical, secretory or mechanical effects, is unidirectional and anterograde. However, there are other types of "synaptic traffic" which are bidirectional (Fig. 24.8). Fast two-way transmission occurs in "electrical synapses" via gap junctions (Fig. 24.8a1), or in juxtaposed dendro-dendritic chemical synapses (Fig. 24.8a2). Activation of a target cell may cause it to release modulatory signals, e.g. adenosine or NO, which diffuse across the synaptic cleft to the nerve terminal and may either depress or enhance transmitter release (Fig. 24.8b). Specific proteins released from large dense core vesicles exert long-term effects on the distribution of transmitter receptors on the surface of the target cell (Fig. 24.8c). Growth factors or other substances released from target cells, taken up into nerve terminals and retrogradely transported to the cell body, induce growth and differentiation of the neuron and may determine its transmitter choice (Fig. 24.8d).

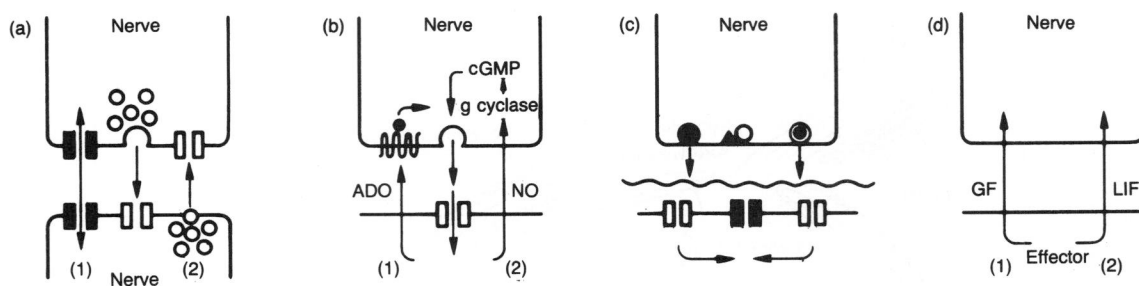

FIGURE 24.8(a) (1) Bidirectional electrical transmission via a gap junction. (2) Bidirectional chemical transmission in a dendro-dendritic synapse. (b) Two examples of trans-synaptic feedback modulation of transmitter release. (1) Transmitter-induced activation of the target cell causes it to release adenosine (ADO). Adenosine depresses $Ca^{2+}$ influx and promotes $K^+$ efflux via G-protein-coupled receptors on the nerve terminals and, at least in part by these mechanisms, inhibits transmitter release. (2) A rise in the intracellular concentration of $Ca^{2+}$ in the target cell induces formation of nitric oxide (NO) which diffuses into the nerve terminal, activates soluble guanylyl cyclase (g cyclase), increases formation of cGMP and causes a prolonged enhancement of per pulse transmitter release. This mechanism is a presynaptic component of long-term potentiation (LTP) of transmission in hippo-campal synapses, a mechanism believed to play a vital role in learning and memory. (c) In the skeletal neuromuscular junction proteins such as agrin released from large dense core vesicles are immobilized in the basal lamina, bind to a receptor on the postsynaptic membrane and induce nicotinic acetylcholine receptors to cluster on the intrasynaptic membrane. (d) Two examples of slow retrograde signaling from target cell to neuron. (1) Growth factors (GF) taken up into the nerve terminals and transported to the cell soma control growth and differentiation of the neuron. (2) Uptake of released leukemia inhibitory factor (LIF) causes a sympathetic neuron to use acetylcholine instead of noradrenaline as its transmitter.

## NEUROTRANSMITTERS

Presently known neurotransmitters belong to five different classes:

- Specialized compounds, e.g. acetylcholine, catecholamines (dopamine, norepinephrine and epinephrine), and 5-hydroxytryptamine.
- Nucleotides, e.g. ATP.
- Amino acids, e.g. glutamate, GABA and glycine.
- NO.
- Neuropeptides.

The neuropeptides are synthesized and packaged into large dense core vesicles in the cell soma and carried to the terminals by fast axonal transport at a rate of up to 15 mm/h. Members of the other classes are synthesized locally in the nerve terminals.

## Neurotransmitter release

Nerve impulses release neurotransmitters by exocytosis of multimolecular packets, i.e. as quanta. Exocytosis of transmitters in synaptic vesicles is triggered by a focal rise in free intraterminal $[Ca^{2+}]$ to $\geq 100$ μM and occurs from specialized release sites, active zones. This release contrasts with exocytosis of neuropeptides in large dense core vesicles which is triggered by a global rise in free $[Ca^{2+}]$ to $\leq 10$ μM and occurs from random sites (Fig. 24.7). Transmitter is also released under resting conditions, both by spontaneous exocytosis and by molecular leakage of cytosolic transmitter. Molecular leakage may occur by reversal of the plasma membrane transporter which normally takes up transmitters from the extracellular space, or may utilize the transporters of vesicle membrane patches incorporated into the plasma membrane (Fig. 24.9a). The physiological role of molecular leakage is unclear, but drug-induced acceleration of this process, e.g. the increased efflux of monoamines induced by amphetamine, underlies most of the clinical effects of such drugs.

## Rate-limiting factors

The majority of synaptic vesicles are not releasable because the vesicle membrane phosphoprotein, Synapsin 1, in its dephosphorylated state crosslinks with actin filaments in the cytoskeleton. The four steps involved in quantal release of transmitter from an active zone of the presynaptic membrane are described in Fig. 24.9b. The first step is triggered by a rise in global intraterminal $[Ca^{2+}]$ to $\geq 0.5$ μM on arrival of a high frequency train of nerve impulses. This activates calcium calmodulin protein kinase II in the vesicle membrane causing phosphorylation of Synapsin 1. The resulting liberation of the vesicle from its bond to actin allows it to migrate to and dock at the active zone. The second step, the activation (or priming) required to make the vesicle releasable, is as yet poorly understood. The third step, exocytosis of a primed vesicle, is triggered by the action potential-which opens $Ca^{2+}$ channels at the active zone and causes intraterminal $[Ca^{2+}$ within 10 nm of the channel mouth to rise, for some 10 μs, to $\geq 100$ μM. The fourth step is retrieval of the vesicle membrane,

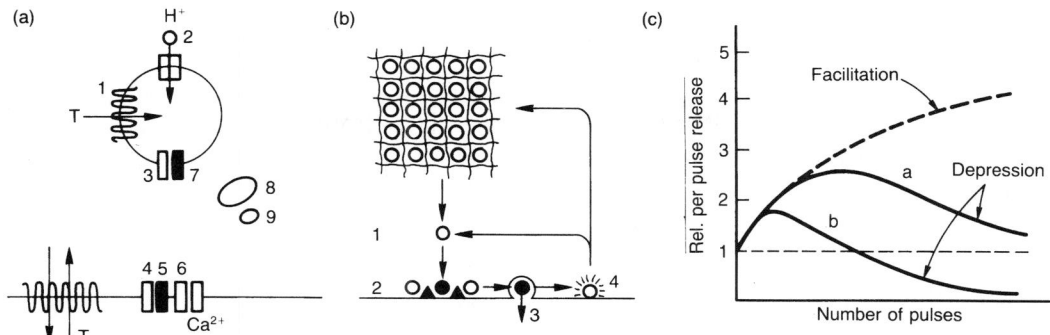

FIGURE 24.9(a) Synaptic proteins are involved in exocytotic quantal release or molecular leakage of a transmitter (T). The synaptic vesicle membrane transporter (1) takes up T from the cytosol. An ATP-driven proton pump (2) in the vesicle membrane provides the energy. The synaptic vesicle destination tag VAMP (3) helps the vesicle find its docking site. The plasma membrane proteins, SNAP-25 (4) and syntaxin (5), are vesicle recognition and docking sites (*see also* page 331). Depolarization of the nerve terminal opens $Ca^{2+}$ channels (6) at the active zone, transiently raises $[Ca^{2+}]$ locally to $\geq 100$ μM and triggers exocytosis. The low affinity receptor for this intense $Ca^{2+}$ signal is the synaptic vesicle membrane protein, synaptotagmin (7), which is also thought to restrict release, i.e. act as a fusion clamp. The cytosolic proteins, NSF (8) and soluble NSF attachment protein SNAP (9), displace synaptotagmin and form the fusion complex, (3)+(4)+(5)+(8)+(9), which allows the rise in $[Ca^{2+}]$ to trigger exocytosis. The plasma membrane T transporter normally takes up T extraneuronal; reversal of this transport causes molecular leakage of T to the extracellular space. (1) is the target of reserpine; (3),(4) and (5) are targets of botulinum or tetanus neurotoxins which block transmitter release; the uptake of extraneuronal T is the target of amphetamine, cocaine, tricyclic antidepressants and blockers of 5-hydroxytryptamine reuptake (e.g. Prozac). (b) Rate limiting steps for quantal release from an active zone: (1) Liberation of a synaptic vesicle in the large reserve pool from actin filaments in the cytoskeleton allows it to migrate to and dock at the active zone. (2) Activation of one of the docked vesicles makes it releasable. (3) $Ca^{2+}$ entry through channels at the active zone of the presynaptic membrane triggers exocytosis of the vesicle. (4) The vesicle membrane is retrieved by a clathrin-dependent mechanism, recycled, refilled with transmitter and reused. (c) The rise in global intraterminal $[Ca^{2+}]$ during a short high-frequency train of nerve impulses progressively increases the release probability (facilitation), but hence may deplete the small pool of releasable vesicles and later reduce the per pulse release of transmitter (depression). Note that the relative proportions of facilitation and depression are different in different tissues (represented by curves a and b) probably due to differences in the size of their releasable pools.

possibly by a clathrin-dependent mechanism, recycling, refilling and reuse. The entire cycle takes less than 60 seconds (*see* page 331).

Each of the four steps is $Ca^{2+}$-dependent but involves different receptors, all in different modes. Steps 1 and 2 are promoted via high affinity $Ca^{2+}$ receptors (e.g. calcium/calmodulin protein kinase II, or protein kinase C). Step 3 is triggered by low affinity $Ca^{2+}$ receptors (probably synaptotagmin in the vesicle membrane). In contrast, step 4 is inhibited by the rise in global $[Ca^{2+}]$ during a high frequency train. As illustrated in Fig. 24.9, the amount of transmitter released at each impulse increases during the early phase of a stimulus train (facilitation); it declines progressively as the releasable pool becomes depleted (depression). When the stimulus train is switched from high frequency to low frequency the amount of transmitter release at each impulse may now be increased (post-tetanic potentiation).

Presently available data suggest that active zones may behave as binary units, i.e. they either ignore the action potential or respond by releasing a single quantum and obey the following rules:

- The overall probability (P) of monoquantal release from an active zone is a product of each of the four steps described above (i.e. $P = P_1 \times P_2 \times P_3 \times P_4$).
- The probability that a primed vesicle is released ($P_3$) may approach unity.
- The probability ($P_1 \times P_2$) of having a primed vesicle at the active zone may determine P for release by a single pulse.
- The probability that a vesicle in the reserve pool will migrate to the active zone ($P_1$) and/or that an "emptied" vesicle will be recycled and ready for reuse ($P_4$) may increasingly become rate-limiting for release during high frequency trains.

## MOLECULAR MECHANISMS OF NERVE IMPULSE-INDUCED EXOCYTOSIS

During recent years many protein components of the synaptic vesicle and plasma membranes have been identified and cloned but their functional roles have remained poorly understood. A major breakthrough in this field was the recent discovery that the protein components of the molecular machinery of transmitter exocytosis from small synaptic vesicles are homologous with those mediating constitutive exocytosis, the main mechanism of transport of material between intracellular compartments (e.g. endoplasmic reticulum and Golgi cisternae) in all eukaryotic cells. Hence, many of the molecular mechanisms of neurotransmitter release in human brain can be studied in cell-free preparations of yeast. The hypothesis described in Fig. 24.9a appears compatible with existing data but will need modification as new facts emerge. Its value is that it may help explain (1) how the nerve terminal action potential triggers exocytosis, (2) how most potential release sites are enabled to ignore the action potential, (3) the molecular targets and mechanisms of action of many drugs which profoundly alter neurotransmission, e.g. reserpine, neurotoxins, and addictive and antidepressant drugs.

## TRANSMISSION STRATEGIES

The efficacy of synaptic transmission is a function of (1) transmitter release per pulse, (2) the rate of clearance of the transmitter, and (3) the sensitivity of the target to the released transmitter. As shown in the three examples in Fig. 24.10, tissues differ tremendously in the mode with which they utilize the transmitter in a single quantum. The first synapse (Fig. 24.10a) is designed for extremely fast, effective transmission

exclusively mediated via intrajunctional ionotrophic receptors. The second synapse (Fig. 24.10b) is designed to virtually ignore transmitter quanta released by nerve impulses in a single spike mode, but to respond powerfully and in a maintained fashion to firing in a high frequency mode. The third synapse (Fig. 24.10c) is designed for mainly or exclusively peri- or non-synaptic transmission.

## SELECTED READING

Burgoyne RD, Morgan A. $Ca^{2+}$ and secretory-vesicle dynamics. *Trends Neurosci* 1995; **18**: 191.

De Bello WM, O'Connor V, Dresbach T *et al.* SNAP-mediated protein–protein interactions essential for neurotransmitter release. *Nature* 1995; **373**: 626.

Garris PA, Ciolkowski EL, Pastore P *et al.* Efflux of dopamine from the synaptic cleft in the nucleus accumbens of the rat brain. *J Neurosci* 1994; **14**: 6084.

Jessell TM, Kandel ER. Synaptic transmission: a bidirectional and self-modifiable form of cell–cell communication. *Neuron* 1993; **10**: 1.

Söllner T, Rothman JE. Neurotransmission: harnessing fusion machinery at the synapse. *Trends Neurosci* 1994; **17**: 344.

Stjärne L, Stjärne E. Geometry, kinetics and plasticity of release and clearance of ATP and noradrenaline as sympathetic cotransmitters: roles for the neurogenic contraction. *Prog Neurobiol* 1995; **47**: 45.

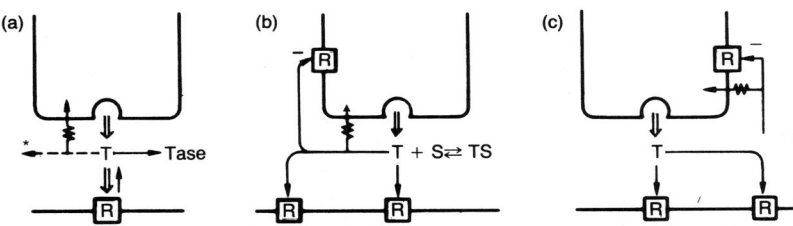

FIGURE 24.10 Three strategies of synaptic transmission mediated by release of a single quantum. (a) In this synapse the released transmitter (T) may be acetylcholine (ACh) in skeletal neuromuscular junction. The life-time of released ACh is a few milliseconds. At least one third of ACh molecules in the quantum are degraded by acetylcholinesterase (T-ase), a low affinity ACh binding protein with powerful destructive properties located in the basal lamina (*see* Fig. 24.6). Two-thirds of ACh molecules bind at least once to nicotinic receptors R ($Kd \geq 50$ μM) in the muscle membrane patch opposite to the release site. Dissociation from the receptors is asynchronous, and back-diffusing single ACh molecules are quantitatively degraded by T-ase. The metabolite, choline, is either taken up by a transporter in the presynaptic nerve membrane (*) or diffuses out of the synaptic cleft. (b). In this synapse the transmitter (T) may be norepinephrine (NE) released from a sympathetic nerve varicosity in rat tail artery. Here the life-time of released NE is $\geq 1500$ milliseconds. Free equilibration of the NE molecules in a single quantum throughout the junctional space would give a NE concentration of $\geq 200$ μM. The intrajunctional concentration of free NE is probably much lower, however, suggesting that it is buffered by reversible binding to as yet unidentified low affinity sites (S). Such a mechanism would explain (1) that the neuronal reuptake ($K_m$ 1 μM) removes $\geq 95$ per cent of NE in single quanta, probably into the releasing varicosity, but is rapidly saturated by repeated release of NE quanta into the same junctional cleft during a high frequency train, (2) that the contractile response to a single pulse mediated by $\alpha_2$-adrenoceptors is blocked by low concentrations ($\leq 0.1$ μM) of the competitive $\alpha_2$-antagonist yohimbine, and (3) that the NE concentration at extrajunctional $\alpha_1$-adrenoceptors or at a carbon fiber electrode is well maintained during a high frequency train, in spite of a declining per pulse release. In this synapse a high frequency train increases the diffusion of released NE out of the junction to the surround, recruits perijunctional $\alpha_1$-adrenoceptors and thereby greatly amplifies the contraction, but also activates perijunctional $\alpha_2$-adrenoceptors on the presynaptic nerve terminal and thereby restricts transmitter release. (c) In this synapse the transmitter (T) may be dopamine (DA) released from nerve terminals in the nucleus accumbens of the rat. Clearance of the released DA molecules from the synaptic cleft has been reported to be unhindered by binding to intrasynaptic proteins and extremely rapid, essentially complete within 1 ms. Here most of the pre- and postsynaptic effects as well as the neuronal reuptake of DA appear to occur outside the synaptic cleft.

# NEUROTRANSMITTERS AND NEUROMODULATORS

A neurotransmitter is a substance that is released at a synapse by one neuron to have a specific effect on a second neuron. A neuromodulator is a substance released by a neuron and has an effect at more distant neurons, often by modulating synaptic function. A developing neuron may synthesize and release more than one transmitter substance but a mature neuron makes use of the same combination of chemical messengers at all its synapses. The classical low-molecular-weight transmitter substances, acetylcholine, dopamine, norepinephrine, epinephrine, serotonin, histamine, γ-aminobutyric acid (GABA), glycine, aspartate and glutamate, are synthesized from precursors derived from intermediary carbohydrate metabolism. ATP and adenosine may also act as transmitters at some synapses. Peptides such as somatostatin, thyrotrophin releasing hormone (TRH) and enkephalins may also act as neurotransmitters. The synthesis and intraneuronal transport of transmitter substances are described above (see page 336). The packaging of transmitters and release at the synapse are also described in detail earlier (see page 336).

Motor neurons of the spinal cord use acetylcholine as the transmitter at the neuromuscular junction (see page 340) and at the recurrent central branch synapse with a Renshaw cell (see page 404). Acetylcholine is also the neurotransmitter at many synapses throughout the brain and, in the autonomic nervous system, is the transmitter for all preganglionic neurons and all parasympathetic postganglionic neurons (see page 428). The catecholamines include norepinephrine, epinephrine and dopamine. Norepinephrine is the transmitter of cells in the locus ceruleus which project throughout the cortex, cerebellum and spinal cord. In the autonomic nervous system norepinephrine is the transmitter of sympathetic postganglionic neurons (see page 428). The indole, serotonin, is found in neurons of the midline raphe nuclei of the brainstem which project widely throughout the brain and spinal cord. Histamine, an imidazole, is a putative transmitter in the vertebrate brain concentrated in the hypothalamus. The amino acid transmitters, glycine, glutamate and aspartate are universal cell constituents. Glycine is a transmitter in spinal cord inhibitory interneurons. Glutamate is the major excitatory transmitter in brain and spinal cord; it is discussed in detail below. The role of aspartate as a transmitter remains uncertain. GABA is synthesized from glutamate; it is an important inhibitory transmitter of interneurons in the spinal cord and brain, e.g granule cells in the olfactory bulb (see page 400), amacrine cells of the retina (see page 392), and Purkinje cells of the cerebellum (see page 405).

Neurotransmitters are further classified on the basis of their signal transduction mechanisms. Ligand-gated ion channel, neurotransmitter or ionophore receptors (see page 336) can be either cation-selective (excitatory), e.g. the nicotinic acetylcholine and N-methyl-D-aspartate (NMDA) receptors, or anion-selective (inhibitory), e.g. the GABA and glycine receptors. Ligand-gated ion channel receptors recognize and bind the transmitter and also effect a response at a different domain of the same macromolecule. On the other hand, for G-protein-coupled receptors, recognition and binding of the transmitter is distinct from the activation of a response (see page 336). This family includes α- and β-adrenergic, serotonin, dopamine, muscarinic acetylcholine and metabotrophic glutamate receptors. The G-protein couples the receptor to an enzyme that produces a diffusible second messenger, e.g cAMP (cyclic adenosine monophosphate), diacylglycerol, or an inositol polyphosphate. The second messages trigger a cascade by either activating specific protein kinases or mobilizing intracellular $Ca^{2+}$. Protein phosphorylation activated by second messengers can either open ion channels that are closed at resting potential, or alternatively close ion channels that are open at resting potential, e.g. transmitters that close $K^+$ leakage channels depolarize the neuron. The time-course of second messenger mediated synaptic action is much longer than that of direct ion channel mediated transmission. Furthermore, diffusible second messengers may act at postsynaptic sites distant from the receptors as neuromodulators in that they may modulate the excitability of neurons. Modulatory transmitters may act on voltage-sensitive ion channels involved in action potential generation to influence spike generation, and the amplitude and duration of the action potential. Some G-proteins and second messengers act directly on ion channels, e.g the cation-selective ion channels on photoreceptors (see page 392). Second messengers can regulate gene expression via phosphorylation of transcriptional regulatory proteins (see page 364). This action is likely to play a role in neuronal development (see page 365) and long-term memory.

Individual neurotransmitters will not be discussed further in this chapter but can be reviewed in the references included in the selected reading. This chapter highlights current information about excitatory amino acid neurotransmitter (EAA) physiology and pharmacology to provide a framework for understanding the role of EAA synapses in normal central nervous system (CNS) development. It must also be emphasized that EAA receptor over-activation is a major mechanism of neurodegeneration in a variety of acute and chronic neurological disorders; this important topic is discussed in the context of mechanisms of perinatal ischemic brain injury in Chapter 31 (see page 443).

## EXCITATORY AMINO ACID TRANSMITTERS

### EAA synapses

In glutamatergic nerve terminals, glutamate is concentrated in presynaptic vesicles. In contrast with some other neurotransmitters, such as dopamine and acetylcholine, synthesis/availability are not rate-limiting factors for glutamate neurotransmission. Relatively little is known about distinctive factors that regulate physiological glutamate release into the synaptic cleft, and whether there are developmental stage specific presynaptic regulatory mechanisms. Several novel experimental methods are in use currently to study glutamate release *in vivo*. Microdialysis probes can be inserted stereotaxically directly into the brain, and the concentrations of glutamate and related amino acids in the dialyzed fluid can be readily quantified. Microdialysis, coupled with sensitive analytical methods, enables measurement of brain extracellular fluid (ECF) glutamate concentrations, which are believed to accurately reflect cumulative regional synaptic glutamate concentrations. In experimental animals, microdialysis data indicate that ECF concentrations of EAA are somewhat lower in the immature than in adult brain. Magnetic resonance spectroscopy-based methods to measure changes in brain glutamate content may provide a clinically applicable non-invasive method to measure regional changes in brain content of glutamate.

Released glutamate is not degraded but, instead, is quickly removed from the synaptic cleft by energy-dependent reuptake transporters which are concentrated in both neurons and adjacent glia (*see* page 345). Standardized assays of EAA reuptake activity in tissue homogenates reveal lower levels in immature than adult brain; this developmental difference has been interpreted as primarily reflecting lower synaptic density, rather than decreased efficiency of transporters in immature brain. Several distinct high affinity glutamate transporters have been cloned, and it is possible that there are important developmental differences in their expression and regulation. Suppression of EAA reuptake, resulting from inadequate energy supply or intrinsic abnormalities of the transporters, may be a pathophysiologically important mechanism leading to increased accumulation of glutamate within the synaptic cleft and thereby contribute to EAA receptor over-activation in disease or injury.

### EAA receptors

There are two major classification schemes for EAA receptors based either on their selective responses to pharmacological agonists or on their signal transduction mechanisms. Three major groups of EAA receptors are activated by the distinct ligands NMDA, kainate, and quisqualate. The alternate classification scheme, based on signal transduction mechanisms, includes two major categories, ionotrophic receptors [NMDA, kainate, and the α-amino-3-hydroxy-5-methyl-4-isoxazole propionic acid (AMPA) responsive subgroup of quisqualate receptors] and metabotrophic receptors (non-AMPA quisqualate receptors). Ionotrophic EAA receptors, which are permeable to sodium and calcium, belong to the superfamily of ligand-gated ion channel neurotransmitter receptors (*see* page 336). Eight metabotrophic receptors have to date been cloned. Metabotrophic receptors are linked by G-proteins to second messenger cascades; the best-characterized EAA metabotrophic receptor signal transduction mechanism involves activation of phospholipase C, eliciting phosphoinositide hydrolysis with formation of inositol trisphosphate and diacylglycerol (*see* page 336).

*In vitro* autoradiography assays have enabled delineation of the regional distribution and density of EAA receptors in mammalian brain; studies of the ontogeny of EAA receptor anatomy and pharmacology demonstrated distinct regional and developmental differences in expression of NMDA and non-NMDA type EAA receptors. In some brain regions, EAA receptor densities peak in the early postnatal period. Autoradiography assays of postmortem human brain tissue demonstrated that EAA receptors are expressed early in human fetal brain development. It is clear that EAA receptor expression often precedes synapse formation.

In 1989, the first EAA receptor subunit was cloned; subsequent studies demonstrated unanticipated diversity of isoforms for each group of EAA receptors. *In situ* hybridization studies of EAA receptor ontogeny have revealed complex developmental regulation of expression of specific isoforms and their splice variants, as well as marked regional differences in receptor ontogeny. The functional consequences of these developmental patterns are currently not fully understood.

## EAA ionotrophic receptor pharmacology

The receptor-channel complex includes a neurotransmitter recognition site, a voltage-dependent calcium-permeant ion channel that is blocked by physiological concentrations of magnesium, and adjacent allosteric regulatory sites that recognize endogenous modulators such as glycine, zinc, and polyamines (Fig. 24.11). The NMDA receptor channel complex is composed of multiple subunits, encoded by distinct genes. Based on studies in rat brain, there are two families of subunits of the NMDA receptor, termed NMDAR1 and NMDAR2; functional receptors invariably include NMDAR1 subunits.

The availability of a wide range of drugs that modulate receptor activity by specific actions at these sites has greatly facilitated functional analysis of the

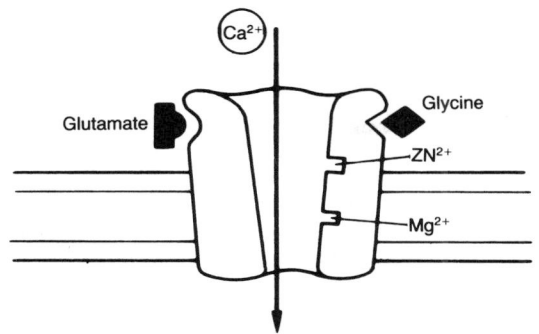

FIGURE 24.11 Scheme of the receptor-channel complex for the NMDA class of glutamate receptor. The complex includes a recognition site for glutamate and a voltage dependent calcium permeant ion channel. Binding of glutamate leads to opening of the $Ca^{2+}$ channel. There are adjacent allosteric regulatory sites that recognize glycine, magnesium, zinc and polyamines that modify NMDA receptor activation. $Mg^{2+}$ and $Zn^{2+}$ inhibit the opening of the NMDA channel. Binding to the glycine site plays a key role in opening the channel in response to endogenous agonists.

receptor channel complex *in vitro* and *in vivo*. Competitive antagonists, such as aminophosphonovaleric acid, block receptor activation by binding to the neurotransmitter recognition site. Non-competitive antagonists such as dizocilpine (MK-801) bind to a site within the ion channel and thereby block activation. In addition, specific drugs with agonist and antagonist actions at the glycine and polyamine sites modulate NMDA receptor activation. Sustained NMDA receptor activation raises intracellular calcium concentrations. Both physiological actions and the pathological effects of NMDA receptor overactivation appear to be initiated by increased intracellular calcium concentrations. Recent studies also suggest that nitric oxide (NO), produced in postsynaptic neurons by a calcium-dependent isoform of nitric oxide synthase, is an important mediator of both physiological and pathological effects of NMDA receptor activation; this highly diffusible compound may also act as a retrograde messenger and influence presynaptic neurotransmitter release.

The pharmacology of AMPA receptors is not as well-characterized. A focus of much current study of AMPA receptors is on the critical role of desensitization, as an intrinsic regulatory mechanism.

## Studies of NMDA receptor activation in normal CNS development

Activation of NMDA receptors appears to play critical roles in many aspects of central nervous system (CNS) development, including neuronal differentiation, migration, synapse formation and elimination. A wide range of complementary *in vivo* and *in vitro* experimental approaches have been used to begin to delineate these roles. In general, results indicate that low levels of agonists promote neuronal maturation (e.g. neurite outgrowth) whereas high agonist concentrations are toxic. The trophic and toxic effects of NMDA receptor activation may both be mediated by varying degrees of duration of increases in intracellular calcium. Evidence that NMDA receptor activity plays a pivotal role in neuronal migration (*see* page 362) included the observations that administration of NMDA antagonists can disrupt migration of granule cells in the developing mouse cerebellum and that pharmacological enhancement of NMDA receptor activity can increase the rate of cell migration.

There is considerable evidence of critical periods in CNS development that involve synapse stabilization and elimination (*see* page 366). Studies in the visual system have provided substantial evidence of the role of NMDA receptors in experience-dependent synaptic plasticity in early postnatal life. A range of complementary experimental strategies have been exploited to demonstrate that NMDA receptor blockade at critical periods can prevent formation of the normal pattern of synaptic maturation in mammalian visual cortex. In addition a recent study provided convincing evidence of the role of NMDA receptor activation in maturation of synaptic circuitry. In the developing mouse brain, surgical implantation of a polymer that slowly released a competitive antagonist of NMDA prevented normal synapse elimination during cerebellar development; this observation provided confirmation of the essential role of NMDA receptor activation in this critical aspect of cerebellar development. Neurochemical, neurophysiological and behavioral data strongly suggest that NMDA receptors play major roles in activity-dependent neuronal plasticity both in the developing and mature nervous system.

## Clinical implications

No developmental disorders or inborn errors of metabolism have been directly linked with EAA receptor abnormalities; in fact, it is conceivable that, in view of the critical roles of EAA receptors in the CNS, these would be lethal mutants. Considerable experimental data indicate that there are major developmental changes in the mechanisms of receptor regulation, in particular with respect to actions of drugs that modulate NMDA receptor activation. A practical implication of these findings is that drugs developed to modulate glutamatergic synaptic activity may have different effects in infants and children from the effects in adults. Based on the evidence presented of the critical role of EAA synapses in CNS development, it is likely that agents that interfere with EAA receptor function could disrupt brain development. For example, experimental data indicate that alcohol attenuates NMDA receptor activity. Thus, it is possible that one of the mechanisms by which alcohol is teratogenic to the developing brain involves blockade of critical aspects of brain development that depend on NMDA receptor activity. Similarly, there is experimental evidence that drugs with EAA receptor antagonist properties may have therapeutic utility as neuroprotective agents (*see* page 444). A potential implication of the critical role of EAA receptors in the developing brain, is that even transient blockade of EAA receptors may have long-lasting impact on CNS development. As more is understood about the complex roles of EAA receptors in CNS development, it will be possible to more effectively weigh the potential risks and benefits of acute or chronic treatment with drugs that block EAA receptors in infants and children.

## NEUROACTIVE PEPTIDES

Neuroactive peptides are transported from the cell body to the synapse by fast axonal transport (*see* page 331). More than 50 peptides found in neurons have been found to be pharmacologically active. They can be grouped in families based on their structures including:

- opioids, e.g. enkephalins;
- tachykinins, e.g. substance P and bombesin;
- secretins, e.g. vasoactive intestinal peptide;
- neurohypophyseal hormones, e.g. vasopressin.

Neuroactive peptides are frequently co-released with neurotransmitters from the presynaptic membrane and hence enhance or modulate the action of the transmitter.

## PURINES

ATP is co-released with both neurotransmitters and neuroactive peptides from the presynaptic membrane. Both ATP and its degradation product, adenosine, may act as neurotransmitters/neuromodulators on post-synaptic membranes depending on the presence of specific purine receptors. Presynaptic receptors for denosine have been characterized.

## SELECTED READING

Collingridge G, Lester RA. Excitatory amino acid receptors in the vertebrate central nervous system. *Pharmacol Rev* 1989; **40**: 143.

Collingridge GL, Singer W. Excitatory amino acid receptors and synaptic plasticity. *Trends Pharmacol Sci* 1990; **11**: 290.

Constantine-Paton M, Cline HT, Debski E. 1990. Patterned activity, synaptic convergence, and the NMDA receptor in developing visual pathways. *Annu Rev Neurosci* 1990; **13**: 129.

Cooper JR, Bloom FE, Roth RH. *The biochemical basis of neuropharmacology*, 6th edn. New York: Oxford University Press, 1991.

Hollmann M, Heinemann S. Cloned glutamate receptors. *Annu Rev Neurosci* 1994; **17**: 31.

Komuro H, Rakic R. Modulation of neuronal migration by NMDA receptors. *Science* 1993; **260**: 95.

Malenka R, Nicoll RA. NMDA receptor-dependent synaptic plasticity: multiple forms and mechanisms. *Trends Neurosci* 1993; **16**: 521.

Nakanishi S. Molecular diversity of glutamate receptors and implications for brain function. *Science* 1992; **258**: 597.

Rabacchi S, Bailly Y, Delhaye-Bouchard N, Mariani J. Involvement of the *N*-methyl-D-aspartate (NMDA) receptor in synapse elimination during cerebellar development. *Science* 1992; **256**: 1823.

Sternweis PC, Pang I-H. The G protein-channel connection. *Trends Neurosci* 1990; **13**: 122.

Stevens CF. Molecular neurobiology: Channel families in the brain. *Nature* 1987; **328**: 198.

# GLIAL CELL BIOLOGY – ASTROCYTES

Neurons are wholly surrounded and supported by glial ("glue") cells which present in numbers 10 to 50 times greater than the number of neurons. The macroglia or neuroglia include astrocytes and oligodendrocytes/Schwann cells. Astrocytes have an irregular oval nucleus, small cell body and star-shaped radiation of astrocytic processes. Astrocytic processes form end-feet adjacent to the surface of neurons, the pial surface of the brain and spinal cord, and blood vessels. The end-feet adjacent to the vascular endothelium induce the endothelial cells to form tight junctions which play a role in the blood–brain barrier (*see* page 350 for more details). Two types of astrocytes may be distinguished by surface antibody expression. Type I or fibrous astrocytes provide the structural framework of the nerve, while type II or protoplasmic astrocytes ensheathe axons and surround neuronal synapses. In addition to providing structural support and repair after injury, astrocytes have several important physiological roles including the modulation of neuronal activity. Astrocytes can selectively take up substances through the blood–brain barrier and so regulate nearly all aspects of the neuronal environment. There are a large number of imperfectly understood signals, both from direct contact and through soluble factors, that determine the relationship between astrocytes and their neurons; even in the adult brain, background production by astrocytes of growth factors such as IGF-I (insulin-like growth factor I) help promote the survival and function of neurons.

# THE ROLE OF ASTROCYTES IN NEURAL HOMEOSTASIS

## Ion homeostasis

Astrocytes have a high capacity for transport of potassium ions which appears to be the basis for the clearance of $K^+$ from the synaptic cleft during neuronal activity. Astrocyte uptake of $K^+$ is able to buffer the extracellular $K^+$ concentration in such a way that even during excessive neuronal activity the extracellular $K^+$ concentration does not exceed 10–12 mM.

## Homeostasis of neurotransmitters

### Monoamines

Inactivation of neurotransmission mediated by the monoamines, catecholamines and serotonin normally occurs by reuptake of the transmitter into the presynaptic nerve ending. Astrocytes also possess high affinity transport systems for the monoamines, express the enzymes (monamine oxidase and catechol-O-methyltransferase) responsible for monoamine metabolism and probably participate in the uptake and metabolism of monoamine neurotransmitters. Monoamine oxidase B, which is responsible for oxidation of MPTP to the neurotoxin $MPP^+$ is located primarily in astrocytes.

### Amino acids

The two amino acids, glutamate and γ-aminobutyric acid (GABA), act as neurotramsmitters at the vast majority of synapses in the brain (*see* page 341). Astrocytes express high affinity transport systems for

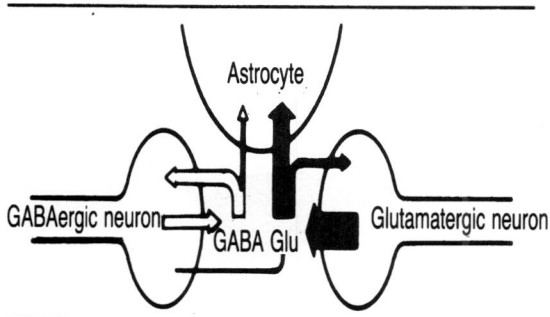

FIGURE 24.12 Schematic drawing of evoked release and uptake of glutamate and GABA in or glutaminergic GABAergic neurons and in astrocytes. The sizes of the arrows give an estimate of the relative magnitudes of the respective fluxes. Neuronally released glutamate to a major extent is accumulated in astrocytes, whereas most of the released GABA is reaccumulated into neurons. (From Hertz L, Schousboe A. In Vernadakis A ed. *Model systems of development and aging of the nervous system*. Boston: M Nijhoff Publishing Co, 1987: 19, with permission.)

both glutamate and GABA. In the case of glutamate transport into astrocytes is more efficient than transport into nerve endings (Fig. 24.12). Removal of glutamate from the synaptic cleft by an astrocytic high affinity glutamate carrier is important in the maintenance of low extrasynaptic glutamate levels. Excess glutamate is a powerful neurotoxin (*see* page 344). Failure of glutamate uptake and metabolism occurs in *olivopontocerebellar atrophy* and possibly in other neurodegenerative disorders. Reuptake of GABA into GABAergic presynaptic nerve endings appears to be important for sustained function (Fig. 24.12). Therefore excessive uptake of GABA into astrocytes may lead to loss of inhibitory transmission (e.g. seizure activity). In some cases seizures may be prevented by administration of inhibitors of astrocytic GABA uptake, e.g. the new antiepileptic drug, tiagabine.

# ASTROCYTES AS BIOSENSORS

Astrocytes express receptors for a large number of neurotransmitters, neuromodulators and neurohormones. Therefore, astrocytes can monitor neuronal activity and also act as biosensors, a function that may facilitate the role of astrocytes in the supply of important metabolites to neurons.

# ASTROCYTES SUPPLY NEUROTRANSMITTER PRECURSORS TO NEURONS

Neurons contain essentially all enzymes pertinent for metabolism of glucose and lactate. It should be underlined, however, that two important enzymes are not expressed in neurons. These are glutamine synthetase (GS) and pyruvate carboxylase (PC), both of which are present only in astrocytes and possibly other types of glial cells (see below). The functional consequence of the lack of GS is that neurons are unable to synthesize glutamine and therefore are dependent on a supply of this amino acid from astrocytes since supply from blood appears to be negligible. This is particularly important in case of glutamatergic and GABAergic neurons since glutamine serves as the precursor for these neurotransmitter amino acids. These neurons are dependent on astrocytes with regard to supply of the substrate for biosynthesis of their neurotransmitters. Neurons also lack PC. This enzyme which by fixation of $CO_2$ converts pyruvate to oxaloacetate, a Krebs (tricarboxylic acid; TCA) cycle constituent, is necessary in order for a cell to maintain normal levels of TCA cycle constituents. Since glutamate and GABA could be synthesized not only from glutamine but alternatively also from α-ketoglutarate, a TCA cycle constituent, neurons could have overcome the dependency on the astrocytes concerning glutamine supply if they had the ability to perform a net synthesis of TCA cycle intermediates from glucose. However, due to the lack of PC, the neurons are also totally dependent on astrocytes as far as this alternative pathway for neurotransmitter amino acid biosynthesis is concerned, since again supply from the circulatory blood appears to be negligible. The implication of this functional metabolic compartmentation is not clear, but is the topic of active research.

Astrocytes also produce a net synthesis of citrate, an intermediate of the TCA cycle. Citrate exerts an important action extracellularly by modulating the excitation of neurons via the N-methyl-D-aspartate (NMDA) glutamate receptor subtype. This action of citrate is related to its ability to chelate $Zn^{2+}$, an endogenous inhibitor of NMDA receptor activity, and represents a novel aspect of astrocytic modulation of neuronal activity.

## RESPONSE OF ASTROCYTES TO INJURY

Astrocytes become "activated" by acute brain injury and express a number of cytokines and glial fibrillary acidic protein (GFAP), and replicate. They may assume a phagocytic appearance and are presumed to have an active phagocytic role removing neuronal debris. The invasion of astrocytes separate pre- and postsynaptic terminals ("synaptic stripping"). The proliferation of astrocytes in the region of injury leads to an astrocytic scar (sclerosis). The production of cytokines may regulate the microglial reaction. The production of growth factors may provide trophic support to damaged neurons.

## SELECTED READING

Norenberg MD, Hertz L, Schousbe A, eds. *Biochemical pathology of astrocytes.* New York: Alan Liss, 1988.

Schousbe A. Neurochemical alterations associated with epilepsy or seizure activity. In Dam M, Gram L, eds. *Comprehensive epileptology.* New York: Raven Press, 1990.

Schousboe A, Westergaard N. Pathologic consequences in hippocampus of aberrations in the metabolic trafficking between neurons and glial cells necessary for normal glutamate homeostasis. *Hippocampus* 1993; 3: 165.

Westergaard N, Banke T, Wahl P *et al.* Citrate modulates the regulation by $Zn^{2+}$ of N-methyl-D-aspartate receptor-mediated channel current and neurotransmitter release. *Proc Natl Acad Sci USA* 1995; **92**: 3367

# GLIAL CELL BIOLOGY — OLIGODENDROCYTES

Oligodendrocytes (and the related Schwann cells in the peripheral nervous system) produce an insulating sheath, myelin, formed from up to 300 concentric layers of plasma membrane, around large axons.

These membranes have high proportions of complex lipids, including cholesterol, sphingomyelin and cerebrosides. These cells contain round, dark nuclei with no distinct cytoplasm (Fig. 24.13). They predominate in white matter but also surround neuronal bodies in gray matter. The oligodendrocyte may myelinate multiple axons for up to 1 mm along each axon. There are 0.5 μm gaps between segments of myelin, the nodes of Ranvier. Myelin reduces the capacitance of the axon membrane while preventing all current leakage across it, so that the action potentials are restricted to the nodes of Ranvier (*see* pages 334 for details about axonal conduction). Myelination thus markedly increases conduction velocity and reduces metabolic energy required for signal transmission along the axon.

The myelin sheath in the peripheral nervous system differs only slightly from that in the central nervous system (CNS). The Schwann cells each wrap only a single axon, and the myelination begins later: whereas the first myelin tubules in the central nervous system are seen from as early as 15 weeks' gestation, myelination of most peripheral nerves begins around the time of birth. The bulk of both central and peripheral myelination is completed in the first 18 months of life. This is most clearly shown by the increase in nerve conduction velocity (*see* page 373). Smaller nerve fibers, such as those involved in pain and temperature sensation never become myelinated.

Myelination of the peripheral nerve commences with the axon being protected by an enveloping trough formed by the Schwann cells. The external cell membrane of each Schwann cell surrounds the axon and then spirals around it many times. This extended cell membrane is termed the mesaxon. The cytoplasm is extruded to allow the mesaxon to compact. Peripheral myelin contains characteristic glycoproteins. An important component of both central and

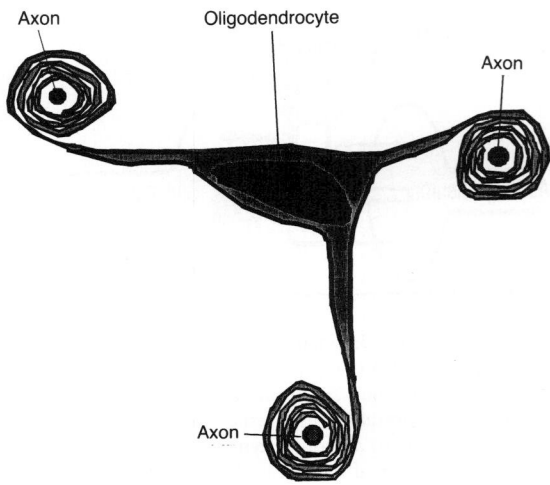

FIGURE 24.13 Schematic figure showing the stellate appearance of the mature oligodendrocyte which is wrapping multiple axons in myelin

peripheral myelin is myelin basic protein (MBP). MBP is 18 kD and is highly antigenic and has been suggested as the primary antigen in *multiple sclerosis.*

# MICROGLIA AND IMMUNE FUNCTION

Microglia represent the major source of macrophages in the central nervous system (CNS) where they participate in the response to trauma, inflammation and degenerative processes. They can be regarded as the parenchymal CNS defense cells and are likely to modulate the activity and survival of neuroglia and neurons both in normal and disease states.

## ORIGIN OF MICROGLIA

The cellular origin of microglia remains unresolved. Whether these cells are derived from neuroepithelial stem cells similar to neurons and other glial cells, or from blood monocytes that migrate into the brain tissue during fetal development has been the subject of debate for many years. Recent studies using rat bone marrow chimeras and developmental studies on retinal tissue, however, support the prevailing concept of the monocytic origin of microglia.

## MORPHOLOGY

Ameboid microglia are found in the brain from late prenatal to early postnatal periods. These cells present with a broad flat morphology with pseudopodia and in general they display many ultrastructural features typical of monocyte-derived phagocytes. However, the ameboid form represents only a transitory phase as they differentiate into a phenotypically and morphologically altered ramified form within two weeks postnatally. These cells have a small cell body (5–10 μm) from which project several thin branching processes but are quite distinct from astrocytes and oligodendrocytes. This transformation is considered to be a regressive phenomenon since there is decreased content of hydrolytic enzymes, down regulation of surface antigens and a loss of phagocytic activity. The resulting ramified microglia are the predominant parenchymal form of microglia in the resting state and constitute up to 20 per cent of the total population of glial cells. They are found lying between neurons in the gray matter and parallel to axons in the white matter but they do not make contact with each other.

Apart from the ramified microglia, distinct populations of macrophages are also associated with the brain. These are predominant in the leptomeninges and choroid plexus but their difference in morphology and phenotype suggests different functions to microglia. Small numbers of macrophages are also present in cerebrospinal fluid indicating traffic of macrophages through the choroid plexus to the cerebrospinal fluid in normal brain.

## ACTIVATION OF MICROGLIA

In response to a pathological event, quiescent ramified microglia exhibit an activation program that allows them to participate in tissue defense (Fig. 24.14). This activation is characterized initially by an alteration in morphology as the microglia draw in their branches and revert to the ameboid state. Conversion appears to occur non-specifically in response to any perturbance and the so called "reactive microglia" then rapidly proliferate and migrate to the site of injury. Activation is characterized by the upregulation of cell surface antigen molecules, e.g. leukocyte common antigen (CD4), complement receptor (CR3) and the major histocompatibility (MHC) class I and II antigens. Other marker molecules include vimentin and amyloid precursor protein and there is also upregulation of the expression of cytokines, in particular, transforming growth factor β (TGFβ). Activation is graded depending on the severity of the insult and it is only when neuronal death and degeneration occurs that activated microglia become phagocytic. Conversion to fully phagocytic macrophages is accompanied by a further increase in MHC Ia antigen and *de novo* expression of ED1 and ED3 macrophage specific antigens.

The signals involved in activation remain unclear. Presumably damaged neurons produce signals which regulate this process. There is evidence for a role for cytokines, particularly the colony-stimulating factors, and even more subtle signals such as changes in extracellular $K^+$ or ATP.

## FUNCTIONS OF MICROGLIA

Once activated, the microglia rapidly recruit to the site of injury. Under conditions where they are non-phagocytic, as following axotomy, the microglia migrate to a close perineuronal position and begin a process of "synaptic stripping" whereby the afferent terminals are separated from the postsynaptic sites of the damaged neuron. Although this interferes with information processing, the prevention of synaptic drive isolates the damaged neuron to allow it to undergo repair. In response to more severe injury where neuronal death occurs, the microglia become phagocytic and engulf cellular debris that are then transported to the vascular system. Typically, phagocytes produce large quantities of reactive oxygen species and nitric oxide as well as releasing proteolytic enzymes. At this stage, the microglial response can aggravate the injury by promoting inflammation and/ or necrosis rather than providing protection.

(a)

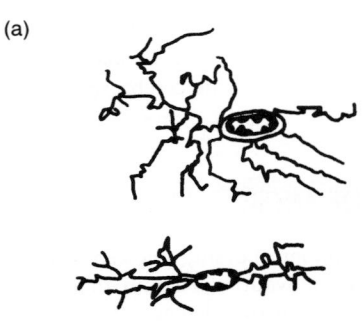

(b)

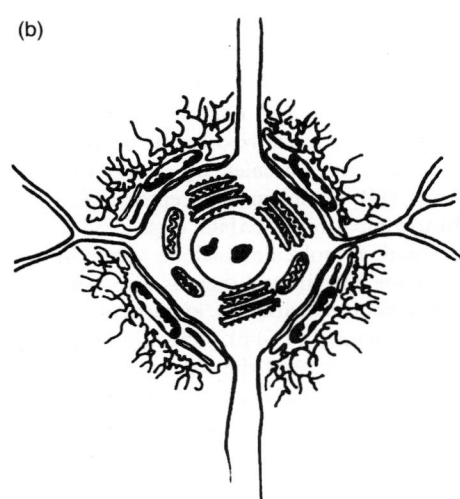

(c)

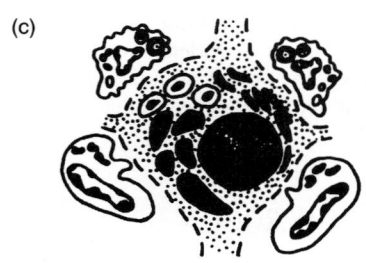

FIGURE 24.14(a) Resting microglia. (b) Activated microglia surrounding an axotomized neuron. (c) Phagocytic microglia surrounding a dying neuron. (From Feistle K. *Clin Neuropath* 1993; **12**: 301 with permission.)

The interactions between neurons and microglia are not restricted to the removal of cell debris. Once activated, microglia produce various growth factors and cytokines that can mediate post-injury events such as astrogliosis and later wound healing. In addition, activated microglia can also secrete factors that promote neuronal survival and growth. Most significant perhaps is the ability of these cells to rapidly upregulate MHC antigens and to activate the complement cascade. In this respect, microglia behave as the primary immunocompetent accessory cell population in the CNS. A T cell-mediated immune response is possible since activated T lymphocytes can enter the CNS and survey the parenchyma for any antigen presenting cells. Thus, both immune and autoimmune reactions can take place in the CNS despite the conception that the brain is an "immunologically privileged" site.

While activated microglia appear to serve a variety of functional roles, the ramified microglia in normal tissue were originally thought to be functionally inert. However, recent time-lapse photography studies show that individual ramified microglia possess firstly a high level of endocytic activity corresponding to pinocytosis and secondly exhibit high motility within a local area. These properties suggest that resting microglia may play an active role in tissue maintenance by removing cellular metabolites and waste by-products.

## MICROGLIA IN DISEASE STATES

The involvement of microglia has been identified in an increasing number of neurological disorders. Microglia are the only cell type in the brain that are known to be infected with human immunodeficiency virus (HIV) and so may be selectively involved in *acquired immune deficiency syndrome >(AIDS) dementia complex*. Entry of HIV-1 into the microglia is facilitated by the CD4 antigen which serves as a receptor for the virus. Although neurons are not directly infected by HIV, their degeneration is thought to be due in part to the release of neurotoxic factors by infected microglial cells. In *Alzheimer disease*, microglia are implicated as the primary source of amyloid precursor protein that is responsible for the deposition of insoluble amyloid plaques and in the subsequent inflammatory reaction within these plaques. Ongoing demyelination in *multiple sclerosis* is characterized by the presence of microglia which act as antigen presenting cells and to some extent degrade myelin.

The activation of microglia may be a common feature in all neurological conditions irrespective of the etiology. Activation is likely to contribute to further damage through immune-mediated cellular reaction and although microglia activation is beneficial in the initiation of wound healing, scar formation may inadvertently contribute to further dysfunction by blockade of synapse reformation.

## SELECTED READING

Davies EJ, Foster TD, Thomas WE. Cellular forms and functions of brain microglia. *Brain Res Bull* 1994; **34**: 73.

Ling EA. The origin and nature of microglia. In Fedoroff S and Hertz L, eds. *Advances in cellular neurobiology*, Vol. 2. New York: Academic Press, 1981: 33.

Perry VH, Gordon S. Macrophages and microglia in the nervous system. *Trends Neurosci* 1988; **11**: 273.

Thomas WE. Brain macrophages: evaluation of microglia and their functions. *Brain Res Rev* 1992; **17**: 61.

# NUTRITION OF NEURONS

## ENERGY METABOLISM

### Neurons

Under normal conditions the main substrate for energy metabolism in neurons is glucose. Neurons contain all enzymes necessary for conversion of glucose to either lactate or carbon dioxide ($CO_2$) and water via the pyruvate dehydrogenase reaction and the Krebs (tricarboxylic acid; TCA) cycle. While oxidation of glucose to $CO_2$ yields 36–38 molecules of adenosine triphosphate (ATP) per glucose, its conversion to lactate via anaerobic glycolysis leads to production of only two molecules of ATP per glucose. Under conditions with an adequate oxygen supply, lactate production is small and glucose is oxidized almost entirely through pyruvate dehydrogenase and the TCA cycle. Under conditions where the supply of glucose is inadequate, neuronal energy metabolism can utilize ketone bodies (acetoacetate and β-hydroxybutyrate) when present in high concentrations, or amino acids such as glutamine and branched-chain amino acids (valine, leucine and isoleucine). With regard to ketone bodies, it has been shown that the metabolic rate of neurons in culture is similar when acetoacetate is substituted for glucose. Acetoacetate also appears to be an excellent substrate to maintain oxidative metabolism in most neurons. It should, however, be emphasized that in glutamatergic neurons, glutamine serves as an energy source only under extreme conditions of glucose deprivation because it is acting as the precursor for neurotransmitter glutamate. The branched-chain amino acids, although being metabolized in neurons, are unlikely to play any major role in the maintenance of ATP levels in neurons.

### Astrocytes

Like neurons, astrocytic energy metabolism is normally maintained with glucose as the major substrate and, like neurons, astrocytes are capable of utilizing other substrates such as ketone bodies and amino acids when they are present at high concentration. Compared to neurons, astrocytes in culture have much more active glycolysis, leading to lactate production. However, in the brain *in vivo* this is unlikely to occur, since the overall lactate formation of the brain is rather modest.

Glycogen which is exclusively stored in astrocytes can be converted to glucose or lactate on stimulation of astrocytes by certain neurotransmitters/neuromodulators, e.g. vasoactive intestinal polypeptide (VIP) and norepinephrine. Thus neurons can utilize such molecules to signal surrounding astrocytes to mobilize glucose or lactate. This requires the hydrolysis of glucose

6-phosphate to glucose by glucose 6-phosphatase, an enzyme present in astrocytes although of low activity. It is likely that the main product of glycogen metabolism is lactate. The amount of glycogen stored is, however, modest compared with other glycogen storing tissues like muscle and liver and it is not clear to what extent glycogen plays a functional metabolic role in brain energy metabolism. In this context it may be of functional importance that astrocytes can metabolize glutamate to lactate via the TCA cycle and malic enzyme which is only expressed in astrocytes and not in neurons.

## ONTOGENETIC ASPECTS

Regulation of the metabolism of glucose to either lactate or (acetyl coenzyme A) acetyl-CoA is dependent among other factors on pyruvate dehydrogenase and the subunit composition of lactate dehydrogenase (LDH). This latter enzyme consists of five isoforms known as LDH 1–5 and the relative amount of each one of these five isoenzymes appears to influence whether pyruvate will be converted to lactate or will be oxidized to acetyl-CoA. Other key factors are the regulation of pyruvate dehydrogenase and the redox state of the cytosol, i.e. the $NAD^+$/NADH ratio (NAD; nicotinamide adenine dinucleotide). In adult brain, the LDH isoenzyme composition appears to favor oxidative metabolism but at early ontogenetic stages the LDH isoenzyme composition favors anaerobic glycolysis, i.e. lactate formation. This means that in newborns the brain is better equipped for ATP production via anaerobic glycolysis during hypoxia. However, significant lactate production takes place only to the extent that there is a net NADH production in the cell which is not compensated for by oxidative phosphorylation in the mitochondria. This change in the LDH isoenzyme composition during development appears to take place both in neurons and astrocytes. The lactate production of the newborn is an efficient ATP generating pathway only because here the lactate release from the brain is more efficient than in the adult brain probably due to a higher permeability of the blood–brain barrier to small molecules (*see* page 350).

## GLUCOSE UTILIZATION BY THE BRAIN

Normally in the brain there is a distinct regional heterogeneity of blood flow and a tight coupling between blood flow and metabolic activity. However, this coupling may be disrupted during ischemia and during a phase of reperfusion following ischemia where low flow regions may exhibit a very high glycolytic activity. This mismatch is associated with histological evidence of damage. In fact, a deranged ratio of glucose metabolism to blood flow on a regional basis has been suggested as one general mechanism of neuronal injury.

## SELECTED READING

Ginsberg MD. Local metabolism responses to cerebral ischemia. *Cerebrovasc Brain Metab Rev* 1990; **2**: 58.

Hertz L, Drejer J, Schousboe A. Energy metabolism in gluta-matergic neurons, GABAergic neurons and astrocytes in primary cultures. *Neurochem Res* 1988; **13**: 605.

Lassen NA, Ingvar DH, Raichler ME *et al.* eds. *Brain work imaging.* Alfred Benzon Symposium 31, Munksgaard, Copenhagen, 1991.

# BLOOD–BRAIN BARRIER AND OTHER BARRIERS IN THE DEVELOPING BRAIN

The concept of a blood–brain barrier arose more than 100 years ago from investigations which demonstrated that certain dyes injected intravenously in experimental animals stained most tissues but not the brain. Later it was shown that these dyes were bound to plasma proteins so that the barrier to the dyes was actually a barrier to dye–protein complexes. More recently the concept has been extended to include a series of mechanisms that control the internal environment of the brain. Although the term blood–brain barrier implies an overall impermeability, it is best considered as selectively permeable to a range of molecules, the degree of permeability depending upon a combination of the physical properties of the molecules and the presence of specialized mechanisms at the blood–brain interfaces. The lipid solubility of the molecule is of overriding importance in determining its ability to penetrate from the blood into the brain. Substances of high lipid solubility, e.g. theophylline, will penetrate freely into brain, although the kinetics of their penetration becomes complicated if they are bound to proteins in plasma (see below). For lipid-insoluble molecules, size, charge and presence or absence of specific transfer mechanisms between blood and brain are the important determinants of barrier permeability.

An important mechanism of the blood–brain barrier is a diffusion restraint provided by membrane specializations, tight junctions. Tight junctions are present at three main sites: (1) between the non-fenestrated endothelial cells of cerebral blood vessels (the blood–brain barrier), (2) between epithelial cells of the choroid plexus (the blood–cerebrospinal fluid (CSF) barrier), and (3) between the cells of the arachnoid (the blood–arachnoid barrier). Tight junctions exclude blood-borne macromolecules such as proteins from brain extracellular fluid and CSF. They also restrict penetration into brain and CSF of smaller lipid-insoluble molecules such as insulin and sucrose.

Various "active" mechanisms (e.g. carrier-mediated transport and receptor-mediated transcytosis) are also responsible for selective permeability of the blood–brain barrier. These mechanisms reside in luminal and abluminal cell membranes and depend upon intracellular properties of cerebral endothelial cells, choroid plexus epithelial cells and arachnoid cells. They are responsible for the transport of essential materials (e.g. glucose, amino acids and electrolytes) into and out of the brain leading to the build up of gradients between brain and plasma, and brain and CSF. Thus the blood–brain barrier has important functions in maintenance of brain electrolyte levels, modulation of substrate entry (saturable transport systems, endothelial cell enzymes), protection from systemic neurotransmitters and hormones and exclusion of blood-borne toxic substances.

The basement membrane surrounding capillary endothelial cells provides restraint to overdistention of the capillary but offers no impediment to the diffusion of even large tracer molecules. Astrocytes induce and maintain some of the specific functions of the brain endothelial cells, including development of tight junctions, via their end-feet that contact the endothelial cell basement membrane. Brain capillaries may undergo structural changes in pathological conditions, where this role of astrocytes is lost, to become generally permeable like systemic capillaries.

In several regions of the brain the normal non-fenestrated endothelial cells are replaced by highly permeable fenestrated capillaries that permit neurons to monitor substances in the blood and allow neurosecretory neurons to release secretory material into the systemic circulation. Such regions, devoid of a blood–brain barrier but with an intact blood–CSF barrier, include the pineal gland, the subfornical organ, the organum vasculosum of the lamina terminalis, the median eminence, the neurohypophysis, and the area postrema. These structures are collectively referred to as the circumventricular organs.

## BARRIERS IN THE DEVELOPING BRAIN

The mechanisms that control the internal environment of the human brain appear sequentially during development. Tight junctions appear early, probably as soon as blood vessels invade the brain and the choroid plexus begins to differentiate. Although these junctions are probably "tight" to protein as soon as they form, recent tissue culture evidence suggests that they may be initially more permeable to smaller molecules.

In addition to the blood–brain, blood–CSF and blood–arachnoid barriers to proteins, there is a barrier at the CSF–brain interface in the immature brain that is not present in the adult. This CSF–brain barrier is dependent on specialized intercellular junctions (strap junctions) between adjacent neuroepithelial cells which prevent intercellular passage of protein from CSF to the brain extracellular space. The presence of this barrier correlates with very high concentrations of plasma proteins in CSF of the immature brain. These proteins enter the CSF from plasma via transcellular protein-specific transfer mechanisms in the choroid plexus. In the human, the clinical significance of this recent finding is that drugs administered to pregnant women, that reach the fetus and bind to albumin or other plasma proteins, will penetrate into the immature brain. The same will also be the case for heavy metal exposure, since most heavy metals bind to plasma proteins. This mechanism is likely to be important in the first half of gestation and may still be present to some extent in the preterm neonate.

The high concentration of proteins in immature CSF may be essential to cell proliferation in the ventricular zone. The relative isolation of the developing brain from extracellular protein may be an important prerequisite for normal neuronal migration and differentiation and for establishing the initial neuronal networks.

Many low-molecular-weight compounds, including nutritionally important compounds such as amino acids, penetrate to a greater extent into the developing brain than into the adult brain. Whether this greater permeability to certain compounds early in brain development is a reflection of "immaturity," or is due to developmental specialization is not clear. The fact that it is selective suggests that the latter is more likely.

## CIRCUMVENTION OF BRAIN BARRIERS VIA RETROGRADE AXONAL TRANSPORT

In addition to the active transport of proteins from plasma to CSF in the developing brain described above, the barrier systems in the brain, both mature and developing, can be circumvented by transport via axons of motor neurons in the spinal cord and brainstem. Substances such as viruses, bacterial toxins, and various plasma protein-bound ligands (e.g. heavy metals and dyes) can reach the neuronal perikarya within the brain by both receptor-mediated uptake and endocytosis followed by retrograde axonal transport.

## PATHOPHYSIOLOGY OF BARRIERS IN THE DEVELOPING BRAIN

*Kernicterus* occurs in infants exposed to high levels of unconjugated bilirubin. Accumulation of unconjugated bilirubin beyond the neonatal period is very unusual but is found in the rare congenital deficiency of glucuronyl transferase, *Crigler–Najjar syndrome*; such patients may show clinical signs of bilirubin encephalopathy as adults. Unconjugated bilirubin binds to albumin; kernicterus only occurs when the binding capacity of albumin for bilirubin is exceeded. Unbound bilirubin is lipid soluble and able to penetrate easily into the brain. Kernicterus occurs when the rate of bilirubin deposition becomes very high as a result of a number of factors including high bilirubin concentrations, low albumin reserve binding sites, low pH, administration of drugs that displace bilirubin from albumin, and when the bilirubin oxidase system has been affected by asphyxia. Such a complex pathophysiology would appear to account for many clinical findings that have previously appeared contradictory.

High $CO_2$ levels in the blood increase penetration of various molecules such as albumin and sucrose into both brain and CSF in the adult. As indicated above the blood–brain and blood–CSF barriers to low-molecular weight substances are much more permeable in the immature than in the mature brain. The effect of hypercapnia superimposed upon the intrinsically high normal permeability results in a considerable penetration of smaller molecules into brain and CSF. In newborn rats the penetration of L-glucose was increased substantially, whereas that for theophylline was scarcely affected during hypercapnia. These results from animal experiments have important implications for the newborn infant with a respiratory disorder to whom drugs may be administered. Lipid soluble drugs are probably not affected by this mechanism, although there may be a secondary increase in penetration into the brain due to effects of low pH on drug binding to albumin or other plasma proteins.

## SELECTED READING

Dziegielewska KM, Habgood MD, Møllgård K *et al.* Species specific transfer of albumin from blood into different cerebrospinal fluid compartments in the immature fetal sheep. *J Physiol* 1991; **439**: 215.

Dziegielewska KM, Møllgård K, Saunders NR *et al.* Fetuin synthesis in cells of the immature neocortex. *J Neurocytol* 1993; **22**: 266.

Habgood MD. The nature of increased blood–cerebrospinal fluid barrier exchange during $CO_2$ inhalation in newborn and adult rats. *Exp Physiol* 1995; **80**: 117.

Habgood MD, Sedgwick JEC, Dziegielewska KM *et al.* A developmentally regulated blood–CSF transfer of albumin in immature rats. *J Physiol* 1992; **456**: 181.

Saunders, NR. Ontogenetic development of brain barrier mechanisms. In Bradbury MWB, ed. *Physiology and pharmacology of the blood–brain barrier*. Berlin: Springer-Verlag, 1992: 327.

# CEREBROSPINAL FLUID AND VOLUME CONDUCTION

## CEREBROSPINAL FLUID CIRCULATION

The view generally presented in modern textbooks is that the cerebrospinal fluid (CSF) flows from its production site in the choroid plexus of the cerebral ventricles and is absorbed in the Pacchionian granulations within the sagittal sinus. According to this bulk flow model (Fig. 24.15c) only a minor portion of the CSF is produced and absorbed elsewhere in the subarachnoid space; *hydrocephalus* is regarded as an imbalance between the production and absorption of CSF and *communicating hydrocephalus* is thought to be a result of obstruction of absorption of CSF at the Pacchionian granulations.

Information gained from gated magnetic resonance imaging (MRI) has called for a reconsideration of the bulk flow model. Studies indicate that CSF production occurs within the ventricular system and CSF absorption takes place through capillaries throughout the neuraxis. As a result, outside the ventricles no net flow can be demonstrated but pulsations lead to rapid mixing of CSF.

The lateral lacunae and Pacchionian granulations are not present at birth and develop in infants at the time of closure of the fontanelles. Therefore the bulk flow model cannot be directly applied to early childhood. The Pacchionian granulations are compressible structures which can be displaced into the veins. They probably serve as regulators of pulse pressure thereby taking over the function of the fontanelles when the skull has been closed.

## CEREBRAL BLOOD FLOW AND CSF VOLUME CONDUCTION

It is apparent that the pulsatile nature of cerebral blood flow has major effects on CSF flow. The new view on the CSF circulation including pulsatile and bulk flow is summarized in Fig. 24.15a,b. In systole, blood pressure increases simultaneously in the carotid and basilar arteries. In the closed circuit cavity this systolic pressure peak is instantaneously transmitted to the subarachnoid spaces and hence to the cortical veins. This transmission results in an immediate systolic increase in the flow in the sinus due to compression of the veins close to their outlet to the sinus. The ensuing increase in the resistance in the outlets causes a venom "counter pressure" and probably contributes to the maintenance of cerebral blood flow by keeping

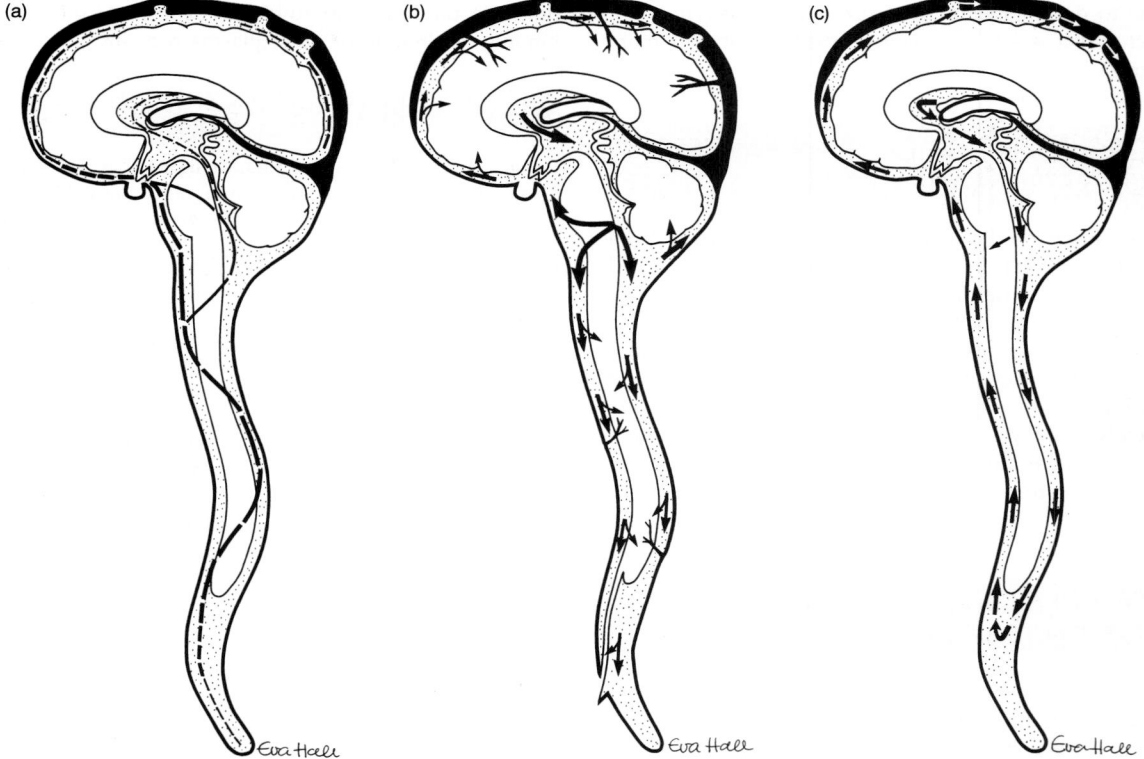

FIGURE 24.15 Diagram of CSF circulation. In (a) the amplitude and velocity of pulsatile flow are indicated by the length of segments of the dotted line. There is a dominant pulsatile flow with fast velocity in the brainstem and spinal cord compartments and slower velocities at the upper and lower reaches of the subarachnoid space. The systolic and diastolic flows in the spinal canal follow one main channel located towards the convexities showing a meandering S-shaped route due to centrifugal forces and lower resistance at the points where the CSF space is wider. In (b) the minute bulk flows are exaggerated for more clear illustration. The thickness of the arrows is related to the magnitude of the bulk flow, which decreases both above and below the foramen magnum. The CSF is resorbed throughout the nervous system by circulating blood. The cauda equina and spinal nerves are represented by only one nerve in the schematic drawing. In (c) the commonly accepted bulk flow model is shown. (From Greitz D, Hannerz J. *Am J Neuroradiol* 1996; 17: 431–8 with permission.)

intracerebral veins distended. A second rise in sinus flow during diastole results from inflow of blood from the brain. Such pressure changes affect CSF flow (Figs 24.15 and 24.16). A relatively large outflow of CSF through the foramen magnum into the spinal canal during systole results from expansion of intracranial arteries directly. Flow through the foramen magnum is reversed during late systole. A small outflow of CSF through the aqueduct during systole results from transmission of pressure resulting from brain expansion during systole inwards to the ventricles.

## RECLASSIFICATION OF HYDROCEPHALUS

Such a model of CSF flow leads to a new classification of *hydrocephalus* (Table 24.1).

## Obstructive hydrocephalus (VC-hydrocephalus)

*Obstructive hydrocephalus* is called *venous congestion hydrocephalus* (VCP-hydrocephalus). Obstructive

hydrocephalus is initiated by a hindrance to CSF flow within the ventricular system. An imbalance between production and absorption of CSF is a result of decreased outflow from the ventricular system. The enlarged ventricles act as an expanding mass and cause compression of cerebral veins. From the hemodynamic perspective the consequences of obstructive hydrocephalus are due to venous obstruction and raised venous pressure.

## Communicating hydrocephalus (RAP hydrocephalus)

*Communicating hydrocephalus*, which may be caused by any process that restricts arterial pulsations, is now termed *restricted arterial pulsation hydrocephalus* (RAP hydrocephalus). In cases of communicating hydrocephalus, an invariable finding on MRI is decreased pusilile CSF flow at the foramen magnum. Hence, communicating hydrocephalus is caused by decreased arterial expansion during systole as a result of either decreased compliance in the arterial wall or in the arachnoid compartment. The etiology may be primary changes in the arterial wall, e.g. spasm, arteritis

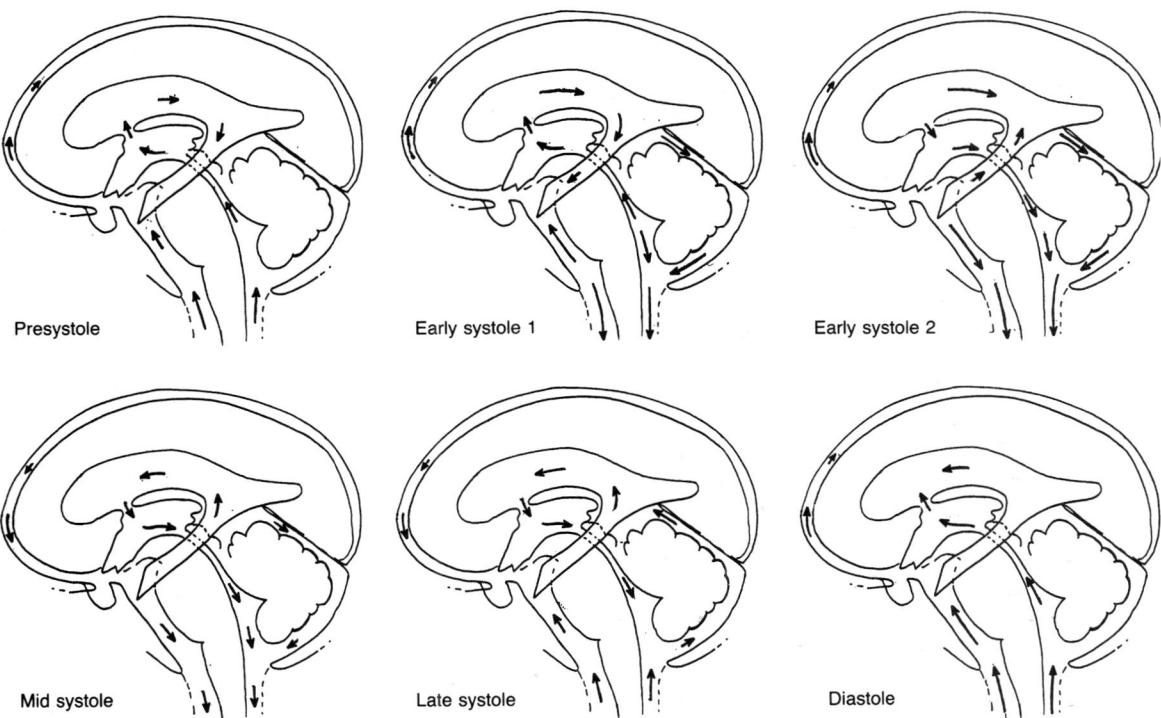

FIGURE 24.16 Pulsatile CSF flow during the cardiac cycle. CSF flow is caused by dynamic pressure gradients; the largest gradient located at the foramen magnum. The magnitude and direction of flow is indicated by the size and direction of the arrows. No flow is seen at the upper convexity. Presystole (late diastole): There is flow of CSF from the spinal canal into the cranial cavity, including the ventricular system. Early systole 1: Arterial expansion causes a flow reversal at the foramen magnum and foramen of Magendie and enhanced backflow in the cella media. There are counter-directed flows in the fourth ventricle and prepontine–medullary spaces. Early systole 2: There is reversal of flow in the aqueduct beginning 30 ms after flow reversal in the pontine cistern. Mid systole: All flow is directed out of the cranial cavity into the spinal canal. Late systole: CSF begins to re-enter the cranial cavity at the foramen magnum. Diastole: All flow is directed into the cranial cavity. (From Greitz D. *Acta Radiol Suppl* 1993; **386**: 1, with permission.)

TABLE 24.1 **Classification of hydrocephalus**

| | |
|---|---|
| **A. Primary hemodynamic disturbance: restricted arterial pulsation (RAP) hydrocephalus** | |
| Pathophysiology | Any process that restricts the expansion of cerebral arteries. |
| Etiology: | Primary arterial disease – arteritis, spasm or small vessel disease. |
| | Arachnoiditis – subarachnoid hemorrhage, trauma or craniotomy. |
| | Meningitis. |
| | Chiari malformation I and II – small posterior fossa. |
| | Achondroplasia – small foramen magnum. |
| | Cervical spinal stenosis. |
| | Slit ventricle syndrome? |
| Morphology | Communicating hydrocephalus |
| Intracranial Pressure | Intermittent pressure hydrocephalus (IPH). |
| | Normal or slightly increased ventricular pressure with increased pulsations and intermittent high pressure waves. |
| **B. Secondary hemodynamic disturbance: venous congestion (VC) hydrocephalus.** | |
| Pathophysiology | An intraventricular obstruction causing hydrocephalus with secondary venous obstruction and raised intracranial pressure. |
| Etiology | Block by a mass in the ventricular system. |
| | Block by an adhesion in the ventricular system. |
| | Slit ventricule syndrome? |
| Morphology | Obstructive hydrocephalus. |
| Intracranial Pressure | High pressure hydrocephalus (HPH). |
| | Increased intraventricular pressure with intermittent plateau waves. |

or small vessel disease or more commonly changes in the arachnoid space, e.g. following *subarachnoid hemorrhage* or *meningitis*. The same mechanism, also restricting arterial expansion, may operate when there are anatomical obstructions in the subarachnoid space at the level of the foramen magnum as with *Chiari I and II malformations*, *achondroplasia* and *cervical spinal stenosis*.

Classical physics states that static pressure gradients cannot exist in a closed space such as the cranial cavity. However, a dynamic pressure gradient may arise providing volume conduction is allowed for by flow changes. In the cranial cavity this is made possible by the compression of cerebral veins and the venting of CSF through the foramen magnum. The dilatation of the ventricular system may be due to an increase in the normal dynamic pressure gradient, which implies a higher pressure within the ventricular system than within the subarachnoid space. This "transmantle pressure gradient" has been regarded as static but should be considered as dynamic, since it is related to, and changes with, the amplitude of the intracranial pressure pulse. Because intraventricular arteries cannot expand in the case of RAP hydrocephalus, the systolic pressure wave is transmitted undamped to brain giving rise to a higher pressure in the brain tissue and ventricles than outside the brain, i.e. an increased transmantle pressure gradient. This explains the ventricular dilatation and the increased intraventricular pulsations observed both by direct pressure measurements and by MR techniques.

The decreased venous counter pressure and the increased transmantle pressure gradient in RAP hydrocephalus leads to both decreased cerebral blood volume and reduced cerebral blood flow. Symptomatic improvement following placement of a shunt depends on the restoration of cerebral blood flow by dilatation of cerebral vessels and increase in intracranial compliance. This also leads to a decrease in the transmantle pressure gradient.

## HYDROCEPHALUS IN CHILDREN

The phenomenon of "shunt dependence" in children treated for hydrocephalus may be explained by changes which occur in the regulation of venous tone. Very little is known about the regulation of tone in cerebral veins and impairment of their vasomotor control, which have a thin smooth muscle layer in the tunica adventitia. It is postulated that when a shunt takes over regulation of intracranial pressure by draining CSF, there is persistent dilatation of cerebral veins and impairment of their varomotor control. Regulation of intracranial pressure will hence depend on constriction of arterioli and the mechanics of the shunt. A related problem may occur in children with Chiari II malformation who may already be "shunt" dependent *in utero* when CSF drains via a *meningomyelocele* into the amniotic fluid. Hydrocephalus frequently becomes apparent following closure of the meningomyelocele.

Symptoms of increased intracranial pressure may arise despite a functioning shunt in the *slit ventricle syndrome*. Excessive drainage of CSF results in a decrease in the venting of CSF through the foramen magnum in systole and decrease in intracranial venous pressure in diastole. Therefore the same hemodynamic disturbances may develop in the slit ventricle syndrome as in communicating hydrocephalus. Excessive CSF drainage has a direct effect on dilatation of cerebral veins. This in turn may lead to increased intracranial pressure with intermittent increases in pressure (plateau waves) compatible with both a primary and secondary hemodynamic disturbance (Table 24.1). To maintain normal regulation of venous counter pressure it seems to be important to place a shunt that will maintain normal or slightly raised intracranial pressure.

Patients with small ventricles who have a shunt malfunction and decreased intracranial compliance causing increased intracranial pressure cannot be easily differentiated from slit ventricle syndrome (Table 24.1). Improved shunt devices which enable long-term pressure monitoring and pressure regulation will assist in the differentiation and management of these conditions.

## SELECTED READING

Davson H, Welch K, Segal MB, eds. *Physiology and pathophysiology of cerebrospinal fluid*. London: Churchill Livingstone, 1987.

Di Rocco C. Is the slit ventricle syndrome always a slit ventricle syndrome? *Child's Nerv Syst* 1994; 10: 49.

Greitz D. Cerebrospinal fluid circulation and associated intracranial dynamics. A radiologic investigation using MR imaging and radionuclide cisternography. *Acta Radiol Suppl* 1993; 386: 1.

Greitz D, Hannerz J. A proposed model of cerebrospinal fluid circulation: observations with radionuclide cisternography. *Am J Neuroradiol* 1996; 17: 431,

Greitz D, Hannerz J, Rahn T *et al.* MR imaging of cerebrospinal fluid dynamics in health and disease. On the vascular pathogenesis of communicating hydrocephalus and benign intracranial hypertension. *Acta Radiol* 1994; 35: 204.

Greitz D, Hannerz J, Bellander B-M *et al.* Restricted arterial expansion as a universal causative factor in communicating hydrocephalus. *Neuroradiology* 1995; 37: 14.

McComb JG. Recent research into the nature of the cerebrospinal fluid formation and absorption. *J Neurosurg* 1983; 59: 369.

# 25

# Development of the Central Nervous System

## GENETIC CONTROL OF EARLY CENTRAL NERVOUS SYSTEM DEVELOPMENT

There is an ordered progression from a relatively simple ectodermal cell layer to the complex adult central nervous system (CNS) with its billions of functionally interacting cells. This development proceeds through a series of distinct steps. First, the dorsal ectoderm is induced by underlying mesoderm to become neuro-ectoderm in the neural plate. Next, the plate folds to form the neural groove, which eventually pinches off from the dorsal ectoderm to generate the neural tube (*see* page 359). The neuroepithelial cells in the neural tube, CNS progenitor cells, proliferate transiently according to a strictly controlled scheme and give rise to neurons and glial cells in the adult CNS. Neural crest cells from the dorsal aspect of the neural tube migrate out to form the peripheral nervous system (PNS). At later stages during embryogenesis, CNS progenitor cells become confined to the inner ventricular and subventricular layers and neurons populate the outer mantle layers (*see* page 360).

This chapter summarizes: (1) the characteristics of the CNS progenitor cells, their developmental plasticity and possible self-renewing capacity; (2) the recent identification of genes important for CNS development and the high degree of evolutionary conservation of these genes and (3) *in vivo* experimental techniques that address these issues *in vivo*.

### CELL LINEAGE IN THE CNS

Various models have been proposed to explain how the relatively simple neuroepithelium transforms into the mature, organized CNS. In some models, the CNS progenitor cells are uncommitted until very late stages of development and their maturation is driven by cellular interactions at late differentiation stages; i.e. the CNS is largely a self-organizing system. In other models, the organization is laid down very early in CNS development, possibly already at the neural plate stage, which then would form a "proto-cortex." To learn which cells are the direct descendants to a particular progenitor cell, cell lineage analysis is used. An individual progenitor cell is labeled in a way that all cell progeny derived from this cell can be uniquely identified:

- Single cells can be labeled with a dye which is distributed to all daughter cells.
- Single cells can be labeled with a retrovirus carrying a foreign gene referred to as a "reporter gene" which is introduced into the genome of the infected cell and is replicated when two daughter cells are produced. In this way, all cells that are clonally related will carry the gene and can be identified by expression of the gene, i.e. production of RNA and protein.

Cell lineage analysis has been used to investigate whether a single cell can give rise to more than one type of daughter cell and if the clonal offspring can migrate and become dispersed in the mature CNS. The emerging picture is complex. Some data clearly show that progenitor cells in certain regions such as the retina are multipotent and can give rise to both neurons and glial cells. Progenitor cells in other regions appear to be more determined and generally only produce one type of cell progeny. A clone of cells can be widely dispersed in the adult cortex. There is a fair degree of lateral movement in the ventricular zone during embryogenesis, which supports the concept that there is greater plasticity at these early stages of development.

## CNS STEM CELLS

Many organs in the body replace lost cells by proliferation from stem cells, which are defined as cells that can give rise to both differentiated progeny and additional copies of themselves. The traditional view holds that this is not the case in the CNS; however, cells have recently been identified in both embryonic and postnatal CNS, which show characteristics of stem cells. Thus, if cells from the developing rat cortex at embryonic day 16 (E16) are cultured in vitro at single cell dilution, they can give rise to neurons, glial cells, and cells which retain the capacity to divide and later generate neurons and glial cells, i.e. stem cells. Furthermore, cells from adult rat striatum also show stem cell characteristics and the ability of generating neurons and glial cells in vitro. These adult CNS stem cells have been localized to the subventricular region of the lateral ventricles. Transplant experiments have demonstrated that they can proliferate, migrate long distances in the brain, and differentiate into neurons. Needless to say the possibility of culturing adult CNS stem cells, to generate new neurons and glial cells in vitro, opens up exciting potential therapeutic possibilities.

## GENES THAT CONTROL CNS DEVELOPMENT

A subset of the genes in the genome of our cells play important roles in the control of CNS development. Most fundamental and basic genetic mechanisms for generating a tissue are subject to strong selective pressure and are therefore evolutionarily very stable. Genes involved in these fundamental processes are sufficiently similar to be identified even in widely diverged species. Because of the relative ease by which genetic mutants can be obtained and analyzed in the fruit fly, Drosophila melanogaster, large numbers of mutants affecting nervous system development have been characterized. Despite the fact that 600 million years of evolution separates Drosophila from the mammalian lineage, mammalian homologs to many of the genes important for Drosophila nervous system development have been identified.

## Proneural and neurogenic genes

During the earliest phases of nervous system development some cells from the ectoderm of Drosophila embryos are sorted out to become neural cells, whereas other cells remain in the ectoderm and become epidermis. Proneural genes, e.g. genes in the Achaete–Scute complex, are required to potentiate cells over broad regions to a neural fate. Within these regions neurogenic genes, e.g. Notch and Delta, determine which cells adopt the neural fate, allowing some cells to do so and inhibiting others. Loss of neurogenic genes leads to an overcommitment of neural cells at the expense of epidermal cells. Recently, two mammalian gene homologs to the Achaete–Scute genes have been identified (MASH 1 and 2). The MASH 1 gene, which encodes a transcription factor, has been shown to be important in mammalian CNS development. A family of genes has been identified in mammals which are clonally related to the Notch and Delta genes which encode a receptor and the corresponding ligand.

## Genetic control of the dorso–ventral body axis

It is clearly important for cells in the nervous system to have a positional value, i.e. where they are along the dorso–ventral (D–V) and the anterior–posterior (A–P) body axis. Several genes important for the D–V organization have recently been identified, again on the basis of homology to *Drosophila* genes. Three mammalian genes that are homologs to the *Drosophila* "Hedgehog gene" have been identified: "*Sonic Hedgehog*," "*Indian Hedgehog*," and "*Desert Hedgehog*." The *Sonic Hedgehog* gene, which encodes a secreted protein, is expressed in the notochord, ventral to the neural tube, and is important for the formation of the neural tube. High levels of the secreted Sonic Hedgehog protein induce the formation of the most ventral cells of the neural plate, the floor plate (*see* page 360), while lower levels induce motor neuron formation. The Sonic Hedgehog protein thus acts as an endogenous morphogen for CNS development.

The dorsal and ventral regions of the neural tube differ also in terms of expression of certain transcription factors. The *Pax* genes are a family of genes encoding transcription factors. The name Pax is derived from "paired box," describing a conserved motif in the genes, and which was first identified in the *Drosophila* "Paired gene." The mouse *Pax* genes exhibit transient expression patterns during CNS development, and expression appears to be confined to specific domains along the D-V axis. Thus, *Pax3* and *Pax7* are predominantly expressed in the dorsal aspects and *Pax6* in the ventral parts of the neural tube. Mice mutant in *Pax3* are called Splotch and show neural tube defects of the spina bifida type, hearing defects and abnormal pigmentation. Human mutations in *PAX3* are the genetic cause of the *Waardenburg syndrome*. Mice mutant for *Pax6* develop the Small eye phenotype. Similarly, *PAX6* mutations have been detected in several patients with aniridia.

## Genetic control of the anterior–posterior axis

In 1894 Bateson coined the term homeotic mutation, which implies that one body part is replaced by another as a consequence of a particular mutation. A wealth of data from *Drosophila* has enabled us to identify genes involved in these processes. Some of the most important genes encode transcription factors of the homeobox type. These genes are so named because they contain a common sequence of about 180 nucleotide pairs, called the homeobox. Over 20 such genes have been identified; nearly all playing a role in determining the A–P pattern of the body. They include the egg polarity gene, *Bicoid*. In *Drosophila* several of these genes form a cluster on one of the chromosomes. The presence of similar gene clusters in mammals represents one of the most dramatic examples of evolutionary conservation. Not only are the structures of the genes highly conserved, but also their relative order on the chromosome and their expression patterns. In *Drosophila* and in mammals, genes located at one end of the cluster are expressed in the most posterior parts of the body, while genes progressively closer to the other end of the cluster show more and more anterior expression boundaries. Genetic data from *Drosophila* and from transgenic experiments in mice indicate the different combinations of Hox proteins are present at different segments; this is termed the "Hox code." Thus, cells expressing many Hox proteins develop posterior structures, whereas cells with fewer Hox proteins develop to more anterior structures. Mice in which the *Hoxa-2* gene is functionally inactivated show anterior transformations of skeletal elements derived from the second branchial arch. Overexpression of *Hoxa-7* leads to craniofacial abnormalities, such as cleft palate and open eyes.

The *LIM* homeobox genes are a gene family related to the *Hox* genes. They are also evolutionarily conserved and encode transcription factors. It has recently been shown that the *LIM* homeobox genes *Islet-1*, *Islet-2*, *Lim-1* and *Lim-3* are differently expressed in the young motor neurons before motor columns appear. Expression patterns of *LIM* homeobox genes uniquely identify subpopulations of motor neurons which later choose distinct axonal pathways.

## Genes controlling growth cone attraction and repulsion

The axon and dendrites grow from irregular spiky enlargements at the tip of each developing nerve cell process known as a growth cone. Growth guidance, by attraction and repulsion, appears to be vital for the control of axonal outgrowth. In 1994 two proteins, Netrin-1 and Netrin-2, which are secreted and have chemoattractive effects on neurons were identified. Netrin-1 is produced from the ventral part of the neural tube, the floor plate, and attracts growth cones from commissural neurons. A homolog to the *Netrin-1* gene is found in the nematode *Caenorhabditis elegans*, and this homolog, called *unc-6*, performs similar functions in the worm. A gene encoding a repulsion effect on growth cones was recently identified. Expression of this gene, *Collapsin*, mediates growth cone collapse. The structural homologs in *Drosophila*, the *Semaphorin* genes, have similar functions.

## SELECTED READING

Artavanis-Tsakonas S, Matsuno K, Fortini ME. Notch signaling. *Science* 1995; 268: 225.
Goodman CS. The likeness of being: phylogenetically conserved molecular mechanisms of growth cone guidance. *Cell* 1994; 78: 353.
Jacobson M. *Developmental neurobiology*. New York: Plenum Publishing Corp., 1991.
Johnson RL, Tabin C. The long and short of hedgehog signaling. *Cell* 1995; 81: 313.

Kilpatrick TJ, Richards LJ, Bartlett PF. The regulation of neural precursor cells within the mammalian brain. *Mol Cell Neurosci* 1995; **6**: 2.

Manak JR, Scott MP. A class act: conservation of homeo-domain protein functions. *Development.* 1994; Suppl: 61.

Strachan T, Read, AP. *PAX* genes. *Curr Op Gen Dev* 1994; **4**: 427.

Tsuchida T, Ensini M, Morton SB *et al.* Topographic organization of embryonic motor neurons defined by expression of *LIM* homeobox genes. *Cell* 1994; **79**: 959.

# EARLY DEVELOPMENT OF THE NERVOUS SYSTEM: CELL PROLIFERATION AND NEURONAL MIGRATION

## NEURULATION

Early during the development of a vertebrate embryo, the structures that will give rise to the central nervous system (CNS) are formed from the primitive ectoderm by a process known as neurulation which begins by the end of the third week after conception. During neurulation, the neural tube and neural crest are formed by the folding in upon itself of the ectoderm, the outer surface of the embryo. A shallow neural groove just above the notochord marks the position of the neural plate (Fig. 25.1a). As the neural groove deepens (Fig. 25.1b), the lateral edges of the neural plate fuse to form the neural tube (Fig. 25.1c). The lumen of the neural tube will become the ventricular system of the mature CNS. Cells just lateral to the neural plate and some cells in the dorsal neural tube become the neural crest which produces most of the peripheral nervous system.

Developmental errors in neural tube closure lead to severe malformations of the CNS as these are two of the earliest events of CNS development. The most common places for failure of the neural tube closure are at its two ends, i.e. in the spinal cord and prosencephalon. Failure of the neural tube to close at its caudal end results in a severe form of *spina bifida* known as *rachischisis*. In rachischisis, the spinal cord, vertebrae and the overlying skin are malformed such that the central canal of the spinal cord remains open to the skin surface. This malformation is detectable by ultrasonography and by measurement of serum α-fetoprotein. Failure at later stages of closure result in less severe forms of spina bifida. Failure of neural tube closure at the rostral end of the neural tube results in *anencephaly*, a malformation in which the derivatives of the prosencephalon do not form. In the mouse, mutations (at the *Splotch* locus and at the *T*-locus) produce neural tube defects which resemble those seen in some human disorders.

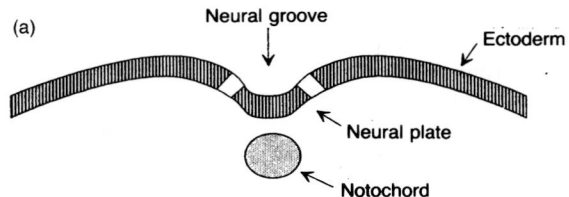

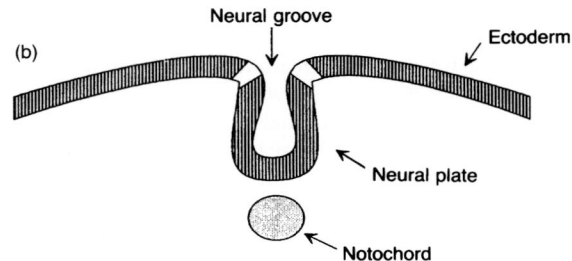

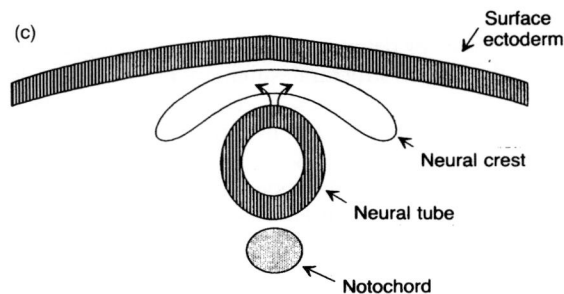

FIGURE 25.1 Neurulation. (a) At the beginning of neurulation there is a shallow groove just above the notochord; this groove marks the position of the neural plate. As the neural groove deepens (b), the lateral edges of the neural plate fuse to form the neural tube (c). The cells just lateral to the edge of the neural plate and some of the cells (arrows) from the dorsal portion of the neural tube become the neural crest.

## DIFFERENTIATION OF THE NEURAL TUBE

Differential differentiation along the anterior–posterior (A–P) dimension of the neural tube produces the major subdivisions of the CNS. Within each of these major subdivisions, differential differentiation in the dorso–ventral (D–V) dimension gives rise to structurally and functionally distinct areas. Along the radial dimension the wall of the neural tube develops laminae or nuclei that are distinct for each subdivision.

## Differentiation along the A–P dimension

The head and tail ends of the embryo have already been determined before the beginning of neurulation. About 50 per cent of the neural tube at the caudal end becomes the spinal cord and acquires a segmental organization, i.e. it is organized in repeating segments. Each segment is associated with sensory and motor innervation of one part of the body. The cephalic portion of the neural tube acquires a mostly "suprasegmental" organization and becomes the brain. The brainstem, which develops from intermediate portions of the neural tube, acquires a pattern of organization which is in part segmental (i.e. motor and sensory components of the cranial nerves) and in part suprasegmental.

The cephalic neural tube exhibits tremendous growth relative to the remainder of the neural tube; this disproportionate growth is referred to as "encephalization." The cephalic neural tube differentiates into three primary vesicles, the prosencephalon (forebrain), the mesencephalon (midbrain) and the rhombencephalon (hindbrain). The prosencephalon subdivides into the telencephalon rostrally and the diencephalon caudally; the rhombencephalon subdivides into the metencephalon rostrally and myelencephalon caudally. These five secondary vesicles are recognizable at 5 weeks' gestation in the human embryo, thereby defining at a very early developmental stage the major structural subdivisions of the adult brain. The cerebral cortex is derived from the telencephalon; the thalamus and hypothalamus are derived from the diencephalon; the midbrain is derived from the mesencephalon; the pons and cerebellum are derived from the metencephalon; and the medulla is derived from the myelencephalon.

The differentiation of the embryonic nervous system is under the apparent control of a family of genes originally identified in *Drosophila*, i.e. the *Hox* and *Hox*-related genes (*see* page 358).

## Differentiation in the D–V dimension

D-V differentiation of the neural tube (*see* page 357) is present in its most simple form in the region of the tube destined to become the spinal cord. The neural tube is divided into four zones or "plates," the floor plate, paired lateral plates, and the roof plate. Each of the two lateral plates is divided into a basal plate and an alar plate on either side of the sulcus limitans (Fig. 25.2a). The dorsal horn (sensory) of the adult spinal cord develops predominantly from the alar plate; the ventral horn (motor) develops predominantly from the basal plate (Fig. 25.2b). The four subdivisions exist in the brainstem where the relationship of sensory and motor derivatives of the alar and basal plates to the sulcus limitans is retained (Fig. 25.2c, d), although growth and expansion of the roof and floor plates alter the shape of the neural tube. Differentiation in the D–V dimension is still obvious in the prosencephalon although the correspondence to alar, basal, roof and floor plates is not applicable. For example, three sulci divide the wall of the diencephalon into four zones that become, from dorsal to ventral, the epitha-

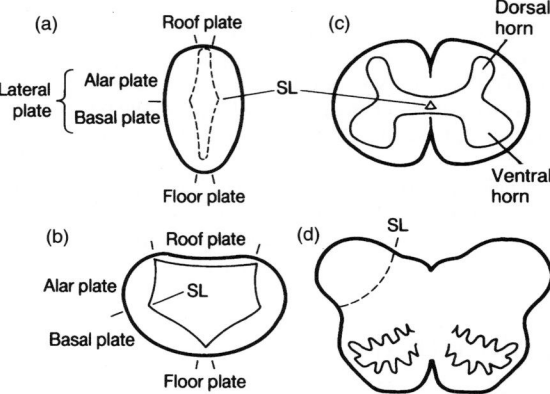

FIGURE 25.2 Dorso–ventral differentiation of the neural tube. In the spinal cord (a and b) there are four zones: a roof plate, an alar plate, a basal plate, and a floor plate. In the medulla (c and d), the alar and basal plates are displaced laterally by widening and attenuation of the roof plate. In both the spinal cord and medulla the sulcus limitans (SL) marks the border between the alar and basal plates. In the adult cord the morphological relationship between the sensory and motor derivatives of these plates is similar although their orientation around the sulcus limitans shifts from dorsoventral in the spinal cord (b) to mediolateral in the medulla (d).

lamus, dorsal thalamus, ventral thalamus and hypothalamus. Similarly, in the telencephalon cortical subtypes are derived from different regions of the wall of the hemisphere. The archicortex is derived from the medial wall of the lateral hemisphere, the neocortex from the dorsolateral wall and the paleocortex from the lateral wall of the hemisphere.

The variation of the development of the dorsal and ventral regions of the spinal cord portion of the neural tube has recently been shown to involve families of secreted signaling molecules derived from the *Hedgehog* gene and *Pax* gene families (*see* page 358). Molecules from these gene families are specifically expressed in limited regions of the neural tube and appear to control the differentiation and fate of the cells of these regions.

## CELL PROLIFERATION

Within each division of the developing CNS, cell proliferation, cell migration, and cell differentiation occur simultaneously. For a single cell these steps represent a cascade of developmental events. Cells which pass through the cascade early can influence the fate of those cells which pass through the cascade at subsequent times. In any part of the nervous system cells in the same or in different states of maturation can interact and affect each other's fate.

Cell proliferation in the developing CNS occurs in two specialized zones adjacent to the lumen of the neural tube; the ventricular zone immediately adjacent to the ventricular surface, and the subventricular zone.

The ventricular zone appears first and is present in all regions of the developing CNS. The cells of the ventricular zone form a pseudostratified columnar epithelium; they are attached to the ventricular surface and have a long, pially directed process which ends either on the pial surface or on a blood vessel. Mitosis occurs in a nucleus adjacent to the ventricular surface. The nucleus of the newly divided cell moves radially to the border of the ventricular zone, where it re-enters the DNA-synthetic phase (S-phase) of the cell cycle, and begins to move back towards the ventricular surface (Fig. 25.3a). This "to-and-fro" movement is known as interkinetic nuclear migration. The subventricular zone appears in phylogenetically "newer" regions of the developing CNS such as the neocortex. Cells in the subventricular zone are not attached to either the ventricular or pial surface (Fig. 25.3e, g); their nuclei do not undergo a "to-and-fro" movement with different phases of the cell cycle. In regions of the nervous system (e.g. the neocortex) in which both the ventricular zone and subventricular zone occur, the ventricular zone produces most of the neurons, and the subventricular zone produces most of the glial cells. In other regions of the CNS in which only the ventricular zone occurs (e.g. the hippocampus and retina) this proliferative population must produce both neurons and glia. Lineage analysis using retroviral and other cell markers is beginning to reveal the details and complexity of cell production (*see* page 357).

The proliferative zones are present transiently during the development. Both the duration of neuronal production and the time of its occurrence are characteristic of a specific region of the CNS. For example, in the mouse the neurons of the neocortex are produced in the ventricular zone during a 6-day period lasting from the 11th through the 17th embryonic day. This period contains 11 cell cycles which increase in length from 8–20 hours. The similar period in the human lasts almost 100 days from 10–22 weeks' gestation and is estimated to contain 34–35 cell cycles. Glial cell proliferation in the subventricular zone in both species

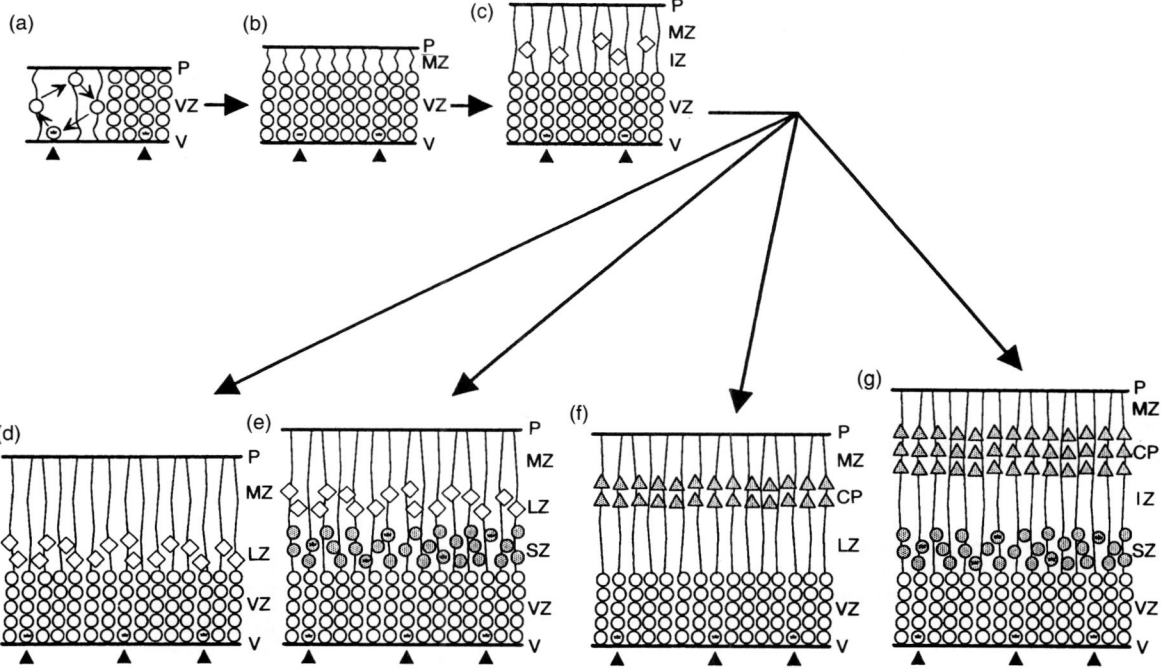

FIGURE 25.3 Differentiation in the radial dimension. (a, b and c) All parts of the early developing CNS have a ventricular zone (VZ) and eventually develop a marginal zone (MZ) just subjacent to the pial surface (P). The VZ is a pseudostratified columnar epithelium so that each cell contact the ventricular (V) and pial surfaces of the neural tube. (a) Illustration of the movement of the nucleus of a single cell as it passes through the various phases of the cell cycle; DNA synthesis occurs in the outer half of the VZ and mitosis occurs adjacent to the ventricular surface. Shortly after neurulation the neural tube consists of only the VZ. (b) The next zone to appear is the MZ, which is an almost cell-free zone just subjacent to the pial surface. (c) Shortly after the appearance of the MZ an intermediate zone (IZ) develops. IZ contains the first postmitotic cells of the nervous system. (d, e, f, g) After achieving the stage represented in c, the development of different regions of the CNS varies. Movement of postmitotic neurons is by passive displacement (d, e) or active migration (f, g). There may be one (d, f) or two (e, g) proliferative zones. (d) In parts of the neural tube in which VZ is the only proliferative zone, e.g. the spinal cord, postmitotic cells aggregate and mature in the IZ, immediately adjacent to the VZ. (e) In other regions, e.g. the dorsal thalamus, postmitotic cells also aggregate in the IZ and differentiate there, but may be derived from the subventricular zone, SZ. (f) In the hippocampus (archicortex) all postmitotic cells are derived from the VZ. They migrate across the sparsely populated IZ and form the cortical plate (CP). (g) In the neocortex both a VZ and a SZ are present; derivatives of these two proliferative zones migrate across the IZ to form the CP.

continues long after birth. Neuronal production is not, however, confined to the prenatal period in all brain areas. For example, the neurons of the human cerebellar cortex are produced over a much longer period that begins for Purkinje cells at about 10 weeks and ends for the cerebellar granule cells at about the third postnatal month. In addition, in each region, neurons are produced in a characteristic sequence, such that there is a correlation between neuronal birthdays and cell class and distribution. In general, the first neurons to be produced in each region are the large projection neurons. Also among the first cells to be produced are a population of astrocyte-like cells called radial glial cells that play an important role in neuronal migration.

Studies of mental retardation in children who were exposed *in utero* to the high radiation levels associated with the atomic bombs dropped on Hiroshima and Nagasaki and the gestational age of the fetuses at the time of the exposure indicate a critical period lasting from 8–15 weeks' gestation. During the critical period the risk of mental retardation was directly proportional to the dose of radiation received. However, if the exposure occurred before the eighth week the risk of mental retardation was no greater than in the general population, and if it occurred after the fifteenth week the risk of mental retardation was less than one-fifth of the risk associated with exposure during the critical period. The time of occurrence of this critical period implicates a radiation-induced compromise in the proliferation of neurons destined for the cerebral cortex.

## NEURONAL MIGRATION

The patterns of movement of postmitotic neurons vary between different regions of the CNS. In some regions, neurons leaving the proliferative population remain in an "intermediate zone" immediately adjacent to the proliferative zones (Fig. 25.3c, d, e). In other regions, neurons leaving the proliferative population move some distance away from the proliferative zones and eventually coalesce to form an incipient cortex, the "cortical plate" (Fig. 25.3f, g).

There are different mechanisms by which neurons move from the sites of cell proliferation to their final position. For both passive cell displacement and active neuronal migration there is a correlation between a neuron's final position and its time of origin. Passive cell displacement does not require active locomotory movement by the postmitotic neuron; a neuron leaves the proliferative population and is displaced a short distance from the edge of the proliferative zone (Fig. 25.4a). Thereafter, as the new postmitotic neurons move outward, the original cells are passively displaced further from the proliferative zone by the interposition of the subsequently generated neurons (Fig. 25.4b, c). Passive cell displacement produces a spatiotemporal gradient in which the earlier a cell is produced the closer it is to the pial surface. This gradient is manifest in the thalamus, hypothalamus, spinal cord, many regions of the brainstem, retina, and dentate gyrus of the hippocampus. The gradient is reversed in the cerebellum where granule cell proliferation occurs adjacent to the pia.

In active migration neurons are displaced distant from their proliferative zones, and during migration bypass earlier generated neurons and occupy positions sequentially closer to the pial surface (Fig. 25.5a, b, c). This process results in a spatiotemporal gradient in which the earlier a cell is produced the further it is from the pial surface. This gradient is found in most regions of the cerebral cortex and in several subcortical areas; regions which are, in general, well-laminated structures with layers oriented tangential to the radial dimension of the CNS, i.e. that run parallel with the surface of the proliferative zones.

The granule cells of the cerebellar cortex and the granule cells of the dentate gyrus, actively participate

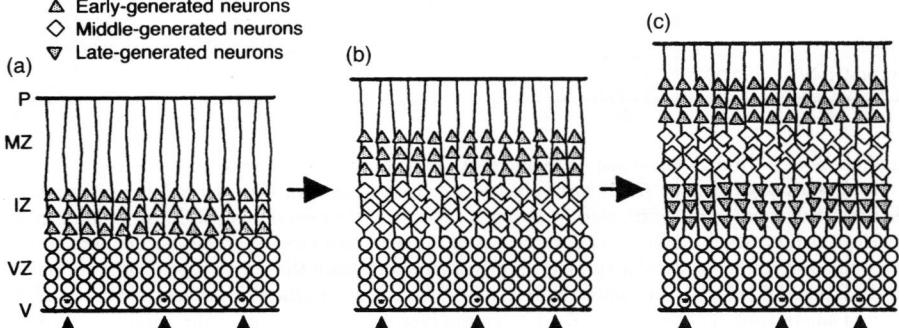

FIGURE 25.4 The sequence of events associated with passive displacement. (a) The earliest generated neurons which leave the ventricular zone (VZ) and enter the intermediate zone (IZ) are shown as triangles. (b) The next group of neurons to be generated are represented by diamonds. Their movement out of the VZ displaces the earlier generated neurons away from the ventricular surface (V) toward the marginal zone (MZ) and pial surface (P). (c) The last neurons generated, represented by inverted triangles, displace both of the earlier generated populations of neurons. This sequence of events produces a specific spatiotemporal gradient of neurons.

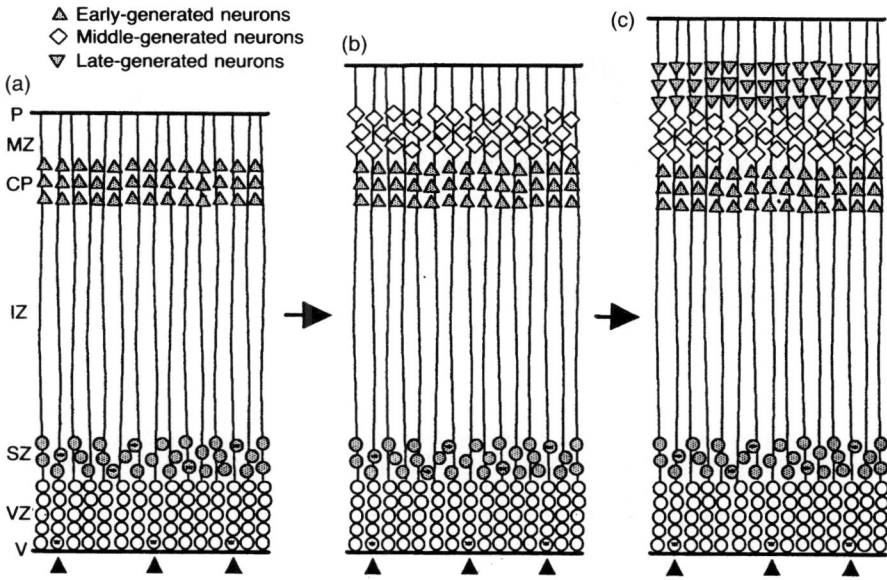

△ Early-generated neurons
◇ Middle-generated neurons
▽ Late-generated neurons

FIGURE 25.5 The sequence of events associated with active neuronal migration. (a) The early-generated neurons (triangles) leave the proliferative ventricular (VZ) and subventricular (SZ) zones and assemble in the cortical plate (CP), which is situated between the intermediate (IZ) and marginal zones (MZ). (b) Later-generated groups of neurons (diamonds) leave the proliferative population, traverse the IZ and pass the earlier generated cells to take up a position between the existing CP and the marginal zone (MZ). (c) The last generated neurons (inverted triangles) migrate across the IZ, past both groups of earlier generated cells and take up residence at pial aspect of the CP. This sequence of events produces a specific spatiotemporal gradient of neurons.

in the initial migration as they leave the proliferative zone. However, at their destination they do not bypass the earlier generated cells but push them further away from the proliferative zone.

## Active neuronal migration and radial glial fibers

During active migration many neurons are guided to their final position by radial glial fibers, which provide the "scaffolding" for the future adult neocortex as well as for other cortical and non-cortical structures. The radial glial fibers are the long, pially directed processes of an astrocyte-like cell whose soma is usually found in the ventricular or subventricular zone (Fig. 25.6). During early development the radial glial cells have an attachment to both the ventricular surface and the pial surface. With differential growth of regions of the cortex the radial glial fibers become a curved or even tortuous path. In principle the neurons that are produced by the proliferating cells from a small area of the ventricular zone will migrate along the surface of the same, or adjacent, radial glial fibers and will end up in close proximity to each other in the mature CNS.

The process of neuronal migration consists of three phases: an initiation phase, a locomotory phase, and a termination phase. During the initiation phase a newly divided cell makes the transition from neuroblast (i.e. a

proliferating cell) to young neuron (i.e. a non-proliferating, permanently postmitotic cell) and leaves the proliferative population. The young neuron then becomes apposed along its length to a radial glial fiber, thus establishing an axis of polarity away from the ventricular surface. The locomotory phase of migration begins once the young neuron is aligned with the radial glial fiber. During this phase a young neuron moves actively along the surface of a radial glial cell, retaining its apposition to the radial glial fiber and its axis of polarity. Upon reaching the vicinity of its final position at the border of the cortical plate and the marginal zone, a young neuron stops its migration and becomes detached from the radial glial fiber, thus freeing up space on the radial glial fiber for subsequently generated neurons. Its migration completed, the young neuron continues its differentiation process by growing dendrites and sending out an axon that eventually makes contact with other neurons. The locomotory phase can be very long, for example, in the cerebral cortex where a migrating neuron can move along a radial glial fiber which may be tens of millimeters long.

## Disruptions of migration

Neurons which fail to reach their appropriate final positions are said to be ectopic (or heterotopic). In humans, the best studied examples of defects in

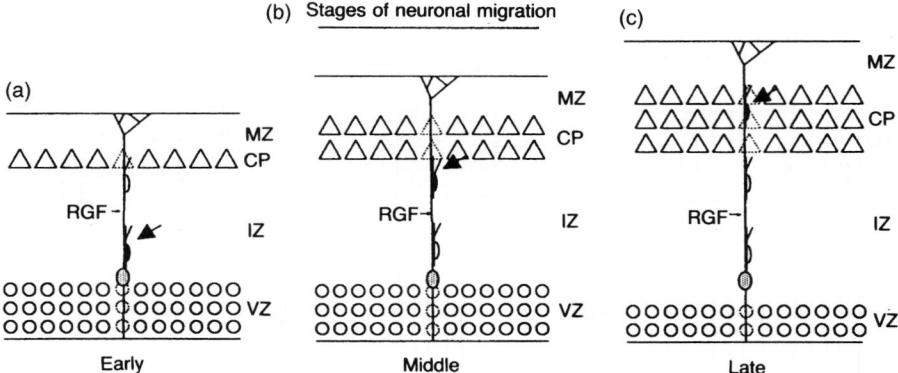

FIGURE 25.6 A schematic illustration of the interaction between migrating neurons and radial glial fibers. After leaving the proliferative zone (VZ), a young neuron moves toward its final position in the cortical plate (CP) along a radially aligned glial cell (shaded ellipse) which has attachments to both ventricular and pial surfaces. The progression of one such young neuron from the VZ through the intermediate zone (IZ) to the CP is illustrated by a single black cell marked by an arrow in each of the three drawings (a), (b) and (c). (a) As a neuron leaves the proliferative zone it becomes apposed to a radial glial fiber (RGF) and acquires a polarity directed toward the pial surface. (b) Next, the neuron enters the locomotory phase and traverses the IZ, maintaining its apposition to the RGF and its polarity. (c) When the neuron reaches pial aspect of the CP, it loses its apposition to the RGF and reorganizes its polarity in order to differentiate into a mature neuron. Disruption of any of the three steps of the migratory process can result in ectopic neurons.

neuronal positioning are in the cerebral cortex where abnormalities in neuronal migration have been associated with a variety of disorders and syndromes ranging from severe mental retardation to minimal behavior disorders. The presence of ectopic neurons and disruptions of the migratory process has been associated with the sequelae of *hydrocephalus*, *lissencephaly*, methylmercury poisoning, methanol exposure, some craniofacial anomalies, and a variety of other conditions. In addition, ectopic neurons have been found in some patients with mental retardation and seizures and in area CA1 of the hippocampus of patients with *schizophrenia* and in the language areas of patients with *dyslexia*. It is difficult to assess in such human pathological material the developmental fate of neurons that fail to migrate to their proper positions. It is not known, for example, whether the connections made by these abnormally positioned neurons are with their normal targets or with some other targets. Most importantly it is not known how such abnormalities in connectivity (if they exist) might affect the function of the area of the brain in which the ectopic cells were normally destined to reside. Some insight into these issues is beginning to emerge from studies in mutant mice that have defects in neuronal migration and from experimental disruptions of the migratory process.

## VARIATION IN BRAIN MATURATION BETWEEN SPECIES

The relative maturity of the brain at the time of birth varies from species to species. For example, in rats and mice most of the cells destined to comprise the cerebral cortex are generated during the second half of gestation, during a period that ends only a few days before birth. In contrast, in monkeys and humans these same events are completed towards the end of the second trimester, well before birth. In humans the brain weighs about 350 g at birth. After birth the brain continues to grow, mostly by modifications of the numbers, size and connections of the neurons generated before birth, reaching about 1350 g at 20 years. Most of the postnatal growth occurs within the first 3–4 years after birth, but changes in myelination and in other measures of maturation (e.g. cortical surface area, numbers of glial cells) continue even at 70–80 years of age.

## SELECTED READING

Barbe MF, Levitt P. The early commitment of fetal neurons to the limbic cortex. *J Neurosci* 1991; **11**: 519.

Jacobson M. *Developmental neurobiology*. 3rd edn. New York: Plenum, 1991.

Keynes R, Lumsden A. Segmentation and the origin of regional diversity in the vertebrate central nervous system. *Neuron* 1990; **2**: 1.

Nowakowski RS. Basic concepts of CNS development. *Child Dev* 1987; **58**: 568.

O'Leary DDM. Do cortical areas emerge from a protocortex? *Trends Neurosci* 1989; **12**: 400.

Rakic P. Cell migration and neuronal ectopias in the brain. *Birth defects* 1975; **11**: 95.

Rakic P. Specification of cerebral cortical areas. *Science* 1988; **241**: 170.

Sidman RL, Rakic P. Development of the human central nervous system. In Haymaker W, Adams RD, eds. *Histology and histopathology of the nervous system*. Springfield, IL: CC Thomas, 1982: 3.

Walsh C, Cepko C. Widespread dispersion of neuronal clones across functional regions of the cerebral cortex. *Science* 1992; **255**: 434.

# DEVELOPMENT OF NEURONAL AND NEUROMUSCULAR CONNECTIVITY

## Polarization of neurons

Neurons are highly polarized cells with two types of extensions from the cell body; the axon which mediates electrical signals from the neuron to other nerve cells, and the dendrites which receive electrically mediated information from other neurons. There are clear structural differences between axons and dendrites, particularly in the organization of the cell membrane and the cytoskeleton (*see* page 330). Neurons are initially non-polarized in that all processes extending from the cell body have the same undifferentiated characteristics. Initial outgrowth of the axon is predetermined in the neuron, but the direction of further elongation is determined by factors in the tissue through which the axon is growing.

## Axon growth

There are two stages in the formation of precise connections between neurons. First, outgrowing axons are led by various molecular guidance cues from specific areas to broadly defined target regions. The axon extends at its growing tip by means of a specialized enlargement of the axon shaft called the growth cone. The directed growth of the axon is accomplished by interactions between the growth cone and its environment. Such interactive mechanisms may include:

■ mechanical routing by specifically oriented structures in the pathways.
■ differential adhesiveness between the growing axon and molecules of surrounding tissue elements.
■ influence from electrical fields in the tissue.
■ release of factors promoting or inhibiting axon growth by cells in the axonal pathways and by axonal targets.

None of these factors can by itself explain all features of axon growth. Multiple mechanisms most likely act together with a specific timing to lead axons to their targets.

The second stage includes an exact point-to-point matching between each axon and the specific target neurons. This matching is achieved by intricate inter-actions between the cells and leads to the formation of synapses between neurons. A synaptic contact has a number of ultrastructural features, including opposed plasma membranes of the pre- and postsynaptic elements, a synaptic cleft between the membranes, and synaptic vesicles containing transmitter substances, close to or in contact with the presynaptic membrane. Receptors for the transmitters are located in the postsynaptic membrane. By the release of transmitters the presynaptic neuron may induce electrical and/or chemical short- and/or long-term changes in the postsynaptic cell.

The development of the synapse involves an interaction between the pre- and postsynaptic elements. A number of factors may act in combination to achieve functional development of a synapse. One obvious such factor is that the two elements involved come into close proximity at the appropriate time for establishment of the connection. A biochemical compatibility or affinity between pre- and postsynaptic elements must also exist.

This interplay between developing pre- and postsynaptic structures has been most extensively studied at the neuromuscular junction where it has been shown that the presynaptic motor nerve terminal, using acetylcholine (ACh) as transmitter substance, has a major role in the formation of synaptic contacts. Thus, before the arrival of the motor nerve, nicotinic ACh receptors are distributed rather uniformly over the surface of muscle fibers (Fig. 25.7). After innervation of the muscle fiber, the density of receptors is increased at the site of innervation, and decreased at extrasynaptic sites. This effect seems to be mediated by electrical activity and diffusible factors other than ACh; e.g. calcitonin gene-related peptide (CGRP), released by the presynaptic nerve terminal. Initially, the newly formed synapse is rather labile, as exemplified by the short half-life of ACh receptors in the postsynaptic membrane. With increasing time, a stabilization of the synapse occurs, with a decreasing lateral mobility and a longer half-life of the receptors. The functional channel properties of the receptors also show a progressive change following initial innervation.

Substances released from the presynaptic motor-neuron nerve terminal may have an influence on the production of postsynaptic receptors. There is also evidence of an influence in the reverse, retrograde direction. An example of such a retrograde influence is motorneuron death during the period of muscle innervation when about half the population of spinal motorneurons die by apoptosis. There is ample evidence that the number of surviving motorneurons depends on the number of muscle fibers available for innervation. Thus, early limb amputation results in greater loss of motorneurons than normal, whereas

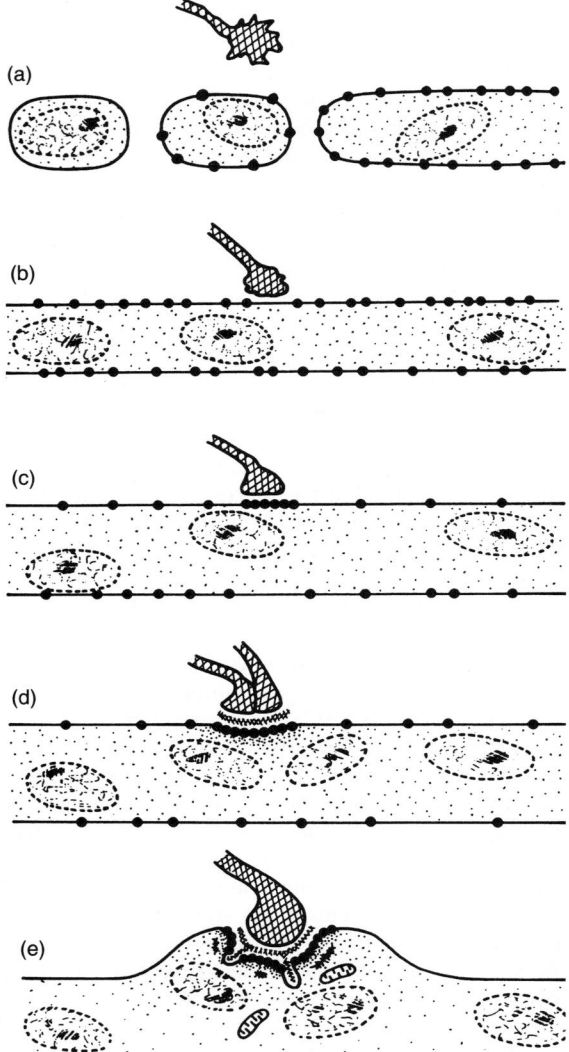

FIGURE 25.7 Schematic illustration of the formation of a synapse between a nerve and a skeletal muscle during development in the rat. (a) The growth cone arrives at the surface of mononucleated myoblasts, which have started to express acetylcholine receptor (AChR) molecules (filled circles) all over the surface of their cytoplasmic membranes. (b) Fusion of myoblasts into myotubes is accompanied by an increase of AChR biosynthesis. (c) The growth cone is immobilized and receptor molecules are accumulated beneath the nerve terminal. The expression of the genes encoding the AChR subunits becomes restricted to fundamental nuclei under the end plate. (d) Multiple innervation is transiently seen and receptors outside the synapse are gradually disappearing. (e) The maturation of the motor end plate includes stabilization of the receptor and change in the mean opening time of ion channels. (By courtesy of Professor Jean-Pierre Changeux, Institut Pasteur, Paris.)

grafting an additional limb increases the number of surviving neurons. It appears that the motorneurons, after the initial axon outgrowth, compete for trophic factors which are essential for the survival of developing motoneurons.

## TROPHIC EFFECTS ON THE PRESYNAPTIC ELEMENT

Trophic effects of the postsynaptic muscle fiber on the presynaptic motorneuron are exerted by at least two mechanisms. First, the muscle releases factors which induce the terminal motor axon to arborize or sprout. Second, trophic factors are released locally at the synaptic site and then transported retrogradely to the motorneuron cell body. The level of neural activity may be important for the production of trophic factors. Pharmacological blockade of neuromuscular transmission during a critical stage of development may result in survival of motorneurons that otherwise would have died. This may be explained by a greater production of neurotrophic substances by inactive muscle fibers.

## SYNAPSE ELIMINATION

A key feature of normal neural development is programmed neuronal death. A large percentage of neurons formed are programmed to die by an apoptotic process before birth. In mammals, motorneuron apoptosis is complete before birth. However, at birth each muscle fiber may still be innervated by several motorneurons and this polyneuronal innervation is eliminated during the first few weeks of postnatal life so that in the adult a muscle fiber is innervated by one motorneuron only (Fig. 25.8). The mechanism for this elimination is a withdrawal of the presynaptic branch into the parent motor axon. Although the number of neuronal inputs to a muscle fiber decreases during development the complexity of the remaining motorneuron contacts increases with the formation of a large number of synaptic boutons and release sites. Synapse overproduction followed by synapse elimination has been shown in peripheral ganglia (Fig. 25.8), as well as in the cerebellar and cerebral cortices.

# Regulation of synapse elimination

The elimination of neuromuscular synapses is dependent on muscle contraction and is delayed after transection of a muscle tendon or after blocking the synaptic transmission. The mechanism of this activity-dependent synapse elimination is not known. It has been speculated that the release of trophic factors only occurs during depolarization of the muscle fibers and that these factors can only be taken up by simultaneously active terminals. Thus, asynchronous activation of the nerve terminal and muscle fiber would lead to a lack of trophic support to the terminal, thereby triggering a withdrawal of the presynaptic branch. The overall purpose of these mechanisms would be to match an appropriate number of innervating axons to each target cell and vice versa.

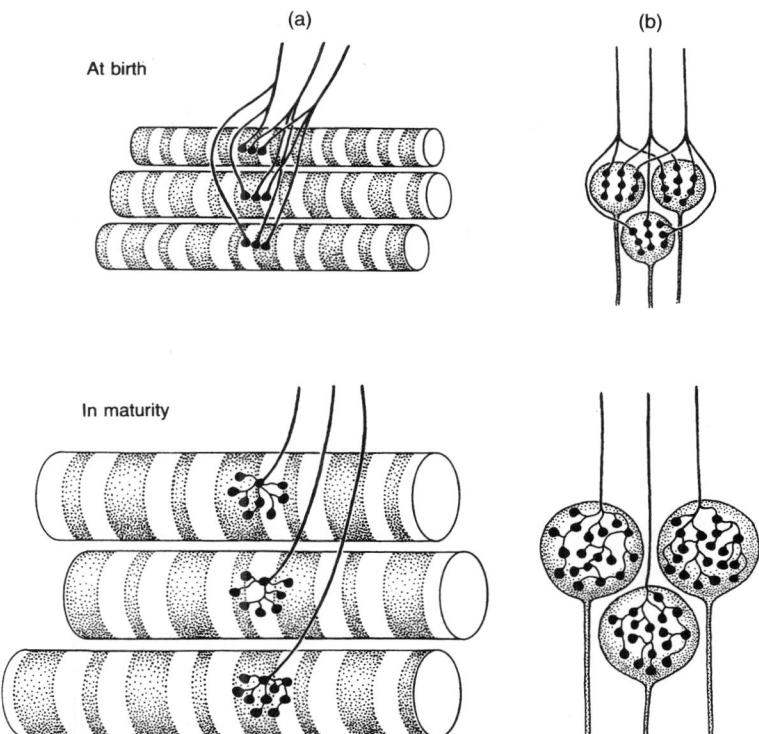

FIGURE 25.8 Schematic illustrations of postnatal synaptic rearrangements in mammalian muscle (a) and ganglia (b). At birth, each axon innervates more target cells than in maturity, but the terminal arborizations display a larger complexity in the adult animal. (From Purves D. *Body and brain: a trophic theory of neural connections.* Cambridge, MA: Harvard University Press, 1988, with permission.)

## SYNAPTIC REARRANGEMENTS IN NEURONS WITH A COMPLEX CONNECTIVITY

Experiments which form the basis for the above hypothesis were performed on simple systems. Since most central neurons are geometrically complex, it may be very difficult to verify synaptic rearrangement in these cases. Attempts to study the development of the synaptic connectivity of a richly innervated neuron, the spinal motorneuron, have revealed a much more intricate rearrangement of the synaptic input.

Synaptic boutons are present on the initial axon segment of the spinal motorneuron at birth, but disappear from that region during the first few weeks of life. There is also postnatal loss of boutons from the cell body and the motor axon collaterals with projections in the cord lose terminal branches. In these regions, elimination of synapses is parallel with that in the periphery. However, the total number of synapses on the dendrites appears the same, about 50 000, irrespective of postnatal age. This constant number seems to be the result of an elimination of some inputs and a formation of others (Fig. 25.9). This process may be explained by the trophism hypothesis, but it certainly requires a

much more complex set of events, probably involving a number of different trophic substances. It has been proposed that these changes reflect a shift in the control of the spinal motorneuron from local to supraspinal levels. It has also been suggested that the central parts of the motorneuron may be under an inhibitory influence during the rearrangement period.

## SELECTED READING

Dan Y, Poo MM. Retrograde interactions during formation and elimination of neuromuscular synapses. *Curr Opin Neurobiol* 1994; 4: 95.

Jacobson M. *Developmental neurobiology.* 3rd edn. New York: Plenum Press, 1991.

Jessell TM. Neuronal survival and synapse formation. In Kandel ER, Schwartz JH, Jessell TM, eds. *Principles of neural science.* 3rd edn. East Norwalk CT: Appleton and Lange, 1991.

Kandel ER, Jessell TM. Early experience and the fine tuning of synaptic connections. In Kandel ER, Schwartz JH, Jessell TM, eds. *Principles of neural science.* 3rd edn. East Norwalk CT: Appleton and Lange, 1991: 945.

Purves D. *Body and brain. A trophic theory of neural connections.* Cambridge MA: Harvard University Press, 1988.

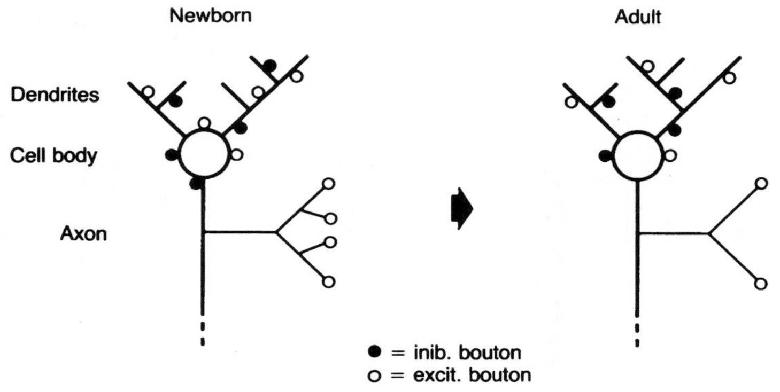

FIGURE 25.9 Scheme for intramedullary synaptic rearrangements in cat α-motorneurons postnatally. The number of synaptic terminals of the axon collateral system is reduced by half within a constant terminal field. Half the number of synapses on the cell body and all synapses (predominantly inhibitory) on the initial axon segment are removed. The dendrites are apposed by a constant number of synaptic boutons reflecting a balance between the establishment and removal of synaptic connections. The dendrites are to some degree remodeled during their invasion of new territories, but the total number of dendritic end branches remains constant. (From Cullheim S, Ulfhake B. In *Neurobiology of early infant behaviour*. London: The Macmillan Press, 1988, with permission.)

# NEUROTROPHIC FACTORS

## INTRODUCTION

Neurotrophic factors support the growth, differentiation, and survival of neurons in the developing nervous system and maintain neurons in the mature nervous system. Their existence was discovered over 40 years ago in experiments investigating developmental death of neurons. There is a large and rapidly growing number of identified neurotrophic factors.

Neurotrophins are an important family of structurally related neurotrophic factors. Nerve growth factor (NGF) was the first discovered and best characterized neurotrophin. More recently identified members of the neurotrophin family include brain-derived neurotrophic factor (BDNF), neurotrophin-3 (NT-3), and neurotrophin-4/5 (NT-4/5). Neurotrophins exert their effects by binding to and activating specific cell surface receptors. Activated receptors initiate a cascade of intracellular events which result in induction of gene expression and changes in neuronal morphology and differentiation. Neurotrophins are critical regulators of normal neuronal development and maintenance.

The neurotrophins are one important class of neurotrophic factors. Other neurotrophic factors include ciliary neurotrophic factor (CNTF), the insulin-like growth factors (IGFs), the fibroblast growth factors (FGFs), and glial cell line-derived nerve factor (GDNF). These factors will not be discussed individually in this chapter but can be reviewed in the references included in the reading list.

Although each neurotrophic factor has a unique pattern of expression and actions, one can nevertheless propose a "neurotrophic factor hypothesis" to broadly describe the biology of these molecules. Neurotrophic factors are diffusible polypeptides released from neuronal and non-neuronal cells that act via specific receptors on neuronal progenitor cells and neurons to enhance survival (i.e. to prevent apoptosis) and promote function. Neurotrophic factor actions include target-derived, autocrine and paracrine effects. In some neuronal populations, multiple neurotrophic factors acting together or in sequence may be required. Finally, neurotrophic factors continue to exert important actions in the mature nervous system and in the setting of injury and disease.

## NERVE GROWTH FACTOR (NGF)

NGF was discovered in the early 1950s by Levi-Montalcini and Hamburger in experiments exploring the regulation of neuronal death during embryonic development. NGF is synthesized by and released from target tissues of NGF-responsive developing and mature neurons in the central and peripheral nervous systems. It acts by binding to and activating specific receptors on the surface of cell bodies, axons, and dendrites of responsive neurons. Through activating its receptors, NGF initiates and maintains trophic relationships. NGF binds to two distinct receptors; the p75 receptor and the trkA receptor. The p75 receptor is a transmembrane glycoprotein that appears to modulate signaling by enhancing NGF binding to trkA and by increasing neuronal responsiveness to NGF. trkA is a receptor tyrosine kinase whose activation is essential for most aspects of NGF signaling. The trkA receptor contains an extracellular amino-terminal domain that binds NGF, a single transmembrane domain, and a cytoplasmic region that features the functionally important tyrosine kinase catalytic domain (Fig. 25.10). NGF

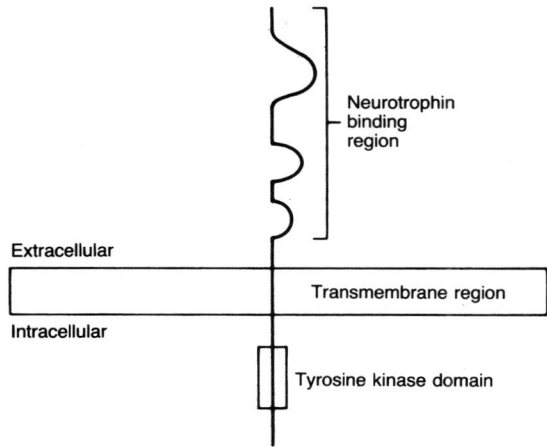

FIGURE 25.10 Schematic structure of members of the trk receptor family. Neurotrophins bind to an extracellular region. The transmembrane domain lodges the receptor in the membrane. Signaling occurs as a result of activating the intracellular tyrosine kinase.

binding to trkA results in receptor dimerization, activation of the trkA tyrosine kinase, and receptor autophosphorylation and activation. The activated receptor initiates a cascade of intracellular events which include activation of signaling intermediate proteins, generation of second messengers, changes in phospholipid metabolism, and induction of gene expression. These events ultimately result in changes in neuronal morphology and function, and improved neuronal growth and survival (Fig. 25.11).

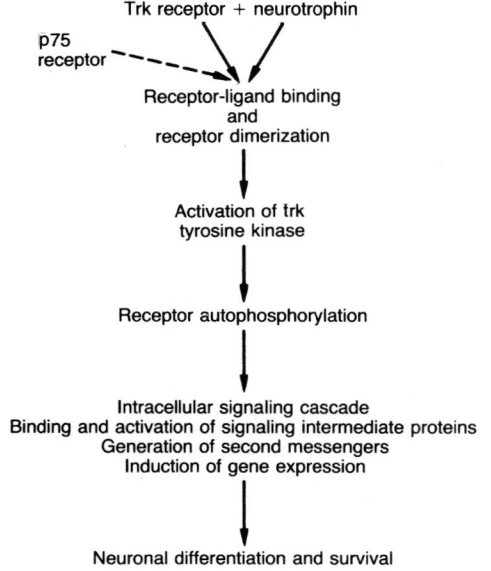

FIGURE 25.11 Neurotrophins bind and activate trk receptors to initiate a cascade of intracellular events resulting in induction of gene expression, changes in neuronal morphology and differentiation, and enhanced survival

Expression of *trkA* occurs in well-defined populations of central and peripheral neurons. NGF-responsive cells in the central nervous system include cholinergic neurons of the basal forebrain and striatum, and certain neuronal populations in the thalamus and brainstem. NGF-responsive cells in the peripheral nervous system include neurons in the sympathetic ganglia, and sensory neurons in the trigeminal and dorsal root ganglia. To date, all *trkA*-expressing neurons have been shown to be NGF-responsive. Expression of *NGF* and *trkA* is developmentally regulated. Most studies have reported little or no overlap in the location of gene expression NGF and *trkA*. These data favor the view that NGF is produced in the target of responsive neurons.

The physiologic importance of NGF to developing sensory and sympathetic neurons in the peripheral nervous system has been persuasively documented in a number of studies. In rodents, Ngf deprivation by injection of NGF antibodies during fetal life results in death of peripheral sensory neurons, whereas during early postnatal life it results in sympathetic neuronal loss. In addition, administration of exogenous Ngf reduces the developmental death of sympathetic neurons in postnatal animals. In recent studies, mutant mice lacking the gene encoding Ngf or the gene for the *trkA* receptor provide dramatic evidence for a critical role of NGF in regulating nervous system development. *Ngf* null mutant mice are growth-retarded at birth, fail to thrive, and die within the first few days to weeks after birth. *trkA* null mutant mice are normal at birth but also fail to thrive. Both the *Ngf* and *trkA* mutants have markedly impaired pain and temperature sensitivity, and develop abnormalities indicative of deficient sympathetic innervation including ptosis and miosis. Consistent with these abnormalities, mutant mice have profoundly reduced numbers of thermoceptive and nociceptive dorsal root ganglia neurons and experience progressive death of sympathetic neurons. Thus, NGF deprivation during development results in marked abnormalities in NGF-responsive sensory and sympathetic neurons. The exact role of NGF during central nervous system development is not yet established. NGF promotes growth and differentiation of basal forebrain cholinergic neurons. In addition, antibody-mediated NGF deprivation results in delayed morphological and biochemical differentiation of these neurons. Despite these actions, NGF may not be a survival factor for these neurons. NGF mutant mice have basal forebrain cholinergic neurons that are smaller than normal, and *trkA* mutant mice show incomplete differentiation of these cells. However, these neurons appear to be present in normal numbers in both mutants. Thus, NGF actions during brain development are important for neuronal differentiation but perhaps not for cell survival. Further studies are necessary to establish the precise role of NGF in the developing central nervous system.

## BRAIN-DERIVED NEUROTROPHIC FACTOR (BDNF)

BDNF was the second neurotrophin to be identified. Its discovery in 1982 by Barde and colleagues suggested the existence of a larger neurotrophin gene family. Subsequently identified members of this neurotrophin family include NT-3 and NT-4/5. Neurotrophins have extensive amino acid sequence homology which is clustered in several conserved regions. They exert their actions by binding to specific members of the trk tyrosine kinase family of cell surface receptors (Fig. 25.12). The neurotrophins also bind the p75 receptor. Although the precise role of p75 in neurotrophin signaling is not clear, co-expression of p75 with trk family members appears to increase the affinity and specificity of neurotrophin binding and signal transduction, and may increase neuronal responsiveness to neurotrophins.

BDNF exerts its effects in the central and peripheral nervous systems by binding to and activating the trkB tyrosine kinase receptor which, like the trkA receptor, dimerizes on ligand association. Two classes of trkB receptors have been identified. There is a catalytic form which contains an intracellular cytoplasmic tyrosine kinase region. This molecule closely resembles the trkA receptor. There is also a truncated class of trkB receptors which lack the cytoplasmic tyrosine kinase region. Most aspects of BDNF signal transduction appear to be mediated by the catalytic form of the trkB receptor. Whether the truncated form of the receptor has a signaling function is uncertain.

*BDNF* and *trkB* expression are widely distributed in the nervous system. BDNF-responsive cells in the central nervous system include hippocampal neurons, cholinergic and GABAergic neurons in the basal forebrain, mesencephalic dopaminergic neurons, cerebellar granule neurons, retinal ganglion neurons, and motor neurons in the facial nucleus and spinal cord. BDNF-responsive cells in the peripheral nervous system include sensory neurons in the vestibular, nodose, trigeminal, and dorsal root ganglia.

The biology of BDNF signaling appears more complex than that observed for NGF. Although in some neuronal circuits expression of BDNF and its trkB receptor occur in distinct cells, in other neuronal populations there is co-expression. Thus, BDNF may act as a target-derived neurotrophic factor for some neuronal populations and via autocrine or paracrine mechanisms for others. Interestingly, in some neurons there is a developmental change in neurotrophin responsiveness. For example, trigeminal sensory neurons which ultimately become NGF-dependent appear to respond to BDNF earlier in development. *In vitro* studies suggest that BDNF can enhance the differentiation of immature dorsal root ganglion neurons prior to the time of target contact and prior to their dependence on neurotrophins for survival. BDNF signaling is also complicated by the synthesis of truncated receptors through which certain signaling events may be modified or precluded. The observed increased expression of these truncated receptors during development may be important in the decreased responsiveness of central nervous system neurons to BDNF during postnatal life.

A critical role for BDNF during peripheral nervous system development has been demonstrated by the phenotypic abnormalities exhibited by null mutant mice lacking the gene encoding this neurotrophin. BDNF null mutant mice are born alive but most die within 48 hours of birth. Survivors exhibit abnormal respiratory patterns and alternating periods of hyperactivity and inactivity. They show progressively severe movement abnormalities including head bobbing and tilting, spinning and circling, and ataxia. These abnormalities may be explained by loss of sensory neurons in the petrosal, nodose, vestibular, trigeminal, and dorsal root ganglia. Although *Bdnf* null mutant mice have profound peripheral nervous system deficiencies, their central nervous system abnormalities are relatively mild and include decreased expression of certain proteins in some neuronal populations. As with NGF, it appears that BDNF is a critical factor in peripheral nervous system development. Further studies are important to clarify its actions during central nervous system development.

## NEUROTROPHIN-3 (NT-3)

NT-3 was the third member of the neurotrophin family to be identified. Like the other neurotrophins, NT-3 exerts its actions by binding to and activating members of the trk family of tyrosine kinase receptors. NT-3 is somewhat promiscuous in its receptor binding. NT-3 activates the trkC receptor with maximal potency. However, in certain cells it can also activate trkA and trkB receptors (Fig. 25.12).

*NT-3* and *trkC* are widely expressed in the central and peripheral nervous systems. NT-3-responsive cells in the central nervous system include neurons in the trigeminal mesencephalic nucleus, hippocampal neurons, dopaminergic and GABAergic neurons in the ventral mesencephalon, and motor neurons in the spinal cord. NT-3-responsive cells in the peripheral nervous system include sensory neurons in the nodose and dorsal root ganglia, and sympathetic neurons.

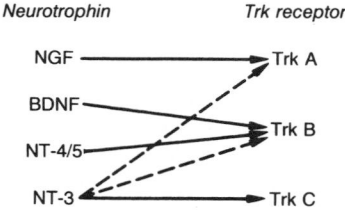

FIGURE 25.12 Neurotrophins bind with high affinity to specific members of the trk family of cell surface receptors

Like BDNF, the biology of NT-3 appears to be more complex than that for NGF. NT-3 functions as a target-derived neurotrophic factor in some neuronal populations and probably via autocrine or paracrine modes in others. In addition, there is evidence that NT-3 mediates events during early development, some of which may occur prior to neuronal innervation of target tissues. In the central nervous system, there is extensive NT-3 expression during early development. In addition, there is widespread expression of the trkC receptor and marked neuronal responsiveness to NT-3 during embryonic and early postnatal development. These data suggest that NT-3 may have a role in regulating early central nervous system developmental events such as neuronal migration and differentiation. In the peripheral nervous system, dorsal root ganglia neurons that have not yet achieved target contact respond to NT-3 with enhanced differentiation. In addition, NT-3 enhances the survival of dividing sympathetic neuroblasts and young sympathetic neurons. Survival dependence in sympathetic neurons subsequently switches to NGF. This change correlates with a switch in neurotrophin receptor expression from trkC to trkA. Thus, the development of certain neuronal populations appears to require the sequential actions of multiple neurotrophins. Like BDNF, NT-3 signaling is complicated by the synthesis of both catalytic and truncated trkC receptors. In addition, there are transcripts for alternative forms of each class of the trkC receptor. The function of these receptor isoforms is uncertain. Expression of truncated and alternative forms of the trkC receptor may be important in modifying neuronal responsiveness during development.

The phenotypic abnormalities observed in mutant mice deficient for the gene encoding Nt-3 provide dramatic evidence for a critical role of NT-3 during normal development. Nt-3 mutant mice are born alive and appear healthy at birth. However, they have reduced growth rates and severely shortened life spans. In addition, they display abnormal movements and postures. The neurologic basis of these abnormalities is a severe reduction in peripheral sensory neurons required for proprioception. Preliminary observations indicate that the central nervous system of Nt-3 mutant mice is relatively unaffected. More detailed studies, especially in older animals, are necessary to define the central nervous system actions of NT-3.

## NEUROTROPHIN-4/5 (NT-4/5)

NT-4/5 is the most recently identified and least well-characterized member of the neurotrophin family. Like BDNF, NT-4/5 exerts its effects by binding to and activating the trkB receptor. This shared signaling pathway and the overlapping expression of NT-4/5 and BDNF have made it difficult to define the precise role of NT-4/5 in the nervous system.

The gene for NT-4/5 is expressed in both the central and peripheral nervous systems, and NT-4/5 acts on neurons throughout the nervous system. NT-4/5-responsive cells in the central nervous system include neurons in the hippocampus and ventral mesencephalon, as well as motorneurons in the facial nucleus and spinal cord. NT-4/5-responsive cells in the peripheral nervous system include sensory neurons in the dorsal root, nodose, trigeminal, and jugular ganglia.

The recent generation of mutant mice deficient for the gene encoding Nt-4/5 has provided information for the physiologic role of this neurotrophin. Compared with mice mutant for other neurotrophins, Nt-4/5 null mutant mice have relatively mild defects. They are born alive and appear healthy. They have normal growth and behavior, and produce viable offspring. Their primary anatomic defect is loss of cranial sensory neurons. Thus far, no abnormalities have been identified in the central nervous system of these mice. Since both NT-4/5 and BDNF act through the trkB receptor, it has been suggested that a deficiency of either factor may be compensated for by the other. Mutant mice lacking the genes for both Nt-4/5 and Bdnf have recently been examined. These double mutant mice have some deficits which are much more marked than those seen in mice with either mutation alone. Interestingly, there was no loss of motorneurons in either the Nt-4/5 or the double mutant mouse.

## THERAPEUTIC IMPLICATIONS AND CLINICAL APPLICATIONS

The therapeutic use of neurotrophins is the subject of intense investigation. Neurotrophins have potent neuroprotective effects in vitro and in vivo. Significantly, neurotrophins ameliorate neuronal dysfunction and death in animal models of peripheral neuropathy, motor neuron disease, and neurodegenerative diseases. Their therapeutic potential in human disease is being investigated in several clinical trials. Thus far, little attention has been paid to a role for neurotrophins in the treatment of pediatric neurologic disease. However, one can speculate that neurotrophins may ameliorate, reverse, or prevent disorders in which the viability or function of specific developing neuronal populations is threatened.

## SELECTED READING

Barbacid M. The Trk family of neurotrophin receptors. *J Neurobiol* 1994; **25**: 1386.

Chao, MV. The p75 receptor. *J Neurobiol* 1994; **25**: 1373.

Davies AM. The role of neurotrophins in the developing nervous system. *J Neurobiol* 1994; **25**: 1334.

Escandon E, Soppet D, Rosenthal A et al. Regulation of neurotrophin receptor expression during embryonic and postnatal development. *J Neurosci* 1994; **14**: 2054.

Holtzman DM, Mobley WC. Neurotrophic factors and neurologic disease. *Western J Med* 1994; **161**: 246.

Kaplan DR, Stephens RM. Neurotrophin signal transduction by the Trk receptor. *J Neurobiol* 1994; **25**: 1404.

Klein R. Role of neurotrophins in mouse neuronal development. *FASEB J* 1994; **8**: 738.

Knusel B, Rabin SJ, Hefti F, Kaplan DR. Regulated neurotrophin receptor responsiveness during neuronal migration and early differentiation. *J Neurosci* 1994; **14**: 1542.

Korsching S. The neurotrophic factor concept: A re-examination. *J Neurosci* 1993; **13**: 2739.

Longo FM, Holtzman DM, Grimes ML, Mobley WC. Nerve growth factor: Actions in the peripheral and central nervous system. In: Loughlin S, Fallon J, eds. *Neurotrophic factors*. New York: Academic Press, 1993: 209.

Snider WD. Functions of the neurotrophins during nervous system development: What the knockouts are teaching us. *Cell* 1994; **77**: 627.

# DEVELOPMENT OF NEUROGLIA

The nervous system is derived during embryogenesis from a columnar layer of cells known as the neuroepithelium, which forms the neural tube (*see* page 359). In rodents primordial precursor cells are first committed to become either neurons or glia at approximately midgestation, with neurogenesis preceding the bulk of gliogenesis. In the rat terminally differentiated neurons appear at E11, while proliferation continues until E20. Although most glial cells do not appear until somewhat later, a specialized type of glia, the radial glia, appear shortly prior to neurogenesis. These cells provide a framework to guide first neural precursors, and later glial precursors, from a germinal zone surrounding the ventricles to their eventual sites of terminal differentiation (*see* page 361).

The exact sequence of subsequent gliogenesis remains controversial, however, the following hypothesis is supported by evidence from recent experiments in rats (Fig. 25.13). The radial glia in the rat transform into type I astrocytes in the first week postnatally. Most mature glia, however, are derived from glial precursor cells directly. Astrocyte (type I) differentiation commences at E16, and continues postnatally. A bipotential glial progenitor (dubbed the O-2A progenitor) emerges a few days before birth, to generate first oligodendrocytes around birth, and then type II astrocytes during the second postnatal week.

In contrast to this stereotyped developmental sequence *in situ*, precursor cells sampled at different ages show a similar potential for producing different glial lineages *in vitro*. Thus, there is a progressive developmental restriction *in situ*, which is related to environmental signals such as growth factors, as well as extracellular matrix signals, and direct cellular contact. Basic fibroblast growth factor (bFGF) promotes the proliferation of the precursors and is potentiated by other growth factors, e.g. nerve growth factor (NGF). Platelet-derived growth factor (PDGF) is a proliferative factor for the O-2A progenitor in the rat optic nerve. Subsequent differentiation may be related to a reduction in bFGF, with continuing PDGF, and increasing insulin like growth factor (IGF)-I and IGF-II expression, as well as, as yet unidentified neuronal derived factors. Ciliary neurotrophic factor (CTNF) and leukemia inhibitory factor (LIF) both promote the dif-

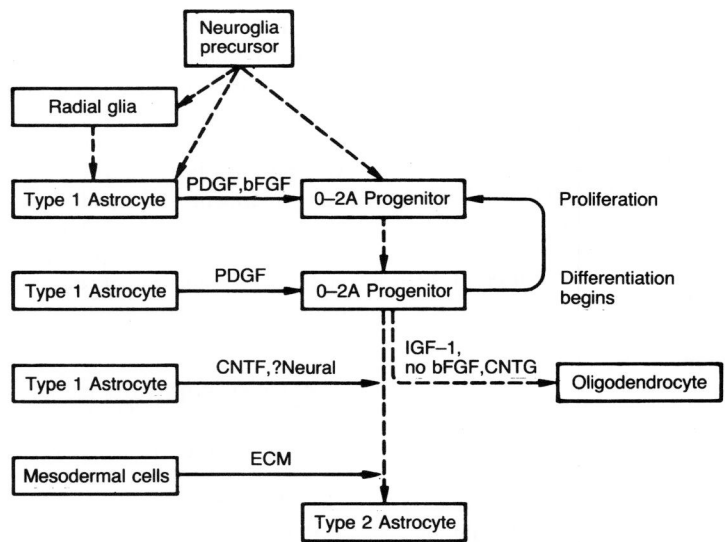

FIGURE 25.13 Proposed scheme of glial development. During embryogenesis basic fibroblast growth factor (bFGF) and platelet derived growth factor (PDGF) secretion by type I astrocytes promote O-2A progenitor proliferation. With time, the O-2A cells begin to differentiate as well as continuing to proliferate; this has been related to a fall in bFGF production, in the presence of continued PDGF secretion. The type I astrocyte may then secrete either ciliary neurotrophic factor (CNTF) which initiates the differentiation of type II astrocytes, or IGF-I and IGF-II which promote oligodendrocyte production. Unidentified molecules (probably extracellular matrix proteins) secreted by mesenchymal cells appear to be necessary to complete type II astrocyte differentiation.

ferentiation of oligodendrocytes in isolation, but promote differentiation into type II astrocytes in presence of endothelial cell derived extracellular matrix proteins. CNTF and LIF have equivalent potency to IGF-I in promoting glial survival *in vitro*. There is evidence of an intermediate, pro-oligodendrocyte form, that inhibits the proliferation of O-2A progenitors. Thus autocrine inhibitory mechanisms may also have an important role in regulating cell proliferation.

Gliogenesis in primates is similar but is not so clearly documented. In the monkey radial glia appear in parallel with neurogenesis, from E47 (gestation in the monkey is 165 days). Similarly, radial glia have been found in the human fetus at 8–10 weeks' gestation. In the spinal cord of the human fetus early myelin

tubules, identified using antibodies to myelin basic protein, are found at 15–18 weeks' gestation; myelination continues throughout fetal life and the rate of myelination peaks in the first year postnatally. Neuronal conduction velocities show a parallel increase. Peripheral nerve conduction velocities, e.g. in the ulnar nerve, increase rapidly in the first year of life, with further marginal increases until mid-childhood (Fig. 25.14). Central conduction times have been determined using somatosensory evoked potentials for afferent pathways and magneto-electric motor evoked potentials for efferent pathways. Central conduction velocity increases very rapidly in the first 6–12 months after birth, but adult values are not reached until the end of the first decade (Fig. 25.15).

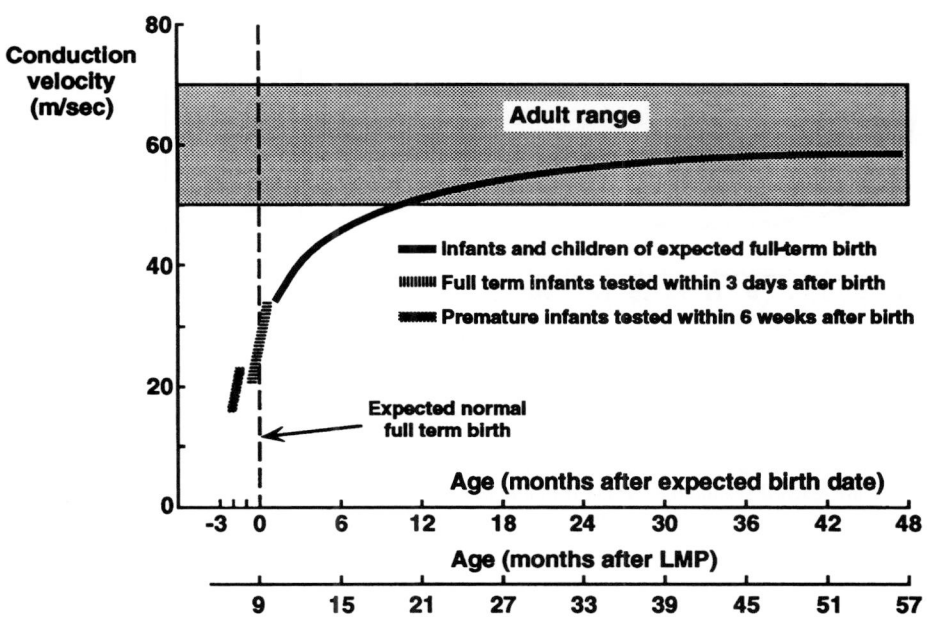

FIGURE 25.14 Maturation of motor conduction velocity in the ulnar nerve between the elbow and the wrist. Velocities in normal young adults range from 47 to 73 m/s. (From Thomas JE, Lambert EH. *J Appl Physiol* 1960; 15: 1, with permission.)

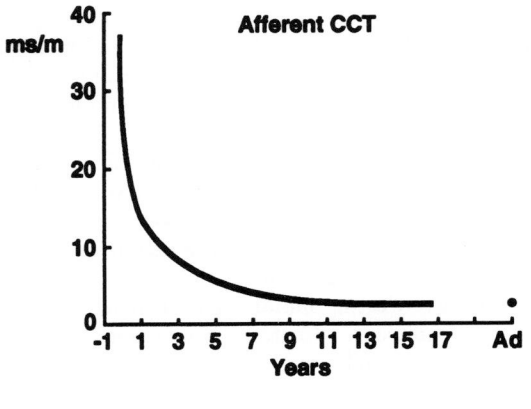
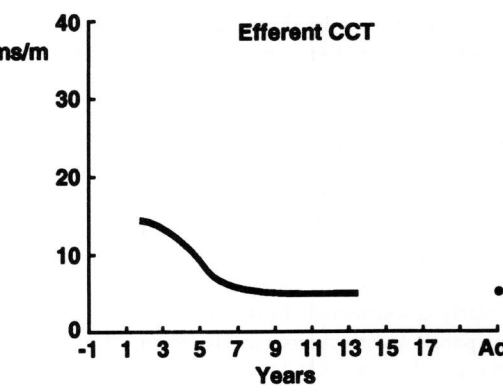
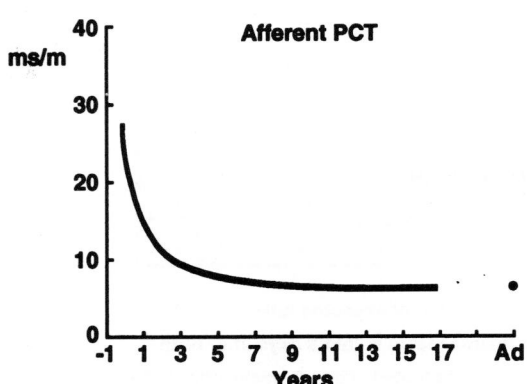
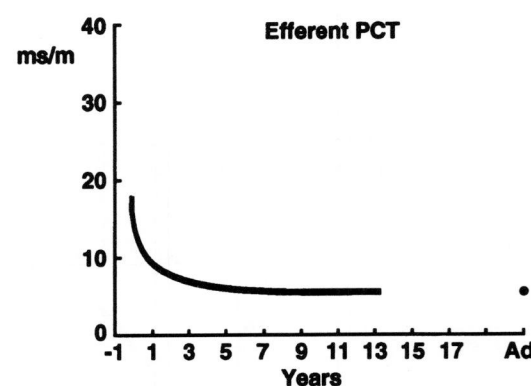

FIGURE 25.15 Maturation of afferent and efferent central (CCT) and peripheral (PCT) conduction times. Afferent conduction times (CCT and PCT) were derived from median nerve somatosensory evoked potentials. Efferent conduction times (CCT and PCT) were derived from motor evoked potentials (MEP) recorded at the thenar eminence following stimulation at the vertex and upper cervical region. Because stimulation thresholds for MEP are too high during the first year of life efferent conduction times could be measured only after the age of 13 months. The pace of maturation is different in the central and peripheral nervous system. Adult values (Ad) of PCT are reached around the third year of life, whereas CCTs show a prolonged maturation. (From Müller K, Ebner B, Hömberg V. *Neurosci Lett* 1994; **166**: 9, with permission.)

## SELECTED READING

Bartlett PF, Kilpatrick TJ, Richards LJ *et al.* Regulation of the early development of the nervous system by growth factors. *Pharmacol Ther* 1994; **64**: 371.

Goldman JE. Regulation of oligodendrocyte differentiation. *TINS* 1992; **15**: 359.

Kandel ER, Schwartz JH, Jessel TM, eds. *Principles of neural science*. East Norwalk CT: Appleton and Lange, 1991.

Levison SW, Chuang C, Abramson BJ *et al.* The migrational patterns and developmental fates of glial precursors in the rat subventricular zone are temporally regulated. *Development* 1993; **119**: 611.

# 26

# Sensory Systems

# SOMATOSENSORY SYSTEMS

## SOMATOSENSORY SYSTEM PHYSIOLOGY

The somatosensory system enables us to perceive a wide range of tactile, thermal and nociceptive stimuli over the entire body surface. We are also aware of the positions and movements of our skeletal body parts and use this information for the control of posture and movement.

## CUTANEOUS RECEPTORS

The entire body surface is covered with skin which contains a variety of receptors providing information to the central nervous system. Most of the body is covered by hairy skin. The ventral surfaces of the hands and the soles of the feet are covered by glabrous skin which has a different structure and innervation to hairy skin. Glabrous skin is characterized by a regular arrangement of dermal papillae with interlocking epidermal protrusions; the outer layers of the epidermis are keratinized (Fig. 26.1). This regular arrangement gives glabrous skin its ridged appearance, most spectacular in the fingertips where the result is a fingerprint pattern unique to the individual. There are four classes of mechanoreceptors in the glabrous skin. Meissner corpuscles in the dermal papillae and Merkel cell–

neurite complexes at the epidermal–dermal junction are relatively superficial. Ruffini endings are located deeper in the skin, as are Pacinian corpuscles which are also found in subcutaneous tissue. In hairy skin there are no Meissner corpuscles, and the Merkel complexes are clustered together in specialized epidermal protrusions (up to 0.5 mm in diameter) known as touch domes. Ruffini organs and Pacinian corpuscles are present in hairy skin. In addition, fibers innervating hair follicles respond to mechanical stimulation. Both glabrous and hairy skin have free nerve endings in the dermis and epidermis; these act as receptors for thermal and noxious stimuli.

## PROPERTIES OF PRIMARY AFFERENTS

The low threshold mechanoreceptors in glabrous skin (Meissner, Merkel, Ruffini and Pacinian) are innervated by large myelinated fibers of the Aβ group in the peripheral nerve. These respond to gentle mechanical stimulation of an area of skin which forms the receptive field. Afferents from Merkel and Ruffini endings have a static response; action potentials are elicited as long as deformation of the receptive field is maintained. Ruffini endings are particularly sensitive to lateral stretch of the skin, presumably because of the horizontal orientation of the elongated Ruffini organ. Fibers from Merkel endings are known as slowly adapting type I; from Ruffini endings as type II. Afferents from Meissner and Pacinian endings

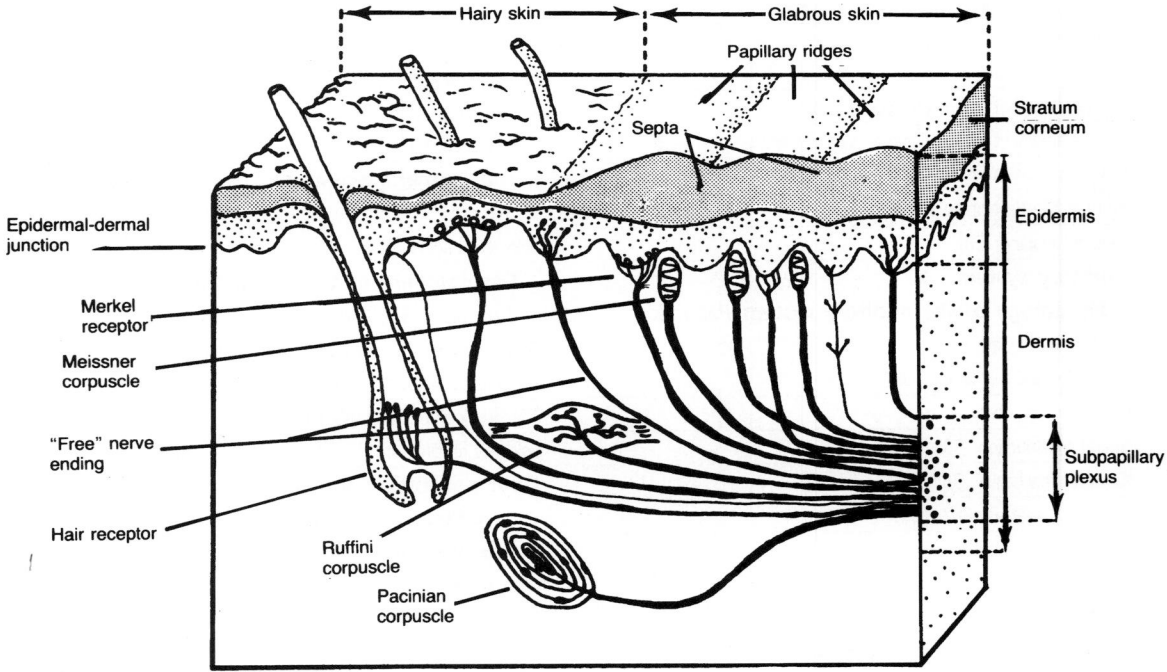

FIGURE 26.1 Innervation of glabrous and hairy skin. In glabrous skin the Meissner and Merkel endings are closer to the surface than the Ruffini and Pacinian endings. All afferent fibers are myelinated (thick lines) except for the C fibers shown by thin lines. (Adapted from Light AR, Perl ER. In Dyck PJ, Thomas PK, Lambert EH, Burge R. eds. *Peripheral neuropathy*, 2nd edn. Vol. 1. Philadelphia: Saunders, 1984: 210, with permission.)

(which are encapsulated and have an alternating lamella structure) have a dynamic response; action potentials are elicited only when deformations of the receptive field are changing. Meissner afferents (rapidly adapting type I) respond preferentially to stimuli that are changing relatively slowly (for a vibratory stimulus their optimum frequency is about 30 Hz). Pacinian afferents (rapidly adapting type II) are most sensitive to rapidly changing stimuli (optimum vibratory frequency about 300 Hz). Because of their more superficial location, Meissner and Merkel afferents have smaller receptive fields than Ruffini and Pacinian afferents.

In hairy skin, there are two further classes of afferents both of which have large receptive fields and both of which are rapidly adapting. Hair units are associated with the hair follicles, and field units are of unknown origin. Recently, unmyelinated fibers from hairy skin responding to low threshold mechanical stimuli have been found; their endings and their function are not known.

There are two classes of thermoreceptors in skin. Cold receptors are activated by a decrease in skin temperature and are innervated by small myelinated Aδ axons. Warm receptors respond to an increase in temperature and are innervated by unmyelinated C fibers. These receptors respond to changes in temperature of a fraction of a degree centigrade, and have both a static and a dynamic component to their response. Finally there are three classes of nociceptors; mechanical nociceptors innervated by Aδ fibers, mechano-thermal nociceptors innervated by Aδ and C fibers, and polymodal nociceptors innervated by C fibers. The thermoreceptors and nociceptors are presumed to be free nerve endings.

## PROPRIOCEPTION

Throughout the body there are receptors which provide information about the positions and movements of the limbs. There are receptors in the joint capsule which signal joint angle, but they are sparse and many respond only at extremes of joint angle. Responses of cutaneous afferents around the joints change systematically with changes in joint angle. Muscles are richly innervated with spindles (*see* page 403) which provide precise signals about the lengths of the muscles and the velocities of stretch and hence about the positions and movements of the attached limbs. Golgi tendon organs at the musculo-tendinous junction (*see* page 403) signal tension in the muscles and hence forces in the limbs.

## HAND FUNCTION

Classically, the skin is thought of as supplying the brain with information of a relatively simple nature with low spatial and temporal resolution. While this may apply to hairy skin, it is not true in the glabrous skin of the hand where complex information is relayed with high spatiotemporal fidelity and without which hand function would not be possible. The hand is an organ which has evolved in primates and is critical to everyday human life. The cutaneous afferents, which have a far higher innervation density in the fingerpad (e.g. $140/cm^2$ for the Meissner afferents) than in the rest of the body, provide detailed information about the surface texture, the local shape, the contact force and the position on the fingers of objects we handle. This information is used in conjunction with signals from the joints and muscles. Thus, when handling objects, we can differentiate the texture of silk and cotton, the compliance of a ripe or green peach; we can manipulate a fragile egg or a stiff tap.

## CENTRAL PATHWAYS

The peripheral nerve fibers have cell bodies in the dorsal root ganglia and enter the spinal cord via the dorsal roots forming two principal pathways for relaying signals to the brain. The high spatial and temporal resolution signals that we alluded to in discussing hand function are often referred to as "fine touch." Fibers conveying fine touch information travel up the dorsal columns of the spinal cord (Fig. 26.2a) and synapse in the dorsal column nuclei in the medulla; these are the gracile nucleus for the lower limbs and lower body and the cuneate nucleus for the upper limbs and upper body. Axons from cells in these nuclei cross to the contralateral side as the internal arcuate fibers and ascend the brainstem as the medial lemniscus terminating in the thalamus, mainly in the ventral posterior lateral nucleus (also in the posterior nucleus). The thalamic cells project to the somatosensory cortex.

Fibers conveying thermal and nociceptive signals enter the dorsal roots and synapse in the dorsal horn (Fig. 26.2b). Second order fibers cross in the spinal cord and travel up the contralateral anterolateral columns. On reaching the brainstem, these fibers form three separate groups. Many terminate in the thalamus (ventral posterior, posterior and intralaminar nuclei) forming the spinothalamic fibers, some terminate in the reticular formation (the spinoreticular fibers) and some in the midbrain (the spinomesencephalic fibers). The anterolateral system conveys pain and thermal sensation as well as some touch sensation.

The distinction between the two pathways is important clinically, as they cross the nervous system at quite different levels; lesions of the anterolateral system lead principally to pain and temperature deficits and lesions of the medial lemniscal system result mainly in disturbances of fine touch and position sense. There is an analogous dual pathway for sensations from the head via the trigeminal nerve; the principal thalamic nucleus for the head is the ventral posterior medial nucleus.

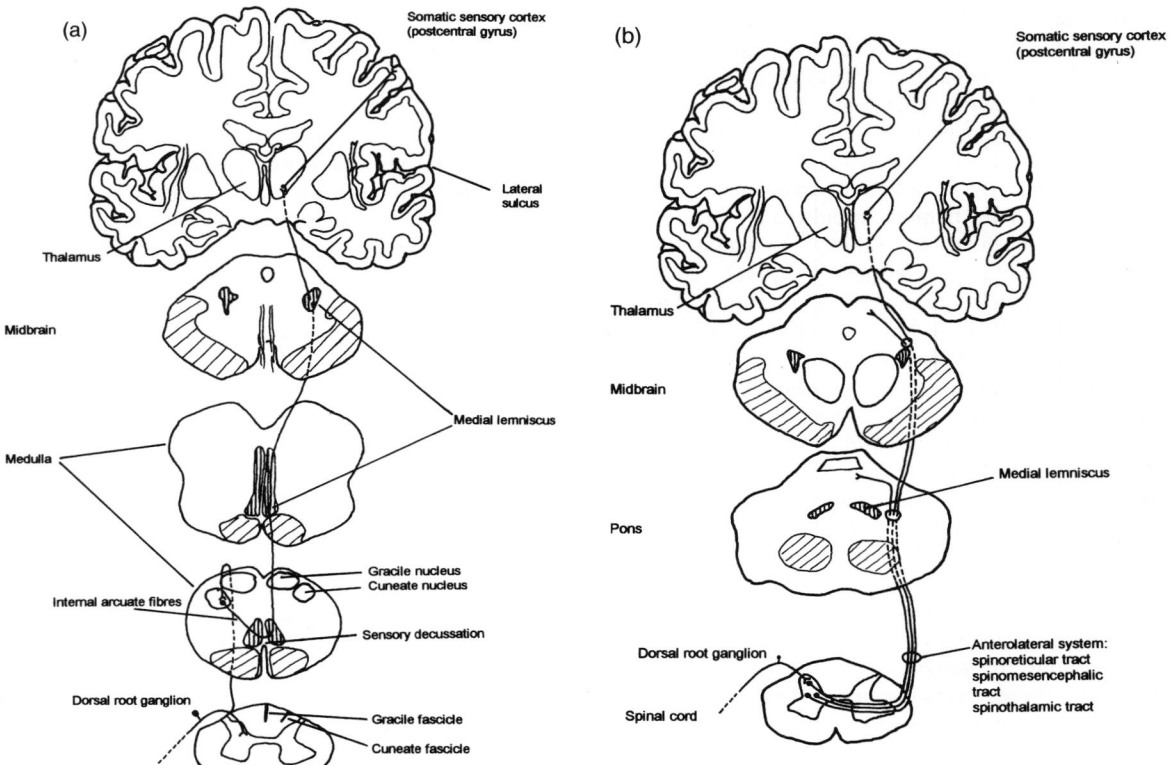

FIGURE 26.2 Pathways for the dorsal column or medial lemniscal system, which conveys fine touch (a), and for the anterolateral system, which conveys thermal and nociceptive signals (b). Both pathways project to the contralateral somatosensory cortex, but they cross at different levels of the nervous system.

## SOMATOSENSORY CORTEX

The principal site of termination of sensory pathway fibers leaving the thalamus is the postcentral gyrus (Fig. 26.3a) known as somatosensory area I (SI). SI comprises four cytoarchitectonically distinct but interconnected regions referred to as areas 3a, 3b, 1 and 2 lying in a rostral–caudal relationship across the gyrus. The relative contributions of the different classes of peripheral receptors to each of these four areas are different; different areas appear to serve different functions, e.g. texture discrimination in area 1, and size and shape discrimination in area 2, but the differences are not clear cut and not well understood. The receptive field properties of cortical cells have not been characterized as thoroughly as those in the visual and auditory cortices. Nevertheless, properties such as inhibitory regions and direction selectivity have been demonstrated. A second somatosensory area, SII, located on the upper bank of the lateral sulcus receives input from SI and from the thalamus. There are additional somatosensory areas in the insula region. The somatosensory cortex is topographically organized circumferentially as shown by the classic "homunculus" of Penfield (Fig. 26.3b). The two features of the map are an ordered representation of the body surface and

a disproportionately large representation of parts requiring greater resolution, like the fingers and lips. Each of the four areas 3a, 3b, 1 and 2 which lie in parallel along the length of the gyrus has a separate complete representation or map of the body. This topographic arrangement is in fact preserved throughout the somatosensory system from the dermatomes to the cortex.

Further elaboration of somatosensory processing occurs in the association cortex, in particular the posterior parietal cortex where complex sensations such as three-dimensional shape, and movements in extrapersonal space appear to be dealt with. Other areas of the brain, such as motor, premotor and supplementary motor cortex are linked with somatosensory cortex to implement sensorimotor integration. There are also links between somatosensory cortex and areas of the brain serving other senses. Everyday tasks such as viewing an object and then reaching out to grasp and handle it require complex integration of multiple sensory signals and motor commands.

## SOMATOSENSORY EVOKED POTENTIALS

The somatosensory evoked potentials (SEP) are used in the evaluation of central somatosensory pathways. A

(a)

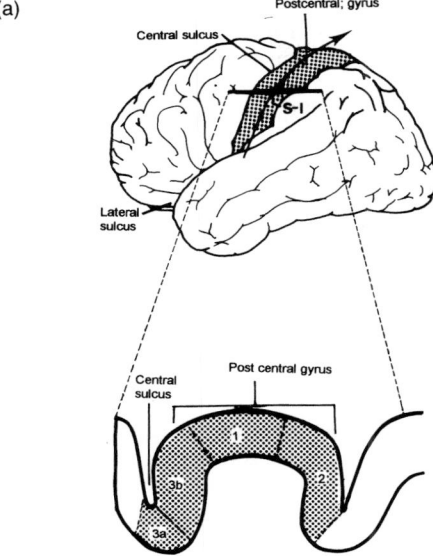

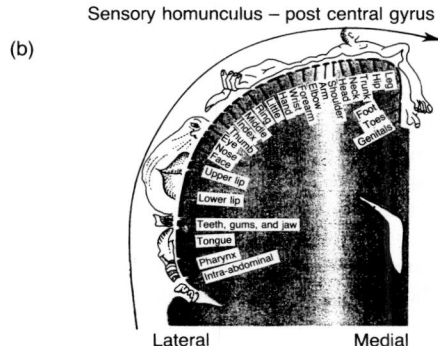

Sensory homunculus – post central gyrus

(b)

FIGURE 26.3 (a) The SI somatosensory cortex, located in the postcentral gyrus, consists of four distinct cytoarchitectonic areas. (b) The representation or map of the body surface on the postcentral gyrus is shown by the homunculus. The map is ordered, and more sensitive body parts have a proportionately greater representation. (Adapted from Penfield W, Rassmusen T. *The cerebral cortex of man: a clinical study of localization of function*. New York: Macmillan, 1950, with permission.)

peripheral nerve, commonly the ulnar or median at the wrist or posterior tibial at the ankle, is stimulated electrically at a level that produces a motor response. Following median nerve stimulation the action potential in large rapidly conducting myelinated fibers is recorded by an electrode placed on the neck over the brachial plexus. Responses are also recorded from the posterior cervical region and the scalp. Low amplitude responses from the cervical cord, brainstem and cortex are recorded with the aid of computer averaging from the posterior neck and scalp. The central conduction time, the interval between the response recorded from the brainstem, P14, and that recorded from the primary somatosensory cortex, N20, over the contralateral central parietal scalp, is used in a number of clinical settings to estimate function in central pathways, e.g. in the assessment of head injury.

## SELECTED READING

Carlson M. Development of tactile discrimination capacity in *Macaca mulatta* II. Effects of partial removal of primary somatic sensory cortex (SmI) in infants and juveniles. *Dev Brain Res* 1984; **16**: 83.

Darian-Smith I. The sense of touch: performance and peripheral neural processes. In Brookhart JM, Mountcastle VB, Darian-Smith I, Geiger SR, eds. *Handbook of physiology – the nervous system, III*. Bethesda: American Physiological Society, 1984: 739.

Gandevia SC, McCloskey DI, Burke D. Kinaesthetic signals and muscle contraction. *Trends Neurosci* 1992; **15**: 62.

Goodwin AW. Touch: The code for roughness. *Curr Biol* 1993; **3**: 378.

Johnson KO, Hsiao SS. Neural mechanisms of tactual form and texture perception. *Annu Rev Neurosci* 1992; **15**: 226.

Light AR, Perl ER. Peripheral sensory systems. In Dyck PJ, Thomas PK, Lambert EH, Burge R. eds. *Peripheral neuropathy*, 2nd edn. Vol. 1. Philadelphia: Saunders, 1984: 210.

Mountcastle VB. Central nervous mechanisms in mechanoreceptive sensibility. In Brookhart JM, Mountcastle VB, Darian-Smith I, Geiger SR, eds. *Handbook of physiology – the nervous system, III*. Bethesda: American Physiological Society, 1984: 789.

Nelson RJ, Sur M, Felleman DJ, Kaas JH. Representations of the body surface in postcentral parietal cortex of *Macaca fascicularis*. *J Comp Neurol* 1980; **192**: 611.

Penfield W, Rassmusen T. *The cerebral cortex of man: a clinical study of localization of function*. New York: Macmillan, 1950.

Rees S, Nitsos I, Rawson J. The development of cutaneous afferent pathways in fetal sheep: a structural and functional study. *Brain Res* 1994; **661**: 207.

Vallbo AB, Johansson RS. Properties of cutaneous mechanoreceptors in the human hand related to touch sensation. *Human Neurobiol* 1984; **3**: 3.

Willis WD, Coggeshall RE. *Sensory mechanisms of the spinal cord*. New York: Plenum, 1991.

# DEVELOPMENT OF SOMATOSENSORY FUNCTION

The somatosensory system begins to develop early in fetal life, before either the auditory or the visual systems. At 7–8 weeks' gestation in the human and 15 embryonic days in the rat (E15) the primary sensory neurons in the trigeminal ganglion make the first connections between their peripheral processes and their targets in skin and muscle, and between their central processes in cranial nerve V and neurons in the brainstem. Motoneurons make contact with muscles at about the same time, thus completing the components of a reflex arc. Stroking the upper or lower lip with a light hair causes a reflex response in the 8-week human fetus. These first sensory connections develop in a rostrocaudal sequence; at 10.5 weeks the hands are sensitive and by 14 weeks stimulation of any part of the body surface can evoke reflex responses. A similar sequence is observed in the fetal rat over E14–17.

The onset of somatosensory reflexes indicates the formation of sensory connections at the segmental level. In the rat, projection fibers from the spinal cord and brainstem begin to grow into the thalamus in the late fetal period and continue to do so over the early postnatal period. Somewhat later, perhaps triggered by the sensory input, descending cortical fibers reach the thalamus and arrange themselves in a lattice around spinothalamic and trigeminothalamic terminals. Thalamic projection fibers arrive at the cortical plate at birth making an organized pattern of terminals by postnatal day 4 (P4) in the rat and approximately 29 weeks in the human fetus, coinciding with the appearance of somatosensory evoked potentials (*see* page 378). The maturation of thalamic and cortical connections takes place postnatally. In order to understand somatosensory function during development, it is not enough to establish when appropriate sensory connections are made. We need to study how the signals are transmitted from the periphery and how they are processed centrally at each developmental stage.

## DEVELOPMENT OF PERIPHERAL SENSORY RECEPTORS

Information about the nature of a peripheral stimulus is provided by specific sensory afferents, each responding to a particular stimulus. At the time sensory nerves first reach the skin all the sensory nerve endings are homogeneously distributed in a plexus of free nerve endings; it is already possible to distinguish low threshold, rapidly adapting "touch" receptors, high threshold, slowly adapting "pressure" receptors and polymodal nociceptors. The sensory modality is intrinsic to the sensory afferents and not imposed on them by anatomical receptors in the target skin. The extent to which this specificity is transmitted centrally in the fetus is not clear.

The ability of peripheral sensory afferents to accurately reflect stimulus intensity in terms of frequency of firing matures during fetal life and infancy. In the adult, very fine alterations in stimulus intensity can be accurately monitored by alterations in firing frequencies of low threshold receptors. Such receptors may fire at 500 Hz or more. Such fine tuning is not present in the fetus and develops gradually, partly with myelination of the axons but especially with the growth and innervation of peripheral end organs (*see* page 376). End organs, such as hair follicles and Meissner corpuscles act as amplifiers to improve the frequency response of primary afferents. Primary afferents that do not innervate specialized end organs and remain unmyelinated do not change their firing properties from fetal life, e.g. C-fiber nociceptors. They are polymodal receptors, responding to mechanical, ther-

mal and chemical noxious stimuli with a characteristic low frequency of firing and fairly slow onset and long after-discharge. As such, these properties appear to be fairly "primitive" and are established in the fetus with no further need for maturation. Aδ-nociceptors, which are mechanical and heat nociceptors with thinly myelinated axons, do change over the postnatal period but only in their frequency of firing rather than in a fundamental change in sensitivity.

## MATURATION OF CENTRAL SENSORY PROCESSING IN THE SPINAL CORD AND BRAINSTEM

Slow maturation of central synapses in somatosensory pathways restricts the transfer of information into the central nervous system in the newborn rat. The ability of neurons in the spinal cord to code information about the temporal nature of the stimulus is limited. In the rat, myelinated sensory afferents grow into the cord before birth and rapidly make effective synaptic connections. Although C-fibers grow into the spinal cord at birth, they do not make connections for at least a week after this; C-fiber terminals present in the spinal cord are capable of releasing neurotransmitter when stimulated, but cannot evoke action potentials in spinal cord neurons to allow information to be transmitted to higher centers. In this immature state, the release of neurotransmitters by C-fibers in response to noxious stimulation may raise the overall excitability of the spinal cord. This suggests that responses to noxious stimuli in the human infant, particularly those involving tissue damage and inflammation that activate C-fibers, may be present but more diffuse and less specific than in the adult. Substance P and other neuropeptides appear in small diameter C-fiber afferents before birth in the rat and can be released into the spinal cord on electrical stimulation. Levels of substance P do not reach those in the adult, however, until postnatal P15. In the neonatal rat, substance P binding sites are diffusely distributed at high density all over the spinal gray matter and only by P21 do they become organized into discrete areas in superficial dorsal horn and ventral nuclei. In the human spinal cord, substance P appears at about 9 weeks, gestation but levels remain low until birth. Enkephalin is one of the last peptides to appear at 14 weeks in the human cord and in the rat at birth. Opiate receptors also undergo considerable postnatal maturation. The appearance of functionally active κ receptors precedes the appearance of μ receptors, and both correspond to the onset of κ- and μ-mediated analgesia in rat spinal cord.

## THE DEVELOPMENT OF SOMATOTROPHIC MAPS

In the adult, inhibitory processes act to focus the somatotrophic map (*see* page 378), reducing the size of the receptive fields of spinal neurons and reducing the overlap of the receptive fields of neighboring cells. This inhibition is lacking in the fetus and neonate, thus receptive fields are larger and the map less focused. In the newborn the increased chance of activation of a spinal neuron by a peripheral stimulus is at the expense of accurate information on stimulus location.

## THE DEVELOPMENT OF ASCENDING AND DESCENDING PATHWAYS

Recent investigations have shown that thalamic afferents reach the cortical plate at birth in the rat. These terminals organize themselves into the adult form by P4. There is good evidence that the pattern of thalamocortical afferent projections and organization of cortical sensory cells is determined by the periphery. Experiments using the development of the highly organized sensory pathways for the vibrissae show that a blueprint for constructing an organized "barrel" of cortical cells related to a single vibrissa is initiated in the periphery. This is transferred to the cortex via a sequentially developing chain of afferent connections, through trigeminal axons, brainstem projections and thalamocortical axons through to the cortical cells. The physiological maturation of the receptive fields of cortical neurons takes some time. By P7 cells have a clear columnar organization but receptive fields are larger than in the adult, latencies very long and frequency following poor. The same processes almost certainly take place in human infants over months following the arrival of thalamic afferents in the cortex at 29 weeks.

A particularly important pathway in pain processing is the descending axons that travel down from brainstem control centers onto sensory cells of the spinal cord and trigeminal system. Such descending fibers form an important part of the endogenous pain control system in adults, whereby a noxious input is inhibited at spinal cord level and the resultant pain transmission to higher levels greatly reduced. These descending fibers are present from before birth in the rat but do not become effective until the second postnatal week. As a result, there is no endogenous dampening down of noxious inputs to the central nervous system in the infant rat. This may be partly due to the low levels of the transmitters 5-hydroxytryptamine and norepinephrine in these descending inhibitory axons at this time, but also due to immature interneurons in the spinal cord.

## PAIN RESPONSES IN INFANTS

From the above discussion it is not surprising that even premature human neonates display responses to painful stimuli. Measures of pain responses in infants use facial expression, body movement and cry. Of these, facial expression is the most reliable, characterized by a "cluster" of facial actions comprising brow bulging, eyes squeezed shut, deepening of the nasolateral furrow and open mouth. Physiological measures such as heart rate, blood pressure and palmar sweating have also been shown to be useful although the immaturity of the autonomic nervous system may confound assessment. Considering the wealth of evidence for such reactions to infant pain and the clear physiological evidence for functional pain pathways, it is interesting that infant pain was ignored and denied for so long. Many reports demonstrate the inherent inter- and intrasubject variability in response to such brief noxious stimuli such as that evoked by a heel lance. Such short, sharp pain may have little relation to pain in a clinical setting such as postoperatively or during intensive care procedures. Hormonal and metabolic responses provide very clear indication of pain in infants following surgery for ligation of a patent ductus arteriosus and support the use of fentanyl in both pain relief and reducing postoperative complications. Studies using sensory reflex thresholds after repeated (rather than single) heel lances show that a clear hyperalgesia or tenderness develops in the site of a local skin injury in premature infants.

## INJURY IN THE DEVELOPING SOMATOSENSORY SYSTEM

Peripheral sensory nerves are highly sensitive to injury up to P10 in the rat. Damage to peripheral axons will result in irreversible cell death in the dorsal root ganglion and permanent denervation to that body region. The development of central cells is dependent on primary afferent input; deafferentation of the neonatal rat spinal cord results in permanent growth retardation of spinal cord cells. Central adjustments are made to this peripheral loss. Dorsal roots from nearby intact sensory afferents sprout into the deafferented region resulting in a permanent distortion of the somatotopic map. This phenomenon is seen right up to the cortical level; reorganization of connections within the cortex after peripheral injury results in a disproportionately large amount of the sensory cortex connected to neighboring innervated skin at the expense of the denervated region. Excessive or noxious inputs may be equally powerful in altering the pattern of connections in the developing nervous system.

## SELECTED READING

Anand KJS, Sippell WG, Aynsley-Green A. Randomized trial of fentanyl anaesthesia in preterm babies undergoing surgery: effects on the stress response. *Lancet* 1987; i: 243.

Coleman JR, ed. *Development of sensory systems in mammals*. Chichester: John Wiley & Sons Inc., 1990.

Fitzgerald M. Development of pain mechanisms. *Br Med Bull* 1991; 47: 667.

Fitzgerald M. The developmental neurobiology of pain. In Bond MR, Charlton JE, Woolf CJ, eds. *Pain research and clinical management*. Amsterdam: Elsevier, 1991: 253.

Fitzgerald, M. Pain in infancy: some unanswered questions. *Pain Rev* 1995; **2**: 77.

Fitzgerald M, Shaw A, MacIntosh N. Postnatal development of the cutaneous flexor reflex: comparative study of pre-term infants and newborn rat pups. *Dev Med Child Neurol* 1988; **30**: 520.

Hanson MA, ed. *The fetal and neonatal brain-stem – developmental and clinical issues*. Cambridge: Cambridge University Press, 1991.

McGrath P. *Pain in children*. New York: The Guilford Press, 1990.

McGrath PJ, Unruh AM. Pain in children and adolescents. In Bond MR, Charlton JE, Woolf CJ, eds. *Pain research and clinical management*. Vol. 1. Amsterdam: Elsevier, 1987.

Rowe M, Willis WD, eds. *Development and plasticity of somatosensory brain maps*. New York: Alan Liss, 1985.

Schechter N, Berde C, Yaster M. *Pain management in children and adolescents*. Baltimore: Williams & Wilkins, 1993.

Willis WD, Coggeshall RE, eds. *Sensory mechanisms of the spinal cord*, 2nd edn. New York: Plenum Press, 1991.

# AUDITORY SYSTEM

# PHYSIOLOGY OF THE AUDITORY SYSTEM

The human auditory sense has remarkable performance characteristics. The ear is capable of detecting sounds ranging in frequency from approximately 20–20 000 Hz, over an intensity range of 0 dBSPL (decibels sound pressure level) to 140 dBSPL, the level at which pain and certain damage to the ear occurs. This dynamic range corresponds to a ratio of sound pressure of $1:10^7$ or a ten million-fold difference between the levels of the softest and loudest sounds that are perceivable. These upper limits, however, vary between subjects with feelings of tickle or uncomfortable loudness occurring at intensities between 100–120 dBSPL.

Auditory sensitivity (the auditory threshold) differs with frequency, showing a maximum between approximately 750–4000 Hz (Fig. 26.4). For humans, the ability to detect sounds in this range is particularly important as the acoustic energy in speech sounds is concentrated in the region of 250 to 4000 Hz.

The auditory system can be divided structurally and functionally into three components: the peripheral system, comprising the outer, middle and inner ears; the auditory nerve (VIIIth cranial or vestibulocochlear nerve); and the auditory centers in the brain. Briefly, the process of sound detection involves the transmission of sound through the middle ear to the inner ear where the mechanical vibrations are transduced into neural activity by the auditory sensory cells. The structural and functional features of these different components and their involvement in the transduction of sound are discussed briefly below.

## THE OUTER AND MIDDLE EAR

The outer ear consists of the pinna and the external auditory meatus (EAM), the latter being separated from the structures of the middle ear by the thin, conically-shaped tympanic membrane (Fig. 26.5). The tympanic membrane comprises three tissue layers: an

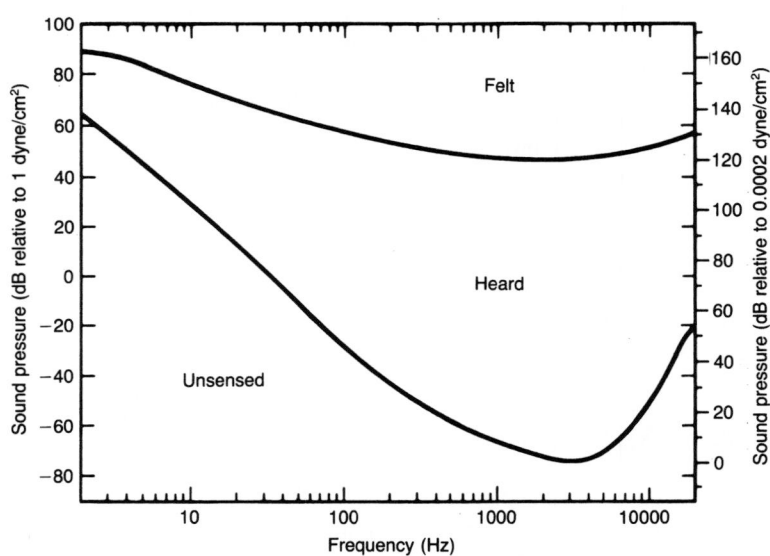

FIGURE 26.4 The range of human hearing. The threshold of hearing and the threshold of feeling (dB sound pressure level (dBSPL)) for sounds of different frequency. It shows a greater sensitivity to sounds in the range 750–6000 Hz.

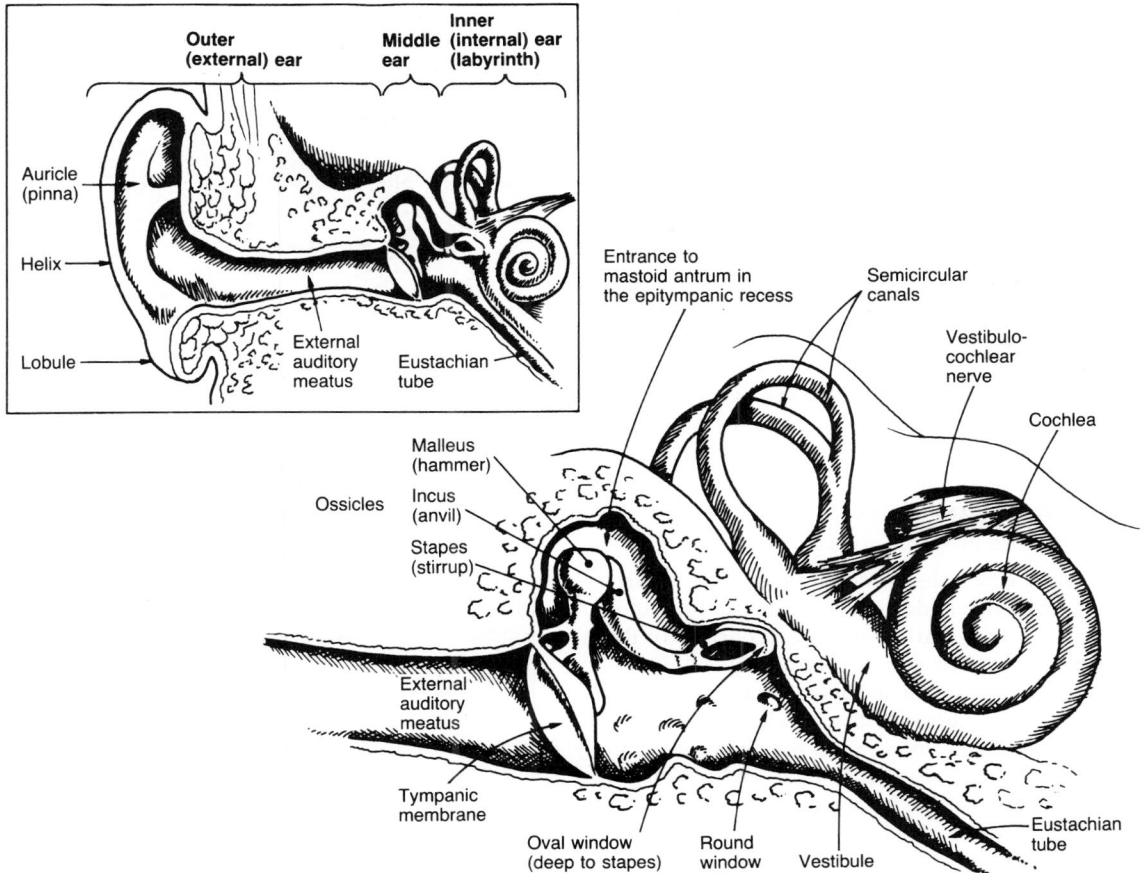

FIGURE 26.5 Schematic diagram showing the structure of the human ear. Note the three parts of the ear; the outer, middle and inner ear, the latter formed by the cochlea, semicircular canals and the vestibule. (From Marieb EN, ed. *Human anatomy and physiology*, 2nd edn. New York: Benjamin-Cummings, 1992; 522, with permission.)

epithelial layer continuous with the skin of the ear canal; an intervening fibrous layer; and a medial mucosal layer continuous with the mucosa of the middle ear. The middle ear is an air-filled space within the temporal bone approximately 2 mm deep, 4 mm wide and 6–8 mm high. The Eustachian tube descends anteriorly and inferiorly to open into the nasopharynx. This tube normally opens and closes during swallowing thus maintaining the middle ear pressure similar to ambient air pressure.

Within the middle ear lie the three bones of the ossicular chain, the malleus, incus and stapes, suspended in the middle ear cavity (tympanum) by ligaments. The long arm of the malleus is embedded in the fibrous layer of the tympanic membrane while the footplate of the stapes terminates in the oval window of the inner ear. A fast skeletal muscle, the stapedius muscle, is attached to the posterior crus of the stapes and upon contraction, initiated by activity of the motor division of the facial nerve, serves to stiffen the ossicular chain and reduce sound transmission to the inner ear.

Airborne sound is transmitted from the environment to the inner ear via the vibration of the tympanic membrane and the movement of the ossicular chain in the middle ear. The pinna and the ear canal have a profound effect on the spectral characteristics of the sound that finally impinges on the tympanic membrane. Ridges and hollows on the pinna can cause significant reflections of the sound and, acting as a 1/4 wave resonant cavity, the external auditory meatus serves to modify the incoming sound, enhancing frequencies in the 2–5 kHz region by up to 20 dBSPL. This modification of the sound, or the outer ear transfer function is direction dependent, which may be important for sound localization. For example, differences in the spectral characteristics of sounds depending on their location may provide important cues for localizing a sound in space.

In transferring airborne sound to the inner ear, via the ossicular chain, the middle ear also acts as an impedance transformer. This is essential to overcome the mismatch between the low acoustic impedance of the air at the tympanic membrane (approximately 400 N s/m$^2$) and the high acoustic impedance of the fluid-filled inner ear (approximately $1 \times 10^6$ N s/m$^2$). Without the transforming action of the middle ear, a significant proportion of the sound energy (approximately 99.7 per cent) would be reflected at the oval window resulting in a transmission loss of about 30–36 dB. The middle ear overcomes this impedance mismatch in three ways:

- The large ratio (35:1) of the effective area of the tympanic membrane to the smaller oval window results in a greatly increased sound pressure level at the oval window.
- 2  The lever ratio (1.15:1) of the manubrium of the malleus to the long arm of the incus results in an increased force and reduced velocity of sound at the oval window.
- The tympanic membrane lever ratio (4:1); the concave shape of the tympanic membrane acts as a lever allowing the sound-induced displacements in the periphery of the tympanic membrane to be transformed into smaller displacements with greater force at the malleus.

The extent to which the impedance mismatch is overcome by the human middle ear is still debatable, but it has been calculated that the transformer action of the middle ear reduces the energy loss to only 3–4 dB.

Transmission through the middle ear is also frequency-dependent. Because the middle ear contains mass (the ossicles), stiffness (air in the middle ear cavity, ligaments and ossicular joints) and resistance (cochlear fluids), it has a frequency response given by its transfer function. The transfer function of the human middle ear is complex but shows a major resonant frequency at 0.7–1.5 kHz with transmission declining at approximately 6 dB/octave above and below this frequency range. This characteristic of the middle ear, together with the frequency gain provided by the outer ear canal are the main determinants of the frequency range of human hearing.

## THE INNER EAR

The inner ear contains the auditory and vestibular sense organs. It comprises a series of cavities within the temporal bone, filled with fluid which form the vestibule and semicircular canals of the vestibular system, and the cochlea of the auditory system (Fig. 26.6).

The bony cochlea comprises a tube which spirals around a central core, the modiolus, containing the auditory nerve and cochlear vascular supply. This bony cochlea is filled with a fluid, perilymph, which has a composition similar to extracellular fluid being high in Na$^+$ (140 mM) and low in K$^+$ (5–10 mM). Within the perilymphatic cavity, lies a tube, termed the cochlear duct or membranous cochlea. The floor of this tube is the basilar membrane, a fibrous structure which extends from its medial attachment on a shelf of bone, the osseous spiral lamina which projects from the modiolus to the spiral ligament, a thickened region of the bony endosteum on the lateral wall of the cochlea. The cochlear duct is bounded on its medial

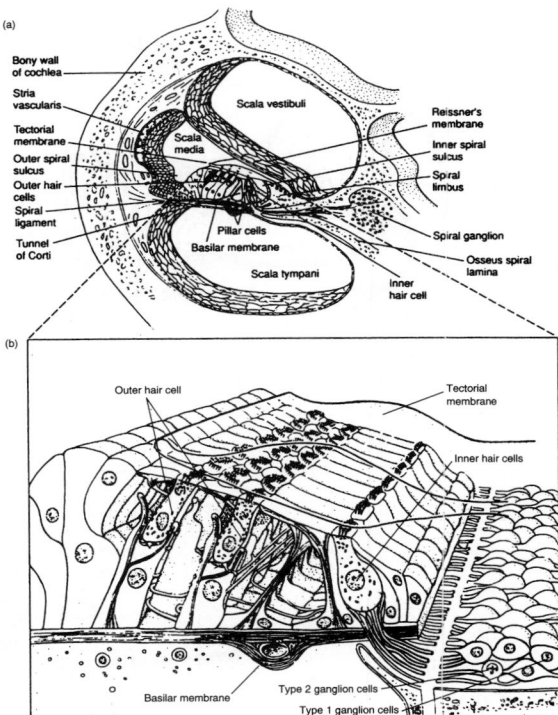

FIGURE 26.6 Schematic diagrams showing the structure of the cochlea (a) and the organ of Corti (b). (From Kandel ER, Schwartz JH, Jessell TM, eds. *Principles of neural science.* East Norwalk, CT: Appleton and Lange, 1991; 484, with permission.)

side by a thin, bicellular membrane with an intervening basal lamina, known as the Reissner membrane.

The cochlear duct is filled with endolymph, an extraordinary extracellular fluid as it has an ionic composition more similar to intracellular fluid, being high in K$^+$ (140–150 mM) and low in Na$^+$ (4 mM). This duct (also termed scala media) essentially divides the perilymphatic fluid space into two separate fluid compartments: the scala vestibuli above which communicates with the vestibule; and the scala tympani below which terminates at the round window. Perilymph is in communication with the subarachnoid space and cerebrospinal fluid (CSF) through the cochlear aqueduct. However, it is probably derived from cells lining the perilymphatic compartment rather than being an ultrafiltrate of CSF, as was originally thought. Endolymph is produced by a highly vascular and metabolic region of the lateral wall of the cochlear duct, known as the stria vascularis. The stria vascularis is also responsible for the production of a positive electrical potential in the endolymph, the endocochlear potential (+60 to +90 mV). While the mechanism of production of this unusual extracellular potential is not clear, it is likely to be derived from the special epithelial cells, the marginal cells on the luminal surface of the stria vascularis. Interestingly, marginal cells have a positive intracellular potential which is higher than endolymph. These cells have ion pumps on their basolateral margins moving $K^+$ into the cell which then diffuses into the endolymph. As will be discussed later, this endocochlear potential is essential to cochlear function as it provides the driving potential for the hair cells.

Within the cochlear duct lies the auditory sense organ, the organ of Corti containing the auditory sensory cells, the hair cells. There are approximately 20 000 hair cells, so-called because of the sensory hairs or stereocilia which project from their apical surface. There are two types of hair cell: the outer hair cells (OHC), cylindrically-shaped cells which comprise approximately 75 per cent of the hair cell population; and inner hair cells (IHC), more flask-shaped cells which comprise the remainder of the hair cell population. These cells are surrounded by a matrix of supporting cells which provide the integral structural support for the organ of Corti.

The organ of Corti receives both an afferent and efferent innervation. Afferent fibers of the VIIIth cranial nerve have their cell bodies in the spiral ganglion in the modiolus of the cochlea. There are two types; the myelinated Type I ganglion cells which constitute 90–95 per cent of the neural population and which innervate the IHC and project to the cochlear nucleus in the brainstem; and the smaller unmyelinated Type II ganglion cells, comprising the remaining 5–10 per cent of auditory nerve fibers and which innervate the OHC. These fibers also project to the cochlear nucleus in the brainstem although their target cells are less well defined. Each Type I afferent fibre only innervates one IHC, and each IHC receives up to 20 afferent fibers. On the other hand, the innervation of OHC is sparser with a single Type II fibre innervating up to 20 OHC.

In contrast to the afferent innervation patterns, descending nerves, which arise in the ipsilateral and contralateral superior olivary nucleus and pass to the cochlea in the olivocochlear bundle, innervate predominantly the OHC. There is an efferent innervation of the Type I afferent boutons but the IHC do not receive any efferent fibers directly.

Because of their extensive afferent innervation, IHC are clearly the major auditory sensory cells, detecting the acoustic stimulus and signaling the response to the central nervous system. Outer hair cells, however, are effector cells which have limited input to the central nervous system but appear to modify the mechanical activity of the organ of Corti and control the input to the IHC, particularly at low stimulus levels. The complex descending innervation of these cells implies that their activity is under considerable central control although the precise functions of these descending pathways are not yet understood.

## SOUND TRANSDUCTION

Displacement of the stapes in the oval window of the cochlea is transferred through the cochlear fluids and causes the displacement of the basilar membrane and organ of Corti. This mechanical stimulus is detected by the hair cell through the deflection of the stereocilia, either by the direct displacement of the fluids or a shearing force against the tectorial membrane, resulting in the generation of a receptor potential in the cell and release of neurotransmitter at its base.

The hair cell transduction process is mediated by the mechanical operation of mechanical-to-electrical transduction (MET) channels in the stereocilia. These channels are located at the tips of the individual stereocilia and are mechanically-gated by fine filamentous linkages (known as the "tip links") attaching the channel to an adjacent stereocilium. Displacement of stereocilia initiates a shearing action between the stereocilia pulling on the linkages and opening the channels. Transduction currents in the cells follow the stereocilia deflection by about 20–40 μs, supporting the view that transduction involves a direct mechanical rather than second messenger process. Such direct mechanical gating of an ion channel in the membrane presumably ensures that hair cells can detect rapid deflections, which is necessary for detection of high acoustic frequencies. Tension of the linkage can be altered to affect channel sensitivity, perhaps by contractile protein molecules (possibly myosin) attached to its intracellular portion.

It is now recognized that there are approximately 100 channels per hair cell which amounts to 1 per stereocilium each with a conductance of 3–5 nS. The MET channels are non-specific cation channels but the current is carried by $K^+$ because this is the predominant ion in endolymph. There is a very large potential difference across the apical pole of the hair cell produced by the high positive potential of the endolymph (+60–90 mV) and the resting membrane potential of the hair cell (−45 to 70 mV).

In the absence of any acoustic stimulus hair cells exhibit a standing current (the silent current) as a small proportion of the MET channels are maintained open. Hair cells are polarized such that displacement of the stereocilia laterally (away from the modiolus) causes depolarization and neurotransmitter release, whereas deflection medially results in hyperpolarization and a reduction in neurotransmitter release (Fig. 26.7). Deflection of stereocilia thus essentially modulates the current through the hair cell by increasing and decreasing the number of channels open. Movement of the stereocilia in an excitatory direction opens more channels and increases current flow through the hair cell. Displacement in the opposite direction closes the ion channels and decreases current flow.

A variety of neurotransmitters have been identified in the cochlea. There is strong evidence for glutamate as the afferent transmitter and acetylcholine and γ-amino butyric acid (GABA) as the efferent neurotransmitters.

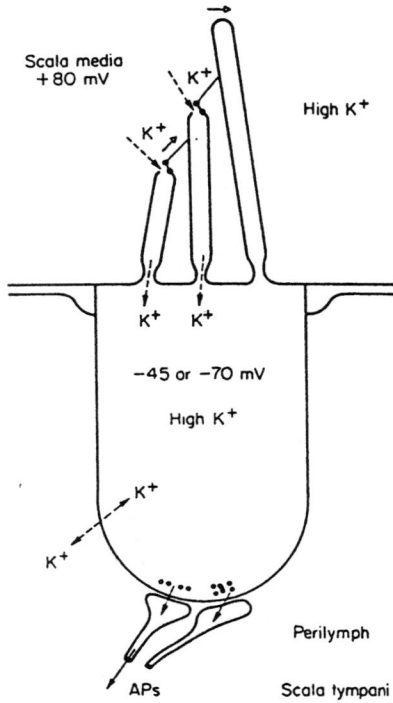

Scala media
+80 mV

High K⁺

K⁺
K⁺
K⁺

K⁺   K⁺

−45 or −70 mV

High K⁺

K⁺

K⁺

Perilymph

APs          Scala tympani

FIGURE 26.7 A schematic diagram of the cochlear hair cell showing the essential features of the sound transduction process. The transducer channels at the tips of the stereocilia are opened by deflection of the stereocilia, enabling potassium ions to flow into the cell from scala media. Intracellular depolarization leads to release of neurotransmitter at the base of the cell and activation of the auditory nerve. The resting potentials (−45 and −70 mV) are for inner and outer hair cells, respectively. APS, action potentials. (From Pickles JO. *An introduction to the physiology of hearing*, 2nd edn. London: Academic Press, 1988: 60, with permission.)

## COCHLEAR MECHANICS

The transfer of the stimulus to the hair cell and its mechanical stimulation is the field of cochlear mechanics, and is an important basis of the peripheral processing of sound. Movement of the stapes in the oval window in scala vestibuli initiates a traveling wave of displacement along the basilar membrane and organ of Corti. There is a gradient of decreasing stiffness and increasing mass of the basilar membrane and organ of Corti from the basal end to the apex of the cochlea. Because a stiffness-limited region will move before a mass-limited region, this wave travels from the base to apex of the cochlea, increasing in amplitude and decreasing in velocity as it reaches a region of resonance. There is a strong relationship between the position of maximum amplitude and the frequency of the stimulus, such that tones of increasing frequency stimulate regions progressively closer to the stapes. Thus the cochlea separates frequency by vibration patterns at different locations depending on the sound frequency. Tones of low frequency tend to stimulate towards the apex while higher frequency tones stimulate toward the base of the cochlea.

Each receptive region of the basilar membrane is mechanically tuned to a very narrow frequency band. At threshold the vibration pattern for a given frequency is probably localized to a region of approximately 500 μm and the basilar membrane displacement is approximately 0.3 nm producing a deflection of the stereocilia of about 0.02 degrees. The remarkable sensitivity and frequency selectivity of the basilar membrane is not related solely to the passive mechanical characteristics of these structures. This mechanical tuning and sensitivity is extremely labile showing considerable susceptibility to metabolic insult and damage from ototoxic drugs and hypoxia. Indeed there is now evidence for an intriguing active, metabolically labile mechanism in the cochlea which enhances the mechanical sensitivity and frequency response of the basilar membrane to overcome the viscous damping of the cochlear fluids. This is the so-called "cochlear amplifier" which operates to boost the motion of the basilar membrane but only at low intensities, becoming saturated above approximately 50 dBSPL.

The cochlear amplifier appears to involve the OHC. These cells are postulated to act as force generators, acting as part of a feedback loop to actively injecting mechanical energy into the traveling wave as it passes along the organ of Corti in a frequency specific manner. This serves to boost the mechanical displacement of the organ of Corti, thereby enhancing the sensitivity and frequency specificity of the mechanical response of the basilar membrane which is transmitted to the IHC. This process may involve rapid changes in OHC length in proportion to the transmembrane voltage; a process of reverse transduction. Support for such a process has been provided by the numerous observations that single isolated OHC mechanically oscillate at acoustic frequencies upon electrical stimulation, and that electrical stimulation of the cochlea can elicit a traveling wave along the organ of Corti. This latter finding implies an electrically-generated motile system within the organ of Corti. Additional support for an active process in the cochlea arises from the observation that the cochlea produces sounds (otoacoustic emissions) either spontaneously or when stimulated. These sounds which can be measured in the ear canal, are postulated to be caused by the biomechanical activity in the organ of Corti dependent on OHC function. Outer hair cell activity and length changes can be modulated by the application of acetylcholine, the putative efferent neurotransmitter in the cochlea. Cochlear efferents may thus modulate the activity of OHC and hence hearing sensitivity. It is interesting that the appearance of the motile response of OHC in the developing ear is generally associated with the onset of hearing.

The mechanisms of the OHC force generation are not clear. The changes in cell length are too fast for conventional contractile mechanisms involving actin–myosin interactions. Recently evidence has been provided for a unique "motor" protein within the plasma membrane of the OHC which undergoes conformational changes with electrical stimulation. These could be transmitted into length changes via a cytoskeletal network beneath the membrane.

## FREQUENCY ANALYSIS

The tonotopic organization of the cochlea is the basis of the "place theory" of frequency or pitch detection. This theory attributes the detection of individual frequency components to discrete places in the cochlea. Nerves innervating the cochlea project to auditory centers in the brain which are also tonotopically organized. Frequency detection, at least at frequencies below 1000 Hz may also be determined by the temporal characteristics of the stimulus. At these frequencies, individual afferent nerve fibers are firing in phase with each cycle of the stimulus. Thus frequency information may also be coded by the frequency of discharges in the auditory nerve. This phenomenon, referred to as "phase locking," diminishes with increasing stimulus frequency, mainly because of the refractoriness of the nerve and the frequency response of the sensory cell. It is thus likely that the temporal coding or "phase locking" is important in detection of low frequencies whereas the place information becomes more important for detection of frequencies greater than 1000 Hz.

## CENTRAL AUDITORY PATHWAYS

Ascending auditory pathways involve a number of auditory nuclei in the brain stem which then project via the thalamic nuclei to the auditory cortex (Fig. 26.8). The auditory nerve, with its cell bodies in the spiral ganglion within the cochlear modiolus, passes from the cochlea combining with the vestibular and facial nerve within the internal auditory meatus. Auditory nerve axons project to the cochlear nucleus in the brainstem medulla. This nucleus comprises two main divisions: the dorsal (DCN) and ventral (VCN) cochlear nucleus. The DCN sends projections mainly contralaterally via the stria of Held to the inferior colliculus (IC). Neurons from the VCN project ipsilaterally and contralaterally to the superior olivary complex which in turn sends projections to the inferior colliculi via the lateral lemniscus. Both inferior colliculi project via the medial geniculate bodies to the auditory cortex in the Sylvian fissure of the temporal lobe.

Considerable processing of auditory information occurs in the brainstem nuclei. Binaural interactions occur at the level of the superior olivary complex and inferior colliculus which are considered to underlie the ability to localize sound in space. Cells within these nuclei are sensitive to differences between the ears in

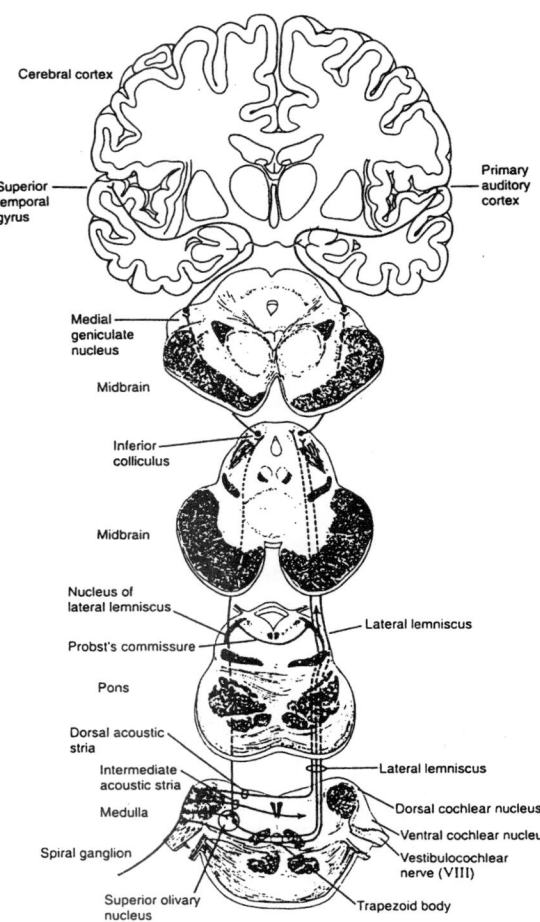

FIGURE 26.8 The central auditory pathways extending from the cochlear nucleus to the auditory cortex. (From Kandel ER, Schwartz JH, Jessell, TM, eds. *Principles of neural science*. East Norwalk, CT: Appleton and Lange, 1991; 495, with permission.)

time of arrival and intensity of sounds which are major cues used to localize a sound.

## ASSESSMENT OF HEARING ABILITY

Hearing and the integrity of the auditory system is assessed by behavioral and objective, physiological methods. There are numerous behavioral audiometric techniques which assist to define the hearing ability of an individual. These include standard pure tone and speech audiometry which enable the determination of auditory thresholds to pure tones and the performance of the system in the detection and understanding of complex speech signals. Pure tone auditory thresholds are conventionally displayed in an audiogram which graphs the hearing level, relative to a normally hearing population, against frequency.

Objective methods include tympanometry, auditory evoked response audiometry (ERA) and, more recently, otoacoustic emission measurement (OAE).

These techniques are important for determining the integrity of different parts of the auditory pathways, particularly for isolating the site of any lesion (e.g. an VIIIth nerve tumor) or for assessing hearing in special populations such as neonates, where behavioral techniques cannot be used with confidence. Tympanommetry is a technique which measures the mobility of the eardrum and can be used to determine the presence of middle ear disease, such as *otitis media with effusion* (OME). Evoked activity in the auditory pathways is recorded from scalp electrodes and can be used to assess the integrity of these pathways or to determine estimates of auditory threshold. The variety of auditory evoked electrical potentials recorded are classified according to their latencies. These are the short latency brainstem auditory evoked response (BAER) originating in the eighth nerve and brainstem auditory centers (Fig. 26.9), the middle latency response (MLR) and the late potentials, arising from the auditory cortex. The BAER is often used to diagnose deafness in neonates or young children and cor-

tical potentials to frequency specific stimuli can be used to estimate auditory thresholds in children and adults.

Otoacoustic emissions are sounds which are generated by the healthy inner ear. As described earlier energy is produced by the hair cells in the cochlea during the acoustic transduction process. This energy is emitted from the ear and can be measured as faint sound in the ear canal, using a miniature microphone. These emissions are absent if there is a hearing loss greater than 30–40 dBHL due to cochlear damage. Thus their presence or absence can be used clinically to assess ear function. There is considerable worldwide interest in using OAE measurement as a screening technique for deafness in neonates as it is a relatively quick and non-invasive test. A number of clinical centers around the world are testing this technique as a screening method for deafness.

## SELECTED READING

Ashmore JF. The cellular machinery of the cochlea. *Exp Physiol* 1994; **79**: 113.

Gelfand SA. *Hearing: an introduction to psychological and physiological acoustics*, 2nd edn. New York: Marcel Dekker Inc., 1990.

Hudspeth AJ. How the ear's works work. *Nature* 1989; **341**: 397.

Patuzzi R, Robertson D. Tuning in the mammalian cochlea. *Physiol Rev* 1988; **68**: 1009.

Pickles JO. *An introduction to the physiology of hearing*, 2nd edn. New York: Academic Press, 1988.

Santos-Sacchi J. Cochlear physiology. In Jahn AF, Santos-Sacchi J, eds. *Physiology of the ear*. New York: Raven Press, 1988: 271.

# DEVELOPMENT OF AUDITORY FUNCTION

The development of speech and language depend on adequate auditory function from a very early age. The auditory system is, however, vulnerable to adverse prenatal and postnatal influences and these factors can have long-term consequences on the behavior and function of the individual.

## DEVELOPMENT OF THE PERIPHERAL AUDITORY SYSTEM

The human pinna achieves an adult-like shape by 20 weeks' gestation and continues to grow until about the age of 10 years. The ear canal in the newborn infant is only slightly shorter than that of the adult, but it is narrower, more oval in shape, and because it is surrounded by only a thin layer of cartilage it is very soft. This feature has important implications for auditory assessment in neonates because false diagnosis of audi-

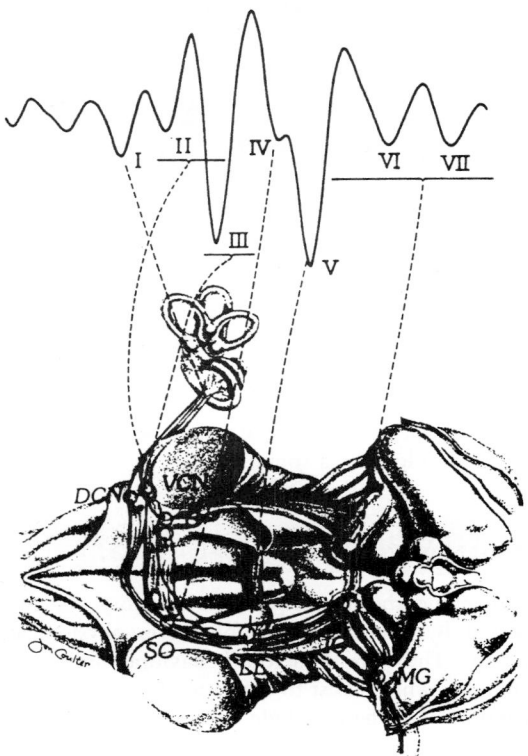

FIGURE 26.9 A recording of the auditory evoked brainstem response in a human. It shows the five distinct waves of the BAEP (I–VII) with their approximate origins in the auditory brainstem nuclei. Abbreviations: DCN, dorsal cochlear nucleus; IC, inferior colliculus; LL, lateral lemniscus; MG, medial geniculate nucleus; SO, superior olive; VCN, ventral cochlear nucleus. (From Jacobson JT. *The auditory brainstem response*. Boston: College-Hill Press, 1985: 27, with permission.)

tory deficit can arise from compression of the outer canal. During infancy, the canal wall and the cartilage thicken to produce a more rigid meatus and the position of the tympanic membrane changes relative to the wall of the canal.

The ossicles of the middle ear cavity and the tympanic ring (which supports the tympanic membrane) grow to adult size between 10–22 weeks' gestation. At this age the ossicles are cartilaginous, but ossification is completed by 32 weeks' gestation. The maturation of the tympanic ring is protracted and includes completion of the ring structure and growth of lateral processes which contribute to the outer canal. The middle ear muscles mature during the fourth month of gestation. The maturation of the tympanic membrane is completed by 6–7 months' gestation although slight changes in its orientation occur postnatally. Clearance of fluid from the middle ear cavity occurs during the last month of gestation but the cavity becomes enlarged postnatally. All of these changes contribute to the development of middle ear function and an increase in middle ear compliance in the neonatal period. The functional development of the middle ear is probably the determining factor in the development of auditory sensitivity.

## DEVELOPMENT OF THE COCHLEA

In the human the cochlea begins to develop at 3 weeks after conception. The organ of Corti differentiates between 10–25 weeks' gestation, by which time it has reached its adult form. The inner hair cells differentiate prior to the outer hair cells; this occurs first in the middle of the basal turn of the cochlea and then proceeds to the remaining part of the basal turn and towards the apex. The axons of cochlear ganglion cells enter the developing cochlea very early and innervate the hair cells in a basal to apical sequence soon after they differentiate. Synaptogenesis between the axons and the hair cells occurs at 15 weeks prior to formation of the stereocilia at 22 weeks. The growth and myelination of the cochlear axons occurs in the same basal to apical sequence, myelination having begun at 6 months' gestation.

## DEVELOPMENT OF THE AUDITORY PATHWAY

The central axons of the cochlear ganglion cells penetrate the medulla at 8 weeks' gestation, just after the differentiation of the brainstem auditory nuclei. The differentiation of the higher nuclei of the central auditory pathway occurs over the next few weeks and myelination of the central pathway begins in the brainstem at about 6 months' gestation and slightly later at higher levels of the pathway.

## ONSET OF FUNCTION

It has been estimated that the human cochlea has sufficient structural development at 18 weeks to provide auditory input. However, the onset of hearing in the human probably occurs at 26–27 weeks' gestation. It is at or soon after this age that acceleration of the heart rate, movements of the body and eye-blinks of the fetus *in utero* can be detected in response to loud sounds delivered to the maternal abdomen. These responses are best evoked using tones below 2 kHz; responses to tones of higher frequency appear to develop later. It is also at 27–28 weeks' post-conception that neurophysiological evidence of central neuronal activity in response to brief sounds can be recorded in premature infants.

## DEVELOPMENT OF AUDITORY SENSITIVITY

Several methods have been developed to assess the auditory sensitivity of newborn infants. Some of these methods rely on the behavioral response of the infant to a sound. While these techniques are relatively simple, the interpretation of data can be complicated by changes in the state of arousal of the infant. The most popular objective method for determining the auditory sensitivity of a neonate is to record brainstem auditory evoked responses (BAER) (*see* page 388). The BAER is unaffected by the state of arousal of the infant, is a highly reproducible response and is ideal for determining the auditory sensitivity of an infant. Thresholds for sounds of various types probably are higher in preterm neonates than in older infants and adults. Relatively few studies, however, have examined the development of auditory sensitivity in neonates in detail. Steps to facilitate the earliest possible detection of hearing deficit in infants must be considered relative to the time course of normal auditory development.

## FUNCTIONAL CAPACITY OF THE AUDITORY SYSTEM IN THE NEWBORN

### Sound localization

Provided certain procedural and stimulus conditions are observed, it is possible to demonstrate that infants of only a few days of age are capable of orienting their head toward an off-center sound such as that of a rattle. This ability is lost after about the first month postnatal, and re-emerges at 4–5 months. It has been proposed that the first period of orientation ability is associated with reflex mechanisms in the brainstem and that the subsequent decrease and re-emergence of orientation ability reflects changes in cortical control of the behavior. This possibility has received support from studies in which the precedence effect was used to examine the role of cortical processing in auditory localization in infants. Infants were only able to localize sounds under these conditions during the second phase of orientation responses to simpler sounds. Even though other explanations of this age-related change in behavior can be proposed, the data indicate that the use of orientation responses for testing auditory sensitivity in young infants must be made with care.

## Speech discrimination

It has been established for some time that infants can discriminate between speech sounds which differ in vowel content, voicing and initial or final consonants. Indeed, behavioral studies suggest that the processing of auditory signals by infants at 1 month of age may be adequate for speech perception and language comprehension. Recent research has also shown that infants as young as 2 days of age exhibit a preference for so-called child-directed speech ("motherese"), which is characterized in comparison to adult-directed speech by higher overall pitch, wider excursions in pitch, and slower tempo. Newborn infants also prefer their mother's voice to that of another female saying the same words and they can discriminate two languages when one of the languages is native to their culture. These abilities have been attributed to the capacity of the auditory system in the newborn to respond to psychophysical properties of speech sounds. Infants at this age also show left–right preferences for tones and syllables. These and other behavioral observations indicate that auditory function during the last stages of gestation and in the newborn period is well developed and exerts an important influence on behavior. The recording of averaged cortical potentials evoked by different speech sounds during development of newborn infants has also been undertaken and variations in the responses with electrode location, stimulus content, arousal and maturation have been reported.

## TESTS FOR AUDITORY DYSFUNCTION IN NEONATES

Whilst some preterm neonates can have BAER (see page 388) thresholds to click stimuli of 40 dB hearing level at 28–34 weeks' gestation, other preterm infants, who subsequently have normal hearing, have BAER thresholds at considerably higher levels (70–80 dB hearing level) at this early age. On the other hand, a small percentage of preterm infants who have thresholds at this level at this age can exhibit long-lasting moderate to profound hearing deficits. On the basis of longitudinal and cross-sectional studies of preterm and term infants using BAERs, it appears that those infants who achieve thresholds of 30 dB hearing level or better by term equivalent age can be expected to have normal auditory sensitivity. Furthermore, it has been recommended that any screening procedure for early detection of auditory deficits is best performed at or as close as possible to term equivalent age. Tests prior to this age can reveal thresholds that are elevated but which subsequently resolve over as little as 2 days, and the infants subsequently have normal hearing. It has also been recommended that any evidence of elevated auditory thresholds at term age be confirmed by follow-up testing using BAERs and behavioral methods.

Methods such as the auditory cradle or "crib-o-gram" and habituation techniques, which rely on infant movement following a sound, have been used and provide a relatively inexpensive first level screen for auditory dysfunction. Follow-up assessment of infants who have failed to reach criteria with these and other behavioral methods are essential.

The otoacoustic emission technique (see page 388) has been recommended for auditory screening but when a negative result is detected, hearing should also be assessed using BAERs.

## FACTORS THAT INFLUENCE AUDITORY DEVELOPMENT

Certain perinatal factors place an infant at risk of auditory dysfunction. The list of these factors most often includes: (1) family history of deafness, (2) maternal infection during pregnancy (toxoplasmosis, rubella, cytomegalovirus, or herpes simplex), (3) neonatal infection (especially meningitis), (4) congenital malformations and (5) complications commonly associated with preterm delivery. The possibility that auditory deficits in older infants may have followed exposure to loud sounds for extended periods should also not be overlooked.

The highest incidence of auditory deficit is consistently reported to be amongst infants who have survived very early preterm delivery, and in particular those preterm infants who have suffered severe hyperbilirubinemia and relatively long-term exposure to ototoxic antibiotics. However, just as one factor might be prominent for one infant, another infant with the same insult can have normal hearing. Thus the general view has been put that auditory deficits in preterm infants are associated with a complex interaction of factors which occurs during a less-than-optimal perinatal course.

Growth retarded neonates and experimental animals may show evidence of transient neural precocity. This may be reflected in the BAER as well as in classical neurological developmental examination but the relative advance is only transient. The factors underlying this dysmaturation are not understood.

## CHANGES IN THE AUDITORY PATHWAY WITH ABNORMAL DEVELOPMENT

The development of neuronal populations and the interconnection between neurons within the auditory system can be severely disrupted by abnormal development of the peripheral auditory system. For example, lesions of the cochlea at a very young age are associated with substantial loss of neurons in the cochlear nucleus and rearrangement of connections between neurons in these and other brainstem auditory nuclei. On the other hand, unilateral conductive hearing loss does not appear to affect the number of neurons in the cochlear nucleus on the affected side, but it does interfere with the organization of connections between the cochlear nuclei and the inferior colliculus. Several studies also indicate that activity within the auditory axons has an important influence on the transneuronal regulation of cell size in the auditory nuclei. These experimental data should be borne in mind when the development of the auditory system in neonates is under threat. It cannot be assumed that strategies for the alleviation of auditory deficits in newborn infants and young children will be operating through a normal auditory pathway.

## SELECTED READING

Edelman GM, Gall WE, Cowan WM, eds. *Auditory function. Neurobiological bases of hearing.* New York: John Wiley & Sons, 1988.
Moore DR. Anatomy and physiology of binaural hearing. *Audiology* 1991; 30: 25.
Muir DW, Clifton RK, Clarkson MG. The development of a motor action? The deficit in development could be in any human auditory localization response: a U-shaped function. *Can J Psychol* 1989; 43: 199.
Pettigrew AG, Edwards DA, Henderson-Smart DJ. Screening for auditory dysfunction in high risk neonates. *Early Hum Dev* 1986; 14: 109.
Pettigrew AG, Edwards DA, Henderson-Smart DJ. Perinatal risk factors in preterm infants with moderate-to-profound hearing deficits. *Med J Aust* 1988; 148: 174.
Romand R, ed. *Development of auditory and vestibular systems.* New York: Academic Press, 1983.
Stevens JC, Webb HD, Hutchinson J *et al.* Evaluation of click-evoked oto-acoustic emissions in the newborn. *Br J Audiol* 1991; 25: 11.

# VISUAL SYSTEM

# PHYSIOLOGY OF THE VISUAL SYSTEM

The visual system takes a two-dimensional image projected onto the retina and creates the perception of a three-dimensional world full of color, movement and precision over a wide range of ambient light conditions and level of contrast between an object of interest and its surroundings. This is accomplished by amplification of signals and parallel processing of multiple channels of sensory information. The visual system can be divided structurally and functionally into two components: (1) the peripheral system comprising the eye in which light entering the cornea is projected onto the retina and converted into electrical signals; (2) the neural pathways connecting the retinal ganglion cells to central structures where successive levels of signal processing take place.

## THE RETINA

### Photoreceptors

The retina, derived from the neural ectoderm, contains photoreceptors, cones and rods, which transduce light into electrical signals and layers of translucent neurons and neuronal processes. The photoreceptors lie adjacent to the pigment epithelium containing melanin which absorbs light and prevents reflection of any light not absorbed by the photoreceptors. The system of cones functions at day-time levels of light; it mediates color vision and responds with a high level of spatial and temporal resolution. The system of rods functions at low light levels at dusk or at night. Rods contain more light sensitive pigment than cones and neural connections within the retina amplify signals derived from the rods thereby enabling the rod system to detect light down to the level of a single photon. The photoreceptors consist of an outer segment containing densely packed visual pigment, an inner segment containing cell nuclei and mitochondria, and a synaptic terminal. In the outer segment visual pigment is attached to a large transmembrane $Na^+$ channel protein; the membrane is invaginated to form layers of discs oriented vertically within the retina. The discs are continuously recycled; new discs formed at the base of the outer segment migrate outward; discs are phagocytosed by the pigment epithelium as they are shed from the tip. In *retinitis pigmentosa* turnover of these discs is impaired.

### Phototransduction

In rods the visual pigment is rhodopsin which consists of a protein, opsin, embedded in the disc membrane and a non-covalently bound sterol, retinal. Retinal is a chromophone, a light-absorbing molecule. There are about $10^9$ rhodopsin molecules in each rod cell. The 11-*cis* isomer of retinal fits the opsin binding site. In the presence of light retinal converts to the all-*trans* configuration which no longer fits the opsin binding site and leads to the conformational change in opsin that triggers the next step in the transduction cascade (Fig. 26.10). After the linkage between opsin and retinal is hydrolyzed the all-*trans* retinal is transported to the pigment epithelium to be recycled to the 11-*cis* form. All-*trans* retinol (vitamin A), the precursor of 11-*cis* retinal in its conversion from all-*trans* retinal, cannot be synthesized by humans. Nutritional deficiency in vitamin A can lead to rod dysfunction and

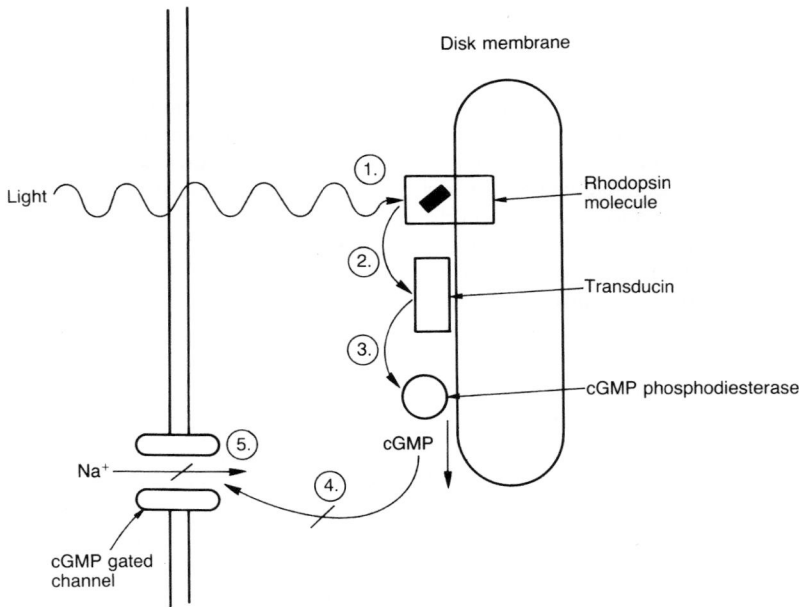

FIGURE 26.10 Phototransduction in rod photoreceptors. The outer segment of a rod is represented in the diagram. At (1) light passing through the outer segment membrane is absorbed by rhodopsin embedded in the disc membrane. In the presence of light 11-*cis* retinal attached to rhodopsin molecule converts to the all-*trans* configuration. (2) A G-protein, transducin, is induced to activate cGMP diphosphodiesterase which hydrolyzes cGMP to 5'GMP (3). The consequent fall in cGMP allows Na$^+$ channels in the outer segment membrane to close (4). Cessation of Na$^+$ flux (dark current) in the outer segment (5) results in hyperpolarization of the receptor.

night-blindness. Exposure to very bright light reduces rhodopsin concentrations and it takes about one hour for resynthesis. This phenomenon is termed photochemical adaptation. The electrical response is also reduced by bright light (neural adaptation). These two processes regulate the sensitivity of the rod to ambient light.

In cone cells the visual pigment is also composed of two parts – a protein termed cone opsin and the sterol, retinal. In primates there are three cone opsins which each react with 11-*cis* retinal to cause it to be differentially sensitive to the wavelength of light absorbed. The B (blue) pigment absorbs most strongly at 420 nm; the G (green) pigment absorbs at 531 nm; the R (red) pigment at 558 nm. Only G and R cones are present at the fovea. The most common causes of color blindness, defects of red or green cone pigments, are recessive mutations located on the X chromosome.

The transformation of rhodopsin or cone opsin by light activates cGMP (cyclic guanosine monophosphate) phosphodiesterase, an enzyme which hydrolyzes cGMP to 5'GMP, via a G-protein, transducin (*see* page 60). The consequent fall in cGMP results in a reduction in current flowing through cGMP-gated Na$^+$ channels in the outer segment membrane. Thus a remarkable feature of photoreceptor cells is that light inhibits and dark stimulates neurotransmitter release at the synaptic terminal. In addition to cGMP-gated channels, the photoreceptor membrane potential is also determined by K$^+$-selective, non-gated channels located in the inner segment. In darkness the photoreceptor membrane potential is maintained at about $-40$ mV. When light reduces cGMP and cGMP-gated channels close the cell is hyperpolarized to a potential between $-40$ and $-70$ mV depending on light intensity. Rapid adaptation to bright light is mediated by a release from Ca$^{2+}$-dependent inhibition of guanylate cyclase, the enzyme that synthesizes cGMP from GTP.

## Signal processing in the retina

The visual information, having being transduced into electrical signals by the photoreceptors, is then transferred to the ganglion cells via the bipolar cells. The ganglion cells in turn project to the brain. There are three layers of nuclei within the retina; the outer nuclear layer containing photoreceptors, the inner nuclear layer containing the interneurons, bipolar, horizontal and amacrine cells, and the ganglion cell layer (Fig. 26.11). The outer plexiform layer contains processes of receptor, bipolar and horizontal cells; the inner plexiform layer contains processes of the bipolar, amacrine and ganglion cells. Hence, some bipolar cells form a direct bridge between photoreceptors and gang-

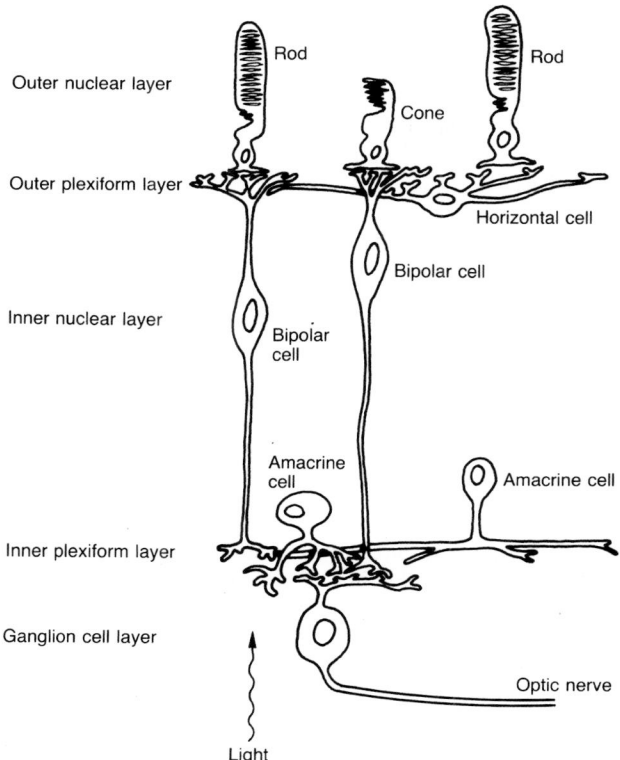

FIGURE 26.11 The retina has five classes of neurons which are arranged in the three nuclear layers of the retina. Photoreceptors, bipolar cells and horizontal cells make connections in the outer plexiform layer. Bipolar cells, amacrine cells and ganglion cells make connections in the inner plexiform layer. Bipolar cells form a vertical link between the outer plexiform layer and the ganglion cells layer. Bipolar, amacrine and horizontal cells form horizontal connections within the plexiform layers.

lion cells; horizontal cells are interneurons between distant photoreceptors and bipolar cells; amacrine cells are interneurons between distant bipolar cells and ganglion cells. Hyperpolarization of a cone in response to illumination reduces the rate of glutamate release at its synapse with a bipolar cell. There are two classes of bipolar cells differing in the type of ion channels gated by glutamate the neurotransmitter of the photoreceptor cell; they are either hyperpolarized by glutamate (by closing Na$^+$ channels), on-center cells, or depolarized by glutamate (by opening Na$^+$ channels), off-center cells. Each cone forms synapses with both types of bipolar cell. In turn bipolar cells synapse with either off-center or on-center ganglion cells.

Several subsets of ganglion cells connect to the same photoreceptors in parallel and serve different functions. In the primate M ganglion cells have large receptive fields and are sensitive to orientation; the more numerous P ganglion cells have small receptive fields and are responsive to the wavelength of incident light. The axons of both M and P ganglion cells are continuously active even in the dark; the rate of spontaneous activity is modulated by light reaching the receptive field of each cell. The receptive field is circular with a central region and a surrounding peripheral region.

Two classes of ganglion cells account for parallel output systems from the retina. On-center ganglion cells are excited by on-center bipolar cells to increase activity when light is incident at the central field region and decrease activity when light is incident at the surround. Off-center ganglion cells are excited by off-center bipolar cells and respond in a reciprocal manner such that their activity is highest immediately light ceases at the center field region. For both classes of cells activity is minimal when light is constant over the entire receptive field. G and R cones provide input to ganglion cells with the center-surround receptive field organization. Color opponent ganglion cells respond maximally to either a red center and more extensive green surround in their receptive field or conversely to a green center and red surround. Information from B cones is transmitted via co-extensive opponent ganglion cells which have uniform receptive field in which inputs from B cones antagonize combined inputs from R and G cones. This interaction between outputs of the three cone types underlies the phenomenon of color opponency (e.g. red and green combine to give the perception of yellow).

During dark adaptation to a moderate level, e.g. at dusk, rod signals are transmitted to adjacent cones via gap junctions and the receptive field characteristics of ganglion cells do not change. Dark adaptation to very dim light involves a loss of ganglion cell surround inhibition; gap junctions between cones and rods close, rod bipolar cells receive direct synaptic input from rods and connect to ganglion cells via amacrine cells.

A third class of ganglion cell that lacks center-surround field organization responds to overall luminance of their visual field and provides input to the pupillary reflex and via the retino-hypothalamic tract to the suprachiasmatic nucleus.

## CENTRAL VISUAL PATHWAYS

Ganglion cell axons are myelinated as they reach the optic disc and pass into the optic nerve. At the optic chiasm axons arising from nasal hemiretina, corresponding to the temporal hemifield, cross to the contralateral optic tract; axons arising in the temporal hemiretina, corresponding to the nasal hemifield, pass into the ipsilateral optic tract. The retina projects to three subcortical areas.

■ Ganglion cells that project to the pretectal area of the midbrain respond to overall retinal illumination. Pretectal cells project bilaterally to preganglionic parasympathetic neurons that innervate the ciliary ganglion subserving the pupillary light reflex (Fig. 26.12).
■ The superior colliculus receives visual information from the retina and visual cortex and projects to areas that control eye and head movements (*see* page 410).

■ The optic tracts project to the lateral geniculate nuclei of the thalamus in a manner that retains a visuotopic representation of the contralateral visual hemifield at each nucleus.

The fovea has proportionately the greatest representation in lateral geniculate nuclei. In primates there are six layers of cell bodies in the lateral geniculate nuclei; individual layers receiving input from one eye only (Fig. 26.13). The ventral layers of relatively large cells, magnocellular, receive input from M ganglion cells and are involved in achromatic vision. The dorsal layers, parvocellular, receive input from P ganglion cells and relay information about color as well as achromatic detail.

## PRIMARY VISUAL CORTEX (V1)

The lateral geniculate ganglia project to the primary visual cortex, V1, where there is further development in visual field receptive properties. V1 is distinguished by the presence of myelinated axons in layer 4 giving it a striate appearance. Axons from cells in the lateral geniculate terminate on spiny stellate cells (excitatory interneurons) in layer 4; M cells terminate in sublamina 4Cα; some P cells terminate in sublamina 4Cβ.

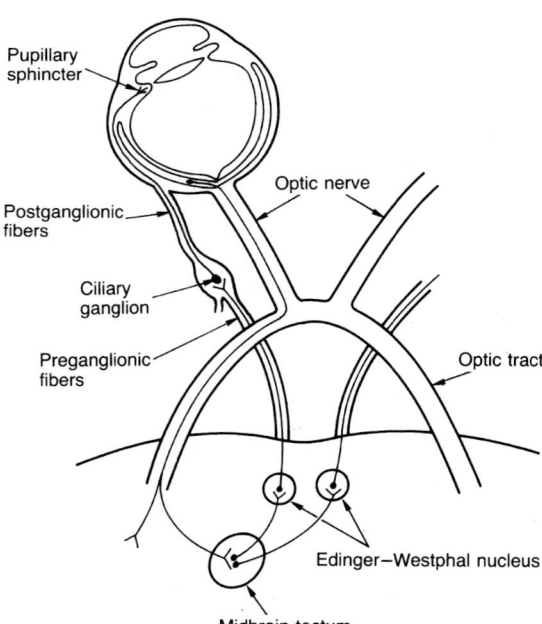

FIGURE 26.12 The pathway mediating pupil constriction to light. Light signals pass via the optic nerve to the midbrain tectum. In the tectum connections are made to the ipsilateral and contralateral Edinger-Westphal nuclei which send preganglionic fibers via the oculomotor nerve to the ciliary ganglion. Postganglionic fibers innervate smooth muscle fibers in the pupillary sphincter.

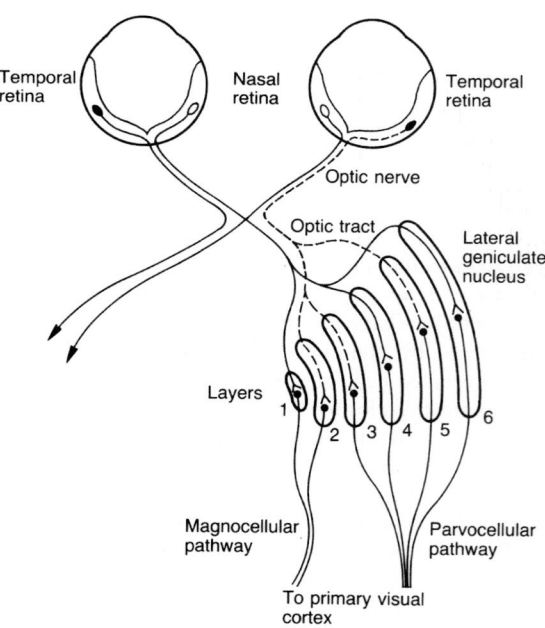

FIGURE 26.13 Central visual pathways. In the diagram the right hemiretina of each eye projects to the right lateral geniculate nucleus (LGN). The LGN consists of six layers: layers 1 and 2 are termed magnocellular layers; layers 3 to 6 are termed parvocellular layers. Three major pathways project from the LGN to the primary visual cortex, V1. One magnocellular, M, pathway subserves movement and gross features of the visual stimulus; one parvocellular pathway subserves fine details of the stimulus; the second parvocellular pathway subserves color perception.

Spiny stellate cells project to layers 4B, 2 and 3. Cells in layers 2 and 3 project to pyramidal cells (excitatory projection neurons) in layer 5 which in turn send axon collaterals to pyramidal cells in layer 6. Pyramidal cells in layer 6 send axon collaterals to smooth stellate cells in layer 4. Inhibitory smooth stellate cells modulate activity of spiny stellate cells in layer 4, completing an inhibitory feedback loop.

Cells in the interlaminar nucleus of the lateral geniculate terminate in layers 2 and 3 on groups of cells called blobs which are concerned with color vision. Inputs from single-opponent cells are combined on double-opponent cells within the blobs. These cells maintain an antagonistic center-surround receptive field organization but are even more sensitive to chromatic stimuli than the single-opponent cells. There are four classes of double-opponent cells. Cells of one class are excited by R cones in the center and inhibited in the surround, and respond in a reverse fashion to G cones, i.e. they respond maximally to a red object on a green background. Other classes of double-opponent cells respond maximally to a green spot on a red background, or blue spot on a yellow background, or a yellow spot on a blue background. This organization of cortical cells provides a mechanism for the psychological phenomenon of color opponency and helps explain color contrast and color constancy in which an object appears as the same color when the wavelength of ambient light changes.

In contrast the circular receptive fields of cells in the retina and thalamus cells in the visual cortex, except for blobs, respond to lines and bars. Simple cortical cells have rectangular "on" zone with a specific axis

of orientation flanked by a rectangular "off" zone. All axes of orientation and positions in the retina are represented in the cortex (Fig. 26.14). Complex cortical cells also have a critical axis of orientation but may also respond to movement across the receptive field and are sensitive to orientation over a wide range of retinal positions. The two distinct functional pathways, represented by M and C cells in the lateral geniculate, persist in V1. As in the somatosensory cortex (*see* page 378), V1 consists of vertical columns of cells. Each column contains cells with the same orientation axis. Adjacent columns correspond to a shift in axis of approximately 10°. Ocular dominance columns also alternate across V1; they are specific to each eye and function in binocular depth vision. "Hypercolumns," each occupying about 1 mm$^2$ of the cortex, combine columns from both eyes which correspond to lines of all orientations in one position of the visual field and include blobs.

Pyramidal cells from all layers except layer 4 project beyond V1; cells in layers 2 and 3 project to association cortex, e.g. area 18, and via the corpus callosum to the other side; cells in layer 4B project to the median temporal lobe; cells in layer 5 project to the superior colliculus, pons and pulvinar; cells in layer 6 project to the lateral geniculate and claustrum. The claustrum and pulvinar play a role in visual attention.

## OTHER VISUAL CORTICAL AREAS

In addition to V1 other areas of the occipital cortex contain retinotopic maps; V2 and V3 are in area 18; V3a, V4 and V5 are in area 19. Different features of the visual image are processed in each area, e.g. depth and motion in V5, color and orientation in V6.

The pathway from M ganglion cells to magnocellular neurons in the lateral geniculate to layers 4Cα, 4B and 6 in V1 and to V5 in the superior temporal gyrus, subserves movement perception and direction of eye movements towards a moving target; lesions in the superior temporal gyrus result in a selective deficit in movement perception (*movement agnosia*). The pathway from small P ganglion cells to parvocellular neurons in the lateral geniculate to layers 4Cβ, 2 and 3 in V1 and to V2, V4 and the inferior temporal cortex, subserves object recognition; lesions in the inferior temporal cortex result in deficits in the recognition of objects, e.g. in the recognition of faces (*prosopagnosia*). The pathway from P ganglion cells to parvocellular neurons in the lateral geniculate to blobs of layers 2 and 3 in V1 and to V2, V4 and the inferior temporal cortex subserve color vision; lesions in this pathway result in deficits in color perception (*achromatopsia*).

## VISUAL EVOKED POTENTIALS

The visual system, including central pathways and primary visual cortex, is often assessed by the technique

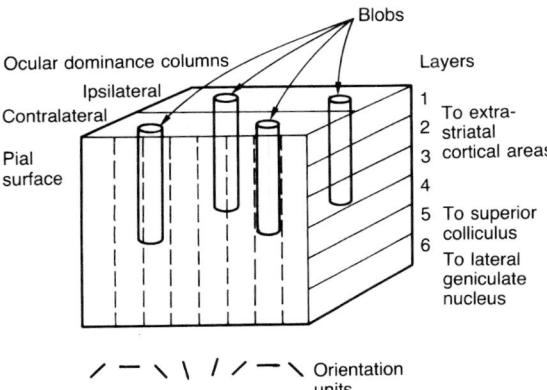

FIGURE 26.14 The primary visual cortex (V1) is organized into complex functional units called hypercolumns represented in the diagram by a cube. Each hypercolumn analyses a discrete area of the visual field including right and left ocular dominance column (receiving input from either the right or left eye), a complete set of orientation columns (representing 180 degrees of stimulus orientation) and several blobs which are involved in color vision. Layers 2 and 3 project to visual cortical areas outside V1; layer 5 sends fibers to the superior colliculus involved in eye movements; layer 6 projects back to the lateral geniculate nucleus.

of visual evoked potentials (VEP). An averaged electrical response is recorded from the occipital scalp (at approximately 100 ms in the adult) to a visual stimulus which may be presented to one or both eyes. An alternating checkerboard pattern, which may be varied in contrast and size, is most often used clinically although a variety of stimuli will produce a detectable response.

## SELECTED READING

Daw NW. The psychology and physiology of color vision. *Trends Neurosci* 1984; **7**: 330.
Hubel DH. *Eye, brain and vision.* New York: Scientific American Library, 1988.
Livingstone M, Hubel DH. Segregation of form, color, movement, and depth: Anatomy, physiology and perception. *Science* 1988; **240**: 740.
Nathans J. Molecular biology of visual pigments. *Ann Rev Neurosci* 1987; **10**: 187.
Ts'o DY, Frostig RD, Lieke EE *et al.* Functional organization of the primate visual cortex revealed by high resolution optical imaging. *Science* 1990; **249**: 417.

# THE RETINAL VASCULATURE

Retinal development, including neural components, supporting tissues and blood vessels, proceeds centrifugally from the optic disc towards the periphery of the eye. There are three vascular systems in the developing eye. The hyaloid vasculature which mainly nourishes the developing lens, undergoes atrophy during the last five months of gestation in the human fetus. The choroidal vasculature, on the outer surface of the retina, develops early and, by diffusion, nourishes the very immature sensory retina; the sensory retina itself remains avascular until later. In the sixteenth week of gestation, spindle-shaped cells, of mesenchymal origin, spread centrifugally from the optic disc towards the periphery of the eye. They create a primitive capillary net, which is subsequently differentiated into the definitive pattern of retinal arteries, veins and capillaries. The development of this retinal vasculature parallels the development of the photoreceptors and their increased oxygen demand. At 35 weeks the nasal retina becomes fully vascularized and at term the vascularization of the temporal retina is completed.

*Retinopathy of prematurity* (ROP) is a disease of the immature retinal vessels. Compared to *in utero*, the environment becomes relatively hyperoxic at birth. Oxygen then diffuses freely from the choroidal vasculature, that cannot constrict. The spindle-shaped cells become stressed by increased exposition of oxygen. They stop migrating peripherally and the retinal development is interrupted. The spindle cells synthesize angiogenic factors, that simulate the development of neovascularization at the boundary between vascularized and unvascularized retina. The boundary becomes

a shunt of blood. Later in the disease process, myofibroblasts invade the vitreous and contribute to contraction of the vitreous, which may result in traction and detachment of the retina.

## SELECTED READING

Flynn JT, Tasman W, *Retinopathy of prematurity*, New York: Springer-Verlag, 1992

# DEVELOPMENT OF VISUAL FUNCTION

The development of the visual system can be thought of as consisting of three overlapping and interacting facets:

■ Increasing sensitivity to different visual attributes such as contrast, detail, velocity of motion, orientation and slant resulting from developmental changes in the retina, central pathways and cortex;
■ Improvements in the eye movement control systems, linked in many instances to mechanisms responsible for selective attention;
■ Development of interpretive mechanisms to understand incoming information and initiate appropriate motor actions.

It is not always possible to separate these three facets in any observable overt visual behavior. For example, if a 9-month-old child learning to crawl falls down a step, is this because the child cannot detect and perceive depth changes, or because he can analyze disparity cues but cannot interpret them, or merely because he has poor integration between perceptual and motor actions?

## ASSESSMENT OF THE DEVELOPING VISUAL SYSTEM

A number of different techniques and methodologies have been developed to dissociate different sensory, perceptual, cognitive and motor operations. These can be broadly specified as behavioral, electrophysiological or photorefractive.

In behavioral assessment overt visual behavior is observed and measured. In "preferential looking" the ability to detect differences between two simultaneously presented displays is gauged from the child's preference for looking at one display rather than the other. Preferential looking has been used extensively to measure acuity. More complex visual and cognitive discriminations, e.g. between different textures, have been tested in infants using habituation/dishabituation paradigms. When the same pattern is presented repeatedly an infant's responsiveness (assessed either by looking time or measures of arousal) declines; the infant is said to be "habituated" to the pattern when a certain criterion or decrement in responsiveness is reached. When a novel pattern is presented and responsiveness increases the infant must have been able to detect a difference between the old and the new patterns; the infant is now "dishabituated." In electrophysiological assessment of visual function in the infant or child the visual evoked potential (VEP) to a reversed checkerboard pattern is often used (*see* page 395). "Designer" stimuli which may dissociate cortical from subcortical responses are described below. Recently a family of techniques has been devised for measuring the optics of the eyes in infants and young children; these are called photorefraction or videorefraction. The technique depends on measurement of a light reflex on the retina from a small flash source.

## THEORIES OF VISUAL DEVELOPMENT

Data obtained over the last 20 years using the above techniques have led to several theoretical models of visual development. The idea of "two visual systems" arose out of comparative studies of vision across different species. It was suggested that subcortical systems control orienting responses which define crudely "where" an object is located and trigger foveation to this location, while cortical mechanisms are used to define "what" is actually in the foveated area. Atkinson (1984) put forward a modified "two visual systems" model suggesting that the newborn visual system was "largely" subcortically controlled, with different cortical mechanisms starting to function at different times postnatally.

Anatomical and physiological findings in primates have allowed identification of populations of neurons specific for detection of certain visual attributes within two parallel visual pathways: (1) from M ganglion cells to magnocellular neurons in the lateral geniculate and the cortex, V1, subserving movement perception and some aspects of stereoscopic vision, and (2) from P ganglion cells to parvocellular neurons in the lateral geniculate and the cortex, V1, subserving detailed form vision and color (*see* page 394). It is possible to consider infant development in terms of onset of function in specific visual pathways and their cortical connections.

## THE DEVELOPMENT OF VISUAL FUNCTION

### Visual acuity and contrast sensitivity

The commonest clinical measure of visual function is that of visual acuity. Three functions can be defined:

- Detection acuity, the smallest object or line that can be detected;
- Resolution acuity, the finest detail that can be resolved, is often measured in infants and young

children with limited communication skills by means of preferential looking;
- Recognition acuity, the smallest letter stroke width to allow correct letter identification.

The Snellen test is universally used to measure adult visual acuity (expressed as a fraction of a standard adult ability to detect a stroke width equal to 1-minute arc). Modifications using letter matching in preschool children have been devised. Recognition acuity in adults is slightly lower for letters in a crowded array than for isolated single letters. This "crowding effect" is more marked in preschool children, *amblyopes* and some *dyslexics*.

Visual acuity specifies only how well the system handles fine detail. The quality of functional vision depends also on how well more coarse, but possibly fainter, patterns of light and dark can be detected, measured in the contrast sensitivity function. Grating patterns with sinusoidal luminance profiles are used, varying both spatial frequency (broadness of the stripes) and contrast (the intensity difference between the brightest and darkest points of the grating). In adults the contrast sensitivity function is approximately U-shaped, with lower sensitivity at both low and very high spatial frequencies. Resolution acuity represents the special point on this function where even a grating of 100 per cent contrast can only just be detected. There is very rapid development of both acuity and contrast sensitivity over the first 6 postnatal months (simulated in Fig. 26.15). This is followed by gradual increases in function up to adult levels for resolution acuity by 3–5 years and for recognition acuity of single letters by 5–6 years. Newborn acuity, measured at near distances, has been estimated at around the 30-minute arc.

Three processes, the differentiation of the fovea, myelination of the visual pathways, and increases in the number of synapses, which develop over the first year are likely to be limiting factors in the development of visual acuity and contrast sensitivity. In addition, optical refractive errors (in particular *astigmatism*) may be a major limiting factor in infants over 6 months of age.

### Orientation or slant

There is now general agreement that infants can discriminate between static grating patterns, differing in orientation or slant of the lines. A reliable steady state VEP can be elicited by a 90° change in orientation (OR–VEP). This is taken as evidence for orientation-selective mechanisms which are found in the visual cortex and not subcortically. At a rapid rate of alternation between the two orientations (e.g. eight reversals per second) the OR–VEP may be recorded in the second postnatal month. With slower alternations (e.g. three reversals per second), the median age for the response is 3 weeks. This rapid development in tem-

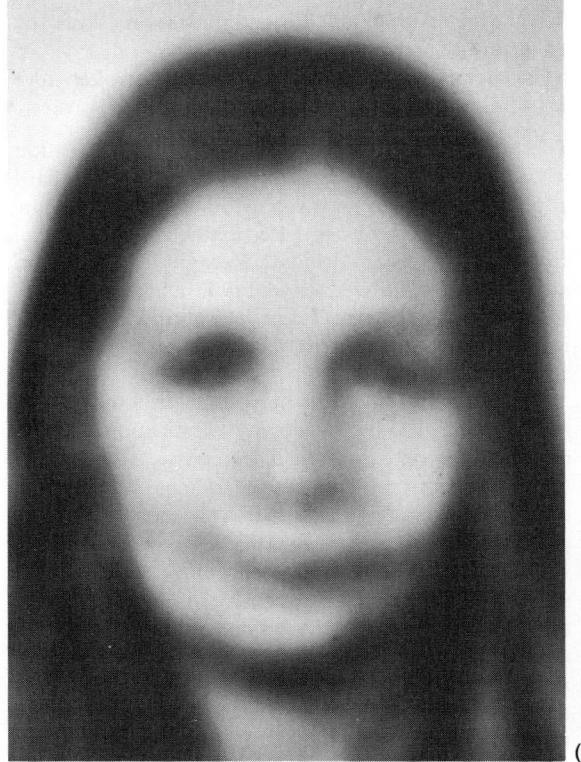

(a)

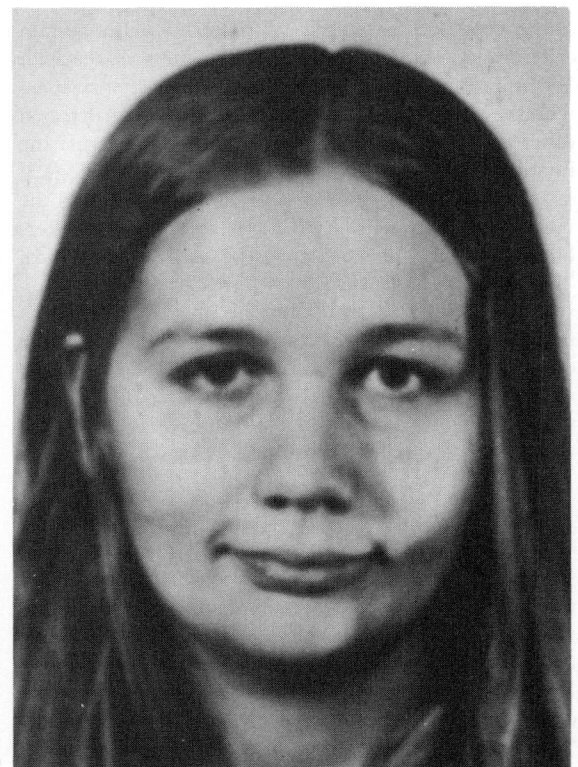

(b)

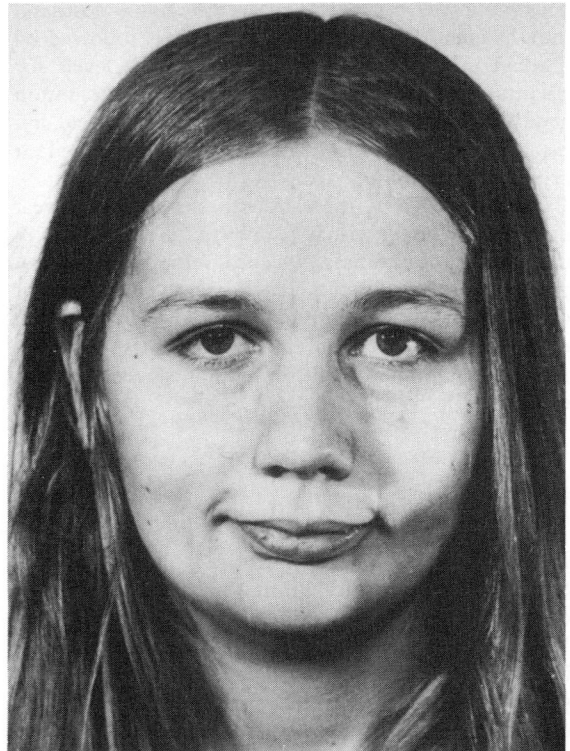

(c)

FIGURE 26.15 (a) Simulation, using experimental acuity values and an optical blur function, of the image a newborn would have of a face, viewed at 25 cm distance. (b) Similar simulation for 3-month infant. (c) Fully focused image seen by an adult.

poral sensitivity in the first month appears to be specific to the orientation response and not to non-orientational mechanisms.

## Directional motion

It is well established that young infants prefer moving to static visual displays. However, this in itself cannot be taken as evidence of the operation of true motion mechanisms. Any moving stimulus also produces a temporal modulation and it is well known that infants show a preference for full field flicker, i.e. temporal modulation without coherent motion. In general, true motion detectors are in evidence if a differential response to different directions of motion can be demonstrated. To measure such mechanisms "designer" stimuli are used, consisting of two-dimensional random dot displays, which can have a particular direction of motion without the confounding presence of any dominant orientation component. In a similar way to the OR–VEP, a VEP can thus be generated to a change in the direction of motion of a set of random dots. The first significant motion VEP for a velocity of five degrees per second appears at around 2 months of age, with onset for higher velocities occurring later. Parallel behavioral studies show once again that the velocity is a critical determinant in obtaining discrimination of relative motion at different ages.

As discussed previously, some discrimination of orientations is possible at birth and it seems strange that information about direction of movement should not also be a built-in capability of the newborn. Indeed the newborn does have a crude directional system already operating as is evidenced by the optokinetic system. Optokinetic nystagmus (OKN) is a largely subcortical stabilizing mechanism which is present in the visual system of virtually every species. Thus it seems that the infant has at least two potential "where" systems – the OKN mechanism (operating maximally when the whole visual field is moving in a uniform direction) and a cortically controlled system (to fixate and smoothly track a single object in the field of view). This later cortical system presumably operates within the magnocellular pathway (*see* page 394) and in developmental terms becomes functional later than the subcortical system.

## Binocularity

As signals from the two eyes first interact at the cortex, any response dependent on detection of binocular correlation or disparity must be dependent on the operation of cortical rather than subcortical mechanisms. Such responses are first seen on average around 3–4 months post-term with adult values in stereoacuity being reached by 4–5 years, or possibly a little earlier. These studies and models indicate that the onset of functioning of cortical binocular mechanisms is post-

natal and such mechanisms cannot be used in any depth or distance judgements involved in spatial localization made prior to 3 months of age. The magnocellular pathway is thought to be the predominant location of disparity-selective neurons.

## Differential development of magnocellular and parvocellular pathways

The findings on development of three types of cortical detectors have been considered above. Each type is specific for coding information concerning a particular spatial attribute: orientation (necessary for shape analysis), directional movement (for analyzing an object's trajectory), and correlation/disparity detection (for judging the object's relative depth or distance from other objects). Development of sensitivity to these attributes takes place postnatally and must depend on cortical, rather than subcortical, analysis.

Infants show sensitivity to changes of orientation before they show differential responses to the direction of movement and before they detect disparity change. Although not discussed here, infants in the first few weeks after birth show relatively sophisticated ability to detect differences based on color alone, using isoluminant displays. The above data suggest that certain parts of the parvocellular system become functional slightly before parts of the magnocellular system.

## Development of eye movement systems and attentional control mechanisms

Many eye movement control systems are subcortical. However, effective oculomotor behavior requires not only selection of a fixation target but also disengagement of attention from one object to switch to another. These abilities, involving cortical control of subcortical circuitry, show striking improvements in the first few postnatal months. The newborn has difficulty disengaging fixation from a continuously present central target to a second one in the peripheral field. This "sticky" fixation can be likened to patients with bilateral parietal damage (*Balint syndrome*). Difficulties in shifting attention, detected by photorefraction techniques, show that the newborn change their focus for targets over a fairly narrow near range (60–90 cm). However, by 6 months this ability is almost adultlike.

## Changes in refraction with age, abnormal refractions and links to strabismus

Statements about refraction and refractive errors usually refer to the focusing power of the eye when accommodation is completely relaxed, for instance by a cycloplegic drug. Where the eyes are focused in normal vision depends on whether the eyes are *myopic*, *emmetropic* or *hyperopic* when relaxed, and on the degree of active accommodation at that instance. Two different refractive states are seen in the newborn depending on whether cycloplegia is used or not; the average cycloplegic refraction is slightly hyperopic while the newborn tends to accommodate freely myopically. Very few marked spherical myopic cycloplegic refractions are seen in the first few years of life, although there is a high incidence of both *myopic* and *hyperopic astigmatisms* and *spherical hyperopia*. These errors tend to reduce in most infants by 2 years of age. Any marked error persisting beyond 2 years may lead to *amblyopia*.

Marked hyperopia in the first year of life is predictive for strabismus and amblyopia in the preschool years. Successful prevention of strabismus and amblyopia may be achieved by spectacle correction for refractive errors in infancy. Disruption of normal vision in one eye early in life can seriously disrupt development of binocular vision. The resulting amblyopia means that this eye cannot perceive forms and shapes normally. Misalignment of the two eyes (*strabismus*) usually results in the visual cortex not encoding the information from the deviating eye (suppression). If a strabismus is present early in life and left untreated for years, late surgery will be largely cosmetic with little vision recovered. Very few squints are manifest at birth, although the newborn can be intermittently strabismic for several months. It is possible that some infants develop strabismus because of a congenital lack of potential binocularity; e.g. albinos lack the uncrossed visual pathways so information from the two eyes is not combined in the cortex. Others develop normal disparity detection at four months postnatally, but lose it as the result of a developing strabismus. Early surgery is thought more likely to restore normal binocular development, although even with early treatment good stereoacuity is rarely achieved.

Here visual development has been considered largely in isolation from other developing systems. However, sensory, perceptual, cognitive, and social development is heavily linked. It may be that delays in the development of one visual mechanism affect not only other visual circuitry, but also other integrative systems cross-modally. It may be that there are often delays common to all brain mechanisms in a single individual. As yet there is debate about whether these relationships are correlations or causations.

## SELECTED READING

Atkinson J. Human visual development over the first six months of life: a review and a hypothesis. *Hum Neurobiol* 1984; 3: 61.

Atkinson J. Assessment of vision in infants and young children. In Harel S, Anastasiow NJ, eds. *The at-risk infant: psycho/socio/medical aspects.* Baltimore: Paul H Brookes Publishing Co. Inc., 1985.

Atkinson J. Infant vision screening: prediction and prevention of strabismus and amblyopia from refractive screening in the Cambridge photorefraction program. In Simons K, ed. *Infant vision: basic and clinical research committee on vision.* Commission on Behavioral and Social Sciences and Education, National Research Council. New York: Oxford University Press, in press.

# ODOR PERCEPTION AND DEVELOPMENT OF RESPONSES TO OLFACTORY CUES

Receptors for smell and taste use mechanisms for transduction that are similar to the other sensory systems. However, they are phylogenetically primitive sensibilities, e.g. the central pathway for smell projects initially to the paleocortex. The ability to distinguish thousands of different odors and flavors is achieved through the action of specific receptors.

## ODOR PERCEPTION

### Odor receptors

In humans the olfactory epithelium covers a 5-cm$^2$ area of the turbinate cartilage high in the nasal cavity; it contains receptor, supporting and basal cells. The receptor cell has a short process which extends to the mucosal surface and ends in an expanded knob from which cilia protrude into the surface layer of mucus. Olfactory binding protein secreted by the lateral nasal gland is thought to trap odorants and concentrate them at the receptor sites. Receptor transduction in the olfactory epithelium has many similarities to phototransduction in the retina (*see* page 391). The cilia are the primary sites of signal transduction. The odor receptors belong to the G-protein-linked receptor family which includes rhodopsin and a number of neurotransmitter receptors. The odor receptors show marked sequence diversity within the transmembrane segments III, IV and V; it is this diversity that indicates a multigene family with at least 100, and possibly up to 2000, members. Blocks of non-conserved residues on the receptor molecule probably represent sites of contact with odorous ligands. Each member of the receptor family recognizes only one or a small family of odorants. The binding of an odorant opens a cation channel selective for Na$^+$ which is gated by second messengers, cAMP and cGMP.

### Central pathways

The central extensions of the receptor cells are unmyelinated axons which form bundles and pass from the nasal cavity through the cribriform plate and end in specialized synapses within the paired olfactory bulbs called glomeruli. Exposure of an awake rat to a specific odor elicits a distinct pattern of 2-dexoyglucose on the glomerular layer of the bulb. The domain of highest uptake for a given odor is reproducible from animal to animal; it characteristically overlaps those for other odors but is distinct from them. The extent of activity varies with odor concentration. Thus the first synaptic relay in the olfactory pathway abstracts a "molecular image" analogous to the visual image at the earliest stage of visual processing. Processing at the level of the glomeruli "microcircuits" involves synaptic connections between sets of mitral, tufted and periglomeruli cell dendrites. They have several functions, e.g. intraglomerular inhibitory interactions may sharpen the discrimination of dissimilar inputs; interglomerular excitatory interactions may bind together activity of glomeruli receiving similar inputs.

Axons of large mitral and small tufted cells in the olfactory bulbs project via the olfactory tract to the anterior olfactory nucleus, the olfactory tubercle, the pyriform cortex, the cortical nucleus of the amygdala, and the entorhinal area which projects to the hippocampus. The olfactory tubercle projects to the medial dorsal nucleus of the thalamus, which in turn projects to the orbitofrontal cortex, the area involved in the conscious perception of smell. Pathways to the limbic system (amygdala and hippocampus) mediate the affective response to smells.

## DEVELOPMENT OF ODOR PERCEPTION

The sense of smell is functional at birth, possibly even *in utero*. Recent research indicates that the newborn infant is especially sensitive to odors, and that such cues exert an important influence on neonatal behavior.

## Prenatal development

Olfactory receptors, as well as receptors of the anatomically distinct vomeronasal and trigeminal systems, are sufficiently mature to respond to chemical stimuli by the third trimester of gestation. Epithelial plugs blocking the nostrils of the fetus resolve at 4–6 months post-conception. Odorous substances in the amniotic fluid may then come into contact with nasal chemoreceptors as that fluid is inhaled by the fetus. Odors may also gain access to fetal olfactory receptors by diffusion from nasal blood vessels. Clear behavioral responses to strong odorants have been reported in preterm infants born at 29 weeks' gestation. At this stage of prenatal development, olfactory marker protein, considered to indicate olfactory neuron maturity, first becomes evident. It has not been determined whether human fetuses are capable of perceiving odors in their uterine environment. It has been demon-

strated in laboratory rodents that prenatal exposure to specific odorants influences subsequent long-term responses to those same scents after birth. A similar process could account for the newborn human infant's attraction to the odor of amniotic fluid.

## Postnatal responsiveness to odors

Healthy, full-term neonates respond to a wide range of olfactory stimuli, including food odors, artificial odorants, and natural scents emanating from their mother. Physiological and behavioral responses to odors, e.g. changes in respiratory rate and facial expressions, body movements, directional orientation, have been described during the first few days following birth. Repeated presentations of the same odorant under the infant's nostrils results in reduced responsiveness, habituation. Infants develop learned preferences for artifical odors that are associated with positive reinforcement, e.g. body stroking, or even as a function of mere exposure. Thus, infants less than 2 days old oriented preferentially toward an odor that had been present in their nursery bassinet for the preceding 24 hours, rather than in the direction of a completely novel scent. Similar exposure treatments restricted to the first 1–2 days postpartum resulted in specific olfactory preferences that were still evident 2 weeks after the odor exposure was discontinued.

## ATTRACTION TO BREAST ODORS

Breast odors produced by lactating women appear to be highly salient for neonates. The nipple and areola are rich sources of substances that could serve as olfactory signals, e.g. milk, colostrum, and secretions of densely concentrated sebaceous and apocrine glands. Diffusion of odorous molecules may be further enhanced by the elevated surface temperature of the areola region. In a series of two-choice odor-preference tests, 2-week-old bottle-fed babies oriented preferentially to an odorized breast pad from a nursing woman when paired with either that same woman's axillary pad or a breast pad from a non-parturient female. Similar positive responses to breast odors from unfamiliar lactating women were displayed by infants of this same age that had been nursed by their own mother since birth, indicating that such cues may function as general attractants for neonates. An additional sample of exclusively bottle-fed infants spent more time turned toward odors emanating from the breast of an unfamiliar lactating woman than to the scent of their own familiar formula. These latter babies thus preferred an odor to which they had no obvious postnatal exposure over an odor that they had encountered repeatedly in the context of feeding, which suggests that the observed preferences were either unlearned, i.e. genetically determined, or learned prior to birth.

## RECOGNITION OF THE MOTHER'S UNIQUE ODOR SIGNATURE

There is considerable evidence that members of our own species have distinct individual odors, i.e. olfactory signatures. In the initial experiment demonstrating that infants recognize their own mother's odor, breast pads from the nursing mother and an unfamiliar lactating woman were suspended along either side of each subject baby's face. Significantly more 6-day-old breast-fed infants turned preferentially in the direction of their own mother's odor pad rather than toward an alien breast odor. Production of recognizable maternal signatures is not restricted to the breast region alone. Breast-fed infants have also been reported to orient discriminatively toward their mother's axillary odor when paired with axillary odors from either a strange lactating woman or a non-parturient female. Unlike breast-fed babies, formula-fed infants of the same age show no evidence of recognizing their own mother's axillary scent. The observed difference between breast versus bottle-fed babies is most likely a function of their differential familiarity with the characteristic odor of their mother.

## OLFACTORY FUNCTION IN NEUROLOGICAL DISORDERS

Neurological screening procedures for newborn babies typically ignore olfactory functioning. However, assessment of the integrity of this sensory modality could have considerable diagnostic value. Failure to respond to salient odors might be a reflection of pathological conditions ranging from nasal obstructions and infections to genetic and central nervous systems anomalies. Congential deficits are associated with *bulbar agenesis*, *trisomy* -13, diabetic pregnancies, *Kallmann syndrome*, and other developmental disorders.

## SELECTED READING

Beuchamp GK, Cowart BJ, Schmidt HJ. Development of chemosensory sensitivity and preference. In Getchell TV, Doty RL, Bartoshuk LM, Snow JB, eds. *Smell and taste in health and disease*. New York: Raven Press, 1991: 405.

Brand JG, Teeter JH, Cagan RH, Kare MR, eds. *Chemical senses, vol. 1: Receptor events and transduction in taste and olfaction*. New York: Marcel Dekker, 1989.

Chuah MI, Farbman AI. Developmental anatomy of the olfactory system. In Doty RL, ed. *Handbook of olfaction and gustation*. New York: Marcel Dekker, 1995: 147.

Porter RH, Schaal B. Olfaction and development of social preferences in neonatal organisms. In Doty RL, ed. *Handbook of olfaction and gustation*. New York: Marcel Dekker, 1995: 299.

Shepherd GM, Firestein S. Toward a pharmacology of odor receptors and the processing of odor images. *J Steroid Biochem Molec Biol* 1991: 39: 583.

Varendi H, Porter RH, Winberg J. Does the newborn baby find the nipple by smell? *Lancet* 1994; 344: 989.

# 27

# Motor Systems

## PHYSIOLOGY OF MOTOR SYSTEMS

The cerebral cortex, brainstem and spinal cord form a hierarchy of structures that subserve motor function (see Fig. 27.1). The spinal cord has the capacity to generate complex patterns of activity that make up reflexes and rhythmic motor patterns. Motor areas of the cortex and descending systems of the brainstem both project in parallel to the spinal cord. Each level receives independent sensory input from the periphery. The basal ganglia and cerebellum modulate cortical and brainstem activity. Like the sensory system, those areas involved in control of movement are organized somatotopically.

## SPINAL CORD

### Motorneurons

Cell bodies of α-motorneurons that innervate a single muscle cluster in a longitudinal column that extends over up to four spinal segments. Motorneurons innervating the muscles of the neck and back are grouped in the medial part of the ventral horn where local interneurons project bilaterally. At cervical and lumbosa-

cral segments, neurons sited laterally innervate proximal muscles of the shoulder and pelvis, and those sited more laterally innervate distal limb muscles. In these lateral areas local interneurons project only ipsilaterally.

### Muscle afferents

Muscle spindles and Golgi organs are structures distributed extensively throughout skeletal muscles. They signal the state of the muscle, in terms of length and tension, to all levels of the motor system. There are two types of sensory endings in muscle spindles; primary endings which discharge at a high rate during the dynamic phase of muscle contraction, and secondary endings which increase their discharge rate slowly at the onset of muscle contraction. Primary endings subserve velocity sensitivity during both active muscle shortening and passive lengthening and respond transiently to brief taps or vibration of the muscle. The sensitivity of muscle spindles to the length of a muscle is continuously modified by segmental and suprasegmental mechanisms via the γ-efferent system which innervates intrafusal fibers. Sensitivity to changes in muscle length is retained during muscle contraction by α–γ-coactivation. Two classes of γ-efferents influ-

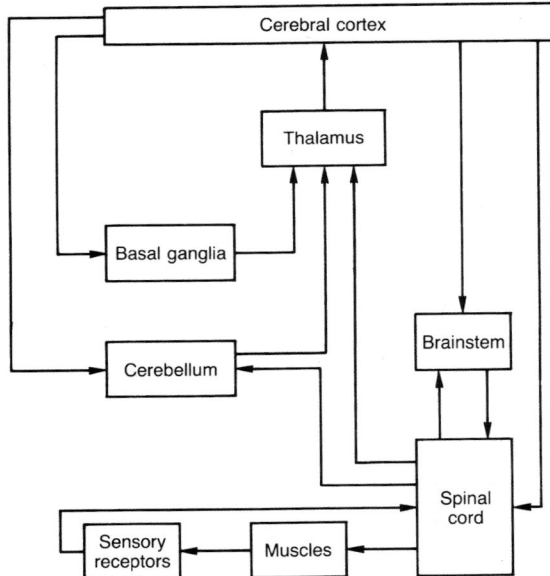

FIGURE 27.1 A scheme of the motor system with functional units that are connected both hierarchically and in parallel. The motor cortex projects directly to the spinal cord (corticospinal tract) and brainstem (corticobulbar tract) and indirectly to the spinal cord. Two subcortical systems located in the basal ganglia and cerebellum modify activity of the motor cortex. The cerebellum, brainstem and thalamus receive direct input from the spinal cord to monitor somatosensory feedback from movement. Sensory feedback reaches the cortex via the thalamus.

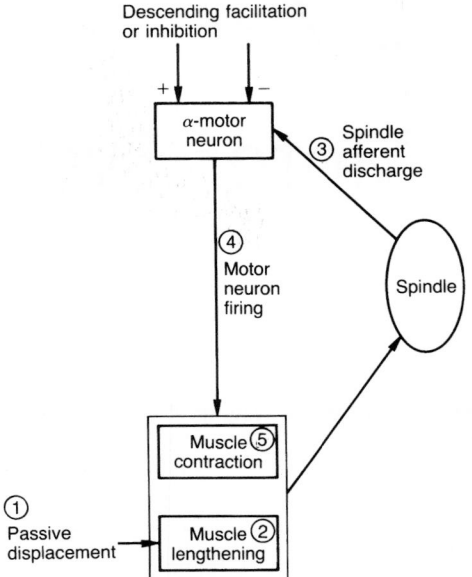

FIGURE 27.2 A scheme of the stretch reflex. Descending signals acting on the α motorneuron regulate muscle length. When a passive joint displacement (1) causes muscle lengthening (2) the afferent discharge from muscle spindles (3) has a direct excitatory input on the α-motorneuron. The motoneuron response (4) which leads to corrective muscle contraction (5) is modulated by both excitatory and inhibitory descending inputs.

ence the dynamic and static responsiveness of the spindles. Both types of γ-efferents are activated to a higher level relative to α-efferent activation as the speed and difficulty of a motor task increase. Golgi tendon organs, situated at the junction of muscle and tendon, discharge as tension generated by muscle contraction distorts nerve endings entwined between collagen fibers.

## Spinal reflexes

Spinal reflexes are organized entirely with the spinal cord but are under the influence of descending pathways. The stretch reflex consists of a monosynaptic connection between afferent fibers from a muscle spindle and α-motorneurons innervating the same and synergistic muscles (Fig. 27.2). This is the basis of the tendon jerk in which a brisk tap on a muscle tendon produces rapid phasic contraction of the same muscle. Lesions of any component of the reflex arc can result in an absent or weak tendon jerk. Hypoactive tendon jerks also result from a reduction in excitatory descending influences. Hyperactive tendon jerks, manifested by a spread of the motor response widely to synergistic muscles, occur when there is a net increase in excitatory input to the motorneuron pool. The gain setting of stretch reflexes contributes to muscle tone,

i.e. the set value of muscle length. Spasticity is a common form of hypertonia in which muscles show abnormally high resistance to rapid stretch.

Most spinal reflexes are polysynaptic and coordinate the activity of groups of muscles. Tactile stimulation of skin can produce reflex contraction of specific muscles. Examples of cutaneous reflexes involving stimulation of the lower extremity are the plantar reflex, evoked by stroking the plantar surface of the foot, the extensor thrust, evoked by light pressure on the plantar surface, and flexion withdrawal, evoked by painful stimulation. Rhythmic motor patterns of locomotion are generated by intrinsic circuits of the spinal cord which require activation by brainstem centers.

## BRAINSTEM

The brainstem contains three neuronal systems that project to segmental networks of interneurons in the spinal cord and play an important role in the control of posture. Medial pathways connect to motorneurons that innervate axial and limb girdle muscles; the vestibulospinal tract is involved in the reflex control of balance; the reticulospinal tract is involved in regulation of posture and modulation of spinal reflexes; the tectospinal tract projects only to the cervical segments and is involved in the coordination of head and eye movements. The main lateral pathway, the rubrospinal tract, influences motorneurons that control distal limb muscles but is vestigial in humans. A third system originates in the locus ceruleus (noradrenergic), and raphe nuclei (serotonergic), and reaches all levels of the spinal cord.

## CORTEX

The primary motor cortex (immediately anterior to the central sulcus), premotor cortex (on the lateral surface of the frontal lobe) and supplementary motor area (on the superior and medial aspects of the frontal lobe) all have a somatotopic organization.

The primary and premotor cortex receive input directly from the thalamus (ventroposterolateral and ventrolateral nuclei). Input from the cerebellum basal ganglia and spinal cord are routed through the thalamus (Fig. 27.1). The motor cortex also receive input from the somatosensory and sensory association areas. There also are intracortical connections between the primary and premotor cortical areas and between premotor cortex and posterior parietal and prefrontal association areas.

The primary motor cortex is distinctive for giant pyramidal neurons in layer 5. Axons of pyramidal neurons join axons arising from the other motor cortical areas to project to the spinal cord directly via the corticospinal tract. There also are important indirect connections via brainstem pathways. Corticospinal and corticobulbar fibers pass through the posterior limb of the internal capsule to the ventral midbrain. Corticobulbar fibers project to trigeminal, facial and hypoglossal nuclei in the brainstem. Projections to the facial nuclei are bilateral but neurons innervating the lower face receive predominantly contralateral fibers. Corticospinal fibers pass through ventral pons and medulla to the medullary-spinal junction where three-quarters of the fibers decussate. The uncrossed fibers form the ventral corticospinal tract and project to the ventromedial area which contains motorneurons innervating axial muscles. Crossed fibers form the lateral corticospinal tract in the dorso-lateral column and project to motorneurons innervating limb muscles.

The discharge frequency of a corticospinal tract neuron encodes the amount of force used to carry out a movement. Some neurons of the primary motor cortex encode the rate of change of force. Individual neurons within a column of the primary motor cortex fire in movements of similar direction. The activity of neurons in the motor cortex during a movement depends on the nature of the task being performed, e.g. they are active during an arm movement performed to reach an object, but are silent during a similar movement performed as an emotional gesture. The time it takes to prepare for a voluntary movement varies with the complexity and difficulty of the task. The supplementary motor area is activated during the planning of a motor task. Blood flow studies have demonstrated increased activity of this area during rehearsal of a sequence of movements. The supplementary motor area has bilateral connections and plays a role in the coordination of posture and voluntary movements. The lateral premotor cortex receives input from the posterior parietal cortex and is thought to play a role in stabilizing axial and proximal muscles during the planning of a movement.

As the corticospinal system provides the only descending input to distal limb muscles, isolated movements of the digits or at the wrist are lost following lesions of this pathway. Lesions of the premotor areas impair the ability to plan a movement.

## CEREBELLUM

The cerebellum monitors activity in cortical and brainstem motor pathways and compares this activity against sensory feedback from movements. To do this the cerebellum receives input about motor planning from the motor and premotor cortex, the spinal motorneurons and spinal interneurons. It also receives somatosensory feedback from movement via the spinocerebellar tracts, as well as input from the auditory, visual and vestibular systems.

Subdivisions of the cerebellum have distinct functions. In the anterior and posterior lobes the midline vermis receives sensory information from the periphery and projects via the fastigial nuclei to cortical and brainstem regions and to descending pathways that control proximal muscles. The intermediate zones of each hemisphere project via the interposed nuclei to regions that control distal limb muscles. The vermis, intermediate zones of the hemispheres and associated deep nuclei contain complete somatotopic maps of the body. The lateral zone of each hemisphere receives input only from the cerebropontocerebellar pathway and projects via the dentate nuclei to the thalamus and hence to the motor and premotor cortex. The phylogenetically older flocculonodular lobe both receives input and projects to the brainstem vestibular nuclei to function in the control of eye movements and balance.

The cerebellar cortex has three layers. The outer molecular layer contains the interneurons, stellate and basket cells, axons of granule calls and dendrites of Purkinje cells. The Purkinje cell layer contains cell bodies of the sole output cells of the cortex which are inhibitory, i.e. use γ-amino butyric acid (GABA) as their transmitter. The inner granular layer contains mostly small granule cells which form complex synaptic contacts (glomeruli) with afferent mossy axons. Golgi cells are present in the outer margin of the granular layer. Connections between the two excitatory input systems to the cerebellar cortex, the mossy fibers (from the spinocerebellar tract) and climbing fibers (originating in the inferior olivary nuclei), and the Purkinje cell output of the cortex are illustrated in Fig. 27.3. The cerebellum has the capacity to alter its function based on experience, giving it a role in learned motor tasks.

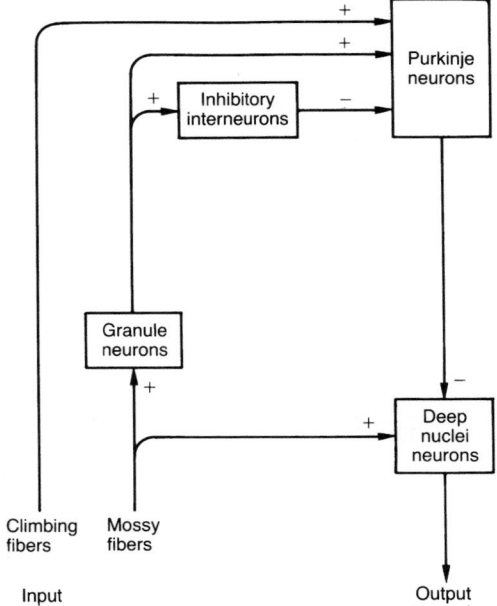

Figure 27.3 A scheme of the primary circuit of cerebellar connections. Excitatory input from mossy fibers acts through excitatory–inhibitory interneurons and granule cells (each granule cell connects input from many mossy fibers). Granule cell axons bifurcate and make excitatory connections with many Purkinje cells along the long axis of the cerebellar folia. The second excitatory input, climbing fibers, enter the cortex directly to contact the soma and dendrites of Purkinje cells (each climbing fiber contacts only 1–10 Purkinje cells). Granule cell axons contact inhibitory interneurons, stellate, basket and Golgi cells, which are connected to Purkinje cells in a manner to produce a center-surround antagonism across the Purkinje cell layer.

Lesions of the cerebellum do not impair the strength or speed of muscle contractions but lead to hypotonia, via reduced activity of γ-motorneurons (*see* page 403), and impair balance and coordination of movements (ataxia). Lesions of the intermediate zone of the cerebellar cortex impair movements on the same side of the body. Lesions of the lateral hemispheres and/or dentate nuclei lead to delays in movement initiation, terminal tremor, and in coordination of movements about multiple joints.

## BASAL GANGLIA

The basal ganglia are composed of five paired nuclei; the caudate and putamen forming the neostriatum (striatum), the globus pallidus derived from the diencephalon, and the subthalamic nuclei and substantia nigra. The striatum are the major input nuclei receiving afferent fibers directly from the cerebral cortex via the corticostriate projection and indirectly via the intralaminar nuclei of the thalamus (Fig. 27.4). The striatum projects to the globus pallidus via the striatopallidal pathway and to the substantia nigra via the striato-

nigral pathway. The external segment of the globus pallidus projects to the subthalamic nucleus which also receives direct input from the cerebral cortex. The pars compacta of the substantia nigra has a dopaminergic projection to the neostriatum. These connections into and within the basal ganglia are all topographically organized. The major output nuclei of the basal ganglia, the globus pallidus and pars reticulata of the substantia nigra project to the ventral lateral, ventral anterior and mediodorsal nuclei of the thalamus. The thalamic nuclei receiving input from the basal ganglia in turn project to the prefrontal cortex, premotor cortex, the supplemental motor area and the primary motor cortex. The pars reticulata of the substantia nigra also projects to the superior colliculus in a pathway which influences eye movements.

The basal ganglia are connected to all areas of the cerebral cortex and are involved in functions outside the motor system, e.g. aspects of memory and beha-

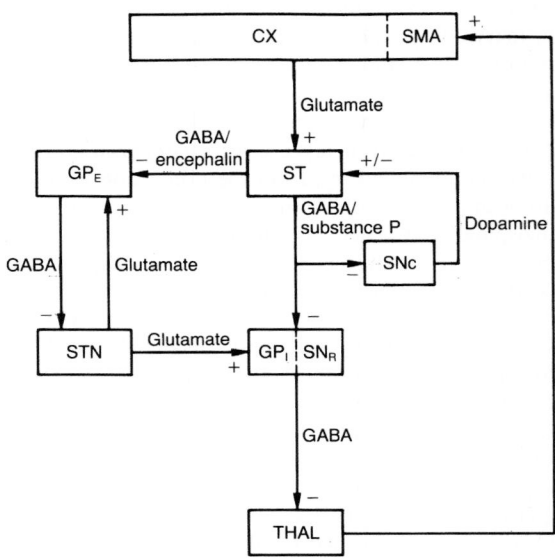

FIGURE 27.4 A scheme of the pathways within the basal ganglia including their putative neurotransmitters. Afferents (excitatory) from the cortex (CX) to the striatum (ST) are mediated by glutamate. In the direct pathway to the thalamus (THAL) via the internal segment of the globus pallidus (GPi) and pars reticulata of the substantia nigra (SNr) both segments are inhibitory mediated by GABA and substance P. In this pathway excitatory input from the cortex leads to disinhibition of thalamocortical neurons and facilitation of movement. In the indirect pathway corticostriatal excitation leads to inhibition of the external segment of the globus pallidus (GPe) mediated by GABA and enkephalin, and disinhibition of the subthalamic nucleus (STN) mediated by GABA. This excites the output nuclei (mediated by glutamate) with subsequent inhibition of the thalamus and a decrease in input to the supplementary motor area (SMA). The dopaminergic pathways from the pars compacta of the substantia nigra (SNc) have a dual action in the striatum; they excite neurons projecting via the direct pathway; they inhibit neurons projecting via the indirect pathway. The net effect of dopamine is to facilitate movement.

vioral set. Impairment of function in the basal ganglia can lead to involuntary movements, e.g. tremor, athetosis, chorea, ballism or dystonia, or impairment of movement, e.g. akinesia or bradykinesia. Disturbances of cognition in addition to a motor disorder are seen in diseases of the basal ganglia, e.g. *kernicterus*, *Parkinson* and *Wilson diseases*.

## SELECTED READING

Alexander GE, Crutcher MD. Functional architecture of basal ganglia circuits: Neural substrates of parallel functioning. *Trends Neurosci* 1990; **13**: 266.

Hepp-Reymond MC. Functional organization of the motor cortex and its participation in voluntary movements. In Steklis HD, Irwin J, eds. *Comparative primate biology*, Vol 4. *Neurosciences*. New York: Liss, 1988: 501.

Kandel ER, Schwartz JH, Jessel TM. *Principles of neural science*, 3rd edn. East Norwalk CT: Appleton and Lange, 1991.

Kuypers HGJM. The anatomical and functional organization of the motor system. In Swash M, Kennard C, eds. *Scientific basis of clinical neurology*. New York: Churchill Livingstone, 1985.

Gilman S. The cerebellum: Its role in posture and movement. In Swash M, Kennard C, eds. *Scientific basis of clinical neurology*. New York: Churchill Livingstone, 1985.

# DEVELOPMENT OF MOTOR FUNCTION

## INNATE MOTOR PATTERNS

Innate motor patterns are crucial for survival of many species at birth providing vital functions (e.g. breathing, sucking and swallowing), and body movements (e.g. locomotion and posture). In primates, some sophisticated movements are innate, for example facial expression of emotions. Innate motor patterns are controlled by neural networks in the brainstem and spinal cord. Central pattern generators that produce movements that are cyclically repeated (e.g. breathing and locomotion), are organized to generate an oscillatory activity and are capable of generating motor patterns without sensory input. However, motor patterns are modified by sensory feedback during the movement, for example after perturbation of an ongoing movement arising from the environment. Reflex patterns of movement such as swallowing or grasping are elicited in response to specific sensory input, or arise voluntarily. In the fetus early movement patterns are present before sensory connections are established, indicating that innate movement may be genetically determined.

## MOVEMENTS IN THE NEWBORN

The term infant has a repertoire of innate motor patterns, e.g. respiration and swallowing, that have been practiced during most of fetal life. Complex reflexes that are elicited by sensory stimulation, e.g. the swallow and blink reflexes, are present in their mature form at birth. Several developmental reflexes are overt only in the young infant and disappear as the motor system matures. The majority of neonatal movements are spontaneously generated, and as they involve the head and all extremities, are called general movements. Protective reflexes, e.g. the blink, cough and sneeze, are present at birth and remain essentially unchanged throughout life. Painful stimulation of a limb produces a flexion reflex in the infant. The flexor reflex, responding with a flexion of the limb after a noxious stimulus, is also present after birth.

## MUSCLE TONE

The muscle tone (i.e. the tension of the muscles at rest), is modified during the last trimester of fetal life and during the first months of postnatal life. The muscles are flaccid before 28 weeks' gestation. Tone first increases in distal segments and in flexor muscles compared to extensors, resulting in flexion of the limbs. The progress of flexor tone in the preterm infant is one measure used to estimate gestational age. Muscle tone results from both resting activity of the α-motorneuron (*see* page 403) and from passive mechanical components, i.e. muscle fibers, tendons and ligaments. Post-term extensor tone increases in a craniocaudal gradient, along with supraspinal inhibition of inhibitory interneurons acting on motorneurons innervating extensor muscles. Recent injury to the central nervous system usually results in decreased muscle tone. Subsequent increases in extensor tone may be an early predictor of permanent motor disability.

## DEVELOPMENTAL REFLEXES

Several reflexes appear transiently during the newborn period, e.g. stepping. The threshold to elicit a reflex varies with the behavioral state of the infant. The Moro reflex consists of an abduction–extension movement of the upper extremities followed by adduction and flexion. It is elicited by vestibular stimulation, i.e. following sudden extension of the neck. The reaction is modified if the child is grasping an object, i.e. a mild passive stretching of the arms changes the pattern into flexion–adduction. In human infants the Moro reflex has no obvious function, while a similar movement in the monkey infant enables the infant to attach to the mother during her movements.

The asymmetric tonic neck reflex (ATNR) is elicited by activation of stretch receptors in the neck muscles on rotation of the head. The response is controlled by neural networks in the brainstem since it can be elicited after decerebration. The ATNR is usually not present in the newborn but appears at 2–4 weeks. It is most prominent during the second postnatal month and disappears by 5 months. The ATNR is transient and is usually terminated by spontaneous general movements. When the ATNR persists it is pathological and is a sensitive indicator of motor system abnormalities. There are several other neck righting reflexes, initiated by neck muscle receptors or by vestibular stimulation, which influence the position of the head and body.

The palmar grasp reflex is elicited by tactile stimulation of the palm in addition to proprioceptive stimulation achieved by stretching the arm. It involves both finger flexors and proximal arm muscles which are activated in flexor synergy, i.e. all flexor muscles at all joints are activated *en bloc*. The grasp reflex is difficult to elicit once the child starts to grip voluntarily.

The threshold and intensity of rooting and sucking reflexes are dependent on hunger and satiation. Rooting is initiated by tactile stimuli around the mouth and becomes totally directed. Sucking is elicited by lip and mouth stimulation. Both reflex patterns also occur spontaneously.

Infant stepping can be induced by holding the infant erect with the feet placed on a horizontal surface supporting some of the body weight. Alternating stepping movements occur when the infant is slowly pulled forward. Stepping movements are usually elicited only in the first month. Some children may maintain reflex stepping until they start walking with support. Infant supine kicking with alternating leg movements resembles stepping movements. Tactile placing reactions are elicited when the dorsal aspect of a foot contacts, for example, the edge of a table. It consists of a flexion and forward movement of the leg followed by a placing of the foot. Both tactile and proprioceptive stimuli elicit the response.

The presence or absence of reflex motor patterns in infancy do not predict developmental outcome. However, persistence of neonatal reflexes often indicates brain injury. Responses resembling the infantile reflexes, e.g. rooting, sucking, and the grasp reflex, often reappear in adults in association with dementing illnesses or diffuse brain injury.

## POSTURAL CONTROL

Postural control implies: (1) ability to maintain a position against gravity, (2) maintenance of the relative position of the body segments, and (3) maintenance of equilibrium. Antigravity muscle tone and righting reflexes develop in a craniocaudal sequence; most infants gain head control by 3 months. The extensor muscles of the legs are usually strong enough to carry the body by 4–6 months of age. Independent sitting

and standing require further development of extensor tone in the spine and hips.

The vestibular, visual and somatosensory systems provide continuous information about body position. A deviation of the body is immediately monitored and initiates postural adjustments. In the standing adult the somatosensory system responds first and initiates sharp bursts of muscle activity 90–100 ms after the perturbation. This is followed by responses evoked by the vestibular system (latency about 180–200 ms). Motor activity evoked by the visual system is slower and is important for achieving the final position. The responses have specific muscle activation patterns for certain disturbances and contain a whole set of muscle contractions, for example a forward sway of the standing body is counteracted by a wave of muscle contractions on the dorsal side of the body beginning in the calf muscles and spreading upwards to the neck muscles. The responses can be adapted and modified depending on the nature of the disturbance, for example if the support phase is rotated or translated or during weightlessness. The adaptation is a function of an integration between the three sensory systems and requires an intact cerebellum. The vestibular, visual, and somatosensory systems are functioning in the term newborn, but it is only after several weeks that postural adjustments can be elicited by external perturbations. Side-fall reflexes and parachute reactions first develop after 6 months. The development of neural networks responding to sensory stimuli and producing the adequate motor pattern is the factor limiting their appearance.

Abnormal development of postural control in children with cerebral palsy results in muscle activation patterns that deviate from the normal sequence and are accompanied by an excess of antagonist coactivation in neck and leg muscles.

## INTEGRATION BETWEEN POSTURE AND MOVEMENT

During voluntary movements the moving limb causes a change in the center of mass. In adults, voluntary movements are accompanied by activation of postural muscles, counteracting the perturbation evoked by the movement. This activity is initiated prior to the movement and is called anticipatory postural activity. Postural control is present by the second year. In children with mental retardation and delayed motor development the emergence of anticipatory postural control may be delayed.

## LOCOMOTION

The development of locomotion is divided into six phases. In the majority of infants the stepping movements are only elicited during the first postnatal months. This is followed by an inhibitory period until supported locomotion occurs at 6–9 months.

During this stage the infants can voluntarily walk and direct the direction of their gait. They also can support their body weight on one leg but need support to maintain equilibrium. During this stage they are also usually able to crawl on all four limbs. At 18–19 months the child can maintain balance while walking. The gait pattern is subsequently transformed into the adult plantigrade form. There are several specific adaptations to a bipedal, plantigrade gait, which reduce the vertical oscillation of the body and increase the step length resulting in lower energy expenditure. The prominent heel strike results from active dorsiflexion of the foot, provided by contractions of the pretibial muscles and inhibition of the calf muscle activity during the end of the swing phase. This is achieved by a specific individualized pattern of muscle activity and rotates the ankle joint out of phase with the knee and hip. None of the plantigrade determinants are present in the early stages of locomotion when all muscles are activated in conjunction. Many infants are still walking on their toes (never contacting the floor with the heel) when they start to walk independently. A slow transformation of the gait pattern occurs after independent gait is established. At the same time muscle strength and postural control develop, the child takes longer steps, and the gait increases in speed, the base narrows, and later, around 2 years, the child can run.

At the time when children normally transform their locomotor pattern into a plantigrade gait, children with cerebral palsy retain the immature non-plantigrade pattern. All muscles are activated together in a uniform pattern with a high degree of antagonistic coactivation. Children may continue to walk on their toes as a result of premature activation of the calf muscles during the swing phase. In addition to the disturbed coordination of locomotor movements, the gait of these children is also disturbed by muscle weakness (paresis) and spasticity. An immature gait pattern may also be seen in association with mental retardation. In habitual toe walkers the immature gait pattern is retained up to school age, without other neurological symptoms.

## EYE–HAND COORDINATION AND REACHING

Movements in extrapersonal space require information from several sensory modalities. When a hand movement to a visible target is generated the position of the target is defined in a visual coordinate system while the hand position is derived from somatosensory information fed into a body-oriented coordinate system. The sensory information and motor commands must be coordinated. This type of integration and transformation is present in an immature form in the newborn infant, who may perform pre-reaching movements, e.g. moving the hand toward an object without grasping. This implies that components of the mechanisms are innate. At 4 months when the infant can first reach out

and grasp an object, movement consists of several segments of acceleration and deceleration. By 12 months this movement usually consists of only one large initial segment followed by a few small segments.

The development of the movement trajectory reflects a transition from several small motor commands, each moving the hand a bit closer to the target, to a single motor program bringing the hand the entire distance. There is thus a change in the strategy from a feedback controlled movement in which the trajectory is continuously monitored to a feedforward controlled program, in which the entire movement is programmed in advance of the movement being initiated. The small segments at the end of the movement are correcting movements based on visual information during the movement. When an infant first reaches for objects the movement trajectory of the hand may vary from direct to circumferential. The body is also moved forward and rotated to be closer to the object. Initially the hand is open until the object is contacted. At 9 months the infant will shape the hand according to the form of the object; during the second year the hand starts to close before it contacts the object. When mature, the reaching movements thus involve two motor programs activated in parallel.

"Clumsy children" often have a reduced capability to process and utilize the sensory information required to program movements to targets in the extrapersonal space. Similar deficits may be seen in children with cerebral palsy. Children with congenital blindness are delayed in performing movements in extrapersonal space. They do not use their hands as perceptual organs to obtain information about external objects, but use them to eat and pull objects, so-called "blind hands." Motor development in blind children is generally delayed. This delay includes tasks that do not directly rely on visual information.

## MANIPULATION AND GRASPING

When voluntary grasping emerges at 3–4 months, it is in the form of the immature power grasp, i.e. all fingers and joints of the arm are flexed. Subsequent development is characterized by a fractionation of the grasp, i.e. the thumb and fingers can be individually controlled. At 9–11 months a precision grip develops, i.e. a small object can be picked up between the tips of the thumb and index finger. This development parallels maturation of the motor cortex and corticospinal tracts.

Manipulation of objects requires precise control of the grasping and lifting actions. The grip force is adjusted by the detection of microslips of the object by cutaneous mechanoreceptors in the finger tips. If the object starts to slip, grip reflexes instantly (60 ms) increase the force of the grip. Similarly, short loading reflexes adjust vertical lift force. When infants first use the precision grip, the grip force is excessive. They squeeze the object before lifting, i.e. the grip force is initiated well before the lift force. At 2 years the child can adapt grip force to the friction of the object. Grip reflex latencies continue to shorten up to 5–6 years.

When small children lift objects with the precision grip, they increase the isometric force in segments until the lift force overcomes the gravitational force of the object. The force increase is terminated by sensory feedback that indicates lift-off. During the second year, children gradually change to feedforward strategy. The grip force and load force are initiated together, i.e. the motor command is programmed in advance. The ability to program motor actions continues to develop until 10 years of age. Proprioceptive information about the weight of an object can be used by the 2-year-old while visual size information (transformed into weight) can be used first after 3 years.

The inability to perform task-related individual finger movements is common in children with cerebral palsy. These children may retain a sequential initiation of action. They may use excessive grip force and continue to use a feedback strategy with inefficient sensorimotor integration.

## LEARNED MOTOR SKILLS

Complex motor skills, such as writing and playing instruments, require practice before they can be skillfully performed. They can eventually become automated and performed without specific attention. During practice, sensory feedback from the movement is compared to the "ideal" movement; the next time the movement is executed the previous sensory information is used for programming of the next movement. As training advances, a central motor program is shaped. After a motor program has been established, sensory information is no longer crucial. Hence, learned movements may continue to be performed following deafferentation. The afferent information is, however, normally used to parameterize the movement, i.e. to scale the strength and duration of the motor program. Afferents compensate for perturbations of the movement. Often learning implies a change from segmented movement trajectories into faster one-segment movements. This is usually accompanied by a transformation from coactivation of antagonistic muscles to reciprocal muscle activity, often in a triphasic pattern. A complex program contains several parts, or subprograms, which are activated together or in sequence. These subprograms may be innate or learned movements, integrated into the learned movement complex. In certain motor patterns, several complex motor programs are successively initiated, for example, picking up an object from the floor, walking a couple of steps and putting the object on a shelf. To achieve such a smooth movement the motor programs are coordinated into a motor plan.

The neural substrate for learned motor programs and motor plans are not known, but the control is likely distributed between several systems. Learned sequences of finger movements are controlled from the premotor area via the motor cortex (*see* page 405). The cerebellum is crucial for other learned movements, while motor planning and procedural memories are disturbed after dysfunction of the basal ganglia.

Development of motor skills during childhood is a result of neural maturation as well as of learning processes. Often it is not possible to separate the two mechanisms. Generally the motor patterns during early development depend mainly on maturation (i.e. innate movements), while movements developing later are achieved with learning and practice. Complex motor skills are the most vulnerable and dysco-ordination or clumsiness is a common motor problem in children without other neurological impairments.

## SELECTED READING

Euler C, Forssberg H, Lagercrantz H. In *Neurobiology of early infant behavior*. Wenner-Gren International Series. London: Macmillan, 1989.

Forssberg H, Hirschfeld H. In *Children with movement disorders: motor control theories and therapeutic concepts*. Basel: Karger, 1992.

Forssberg H, Stokes VP, Hirschfeld H. Basic mechanisms of human locomotion development. In Gunnar M, Nelson C, eds. *The Minnesota Symposia on Child Psychology*. Vol. 24. New Jersey: Erlbaum and Associates, 1992: 37.

Prechtl HFR, ed. *Continuity of neural functions from prenatal to postnatal life. Clinics in Developmental Medicine*. Oxford: Blackwell, 1984.

Prechtl HFR, ed. *The neurological examination of the fullterm newborn infant*. 2nd edn. *Clinics in Developmental Medicine* 63. London: Heinemann, 1977.

# OCULAR MOTOR CONTROL

Eye movements carry out two important functions related to vision. First, the ocular motor system allows the visual system to perform optimally with the image steady on the retina. Since the head and body are in motion most of the time, eye movements must compensate to maintain stable vision. The vestibulo-ocular reflex (VOR) and optokinetic system serve this function. Secondly, eye movements are needed to bring the object of interest onto the fovea where the highest visual acuity resides. The saccadic system serves this function. When at the fovea, the smooth pursuit system holds moving targets in a stable position.

Although much is known about ocular motor control in general, very little attention has been given to the development of ocular motor function, despite the fact that such knowledge is crucial for the understanding of many neurological and ophthalmological disorders in infants and children. Studies on eye movements in adults are extensive, but only recently has it been possible to record eye movements in infants. This is due to the development of accurate new techniques such as the infrared reflection technique and video based systems. Both techniques are only moderately intrusive and do not require much cooperation on part of the child; they usually are more sensitive than the, until now, most commonly used technique, electro-oculography (EOG).

## DEVELOPMENT OF OCULAR MOTOR FUNCTION

Eye muscles and their motor nerves are formed during the sixth week of fetal life. Fetal eye movements have been demonstrated with ultrasound in the fourteenth week of gestation. These eye movements are at first slow changes in eye position; they are more related to fetal behavior by the end of the third trimester. Thus the relationship of eye movements to other behavioral patterns may be used to give information about the integration of central nervous system function. The eye muscles are functioning at birth in a manner similar to that of the adult, with the exception of speed of contraction which is slower. Very little is known about the development of the brainstem mechanisms for the control of eye movements.

Congenital defects of eye muscles, motor nuclei and nerves are uncommon. Aplasia of the abducens nucleus leads to misdirected innervation of the lateral rectus muscle by the ocular motor nerve in the *eye retraction syndrome of Stilling–Turk–Duane*. Eye motor defects may result from congenital brainstem or cerebellar anomalies such as *myelomeningocele with the Chiari malformation*. The defects include horizontal gaze palsy, strabismus and nystagmus.

### The vestibulo-ocular reflex (VOR)

Existing data indicate that the VOR time constant undergoes an increase during the first 3–5 months before reaching adult values. The gain of the VOR is larger in infancy and declines during childhood and adolescence to adult rates.

Ophthalmological nystagmus of the fixation type such as *congenital nystagmus* is probably not connected with VOR dysfunction but more likely with other abnormalities of the brainstem or of cerebellar control of eye movements.

### Optokinetic nystagmus (OKN)

Since OKN can be evoked very early after birth (within a few hours) it has been used for a long time to study various aspects of perception, including visual acuity. The early form of OKN, however, exhibits subnormal slow phase velocity. With monocular testing there is a clear directional preponderance in the infant less than 4 months of age, and nasally directed stimuli elicit stronger and earlier OKN than temporally directed ones. The asymmetry disappears with the development of binocular vision, but is retained in individuals with early onset *convergent strabismus* (see below) who do not develop proper binocularity. An OKN abnormality is also believed to be an important factor for the development of *latent nystagmus* in children with this type of strabismus.

### Saccades

Saccades, the fastest of all eye movements, serve to redirect the line of sight to a new target of interest. During the first postnatal months the tendency to change fixation increases and older infants become more attentive to peripherally located visual stimuli. The saccadic latencies are longer in infants than in adults and increase with target eccentricity. Large saccades are usually hypometric in infants and seem to be programmed in smaller, stepwise movements due to some motor or sensory constraint. However, the saccadic system in infancy can function without hypometria if appropriate targets are supplied. Infants' saccades are also known to follow a main sequence when free scanning of the visual scene is allowed. The saccadic system thus appears to be the first well coordinated motor system of human development. However, the age at which the size, the latency and the sequencing of saccades reach adult levels is not known.

Saccades are among the few eye movements that can be executed voluntarily. *Congenital oculomotor apraxia* is a defect of horizontal but not vertical saccadic movements. Refixations are elicited instead with head thrusts, which are very characteristic of the condition.

### Pursuit

The smooth pursuit system serves to track an object of interest and to keep that target on the fovea. Pursuit is generally believed to reflect foveal function, and infants are known to have immature foveas. Smooth pursuit in young infants is dependent on the size and the speed of the moving target. Stimulation with large targets at low speed may activate not only the fovea but also parafoveal retinal areas and therefore elicit optokinetic responses and not actual pursuit movements. Saccadic pursuit or "cog-wheeling" is easily evoked in infants, as are combinations of the eye and head movements. At 2 months of age smooth pursuit movements are seen but they lag the stimulus. An adult-like smooth pursuit has not evolved even at 8 months of age, but the exact age of maturation is not known. However, horizontal pursuit movements seem to develop earlier than vertical movements.

# Vergence movements

Proper vergence movements are the requirements for normal development of binocular function. The system is already functioning in the newborn although with limitations in range and accuracy. Sensory constraints in the form of low accommodation accuracy and poor disparity detection limit vergence functions in the first months of life. However, there is a gradual improvement and at 6 months consistent responses to changes in binocular parallax and retinal disparity are obtained. Dysfunction of the vergence system is a hallmark of *strabismus*, but it is unclear if the initial defect in this group of diseases is in the vergence system or in the binocular functions that supply the command signals for vergence movements.

There is a strong coupling between the vergence system and accommodation (increase in refractive power of the lens in order to allow proper near vision). Abnormalities of vergence movements without strabismus are usually of psychogenic origin, but can also be due to accommodation deficits.

## STRABISMUS

Strabismus is defined as a pathological deviation of one eye with respect to the other. It is generally a childhood disease with a strong familial trait. Binocular functions always suffer in childhood strabismus, but it is mainly in its effects on monocular vision, i.e. as a creator of *amblyopia* that strabismus causes ophthalmological concern. The cause or causes of manifest childhood strabismus are known to a very limited extent. Interference with the mechanisms to fuse the images of the two eyes into one is an established factor, but how this inadequacy comes about in childhood strabismus is a matter of controversy, particularly whether the fusion defect is congenital or acquired, or if it is sensory or motor (vergence disturbance). In children with brain abnormalities, for instance those with Down syndrome, cerebral palsy, hydrocephalus and other more general brain disease, strabismus is common (40–60 per cent) in addition to other abnormalities of ocular motility. Anatomical factors are most likely the cause of strabismus in cranio-facial malformations but not otherwise. Sometimes specific brainstem lesions can be connected with strabismus (e.g. the *Duane* and *Möbius syndromes*).

Refractive errors play an important part in the etiology of squint since there is a close relationship between accommodation and convergence. For example, uncorrected hyperopia may cause a disproportionately large convergence impulse and convergent strabismus. However, it does not account for more than 20–30 per cent of strabismus cases.

## SELECTED READING

Aslin RN. Normative oculomotor development in human infants. In Lennerstrand G, von Noorden GK, Campos E, eds. *Strabismus and amblyopia*. London: Macmillan, 1988: 133.

Leigh RJ, Zee DS. *The neurology of eye movements*, 2nd edn. Philadelphia: FA Davies Co, 1991.

Sharpest C, Fuchs, AF. Minireview: Development of conjugate eye movements. *Vision Res* 1988; **28**: 585.

Taylor D, Avetisov E, Baraitser M *et al. Pediatric ophthalmology*. Boston: Blackwell Scientific Publications, 1990.

von Noorden GK. *Burian and von Noorden's binocular vision and ocular motility*. St Louis: CV Mosby, 1995.

# 28

# Biological Rhythms, Sleep and Psychological Development

## BIOLOGICAL RHYTHMS

### DEFINITIONS

In biology there are a wide range of processes which repeat in a predictable manner. "Circannual rhythms" such as the reproductive rhythms in seasonally breeding animals have a period of about a year. "Infradian rhythms" are biological rhythms with a periodicity of more than 28 hours, whereas "circadian rhythms" are approximately 24 hours in length. "Ultradian rhythms" are rhythms which recur with a periodicity of less than 20 hours. This section will review the biology of circadian rhythms, then focus on their development and review the evidence that the circadian rhythm generating system is functional before birth. Changes which occur in the circadian system in the 3–6 months immediately after birth will also be reviewed.

### CIRCADIAN RHYTHMS

The pattern of activity of many normal physiological functions (such as sleep and wakefulness, body temperature, urinary electrolyte excretion, melatonin and cortisol secretion) follow a circadian rhythm. Circadian rhythms are endogenously generated by a "body clock" or circadian "pacemaker" which oscillates with an inherent periodicity within the central nervous system. In the absence of any information about the external environment, circadian pacemakers oscillate with a periodicity of around, but not exactly, 24 hours, i.e. their activity and the activity of the rhythms they generate are said to "free run." In the presence of external time cues, e.g. light and dark cycles, the activity of the pacemakers is entrained to an exact 24-hour cycle. Whilst the main external time cue (or *zeitgeber*) is considered to be the light/dark cycle, other cues, including external temperature variations and social cues, are also thought to be important in the entrainment of circadian pacemaker activity. It has been found that in human subjects kept isolated from the range of daily time cues, two main groups of endogenous circadian rhythms maintain different periodicities over several months. The rhythms of rapid eye movement (REM) sleep, urinary $K^+$ excretion, plasma cortisol concentrations and core body temperatures are linked; the periodicity of these rhythms under conditions of temporal isolation is different from that of the rhythms in skin temperature, urinary $Ca^{2+}$ excretion and slow wave sleep. This phenomenon of internal desynchronization of rhythmic functions suggests that there are at least two circadian oscillators which control circadian rhythm generation in the human. In the presence of external time cues the pattern of activity of these oscillators must be coordinated to maintain an exact 24-hour periodicity of all physiological functions which show circadian rhythmicity.

## THE CIRCADIAN PACEMAKER AND ENTRAINMENT

The period (*per*) gene in the fly, *Drosophila*, is critical to circadian pacemaker function. Levels of *per* messenger RNA and *per*-encoded protein in the fly head undergo circadian oscillation which persists in constant darkness. per protein activity is involved in a feedback loop that influences the cycling of its own messenger RNA. An antibody against a small domain of the *Drosophila* per protein labels cell bodies in the rat suprachiasmatic nucleus (SCN). The region of the per protein recognized by this antibody is apparently widely conserved in neuronal circadian pacemakers.

The paired SCN located in the anterior hypothalamus have been identified as the site of a circadian pacemaker in mammalian species. The SCN contain several cell groups defined by their cytoarchitecture and expression of peptides. Vasoactive intestinal peptide (VIP) containing neurons are located in the ventrolateral SCN. Neuropeptide Y cells synapse on dendrites of VIP cells. The dorsomedial SCN contains clusters of parvocellular neurons expressing vasopressin (VP) and somatostatin, and receive VIP fibers from the ventrolateral SCN. γ-Amino butyric acid (GABA) containing neurons are present throughout the SCN. Circadian rhythms in VP content and in somatostatin in the rat dorsomedial SCN are not directly influenced by light. In contrast, VIP levels in ventrolateral SCN exhibit no circadian rhythmicity but respond to ambient light. These findings support the hypothesis that the ventrolateral SCN mediate information about environmental light and the dorsomedial SCN transmit the pacemaker signal to other areas of the brain.

The SCN project to and receive projections from the anterior hypothalamus, retrochiasmatic area and ventromedial nucleus of the tuber cinereum of the hypothalamus. Pathways project from the SCN to the hypothalamus; descending projections from the hypothalamus reach the intermediolateral column of the spinal cord which innervates the superior cervical ganglion (SCG); adrenergic postganglionic fibers from the SCG supply the pineal gland.

Entrainment to the light–dark cycle is mediated by the retina and by neural pathways from the retina to the brain, the retinohypothalamic tracts (RHT), which terminate in the SCN. The mechanism of entrainment at the cellular level is unknown; it occurs by a nonneuronal mechanism related to maternal influences in the late prenatal rat; by direct retinal connections to the SCN postnatally. Exposure of animals to phase-shifting light pulses is associated with induction of proto-oncogene, *c-fos*, in neurons in the retino-recipient zone of the SCN. *c-fos* and other immediate–early genes encode DNA-binding proteins that couple short-term membrane events to the long-term modification of gene transcription. There is a partitioning of retino-receptive neurons between those responsive to glutamate and involved in entrainment in ventral SCN, and those activated by other non-photic mechanisms in dorsal SCN.

Retinal illumination causes a reduction in norepinephrine release at postganglionic nerve endings in the pineal. Effects are modulated via cyclic AMP and inactivation of *n*-acetyltransferase, the rate limiting enzyme in melatonin production. Melatonin inhibits metabolic activity in the rat SCN and can reset the SCN electrical activity rhythm during the period of day–night transition *in vitro*. This transition coincides with time of maximal density of low-affinity melatonin binding sites in the rat SCN. Melatonin also induces *c-fos* in the SCN in a phase-dependent manner. Thus melatonin synthesis in the pineal is regulated by SCN output and SCN output is, in turn, modulated by melatonin in a feedback loop. This feedback loop may serve the function of synchronizing the SCN circadian clock to the time of nightfall and contribute to seasonal adjustments to the clock that occur with changing length in hours of darkness.

## DEVELOPMENT OF THE CIRCADIAN PACEMAKERS

The developing circadian system has been studied extensively in the rat. The SCN are formed by migration of cells from the ventral diencephalic zone of the germinal matrix immediately dorsal to the optic chiasm on embryonic days 14–16 (E14–16). VIP-immunoreactivity is present from E18 but VP-immunoreactivity does not appear until postnatal day 2 (P2). The adult pattern is approximated by P10 for both groups of neurons. Few synapses are present at E18 and active synaptogenesis occurs postnatally up to

P10. The RHT forms as collaterals of fibers already present in the optic chiasm. No RHT projection is present at P3 and by P10 the RHT extends to occupy the entire visual SCN. In the human fetus the SCN are already formed by the 18th week of gestation. [$^{128}$I]iodomelatonin binding sites (putative melatonin receptors) are present in the human fetal hypothalamus at 20–22 weeks' gestation. Immunocytochemical studies of neurons in the SCN which express VP show clear staining at 31 weeks' gestation. The number of VP cells rises rapidly in the neonatal period.

In the fetal rat there is a circadian rhythm in metabolic activity in the SCN from E19. The rhythm in the fetal SCN is entrained to the activity rhythm in the maternal SCN. Whilst it is clear that activity of the fetal SCN has an endogenous circadian rhythm, this rhythm is present at a time when the SCN are morphologically immature and have few synaptic connections. Hormonal and behavioral rhythms are only present in the newborn rat from the end of the first postnatal week. Therefore it is unclear whether the activity rhythm in the fetal rat SCN has any role in prenatal life. In longer gestation species, including man, there is limited information on the structure of the developing circadian pacemakers. In the human there are 24-hour rhythms in a range of fetal physiological parameters which are present during late gestation. A key question is whether these fetal rhythms are endogenously generated by the fetal circadian pacemakers which are entrained by the influence of external times cues. Such time cues could be maternal in origin, e.g. hormonal signals generated by the maternal circadian pacemaker which is itself entrained to the external day–night cycle. The presence of some fetal rhythms may, however, simply reflect the fetal behavioral or hormonal responses to certain stimuli (e.g. the metabolic consequences of maternal feeding) which tend to occur at the same time each day. In order to understand the origin and source of fetal rhythms it is necessary to compare data from studies in the human with those in the experimental animal, the sheep.

## DAILY FETAL RHYTHMS

Daily rhythms are found in the human fetus from around 20 weeks' gestation. The fetal heart rate shows a clear 24-hour rhythm from as early as 22 weeks' gestation and the incidence of human fetal body movements peaks in the early hours of the morning (02:00–04:00 hours) during the last 10 weeks of pregnancy. In fetal sheep, there is a daily variation in the incidence and amplitude of breathing movements which is present from around 125 days' gestation (gestational length of 147 days). This fetal rhythm is not a consequence of the maternal feeding regimen or of diurnal changes in fetal plasma glucose or prostaglandin concentrations. An eight-hour phase advance in the time onset of external darkness (i.e. from 19:00–11:00 hours) produces a shift in the phase of the

rhythm in breathing movements in the fetal sheep. This change in the time of darkness is associated with a change in the phase of the maternal and fetal plasma melatonin rhythms; it has been suggested that the maternal melatonin rhythm may act as a transplacental signal to entrain fetal behavioral activity to the external day–night cycle. Fetal melatonin rhythm is derived entirely by transplacental passage of maternal melatonin. It is not known whether melatonin acts to entrain the activity of the fetal SCN to the external day–night cycle or whether it acts directly at the respiratory centers in the fetal brainstem.

While there is some evidence that fetal behavioral rhythms are endogenously generated, there is no evidence that the rhythm in human fetal adrenal function is endogenously generated. In late pregnancy there is an inverse relationship between the 24-hour profiles of maternal plasma concentrations of cortisol and estriol. Measurements of maternal estriol provide a useful measure of fetal adreno-placental function (*see* page 211). The presence of an inverse relationship between the 24-hour rhythms of cortisol and estriol in late pregnancy is consistent with the hypothesis that maternally derived glucocorticoids act via negative feedback in the fetal hypothalamic–pituitary axis. This is supported by the observation that exogenous glucocorticoids suppress the maternal cortisol rhythm and also abolish the diurnal rhythm in maternal estriol. These observations indicate that while there are a range of 24-hour rhythms in fetal behavioral and hormonal patterns, each rhythm may be generated by a different fetal or maternal mechanism. The presence of such rhythms is not unequivocal evidence that the human fetal circadian pacemakers are active before birth.

## POSTNATAL CIRCADIAN RHYTHMS

There is a delay after birth in the emergence of entrained circadian behavioral and hormonal rhythms. The earliest age at which entrained rhythms in sleep and wakefulness and in plasma cortisol and melatonin concentrations emerge is at 8–12 weeks after birth. It is not known if the emergence of entrained circadian rhythms is a consequence of maturation of central pathways which carry information about the light–dark cycle to the circadian pacemaker or maturation of the synaptic connections of the circadian pacemaker. It is possible that exposure to external time cues, such as the daily light–dark cycle, determines the rate at which circadian entrainment develops. The emergence of an entrained sleep–wake profile in the human infant is thought to be predominantly the result of maturation of the central nervous system (CNS). This is supported by the demonstration using spectral analysis that sleep–wake activity has a more prominent 24-hour component in term infants when compared with preterm infants at the same postnatal age. However, it may be misleading to compare the development of sleep–wake rhythms in pre- and full-term infants without taking into account that after birth the preterm infant will spend some time in a hospital neonatal nursery where there is often constant illumination through the day and night and where there are several different caregivers in any 24-hour period. In one study the circadian sleep–wake rhythm in a group of preterm infants entrained after a similar time of exposure to an environment with daily time cues (i.e. light–dark cycles and a single caregiver) but at an earlier post-conceptional age when compared with a group of term infants. The length of exposure to environmental time cues may be as important as neurological maturity in determining the development of entrainment of circadian rhythms in the human infant.

## SELECTED READING

Miller JD. On the nature of the circadian clock in mammals. *Am J Physiol* 1993; **264**: R821.

Reppert SM, ed. *Development of circadian rhythmicity and photoperiodism in mammals*. Ithaca, NY: Perinatology Press, 1989.

# SLEEP

## PHYSIOLOGY OF SLEEP

In the human adult the waking state is defined by the purposeful quality of responses to the environment and by the presence of intact memory. However, any behavioral definition of the transition between waking and sleep is difficult to apply in practice and for clinical purposes this transition is defined by the electroencephalogram (EEG). The waking EEG is characterized by rhythmic activity in the α frequency range (8–12 Hz). Drowsiness (Stage 1 sleep), with loss of visual fixation and appearance of slow eye movements, is accompanied by the reduction in amplitude of alpha activity and the intrusion of theta frequency activity (4–7 Hz). Specific EEG transients, spindles and K-complexes, define the onset of true sleep and are characteristic of Stage 2 sleep. If sleep is maintained, high voltage delta activity (0.5–3 Hz) becomes increasingly prominent. Stage 3 sleep is defined by the presence of high voltage delta activity during 30–70 per cent of the record; Stage 4 sleep by the presence of high voltage delta activity during greater than 70 per cent of the record. The quality and duration of delta sleep is dependent to some degree on the time of day but is mostly influenced by the sleep history, i.e. the amount of delta activity is determined by the duration of waking prior to sleep onset and tends to decline as sleep continues. Behaviorally, sleep Stages 2, 3 and 4 are characterized as non-rapid eye movement sleep (non-REM). In non-REM sleep postural (tonic) muscle tone

is high, especially in antigravity muscles of the jaw and neck including muscles that maintain the patency of the upper airway. In contrast, phasic muscle activity including eye and limb movement, is absent.

When sleep is maintained for more than 90 minutes, a transition to rapid eye movement sleep (REM) may occur, especially during the night. This transition is often heralded by isolated rapid eye movements. At REM sleep onset, a body movement is followed by a sudden fall in postural muscle tone. Bursts of rapid eye movements then become prominent. The EEG reverts to a low voltage pattern resembling that seen in the drowsy state. REM sleep persists for up to 30 minutes before tonic muscle activity is reinstated following a body movement and Stage 2 sleep transients reappear; a second sleep cycle begins. Both the propensity for REM sleep and the duration of REM sleep episodes are determined by an endogenous circadian rhythm (*see* page 413) and are linked to the nadir of the body temperature cycle.

An individual entrained to the day–night environment and sleeping 7–9 hours per night experiences most delta sleep in the first 2–4 hours of the sleep period and most REM sleep in the early morning hours just prior to waking. This is in accordance with the association of delta sleep with prior waking and the linkage between REM sleep and the nadir of the body temperature rhythm. There is a circadian rhythm of sleep propensity evident in the latency to sleep onset of individuals studied in a constant environment and in the proportion of sleep achieved by individuals studied using an ultradian (e.g. 30-minute) sleep–wake schedule. There is a peak of sleep propensity in the mid-afternoon followed by a period of wake maintenance in the early evening when sleep initiation is impossible. The wake maintenance zone is followed by a "gate" after which the nocturnal increase in sleep propensity is expressed.

## DEVELOPMENT OF SLEEP AND WAKING STATES

### Preterm infant

The developmental aspects of sleep physiology are highly related to brain maturity and to a lesser degree are affected by experience. Therefore, it may be appropriate to extrapolate information gained from the study of infants born prematurely to the fetus *in utero*.

The behavioral and EEG characteristics of sleep states in infancy are summarized in Table 28.1. Prior to 28 weeks' gestation the preterm infant displays little temporal organization of behaviors although there may be some clustering of eye and limb movements after 22 weeks. The EEG shows an invariate discontinuous pattern of low-amplitude activity intermittently interrupted by bursts of high

TABLE 28.1 Summary of human infant sleep states

| GESTATIONAL AGE (WEEKS) | ACTIVE SLEEP | QUIET SLEEP |
|---|---|---|
| 28–36 | Coalescence of body, limb and eye movements | No movements |
| | High heart rate variability | Low heart rate variability |
| | Irregular breathing | Regular breathing |
| 36–40 | Continuous EEG | Discontinuous EEG |
| 40–44 | Absent tonic activity in postural muscles (REM sleep) | Sustained tonic muscle activity in postural muscles (non-REM sleep) |
| | | Discontinuous EEG (tracé alternans) or continuous low voltage slow EEG |
| Postnatal 1–6 months | | Continuous low voltage slow EEG with sleep spindles after 6 weeks |
| 6 months to adult | | Stage 2 non-REM sleep (EEG – spindles, K-complexes) |
| | | Stages 3 and 4 non-REM sleep (EEG – high voltage delta) |

voltage sharp and slow activity (*tracé discontinu*). At 28–32 weeks' gestation periods of activity alternating with periods of relative quiescence become synchronized with fluctuations in the variability of heart rate and respiratory efforts. The state of relative inactivity with regular heart rate and breathing is clearly a precursor of the non-REM sleep state. Between 28–36 weeks' gestation the behavioral differences between active and quiet sleep states become increasingly clear-cut and the association between the specific EEG patterns and behavior increasingly distinct. At 36 weeks' gestation the discontinuous EEG pattern has matured manifesting an increase in voltage of activity between bursts and decreased interburst interval compared to the more immature pattern, and is uniquely linked to the quiet sleep state. Active sleep, characterized by bursts of rapid eye movements superimposed on rolling slow eye movements, frequent fine face and limb movements and occasional body movements, is a precursor of the REM sleep state. By 36 weeks this behavioral state is closely associated with a continuous EEG pattern similar to that seen in drowsy waking. A significant proportion of sleep time in the preterm remains unclassified, with incomplete coordination between behavior, cardio-respiratory patterns and EEG.

There is little information yet available regarding a diurnal variation in behavioral states in the human fetus or preterm infant; however, a diurnal rhythm in heart rate variability, not apparently determined by maternal food intake or sleep state, has been reported.

## Term infant

In the term infant, waking is recognized by eye opening to stimulation and visual fixation (State 3 of Prechtl). However, states of high activity (State 4) and crying (State 5) are also classified as waking. The transition from waking to sleep cannot be clearly defined in the newborn; slow eye movements appear with the onset of drowsiness; superimposed rapid eye movements that appear at the transition to a sleep-onset active sleep state are not always readily distinguished from saccadic movements seen in waking. The EEG pattern during the transition from quiet waking, to drowsiness, to active sleep demonstrates an increasing amount of low voltage slow activity without a clear distinction between states. After an interval of active sleep usually lasting up to 10 minutes, eye movements cease and the EEG progresses to an alternating pattern of high and low amplitude activity with a periodicity of 3–8 seconds (*tracé alternans*) characteristic of quiet sleep (State 1) After 10–20 minutes of quiet sleep there may be a transition to waking marked by movement, eye opening or crying, or if sleep is maintained, to active sleep (State 2). At term, active sleep has all of the characteristics of REM sleep as described above; there are phasic movements of eyes and limbs on a background of reduced tone in postural muscles; the EEG shows a low-voltage continuous pattern.

The cycle of alternating quiet and active states has a periodicity of approximately 60 minutes in the newborn. The infant sleeps 16–17 hours out of 24 hours. There is usually no diurnal clustering of waking and sleep at birth, although some infants may already demonstrate some prolongation of sleep periods at night and of waking periods during the day in the first week of life.

## Birth to 6 months

The character and timing of sleep changes dramatically during the first 6 months of infancy. A mature non-REM sleep state evolves and a diurnal rhythm of sleep and waking is established. In quiet sleep a continuous EEG pattern characterized by low to moderate voltage 2–4 Hz delta activity emerges after birth and gradually replaces the alternating EEG pattern over the next 4 weeks. From 6 weeks sleep spindle-like activity appears and becomes increasingly prominent during quiet sleep. The EEG pattern of Stages 3 and 4 sleep, characterized by high voltage slowing, emerges between 3–6 months. At 6 months, with the appearance of K-complexes in association with sleep spindles during Stage 2 sleep, non-REM can be adequately described in terms of the adult EEG stages. The mature pattern of sleep onset, via quiet sleep, is increasingly frequent, especially in the laboratory setting, between 3–6 months. However, in a familiar environment the transition from drowsy to an active sleep state at sleep onset is frequently seen throughout the first year.

There is a high degree of interindividual variation in the age of appearance of a diurnal rhythm. Term-born infants living in the home environment typical of westernized countries will achieve a higher propensity for sleep during the hours of darkness by 6 weeks. The prolongation of periods of waking during the daylight hours and shortening of waking duration at night play a major role in the evolution of a diurnal rhythm. Night-time consolidation of 2 to 4-hour sleep periods characteristic of the newborn to form sleep periods of duration 6–8 hours occurs subsequently as an infant learns to re-enter sleep after brief waking without intervention of the caregiver. It must be noted that the timing of sleep and waking in infancy is highly dependent on culturally determined environmental factors and on the timing of the behavior of infant caregivers (see page 415). The influences of an endogenous rhythm of sleep propensity and of behavioral conditioning are probably both additive and interdependent.

## Infancy and childhood

Sleep Stages 3 and 4 become increasingly prominent after 6 months and reach a lifetime peak at 2–4 years in both duration per sleep cycle and in a tendency to recur in successive cycles. The duration of the non-REM–REM sleep cycle lengthens from 60 minutes to 90 minutes during childhood with prolongation of non-REM sleep duration. After 6 months sleep is usually maintained for at least 6 hours at night but a high propensity for sleep continues during the daytime. Multiple daytime naps consisting of one to two sleep cycles gradually consolidate into a single afternoon nap which persists at least to the age of school entry. This increase in sleep propensity in the mid-afternoon is analogous to that experienced by the adult especially under conditions of sleep deprivation or fragmentation.

## STATE-RELATED PHENOMENA

### Breathing

In the human infant the regulation of breathing is strongly influenced by state from 28 weeks' gestation. In the human fetus, breathing movements detected by ultrasound are linked to the behavioral state characterized by the presence of activity, eye movements and high heart rate variability and are otherwise infrequent. Studies of breathing in the ovine fetus indicate that breathing movements are inhibited in association with the high-voltage EEG state and that this inhibition is released by a lesion of the pons (see page 838).

This inhibition is also released at birth when breathing becomes continuous throughout waking and sleep. However, there remain fundamental differences in the regulation of breathing between waking and REM sleep, and non-REM sleep. In non-REM sleep respiratory drive is dependent on metabolic factors, e.g. $O_2$ and $CO_2$ tensions and pH, and stretch reflexes. In waking and REM sleep there is an additional "waking" drive arising from supramedullary centers. Hence, in the *congenital hypoventilation syndrome* (*Ondine's curse*), in which metabolic drive is defective (see page 843), ventilatory failure characteristically occurs in non-REM sleep. On the other hand, the atonia of postural muscles which include intercostal and upper airway maintaining muscles, may have profound effects on breathing during REM sleep in infancy. Upper airway dysfunction may be exacerbated in REM sleep and paradoxical movements of the chest wall are commonly seen in this state in young infants.

## Thermal regulation

The regulation of body temperature (see Chapter 48) is influenced by an endogenous circadian rhythm (see page 413) and by sleep state. Conversely, both diurnal variations in body temperature and sleep state organization are influenced by environmental temperature and by the history of thermal exposure.

In mammalian species basal metabolism and consequently heat production falls and the hypothalamic temperature set point is adjusted downwards at the onset of non-REM sleep (see page 424). In a thermoneutral environment there is an overall decrease in body thermal conductance associated with vasoconstriction of superficial blood vessels. In a high thermal environment an increase in body conductance may be necessary to adjust body temperature downwards during non-REM sleep. In many mammalian species REM sleep is associated with a loss of hypothalamic temperature regulation, so that body temperature changes passively with environmental temperature during brief REM sleep episodes. The situation is not clear in the human infant, but there is some evidence that active thermoregulation is maintained during REM sleep. A circadian rhythm of body thermal conductance causes a fall in body temperature and in trunk skin temperature, and a rise in peripheral skin temperature, during the night in an entrained individual in a thermoneutral environment. The changes in body and skin temperature associated with sleep are superimposed onto these diurnal rhythms. The night-time fall in body temperature is minimal in the first weeks of infancy and becomes clearly present and independent of environmental temperatures after 6–12 weeks.

## SLEEP DISORDERS

### Insomnia

When sleep is delayed or interrupted by pain, illness or environmental stimuli the effects are two-fold. First, there is a cumulative loss of sleep and secondly, there is a disruption of circadian regulation. Sustained sleep loss can have profound effects on behavior, cardiovascular function, thermoregulation and breathing. Irritability, hyperactivity and deficits in attention are prominent in the infant and young child who is sleep deprived. The direct relationship between waking duration and delta sleep propensity means that Stages 3 and 4 sleep occur earlier and persist for longer when sleep has been disturbed. Breathing disorders related to reduced respiratory drive during sleep which include *congenital hypoventilation syndrome* and *obstructive sleep apnea syndrome* (*see* page 843) are exacerbated by sleep loss and by sleep fragmentation. The loss of the diurnal rhythm that facilitates sustained sleep at night places great stress on the families and caregivers of infants and young children. The desynchronization of endogenous circadian rhythms has possibly more wide ranging effects, e.g. disrupting the response to thermal stress or infection.

Some infants who have demonstrated age appropriate sleep behavior in the first 6 months after birth subsequently experience difficulty initiating sleep and in maintaining sleep beyond 2–4 hours. Parents of such infants have often determined that sleep can only be initiated or reinstated if the infant is held, rocked, walked or driven in the car. These requirements may dominate the family's activities. It has been postulated that in these circumstances the infants have been conditioned to initiate sleep only with the specific assistance of the caregivers and that the infants need to relearn how to relax and enter sleep using their own resources. Various regimens have been advocated which require the parents to gradually withdraw their interventions.

### Parasomnias

Several sleep disorders that are common to the preschool child are associated with defective arousal from extreme delta sleep. Stage 4 sleep is most prominent in the child at 2–4 years of age and many sleep problems resolve spontaneously with advancing age. These disorders include *night terrors*, *sleep walking* and *enuresis*. They are all exacerbated by factors which increase the amount and depth of delta sleep and include sleep loss, excitement and physical activity on the preceding day. They are ameliorated by the avoidance of these precipitating factors.

### Sleep-related upper airway dysfunction

When the upper airway is anatomically altered in the presence of craniofacial anomalies, hypertrophy of lymphatic tissue, presence of mucosal swelling or airway secretions to produce luminal narrowing, the pressures generated in order to maintain tidal volume increase disproportionately. In this situation upper airway maintaining muscles may be acting maximally to maintain airway patency during quiet breathing. Any decrease in respiratory drive, as occurs at sleep onset, may then result in a tendency for the airway to narrow on inspiration, causing flow limitation and hypopnea, or in complete airway collapse on inspiration, causing obstructive apnea (*see* page 843). Flow limitation is frequently associated with vibration of the airway structures and snoring. Obstructive apnea may be silent but is usually interrupted by snorting as the airway reopens in association with arousal. Both hypopnea and apnea disrupt sleep and may become more prolonged as sleep loss accumulates; they are both accompanied by marked increases in negative inspiratory intrathoracic pressures and pulsus paradoxus; they may be associated with significant hypoxemia. Many children snore when they suffer from upper respiratory tract infections. A child who snores consistently over months or years warrants otolaryngologic examination for enlarged tonsils and adenoids. Children with craniofacial anomalies, large tongues (e.g. in *mucopolysaccharidoses*), obesity (e.g. in *Prader–Willi syndrome*) may be prone to sleep-related upper airway dysfunction.

## SELECTED READING

Guilleminault C, ed. *Sleep and its disorders in children*. New York: Raven Press, 1987.

Reppert SM, Rivkees SA. Development of human circadian rhythms: implications for health and disease. In Reppert SM, ed. *Research in perinatal medicine*. Vol. IX. *Development of circadian rhythmicity and photoperiodism in mammals*. Ithaca, New York: Perinatology Press, 1989: 245.

Thorpy M, ed. *Handbook of sleep disorders*. New York: Marcel Dekker Inc., 1990.

# FETAL BEHAVIOR

Human fetal movements are recorded using ultrasound techniques, include body, limb and eye movements and breathing (Table 28.2). The fetal heart rate pattern is recorded using cardiotocography (CTG). Four distinct fetal behavioral states have been described which are similar to the neonatal behavioral states described by Prechtl. The fetal states are State 1F, analogous to Prechtl State 1 or quiet sleep; State 2F, analogous to Prechtl State 2 or active sleep; State 3F, analogous

TABLE 28.2 Fetal movements observed ultrasonographically and age of first appearance

| MOVEMENT OBSERVED | GESTATIONAL AGE (WEEKS) |
|---|---|
| First discernible movements | 7–8 |
| General body movements | 8–9 |
| Isolated movements of a limb | 9–11 |
| Breathing movements | 10–12 |
| Yawning | 12–15 |
| Sucking movements/swallowing | 13–15 |
| Eye movements | 16–17 |

to Prechtl State 3 or quiet awake; State 4F, analogous to Prechtl State 4 or active awake. Each fetal behavioral state has a corresponding specific fetal heart rate pattern (Table 28.3). Fetal heart rate pattern A, observed in State 1F, is a stable pattern with a small oscillation bandwidth and only isolated accelerations; fetal heart rate pattern B, observed in State 2F, has a wider bandwidth and frequent accelerations; fetal heart rate pattern C, observed in State 3F, has a wide oscillation bandwidth and no accelerations; fetal heart rate pattern D, observed in State 4F, has long lasting accelerations. Both the frequency and regularity of fetal breathing movements are state dependent. In State 1F fetal breathing movements are usually absent, but when present tend to be regular. Many other fetal functions are also state dependent (e.g. voiding, sucking and swallowing). Fetal behavioral states are most recognizable in the last 4 weeks of pregnancy. Before 36 weeks' gestation fetal behavior is less well organized, although some linkage between movements and heart rate pattern or between eye and body movements can often be observed. The concept of fetal behavioral states is therefore not applicable to earlier gestational ages.

## CONSEQUENCES FOR CLINICAL PRACTICE

The CTG is widely used for fetal surveillance. Awareness of the character and timing of fetal behavioral states is necessary for appropriate interpretation of the CTG. The silent CTG is the most frequently recorded "suspect" tracing. The CTG may be silent, or non-reactive, for up to 45 minutes during fetal State 1 with fetal heart rate pattern A before transition to the more reactive fetal heart rate pattern B occurs. Thus to further assess this phenomenon, the initial

recording time should be extended rather than a second recording commenced at another time. Other suspect CTG patterns include a sinusoidal heart rate pattern seen during fetal sucking, and tachycardia with decelerations which can be recorded during "fetal jogging" in State 4F.

Although the organization of fetal behavior into defined states is a function of the developing CNS, it is not a useful measure of CNS function in the clinical setting because of the large variation in both incidence and duration of individual behavioral states in the healthy fetus. The similarity of fetal behavioral states to behavioral states observed in the newborn infant is evidence that this manifestation of CNS maturation is not affected by the timing of delivery.

## SELECTED READING

Arduini D, Rizzo G, Caforio L, Boccolini MR, Romanini C, Mancuso S. Behavioral state transitions in healthy and growth retarded fetuses. *Early Hum Dev* 1989; **19**: 155.

Bekedam DJ, Visser GHA, Vries JJ de, Prechtl HFR. Motor behavior in the growth retarded fetus. *Early Hum Dev* 1985; **12**: 155.

Nijhuis JG. Behavioral states: concomitants, clinical implications and the assessment of the condition of the nervous system. *Eur J Obstet Gynecol Reprod Biol* 1986; **21**: 301.

Prechtl HFR. The behavioral states of the newborn infant (a review). *Brain Res* 1974; **76**: 185.

Nijhuis JG, ed. *Fetal behavior. Developmental and perinatal aspects.* Oxford: Oxford University Press, 1992.

# PSYCHOLOGICAL DEVELOPMENT DURING THE FIRST YEARS OF LIFE

## THE EARLY COMPETENCE OF THE HUMAN INFANT

The newborn child has several capacities that prepare it to participate in early social interactions. These capacities might be considered early social "building blocks" that are used within the emerging relationship with the parent. Some basic biological assumptions concerning the early development are:

■ The cortex is immature but not non-functional at birth. Some processing within cortical areas can take place very early in life.

TABLE 28.3 Summary of fetal state criteria

| | BODY MOVEMENTS | EYE MOVEMENTS | HEART RATE PATTERN |
|---|---|---|---|
| State 1F | Incidental | Absent | Small oscillation bandwidth, isolated accelerations |
| State 2F | Present | Present | Wider oscillation bandwidth, frequent accelerations |
| State 3F | Absent | Present | Wider oscillation bandwidth, no accelerations |
| State 4F | Continuous | Present | Long accelerations |

- Subcortical areas can govern complex behavioral responses. Animal studies have clearly demonstrated that a complex response can be controlled by subcortical areas during infancy, while at later stages cortical areas "take over" control of the behavior.
- There is a relationship between psychological and biological growth, e.g. a change in visual attention during the second and third months of life parallels a rapid increase in myelination within the central nervous system.
- 4  All senses are functional to some degree at birth. The infant is able to respond to sensory information received, e.g. the newborn child has reduced visual acuity compared to the adult but is able to focus on an image at a distance of 15–25 cm (*see* page 397).

The visual system develops rapidly over the first year and visual acuity reaches adult levels before the first birthday.

The following presentation focuses on some of the more important "building blocks" for early social development: the development of cognitive and communication skills during the first years of life.

## EARLY SOCIAL DEVELOPMENT

### Voice recognition

The neonate is capable of differentiating the mother's voice from another woman's voice at 2–3 days and prefers the mother's voice. A female voice is preferred to a male voice. The infant most probably has learned to recognize the mother's voice while still *in utero*. When the voice of the mother is filtered so that it sounds as it might to the infant *in utero*, the infant less than 1 day old prefers the filtered to the unfiltered voice. Recent observations suggest that repeated exposure to maternal speech during the third trimester (e.g. a short nursery rhyme) affect fetal responses to those sounds. The fetal heart rate decreases significantly when the mother recites a "familiar rhyme" versus an "unfamiliar rhyme."

### Face recognition

Newborn infants, as early as 37 minutes after birth, display an increasing selectivity for face-like forms. Neonates show a preference for following a slowly moving face as compared with a scrambled face pattern or blank stimulus. This preferential tracking is most evident during the first month of life. The capacity declines between 4–6 weeks. The capacity demonstrated by the newborn infant is probably governed by non-cortical systems. Thus, the decline is explained by the maturation of cortical systems aimed at more sophisticated face recognition processes. As the child grows older, moving stimuli as well as real faces become more salient and more motivating. Infants aged 1–2 days can detect the difference between the mother's face and that of another woman.

### Neonatal imitation

The newborn will imitate mouth opening and tongue protrusion, head turning, finger movements, lip protrusion and sounds. This imitative capacity seen at birth, however, is not the same as the more mature imitative capacity that emerges around 9 months. There are some cues as to the nature of imitation:

- Imitation is observed for a wide range of gestures; reflex mechanisms do not explain the phenomena.
- There is a decline in imitation around 3 months of age.
- There are large variations in imitation between individual neonates.
- The imitative capacity observed during the first months of life has been linked to the mother–child interaction.

Infants displaying a strong tendency to imitate, avert their gaze to a lesser degree while interacting with the mother than do infants with a weak tendency to imitate. Neonatal imitation might also help the very young infant to confirm the identity of a person they have previously interacted with. In one study, 6-week-old infants were able to imitate a person after a delay of 24 hours. If shown a tongue protrusion on day 1 they displayed tongue protrusion when brought back to the experiment on day 2.

Neonatal imitation is a robust phenomenon but there is insufficient information to date to allow inclusion of neonatal imitation in any assessment of the psychological wellbeing of a young infant. One can speculate on a possible social function for neonatal imitation. This early imitative capacity can be viewed as a factor that facilitates each participating individual's sensitivity to social cues within an ongoing interaction.

### Eye-to-eye contact

An increased level of alertness at birth in many infants, thought to relate to high levels of catecholamines, enables the parents to interact with a visually active and attentive newborn. This early visual contact between parents and child is often a strong emotional experience. Extended contact between mother and infant directly after delivery tends to have some short-term effects (the physical contact and the time spent in eye-to-eye contact increases) but no clear or consistent effects are seen beyond the first 3 months of life. The importance of eye-to-eye contact increases dramatically as the child grows older. Mothers interacting face to face with their infants find that visual contact dominates during the first 2–3 months. The interaction is primarily regulated by the mother during this early phase since the infant is incapable of sustaining contact for a long period of time. However at 2 months infants interacting with their mother spend 80–90 per cent of their time looking at the mother's face. This intensive eye-to-eye contact is easily interrupted; e.g. if another adult enters the room or if the mother displays a "passive face." The infant will try to keep eye-to-eye contact using movements and vocalizations, but will grow more passive and uninterested if not successful. Thus, the infant knows already at 2 months what to expect from interaction with an adult.

Visual contact continues to be important throughout the child's psychological development, but the amount of time spent in actual eye-to-eye contact diminishes rapidly between 3–6 months. The infant becomes more and more interested in exploring objects and the broader environment, and the focus of the dyadic interaction between mother and child slowly expands to include an increasing number of objects.

## Smiling

Smiling can be observed as early as the first days or weeks of life. This early smile is incomplete, includes only parts of the infant's face (e.g. the mouth region) and it is not elicited by external stimulation. It is frequently observed during sleep especially during REM sleep phases. In the second and third weeks of life a smile can be easily elicited by external stimulation, by a touch while awake or by a soft high-pitched voice.

The human face becomes the most salient stimulus early in the second month making the smile a more obvious "social" response. This later emerging smile resembles the adult smile in that it includes the whole face, both the mouth region and the eyes. The early social smile is elicited by a person interacting with the infant. A clear change can be observed between 3–6 months as the child gradually limits the response to familiar persons.

## Motor development

Several observations during the last 10–15 years make it clear that neonatal movement is far from only reflexive and involuntary:

- One-day-old infants move their hands and body differently when in front of a person as compared with being in front of an object (e.g. a ball).
- The newborn tries to reach for an object that either is placed within the infant's gaze or is moved slowly along a trajectory close to the infant's body (prereaching) although a fully competent reach that includes actual grasping is not seen before four months of age.

- Newborns only counteract an external force (e.g. a light weight attached to the wrist) if they can see the movements of their own arm. Feedback through real-time video is sufficient whereas only kinesthetic information without vision is not.

Newborns have several other areas of competence that can be used in a social context, e.g. the capacity to recognize the mother's odor (see page 401), to show differential crying and to use early vocalization ("cooing") within a face-to-face interaction.

## SOME MILESTONES IN EARLY COGNITIVE DEVELOPMENT

Cognitive development during the first 6 years of life is traditionally divided into two periods. First, the sensorimotor period which covers the first 18–24 months of life and in which the child responds to the stimuli that are present. There is no planning of behavior and there are no internal representations (no words or mental pictures representing the world). Secondly, the preoperational period starts toward the end of the second year and continues until 6–7 years of age. Two early milestones within this period are the fast emerging capacity for symbolic activity, e.g. role-playing and make-believe plays, and the rapidly increasing language skills. The child's way of thinking is, however, primarily egocentric in that the child has difficulties in taking the perspective of someone else. The child also cannot solve tasks requiring the use of general principles or rules.

## Object permanence

In order to understand and interpret the world as adults or older children do, the very young child must develop a set of rules called "perceptual constancies." These rules enable the child to understand that a certain image reflects the same object even when the object moves away from the child. Size constancy develops early so that a child can interpret and act upon depth cues when 6 months old; some size constancy is already evident at 2 months. Shape constancy exists in rudimentary form at 2–3 months. Color constancy is mastered at a basic level at 4 months.

These constancies form the basis for the development of an "object concept." An important milestone in the development of the object concept is the understanding that an object continues to exist when not visible. This "object permanence" develops over the first year. The first sign of object permanence can be observed at 2 months; the infant displays a surprise reaction when a toy suddenly disappears. However, the child does not try to search for the toy before 6–8 months and it is not until 9–12 months that the child actively and successfully searches for a completely hidden toy. This developmental sequence might be partly dependent on or related to parallel development of the cortex, especially the frontal regions.

## Infant cognition

Infant cognition (e.g. visual preference, visual fixation or reaction time) seems to be based on two underlying factors, speed of processing and memory. Testing based on these processes (e.g. Fagan test of infant intelligence) when the child is between 6–12 months better predicts IQ at 3 years of age than traditional infant tests (e.g. Bayley test of infant development).

## Multimodal perception

An infant is able to combine information from different senses very early in life. Four-week-old infants combine tactile and visual information, and 4–5-month-old infants connect sound rhythms with movements and are able to look at a person mouthing a sound that corresponds to a sound they are hearing. Furthermore, the neonate's ability to imitate mouth opening and tongue protrusion indicates that a multimodal capacity is already present at birth.

## Deferred imitation

It was previously thought that the infant's capacity to imitate after a delay of several hours or days (deferred imitation) did not emerge until 18–24 months. However, recent reports indicate that 9-month-old infants can imitate novel actions on objects after a 24-hour delay. Thus, we must assume that both the memory and representational capacities necessary for deferred imitation and recall memory are within the child's ability much earlier than previously thought. Recall for novel actions has been demonstrated over a 4-month period during the second year of life. An act presented to a child when 16 months old was remembered 4 months later.

## Internal representation

The capacity to form internal representations means that the child can form inner mental pictures about the world and is able to manipulate those images or words mentally. It was previously thought that this ability evolved at 18–24 months, but new findings indicate that some capacity for forming internal representations occurs much earlier. The data on deferred imitation is but one of these new pieces of evidence. Three-month-old infants also can visually recognize an object they have previously only felt. This comparison requires at least some rudimentary representational ability.

## Pretend play

The first signs of pretend play are seen around the child's first birthday. A common example is the child that takes a toy spoon and pretends to feed himself. The capacity to play develops rapidly over the second year and a change can be observed at around 15–21 months when the child begins to incorporate other actions or toys, e.g. when the 18-month-old child takes a cup and gives her doll something "to drink."

The child starts to manipulate objects in a more complex manner, e.g. using a baby bottle to comb the doll's hair, between the second and third birthday. This ability is called "substitute pretend play" and continues to develop throughout the preschool years.

Another type of play emerges between 4–5 years. The child is now able to role-play and this is a period when many parents are astonished at the vivid imagination displayed in the play. By 6–7 years this "sociodramatic play" is gradually decreasing, although it does not disappear. At this age games with specific rules become more popular.

## DEVELOPMENT OF COMMUNICATION

### Prelinguistic development

The infant is equipped with several behaviors that communicate to the parents. The neonate can discriminate between different human voices and by 3–4 months discriminates between different language sounds, e.g. letters, syllables, intonation patterns, to a higher degree than most adults. In contrast, the child's own sounds are limited; crying is the most common sound during the first weeks of life, cooing sounds, i.e. sounds made up of single vowels like "uuuu" are heard by 1 month. New vowels are added and the child becomes more and more competent in changing the intonation pattern during the next couple of months.

Between 6–10 months the infant starts to combine vowels and consonants to produce new and different syllables, e.g. "dah dah." This babbling becomes frequent and by 9–10 months the intonation pattern becomes more like the pattern of language the child hears. At this age the child also starts to use gestures in trying to communicate. The child might stretch the arm and hand toward a wanted toy and make whining sounds. Pointing is a gesture first observed between 9–12 months. Categories for language specific sounds have been formed well before 6 months.

# Verbal language

There are large variations in normal children so that speaking the first word occurs generally between 8–18 months. The first word is quite often an idiosyncratic utterance that the child has made up. It is important that it is used consistently to mean something, e.g. naming a toy or a person or indicating a specific request.

Language progresses relatively slowly in the beginning. It takes the child approximately 3 months to add the next 10 words to the vocabulary. Language development proceeds very quickly after the 50-word point at 16–20 months old. On average, the 2-year-old child knows 300 words; the 3-year-old has a vocabulary of some 1000 words; and the six-year-old has a vocabulary of about 14 000 words.

The first sentence is uttered before the second birthday. Early sentences are short and usually consist of two words like "I do" or "eat cookie." However, the child has conveyed complex requests before this happens. A child of 17 months might grab the hand of his mother and say "cookie" meaning "give me a cookie." This communicative strategy of combining a word and a gesture is often called a "holophrase."

The child's first sentences are grammatically short and simple. Since only words critical to the message are included this is called "telegraphic speech." More complex structures like plurals, auxiliary verbs and prepositions are added as the child grows older. The first signs of complexity come as early as 24 months. The child's language continues to be immature for a long period and not before 4 years is it similar to adult language. However, it must be underscored that children display large individual differences in the way they learn language.

## CONCLUDING REMARKS

This chapter has emphasized development taking place within the social, cognitive and language domains during a child's first year. The neonate is already equipped with important competencies that help the child and parents build a mutual relationship. However, compared with later achievements the newborn is immature and in many ways helpless. The first relationship starts to develop immediately after birth, but it is not until the child is 6–12 months old that we can observe formation of a strong affectional bond. Functionally, the early attachment between parent and child serves to give the child security and protection. Thus it is most often in situations of distress or separation when we observe that the child has developed a strong attachment.

Increased separation anxiety and a fear of strangers is seen between 6–8 months. A secure relationship succeeds in comforting the infant after a short separation period. An increase in behaviors in which the child checks out where the mother or father are can be seen around 10 months. One example of this social referencing is when a child looks in the mother's face to try to understand emotional expressions. Thus, by interpreting the mother's cues, the child can judge if a new object or an unfamiliar situation is fearful or not.

## SELECTED READING

Berk LE. *Child development*. Boston: Allyn and Bacon, 1989.

Heimann M. Neonatal imitation: a social and biological phenomenon. In Archer T, Hansen S, eds. *Behavioral biology: neuroendocrine axis*. Hillsdale NJ: Lawrence Erlbaum Associates, 1991: 173.

Colombo J. *Infant cognition*. London: Sage, 1993.

Dawson G, Fischer KW, eds. *Human behavior and the developing brain*. New York: Guilford, 1994.

Johnson MH, Morton J. *Biology and cognitive development: the case of face recognition*. Oxford: Blackwell, 1991.

Kolb B, Fante B. Development of the child's brain and behavior. In Reynolds CR, Fletcher-Jantzen E, eds. *Handbook of clinical child neuropsychology*. New York: Plenum Press, 1989: 17.

Meehler J, Fox R, eds. *Neonate cognition: beyond the blooming buzzing confusion*. Hillsdale, NJ: Erlbaum, 1985.

van der Meer ALH, van der Weel FR, Lee DN. The functional significance of arm movements in neonates. *Science* 1995; 267: 693.

# 29

# Vegetative Functions

## THIRST AND HUNGER

### THIRST (*see also* page 517)

A dynamic balance between intake and output of water normally keeps the body fluid content and tonicity within narrow limits. The maintenance of water balance depends on the ability to alter renal water excretion via changes in antidiuretic hormone (arginine vasopressin, AVP) release (*see* page 516) and an efficient thirst mechanism which ensures that inevitable water loss is replenished. Water intake, induced by absolute or relative lack of water in one of the fluid compartments, is called "primary drinking," while water and/or fluid intake not associated with any water deficit is called "secondary drinking." The latter is the usual manner in which water is supplied, i.e. we drink in advance of apparent need. This terminology is not to be confused with primary and secondary polydipsia which means respectively, augmented water intake without or with preceding increased fluid loss.

Thirst is a general sensation and in its genuine form (i.e. caused by water deficit) one of our strongest motivational drives. The feeling of thirst is usually associated with dryness of the mouth and throat, but local moistening of these parts gives only partial and transient relief of the sensation. Damage to the hypothalamic region of the brain (e.g. trauma, tumor, infarction, hemorrhage) may cause various degrees of thirst deficit (hypodipsia, adipsia) resulting in chronic dehydration and hypernatremia. Selective injuries to the hypothalamo-neurohypophyseal vasopressin system (*central diabetes insipidus*) lead to excessive renal water loss with compensatory secondary polydipsia. Sometimes pathological processes in the anterior hypothalamic region (e.g. tumors, third ventricle cysts) are associated with *primary polydipsia*, apparently due to non-specific irritative stimulation of neuronal circuits involved in thirst control. However, in most cases of primary polydipsia the cause is unknown.

## Regulation

Primary drinking and increased AVP release are elicited by absolute and relative dehydration. Hyperosmolality is the most important stimulus in both conditions and about 1–2 per cent change in plasma tonicity is sufficient to activate these water conserving mechanisms. The threshold for thirst is at a somewhat higher plasma osmolality than for AVP secretion, i.e. water loss is reduced before the urge to drink is aroused, which seems a suitable arrangement for terrestrial life. The hyperosmolality is detected by sensors in or close to the anterior wall of the third cerebral ventricle. The sensors have not been identified histologically and controversies exist whether they are osmoreceptors in a general sense (i.e. activated by cell dehydration) or in some manner specifically sensitive

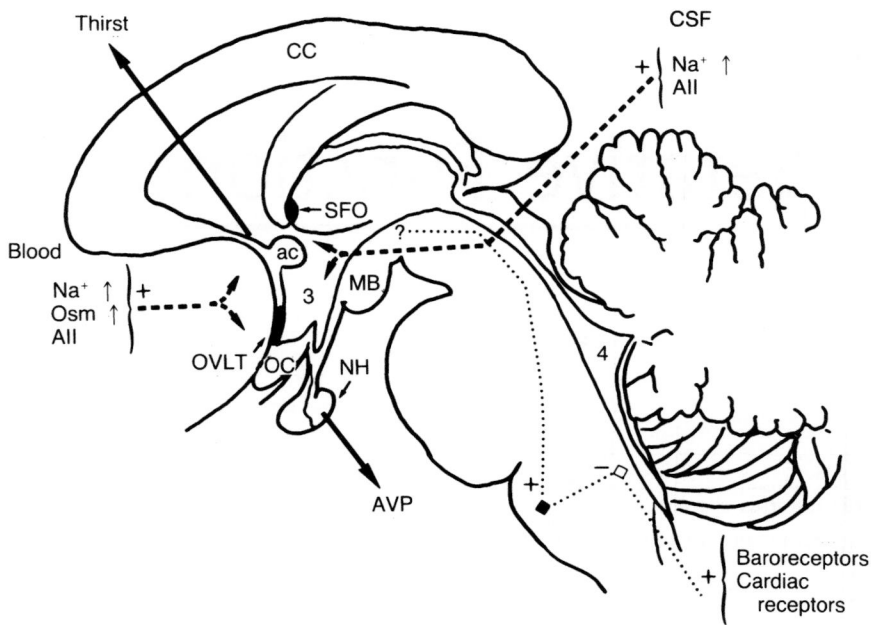

FIGURE 29.1 Cerebral control of water balance. The indicated changes in blood and CSF composition are thought to act on sensors close to the anterior wall of the third ventricle. The two circumventricular organs (OVLT and SFO) in this region may play a key role in this respect. Baroreceptor afferents are relayed in the medulla, from where second- or third-order neurons influence both water intake and AVP release, the latter via projections to the AVP-secreting neurons in the hypothalamus. + = stimulatory influence; – = inhibitory influence. Abbreviations: ac, anterior commissure; AII, angiotensin II; AVP, vasopressin; CC, corpus callosum; CSF, cerebrospinal fluid; NH, neurohypophysis; OC, optic chiasm; Osm, osmolality; OVLT, organum vasculosum of the lamina terminalis; SFO, subfornical organ; 3, third ventricle; 4, fourth ventricle.

to the extracellular sodium concentration. Osmotic changes on either side of the blood–brain barrier (BBB) (i.e. in the vascular and cerebroventricular compartments) influence the apparent activity of the sensors. Recent evidence indicates that they may be located in some of the circumventricular organs, i.e. structures lacking an effective BBB (see Fig. 29.1). The extracellular fluid (ECF) volume is another major determinant of primary drinking. The hypovolemia accompanying absolute dehydration (water deficit) may account for up to 30 per cent of the dipsogenic stimulus in this situation depending on species and degree of dehydration. Intense thirst is also commonly experienced during isotonic hypovolemia (e.g. during hemorrhage). Hypovolemia and/or hypotension may stimulate thirst via both reflex and humoral mechanisms. In the former instance, release of reflex inhibition from arterial baroreceptors and cardiopulmonary distention receptors is thought to increase water intake. However, this kind of influence on thirst is less apparent than for the AVP release. Reduced ECF volume may also stimulate thirst via the elevated plasma levels of angiotensin II (AII) which, at least in experimental conditions, is a potent dipsogen. Circulating AII is thought to stimulate water intake via the circumventricular organs mentioned above. The central AII system may also be involved (see page 524). The physiological and pathophysiological roles of AII in thirst control still remain to be defined, however.

The neuronal circuits involved in relaying different relevant stimuli for thirst are only partially resolved and the cerebral site(s) where these signals are integrated into an urge to drink water is unknown. Current ideas about the cerebral organization of control of primary drinking are summarized in Fig. 29.1.

Secondary drinking is commonly associated with meals and after spicy food. This intake of various beverages is evoked by oropharyngeal factors or specific appetite drives and not by any particular urge for water. Thus, secondary drinking may be influenced by a multitude of factors characteristic of ingestive behavior in general and it is largely unknown whether this is under any regulatory control. However, in certain conditions a specific urge for water is apparent, like the thirst felt by the mother just before or at the onset of breast feeding and thirst often experienced during hemodialysis. This may well be caused by hitherto unknown factors or hormonal or volumetric influences unappreciated in these particular situations.

## Satiation of thirst

Afferent information of, as yet, poorly defined modalities (e.g. osmolality, distention, temperature) from several orogastrointestinal levels contributes to an early preabsorptive termination of drinking. However, ingested water has effects on plasma osmolality within minutes, and diminished osmotic stimulation of thirst may be of importance to satisfy the urge to drink in humans who restore a water deficit rather slowly compared to many other mammalian species. Although the preabsorptive inhibitory signals in dehydrative thirst are exact and potent they appear insufficient to affect the fluid intake in most instances of secondary drinking when a surplus of water is commonly ingested.

## Specific developmental aspects

Water drinking appears to be an innate behavioral capacity although initial control of thirst mechanisms is not critical for survival in mammals since the mother's milk is sufficient for maintenance of water balance. At the time of weaning, however, it is essential that a regulatory control of water intake is functional. Rat pups respond to thirst challenges such as hypertonic saline, hypovolemia and angiotensin II during the first week of life, i.e. 2 weeks before weaning. Still, the suckling of milk is not influenced by dehydration in this species, but rather is governed by feeding control. Little is known about the maturation of thirst control in humans. Water is usually aversive to newborn babies, but may be readily taken by a few weeks of age. Severe forms of congenital diabetes insipidus (*central* or *nephrogenic*) may cause extreme dehydration leading to neonatal death or mental retardation, but the inability to match water intake with the fluid losses in these situations is usually not a manifestation of immature thirst control. It is important to understand more about the development of thirst control in infants, not only because dehydration is common but also since hypertonicity itself, by causing vomiting and diarrhea, may contribute to further fluid loss, possibly leading to brain damage.

Several disorders (e.g. congenital cerebral malformations, hydrocephalus, intraventricular cysts, craniopharyngioma) may cause severe damage to the hypothalamic region with consequent effects on many autonomic functions, causing a plethora of clinical symptoms. Both polydipsia and hypodipsia/adipsia may appear. In the former it is essential to judge whether the increased water intake is secondary to augmented renal fluid loss or not. Reduced or absent thirst is a prerequisite for the occurrence of chronic hypernatremia if water is available and there are no motor deficits to disable fluid ingestion. The plasma $Na^+$ concentration is commonly higher than expected from the estimated water deficit in these patients who in response to dehydration, may fail to increase $Na^+$ excretion which normally "buffers" the degree of developing hypernatremia.

## HUNGER

Hunger provides the motivational drive for the complex act of feeding which involves seeking and ingesting (and preparing) of food. Feeding is part of the homeostatic control of energy balance by providing the metabolic fuel (calories). Like water drinking, food intake also is influenced by psychological and sociocultural factors. Quite often we experience a more or less strong desire (i.e. appetite) for food and/or drink of a certain flavor, which sometimes may reflect an actual need for specific substances (e.g. salt appetite in $Na^+$ deficiency). Despite stronger psychological influences and specific appetite drives on food intake than on water drinking, humans (like other mammalian species) often maintain a constant body weight over long periods of time. Since small differences in daily caloric intake and energy expenditure would result in change of body weight, the nutrient intake (and metabolism) is apparently under homeostatic control.

## Regulation

The classical concept of the cerebral control of food intake with dual feeding (or hunger) and satiety centers in the lateral and ventromedial hypothalamus respectively, has been revised. It has become apparent that relevant visceral information (mainly gastrointestinal and hepatic afferents) and visual, gustatory and olfactory stimuli project to several cortical and subcortical areas; including most parts of the limbic system. Additionally, the strong influence of associative factors, e.g. learned behavior and stress, on food intake implicates a rather widespread cerebral involvement in hunger and satiety control. However, the hypothalamus is crucially involved in the cerebral regulation of feeding and damage to the ventromedial parts, without apparent effects on pituitary function, causes hyperphagia and obesity (*hypothalamic obesity*). Large lesions in the lateral hypothalamus induce aphagia, and also other behavioral deficits. Further analysis of hypothalamic lesions has revealed that these effects largely, but not exclusively, are caused by destruction of fibers of passage rather than of "integrating centers." Damage to other parts of the limbic system may cause similar disturbances in feeding control (particularly *aphagia*) but the effects are usually less dramatic.

Plasma glucose concentrations, or rather cellular glucose metabolism, are normally inversely correlated with hunger feelings. However, the strong reinforcement of hunger by the sight, smell, taste and initial intake of palatable food hints at the complex constellation of non-metabolic factors which makes it difficult to identify the relative importance of possible metabolically related "signals" for initiation of feeding. Peripheral, as well as central, administration of a number of endogenous substances, such as neurotransmitters and neuropeptides, causes satiated animals to eat; this probably reflects pharmacological activation or inhibition of neuronal systems involved in feeding behavior rather than indicating roles as messengers from deprived energy depots for the arousal of hunger. Regardless of the possible functional role of such substances in feeding control, it is interesting to note that local cerebral injection of certain neurotransmitters and peptides may selectively enhance consumption of carbohydrates, fats or proteins.

Eating is terminated before any significant uptake of nutrients has occurred. Both stomach fullness and the composition of ingested food are of importance for the degree of satiety. Additionally, gustatory and olfactory influences and the act of swallowing seem to contribute, since direct intragastric administration of food is less satiating than an orally ingested meal. Several gastrointestinal peptides appear to be involved in mediating "satiety signals" between the gut and brain, but the experimental evidence for such a role is conflicting for each of them. Cholecystokinin (CCK) inhibits feeding after peripheral as well as central administration. Recent evidence suggests that CCK activates vagal afferents peripherally, which in turn, via unknown mechanisms, lead to release of CCK in the brain where it acts as a satiety agent.

## Specific developmental aspects

Initial feeding behavior is probably mainly governed by the sucking reflex since this capacity is present in anencephalic babies and in decerebrate animal pups. However, it is generally believed that crying babies who eagerly take the breast and suck intensely express hunger. Little is known about whether the caloric intake is under any regulatory control during the early stages of life when large amounts of nutrients are needed for the rapid rate of growth. Apparently, insufficient feeding in newborn full-term or preterm babies is commonly due to a poorly developed sucking reflex, general weakness or respiratory problems. During development the control mechanisms of feeding go through several stages of encephalization with a gradual change to food which, at least initially, appears to be less palatable.

Feeding disorders (e.g. *anorexia nervosa*, *obesity*, *bulimia nervosa*) appear during childhood and adolescence. The neural and "humoral" basis for hunger and satiety control briefly summarized above has offered relatively little to the understanding of etiological factors for these disturbances. Hypothalamic damage of various causes (see above under thirst) may, depending on its extent and location, induce hyperphagia and obesity as well as anorexia. However, in most instances of these conditions the possible involvement of hypothalamic or other neural malfunction is unknown.

## SELECTED READING

Andersson B. Regulation of water intake. *Physiol Rev* 1978; 58: 582.

Booth DA, ed. *Neurophysiology of ingestion*. Oxford: Pergamon Press, 1993.

Fitzsimons JT. Thirst and sodium appetite. In Lightman SL, Everitt BJ, eds. *Neuroendocrinology*. Oxford: Blackwell Scientific, 1986: 207.

Le Magnen J. *Neurobiology of feeding and nutrition*. New York: Academic Press, 1992.

Robbins TW. Hunger. In Lightman SL, Everitt BJ, eds. *Neuroendocrinology*. Oxford: Blackwell Scientific, 1986: 252.

Robertson GL, Berl T. Pathophysiology of water metabolism. In Brenner BM, Rector Jr FC, eds. *The kidney*, Vol I. Philadelphia: Saunders, 1991: 677.

Rolls BJ, Rolls ET. *Thirst*. Cambridge: Cambridge University Press, 1982.

Shepherd R, ed. *Handbook of the psychophysiology of human eating*. Chichester: Wiley, 1989.

# THE AUTONOMIC NERVOUS SYSTEM (*see also* page 531)

## INTRODUCTION

The sympathetic and parasympathetic nervous systems, together with the chromaffin cells of the paraganglia, the adrenal medulla and enteric innervations comprise the autonomic nervous system. Other structures, both on embryological and functional grounds, e.g. the glomus cells of the arterial chemoreceptors, are candidates for inclusion.

Sympathetic and parasympathetic pathways consist of two-neuron chains. All autonomic preganglionic neurons release acetylcholine. Parasympathetic postganglionic neurons also release acetylcholine, whereas most, but not all, sympathetic postganglionic neurons release noradrenaline. A small subset of sympathetic neurons release dopamine (e.g renal nerve), and others release acetylcholine (e.g. innervation of the skin vasodilator and sweat glands). The innervation of the wall of the gut is non-adrenergic and non-cholinergic (NANC) and releases the purine nucleotide adenosine 5'-triphosphate (ATP) and possibly also nitric oxide (NO). The enteric innervation is now often regarded as a third, separate part of the autonomic system with a high degree of internal complexity, organization and local functional control.

## CENTRAL CONTROL

The autonomic system is controlled in two ways: first, by reflex arcs involving relatively few neurons, e.g. the baroreceptor reflex and reflexes controlling sweating and emptying of the bladder and the bowel; second, by central networks producing widespread responses or mass discharge as seen during stress. Most of the sensory input (via cranial nerves VII, IX and X) to the autonomic nervous system is relayed through the nucleus tractus solitarius (NTS) in the brainstem. The NTS receives visceral afferents from the respiratory, cardiovascular and gastrointestinal systems (Fig. 29.2). There are projections from the NTS to the brainstem and forebrain nuclei, e.g. the amygdala and paraventricular hypothalamic nuclei which project back to the nTS (Fig. 29.3). Information about the internal environment of the body is processed in this central autonomic network. The resulting efferent signals, particularly to the vagal motor nucleus and the sympathetic preganglionic neurons, cause reflex adjustment of the end organs.

Many of the brainstem neuron clusters controlling the autonomic nervous system are monoaminergic. The NTS contains norepinephrine and is also classified as A2 among the noradrenergic nuclei. A ventrolateral group controlling the sympathetic outflow contains mainly epinephrine (C1). The locus ceruleus (A6) itself is a noradrenergic cell group within the brainstem with massive projections to all levels of the neuraxis and is crucially important in producing central nervous system (CNS) arousal. A5 has a similar function controlling the visceral organs. These CNS cell groups form the central component of the sympathetic nervous system. Likewise, the vagal preganglionic neurons in the nucleus ambiguus and

dorsal vagal nucleus are the central components of the parasympathetic nervous system.

## DEVELOPMENT

Preganglionic neurons originate from the neural tube; postganglionic neurons develop from the neural crest. The sympathetic chain including the adrenal medulla, develops from the entire length of the neural crest. Enteric neurons migrate from the cranial part of the neural crest to the foregut where they give rise to the Meissner and Auerbach plexi. The vagal innervation of organs in the thorax and abdomen is derived from cells originating from both the hindbrain and the vagal ganglia within the cranium. These cells innervate the heart, lungs, stomach and upper intestines.

The sympathetic nerve trunk is formed by about the seventh week of conception in the human. The adrenal medulla and the paraganglia start to differentiate from 10–12 weeks. Sympathetic innervation of visceral organs matures after birth in the immature rat, but starts around midgestation in the fetal sheep. By extrapolation we assume that in the human innervation of the viscera is not fully developed at birth. Cardiac innervation is described on page 729.

## Differentiation and plasticity

An important question is whether the ultimate fate of the cells is already determined by the position they

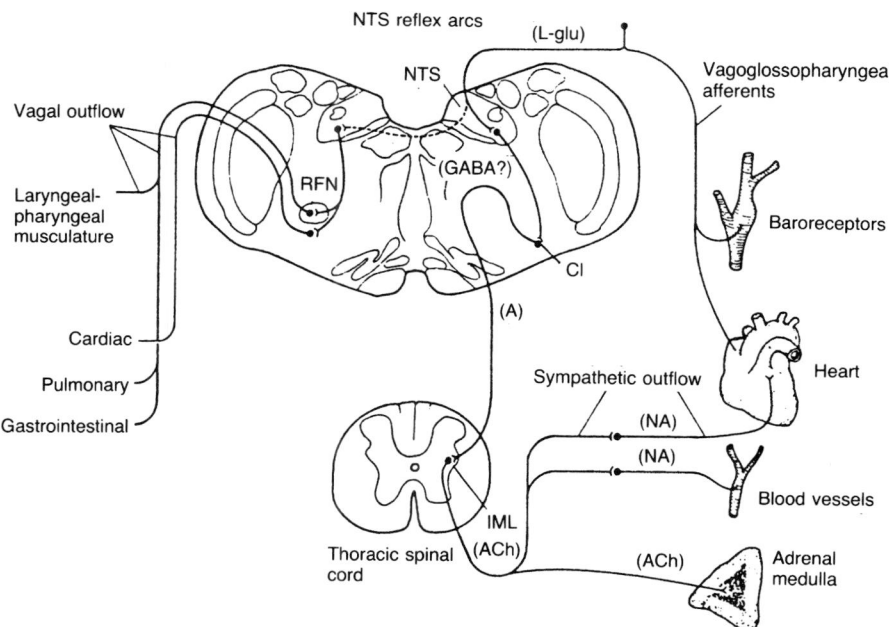

FIGURE 29.2 Baroreceptor and other visceral autonomic reflexes. Cranial nerves IX and X terminate in the nucleus tractus solitarius (NTS), which projects to the ventrolateral medulla (C1) controlling the sympathetic outflow via the intermediolateral cell column (IML) in the spinal cord. The NTS also projects to the vagal complex controlling parasympathetic outflow (From Bannister R, Mathias CJ. *Autonomic failure*, 3rd edn. Oxford: Oxford University Press, 1992, 953 with permission.)

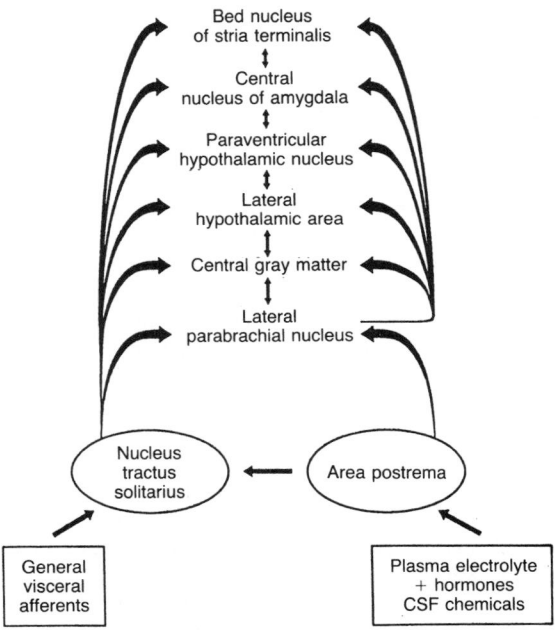

FIGURE 29.3 Afferent information from the internal environment of the body transmitted in the central autonomic network of the brain. (From Loewg AD, Spyer KM. Central regulation of autonomic function. New York: Oxford University Press, 1990: 93, with permission)

initially occupy along the axis of the neural crest, or whether their differentiation is determined by their route of migration and the position they finally occupy in the body. Transplantation of neuroblasts between chick and quail embryos has given invaluable insight into this question. When cells from the vagal neural crest of the quail were introduced into adrenomedullary region of the chick neural crest the cells become adrenomedullary in phenotype. Conversely, when quail cells from the adrenomedullary region were placed in the vagal region of the chick embryo neural crest, these cells colonized the gut and were transformed into cholinergic ganglia and peptidergic neurons. Thus neural crest cells are "pluripotent" and the phenotype expressed is determined by signals received during migration and/or by the target tissue in which the cell is ultimately embedded.

The microenvironment is important for the differentiation and choice of transmitters that a neuron will develop. For example, immature sympathetic ganglion cells in tissue culture first contain norepinephrine, but change their transmitter production to acetylcholine in the presence of a cytoplasmic factor in the culture medium. In the absence of this crucial substance the ganglia retain norepinephrine as their principal transmitter.

## RECEPTORS

The catecholamine receptors are classified into four types: $\alpha_1$, $\alpha_2$, $\beta_1$ and $\beta_2$. They act through two different second messenger and amplifying systems: the $\alpha$-recep-

tors are coupled to the metabolism of phosphatidylinositol in the cell membrane; $\beta$-receptors activate the adenylyl cyclase system. The two types of $\beta$-adrenoreceptors act like isoreceptors, since the only difference between them seems to be their order of potency. Epinephrine is a more potent stimulator of $\beta_2$-receptors than norepinephrine while both catecholamines are equipotent $\beta_1$-adrenoreceptor agonists. There are different proportions of adrenergic receptors in various organs, and the proportions change during development. All adrenoreceptors are coupled to G-proteins (see page 55). $G_s$-proteins (s, stimulatory) are coupled to $\beta_1$- and $\beta_2$-adrenoreceptors and the protein $G_i$ (i, inhibitory) is coupled to $\alpha_2$-adrenoreceptors. The number of adrenoreceptors in target cells shows marked organ-specific alterations during fetal and neonatal life. In the rat heart, the $\beta$-adrenoreceptor number is fairly constant from birth to adult life, whereas there is a marked increase in receptor number in the lung from day 1 to day 20. There is no correlation between the development of sympathetic innervation and the numbers of receptors in these organs. During development there is not a proportional one-to-one relationship between the number of occupied receptors and the biological effect. The unoccupied receptors are called "spare receptors" and they seem to increase in number during development. This and other factors might explain the higher the sensitivity of the fetal heart to respond to exogenous catecholamines.

## Cholinergic receptors

Cholinergic receptors occur as "nicotinic" and "muscarinic" subtypes, a distinction originally made on the basis of the selective effects of nicotine and muscarine-like substances, but more recently confirmed at the molecular level. Nicotinic receptors occur at the neuromuscular junction and in all autonomic ganglia, and muscarinic receptors occur at the synapse of postganglionic parasympathetic neurons with tissues. Nicotinic receptors are a single class of membrane bound excitatory receptors. In contrast, at least three subtypes of muscarinic receptors have been identified pharmacologically ($M_1$, $M_2$, $M_3$), and five subtypes have been identified using molecular cloning techniques ($m_1$, $m_2$, $m_3$, $m_4$, $m_5$). The M1, M2 and M3 pharmacological subtypes probably correspond to the $m_1$, $m_2$, $m_3$ molecular subtypes, while the $m_4$ and $m_5$ variants are presently of unknown function. $M_1$, $M_3$ and $M_5$ activate phosphatidylinoside hydrolysis and $M_2$ and $M_4$ inhibit adenylyl cyclase.

## FUNCTIONAL ROLE DURING FETAL LIFE

Knock-out experiments targeting the genes encoding tyrosine hydroxylase (TH) or dopamine $\beta$-hydroxylase (DBH) (see page 132) of the mouse embryonic cells have shown that the catecholamine system is essential for fetal development. Most TH-deficient mice die *in utero* after about 12 embryonic days and if they survived after birth they were severely runted, had abnormal motor function and died within weeks. If L-dopa was given to the pregnant mice, their knock-out fetuses could be rescued. Most of DBH-deficient mice also died *in utero* and survival probably was dependent on placental transfer of noradrenaline. Furthermore, if norepinephrine was provided by giving a precursor which could be converted to norepinephrine without DBH, the knock-out fetuses could be rescued. The noradrenergic system is essential for heart contractility during fetal life. Knock-out fetuses have markedly dilated atria and congested livers and major vessels. The catecholamines also have been shown to be important growth inducers of cardiac and others cells in tissue cultures.

Knocking-out the TH gene also results in bradycardia of mouse fetuses. However, adrenergic blockade with propranolol, chemical sympathectomy with guanethidine or adrenal demedullation in fetal sheep results in little or no decrease of heart rate indicating that the fetal heart rate is only minimally dependent on sympathetic tone.

The decline of the heart rate in the human fetus during gestation is assumed to be due to increased vagal tone toward the end of gestation. By giving atropine to the fetal sheep the increasing vagal tone can also be demonstrated.

## FUNCTIONAL ROLE DURING THE PERINATAL PERIOD

The sympathoadrenal system is considerably activated during birth as indicated by the remarkable surge of plasma catecholamine concentrations (see also page 532). Before birth the concentrations are lower than in resting adults, but increase 20–30-fold during normal vaginal delivery. The concentration of catecholamines is two-fold higher in the umbilical artery than in the umbilical vein indicating that they mainly originate from the fetus. The proportion of norepinephrine to epinephrine is about 6:1, which is higher than in the adult.

The parasympathetic nervous system is also activated, particularly if the delivery is complicated. The early heart rate decelerations seen during uterine contractions may be due to pressure on the fetal head activating nuclei in the brainstem. By determining the P–Q time interval of the fetal ECG in relation to the R–R interval, a considerable level of vagal input to the fetal heart can be demonstrated in the hypoxic fetus.

There also seems to be a parallel central activation of the brainstem immediately after birth. A three-fold increase of norepinephrine turnover was found in the brainstem of 1-hour-old rats compared with mature fetuses. The change of behavior of the infant from the sleep-like state observed *in utero*, to wide awake,

aroused state immediately at birth, has been attributed to activation of central noradrenaline pathways, especially those arising from the locus ceruleus in the brainstem.

## FUNCTIONAL ROLE AFTER BIRTH

The newborn infant is subject to a high level of sympathoadrenal activity in the first hours after birth. The heart rate is elevated, the pupils are dilated, the intestines have little motility. The catecholamine surge at birth is of importance for the neonatal adaptation. This has been demonstrated in animal experiments by comparing cortisol infused adrenalectomized newborn lambs with sham-operated controls (*see* page 532).

## FUNCTIONAL ROLE IN THE INFANT AND CHILD

The maturation of the parasympathetic nervous system lags behind the sympathoadrenal one. This is reflected in the decrease in fetal and newborn heart rates from 120 to 160 b.p.m. to about 100 b.p.m. in the infant and 70 b.p.m. in the adult. The parasympathetic system plays a greater role when the infant begins to gain weight rapidly a few weeks after birth; it is then of great importance for optimal gastrointestinal function. The sympathetic paraganglia atrophy and the relative size of the adrenals is reduced after 2–3 months. The organism is more dependent on the norepinephrine released from sprouting sympathetic nerve terminals in the target organ than on hormonal catecholamines.

## ALARM OR STRESS RESPONSE OF THE AUTONOMIC NERVOUS SYSTEM

The adult usually responds to physical or mental stress with an alarm reaction corresponding to the "fight and flight" response in most mammals. This response includes increased blood pressure and heart rate, shunting of blood from the kidneys and gastrointestinal tract to the muscles, increased glycolysis and blood glucose concentrations and increased muscle strength. The fetus and the infant usually react with a reversed or paradoxical stress response, i.e. bradycardia, decreased muscle blood flow and paralysis. This "playing dead reaction" is more appropriate for the fetus or the neonate. It can be observed in rabbit and mink pups and in reindeer, who can succumb in asystole if the response is very strong.

The defense reaction can be elicited by electrical or chemical stimulation of the amygdala, hypothalamus, midbrain and the medulla. The amygdala seems to be important for assessing the emotional significance of the stimuli. The paradoxical response seen in the fetus and infant indicates that there is not only a massive discharge of the sympathoadrenal, but also of the parasympathetic nervous system.

## AUTONOMIC REFLEX RESPONSES IN INFANTS

A battery of clinical physiological tests to assess autonomic function is available.

- Postural challenge. The infant responds first with a brief tachycardia and then bradycardia. The ratio between these two responses crudely reflects the sympathetic versus the vagal input to the heart.
- Bulbar compression.
- Cold face test. This is a more gentle way of testing parasympathetic overactivity in infants. However, the responses are not very consistent.
- Sweat excretion. This reflects parasympathetic activity and can be determined accurately by using a special evaporation probe.
- Autonomic score.
- Spectral analyses of ECG. This is probably a superior method to those detailed above as it is noninvasive. The amplitude of respiratory sinus arrhythmia can be used as an index of vagally mediated heart-rate pattern. By spectral analyses of the R–R intervals, high (HF) and low frequency (LF) peaks can

be identified. These crudely reflect parasympathetic versus sympathetic activity respectively.

These tests may be used in the investigation of preterm infants with recurrent apnea and bradycardia, infants with *apparent life threatening events* (ALTE), children with affection spells and *dysautonomia*.

## SELECTED READING

Bannister R, Mathias CJ. *Autonomic failure*, 3rd edn. Oxford: Oxford University Press, 1992: 953.

Cooper JR, Bloom FE, Roth RH. *The biochemical basis of neuropharmacology*, 6th edn. Oxford: Oxford University Press, 1991: 454.

Gootman PM, Gootman N. *The assessment of the autonomic nervous system*. In Eyre JA, ed. *The neurophysiological examination of the newborn infant*. London: MacKeith Press, 1992: 168.

Lagercrantz H. Stress, arousal and gene activation at birth. *News Physiol Sci* (in press).

Loewy AD, Spyer KM. *Central regulation of autonomic function*. New York: Oxford University Press 1990; 390.

Porges S. Vagal tone: A physiological marker of stress vulnerability. *Pediatrics* 1992; 90: 498.

Thomas SA, Matsumoto AM, Palmiter RD. Noradrenaline is essential for mouse fetal development. *Nature* 1995; 374: 643.

# 30

# Cerebrovascular Regulation

William J. Pearce

## INTRODUCTION

The blood vessels of the brain are immature at birth, particularly in preterm infants. At about 26 weeks' gestation, human cerebral blood vessels begin to grow rapidly, increasing in both density and diameter, and reach peak numbers and size by 35 weeks. Thereafter, the composition and function of the arteries change most dramatically, while their numbers and size change relatively little.

A key maturational change in the composition of cerebral arteries is a progressive increase in mechanical stiffness after birth. This is primarily due to changes in connective tissue but also is associated with some reduction in extracellular water during the first few days of extrauterine life. Subsequently the arterial walls thicken due to the synthesis and extracellular deposition of collagen and elastin. As maturation proceeds, connective tissue turnover continues with the production of relatively more type III and less type I collagen, and increases in the collagen to elastin ratio, with the greatest increases in the largest arteries.

Accompanying these changes in stiffness and composition are important changes in cerebrovascular reactivity, many of which coincide with changes in circulating hormone concentrations in the perinatal period. For example, plasma renin activity and concentrations of angiotensin II, arginine vasopressin, $T_3$, and $T_4$ are all higher in newborns than adults. Although a causal link between changes in circulating hormone concentrations and changes in cerebrovascular reactivity has yet to be demonstrated, the connection seems probable in light of the well documented ability of steroid hormones to change tissue levels of key enzymes such as $Na^+/K^+$–ATPase and guanylyl cyclase.

## CEREBRAL ARTERY REACTIVITY

Differences in contractile characteristics exist not only between arteries and veins, but also between large and small arteries, between arteries of the brainstem and those of the cortex, and between pial and parenchymal arterioles. It is important to bear in mind both the species and the specific artery under study when considering cerebrovascular reactivity.

Perinatal studies of the cerebral circulation have chiefly employed puppies, piglets, and lambs. Of these, cerebral development at birth is least mature in puppies and most mature in term lambs. Nonetheless, certain characteristics are common to the cerebral arteries of all three species.

- Maximum contractile force increases with advancing age.
- Sensitivity to the nitro-vasodilators, such as nitroglycerine and nitroprusside, is present at birth.
- Sensitivity to the vasodilating effects of adenosine is also present at birth. In general, each of these

characteristics is also present in the cerebral arteries of term human infants (Fig. 30.1).

The reactivity of the cerebral arteries to receptor-dependent agonists changes dramatically between fetal and newborn life. For example, cerebral artery contractile responses to serotonin are greater in term fetuses than in newborn lambs, and both are greater than in adult sheep. There are differences in the vascular responses between immature and adult animals for many agents including norepinephrine, acetylcholine and vasoactive peptides. Such differences suggest that the type and number of receptors populating the cerebral arteries are dynamic and under developmental, and probably hormonal, control. These populations are also subject to environmental modulation; there are different patterns of receptor-dependent cerebrovascular reactivity in fetal lambs at sea level and those born at high altitude.

## PROSTAGLANDINS AND THE CEREBRAL CIRCULATION

One group of receptor-dependent vasoactive compounds, the prostaglandins (PGs), play an important role both by maintaining patency of the ductus arteriosus, and by influencing vascular resistance in many organs, including the brain in the perinatal period (*see* page 166). PGs are synthesized perivascularly and act predominantly as mediators and/or modulators of adaptive responses to a variety of stimuli such as changes in blood pressure or hypoxia, and to some receptor-dependent agents such as opioids. Most cell types within the brain can produce and release prosta-

glandins, and the metabolism of these compounds appears to be particularly important in the glia. Indeed, certain perturbations may influence cerebral perfusion by stimulating glial elements to release vasoactive prostanoids. In turn, these prostanoids may also stimulate other glial cells to release additional vasoactive compounds.

PGs appear to be net cerebral vasodilators in the perinatal period, since indomethacin, an inhibitor of cyclo-oxygenase (a key enzyme in PG synthesis), produces a fall in cerebral blood flow (CBF) in almost all species. However, in piglets, ibuprofen (another cyclo-oxygenase inhibitor) does not alter basal CBF, but actually widens the range of autoregulation so that it more closely approximates the range found in adults (Fig. 30.2). Thus indomethacin may have additional mechanisms of action not mediated by PGs. This tendency to widen the range of effective autoregulation may explain the proposed reduced incidence of *intraventricular hemorrhage* (IVH) associated with cyclo-oxygenase inhibitors.

Prostaglandin $E_2$ ($PGE_2$) is a potent vasodilator in both the piglet and the fetal baboon. Because plasma $PGE_2$ concentrations are higher in the baboon fetus than in the mother, and its vasodilator potency is greater in newborns than adults, $PGE_2$ has been proposed to contribute to the lower cerebrovascular resistance characteristic of fetal life. Prostaglandin $E_1$ ($PGE_1$) is also a potent vasodilator of cerebral arteries of the fetal baboon and, as is true of $PGE_2$, sensitivity to $PGE_1$ appears to diminish with maturity.

During the perinatal period, another important prostanoid, prostacyclin ($PGI_2$) reduces tone in cerebral, mesenteric, and pulmonary arteries of both pig-

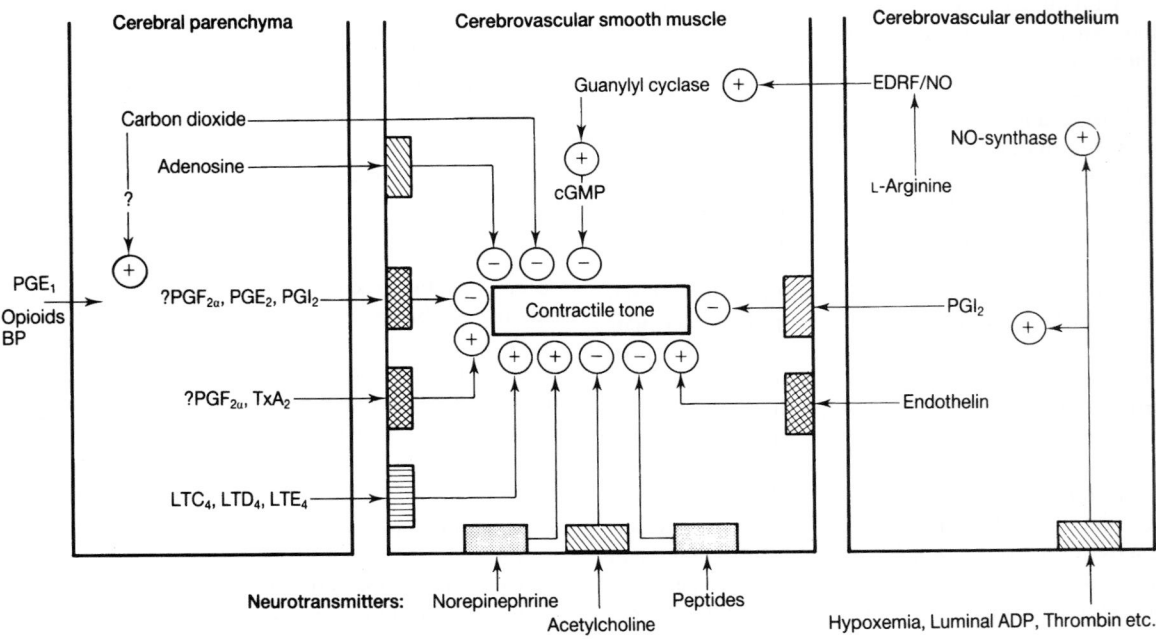

FIGURE 30.1 Diagrammatic scheme of factors effecting cerebrovascular tone. See text for abbreviations.

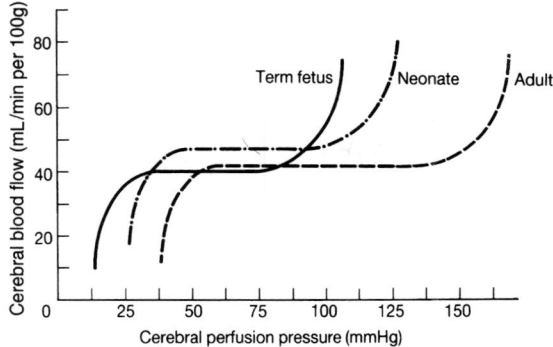

FIGURE 30.2 Patterns of autoregulation in the term fetal, neonatal and adult cerebral circulations

lets and baboons. In addition, the synthesis of, and sensitivity to, $PGI_2$ appears to be greater in newborns than adults in many artery types, suggesting that $PGI_2$ may be uniquely important in the immature cerebral circulation and may also contribute to age-related differences in cerebrovascular regulation.

Prostaglandin $F_{2\alpha}$ ($PGF_{2\alpha}$), a potent cerebral vasoconstrictor in adult cerebral arteries of most species, appears to promote vasodilatation at low concentrations in cerebral arteries of fetal baboons and newborn piglets. Again, this important age-related difference in reactivity suggests major differences in the density and intracellular coupling of prostaglandin receptors between immature and mature cerebral arteries. Such differences are not universal for all arachidonate derivatives however; the leukotrienes, $C_4$, $D_4$, and $E_4$, all promote cerebral vasoconstriction in both newborns and adults, as do all thromboxane analogs.

As indicated above, an important feature of prostanoid metabolism is that it mediates and/or modulates the cerebrovascular responses to a wide variety of both physiological and pharmacological stimuli. Opioids, such as enkephalins and dynorphins, promote the synthesis and release of vasodilator PGs, which mediate the vasodilator effects of these opioids. Lysine vasopressin also promotes the release of vasodilator PGs. Conversely, the contractile responses of piglet cerebral arteries to the free radicals released by hydrogen peroxide involve the synthesis and release of vasoconstrictor prostanoids. However, not all cerebrovascular responses in newborn piglets involve prostanoid release; cerebral vasodilator responses to the amino acids $N$-methyl-D-aspartate (NMDA), glutamate, aspartate, and taurine, for example, are all independent of PG release.

## CEREBRAL ENDOTHELIUM

The vascular endothelium is one source of vasodilator PGs, particularly $PGI_2$, in the neonatal cerebral circulation. In the infant, endothelial release of $PGI_2$ mediates the cerebral vasodilatation produced by acetylcholine. With maturation, however, the capacity for endothelial release of $PGI_2$ declines concomitant with an increased capacity for synthesis and release of endothelium-derived relaxing factor (EDRF) (see page 697), now widely held to be nitric oxide (NO) synthesized from L-arginine by the enzyme nitric oxide synthase (NOS). NO released by the cerebral endothelium readily diffuses into the adjacent vascular smooth muscle. There it activates guanylyl cyclase, elevates levels of vascular cGMP, and precipitates vasodilatation through the actions of cGMP-dependent protein kinase on calcium ATPase and membrane potassium channels. Due to the differential effects of maturation on endothelial release of $PGI_2$ and NO, the mechanisms mediating endothelium-dependent relaxation shift from indomethacin-sensitive in the neonate to indomethacin-resistant in the adult and the overall magnitude of this relaxation tends to increase with postnatal age.

Cerebral endothelium can also release the peptide endothelin (ET), which for human endothelium is primarily of the ET-1 isoform (see also page 700). Circulating concentrations of endothelin are elevated in the newborn relative to the adult, and the membrane receptors which mediate the diverse effects of endothelin are regulated during development in terms of both their density and their distribution. Pulmonary hypertension or hypoxia also may be associated with modulation of endothelin receptor expression. In general, the effects of endothelin receptor activation are mediated by an increased influx of extracellular calcium, but the end-effects of endothelin are highly cell-type specific. For example, endothelin can depolarize neurons, modulate astrocyte growth and differentiation, and augment coagulation. In neonatal cerebral arteries, endothelin dilates at low concentrations and constricts at concentrations above 1 ng/ml and both of these effects involve increased prostanoid synthesis. The physiological stimuli which promote the release of endothelin from cerebral arteries during the perinatal period remain controversial but probably include hypoxia, flow-induced shear stress, and stretch of the cerebral arterial wall.

## CEREBROVASCULAR INNERVATION

In adults, the cerebral arteries are innervated by fibers containing adrenergic, cholinergic, and peptidergic neurotransmitters. There are three general phases of nerve development: (1) the outgrowth of new axons, (2) the development of transmitter synthesis and storage capacity, and (3) the growth and differentiation of nerve varicosities. In general, postsynaptic function, reflecting the presence of appropriately coupled receptors, can be demonstrated before presynaptic elements are fully functional. The rate and timing of development of cerebrovascular innervation vary considerably among species and among different neurotransmitter systems.

The neurovascular system best characterized in cerebral arteries during the perinatal period is adrenergic sympathetic innervation. In human fetuses, immature adrenergic nerves with few varicosities can be demonstrated at 19–23 weeks' gestation, and their density is greatest in the more rostral vessels. In baboons, cerebral arteries contract in response to norepinephrine; the strength of these contractions is greatest in fetuses and diminishes with age. Similarly, cerebral arteries of newborn puppies, piglets, and lambs have all been shown to contract with norepinephrine. In newborn piglets, norepinephrine acts predominantly on $\alpha_1$-adrenergic receptors in cerebral resistance vessels and on $\alpha_2$-adrenergic receptors in pial arterioles. In newborn piglets, norepinephrine also stimulates the release of $PGE_2$, which apparently limits the magnitude of the vasoconstrictor response to norepinephrine. In addition, electrical stimulation of the cerebrovascular sympathetic innervation decreases cerebral blood flow by up to 25 per cent in newborn lambs and 15 per cent in newborn piglets. In lambs, as in baboons, the responsiveness to norepinephrine is greatest in fetuses and diminishes with age, suggesting that the functional importance of adrenergic cerebrovascular innervation is probably greater during fetal than adult life.

Nerves containing acetylcholine can also be demonstrated in fetal human cerebral arteries between 19 and 23 weeks' gestation, and as for adrenergic fibers, the fibers generally lack varicosities and are probably functionally immature. In fetal and newborn baboon cerebral arteries, acetylcholine elicits a contractile response that is absent in corresponding arteries from adults. In newborn piglet pial arteries, low concentrations of acetylcholine produce dilatation whereas higher concentrations (100 µM) produce vasoconstriction. Interestingly, indomethacin at 5 mg/kg can block pial artery contractile responses to 100 µM acetylcholine, suggesting that vasoconstrictor prostanoids, such as $PGF_{2\alpha}$ and thromboxane $A_2$, somehow mediate the response.

Although there is some evidence of a serotoninergic innervation supplying arteries of the circle of Willis in term human infants, these findings remain controversial and difficult to corroborate. Certainly, serotonin receptors are present in the cerebral arteries of most species at birth, but the pharmacological identity and cross-reactivity of serotonin with these receptors and $\alpha$-adrenergic receptors in the neonatal cerebral circulation remains uncertain. On the other hand, the presence of a peptidergic innervation supplying human fetal cerebral arteries is more widely accepted. These peptidergic systems supply separate nerves containing neuropeptide Y and vasoactive intestinal peptide (VIP) to the major arteries of the circle of Willis and the large pial arteries. In fetal rats, the cerebral arteries are innervated by sensory fibers from the trigeminal ganglion that contain substance P, VIP, cholecystokinin, somatostatin, and calcitonin gene-related peptide (CGRP). In adults, these peptides are all vasodilators. Their effects on cerebral arteries during the perinatal period, however, remain largely undocumented, as do the physiological stimuli that elicit their release.

## AGE-RELATED CHANGES IN CEREBRAL PERFUSION AND METABOLISM

In all mammalian species, cerebral perfusion and cerebral metabolic rate (CMR) are closely coupled. Although the exact mechanisms responsible for this coupling remain elusive, this matching between flow and metabolism remains a characteristic feature of cerebrovascular regulation, even during the perinatal period. Thus, the key to understanding age-related changes in cerebral blood flow is to focus first on the developmental changes in cerebral metabolic rate. In newborn puppies, the brain is relatively immature at birth, and cerebral metabolic rate is low, as is cerebral perfusion. With postnatal maturation in the puppy, both cerebral metabolic rate and cerebral blood flow rise to reach adult levels. In contrast, the lamb cerebrum is largely mature at birth, the reticular activating system is fully functional, and cerebral blood flow is higher than in adults. The pattern in term human infants is somewhere between these two. At birth, human cerebral blood flow and cerebral metabolic rate are low, and both variables increase steadily through the first six years of life, after which cerebral flow and metabolism gradually decline throughout the remainder of life.

Cerebral metabolic rate is not the only factor influencing cerebral perfusion in the neonate. As shown in an extensive series of studies in fetal and newborn lambs, cerebral $O_2$ delivery is an actively regulated variable (Fig. 30.3).

Cerebral $O_2$ delivery = cerebral blood flow × arterial blood $O_2$ content ($CaO_2$)

Because the position of the oxyhemoglobin dissociation curve directly determines the amount of $O_2$ that can be extracted from blood by the tissue (see page 785), shifts in the hemoglobin $P_{50}$ produce corresponding shifts in the rate of cerebral perfusion; leftward shifts in the oxyhemoglobin dissociation curve decrease the amount of tissue extractable $O_2$ and produce an increase in flow. Correspondingly, other maneuvers that alter $O_2$ carrying capacity, such as hemodilution or carbon monoxide poisoning, also alter the ratio of cerebral perfusion to metabolism. Central to the concept of the regulation of $O_2$ delivery is the assumption of a feedback mechanism matching tissue $O_2$ supply and demand. Although the mechanisms mediating this matching remain elusive, the "$O_2$ coupling hypothesis" remains of great value in predicting the behavior of cerebral perfusion in response to a wide variety of physiological stimuli.

Other stimuli that influence cerebral perfusion include direct vascular stimuli, such as neurotransmitters or PGs, which act primarily on vascular smooth

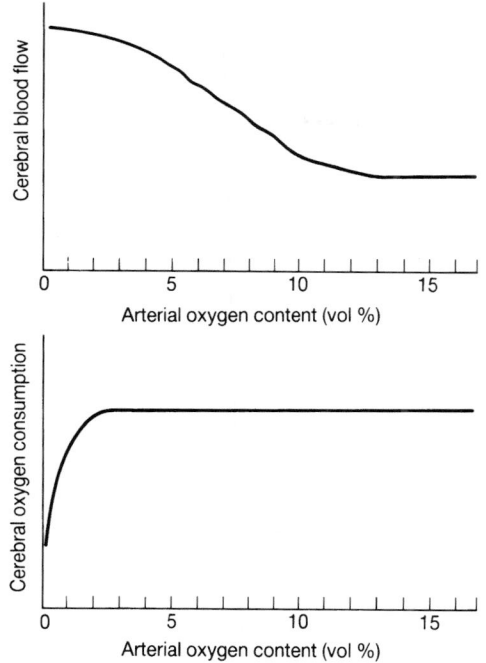

FIGURE 30.3 Relationship of arterial blood $O_2$ content and cerebral blood flow (top panel) and cerebral $O_2$ consumption (lower panel)

muscle, and metabolic stimuli, such as catabolic hormones or anesthetics, which act primarily to alter cerebral metabolic rate. For both classes of stimuli, the net effect is determined by how the stimulus affects the cerebral $O_2$ supply/demand ratio, and how the mechanisms maintaining this coupling compensate. As with most biological control systems, compensation is often not complete, and some "steady-state error" will remain at equilibrium. Thus, the high $CO_2$ and $PGE_2$ levels typical of fetal life may contribute to a relative overperfusion of the fetal brain, at least in the ovine species. In human infants, the mechanisms matching tissue $O_2$ supply and demand appear fully intact at birth.

## CEREBROVASCULAR AUTOREGULATION

Another feature of cerebrovascular regulation in both neonates and adults is autoregulation, defined as the ability to maintain a constant rate of cerebral perfusion despite changes in cerebral perfusion pressure.

> Cerebral perfusion pressure = arterial blood pressure − cerebrospinal fluid pressure

A key characteristic of autoregulation is the range of perfusion pressures over which autoregulation is effective (Fig. 30.2). In adults, this range extends from a lower limit of approximately 50–60 mmHg (6.6–8.0 kPa) to an upper limit of approximately 140–

150 mmHg (18.62–19.95 kPa). In fetuses and neonates, cerebral perfusion pressure is considerably lower than in adults (largely due to a lower mean arterial pressure), and correspondingly, the lower limit of autoregulation extends to lower perfusion pressures of 30–40 mmHg (3.99–5.32 kPa) in most species, including human infants. Similarly, the upper limit of autoregulation is also lower in neonates (70–100 mmHg; 9.31–13.3 kPa), rendering the neonates of most species, including human infants, more vulnerable than adults to hypertensive transients. In most species, including humans, cerebral autoregulation is fully functional at birth.

One possible mediator of autoregulatory cerebral vasodilatation induced by hypotension is tissue adenosine, which is a potent vasodilator. Cerebral adenosine (a vasodilator) production increases as cerebral perfusion pressure is lowered. In addition, cerebral adenosine production increases as cerebral $O_2$ supply is decreased, suggesting a possible common mechanism for the coupling of cerebral flow and metabolism, and cerebral autoregulation. However, hypotension also increases the cerebrospinal fluid concentrations of a variety of other compounds including both vasodilator and vasoconstrictor PGs, thromboxane and opioids. At the other end of the autoregulatory range, sympathetic vasoconstriction limits the increases in cerebral perfusion caused by elevated perfusion pressure in newborn piglets, and thus extends the upper limit of cerebral autoregulation. Clearly, cerebral autoregulation is a complex response involving multiple mechanisms, which may explain why it is vulnerable to a wide variety of insults including metabolic acidosis, severe hypoxia or asphyxia, cerebral ischemia, and intracranial hemorrhage.

## HYPERCAPNIC AND HYPOXIC CEREBRAL VASODILATATION

One of the oldest known cerebral vasodilators in adults is $CO_2$. *Hypercapnia* can increase cerebral perfusion in both newborn and fetal lambs, as well as in newborn and preterm human infants. In general, hypercapnia is a less potent vasodilator in newborns and infants than in adults; the reasons for this difference remain unclear. Some of this difference might be due to acidosis which, in the range which typically accompanies hypercapnia, is a better vasodilator in adult than in newborn cerebral arteries. Age-related changes in hematocrit also may be involved, as hematocrit is inversely proportional to cerebral $CO_2$ reactivity in newborn baboons.

Numerous studies now suggest that NO, released from non-vascular cerebral tissues, plays a key intermediary role in hypercapnic vasodilatation of adult rat cerebral arteries. Although this mechanism has yet to be explored in the neonatal cerebral circulation of any species, the fact that overall cerebral NOS activity increases with maturation suggests that age-related changes in this pathway may be involved in the corresponding age-related differences in hypercapnic cerebral reactivity.

In addition to a possible age-related role of NO in hypercapnic cerebral vasodilatation, vasodilator prostanoids also mediate up to 50 per cent of this response in both newborn piglets and human infants. The key observations supporting this view are that hypercapnia increases $PGI_2$ release into the cerebrospinal fluid and that indomethacin blocks both the rise in $PGI_2$ levels and the attendant vasodilatation. Because endothelial damage attenuates local responsiveness to hypercapnia, and hypercapnia promotes the release of $PGI_2$ from endothelial but not smooth muscle or glial cells in culture, the source of the $PGI_2$ involved in hypercapnic cerebral vasodilatation appears to be the vascular endothelium. Interestingly, addition of $PGI_2$ receptor agonists to pial arteries pretreated with indomethacin restores their ability to respond to hypercapnia, suggesting that $PGI_2$ is not the final mediator of hypercapnic cerebral vasodilatation, but rather plays an intermediary or permissive role in the overall response. The identity of the final mediator is currently unknown, but has been shown not to be an activated oxygen radical and its production is independent of reflex changes in sympathetic discharge or of changes in cerebral metabolic rate.

Acute hypoxia also elicits cerebral vasodilatation in neonates of most mammalian species, including rats, piglets, puppies and fetal and newborn lambs. In newborn lambs, the response is greater than in adults, but in newborn puppies it is less, suggesting that the magnitude of response may be related to the extent of cerebral maturation and/or cerebral metabolic rate. Consistent with this view, the brainstem regions of both lambs and puppies, which are generally the most mature of any brain region at birth and have the highest metabolic rates, also exhibit greater responsiveness to hypoxia than do other brain regions.

With the onset of cerebral hypoxia, the cerebrovascular response first involves a pronounced vasodilatation, which serves to increase cerebral perfusion and maintain $O_2$ delivery with little change in the $O_2$ extraction fraction ($O_2$ uptake/$O_2$ delivery) (Fig. 30.3). With increasing hypoxia, the cerebral $O_2$ extraction fraction begins to increase until maximum $O_2$ extraction is attained. If hypoxia becomes even more severe, then cerebral $O_2$ consumption may decrease and anaerobic glycolysis may ensue with attendant lactic acidosis. Thus hypoxic vasodilatation may be viewed as an intrinsic extension of the autoregulatory mechanisms coupling cerebral $O_2$ supply and demand. As stated above, adenosine is a possible mediator of hypoxic cerebral vasodilatation because acute hypoxia increases cerebral adenosine in adult and newborn rats and pigs. In newborn puppies, however, acute hypoxia also increases vasodilator PGs. Furthermore, hypoxia may also directly affect

vascular smooth muscle and endothelium of cerebral arteries. Clearly, hypoxia is a complex stimulus that elicits multiple mechanisms of cerebrovascular response in both neonates and adults.

## CEREBROVASCULAR CHANGES DURING HYPOXIA–ISCHEMIA

Hypoxia–ischemia (HI) is a common insult during the perinatal period, in which a number of stimuli are combined. Initially there is hypoxia and hypercapnia (asphyxia), which increase cerebral perfusion and, at least in piglets, simultaneously increase adenosine and vasodilator PGs. During prolonged or severe insults, there often is relative hypoperfusion due to redistribution of CBF, or overt ischemia due to hypotension. During asphyxia, in all species studied, neonates show a preferential increase in perfusion to the brainstem relative to the cerebral hemispheres; this response may be related to reflex sympathetic cerebral vasoconstriction in the latter regions. This pattern is in marked contrast to adults where increases in CBF are more evenly distributed. This difference may improve neonatal resistance to asphyxia while increasing the risk of survival with hemispheric damage (*hypoxemic–ischemic encephalopathy*). In human newborns, the threshold rate of CBF below which irreversible ischemic damage is certain is lower than in adults and is between 10 and 15 mL/(min·100 g). In lambs cerebrovascular regulatory mechanisms will maintain $O_2$ delivery until a $Ca_{O_2}$ of below 1 mM is reached. In both newborn lambs and humans, the mechanisms responsible for matching cerebral $O_2$ supply and demand and of cerebral autoregulation may be reversibly impaired during, and for variable periods after, asphyxia. Thus during a severe HI insult, CBF may become "pressure passive," i.e. directly related to blood pressure, explaining the critical importance of hypotension in promoting post-asphyxial cerebral damage (*see also* page 443).

## INTRACRANIAL HEMORRHAGE

*Intraventricular hemorrhage* is a common neurological occurrence in most neonatal intensive care units, with a significant incidence of *periventricular hemorrhage* in infants less than 35 weeks' gestation. There is a tendency for intraventricular hemorrhage to occur predominantly in the germinal matrix region, a finding attributed to the relative immaturity of blood vessels located there. Multiple factors, including cerebral venous infarction, altered coagulation characteristics, fluctuating blood pressure, acid–base imbalance, and deranged prostanoid metabolism, probably are involved.

When administered postnatally, indomethacin has been thought to reduce the short-term risk for intraventricular hemorrhage and over the long term to even accelerate germinal matrix microvessel maturation by increasing basement membrane laminin deposition in the immature cerebral arteries. The potential of indomethacin to reduce the risk of intraventricular hemorrhage likely is related to its ability to reduce cerebral blood flow and to extend the upper limit of autoregulation. Interestingly, the doses of indomethacin associated with reduced risk for intraventricular hemorrhage appear to have minimal effects on fetal prostaglandin metabolism, which suggests a possible cyclo-oxygenase-independent mechanism of action.

Whatever the mechanisms that together precipitate intraventricular hemorrhage, it is clear that once periventricular blood appears, most normal cerebrovascular regulation is compromised. Perivascular blood attenuates adrenergic vasoconstriction, endothelium-mediated relaxation, hypercapnic vasodilatation, autoregulation, and a host of other responses. The primary goal for management of periventricular hemorrhage is to attempt to minimize the influences which predispose its occurrence.

## SELECTED READING

Altman DI, Perlman JM, Volpe JJ, Powers WJ. Cerebral oxygen metabolism in newborns. *Pediatrics* 1993; **92**: 99.

Ball WS Jr. Cerebrovascular occlusive disease in childhood. *Neuroimaging Clin N Am* 1994; **4**: 393.

Del Toro J, Louis PT, Goddard Finegold J. Cerebrovascular regulation and neonatal brain injury. *Pediatr Neurol* 1991; **7**: 3.

Greisen G. Effect of cerebral blood flow and cerebrovascular autoregulation on the distribution, type and extent of cerebral injury. *Brain Pathol* 1992; **2**: 223.

Ment LR, Oh W, Ehrenkranz RA *et al*. Low-dose indomethacin therapy and prevention of intraventricular hemorrhage: a multicenter randomized trial. *Pediatrics* 1994; **93**: 543.

Palmer C, Vannucci RC. Potential new therapies for perinatal cerebral hypoxia–ischemia. *Clin Perinatol* 1993; **20**: 411.

Phillis JW. *The regulation of cerebral blood flow*. Ann Arbor: CRC Press, 1993; 425.

Pryds O. Control of cerebral circulation in the high-risk neonate. *Ann Neurol* 1991; **30**: 321.

Rivkin MJ, Volpe JJ. Hypoxic–ischemic brain injury in the newborn. *Semin Neurol* 1993; **13**: 30.

Volpe JJ. Brain injury in the premature infant – current concepts of pathogenesis and prevention. *Biol Neonate* 1992; **62**: 231.

Wood JH. *Cerebral blood flow: physiologic and clinical aspects*. New York: McGraw-Hill, 1987: 792.

Zuckerman SL, Leffler CW, Shibata M. Recent advances and controversies in cerebrovascular physiology in the newborn. *Curr Opin Pediatr* 1993; **5**: 162.

# 31

# Nervous System Pathophysiology

## PATHOPHYSIOLOGY OF SEIZURES

*Epilepsy* is defined as a paroxysmal disturbance of the central nervous system (CNS) which is recurrent, stereotyped and associated with an excessive synchronous and self-limiting neuronal discharge.

### NEUROCHEMICAL AND MORPHOLOGICAL CHANGES IN PARTIAL EPILEPSY

This section is mainly concerned with *partial epilepsy* particularly that arising in the temporal lobe and associated with neuronal hyperexcitability and selective loss of certain neuronal populations in the hippocampus. The typical seizure of temporal lobe origin is the *complex partial seizure* (CPS).

No single model exists which possesses all of the characteristics of human epilepsy. Kindling has traditionally been the paradigm used to model *temporal lobe epilepsy*; it is the phenomenon whereby brief bursts of localized non-polarizing electrical brain stimulation are presented at regular intervals at a constant intensity. Initially these stimuli have little effect

on behavior; however, with repetition, focal afterdischarges and eventually generalized convulsions will develop. Once induced, these latter changes in brain function appear to be permanent. Kindling is conceivably a mechanism by which epileptogenesis is established in humans. *Temporal lobe epilepsy* (TLE) is often a progressive disease in which early, subtle seizure manifestations may escape attention; however, with time, as generalized convulsions emerge, the epileptic engram becomes permanently engraved in the brain and the seizures become intractable. A key criterion for an animal model of chronic epilepsy is that seizures occur spontaneously. In general kindled seizures do not occur spontaneously, but rather are triggered by experimenter-controlled stimulation. However, extensive stimulation of the amygdala, hippocampus, or entorhinal cortex will lead to the appearance of spontaneous seizures.

An alternative model of TLE is the continuous hippocampal stimulation (CHS) model in which electrical stimuli are delivered frequently or nearly continuously and for at least 30 min. This results in the generation of self-sustaining *status epilepticus* (SE) that can continue for several hours and is followed by spontaneous recurrent seizures. In rats these are recorded from approximately one month following the initial stimulation.

The most common pathological finding in human temporal lobes removed in the course of surgical treatment for TLE is hippocampal or Ammon's horn sclerosis (AHS). In AHS the distribution of neuron loss and gliosis in the hippocampus is relatively stereotyped and is characterized by extensive loss of dentate hilar neurons and pyramidal cells in CA1, with a lesser loss in the CA3 and fascia dentata regions, and relative preservation of the CA2 subfield of the hippocampus. This pattern of cell loss has been identified in the brains of many chronic epileptic patients and in those having experienced prolonged status. Loss of dentate hilar neurons (end-folium sclerosis) occurs in all epileptic patients with hippocampal cell loss. Furthermore, end-folium sclerosis is often the only apparent hippocampal lesion. Many individuals with AHS have experienced prolonged *febrile seizures* or SE in childhood, followed by the development of TLE later in childhood or adolescence.

Gamma-amino butyric acid (GABA)ergic dentate basket cells are more resistant to seizure induced neuronal death than other hippocampal neurons. Glutamatergic mossy cells in the dentate hilus, the region between the blades of the granule cell layers, characteristically degenerate in human epilepsy. The mossy cells receive synaptic input from both dentate granule cells and the perforant path, and project to the stratum moleculare of the dentate gyrus, which contains the dendrites of granule cells and interneurons. The preservation of GABAergic interneurons in the epileptic hippocampus, together with a diminution of GABA-mediated inhibition in animals models of TLE has led to the hypothesis that inhibitory GABAergic neurons in the hippocampus are dormant in TLE as a result of being disconnected from their excitatory inputs. The loss of inhibitory basket cell activity would therefore lead to excessive firing of the granule cells, progression of cell death, and the development of an epileptic condition.

The loss of mossy cells also might account for the mossy fiber sprouting observed in both animal models and in human epilepsy. The mossy fibers are the axonic pathway from the dentate gyrus to CA3/CA4. In many animal models of epilepsy there is synaptic re-organization in the mossy fiber pathway. Findings in resected human brain suggest a projection of the mossy fibers to the supragranular region of the inner molecular layer of the dentate gyrus. The mossy fiber pathways in normal human hippocampus do not have a significant projection into the inner molecular layer of the dentate gyrus. The reason for the mossy fiber sprouting into the supragranular layer of the dentate molecular layer appears to be loss of hilar mossy neurons which normally commissurally innervate this region. On the other hand, it is possible that mossy fiber sprouting is generated by seizure-induced changes in granule cell biochemistry.

A strong correlation between mossy fiber synaptic reorganization and the development, progression and permanence of kindling has been demonstrated. These experiments showing mossy fiber reorganization suggest that excitatory plasticity of the hippocampus may contribute to the evolution of epileptic seizures in humans through the development of a recurrent excitatory circuit. In humans the intensity of sprouting shows a positive correlation to the severity of seizures and the severity of hilar cell loss. The findings suggest that early insults, e.g. prolonged febrile seizures, may lead to mossy fiber sprouting, which causes hippocampal hyperexcitability and spontaneous partial seizures. With time, partial seizures become secondarily generalized through a kindling-type mechanism.

## STATUS EPILEPTICUS

Status epilepticus (SE) is a condition of prolonged and/or recurrent seizures that persist for 20 minutes or longer. Mortality and the risk of permanent brain injury increases with the length of status. Convulsive SE is the most common form of SE and one in which seizures are either secondarily generalized from partial seizures or primarily generalized from the start.

In chemically-induced SE, neuronal pathways involved in the initiation and propagation of seizures cannot be specifically defined due to the continued presence of the drug. Repeated trains of electrical stimuli or continuous electrical stimulation delivered through chronically implanted hippocampal or amygdala electrodes produce self-sustaining generalized or limbic SE. Thus in these models, the seizures generate from the site of stimulation.

## What initiates SE?

### Enhancement of excitatory systems

The *N*-methyl-D-aspartate (NMDA) subtype of glutamate receptors (*see* page 342) may be involved in SE initiation; administration of the non-competitive NMDA receptor blocker, MK-801, prevents SE generated in a number of chemical convulsant models. Activation of muscarinic receptors by the administration of high doses of the muscarinic agonist, pilocarpine, can also initiate SE. This effect is suppressed by co-administration of the receptor blockers. Thus chemically-induced SE may be initiated by activation of both glutamate and muscarinic receptors. However, while blockade of NMDA receptors also prevents electrically-induced SE, muscarinic receptor antagonists do not suppress electrically-induced SE. 6-Nitro-7-sulfamoylbenzo (f)-quinoxaline-2,3-dione (NBQX), a blocker of non-NMDA ionotropic α-amino-3-hydroxy-5-methyl-4-isoxazole propionic acid (AMPA) and kainate receptors, prevents electrically-induced SE, suggesting that AMPA and kainate receptors also may have a role in SE initiation. This effect may, however, result from blockage of the receptors involved in SE maintenance (see below). Thus, activation of NMDA and possibly non-NMDA ionotropic glutamate receptors play a major role in SE initiation.

## A blockade of inhibitory mechanisms

Administration of GABA$_A$ antagonists such as bicuculline to experimental animals can cause SE; barbiturates and benzodiazepines which augment GABAergic function are very effective anticonvulsants in SE in humans. However, blocking GABA$_A$ receptors with benzodiazepine inverse agonists or with GABA$_A$ antagonists does not transform brief hippocampal seizures into SE. It is unclear whether GABA levels change prior to SE, although recent studies have shown low GABA levels in human epileptogenic hippocampi and these levels remain unchanged with seizure onset. Thus, although block of GABA$_A$ receptors can generate SE and activation of these receptors can block SE, an unequivocal role for the GABAergic systems in SE generation has not been established.

## Failure of seizure termination mechanisms

Epileptic seizures are usually brief (lasting one to two minutes) and self-limiting, even in the absence of anticonvulsant medication. The nervous system remains refractory to further seizures for a period of time after an epileptic attack. Therefore, if the brain has an endogenous anticonvulsant system which normally terminates seizures and protects the brain postictally from further attacks, then perhaps an alteration or loss of this mechanism results in SE. The strongest evidence points to the involvement of specific anticonvulsant neurochemicals that are liberated during and after the seizure itself. In particular, recent experimental evidence suggests that the purine neuromodulator, adenosine, may play a major role in seizure termination. Within 10 s of the initiation of a seizure in rat and human brain, adenosine levels rise rapidly and reach a peak at times that coincide with seizure arrest. Furthermore, blockers of adenosine receptors can prolong seizures in rat and human brain, suggesting that this dramatic rise in endogenous adenosine is involved in seizure termination. Other endogenous neurochemicals such as opioids and prostaglandins may also play an anticonvulsant role in the brain. However, block of opioid receptors or prostaglandin production does not result in SE.

High doses of methylxanthine adenosine receptor antagonists such as caffeine and theophylline produce SE, as does homocysteine, a drug which depletes adenosine levels in the brain. Blockade of adenosine receptors with caffeine and theophylline transforms brief partial electrically-induced seizures into SE in rats and humans. Similar effects have been shown using the specific A$_1$-adenosine receptor antagonist 8-cyclopentyltheophylline. Pertussis toxin, which uncouples A$_1$-adenosine receptors from G$_i$-proteins, also causes SE in rats, which suggests that block of G$_i$-protein-coupled A$_1$-adenosine receptors causes convulsive SE. Although it is clear that loss of adenosine action can generate SE, it is not known whether convulsive SE occurring spontaneously in human brain involves a loss of this endogenous anticonvulsant system. The NMDA antagonist, MK-801, can prevent 8-cyclopentyltheophylline-induced SE, as well as preventing SE induced by continuous hippocampal stimulation. This suggests that SE could result from a block of adenosine's modulatory effects on glutamate neurotransmission.

## What maintains seizures during SE?

Experimental evidence indicates that SE is not maintained by a single receptor subtype and there are regional differences in receptor subtypes involved. In a number of chemically-induced SE models and after electrically-induced generalized SE, administration of the NMDA receptor antagonist, MK-801, after SE onset inhibits the motor manifestations shown by these animals but does not arrest SE in limbic regions. The suppression of neocortical seizures suggests NMDA receptors maintain seizures in this region but that another glutamate receptor subtype must be involved in maintaining seizures in limbic circuits. These receptors have recently been identified in an electrically-induced SE model as the non-NMDA ionotropic AMPA/kainate receptors; as blockers such as NBQX terminated SE in all regions when administered directly into the brain. This suggests that AMPA/kainate receptors maintain seizures in limbic regions whereas both NMDA and non-NMDA ionotropic AMPA/kainate receptors maintain seizures in neocortical regions. Metabotropic (i.e. G-protein-linked) glutamate receptor blockers were also shown to have effect against electrically-induced SE.

These results suggest that SE is maintained mainly by activation of non-NMDA glutamate type receptors in the brain, although NMDA receptors play a role in maintaining neocortical seizures. The neurotransmitter(s) acting on these receptors to maintain SE remain unclear because there is a controversy as to whether levels of glutamate or aspartate rise during SE, although there is a dramatic rise in glutamate in human brain following brief seizures. Available non-NMDA blocking agents have limitations for clinical use due to limited penetrability into the brain.

## SELECTED READING

Dragunow M. Endogenous anticonvulsant substances. *Neurosci Biobehav Rev* 1986; 10: 229.

Sloviter RS. The functional organization of the hippocampal dentate gyrus and its relevance to the pathogenesis of temporal lobe epilepsy. *Ann Neurol* 1995; 35: 650.

Young D, Dragunow M. Status epilepticus may be caused by loss of adenosine anticonvulsant mechanisms. *Neuroscience* 1994; 58: 245.

# CENTRAL NERVOUS SYSTEM RESPONSE TO INJURY

## HYPOXIC–ISCHEMIC ENCEPHALOPATHY

### Primary and secondary phases of injury

There is experimental, and now clinical evidence, that cerebral injury occurs in two phases after a global hypoxic–ischemic insult: a primary phase during the insult, followed by a secondary phase many hours later. The exact delay between the primary and secondary phases is highly variable, between 30 min and 72 hours, depending on the severity of the injury and the cell population injured. Thus the amount of neuronal loss in the hippocampus increases for many days in patients resuscitated following cardiac arrest. In general, as the insult becomes increasingly severe, the greater the proportion of cell death in the primary phase, and usually the shorter the interval between the phases.

The time course of DNA degradation in the immature rat and the piglet has been studied after moderate hypoxia–ischemia. At 5 hours the DNA is still intact and degradation is noted in the striatum only at 24 hours and in the cortex and CA1 region of the hippocampus by 3 days. The morphology of some of the neurons is consistent with apoptosis (*see* page 365) while others show a necrotic pattern. This implies that at least some of the neuronal damage is due to initiation of complex signals which effectively leads to cells "committing suicide" (i.e. apoptosis) rather than being directly killed by the insult.

The effects of varying periods of reversible global cerebral ischemia and systemic asphyxia have been studied in the fetal sheep using continuous parietal electroencephalogram (EEG) and impedance monitoring. Cortical impedance is a measure of intracellular or cytotoxic edema. The time course of changes after 30 min of cerebral ischemia *in utero* is shown in Fig. 31.1.

Four phases of injury are evident:

■ The primary insult: during ischemia the EEG rapidly becomes isoelectric, while impedance, reflecting cells swelling with depolarization rises dramatically.
■ The phase of suppression: the EEG intensity recovers partially after reperfusion and remains reduced for approximately 10 hours after the insult. In contrast, the impedance signal continues to rise for up to 10 min after reperfusion, then

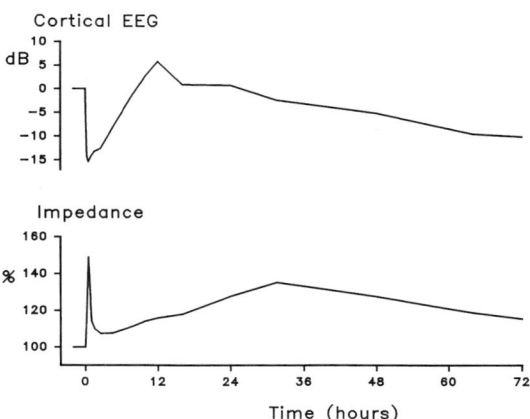

FIGURE 31.1 The consequences of a 30 min episode of cerebral ischemia in fetal sheep. Cortical impedance (upper plot) is a measure of intracellular swelling. The two phases of injury are clearly seen. There is an initial rise in impedance during ischemia which partially resolves during reperfusion. Approximately 9 hours following reperfusion there is a period of secondary EEG hyperactivity, which correlates with seizures, and a rise in impedance.

rapidly recovers, with only minimal residual elevation.
■ Phase of secondary edema: an abrupt increase in EEG intensity occurs about 10 hours after the insult and peaks by 12 hours. This EEG hyperactivity (intensity rises above the preinsult level) corresponds to high voltage spike, polyspike and spike-wave discharges in the EEG. The seizures of phase 3 resolve between 48 and 72 hours. A secondary rise in impedance parallels the onset of seizures, and peaks later, between 36 and 48 hours after the insult, then returns toward the preinsult level by 72 hours.
■ The phase of resolution: the EEG remains markedly suppressed; the degree of suppression is related to the amount of cortical neuronal loss. A recovery of sleep state cycles may occur by 3–5 days.

The effects of increasing duration/severity of cerebral ischemia are not linear. A minimal, 10-min insult in the fetal sheep leads to the acute changes in EEG and impedance. The EEG, however, recovers rapidly (within 4–6 hours), with no secondary phase of hyperactivity; the impedance change resolves fully and there is only minimal selective neuronal loss, mainly in the hippocampus and the parasagittal sulci. As the duration of the insult is increased a fetus is more likely to demonstrate the pattern of delayed EEG hyperactivity, and develop localized infarction in the parasagittal cortical regions. After 40 min of ischemia the increase in impedance persists at the end of the insult. Although a secondary rise in impedance occurs it is attenuated in amplitude relative to that seen after 30 min of ischemia. This suggests that over a critical threshold much of the cerebral damage is occurring in the primary insult, with many fewer cells surviving to die in the secondary phase; global cortical infarction is evident on examination of the brain at 3 days.

Microdialysis studies of amino acid neurotransmitters following ischemia have demonstrated a striking secondary rise in the combined concentration of glutamate and glycine relative to γ-amino butyric acid (GABA) and of byproducts of nitric oxide (NO) in parallel with the secondary rise in cortical impedance.

Magnetic resonance spectroscopy (MRS) provides direct evidence of secondary failure of energy metabolism (associated primarily with mitochondrial function). MRS can indirectly evaluate the relationship of ATP generation to consumption by measuring the ratio of phosphocreatine to inorganic orthophosphate (PCr/$P_i$). A relative fall in the amount of PCr suggests a failure of oxidative phosphorylation. After an hypoxic–ischemic insult in the newborn piglet, the PCr/$P_i$ ratio initially recovers, to return to preinsult levels by 2 hours; it falls again to very low levels by 24 hours postinsult. A similar time course of MRS changes are described in neonates with moderate to severe hypoxic–ischemic encephalopathy (HIE); the decline in PCr/$P_i$ ratio after 24 hours is strongly correlated with the neurodevelopmental outcome at 1 year.

# Mechanisms of neuronal loss

Different, but overlapping multiple mechanisms are involved in the primary and secondary phases of neuronal loss. The major mechanisms implicated in primary neuronal loss are cytotoxic edema, free radical induced cell membrane injury, cytotoxic intracellular calcium accumulation and the excitotoxic effects of glutamate (excitotoxins). Secondary cell death involves primary apoptosis and excitotoxicity. In addition microglial activation may aggravate neuronal injury. Knowledge of these mechanisms may lead to strategic approaches to neuroprotection therapy.

## Cytotoxic edema

Cytotoxic intracellular edema occurs by several mechanisms. Hypoxia induced depolarization leads to $Na^+$ flux into the cell and $K^+$ efflux. Failure of energy-dependent $Na^+$ export prevents maintenance of low intracellular $Na^+$ concentrations. Passive water and $Cl^-$ flux accompanies the increase in intracellular $Na^+$. In addition glutamate acting on the kainate/ α-amino-3-hydroxy-5-methyl-4-isoxazole propionic acid (AMPA) receptor increases $Na^+$ influx via the associated $Na^+$ channel. The cell membrane may be further destabilized by free radical production and consequent membrane lipid peroxidation.

## Free radical-induced cell membrane injury

Oxygen free radical production occurs particularly during the reoxygenation/reperfusion/resuscitation phase. Oxygen free radicals are produced if the reduction of oxygen to water is incomplete, as occurs in asphyxia, and leads to a production of highly reactive chemical intermediates, such as hydroxyl species (*see* page 168). Normally such free radicals are inactivated by scavenger enzymes including superoxide dismutase, catalase and glutathione peroxidase. Increased ADP production leads to increasing concentrations of hypoxanthine which, when oxidized to uric acid by xanthine oxidase, produces oxygen free radicals. Nitric oxide (NO) is a potential further free radical which is also implicated, leading to the formation of highly toxic species. In asphyxial injury free radical production exceeds the endogenous scavenger capacity. Free radicals induce cell loss by inducing lipid peroxidation, affecting mitochondrial and cell membrane integrity.

## Cytotoxic intracellular calcium accumulation

This occurs for three major reasons:

- Failure of energy dependent pumps that maintain the low intracellular free calcium concentrations.
- Failure of sequestration of intracellular calcium in protein bound forms.
- Increased entry to the cell via the N-methyl-D-aspartate (NMDA)-associated calcium conductance.

Calcium accumulation can inappropriately activate a number of enzymes including phospholipase C, leading to cell membrane degradation, liberation of free fatty acids and prostanoid accumulation. These disrupt cellular metabolic pathways and, as some products are vasoactive (*see* page 700), lead to microperfusion changes. In addition, intracellular hydroxyapatite may crystallize secondary to the high free $Ca^{2+}$ irreversibly damaging the cell.

## Excitotoxins

Glutamate and perhaps aspartate accumulate in the synapse during asphyxial injury, in part because of failure of energy dependent reuptake via the glutamate transporters into glia. Glutamate acts on NMDA and non-NMDA receptors, increasing intracellular $Ca^{2+}$ and $Na^+$ concentrations. In addition, the excitatory stimulus increases energetic demands. Excitotoxicity contributes to both primary and delayed cell death. In the latter phase, this is associated with postasphyxial seizures perhaps initiated by the creation of dysfunctional neuronal circuits by neuronal loss during the primary phase. These seizures themselves create additional energetic demands. *Postasphyxial seizures* may contribute to some experimental insults and in neonates seem to be bad prognostically.

## Apoptosis

Neuronal apoptosis is a normal developmental process. It involves the activation and deactivation of a complex cascade of factors (*see* page 100). Transgenic animals over-expressing Bcl-2 (an antiapoptotic protein) are more resistant to asphyxial brain injury. Apoptotic neurons have a characteristic appearance and can be demonstrated both in human neonatal brains after birth asphyxia and in experimental brain injury. It is generally thought that apoptosis is the primary mechanism of delayed cell death. Neurotrophic factors such as insulin-like growth factor (IGF-I) which inhibit developmental neuronal apoptosis will also limit experimental brain injury.

## Microglial activation

Microglia are brain resident macrophages (*see* page 347). If activated excessively, they may produce cytotoxins such as tumor necrosis factor α (TNFα) and NO which may contribute to the death of already injured neurons.

## PATHOPHYSIOLOGY OF ASPHYXIAL INJURY

At the simplest level cerebral injury is due to inadequate delivery of oxygen to the brain. In cardiac arrest, neurons depolarize within seconds. During hypoxia a number of central and peripheral mechanisms act together to maintain oxygen delivery to the brain. The cerebral vascular resistance falls while the total peripheral resistance rises; thus cerebral blood flow is increased (*see* page 437). As well as a direct effect of hypoxia, hypercapnia in asphyxia contributes to this vasodilatation. Furthermore, the extraction of oxygen by the brain increases. These factors allow the cerebral oxygen consumption ($CMRO_2$) to remain constant over a $PaO_2$ range of 14–36 mmHg (1.86–4.78 kPa). In severe asphyxia cerebral blood flow (CBF) can no longer be increased; $CMRO_2$ begins to fall when oxygen content falls to less than about 1 mM.

If oxygen uptake was the only important factor the amount of damage should clearly be proportional to the total "oxygen debit," i.e. duration × reduction in $CMRO_2$. For many years, however, it has been clear that there are major differences in the amount of damage seen in different regions of the brain after any given insult, and that most neurons can survive periods of complete loss of high energy phosphates. Susceptibility may vary with differing cell populations, stage of development, the pattern and type of insult, and the pre-existing metabolic condition of the fetus.

## FACTORS AFFECTING THE PATTERN OF DAMAGE

## Cell populations

A brief period of dense forebrain ischemia in the adult rat or gerbil is associated with selective loss of pyramidal neurons of CA1, medium sized striatal neurons, and neocortical neurons in layers 3, 5 and 6. That this selective vulnerability does not correlate with differential CBF during global ischemia, implies that additional metabolic factors must be considered. Vulnerable neurons tend to be metabolically active, do not express nitric oxide synthetase (NOS), and tend to have large inputs of excitatory neurotransmitters (*see* page 342).

## Developmental age

The relationship between developmental age, different insults and the different lesions seen at postmortem or by modern imaging techniques is still unclear. Total CBF increases with age, more so in the cortex than the hindbrain and the hypoxic increase in CBF increases with age, although the response to hypercapnia matures earlier. Further, a preferential increase in the CBF to the brainstem relative to the cortex is seen during hypoxic–ischemic insults in all immature species studied compared to that seen in adults. This differential perfusion may explain the frequent pattern of parasagittal necrosis of the cortex, and dorsal hippocampus seen in term infants.

Preterm infants appear to preferentially suffer lesions of the periventricular white matter (and of the brainstem) although this may occur at term as well. This may be related to a relative reduction in CBF to this region in immature animals. Areas of the brain that are undergoing rapid developmental changes may have increased susceptibility, but detailed relationships have not been established.

Neuronal tolerance to anoxia varies dramatically with age. In all species studied the fetus or immature animal can tolerate greater durations of anoxia or ischemia without damage compared to adult animals. This is not a simple phenomenon however. Preliminary data have been presented suggesting that while the midgestation fetal sheep may have much less damage after a moderate insult, they may show much greater damage with a slightly more severe insult, once some threshold has been crossed; these changes in susceptibility may also show regional variations.

## Patterns of insult

A purely hypotensive insult tends to cause a watershed pattern of injury, often with damage restricted to vulnerable groups of neurons. Venous or arterial obstruction, whether thrombotic or hemorrhagic, of a single vessel causes a stroke-like infarction in the territory of that vessel. Not all damage is, however, caused by a single long insult. Short insults which individually cause little or no damage, repeated before the neurons have fully recovered membrane function, produce synergistic injury in the hippocampus and parietal cortex of the adult rat and gerbil, such that several short insults an hour apart cause a similar amount of damage to a single long insult. The pattern of injury may be altered as well, with a relative increase in damage to the ventral thalamus, but reduced in the substantia nigra and inferior colliculus. In fetal sheep, repeated periods of ischemia produce a disproportionate increase in striatal injury, compared with the cortex. When the interval between insults was only 1 hour, three 10-min insults produced a similar degree of hippocampal and cortical injury to a single 30-min insult. When the interval was increased to 5 hours, cortical damage was only trivially greater than after a single 10-min insult, but striatal damage was still as great as that seen after a single 30-min insult. This relative augmentation of damage to the basal ganglia by many short insults is also seen in studies of repeated brief episodes of complete umbilical occlusion in the sheep, and in prolonged partial asphyxia, with episodes of hypotension.

The increased susceptibility of the striatum suggests a longer latency of recovery in the striatum at this age, which requires further investigation. In view of the often intermittent nature of intrapartum asphyxia, with acute compromise during contractions, this mechanism may be a common precursor of striatal damage; different spacing between insults would account for the variable amount of associated cortical damage. These studies shed light on the very poor correlation between cord pH and base deficit and any subsequent encephalopathy.

## Effects of fetal wellbeing/growth

The fetus with intrauterine growth retardation (IUGR) appears to be more vulnerable to asphyxial injury; the limited experimental evidence supports this. The IUGR fetus may be compromised by reduced reserve capacity for cerebral oxygen delivery, reduced metabolic reserves and altered neurotransmitter activity. One major confounding variable, however, is that IUGR also affects cerebral development. Although cerebral oxidative metabolism is reported to be normal, IUGR has been associated with accelerated maturation of cortical structures and of brainstem function (using brainstem auditory evoked potentials) in the fetal sheep and human neonate. Accompanying this developmental change is reduced cerebral myelination, altered synaptogenesis and smaller brain size in the rat and sheep. Retardation of the maturation of EEG

spectra occurs in the rat subjected to protein deprivation, as well as perturbations of neuromodulator expression.

## The effects of remodeling of cerebral function

Although neuronal proliferation does not occur after birth, a considerable amount of recovery can take place following injury; recovery is probably greater in the immature brain. The redundancy of motorneuron innervation, for example, which is eliminated during development, seems to allow better recovery from a purely unilateral injury than from a more diffuse injury. Much short-term recovery is due to reversal of functional depression in undamaged structures that are interconnected with damaged regions. Both peptide growth factors and spontaneous electrical activity influence recovery, and are closely connected. The main cellular events following loss of targets or inputs include dendritic stripping, followed by sprouting and re-establishment of interconnections. Invading glial cells separate the synapses during the first 5 days following injury in the hippocampus, with closely paralleled electrophysiologic changes.

Global neurotrophic activity begins to increase around 3–5 days after central nervous system (CNS) injury particularly in the developing brain, reaching a maximum at 8–15 days. Their function at this late period, well removed from the injury, may be to promote repair and neurite outgrowth. Intracerebral grafts of fetal CNS tissue or cultured astrocytes probably promote functional recovery by supplying neurotrophic factors. Putative neurotrophic factors include basic fibroblast growth factor (FGF) and IGF-I.

Growth factor activity is high in the developing brain compared with adults, both in basal conditions and in response to injury with differential expression of some factors (see page 368). There is now increasing experimental evidence that some exogenous growth factors (e.g. IGF-I) markedly reduce neuronal death during the suppression phase after injury. Endogenous growth factors may support neuronal survival *in vitro* or *in vivo*. The role of electrical activity is complex; it may directly help maintain homeostasis in target neurons but also may stimulate the release of neurotrophic factors. This may be one mechanism by which glia protect neurons *in vitro* from excitotoxins.

In conclusion, experimental studies based on the data presented above suggest that a range of potential treatments several hours postinsult, including exogenous neurotrophic growth factors, hypothermia, and antioxidant and antiexcitotoxic agents can reduce the degree of cerebral damage following ischemic injury, confirming that a therapeutic window of opportunity does exist, and that such interventions may have clinical benefit.

## SELECTED READING

Choi DW. Calcium: Still center-stage in hypoxic–ischemic neuronal death. *Trends Neurosci* 1995; **18**: 58.

Gluckman PD, Beilharz EJ, Johnston BM *et al*. Growth factors and perinatal asphyxia. *Dev Endocrinol* 1994; **6**: 185.

Roth SC, Azzopardi D, Edwards AD *et al*. Relation between cerebral oxidative metabolism following birth asphyxia and neurodevelopmental outcome and brain growth at one year. *Dev Med Child Neurol* 1992; **34**: 285.

Williams CE, Mallard EC, Tan WKM, Gluckman PD. Pathophysiology of perinatal asphyxia. *Clin Perinatol* 1993; **20**: 305.

# PERIPHERAL NERVE INJURY AND REGENERATION

Most peripheral nerves contain both motor and sensory nerve fibers. The motor component of a peripheral nerve may be regarded as a final common pathway, connecting motorneurons and autonomic postganglionic axons with their peripheral targets. The sensory component conveys pain stimuli (from nerve endings in the skin, internal organs and tendons), vibration and touch sensibility from specialized receptors (e.g. Pacinian and Meissner corpuscles) (*see* page 376) and proprioceptive information from the muscle spindles and the Golgi tendon organs (*see* page 403). Axons are contained in slender nerve trunks together with specialized connective tissue structures and blood vessels which provide protection and nutrition to the nerve fibers. A nerve lesion may induce paralysis, and anesthesia, and widespread metabolic effects and/or cell death of distant nerve cell groups and target organs. Although restoration of function after injury is more complete in the peripheral (PNS) than in the central nervous system (CNS), traumatic lesions in the PNS are often associated with permanent sequelae such as chronic pain, impaired activation of sweat glands, loss of stereognosis or inappropriate muscle control. Reactions in the nervous system to injury differ in several respects in the immature and the mature individual. Although the immature nervous system is more susceptible to neuronal death after a lesion, both experimental and clinical observations indicate that regeneration and recovery of function is much better before maturity. It has been suggested that the regrowing axons have a greater ability to orient due to persisting diffusible or surface bound cues in targets and satellite cells in the young individual in combination with a greater degree of cerebral plasticity that will allow adaptation for misdirected axons.

## The axon reaction

Transection of the axon induces rapid metabolic and morphological changes in the affected neuron. A dissolution of Nissl bodies (i.e. cromatolysis, due to a changed configuration of the granular endoplastic reticulum), swelling of cell body, retraction of dendrites, loss of synaptic boutons and an excentric position of the nucleus are accompanied by a decrease in neurotransmitter production and an upregulation of the synthesis of neurotrophic proteins. Many neurons show altered expression of neuropeptides in the acute phase after the lesion. The amount of substance P and calcitonin gene-related peptide (CGRP) is decreased in injured primary sensory neurons; vasoactive intestinal peptide (VIP) is upregulated. Spinal motorneurons show an increased content of CGRP. Some changes are transient while others are reversed only if the neuron can successfully re-establish its contact with an appropriate target. Neurons which fail to regenerate the axon become atrophic or die by retrograde degeneration.

## Retrograde neuronal death

With the exception for the neurons of the olfactory epithelium, axotomy-induced retrograde cell death represents a permanent impediment for re-establishment of function. Unlike apoptosis, during prenatal development and axotomy-induced cell death in the olfactory system, retrograde cell death does not activate a suicidal program in affected cells. Instead of DNA fragmentation, cell shrinkage and pyknosis (the characteristics of apoptosis), these neurons show signs of necrosis. It is not fully understood why some neurons die from lesion-induced cell death, but interruption of the retrograde transport of neurotrophins may be a factor of importance. Motorneurons can be rescued from retrograde cell death by the addition of ciliary neurotrophic factor (CNTF) and brain-derived neurotrophic factor (BDNF); retrograde cell death is more widespread in young individuals than in adults. The incidence of retrograde cell death is higher after severance of the nerve trunk (neurotmesis) than after interruption of the neurites in a continuous nerve trunk (axonotmesis). In addition, the magnitude of cell death is dependent on the proximity of the lesion. Thus, an injury close to the cell body may result in the death of a neuron which would survive a distal lesion. There are some considerable differences in the reactions of different types of neurons. Primary sensory neurons seem generally more susceptible than motorneurons. The small pain-transducing primary sensory neurons appear to be more vulnerable than larger sensory

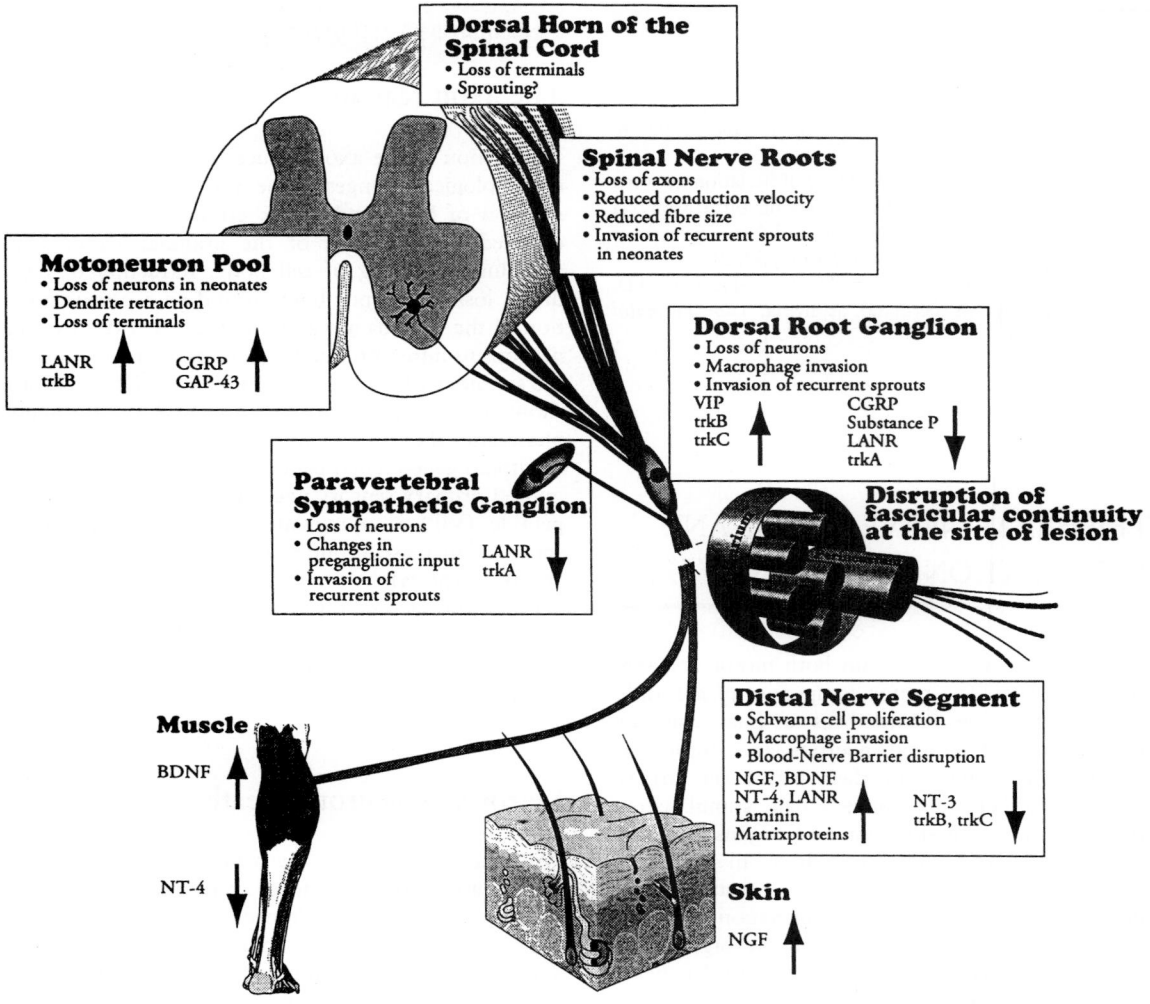

**Dorsal Horn of the Spinal Cord**
• Loss of terminals
• Sprouting?

**Spinal Nerve Roots**
• Loss of axons
• Reduced conduction velocity
• Reduced fibre size
• Invasion of recurrent sprouts in neonates

**Motoneuron Pool**
• Loss of neurons in neonates
• Dendrite retraction
• Loss of terminals

LANR        CGRP
trkB        GAP-43

**Dorsal Root Ganglion**
• Loss of neurons
• Macrophage invasion
• Invasion of recurrent sprouts
VIP         CGRP
trkB        Substance P
trkC        LANR
            trkA

**Paravertebral Sympathetic Ganglion**
• Loss of neurons
• Changes in preganglionic input
• Invasion of recurrent sprouts
LANR
trkA

**Disruption of fascicular continuity at the site of lesion**

**Muscle**
BDNF

NT-4

**Distal Nerve Segment**
• Schwann cell proliferation
• Macrophage invasion
• Blood-Nerve Barrier disruption
NGF, BDNF
NT-4, LANR        NT-3
Laminin           trkB, trkC
Matrixproteins

**Skin**
NGF

FIGURE 31.2 Schematic drawing illustrating alterations in cell numbers, transmitter content as well as immunoreactivity and/or mRNA levels for neurotrophins and neurotrophin receptors after peripheral nerve injury. Abbreviations: CGRP, calcitonin gene-related peptide; VIP, vasoactive intestinal peptide; GAP-43, a growth-associated protein; NGF, nerve growth factor; BDNF, brain-derived neurotrophic factor; NT-3, neurotrophin 3; NT-4, neurotrophin 4; LANR, low-affinity neurotrophin receptor; trkA, high affinity receptor for NGF; trkB, the high affinity receptor for BDNF and NT-4; trkC, the high-affinity receptor for NT-3.

neurons. The $\gamma$ motoneurons which innervate the muscle spindles (*see* page 403) may die from retrograde cell death whereas the larger $\alpha$-motorneurons usually resist the same type of lesion.

The death of a number of primary sensory neurons is followed by a so-called transganglionic loss of axon terminals within the CNS. Retrograde cell death in a paravertebral sympathetic ganglion or in motorneurons may elicit transneuronal changes in the impinging presynaptic neurons.

## Acute reactions at the site of lesion

(Fig. 31.3)

The peripheral nerve trunks are surrounded by the epineurial sheath. The nerve fibers aggregate in nerve fascicles which also contain endoneurial collagen fibers and blood vessels. These fascicles are separated from the loose epineurial connective tissue and blood vessels by the tough perineurial sheaths, which also form a

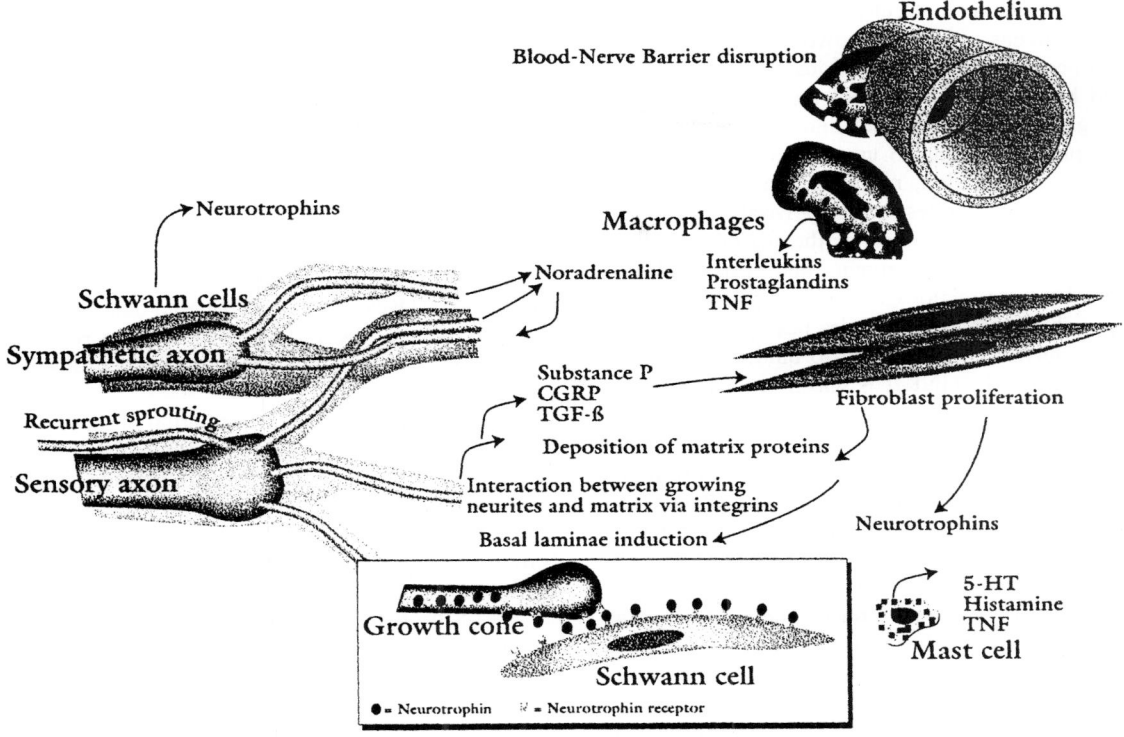

FIGURE 31.3 Schematic drawing illustrating possible interactions between neural mediators/transmitters, cytokines, growth factors and matrix molecules at the site of a peripheral nerve injury. Abbreviations: TGF, transforming growth factor; TNF, tumor necrosis factor; 5-HT, 5-hydroxytryptamine; and CGRP, calcitonin gene-related peptide.

diffusion barrier between the epineurium and endoneurium. The endoneurial blood vessels have a very restricted permeability, i.e. the blood–nerve barrier (BNB), which creates a privileged internal milieu inside the nerve fascicles. The BNB, for example, prevents the influx of proteins and the spread of epineurial edema. After nerve lesions the permeability in the endoneurial blood vessels is increased. This BNB dysfunction results in the invasion of macrophages and other inflammatory cells which contribute to the removal of debris resulting from Wallerian degeneration of the nerve fibers. These cells also represent important sources of interleukins (ILs), transforming factor β (TGFβ) and prostaglandins (PGs). These molecules may induce a cascade of reactions and regulate the synthesis of neurotrophins and matrix molecules in Schwann cells and endoneurial fibroblasts. The deposition of matrix proteins may require the interaction of different cell types. For instance, basal laminae formation in Schwann cells is dependant on the presence of fibroblasts. The functional anatomy of the perineurium and endoneurial blood vessels may be affected for a prolonged time, due to fibroblast invasion and scar formation at the lesion site.

## AXONAL REGROWTH AND TARGET REINNERVATION

## Role of recognition molecules and neurotrophins

The division of a peripheral nerve results in the unavoidable degradation and removal of the distal axon segment and associated myelin sheaths by Wallerian degeneration. Proliferating Schwann cells and persisting basal laminae form the so-called bands of Büngner. Multiple axonal sprouts emerge at the lesion site or from nodes of Ranvier in the proximal axon segment. Growth cones at the front end of the sprouts elongate after sending out thin filopodia which respond to environmental signals and either retract or dilate. This type of growth cone navigation is dependent on guidance cues in the environment. Possible mechanisms for pathfinding include differential substrate adhesivity or activation of intracellular messengers via specific transmembrane receptors. Of importance in this context are the different groups of recognition molecules including the cadherins, proteoglycans and integrins as well as molecules containing immunoglobin-like domains, epidermal growth factor-like repeats or fibronectin type III-like domains. Signaling accomplished by punctate deposits of matrix proteins may induce growth cone navigation and redirection by protein to protein binding to integrins associated to the axolemma. In addition, neural-recognition molecules may carry carbohydrates such as polysialic acid or oligomannosidic glycans indicating the possible contribution of carbohydrate–protein and carbohydrate–carbohydrate interactions to the recognition process. Of special interest are molecules bearing the HNK-1 glycan (which was first known to bind to the human natural killer cell). HNK-1 is selectively expressed by myelinating Schwann cells that are associated with motor axons and has been suggested to play a role in motor axon-specific reinnervation of original targets.

The target-derived neurotrophins, which conceivably have an important function in maintaining neuronal survival and phenotype, can also induce a powerful neurite outgrowth. Gradients of neurotrophins may attract and direct growth cones. The neurotrophins of the nerve growth factor (NGF) family (see page 368) show a time-dependent expression in reactive Schwann cells and denervated targets. NGF is up-regulated in Schwann cells and skin, whereas the content of brain-derived neurotrophic factor (BDNF) is increased in Schwann cells and muscle. Neurotrophin 4 (NT-4) is down-regulated in muscle, but up-regulated in Schwann cells, and neurotrophin 3 (NT-3) is decreased in Schwann cells. The low affinity neurotrophin receptor (LANR or p75) which can bind all these neurotrophins is up-regulated in Schwann cells and lesioned motorneurons, but down-regulated in primary sensory neurons and paravertebral sympathetic neurons after nerve injury. The tyrosine kinase receptor trkA is a transmembrane high affinity signal transducing receptor for NGF; trkB is the receptor for BDNF and NT-4, whereas NT-3 is thought to exert its effects via interaction with trkC. These high affinity neurotrophin receptors show a dynamic regulation after lesions. trkB is up-regulated in lesioned motorneurons and trkB and trkC are increased in primary sensory neurons. trkA is down-regulated in primary sensory neurons while trkB and trkC are down-regulated in the distal nerve stump. LANR on the surface of reactive Schwann cells has been suggested to concentrate and present NGF or BDNF to the growth cones.

# Regrowth of immature axons

A period of natural cell death in prenatal motorneuron development is followed by a postnatal period of sensitivity to axonal injury. This period of vulnerability coincides with very low ciliary neurotrophic factor (CNTF) levels in the sciatic nerve before CNTF increases to adult levels. It has been demonstrated that local application of CNTF prevents lesion-induced degeneration of newborn rat motorneurons. The time course of CNTF expression, its regional tissue distribution and its cytosolic localization indicate a role as a lesion factor rather than a target-derived neurotrophic molecule.

In young individuals, a large fraction of the sprouts are misdirected and grow for considerable distances along the proximal nerve. Such retrograde sprouts may even invade the spinal nerve roots, the pia mater and paravertebral sympathetic ganglia. Strands of Schwann cells, vacant after retrograde neuronal degeneration, can facilitate retrograde sprouting.

Matrix proteins such as laminin, collagen type IV and tenascin may also play a role in axonal maturation since they are known to induce both neurite elongation and axonal polarization in vitro. Sprouts which enter the bands of Büngner may eventually reach targets and myelinate. Even after successful reinnervation, the axons in the distal nerve segment exhibit reduced conduction velocities and decreased internodal spacing. In young individuals, neurons may be affected by a lesion-induced non-reversible growth retardation which affects axon diameter and conduction velocity also in the proximal axon segment. In addition, specialized sensory receptors such as the Pacinian corpuscles may show signs of maldevelopment after early postnatal injuries. Autonomic efferent systems, such as the sweat gland innervation, can be severely affected.

## SELECTED READING

Korsching S. The neurotrophic factor concept: A reexamination. J Neurosci 1993; 13: 2739.

Rothwell NJ, Hopkins SJ. Cytokines and the nervous system II. Trends Neurosci 1995; 18: 130.

Schachner M, Martini R. Glycans and the modulation of neural-recognition molecule function. Trends Neurosci 1995; 18: 183.

Sunderland S. Nerves and nerve injuries. Edinburgh: Churchill Livingstone, 1978.

Thoenen H. The changing scene of neurotrophic factors. Trends Neurosci 1991; 14: 165.

# 32

# Muscle Physiology and Development

Thomas Sejersen, Lars Edström and
Lars-Erik Thornell

## THE MUSCLE FIBER

The vertebrate muscle fiber is a single, multinucleated (syncytial) cell, typically 10–100 mm in diameter and several centimeters long. Its cell membrane, sarcolemma, is composed of a plasma membrane to which a basal lamina is attached. The main muscle fiber constituents are myofibrils 1–3 mm in diameter, nuclei, sarcoplasmic reticulum, the T-system, mitochondria and cytoskeletal organelles. Each muscle fiber is innervated by a terminal motor axon at a specialized synapse, the neuromuscular junction. The postsynaptic membrane, the motor end plate, is a specialized area of the sarcolemma containing acetylcholine receptors (*see* page 366). In immature muscle fibers acetylcholine receptors are widely distributed over the sarcolemma; this distribution is also reproduced in denervated mature muscle fibers. One single motorneuron and its muscle fibers constitute the motor unit, the smallest functional unit of the motor system.

## Muscle fiber structure and physiology of muscle contraction

The ultrastructure of the myofibril is demonstrated in Fig. 32.1. The striation pattern of dark and light bands of the myofibril repeats with a periodicity of 2–3 μm. Each unit is called a sarcomere, the fundamental contractile element of the striated muscle fiber. The band pattern is determined by a precisely ordered arrangement of contractile filaments within the myofibril. The A-band contains an array of thick (15 nm diameter) myofilaments, in longitudinal register parallel to the fibril axis. The thick filaments are interconnected by the M-line. The I-bands contain the thin (8 nm diameter) filaments which are anchored to the Z-discs. The thin filaments also overlap the thick filaments in the A-band. The H-zone is less dense than the rest of the A-band owing to the absence of overlapping thin filaments. The thick filaments are composed of actin, troponin and tropomyosin molecules. The myosin molecules contain six polypeptide chains: two heavy chains (myosin heavy chain, MHC, 200 kD) and two pairs of light chains (myosin light chain, MLC, 15–27 kD). The myosin heavy chains form a rod and a head portion. The head has both a functional and a structural domain, i.e. it contains the actin binding site and the myosin ATPase activity. The T-system of a muscle cell is a network of tubular invaginations of the plasma membrane. Specific functional associations, triads, are formed with the sarcoplasmic reticulum (SR). The SR is equivalent to the endoplasmic reticulum of other cells and thus represents an intracellular tubular system. It captures, stores and releases $Ca^{2+}$. The T-system has the function of carrying electrical depolarization into the cell to activate contraction by causing $Ca^{2+}$ release from the SR. The myofibrillar proteins, actin and myosin, are responsible for the transduction of chemical energy into mechanical work when muscle contracts. The actin–myosin complex hydrolyzes ATP. Troponin is a $Ca^{2+}$-binding protein. In combination with tropomyosin it is a regulator of the contractile activity of muscle. At low levels of $Ca^{2+}$ the actin–myosin interaction is inhibited by tro-

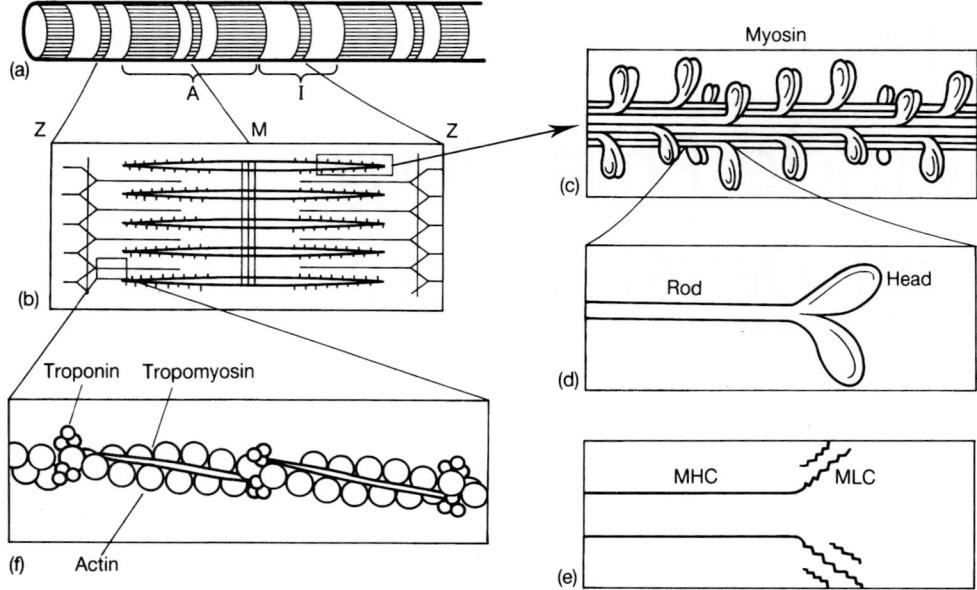

FIGURE 32.1 Schematic model of the structure and composition of the thick and thin filaments. (a) Myofibril. (b) A sarcomere interdigitating thick and thin filaments. The thick filaments are anchored in the M-band and the thin filaments in the Z-discs. (c) The thick filaments are composed of myosin molecules which have two heads and a rod portion (d). (e) Two myosin heavy chains (MHC) form the rod and the major portion of the heads, which in addition contain two pairs of myosin light chains (MLC). (f) The thin filaments are composed of a helix of ball-shaped actin molecules with thin strands of tropomyosin and troponin molecules located at regular intervals.

ponin–tropomyosin resulting in low ATPase activity and a relaxed muscle. When the muscle is stimulated to contract, $Ca^{2+}$ is released from the SR, increasing the concentration of $Ca^{2+}$ in the sarcoplasm. Troponin then binds $Ca^{2+}$, the inhibitory effect of troponin–tropomyosin is removed, actin and myosin are able to interact, ATPase activity increases and the muscle contracts.

Skeletal muscle fibers can be described as slow and fast twitch, based on physiological, morphological, histochemical and biochemical characteristics. Fast twitch and slow twitch fibers are organized into separate motor units where the muscle fibre type is matched to the motorneuron discharge properties. Thus typical slow twitch motor units are responsible for postural muscle function and typical fast twitch motor units are responsible for rapid movements. There are structural differences between typical slow twitch and fast twitch fibers. The Z-discs are broader in the former than in the latter and the M-line morphology is specific to fiber type.

The speed of contraction of individual muscle fibers is related to the myosin ATPase content of the fiber and properties of the heavy chain of the myosin molecule. Thus separate myosin isoforms (slow, or fast subtype e.g. type IIA, IIB, IIX) are related to slow twitch and fast twitch fiber types. Embryonic and fetal isoforms of MHC are found in immature muscle fibers but may be up-regulated in adult fibers under pathological conditions. The physiological impact of differ-

ent fiber types is related to their differences in frequency–force relation. Thus a slow twitch fiber produces maximal force in full fusion at a lower contraction frequency than a fast twitch type and at a lower energy cost. The contraction properties are not only dependent on the isoform of myosin molecule but also on the properties of the SR.

Many neuromuscular disorders result in a mismatch between contractile properties of muscle fibers and the discharge pattern of their motorneuron, which alter the functional prerequisites for the motor units. Specific ion channels are responsible for the conductance of $K^+$, $Na^+$, $Cl^-$ and $Ca^{2+}$, and for the excitation of the muscle plasma membrane which elicits muscle contraction by an excitation–contraction coupling process. In hereditary neuromuscular disorders mutations are related to defects in specific ion channels. Thus, *hypokalemic periodic paralysis* and *paramyotonia congenita* are caused by a mutation (17q13.1–13.3) affecting an α-subunit of the sodium channel (SCN4A). These two clinical entities are thus allelic. In *congenital myotonia (Thomsen* and *Becker myotonia)* a mutation (7q35) affects a chloride channel component (CLC-1). In the autosomal form of *hypokalemic periodic paralysis*, a mutation (1q31–32) affects the dihydropyridine receptor of the $Ca^{2+}$ channel. A mutation of the ryanodine receptor gene of the $Ca^{2+}$-release channel located in the SR is responsible for *central core disease* and some cases of *malignant hyperthermia*.

# EMBRYONIC ORIGIN OF SKELETAL MUSCLE

The majority of skeletal muscle cells originate from mesodermal cells in the somites of the early developing embryo (Fig. 32.2a). In human development, somite pairs begin to form adjacent to the notochord and the neural tube around day 20. It continues in a caudal direction to reach the final approximately 37 somite pairs around day 30. This rostral-to-caudal order of somite formation eventually affects the later temporal order of muscle development. The somites depend on interaction with the notochord and/or neural tube for correct formation of vertebral muscle, whereas limb and body wall muscle development is independent of this interaction.

Within one day after formation, cells in the ventral region of somites form the sclerotome (future vertebrae and ribs), and cells in the dorsal–lateral region develop into the dermamyotome. Subsequently, myotomal cells form beneath the dermamyotome, elongate caudally to the end of each somite, and eventually give rise to the vertebral muscles. The skeletal muscle of the trunk and limbs are derived from precursor cells that migrate out from the lateral region of the dermamyotome. In humans, limb buds appear around 28 days' gestation. Two major muscle masses are formed initially, separated by precursors of bones and tendons. The ventral muscle mass gives rise to extensors, supinators, and abductors; the dorsal muscle mass gives rise to flexors, pronators, and adductors. Extracellular matrix (ECM) components and the integrin-family of ECM-binding cell membrane proteins are essential for successful migration of muscle precursor cells distally into the limb buds. The migrating myogenic cells undergo rapid proliferation before they eventually withdraw from the cell cycle, fuse into multinucleated myotubes, and undergo further maturation to form mature muscle fibers. In the gastrocnemius muscle, the first myotubes appear around 45 days' gestation in the human. By 95 days' gestation more than 80 per cent of the nuclei in the muscle are present in multinucleated myo-

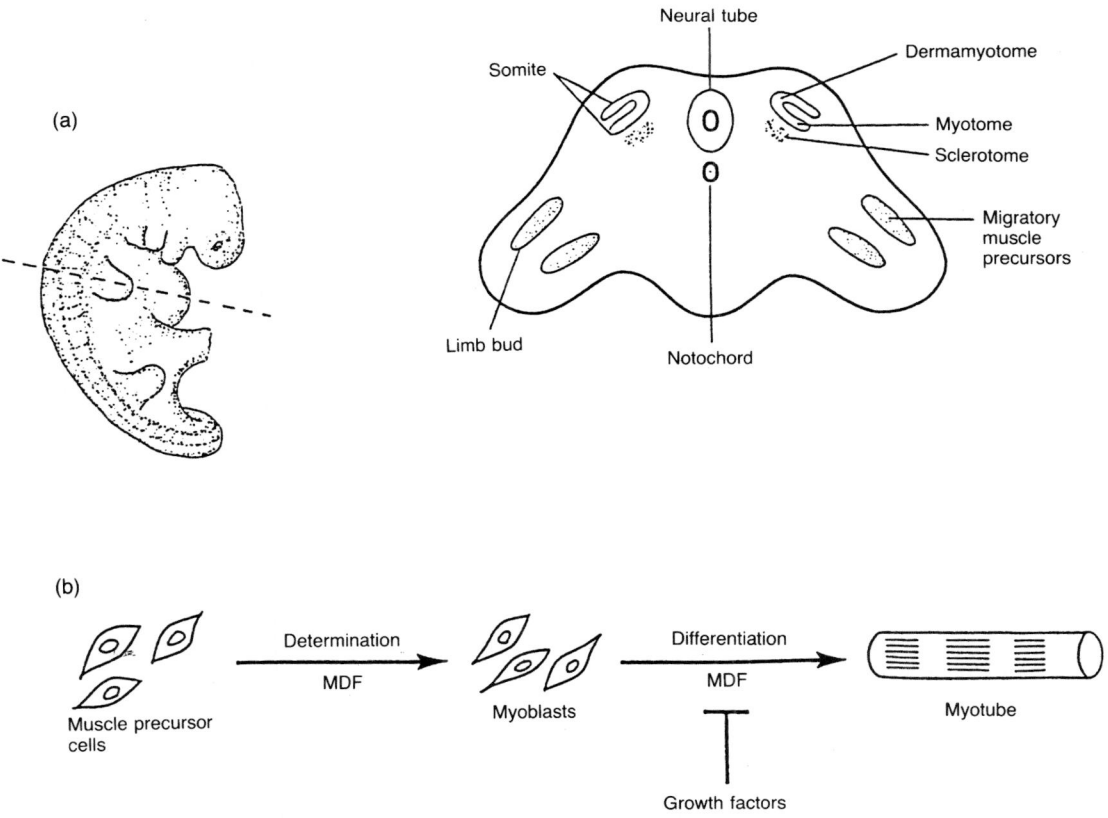

FIGURE 32.2 (a) Side view (left) and cross-section (right) of a human embryo at the end of the fourth week. At this stage the somite is subdivided into dermamyotome, myotome, and sclerotome. Muscle precursor cells migrate into the limb buds. (b) Myogenic determination factors (MDF) predestine somitic mesodermal cells to become determined for the myogenic pathway. MDF also affect subsequent differentiation including myotube formation and activation of muscle-specific genes, a process inhibited by growth factors. (Illustration made by Eva Hall, Karolinska Institute.)

tubes; by the 20th week few mononucleate cells persist. The formation of myotubes is not constant, but rather takes place in at least three waves, called primary, secondary, and tertiary. Myofibers derived from primary, secondary and tertiary myotubes eventually become indistinguishable in the adult, but their phenotypes and neural dependence differ transiently. They most likely represent distinct myogenic lineages.

During maturation of the myofibers the nuclei shift to a subsarcolemmal position typical of the mature cell. Central nuclei are commonly found in association with pathological processes, e.g. *centronuclear myopathy* and *myotonic dystrophy*.

Not all myoblasts differentiate to myotubes in fetal life. Mononucleate myoblasts persist as so-called satellite cells in adult muscle, where they account for 2–5 per cent of the number of nuclei. If the muscle fiber is damaged, such satellite cells are activated and initiate regeneration, e.g. in early phases of muscular dystrophies.

## MUSCLE FIBER DEVELOPMENT

Concomitant with withdrawal from the replicative cell cycle and myotube formation, a number of muscle-specific proteins accumulate. Among them are proteins of the myofibril, the sarcolemma, the sarcoplasmic reticulum, and enzymes essential in muscle metabolism. Failure to produce correct proteins in these structures have been associated with hereditary neuromuscular diseases, e.g. muscular dystrophies and ion channel diseases (sarcolemmal defects), and glycogenoses and mitochondrial myopathies (defects in muscle metabolism).

Skeletal muscle genes are subject to complex differences in their regulation. An important developmental aspect of the regulation of muscle specific genes is the great variety of isoforms due to the existence of multigene families. Most of the major myofibrillar components, e.g. myosin, actin, tropomyosin, and troponin, exist in fast, slow, cardiac and developmental isoforms, encoded by different genes. Another important level of isoform regulation is the existence of alternative RNA splicing.

Several of the muscle-specific genes encode myofibrillar and cytoskeletal proteins. Myofibrillogenesis starts with the formation of Z-brushes composed of α-actinin and actin to which titin and intermediate filaments become linked. The primitive A-bands are formed independently, and at a later developmental stage the interaction of the Z-brushes and the A-bands occur to form the sarcomeres in the myofibrils. Mutated forms of myofibrilla proteins have been identified in *familiar hypertrophic cardiomyopathy* (cardiac β-myosin heavy chain) and in *nemaline myopathy* (tropomyosin).

The dystrophin–glycoprotein complex is a trans-sarcolemmal structure consisting of several proteins considered to form a linkage between the myofibrils and the extracellular matrix component laminin. Deficiency of proteins in this linkage chain play an important role in the molecular pathogenesis of several forms of muscular dystrophy. In *Duchenne muscular dystrophy* there is an almost total lack of dystrophin. In *Becker muscular dystrophy* the dystrophin expression is reduced, and/or leads to an abnormal protein. Collectively, Duchenne and Becker muscular dystrophies are denoted *dystrophinopathies. Severe congenital autosomal recessive muscular dystrophy* (SCARMD) is associated with mutations in the gene for adhalin, a dystrophin-associated glycoprotein. Finally, a large proportion of cases of *congenital muscular dystrophy* are associated with mutations in merosin, a subunit of laminin in the extracellular matrix.

The sarcoplasmic reticulum (SR) and transverse (T) tubules are formed in parallel with myofibrillogenesis. In embryonic muscle cells the early SR is seen as tubular extrusions from the endoplasmic reticulum, which forms reticular networks around the developing myofibrils. An early association between the Z-disc of the myofibril and the SR has been observed. At first, early SR form irregular associations with the developing T-tubules. Later on there is formation of triads which are composed of SR and T-system components.

## DEVELOPMENT OF MUSCLE FIBER INNERVATION

Motorneurons establish contacts with muscle fibers at synapses (neuromuscular junctions), a process beginning around gestational week 10. Early interaction with neural tissue is important in the formation of some myoblasts from non-myogenic precursor cells. Later there are two phases in myogenesis; first, where myogenesis and fiber type formation is independent of innervation, and later a phase where further development of fiber types is motorneuron-dependent.

Developmental failure to form motorneurons results in *spinal muscular atrophy* (SMA). Mutations in two different genes within the locus (5q13), both implied to be important for motorneuron development, have recently been identified in patients with SMA.

## REGULATION OF MUSCLE DEVELOPMENT

Knowledge about molecular events that underlie the formation of skeletal muscle has increased considerably the past few years. Most notably, the importance of myogenic determination factors (MDFs) in myogenic regulation has been recognized. In vertebrate embryos, skeletal muscle formation is controlled by the MDF family of muscle-specific basic-helix–loop-helix proteins, which includes MyoD (Myf-3 in human), myogenin (Myf-4 in human), Myf-5, and MRF4 (Myf-6 in human). The MDFs regulate both the determination of early somite cells for the myogenic differentiation pathway, and the subsequent transcription of muscle-specific genes (Fig. 32.2b). All four MDFs have the ability to initiate transcription of muscle-specific genes when transfected into a variety of non-muscle cells. Normal MDF expression is restricted to muscle precursor cells in the somite and to its descending cells of the myogenic lineage. The four MDFs appear to control muscle development at different points in the myogenic pathway. All four MDFs act as transcription factors, and bind to the consensus sequence CANNTG (so-called E-box) present in regulatory regions of most studied muscle-specific genes.

Other major control element families have been identified in muscle genes to which other muscle transcription factors bind: these include A/T-rich elements (homeodomain factors), MEF-2 sites (myocyte-specific enhancer binding factor MEF-2), M-CAT (M-CAT binding factor), and CArG sites (a variety of factors, many of which are regulated by growth factors).

Skeletal muscle cell proliferation and differentiation are mutually exclusive processes, and *in vitro* studies have demonstrated differentiation inhibiting properties of serum and isolated growth factors. The effects of fibroblast growth factors (FGFs), transforming growth factor-β, platelet-derived growth factor (PDGF), and insulin-like growth factors (IGFs) on myogenic differentiation have been most extensively studied. It is generally believed that growth factors while stimulating proliferation inhibit myoblasts from initiating differentiation by inhibitory effects on the MDFs (Fig. 32.2b). Two other factors, Id (inhibitor of differentiation) and Notch, are also implied to repress muscle differentiation by inhibitory interaction with the MDFs.

## INTRAFUSAL MUSCLE FIBERS

Muscle spindles are stretch–tension receptor organs in muscles (*see* page 403). They are composed of long fibers of small diameter, intrafusal muscle fibers, innervated by both afferent and efferent nerves and surrounded by a capsule. Nuclear bag fibers contain a bag of nuclei at the central part of the fiber whereas nuclear chain fibers have their nuclei in a chain. Three types of intrafusal fibers can be distinguished on the basis of their expression of myosin heavy chains. Bag fibers are of two types expressing predominantly slow types of MHC whereas chain fibers express fast isoforms. A special MHC isoform, slow tonic myosin, is regionally expressed in the bag fibers and is never expressed in extrafusal fibers in mammalian limb muscle. By 10 weeks' gestation a subpopulation of the primary generation of myotubes express the slow tonic MHC and seem destined to become intrafusal muscle spindle fibers. Second generation fibers found in close relation to each spindle precursor initially express only fetal and embryonic MHC. Later one or more of these secondary myotubes express slow tonic and slow twitch MHC and give rise to nuclear bag fibers. The rest become nuclear chain fibers.

The afferent innervation seems to be of ultimate importance for the initiation of muscle spindle differentiation. Defective spindle function during development might be one causative factor in *arthrogryposis*.

## SELECTED READING

Barbet JP, Thornell LE, Butler-Browne GS. Immunocytochemical characterization of two generations of fibers during the development of the human quadriceps muscle. *Mech Dev* 1991; **35**: 3.

Fischman DA. Myofibrillogenesis and morphogenesis of skeletal muscle. In Engel AG, Banker BQ, eds. *Myology*. New York: McGraw-Hill, 1986: 5.

Konisberg IR. The embryonic origin of muscle. In Engel AG, Banker BQ, eds. *Myology*. New York: McGraw-Hill, 1986: 39.

Miller JB. Myoblasts, myosins, myoDs and the diversification of muscle fibers. *Neuromusc Dis* 1991; **1**: 7.

Pette D, Staron RS. Cellular and molecular diversities of mammalian skeletal muscle fibers. *Rev Physiol Biochem Pharmacol* 1990; **116**: 2.

# PART SEVEN

# The Endocrine System

**Editor: Peter D. Gluckman**

# 33

# General Principles of Endocrinology

Peter D. Gluckman and Michael Bauer

## Overview

As one of the two systems of extracellular communication, the endocrine system has classically been defined in terms of hormones secreted into the blood stream acting at sites distal to their production. This is no longer an appropriate definition. Chemical messengers may act either on their own cells of production in an "autocrine" manner or on neighboring cells in a "paracrine" manner (Fig. 33.1). The possibility of some hormones acting on their own cells of production without extracellular secretion in an "intracrine" manner has also been raised. This expanded hormonal system is critically involved in the processes of growth, reproduction, cellular nutrition and energy homeostasis as well as in other physiological mechanisms such as thermal, cardiovascular and fluid homeostasis. Thus it is not surprising that there are marked ontogenetic changes in all endocrine axes and that many disorders of the endocrine system in childhood manifest with altered growth.

The endocrine system is characterized by interactions such as feed-back loops which may be inhibitory or stimulatory (*see* page 468). In addition, hormones may regulate the number or affinity of their own or heterologous receptors, e.g. pituitary growth hormone (GH) up-regulates the concentration of high affinity GH receptors (*see* page 462), insulin up-regulates the type II insulin-like growth factor (IGF) receptor (which is a clearance receptor for IGF-II) but down-regulates its own receptor. Hormones also may compete with heterologous receptors, e.g. most actions of testosterone in the brain are due to binding to the estradiol receptor and it has recently been recognized that in the epiphysis, epiphyseal closure is dependent on testosterone being aromatized to estradiol-17β and acting on the estrogen receptor (*see* page 495). Similarly,

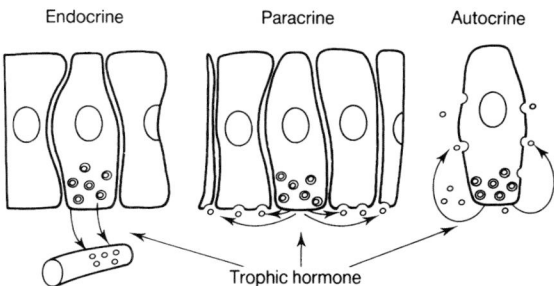

FIGURE 33.1 Schematic representation of modalities by which hormones and growth factors reach target tissues. Whereas traditional hormones are formed in glands of internal secretion and are transported to distant sites of action through the blood stream (endocrine modality), peptide growth factors are more often produced locally by the target cells themselves (autocrine modality) or by neighboring cells (paracrine modality). Regardless of where they are formed, production is regulated in a similar fashion by trophic hormones and other regulatory influences. (From Underwood LE, Van Wyk JJ. Peptide growth factors other than somatomedins. The relationship to traditional hormones: paracrine and autocrine versus endocrine modes of action. In Wilson JD, Foster DW, eds. *Williams' Textbook of Endocrinology*. 8th edn. Philadelphia: WB Saunders Co., 1992: 1087. Reproduced by permission of WB Saunders Co.)

while testosterone acts on its own receptor to promote Wolffian duct development, development of the external genitalia is dependent on enzymatic reduction to dihydrotestosterone (DHT) (*see* page 198). Several hormones are obviously trophic to the release of others in well defined axes (e.g. the thyrotrophin releasing hormone (TRH)–thyroid stimulating hormone (TSH)-thyroid axis), but other hormones can have indirect effects on other components of the endocrine system.

For example, the action of follicle stimulating hormone (FSH) on granulosa cell proliferation involves stimulation of autocrine production of IGF-I (*see* page 494).

Hormone action depends on the interaction of the hormone with a receptor which may be either membrane-bound, cytosolic or nuclear. A number of distinct signaling systems are then utilized which then manifest in hormone action. There are two major groups of hormones: those that are peptides or amino acids, and those that are steroids or sterol-derived (e.g. vitamin D).

Polypeptide/amino acid hormones, with the exception of thyroid hormones, bind to membrane-bound receptors. As with the hormones there can be close evolutionary relationships between hormone receptors which can be classified into receptor superfamilies. The three major families of membrane-associated receptors are the tyrosine kinase-associated receptors, the G-protein-related receptors and the cytokine receptor superfamily which includes GH and prolactin (PRL) receptors. Activation of each of these classes of receptor leads to a variety of cytosolic "signal transduction" or "second messenger" systems which act through complex cascades leading generally to alterations in gene transcription (*see* page 60). However, as many peptide hormones (e.g. insulin) are internalized in association with their membrane receptor after binding, the possibility that such internalization may be part of signal transduction as well as a degradation cannot be ignored. Steroid/sterol hormones and thyroid hormones diffuse into cells and act primarily on intracellular receptors of the steroid/retinoic acid receptor superfamily.

Not all hormonal "receptors" are associated with signal transduction. For example, while IGF-II exerts its biological effects via the IGF-I receptor, which is a member of the insulin family of tyrosine kinase receptors, it in addition binds to a specific IGF-II receptor which has no obvious intracellular signaling system. This receptor is the same protein as the mannose-6-phosphate cation-independent receptor which is used intracellularly to regulate trafficking of lysosomal enzymes. This receptor appears to act to internalize IGF-II to the lysozyme for clearance. Similarly "clearance" receptors have been described for atrial natriuretic peptide (ANP) and for the short form of the PRL receptor.

A number of "orphan" receptors have been described. These are receptors for which no ligand has yet been identified. These have been identified by molecular biological examination of the receptor superfamilies. The insulin receptor-related receptor is one such receptor: it is highly homologous to the insulin and IGF-I receptors, yet has no known ligand. Many orphan receptors have been identified within the steroid receptor superfamily.

For some hormones the receptor remains to be identified. In other cases one receptor is responsible for signaling of closely related hormones. For example, it is not certain through which receptor placental lacto-gen (PL) exerts its biological effects. They may be primarily mediated by the GH and PRL receptors, or PL may have an as yet undiscovered unique receptor. IGF-I and -II both act to promote cell proliferation via the IGF-I receptor: in this case the differing affinity for the IGF binding protein (IGFBP) may modulate action at the receptor (*see* page 317).

Hormone action is targeted. In large part this is achieved by tissue-specific expression of hormone receptors. However, other mechanisms exist. Some hormones are localized by virtue of secretion into the hypophyseal or gastrointestinal portal vessels. Circulating and tissue-binding proteins may prevent high levels of free hormone acting at inappropriate sites. Thus many steroid hormones and some peptide hormones (e.g. IGF-I, GH, thyroid hormones) have specific binding proteins. There is evidence that the IGFBPs may target IGFs to specific cell types. The paracrine route of secretion is increasingly recognized as a major means of hormone targeting and specificity of action. Under some circumstances the "hormone" is metabolized to its active derivative within the target tissue (e.g. brown fat converts thyroxine to triiodothyronine, genital tissue converts testosterone to dihydrotestosterone).

It thus is not surprising that there can be complex dose–response relationships in endocrinology. For example IGF-I probably only exerts insulin-like actions *in vivo* at very high doses when the IGFBPs have been saturated and free IGF-I concentrations rise to be significant at the insulin receptor. In some cases an inverse bell-shape dose response may be observed. Many of the classical actions of transforming growth factor β (TGFβ) are demonstrated only within a narrow range of concentrations and not at higher or lower concentrations, and indeed at extreme doses the biological action may be contrary to that at a middle dose. This bell-shaped dose–response curve may be the consequence of activating a different subset of receptors, of intracellular "cross-talk" between signal transduction mechanisms or of extracellular processes (e.g. saturation of matrix binding sites).

## ENDOCRINE PATHOPHYSIOLOGY

Pathophysiological disturbance of the endocrine system may be due to hormone excess or deficiency, or to abnormalities of the receptor/postreceptor mechanisms leading to hormone resistance. Abnormalities of hormone secretion also may be due to the secretion of an abnormal hormone, e.g. single point mutations in the vasopressin prohormone may lead to inherited forms of diabetes insipidus. In malignancy, incompletely or incorrectly processed hormones may be secreted. Tumors may inappropriately express hormones ectopically. Another form of inappropriate hormone receptor stimulation can occur when an immunoglobulin capable of binding to the receptor and activating signal transduction is circulating (e.g. thyroid stimulating antibodies in thyrotoxicosis).

The interpretation of a hormone concentration in blood is not always straightforward. Many hormones are sensitive to stress (e.g. PRL, catecholamines) or to changes in posture (e.g. renin) or to acute (e.g. insulin) or chronic (e.g. IGF-I) changes in nutrition. High plasma concentrations of a hormone may reflect inappropriate and pathological hypersecretion (e.g. high luteinizing hormone [LH] and FSH concentrations in central precocious puberty); they may be appropriate because the changes are secondary to abnormalities of binding proteins and the effective free concentration is normal (e.g. the high thyroxine concentrations associated with hereditary excess of thyroid-binding globulin [TBG] or a high concentration may be secondary to a defect in feed-back – either as a consequence of receptor or postreceptor defects (e.g. high concentrations of GH in *Laron syndrome*) or of end organ failure (e.g. high gonadotrophin concentrations in *Turner syndrome*).

Many hormones are secreted in characteristic temporal patterns. Some are markedly pulsatile (e.g. adrenocorticotrophic hormone [ACTH], GH), making single time point measurement uninterpretable. Some show diurnal rhythms (e.g. melatonin, cortisol, GH, PRL) and others show longer cycles (e.g. menstrually-related changes in LH, FSH, estradiol, progesterone, PRL).

Given these complexities and the problems of interpretation of isolated hormone measurements, the assessment of the endocrine system generally involves carefully standardized tests of the dynamic interplay between different components of the axis.

## PEPTIDE HORMONE SECRETION AND ACTION

## Synthesis and secretion

The synthesis of peptide hormones, as for other proteins, involves first transcription of DNA to pre-mRNA followed by post-transcriptional processing by way of excision of introns, polyadenylation of the $3'$ end and capping of the $5'$ end. At this step diversity may occur. Several hormones arise as a result of alternate splicing during post-transcriptional processing (e.g. the 20 kD variant of GH arises from alternate splicing of the pituitary GH gene, calcitonin gene-related peptide [CGRP] is formed by alternate splicing of the calcitonin gene). Some hormone genes show remarkable complexity with long sequences of uncoded $5'$ or $3'$ nucleotides, complex intron/exon structures with multiple splicing alternatives, multiple promoter and polyadenylation sites. Such complexity is particularly notable for IGF-I and IGF-II genes presumably reflecting their diverse paracrine, autocrine and endocrine roles and the consequent need for multiple sites of regulation (*see* page 314). The $5'$ region of the gene contains the regulatory sequences including tissue specific and metabolic/hormone response elements which are specific binding sites for regulatory proteins. In the case of metabolic/hormone response promoters these may be the intracellular hormone receptors themselves (e.g. steroid hormone receptors) or trans-acting factors whose production is under hormonal regulation, e.g. the cAMP response element (CRE) is activated by the CRE-binding protein (CREB) which in turn is regulated by a cAMP-dependent cascade. Introns may also contain regulatory elements.

The translation of the genetic information from mRNA into a peptide occurs on the endoplasmic reticulum. The peptide formed is not the mature peptide but is a prepeptide with an amino terminal signal sequence. This prepeptide then undergoes post-translational processing before secretion. The presence of a signal peptide is an essential characteristic of a peptide that is to be secreted as it enables its sequestration in the cisterna of the endoplasmic reticulum which is the first step in the export from the cell of a secreted protein. The signal peptide is 15–30 amino acids in length, is hydrophobic and recognizes specific sequences on the endoplasmic reticulum to allow translocation into the cisterna. Most post-translational processing then occurs in the Golgi region. If, after removal of the signal peptide by proteolytic cleavage, the remaining peptide is active the prepeptide is known as a prehormone; however, most hormones are synthesized as preprohormones, i.e. after cleavage of the signal peptide the remaining peptide will require further post-translational cleavage to release the mature hormone. This may lead to the release from the prohormone of other peptides of unknown biological significance (e.g. neurophysin is coreleased with arginine vasopressin [AVP]). A single preprohormone may be the precursor to one (e.g. preproinsulin) or several hormones (e.g. prepro-opiomelanocortin is the precursor of β-endorphin and ACTH; preproenkephalin contains multiple copies of both met- and leu-enkephalin). Other forms of post-translational modification include glycosylation, phosphorylation, sulfation, acetylation and finally folding into tertiary structure. In rare cases the post-translational steps may vary for a single prohormone (e.g. in the anterior lobe of the pituitary pro-opiomelanocortin is cleaved to ACTH and β-endorphin, whereas in the intermediate lobe ACTH is processed further to α-melanocyte stimulating hormone (αMSH) and corticotrophin-like intermediate peptide (CLIP).

Within the Golgi apparatus the prohormones are processed and packaged into secretory vesicles which bud off from the Golgi stack of smooth endoplasmic reticulum. Generally, these mature by condensation of the protein into a more tightly packed granule and the application of a second membrane to the vesicle. Under the appropriate stimuli the granules migrate to the cell surface and by fusing to the cell membrane exocytose their contents from the cell.

The regulation of hormone secretion can take place at each level in this complex process. However, in practice, the major sites of regulation are either translational or at the secretory step. Most hormone secreting cells maintain significant prepacked hormone for release and the primary event is to stimulate secretion. However, in some cases, hormones are not prepackaged ready for release (e.g. IGF-I) and enhanced synthesis is the primary event.

## Membrane-associated receptors

The binding of a hormone to the membrane-bound receptor is rapid and determined by the number and affinity of unoccupied receptors on the cell surface. As hormones generally circulate in low concentrations, hormone receptors must have high affinities to have physiological significance. Further, they must have relatively low capacity to be saturable and have specificity. This specificity is not always absolute (e.g. at high concentration insulin has some affinity for the IGF-1 receptor and this may explain somatic overgrowth in fetal hyperinsulinemia). For most larger peptides the binding structure relies on the three-dimensional structure of the hormone and the receptor.

Membrane-bound receptors can be classed in several superfamilies. Members of these superfamilies have evolutionary relationships and are presumed to have formed by gene duplication. The major classes are reviewed on page 55 and include the G-protein-linked receptors, tyrosine kinase receptor superfamily and the GH/PRL/cytokine receptor superfamily.

Receptor dimerization is a frequently observed characteristic in the latter two classes of receptor. The dimerization may be ligand-activated as in the case of the GH receptor. Other receptors are dimeric in their basal state (e.g. insulin receptors). In some dimeric receptor families, the chains can combine in multiple ways. For example the insulin receptor and the IGF-I receptor are both homodimeric, but a hybrid receptor comprising a dimer of an insulin and IGF-I receptor may be found in some tissues. The neurotrophic hormones (nerve growth factor: NGF, brain-derived neurotrophic factor: BDNF etc.) receptors may form either hetero- or homodimeric receptors (see page 368).

Membrane receptors act through a variety of intracellular mechanisms leading eventually to altered gene transcription. It is now apparent that multiple signal transduction pathways are activated following ligand binding to a single class of receptor. For example binding to a G-protein-linked receptor may activate adenylyl cyclase, alter intracellular $Ca^{2+}$ concentrations, affect phosphorylation of a number of cytosolic signal peptides or affect the phosphatidylinositol cascade. These intracellular signaling pathways are shared by many hormone receptors offering apparent convergence in the endocrine cascade. However, it is these interactions at an intracellular level that lead to the fine tuning of hormone action and to a further level of influence of one hormone on the action of another.

The potential for cross-talk at the postreceptor level makes quite clear that not only is ligand specificity of the receptor very important, but also the receptor population on the cell membrane. Functional enhancement and/or silencing of postreceptor signaling pathways by postreceptor cross-talk between different hormones creates a further complexity to the endocrine system. Thus the relationship between receptor occupancy and hormone action is not linear. Complex mechanisms exist to allow the appropriate response under conditions which would not be favorable for simple linear coupling. These mechanisms involve both changes in binding properties and postreceptor events. In addition, most hormones either up-regulate or, more often, down-regulate their own receptor, thus offering a greater degree of complexity of regulation.

Membrane receptors are in a dynamic state. Like other proteins they are synthesized on the endoplasmic reticulum but lacking the signal peptide they are not processed for exocytosis but following post-translational modification are inserted into the cell membrane by membrane fusion. A characteristic of many membrane-associated receptors is that after ligand binding they aggregate on the cell surface. This appears important for signal transduction. After aggregation the receptor is internalized through special regions known as coated pits. These are clathrin rich and eventually pinch off into the cytoplasm and form endosomes. These carry the receptor–hormone couplet into the cell. These endosomes then fuse with lysosomes, the hormone is degraded and the receptor is either degraded or recycled. This cycle may itself be under endocrine regulation (e.g. insulin enhances cycling of the type II IGF receptor to the cell surface). Not all hormones are degraded in this manner and in many cases membrane-bound or circulating proteases are more important than receptor-mediated degradation.

## The GH/PRL/cytokine receptor superfamily

The GH receptor (GHR) has been identified as a member of a large family of receptors including the PRL receptor and a number of cytokine receptors. These receptors are characterized by evolutionary homologies, indirect activation of intracellular kinases, and in general, by requiring ligand mediated dimerization for activity. In the case of the GH and PRL receptors, the dimerization is of two identical receptor units; in the case of the IL-2 receptor, for example, the dimerization is heterodimeric.

The GH molecule has two binding sites for the GH receptor and after binding to the receptor at site 1 it subsequently binds at site 2 and forms the GH–$(GHR)_2$ dimer complex, which is necessary for signal transduction (*see* page 310). Mutations of the GH receptor that prevent dimerization are one cause of *growth hormone insensitivity syndrome*. However, most mutations causing this syndrome occur in the extracellular GH-binding domain of the receptor.

Ligand binding to a receptor of the cytokine receptor superfamily induces rapid phosphorylation of protein tyrosine kinases. So far 3 kinases of the Janus family (Jaks) and a novel tyrosine kinase 2 (tyk2) have been identified to be involved in signaling of the cytokine receptor superfamily. The GH receptor, as a member of the cytokine receptor superfamily, has been shown to activate Jak2. Once GH has induced the GH receptor dimerization a multitude of postreceptor signaling cascades are activated (Fig. 33.2). The receptor dimerization is thought to increase the affinity of the receptor for Jak2 and the signal transduction is initiated by rapid phosphorylation of Jak2 and the GHR itself. This is followed by a downstream phosphorylation of two smaller proteins, ERK1 and ERK2 (extracellular signal-regulated kinases). In addition Jak2 can activate the S6 kinase (S6K) pathway as well as the mitogen-activated protein kinase (MAPK)-mediated signaling cascade (*see* page 63). Even though these two pathways must be seen as independent sig-

naling cascades, they are able to stimulate phosphorylation of each other, thus enabling further cross-talk after signal transduction has been initiated. ERK1, ERK2, S6K and MAPKs can translocate into the nucleus and phosphorylate nuclear transcription factors which bind to the DNA. The phosphorylated transcription factors then initiate gene transcription, which will eventually lead to the well known anabolic effects of GH. GH is known not only for its anabolic actions, but also for its antidiabetogenic and lipolytic effects. There is evidence that these effects are at least partially mediated by several interactions between GH-induced signal transduction systems and insulin-induced signal transduction systems at an intracellular level (see Fig. 33.2).

### The tyrosine kinase receptor superfamily (*see also* page 56)

There are a large number of receptors of various degrees of evolutionary homology that have intrinsic tyrosine kinase activity in their intracellular domain. On ligand binding, the cytosolic tyrosine kinase domain is activated thus leading to phosphorylation

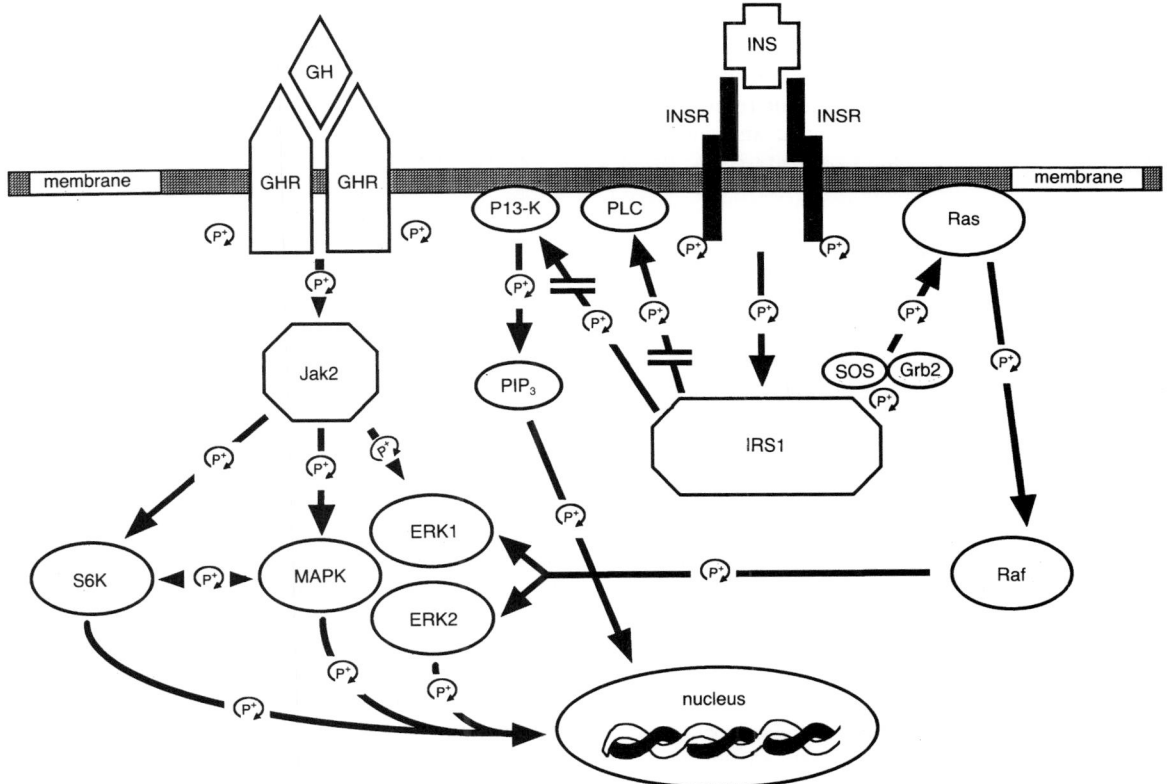

FIGURE 33.2 Illustration of growth hormone (GH) and insulin (INS) postreceptor pathways. GHR, growth hormone receptor; INSR insulin receptor; Jak2, Janus kinase 2; S6K, S6 kinase; ERK1, ERK2, extracellular signal-regulated kinases 1 and 2; MAPK, mitogen-activated protein kinase; IRS1, insulin receptor substrate; PI3-K, phosphatidylinositol-3 kinase; PIP3, phosphatidylinositol-3 phosphate; Grb2, growth factor receptor-bound protein 2; SOS, son of sevenless Ras activating factor (guanine nucleotide exchange factor); PLC, phosphatidylinositol phospholipase C; P+, phosphorylation.

of various intracellular substrates. One typical subfamily of these receptors is the insulin/IGF-I receptor family. It has four members, the insulin receptor, the closely homologous IGF-I receptor, the hybrid insulin-IGF-I receptor and the insulin receptor-related receptor. The latter is an orphan receptor with an unknown ligand. After binding of the insulin, receptor-intrinsic tyrosine kinases are activated by autophosphorylation. In turn this leads to activation of several interacting intracellular cascades by phosphorylating intracellular signaling proteins that come into association with the activated receptor. These are characterized by having $SH_2$ domains. The most clearly defined pathway involves phosphorylation of an intracellular substrate called IRS1 (insulin receptor substrate). IRS1 can be viewed as a "docking protein" that, after phosphorylation at multiple tyrosine sites, further distributes the signal to different cascades. (Fig. 33.2). The first cascade involves phosphatidylinositol-3 kinase (PI3-K). The activation of PI3-K is then followed by the formation of phosphatidylinositol-3-phosphate ($PIP_3$) which, in turn, through a further cascade initiates gene transcription. A second pathway involves a sequential activation of a series of proteins by phosphorylation. The cascade involves the growth factor receptor-bound protein (Grb2), which in turn activates the guanine nucleotide exchange factor, SOS, which in turn activates the GTP-binding protein Ras, which activates Raf, which activates ERK1 and ERK2, which in turn transmit a signal to the nucleus. Activation of IRS1 can also activate alternate intracellular pathways leading to metabolic and mitogenic responses.

### G-protein-linked receptors

Many hormones activate membrane receptors that are linked to the heterotrimeric G-proteins. Binding of the ligand to the receptors leads to a variety of intracellular and intramembranous events including activation or inhibition of adenylyl cyclase, activation of phospholipases or alterations in membrane ion channels. These

TABLE 33.1 Examples of endocrine diseases in children caused by mutations in G-protein or G-protein-linked receptors

| DISEASE | COMMENT |
| --- | --- |
| Pseudohypoparathyroidism type 1a | PTH receptor-linked $G\alpha_s$ dysfunctional |
| McCune–Albright syndrome | A mutation in $G\alpha_s$ inhibits GTPase activity allowing ligand-independent activation |
| Nephrogenic diabetes insipidus | Dysfunctional mutation in $V_2$ vasopressin receptor |
| Familial male precocious puberty (testotoxicosis) | Mutation in LH receptor leading to ligand-independent activation |
| Male-pseudohermaphroditism | Dysfunctional mutation in LH receptor |

mechanisms are described in more detail on page 60. There are a large number of specific G-proteins and mutations in the genes encoding these G-proteins can lead to specific endocrinopathies. Examples of mutations in G-proteins or G-protein-linked receptors leading to endocrine disease are shown in Table 33.1.

## STEROID HORMONES

### Secretion

The regulation of steroid synthesis and secretion is dependent on the provision of cholesterol as the substrate. Most is provided from circulating low-density lipoproteins (LDL). These contain a protein moiety, apolipoprotein B, which binds to a cell-surface receptor and is internalized via a coated pit/endosomal pathway in an identical process to that for other protein hormones and thus liberates cholesterol into the cell. Small amounts of cholesterol may be synthesized *de novo* in the cell from acetate or be mobilized from intracellular cholesterol ester pools. Cytosolic free cholesterol is actively regulated; for example, LDL uptake inhibits *de novo* cholesterol biosynthesis.

The tropic hormones that stimulate steroid synthesis do so primarily by stimulating side-chain cleavage and the formation of pregnenolone, the rate-limiting step in steroid biosynthesis. However, all the relevant enzymes are subject to a degree of endocrine control as are some steps in cholesterol supply (e.g. LDL receptor number is enhanced by ACTH).

### Steroid and other nuclear receptors

Steroids, vitamin D, thyroid hormone and retinoic acids (natural derivatives of vitamin A) are hydrophobic substances which can diffuse through the cell membrane. They all activate nuclear receptors, which belong to the superfamily of ligand inducible transcription factors. Upon binding of the ligand, these receptors modulate gene transcription through DNA response elements. It is thought that in the absence of ligand, some steroid receptors are inactivated by binding in the cytoplasm to heat shock protein 90 (HSP 90). This appears to be most likely for the glucocorticoid receptors, whereas androgen and estrogen receptors are exclusively located in the nucleus. In the presence of ligand the steroid receptors undergo conformational changes which allow them to bind to the steroid response elements of the DNA at the 5' untranslated region. The target gene is then activated and transcription initiated. Steroid receptors contain two binding sites, one for the ligand and a zinc finger motif which binds to the DNA. The synthesis and regulation of steroid receptors is strongly influenced by the endocrine milieu. Steroid receptors and thyroid receptors can up-regulate themselves in the presence of their ligand (autoregulation), but can also influence the regulation of other nuclear receptors (crossregulation; e.g. progesterone can regulate estrogen receptors). Autoregulation of steroid and thyroid hormone receptors has been described in many growth and developmental systems.

It has become clear only very recently that, whereas steroid receptors usually form homodimers, thyroid receptors, retinoic acid receptors (RARs) and the retinoic X receptors (RXRs) require heterodimerization to effectively stimulate their DNA response elements. The RXRs play a central role within this scenario of heterodimer formation, insofar that RXR is always the binding partner for either thyroid receptors or retinoic acid receptors. RXRs can also form homodimers in the presence of excess 9-*cis* retinoic acid (a naturally occurring stereoisomer of *trans* retinoic acid), which leads to the activation of a specific 9-*cis* response element (9-*cis* RE). Even though RXRs are always part of a heterodimer, the RXR does not need to be activated by its ligand for that heterodimer to be able to initiate gene transcription (Fig. 33.3). DNA binding of heterodimers is independent of ligand binding. This way the receptor can serve dual functions: initiating gene transcription in the presence of ligand or repressing gene transcription in the absence of ligand. Apart from the activation of a specific response element, the formation of RXRs homodimers is also thought to be involved in the regulation of the availability of RXRs for the formation of heterodimers with other receptors and thus allows further hormonal cross-talk. The phenomena of autoregulation and crossregulation as well as the complex-

ity of heterodimer formation enables a multitude of interactions between several ligands and their response elements. The function of these phenomena is comparable to the membrane receptor signaling cross-talk, described earlier.

# Membrane-mediated effects of steroids – neurosteroids

The brain itself can form "neurosteroids" from steroid hormone precursors or take steroids from the circulation. Many actions are mediated by classical steroid receptors (e.g. the androgenization of the brain is dependent on peripheral testosterone being converted in the brain to estradiol-17β and acting on estrogen receptors). Other actions, however, appear to be independent of cytosolic/nuclear steroid receptors. It has been suggested that they may be incorporated into plasma membranes and alter cell membrane properties. This is one possible mode of action of the steroid derived lazeroids that ameliorate asphyxial brain injury. However, it now is recognized that some actions of neurosteroids are mediated by binding sites on neurotransmitter receptors. The γ-amino butyric acid (GABA) receptor is an oligomeric receptor complex which when activated increases $Cl^-$ conductance and thus membrane hyperpolarization and reduced neuronal excitability. In nerve cell membranes progesterone can activate this receptor thus explaining the anesthetic and sedative properties of progesterone. Its

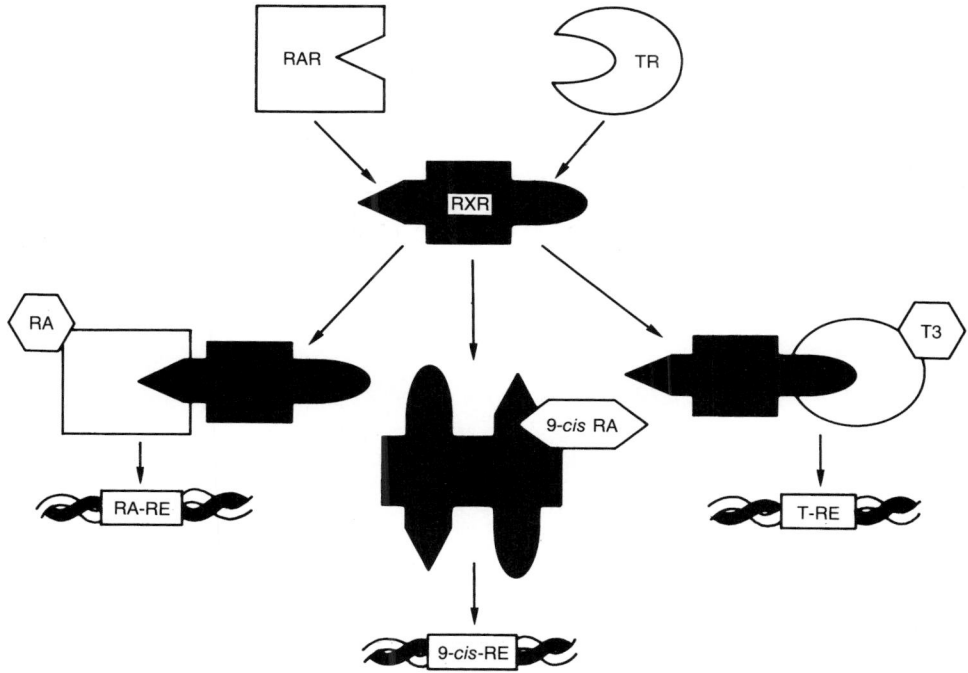

FIGURE 33.2 Illustration of dimer formation and response element (RE) activation by the retinoic acid receptor (RAR), retinoic X receptor (RXR) and thyroid receptor (TR). RA, retinoic acid; 9-*cis* RA, 9-*cis* retinoic acid.

precursor, pregnenolone sulfate, is inhibitory. There is evidence for modulating action by steroids on the glycine and $N$-methyl-D-aspartate (NMDA) (glutamate) receptor also. Neurosteroids are thought to play a neuromodulatory role in pregnancy, the menstrual cycle and in determining sexual behavior.

## SELECTED READING

Habener JF. Genetic control of hormone formation. In Wilson JD, Foster DW, eds. *Williams' textbook of endocrinology*. 8th edn. Philadelphia: WB Saunders, 1992: 9.

Jones JI, Clemmons DR. Insulin-like growth factors and their binding proteins: Biological actions. *Endocr Rev* 1995; **16**: 3.

Robel P, Baulieu EE. Neurosteroids: biosynthesis and function. *Trends Endocrinol Metab* 1994; **5**: 1.

Roupas P, Herrington AC. Postreceptor signalling mechanisms for growth hormone. *Trends Endocrinol Metab* 1994; **5**: 154.

Zhang X-K, Pfahl M. Regulation of retinoid and thyroid hormone action through homodimeric and heterodimeric receptors. *Trends Endocrinol Metab* 1993; **4**: 156.

# 34

# Neuroendocrine Mechanisms

Gail E. Richards

Neuroendocrinology encompasses the processes by which various homeostatic systems are regulated by the central nervous system. Although exceptions exist, the majority of this communication is mediated by the hypothalamus.

## FUNCTIONAL HYPOTHALAMIC–PITUITARY RELATIONSHIPS

Hormonal homeostasis is maintained by multiple interacting regulatory loops which act by determining the secretory activity of several discrete hypothalamic–pituitary regulatory systems. A group of well-developed hypothalamic nuclei at the base of the third ventricle, whose neurons project to the medial eminence and the posterior lobe of the pituitary, is responsible for integration of signals from the brain and body and translation of those signals into an appropriate level of hormone secretion.

Neurons in these areas regulate the hormonal secretions of the pituitary in several ways. Some neurons, such as those of the supraoptic and paraventricular nuclei which secrete vasopressin and oxytocin, project directly to the posterior pituitary. Their cell terminals form the posterior lobe of the pituitary. Thus when a stimulus to oxytocin or vasopressin release occurs in the brain or the periphery, the signal is received in the supraoptic or paraventricular nucleus and hormone is released from the same neuron's terminals within the posterior pituitary (see page 515).

A second type of neuron, found more commonly in the arcuate nucleus, has cell bodies in one of the hypothalamic nuclei and nerve endings abutting on the hypothalamic–pituitary–portal capillaries (primary capillary plexus) in the median eminence. These neurons release their peptide hormone message into the hypophyseal–portal circulation, which ends as a secondary capillary plexus among the pituicytes of the anterior lobe of the pituitary. The unique anatomical features of this portal system are the small distance traversed and the complexity of the multihormonal milieu of the anterior pituitary.

A third type of hypothalamic neuron which plays an important role in hormonal regulation has its cell body in one nucleus and its terminal on another neuropeptide secretory neuron in the same or another nucleus. These neurons probably have modulatory and integrational roles in hormone secretion.

These three kinds of neuronal connections describe the functional relationship of the hypothalamus and pituitary. The pituitary itself consists of the anterior lobe, whose cells produce and secrete growth hormone (GH), luteinizing hormone (LH), follicle-stimulating hormone (FSH), prolactin (PRL), thyroid-stimulating hormone (TSH), and adrenocorticotrophic hormone (ACTH). The posterior pituitary secretes vasopressin (AVP) and oxytocin (OT).

In the fetus a distinct intermediate lobe forms from the posterior limb of the Rathke pouch. This is corticotrope rich but, in contrast to the adenohypophysis, it appears to be regulated by direct innervation by dopaminergic neurons arising in the arcuate nucleus. The post-translational processing of the pro-opiomelanocortin (see page 504) also differs in the intermediate lobe. The intermediate lobe is less apparent postnatally and its biological significance is unknown.

## PATTERNS OF HORMONAL REGULATION
(Fig. 34.1)

Input from both the internal and external environment affects hypothalamic–pituitary functioning through combinations of open loop and feedback loop systems to integrate the effects of nutrition, temperature, day/night light cycles, pain, affective factors and different schedules of intrinsic rhythms. The regulation of individual pituitary hormones is discussed in more depth in subsequent chapters.

## Feedback loops

To maintain homeostasis, hormone release must be closely regulated by a series of feedback systems. For such a system to work there must be discrete outputs to be regulated, receptors and processors to receive

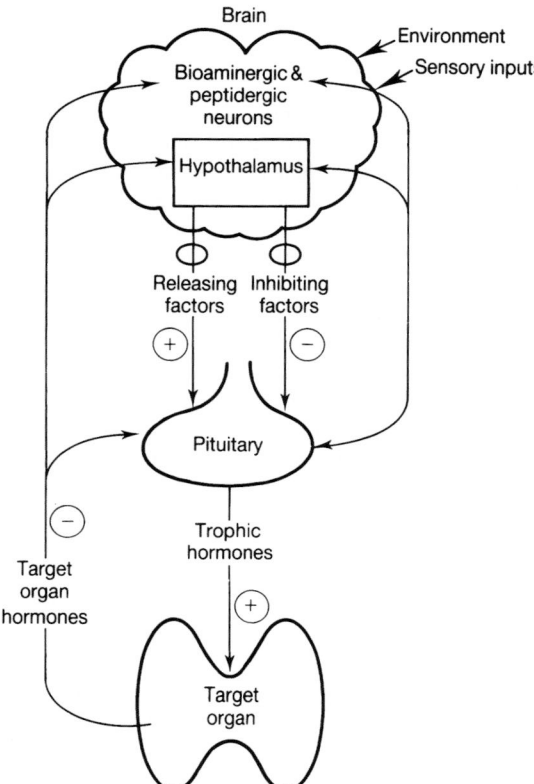

FIGURE 34.1 Regulatory feedback loops of the hypothalamic–pituitary–target organ axis. Being a combination of both stimulatory and inhibitory factors, hormones often act in concert to maintain homeostatic balance in the face of physiological or pathophysiological perturbations. (From Habener JF. Genetic control of hormone formation. In Wilson JD, Foster DW, eds. *Williams' textbook of endocrinology.* Philadelphia: WB Saunders Co., 1992: 16. Reprinted with permission of WB Saunders Co.)

signals and recognize discrepancies between a set point and current amount of activity. Four examples of feedback mechanisms can be used to illustrate these general principles.

*Long loop feedback* mechanisms typically involve a three-step signaling sequence, such as hypothalamus–pituitary–target organ. In this type of system, the output of the target organ signals the hypothalamus to decrease (negative feedback) or increase (positive feedback) its specific output to the pituitary. Most anterior pituitary hormones have a long loop feedback system. For example, thyrotrophin-releasing hormone (TRH) from the hypothalamus stimulates the pituitary to secrete TSH which in turn stimulates the thyroid gland to secrete thyroxine. When circulating thyroxine decreases, the secretion of TRH and subsequently TSH increases, encouraging more secretion of thyroxine from the thyroid gland.

*Short loop feedback* is a direct signal from a target organ to the source of that organ's regulation. An example of this mechanism is the ability of GH to influence the output of growth hormone releasing hormone and somatostatin (somatotrophin release-inhibiting factor, SRIF).

*Ultrashort (paracrine) feedback* is the ability of a cell to influence the output of cells of a similar cell type; for example, prolactin can decrease further the secretion of prolactin by lactotropes in the pituitary. A variant of this mechanism is hormonal secretion which subsequently regulates further secretion by the same secretory cell (*autocrine feedback*).

Many hormonal feedback systems involve several of these mechanisms. In addition, there are distinct inputs from many parts of the central nervous system which are not known to be regulated in any manner by the hormones which are affected (for example the effect of cold on TSH release). This situation is known as *open loop input*. Further molecular levels of regulation exist through regulation of gene translation, differential production of alternative gene products, post-translational processing and other mechanisms.

## Neuroendocrine rhythms

Most pituitary hormones are released by periodic bursts of active secretion with, or without, a background amount of constant (or tonic) secretion. Onto this short-term rhythm of secretion may be imposed ultradian or circadian (e.g. ACTH) patterns of medium-term increases and decreases in activity of the loop. In some instances an even longer term pattern of seasonal activity (e.g. prolactin) or developmentally regulated activity of the loop (e.g. gonadotrophins) exists. Further regulatory influences such as nutrition, exercise and affective factors can modulate the activity of a feedback system.

## DEVELOPMENT OF THE HYPOTHALAMIC–PITUITARY UNIT

### Anatomy

The human anterior pituitary takes shape by 5 weeks of gestation with the formation of the Rathke pouch. Although classical teaching has been that the Rathke pouch and the anterior pituitary arise from the oral ectoderm, an alternative hypothesis is their derivation directly from the neural ridge. The hypothalamus, pituitary stalk and posterior pituitary have formed from the primitive ventral neural ridges by 7 weeks. By 9 weeks of gestation capillaries have begun to develop around the portion of the diencephalon adjacent to the Rathke pouch. These capillaries differentiate into the hypothalamic–hypophyseal–portal system by about 11 weeks of gestation. The Rathke pouch will form the anterior and intermediate lobes of the pituitary gland. The area known as the hypothalamus at maturity is recognizable as discrete nuclei by about 15 weeks. The functional integrity of both the portal system and hypothalamic nuclei continues to mature until late in gestation. The general scheme by which these nuclei are formed is by migration of neurons from the outside of the primitive brain anlage inward to the place of nuclear organization. Further organization and interconnection of nuclei occurs until about 18 weeks. By this time the fetus is able to regulate its internal environment in a sophisticated and autonomous manner. The differentiation of anterior pituitary cells into hormone-specific cell lines probably occurs under the influence of a number of transcription factors such as pituitary-specific differentiation and transcription factor (Pit-1) and differentiation factors such as gonadotrophin-releasing hormone (GnRH), TRH, triiodothyronine ($T_3$) and others. The details of regulation of specific hormones will be discussed in subsequent sections.

Several clinical syndromes can result from incomplete development of the hypothalamic–pituitary unit. For example, *anencephaly* deprives the fetus of any hypothalamic function, although the pituitary gland itself forms normally. More subtle functional abnormalities of the hypothalamus are observed in children with the syndrome of *septo-optic dysplasia* and other mid-line anatomical abnormalities. Failure of Rathke pouch migration can result in a pituitary gland which is not connected to its regulatory input. This isolated pituitary syndrome is probably the most common cause of *congenital hypopituitarism* and can be detected by magnetic resonance imaging. The differentiation of specific cell types within the anterior pituitary is dependent on extrinsic and intrinsic factors. Abnormalities of Pit-1 may result in abnormal formation not only of GH-producing cells, but of TSH- and PRL-producing cells for which Pit-1 is also a necessary transcription factor. This results in a rare autosomal recessive form of *congenital hypopituitarism* with GH, PRL and variable TSH deficiency. Tumors of the cells of the Rathke pouch (*craniopharyngioma*), can disrupt the normal hypothalamic–pituitary anatomical relationship and cause pituitary dysfunction.

## The development of neuroendocrine sexual dimorphism

The human, as many other species, has a sexually dimorphic brain. Differences between males and females include the preoptic hypothalamic area, in which females undergo loss of cells between the ages of 4 and 10 years; the functional significance of this region is not known. The factors responsible for the multiple sexually dimorphic features of the brain are not well understood. It is possible that the pattern of sex steroid secretion in the perinatal period and the selective presence of receptors for steroids on specific neurons combine to orchestrate different patterns of cell development and cell death in males and females. The observation that male and female fetuses regulate gonadotrophins differently suggests that these sex differences may be programmed very early in development. GH regulation is likewise sexually dimorphic. There are numerous examples in animals of anatomical and behavioral changes induced by manipulation of the sex steroid milieu during a critical period of development.

## Functional maturation of neuroendocrine regulation

Hypothalamic–hypophyseal function requires the completion of a large number of developmental processes, which are only beginning to be understood. The ability to communicate by neurosecretion presupposes that the neuron has the ability to synthesize a specific neurotransmitter and/or neuropeptide. The message emitted by one cell must be received by another cell or cells, which is dependent upon the development of specific receptors. Furthermore, the appropriate intracellular second messenger systems must be sufficiently mature to effect the appropriate cellular response. These receptors and intracellular elements must be functional at all levels of the feedback loops described above. Thus the development of one receptor (or any one particular element) in a feedback regulatory system can be the developmental regulator of the function of the entire system. It is more likely that the components of a feedback system are individually developmentally regulated in such a way that the system functions differently at different times to suit the needs of the organism as a whole. Understanding of this complex developmental orchestration is primitive.

Although there are significant differences in the signals for neuroendocrine regulation among the pituitary hormone systems, which will be discussed in later sections, there are common developmental patterns which suggest an overall scheme by which regulatory systems are built. The first of these patterns is the increasing pituitary content of hormone as development progresses. The second is a tendency for plasma hormone concentrations to increase during gestation, sometimes with a subsequent decrease toward term. These two patterns together imply gradual acquisition by the fetus of the ability to restrain pituitary secretion. The time during the second half of gestation when these phenomena can occur corresponds in the human with the progressive development of the hypothalamic nuclei and neuronal tracts which have been demonstrated to modulate neuroendocrine function in the mature animal. The third pattern is the asynchronous development of specific hypothalamic inputs which either stimulate or suppress pituitary hormonal secretion. For example, the responses of both PRL and GH to various pharmacological stimulants and suppressants do not develop all at once, but follow a program specific to both the stimulus and responding hormone. The result is a gradual accumulation of an increasing number of modulating inputs to hormone secretion. A fourth consideration is the asynchronous development of the ability to manufacture and secrete a hormone and of the receptors for that hormone. For example, the role of GH in regulating growth is relatively less in the neonate because of receptor immaturity; thus in *congenital growth hormone deficiency*, birth length is only slightly reduced (see page 288).

## Role of the maternal–placental unit

A final influence on the development of neuroendocrine regulatory systems to consider is the effect of the fetal hormonal milieu resulting from maternal and placental hormone production. This influence includes placental production of a wide variety of both steroid and protein hormones, some of which (chorionic gonadotrophin, estrogen, etc.) are integral parts of developing feedback systems. The placenta may perform other functions which modulate fetal neuroendocrinology, such as metabolizing hormones to inactive compounds, selectively regulating fetal exposure to maternal hormones, production of growth factors and specific regulation of nutrient availability.

## NEUROIMMUNOENDOCRINOLOGY

There are three major ways in which the neuroendocrine and immunological systems interact. It is well recognized that many hormones have dramatic effects on immune function. The effects of glucocorticoids on all aspects of lymphokine synthesis and action are the most obvious example. Second, the lymphokines produced by the immune system have significant effects on neuroendocrine function. The multiple actions of interleukin-1 on the adrenocorticotrophic and gonadotrophic axes are examples. Third, cells of the immune system produce hormones and peptides which have been associated with classic neuroendocrinology, such as ACTH, GH, TSH and enkephalins. The developmental aspects and teleology of these findings are not well understood, however there is preliminary evidence for the existence of feedback regulation of hypothalamic/pituitary hormones by immunocyte derived neuropeptides.

## SELECTED READING

Fisher DA. Endocrinology of fetal development. In Wilson JD, Foster DW, eds. *Williams' textbook of endocrinology*. Philadelphia: WB Saunders Co., 1992: 1049.

Gluckman PD, Grumbach MM, Kaplan SL. The neuroendocrine regulation and function of growth hormone and prolactin in the mammalian fetus. *Endocr Rev* 1981; 2: 363.

Hokfelt T, Meister B, Villar MJ *et al*. Hypothalamic neurosecretory systems and their messenger molecules. *Acta Physiol Scand Suppl* 1989; 583: 105.

Jacobson M. *Developmental neurobiology*. 3rd edn. New York: Plenum Press, 1991: Chapters 7 and 8.

Mulchahey JJ, Di Blasio AM, Martin MC *et al*. Hormone production and peptide regulation of the human fetal pituitary gland. *Endocr Rev* 1987; 8: 406.

# 35

# Growth Hormone

Francis de Zegher

Growth hormone (GH) is the principal hormone regulating longitudinal growth during childhood (see Fig. 35.1). The assessment of GH secretion is important in the evaluation of children with growth disorders. Recombinant human GH is therapeutically used in an increasing range of disorders. This section will focus on the regulation of GH secretion; GH receptors and GH action are discussed further in Chapter 23 page 309.

## ORIGIN, BIOCHEMISTRY, CIRCULATION

The GH and prolactin gene evolved from a common precursor gene. The GH gene is part of a cluster of related genes, located on chromosome 17. This cluster also codes for other members of the GH gene family, namely placental lactogen and placental GH. Deletions of the gene are responsible for type Ia form of *familial growth hormone deficiency*. GH is a single chain 22 kD peptide of 191 amino acids synthesized and secreted from storage granules by the somatotropes of the anterior pituitary. Somatotropes, lactotropes and thyrotropes are derived from a common ontogenetic precursor cell: they depend on the activity of the pituitary-specific transcription factor (Pit-1) for differentiation, proliferation and maintenance. Defects in Pit-1 expression result in congenital deficiency of GH, prolactin (PRL) and thyroid stimulating hormone (TSH). GH is stored in somatotropes in vesicles as a $(Zn^{2+}, hGH)_2$ complex. On release it dissociates into a monomeric form. Variant forms of GH may also be secreted by the adenohypophysis. The most important is 20 kD GH which represents about 10 per cent of secreted GH and is a consequence of alternate splicing of the GH gene such that a second mRNA species coding for a GH missing 15 residues is formed. Its biological significance is unclear but it may have different affinity for the GH receptor.

GH circulates in the blood partly complexed with a binding protein that is structurally similar to the extracellular domain of the GH receptor. The human GH-binding protein is formed by proteolytic cleavage of the extramembranous portion of the GH receptor rather than by alternate splicing of the GH receptor gene. This GH-binding protein modulates the half-life of circulating GH which is approximately 7 minutes for free GH, 27 minutes for bound GH and 18 minutes for total GH. In those cases of *Laron syndrome* where the mutation affects the binding domain of the GH receptor, the GH-binding protein is less abundant or absent in the circulation. Serum GH-binding protein concentrations also may be low in children with *renal failure, cirrhosis, diabetes mellitus, malnutrition* and severe acute illness.

## REGULATION OF GH SECRETION

GH secretion is under the regulatory control of the central nervous system. Complex networks of neurotransmitter neurons modulate the release of two hypothalamic hormones, the stimulatory GH-releasing hormone (GHRH) and the inhibitory somatostatin (somatotrophin release-inhibiting factor, SRIF); these are the principal final mediators of metabolic, endo-

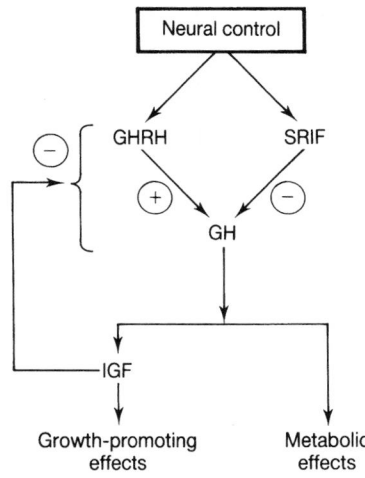

FIGURE 35.1 Simplified concept of the somatotrophic axis

crine and neural influences on GH secretion. The net effect of these hypothalamic influences is stimulatory and in structural or functional disorders of the hypothalamic–pituitary connection such as in congenital hypopituitarism, GH secretion is deficient.

A host of neuropeptides and neurotransmitters are capable of modulating GH secretion. Many of them, including enkephalins, neurotensin, γ-amino butyric acid (GABA), dopamine and neuropeptide Y, have been localized in the hypothalamic arcuate nucleus–median eminence complex. They may act at the level of the GHRH and/or SRIF producing neurons; some may also directly influence GH secretion at the pituitary level.

GHRH is a 44-amino-acid amide. The GHRH gene is located on chromosome 20. *In vivo*, GHRH is rapidly degraded to a biologically inactive product through cleavage at the N-terminus. In the brain, GHRH is found only in cell bodies of the ventromedial and arcuate nuclei from where fibers project to the median eminence and make contact with portal vessels. Some GHRH neurons also produce galanin. Serum immunoreactive GHRH appears to be mainly from extrahypothalamic origin, probably from the gut and pancreas. Hypothalamic GHRH synthesis and/or release is stimulated by $\alpha_2$-adrenergic receptor agonists, opioids, thyroid hormones and GABA, and is inhibited by SRIF, GH, and insulin-like growth factor I (IGF-I). The actions of GHRH on the somatotrope are mediated by G-protein-linked membrane receptors, that are up-regulated by Pit-1 and glucocorticoids, and down-regulated by GHRH itself. GHRH elicits an immediate release of preformed GH through its intramembranous G-protein-linked receptor which activates adenylyl cyclase. In contrast SRIF exerts an inhibitory effect on adenylyl cyclase. The activated adenylyl cyclase converts ATP to cAMP, that stimulates GH release. $Ca^{2+}$ mobilization participates in GHRH-mediated GH release, either at the adenylyl cyclase level or at a step distal to cAMP. GHRH stimulates GH gene transcription and GH synthesis in the somatotropes; these actions appear to be independent of $Ca^{2+}$ mobilization and GH release. GHRH is also able to induce somatotrope proliferation.

SRIF-14, a cyclic tetradecapeptide, is the most important product processed from preproSRIF in SRIF-containing cells. A larger-molecular-weight form, SRIF-28 may also play some physiological role, as it has a distinct receptor. SRIF is an important inhibitory neurotransmitter widely distributed in the brain, but also in the gastrointestinal tract. The highest density of SRIF-containing cells is found in the anterior periventricular region of the hypothalamus. Axons of a major part of the periventricular SRIF cells sweep laterally, then caudally and again toward the midline, thus forming an SRIF pathway ending in the median eminence at the level of the ventromedial nucleus. Hypothalamic SRIF release is $Ca^{2+}$-dependent with the neurotransmitters dopamine, acetylcholine and norepinephrine enhancing SRIF release, and β-adrener-

gic blockers, GABA and serotonin inhibiting SRIF release. Similarly, the peptides glucagon, insulin, neurotensin, GHRH and bombesin stimulate, whereas opiates and galanin inhibit SRIF secretion. GHRH, GH and IGF-I all stimulate hypothalamic SRIF release and SRIF inhibits its own release. Binding of SRIF to the G-protein-linked membrane SRIF receptors of the somatotropes inhibits the catalytic subunit of the adenylyl cyclase system, which results in an inhibition of basal and GHRH-stimulated GH release. However, SRIF does not inhibit GH gene transcription and GH synthesis. SRIF can partly inhibit GHRH-stimulated somatotrope proliferation. SRIF also is able to down-regulate its own pituitary binding sites. In other tissues SRIF binds to closely related but distinct forms of the SRIF receptor.

GHRH and SRIF are released into the hypophyseal portal system in a reciprocal manner. Their complex interaction on the somatotropes results in an intermittent release of GH into the circulation, thus eliciting a pulsatile plasma GH profile. The regulation of GH secretion is completed by a variety of feedback loops at both the hypothalamic and the pituitary level, in which at least GHRH, SRIF, GH itself, IGFs and intrapituitary paracrine modulators (e.g. acetylcholine) are involved. Finally, some metabolic substrates and circulating cytokines are also known to participate in the regulation of GH secretion: free fatty acids decrease GH release, whereas hypoglycemia and interleukin-1 induce GH secretion.

The normal pulsatile profile of plasma GH in children consists of long trough episodes with low or undetectable GH concentrations, alternating with shorter bursts during which GH concentrations are elevated (see page 309). Throughout childhood, these GH pulses of variable amplitude occur approximately over every 3 hours. Augmented GH peaks are associated with slow wave sleep (stages 3 and 4) possibly through a serotoninergic mechanism. GH pulses provoked by vigorous exercise and by physical or emotional stress are probably of adrenergic origin. Sex steroids, thyroid hormone and low amounts of glucocorticoids increase the amplitude of GH peaks. Spontaneous GH secretion is decreased in alimentary obesity and increased in conditions of starvation, kwashiorkor and marasmus, in part through modulation of the feedback actions by IGFs and their binding proteins.

## ASSESSMENT OF GH SECRETION

The usual indication for the assessment of GH secretion is a growth disorder. Growth velocity appears to be related to GH secretion, particularly to the amplitude of endogenous GH pulses. However, the spectra of normal variation with both growth and GH secretion are very wide. Pathological GH deficiency and GH hypersecretion are rare disorders. Any engagement into the assessment of GH secretion of an individual child should be underbuilt by an auxological evaluation and a complete pediatric examination. *Hypothyroidism, celiac disease, psychosocial deprivation* and tumors of the central nervous system, including *craniopharyngioma*, are well-known causes of growth failure and inappropriate GH secretion, but each needs a different diagnostic and therapeutic approach. GH is measured in plasma, usually by radioimmunoassay. An instructive but laborious way to assess endogenous GH secretion is to measure GH in consecutively obtained plasma samples over 24 hours or during sleep overnight. In view of the short half-life of GH, intermittent sampling, at intervals of maximum 20 minutes, is required to detect major GH peaks accurately. GH profiles obtained with continuous withdrawal methods are less informative because GH pulses are lost or smoothed by the addition of lower basal concentrations which contribute around 80 per cent of the levels measured over a 24-hour period. The latter also explains the poor diagnostic value of GH measurements in randomly obtained plasma samples. This diagnostic value increases when the sampling occurs after a vigorous physical effort (exercise test) or during the onset of slow wave sleep.

The classic and less difficult approach of assessing GH secretion is to verify whether a GH pulse can be elicited by standard provocative stimuli applied either separately or in combination. The β-adrenergic receptor blocker propranolol and the amino acid arginine normally evoke a burst of GH release by inhibiting the hypothalamic secretion of SRIF. The same mechanism is thought to be activated by insulin-induced hypoglycemia and by the relative hypoglycemia following glucagon-induced hyperglycemia. In contrast, the α-adrenergic precursor L-DOPA and the α-adrenergic receptor agonist clonidine appear to provoke GH release through stimulation of hypothalamic GHRH secretion. A definite GH response in these controlled circumstances strongly suggests functional integrity of the hypothalamic–pituitary–somatotrophic axis, but offers no guarantee for normal spontaneous GH secretion. Some children, fulfilling the auxological criteria of GH deficiency, respond normally to provocative puberty stimuli but fail to secrete sufficient GH spontaneously (so-called *neurosecretory GH dysfunction*). Conversely, normal subjects may occasionally fail to respond to a pharmacological stimulus. Therefore, the diagnosis of true *GH deficiency* cannot be based on a single test. The administration of GHRH may be helpful to localize the origin of GH deficiency in the hypothalamus (GH response to GHRH present) or at the pituitary level (GH response absent). In childhood, *GH deficiency* is most often of hypothalamic origin. GH hypersecretion during childhood, resulting in *gigantism*, is excessively rare and most likely due to a pituitary adenoma. In these cases, plasma GH levels are continuously elevated, are not suppressible by hyperglycemia and are responsive to stimulation with thyrotrophin-releasing hormone. Abnormal GH secretion is an indication for morphological studies of the hypothalamo–pituitary complex, preferably by magnetic resonance imaging.

## DEVELOPMENTAL ASPECTS

### The fetus and newborn

GH does not cross the placenta and the GH that appears in fetal plasma at about 10 weeks of gestation is exclusively of fetal pituitary origin. The fetal somatotropes secrete large amounts of GH in response to hypothalamic GHRH and appear to experience little inhibitory effect from SRIF and IGF-I. By midgestation, this results in markedly elevated plasma GH concentrations (>100 ng/mL) with intermittent GH pulses of an exaggerated amplitude. Inhibitory influences on the somatotropes become more effective toward term and certainly after birth, resulting in a gradual decrease of GH baseline concentrations and GH pulses. In the newborn, the GH pulse frequency approximates one per hour. GH secretion is relatively increased in premature and dysmature infants and is decreased in the newborn with hypopituitarism or primary hypothyroidism. Paradoxically, glucose infusion elicits a GH response in the newborn, whereas dopamine inhibits GH secretion. Sleep-associated GH release develops shortly after the neonatal period. Placental GH, a GH variant synthesized by the placenta by a separate gene to pituitary GH, is not secreted into the fetal circulation but only into the maternal compartment. Plasma GH-binding protein concentrations are low in the fetus and increase during early infancy, possibly reflecting an increase in GH receptor number postnatally (see page 288).

### Puberty

At the end of the prepubertal period, GH secretion may be transiently low, particularly when the onset of puberty is delayed. GH secretion during midpuberty is two- to three-fold increased compared to childhood. This change consists principally of an increase in GH burst amplitude. It is provoked by the circulating sex steroids and is probably mediated by an augmented hypothalamic GHRH release. After puberty, GH secretion decreases slowly throughout adult life. Because sex steroids increase GH secretion, sex steroid priming has been used in the evaluation of GH secretion when puberty is delayed.

### Pregnancy

The secretion of pituitary GH by the pregnant woman decreases with advancing gestation, due to increased inhibition of GH release at the pituitary level by placental lactogen and placental growth hormone. The pulsatile presence of pituitary GH in the maternal circulation is gradually replaced by constantly elevated concentrations of placental GH, which fall immediately after birth; maternal concentrations of placental GH are lower in pregnancies associated with intrauterine growth retardation. The puerperal recovery of pituitary GH secretion is delayed by lactation.

## GH ACTIONS (*see* page 309)

GH acts through ubiquitously distributed GH-membrane receptors (see page 310). These receptors are structurally related to prolactin receptors. The principal actions of GH are metabolic and growth promoting. The effects of GH on intermediary metabolism are complex and depend in part on the age, the nutritional status, and the endocrine equilibrium of the considered individual. GH appears to have net anabolic effects on protein metabolism and has insulin-antagonizing effects on lipid and carbohydrate metabolism, as GH has lipolytic, glycogenolytic and gluconeogenic characteristics. The growth-promoting properties of GH are thought to be mediated by IGFs and to be facilitated by thyroid hormones. GH is currently recommended to be administered subcutaneously, once daily, in the evening. Although this practice results in a single, large, plasma GH peak during the night, a profile differing markedly from the physiological pulsatile pattern. The resulting GH effects appear to mimic closely the effects of normal GH secretion. The classic indication for treatment with exogenous GH is *GH deficiency* during infancy, childhood and adolescence. However, the metabolic and growth-promoting properties of GH are increasingly explored in a variety of conditions associated with catabolic status or growth failure.

The latter include *Turner syndrome* and *short stature of prenatal onset*.

## SELECTED READING

Baumann G. Growth hormone heterogeneity: genes, isohormones, variants and binding proteins. *Endocr Rev* 1991; **12**: 424.

Evain-Brion D, Alsat E, Igout A *et al*. Placental growth hormone variant: assay and clinical aspects. *Acta Paediatr Suppl* 1994; **399**: 49.

Gluckman PD, Grumbach MM, Kaplan SL. The neuroendocrine regulation and function of growth hormone and prolactin in the mammalian fetus. *Endocr Rev* 1981; **2**: 363.

Mason WT, Dickson SL, Leng G. Control of growth hormone secretion at the single cell level. *Acta Paediatr Suppl* 1993; **388**: 84.

Parks JS, Abdul-Latif H, Kinoshita E. Genetics of growth hormone gene expression. *Horm Res* 1993; **40**: 54.

Phillips JA, Cogan JD. Molecular basis of familial human growth hormone deficiency. *J Clin Endocrinol Metab* 1994; **78**: 11.

Plotsky PM, Vale W. Patterns of growth hormone-releasing factor and somatostatin secretion into the hypophysial–portal circulation of the rat. *Science* 1985; **230**: 461.

Robinson ICAF. The growth hormone secretory pattern: a response to neuroendocrine signals. *Acta Paediatr Suppl* 1991; **372**: 70.

Rogol AD. Growth and growth hormone secretion at puberty: the role of gonadal steroid hormones. *Acta Paediatr Suppl* 1992; **383**: 15.

Tannenbaum GS. Neuroendocrine control of growth hormone secretion. *Acta Paediatr Suppl* 1991; **372**: 5.

Theill LE, Karin M. Transcriptional control of growth hormone expression and anterior pituitary development. *Endocr Rev* 1993; **14**: 670.

de Zegher F, Devlieger H, Veldhuis JD. Properties of growth hormone and prolactin hypersecretion by the human infant on the day of birth. *J Clin Endocrinol Metab* 1993; **76**: 1177.

# 36

# Prolactin

Peter D. Gluckman

The biological significance of prolactin (PRL) in man remains poorly defined. PRL stimulates milk secretion, provided the mammary gland has been primed with other hormones including estrogens. In hyperprolactinemic states (e.g. *pituitary microadenoma*), galactorrhea is frequently the presenting symptom. Pituitary infarction (*Sheehan syndrome*) is associated with lactational failure. Hyperprolactinemia inhibits the human gonadotrophic axis. PRL secreting tumors are rare in childhood but may present in adolescence as delayed puberty or amenorrhea.

PRL may be associated with specific functions in the perinatal period, including effects on lung maturation and fluid and electrolyte homeostasis. The latter may reflect a similar role for PRL in amphibia and fish.

## BIOCHEMISTRY

PRL is a single chain peptide of 198 amino acids, evolutionarily related to growth hormone (GH) and placental lactogen. It is secreted from storage granules by the lactotrope, an eosinophilic adenohypophyseal cell. In the fetus a proportion of PRL is secreted by a somatolactotrope, a cell that can secrete both GH and PRL and may be the precursor to both mature somatotrope and lactotrope forms of eosinophilic cells. It is now recognized that, as with GH, a number of isoforms are secreted by the pituitary. These include oligomeric, phosphorylated, deamidated and glycosylated forms as well as the classic dominant monomeric 24 kD form. These various forms of post-translational modification appear to be physiologically regulated as the different forms have various levels of biological activity. This offers a further level of regulatory complexity.

## REGULATION

Pituitary PRL, unlike other anterior pituitary hormones, is under a tonic inhibitory hypothalamic influence (Fig. 36.1). Thus, following hypothalamic–pituitary functional disconnection (e.g. trauma, hypothalamic tumor), PRL secretion is maintained or increased. Only if the pituitary itself is destroyed (e.g. *congenital pituitary aplasia*), is PRL secretion diminished.

Dopamine, the major PRL inhibitory neurohormone, originates in tuberoinfundibular neurons, with cell bodies in the hypothalamic arcuate nucleus, and secretes into the primary hypophyseal–portal plexus. Thus dopaminergic antagonists, including many psychotrophic agents (e.g. chlorpromazine, reserpine, angel dust), increase circulating PRL concentrations. Dopaminergic agonists (e.g. bromocriptine) reduce PRL secretion. The primary hypothalamic stimulatory factor is thyrotrophin releasing hormone (TRH) which also stimulates thyroid stimulating hormone (TSH) release. Thus in *primary hypothyroidism*, hyperprolactinemia may result from this overlap. Putative peptidergic specific PRL-releasing and inhibitory factors have been suggested. PRL is considerably influenced by other neurotransmitter and neuropeptidergic systems. Most operate through alterations in the secretion of the relevant neurohormones (dopamine and TRH). However, direct secretion of some, such as vasoactive intestinal peptide (VIP), into the portal circulation and intrapituitary paracrine mechanisms provides greater complexity of control. PRL secretion is very sensitive to external stimuli. Stress of any type including pain, exercise, or fear, elevates PRL secretion hindering interpretation of random samples. PRL secretion prob-

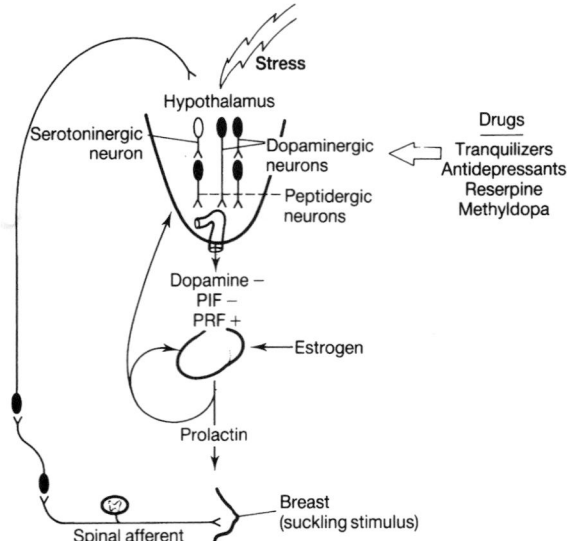

FIGURE 36.1 Hypothalamic regulation of PRL secretion. The predominant effect of the hypothalamus is inhibitory, an effect mediated principally by dopamine secreted by the tuberohypophyseal dopaminergic neuron system. One or more prolactin releasing factors (PRFs) probably mediate acute release of PRL as in suckling and stress. There are several candidate PRFs, including TRH and vasoactive intestinal peptide (VIP). Estrogen sensitizes the pituitary to release PRL. PRL feeds back on the pituitary to regulate its own secretion (short loop feedback). Short loop feedback is probably mediated indirectly by modifications of hypothalamic catecholamine secretion and turnover. Direct ultrashort feedback inhibition probably also occurs. (Modified from Reichlin S. Neuroendocrinology. In Wilson JD, Foster DW, eds. *Williams' textbook of endocrinology*, 8th edns. Philadelphia: WB Saunders Co., 1992: 174. Reprinted with permission of WB Saunders Co.)

ably follows a diurnal rhythm in man, increasing in the early morning.

The other major influence on PRL secretion is estrogen, which stimulates PRL release by a number of actions at both hypothalamic and pituitary levels; these include inhibition of dopamine release and action, and an increase in mRNA coding for PRL synthesis. PRL levels surge at ovulation.

## ACTIONS

Prolactin acts via cell-membrane receptors, members of the GH/cytokine receptor superfamily (*see* page 462). These lactogenic receptors have a long extracellular portion, a short single transmembrane domain, and an intracellular region. Two major forms are described, at least in rodents, one with a short cytoplasmic tail of <60 amino acids and one with a long cytoplasmic tail of 358 amino acids. The shorter form dominates in the liver and appears to be a clearance receptor. Alternate splicing appears to give rise to the different intracellular domains in different tissues.

Receptor homodimerization is required for signal transduction which appears to involve activation of Jak2 kinase. The extracellular region has high homology to the somatotrophic (GH) receptor; therefore, GH has weak affinity for the lactogenic receptor and vice versa. In contrast, the intracellular region of the somatogenic receptor is not homologous, providing the basis for the different spectra of activities.

## EVALUATION OF PRL SECRETION

PRL is measured by radioimmunoassay. In childhood there is little clinical indication for the measurement of PRL. Hypersecretion is determined from random measurement in non-stressed patients, by an enhanced response to TRH or dopaminergic antagonists and by incomplete suppression in response to bromocriptine. Pathophysiological hyperprolactinemia is most likely due to *pituitary microadenoma*. Hyposecretion is seen as a deficient response to TRH. This is useful in *neonatal hypopituitarism* to distinguish *pituitary agenesis* (an autosomal recessive condition) from more common, sporadic hypothalamic causes.

## SPECIFIC DEVELOPMENTAL ASPECTS

### Fetal life

PRL does not pass across the placenta. PRL is first detectable in fetal plasma at about 10 weeks of gestation. After 30 weeks concentrations rise progressively, peaking at delivery with levels 20-fold above adult values. This developmental hyperprolactinemia is likely secondary to high circulating estrogens of placental origin in the fetal circulation. A diurnal rhythm in fetal PRL levels, perhaps due to transplacental melatonin, is seen experimentally.

### Changes at birth

PRL concentrations are very high in umbilical cord blood. They decline rapidly over the first neonatal week, then more slowly over the next 2 months, perhaps as residual effects wane.

### Pregnancy and amniotic fluid

PRL concentrations also rise in the mother throughout pregnancy, presumably secondary to the estrogenic influences. This rise plays a part in mammary development. PRL remains elevated into the puerperium and can be maintained by suckling.

The endometrium, which in pregnancy becomes the decidua, is a further source of PRL. Unknown local factors regulate decidual PRL which enters amniotic fluid but not the blood stream. It may influence amniotic fluid volume and osmolality by affecting fluid and electrolyte transfer across the amnion and possibly the fetal skin. Decidual PRL may also play a role in inhibiting myometrial contractility.

## The role of PRL in the fetal and neonatal period

PRL may be important in regulating fetal fluid balance through antidiuretic actions on the fetal kidney. The reduction in total body water after birth may reflect the decline in PRL secretion. Most interest has focused on the role of fetal PRL in maturation of the pulmonary surfactant system. Cord blood PRL concentrations are low in infants who develop *respiratory distress syndrome*.

While PRL alone has little effect on fetal pulmonary maturation, in conjunction with glucocorticoids and thyroid hormones it has pronounced effects experimentally. TRH crosses the human placenta and stimulates both PRL and thyroid hormone release *in utero*. This is the basis of current trials of maternal TRH administration to enhance lung maturation.

## SELECTED READING

Gluckman PD, Bassett NS. The development of hypothalamic function in the perinatal period. In Meisami E, Timeras P, eds. *Handbook of human growth and developmental biology*. Vol. II, Part A. Boca Raton: CRC Press, 1989: 3.

Gluckman PD, Grumbach MM, Kaplan SL. The neuroendocrine regulation and function of growth hormone and prolactin in the mammalian fetus. *Endocr Rev* 1981; 2: 363.

Kelly PA, Djiane J, Edery M. Different forms of the prolactin receptor. Insights into the mechanism of prolactin action. *Trends Endocrinol Metab* 1992; 3: 54.

# 37

# The Thyroid Gland

Jossi Sack

The secretion and metabolism of thyroid hormones are controlled by an autoregulated, negative feedback system that involves the central nervous system (CNS), hypothalamus, pituitary gland, thyroid and peripheral tissues. The system is initiated by CNS activation of the hypothalamus to release thyrotrophin-releasing hormone (TRH), to stimulate thyroid-stimulating hormone (thyrotrophin, TSH) secretion, which in turn, provides the signal for synthesis and secretion of thyroid hormones from thyroid follicular cells (Fig. 37.1).

## THYROTROPHIN-RELEASING HORMONE

TRH is a tripeptide, (pyro) Glu-His-Pro($NH_2$), derived from a prohormone that undergoes extensive post-translational processing. In response to neural stimulation it is secreted into the adenohypophyseal–portal circulation. Somatostatin, norepinephrine and dopaminergic drugs increase TRH release.

TRH is widely distributed throughout the nervous system. Some studies have shown an association between TRH administration and mood elevation, suggesting that this tripeptide may act as a neurotransmitter in addition to regulating TSH and prolactin (PRL) secretion by acting on the thyrotrope and lactotrope respectively.

TRH belongs to the group of G-protein-linked cell-surface interacting hormones. The binding of TRH to its receptor in the cell-surface membrane activates the guanine nucleotide-binding regulatory proteins of the receptor. This binds guanine triphosphate (GTP), which in turn binds to phospholipase C, and activates the enzyme which catalyzes the hydrolysis of phosphatidylinositol-4,5 bisphosphate. This hydrolysis generates two intracellular mediators, inositol trisphosphate ($IP_3$) and 1,2-diacylglycerol (DAG) in the target cell, resulting in a rapid rise in the concentration of free $Ca^{2+}$ ions in the cell cytoplasm. The sudden elevation of free $Ca^{2+}$ ions activates the movement of secretory granules to the cell surface and their fusion with the cell-surface membrane, followed by exocytosis and

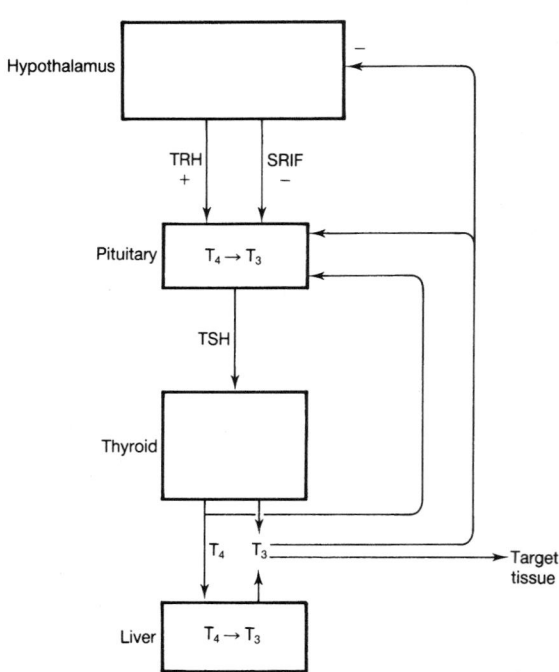

FIGURE 37.1 Schema of the hypothalamic–pituitary–thyroidal axis showing the major factors regulating the generation of $T_4$ and $T_3$. TSH stimulates thyroidal secretion of $T_4$ and some $T_3$. However, 85 per cent of circulating $T_3$ is derived from hepatic and other peripheral deiodination of $T_4$. Circulating $T_3$ and $T_4$ inhibit pituitary TSH release. The $T_4$ acts after intrapituitary conversion to $T_3$. $T_3$ may also exert negative feedback at the hypothalamic level either by inhibiting TRF release or stimulating SRIF release.

TSH release. The simultaneous activation of protein kinase C by DAG leads to phosphorylation of proteins, involved in exocytosis, that mediate the sustained phase of secretion.

TRH profoundly stimulates TSH secretion and is the major positive regulator of TSH secretion.

Exogenous TRH increases serum TSH and PRL, with a peak at 10–15 minutes. Intravenous administration of TRH is the only test available to distinguish between *pituitary* (secondary) and *hypothalamic* (tertiary) *hypothyroidism*. In *pituitary hypothyroidism* the TSH response to TRH is decreased or absent while in *hypothalamic hypothyroidism* TSH response to intravenous TRH is adequate, but often with a delayed peak response because of an abnormal inhibitory control. This test can be used diagnostically as early as the neonatal period.

## Fetal life

TRH is detectable in the hypothalamus at 9–10 weeks' gestation, at a time when the hypothalamic–hypophyseal–portal vascular system is functioning. By the 13th week of gestation, TSH-producing cells are identified.

## THYROID-STIMULATING HORMONE

The pituitary glycoprotein hormone, TSH, is synthesized and secreted by the thyrotropes in the anterior pituitary. TSH increases thyroid gland production of the thyroid hormones thyroxine ($T_4$) and triiodothyronine ($T_3$) which then act on organs throughout the body to modulate growth and various metabolic functions.

## Biochemistry

TSH, a pituitary-derived glycoprotein of 28–30 kD, is composed of two non-covalently linked subunits. The α-subunit is a glycoprotein: the protein core is identical to that of the α-subunit of pituitary luteinizing hormone (LH) and follicle stimulating hormone (FSH) and chorionic gonadotrophin, but with different glycosylation. The β-subunits of these hormones are also glycoproteins and show considerable homology. Unlike most glycoproteins, the oligosaccharides of TSH appear to play vital functional roles. Precursor forms of the oligosaccharides allow nascent subunits to fold properly during biosynthesis, and prevent degradation and aggregation of the subunits. The structure of the oligosaccharides may be regulated by endocrine factors during TSH biosynthesis, so that qualitatively different forms of TSH are secreted in different physiological states. TSH is more sialated in hypothyroid patients than in euthyroid patients. The biological activity or significance of free α-subunits is unknown, but the abundance of α-subunit has led to the speculation that regulation of TSH β-subunits is the limiting step in modulating hormone levels. Production of the intact hormone involves the coordinated synthesis of TSH β- and α-subunits.

## Regulation

Negative feedback by thyroid hormones is the most important physiological regulator of TSH levels. High levels of thyroid hormones act at the pituitary to suppress synthesis and secretion of TSH. $T_3$ treatment decreases the TSH response to TRH, an effect which may be at least partially due to the decreased numbers of pituitary TRH receptors. $T_3$-mediated feedback also regulates both TSH subunits. The β-subunit, which is responsible for the distinctive biological effect of TSH, is more closely and rapidly inhibited by $T_3$ than is the α-subunit.

Circulating TSH concentrations are also modulated, by neurotransmitters released by the hypothalamus. The most prominent are TRH which is stimulatory, and somatostatin (SRIF) and dopamine which are inhibitory. The effect of TRH on TSH can be modified by the thyroid state with more pronounced stimulatory effects in hypothyroidism. TRH administration to *growth hormone* (GH) *deficient* children is associated with a greater TSH response. This effect can also be explained by lower somatostatin tone in GH deficiency. Increased responsiveness to TRH can also be induced by estrogens. This may be due to an increase in the concentration of TRH receptors in the pituitary.

## Actions of TSH

TSH binds to specific receptors on the thyroid plasma membrane. TSH activation of adenylyl cyclase leads to increased cAMP formation, and in turn to the activation of protein kinase. In the rare condition of *TSH unresponsiveness* there is a defect in coupling the receptor to cAMP generation.

TSH may stimulate growth as well as differentiation of the thyroid. This may be indirect via intermediary growth factors including insulin-like growth factor I (IGF-I) and epidermal growth factor. TSH stimulates iodine uptake by the thyroid follicular cell, but the mechanism of iodine ion transport across the thyroid cell membrane is as yet speculative. Iodine transport from the extracellular fluid into the thyroid cell is an energy-requiring process which concentrates iodine against an electrochemical gradient and involves oxidative metabolism and phosphorylation. Concentration gradients of iodine across the cell membrane higher than 20:1 are achieved by TSH stimulation. The response to TSH is biphasic, iodine transport first decreasing then increasing, and there is new protein synthesis in this process. Iodine transport mechanisms which are independent of TSH stimulation have been observed in the gastric mucosa, salivary and mammary glands, the choroid plexus and the placenta.

# Human chorionic gonadotrophin (hCG)

Chorionic gonadotrophin bears structural similarity to pituitary TSH. It also is a glycoprotein hormone with an identical α-subunit and a similar β-subunit (see page 207). In patients with trophoblastic tumors with very high circulating hCG concentrations, thyrotoxicosis may occur. Even in the absence of hyperthyroidism, changes in thyroid function have been noted. hCG has been shown to bind to, and compete with, TSH for receptor-binding sites, and to stimulate the membrane-bound adenylyl cyclase. The potency of hCG as a thyroid stimulator is relatively low; however, hCG may be a regulator of the thyroid gland in early pregnancy.

## THE THYROID GLAND

The thyroid gland is unique among the endocrine glands because of its large store of preformed hormone. The first endocrine gland in embryonic development, it appears at 3 weeks of gestation as a single median endodermal placode in the primitive pharynx, caudal to the oropharyngeal membrane, between the first and the second branchial arches. This placode is lined by epithelium which forms the primordia of the thyroid gland and the thyroglossal duct. The placode evaginates into the vertical mesoderm. Then the opening in the pharynx closes and the duct elongates. At this stage the primordial thyroid is located close to the developing heart. The relatively high incidence of congenital heart defects associated with congenital hypothyroidism may be explained by the anatomical proximity of the developing thyroid to the fetal heart.

During subsequent downgrowth there is bifurcation of the thyroid into two lobes. At about 5 weeks the thyroglossal ducts atrophy, the thyrocytes are arranged in epithelial cords and the follicular structure begins to form. At 10 weeks the colloid in the follicle appears. At this stage the thyroid gland can accumulate iodine, organify it and secrete thyroglobulin (Tg) into the colloid. Defects in the embryogenesis of the thyroid are not uncommon, leading to congenital hypothyroidism associated with hypoplasia/atresia. Thyroglossal duct remnants may persist.

## Secretion of the thyroid hormones (see Fig. 37.2)

The first step in thyroid hormone synthesis is iodide trapping by the thyroid gland. This is a rate-limiting energy-dependent process and accumulates iodide against a marked concentration gradient. Similar mechanisms exist in the salivary gland, mammary gland, placenta and gastric mucosa. Rare iodide trapping defects are reported.

Tg is synthesized in the thyroid follicular cells. Its tyrosol residues are iodinated by the enzyme thyroid peroxidase (TPO). The iodide must be oxidized in the presence of $H_2O_2$ before it is organified. Congenital peroxidase deficiency causes goitrous hypothyroidism or cretinism. Iodide also transiently blocks this step and this is the basis of the therapeutic use of iodide in acute thyrotoxicosis. The iodinated tyrosyl residues within the thyroglobulin are coupled to form tri-iodothyronine ($T_3$) and thyroxine ($T_4$). Congenital defects of coupling enzymes also cause goitrous hypothyroidism. Then vesicles containing Tg fuse with the cytoplasmic lysosomes that contain enzymes which degrade Tg to amino acids, diiodothyronine ($T_2$), monoiodothyronine ($T_1$) and $T_4$ and $T_3$. The $T_2$ and $T_1$ are deiodinased to recycle iodine. Deiodinase defects cause goitrous hypothyroidism due to inability to efficiently conserve iodine. Following hydrolysis, $T_4$ and $T_3$ migrate toward the basal surface of the follicle, where they are secreted into the circulation. Excess iodide also inhibits this step. Defects in Tg synthesis or transport present as familial goitrous hypothyroidism.

Thyroxine is the major thyroid hormone released by the thyroid gland and while $T_3$ is the active thyroid hormone only a small portion of $T_3$ is secreted by the gland: the rest being formed by deiodination from $T_4$ in peripheral tissues. The peripheral turnover (half-life) of the two major iodothyronines $T_4$ and $T_3$ is relatively slow, at 7 days and 1 day, respectively, due to the tight binding of the hormones to circulating plasma proteins. Approximately 99 per cent of $T_4$ is bound to three major binding proteins: thyroxine-binding globulin (TBG), $T_4$-binding prealbumin, transthyretin (TTR), and albumin. About 77 per cent of the $T_4$ is strongly bound to TBG, 15 per cent is bound to TTR, and 10 per cent is loosely bound to albumin. About 99 per cent of $T_3$ is bound to plasma proteins; 75 per cent to TBG and some 25 per cent to albumin. The bound hormone may serve as a reservoir of hormone, available to the peripheral tissues for metabolic action and metabolism. Many drugs, including salicylates, sulfonylureas and phenytoin, can interfere with the binding of thyroid hormones to these binding proteins. The concentration of binding protein is increased by estrogens, and inhibited by androgens and glucocorticoids. In addition, genetic hyper- or hypo-TBGemia may occur. Thus the interpretation of an abnormal thyroid hormone concentration depends firstly on elucidating the bound versus free hormone and secondly on assessing for evidence of abnormal thyroid function (e.g. altered plasma TSH concentrations, altered response to TRH).

Once secreted, $T_4$ is metabolized by several pathways including deiodination, deamination, decarboxylation, conjugation of metabolites, and ether link cleavage. The most important pathway is deiodination, which may account for 80 per cent of $T_4$ metabolism.

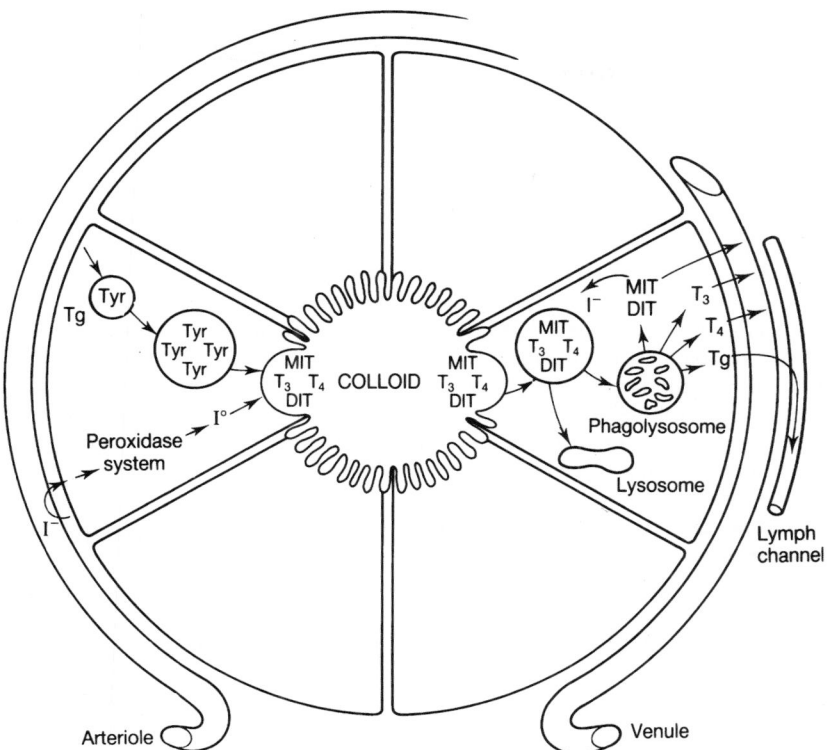

FIGURE 37.2 Thyroid hormone synthesis and secretion by thyroid follicular cells. Synthesis and secretion are shown separately, but occur in the same cell. The thyroid follicular cells form spherules with a storage pool of colloid in the center; this drawing shows a cross-section of a spheroid follicle (Tg, thyroglobulin; $I^-$, iodide; $I^\circ$, oxidized reactive iodine; Tyr, tyrosine; MIT, monoiodotyrosine; DIT, diiodotyrosine; $T_3$, triiodothyronine; $T_4$, thyroxine). Thyroglobulin, containing tyrosine residues, is synthesized within the cell and is transported to the luminal membrane, where it is exposed to oxidized, reactive iodine. The exposed tyrosine molecules within the Tg are iodinated to MIT or DIT and those MIT and DIT molecules are spatially oriented for coupling to form $T_3$ or $T_4$ molecules. The iodinated thyroglobulin is stored as colloid. Activation of secretion by TSH stimulates colloid endocytosis. Infolding colloid droplets fuse with cell lysosomes to form phagolysosomes within which thyroglobulin is degraded to release iodotyrosines $T_3$ and $T_4$. Some thyroglobulin escapes from the cell to the circulation predominantly via lymphatics. (From Fisher DA. The thyroid. In Kaplan SA, ed. *Clinical pediatric endocrinology*. Philadelphia: WB Saunders Co., 1990: 87. Reprinted with permission from WB Saunders Co.)

Postnatally, 70–90 per cent of the circulating $T_3$ is derived from peripheral monodeiodination of the outer phenolic ring of $T_4$. Monoiodination of the inner tyrosyl ring of $T_4$ produces reverse $T_3$ ($rT_3$), an inactive metabolite. Over 85 per cent of circulating $T_3$ is derived by peripheral deiodination of secreted $T_4$ rather than by direct secretion of $T_3$. About 30 per cent of $T_4$ secreted each day is converted to $T_3$. The most important sites are the liver and kidney and in the newborn, brown fat. In addition deiodination occurs in the CNS and in the pituitary gland; the latter is key to the negative feedback by thyroxine on TSH release. Many syndromes are associated with a decreased conversion of $T_4$ to $T_3$. These include starvation, use of glucocorticoids, chronic or acute illness, e.g. burns, diabetic ketoacidosis. They produce the *low $T_3$* or *euthyroid sick* syndrome. This can be differentiated from *true hypothyroidism* by the normal $T_4$ and often elevated $rT_3$ concentrations.

Generally the circulating $T_4$ concentration is sufficient to prevent clinical hypothyroidism. A particularly confusing situation is the sick premature neonate where, for ontogenetic reasons, $T_4$ and $T_3$ concentrations are lower than in term infants.

Degradation of $T_3$ and $rT_3$ produces three separate $T_2$s; further metabolism leads to the formation of two $T_1$s, and finally terminal deiodination yields thyronine. Peripheral deiodinase deficiency may be isolated or be associated with thyroidal deiodinase deficiency and lead to goiter. The monodeiodination of $T_4$ can be affected by a multitude of physiological conditions, clinical disorders and pharmacological agents. Inhibition of the conversion of $T_4$ to $T_3$ may be a protective mechanism as it reduces the level of active $T_3$ hormone. Pregnant women have increased levels of $T_2$ and $T_1$, probably because of high TBG levels. Newborn infants have low $T_3$ and high $rT_3$ levels.

## Thyroglobulin

Thyroglobulin is an important precursor protein for the synthesis of the thyroid hormones. It is a 660 kD glycoprotein, composed of two identical subunits and containing about 10 per cent carbohydrate. It can be found in the blood in low but detectable concentrations; its physiological role outside the thyroid gland is unknown. Elevated levels are observed with increased TSH stimulation of the thyroid gland. In subjects receiving suppressive doses of thyroid hormone, or in children who have ingested high doses of L-thyroxine, serum Tg may be undetectable (less than 3 ng/mL). In congenital hypothyroidism secondary to *thyroid atresia*, Tg in the serum is undetectable. In patients with congenital hypothyroidism due to a small *ectopic thyroid gland*, Tg can be detected many years after the initiation of treatment with L-thyroxine. Tg is also found in the serum of children with *congenital hypothyroidism* resulting from dyshormonogenesis.

## THYROID HORMONE ACTION

## Nuclear level

A full understanding of the nuclear site of initiation of thyroid hormone action depends on the recognition that $T_3$ is the active hormone and that $T_4$ serves largely as a precursor. There is now general agreement about the nature of the high-affinity, low-capacity nuclear receptors and which are the primary sites of $T_3$ action. Extranuclear binding sites for $T_3$ have been identified, but there is no convincing evidence to date that their binding results in recognized hormonal action.

The c-*erb*-A proto-oncogenes encode a high affinity receptor for $T_3$ and $T_4$. The c-*erb*-A gene products are related to the superfamily of steroid hormone receptors (*see* page 464). Each of these receptors is characterized by a carboxyl terminal ligand-binding domain, and by a highly conserved cysteine-rich, DNA-binding domain situated closer to the amino terminus. The DNA-binding domain is characterized by a cysteine-rich amino acid sequence that is believed to chelate zinc. These structures are therefore referred to as zinc fingers and are the DNA-binding regions. By analogy to other transcription factors, these receptors are also likely to contain activation domains which interact with cellular transcription machinery. Three distinct thyroid receptors (TRs), $\alpha_1$, $\beta_1$, and $\beta_2$, are expressed in pituitary cell culture. TR $\alpha_1$ is the product of the c-*erb*-A $\alpha$ gene. The c-*erb*-A $\beta$ gene encodes TR $\beta_1$ and TR $\beta_2$, which differ from one another only in their amino terminus. The human TR cDNA isolated from the placenta is designated $\beta_1$, and the pituitary specific form $\beta_2$.

Although the existence of multiple TRs and their differential expression suggests unique biological roles for each, studies have not revealed important functional differences. The syndrome of *generalized resistance to thyroid hormone* is characterized by high serum concentrations of free thyroid hormones in the absence of increased basal metabolism and TSH suppression. Such patients have high $T_4$ concentrations with persistently elevated TSH values. They may present with mixed clinical signs of hypo- and hyperthyroidism. There are both autosomal dominant and recessive modes of inheritance. In severely affected homozygous patients there is a major deletion in both c-*erb*-A $\beta$-alleles resulting in the absence of $\beta$-receptor. The signs of extreme resistance include a delay in brain development and skeletal maturation, while persistent tachycardia and lack of weight gain suggest hyperthyroidism. Thus the $\beta$-receptor appears to play a crucial role in the pituitary, the brain, and bone, whereas the $\alpha$-receptor may be more significant in mediating thyroid hormone action in cardiac tissue.

## Action at the cell, tissue and organ level

Information concerning the effects of thyroid hormones on target tissues derives mostly from clinical and experimental observations on the effects of the excess or deficiency of thyroid hormones. However, much of the molecular basis for the clinical symptoms in hypo- and hyperthyroidism remains unexplained. In general, thyroid hormone effects resemble those of catecholamines: increase in the basal metabolic rate, in $O_2$ consumption and in thermogenesis.

Although the exact mechanism involved in the maintenance of constant body temperature is unknown there is no doubt that $T_3$ plays a critical role (*see* page 588). Thyroid hormone may exert its thermogenic effect by stimulating futile biochemical cycles. The synthesis of fatty acids requires high energy phosphate, and since such high energy phosphate can be obtained in large part from that released in the course of fatty acid oxidation, the fatty acid synthesis–degradation cycle appears to be the thermogenic futile cycle stimulated by thyroid hormone action. The increase in thermogenesis by thyroid hormones may occur partly by increasing the metabolic response to catecholamines; thyroid hormones increase primarily the basal metabolic rate, while catecholamines increase the metabolic rate above the basal rate in response to environmental stimuli.

The abnormalities associated with thyroid hormone deficiency also involve retardation of body growth, and retarded maturation of individual cells and tissues. Thyroid hormone appears to function both by stimulation of growth and by accelerating the differentiation of specific cell types. Thus whereas in adult onset hypothyroidism most of the effects of thyroid hormone deficiency can be easily reversed; this is not the case in neonates.

## Thyroid hormone and the CNS

Specific nuclear $T_3$ receptors are present in the fetal, neonatal and adult brain. In the neonatal rat hypothyroid brain there is reduction in the branching of dendrites and axons, as well as a deficiency in axonal myelin formation. The primary effect of thyroid hormone in the brain is probably to switch the cells from a proliferative to a differentiative state. Some of its effects may be mediated by stimulating the production of nerve growth factor and other neurotrophic factors.

After the introduction of neonatal screening for *congenital hypothyroidism*, preliminary studies of the outcome in affected fetuses were very encouraging. However, evidence is now accumulating that not all the effects of fetal hypothyroidism are reversed by early postnatal treatment, and some neurological deficit may persist. Thus, complete prevention of neurological damage may be achieved only if hypothyroidism is diagnosed *in utero*, and treatment initiated either by intra-amniotic or cord injections of $T_4$ before birth.

## Thyroid hormone and the skeleton

The absence of femoral, tibial and cuboid bone nuclei epiphyses in hypothyroid infants stresses the importance of thyroid hormone in bone maturation. Lack of thyroid hormone in the fetus and neonate also causes a depressed nasal bridge and delay in closure of the fontanelles, while hyperthyroidism can cause craniosynostosis and premature closure of the skull sutures. Thyroid hormones stimulate endochondrial ossification and bone cell maturation, and also increase cartilage cell proliferation via stimulation of GH secretion and IGF-I function. Hypothyroidism therefore can cause extreme bone age retardation, as seen on X-ray, while hyperthyroidism accelerates bone age. Hyperthyroidism increases and hypothyroidism decreases bone turnover. The hypercalcemia observed in the hyperthyroid state is the result of increased bone destruction as well as increased $Ca^{2+}$ absorption in the gut. $T_4$ administration in congenital hypothyroid children is followed by hypercalciuria, probably due to increased formation of 1,25-dihydroxyvitamin D from its precursors.

## Thyroid hormone and the heart

The cardiovascular effects of thyroid hormone are similar to those of catecholamines. However, in hyperthyroid states, there is no increase in circulating catecholamines. An increase in the number of β-adrenergic receptors, and a concomitant increase in myocardial responses to catecholamines may be an explanation. β-Adrenergic receptor blockers are effective in the amelioration of hyperthyroidism.

## Effects on carbohydrate, lipid and protein metabolism

Thyroid hormone stimulates both glycolysis and gluconeogenesis. Key gluconeogenic enzymes, phosphoenolpyruvate carboxykinase, pyruvate carboxylase and glucose 6-phosphatase, are stimulated by thyroid hormones.

Thyroid hormones also increase the secretion of mitochondrial enzymes, thus increasing pyruvate to glucose conversion. In muscle there is also an increase in lactate formation and conversion to glucose. The glycogen content in the liver is diminished in both hyper- and hypothyroidism: in hyperthyroidism this is due to increased degradation, while in hypothyroidism the rate of synthesis is lowered.

Thyroid hormone increases lipogenesis and fat tissue lipolysis. Again, these effects may involve changes in catecholamine action via the cAMP pathway. Clinically, in hypothyroidism there is hypercholesterolemia and increased concentrations of low-density lipoproteins (LDL), whereas the concentrations of both are low in hyperthyroidism. Thyroid hormone normally increases body growth and induces a net positive nitrogen balance. In hyperthyroidism, there is weight loss and a net negative nitrogen balance.

## Thyroid function during development

### Changes during fetal life

Serum concentrations of thyroid hormones are higher in pregnant than in non-pregnant women primarily due to elevation of serum thyroxine-binding globulin concentrations. In the mother hCG has a thyrotrophic effect, probably contributing to the increase in total $T_4$ and $T_3$ concentrations. The placenta is impermeable to TSH. Maternal $T_4$ and $T_3$ do not cross the placenta in sufficient quantity to maintain fetal euthyroidism. This is most probably due to the presence of an active inner ring iodothyronine deiodinase, which deiodinates $T_4$ to inactive $rT_3$, and deiodinates $T_3$ to inactive $T_2$. The fetus therefore is dependent upon its own pituitary hormones and thyroid. Thus, the fetal pituitary–thyroid axis develops independently of the maternal system.

While TRH is not normally found in significant amounts in the circulation, TRH given to the mother, will cross the placenta and stimulate fetal TSH and prolactin release. This has been used therapeutically to promote lung maturation.

TRH can be detected in the fetal pituitary and hypothalamus from about 10 weeks' gestation, and thyroxine and thyrotrophin appear in the circulation from 12 weeks. Recently, studies of fetal serum obtained by percutaneous umbilical blood sampling have confirmed that the fetal pituitary secretes thyrotrophin and the thyroid secretes $T_4$ as early as 12 weeks of gestation. Fetal serum concentrations of $T_4$, free $T_4$ ($FT_4$), TSH, TBG and albumin increase significantly between 12 and 36 weeks' gestation, while the maternal levels of these hormones and binding protein do not change. Fetal $T_4$ increases throughout gestation, although at 28 weeks concentrations are still lower than the adult range, suggesting that the fetal thyroid gland is as yet immature. On the other hand, $FT_4$ concentrations are within the normal adult range as early as 28 weeks' gestation. The difference between the changes in $T_4$ and $FT_4$ concentrations is probably due to changes in serum-binding proteins.

Although circulating $T_4$ and $FT_4$ concentrations are at adult levels by 36 weeks' gestation, fetal serum $T_3$ and free $T_3$ ($FT_3$) concentrations are always less than 50 per cent of the maternal levels. These low levels of $T_3$ and $FT_3$ most probably are due to low conversion of $T_4$ to $T_3$, or increased rapid degradation of $T_3$ to $T_2$ by the placenta.

The rising concentrations of both fetal $T_4$ and TSH in late gestation suggests immaturity of the negative feedback loop. This deficient inhibition of TSH by $T_4$ in the fetus associated with $FT_4$ concentrations within the adult range suggests that the fetal pituitary is relatively insensitive to negative feedback. After birth $T_3$, produced mainly by intrapituitary local monodeiodination of $T_4$, is responsible for suppression of TSH. It is possible that because of the low circulating $T_3$ and $FT_3$ concentrations, the negative feedback threshold is never reached *in utero*. Alternative explanations are delayed maturation of intracellular mechanisms for conversion of $T_4$ to $T_3$, or of $T_3$ receptor/postreceptor infant mechanisms in the pituitary.

Ultrasound guided umbilical cord blood sampling (cordocentesis) has made it possible to study fetal thyroid hormone status during the last two trimesters of gestation. Cord blood $T_4$ and TSH concentrations are the most reliable indicators available for assessment of thyroid function *in utero*. Up to 10 weeks of gestation the amniotic cavity containing the developing embryo is completely surrounded by an exocelomic cavity and by the placenta. By sampling, using the transvaginal ultrasonographically-guided approach, it has been shown that thyroxine can reach these cavities as early as the 4th–6th week after conception, before the fetal thyroid has begun to function. Measurements of $T_4$, $T_3$ and $rT_3$ in the amniotic fluid are of little value because the concentrations are low and do not reflect the thyroid status of the fetus. On the other hand, amniotic fluid TSH reflects fetal rather than maternal thyroid function and may be helpful in fetal assessment. Similarly, injection of thyroxine into the amniotic fluid results in increased concentrations of $T_4$, $T_3$ and $rT_3$ in both amniotic fluid and cord blood without affecting maternal serum values and this may have therapeutic usefulness.

In the hypothyroid fetus although a little $T_4$ may cross the placenta from the mother, persistently low $T_4$ concentrations nevertheless lead to a rise in TSH. This in turn stimulates thyroid growth as shown by the goiter that sometimes develops in infants with defects of thyroid hormone biosynthesis (e.g. organification defects) or in the presence of excess iodide or goitrogens. The insufficient transfer of maternal $T_4$ to the fetus is also reflected by more severe manifestation of clinical hypothyroidism in infants with *agenesis of the thyroid gland*.

Intra-amniotic administration of $T_4$ to the human preterm fetus has been shown to accelerate lung maturation as measured by various amniotic fluid indicators, such as lecithin/sphingomyelin (L/S) ratio and phosphatidylglycerol (PG) levels. Furthermore, injection of $T_4$ intra-amniotically reduces the size of fetal goiter due to organification defects or iodine deficiency and suppresses fetal TSH levels. Thus, intra-amniotic injection of thyroxine can be useful in treating *in utero* hypothyroidism.

## Changes at birth

Umbilical cord blood TSH concentrations are low at birth, and after the cord is cut there is a rapid excretion of TSH which results in peak serum concentrations of 50–100 mU/L about 10–15 minutes after birth. This surge of TSH may constitute an adaptive mechanism to the cooler environment outside the uterus.

In a recent study, the lipolytic effect of several hormones on isolated human adipocytes obtained at different donor ages was examined. In neonates, norepinephrine and epinephrine had an insignificant lipolytic effect, while TSH had a significant effect in physiological concentrations. TSH may thus be an important lipolytic hormone during the neonatal period, and the TSH surge after birth may be essential for lipolysis during this period of life. During childhood and in adults the lipolytic effect of TSH gradually decreases.

In response to the rapid surge in TSH after birth, $T_4$ and $T_3$ secretion from the thyroid gland are stimulated. $T_4$ peaks at 48 hours; $T_3$ rises abruptly between 1 and 4 hours after birth. A further progressive increase in $T_3$ occurs between 4 and 24 hours, because of the augmented conversion of $T_4$ to $T_3$ in peripheral tissues resulting from an accelerated increase in hepatic 5'-monoiododeiodinase (outer ring deiodinase) activity. Separation from the placenta and its active enzyme iodothyronine deiodinase also may contribute to the abrupt rise in $T_3$. Brown fat also is rich in 5'-monoiododeiodinase activity leading to increased conversion of $T_4$ to $T_3$ levels in brown fat, thus promoting thermogenesis. Because the biological half-life of $T_4$ in the neonatal period is considerably shorter than in older children and adults, the $T_4$ requirement in the neonate (per kg body weight) is five times higher than in adults. Reverse $T_3$ production by fetal and neonatal tissues decreases by 1 month at which time serum $rT_3$ concentrations fall to childhood and adult concentrations.

## Thyroid function in the premature infant

In the premature infant the hypothalamic–pituitary–thyroid axis is immature at birth. The early neonatal TSH rise and the postnatal increase in $T_4$ and $T_3$ concentrations are less than in term infants. In premature infants at 25 weeks' gestation, mean TSH concentrations increase from a very low value of <1 mU/L at 5 days to 6 mU/L by 5 weeks of age. The thyroid hormone feedback control of pituitary TSH release in the extremely premature infants begins to mature after 6 weeks of postnatal life, suggesting a delay in maturation of the axis. Thus, the maturational pattern of the thyroid axis in premature infants is similar to that of the intrauterine fetus. The relatively hypothyroid state of premature infants is probably due to the immaturity of the hypothalamic–pituitary–thyroid axis, relatively low activity of the outer ring deiodinase enzyme system, and resultant reduced conversion of $T_4$ and $T_3$. As discussed earlier, the interpretation of $T_3$ concentrations in the sick neonate is further confounded by systemic factors which may compromise peripheral conversion of $T_4$ to $T_3$.

## Thyroid function in children

In healthy boys and girls serum TSH concentrations remain essentially constant from 1 month of age throughout childhood. On the other hand, serum $T_4$ and $T_3$ concentrations decrease progressively with increasing age due to the decrease in serum TBG concentrations which fall by about 30 per cent between 1 and 15 years. The progressive decrease in the serum concentration of thyroid hormones during childhood is not associated with changes in TSH concentrations. As there is a progressive and proportionate increase in the absolute size of the thyroid gland during childhood this might suggest that a decrease in TSH responsiveness with age would be likely. This could be due to a progressive decrease in TSH receptors per cell or to a decrease in the thyroid follicular cell response to TSH or to cAMP.

## Thyroid function during puberty

Only a few studies correlate the thyroid hormone concentrations and the stage of puberty. Estrogen is known to increase the concentration of serum TBG, while testosterone lowers it. On the other hand, serum $T_4$ concentrations decrease during puberty in both boys and girls. Serum $T_3$ does not change significantly during the pubertal stages, but toward adulthood it decreases.

## SELECTED READING

Contempre B, Jauniaux E, Calvo R et al. Detection of thyroid hormones in human embryonic cavities during the first trimester of pregnancy. *J Clin Endocrinol Metab* 1993; 77: 1719.

Lazar MA, Berrodin TJ. Thyroid hormone receptors form distinct nuclear protein dependent and independent complexes with a thyroid hormone response element. *Mol Endocrinol* 1990; 4: 1627.

Lever EG, Medeiros-Neto GA, De Groot LJ. Inherited disorders of thyroid metabolism. *Endocr Rev* 1983; 4: 213.

Oppenheimer J. Tissue and cellular effects of thyroid hormones and their mechanism of action. In Burrow GN, Oppenheimer JH, Volpe R eds. *Thyroid function and disease*. Philadelphia: WB Saunders, 1989: 90.

Perelman AH, Johnson RL, Clemons RD et al. Intrauterine diagnosis and treatment of fetal goitrous hypothyroidism. *J Clin Endocrinol Metab* 1990; 71: 618.

Sack J, Kaiserman I, Siebner R. Maternal–fetal $R_4$ transfer does not suffice to prevent the effects of *in utero* hypothyroidism. *Horm Res* 1993; 39: 1.

Shupnik MA, Ridgway EC, Chin WW. Molecular biology of thyrotrophin. *Endocr Rev* 1990; 10: 459.

Thorpe-Beeston JG, Nicolaides KH, Felton CV et al. Maturation of the secretion of thyroid hormone and thyroid stimulating hormone in the fetus. *N Engl J Med* 1991; 324: 532.

# 38

# Gonads and Gonadotrophins

## THE GONADOTROPHINS

The hypothalamic–pituitary–gonadal (HPG) axis is responsible for some aspects of sexual differentiation and for orchestrating an orderly progression toward sexual maturity and reproductive capacity. This section reviews the physiology of the gonadotrophic axis in the male and female. Gonadal function is discussed in the following section. For further discussion refer also to the section on puberty (page 255).

### THE GONADOTROPHIC AXIS (*see* Fig. 38.1)

#### The control of gonadotrophin release

Several neurotransmitters within the central nervous system (such as norepinephrine, dopamine and endogenous opiates) modulate the pulsatile release of gonadotrophin releasing hormone (GnRH) from neurons which are located primarily in the medial preoptic area and the arcuate nucleus of the hypothalamus. The precise role of these central nervous system (CNS) signals under physiological conditions is not well understood. GnRH is cleaved from its prohormone to yield GnRH and GAP (gonadotrophin releasing hormone-associated peptide). The biological significance of GAP, which stimulates gonadotrophin secretion and inhibits prolactin *in vitro*, is not clear.

GnRH, a peptide of 10 amino acids also known as luteinizing releasing hormone (LHRH), is discharged from nerve terminals in the median eminence into the hypothalamic portal system by which it reaches pituitary gonadotropes and binds to specific receptors. GnRH stimulates both gonadotrophin synthesis within the cell and also gonadotrophin release from the pituitary into the general circulation. Pituitary gonadotropes may contain luteinizing hormone (LH), follicle stimulating hormone (FSH) or both gonadotrophins. *Kallmann syndrome*, isolated gonadotrophin deficiency due to GnRH deficiency, is associated with olfactory bulb abnormalities. GnRH deficiency may also be part of a more extensive defect in *congenital hypothalamic hypopituitarism*.

GnRH containing neurons are found primarily in the periventricular and arcuate nuclei and the medial preoptic area of the hypothalamus. These neurons provide a pulse of GnRH to the pituitary, by means of the hypophyseal–portal system, approximately every 90 minutes. The GnRH receptor is G-protein-linked. If the pituitary is stimulated by more frequent pulses or continuous administration of GnRH, a decrease in gonadotrophin secretion occurs as a result of desensitization of GnRH receptors. Similarly, pharmacological agonists of GnRH, which remain bound to the GnRH receptor longer than native GnRH, have a suppressive effect on gonadotrophin secretion. This explains the apparently paradoxical use of GnRH superagonists in treatment of *central precocious puberty*.

LH and FSH reach the gonads through the general circulation and bind to specific receptors to exert their effects. These gonadotrophins are dimeric glycoproteins. Each contains an α-subunit of 89 amino acids that has a molecular weight of 14 kD and is identical to the α-subunit of TSH and human chorio-

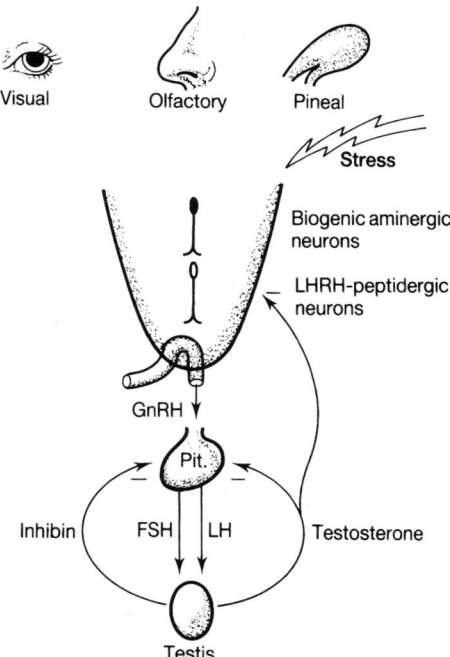

FIGURE 38.1 Regulation of gonadotrophin secretion in the human male. Schematic diagram of gonadotrophin control system in the male, showing the interaction of neural and hormonal feedback controls. Pituitary and testis are connected by a negative feedback link. Secretion of testosterone by the testis is stimulated by LH, whereas maturation and growth of the tubule cells are stimulated by FSH. The secretion of testosterone in turn inhibits the secretion of LH and FSH. Inhibin is secreted by Sertoli cells and exerts a direct inhibitory effect on FSH secretion. The LHRH peptidergic neurons are in turn regulated by a biogenic aminergic system that links gonadotrophin regulation to the remainder of the brain. Through this system a wide variety of impulses can be exerted on reproductive function. Stimuli affecting male gonadotrophic secretion have been well demonstrated in experimental animals, although they are not as well worked out in the human. Visual influences include light-induced changes in seasonal breeders such as domestic cattle, deer and birds. Olfactory signals in male rats influence gonadal function. The pineal gland in many species of animals inhibits gonadotrophin secretion by direct effects of pineal secretions on either the hypothalamus or the pituitary. The role of the pineal in human reproduction control has not been established. (Modified from Martin JB, Reichlin S, Brown GM. Neuroendocrinology of reproduction. In *Clinical neuroendocrinology*. Philadelphia: FA Davis, 1977: 93.)

nic gonadotrophin (hCG). The β-subunits of 115 amino acids determine the specific function of the molecule. The complete molecular weight of each gonadotrophin is about 29 kD. These weights are approximate because of the extensive and variable carbohydrate side-chains which complete the glycoprotein structure.

## Gonadal function (*see also* page 490)

The gonads have specific gonadotrophin receptors, through which the gonadotrophins stimulate sex steroid production and gamete maturation. Both LH and FSH receptors are G-protein-linked and act via increased cAMP production. GnRH receptors are also present in the gonads but their significance is uncertain. In general LH stimulates steroid biosynthesis and FSH is responsible for gamete maturation but there are complex interactions which prevent complete separation of the function of the two gonadotrophins. The gonads complete the feedback loop by signaling the hypothalamus and pituitary, and possibly higher brain centers, in both a negative and positive feedback fashion, the sensitivity of which is developmentally regulated.

### The testis (*see also* page 493)

In the male testosterone production is from the Leydig cell, the Sertoli cell producing inhibin and, in fetal life, anti-Müllerian hormone. The Leydig cell responds to LH by increasing testosterone release. In early fetal life hCG performs the same function. A defect in the common LH/hCG receptor is one cause of abnormal sexual differentiation. The seminiferous tubules which are the main site of FSH action are comprised of Sertoli cells and germ cells; spermatocytes mature from the latter. However, FSH may have indirect effects on testosterone production via increasing Leydig cell maturation or by increasing the number of LH receptors on Leydig cells.

### The ovary

Ovarian steroid production depends on the developmental stage of the female and, if mature, the stage of the menstrual cycle. Ovarian follicles are embedded in the stroma of the ovarian cortex. Only a few are recruited each cycle. The primordial follicle is composed of an oocyte surrounded by a single layer of granulosa cells surrounded in turn by a basement membrane. Follicular development involves the formation of a primary follicle by the proliferation of granulosa cells associated with maturation of the oocyte which enlarges and secretes a glycoprotein coat (zona pellucida). FSH is responsible for this proliferation, perhaps operating via local insulin-like growth factor I (IGF-I) production. Further granulosa cell proliferation occurs and the surrounding stroma begins to organize into the theca interna and externa to form first a secondary, then a tertiary, follicle as the theca further organizes and an antrum appears in the granulosa cell. Gap junctions form between the granulosa and thecal cells which may be essential for the coordinated synthesis of estrogens and progesterone. A further rapid increase in follicular size leads to formation of the

Graafian follicle. Only one or two recruited primordial follicles per cycle fully mature; the remainder become atretic at an earlier stage.

Estrogens are the major product of the granulosa cell. The primary estrogen is 17β-estradiol, but estrone and estriol are also formed. Both thecal and granulosa cells produce progesterone, but granulosa cell progesterone is largely used as a substrate for conversion to estrogen. Some androgens are also secreted by the ovary but, except in enzyme disorders, these are of minor significance. For a further discussion of sex steroid synthesis by the ovary, (see page 494). The granulosa cell produces primarily estrogens, the luteal cells produce primarily progesterone and the thecal cells and stroma produce androgens. LH primarily stimulates the initial conversion of cholesterol to pregnenolone whereas FSH has a major effect on aromatase, the enzyme that converts testosterone to estradiol. It has therefore been suggested that FSH and LH act in concert on the thecal and granulosa cells to maximize estradiol production; LH stimulates androstenedione production by the thecal origin which is provided to the granulosa cell for FSH-stimulated aromatization.

## Inhibin and activin (see also page 497)

In addition to sex steroid-mediated feedback, both the testis (Sertoli cell) and ovary (granulosa cell) produce inhibin, a heterodimeric protein which selectively decreases FSH secretion. Two covalently linked β-subunits of inhibin form activin which has reciprocal actions to those of inhibin at both the pituitary and gonadal level. Activin stimulates pituitary FSH secretion and inhibits gonadal steroid production and cell multiplication. Inhibin, by contrast, stimulates gonadal steroidogenesis and cell proliferation in the gonad. The placenta produces inhibin, and this may be one mechanism by which the maternal gonadotrophic axis is suppressed during pregnancy. Activin also is formed in the central nervous system where it is neurotrophic and in the bone marrow where it is a potent stimulator of erythropoiesis.

## THE MENSTRUAL CYCLE

The pubertal process (see page 256) results in a mature HPG axis, which functions in a cyclic fashion in females. The cycle involves orchestrated changes in gonadotrophins and sex steroids, ovarian and endometrial structure as summarized in Fig. 38.2. During the early follicular phase, the ovary is stimulated by FSH to recruit follicles for the next cycle. Eventually one follicle is selected as the dominant or ovulatory follicle; the others undergo atresia. As this follicle grows, estrogen secretion increases. At a critical concentration and duration of estrogen secretion, positive feedback results in a burst of gonadotrophin secretion and ovulation. After ovulation the follicle changes its steroidogenic characteristics and begins to function as the

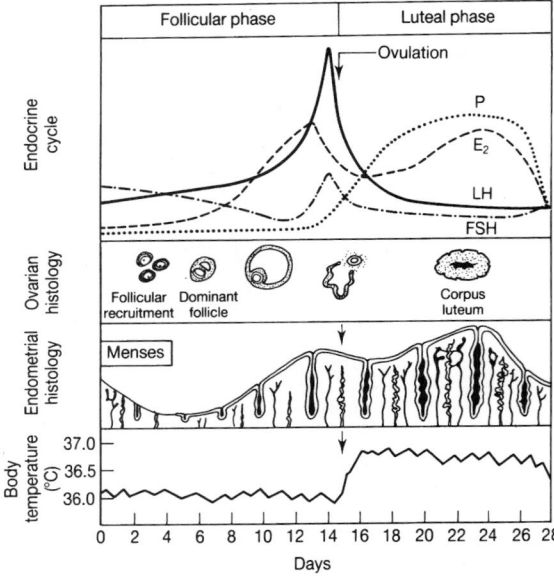

FIGURE 38.2 Hormonal, ovarian, endometrial, and basal body temperature changes and relationships throughout the normal menstrual cycle. (From Carr BR, Wilson JD. Disorders of the ovary and female reproductive tract. In Braunwald E, Isselbacher KJ, Petersdorf RG *et al.* eds. *Harrison's principles of internal medicine.* 11th edn. New York: McGraw-Hill, 1987: 1818. Reproduced with permission of McGraw-Hill Inc.)

corpus luteum, producing large amounts of progesterone as well as estradiol. These high steroid concentrations cause gonadotrophins to decrease. Eventually, in the absence of pregnancy, the corpus luteum undergoes luteolysis. The withdrawal of hormonal support triggers shedding of the endometrium at the time of menses. The cycle begins again with increases in FSH secretion and follicle recruitment for the next cycle even as estradiol and progesterone concentrations reach their lowest concentrations before menses occur. It is very common for follicular development to be inadequate at the ends of the reproductive spectrum of mid-puberty and the premenopausal years.

## DEVELOPMENTAL ASPECTS

The hypothalamic–pituitary–gonadal axis undergoes several developmental phases. Each phase can be thought of in a teleological sense as accomplishing a purpose to convey an evolutionary advantage.

### Intrauterine phase (see Figs. 38.3 and 38.4)

The tasks accomplished during the intrauterine phase of development of the HPG axis are sexual differentiation (see page 197) and establishment of a sexually dimorphic regulatory system which has certain pro-

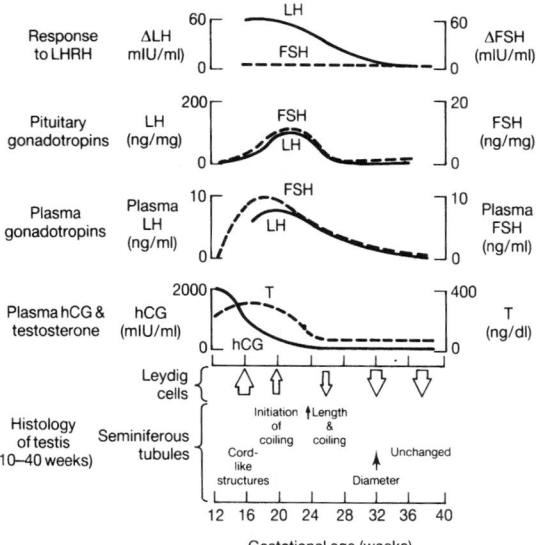

FIGURE 38.3 Comparison of the pattern of change of serum testosterone, hCG, and serum and pituitary LH and FSH concentrations in the human male fetus during gestation in relation to the morphological changes in fetal testis. The top graph illustrates the regression curve for the increment (Δ) between a baseline plasma LH and FSH concentration and the 15 minute response to administration of GnRH to the male fetus plotted as a function of gestational age. The scale masks the slight increase in plasma FSH. The evidence supports the hypothesis that the hypothalamic GnRH pulse generator is functional early in gestation and mediates the rise in serum concentration of fetal pituitary gonadotropes. (From Grumbach MM, Styne DM. Puberty: ontogeny, neuroendocrinology, physiology, and disorders. In Wilson JD, Foster DW eds. *Williams' textbook of endocrinology*. 8th edn. Philadelphia: WB Saunders Co., 1992: 1157. Reproduced by permission of WB Saunders Co.)

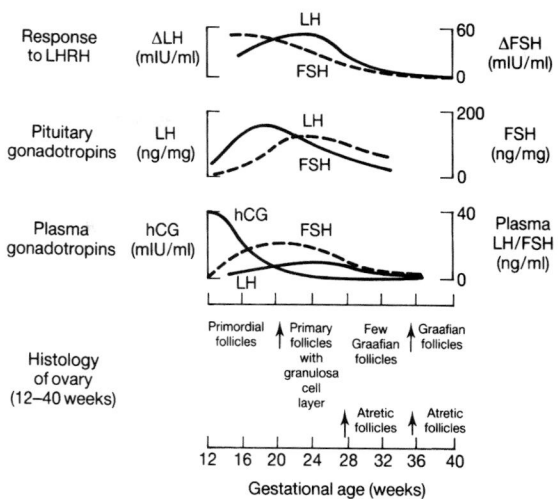

FIGURE 38.4 Pattern of change of serum FSH, LH and hCG concentrations; concentration of pituitary FSH and LH; and increment (Δ) between baseline FSH and LH and the 15-minute response to administration of GnRH in human female fetus during gestation with the development of the fetal ovary. (From Grumbach MM, Styne DM. Puberty: ontogeny, neuroendocrinology, physiology, and disorders. In Wilson JD, Foster DW, eds. *Williams' textbook of endocrinology*. 8th edn. Philadelphia: WB Saunders Co., 1992: 1157. Reproduced by permission of WB Saunders Co.)

grammed aspects but retains the ability to respond to internal and external environmental conditions.

Gonadotrophin releasing hormone (GnRH) is detectable in the hypothalamus by 8 weeks' gestation. The anatomical conditions necessary for regulation of the HPG axis are established in the fetus by 11–12 weeks' gestation. By this time LH and FSH are detectable in the pituitary gland, implying that some form of relationship has been established. Regulation of pituitary secretion by the hypothalamus at this time could include an ultra-short loop or paracrine mechanism as the hypophyseal–portal system becomes fully functional. Hypothalamic GnRH increases, as do pituitary and serum LH and FSH until mid-gestation (weeks 20–24). By this time, there is evidence for sexual dimorphism in the regulation of this axis. Female fetuses have higher serum FSH concentrations than males, a pattern which persists, at least in response to GnRH. Evidence from animal studies indicates that castration of a male fetus during gestation results in decreased serum testosterone and increased LH and FSH, whereas ovariectomy does not have the same consequence. Thus a

difference in sensitivity of the feedback mechanism between male and female fetuses can be inferred.

By early in the third trimester the ovine fetus has established pulsatile gonadotrophin secretion, responsiveness of gonadotropes to GnRH and GnRH super-agonists, confirming the presence of a regulated system. Changes in the sensitivity of the feedback set points seem to be important to the phenomena observed in this and subsequent phases of development. As gestation progresses, GnRH content of the hypothalamus, LH and FSH content of the pituitary and serum LH and FSH decrease.

Gonadal function is not entirely dependent upon the integrity of the fetal HPG axis, as human chorionic gonadotrophin (hCG), produced from the beginning of gestation, can stimulate LH receptors on the gonad which in turn stimulate sex steroid synthesis. Thus by 6–8 weeks' gestation, Sertoli and Leydig cells are both present and testosterone synthesis begins. Within the testis, testosterone content is maximal at 12–14 weeks. The fetal ovary, in contrast, has very little activity of the steroidogenic enzymes and lacks hCG receptors. The development of the gonads is described in the following chapter.

## Neonatal phase

Serum LH and FSH are low in cord blood, presumably because a sufficiently sensitive negative feedback system has developed to respond to the high estrogen concentration of the intrauterine environment. Released from this estrogenic inhibition, LH and FSH increase for a few months and subsequently decrease. Thus infants in the first few months of life can have gonadotrophin and sex steroid concentrations in plasma, and pulsatile secretory patterns, that are comparable to pubertal individuals. During this time, the gonadotrophin response to exogenous GnRH is also comparable to the response seen at the time of puberty.

Gonadotrophins and sex steroids decrease to very low concentrations, generally by 6–12 months of age. This decrease is thought to be due to both intrinsic development of central nervous system factors which restrain puberty, and to increasing sensitivity of the negative feedback loop to small concentrations of sex steroids. A schematic representation of postnatal gonadotrophin secretion patterns is described in Fig. 38.5.

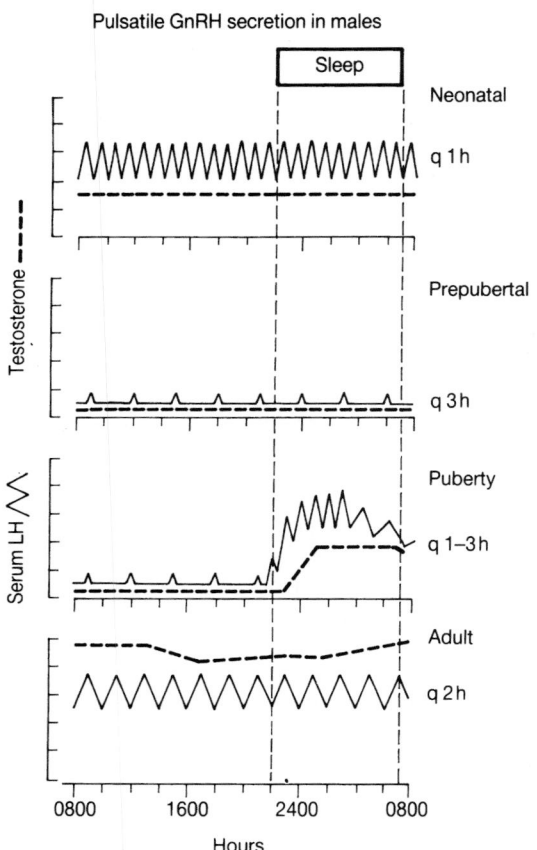

FIGURE 38.5 Schematic diagram of presumed changes in the pulsatile secretion of GnRH as inferred by the pulsatile secretory patterns of LH throughout male sexual maturation. (From Kelch RP, Foster CM, Kletter GB *et al*. Neuroendocrine regulation of puberty in boys. In Aubert ML, Sizonenko PC eds. *Developmental endocrinology*. Serona Symposia, Vol. 67. New York: Raven Press, 1990: 104. Reproduced by permission of Raven Press, New York.)

## Juvenile pause

After the neonatal increase in activity of the gonadotrophic axis, the entire system subsides into a period of apparent quiescence which lasts until the hormonal changes of early puberty occur. The length of this juvenile pause is extremely important in an evolutionary sense. This time of prolonged dependence with freedom from reproductive pressures is thought to correlate with the ability of a species to provide extensive education to its young.

The physiological reasons for the juvenile pause are elusive. The occurrence of precocious puberty when portions of the brain are damaged by tumor or other pathology provides evidence that the central nervous system somehow restrains puberty. The search for a hormonal mediator of this period of restraint has not yielded results that are directly applicable to humans.

## Puberty

Puberty is a period of several years during which the transition from sexual immaturity to reproductive competence occurs. This process involves changes in the activity of each level of the HPG axis. For details refer to Chapter 16.

### SELECTED READING

Burger HG, de Kretser DM eds. *The testis*. 2nd edn. New York: Raven Press Ltd, 1989.

Gluckman PD, Grumbach MM, Kaplan SL. The human fetal hypothalamus and pituitary gland. In Tulchinsky D, Ryan KJ eds. *Maternal–fetal endocrinology*. Philadelphia: WB Saunders, 1980: 196.

Grumbach MM, Styne DM. Puberty: ontogeny, neuroendocrinology, physiology and disorders. In Wilson JD, Foster DW, eds. *Williams' textbook of endocrinology, 8th edn.* Philadelphia: WB Saunders Co, 1992: 1155.

Kelch RP, Foster CM, Kletter GB, Marshall JC. Neuroendocrine regulation of puberty in boys. In Sizonenko PC, Aubert ML eds. *Developmental endocrinology*. New York: Raven Press, 1990.

Ravinovici J, Jaffe RB. Development and regulation of growth and differentiated function in human and subhuman primate fetal gonads. *Endocr Rev* 1990; 11: 532.

Richards JS, Jahnsen T, Hedin L *et al*. Ovarian follicular development from physiology to molecular biology. *Recent Prog Horm Res* 1987; 43: 231.

## THE OVARY AND TESTIS

The gonads are both endocrine glands producing sex hormones, and exocrine glands secreting gametes.

## FUNCTIONAL ANATOMY

### The ovary

The ovary contains two compartments organized within the ovarian "cortex"; the ovarian follicles and the stroma within which the follicles are imbedded. A follicle is a structure composed of a membrane surrounding one oocyte or ovule (depending on the maturational stage) and other cells, mainly granulosa and theca cells that secrete the sex hormones. A limited number of follicles are activated and mature through each menstrual cycle, progressing from the primordial follicle to either Graafian or atretic follicles. Most of the follicles activated in a cycle will become atretic at an early stage of maturation.

The primordial follicle contains, inside a surrounding basement membrane, one oocyte and a single layer of granulosa cells. During the follicle stimulating hormone (FSH)-dependent maturational process the granulosa cells proliferate and the oocyte enlarges while it becomes surrounded by the zona pellucida. The oocyte is separated from the granulosa cells by a basal lamina.

During the secondary and tertiary phase of follicle development, both the theca interna (richly vascularized) and theca externa differentiate from the stroma around the granulosa cells. These two thecal cell types develop gap junctions which are of probable importance for the paracrine regulation of steroidogenesis.

Both granulosa and thecal cells play a coordinating role in the synthesis and secretion of sex steroids. It is postulated that thecal cells, expressing only luteinizing hormone (LH) receptors, and granulosa cells expressing both LH and FSH receptors cooperate for synthesis of both estrogen and progesterone. A rapid follicullar growth phase leads to the formation of the graafian follicle with follicular fluid which contains sex steroids accumulating in the antrum. Preovulatory follicles measure 10–20 mm in diameter. Ovulation occurs by rupture of one mature graafian follicle letting the ovule free with some cells from the cumulus. The residual follicle then transforms into the corpus luteum.

### The testis

The testis has two compartments: the tubular and the interstitial. These two compartments are separated by a basement membrane, the basal lamina. The interstitial compartment is vascularized; a route that brings to the testis endocrine hormones, including the gonadatrophins. Two important cell types lie in this interstitial compartment: the Leydig cells, responsible for LH-dependent steroidogenesis and in particular the production of testosterone, and the myoid or peritubular cells that lie along the basal lamina (Fig. 38.6). The tubular compartment, where sperma-

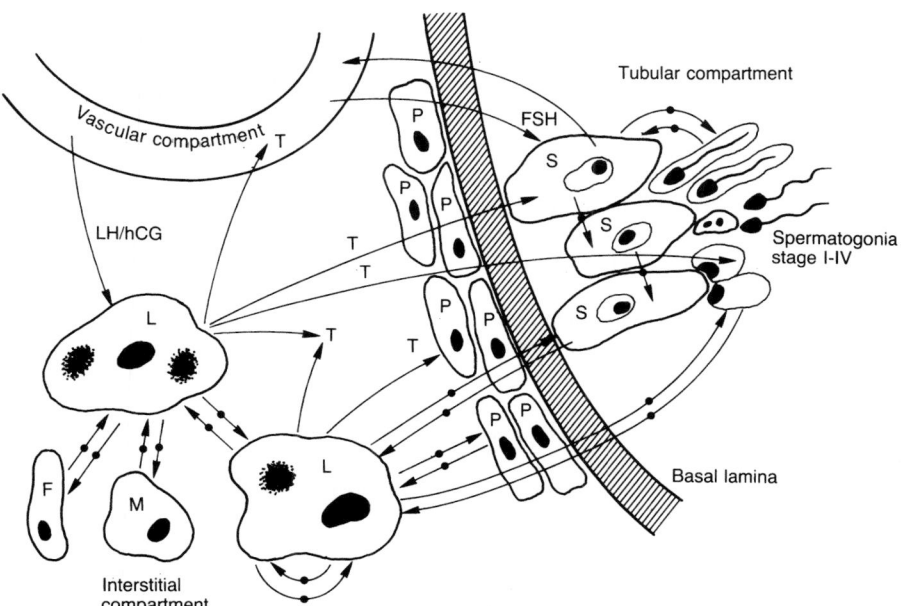

FIGURE 38.6 Schematic representation of the three compartments of the testis showing the endocrine and paracrine relationships. LH (hCG) and FSH enter the testis from the bloodstream and the testis secretes testosterone (T), inhibin (I) and activin (A) into the bloodstream. The myoid/peritubular cells (P) and basal lamina form the blood–testis barrier. The Sertoli cells (S) are the main target for FSH and the Leydig cells (L), which are the source of testosterone, are the target for LH/hCG. Testosterone acts on the Sertoli cells, spermatogonia and myoid cells. Other cell types in the interstitial compartment include macrophages (M) and fibroblasts (F). All cell types may be the source of autocrine and paracrine factors such as IGF-I, bFGF, TGFβ, IL-1 which act within the testis. Such actions are indicated ──●──▶.

togenesis and spermiogenesis occur, has a cylindrical shape, surrounded by the basal lamina and is avascular lying within the "blood–testis barrier." On the inner side of the basal lamina in the tubular compartment lie the Sertoli and the germ cells. The Sertoli cells are in contact with the basal lamina. The Sertoli cells develop Sertoli–Sertoli tight junctions and influence the development of the germ cells in the germinal epithelium, through their secretion of paracrine factors. Gap junctions also may form between the Sertoli and the germ cells. The germ cells develop, by multiplication and maturation in six stages, to fully mature spermatozoa. The germ cells also influence Sertoli cell function. There are exchanges through the basal lamina in both directions between the institutional and tubular compartments, which involve both sex hormones and protein factors. These structures account for the endocrine, paracrine and autocrine interactions described later.

## DEVELOPMENT AND ONTOGENY

Sexual differentiation is described in Chapter 12.

## The ovary

### The fetal ovary

The undifferentiated gonadal blastema derives from the celomic epithelium, the mesenchyme and the primordial germ cells. By 5 weeks' gestation it has developed an outer cortex and inner medulla. The presence of an XX karyotype results in the persistence of the cortex and regression of the medulla. The primitive ovary thus develops with a cortex and a hilum. The cortex includes the external cellular layer, known as the germinal epithelium, the stroma, containing three cell types (connective tissue, interstitial and contractile cells) and the follicular complex. The follicular complex contains the oocytes. By the end of the third week, primordial germ cells (oogonia) are identified in the fetal ovary. They divide by the fifth week, a process that can persist until 24–28 weeks' gestation when 6–7 million oogonia are present, after which time the numbers decrease through atresia so that only 1 million are present at birth. The maturation of oogonia leads to the appearance of primary oocytes (8–13 weeks). Meiosis begins 2–3 weeks after fetal ovary differentiation. In the first meiotic division of germ cells, paternal and maternal genes are exchanged and chromosome pairs are divided to give two daughter cells. These cells subsequently divide without DNA synthesis resulting in haploid cells. Meiosis is then blocked in late prophase (*see* page 109). The division process restarts with ovulatory cycles at puberty: the ovulatory oocyte is activated and meiosis is completed resulting in one ovule and two or three polar bodies (*see* page 110).

The primary steroidogenic cells (ultimately the granulosa cells) are observed from 12 weeks' gestation in the cortex of the fetal ovary. Steroidogenic enzyme activity is present at 14 weeks. Granulosa cells normally develop in several layers as encountered by 150 days' gestation. Follicles are formed by 90 days' gestation. Follicular formation seems partially gonadotrophin-dependent since the process is retarded in anencephalic fetuses who have hypoplasic ovaries containing a decreased number of follicles.

Steroidogenic enzymatic activity, such as aromatase activity, is present by 8 weeks' gestation, 3β-hydroxysteroid dehydrogenase (3β-HSD) activity at 14 weeks. By 12 weeks' gestation, dehydroepiandrosterone is secreted, although there is little estrogen and testosterone and the ovary produces significant amounts of sex steroids only late in gestation. The regulation of fetal ovarian steroidogenesis is still poorly understood. Human chorionic gonadotrophin (hCG) and LH receptors seem not to be present in the human ovary during fetal life. FSH receptors are expressed by 8–14 weeks. However, there is continuous maturation of follicles from late fetal gestation to menopause.

### The postnatal and prepubertal ovary

Ovule number decreases from around 1–2 million at birth to approximately 300 000 at puberty. From the first year of life up to the end of the prepubertal phase, the ovary is relatively quiescent and usually only primordial follicles are observed. However, the maturation of occasional non-ovulatory follicles up to graafian phase is not exceptional and is commonly observed by ultrasonography in some prepubertal age girls. However, there is usually no evidence of follicular rupture and therefore no ovulation.

Postnatally there is a peak of 17α-hydroxyprogesterone by 1 month of age. Circulating sex steroid concentrations stay very low from 6 months until the onset of puberty. This pattern parallels changed activity of gonadotrophin secretion (*see* page 490). In part as a consequence of placental production there are high concentrations of estradiol, progesterone, testosterone, androstenedione and dehydroepiandrosterone at birth, but these then fall rapidly in the neonate.

### The ovary at puberty

At puberty, ovarian function is marked by the appearance of cyclic secretion of estrogens and progesterone and maturation of one follicle leading to ovulation at mid-cycle ending with menstruation. Thus of the 400 000 germ cells present at the onset of puberty, only 400–500 will undergo ovulation during the lifetime of the female. The maturation from primordial to graafian follicles starts, and is accompanied by a progressive increase in sex steroids during the follicular phase, followed by formation of the corpus luteum and progesterone production during the luteal phase. Ovulation occurs by rupture of one mature graafian follicle, letting the ovule free ready for fertilization. The pubertal process and its regulation is described in Chapter 16.

## The testis

### The fetal testis

In the presence of a Y chromosome with a normal sex-determining region that contains the SRY gene, the major testicular differentiating factor (see page 194), testicular differentiation begins by 6 weeks of gestation with the gradual development of the gonadal blastema into the testicular cords and the interstitium. Male genital differentiation begins with the differentiation of Sertoli cells in the medullary sex cords. During weeks 6–7 of gestation, Sertoli cells proliferate and aggregate to form the seminiferous cords. Later this structure will enclose the germ cells. The fetal Leydig precursors arise from undifferentiated mesenchymal cells during week 8. A "fetal-type" Leydig cell is responsible for testosterone production, and thus masculinization, of the internal and external genitalia during fetal and neonatal life. These cells seem to regress thereafter. This is followed by the emergence of an adult-type population of Leydig cells which is responsible for pubertal masculinization. Testosterone is detected in the fetal human testis at 6–7 weeks' gestation. As Leydig cells proliferate, androgen concentrations in testicular tissue, blood and amniotic fluid rise to peak by 15–18 weeks. These developments seem to correlate with an increase in plasma hCG concentrations (see page 207). From week 16 of gestation to birth, Leydig cell numbers decrease by 60 per cent. This decrease is associated with a parallel decrease in plasma hCG concentrations. In the human, pituitary LH does not seem to control fetal Leydig cell differentiation. Immunoreactive gonadotrophins are not detected in the fetal pituitary before 10 weeks of gestation, that is 3–4 weeks after the onset of testosterone production by the testis. Data presently available indicate that the secretion of testosterone by the fetal human testis during the first 15 weeks is under hCG control. The pituitary control of testicular steroidogenesis is however significant in the second part of gestation since anencephalic fetuses have reduced Leydig cell numbers and have altered testicular steroidogenesis.

### The postnatal and prepubertal testis

After birth a second testosterone surge is observed, with a peak around 2 months postnatally that reaches a value above 10 nmol/L in the normal male (normal range in the normal fully mature young adult is 11–29 nmol/L). This phenomenon is driven by pituitary LH and is associated with the development of a second wave of Leydig cells. Thus in a child with either a testicular problem (such as undescended testis) or incomplete masculinization (such as hypospadias), testosterone measurement between 1–2 months of age may provide reliable evidence of endogenous LH-driven testicular steroidogenesis. The number of Leydig cells then decreases again until very few Leydig cells remain by the first year of postnatal life.

### The testis at puberty

At puberty (see page 255) there is the third phase of Leydig cell development. Mesenchymal cells start to differentiate into adult-type Leydig cells under the control of LH. The seminiferous tubules develop, resulting in the large pubertal increase in testicular volume. There is a progressive gonadotrophin releasing hormone (GnRH)-dependent increase in pituitary gonadotrophin secretion (see page 490). This results in both a progressive maturation of Leydig cell function, with an increase in plasma testosterone concentration to adult levels and a maturation of Sertoli cell function contributing to the maturation of the germinal epithelium and the development of spermatogenesis and spermiogenesis. There also is a pubertal increase in GH secretion and plasma insulin-like growth factor I (IGF-I) concentrations which may be sex steroid dependent and may contribute to the maturation of Leydig and Sertoli cell function. Therefore, normal pubertal development is not only dependent on a normal pituitary–gonadotrophic axis but also a normal somatotroph function and pubertal development is abnormal in growth hormone deficiency.

LH is required for the maintenance of Leydig cell specific functions and is the main factor controlling Leydig cell steroidogenesis. FSH is required for the maintenance of Sertoli cell specific functions. The maintenance of spermatogenesis is dependent upon both androgen production and FSH. For further discussion of the endocrine aspects of puberty see page 255.

## Endocrine dimorphism in the early postnatal period

During the first 3 postnatal months there is a sexual dimorphism in the endocrine function of the gonads. Females are characterized by high FSH secretion and a low LH secretion and a peak of plasma 17α-hydroxyprogesterone concentrations at 1 month, mainly of ovarian origin. In contrast, males present with a peak in testosterone concentrations between 1 and 2 months postnatally and high LH but low FSH concentrations.

## THE ENDOCRINE, PARACRINE AND AUTOCRINE GONADAL SYSTEMS

Much of our recent understanding of gonadal endocrine function comes from data showing that the regulation of sex hormone synthesis is under the control of paracrine and autocrine factors acting synergistically with the classical endocrine factors. These paracrine and autocrine factors are known to be peptide growth factors, whose genes are expressed by some gonadal cell types and are secreted locally. Their actions control the gonadal cell function by stimulating or inhibiting the differentiation of these cells. These actions are exerted in concert with the endocrine hormones, the gonadotrophins and the sex hormones. Furthermore these growth factors control gonadal cell multiplication and influence gonadal development and maturation.

## The ovary

Sex steroids are produced by granulosa cells, thecal cells and the corpus luteum. The principal pathway of steroid hormone synthesis in the ovary is shown in Fig. 38.7. Steroidal biosynthesis is initiated from and by the uptake of low density lipoprotein (LDL) cholesterol. The two main synthetic pathways involve either the $\Delta^5$ pathway or the $\Delta^4$ pathway which utilize the same enzymes, albeit in a different sequence. In the $\Delta^5$ pathway 17$\alpha$-hydroxylation of pregnenolone is the first step which then proceeds to dehydroepiandrosterone (DHEA), androstenedione, and then to testosterone for aromatization to estradiol. The $\Delta^4$ pathway involves first conversion by 3$\beta$-HSD of pregnenolone to progesterone, and thence via 17$\alpha$-hydroxyprogesterone, androstenedione and testosterone, to estradiol. Both pathways are utilized to different extents by granulosa, thecal and luteal cells. The major source of estrogen production is the granulosa cell. Progesterone essentially is produced by the corpus luteum and androgens are produced by the thecal cells. LH primarily stimulates the initial conversion of cholesterol to pregnenolone. An important enzyme in the production of estrogen is FSH-modulated aromatase that transforms both testosterone and androstenedione of thecal origin to estradiol and estrone, respectively, within the granulosa cells. Thus LH and FSH act in concert on the thecal and granulosa cells to maximize estradiol production. LH stimulates thecal cell production of androstenedione which then is provided to the granulosa cell for FSH induced aromatization. Virilization is observed in the genotypic 46XX virilized female presenting with *aromatase deficiency*.

The local growth and differentiating factors that contribute to the development and maintenance of fully mature steroidogenesis will be discussed in relationship to the testis. However, the same growth factors are involved in the ovary and include insulin-like growth factor I (IGF-I), transforming growth factor (TGF)$\beta$, basic fibroblast growth factor (bFGF), epidermal growth factor (EGF)/TGF$\alpha$ and several cytokines (see Table 38.1). IGF-I is synthesized by the granulosa cells and is secreted into the follicular fluid. It acts as a differentiating and maintenance factor for granulosa cells by potentiating several key enzymes of steroidogenesis. IGF-I potentiates estrogen production in response to LH stimulation *in vitro*. Both severe *isolated growth-hormone-deficient* female patients and growth hormone (GH)-resistant female patients (*Laron dwarfism*) present with markedly delayed puberty although they do not have gonadotrophin deficiency. These observations suggest that the GH-dependent IGF-I is involved in the final maturation of ovarian endocrine function. Estrogen is responsible for the development of the main secondary female sex characteristics, breast development and uterine growth. Progesterone acts mainly on endometrial maturation. It also has a key role in implantation as well as in the maintenance of early pregnancy.

## The testis

Paracrine and autocrine interactions have recently emerged as sophisticated systems through which the subtle regulation of testicular function, in particular that of Leydig cells, is achieved. The description of these paracrine and autocrine interactions has become critical to our understanding of testicular differentiation and function.

Almost all testicular androgens are synthesized and secreted by the Leydig cells. The seminiferous tubular cells may contribute by using steroids formed in the Leydig cells for further derivative production. The testis also produces small amount of estrogens mainly in the Leydig cell.

The pathway of testosterone synthesis in the testis is shown in Fig. 38.8. The Leydig cell utilizes both *de novo* synthesis of cholesterol and cholesterol of low density lipoprotein origin as the substrate for testosterone synthesis. Cholesterol transfer to the inner mitochondrial membrane involves several factors. Enzymes of the steroidogenic pathway modify the cholesterol molecule step by step. The steps are similar to those in the adrenal. The enzymes are described in detail on p. 502. The rate limiting step, as for cortisol synthesis, is side-chain cleavage to form pregnenolone. The primary pathway is the $\Delta^5$ pathway via 17$\alpha$-hydroxypregnenolone to DHEA to androstenediol to testosterone.

Conversion of 3-hydroxysteroids (17$\alpha$-OH-pregnenolone, DHEA) into 3-ketosteroids (17$\alpha$-OH-progesterone, androstenedione) is performed by 3$\beta$-hydroxysteroid dehydrogenase/$\Delta^5$–$\Delta^5$-isomerase (3$\beta$-HSD). Two human genes, type I and II, and three pseudogenes have been cloned for this enzyme. The type I mRNA is almost exclusively present in the

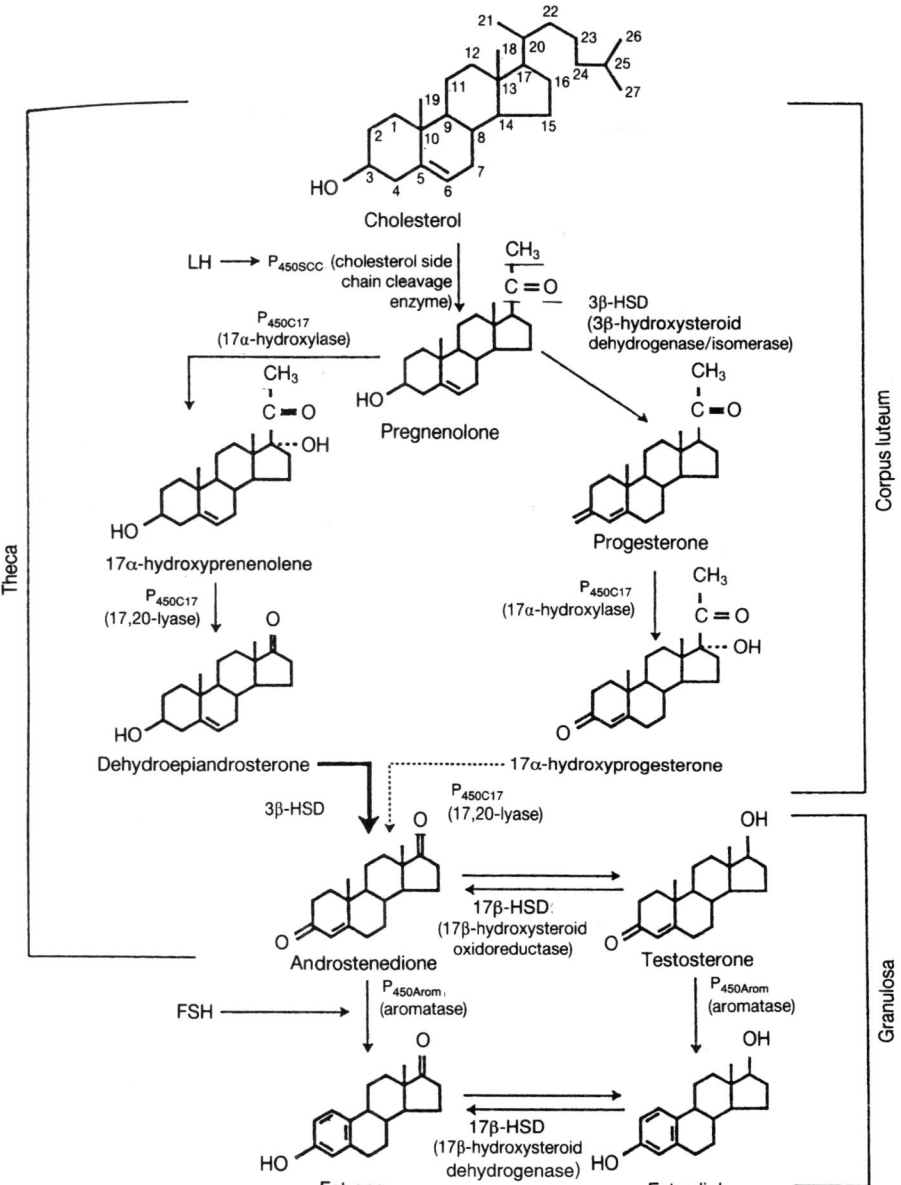

FIGURE 38.7 Principal pathways of steroid hormone biosynthesis in the human ovary. Although each cell type of the ovary contains the complete enzyme complement required for the formation of estradiol from cholesterol, the amounts of the various enzymes and consequently the predominant hormones formed differ among the cell types. The major enzyme complements for the corpus luteum, theca, and granulosa cells are shown in parentheses; these cells produce predominantly progesterone and 17α-hydroxy-progesterone (corpus luteum); androgen (theca), and estrogen (granulosa). The major sites of action of LH and FSH in mediating this pathway are shown by the horizontal arrows. The dotted line emphasizes that the metabolism of 17α-hydroxyprogesterone is limited in the human ovary. (From Carr BR. Disorders of the ovary. In Wilson JD, Foster DW eds. *Williams' textbook of endocrinology*. 8th edn. Philadelphia: WB Saunders Co., 1992: 745. Reproduced by permission of WB Saunders Co.)

placenta and in skin, while type II is the predominant form expressed in the adrenal, ovary and testis. The conversion of C-21 steroids into C-19 steroids proceeds in two steps catalyzed by a single enzyme, cytochrome $P_{450c17}$. Full-length human cDNA probes isolated from testis and adrenal have confirmed that the enzyme structure at both steps is identical and that $P_{450c17}$ can catalyze both 17α-hydroxylase and 17,20 lyase reactions. Defects of 3β-HSD or $P_{450c17}$ lead to rare forms of *congenital adrenal hyperplasia* with incomplete virilization in the male (*see* page 512). The microsomal enzyme 17β-hydroxysteroid dehydrogenase (17β-HSD) catalyzes the interconversion of the steroid pairs: androstenedione and testosterone, DHEA and 5-androstene-3β 17β-diol, and estrone and estradiol. The gene has been localized to chromo-

TABLE 38.1 Intra-testicular paracrine factors

| PEPTIDE AND/OR GROWTH FACTORS | SITE OF CELL PRODUCTION | EFFECTS ON LEYDIG CELL | EFFECTS ON SERTOLI CELLS | EFFECTS ON GERM CELLS | REGULATION |
|---|---|---|---|---|---|
| IGF-I | L<br>S | ↑ Differentiated function and potentiates steroidogenesis | ↑ Differentiated function | Mitogen | FSH ↑ (S)<br>hCG ↑ (L) |
| TGFβ | L,S,P | ↓ Differentiated function | ↓ Plasminogen activator | | FSH ↓ (S) |
| EGF/TGFα | L,S,P,G | ↑ Differentiated function and steroidogenesis | ↑ Plasminogen activator | Mitogen | ? |
| bFGF | L,S,P,G | ↑ Differentiated function and steroidogenesis | | | FSH ↑ (S) |
| Inhibin/activin | L,S | Inhibin:<br>↑ steroidogenesis<br>Activin:<br>↓ steroidogenesis | Activin:<br>↑ pseudotubular aggregation | | FSH ↑ (S)<br><br>hCG ↑ (L) |
| Interleukin 1 | L,S,M | hCG ↑ (L) | | Mitogen | |
| CRF | L | ↓ LH stimulated steroidogenesis | | | |
| TNFα | G | | ↓ Differentiated function | | |
| POMC | L | | ↓ Differentiated function | | LH ↑ (L) |
| Interleukin 6 | L,S,M | | | ↓ Multiplication | IL-1 ↑ (S)<br>FSH ↑ (S)<br>hCG ↑ (L) |

S, Sertoli; L, Leydig; P, peritubular or myoid; G, germ; M, macrophage; IGF-I, insulin-like growth factor I; TGFβ, transforming growth factor β; TGFα, transforming growth factor α; EGF, epidermal growth factor; bFGF, basic fibroblast growth factor; TNFα, tumor necrosis factor α; POMC, pro-opiomelanocortin; CRF, corticotrophin-releasing factor. ↑: up-regulates or stimulates; ↓: down-regulates or inhibits.

some 17. In human testis, the interconversion of androstenedione and testosterone is higher than that of estrone and estradiol, while the contrary is observed in the ovary.

The aromatization of androgens to estrogens is mediated by cytochrome $P_{450}$ aromatase ($P_{450arom}$) which is located in microsomes. The testes are thus able to produce estrogens. A microsomal enzyme, $5\alpha$-reductase, catalyzes the conversion of testosterone into dihydrotestosterone, the most potent androgen responsible for differentiation of the male external genitalia and prostate as well as for virilization at puberty. Most peripheral tissues convert testosterone into dihydrotestosterone; in particular in androgen-responsive tissues. Some activity is also present in the testis.

There is abundant evidence for local regulation of Leydig cell function. There is communication between Leydig cells with gap junctions allowing exchange of low molecular weight molecules (MW < 1 kD) to pass through. There is also experimental evidence for Sertoli cell secreted proteins that modulate Leydig cell function. *In vitro* co-culture of Leydig and Sertoli cells demonstrates potentiation of both cell type specific functions; the phenomenon being further modu-lated by LH and FSH. These growth factors most likely act in a paracrine fashion. In addition the myoid/peritubular cells form tight junctions and represent a component of the blood–testis barrier. Whereas there is strong experimental evidence indicating cooperation between Sertoli cells and myoid/peritubular cells there is little data concerning the interaction between Leydig cells and myoid/peritubular cells. There is also strong evidence of cooperation between germ cells and Sertoli cells in a reciprocal manner. Macrophages have been documented within the interstitial compartment of the testis and also could play a role in these local interactions. Locally produced growth factors are key regulators of Leydig cells, Sertoli cells, and to some degree, germ cells. A long, although limited, list of these growth factors and their source and functions that are either present or produced within the testis is presented in Table 38.1.

One example is the action on testicular function of the growth hormone-dependent somatomedin, IGF-I. Both *isolated severe (congenital) GH deficiency* and *Laron dwarfism* are associated with delayed puberty and poor response to exogenous hCG. When GH deficiency is treated with GH, normalization of the

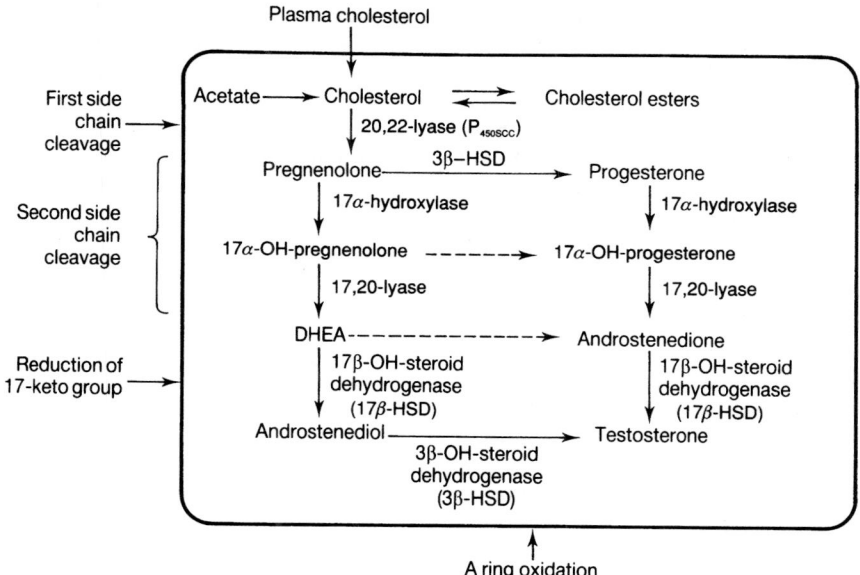

Plasma cholesterol

FIGURE 38.8 Pathways of testosterone synthesis in human testis. The three potential sources of cholesterol for testosterone synthesis are (1) plasma cholesterol; (2) cholesterol synthesized within the cell; and (3) cholesterol stored in the form of cholesterol esters. The first side-chain cleavage of cholesterol to pregnenolone is the rate-limiting reaction in the process and is probably the process that is regulated by luteinizing hormone. Conversion of pregnenolone to testosterone can take place by two theoretical pathways – one in which side-chain cleavage and reduction of the 17-keto group are accomplished before A ring oxidation ($\Delta^5$ pathway, left-hand pathway), and the other in which this sequence is reversed ($\Delta^4$ pathway, right-hand pathway). (From Griffin JE, Wilson JD. The testis. In Bondy PK, Rosenberg LE, eds. *Metabolic control and disease*. 8th edn. Philadelphia: WB Saunders Co., 1980: 1535. Reproduced by permission of WB Saunders Co.)

onset and duration of puberty and the response to hCG are observed, suggesting that GH is involved in the maturation and maintenance of Leydig cell steroidogenesis and responsiveness to hCG. Most of the actions of GH on Leydig cells *in vivo* are thought to be mediated by IGF-I since a direct effect of GH on cultured Leydig cells has not been reported.

## Inhibin and activin

Inhibin and activin are proteins of a structurally related superfamily that includes transforming growth factor β, anti-Müllerian hormone and bone morphogenic protein (BMP) among others; they are endocrine hormones as well as paracrine factors. Inhibin inhibits, and activin stimulates, the secretion of FSH by the adenohypophysis. Gonadal inhibin thus provides a compartment of negative feedback, in addition to that contributed to by sex steroids, on gonadotrophin secretion. Sex steroids exert their dominant inhibiting effect on LH release.

Inhibin is a heterodimeric protein of one β plus either one A or one B (βA or βB) subunit, whereas activins are dimers of two β subunits (βA–βA, βA–βB or βB–βB). Inhibin and activin act as paracrine/autocrine factors in the testis. Sertoli cells appear to be able to secrete both inhibin and activins. In addition some

inhibin subunit expression is regulated by germ cells. Leydig cells also produce both activin and inhibin. Granulosa cell production of inhibin in conjunction with estradiol is responsible for inhibiting pituitary FSH production to prevent other follicles from maturing.

## GAMETOGENESIS

The ultimate goal of the gonadotrophic axis is the production of functional gametes. In the male, germ cells increase in number under the influence of FSH facilitated by LH-mediated testosterone production in nearby Leydig cells. At the time of puberty maturation of spermatogonia to spermatozoa occurs in coordinated groups of contiguous cells over a period of about 70 days such that about 200 million sperm are produced each day. Further development during epididymal passage, a process requiring 12–21 days, results in improved motility by changes in both nuclear chromatin and tail organelles. Although it is clear that spermatogenesis depends on gonadotrophins there is evidence that testosterone and IGF-I are important for normal testicular function as well. The hormonal requirements for initiation of spermatogenesis differ from those required for its maintenance. *Klinefelter syndrome*, or *seminiferous tubule dysgenesis*, is an example of failure of spermatogenesis which results from an extra X chromosome.

The ovary, by contrast, generates oogonia from primordial cells during gestation, with a maximal number of 6 or 7 million around mid-gestation. Germ cell numbers decrease rapidly through atresia so that about 1 million are present at the time of birth. These primary oocytes undergo meiosis, but division is arrested in the diplotene phase of the first meiotic division, to be continued only as ovulation occurs in later years. By the time of menarche further atresia has occurred so that only about 400 000 germ cells are present, of which 400–500 undergo ovulation. Follicular growth and atresia occurs constantly during childhood, a phenomenon which may be responsible for the common occurrence of transient breast development in prepubertal girls. This constant process of atresia probably occurs through apoptosis or programmed cell death, although the ambient androgen environment is also an important influence.

## PATHOPHYSIOLOGY OF THE GONADS

Alteration of gonadal function may be due to chromosomal anomalies, environmental factors during embryonic development (such as viral or toxic agents), or genetic defects altering the expression and/or action of the substances involved in the control of sex differentiation (see Chapter 12).

## Pathology of the ovary

Gonadal dysgenesis is observed in females with *Turner syndrome* resulting from the lack (total or partial) of one X chromosome (see Chapter 12). *Pure gonadal dysgenesis* without Turner features, with a normal female phenotype, normal (so far) 46XX karyotype and normal growth can be observed. These patients present with absence of puberty. Internal genitalia show a normal uterus and vagina. No gonadal tissue is seen but instead a streak of tissue similar to that in Turner syndrome. *Mixed gonadal dysgenesis* is rare and results from unilateral testicular differentiation with 45XO/46XY karyotype. Clinically external genitalia are present with variable ambiguity (limited clitoral hypertrophy) and often asymmetry. Internal genitalia show a uterus, a vagina, a streak ovary on one side and a testis on the other side. This male gonad is usually located in the labia major.

Girls may present at birth with virilization. As long as the genetic sex is 46XX this condition is named *female pseudohermaphroditism* (see Chapter 12). This situation may rise from several etiologies. The most common is excessive adrenal androgen secretion due to *congenital adrenal hyperplasia* (*see* page 508). A very rare condition is virilization due to aromatase deficiency resulting in lack of testosterone transformation into estrogen and thus virilization during fetal develop-

ment. Ovarian function can suffer if there is persistent androgen excess, often due to more subtle enzymatic defects as in the cryptic forms of *21-hydroxylase deficiency*, and lead to *polycystic ovary syndrome*.

*Precocious puberty* (see Chapter 16) can be truly central (gonadotrophin releasing hormone (GnRH)/ LH/FSH driven) or associated with autonomous ovarian function as observed in *McCune–Albright syndrome* due to an activating mutation of the G-α-s protein.

Microcysts or follicular cysts physiologically occur in the maturing ovary in the fetus, the neonate and at the time of puberty. A cyst can be considered abnormal if it is large and/or if it is associated with signs of sexual development and/or if it is associated with persistent pain.

Ovarian insufficiency can be seen with or without androgen excess. *Primary amenorrhea or oligomenorrhea* is present. At or after the age of 13 years, basal plasma FSH and LH are most often elevated. Both FSH and LH response to luteinizing hormone releasing hormone (LHRH) testing is abnormally high. In contrast plasma sex steroid concentrations (17β-estradiol and progesterone) are low for age. In the absence of virilization, *Turner syndrome* or other chromosomal abnormalities, *primary ovarian failure* or resistant ovary syndrome should be considered. *Resistant ovary syndrome* secondary to radiation therapy and/ or chemotherapy has become an increasing cause of ovarian failure. *Autoimmune ovarian insufficiency* with other autoimmune disorders (*hypoparathyroidism, thyroiditis, type II insulin-dependent diabetes, pernicious anemia, juvenile arthritis, vitiligo,* among others) begins during childhood or adolescence. Lack of 17-ketoreductase, a rare enzymatic defect that affects both the adrenals and the ovary can result in delayed puberty. Ovarian insufficiency may be secondary to a metabolic disorder such as *galactosemia*.

Ovarian dysfunction with androgen excess may be encountered in adolescent girls and young women. Signs of androgenization are present. Pubertal development is less affected and symptoms are most often limited to dysmenorrhea or amenorrhea in late puberty. An *androgen secreting tumor* is usually diagnosed due to rapidly progressive virilization. In case of adrenal androgen excess an adrenocorticotropic hormone (ACTH) test will then be performed to elucidate the enzymatic defect, most often *late onset 21-hydroxylase deficiency* or poorly controlled *classical 21-hydroxylase deficiency*. When no adrenal source is involved, "idiopathic" *polycystic ovary syndrome* (*Stein–Leventhal syndrome*) is to be considered. Two ovarian enzyme defects can be found: 3β-HSD and 17β-HSD deficiency.

## Pathophysiology of the testis

*Male pseudohermaphroditism* is defined by chromosomal 46XY males born with a mild to severe incomplete or altered virilization of external genitalia. It extends from moderate hypospadias to complete androgen resistance with female external genitalia. The etiology is either that of partial to severe androgen resistance due to an abnormality of the androgen receptor gene, or testosterone/dihydrotestosterone biosynthesis defects.

Primary tubular dysgenesis is mainly due to *Klinefelter syndrome* and its variants. In addition other conditions such as *cystic fibrosis* and *del Castillo* syndrome may be associated with tubular dysfunction. Secondary tubular dysfunction is seen after chemotherapy and/or radiation therapy.

Prevalence of *cryptorchidism* increases from 2 per cent at term up to 20 per cent in premature babies. Provided that there is no penile abnormality, the endocrine function of the testis can be assessed by the spontaneous postnatal testosterone/LH peak between 1 and 2 months of corrected postnatal age and/or by hCG testing. Bilateral absence of the testis, "vanishing testis" or *congenital anorchia* is a rare condition whose pathophysiology remains unclear.

Simple delayed puberty is a common situation in males. It most often is familial and idiopathic, rarely due to *hypogonadotrophic hypogonadism*, then possibly associated with anosmia (*Kallman syndrome*). The syndrome of *familial autonomous testicular function* or "testotoxicosis" is a rare condition presenting with precocious puberty. Other causes are central (see Chapter 16).

Environmental factors are taking an increasing place in testicular pathology. There is a trend in decrease in semen quality with a decline from 100–150 to 60–80 million spermatozoa per milliliter between 1940 and 1990. Meanwhile the incidence of testicular cancer, cryptorchidism and hypospadias has almost doubled between the 1970s and the 1990s in several western European countries. Among the suspected or identified factors one must consider many chemicals with estrogenic effects.

## SELECTED READING

Adashi EY, Resnick CE, D'Ercole AJ *et al.* Insulin-like growth factors as intra-ovarian regulators of granulosa cell growth and function. *Endocr Rev* 1985; **6**: 400.

Burger HG, Tamada Y, Bangah ML *et al.* Serum gonadotropin, sex steroid and immunoreactive inhibin levels in the first two years of life. *J Clin Endocrinol Metab* 1991; **72**: 682.

Burger HG, de Krester DM eds. *The testis.* 2nd edn. New York: Raven Press, 1989.

Chatelain P, Berlier J, Francois R. Pathology of the ovary. In Bertrand J, Rappaport R, Sizonenko P eds. *Pediatric endocrinology.* Baltimore: Williams & Wilkins, 1993: 420.

Forest MG, Sizonenko PC, Cathiard AM, Bertrand J. Hypophyseal–gonadal function in infants during the first year of life. I. Evidence for testicular activity in early infancy. *J Clin Invest* 1974; **53**: 819.

Forest MG, Saez JM, Bertrand J. Biochemistry and physiology of gonadotropic and gonadal hormones. In Bertrand J, Rappaport R, Sizonenko P. eds. *Pediatric endocrinology.* Baltimore: Williams & Wilkins, 1993: 351.

Kaplan SL, Grumbach MM, Aubert M. The ontogenesis of pituitary hormones and hypothalamic factors in the human fetus: maturation of the central nervous system of the anterior pituitary function. *Rec Prog Horm Res* 1974; **32**: 161.

Larsen WJ. Development of the urogenital system. In Larsen WJ ed. *Human embryology.* New York: Churchill Livingstone, 1993: 235.

Miljoprojekt n 290. Male reproductive health and environmental chemicals with estrogenic effects. DK-1401-Copenhagen, Danish Environmental Protection Agency (Pub), 1995.

Parvinen M. Regulation of the semineferous epithelium. *Endocr Rev* 1982; **3**: 404.

Richard JS, Jahnsen T, Hedin L. Ovarian follicular development: from physiology to molecular biology. *Recent Prog Horm Res* 1987; **43**: 231.

Ross GT, Schreiber JR. The ovary. In Yen S, Jaffe R eds. *Reproductive endocrinology.* London: WB Saunders, 1978: 63.

Saez JM. Leydig cells: endocrine, paracrine and autocrine regulation. *Endocr Rev* 1995; **15**: 574.

Sizonenko PC. Disorders of the testis. In Bertrand J, Rappaport R, Sizonenko P eds. *Pediatric endocrinology.* Baltimore: Williams & Wilkins, 1993: 430.

# 39

# The Adrenal Cortex

Ieuan A. Hughes and Wayne S. Cutfield

## EMBRYOLOGY AND ANATOMY

The adrenal cortex is mesodermal in origin, arising from the cranial end of the mesonephros during the fifth week of fetal development. This cortico-adrenal anlage is then penetrated on its medial aspect by ectoderm from the neural crest to form the adrenal medulla (*see* page 530). While the cortex and medulla are of separate origin and clearly subserve different endocrine functions, there is now abundant evidence of close interweaving of cortical and chromaffin cells on the basis of immunohistochemical markers and ultrastructural analysis. This suggests the operation of intra-adrenal paracrine mechanisms.

The adrenal cortex of the fetus and young infant consists of two distinct layers. The inner layer develops first to become the fetal cortex (or zone), which rapidly increases in size from the seventh month of life to occupy 80 per cent of the adrenal cortex at birth. The adult or definitive cortex forms as a thin, irregular outer layer and contains the zona glomerulosa and zona fasciculata. High-resolution transvaginal ultrasonography shows a linear increase in fetal adrenal size in early gestation with the fetal adrenal gland being detected as early as 10 weeks. The mean combined adrenal weight increases from about 0.5 g at 14 weeks' gestation to 2.9 g by 27 weeks. In contrast, the adrenal glands are already small in anencephaly by the end of the first trimester and do not exceed a combined weight of 1 g by 26 weeks. In *congenital adrenal hyperplasia*, the combined adrenal weight at comparable gestational ages in those fetuses where the pregnancy was terminated was considerably above the normal range. These observations together with data on amniotic fluid steroid concentrations illustrate the role of fetal pituitary adrenocorticotrophic hormone (ACTH) in the control of differentiation and development of the fetal adrenal cortex. After birth, the fetal cortex involutes quite rapidly to occupy only about 20 per cent of the combined cortical zones.

The outer zone of the adrenal cortex is the zona glomerulosa and comprises 10 per cent of the cortex during childhood. The zona fasciculata occupies the remainder of the definitive cortex until the development of the zona reticularis which first appears in early childhood. The zona reticularis forms the inner zone of the adrenal cortex, and is the primary source of androgen secretion in adrenarche. It ultimately occupies 10 per cent of the cortex by the end of puberty, at which time the adrenal cortex is fully mature. The combined adrenal weight at this stage is 10–12 g.

## FETAL ADRENOCORTICAL FUNCTION

The anatomical subdivision of the cortex is rather artificial, particularly in fetal life where there is evidence of functional zonation on the basis of the ontogeny of steroidogenic enzyme expression. Fetal and transitional zones can be defined by $P_{450scc}$ and $P_{450c17}$ expression in mid-gestation with additional expression of 3β-hydroxysteroid dehydrogenase (3β-HSD) activity in late gestation indicating the appearance of a definitive zone. These three zones produce androgens, glucocorticoids and mineralocorticoids, respectively, and correspond to the traditional zonae reticularis, fasciculata and glomerulosa, respectively.

The fetal adrenal cortex and placenta are termed the "fetoplacental unit" as these two organs interact to produce essential hormones for the mother and fetus (Fig. 39.1) (*see also* page 211 and page 244). The fetal adrenal has two unique functions: to provide precursors for maternal estrogen production and to facilitate, via the action of cortisol, maturation of certain organ systems, particularly the lungs. 3β-HSD activity is not expressed until after 22–24 weeks' gestation and thereafter it is functionally inactivated by placental estrogen. This provides placental control of steroid production by the fetal zone of the adrenal and ensures the major product is dehydroepiandrosterone sulfate (DHEAS). Placental progesterone and pregnenolone are the major substrates for adrenal steroidogenesis by the fetal adrenal cortex. The human placenta lacks 17α-hydroxylase, 17,20 lyase and 16α-hydroxylase enzyme activities. From approximately 8 weeks' gestation, pregnenolone is converted principally to DHEAS which is hydroxylated in other fetal tissues, particularly the liver, to 16-hydroxyDHEAS. Both maternal and fetal 16-hydroxyDHEAS are cleaved to unconjugated steroids by placental sulfatase to provide substrates for androstenedione and 16-hydroxyandrostenedione, and testosterone and 16-hydroxytestosterone production using the enzymes 3β-HSD and 17β-hydroxysteroid dehydrogenase (17β-HSD), respectively. This vast amount of C19 androgens is equivalent to the daily quantity of estrogens produced by the pregnant mother so a mechanism must be in place to protect the fetus from virilizing side effects. This is provided by an efficient placental aromatization system which converts the C19 steroids to estrone, estradiol and estriol. Recently described cases of *placental aromatase deficiency* highlight this protective role since both the mother and female fetuses in such pregnancies are severely virilized. The role of the fetal adrenal gland in the initiation of parturition in the human is not as clearly defined as it is in other species such as the sheep (see Chapter 15). Certainly, the onset of labor may be delayed in pregnancies associated with placental sulfatase and aromatase deficiencies or when the fetus is *anencephalic* or has *congenital adrenal hypoplasia*.

Late in gestation fetal ACTH and cortisol concentrations rise, influencing the maturation of a number of organs including the lungs, gastrointestinal tract, liver and pancreas. Surfactant production is increased by glucocorticoids with evidence of enhanced surfactant-associated protein (SP-A,B,C,D) gene expression. The primary source of fetal cortisol production is the definitive cortex in late gestation with only a small contribution from the fetal zone since 3β-HSD expression is reduced in this zone.

Maternal cortisol would be expected to cross the placenta and in high concentrations may adversely affect fetal growth. The placenta provides another protective system through the operation of an efficient 11β-hydroxysteroid dehydrogenase (11β-HSD) enzyme which converts cortisol to inactive cortisone. This is a shuttle enzyme system so that 11-oxidoreductase activity which interconverts cortisone back to cortisol becomes more active near term in order to expose critical organs such as the lung to glucocorticoid action. There is accumulating evidence of an association between decreased placental 11β-HSD activity and *intrauterine growth retardation*.

The fetal adrenal initially may be independent of fetal hypothalamic–pituitary control, with perhaps human chorionic gonadotrophin (hCG), pro-opiomelanocortin (POMC) cleavage products or insulin-like growth factors (IGFs) acting as trophic factors. However, there is abundant evidence on morphological and functional grounds to indicate that fetal ACTH is the predominant trophic regulator of the fetal adrenal. The placenta also secretes corticotrophin-releasing hormone (CRH) and maternal plasma CRH concentrations rise exponentially with advancing gestation. CRH also is present in amniotic fluid and the fetal circulation, and so presumably influences fetal ACTH regulation of the fetal adrenal gland. A CRH-binding protein (CRH-BP) blocks binding of CRH to its

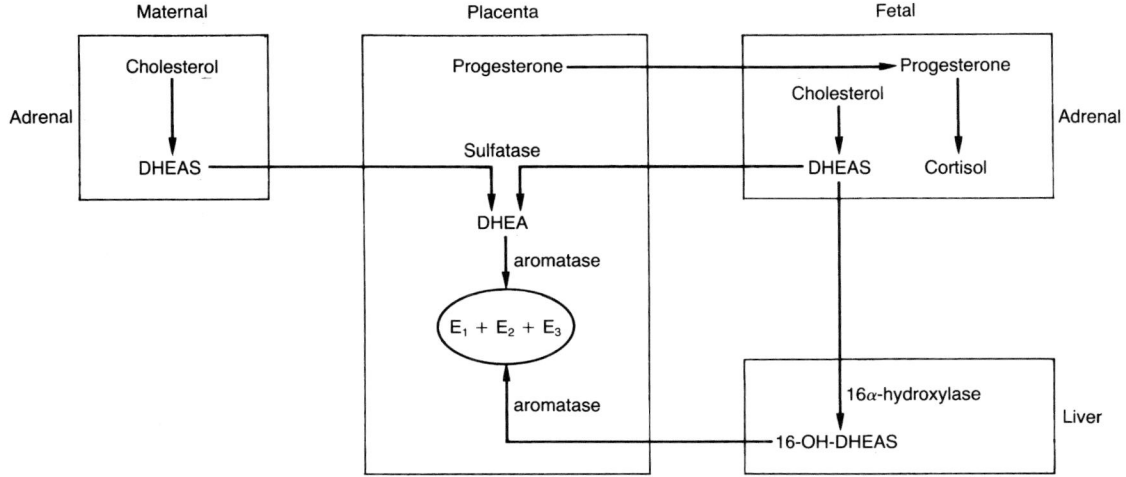

FIGURE 39.1 Schematic representation of the steroid inter-relationships constituting a fetoplacental unit. Key enzymes are placental sulfatase and aromatase. E₁, estrone; E₂, estradiol; E₃, estriol; DHEAS, dehydroepiandrosterone sulfate

receptor, but CRH-BP concentrations fall abruptly about 3 weeks before the onset of spontaneous labor. Thus, there is a temporal association between enhanced CRH bioavailability toward the end of pregnancy and the onset of parturition (see Chapter 15). This suggests the presence of a "placental clock," in the form of CRH bioavailability, which is activated in early pregnancy and which determines gestational length and the timing of parturition rather than other events which occur in late pregnancy.

## PATHWAY OF ADRENAL STEROIDOGENESIS

Steroidogenesis occurs in all three zones of the definitive adrenal cortex, with each zone principally responsible for producing a single class of steroids. Mineralocorticoids are produced in the outer zona glomerulosa, androgens in the inner zona reticularis and glucocorticoids in the zona fasciculata. Since the zonae fasciculata and reticularis and zona glomerulosa are regulated differently they may be regarded as functionally separate glands but housed within the same organ.

All adrenal steroid hormones are formed from cholesterol derived mainly from low-density lipoprotein (LDL) (see page 464). The basic steroid structure is illustrated in Fig. 39.2. Steroid biosynthesis is complex with intermediates sequentially formed in several sites within the cell (Fig. 39.3). Cortisol biosynthesis is under the control of ACTH which increases cholesterol ester hydroxylase or side chain cleavage activity (Fig.

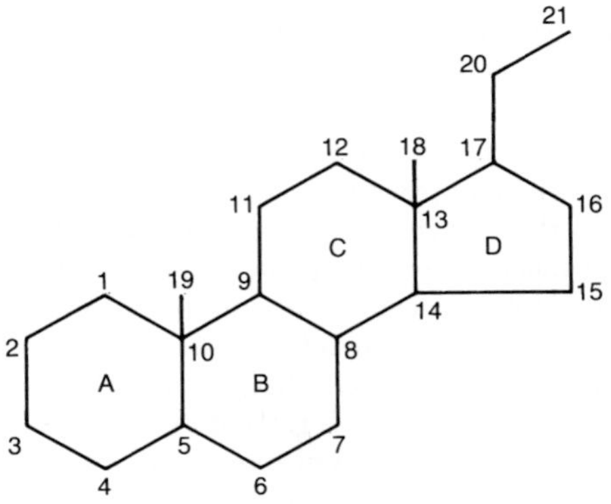

FIGURE 39.2 Basic steroid nucleus represented with 21 carbon atoms. Letters refer to the four rings.

39.3) through adenylyl cyclase activation. All the steroid hydroxylases except 3β-HSD are collectively part of the cytochrome $P_{450}$ system and are b-type cytochrome mixed-function oxidases. The first step common to all steroidogenesis is the cleavage of six carbon atoms from the side chain of cholesterol to form pregnenolone. This is catalyzed by the single side-chain cleavage enzyme $P_{450scc}$, previously known as cholesterol desmolase, and takes place within the mitochondrion. This complex sequence is the rate-limiting step in adrenal steroid synthesis. The reaction requires transfer of electrons from reduced nicotinamide adenine dinucleotide phosphate (NADPH) to adrenodoxin reductase which is a flavoprotein, further transfer to

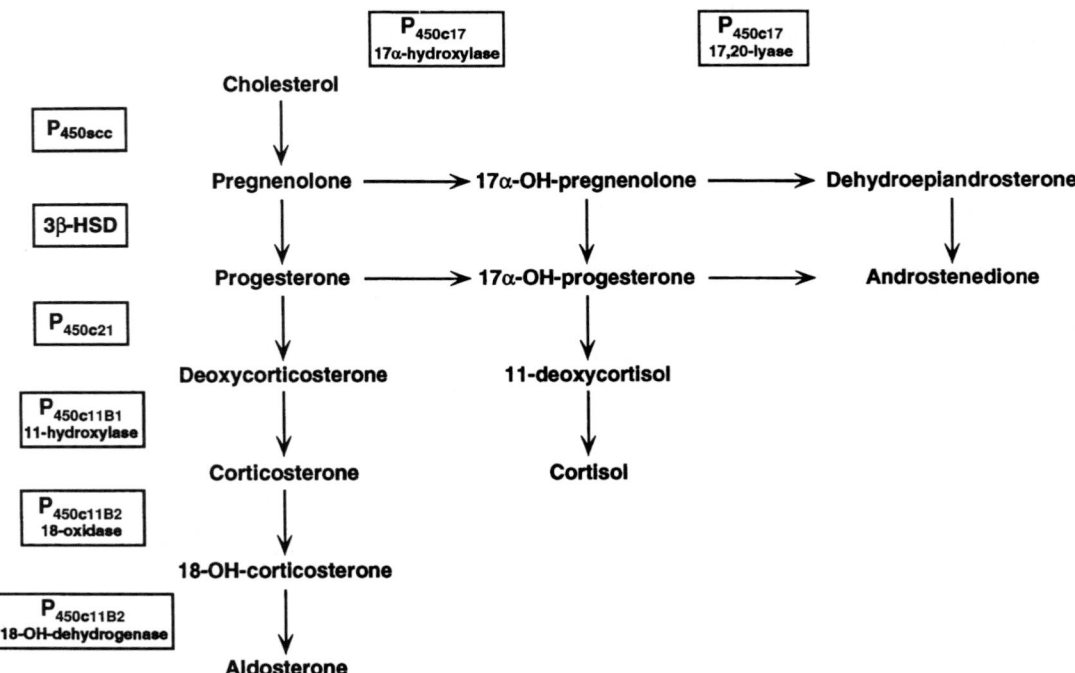

FIGURE 39.3 Pathways of adrenal steroidogenesis. Enzyme activities are boxed. The three separate components of $P_{450C11\beta}$ and the two separate components of $P_{450c17}$ enzyme activities are indicated.

adrenodoxin (an iron–sulfur protein) and thence $P_{450scc}$ reduction.

Pregnenolone passes from the mitochondrion to the endoplasmic reticulum where it either can be converted to progesterone by 3β-HSD activity or can be hydroxylated in the 17α position by $P_{450c17}$ to form 17α-hydroxypregnenolone. This in turn may be converted to 17α-hydroxyprogesterone by the action of 3β-HSD. This enzyme thus transfers a double bond from the B to the A ring of the steroid nucleus in conjunction with a reduction to a ketone group at the carbon 3 position. The $\Delta^5$-hydroxysteroids, pregnenolone, 17α-OH-pregnenolone and dehydroepiandrosterone (DHEA) are converted by 3β-HSD to the $\Delta^4$-3-oxosteroids, progesterone, 17α-OH-progesterone and androstenedione.

A second activity of $P_{450c17}$ is an oxidative cleavage of 17,20 two-carbon side chains (17,20 lyase) yielding either DHEA or androstenedione depending on the substrate. 17,20-Lyase activity is more pronounced in gonads for sex steroid biosynthesis; there is evidence that cytochrome $b_5$ enhances this pathway in the testis as an accessory protein. This dual role enables this single enzyme, $P_{450c17}$, to direct steroid precursors to glucocorticoid or androgen synthesis. This latter function becomes important in disorders such as *21-hydroxylase deficiency* when $P_{450c17}$ acts on increased 17α-OH-progesterone substrate to promote androgen synthesis. Progesterone and 17α-OH-progesterone are hydroxylated in the 21 position by $P_{450c21}$ to form deoxycorticosterone and 11-deoxycortisol, respectively. These products then pass back to the mitochondrion to be 11-hydroxylated by $P_{450c11\beta}$ (isoenzyme type B1, see below) to form corticosterone and cortisol, respectively.

Aldosterone, the principal mineralocorticoid, is produced exclusively in the zona glomerulosa under the control of the renin–angiotensin system (*see* page 523). $P_{450c17}$ is not expressed in this zone so that once progesterone is formed, as in the zona fasciculata, sequential hydroxylation at the 21 and 11β carbon positions occurs. The zona glomerulosa has the further capacity to perform 18-hydroxylation which is an additional function of the second $P_{450c11\beta}$ isoenzyme. The two isoenzymes have been designated B1 and B2, respectively, with the latter also alternatively referred to as $P_{450cmo}$ (corticosterone methyl oxidase) or $P_{450aldo}$ or aldosterone synthase or CYP11B2. Thus $P_{45011B2}$ 18-hydroxylates and 18-oxidizes corticosterone to aldosterone.

Adrenal androgen production is confined to the zona reticularis and once the fetal adrenal involutes after birth, C19 steroid synthesis is insignificant until late childhood. Following adrenarche, DHEA and DHEAS are produced by the adrenals in greatest abundance with plasma concentrations in the micromolar range. The $P_{450c17}$ enzyme with its 17,20 lyase activity is the key switch for adrenal androgen production. Conversion to more potent androgens such as testosterone is extra-adrenal.

The cytochrome $P_{450}$ family of steroidogenic enzymes catalyze more than one function. For example, $P_{450scc}$ mediates 22-hydroxylase, 20-hydroxylase and 20,22 lyase reactions. $P_{450c11\beta}$ displays a unique combination of 11β-hydroxylase, 18-hydroxylase and, in some species, even aromatase activity. Steroidogenic enzyme activity can be inhibited by a number of compounds, some of which have clinical use. Aminoglutethimide inhibits $P_{450scc}$ and has some use in the treatment of autonomous adrenocortical hyperfunction. Metyrapone inhibits $P_{450c11\beta}$ activity and is often used to assess hypothalamo–pituitary–adrenal function as well as for treatment for *Cushing syndrome* due to autonomous adrenocortical hyperfunction. Imidazole-derived antifungal drugs which inhibit fungal $P_{450}$ systems have found a useful role for inhibiting steroidogenesis, through both $P_{450scc}$ and $P_{450c11\beta}$ enzymes. Ketoconazole is one such example, used in some patients with *Cushing syndrome* as well as in *testotoxicosis*, a familial male-limited form of precocious puberty due to constitutively activating mutations of the gene encoding the luteinizing hormone (LH) receptor in the testis (*see* page 197). The genes encoding all the enzymes involved in adrenal steroidogenesis have been cloned so that genetic enzyme deficiencies which result in the general group of conditions called *congenital adrenal hyperplasia* can now be explained on a molecular basis (*see* page 508).

## REGULATION OF CORTISOL SECRETION

The hypothalamus, pituitary and adrenal cortex comprise a neuroendocrine axis which controls cortisol secretion. CRH, a 41-amino-acid peptide, is primarily produced by neurons of the paraventricular nuclei located in the hypothalamus which are apparent by 12 weeks' gestation. CRH is also found in other hypothalamic nuclei, the cerebral and cerebellar cortices, the hippocampus and outside the brain in sites such as the lung, liver, gastrointestinal tract, pancreas, adrenal (mainly medulla), testis and placenta. The CRH gene in humans is located on chromosome 8. CRH is released by the median eminence into the hypophyseal portal circulation to reach the anterior pituitary to stimulate ACTH production and release. The stimulatory effect is brought about by binding of CRH to a receptor on corticotropes which is a transmembrane, G-protein-linked receptor. Circulating CRH is protein bound by CRH-BP which affects the bioavailability. ACTH release is not just regulated by CRH, but also by vasopressin (AVP) and a variety of signals from higher centers whose inputs relay via the hippocampus. This is an area of the brain rich in glucocorticoid receptors where the functional aspects of circadian rhythm, stress responsiveness and glucocorticoid feedback inhibition are modulated. A class of neurosteroids (*see* page 465), with DHEAS predominating, has recently been recognized in the brain and may play a role in CRH regulation. AVP acting in concert with CRH may be important in mediating the rise in ACTH release late in fetal life (*see* page 247). Excitatory neurotransmitters which regulate CRH secretion include catecholamines, serotonin, γ-amino butyric acid (GABA), endogenous opioids, neuropeptide Y (NPY) and cytokines.

The major regulatory factor for ACTH release is the level of negative feedback by circulating cortisol, acting at hippocampal, hypothalamic and pituitary levels. There are both rapid and slow-onset feedback mechanisms. Rapid feedback involves a membrane-mediated, non-genomic mechanism, while the slower response occurs as a result of glucocorticoid inhibition of POMC gene expression.

ACTH is cleaved from the large prohormone, POMC, which contains the sequences of several other peptide hormones (Fig. 39.4). The gene is located on chromosome 2 and comprises three exons separated by two large introns. The cleavage pattern and thereby peptide products of POMC differ according to tissue specificity. In the anterior lobe, the main products are the NH$_2$-terminal peptide, J-peptide, ACTH and β-lipotrophin (β-LPH). In the intermediate lobe which is only active in humans during fetal life and pregnancy, there is further cleavage to include corticotrophin-like intermediate peptide (CLIP), postulated by some workers to be the trophic hormone for the fetal adrenal. Aside from ACTH most of the pituitary POMC products appear to have no major physiological roles. β-LPH has weak steroidogenic, lipolytic and opiate-like activities and may also have melanotrophic activity. β-Endorphin has opiate-like activity as well as effects on feeding and sexual behavior. The NH$_2$-terminal peptide and its products may have weak steroidogenic activity. The melanocyte-stimulating hormones (MSHs) stimulate melanocytes to produce melanin.

ACTH is a 39-amino-acid single-chain polypeptide with a biological half-life of 4–8 minutes. The first N-terminal 24 amino acids confer full steroidogenic activity (synthetic ACTH (Synacthen) has this 24 amino acid sequence) while amino acids 2–12 are conserved throughout most species. ACTH is essential for normal steroidogenesis and has a facilitatory role in maintaining normal adrenal size. ACTH has a weak melanocyte-stimulating effect; however, in pathological states associated with chronically elevated ACTH levels (e.g. *Addison disease*) marked hyperpigmentation may occur. The ACTH receptor is a member of the seven transmembrane domain G-protein-linked receptor superfamily. The actions of ACTH are mediated through adenylyl cyclase activation, increased cAMP levels and activation of cAMP-dependent protein kinases. ACTH has both acute and chronic effects on steroidogenesis. The former involves stimulation of side-chain cleavage activity to convert cholesterol to pregnenolone which requires the transport of cholesterol into the mitochondrion. It is only recently that this process has become better understood, through studying *congenital lipoid adrenal hyperplasia*, a disorder characterized by deficient synthesis of adrenal and gonadal steroids. A 30 kD phosphorylated protein, termed steroidogenic acute regulatory protein (StAR), mediates the rapid, cycloheximide-sensitive response of early steroidogenesis to acute trophic stimulation by transporting cholesterol to the inner mitochondrial membrane where it undergoes side-chain cleavage. The StAR protein is not expressed in the placenta so that other mechanisms must be invoked for cholesterol transport in this tissue, otherwise progesterone production would not take place to maintain viable pregnancies. Chronic exposure to elevated levels of ACTH leads to increased synthesis of all steroidogenic enzymes via cAMP-mediated regulation of gene expression.

## Circadian rhythm of cortisol

Postnatally ACTH is secreted in a pulsatile fashion. Levels start to rise around 03.00 hours, peak at 08.00 hours and gradually decline during the rest of the day. The mature circadian rhythm in cortisol secretion is established by 3 years of age, although there is increasing evidence of circadian rhythmicity from 3 months onwards. The circadian rhythm control center is likely to either be located within, or signal through, the suprachiasmatic nucleus of the hypothalamus (*see* page 413). A form of pulse generator probably also housed in the hypothalamus must also be present to release CRH in a periodic fashion.

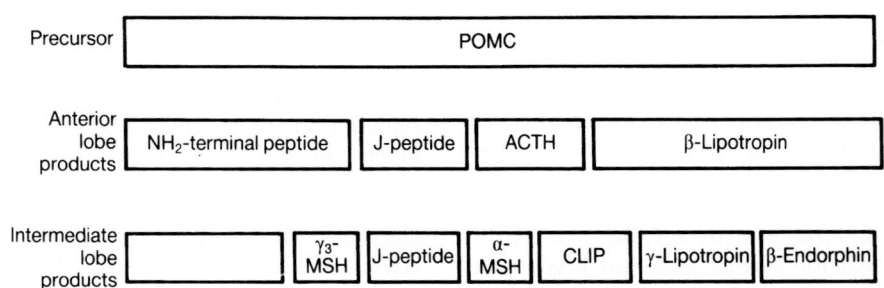

FIGURE 39.4 Pituitary pro-opiomelanocortin and peptide hormone products.

## CONTROL OF ALDOSTERONE SECRETION

The major circulating mineralocorticoid is aldosterone, while its precursors including deoxycorticosterone (DOC), corticosterone and 18-hydroxycorticosterone, possess weak mineralocorticoid activity. The three precursors are synthesized in each of the adrenal zones but 18-hydroxycorticosterone is mainly produced in the zona glomerulosa as is aldosterone. More DOC and corticosterone are synthesized in the zona fasciculata than in the zona glomerulosa, so their production is mainly stimulated by ACTH. Aldosterone is exclusively produced in the zona glomerulosa; the renin–angiotensin system and $K^+$ are the prime regulators. Prolonged elevation of ACTH leads only to a transient increase in aldosterone production. Aldosterone, unlike cortisol, is not secreted in a significant circadian rhythm pattern. Factors that influence aldosterone secretion are listed in Table 39.1. The renin–angiotensin system is reviewed on page 520.

## PLASMA STEROID-BINDING PROTEINS

Steroid hormones are transported predominantly protein-bound in the circulation. The two major specific steroid-binding proteins are corticosteroid-binding globulin (CBG) and sex hormone-binding globulin (SHBG). These carrier proteins have high affinity, but limited capacity for steroid binding. Another major steroid carrier protein is albumin, which operates as a high-capacity, low-affinity binding system.

CBG is an $\alpha_2$-globulin which is a member of the serine protease inhibitor superfamily and includes thyroxine-binding globulin and angiotensinogen. The production of CBG is mainly hepatic and the majority of cortisol in normal circumstances is CBG-bound with the remainder bound to albumin. Synthetic steroids bind poorly to CBG with the exception of prednisolone. Other adrenal C21 steroids bind to CBG but only 60 per cent of aldosterone is protein-bound, the majority to albumin. When total plasma cortisol concentrations exceed about 700 nmol/L, CBG binding sites become saturated so that free cortisol concentrations increase. CBG concentrations are increased by estrogen, are lower in the fetus than in the adult, rise considerably during childhood and then fall to adult levels by puberty.

The weak adrenal androgens bind predominantly to albumin, with minimal binding to SHBG to which testosterone, dihydrotestosterone and estradiol are primarily bound.

## STEROID METABOLISM

The liver is the main site of the production of metabolites. These are produced from reduction of the A ring double bond using $5\alpha/5\beta$-reductases and further reduction at the 3-oxo group by $3\alpha$-hydroxysteroid dehydrogenase to yield tetrahydrocortisols. Cortisol and cortisone may also be reduced by $20\alpha$- and $20\beta$-hydroxysteroid dehydrogenase to produce cortol and cortolone, respectively. Their excretion in the urine as glucuronides accounts for 60–70 per cent of total cortisol production. Cortisol is also metabolized to cortisone in the kidney by 11β-HSD acting as a shuttle system (Fig. 39.5). This enzyme has been described as acting as a "moat" to prevent excess glucocorticoid exposure to both mineralcorticoid and glucocorticoid

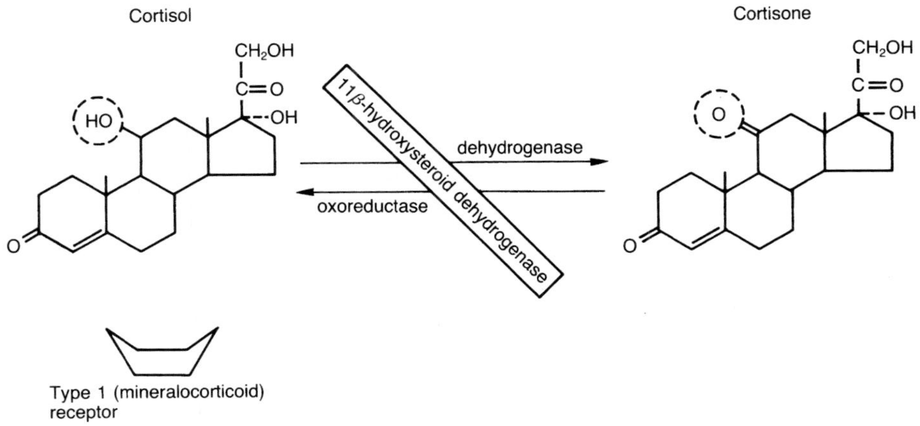

TABLE 39.1 Factors influencing the control of aldosterone secretion

| Stimulatory | Renin–angiotensin, via renal perfusion |
| | Hypokalemia |
| | ACTH |
| | Prostaglandins |
| | β-Adrenergic stimulation |
| | Hypernatremia |
| | Serotonin |
| Inhibitory | Dopamine |
| | Atrial natriuretic peptide |
| | Somatostatin |

FIGURE 39.5 The cortisol:cortisone shuttle and its relation to the mineralocorticoid receptor. Hydroxyl and ketone substitutions at position C11 are highlighted.

receptors. Deficiency of 11β-HSD activity leads to a syndrome of apparent mineralocorticoid excess whereby cortisol is not metabolized sufficiently to cortisone in the renal tubule thereby occupying Type 1 mineralocorticoid receptor sites to function as a mineralocorticoid. There is resulting severe hypokalemic alkalosis, low plasma renin activity and hypertension. A mutation in the Type II 11β-HSD gene expressed in the kidney has now been identified in a patient with this syndrome. Ingestion of licorice, which contains glycyrrhizic acid, can also produce hypertension, in a similar fashion by acting as a competitive inhibitor of 11β-HSD.

The epidemiological studies which relate adult hypertension to a prenatal origin (*see* page 302), based on the combination of a reduced birth weight and a large placenta, may be explained partly on the basis of altered 11β-HSD activity in the placenta resulting in excess fetal exposure to maternal cortisol, with subsequent growth retardation and later hypertension.

## ADRENAL STEROID RECEPTORS (*see also* page 464)

The glucocorticoid and mineralocorticoid receptors are members of a nuclear receptor superfamily which also includes all steroid, thyroid hormone and retinoic acid receptors as well as an increasing number of orphan receptors whose ligands remain to be identified. Nuclear receptors have in common a tripartite functional domain structure comprising a hypervariable N-terminal domain involved in transactivation, a highly conserved central DNA binding domain which recognizes appropriate DNA response elements and a C-terminal domain which mediates ligand binding, nuclear localization, receptor dimerization and heat shock protein binding (Fig. 39.6). Steroid hormones are lipophilic and enter target cells in the unbound form by passive diffusion.

The glucocorticoid receptor is encoded by a 10 exon gene on chromosome 5. The receptor resides in the cytoplasm in the unliganded state in association with heat shock protein 90. This dissociates when glucocorticoids bind to the receptor and permits, in some way, nuclear translocation and subsequent transactivation (Fig. 39.7). The hormone–receptor complex binds to DNA glucocorticoid response elements by virtue of two zinc fingers each of which is coordinated by four cysteines. The receptor binds in a dimeric form to the response element. Glucocorticoid receptors are ubiquitously expressed throughout all tissues in keeping with the wide diversity of glucocorticoid biological effects. An orphan nuclear receptor, designated steroidogenic factor 1 (SF-1) has been identified in mice as a key regulator of steroid hydroxylases in steroidogenic tissues. SF-1 is expressed in the adrenal cortex, Leydig cells, ovary and in the developing urogenital ridge. Remarkably, targeted gene disruption to produce mice deficient in SF-1 led to complete absence of adrenal and gonadal development. An equivalent syndrome has yet to be reported in humans. SF-1 apparently is essential for the formation of the ventromedial hypothalamic nucleus, a region of the brain important in reproductive behavior.

Aldosterone binds to Type I (mineralocorticoid) and Type II (glucocorticoid) receptors. Since cortisol, which circulates at much higher concentrations than aldosterone, also binds to the Type I receptor, the 11β-HSD "moat" mechanism is operative in mineralocorticoid target tissues to convert cortisol to inert cortisone. Such tissues include the kidney, salivary and sweat glands, and the large bowel. Type I receptors are also present in the brain, pituitary, liver and circulating mononuclear cells.

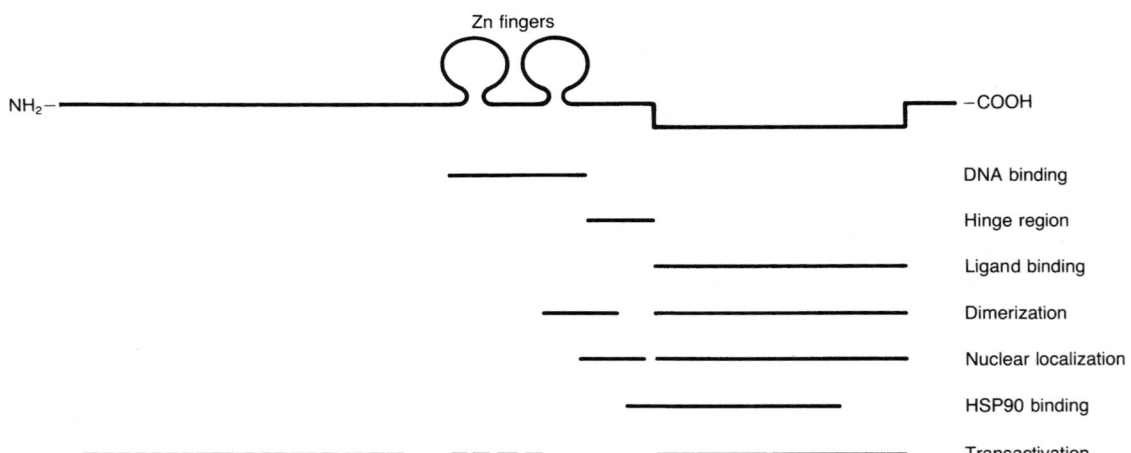

FIGURE 39.6 General structure of a generic steroid receptor. The extent of various functional domains are indicated by the bar lengths.

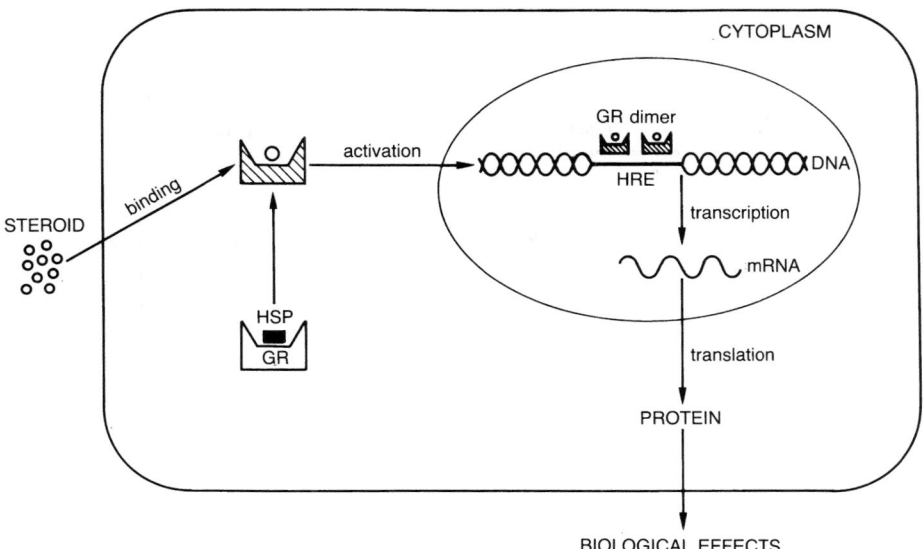

FIGURE 39.7 Schematic representation of glucocorticoid action. HSP, heat shock protein (includes HSP70, HSP90); GR, glucocorticoid receptor; HRE, hormone response element.

## PHYSIOLOGICAL ACTIONS OF GLUCOCORTICOIDS

Glucocorticoids comprise one of the group of counter-regulatory hormones which contribute to glucose homeostasis. They raise blood glucose levels by stimulating hepatic gluconeogenesis, enhancing glycogenolysis by adrenaline, inhibiting peripheral glucose utilization and promoting liver glycogen stores. Gluconeogenesis is achieved through two separate glucocorticoid effects. First, extrahepatic gluconeogenic amino acids are mobilized, principally from skeletal muscle. Second, conversion of these amino acids to glucose is increased in the liver via enhanced activities of phosphoenolpyruvate carboxykinase and glucose-6-phosphatase. Other gluconeogenic hormones such as adrenaline and glucagon are ineffective without the permissive effect of glucocorticoids. Glycogenesis in fetal and postnatal life is promoted by glucocorticoid activation of glycogen synthetase and inhibition of glycogen phosphorylase. Glucocorticoids inhibit peripheral glucose utilization in tissues such as skin, fat, and muscle by reducing glucose uptake through decreased transporter mRNA levels. Glucocorticoids acutely stimulate lipolysis from adipocytes, leading to increased plasma free fatty acids. The effect is permissive only in the presence of other lipolytic agents such as growth hormone. The mechanism of how excess fat is redistributed with chronic glucocorticoid exposure is unknown.

The effects of glucocorticoids on the immune system, inflammatory processes, skeleton and connective tissue are only seen in states of prolonged glucocorticoid excess and therefore are unlikely to constitute normal physiological responses. Excessive and pro-longed treatment with glucocorticoids during childhood has adverse effects on the skeleton. These include impairment of normal bone formation and inhibition of bone growth. Reduced osteoblastic activity with concomitant increased osteoclastic activity leads to reduced new bone formation and osteopenia. Indirect effects include reduced calcium absorption from the gut, increased urinary calcium excretion and direct stimulation of parathyroid hormone secretion. The precise mechanism of glucocorticoid inhibition of bone growth remains to be determined; it is likely to include inhibition of IGF-I action and impairment of procollagen production.

Immunological and inflammatory responses are suppressed by excess glucocorticoids. Circulating lymphocytes (T and B cells) are reduced, due to relocation in extravascular sites. B cell, T cell and macrophage differentiation, proliferation and actions are also inhibited. These adverse events are mediated through effects on cytokines, bradykinin, serotonin, histamine and plasminogen activators.

The mechanisms through which glucocorticoids maintain vascular integrity during stress are poorly understood. Glucocorticoid excess leads to hypertension, whereas glucocorticoid deficiency is associated with hypotension, suggesting that glucocorticoids have either a direct or indirect effect on vascular tone. There is evidence to show that glucocorticoids induce expression of $\alpha_{1\beta}$ and $\beta_2$ adrenergic receptors in smooth muscle cells. Glucocorticoids inhibit AVP and increase atrial natriuretic peptide (ANP) synthesis. Consequently in glucocorticoid deficient states, AVP and ANP concentrations are elevated, leading to increased $Na^+$ and water retention thus limiting the degree of hypotension.

## PHYSIOLOGICAL ACTIONS OF MINERALOCORTICOIDS (*see* page 946)

Mineralocorticoids are essential for life. Aldosterone accounts for 90 per cent of circulating mineralocorticoid activity with most of the remaining 10 per cent provided by cortisol. The prime function of aldosterone is to enhance $Na^+$ absorption and $K^+$ excretion across epithelia in order to maintain electrolyte balance and a normal circulating blood volume. Aldosterone acts in a limited number of tissues including the kidney, sweat glands, salivary glands and the colon.

## NORMAL ADRENAL STEROID SECRETION

### Neonatal

Plasma adrenal steroid precursor levels, especially DHEAS, are higher in preterm compared to term infants owing to delayed expression of 3β-HSD activity and the continuing prominence of the fetal zone. Stressed infants have a remarkable capacity to secrete C21 steroids so that 17α-OH-progesterone levels, for example, can be exceedingly high in a sick, preterm infant. This may lead to a spurious diagnosis of congenital adrenal hyperplasia. Care must be taken with the interpretation of C21 steroid concentrations in the newborn especially if less specific immunoassays are performed using non-extracted plasma. Recent studies using repeated blood sampling and the technique of deconvolution analysis indicate that both preterm and term infants secrete cortisol in a pulsatile fashion although a circadian rhythm is not established until at least 3 months after birth.

Plasma concentrations of cortisol rise abruptly following delivery and return to basal levels within 24 hours. It is quite remarkable to note that the cortisol secretion rate in newborns is about 6–8 mg/m²/day which is similar to values recently revised for older children and adults. Plasma renin and aldosterone concentrations are elevated in both preterm and term infants, yet hyponatremia is a common observation in preterm infants. It has been assumed that a maturational delay in the ligand-induced, mineralocorticoid-receptor-mediated transport of $Na^+$ in the renal tubule underlies this metabolic disturbance (*see* page 940).

### Childhood

After infancy, DHEAS concentrations remain low throughout early childhood. Concentrations of DHEAS and androstenedione begin to rise at 7 years of age reaching adult levels in late puberty. The initiation of the rise in adrenal androgens prior to puberty is termed *adrenarche*, although there is seldom clinical evidence of androgenic effect (*see also* page 260). Careful and detailed growth studies have suggested

there may be a mini-growth spurt accompanying these changes. Some children do have early pubic or labial hair growth and signs of increased body odor. Random measurements of DHEAS may show elevated concentrations. The natural course of events is a sequential and consonant development of the other signs of puberty occurring at a normal age.

The onset of adrenarche in association with increased adrenal androgen production occurs in both sexes and is not accompanied by an increase in cortisol secretion. Thus, there has been considerable debate about what is the trophic factor which causes increased steroidogenic activity in the zona reticularis. Suggestions have included prolactin, an unidentified specific adrenal androgen-stimulating hormone of pituitary origin, or an intra-adrenal modulation of steroidogenesis through changes in vascular supply, neural regulation and even an intra-adrenal CRH–ACTH axis. A compelling piece of evidence to suggest that ACTH does play a role comes from the study of patients with *familial glucocorticoid deficiency* due to ACTH resistance. At the expected age of adrenarche, DHEAS as well as cortisol concentrations are extremely low despite markedly increased ACTH concentrations.

## PATHOPHYSIOLOGY OF ADRENAL STEROIDOGENESIS

The complex network of enzymes and their zonal distribution within the adrenal cortex provides the framework for a sequential series of steps to produce the three classes of adrenocortical hormones. Nowhere are endocrine pathophysiologic mechanisms better illustrated than in the family of disorders which result in congenital adrenal hyperplasia (CAH), which comprises, by far, the bulk of adrenal disorders in infancy and childhood. A defect in one enzyme step results in low end product output, the amplification of a classic negative feedback effect, and enhanced trophic stimulation of intermediary products which act as substrates for abnormally increased steroid production. These diseases will be described in some detail as they illustrate well the role of molecular biology in understanding complex pathophysiology.

The pathways of adrenal steroidogenesis are illustrated in Fig. 39.1. Deficiencies in any one of the enzymes involved in steroid biosynthesis can lead to a specific form of CAH. The pathogenesis of each variant has been more clearly understood in recent years through the cloning and identification of the genes encoding these enzymes. Some details are summarized in Table 39.2.

### 21-Hydroxylase deficiency

Absolute or relative deficiency of $P_{450c21}$ enzyme activity accounts for at least 90 per cent of CAH.

TABLE 39.2 Genes and enzymes involved in adrenal steroidogenesis

| ENZYME ACTIVITY | SITE OF ENZYME | GENE LABEL; CHROMOSOME |
|---|---|---|
| Side chain cleavage ($P_{450scc}$) | Mitochondrion | CYP11A; 15 |
| 3β-hydroxysteroid dehydrogenase/isomerase (3β-HSD) | Endoplasmic reticulum | Type I; 1p13 Type II |
| 17α-hydroxylase ($P_{450c17\alpha}$) | Endoplasmic reticulum | CYP17; 10 |
| 21-hydroxylase ($P_{450c21}$) | Endoplasmic reticulum | CYP21; 6p21 CYP21P |
| 11β-hydroxylase ($P_{450c11\beta}$) | Mitochondrion | CYP11B1; 8q21-q22 CYP11B2 |

The clinical presentation is traditionally subdivided into *classical* and *non-classical* CAH. There are two forms of classical CAH: salt-wasting and simple virilizing. The salt-wasting form has a dramatic presentation in the first months of life with life threatening electrolyte disturbances as a result of the combined effects of aldosterone deficiency, competitive inhibition of binding of mineralocorticoids to the Type 1 renal receptor by elevated steroid precursors (progesterone, 17α-OH-progesterone) and the maturational delay in renal tubular Na+ conservation. It is important to understand this when calculating the proportion of glucocorticoid and mineralocorticoid replacement to obtain optimal growth. In the face of high plasma testosterone concentrations, the absence of virilization at birth in affected males is not fully understood. Elevated levels of estradiol and SHBG could modify the effects of increased total testosterone concentrations, which may partly explain the delayed onset of virilization in untreated males.

The simple virilizing form usually presents at birth in females, while presentation is delayed to the second year of life in boys when penile enlargement, growth of pubic hair and increased stature, reflecting persistent androgen hypersecretion, become apparent. The signs are gonadotrophin-independent as shown by the maintenance of prepubertal size testes. The non-classical or truly late-onset form predominates in females with features such as early onset of pubic hair, or after puberty, with hirsutism and symptoms of menstrual dysfunction.

Plasma concentrations of 17α-OH-progesterone are markedly elevated, making this measurement a reliable diagnostic test. The stress response in sick preterm infants can lead to spuriously high concentrations. Progesterone, androstenedione, testosterone and 21-deoxycortisol concentrations also may be elevated. Aldosterone deficiency is indicated indirectly by a marked increase in plasma renin activity. More direct and immediate evidence of salt-wasting is provided by increased urinary Na+ excretion, hyponatremia, hyperkalemia and acidosis.

## Molecular genetics

Genetic linkage studies indicate that the gene encoding $P_{450c21}$ is closely linked with the genes encoding the major histocompatibility complex on the short arm of chromosome 6. Prior to the availability of mutational analysis, the combination of human leukocyte antigen (HLA) haplotyping and amniotic fluid 17α-OH-progesterone measurements was a fairly reliable method for carrier detection and prenatal diagnosis.

There are two $P_{450c21}$ genes located within the HLA class III region on chromosome 6p21.3 (Fig. 39.8). An active gene CYP21 (or CYP21B), and an inactive gene CYP21P (or CYP21A), which are 98 per cent homologous in nucleotide sequence, and are approximately 30 kb apart. They are adjacent to, and in tandem repeat, with two complement C4A and C4B genes. Both CYP genes comprise 10 exons. This region of the genome is highly recombinant. The spectrum of mutations resulting in 21-hydroxylase deficiency can be subdivided into two main categories. Unequal crossing over during meiosis so that there is a 30-kb deletion involving the 3' end of CYP21P, the whole of C4B and the 5' end of CYP21; gene conversion-like exchanges so that a number of mutations which make the CYP21 gene inactive are transferred to its active counterpart, CYP21. Some are macroconversions where several mutations have been transferred from the inactive to the active gene.

The correlation between the type of mutation and whether the clinical variant is salt-wasting, simple virilizing or late-onset (non-classical) is remarkably close for this single gene autosomal recessive disorder. Deficiency of 21-hydroxylase activity is absolute in gene deletions and macroconversions which together make up 15–30 per cent of cases. The clinical phenotype is salt-wasting in each case. Table 39.3 contains a summary of the deleterious mutations which account for the majority of the remaining cases of 21-hydroxylase deficiency. The clinical phenotype is also listed together with the allele frequency. About 20–25 per cent of alleles are associated with a splice site mutation which results from an A or C to G substitution occurring 13 bp before the end of intron 2. Invariably this leads to salt-wasting in homozygotes or compound heterozygotes; however, some patients with this mutation are simple virilizers which may occur as a result of the phenomenon of a leaky splice-site mutation. A

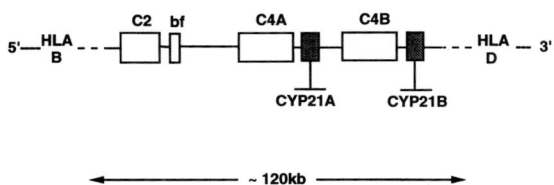

FIGURE 39.8 Location of $P_{450C21}$ genes on chromosome 6. The pseudogene, CYP21A, is also referred to as CYP21P and the active gene, CYP21B, as CYP21.

TABLE 39.3 Mutation type, allele frequency and clinical forms of 21-hydroxylase deficiency

| MUTATION (CYP21) | ALLELE FREQUENCY (%) | CLINICAL STATE |
|---|---|---|
| Gene deletion | 15–20 | SW |
| Gene macroconversions | 8 | SW |
| Intron 2 splice variant | 20–25 | SW (usually) |
| Ile 172 Asn | 20 | SV |
| Val 281 Leu | 6 | NC |
| 8bp deletion | 3–5 | SW |
| Arg 356 Trp | 3 | SV |
| Pro 30 Leu | 2 | NC |
| Cluster (exon 6) | 1 | SW |

Many more mutations of low allele frequency are reported. In about 10 per cent of patients with 21-hydroxylase deficiency, no CYP21 mutation has been identified. SW, salt-wasting; SV, simple virilizing; NC, non-classical.

further 20 per cent of alleles contain an isoleucine to asparagine missense mutation at amino acid position 172 (I172N) encoded in exon 4. The phenotype for this mutation is the simple virilizing form of CAH. The non-classical or late-onset form is associated with a valine to leucine missense mutation (V281L) accounting for 6 per cent of alleles.

Several other missense and nonsense mutations are listed in Table 39.3. These mutations may occur simply or in combination as in compound heterozygotes, or as a cluster in exon 6. How these amino acid changes affect $P_{450C21}$ enzyme function is unclear although predictions can be made on the basis of changes in polarity and hydrophobicity. Mutations associated with salt-wasting exhibit absolutely no enzyme activity; about 1 per cent residual activity appears sufficient to ensure non-salt-wasting (simple virilizing) whereas as much as 50 per cent residual enzyme activity is present in the non-classical variant.

Knowledge of the precise mutation has clear implications for carrier detection, prenatal diagnosis and prediction of the phenotype. However, because more than one mutation may be present, it is important to study the parents to determine how the mutations have segregated and also to ensure that the index case has the mutation expressed on both chromosomes. *De novo* mutations do occur occasionally; this is a further reason to test the parents before a prenatal diagnosis is undertaken.

CAH is unique as an endocrine disorder since it is amenable to treatment before birth. This is given in the form of glucocorticoid (generally dexamethasone) administration to the mother in order to provide transplacental passage of steroids and inhibition of fetal pituitary–adrenal activity. The fetal adrenal cortex synthesizes steroids in early gestation; treatment should start once pregnancy is confirmed with the diagnosis confirmed later by chorionic villus biopsy (around the 10th week of gestation) or amniocentesis (16 weeks). A combination of a karyotype, DNA analysis for $P_{450c21}$, *C4*, *HLA I* and *II* genes, and amniotic

fluid measurements of 17α-OH-progesterone, 21-deoxycortisol, androstenedione and testosterone is used for this purpose. Application of allele-specific polymerase chain reaction techniques can be applied to provide rapid results with a high degree of accuracy for the most common point mutations. Dexamethasone treatment is only continued if the diagnosis is confirmed in a female fetus. Maternal estriol levels are a useful monitor of adequate fetal adrenal suppression (*see* Fig. 39.1).

# 11β-Hydroxylase deficiency

This enzyme deficiency accounts for approximately 5–8 per cent of cases of CAH. The clinical hallmark is virilization which seems to be more profound than in *21-hydroxylase deficiency*. Mineralocorticoid excess due to increased concentrations of deoxycorticosterone (see Fig. 39.3) leads to salt and water retention and the later onset of hypertension. There is a poor correlation between levels of deoxycorticosterone, serum $K^+$ and blood pressure so that the etiology of hypertension in 11β-hydroxylase deficiency is not entirely clear; perhaps metabolites of deoxycorticosterone such as 19-hydroxy derivatives are more potent mineralocorticoids. As with *21-hydroxylase deficiency*, there also is a late-onset form of *11β-hydroxylase deficiency* presenting with signs of adrenarche in late childhood, or hirsutism and menstrual dysfunction in adult females. Blood pressure is usually normal.

The biochemical diagnosis is based on elevated plasma concentrations of 11-deoxycortisol and deoxycortiscosterone, increased urinary excretion of the tetrahydro-metabolites of these precursors, elevated androgen concentrations and suppressed plasma renin activity.

## Molecular genetics

There are two isoenzymes of $P_{450c11β}$, CYP11B1 and CYP11B2, involved in cortisol and aldosterone biosynthesis, respectively. CYP11B1 is highly expressed in the adrenal, is ACTH-regulated, but is unable to convert corticosterone to aldosterone. In contrast, CYP11B2 is expressed at lower levels, is angiotensin II-regulated and possesses 18-hydroxylase and 18-oxidase activities in order to synthesize aldosterone via deoxycorticosterone and corticosterone. The genes for *CYP11B1* and *CYP11B2* are located on chromosome 8q 21-22 approximately 40 kb apart. Each gene contains nine exons and the protein sequences are 93 per cent identical. There is some amino acid sequence homology with $P_{450scc}$, thus grouping these genes together as a sub-group within the cytochrome $P_{450}$ gene superfamily.

A number of mutations have been identified in the *CYP11B1* gene causing classical *11β-hydroxylase deficiency*. The incidence of this enzyme defect is 1 in 6000 in Moroccan Jews in whom nearly all affected alleles have a single mutation (arginine 448 histidine) in exon 8. This alters the heme-binding sequence which is a unique and conserved feature of all cytochrome $P_{450}$ enzymes. Mutations reported in other ethnic groups include nonsense, frameshift and missense mutations. The last group are all in amino acid regions of functional importance and enzyme activity is abolished. Prenatal diagnosis and treatment is possible using similar techniques and management as that described for 21-hydroxylase deficiency.

The $P_{450c11\beta}$ enzyme complex is affected by other mutations which alter aldosterone biosynthesis alone. The final steps in aldosterone biosynthesis are disturbed in two disorders referred to as corticosterone methyloxidase deficiency types I (CMO-I) and II (CMO-II). The biochemistry is characterized by elevated levels of corticosterone in CMO-I and 18-hydroxycorticosterone in CMO-II. The ratio of 18-hydroxycorticosterone to aldosterone is markedly increased in the serum and urine from patients with CMO-II.

Genetic studies so far have identified two separate mutations in the *CYP11B2* gene causing *CMO-I deficiency*. The first, in a consanguineous Amish family, involved a 5-bp deletion in exon 1 which resulted in a frameshift and absent protein synthesis. The second, a point mutation involving exon 7, resulted in substitution of the highly conserved arginine 384 by proline. There is complete loss of 11β- and 18-hydroxylase activities.

In the case of CMO-II deficiency, combined homozygous missense mutations identified as arginine 181 tryptophan and valine 386 alanine have been found in the *CYP11B2* gene of Iranian Jews. The double mutant enzyme needs to be present since individuals who just have either mutation alone, even in the homozygous state, are asymptomatic. It appears that a small amount of 18-oxidase activity is sufficient for normal aldosterone biosynthesis suggesting that milder forms of isolated aldosterone deficiency may exist. The clinical manifestations of CMO-I and CMO-II deficiences vary from severe salt-wasting and circulatory collapse in early infancy to a form characterized by failure to thrive in the older child or virtual asymptomatic features in adulthood.

A unique chimeric gene has now been identified as underlying the pathogenesis of a syndrome associated with excess aldosterone biosynthesis which can be suppressed with glucocorticoid treatment. Hypertension inherited in an autosomal dominant manner is the clinical hallmark. Aldosterone concentrations are moderately elevated, plasma renin activity is suppressed and elevated 18-oxocortisol is the reliable biochemical marker. This steroid, along with 18-hydroxycortisol are 17α-hydroxylated analogs of aldosterone and 18-hydrocorticosterone, respectively. Since 17α-hydroxylation does not occur in the zona glomerulosa, the biochemical profile suggested overexpression of an 18-oxidase type enzyme in the zona fasciculata. The

biochemical changes returned to normal with glucocorticoid suppression, thus suggesting they were ACTH dependent.

Genetic studies in this syndrome show the presence of an additional chimeric gene, linked with the two normal *CYP11B* genes on chromosome 8, which is generated by unequal crossover events (Fig. 39.9). The chimeric gene arises from unequal homologous recombination between exon 2 of the *CYP11B1* gene and exon 4 of the *CYP11B2* (aldosterone synthase) gene. This means that the chimeric gene is under the control of the CYP11B1 (11β-hydroxylase) promoter whose expression is up-regulated and down-regulated by ACTH and glucocorticoid, respectively. This hybrid gene, when expressed in cultured cells, encodes a chimeric enzyme which has sufficient 18-oxidase activity to synthesize aldosterone under the control of ACTH *in vivo*. It is clear, therefore, how glucocorticoid treatment can paradoxically be the potential cure for hypertension in this syndrome. Aldosterone hypersecretion is suppressed and plasma renin activity increases into the normal range.

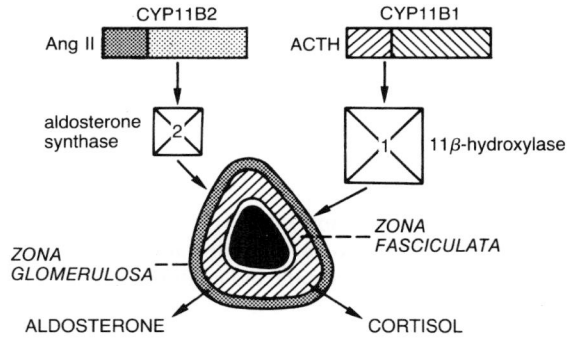

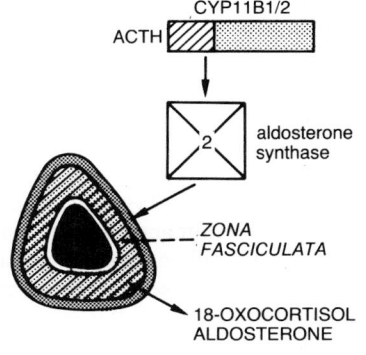

FIGURE 39.9 Diagrammatic representation of the normal functions of *CYP11B1* and *CYP11B2* (top) and the net result of generating a chimeric gene (bottom). The 5′ end of *CYP11B1* (crosshatched) is juxtaposed with the 3′ end of *CYP11B2* (shaded) so that the chimera is under the control of ACTH. This leads to glucocorticoid-suppressible hyperaldosteronism. Ang II, angiotensin II. (From White PC, Curnow KM, Pascoe L. Disorders of steroid 11β-hydroxylase isozymes. *Endocr Rev* 1994; 15: 421. Reproduced by permission of The Endocrine Society, Bethesda.)

# 3β-Hydroxysteroid dehydrogenase deficiency

The 3β-hydroxysteroid dehydrogenase/isomerase (3β-HSD) complex is the only non-$P_{450}$ adrenal enzyme and plays a central role in the production of all three classes of adrenal steroids by its action in transferring a double bond from the B ring to the A ring of the steroid nucleus. The enzyme also is required for gonadal steroidogenesis. The clinical features of *3β-HSD deficiency* are predictable: signs of salt-wasting and hypovolemic shock with hyperkalemia due to glucocorticoid and mineralocorticoid insufficiency; ambiguous genitalia in newborn males due to inadequate fetal testicular testosterone production, while affected females may be mildly virilized as a result of increased production of DHEA. Biochemical indices of 3β-HSD deficiency include elevated plasma concentrations of pregnenolone, 17α-OH-pregnenolone and DHEA. It is useful to express the concentrations of these $\Delta^5$ steroids in relation to their $\Delta^4$ steroid counterparts (progesterone, 17α-OH-progesterone and androstenedione, respectively) especially in the milder forms of 3β-HSD deficiency. The most reliable single diagnostic marker is plasma 17α-OH-pregnenolone.

## Molecular genetics

3β-HSD is expressed not only in the adrenals, gonads and placenta but also in the skin, adipocytes, liver, kidney, lung, brain, prostate and epididymis. Two isoenzymes have been identified in the human. Type I 3β-HSD isoenzyme comprises 372 amino acids and is expressed predominantly in the placenta and peripheral tissues. Type II 3β-HSD shares 93.5 per cent homology with Type I and is the isoenzyme expressed in the adrenals, testis and ovary. The genes encoding 3β-HSD are located on chromosome 1p11-13 and each contain three exons spanning over 8 kb. There is evidence of additional *3β-HSD* genes, which are probably inactive in the human.

Mutations giving rise to *3β-HSD deficiency* have been identified in the *Type II* gene only. They include nonsense, frameshift and missense mutations which, in general, abolish all enzyme activity and consequently are associated with severe salt-wasting. Point mutations can lead to a non-salt losing form when affecting less conserved regions of the gene.

Premature adrenarche in children and hirsutism with menstrual dysfunction in young women are relatively common disorders. Various studies have suggested a proportion of these two clinical disorders are due to mild 3β-HSD deficiency as based on ACTH-stimulated levels of $\Delta^5$-steroid precursors. However, no allelic mutation in either Type I or *Type II 3β-HSD* genes has yet been reported in these two disorders.

# 17α-Hydroxylase deficiency

A single microsomal cytochrome $P_{450C17}$ enzyme catalyses 17α-hydroxylase and 17,20 lyase reactions. Both activities are required for the synthesis of sex steroids whereas only 17α-hydroxylase is needed for cortisol synthesis. The 17,20 lyase activity predominates in the gonads enhanced by the presence of an electron transport protein, cytochrome $b_5$.

Deficiency of 17α-hydroxylase activity is another adrenal cause of hypertension due to ACTH-stimulated increased production of 17-deoxysteroids consequent upon cortisol deficiency. Deoxycorticosterone is the predominant mineralocorticoid leading to a hypokalemic, metabolic alkalosis. Decreased sex hormone production leads to a variable genital phenotype in affected males, while females have normal external genitalia but fail to develop secondary sexual characteristics and menarche. The occasional patient has been reported with either isolated *17α-hydroxylase deficiency* or *isolated 17,20 lyase deficiency*.

A single copy of the human $P_{450c17}$ gene comprising eight exons is located on chromosome 10q 24.3. The protein has 507 amino acids and shares sequence homology with $P_{450c21}$. A range of mutations have been identified in patients with 17α-hydroxylase deficiency. A 4-bp duplication in exon 8 alters the reading frame to create a shortened carboxy-terminal sequence. This was discovered in homozygous form in two unrelated Mennonite families settled in Canada and several families in the Friesland region of the Netherlands where the specific Mennonite religious sect originated. This particular mutation probably reflects a founder effect. Partial enzyme deficiency may result in ambiguous external genitalia in an affected male.

# Congenital lipoid adrenal hyperplasia

*Congenital lipoid adrenal hyperplasia* is a descriptive term for a rare form of CAH associated with massive accumulation of cholesterol and cholesterol esters in the adrenals. The conversion of cholesterol to pregnenolone as the rate-limiting step in the synthesis of all classes of adrenal and gonadal steroids is absent due to an apparent deficiency in cholesterol side-chain cleavage or $P_{450scc}$ activity. No glucocorticoids or mineralocorticoids are produced so that the condition is lethal unless recognized and treated promptly. Since no sex steroids are produced, the phenotype is female regardless of the genotype. Milder cases, which have survived infancy untreated, are recorded. Plasma steroid and urinary metabolite concentrations are low and unresponsive to ACTH stimulation.

## Molecular genetics

A single $P_{450scc}$ gene of nine exons is located on chromosome 15q 23-24 and encodes a mature protein of 482 amino acids. A number of patients with clinical and biochemical features of *lipoid adrenal hyperplasia* have been studied for mutations in the $P_{450scc}$ gene, and none has been found. Furthermore, no mutations were identified in genes encoding adrenodoxin reductase and adrenodoxin, two accessory proteins involved in the transfer of electrons during oxidation of cholesterol to pregnenolone.

This paradox has been partly resolved by the identification of nonsense mutations which lead to premature stop codons in the gene encoding steroidogenic acute regulatory protein (StAR), which appears to mediate the rapid steroidogenic response to ACTH and LH by transporting cholesterol into the mitochondrion. StAR is not expressed in placental tissue. This explains normal placental steroidogenesis in a pregnancy associated with fetal lipoid adrenal hyperplasia. Amniotic fluid progesterone concentrations were almost normal and cord estradiol concentrations were easily detectable. However, products dependent on fetal adrenal steroids as substrate such as estriol, were almost undetectable. Presumably an alternative mechanism exists to transport cholesterol across the mitochondrial membrane in the placenta.

## Other disorders associated with the adrenals

Several other disorders which either involve the control of adrenal steroidogenesis or the mode of steroid action are now better understood as a result of analyses at the molecular level. A few are described briefly as an illustration.

## Familial glucocorticoid deficiency

*Familial glucocorticoid deficiency* is an autosomal recessive disorder of isolated glucocorticoid deficiency with an intact renin–angiotension–aldosterone pathway. Histological examination of the adrenals post mortem shows atrophy of the zona fasciculata and reticularis, with normal preservation of the zona glomerulosa. The cortisol response to ACTH is impaired whereas the normal postural change in aldosterone levels is intact. A number of mutations in the gene encoding for the G-protein-linked ACTH receptor have been described in this condition. However, this does not account for all cases so that a genetic defect at another locus may also give rise to the same phenotype.

A neurodegenerative disease leading predominantly to glucocorticoid deficiency and mainly sparing aldosterone synthesis is *adrenoleukodystrophy* which is X-linked. This has now been ascribed to defects in a perioxisomal membrane transporter gene Xq28 which encodes a protein homologous to the ATP binding cassette family of transporters. The protein is thought to be involved with the activation of the very long chain fatty acid $\omega$ enzyme A synthetase.

## Resistance to glucocorticoids and mineralocorticoids

A number of clinical syndromes are associated with resistance to the action of these hormones.

### Glucocorticoids

Resistance to the action of glucocorticoids is recognized as a rare disorder of hypercortisolism unassociated with features of *Cushing syndrome*. The pathophysiology of this condition illustrates well the negative feedback system involving hypothalamic CRH, pituitary ACTH and adrenal steroidogenesis (Fig. 39.10). ACTH-dependent increase in mineralocorticoid and adrenal androgen production leads to the clinical features characteristic of glucocorticoid resistance. Molecular analysis of the glucocorticoid receptor in this syndrome shows missense mutations affecting the ligand-binding domain of the receptor as well as a splice-site deletion which causes a decrease in glucorticoid receptor numbers. Glucocorticoid resistance cannot be absolute for a receptor which is ubiquitously expressed and involved in such diverse glucocorticoid actions. The effectiveness of dexamethasone treatment is further evidence for partial resistance.

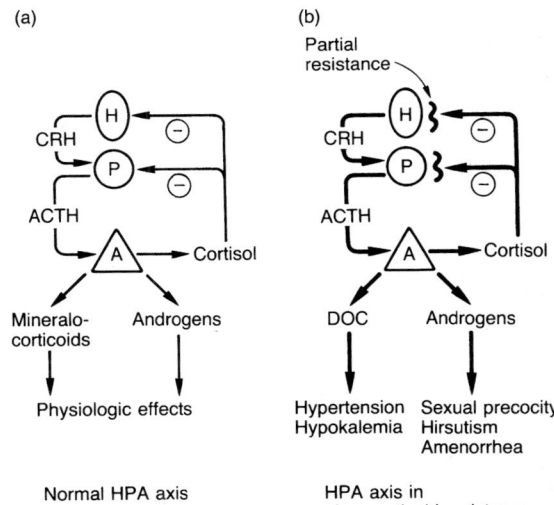

FIGURE 39.10 Hypothalamic–pituitary–adrenal axis in (a) normals and (b) in glucocorticoid resistance. H, hypothalamus; P, pituitary; A, adrenal; DOC, deoxycorticosterone. (From Malchoff CD, Malchoff DM. Glucocorticoid resistance in humans. *TEM* 1995; **6**: 89. Reproduced by permission of Elsevier Science, New York.)

## Mineralocorticoids

The equivalent syndrome associated with mineralocorticoid resistance is *pseudohypoaldosteronism*. This presents in dramatic fashion early in life with profound salt-wasting and circulatory collapse. There is no response to treatment with 9α-fludrocortisone so that replenishment with intravenous saline followed later by a high salt intake is the mainstay of treatment. The tendency to lose salt decreases with time so by 4 years of age salt-wasting is no longer a major clinical problem. Serum concentrations of aldosterone are chronically elevated from activation of the renin–angiotensin system and from elevated $K^+$ concentrations. The disorder displays features consistent with a mineralocorticoid receptor dysfunction. Decreased binding of aldosterone to peripheral mononuclear cells has been demonstrated. The receptor dysfunction appears to affect several target sites including the kidneys, colon, sweat and salivary glands. However, no mutations have been found in the gene encoding for the mineralocorticoid receptor. It is now postulated that the defect may involve some component of the epithelial $Na^+$ channel such as has been described in a subunit of the amiloride-sensitive $Na^+$ channel involved in *Liddle syndrome*.

## Congenital adrenal hypoplasia

This disorder occurs in two separate inherited forms. *Autosomal recessive adrenal hypoplasia* is referred as the miniature form histologically, while an X-linked form is associated with a cytomegalic histological pattern. The genetics of the latter type have now been characterized more fully. The gene has been mapped to a region on chromosome Xp21 based on clinical signs of a contiguous gene deletion syndrome in several patients producing *adrenal hypoplasia congenita* (AHC), *hypogonadotrophic hypogonadism, mental* *retardation, glycerol kinase deficiency* and *Duchenne muscular dystrophy.*

## SELECTED READING

Clark AJL, Weber A. Molecular insights into inherited ACTH resistance syndromes. *TEM* 1994; 5: 209.

Grossman A. Corticotrophin-releasing hormone: basic physiology and clinical applications. In DeGroot LJ, Besser B, Burger HG *et al.*, eds. *Endocrinology*, 3rd edn. Philadelphia: WB Saunders Co., 1995: 341.

Honour JW. The adrenal cortex. In Brook CGD, ed. *Clinical paediatric endocrinology*, 3rd edn. Oxford: Blackwell Science, 1995: 434.

Hughes IA. Congenital adrenal hyperplasia. In Weatherhall D, Ledingham JGG, Warrell DA, eds. *Oxford textbook of medicine*, 3rd edn. Oxford: Oxford University Press 1995.

Komesaroff PA, Funder JW, Fuller PJ. Hormone-nuclear receptor interactions in health and disease. Mineralocorticoid resistance. *Baillière's Clin Endocrinol Metab*. London: Baillière Tindall, 1994; 8: 333.

Lin D, Sugawara T, Strauss III JF *et al*. Role of steroidogenic acute regulatory protein in adrenal and gonadal steroidogenesis. *Science* 1995; 267: 1828.

Malchoff CD, Malchoff DM. Glucocorticoid resistance in humans. *TEM* 1995; 6: 89.

Miller WL. Genetics, diagnosis, and management of 21-hydroxylase deficiency. *J Clin Endocrinol Metab* 1994; 78: 241.

Truss M, Beato M. Steroid hormone receptors: interaction with deoxyribonucleic acid and transcription factors. *Endocr Rev* 1993; 14: 459.

White PC, Curnow KM, Pascoe L. Disorders of steroid 11β-hydroxylase isozymes. *Endocr Rev* 1994; 15: 421.

White PC. Genetic diseases of steroid metabolism. In Litwack G, ed. *Vitamins and hormones. Steroids.* Vol. 49. London: Academic Press, 1994: 131.

Zanaria E, Muscatelli F, Bardoni B *et al*. An unusual member of the nuclear hormone receptor superfamily responsible for X-linked adrenal hypoplasia congenita. *Nature* 1994; 372: 635.

# 40

# Vasopressin and Oxytocin

Peter D. Gluckman

## THE NEUROHYPOPHYSEAL SYSTEM

### Anatomy

The two neurohypophyseal hormones, arginine vasopressin (AVP), or antidiuretic hormone (ADH), and oxytocin (OT) are the secretory products of hypothalamic neurons whose axons terminate in the posterior lobe and secrete directly into the systemic circulation. The cell bodies of these neurons lie within the paraventricular nucleus (PVN) and supraoptic nuclei (SON). Their axons traverse the inner zone of the median eminence to reach the posterior lobe. Also found within the posterior pituitary are glial-like small pituicytes. This direct neurosecretory system is in marked distinction from the hypothalamic control of anterior pituitary secretion (see page 467).

The neurohypophyseal neurons arising in these two nuclei are very large: thus the neurohypophyseal system is often termed the magnocellular system. Both OT and AVP staining neurons are found in both the PVN and SON. While essentially all SON neurons are magnocellular and project to the posterior lobe, there are multiple cell types in the PVN including corticotropin releasing hormone (CRH) neurons and small (parvicellular) AVP containing neurons that project to the median eminence. This subgroup of AVP neurons is believed to function in a manner analogous to other hypothalamic neurons regulating anterior pituitary function. These may costain for CRH and there is good evidence that AVP and CRH both interact in the control of adrenocorticotrophic hormone (ACTH) release, particularly in fetal life. Some AVP-staining neurons also are found in the organum vasculosum of the lamina terminalis (OVLT), one of the circumventricular organs lying outside the blood–brain barrier.

### Biochemistry

In humans, the only two neurohypophyseal hormones are AVP and OT. These are both nonapeptides with cysteines at positions 1 and 6 forming an N-terminal loop by a disulfide bond. Both hormones are synthesized as large prohormones which are transported in neurosecretory granules to the posterior lobe. Final post-translational modification occurs within these granules by proteolytic cleavage to release AVP or OT from the N-terminal. The large (10 kD) other peptide derived from the prohormone is termed a neurophysin. The prohormones for OT and AVP are different. That for AVP is termed propressophysin and gives rise to AVP and neurophysin II; pro-oxyphysin gives rise to OT and neurophysin I. Defects in the propressophysin gene can give rise to autosomal dominant forms of central *diabetes insipidus*. Mutations in both the signal protein and in the neurophysin II portion of the gene are reported. The former will lead to defective packaging in the Golgi and the latter probably leads to defective transport and post-translational processing of the gene product.

### Neurosecretion

There is good evidence that OT and AVP are secreted in response to specific firing patterns of the two respective classes of neurosecretory neurons. The AVP neurons generate action potentials leading to $Ca^{2+}$-dependent exocytosis of the AVP containing granules from the nerve terminals in a manner analogous to neurotransmitter release. Such action potentials are stimulated by hyperosmotic stimuli but the osmoreceptors are at least one synapse removed from the magnocellular neuron. Acetylcholine may be the critical intermediate neurotransmitter, as nicotinic agents directly stimulate and muscarinic agents inhibit, AVP release. This would explain the well known antidiuretic effect of smoking. While the neurophysins are co-released with AVP or OT, their biological significance remains uncertain. Other vasopressinergic neurons project from the PVN to the brainstem and limbic system. Vasopressin has thus been implicated as a neurotransmitter involved in a variety of functions including memory. Vasopressin is also secreted into the cerebrospinal fluid (CSF) from the suprachiasmatic nuclei in a diurnal rhythm – this may provide a wide-ranging cue of the temporal state to the nervous system.

## VASOPRESSIN

## Regulation of secretion

The most important stimulus to AVP release is an increase in plasma osmotic pressure. Osmoreceptors are concentrated in the anterior hypothalamus close to, but not within, the SON. They may be located outside the blood–brain barrier in the OVLT. These osmoreceptors appear to have a critical set point. Below an osmotic threshold of 280 mmol/kg, the secretion of AVP is low, but above this point there is a steep rise in secretion (Fig. 40.1). The sensitivity of this relationship may vary. The system is more sensitive to solutes such as Na$^+$ and mannitol and has little response to glucose and urea. This may reflect the different rate of solute transfer into the cell and thus differential effects on osmoreceptor cell volume. In the *syndrome of inappropriate ADH release* there appears to be a defect in osmoregulatory function.

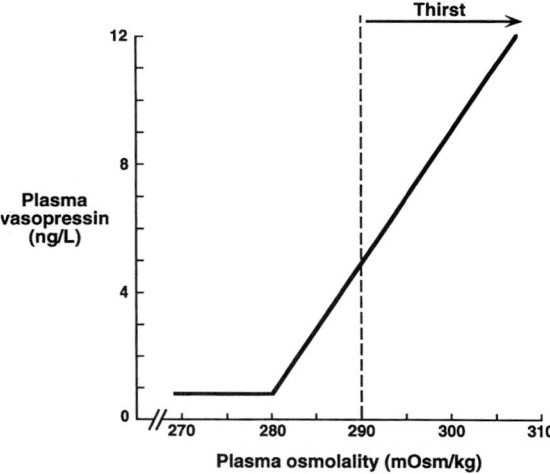

FIGURE 40.1 The relationship between plasma osmolality and plasma AVP concentrations. To convert AVP values to picomoles per liter, divide by 1.1. (Redrawn from Robertson GL, Berl T. Pathophysiology of water metabolism. In Brenner BM, Rector FC. *The kidney.* Philadelphia: WB Saunders Co., 1991: 686. Reprinted with permission from WB Saunders Co.)

Vasopressin release is also affected by changes in blood volume and blood pressure via baroreceptor reflexes. The afferent limb thus passes via the IXth and Xth nerves to the brainstem. The relationship between hypotension and AVP release is not linear, requiring at least a 10 per cent fall in blood pressure before AVP release is enhanced. Any factor which alters blood volume or blood pressure may thus lead to changes in AVP secretion. These include posture, hemorrhage, changes in the renin–aldosterone system, catecholamine release, etc. In addition, the central angiotensin pathway stimulates AVP release. As angiotensin II (AII) is present both in the circumventricular subfornical organ and in the magnocellular nuclei, this neurotransmitter may be an important aspect of the link between peripheral fluid status and AVP release.

Nausea stimulates AVP release by a specific medullary pathway. Stress is also a potent stimulus – whether these effects are primary or mediated by the other mechanisms (e.g. the nausea pathway) or by central catecholaminergic-mediated stimulation of AVP release is not certain.

## Actions of vasopressin

There are three classes of AVP receptor. The V$_{1a}$ receptor is involved in pressor responses and metabolic responses and is found in hepatocytes, glomerular mesangial cells, platelets and vascular smooth muscle cells. Activation of these receptors leads to: contraction of vascular smooth muscle; hepatic glycogenolysis and gluconeogenesis; prostaglandin E$_2$ (PGE$_2$) production by renal collecting duct cells. The V$_{1b}$ receptor is found in the corticotrope and mediates ACTH release in response to AVP. The V$_2$ receptor is found in the collecting ducts of the kidney and mediates the major action of AVP to conserve water. This system is intimately dependent on the countercurrent system of the loop of Henle and the interstitial osmotic gradient of the renal medulla, thus in *primary polydipsia* the efficiency of AVP is reduced (*see* page 957). V$_1$ and V$_2$ receptors are coupled to G-proteins (Fig. 40.2). There is moderate homology between the protein sequences for V$_{1a}$ and V$_2$ receptors which have a molecular weight of 40 kD. The V$_1$ receptor and V$_{1b}$ receptors are both linked to G$_{plc}$ (phospholipase C-coupled G-protein) whereas the V$_2$ receptor is linked to G$_s$. V$_{1a}$ and V$_{1b}$ thus act primarily via the phospholipase C intracellular signaling pathways to induce phosphokinase C and increase intracellular Ca$^{2+}$ levels. V$_2$ acts via the cAMP signaling pathway and protein kinase A.

The gene for the V$_2$ receptor is on the long arm of the X chromosome. A variety of mutations have been described in X-linked *nephrogenic diabetes insipidus*. These include nonsense, missense and frameshift mutations. Alterations in the extracellular domain of the receptor would limit binding of AVP, and alterations in the intracellular domain would affect signal trans-

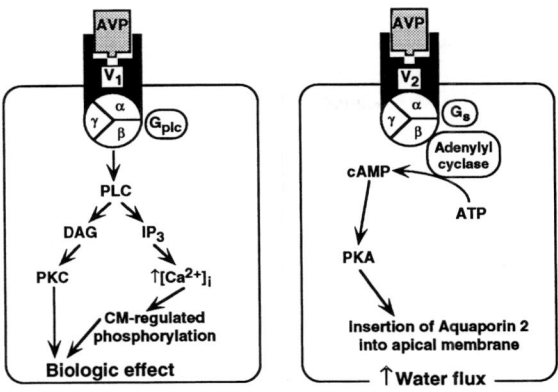

FIGURE 40.2 Second messenger pathways for vasopressin $V_1$ (left) and $V_2$ (right) receptor-mediated intracellular transduction. Abbreviations: CM, calmodulin; PLC, phospholipase C; $G_{plc}$, PLC-coupled G-protein; DAG, 1,2 diacylglycerol; $IP_3$, inositol 1,4,5-triphosphate; $G_s$, adenylyl cyclase stimulatory G-protein; PKA, protein kinase A; PKC, protein kinase C.

duction. Autosomal recessive *nephrogenic diabetes insipidus* is caused by mutations in the aquaporin-2 gene which codes for the AVP-sensitive collecting duct water channel.

Both the $V_1$ and $V_2$ receptors can undergo desensitization. This is most likely due to enhanced receptor mediated endocytosis both in the kidney and in vascular smooth muscle. The major action of AVP is to regulate water permeability in the renal collecting duct, but it also affects the permeability of urea and a number of ions. The effect of AVP on water permeability is restricted to the collecting duct. Activation of the $V_2$ receptor leads to insertion of water channels into the apical membranes of the epithelium of the collecting duct. The collecting duct water channel (also known as aquaporin-2) is a single polypeptide chain protein of 271 amino acids. It is an intrinsic membrane protein with six membrane spanning domains. In the absence of AVP, these water channels remain intracellular in endosomes and AVP, via protein kinase A activation, stimulates their incorporation into the apical surface of collecting duct epithelia. Similarly, AVP has been shown to regulate a urea transporter which has only two transmembrane domains and is expressed only in a more limited region of the collecting duct.

AVP has extrarenal actions which include the stimulation of vascular smooth muscle constriction. This effect appears particularly important in the redistribution of blood flow in the fetal response to asphyxia. This pressor action is mediated by $V_{1a}$ receptors. In the adenohypophysis AVP stimulates ACTH release via actions at the $V_{1b}$ receptor and this appears to be an important aspect of the control of fetal ACTH release late in gestation where it is synergistic with corticotropin releasing factor (*see* page 503).

## Thirst (*see also* page 425)

The related hypothalamic mechanism to preserve osmolality is thirst. This is stimulated by osmoreceptors in the OVLT and neighboring areas. However, they appear to be a distinct population from that involved in AVP regulation. The central AII pathway again appears to be a mediator of the effects of stimulating these osmoreceptors to promote thirst. Satiation of thirst is complex but depends primarily on restoring osmolality. The thirst mechanism is sufficiently powerful that in *diabetes insipidus* hypertonicity will not develop if there is free access to water. If, however, the diabetes insipidus is secondary to a lesion (e.g. *hypothalamic astrocytoma*) impinging on the thirst mechanism, the risk to the individual is severe.

## Regulation of total body water and osmolality (*see also* page 522)

AVP and thirst interact to maintain osmolality. Abnormalities in serum osmolality are more often a consequence of derangements in water balance than in $Na^+$ homeostasis. Normally when osmolality falls below 280 mmol/kg, AVP secretion is minimalized (Fig. 40.1), and the urine is maximally diluted and thirst is suppressed. The ability to excrete free water is such that an adult can ingest 20 L/day without water intoxication. As osmolality increases AVP secretion rises, leading to a reduction in free water clearance and thirst is driven. Thirst is only stimulated above an osmolality of 290 mmol/kg. Thus a standardized water deprivation test is the easiest way of examining the AVP axis. Water deprivation should lead to an increase in AVP once plasma osmolality increases above 280 mmol/kg and urinary osmolality should consequently rise. Failure to increase urinary osmolality may be a reflection of *central diabetes insipidus*, of *nephrogenic diabetes insipidus*, which may be hereditary, usually due to an X-linked defect in $V_2$ receptors, or rarely acquired secondary to certain drugs (e.g. methoxyflurane), or to other electrolyte disturbances (hypercalcemia, hypokalemia) which affect the ability of the renal tubule to respond to AVP. Where renal medullary solute concentrations are reduced, as in *psychogenic polydipsia*, maximal urinary osmolality is also reduced. In *nephrogenic diabetes insipidus*, plasma AVP concentrations will be elevated.

Increases in plasma osmolality are primarily associated with elevations in plasma $Na^+$ which does not cross cell membranes. In *diabetes mellitus* the lack of insulin means that glucose entry is reduced and thus can lead to hyperosmolality. The major causes of hypernatremia are abnormalities of thirst (e.g. *hypothalamic tumors*), excessive fluid loss via the kidney (diabetes insipidus), skin (burns) or gut (diarrhea). Increased solute load, as in *diabetic keto-acidosis* or iatrogenic $Na^+$ loading, can cause hyperosmolality.

Decreases in plasma osmolality can occur if water intake is in excess of the maximal renal excretory capacity (primary polydipsia), or more frequently because the kidney is unable to excrete a maximally dilute urine. This can occur in the *syndrome of inappropriate ADH secretion* where AVP release escapes osmotic control. This may be due to cerebral disorders or ectopic tumor production. Hyponatremia also can be associated with a reduction in $Na^+$ delivery to the renal medulla. This may be associated with either increased or reduced extracellular fluid volume. The former can occur in advanced *heart failure* or *cirrhosis*. The latter may occur with loop diuretic abuse but in pediatrics the most important cause is *adrenal insufficiency* leading to volume depletion, and thus elevated AVP levels, as well as reducing renal $Na^+$ retention. Extrarenal losses of solute via the skin (burns, sweating) or gut can also cause hyponatremia.

## Developmental aspects

The neurohypophyseal system is anatomically mature by the end of the first trimester and AVP is present in the fetal pituitary by 12 weeks. The importance of AVP to fetal cardiovascular hemostasis is reviewed on p. 525. Hypoxemia is a potent stimulus to fetal AVP release and AVP has major effects on the redistribution of fetal blood flow. AVP, while active in the fetal kidney, is less effective because of the reduced medullary osmotic gradient and the low glomerular filtration rate. AVP levels are high immediately after birth. This may be important both to cardiovascular homeostasis during the physiological asphyxia of birth and may also promote fetal lung fluid resorption. While regulatory mechanisms appear fully mature at birth, the ability to maximally concentrate urine is relatively reduced as a consequence of the immaturity in renal medullary osmotic gradient.

In pregnancy, extracellular fluid volume is increased and this is associated with a reduction in plasma osmolality. Despite this, plasma AVP concentrations are normal. Indeed while the regulation of AVP in pregnancy appears normal the set point is different. At any given plasma osmolality, plasma AVP is higher in pregnancy suggesting a resetting of the osmoreceptors. Similarly, thirst is stimulated at a lower plasma osmolality in pregnancy. Late in pregnancy, AVP catabolism is enhanced because of placental vasopressinase. This can lead to *transient diabetes insipidus of pregnancy*.

## OXYTOCIN

## Regulation of secretion

The regulation of OT secretion is coupled tightly to its specific reproductive-related functions. Sucking of the nipple leads, via a neural reflex, to OT release. Similarly, vaginal or cervical distention leads to OT release. The consequent patterns of oxytocinergic neuron firing and thus of OT release differ between these two stimuli. Other factors can impinge on OT release. For example, opioids inhibit OT release, perhaps giving an explanation of how stress can interfere with effective lactation.

## Actions

Oxytocin acts at specific membrane located receptors which are also G-protein linked and which have homology to the AVP receptors. OT receptors in the myometrium are increased late in pregnancy by estrogens. Until labor is imminent the uterus is insensitive to OT. The role of OT in labor appears largely limited to the expulsive phase. There are interactions between the OT system and the prostaglandins (PG). These may increase uterine sensitivity to OT, and OT acts on the decidua to stimulate PG production. There is a rapid decline in uterine OT receptors after birth to reduce uterine sensitivity while maintaining mammary sensitivity. OT receptors in mammary myoepithelial cells are essential to milk ejection. OT receptors are found in other sites, and OT itself is synthesized within other tissues such as the gonads, where a number of possible paracrine roles have been suggested. For example, testicular OT has been suggested to play a role in seminiferous tubule contraction. OT in pharmacological doses can be antidiuretic, leading to water intoxication if used inappropriately in the induction of labor.

## Developmental aspects

OT is present in the fetal pituitary by the end of the first trimester. Its concentrations are markedly elevated in cord blood: the biological significance is unknown.

## SELECTED READING

Carmichael MC, Kumar R. Molecular biology of vasopressin receptors. *Semin Nephrol* 1994; **14**: 341.

Knepper MA, Nielsen S, Chou C-L, Giovanni SR. Mechanism of vasopressin action in the renal collecting duct. *Semin Nephrol* 1994; **14**: 302.

Raymond JR. Hereditary and acquired defects in signaling through the hormone–receptor–G protein complex. *Am J Physiol* 1994; **266**: F163.

Reeves WB, Andreali TE. The posterior pituitary and water metabolism. In Wilson JD, Foster DW, eds. *Williams' textbook of endocrinology*. 8th edn. Philadelphia: WB Saunders, 1992: 311.

Soloff MS, Fuchs A, Fuchs F. Oxytocin receptors and the onset of parturition. In Albrecht E, Pepe G eds. *Perinatal endocrinology*. Ithaca: Perinatology Press, 1985: 289.

# 41

# Neuroendocrine Regulation of Cardiovascular, Fluid and Electrolyte Homeostasis

Harriet S. Iwamoto

## OVERVIEW

Cardiovascular, fluid and electrolyte homeostasis are effectively maintained by precise monitoring and regulation of blood pressure, blood volume and plasma osmolality. A considerable array of central, systemic and local, sensory afferent and efferent mechanisms participate in these functions (Table 41.1). There are four major classes of sensory afferents. These include baroreceptors which monitor arterial blood pressure, cardiopulmonary stretch receptors which monitor blood volume, osmoreceptors that are sensitive to changes in serum tonicity and chemoreceptors which monitor arterial pH and blood gases. Input from these and other sensory mechanisms is integrated in a number of locations in the central nervous system. Output from the central nervous system regulates sympathetic and parasympathetic efferent activity and hormone secretion. The effects of neurohormonal mechanisms are modified by those of local mediators produced in the periphery. The net response is a change in renal function, change in myocardial function and heart rate and a change in vessel caliber. Over 40 substances located in the central nervous system and periphery have been shown to modify one or more of these processes (Table 41.2). Thus, redundancy is a prominent characteristic among mechanisms that regulate cardiovascular and fluid homeostasis. This redundancy helps ensure that blood pressure and volume and plasma osmolality are maintained within narrow limits. Although it is an important feature, one should keep

TABLE 41.1  Basic components of the mechanisms that regulate cardiovascular and fluid and electrolyte homeostasis

| Afferents | Baroreceptors |
|---|---|
| | Volume receptors |
| | Osmoreceptors |
| | Chemoreceptors |
| Central integration | Nucleus of the tractus solitarii |
| | Rostral ventrolateral medulla |
| | Caudal ventrolateral medulla |
| | Nucleus ambiguus |
| | Dorsal motor nucleus of X |
| | Hypothalamus |
| | Circumventricular organs |
| | Cortex and cerebellum |
| Major efferents | Sympathetic nervous system |
| | Parasympathetic nervous system |
| | Arginine vasopressin |
| | Renin–angiotensin system |
| | Atrial natriuretic factor |
| | ACTH, cortisol and opioids |

in mind that redundancy makes it virtually impossible to fully define the entire role for each regulatory mechanism.

TABLE 41.2. Effectors of cardiovascular and fluid and electrolyte homeostasis in the central nervous system and periphery

| | |
|---|---|
| Acetylcholine | Glycine |
| ACTH | Hypoxanthine |
| Adenosine | Insulin |
| Aldosterone | LHRH |
| Angiotensin II | MSH |
| Arginine vasopressin | Motilin |
| Aspartate | Neurotensin |
| Atrial natriuretic peptide | Neurokinin |
| Bombesin | Neuropeptide Y |
| Bradykinin | Nitric oxide |
| Calcitonin | Norepinephrine |
| Calcitonin gene-related peptide | Oxytocin |
| Cholecystokinin | Parathyroid hormone |
| Cortisol | Parathyroid hormone-related peptide |
| Dopamine | Prostaglandins |
| Endorphins | Secretin |
| Endothelin | Serotonin |
| Enkephalins | Somatostatin |
| Epinephrine | Substance P |
| GABA | Thromboxanes |
| Gastrin | TRH |
| Glucagon | VIP |
| Glutamate | |

GABA, γ–amino butyric acid; LHRH, luteinizing hormone-releasing hormone; TRH, thyrotrophin releasing hormone; VIP, vasoactive intestinal peptide.

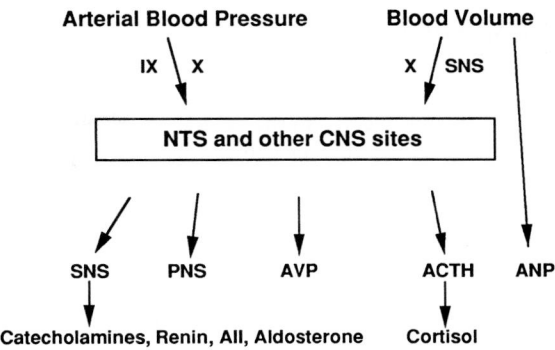

FIGURE 41.1 Regulation of arterial blood pressure and blood volume. IX and X denote afferent transmission of nerve impulses from baroreceptors and volume receptors (via the glossopharyngeal and vagus nerves, respectively) to the nucleus of the tractus solitarius (NTS) and other sites in the central nervous system (CNS). Other abbreviations SNS, sympathetic nervous system; PNS, parasympathetic nervous system; AVP, arginine vasopressin; ACTH, adrenocorticotrophic hormone; ANP, atrial natriuretic peptide; AII, angiotensin II. See text for explanation of the regulatory pathways.

secretion of atrial natriuretic peptide (ANP) decreases. These neurohormonal mechanisms produce increases in heart rate, myocardial contractility, and regional changes in vasomotor tone that restore arterial blood pressure to normal.

# Blood pressure regulation

The basic pathways which regulate cardiovascular, fluid and electrolyte homeostasis are shown in Figs 41.1–41.3. Arterial blood pressure is sensed by arterial baroreceptors located in the aortic arch and carotid sinus (Fig. 41.1). These receptors are activated by stretch and increase their rate of firing when arterial blood pressure increases. Afferent nerve impulses travel from the aortic arch via the vagus nerve and from the carotid sinus via the glossopharyngeal nerve to the nucleus of the tractus solitarius (NTS), located in the medulla. A considerable number of locations in the hypothalamus, midbrain, cortex, cerebellum and brainstem are involved in processing and modulating the primary sensory afferent information. The NTS and other areas relay integrated information to vagal and sympathetic efferent neurons and the hypothalamus. The net response to a decrease in arterial blood pressure is a decrease in parasympathetic activity and increase in sympathetic activity. Secretion of catecholamines, arginine vasopressin (AVP), adrenocorticotrophic hormone (ACTH) and renin increase, while

## Development

Baroreceptor activity has been detected by midgestation in the fetal sheep, in which abrupt increases in arterial blood pressure produce reflex bradycardia mediated by neural mechanisms. Baroreceptor activation also decreases renal nerve sympathetic activity and increases renal excretion of Na⁺. There is disagreement about the maturation of baroreceptors during fetal life. Baroreceptor sensitivity, assessed by heart rate responses to mechanical or pharmacological elevation of arterial blood pressure, has been reported to increase, or not change, throughout the latter half of gestation. Baroreceptor sensitivity, assessed by nerve recordings in the carotid sinus and renal sympathetic nerve, has been reported to decrease during development, being greater in the fetus than in the newborn. Nevertheless, baroreceptor function in the fetus is important for the minute-to-minute regulation of arterial blood pressure and heart rate as baroreceptor denervation greatly increases variability of blood pressure and heart rate. As early as 90 days' gestation in the sheep, electrical stimulation of the hypothalamus produces pressor and heart rate responses that can be inhibited by atropine and adrenergic blockers. Little else is known about central processing pathways and integration during development.

## Blood volume regulation

Blood volume is sensed by primary complex, unencapsulated endings located in the cardiac atria and ventricles and great vessels attached to myelinated fibers in the vagus (Fig. 41.1). Additional afferents in the heart and great vessels carry afferent information via sympathetic afferents. Like the baroreceptors, these receptors are activated by stretch and project to the NTS. Activation of these receptors results in responses similar to activation of baroreceptors which include decreases in AVP, renin, sympathetic activity, decrease in heart rate and contractile force of the myocardium, an increase ANP secretion in sodium and free water clearance by the kidney, and a net decrease in extracellular volume.

### Development

Activation of volume receptors in fetal and newborn sheep demonstrates that volume receptors do not decrease heart rate and renal nerve sympathetic activity or increase urinary $Na^+$ excretion before birth, but do so after birth. However, activation of volume receptors in the fetus increases secretion of ANP and decreases secretion of AVP, renin and cortisol.

## Osmoreceptors

Osmoreceptors are the main mechanisms by which extracellular fluid volume is maintained within narrow limits (Fig. 41.2). Osmoreceptors are sensors located in the anterior wall of the third cerebral ventricle in or near two circumventricular organs, the organum vasculosum of the lamina terminalis and the subfornical organ. These sensors are activated by a 1–2 per cent increase in serum tonicity. Once activated, there is increased c-*fos* gene expression and nerve impulse frequency from the osmoreceptors to the paraventricular (PVN) and supraoptic (SON) nuclei in the hypothalamus which increase AVP and oxytocin secretion from the posterior pituitary. These areas, particularly the subfornical organ, also have an abundance of angiotensin II (AII) receptors. When AII activates these receptors, thirst, AVP and sympathetic nervous system (SNS) activity increase. These responses increase blood volume and blood pressure and return osmolality to normal.

### Development

Osmoreceptors are fairly well-developed during fetal development. An increase in plasma osmolality increases AVP secretion and thirst. Neurons containing AVP are detectable in hypothalamus by 42 days in the sheep, and projections to the anterior and posterior

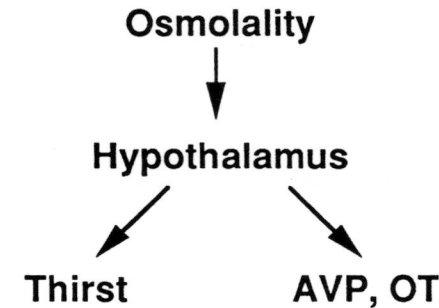

FIGURE 41.2 Regulation of plasma osmolality. An increase in plasma osmolality stimulates osmoreceptors residing in the hypothalamus to increase arginine vasopressin and oxytocin (AVP and OT, respectively) secretion and thirst sensation.

pituitary are abundant by 126 days (term = 145 days). Tyrosine hydroxylase, the rate-limiting enzyme in catecholamine synthesis, is detectable in the hypothalamic anlage at 5 weeks and in the PVN and SON at 28 weeks of gestation in the human. Thus, central integrative control of AVP secretion appears to develop early in gestation.

## Chemoreceptors

Chemoreceptors sense changes in the partial pressures of oxygen ($Po_2$) and carbon dioxide ($Pco_2$) and pH and are important regulators of respiratory ventilation after birth (Fig. 41.3). They are particularly important during intrauterine life when the fetus depends upon appropriate blood flow distribution to the placenta and other vital organs to maintain adequate oxygenation. Chemoreceptors are located in the carotid and aortic bodies and on the ventrolateral surface of the medulla. They send afferent information to the NTS and other central sites via the glossopharyngeal and vagal nerves, respectively. At each stage of development, they have been found to be most sensitive over the normal range of $Po_2$ and $Pco_2$. When arterial $Po_2$ increases abruptly at birth, chemoreceptor sensitivity resets to the higher level over the first 5–10 days after birth. Activation of chemoreceptors causes bradycardia, hypertension, peripheral vasoconstriction mediated by vagal, sympathetic, AVP, ACTH, cortisol, renin and catecholamine mechanisms. Responses to these neurohormonal mediators are modified by the action of locally-produced vasoactive substances which are responsive to local changes in pH and blood gases.

## DEVELOPMENTAL ASPECTS OF HORMONAL EFFERENTS

The discussion in this section is limited to AVP, the renin–angiotensin system, atrial natriuretic peptide

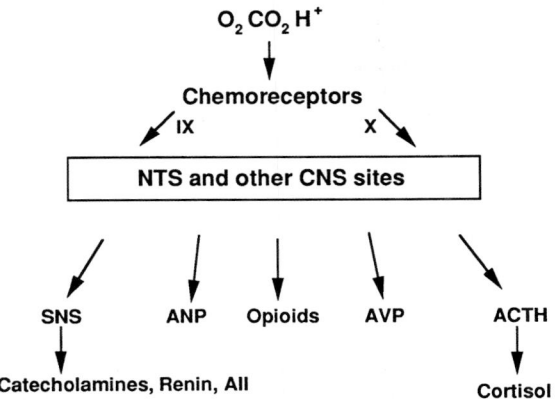

FIGURE 41.3 Chemoreceptor regulatory pathways. A decrease in arterial oxygen tension ($O_2$) and/or an increase in arterial pH or carbon dioxide tension ($CO_2$) stimulates chemoreceptors residing in the carotid and aortic bodies and the ventral surface of the medulla. Signals are processed in the central nervous system and changes in neurohormonal activity result. Abbreviations are as described for Fig. 41.1.

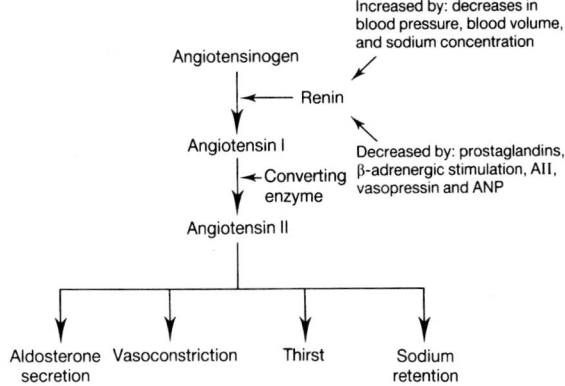

FIGURE 41.4 Basic components of the renin–angiotensin system. See text for details.

(ANP), ACTH and cortisol. Additional mechanisms that affect cardiovascular and fluid and electrolyte homeostasis, i.e. other hormones, neuropeptides, local factors, prostaglandins, and peripheral and central nervous system function, are covered elsewhere (*see* pages 425, 505).

## Renin–angiotensin system

The renin–angiotensin system is generated by a number of components in a cascade of enzymatic reactions (Fig. 41.4). Renin is a highly specific aspartyl protease that converts angiotensinogen, an $\alpha_2$-globulin, to angiotensin I, a decapeptide. Carboxypeptidase converting enzyme or angiotensin converting enzyme (ACE) or kininase II, is a single-chain polypeptide anchored in plasma membranes that cleaves two amino acid residues from angiotensin I to form the octapeptide angiotensin II (AII). AII stimulates zona glomerulosa cells of the adrenal cortex to produce aldosterone. The classic renin–angiotensin system is generated in blood from renin synthesized by juxtaglomerular cells in the kidney, angiotensinogen synthesized by the liver, and converting enzyme residing in endothelial cells, particularly in the lung. Additional, complete systems reside within the brain, kidney, uterus, adrenal, ovary, testes, submaxillary gland, and blood vessels and are believed to act locally near the site of AII generation.

The systemic renin–angiotensin system is regulated by a number of factors. Renin secretion is regulated by the renal baroreceptor, macula densa and the sympathetic nervous system. Renin secretion is increased by small decreases in renal artery pressure, NaCl delivery to the macula densa, and increased $\beta_1$-adrenergic sti-

mulation of juxtaglomerular cells. Renin secretion is also increased by increases in prostaglandin $E_2$ ($PGE_2$) and prostacyclin ($PGI_2$) concentrations, nitric oxide and hypoxia, and decreased by AII, AVP and ANP. Angiotensinogen is available in excess in the adult; however, in pregnant women and preterm and term neonates, renin appears to be available in excess and angiotensinogen, rather than renin, may be rate-limiting. Angiotensinogen secretion is increased by AII, ACTH, estrogens, glucocorticoids, and thyroxin. AII is the primary regulator of aldosterone secretion, but additionally, ACTH stimulates and ANP, high plasma $Na^+$ and low $K^+$ inhibit aldosterone secretion (*see* page 505).

The primary active components of this system are AII and aldosterone. AII is a potent cardiovascular agent that increases blood pressure, heart rate and myocardial contractility. AII mediates some cardiovascular effects through a direct action on the heart (increased $Ca^{2+}$ transport) and blood vessels (vasoconstriction) but also exerts actions via the sympathetic nervous system by facilitating catecholamine release by the adrenal medulla and sympathetic nerve terminals and by activating neural pathways in the central nervous system which increase sympathetic outflow. AII increases extracellular fluid volume by stimulating thirst and aldosterone secretion, and by promoting $Na^+$ reabsorption in the proximal and distal renal tubules. Recently, AII has been shown in a variety of tissues to have potentially important growth-promoting effects mediated by increasing expression of genes and proto-oncogenes (c-*myc*, c-*fos*, c-*jun*) for epidermal growth factor and platelet-derived growth factor. Aldosterone promotes reabsorption of $Na^+$ and secretion of $H^+$ and $K^+$ in the distal renal tubule and alters ion transport in salivary glands, intestine, and sweat glands.

The actions of AII are mediated by at least two specific membrane receptors, AT1 and AT2. AT1 is the most abundant receptor type in the adult and is located in vascular smooth muscle, adrenal and brain. Activation of AT1 receptors activates $G_p$-protein, which increases diacylglycerol and phosphotidylinositol turnover, and $G_i$-protein, which inhibits adenylyl cyclase. AT1 receptors are believed to mediate most of the cardiovascular and fluid actions of AII. Recent evidence suggests that AT1 receptor mechanisms mediate mitogenic responses also. AT1 is widely distributed in the nephrogenic zone and may play a role in nephron growth and development. The second receptor type, AT2 is the most abundant receptor type in the fetus and newborn. They are located in many organs including skeletal muscle, brain, skin, stomach and duodenum, mainly in mesenchymal tissue. They are not coupled to a G-protein and the possibility has been raised that they function as clearance receptors. AT2 is widely distributed and because receptor numbers decrease precipitously after birth, AT2 may be important for cellular differentiation and fetal development.

## Developmental aspects

### Fetus

The renin–angiotensin system is more active during the perinatal period than later in life. Young animals have a superior ability to maintain blood pressure after hemorrhage that is dependent upon intact kidneys, but not intact arterial baroreceptors. In contrast, fetal and neonatal renal responses to aldosterone are less active than in the adult. The components of the renin–angiotensin system in the fetus are derived from fetal sources. Plasma renin activity (PRA), the quantity of angiotensin I generated upon incubation of plasma, is dependent upon renin and angiotensinogen concentrations and is significantly higher and more variable in the fetus than in the adult. Fetal nephrectomy decreases basal levels of PRA and AII concentrations and abolishes responses to furosemide in the fetus, but not in the mother.

The renin–angiotensin–aldosterone system develops early in fetal life. In the human fetus, renin immunoreactivity in the kidney is detectable by 5 weeks of gestation. In fetal rats, renin immunoreactivity and gene expression are initially detectable in the afferent interlobular and arcuate arteries. In the neonate, renin is located only in the afferent arterioles, and by 90 days after birth the amount of renin-specific mRNA decreases and is confined to the juxtaglomerular apparatus. A notable exception occurs in the adult when renin secretion is elevated secondary to converting enzyme inhibition, at which time renin gene expression expands to the arcuate arteries to recruit additional renin-secreting cells. Angiotensinogen immunoreactivity and gene expression are much lower in the fetus than in the newborn and adult.

During the latter portion of gestation in sheep, hemorrhage, hypotension, bilateral carotid occlusion, β-adrenergic stimulation, and hypoxemia stimulate the renin–angiotensin system and increase PRA and AII concentrations. Cortisol inhibits renin release.

Although fetal concentrations of renin and angiotensin exceed those in pregnant and non-pregnant humans or animals, whether the renin–angiotensin system normally regulates fetal cardiovascular function remains undecided. When PRA is elevated slightly, AII in part maintains arterial blood pressure and blood flow to the umbilical–placental circulation. When PRA is low, AII appears to exert little or no cardiovascular effect.

The renin–angiotensin system plays an important role in maintaining cardiovascular homeostasis in response to hemorrhage. Rapid removal of 15–20 per cent of the circulating blood volume produces hypotension and bradycardia, and decreases combined ventricular output and blood flow to the umbilical–placental, peripheral, pulmonary and renal circulations. When AII is inhibited, hemorrhage decreases heart rate, arterial blood pressure, combined ventricular output and blood flow to the umbilical–placental and renal circulations dramatically. Some of these actions may not be direct, but rather mediated via the sympathetic nervous system as AII increases baroreceptor sensitivity in newborn, but not fetal, sheep and may influence sympathetic nerve transmission. AII instilled into cerebral ventricles stimulates thirst, swallowing and AVP secretion. In high doses AII decreases fetal blood volume.

In the fetus, aldosterone responds minimally to AII or ACTH, and has minimal effects on renal function. Aldosterone administration to fetal sheep decreases sodium excretion and the urinary $Na^+/K^+$ ratio, a measure of aldosterone action, but has no effect on $K^+$ excretion. Inhibition of endogenous aldosterone action with spironolactone increases the urinary $Na^+/K^+$ ratio and decreases the fractional excretion of $K^+$. Although these data indicate that aldosterone modifies fetal renal function, the effects are small relative to those in the adult. The possible reasons for the smaller response in the fetus are: (1) fetuses have high concentrations of placental progesterone and deoxycorticosterone that compete for the aldosterone receptor; and (2) the fetal kidney does not retain as great a proportion of filtered $Na^+$ as does the adult kidney (see page 941).

### Neonate

PRA, AII, and aldosterone concentrations increase at birth and fall to low levels within 1 to 3 weeks. The increase at birth is mediated by an increase in renal sympathetic nerve activity and is magnified by prematurity, labor, vaginal delivery, and $Na^+$ depletion. The factors responsible for the increase at birth include stress of labor and delivery, sympathetic stimulation, hypotension, a decrease in metabolic clearance rate, an increase in prostaglandins, low glomerular filtration rate, and renal glomerulotubular imbalance. The increase in PRA may be due in part to an increase in hepatic angiotensinogen gene expression stimulated by the prenatal surge in fetal cortisol secretion, although this is not resolved. The increase in aldosterone concentrations is not related to plasma AII concentrations and may be regulated by another factor such as ACTH.

The renin–angiotensin system appears to be important at birth because captopril, an inhibitor of converting enzyme, reduces arterial blood pressure, glomerular filtration rate and renal blood flow, increases renal vascular resistance, and causes fetal death. Although AII may contribute to the increase in blood pressure that occurs after birth, it does not sustain blood pressure in the infant as basal concentrations decrease while arterial blood pressure remains constant. AII does appear to be important for resetting baroreceptor sensitivity to higher pressures characteristic of the postnatal circulation. Aldosterone increases $Na^+$ reabsorption by the newborn kidney, but overall effectiveness is limited by the relative immaturity of the renal tubule and $Na^+$ transport mechanisms. If aldosterone is not available after birth, plasma $K^+$ and PRA increase. After 2 weeks of aldosterone deprivation, so much $Na^+$ is lost that vasopressin and urine osmolality increase, and hyponatremia, hyperkalemia and acidosis can result. The most common causes of neonatal hypoaldosteronism are associated with adrenogenital syndrome, but isolated disorders of aldosterone synthesis involving the enzymes 18-methyl oxidase I or II, the enzymes involved in converting corticosterone to aldosterone (*see* page 502), may also occur. *Pseudohypoaldosteronism* is a rare salt-losing syndrome of infancy; these infants appear to have defects in the mineralocorticoid receptor.

# Vasopressin

## General

AVP or antidiuretic hormone is synthesized by magnocellular and parvocellular neurons in the SON and PVN, and by parvocellular neurons in the suprachiasmatic nucleus. Magnocellular neurons have nerve endings in the posterior pituitary and release AVP into the blood primarily in response to volume depletion, hypotension, hyperosmolality, AII and stress. Parvocellular neurons project to several areas of the central nervous system, including the NTS. Further details about the biosynthesis and regulation of AVP are provided elsewhere (*see* page 516).

AVP plays important roles in cardiovascular and fluid homeostasis. AVP exerts its actions by interacting with at least three receptor types, $V_{1a}$, $V_{1b}$, and $V_2$. The $V_2$ receptors, located in the collecting duct and thick ascending limb in the kidney, are linked to adenylyl cyclase. Activation of these receptors in the collecting duct increases cAMP generation and promotes aggregation of proteins into water channels in the cell membrane. This permits water to move down its concentration gradient from the tubular lumen to the hypertonic medullary interstitium and decreases free water clearance. Activation of $V_{1a}$ receptors activates $Ca^{2+}$-dependent inositol phosphate turnover which constricts vascular smooth muscle and increases glycogenolysis in hepatocytes. The vasoconstrictor action is not particularly significant under normal conditions, but becomes important when blood volume or blood pressure is reduced or when other regulatory mechanisms are impaired. $V_{1b}$ receptors are located on anterior pituitary cells and influence ACTH secretion by the anterior pituitary. Other actions ascribed to AVP include inhibition of renin secretion, sensitization of baroreceptor input, and increases and decreases in sympathetic nervous activity. The receptor subtypes and intracellular messengers that mediate these responses have not been clearly defined.

## Developmental aspects

### Fetus

AVP is detectable in the human fetal hypothalamus as early as 11 weeks of gestation. Immunocytochemical studies in the human and sheep during the last third of gestation show that AVP-containing neurons in the SON and PVN project a network of fibers of increasing complexity to the posterior and anterior pituitary glands and the median eminence.

Fetal AVP secretion is increased by hyperosmolality, hypovolemia, hypotension, epinephrine, vena caval obstruction, hypoxemia, and acidemia to an extent that increases with gestational age. There is evidence that adenosine is a mediator, the AVP response to hypoxia and that nitric oxide modulates AVP secretion.

Under basal conditions, AVP appears to play little role in circulatory regulation because inhibition of $V_1$ receptors does not alter fetal heart rate, arterial blood pressure or organ blood flow. However, AVP does play an important role in the fetal response to acute intrauterine stress. Producing physiological concentrations of AVP in fetal sheep leads to cardiovascular changes similar to those caused by acute hypoxemia. AVP infusion increases arterial and venous blood pressures and decreases heart rate in a dose-dependent fashion. AVP also decreases blood flow to the intestine and skeletal muscle and increases the proportion of blood flow to the placenta, heart and brain. This redistribution of blood flow accounts for the increases in $O_2$ delivery to the fetus and in fetal blood $O_2$ saturation observed during AVP infusion. Inhibition of $V_1$ receptors in hypoxemic fetuses decreases blood pressure and blood flow to the brain and heart, increases heart rate and blood flow to the placenta and intestine, but does not change blood flow to muscle and bone. However, it is not clear whether these responses are due solely to $V_1$ inhibition or to the local effects of hypoxemia and acidemia. AVP participates in the fetal response to hypotensive hemorrhage by maintaining arterial blood pressure and increasing catecholamine secretion.

AVP also increases ACTH and cortisol secretion through an action in the central nervous system.

### Fluid and Electrolyte Regulation

AVP administration to fetal sheep elicits a prompt decrease in free water clearance and increase in urine osmolality. These responses mediated by activation of $V_2$ receptors. The degree to which urine is maximally concentrated in the fetus is about a quarter that in the adult. This is not related to an inability to respond to AVP but is rather a measure of the low glomerular filtration rate (GFR) and filtration fraction and the shallow medullary interstitial osmotic gradient of the fetal kidney. Low concentrations of AVP increase blood volume, perhaps by increasing precapillary constriction while high concentrations of ANP decrease blood volume by increasing urine flow rate, arterial and venous pressures. AVP influences the acquisition of fluid by the fetus via both placental and extraplacental transfer mechanisms. This is discussed in detail in Chapter 14.

Perinatal AVP treatment has been reported to decrease the number of renal AVP receptors and increase the sensitivity of isolated aortic strips later in life. These effects extend into adult life and support the concept that intrauterine stress may have long-lasting consequences that are mediated by AVP, a concept that should be investigated in more detail.

### Newborn

Plasma AVP concentrations increase after the onset of labor and are greater following vaginal than cesarean delivery. Hypoxemia and acidemia or epinephrine secretion secondary to labor contractions, umbilical cord compression, and head compression may be responsible for the increase. The increase in AVP concentrations may play a role in lung fluid reabsorption at birth, which is necessary for the initiation of breathing and lung gas exchange. AVP infusion has been shown to decrease lung fluid production in late gestation fetal sheep and goats. However, epinephrine is more important in this regard.

At birth, the kidneys assume responsibility for regulating fluid excretion, and total body and extracellular fluid volumes decrease. During the first few days after birth, natriuresis and diuresis normally occur. The extent to which AVP mediates these changes is unknown. AVP, together with epinephrine, may increase hepatic glycogenolysis after birth.

In the newborn, AVP has both pressor and antidiuretic activity. The action of AVP in the newborn does not differ from that in the adult, although maximal responses may be lower due to immaturity of receptors or of ability to activate intracellular response cascades. The increase in plasma AVP concentrations at birth may be responsible, in part, for the increase in arterial blood pressure that occurs at birth. However, plasma concentrations decrease within 2 days after birth, whereas blood pressure continues to rise.

# Atrial natriuretic peptide

The hearts of adult mammals synthesize a substance that produces natriuresis, diuresis, and vasorelaxation and decreases intravascular volume. Although this substance was originally discovered to be synthesized in the cardiac atria, it is also synthesized by other tissues (cardiac ventricles, brain, aortic arch, lung, anterior pituitary, adrenal, thyroid), produces actions in addition to natriuresis, and is a member of a family of peptides. This substance is commonly referred to as atrial natriuretic peptide (ANP, the term used in this section) or atrial natriuretic factor. In the human, plasma ANP is synthesized as preproANP, a 151-amino-acid precursor, which is cleaved to proANP (1–126), the storage (in dense granules) form. The active cardiac form is ANP (99–126), also termed ANP (1–28), which is formed upon secretion. Other natriuretic peptides of this family with biological activity include brain natriuretic peptide (BNP), C-type natriuretic peptide (CNP) urodilatin (ANP 95–126), ANP 31–67, proANP 1–30. Common to most members of this hormone family is a structure that contains a 17-amino-acid loop formed by an intramolecular disulfide linkage.

ANP secretion from the atria is increased by atrial stretch secondary to hypervolemia or tachycardia. ANP is increased also by glucocorticoids, hyperosmolality, hypernatremia, hypoxia, acetylcholine, thyroid hormone, epinephrine, AVP, endothelin and AII. Plasma concentrations are increased considerably prenatally, postnatally, and in pregnancy, three periods when plasma volume is expanded. ANP is also increased in pathological conditions in which ventricular as well as atrial synthesis is increased. This occurs in patients with congenital heart disease in which there is volume loading and congestive heart failure, e.g. patent ductus arteriosus or ventricular septal defect, in systemic hypertension and in human fetuses with immune and nonimmune hydrops, and human fetuses with acidemia and anemia secondary to intrauterine growth retardation.

ANP influences cardiovascular and fluid homeostasis by a variety of direct and indirect mechanisms. Physiological amounts of ANP inhibit ACTH, thyroid hormone, renin, aldosterone and progesterone secretion, and decrease catecholamine synthesis and release from sympathetic nerve terminals. ANP significantly increases sodium chloride excretion by the kidney. ANP dilates afferent renal arterioles and constricts efferent arterioles and opposes AII-induced mesangial cell contraction resulting in increased GFR and filtration fraction. ANP also decreases reabsorption of $Na^+$ in the renal proximal tubule and collecting duct. ANP inhibits renin secretion, AII-mediated aldosterone production, AVP secretion and renal sympathetic nerve activity. Thus, ANP produces diuresis and natriuresis through direct and indirect mechanisms. ANP decreases arterial blood pressure by decreasing blood volume and cardiac output, by relaxing vascular smooth muscle directly, and by opposing the vasoconstrictive effects of other agents. ANP has antiproliferative activity in a number of cell types including vascular smooth muscle, cultured mesangial cells, endothelial cells and astrocytes.

There are two major biochemically and functionally distinct types of receptors, each with a conserved extracellular domain and transmembrane portion. Guanylyl cyclase (GC) receptors, also referred to as R1, type B and type I receptors, have an intracellular domain that activates guanylyl cyclase and thus have cyclic GMP as their second messenger. The GC receptors are classified as GCA or GCB types which have high affinity for ANP or CNP and BNP, respectively. The second type of ANP receptor, C, also known as type R2 and type II receptors, comprise more than 95 per cent of the total receptor population. They bind ANP and BNP with affinities equal to GC; in addition, they also bind ANP fragments with equal affinity. They have been thought of as clearance receptors because they lack a significant intracellular domain. However, recent evidence supports the concept that these receptors possess biological activity in inhibition of adenylyl cyclase and activating phospholipase C and ion channel activity. Thus, there is evidence that cAMP (a decrease) and an increase in phosphotidylinositol turnover and diacylglycerol may be second messengers of ANP. ANP may also exert its actions by decreasing intracellular $Ca^{2+}$ and increasing $K^+$ conductance. Specific receptors have been identified in the kidney, zona glomerulosa of the adrenal, blood vessels, brain, eye, hepatocytes, colon, placenta, anterior pituitary and lung, but their function has not been entirely delineated.

## Developmental aspects

### Fetus

ANP is detectable in cardiac atria and ventricles soon after organogenesis is complete. The concentration of immunoreactive ANP and abundance of ANP specific mRNA is higher in the cardiac ventricles than in the atria. During the neonatal period, ANP content gradually declines in the ventricles and increases in the atria, reaching adult levels by 2 weeks after birth. The significance of this postnatal adjustment is not clear but may be related to an important change in ANP function in the perinatal period. A decrease in right ventricular production following the postnatal decrease in afterload may contribute.

ANP is detectable in fetal blood in concentrations generally greater than those in maternal samples obtained simultaneously or in the non-pregnant adult. ANP clearance and production rates are also greater in the fetus than later in development. The source of ANP in the fetus is primarily myocardial; synthesis is particularly high in the right atrium and ventricle as evidenced by high ANP concentrations in pulmonary arterial blood as compared with carotid arterial and descending aortic blood. Stimuli that increase fetal ANP concentrations include atrial distention, expansion of the blood volume by saline infusion in sheep fetuses, blood transfusion in human fetuses, and blood volume expansion secondary to spontaneous or experimentally-induced hydrops. Fetal ANP also increases in response to hyperosmolality, hypoxemia, endothelin, atrial hypertension secondary to pulmonary artery occlusion, ventilation with $O_2$, and birth. Release of ANP is modified by AVP, cortisol, dexamethasone, catecholamines and the autonomic nervous system.

Specific binding sites for ANP have been identified in fetal blood vessels, brain, lung, adrenal and liver and feto-placental circulation. When ANP is infused at rates that increase plasma concentrations to values observed following volume expansion, ANP has only minimal effects on renal function, arterial blood pressure and heart rate but produces significant increases in blood protein concentration, hematocrit and vascular permeability and decreases in fetal blood volume. ANP in larger amounts increases GFR and urinary excretion of $Na^+$, $K^+$, $Cl^-$, $Ca^{2+}$, and free water. ANP also constricts the umbilical–placental vascular bed and decreases umbilical–placental blood flow and combined ventricular output. BNP also vasoconstricts the placental vasculature, but the physiological consequences are unclear. ANP increases AVP, but not renin, secretion in fetal sheep. Systemic ANP decreases renal blood flow velocity and increases renal vascular resistance by an action attributable not to a direct effect of ANP on the renal vasculature but rather to activation of compensatory vasoconstrictor mechanisms. Presumably these actions are mediated via activation of GC receptors, although there is indirect evidence that C receptors exist in the fetus.

Attempts to determine the role of endogenous ANP during fetal life have been hampered by the absence of a specific inhibitor of ANP action. However, recently endogenous ANP has been neutralized by administration of polyclonal antibodies directed against ANP. Plasma ANP concentrations decreased and remained low following antibody injection. The effects were mostly renal; urine flow rate decreased, as did $Na^+$, $K^+$ and $Cl^-$ excretion, and blood volume increased. There were transient increases in heart rate and arterial blood pressure, probably due to transitory compensation by another cardiovascular regulatory mechanism such as AII. Supraventricular tachycardia (SVT) is associated with abnormalities in fluid and electrolyte distribution. SVT increases ANP secretion postnatally and may contribute to the pathogenesis of non-immune hydrops that develops in fetuses with this syndrome.

### Newborn

At birth, ANP concentrations in plasma increase and remain high for about 10 days. In children with patent ductus arteriosus or other congenital heart diseases with elevated atrial pressures, ANP concentrations remain elevated for an extended period of time. This is probably related to the effects of preload or afterload on right atrial pressure and ANP secretion. ANP may play a role in decreasing pulmonary vascular resistance at birth. In fetal sheep plasma ANP concentrations increase during rhythmic pulmonary ventilation with $O_2$, and intrapulmonary infusion of ANP decreases pulmonary vascular resistance and increases pulmonary blood flow. Further studies are required to determine whether ANP is an important regulator of pulmonary blood flow at birth. Perinatal increases in ANP may also be responsible for the natriuresis that commonly occurs after birth and for the redistribution of body water and electrolytes in the newborn, but further investigation is required to establish this relationship.

## Adrenocortical hormones

Specific details about the biosynthesis, regulation and actions of adrenocortical hormones are discussed in Chapter 39. The effects of ACTH and corticosteroids on cardiovascular and fluid regulation are summarized here. ACTH and corticosteroid concentrations are measurable but low throughout most of fetal life until the last portion of gestation and during labor. Rather early in gestation, plasma concentrations of ACTH and cortisol in the fetus increase in response to hemorrhage, hypotension, hypoxemia, and activation of arterial and atrial baroreceptors and volume receptors but the responses are minimal prior to the last few weeks of gestation.

Cortisol is widely recognized as an important factor in preparing the fetus for birth. In addition to the important effects of cortisol on lung and liver maturation, cortisol also has effects on the cardiovascular system during development. In the adult, glucocorticoids have been shown to be obligatory for the pressor activity of other hormone mechanisms, and there is evidence that cortisol plays such a role in the fetus. Cortisol infusion increases the response of fetal sheep to the pressor actions of AII, but not norepinephrine. Infusion of cortisol within the physiological range for 5 hours, but not apparently for shorter times, increases mean arterial pressure and decreases heart rate and blood volume moderately in fetal sheep. The relative importance of these actions are unclear as heart rate decreases and arterial blood pressure increases with gestational age independently of changes in cortisol concentrations. The marked increase in plasma cortisol concentration at birth may be important for circulatory, metabolic and ventilation changes that occur at birth, as preterm lambs infused with cortisol for 60 hours have these and increased myocardial adenylyl cyclase activity. ACTH appears to mediate the increase in adrenal blood flow in response to acute hypoxemia in the fetal sheep.

More clear-cut are the effects of cortisol on fluid and electrolyte balance in the fetus. Cortisol increases $Na^+$-$K^+$-ATPase activity in the kidney. One study showed that cortisol infusion increased $Na^+$-$Cl^-$ excretion, urine flow rate and GFR while it decreased proximal tubule reabsorption of $Na^+$. Other studies have shown that cortisol increases renal blood flow, GFR, $K^+$ excretion and $Na^+$ reabsorption in the distal tubule and decreases urine flow. Despite subtle differences in experimental results obtained that may be related to differences in study design, it is generally agreed that maturation of renal function is accelerated with corticosteroid treatment.

## Endogenous opioids

Regulation of cardiovascular function is one of the actions ascribed to the opioids in adults. These effects are mediated through specific receptors, μ, κ and δ located in the central nervous system in close proximity to areas which subserve cardiovascular regulatory functions as well as in the periphery. Endogenous opioids appear to participate in circulatory stress responses in the adult because naloxone, when administered to animals in shock, impairs their ability to maintain arterial blood pressure and heart rate.

Different classes of endogenous opioids are present in the fetus. Hormones derived from pro-opiomelanocortin (POMC), β-endorphin, and α-melanocyte stimulating hormone (MSH) have been identified in the anterior pituitary early in the first third of gestation in the human, rhesus monkey, sheep and pig. Derivatives of proenkephalin A, the enkephalins, have been detected in the brain, adrenal, and paraganglia of human fetuses and in the adrenal of the sheep and rhesus monkey. In the human and sheep adrenal medulla, cells stain positively for enkephalin and two enzymes involved in catecholamine synthesis which suggests the possibility of enkephalin and catecholamine cosecretion. However, the importance of this source of opioids is unclear, as adrenalectomy does not significantly alter circulating enkephalins in fetal sheep.

Plasma concentrations of β-endorphin in the fetus are greater than those detected in maternal blood and increase as gestation progresses. β-Endorphin concentrations in the fetus increase in response to acute maternal hypoxemia, large reductions of uterine blood flow and birth. Prolonged intrauterine hypoxemia produces long-lasting changes in the methionine–enkephalin content in certain brain areas in the rabbit.

The effects of endogenous opioids on the developing cardiovascular system have been examined. Administration of morphine to fetal sheep into the peripheral circulation produces a large increase in heart rate and a small increase in arterial blood pressure. Large amounts of α-MSH increases heart rate and blood flow through the ascending aorta and decreases arterial blood pressure in fetal sheep. Methionine–enkephalin injection into fetal sheep produces dose-dependent bradycardia and hypotension that are inhibited with atropine, vagotomy, or ganglionic blockade. β-Endorphin injection produces similar but smaller responses. Central administration of opioids also has effects. Administration of a specific μ-receptor agonist into the cerebral ventricles of fetal sheep produces a large increase in heart rate and a small increase in arterial blood pressure. However, central administration of methionine–enkephalin or β-endorphin elicits no cardiovascular responses but stimulates fetal breathing movements. Several investigators have attempted to define the role of endogenous opioids on fetal cardiovascular function by administering naloxone, a stereospecific opiate antagonist, into fetal sheep. Under basal conditions, naloxone has no effect on resting heart rate or arterial blood pressure which indicates that endogenous opioids have minimal effects on basal cardiovascular function. In fetuses made hypoxemic secondary to maternal hypoxia naloxone decreases heart rate, combined ventricular output and umbilical–placental blood flow markedly which suggests that endogenous opioids improve the ability of the fetus to respond to acute hypoxemia. However, naloxone infusion during umbilical cord compression that results only in hypoxemia has no effect on catecholamine and cardiovascular responses unless the fetuses also become acidemic. In that case, naloxone markedly increases the epinephrine response which suggests that endogenous opioids inhibit the adrenal response to severe stress. Naloxone treatment during uterine artery compression dramatically increases mean arterial pressure and, related to the hypertension, increases blood flow to the brain, heart and adrenals. Taken together, these data suggest a modulatory role of fetal endorphins in the response to acute intrauterine stress but a clear picture has yet to emerge.

## SELECTED READING

Dampney RAL. Functional organization of central pathways regulating the cardiovascular system. *Physiol Rev* 1994; **74**: 323.

Feuillan PP, Millan MA, Aguilera G. Angiotensin-II binding sites in the rat fetus – characterization of receptor subtypes and interaction with guanyl nucleotides. *Regul Peptides* 1993; **44**: 159.

Giussani DA, Spencer JAD, Moore PJ *et al.* Afferent and efferent components of the cardiovascular reflex responses to acute hypoxia in term fetal sheep. *J Physiol* 1993; **461**: 431.

Robillard JE, Guillery EN, Segar JL *et al.* Influence of renal nerves on renal function during development. *Pediatr Nephrol* 1993; **7**: 667.

Robillard JE, Segar JL, Smith FG, Jose PA. Regulation of sodium metabolism and extracellular fluid volume during development. *Clin Perinatol* 1992; **19**: 15.

Smith FG, Sato T, Varille VA, Robillard JE. Atrial natriuretic factor during fetal and postnatal life: a review. *J Dev Physiol* 1989; **12**: 55.

Van Giersbergen PLM, Palkovits M, De Jong W. Involvement of neurotransmitters in the nucleus tractus solitarii in cardiovascular regulation. *Physiol Rev* 1992; **72**: 789.

# 42

# The Adrenal Medulla

James F. Padbury

## EMBRYOLOGY AND DEVELOPMENT

The adrenal medulla is composed of hormone-containing cells and neuronal cells which arise early (8-mm stage in man) in fetal development from neural crest anlage. These neural crest precursors migrate to scattered retroperitoneal locations throughout the abdomen. Primordial neural crest cells are capable of differentiation along primary endocrine (chromaffin) or neuronal (sympathetic) lines. Neuroblastomas arise from these primitive neural crest cells. The chromaffin reaction, a traditional designation, refers to the characteristic appearance of catecholamine containing cells on dichromate staining under light microscopy. The eventual location and local endocrine milieu of these neural crest precursors determines in great measure their final phenotypic expression. Cells residing within the confines of the adrenal and exposed to the high local concentrations of glucocorticoids express the endocrine phenotype and eventually contain high concentrations of epinephrine. Cells located more centrally within the adrenal medulla, and also scattered throughout the medullary tissue, retain neuronal characteristics, are capable of elaborating neurites and do not contain epinephrine.

In the majority of mammalian species, during fetal and early neonatal life there are additional collections of chromaffin-positive cells scattered throughout the retroperitoneum. These extra-adrenal chromaffin cells are unique to early development and involute spontaneously during postnatal life, e.g. by 1 year of age in the human. In some species, e.g. human and rabbit, these cells are discrete glandular structures known as extra-adrenal glands, para-aortic tissue or the organs of Zuckerkandl. The extra-adrenal glands, as distinct from adrenal medullary chromaffin cells, contain high concentrations of norepinephrine but do not express the enzyme phenylethanolamine N-methyltransferase (PNMT) and thus neither synthesize nor contain epinephrine.

## BIOCHEMISTRY

The catecholamines, dopamine (DA), norepinephrine (NE) and epinephrine (E), are synthesized and stored in subcellular organelles known as granules or vesicles. Postganglionic sympathetic neurons, also derived from neural crest, contain small, "dense" noradrenergic vesicles whereas epinephrine-containing adrenal medullary granules are larger and lighter by electron microscopy. The biosynthetic pathway for catecholamines is shown in Fig. 4.4, page 132. Tyrosine hydroxylase is the rate-limiting enzyme in catecholamine biosynthesis. PNMT is the final enzyme in the pathway and catalyzes the conversion of norepinephrine to epinephrine. PNMT is only expressed in adrenal medullary cells and in a few specific nuclei within the brainstem and central nervous system. While adrenal medullary chromaffin cells are differentiated along a final pathway for synthesis and secretion of catecholamines, they also contain other neurotransmitters/neuropeptides. The relative content of each of the other neurotransmitters, neuropeptides, proteins, purines and other molecules from adult bovine tissue is shown in Table 42.1. Thus, while pheochromocytomas, which are chromaffin cell tumors primarily secrete norepinephrine and epinephrine, they may also secrete many other bioactive substances.

During fetal development there are important maturational changes in the relative abundance of the primary catecholamines. PNMT is not expressed until after maturation of the adrenal cortex and production of high local glucocorticoid concentrations. The adrenal epinephrine content is thus a relative marker for maturation and does not become the primary amine until 0.8 gestation in the sheep, 0.7 gestation in the rabbit, 0.8 in the rat. In the human, limited studies suggest that it is comparable to these other species. In contrast, the epinephrine/norepinephrine ratio of extra-adrenal tissue does not exceed 0.1 unless epinephrine synthesis is induced by exogenous glucocorticoid administration.

TABLE 42.1 Relative molecular content in a single chromaffin granule

| CONSTITUENT | CONTENT |
|---|---|
| Total catecholamines (DA, NE, E) | 1000 |
| Purine nucleotides (ATP, adenosine) | 310 |
| $Ca^{2+}$ | 30 |
| Ascorbic acid | 40 |
| Chromogranin A | 1.6 |
| Chromogranin B | 0.03 |
| Total enkephalin (ENK) immunoreactivity | 1.3 |
| Free ENK (penta-, hexa-, hepta-, octapeptides) | 0.09 |
| Neuropeptide Y | 0.1 |
| Dynorphin | 0.003 |
| Neurotensin | 0.0003 |
| Substance P | 0.00015 |
| Dopamine β-hydroxylase | 0.05 |

Adapted from Winkler et al., 1986.

There are relatively few developmental studies of the adrenal medullary content of the other neurotransmitters/peptides. As seen in Table 42.1, proenkephalin derived peptides are the most abundant of the adrenal medullary neuropeptides. In the developing rabbit, the low-molecular-weight (penta-octapeptide) forms of enkephalin represent 40–50 per cent of the total enkephalin immunoreactivity until postnatal life, then the percentage decreases into adulthood when it drops to less than 10 per cent. In sheep, a more precocial species, the low molecular weight pentapeptides increase in relative abundance with advancing gestation. There are no comparable developmental studies in the human. In adults of most species the adrenal medulla and brain striatum contain the highest quantities of enkephalin peptides. The brain content is highly processed (>90 per cent) to the low-molecular-weight forms and the adrenal contains predominantly the prohormone proenkephalin. Interestingly, proenkephalin-derived peptides are colocalized with catecholamines predominantly within cells which express PNMT and contain high quantities of epinephrine. The physiological role of these neuropeptides has not been extensively studied. One of the documented roles of opiate peptides, including enkephalins, is neuromodulation of sympathoadrenal system activity. Opiate receptor blockade during diverse forms of stress, e.g. circulatory shock, hypoglycemia, greatly augments sympathetic neuronal activity and adrenal medullary catecholamine release.

## PHYSIOLOGY

## Intrauterine life

Intrauterine life is characterized by low circulating catecholamine concentrations but a high degree of sympathetic tone. This seeming paradox is explained by a unique adaptation in the fetus. Both intrauterine cate-

cholamine production and clearance rate are two to four-fold higher than in adult animals and humans. Catecholamine clearance represents the integrated summation of reuptake, enzymatic degradation, conjugation and secretion. In most organ systems, reuptake via specific plasma membrane transporters is the predominant mechanism for regulation of extracellular catecholamine concentration. Several plasma membrane transporters have been cloned and sequenced and have been shown to have a high degree of sequence homology. For neurotransmitters like the catecholamines their transporters are expressed predominantly in the central nervous system in nuclei and pathways with dense noradrenergic or dopaminergic innervation. The norepinephrine transporter has recently been shown to be expressed in the placenta with placental reuptake accounting for more than 50 per cent of intrauterine catecholamine turnover. This unique site of expression is vital for maintenance of fetal catecholamine homeostasis and for protection of the fetus from its own high catecholamine production rate. The high intrauterine production and clearance rate also conditions the fetus for the later neonatal period when a sustained high catecholamine production rate is vital to successful transition to postnatal life.

Augmentation of fetal catecholamine release is seen during fetal/neonatal life in response to diverse stimuli including hypoxia, hypoglycemia, hypothermia, hemorrhage, and at the time of labor and delivery. The adrenal medulla is innervated by splanchnic nerves which arise from the celiac ganglion. Immature fetuses, which lack intact splanchnic innervation, cannot activate catecholamine release by the usual neuronal cholinergic-mediated mechanism; however they are able to release catecholamines in response to some direct stimuli like hypoxia. This direct, non-neuronal response results largely in norepinephrine secretion. Later, when splanchnic innervation has been established and epinephrine is the predominant adrenal amine, the response to hypoxia is greater and there is an increase in the proportion of epinephrine released. Splanchnic innervation and acquisition of neuronal control of adrenal epinephrine secretion occurs between 120–125 days' gestation in the fetal sheep (term is about 145 days). Similar findings have been described in neonatal rats where loss of the direct, non-neurogenic response and development of neural control of catecholamine release occurs after the first postnatal week. In calves and foals, development of neural control of catecholamine release and secretion of epinephrine as the predominant amine also occurs postnatally. Humans are presumed to resemble calves more than fetal sheep, with development of splanchnic innervation occurring at, or near, term gestation. However, direct studies in the human are unavailable.

In addition to the absence of glucocorticoid induction of PNMT, extra-adrenal chromaffin tissue differs from adrenal medullary tissue in that it is not innervated by cholinergic neurons. Extra-adrenal secretion is thus solely by direct stimulation. Hypoglycemia and hypoxia both result in depletion of para-aortic norepinephrine content. Thus, this uniquely fetal/neonatal tissue is viewed as a source of catecholamines at a developmental time when dependence on circulating catecholamine concentrations may be greatest and assures the availability of high circulating concentrations of catecholamine during fetal and/or neonatal stress.

Blockade of catecholamine release or of adrenergic receptors in a well, unstressed fetus has little significant effect. In contrast, either receptor blockade or blockade of catecholamine secretion during intrauterine fetal stress (distress) is associated with significant physiological impairment and even death. This observation has been demonstrated most convincingly in animal models but is also recognized increasingly in human fetuses whose mothers had been treated for hypertensive disease with β-receptor blockers. β-Receptor antagonists with some degree of intrinsic agonist activity are not as deleterious for the fetus as non-selective antagonists like propranolol and are thus the drugs of choice for treatment of *maternal hypertension during pregnancy*.

## Role of catecholamine release in the transition to extrauterine life

The immediate transition to extrauterine life is associated with remarkable alterations in a variety of important organ systems. These include:

- closure of fetal vascular shunts and increases in cardiac output and blood pressure;
- the resorption of lung water and the release of pulmonary surfactant to support the onset of effective pulmonary gas exchange;
- the onset of effective central control of breathing;
- important metabolic changes including the mobilization of energy substrates during the early postnatal period.

This time period also is associated with a remarkable increase in the concentrations of several circulating neuroendocrine mediators (catecholamines, angiotensin, vasopressin). For several of these hormones the concentrations associated with this transition period are higher than observed under any other physiological circumstance throughout development and/or life. This is particularly true for catecholamines. Plasma catecholamines begin to rise during the last 2–3 hours of spontaneous labor in the chronically catheterized fetal sheep. Following delivery there is a further, marked increase in circulating catecholamines. The increase in circulating epinephrine and norepinephrine concentrations at birth represents both a generalized increase

in sympathoadrenal system activity and a severance of the placental clearance mechanism. This "surge" in catecholamines at birth has been most carefully investigated in animal models. The precise stimulus for catecholamine release is not clear but probably represents an integrated response to compression, mild asphyxia, vestibular and tactile stimulation, hypothermia and a sudden increase in baroreceptor afferent impulse activity after cord cutting. This results in a sudden, generalized increase in centrally mediated sympathoadrenal activity and adrenal medullary secretion as well as increased postganglionic sympathetic neuronal activity and increased plasma spillover of synaptic norepinephrine.

The increase in sympathoadrenal system activity at birth is vital to successful neonatal adaptation. Adrenergic mechanisms significantly regulate many of the important physiological events at birth including:

- increased myocardial contractility;
- increased peripheral vascular resistance;
- secretion of pulmonary surfactant;
- resorption of lung water;
- onset of non-shivering thermogenesis;
- mobilization of glucose and free fatty acid energy substrates;
- secretion of vasopressin, atrial natriuretic peptide, glucagon and other important hormones.

Abolition of the epinephrine surge at birth following fetal adrenalectomy or blockade of adrenergic receptors severely impairs postnatal cardiovascular, pulmonary, metabolic and endocrine responses.

Thus, fetal and neonatal life are both characterized by unique physiologic adaptations. In the fetus the high catecholamine production rate is modulated by unique placental clearance mechanisms. At birth the exponential increase in circulating catecholamines which occurs is vital to postnatal life. This is unique from older animals and adult humans where circulating catecholamines are accepted merely as a qualitative "index of sympathetic activity."

## SELECTED READING

Lagercrantz H, Marcus, C. Sympathoadrenal mechanisms during development. In Polin RA, Fox WW eds. *Fetal and neonatal physiology*. Vol. I. London: WB Saunders, Harcourt Brace Jovanovich Inc., 1992: 160.

Padbury JF. Functional maturation of the adrenal medulla and peripheral sympathetic nervous system. *Baillière's Clin Endocrinol Metab* 1989; 3: 689.

Winkler H, Apps DK, Fischer-Colbrie R. The molecular function of adrenal chromaffin granules: established facts and unresolved topics. *Neuroscience* 1986; **18**: 261.

# 43

# Calcium, Magnesium and Phosphorus

## REGULATION OF CALCIUM, MAGNESIUM AND PHOSPHATE HOMEOSTASIS

To appreciate the relative importance of $Ca^{2+}$, $Mg^{2+}$ and $PO_4$ in the body it is important to know how much of each is present, and where. Such information is available for the adult only and is shown in a simple form in Table 43.1 to give a sense of perspective. All concentrations are expressed as mmol/L.

## HORMONES OF MINERAL METABOLISM

### Vitamin D

Vitamin D is a secosteroid that plays an important role in the regulation and differentiation of a wide range of tissues. Its principal role is to promote $Ca^{2+}$ and $PO_4$ absorption and facilitate normal bone growth and remodeling. Additional roles consist of:

- Reducing proliferation and promoting differentiation of keratinocytes, hematopoietic cells and intestinal epithelial cells;
- Modulating cardiac contractility and vascular and other smooth muscle tone;
- Inhibition of the growth of certain tumors.

The term vitamin D refers to cholecalciferol (vitamin $D_3$) which is produced in animals and ergocalciferol (vitamin $D_2$) which is synthesized in plants. Only cholecalciferol is produced non-enzymatically in the skin by ultraviolet irradiation of 7-dehydrocholesterol (Fig. 43.1), the last intermediate in the synthesis of cholesterol from acetate. The wavelength (290–320 nm) responsible for photo-oxidation is the same as that causing sunburn. The season, latitude and skin pigmentation are important determinants of vitamin D formation. In excess sunlight, biologically inactive

TABLE 43.1 Representative adult values for normal body content and distribution of divalent cations

| | kg | % BODY WEIGHT | $Ca^{2+}$ (mmol) | % | $PO_4$ (mmol) | % | $Mg^{2+}$ (mmol) | % |
|---|---|---|---|---|---|---|---|---|
| Bone | 7 | 10 | 31 350 | 99.5 | 19 000 | 85 | 600 | 68 |
| Muscle | 32 | 45 | 50 | | 1900 | 9 | 170 | 19 |
| Other | 31 | 45 | 100 | | 1300 | 6 | 112 | 13 |
| Total | 70 | | 31 500 | | 22 200 | | 882 | |

Note: for $Ca^{2+}$ 1 mmol/L = 2 mEq/L = 4 mg/100 ml.

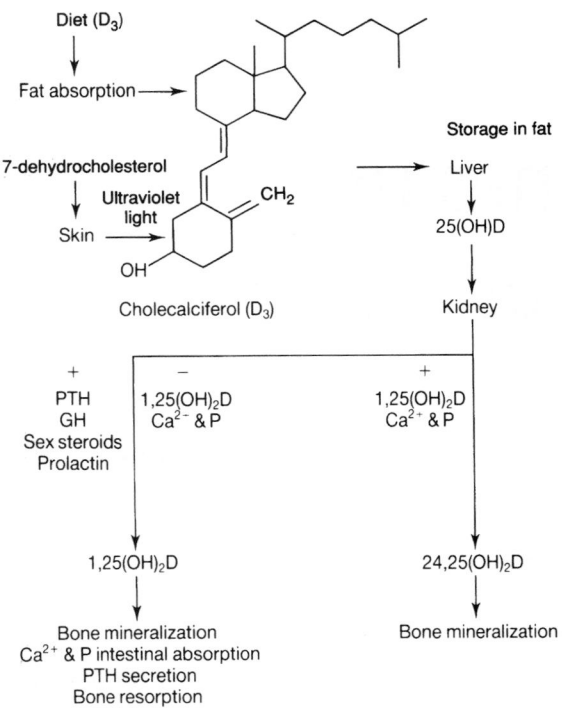

FIGURE 43.1 The major steps in vitamin $D_3$ metabolism and the actions of its metabolites

compounds are synthesized, thus avoiding vitamin D intoxication.

Both forms of vitamin D ($D_2$ and $D_3$) are obtained from the diet, are fat soluble, and are absorbed in the upper intestine with the help of bile salts. The metabolism and biological potency of the two forms are identical in man. Being steroids, the vitamins are transported initially in chylomicrons via the lymphatics. Vitamin D, and all related metabolites in the blood, travel on an $\alpha_2$-globulin of hepatic origin, vitamin D-binding protein (DBP), molecular weight 52 kD. Twenty-five hydroxy (OH) vitamin D (25(OH)D) binds to the DBP with greater avidity than $1,25(OH)_2D$ (see below), thus prolonging the biological half-life of this precursor. DBP synthesis increases during pregnancy and under the influence of oral contraceptives. It is degraded by many different tissues and has a half-life of 1.7 days.

Vitamin D is biologically inactive until it has been hydroxylated (Fig. 43.1). The first step is 25-hydroxylation, which occurs predominantly in hepatic microsomes, but also may take place in the intestine and kidney. 25(OH)D is the major circulating D metabolite (calcidiol) and its concentration is directly proportional to that of vitamin D. The 25-hydroxylation step is high capacity, but the next hydroxylation, which occurs predominantly in the mitochondria of the proximal renal tubule to produce 1,25-dihydroxy-vitamin D[$1,25(OH)_2D$], the active D metabolite (calcitriol), is low capacity and tightly regulated. A

defect in the responsible enzyme, 1-hydroxylase, leads to *vitamin D-dependent rickets type I*, which is usually autosomally recessive. When adequate amounts of circulating $1,25(OH)_2D$ are present 25(OH)D is hydroxylated in the kidney, by 24-hydroxylase, to $24,25(OH)_2D$ which has little or no biological activity. Renal 1-hydroxylation is favored by low circulating concentrations of $Ca^{2+}$, $PO_4$ and 25(OH)D, and by high levels of parathyroid hormone (PTH). When these conditions are reversed, 1-hydroxylase activity diminishes and that of 24-hydroxylase predominates.

Placenta, bone cells and granulomatous tissues can also synthesize $1,25(OH)_2D$. During growth, pregnancy and lactation the 1-hydroxylase is stimulated and more $1,25(OH)_2D$ produced. Normal serum concentrations of 25(OH)D vary with diet and exposure to sunlight, but the concentration of $1,25(OH)_2D$ is not so affected. The average serum concentration of $1,25(OH)_2D$ is about one-thousandth that of 25(OH)D, although the affinity of $1,25(OH)_2D$ for the vitamin D receptor is about 1000-fold greater than that of 25(OH)D. The half-life of circulating $1,25(OH)_2D$ is measured in hours and of 25(OH)D in days. Degradation of $1,25(OH)_2D$ takes place in the liver with biologically inactive metabolites excreted in bile.

The primary action of $1,25(OH)_2D$ in mineral metabolism is to promote $Ca^{2+}$ and $PO_4$ absorption from the intestinal mucosa, thereby providing minerals for incorporation into bone matrix. Although $1,25(OH)_2D$ influences a range of osteoblast-related functions (e.g. modulation of alkaline phosphatase function and increased osteocalcin synthesis), it does not directly influence new bone formation. In general, $1,25(OH)_2D$ reacts with a specific cytosolic receptor, a member of the steroid receptor supergene family (*see* page 464), which is translocated to the nucleus where it regulates gene expression. In *vitamin D-dependent rickets type II* the defect apparently is at this level as plasma $1,25(OH)_2D$ concentrations are elevated. Activation of the vitamin D receptor initiates the synthesis of certain proteins, such as the 8.6-kD $Ca^{2+}$-binding protein (calbindin D), which appears to promote $Ca^{2+}$ transport from the intestinal mucosa into the portal circulation. The role of $1,25(OH)_2D$ in bone remodeling is shown by the opposing effects of facilitating mineralization and increasing osteoclast production.

The $1,25(OH)_2D$ receptor is present in a wide range of cells and may have important actions independent of mineral metabolism. The spectrum of action of vitamin D includes regulation of proliferation, initiation of differentiation, and of hormone secretion from endocrine cells. For example, there are $1,25(OH)_2D$ receptors in the brain and on the pancreatic $\beta$ cell. Immunoregulation and the differentiation of a variety of hematopoietic cells, including monocytes, may involve $1,25(OH)_2D$. The relative importance of these different actions to whole body physiology remains unclear; however, it is conceivable that vitamin D may play a role in hematopoietic disorders and malignancies.

The most prominent influence on $1,25(OH)_2D$ formation is that of PTH. A fall in extracellular $Ca^{2+}$ causes PTH stimulation, which in turn activates the 1-hydroxylase enzyme. An important autoregulatory role is played by $1,25(OH)_2D$, which increases accumulation of 7-dehydrocholesterol in skin, inhibits PTH secretion, hepatic vitamin D 25-hydroxylase and renal 25(OH)D-1-hydroxylase and induces renal 25(OH)D-24-hydroxylase. These are coarse control mechanisms, fine control being in regulation of $1,25(OH)_2D$ receptors on the target cells. Receptors are increased by estradiol and decreased by glucocorticoids. If PTH is seen as the primary link in a simple feedback loop involving $1,25(OH)_2D$ and $Ca^{2+}$, the role of other putative 1-hydroxylase regulators becomes secondary.

*Vitamin D deficiency* remains a clinical problem even in affluent societies. This may be due to either (1) inadequate sunlight exposure in pigmented children with a diet low in vitamin D (e.g. strict vegetarians) or (2) to a low $Ca^{2+}$ intake, possibly related to dietary phytate and fiber. This leads to mild *secondary hyperparathyroidism* and increased production of $1,25(OH)_2D$, which accelerates 25(OH)D metabolism into inactive metabolites. The latter mechanism is responsible for vitamin D deficiency in a variety of conditions characterized by *hyperparathyroidism* or $Ca^{2+}$ malabsorption such as gastrointestinal and chronic liver disease. *Hypervitaminosis D* results from excess vitamin D intake, resulting in elevated 25(OH)D, but normal $1,25(OH)_2D$. In these circumstances the 25(OH)D exerts a pharmacological action and causes hypercalcemia, with soft tissue calcification, vomiting and diarrhea.

## Parathyroid hormone (PTH)

PTH controls the extracellular fluid (ECF) $Ca^{2+}$ concentration by actions on the transfer of $Ca^{2+}$ from bone, glomerular filtrate and intestine to ECF. PTH is made in the chief cells of the four parathyroid glands. The parathyroid glands are derived from endoderm, the lower pair from the third branchial pouch in close association with the thymus and the upper pair from the fourth pouch. The latter pair remain stationary to end up dorsolateral to the thyroid at the isthmus level. *DiGeorge syndrome*, an embryonic failure of the third and fourth pouches, causes thymic and parathyroid hypoplasia and cardiovascular defects.

PTH is a 9.5 kD single polypeptide of 84 amino acids. Full biological activity lies in the 34 amino acids at the amino-terminus. The PTH gene is on the short arm of chromosome 11, very close to the insulin gene. PTH is produced from a 110-amino-acid precursor, preproPTH, by two sequential enzymatic cleavages during transport of the nascent peptide into the cisternal space of the endoplasmic reticulum and

packaging into granules in the Golgi apparatus. Multiple forms of PTH are found in the circulation but the biologically active molecule is exclusively PTH (1–84). PTH is inactivated by cleavage between amino acids 33–43 by cathepsin-like enzymes found in the parathyroid glands, liver and kidney.

Two major mechanisms control PTH secretion: extracellular $Ca^{2+}$ concentration and cAMP, of which $Ca^{2+}$ is the more important. Secretion increases as extracellular $Ca^{2+}$ falls and vice versa. ECF $Ca^{2+}$ concentration is monitored by a parathyroid cell surface $Ca^{2+}$ receptor, mutations of which recently have been identified. Subjects who are heterozygous for such mutations manifest *familial hypocalciuric hypercalcemia* (an asymptomatic condition in which subjects manifest mild hypercalcemia but require no intervention), whereas those who are homozygous for the mutation present with severe *neonatal hyperparathyroidism*. The close link between extracellular and intracellular $Ca^{2+}$ is shown by the fact that $Ca^{2+}$ agonists are potent inhibitors of secretion and $Ca^{2+}$ channel blockers interfere with secretory control mechanisms. $Mg^{2+}$ has a dual effect: hypermagnesemia is inhibitory but less potently so than increased $Ca^{2+}$, but profound hypomagnesemia can also block PTH release. Stimulants of the adenylyl cyclase–cAMP system cause PTH release. These include β-adrenergic agents, secretin, dopamine and E prostaglandins. Conversely prostaglandin F and α-adrenergic catecholamines are inhibitory.

Hyperparathyroidism in childhood is usually inherited. Three forms are recognized: *autosomal recessive parathyroid hyperplasia, autosomal dominant benign hypocalciuric hypercalcemia,* and *autosomal dominant hyperparathyroidism with hypercalciuria. Autosomal recessive parathyroid hyperplasia* begins before birth and there is marked hypercalcemia in the neonatal period resulting in anorexia, vomiting, constipation, renal insufficiency and hypertension, leading to death within months unless the diagnosis is made and appropriate action taken. In contrast, *autosomal dominant benign hypocalciuric hypercalcemia* is usually asymptomatic and detected accidentally as a result of measuring serum $Ca^{2+}$ for another reason, or by family studies after identification of a proband. *Autosomal dominant hyperparathyroidism* with hypercalciuria is characterized by symptoms that are likely to relate to renal stones or kidney failure. Investigation reveals hypercalcemia and hyperparathyroidism in the propositus and family members. Genetically determined hyperparathyroidism may also occur as part of *multiple endocrine (MEN) types I or II. Humoral hypercalcemia of malignancy (HHM)* must be distinguished from hyperparathyroidism with which it shares many clinical features. HHM is characterized by a low plasma $Cl^-$ and $1,25(OH)_2D$, hypokalemia and an equivocally raised plasma immunoreactive PTH concentration. The actual hormone inducing the hypercalcemia is not PTH itself but a PTH-related protein. There are several of these which are produced by alternate splicing of a gene related to the PTH gene. Solid tumors may produce other stimulants of bone resorption such as TGFα.

*Hypoparathyroidism* may be due to inadequate release of PTH or resistance to PTH. Inadequate release may be permanent or transient as in neonatal hypoparathyroidism. If permanent it may be congenital as in *DiGeorge syndrome* or acquired as in autoimmune or idiopathic hypoparathyroidism. Activation of the PTH receptor initiates the adenylyl cyclase/cAMP cascade via a guanine nucleotide regulatory (coupling) protein $G_s$. Resistance to PTH is found in *pseudohypoparathyroidism types I and II*. The molecular defect in pseudohypoparathyroidism type Ia is a deficiency of the α-subunit of $G_s$. In type Ib, the abnormality in the receptor has not been defined but PTH cannot induce cAMP production. In pseudohypoparathyroidism type II, PTH can induce cAMP production, but there is a more distal end-organ resistance.

# Calcitonin

Calcitonin is a 32-amino-acid peptide made by the parafollicular, or C-cells, of the thyroid gland. The C-cells arise embryologically from the fifth branchial pouch and produce the ultimobranchial body which becomes incorporated into the parafollicular interstices of the thyroid. Biological activity of calcitonin depends on the integrity of the molecule. The calcitonin/calcitonin gene-related peptide (CGRP) gene is located on chromosome 11, as is the gene for PTH, and consists of six exons separated by five introns. Coding for calcitonin involves four of the six exons. Another protein, CGRP is expressed by five of the six exons by alternate splicing and is found predominantly in the central nervous system where its physiological significance is uncertain. CGRP is a vasodilator and may play a part in autoregulation of the cerebral and other vasculatures. Expression of the calcitonin gene in the C-cell results in the synthesis of a large precursor polypeptide which is then cleaved to yield three peptides: N-terminal peptide, calcitonin and carboxy-terminal peptide.

Calcitonin secretion, like that of PTH, is controlled by intracellular $Ca^{2+}$ and cAMP. A rise in extracellular $Ca^{2+}$ concentration causes an increase in C-cell calcitonin secretion. The adenylyl cyclase–cAMP system is activated by a number of intestinal hormones including gastrin, cholecystokinin and glucagon. These may play a part in damping potential postprandial surges of $Ca^{2+}$. Calcitonin receptors are found on osteoclasts, and in the medullary ascending thick limb of the nephron. Calcitonin causes hypocalcemia primarily by inhibition of osteoclast activity in bone and by blocking the action of PTH. These actions may be mediated by blocking cAMP. Associated with this are a reduction of alkaline phosphatase and pyrophosphatase activity and inhibition of hydroxyproline produc-

tion. Hypophosphatemia occurs as a result of increased $PO_4$ entry into bone and phosphaturia.

## CALCIUM ($Ca^{2+}$)

The rate of skeletal mineralization approximates the rate of skeletal growth, with the most rapid periods of mineralization occurring during infancy and puberty. Skeletal mass doubles during the first year of life. During adolescence, about 35 per cent of adult skeletal mass is achieved. Bone mineral density of the lumbar spine, an index of trabecular bone, doubles between 1 and 15 years of age.

$Ca^{2+}$ is the most abundant electrolyte in the body. Ninety-nine per cent of skeletal $Ca^{2+}$ is unavailable for immediate homeostasis and only 0.1 per cent total body $Ca^{2+}$ is in the plasma and extravascular fluid. Ionized $Ca^{2+}$, both in the plasma and in the cytosol, plays a central part in regulation of cellular activity, being involved in muscle contraction, nerve conduction, initiation of mitosis and microtubular contraction, as well as enzyme action. Among circulating ions $Ca^{2+}$ is the second most tightly controlled after $Na^+$. The normal plasma $Ca^{2+}$ concentration in children and adults is 2.2–2.6 mmol/L. Approximately 40 per cent is bound to protein. Of the protein-bound $Ca^{2+}$, 60–90 per cent is associated with albumin and the remainder with globulins. $Ca^{2+}$ binding to albumin is strongly pH dependent, being inversely proportional to the $H^+$ concentration. Non-protein-bound $Ca^{2+}$ is a mixture of low molecular weight $Ca^{2+}$ complexes and ionized $Ca^{2+}$. The major fraction of the ultrafilterable $Ca^{2+}$ is ionized and represents about 45–50 per cent of the total $Ca^{2+}$ in normal individuals. $Ca^{2+}$ in other extracellular fluids is technically difficult to measure. There is no reason to assume that the concentration of $Ca^{2+}$ in the interstitial fluid of different organs reflects the circulating $Ca^{2+}$ concentration. There is evidence that local tissue $Ca^{2+}$ kinetics have an important influence.

Osteoblasts are important regulators of bone mineralization (see Chapter 44) and promote $Ca^{2+}$ and $PO_4$ precipitation first in an amorphous form and then as hydroxyapatite crystals. Crystals grow *in vivo* in a similar manner to their behavior in a homogeneous salt solution, by nucleation and surface apposition. Bone matrix collagen has a staggered orientation that may provide nucleation sites and a bone-specific phosphorylated collagen $α_2$-chain has been identified. Bone contains other proteins which have a high affinity for both collagen and apatite, the most avid being osteonectin, which has the capacity to initiate mineralization on type I collagen fibers. Bone also contains a number of molecules that may inhibit mineralization. These include glycosaminoglycans, proteoglycans and pyrophosphate, but the most common, making up 1–2 per cent bone protein, is osteocalcin. Osteocalcin is synthesized and secreted by osteoblasts under the action of $1,25(OH)_2D$. It appears after mineralization and binds to, and stabilizes, apatite crystals. Genetic defects resulting in abnormal collagen formation are responsible for diseases such as *osteogenesis imperfecta* and *Ehlers–Danlos syndrome* (*see* page 561).

## Calcium homeostasis

The major sites of Ca$^{2+}$ transport into and out of the body are the intestinal tract, the kidneys and to a lesser extent the sweat glands. In the healthy adult, renal Ca$^{2+}$ excretion equals net intestinal Ca$^{2+}$ absorption, but in the growing child there is a net Ca$^{2+}$ accumulation by bone. In the adult about 20 mmol Ca$^{2+}$ are ingested each day, the richest source being dairy products. Some plant products (e.g. spinach) have a significant Ca$^{2+}$ content, but the bioavailability of this Ca$^{2+}$ may be lower because of the presence of complexing anions such as oxalate and (in cereals) phytate. Only about 30 per cent is absorbed and 15 per cent secreted into the intestinal lumen, resulting in a net fecal loss of 80 per cent. The other 20 per cent are excreted in the urine. A schematic summary of Ca$^{2+}$ balance is shown in Fig. 43.2. The fractional Ca$^{2+}$ absorption increases as the absolute amount of Ca$^{2+}$ ingested decreases; a net positive Ca$^{2+}$ balance can be maintained with a Ca$^{2+}$ intake as low as 5 mmol/day. Fractional Ca$^{2+}$ absorption is greater in childhood and adolescence than in adulthood, and also is increased during pregnancy and lactation.

Ca$^{2+}$ absorption takes place in all parts of the small intestine distal to the pylorus, and is fastest in the duodenum and jejunum. Ca$^{2+}$ transport is both passive (paracellular) and active (transcellular). The majority of passive Ca$^{2+}$ movement is controlled largely by solvent drag and electrochemical potential differences. Active Ca$^{2+}$ transport varies with both the structure and function of the intestinal and renal epithelium. Active and passive Ca$^{2+}$ transport appear to contribute almost equally to total Ca$^{2+}$ absorption in adults consuming a Western diet; however, at low intakes active absorption will predominate and this route may be the more important in fine tuning whole body homeostasis. The most important regulator of Ca$^{2+}$ uptake by the intestine is 1,25(OH)$_2$D, which is operative from the early neonatal period. The mechanisms of Ca$^{2+}$ transfer to the fetus are discussed on page 540.

The ionized and complexed fractions of plasma Ca$^{2+}$ are filtered at the glomerulus, amounting to approximately 250 mmol/day in adults. Ninety-eight per cent is reabsorbed, two-thirds in the proximal tubule and the remainder along the length of the nephron; proximal tubular reabsorption is an active process closely linked to that of Na$^+$. About 10 per cent of Ca$^{2+}$ reabsorption takes place in the distal nephron and is subject to regulation by PTH. Acidosis and sodium loading promote Ca$^{2+}$ excretion

whereas thiazide diuretics and alkalosis have the opposite effect.

Inhibitors of Ca$^{2+}$ uptake include cellulose, PO$_4$, phytates, anticonvulsants and glucocorticoids. Cellulose and phytate bind Ca$^{2+}$ in the lumen, whereas anticonvulsants interfere with vitamin D metabolism as well as having, together with glucocorticoids, a direct effect on the intestinal epithelial transport mechanism. The pool of circulating Ca$^{2+}$ in the adult is approximately 25 mmol, but when Ca$^{2+}$ is injected, it rapidly equilibrates with a much larger mass, the central miscible pool. Analyses of Ca$^{2+}$ kinetics by pool modeling tend to lack physiological application and only the simplest model is of direct clinical relevance (Fig. 43.2).

Intracellular Ca$^{2+}$ concentrations vary from 0.02 mmol/kg cell water in cells with no organelles, such as erythrocytes, to 510 mmol/kg cell water in muscle. In contrast to extracellular Ca$^{2+}$, intracellular Ca$^{2+}$ is 99.9 per cent bound to a large number of specific binding proteins mainly within the nucleus, mitochondria, endoplasmic reticulum and other special vesicles. The cytosolic concentration is about 10 mmol/L, of which only about 0.1 mmol/L is ionized. This is achieved partly by active transport into the intracellular organelles, but more importantly by energy-dependent pumping of Ca$^{2+}$ out of the cell. Three mechanisms are important: a Ca$^{2+}$–Mg$^{2+}$–ATPase, a Na$^+$–Ca$^{2+}$ pump, and a Ca$^{2+}$–H$^+$ pump. The Ca$^{2+}$–Mg$^{2+}$–ATPase is the principal pump at rest, and the Na$^+$–Ca$^{2+}$ pump operates during cell activity or injury.

*Hypocalcemia* occurs commonly as a transient phenomenon in the newborn, particularly in the premature, the infant of a diabetic mother, or the asphyxiated baby. Hypocalcemia may also occur

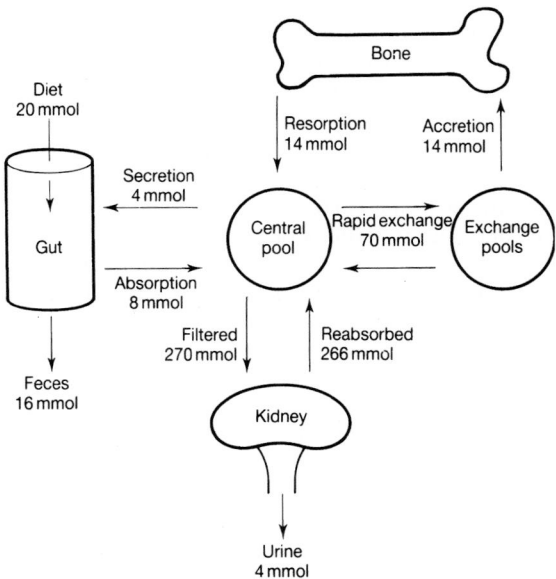

FIGURE 43.2 Calcium balance in a normal 70-kg man

toward the end of the first week of life in infants fed cows' milk with a high $PO_4$ content. In older children the commonest association with hypocalcemia is hypoalbuminemia. In these circumstances the ionized $Ca^{2+}$ is normal and no action regarding $Ca^{2+}$ therapy is indicated. Conditions marked by hyperphosphatemia, such as *chronic renal failure*, parenteral nutrition and *renal tubular acidosis* are all associated with hypocalcemia which resolves upon correction of the plasma $PO_4$. Vitamin D deficiency and hypoparathyroidism also cause hypocalcemia.

*Hypercalcemia* is less common and is most commonly seen in infants and children who have received excess vitamin D. The condition known as *idiopathic hypercalcemia of infancy,* which was diagnosed commonly in the UK but not in the USA, was probably the result of generous supplementation of cows' milk with vitamin D. *Williams syndrome* is characterized by mental retardation, supravalvar aortic stenosis and elfin facies and may be associated with hypercalcemia, but the nature of the link is a mystery. Vitamins D and A are fat soluble and therapeutic preparations often contain both. *Vitamin A toxicity* also causes hypercalcemia as a result of increased osteoclast activity, lysosomal disruption, the release of hydrolytic enzymes and increased bone resorption. If hypercalcemia is discovered unexpectedly, *hyperparathyroidism* or *malignancy* should be suspected. Hypercalcemia associated with malignancy may arise from osteolytic metastases or ectopic hormone production.

## MAGNESIUM (Mg²⁺)

$Mg^{2+}$ is the fourth most abundant cation in the body and, after $K^+$, the second commonest in the intracellular fluid (ICF). Intracellular $Mg^{2+}$ plays a critical role in many metabolic processes including the production and utilization of energy. It also is necessary for a large number of enzymatic reactions, including those involving DNA transcription, RNA aggregation and protein synthesis. Extracellular $Mg^{2+}$ is involved in neuronal activity, neuromuscular transmission and cardiovascular tone. The availability of intracellular $Mg^{2+}$ appears to be the determining factor in $Mg^{2+}$ homeostasis; cellular $Mg^{2+}$ being maintained at the expense of the ECF and bone.

The normal adult body contains about 900 mmol $Mg^{2+}$, of which two-thirds is in bone and one-third in the ICF with only 1 per cent in the ECF. The normal ratio of $Ca^{2+}$ to $Mg^{2+}$ in bone is 50:1. Most bone $Mg^{2+}$ is complexed to the apatite crystal rather than to the bone matrix. The normal intracellular $Mg^{2+}$ concentration varies between 4 and 8 mmol/L and much of it is complexed to proteins and organophosphates. The normal plasma $Mg^{2+}$ concentration is 0.7–1.0 mmol/L, about half of which is ionized.

## Magnesium homeostasis

The normal adult ingests about 12 mmol $Mg^{2+}$ per day and absorbs half of this (Fig. 43.3). The absorbed $Mg^{2+}$ enters an extracellular pool containing 12 mmol $Mg^{2+}$ which is in equilibrium with bone (600 mmol), muscle (170 mmol) and other tissues (100 mmol). Under stable conditions most of the absorbed $Mg^{2+}$ is excreted in the urine and a small amount is secreted into the intestine. $Mg^{2+}$ is absorbed throughout the small intestine but most importantly in the ileum. $Mg^{2+}$ deficiency may occur following small intestine resection.

Absorption takes place by both active and passive routes, but the mechanisms controlling the process are not well understood. Both PTH and vitamin D are alleged to augment $Mg^{2+}$ absorption. Although $Ca^{2+}$ and $Mg^{2+}$ are influenced by similar controls, their pathways of absorption are thought to be independent. Approximately 80 per cent of the plasma $Mg^{2+}$ is filtered at the glomerulus. In the proximal convoluted tubule about 25 per cent of the filtered $Mg^{2+}$ is reabsorbed. Reabsorption occurs in parallel to that of $Na^+$ and $Ca^{2+}$ but at a lower rate, suggesting that the proximal tubular cells are relatively impermeable to $Mg^{2+}$ and the intraluminal concentration rises along the length of the tubule. A further 15 per cent is reabsorbed in the straight proximal tubule which is also relatively impermeable to $Mg^{2+}$. Fifty per cent of $Mg^{2+}$ is reabsorbed in the thick ascending limb of the loop of Henle via an active transport process which apparently is not saturable. About 80 per cent of the delivered load is reabsorbed at all levels of luminal $Mg^{2+}$ concentration, but reabsorption is inversely proportional to the serum $Mg^{2+}$. $Mg^{2+}$ excretion is increased by increased renal perfusion or filtration, as

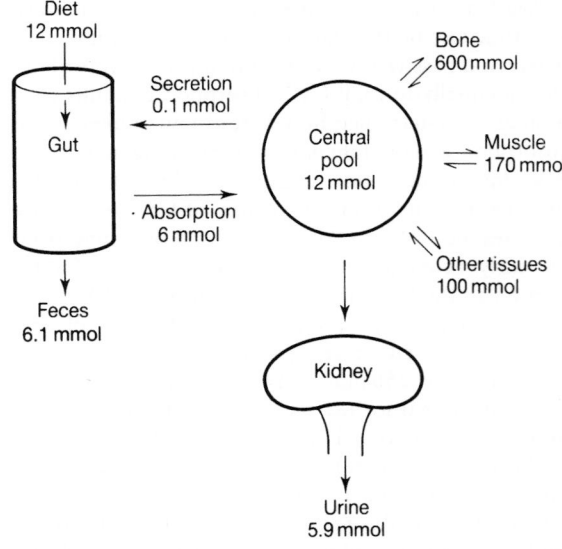

FIGURE 43.3 Magnesium balance in a normal 70-kg man

occurs in volume overload or the use of osmotic diuretics. It also is increased by hypermagnesemia, hypercalcemia, loop diuretics, metabolic acidosis and $PO_4$ depletion. It is decreased by the converse changes and also by PTH and hypothyroidism.

Because $Mg^{2+}$ is principally an intracellular ion, the plasma concentration and body level do not correlate well. Consequently $Mg^{2+}$ depletion can occur in the presence of normomagnesemia, and hypomagnesemia does not necessarily reflect a loss of $Mg^{2+}$ stores. However, it is prudent to assume if a patient has hypomagnesemia there will be some degree of whole body $Mg^{2+}$ depletion. The reduced dietary intake of $Mg^{2+}$ seen in *protein–calorie malnutrition* results in both $Mg^{2+}$ depletion and hypomagnesemia and the latter may persist on refeeding when there is redistribution of total body $Mg^{2+}$ into the intracellular compartment. Any condition characterized by chronic diarrhea or chronic diuretic therapy may be associated with $Mg^{2+}$ losses that are not always reflected in the plasma concentration. The metabolism of $Mg^{2+}$ and $Ca^{2+}$ are closely interrelated and $Mg^{2+}$ is important in $Ca^{2+}$ homeostasis. $Mg^{2+}$ deficiency is always associated with $Ca^{2+}$ deficiency and the latter cannot be corrected by $Ca^{2+}$ alone. It is important to think of $Mg^{2+}$ when considering problems of hypocalcemia.

Inborn errors of $Mg^{2+}$ metabolism occur in both the intestine and kidney. *Hypomagnesemia* may result from a defect in the intestinal active absorptive pathway with preservation of the passive mechanism. $Mg^{2+}$ depletion and hypomagnesemia can be corrected by the administration of $Mg^{2+}$ salts that otherwise would be purgative. Two types of renal $Mg^{2+}$ loss are known: an isolated $Mg^{2+}$ leak, and a combined $Mg^{2+}$ and $K^+$ leak. It is not understood if the isolated defects of renal $Mg^{2+}$ conservation and intestinal $Mg^{2+}$ absorption coexist.

*Hypermagnesemia* occurs rarely. It may be encountered in azotemia and in the newborn infant of a mother treated with intravenous $Mg^{2+}$ for eclampsia or for attempted inhibition of preterm labor.

## PHOSPHATE (PO₄)

The physiologically important circulating $PO_4$ is orthophosphate which is present as $H_2PO_4^-$ and $HPO_4^{2-}$. At pH 7.4 the ratio of $H_2PO_4^-$ to $HPO_4^{2-}$ is 4:1. Since plasma $PO_4$ is a mixture of monovalent and divalent species it has an intermediate valency of 1.8. Plasma $PO_4$ concentration is measured chemically as phosphorus. Phosphate concentrations fluctuate more markedly than those of $Ca^{2+}$, being affected by meals, the time of day, and age. Normal values decline from 1.8–3.2 mmol/L in the first month of life, to 1.4-2.1 mmol/L at one year, 1.2–1.7 mmol/L throughout childhood, reaching the adult range of 0.8–1.4 mmol/L following the cessation of growth. For these reasons, precise evaluation of $PO_4$ concentrations requires standardization of sampling conditions and the use of age-

appropriate normal ranges. The terms plasma phosphorus and plasma $PO_4$ are often used interchangeably, which makes it important to think and work in molar terms to avoid mathematical errors in calculation. Under normal conditions about 15 per cent of plasma $PO_4$ is protein-bound.

## Phosphate homeostasis

Dietary $PO_4$ is both organic and inorganic and most of the organic $PO_4$ is hydrolyzed in the intestinal lumen to yield inorganic $PO_4$ for absorption. Most $PO_4$ is absorbed in the jejunum and in normal subjects net $PO_4$ absorption is not tightly regulated and is approximately two-thirds of dietary intake over a wide range of intakes. Over a normal range of intake net $PO_4$ absorption is linear, whereas net $Ca^{2+}$ absorption is curvilinear, decreasing with increasing absolute $Ca^{2+}$ load. Net $PO_4$ absorption is about double that of $Ca^{2+}$: two-thirds compared to one-third. Intestinal $PO_4$ absorption, like that of $Ca^{2+}$, is both passive and active and under normal circumstances is almost entirely diffusional. The active absorption of both $PO_4$ and $Ca^{2+}$ is stimulated by $1,25(OH)_2D$, but by separate mechanisms. PTH has no direct effect on $PO_4$ absorption. Since most diets contain an abundance of $PO_4$ the quantity of $PO_4$ absorbed always exceeds requirements.

Renal $PO_4$ excretion takes place by filtration and fractional reabsorption; there is no $PO_4$ secretion by the renal tubule. The ionized and complexed fractions of plasma $PO_4$ are filtered at the glomerulus and almost 90 per cent of the filtered load is reabsorbed, resulting in a normal urinary $PO_4$ excretion of about 25 mmol/day in adults. Urinary $PO_4$ excretion is highly dependent on dietary intake, responding within several days to a dietary alteration. Reabsorption takes place principally in the proximal convoluted tubule and more occurs at the beginning than further down. PTH reduces $PO_4$ reabsorption via a mechanism in the straight part of the proximal tubule involving cAMP. This represents the most important physiological effect on renal $PO_4$ excretion and is the major determinant of plasma $PO_4$ concentration. Vitamin D and its metabolites have no direct effect on renal $PO_4$ reabsorption, but influence it profoundly by their overall action on mineral metabolism in different circumstances, being either phosphaturic or antiphosphaturic. Growth hormone (GH) causes $PO_4$ retention by increasing both intestinal and renal absorption of $PO_4$, resulting in hyperphosphatemia. GH has a direct effect on the kidney but the site of action is not clearly defined. Thyroid hormones also have a direct action to stimulate renal $PO_4$ reabsorption but this is masked by their overall effects on $PO_4$ metabolism and their interactions with other hormone systems. Certain *mesenchymal tumors* and *neurocutaneous dysplasias* may be associated with phosphaturia which resolves on removal of the tumor. This has led to the hypothesis that there is a factor released by the pathological tissue which blocks $PO_4$ reabsorption.

Plasma $PO_4$ homeostasis is fundamentally controlled by intestinal $PO_4$ absorption and renal $PO_4$ excretion, with $PO_4$ exchange between the plasma and skeleton and soft tissues playing a secondary role. Whereas the intestine intermittently floods the ECF with $PO_4$, the kidney continuously regulates plasma $PO_4$ and overall $PO_4$ homeostasis by precisely excreting that which is in excess of the body's need. This balance is maintained independently of PTH. There is a pronounced diurnal rhythm in $PO_4$ excretion with a nadir during the morning and a peak in the late evening. This does not appear to be tightly bound to food intake; it may be linked to diurnal changes in glucocorticoid secretion. Increased urine production, for whatever reason, is usually accompanied by increased $PO_4$ excretion due to reduced $PO_4$ reabsorption. The only diuretics that are not phosphaturic are the distal $K^+$-sparing ones such as triamterene, amiloride and spironolactone. Alkalinization of the urine causes phosphaturia.

Whole body $PO_4$ homeostasis is directed more towards the needs of soft tissues than bone. Dietary $PO_4$ restriction is followed immediately by virtual elimination of $PO_4$ from the urine and a sharp reduction in fecal $PO_4$. Growth stops, thereby reducing the need for $PO_4$ and $PO_4$ is mobilized from bone to satisfy the needs of the soft tissues. Dietary $PO_4$ deficiency is responsible for *osteopenia of prematurity*, as seen in preterm infants fed unsupplemented breast milk. Any movement of $PO_4$ into the intracellular compartment or bone can result in *hypophosphatemia* which may be symptomatic or even life threatening. This happens most abruptly during glucose or fructose infusion but is more likely to be serious during total parenteral nutrition if the hyperalimentation fluid is inadequately supplemented with $PO_4$. Phosphaturia can cause hypophosphatemia, and this occurs most commonly as a result of acidosis. The hypophosphatemia of disorders of vitamin D metabolism is due to reduced intestinal absorption of $Ca^{2+}$ and hypocalcemia leading to *secondary hyperparathyroidism* which causes increased renal $PO_4$ excretion and also reduced intestinal $PO_4$ absorption. Increased renal $PO_4$ loss also occurs in primary tubular disorders such as the *Fanconi syndrome*, *renal tubular acidosis*, and *familial X-linked hypophosphatemic rickets*.

*Hyperphosphatemia* occurs whenever the entry of $PO_4$ into the circulation exceeds the renal capacity for $PO_4$ excretion. If renal function is impaired, hyperphosphatemia may occur in the face of normal or even reduced $PO_4$ intake. Excess $PO_4$ enters the circulation as a result of ingestion of $PO_4$-containing enemas, antacid preparations or laxatives, but more commonly in childhood from vitamin D intoxication, stimulating both intestinal $PO_4$ absorption and bone resorption. Acidosis, both metabolic and respiratory, causes hyperphosphatemia. Conditions associated with cellular breakdown, such as *tumor lysis syndrome* or *rhabdomyolysis*, release $PO_4$ into the circulation.

## SELECTED READING

Martin TJ, Raisz LG eds. *Clinical endocrinology of calcium metabolism.* New York: Marcel Dekker, 1987: 410.

Maxwell MH, Kleeman CR, Narins RG eds. *Clinical disorders of fluid and electrolyte metabolism.* 4th edn. New York: McGraw-Hill, 1987: 1268.

Nordin BEC ed. *Calcium in human biology.* London: Springer Verlag, 1988: 481.

Reichel H, Koeffler HP, Norman AW. The role of the Vitamin D endocrine system in health and disease. *N Engl J Med* 1989; 320: 980.

# UNIQUE ASPECTS OF CALCIUM AND VITAMIN D METABOLISM IN THE PLACENTA AND FETUS

## INTRODUCTION

Fetal skeletal calcification occurs late in pregnancy, and approximately two-thirds of the total $Ca^{2+}$ required by the human fetus is acquired from the mother during the third trimester at a rate of up to 150 mg/kg body weight·day. This is used primarily for the calcification of the fetal skeleton. The control of this transplacental $Ca^{2+}$ flux is primarily with the fetus and is intimately involved in the process of fetal $Ca^{2+}$ homeostasis. During this period of gestation the fetal plasma $Ca^{2+}$ ion concentration exceeds that in maternal plasma so that $Ca^{2+}$ transport across the placenta is an active process. This may involve a high affinity $Ca^{2+}$ ion pump situated in the fetal-facing surface of the syncytiotrophoblast. This pump is believed to play a central role in intrauterine $Ca^{2+}$ metabolism (Fig. 43.4).

## PLACENTAL TRANSPORT OF $Ca^{2+}$

During high rates of placental $Ca^{2+}$ passage, the syncytiotrophoblast must maintain a very low $Ca^{2+}$ ion concentration of the order of $10^{-7}$ M. This represents a considerable gradient relative to the extracellular concentration ($10^{-3}$ M). The microvillus membrane participates in the entry of $Ca^{2+}$ ions as the first step in their transfer across the syncytium from mother to fetus. This may occur by facilitated diffusion. The ions must then be carried across the cytoplasm, probably bound to a protein to maintain intracellular $Ca^{2+}$ ion homeostasis, before being exported across the basal surface of the cell into the fetal circulation by the action of an ATP-dependent $Ca^{2+}$ pump.

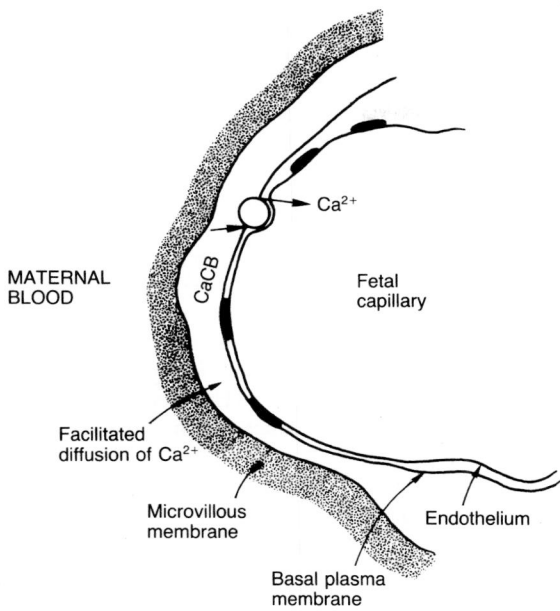

FIGURE 43.4 Maternal–fetal passage of calcium ions across the syncytiotrophoblast during late pregnancy. $\curvearrowright$, ATP-dependent Ca$^{2+}$ pump; CaCB, calbindin-bound calcium.

# Factors regulating the placental transport of Ca$^{2+}$

## Maternal calcemia

Prolonged maternal hypercalcemia, often caused by primary hyperparathyroidism, leads to an increase in the transplacental flux of Ca$^{2+}$ ions which results in an even higher Ca$^{2+}$ ion concentration in fetal plasma. The consequent suppression of the fetal parathyroid glands results in hypocalcemia during the first 3–4 days after birth, when this excessive rate of addition of Ca$^{2+}$ ions has been arrested. Conversely, prolonged maternal hypocalcemia leads to reduced transport of Ca$^{2+}$ ions to the fetus with consequent stimulation of the fetal parathyroid glands in an attempt to maintain normal fetal calcemia.

## 1,25-Dihydroxy vitamin D[1,25(OH)$_2$D]

Under normal circumstances, at least 90 per cent of the vitamin D requirements of the mother are met by endogenous photosynthesis in the skin. After transportation to the liver, bound to the vitamin D binding protein, hydroxylation takes place to yield 25-hydroxy vitamin D [25(OH)D], the principal form that crosses the placenta to the fetus. In both the fetus and the mother, 25(OH)D is converted by a further hydroxylation to either the principal active hormone, 1,25(OH)$_2$D, or the inactive metabolite, 24,25(OH)$_2$D. The major

source of the 1,25(OH)$_2$D circulating in the human fetus is the fetal kidneys, with minor amounts being made in the placenta or transported from the mother. The plasma concentration of 1,25(OH)$_2$D in the human fetus is lower than that in the maternal circulation. The renal production of 1,25(OH)$_2$D is stimulated by hypocalcemia, hypophosphatemia (in the presence of insulin-like growth factor I), parathyroid hormone (1–34) (PTH) and parathyroid hormone-related protein (1–34). Since the first two (hypocalcemia and hypophosphatemia) are reversed in fetal plasma, attention must be focused on the other two factors (see below) when identifying the secretagogs of 1,25(OH)$_2$D in the fetus. A negative feedback exists in which an excessive level of 1,25(OH)$_2$D increases the synthesis of 24,25(OH)$_2$D from 25(OH)D at the expense of the synthesis of more 1,25(OH)$_2$D.

A specific receptor for 1,25(OH)$_2$D has been demonstrated in the human placenta leading to the production of a Ca$^{2+}$-binding protein, calbindin-D9K. In rat, the expression of placental calbindin-D9K mRNA shows a close temporal relationship with the increase in materno-fetal Ca$^{2+}$ clearance found in the last third of pregnancy. However, a gross maternal vitamin D deficiency in pregnant rats has no effect on the Ca$^{2+}$ content of their fetuses nor on the expression of calbindin-D9K in the placenta, and thus it is unclear what exact role calbindin-D9K plays in facilitating Ca$^{2+}$ transport to the fetus. From the rapid effects of 1,25(OH)$_2$D on the rate of placental transport of Ca$^{2+}$ ions, it has been suggested that 1,25(OH)$_2$D has a permissive non-genomic stimulatory effect. This may be exerted by facilitated diffusion at the microvillus membrane of the syncytiotrophoblast. This complements the genomic effect of calbindin-D9K used to buffer the intracellular Ca$^{2+}$ ion concentration during passage across the cell to the Ca$^{2+}$ pump located in the fetal-facing, basal plasma membrane.

## Parathyroid hormone-related protein (PTHrP)

This protein, originally called the hypercalcemic factor of malignancy, has a wide distribution in the human fetus and its specific biological activity is particularly high in the amnion, especially before it ruptures. There is evidence for an umbilical venous–arterial difference in the plasma concentrations of PTHrP, indicative of net secretion of PTHrP from the placenta into the fetal circulation.

Both extracts of fetal parathyroid glands and PTHrP stimulate the rate of transfer of Ca$^{2+}$ ions across the ovine placenta from mother to fetus and conversely, removal of the fetal parathyroid glands reduces the rate of uptake from the mother of $^{45}$Ca into the fetal skeleton. PTHrP, probably a mid-molecular segment, likely exerts this stimulatory effect on placental Ca$^{2+}$ transport via an action on the putative $Ca^{2+}$ pump in the basal plasma membrane of the syncytiotrophoblast.

## DEVELOPMENT OF THE FETAL SKELETON

### Vitamin D

Vitamin D is necessary for both fetal and maternal bone mineralization and turnover. Thus, vitamin D deficiency in the pregnant woman can have drastic sequelae for the calcification of cartilage in the fetal skeleton. Congenital rickets, although rare, has been described in infants born to mothers with vitamin D deficiency. This deficiency must be severe, since the fetal kidney tends to compensate for a small supply of $25(OH)D$ by converting most of it into $1,25(OH)_2D$ with minimal production of $24,25(OH)_2D$.

The mineralization of bone not only is enhanced by $1,25(OH)_2D$ by assisting in the orderly calcification of cartilage during the formation of the endochondral skeleton, but also leads to an increase in number and activity of osteoclasts, so important in the bone remodeling process. In this process, osteoclastic resorption of bone is coupled to neighboring bone accretion.

### Parathyroid hormone-related protein

PTHrP plays a vital role in the development of the endochondral skeleton as shown by homologous recombination experiments to "knock out" the parental gene which encodes for PTHrP. Mice, rendered homologous for the *PTHrP* null mutation, died at birth with widespread developmental abnormalities of endochondral bone involving premature maturation of chondrocytes and consequent accelerated bone formation (e.g. bell-shaped thoracic cage and consequent asphyxia at birth). The rates of maturation of articular cartilage and of development of membranous bone are unaffected. Following short-term fetal parathyroidectomy with the consequent loss of both PTH and some PTHrP, lambs were born with histomorphometric signs of rickets. This was caused not only by the inadequate supply of $Ca^{2+}$ and $PO_4$ ions to maintain a normal rate of bone accretion, but also by defective bone resorption and remodeling. These experiments highlight the essential role of PTHrP in the development of a normal fetal skeleton and contrast with the delivery of live human babies born with hypoparathyroidism (e.g. *DiGeorge syndrome*).

### Parathyroid hormone

In most radioimmunoassays, the circulating plasma concentrations of PTH are undetectable unless the fetus has been rendered hypocalcemic. However, there is evidence in some species that the set-point for PTH secretion is shifted towards a higher plasma $Ca^{2+}$ ion concentration in the fetus. This finding is supported by the results of more sophisticated assays for the biologically active N-terminal region of PTH. Thus, it is now likely that enough PTH circulates in the fetus to play a significant part in development and turnover of the fetal skeleton, similar to, and probably synergistic with, that of the role played by $1,25(OH)_2D$.

### Calcitonin

Calcitonin serves to reduce the motility and biological activity of osteoclasts. Because of the fetal hypercalcemia, the circulating fetal concentrations of calcitonin are higher than in the mother. This implies a level of control of the osteoclastic activity that has been stimulated by the actions of PTH, PTHrP and $1,25(OH)_2D$ which serves to tilt the balance of bone remodeling in favor of net accretion.

## FETAL $Ca^{2+}$ HOMEOSTASIS

The human fetus is maintained hypercalcemic, relative to its mother, by the action of the placental pump. Despite this degree of hypercalcemia, the fetal plasma total concentration of bioactive PTH-like molecules is higher than in maternal plasma. These PTH-like molecules are represented by PTH (1–34), and PTHrP (1–34) both of which share the same receptor in the kidney and in the osteoblast. Both play important roles in bone resorption and turnover whereas a mid-molecular region of PTHrP, which is not present in PTH, is believed to stimulate the transport of $Ca^{2+}$ ions across the placenta to the fetus. This transport is facilitated by $1,25(OH)_2D$. The resultant hypercalcemia promotes net bone accretion as part of the overall growth of the fetus. This is aided by the hypercalcitoninemia which exerts an inhibitory modulatory effect on bone resorption caused by the combined actions of PTH, PTHrP and $1,25(OH)_2D$. The total PTH-like bioactivity in fetal plasma varies inversely with the plasma $Ca^{2+}$ ion concentration and probably plays an important part in fetal $Ca^{2+}$ homeostasis.

## SELECTED READING

Aaron JE, Abbas SK, Colwell A *et al*. Parathyroid gland hormones in the skeletal development of the ovine fetus: the effect of parathyroidectomy with calcium and phosphate infusion. *Bone and Mineral* 1992; **16**: 121.

Bowden SJ, Emly JF, Hughes SV *et al*. Parathyroid hormone-related protein in human term placenta and membranes. *J Endocrinol* 1994; **142**: 217.

Care AD. Development of endocrine pathways in the regulation of calcium homeostasis. *Baillière's Clin. Endocrinol. Metab.*, 1989; 1; 3: 671.

Care AD. The placental transport of calcium. *J Dev Physiol* 1991; **15**: 303.

Kamath GK, Kelley LK, Friedman AF, Smith CH. Transport and binding in calcium uptake by microvillous membrane of human placenta. *Am J Physiol* 1992; **262**: C789.

Karaplis AC, Luz A, Glowacki J *et al.* Lethal skeletal dysplasia from targeted disruption of the parathyroid hormone-related peptide gene. *Genes Dev* 1994; **8**: 277.

Moseley JM, Hayman JA, Danks JA *et al.* Immunohistochemical detection of parathyroid hormone-related protein in human fetal epithelia. *Clin Endocrinol Metab* 1991; **73**: 478.

Sibley CP. Mechanisms of ion transfer by the rat placenta: a model for the human placenta? *Placenta* 1994; **15**: 675.

# PART EIGHT

# Bone, Connective Tissue and Skin

**Editor: R.D.G. Milner**

# 44

# Bone and Cartilage

# HYALINE CARTILAGE IN LONG-BONE DEVELOPMENT

## INTRODUCTION

The perinatal and pediatric development of bone occurs by two separate but interrelated processes, intramembranous and endochondral ossification (*see* page 554 for additional details). *Intramembranous ossification* occurs largely in the bones of the skull, maxilla and mandible, and results in mesenchymal differentiation to produce osteoblasts that elaborate bony trabeculae, that then fuse to form membrane bone. In contrast, *endochondral ossification* relies on the formation of a hyaline cartilage model which acts as a template for the elaboration of both long and short bones, vertebrae and the pelvis.

Endochondral ossification involves two distinct growth patterns: interstitial growth of the cartilage matrix by chondrocytes, and appositional growth by osteoblasts to form primary bone on a calcified cartilage matrix. During growth, primary bone is continuously remodeled by osteoclasts and subsequently is replaced by appositional deposition of secondary bone. Each process occurs simultaneously, the overall increase in bone length and diameter resulting from a finely regulated interplay between these two growth processes.

## DEVELOPMENT OF THE HYALINE CARTILAGE MODEL

The spatial and temporal sequences necessary for limb growth, proximo–distal patterning and musculoskeletal differentiation encompass a complex series of regulatory interactions involving embryonic ectoderm and mesoderm. Three distinct phases have been identified during limb embryogenesis which result in the development of the cartilaginous precursors for the future skeleton.

### Prechondrogenic ectodermal–mesodermal interactions

Limb morphogenesis is initiated by formation of *limb buds*, ectodermal outgrowths which develop on the flank of the embryo during the fifth week of gestation. At the tip of the limb bud, a specialized ectodermal thickening develops known as the apical ectodermal ridge (AER), essential for the continued induction of underlying mesenchymal cells which derive from the somatopleure of the lateral body wall. Mesenchymal cells in turn play a major role in induction and maintenance of the AER, establishing reciprocal ectodermal–mesodermal interactions which ultimately specify the position of hyaline cartilage, muscle differentiation and the patterns of nerve and capillary invasion.

As the limb bud develops, paracrine signals, such as basic fibroblast growth factor released from the AER, promote high rates of mesenchymal cell proliferation and hyaluronan synthesis to facilitate the inductive migration of cells into the region beneath the AER. Thus the initial prechondrogenic phase of limb development is characterized by a homogeneous population of undifferentiated mesenchymal cells surrounded and regulated by ectoderm which at the growing tip forms the AER, proven essential for accurate morphogenesis of musculoskeletal elements in the limb.

## Condensation and patterning

Outward growth of the limb bud leaves behind a trail of mesenchymal cells, released from the inductive influence of the AER, which enter a transient condensation phase. During this period, cells in the proximal center of the mesenchymal mass are the first to condense and form a prechondrogenic core, which subsequently follows the specific spatial and temporal sequences necessary to establish the proximo–distal patterning of the primordial skeleton.

These mesenchymal condensations are characterized by formation of extensive cell–cell and cell–matrix interactions, proven essential to trigger chondrogenic differentiation. These interactions include a functional gradient of gap junction proteins involved in pattern formation along the proximo–distal axis; expression of hyaluronan-binding sites which mediate the endocytosis and degradation of hyaluronan to promote mesenchymal condensation and receptor mediated hyaluronan cross-bridging between cells; and a transient increase in pericellular fibronectin, which forms adhesive interactions with the heparin-like cell surface molecules identified in prechondrogenic mesenchymal cells.

The condensation phase is also accompanied by an increase in cell cycle time, cell rounding and a marked increase in intracellular cAMP. Concurrently, chondrocyte specific gene expression is activated, the initial production of aggrecan core protein and the cartilage collagen types II and IX resulting in the first appearance of pericellular metachromasia in the prechondrogenic core.

Additional mesenchymal condensations form adjacent to the prechondrogenic core, but in contrast, become invested with nerves and blood vessels which promote muscle differentiation. The remaining undifferentiated mesenchymal cells are regulated by transforming growth factor β (TGFβ), released from the ectoderm, which promotes high rates of hyaluronan synthesis and maintains the mesenchymal phenotype essential for differentiation of the perichondrium, tendons, dermis and loose connective tissues. Thus by the end of the condensation phase, prechondrogenic

mesenchymal cells have established the spatial and temporal sequences crucial for proximo–distal patterning, and have acquired the cellular and regulatory mechanisms necessary to proceed with chondrogenesis.

## Chondrogenic differentiation

Overt chondrogenesis is first evident in the most proximal condensations and is accompanied by a marked increase in the synthesis and sequestration of cartilage specific matrix macromolecules such as hyaluronan, aggrecan, and collagen types II and IX. The resulting increase in matrix volume gradually forces the newly differentiated chondrocytes apart, terminating gap junction communication and promoting continued chondrogenesis.

Concomitant with this increased matrix deposition, chondrocytes assume distinctive shapes and orientations within the developing cartilage model. Thus, cells in the center flatten along an axis perpendicular to the proximo–distal axis of growth, while cells in the epiphyses remain rounded. Chondrocyte hypertrophy is initiated in the center of the flattened cell zone, and ultimately signals the location of the mid-diaphysis as the bone collar forms. The three chondrocyte morphologies typical of the hyaline cartilage model are therefore established during chondrogenesis and remain until closure of the epiphyseal plate at skeletal maturity.

## HYALINE CARTILAGE IN LONG-BONE DEVELOPMENT

The role of hyaline cartilage in long-bone development is summarized in Fig. 44.1. Initially, the dumbbell-shaped cartilage model is surrounded by a fibrous perichondrium which contributes to the increase in width by appositional growth as differentiating chondroblasts are added at the periphery of the cartilage model. By contrast, elongation of hyaline cartilage occurs by interstitial growth due to division of chondrocytes and production of additional matrix within the cartilage model (Fig. 44.1a).

By the end of the first trimester capillaries invade the mid-region of the perichondrium, and increased vascularization promotes differentiation of perichondral cells to form osteoblasts which produce a thin collar of bone enclosing the mid-region of the cartilage model (Fig. 44.1b). Thus the perichondrium differentiates to form periosteum, and the bony collar formed increases in width and length by continuous intramembranous ossification. Concurrently, chondrocytes in the mid-region of the cartilage model continue to hypertrophy, creating expanded lacunae separated by thin septa of cartilage matrix, which become calcified (Fig. 44.1c).

At this time, a vascular periosteal bud forms in the mid-region of the periosteum and penetrates the calci-

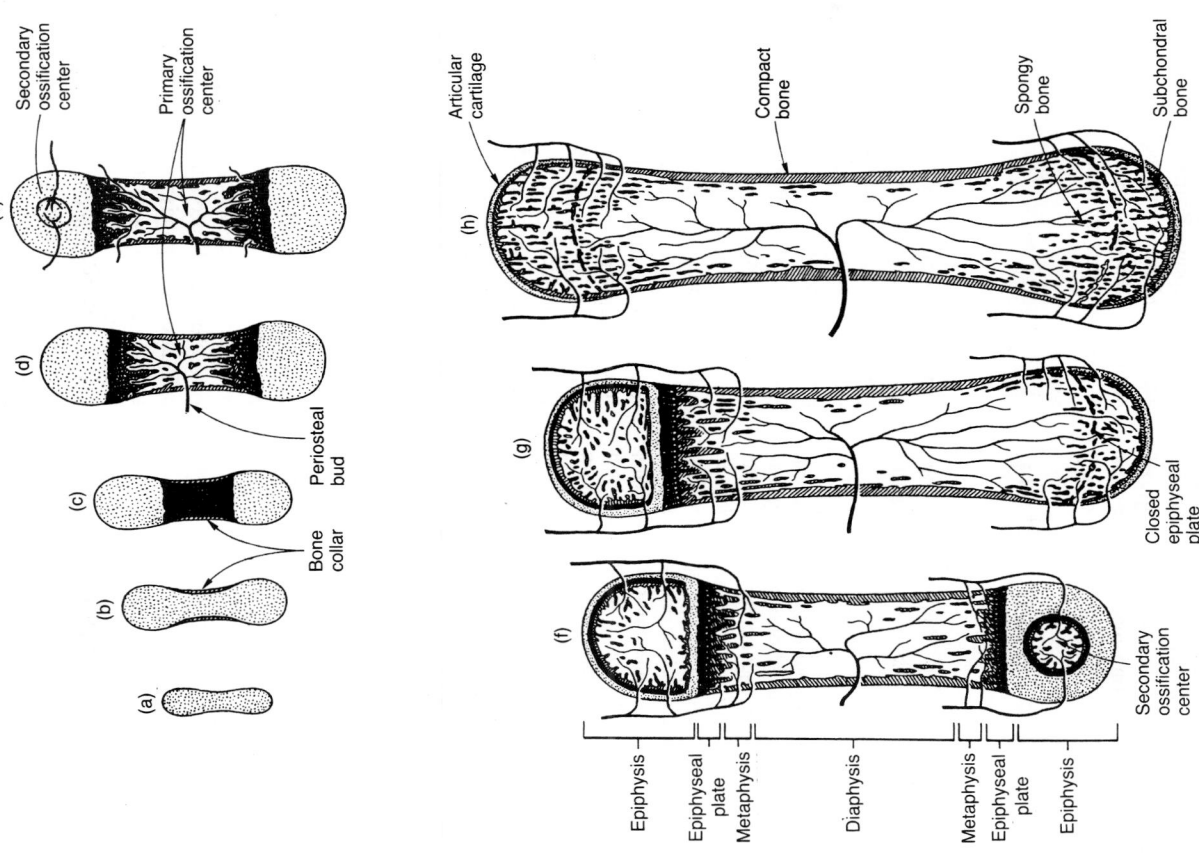

FIGURE 44.1 The hyaline cartilage model and its role in long-bone formation. Hyaline cartilage appears stippled, calcified cartilage is black and bone is defined by hatched lines. (a) to (e) Represent phases of fetal development; (f) to (h) represent pediatric development through to skeletal maturity. Full details are explained in the text. (From Bloom W, Fawcett DW. *A textbook of histology*. 10th edn. Philadelphia: WB Saunders, 1975, with the permission of Chapman & Hall.)

fied cartilage matrix introducing capillary loops, mesenchymal cells, and osteoprogenitor cells to the center of the calcified cartilage model (Fig. 44.1d). Osteogenic cells differentiate into osteoblasts which sequester cancellous bone on the remnants of the calcified cartilage matrix leading to the formation of the *primary ossification center* (Fig. 44.1d). Eventually, the central portion of cancellous bone in the mid-region of the model undergoes resorption creating a central medullary cavity surrounded by cortical bone. At this time the medullary cavity is seeded with circulating

hematopoietic stem cells which give rise to the myeloid tissues typical of the medullary cavity of long bones.

By the third trimester bone consists of two distinct regions, the bony shaft or diaphysis comprising an elongating bony collar and enlarging medullary cavity, and *epiphyseal cartilage* which persists at the ends of the developing bone. Interstitial growth continues in the cartilaginous epiphysis and is precisely coordinated at either end of the diaphysis by cartilage maturation, matrix calcification and continued replacement by bone.

Shortly before parturition at 40 weeks, a secondary ossification center is initiated in the epiphyses of the distal femoral (36 weeks) and proximal tibial (38 weeks) long bones (Fig. 44.1e,f). Chondrocytes in the middle of the epiphysis hypertrophy and the septal matrix calcifies in a similar manner to that seen in the primary ossification center. Capillaries then invade the calcified cartilage introducing osteoprogenitor cells which differentiate into osteoblasts and initiate bone deposition. After birth, ossification spreads from the secondary center in all directions, gradually replacing hyaline cartilage with trabecular bone and associated medullary cavities.

Thus postnatally, the original hyaline cartilage template is significantly remodeled and is retained only as the *articular–epiphyseal cartilage complex* (A–E complex) which covers the articulating surface of the synovial joints, and as a transverse disc of cartilage termed the epiphyseal plate which separates the epiphysis from the metaphysis, that portion of the diaphysis adjacent to the epiphyseal plate (Fig. 44.1f). Typically, the majority of long bones develop two secondary ossification centers, while short bones generally ossify completely from their primary center.

As skeletal maturity approaches, bone replacement on the diaphyseal side of the growth plate eventually overtakes interstitial growth of epiphyseal cartilage and the growth plate is resorbed (Fig. 44.1g,h). This process of epiphyseal closure occurs around age 20 years and signifies the end of longitudinal bone growth at skeletal maturity. The only remnant of the original cartilage model to remain is the articular cartilage of the diarthrodial joint, and this cartilage persists throughout adult life (Fig. 44.1h).

## THE EPIPHYSEAL GROWTH PLATE

The interface between the epiphysis and diaphysis is composed of a distinct hyaline cartilage, variously termed the growth plate, the epiphyseal plate or the physis. This remnant of the cartilage model is characterized by longitudinal columns of chondrocytes and intervening matrix, and is largely responsible for bone elongation. The epiphyseal plate exhibits a highly structured morphology in longitudinal section and is divisible into successive transverse zones which reflect distinct phases of activity in the life cycle of the chondrocytes (Fig. 44.2a).

### The reserve cell zone

Variously known as the stem, germinal or resting cell zone, this zone is located immediately adjacent to the epiphysis and is characterized by flattened chondrocytes exhibiting a slow rate of cell turnover. In addition to an anchoring function, this zone plays a key role in seeding daughter cells into the chondrocyte columns of the proliferative zone, changes in growth rate being

attributed to changes in length of the cell cycle and rate of cell seeding.

### The proliferative cell zone

This zone is characterized by rapid chondrocyte division and alignment into longitudinal columns running parallel with the long axis of the bone. These axial chondrocyte columns represent the functional units of longitudinal growth and continuously replace chondrocytes which undergo apoptosis and disappear on the metaphyseal side of the growth plate.

Daughter chondrocytes in the columns are separated by deposition of a thin matrix in transverse septa, while adjacent columns are separated by thicker longitudinal septa. Cell division contributes to bone growth by insertion of new cells and production of transverse septa in the column, approximately 20 per cent of the increase in bone length being attributed to the proliferative zone.

### The hypertrophic cell zone

Traditionally referred to as the zone of maturation and the zone of calcification, contemporary cryopreservation techniques now indicate that the

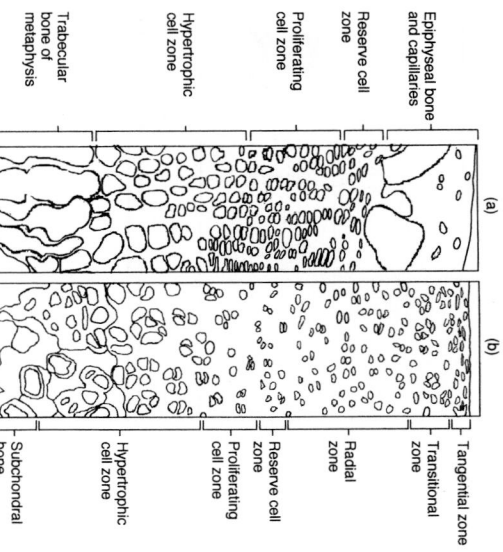

FIGURE 44.2 Schematic comparison of the growth regions in the pediatric long bone. (a) The epiphyseal growth plate is located between the calcified epiphysis and the bony trabecular of the metaphysis. Axial columns represent the functional units of longitudinal growth, while horizontal subdivisions represent distinct phases in the chondrocyte life cycle. See text for details. (b) The articular–epiphyseal cartilage complex of the developing synovial joint. Articular cartilage comprises the upper third of the complex and merges with the epiphyseal growth cartilage which is attached to the subchondral bone of the epiphysis. See text for details.

Epiphyseal bone and capillaries

Reserve cell zone

Proliferating cell zone

Hypertrophic cell zone

Trabecular bone of metaphysis

(a)

(b)

Tangential zone
Transitional zone
Radial zone
Reserve cell zone
Proliferating cell zone
Hypertrophic cell zone
Subchondral bone

hypertrophic zone embraces all cells from the end of proliferation to the elimination of chondrocytes at the metaphysis.

The hypertrophic zone is characterized by chondrocyte hypertrophy, cell volume increasing almost 10-fold and matrix volume doubling. Importantly, chondrocyte hypertrophy is anisotropic, the increase in cell height being significantly greater than transverse expansion. Up to 80 per cent of the increase in longitudinal bone growth is achieved by chondrocyte hypertrophy, and a linear relationship between rate of bone growth and the volume of hypertrophic chondrocytes has been established, indicating chondrocyte hypertrophy is an important variable in the determination of bone growth rates.

The distal portion of the hypertrophic zone is known histologically as the zone of calcification. It is characterized by the terminal hypertrophy and eventual loss of chondrocytes, and coincides with the invasion of metaphyseal blood vessels which occupy the cavity formed by chondrocyte hypertrophy.

Chondrocytes in this region also produce large amounts of alkaline phosphatase, type X collagen and other matrix macromolecules which, in conjunction with matrix vesicles seeded into the longitudinal septa, form a calcified cartilage template for appositional bone deposition. Interestingly, the transverse septa do not calcify, a factor which facilitates capillary invasion from the metaphysis.

## The zone of metaphyseal ossification

While not strictly part of the epiphyseal plate, this zone is characterized by invasion of pluripotent perivascular mesenchymal cells which provide the precursor pool for osteoblasts involved in bone deposition on the surface of the calcified longitudinal septa. The bony trabeculae thus formed define the metaphysis, but are eventually remodeled by osteoclasts to form the medullary cavity of the diaphysis.

Thus bone elongation occurs by proliferation, matrix synthesis and hypertrophy of chondrocytes within the epiphyseal plate and the concurrent loss of hypertrophic chondrocytes, matrix calcification and bone formation on the metaphyseal side of the cartilage model. During growth, the rate of these opposing events is approximately equal, ensuring the thickness of the epiphyseal plate remains constant and is displaced away from the center of the diaphysis. Disruption of the anisotrophic architecture of the epiphyseal plate results in disease states such as *achondroplasia* and the *chondrodystrophies*, while the biomechanical fragility of this region predisposes it to shearing fractures resulting in *osteochondrosis*, particularly during early childhood.

## THE ARTICULAR–EPIPHYSEAL CARTILAGE COMPLEX

Immature joint cartilage is known as the articular–epiphyseal cartilage complex (A–E complex), and represents an additional growth region in developing bones. However the A–E complex does not contribute significantly to longitudinal growth, but rather, is responsible for the proportional enlargement of the epiphyses, and the topographical formation of articular cartilage in the synovial joint. Two regions of growth potential have been identified in the A–E complex, one in the subsurface zone of articular cartilage, the other within a somewhat stunted epiphyseal growth cartilage anchored to the ossified epiphysis.

## Articular cartilage of the A–E complex

During growth and development, articular cartilage has a poorly developed morphology when compared with its adult form, but remains divisible into three transverse layers which merge imperceptibly with each other (Fig. 44.2b).

The tangential zone comprises the articulating surface, and consists of a thin layer of discoid chondrocytes aligned parallel to the articulating surface. Beneath the tangential zone lies a transitional zone characterized by small groups of randomly organized spheroidal chondrocytes. The cells in this region proliferate but do not columnate, resulting in radial rather than longitudinal growth of the articular cartilage.

The third zone of immature articular cartilage comprises the radial zone where small groups of spheroidal chondrocytes show a degree of radial columniation. This zone shows no evidence of cell division, and at skeletal maturity, forms the deep radial layer typical of adult articular cartilage.

The proportion of the A–E complex contributed by articular cartilage varies between species and joints examined, but in general occupies one-third to one-half of A–E complex thickness.

## Epiphyseal cartilage of the A–E complex

The epiphyseal cartilage of the A–E complex and the epiphyseal plate both share a similar pattern of proliferation, hypertrophy and resorption. However, in the A–E complex, proliferating and hypertrophic chondrocytes form truncated, egg-shaped clusters of cells with a resulting excess of radial over longitudinal growth. As with the epiphyseal plate, discrete functional regions can be identified which reflect different phases in endochondral ossification of the epiphyses (Fig. 44.2b).

The reserve cell zone of the A–E complex emerges from the radial zone of the articular cartilage to form a narrow band of discoidal shaped chondrocytes. Beneath this indistinct layer exists the proliferating cell zone, characterized by cells dividing to form egg-shaped clusters which fail to form the extensive longitudinal columns typical of the epiphyseal plate. As with the epiphyseal plate, cell division alone contributes minimally to the radial growth of the epiphyses.

The hypertrophic cell zone is characterized by chondrocyte hypertrophy, although the net increase in cell volume is less than that of equivalent cells of the epiphyseal plate. Moreover, the rounded contour and lack of columnation of these chondrocytes ensures that the epiphysis expands radially rather than longitudinally.

The calcification zone represents the region of terminal chondrocyte hypertrophy and matrix calcification. However, in contrast to the epiphyseal plate where only the longitudinal septa calcify, matrix calcification of the A–E complex totally encloses clusters of hypertrophic chondrocytes. In the final ossification phase, epiphyseal capillaries invade the hypertrophied lacunae, seeding osteoblasts onto the calcified cartilage matrix to initiate bone deposition beneath the growth region. As skeletal maturity approaches, the epiphyseal cartilage of the A–E complex is eventually replaced by bone, forming a continuous and compact subchondral bony plate which delineates the boundary between cancellous bone and the calcified cartilage layer of adult articular cartilage.

## SELECTED READING

Bloom W, Fawcett DW. A textbook of histology, 10th edn. Philadelphia: WB Saunders, 1975; 233.

Breur GJ, Turgai J, VanEnkevort BA et al. Stereological and serial section analysis of chondrocytic enlargement in the proximal tibial growth plate of the rat. Anat Rec 1994; 239; 255.

Dealy CN, Beyer EC, Kosher RA. Expression patterns of mRNAs for the gap junction proteins connexin43 and connexin42 suggest their involvement in chick limb morphogenesis and specification of the arterial vasculature. Dev Dyn 1994; 199; 156.

Hall BK ed. Cartilage, Volume 2: Development, differentiation and growth. New York, London: Academic Press, 1983.

Hill MA, Ruth GR, Van Sickle DC et al. Histochemical morphologic features of growth cartilages in long bones of pigs of various ages. Am J Vet Res 1987; 48; 1477.

Hunziker EB. Mechanism of longitudinal bone growth and its regulation by growth plate chondrocytes. Microscopy Res Tech 1994; 28; 505.

Mankin HJ. The calcified zone (basal layer) of articular cartilage of rabbits. Anat Rec 1963; 145; 73.

O'Rahilly R, Gardner E. The embryology of movable joints. In Sokoloff L ed. The joints and synovial fluid, Vol. 1. New York: Academic Press, 1978; 49.

Poole CA. Structure and function of articular cartilage matrices. In Woessner JF, Howell DS eds. Joint cartilage degradation: basic and clinical aspects. New York: Marcel Dekker, 1993; 1.

Rodriguez JI, Razquin S, Palacios J, Rubio V. Human growth plate development in the fetal and neonatal period. J Orthop Res 1992; 10; 62.

Solursh M. The role of extracellular matrix molecules in early limb development. Semin Dev Biol 1990; 1; 45.

Toole BP. Proteoglycans and hyaluronan in morphogenesis and differentiation. In Hay ED ed. Cell biology of extracellular matrix, 2nd edn. New York: Plenum Press, 1991; 305.

# BONE HOMEOSTASIS

Bone is a tissue of fundamental importance in human biology. It provides protection to other tissues (e.g. the central nervous system), makes respiration possible and is necessary for locomotion and physical interaction with the environment. Non-biologists often regard bone as a structure consisting primarily of mineral, but in reality bone is a tissue containing cellular elements and a connective tissue matrix. Like other tissues, it is metabolically active and responds to demands placed upon it by the organism. Unlike other tissues, it contains crystalline mineral deposits, principally $Ca^{2+}$ and $PO_4$, in the form of hydroxyapatite. The mineral confers compressive strength (tensile strength is provided by the connective tissue matrix) but also provides a vast reservoir of $Ca^{2+}$ and $PO_4$. Thus, bone assumes a central position in the homeostasis of these two minerals and a discussion of bone homeostasis is only possible in the context of an understanding of mineral metabolism (see Chapter 43).

## CALCIUM HOMEOSTASIS (see also Chapter 43)

Calcium also plays major roles outside the skeleton. The extracellular concentration of this ion is critical to maintenance of transmembrane potentials, and thus to central nervous system and cardiovascular function. A number of enzymes are $Ca^{2+}$-dependent, including those involved in blood coagulation, and the $Ca^{2+}$-dependent kinases. The modulation of intracellular $Ca^{2+}$ concentration is an important second messenger system by which extracellular events (e.g. the binding of a hormone to its cell surface receptor) influence intracellular function (e.g. protein phosphorylation or muscle contraction). Cytosolic $Ca^{2+}$ concentrations are maintained between $10^{-6}$ and $10^{-7}$ mol/L, principally by pumps and exchangers in cell membranes.

### Distribution of Ca²⁺

The human adult has a total body $Ca^{2+}$ content of approximately 1 kg, 99 per cent of which is in the skeleton. The typical daily fluxes of $Ca^{2+}$ in a normal

TABLE 44.1 Distribution of plasma $Ca^{2+}$

| PLASMA $Ca^{2+}$ FRACTION | TOTAL PERCENTAGE | CONCENTRATION (mmol/L) |
|---|---|---|
| Ultrafiltrable | 53 | 1.20–1.40 |
| Ionized | 47 | 1.13–1.28 |
| Complexed | 6 | 0.13–0.16 |
| Protein-bound | 47 | 1.03–1.22 |
| Albumin | 37 | 0.81–0.96 |
| Globulin | 10 | 0.22–0.26 |
| Total | 100 | 2.2–2.6 |

adult are shown in Fig. 43.2, page 537. About 1 per cent of skeletal $Ca^{2+}$ is freely exchangeable with that in the extracellular fluid but the bulk of bone $Ca^{2+}$ can only leave the skeleton following bone resorption by osteoclasts. $Ca^{2+}$ ions diffuse freely throughout the extracellular space where their concentration is approximately 1.2 mmol/L. This is equal to the plasma *ionized* $Ca^{2+}$ concentration but the *total* concentration of $Ca^{2+}$ in plasma is approximately two-fold higher as a result of binding to plasma proteins and the formation of complexes with $PO_4$, citrate and bicarbonate (Table 44.1). It is the ionized $Ca^{2+}$ concentration which is physiologically relevant, and therefore closely regulated. The homeostatic priority in $Ca^{2+}$ metabolism is maintenance of the ionized $Ca^{2+}$ concentration in the extracellular fluid within a narrow range, since the function of the nervous and cardiovascular systems is critically dependent upon this.

The three organs which contribute most significantly to the movement of $Ca^{2+}$ in and out of the extracellular fluid (ECF) are the gastrointestinal tract, the kidneys and bone. Further details of gastrointestinal and renal handling of $Ca^{2+}$ are provided in Chapter 43.

One to two per cent of total body $Ca^{2+}$ can be exchanged between bone and the ECF over a period of several days, probably by a passive process. The resorption and subsequent formation of bone which take place as part of the bone remodeling cycle (see below) mobilizes 5–7 per cent of the adult skeleton annually. During growth, formation exceeds resorption and during senescence the opposite is true. Bone turnover is tightly regulated, being stimulated by parathyroid hormone (PTH) and acutely inhibited by calcitonin. Increased osteoclastic bone resorption can contribute to *osteopenia, lytic metastases* or *hypercalcemia* by means of the systemic production of factors which stimulate bone resorption (e.g. parathyroid hormone-related peptide, PTHrP) or paracrine factors activating osteoclasts locally.

## Regulation of $Ca^{2+}$ metabolism

Parathyroid hormone and the vitamin D endocrine systems are the principal regulators of ECF $Ca^{2+}$ concen-

trations (see Chapter 43). Both work to increase $Ca^{2+}$ concentrations. PTH is secreted in response to a falling ECF $Ca^{2+}$ concentration and has two principal sites of action, bone and the kidney. In bone, PTH receptors are found on osteoblasts and their occupancy results in an indirect stimulation of osteoclastic bone resorption and an increase in the number of resorption sites (remodeling units) per unit of skeletal area. In the kidney, PTH increases tubular reabsorption of $Ca^{2+}$ and stimulates activity of 25-hydroxyvitamin D 1α-hydroxylase resulting in increased production of the more active vitamin D metabolite $1,25(OH)_2D$.

The vitamin D endocrine system is illustrated in Fig. 43.1, page 534. The term *vitamin D* is a misnomer since it implies that this substance is an essential dietary ingredient. In fact, most individuals receiving unsupplemented diets produce the greater part of their vitamin D endogenously as a result of the action of ultraviolet light on 7-dehydrocholesterol in the skin. This reaction produces cholecalciferol, which then is hydroxylated to produce 25(OH)D, the principal circulating metabolite and subsequently $1,25(OH)_2D$, the most biologically active metabolite. In bone, $1,25(OH)_2D$ is required for normal osteoclast development and it also may influence renal handling of $Ca^{2+}$ and $PO_4$.

Calcitonin is a peptide produced in the thyroid gland and secreted in response to an increase in ambient $Ca^{2+}$ concentration (see page 536). It acutely inhibits osteoclastic bone resorption and promotes urinary $Ca^{2+}$ loss. Its importance in human $Ca^{2+}$ metabolism is relatively minor and long-term excess or deficiency of this peptide produce no clinically apparent alterations in $Ca^{2+}$ or bone metabolism.

Parathyroid hormone-related peptide (PTHrP) has some similarities in its N-terminal amino acid sequence to PTH and can reproduce the effects of PTH by binding to its receptor. It may have an important role in the regulation of placental $Ca^{2+}$ transfer and the maintenance of circulating $Ca^{2+}$ concentrations in the fetus (see page 541). It is present in very high concentrations in milk and may be involved in the development of tissues such as bone, cartilage and skin.

# PHOSPHATE HOMEOSTASIS

## Distribution of $PO_4$

An adult human contains approximately 600 g of phosphorus, 85 per cent of which is within the skeleton as the inorganic $PO_4$ component of hydroxyapatite. Less than 1 per cent of total body $PO_4$ is in the ECF predominantly as $HPO_4^{2-}$ at pH 7.4. About 10 per cent of plasma $PO_4$ is protein-bound, 35 per cent is complexed to $Na^+$, $Ca^{2+}$ or $Mg^{2+}$ and the balance is ionized. The remainder of body $PO_4$ is within soft tissues in forms such as nucleotides, phospholipids and the $PO_4$ esters involved in intermediary metabolism and intracellular energy transfer. The regulation of many intracellular proteins is mediated by phosphorylation. The transport of $PO_4$ ions across the plasma membrane and the membranes of intracellular organelles is passive, being determined by the movement of cations such as $Ca^{2+}$ (see Chapter 43 for further details).

There are fluxes of $PO_4$ into and out of bone and into and out of the soft tissues, the principal regulation of body $PO_4$ content being dependent upon the kidneys (see Chapter 43). The body responds to falling plasma $PO_4$ concentrations by stimulation of $1,25(OH)_2D$ synthesis in the kidney, an increase in $PO_4$ release from bone and a change in renal tubular reabsorption of $PO_4$ (the precise mechanism of which is unknown). The rise in $1,25(OH)_2D$ increases intestinal absorption of both $Ca^{2+}$ and $PO_4$ and may augment release of these minerals from bone. This results in a fall in PTH secretion which increases urinary $Ca^{2+}$ loss and diminishes phosphaturia. Thus, serum $PO_4$ concentrations are maintained without a change in serum $Ca^{2+}$ concentrations. In the face of rising serum $PO_4$ concentrations this sequence of events is reversed, the hyperphosphatemia leading to a small decrease in circulating $Ca^{2+}$ concentrations which, in turn, stimulates secretion of the phosphaturic substance, PTH.

## MICROANATOMY OF BONE

Bone consists of a protein matrix embedded in mineral (hydroxyapatite). It is maintained and remodeled by the three major cellular elements of bone, osteoblasts (bone-resorbing cells), osteoblasts (bone-forming cells), and osteocytes (inactive osteoblasts seen in mature bone). In addition to these three morphologically distinct cell types, bone has flat surface-lining cells and marrow cells which are thought to be functionally important. The osteoblast is a typical protein-synthesizing cell with a large Golgi apparatus and abundant rough endoplasmic reticulum. Osteoblasts synthesize and secrete type I collagen and also alkaline phosphatase which hydrolyzes pyrophosphate, an inhibitor of $Ca^{2+}$ phosphate crystal growth. When inactive, the osteoblast is thought to become an osteocyte on the surface or inside the bone where it may modulate $Ca^{2+}$ flux between bone and the ECF. The osteoclast is a multinucleated giant cell characterized by a ruffled border, which is a pleated segment of plasma membrane structurally analogous to the brush border of the intestine and kidney. The ruffled border is in contact with resorbing bone and is the site of carbonic anhydrase production responsible for the acid needed to facilitate crystal resorption. A selective deficiency of carbonic anhydrase II is associated histologically with a lack of ruffled borders in osteoclasts and results in osteopetrosis. Ninety per cent of the protein in bone is type I collagen, the balance being made up of a variety of non-collagenous proteins (e.g. osteocalcin) which may be involved in cell attachment and binding to

mineral, though their precise functions remain to be elucidated. The collagen fibers are usually packed in parallel bundles and set in a ground substance of glycoprotein and proteoglycans, which may also be important in the holding together of the various structural elements of bone.

In mature bone, collagen fibers are arranged parallel in layers. The orientation of the fibers alternates from layer to layer. This is known as lamellar bone. When bone is being formed rapidly (e.g. during fracture healing) the collagen fibers are arranged randomly, producing woven bone.

At a higher level of bone architecture, there are two different patterns of arrangement of lamellar bone. The lamellae can be arranged concentrically to form cylinders which are then packed together with no marrow space intervening. This dense form of bone, termed "compact bone," makes up the shafts of long bones. Bone can be arranged as a meshwork of horizontal and vertical trabeculae, with marrow space between. This is known as trabecular or cancellous bone and is seen at the ends of the long bones, in the vertebrae and in the ribs.

## REMODELING

In adult bone, formation and resorption take place in a stereotyped manner which is multifocal rather than diffuse. This remodeling serves to maintain the structural integrity of bone by replacing damaged protein fibers. It begins with osteoclastic bone resorption. The activated, multinucleated osteoclasts become sealed to the bone surface and secrete protons and acid proteases into the space between their cell membrane and bone. This results in the mobilization of mineral and the subsequent digestion of matrix protein. This phase proceeds until a resorption pit has been excavated on the bone surface. The osteoclasts are then replaced by osteoblasts which refill the resorption cavity with new matrix which is subsequently mineralized, forming concentric layers of lamellar bone. In maturity, the quantity of bone formed in this way equals that which has previously been resorbed, and bone mass is maintained. In senescence, there is a net loss of bone at each cycle. There is an enormous research effort at the present time to determine how the balance of formation and resorption within each remodeling unit is determined and also to understand the factors initiating remodeling at a given site on the skeletal surface. Because trabecular bone has a much greater surface-to-volume ratio than cortical bone, it responds more rapidly to diseases or therapies influencing bone mass.

## BONE GROWTH

During embryogenesis, bone tissue can be formed in two ways. Flat bones (e.g. clavicle, skull) are usually formed from an area of connective tissue in which mesenchymal cells differentiate directly into preosteoblasts, and then osteoblasts, with the subsequent formation of organic bone matrix (osteoid). Woven bone is formed which is subsequently remodeled (as described above) into lamellar bone. This process is known as intramembranous ossification.

Long bone development involves the initial formation of a cartilaginous model (endochondral ossification). A ring of woven bone then forms in the area that will become the mid-shaft of the long bone and blood vessels, preceded by osteoclasts, penetrate the central region to create a medullary cavity. The cartilage, which is left at either end of the bone, forms the growth plate, permitting longitudinal growth of the bone until puberty. At the distal (epiphyseal) end of the growth plate, chondrocytes proliferate lengthening the bone. Proximal to these cells, the cartilage becomes calcified. This calcified cartilage is partly resorbed by osteoclasts and subsequently replaced by woven bone. Moving more proximally from the growth plate, there is further remodeling (following the sequence described above) and the woven bone is replaced with lamellar bone.

## REGULATION OF BONE TURNOVER

The importance of PTH and $1,25(OH)_2D$ in regulating skeletal remodeling has already been referred to. Many other hormones, growth factors and cytokines also are involved. Estrogens and androgens have important effects on bone growth during puberty and the reduction in circulating estrogen concentrations at menopause plays a pivotal role in the development of postmenopausal osteoporosis. Estrogens may act by reducing production of osteolytic cytokines such as interleukin-6 from osteoblastic stromal cells. Glucocorticoids at supraphysiological concentrations reduce bone formation and increase resorption resulting in substantially reduced bone density. They also retard the linear growth of bone. Bone is a rich source of a number of growth factors: insulin-like growth factors (IGF)-I and -II, transforming growth factor β, the fibroblast growth factors and platelet-derived growth factor. Some of these are released from bone matrix during osteoclastic resorption and may mediate the coupling of bone formation to its resorption. In addition, systemic growth regulators such as insulin and growth hormone influence bone, the latter by way of local production of IGF-I (see page 312).

Bone cells are derived from precursors which develop in bone marrow, and trabecular bone is in intimate contact with the marrow. It is not surprising, therefore, that cytokines produced in marrow that regulate immune or hematological function also act on bone (e.g. interleukins-1, -6 and -11, leukemia inhibitory factor, tumor necrosis factor -α, the colony stimulating factors and interferon-γ). Local cytokine and growth factor production may be involved in the action of some hormones on bone as well as in the effects of inflammatory and neoplastic diseases on the skeleton. This is an area of active research at present and significant growth of knowledge in this area is expected.

## DISTURBANCES IN BONE HOMEOSTASIS

The most common disturbance of bone homeostasis is *osteoporosis*. This is most commonly a problem of old age and is intimately related to declining sex hormone concentrations at that time. Bone mass is stable in women until the perimenopause. A fall in estrogen concentrations is associated with increased bone resorption — the number of remodelling foci and the depth of the erosion cavities both increase in the absence of estrogen. Biochemical indices of bone formation also increase but not to a sufficient extent to compensate for the more rapid rate of bone removal. Bone is lost at a rate of several per cent per year for the first few years after the menopause. Subsequently the rate of loss decreases but loss continues until the end of life in most regions of the skeleton. In men, bone mass begins to decline in the 60s and continues thereafter. Whether this is related to the gradual decline in serum testosterone concentrations, which begins at this time, remains to be established. In both sexes, sex hormone replacement has beneficial effects on bone density, though this has been much more comprehensively studied in women than it has in men.

Osteoporosis can occur in children. *Idiopathic juvenile osteoporosis* is a rare condition characterized by increased bone turnover, and it often remits at puberty. Anti-resorptive therapies such as bisphosphonates have been used with apparent success in its management. The most common cause of osteoporosis in children, however, is the therapeutic use of *glucocorticoid drugs*, such as prednisone. These compounds result in decreased osteoblast activity, possible an increse in osteoclast uptake in the small intestine and renal tubules. This results in significant negative calcium balance and loss of bone mass and can result in fractures, particularly in trabecular-rich bones such as the vertebral bodies and ribs. Glucocorticoid-induced osteoporosis is best managed by minimization of glucocorticoid dose and the use of local (e.g. inhaled) steroids in preference to systematically administered drugs. In adults, bisphosphonates and calcitriol have shown efficacy in preventing steroid-induced osteoporosis.

In all forms of osteoporosis, the fundamental problem is a diminution in the amount of bone, that is, both matrix and mineral are reduced but the proportion of these two elements is normal. In contrast, *osteomalacia* is characterized by a disproportionate reduction in bone mineral, such that the amount of unmineralized matrix (osteoid) is increased above normal levels. Bone mineralization is dependent upon normal concentrations of calcium and phosphate ions in the extracellular fluid. Thus, osteomalacia can result from any condition which reduces the concentrations of one or other of these ions, and thus their product, worldwide, the commonest cause of *osteomalacia* is *vitamin D deficiency*, which results in malabsorption of both calcium and phosphate. There is no convincing evidence that vitamin D has a direct effect on mineralization other than through control of the concentrations of these two ions. In affluent societies the commonest cause of *osteomalacia is X-linked hypophosphatemia.* This inherited condition results in diminished renal tubular reabsorption of phosphate and, thus, hypophosphatemia. This leads to the characteristic skeletal deformities and linear growth retardation seen in other forms of *rickets.* However, it does not cause the muscle weakness which is seen in rickets attributable to *vitamin D deficiency.* It can be effectively managed with vitamin D metabolites and phosphate supplements. Other rarer causes of osteomalacia are inherited abnormalities of the vitamin D receptor and deficiency of the renal 1α-hydroxylase, which results in reduced levels of 1,25-dihydroxyvitamin D. Osteomalacia can also result from substances which are incorporated into bone and interfere with normal mineralization. This can result from the use of large doses of etidronate or fluoride and from the accumulation of aluminum, which sometimes occurs in patients with renal failure.

Bone disease is a significant complication of *chronic renal failure.* As renal function declines, phosphate excretion falls as does renal production of 1,25-dihydroxyvitamin D. In response to these two changes, secondary hyperparathyroidism develops. The hyperphosphatemia of renal failure can lead to calcium-phosphate deposition, particularly in blood vessels, eyes and skin, resulting sometimes in intense irritation at the latter two sites. Bone density is often reduced, though there can be osteosclerosis in the spine. Linear growth of bones is retarded and bone mineralization can be inhibited, particularly if bone aluminum levels are high as the result of either the use of a dialysate rich in aluminum or the ingestion of aluminum-containing antacids. Renal bone disease is managed by the use of oral calcium supplements to bind phosphate in the gut and thus reduce intestinal phosphate absorption, and the administration of active vitamin D metabolites to increase calcium absorption from the gut and suppress parathyroid hormone secretion.

## SELECTED READING

Favus, MJ ed. *Primer on the metabolic bone diseases and disorders of mineral metabolism.* Raven Press, New York, 1993.

# BONE REPAIR

Bone has a remarkable capacity to modulate its mass and structure in response to changing physical demands. This is epitomized by bone repair which is a process of organ regeneration, not one of scar formation.

## HISTOLOGY

Animal fracture healing models have provided much of our current knowledge on the histology of bone repair. Several distinct histological stages have been defined although these are arbitrary in that they may overlap in different areas of the fracture site. Studies of human tissue suggest that a similar sequence of events is seen in human fracture healing.

## Inflammatory stage

At the moment of injury, there is structural failure of the bone with tearing of adjacent soft tissues and disruption of local blood vessels. The periosteum is extremely resilient in children and strips from the shaft of the bone to some distance from the fracture site. Hemorrhage from endosteal blood vessels, the periosteum and the soft tissue vasculature leads to the formation of a hematoma at the fracture site. This hematoma is largest in fractures involving the shaft of the bone and is limited near the growth plate by the dense attachments of the periosteum in this area. The fracture hematoma contains prostaglandins and other inflammatory mediators, and has a low pH and low $Po_2$. Deprived of a blood supply, the ends of the broken bone become ischemic and undergo localized cell necrosis with release of lysosomal enzymes into the fracture hematoma.

Within the first 24 hours, macrophages, polymorphonuclear neutrophils and other inflammatory cells invade the hematoma organizing it into granulation tissue. At the same time, resorption of the dead bone ends is begun by osteoclasts derived from hematopoietic precursors in the bone marrow. This resorption is seen radiographically 10–14 days later as an apparent widening of the fracture gap. Capillaries from the surrounding soft tissues invade the area, possibly in response to an angiogenic factor secreted by macrophages. Soon the hematoma is organized into fibrovascular tissue containing a collagen matrix, fibroblasts and capillaries. Undifferentiated mesenchymal cells derived either from transformed endothelial cells in the medullary cavity or cells within the surrounding soft tissues begin to proliferate and increase the osteoprogenitor population. This process of expansion and commitment of previously undifferentiated cells is termed osteoinduction.

## Reparative stage

The juxtaposed dead bone ends do not contribute to the repair process. Instead, they act as a passive splint while peripheral connections are formed between separated regions of viable bone. These peripheral bony bridges act to stabilize but bypass the fracture ends. Blood flow to the fracture site peaks early in the reparative phase but, despite this, a state of relative hypoxia exists due to cellular proliferation. This hypoxic state is thought to be favorable for the formation of both cartilage and bone. Cells from the inner or cambial layer of the periosteum proliferate in the first 2 weeks following a fracture and form an external buttress of bone called periosteal callus. This process of direct bone formation without a cartilage intermediate is termed intramembranous ossification. Periosteal callus is particularly extensive in children due to the cellular nature of the periosteum.

## Formation of soft callus

Undifferentiated fibroblastic cells adjacent to the subperiosteal bone acquire a rounded shape and begin to synthesize an avascular basophilic matrix. This matrix is similar in appearance to the cartilaginous matrix in the proliferating zone of the growth plate. Small islands of cartilage first appear within the fracture gap and adjacent to the bone ends. These cartilaginous regions gradually enlarge as more mesenchymal cells differentiate into chondrocytes and eventually all the fibrous tissue is replaced by cartilage. This cartilaginous tissue is known as *soft callus*. Formation of soft callus, between 1–3 weeks after the fracture, is recognized clinically by the subsidence of the initial acute pain and swelling. At this stage, the callus is palpable, but not yet visible on radiograph. The fracture ends are no longer mobile, but soft callus has low resistance to bending forces and will deform with excessive loading.

## Formation of hard callus

The next stage is ossification of the soft callus, a process called endochondral ossification. The chondrocytes hypertrophy and then degenerate with calcification of the extracellular matrix. Capillaries from the adjacent bone invade the calcified matrix. Osteoblasts follow the capillary ingrowth and synthesize osteoid on the calcified cartilage, replacing the cartilage with woven bone, or *hard callus*. Woven bone has a loosely organized haphazard collagen structure and tends to be less dense than lamellar bone. At this point, the fracture ends are healed, but the bone will not recover full biomechanical strength for several months.

While this pathway of healing is most typical for the pediatric fracture treated by cast immobilization, different pathways of healing are seen in operated fractures. Stable fracture fixation by compression plating or external fixation leads to a reduction in interfragmentary movement to a point where cartilage formation does not occur. Instead, healing occurs by direct bony union with internal remodeling in the areas of immediate bony contact. Any gaps are filled by woven bone and later remodeled. This process is slow compared to endochondral ossification and can lead to delayed union and failure of the fixation device.

## Remodeling

This is the longest of the three stages and can theoretically continue until skeletal maturity. During this stage, the newly formed, randomly oriented woven bone is slowly converted into lamellar bone and the medullary canal is reconstituted. Mechanically unnecessary bone is actively reabsorbed by osteoclasts and trabecular bone is reoriented along the lines of stress across the healed bone. In the child, the normal processes of bone replacement and remodeling which occur during longitudinal and appositional growth contribute to the extensive remodeling seen following a fracture. Unlike the adult fracture, in which angular deformities will persist, residual angular deformity can also be corrected by physeal growth. This remodeling of residual angular deformity is most complete when the deformity is both close to a rapidly growing physis, and is in the plane of motion of the adjacent joint.

## BIOCHEMISTRY

The change from undifferentiated mesenchymal cell to cartilage to bone is paralleled by major changes in the expression of extracellular matrix proteins. The initial granulation tissue at the fracture site is rich in type III collagen. The importance of this is not known, however similar production of type III collagen is seen in embryonic limb development just prior to the onset of chondrogenesis. As the soft cartilaginous callus develops, there is increased expression of cartilage specific proteins, type II collagen and proteoglycan core protein. Mineralization of the extracellular matrix is associated with expression of type X collagen by the hypertrophied chondrocytes similar to that seen in the hypertrophic zone of the growth plate. With osteogenesis, there is a switch to the type I collagen found in bone.

Expression of the non-collagenous matrix proteins also varies as bone repair proceeds. Osteonectin, a phosphorylated glycoprotein with both high and low affinity binding sites for $Ca^{2+}$, is expressed in the soft callus by resting and proliferating chondrocytes and by active osteoblasts during both intramembranous and endochondral ossification. Osteonectin can bind both type I collagen and hydroxyapatite suggesting a role in organization of mineral within the newly formed extracellular matrix.

Gene expression of the osteoblastic markers, osteocalcin, osteopontin, and alkaline phosphatase peaks at the onset of mineralization. Osteopontin is a sialic acid-rich, phosphorylated glycoprotein normally present in bone and areas of cartilage to bone transition. The center of the protein contains an arginine–glycine–aspartic acid [RGD] sequence which is characteristically seen in cell binding proteins. Osteopontin is expressed during both intramembranous and endochondral ossification in fracture healing and may act to anchor osteoblasts and osteoclasts to the extracellular matrix.

Osteocalcin, a bone-specific protein present only in mature osteoblasts, is expressed in the hard callus during the later stages of endochondral ossification and bone remodeling but not at any time during intramembranous ossification or in the soft callus. Osteocalcin can bind $Ca^{2+}$ and hydroxyapatite, and may regulate the growth of hydroxyapatite crystals during mineralization. The late expression of osteocalcin in bone repair suggests a role in bone resorption and remodeling.

## MOLECULAR CONTROL OF BONE REPAIR

Multiple growth factors including insulin-like growth factors (IGF-I, IGF-II), transforming growth factor β (TGFβ), basic fibroblast growth factor (bFGF) and platelet derived growth factor (PDGF) are secreted by human bone cells, both in culture and in vivo. These growth factors are stored in the bone matrix and act as autocrine or paracrine regulators of cell proliferation, cell differentiation and matrix synthesis. The expression patterns of these growth factors in fracture healing and their possible functions are summarized in Table 44.2.

Of these factors, only bone morphogenetic proteins (BMPs) have the capacity to induce endochondral ossification in extraskeletal sites when implanted with carrier protein. BMPs are now thought to be the key signaling molecules that initiate cartilage and bone formation during embryonic development. It is speculated that they may also be the primary local factors initiating the cascade of bone formation in fracture repair. A deletion in the BMP 5 gene in mice has been associated

TABLE 44.2 Growth factors expressed during fracture healing

|  | EXPRESSION PATTERN | BIOLOGICAL FUNCTION | |
|---|---|---|---|
|  |  | In vitro | In vivo |
| TGFβ | ■ Released into the fracture hematoma by platelets within 24 hours. ■ Peak expression during soft callus formation. ■ Expression decreases as endochondral ossification occurs. | ■ Regulates chondrocyte proliferation and differentiation. ■ Stimulates osteoblast activity and synthesis of type I collagen. ■ Increases extracellular matrix deposition. | ■ Continuous installation into fracture callus delays calcification of fracture matrix. ■ Subperiosteal injection induces cartilage formation and subsequent endochondral ossification. |
| IGF-I and IGF-II | ■ Expressed in prehypertrophic chondrocytes and active osteoblasts. ■ IGF-II also expressed in proliferating mesenchymal cells and invading capillaries in granulation tissue. | ■ Stimulate replication of cells of osteoblastic lineage. ■ Up-regulate type I collagen synthesis by osteoblasts. | ■ Function not known, may be important in bone remodeling. |
| BMP | ■ Only BMP 4 characterized. ■ Transient expression of BMP 4, 12–72 hours after fracture in proliferating periosteum, medullary cavity and muscles near fracture site. | ■ Chemotactic for monocytes. ■ Stimulates chondrogenesis. ■ Promotes and maintains osteogenic phenotype. | ■ Induces ectopic cartilage and bone formation at extraskeletal sites when injected with carrier protein. |
| bFGF | ■ Expressed early in granulation tissue. ■ Synthesized by chondrocytes and osteoblasts throughout healing process. | ■ Stimulates mesenchymal cell proliferation. ■ Stimulates chondrogenesis. ■ Enhances TGFβ expression in osteoblasts. | ■ Injection at fracture site increases volume and mineral content of callus. |
| PDGF | ■ Released by platelets into fracture hematoma. ■ Synthesized by macrophages in inflammatory stage. | ■ Chemotactic for neutrophils and monocytes. ■ Stimulates bone DNA and protein synthesis but also stimulates bone resorption via prostaglandin pathway. ■ Potent mitogen for mesenchymal cells. | ■ Subperiosteal injection induces intramembranous bone formation. ■ Installation into osteotomy site enhances osteogenic differentiation. |

TGFβ, transforming growth factor β; IGF, insulin-like growth factor; BMP, bone morphogenetic protein; bFGF, basic fibroblast growth factor; PDGF, platelet-derived growth factor.

with reduced callus formation during fracture healing while topical application of BMP 2 can stimulate bone healing in animal fracture non-union models.

BMP 3 and BMP 4 are strongly bound by type IV collagen at physiological levels. This suggests that type IV collagen, which is found on the basement membrane of invading capillaries, may play a role in concentrating and orientating local BMPs in the initial fracture hematoma. BMPs have a high degree of homology within the C-terminal 7-cysteine domain, a characteristic that they share with other members of the TGFβ superfamily. It is speculated that dimerization could occur between the members of the BMP family at this domain explaining the multitude of effects seen in cell and tissue culture.

Mechanical and positional information are also important in bone repair. The end of the bone in a recently amputated limb shows only a limited callus response with early resorption, suggesting that positional signals are required from the opposite end of the fractured bone to continue the callus formation. The nature of these signals is unknown. Early functional weight bearing has been shown to accelerate human fracture healing. Similarly, in animal fracture models, controlled cyclical loading can increase the rate of healing, although variables such as size of fracture gap, magnitude of load, frequency and duration are important. In vitro, osteoblasts respond to cyclical loading by increased cellular proliferation and decreased production of collagen and other non-collagenous matrix proteins. In vivo, mechanical loading of the intact rodent tibia leads to increased transcription of the proto-oncogene c-fos, TGFβ and IGF-I in the periosteum within 4 hours, with concomitant down-regulation of the osteoblastic markers, osteocalcin, osteopontin and alkaline phosphatase. All these findings suggest that mechanical stresses across a fractured bone can be transduced into a coordinated osteogenic response with increased cellular proliferation and production of local growth factors.

## SELECTED READING

Baylink DJ, Finkelman RD, Mohan S. Growth factors to stimulate bone formation. J Bone Min Res 1993; 8: S565.

Cornell CN and Lane JM. Newest factors in fracture healing. Clin Orthop Rel Res 1992; 277: 297.

Elima K. Osteoinductive proteins. Ann Med 1993; 25: 395.

Goodman S, Aspenberg P. Effects of mechanical stimulation on the differentiation of hard tissues. Biomaterials 1993; 14: 563.

McKibbin B. The biology of fracture healing in long bones. J Bone Joint Surg 1978; 60B: 150.

Rosen V, Thies RS. The BMP proteins in bone formation and repair. Trends Genet 1992; 8: 97.

Sandberg MM, Aro HT, Vuorio EI. Gene expression during bone repair. Clin Orthop Rel Res 1993; 289: 292.

Turner CH. Functional determinants of bone structure: Beyond Wolff's law of bone transformation. Bone 1992; 13: 403.

# 45

# Connective Tissues in Development

Stephen J.M. Skinner and Ingrid Winship

## DEVELOPMENTAL BIOLOGY OF CONNECTIVE TISSUE COMPONENTS

(see also Chapters 17 and 18)

Connective tissues are often seen by developmental biologists as the external framework or matrices which provide cells with a solid–liquid gel environment. The different components of the extracellular matrix (ECM) provide the cells of the embryo with cell surface recognition signals which allows them to determine polarity (epithelia), to migrate (neural crest, hematopoietic cells), to grow extensions (neurites) to proliferate or to remain quiescent. The early embryo uses no rigid structures, needing a gel-like environment which allows both rapid expansion of cell mass and plasticity. The rugged fibrous and bony structures are mostly developed after birth and are required for movement and load bearing. However, the mechanical properties of connective tissues become critical after birth, particularly in the requirement for a rib cage which will support the muscular activity of breathing. Many mammals practice movements in utero which will be essential ex utero, and thus the bones which support and resist muscular activity must become relatively rigid even before birth.

Perhaps the first interaction of the embryo with connective tissues is destructive, the conceptus producing factors which induce breakdown of collagens and proteoglycans in the uterine wall, allowing implantation. This plasticity in connective tissues, with intense degradation and synthesis, allows rapid remodeling during normal development and after trauma. The physical barriers which protect the still fragile fetus from outside insults, the fetal membranes and placenta, are very tough structures, rich in collagens and proteoglycans.

Failure in any aspect of connective tissue biosynthesis, due to genetic deletion or mutation, can lead to structural deformation or impaired function. But also, because there is such a comprehensive overlap in the functional properties of connective tissue components, deletion of a single gene product may have no apparent effect. This is perhaps not too surprising when considering that there are multiple gene products for the collagen group of proteins alone.

## CONNECTIVE TISSUE COMPONENTS

### Collagen

The multigene collagen protein family has more than 25 members in 12 chromosomes (Table 45.1). They are composed of trimers of protein chains with approximately 1000 amino acids containing repeats of the sequence GLY(X-Y). Thus GLY constitutes about one-third while PRO (often in the X position) or 4-hydroxy-PRO (often in the Y position), which also are major constituents, comprise about 10 per cent each of all the amino acids.

The fibrillar collagens, collagens I–III (and V and XI) are rod-like fibrillar proteins composed of three molecules coiled in an α-helix (Fig. 45.1). The protein chains, because of all the glycine and proline in the primary structure, are very tightly coiled. Substitution of glycine by site-directed mutagenesis can disrupt the

TABLE 45.1 Table of collagens

| TYPE | COLLAGEN GENES | CHROMOSOME | DISTRIBUTION LOCUS | DISORDER |
|---|---|---|---|---|
| I | COL1A1 | 17q21,31–q22.05 | Bone, skin, tendon, cornea, sclera | OI, EDS VIIA |
|  | COL1A2 | 7q22.1 |  | OI type IV, EDS VIIB |
| II | COL2A1 | 12q 15.11q13.2 | Cartilage | SED congenita, Stickler syndrome, Kniest syndrome, achondrogenesis |
| III | COL3A1 | 2q31–32.3 | Arteries | EDS IV, arterial aneurysms |
| IV | COL4A1 | 13q34 | Basement membrane |  |
|  | COL4A2 | 13q34 |  |  |
|  | COL4A3 | 13q34 |  |  |
|  | COL4A4 | 13q34 |  |  |
|  | COL4A5 | X |  |  |
| V | COL5A2 | 2q31–32.3 |  |  |
| VI | COL6A1 | 21q | Microfibrillar network in ECM of virtually all tissues |  |
|  | COL6A2 | 21q |  |  |
|  | COL6A3 | 6 | Contains 6 repeats of a WF domain |  |
| VII | COL7A1 | 3p21.3 | Dermoepidermal junction | Epidermolysis bullosa (recessive dystrophic) |
| VIII | COL8A1 | 3 | Descemet membrane, corneal epithelium and stroma |  |
|  | COL8A2 | 1 |  |  |
| IX |  |  | Expressed in concert with type II collagen | Cartilage, vitreous humor |
| X |  |  |  |  |
| XI | COL11A1 | 1 | Cartilage |  |
|  | COL11A2 | 6p22 | Cartilage |  |
| XII | COL12A1 |  | Cartilage |  |
| XIV | COL14A1 |  | Cartilage |  |

OI, osteogenis imperfecta; EDS, Ehlers–Danlos syndrome; ECM, extracellular matrix; WF, von Willebrand factor.
The blank spaces in this table no doubt will be filled in by new discoveries. It will be interesting to see which are filled in by the next edition of this book.

coiling ability and cause bone problems (*osteogenesis imperfecta*). The presence of 4-hydroxy-PRO is required for thermal stability. Vitamin C deficiency leads to poor hydroxylation of proline, and collagen can then denature at relatively low temperatures (less than 30°C), whereas the fully hydroxylated form is stable up to 42°C.

The triple helices are held together by hydrogen-bonds and also have intra-molecular cross-links between certain lysines (Fig. 45.2). Other lysyl cross-links are required to link adjacent triple helices. These are essential to form the tri-molecular fibrillar structures in a tension-resisting network. The triple helices are attached to each other in a staggered pattern and are themselves coiled, the networks rolled into rope-like structures which resist tension.

The non-fibrillar collagens are those of basement membrane (type IV), the fibril-associated collagens (types IX, XII and XIV), filament producing collagen (collagen of microfibrils, type VI), network-forming collagens (types VIII and X) and long chain anchoring fibril collagen (type VII). There are also collagenous sequences (GLY-X-Y repeats) in other proteins (lung surfactant apoprotein and the complement component, C1q).

## Collagen synthesis and experimental pathology

The single chains are initially synthesized as preprocollagens. Partial proteolytic cleavage of the globular domains is required to allow the three procollagen chains to correctly associate before α-helix formation (Fig 45.1). The associated globular domains of procollagens hold the three chains in register during proline hydroxylation, and thus allow the three chains to form a stable α-helix. The final coiled native structure is protease resistant and is cleaved only by specific collagenases which slice through all three strands at a specific point. About 10 per cent of most newly-synthesized collagen chains are degraded intracellularly. This is probably because of mistakes in the primary structure or inefficiencies in proline hydroxylation which prevent triple helix formation or lower the denaturation temperature to below 37°C.

Expression of a mutated human procollagen $\alpha_1(I)$ transgene in mice gives rise to a lethal phenotype of fragile bones, used as a model for osteogenesis imperfecta. In normal bone the collagen network and associated molecules hold together the dense accretions of

Chain association and hydroxylation

Triple helix formation

SECRETION

Propeptide cleavage

Assembly and cross-linking of fibrils

FIGURE 45.1 Formation of the collagen fibril networks. The collagen polypeptides are hydroxylated mostly during synthesis on the ribosome (cotranslational modification) and aligned for helix formation by peptide recognition sites on their carboxy terminal (C-terminal) regions. Helix formation proceeds with coiling in the C-to-N direction, and folding is disrupted if glycine is not correctly spaced on every third residue. Sequence mistakes (as in OI) result in poorly aligned chains that do not function properly; most are degraded by proteases before secretion. When properly coiled, the triple helices are secreted and the N- and C-propeptides cleaved off in the extracellular environment before assembly into the "quarter stagger" array and cross-linking into a fibrillar network.

hydroxyapatite. The mutated procollagen $\alpha_1(I)$ couples with the normal mouse $\alpha_1(I)$ and $\alpha_2(I)$ procollagens, producing a type I collagen triple helix which is very poorly aligned and easily subject to denaturation and proteolysis. Thus, the normal collagen synthesis is overwhelmed and rendered nonfunctional by incorporation of the defective strand. The disorder can be "cured" by transfecting with another gene containing antisense coding for human-specific sequences of $\alpha_1(I)$. Expression of the antisense gene gives short sequences of antisense mRNA which complex with the defective human $\alpha_1(I)$ mRNA and prevent the synthesis of the defective protein. The normal mouse type I collagen is then assembled correctly. A similar experimental approach with type II collagen destruction resulted in chondrodysplastic mice with a high incidence of neonatal death. The type I and type II collagens are generally expressed in a mutually exclusive manner. Some of the minor fibrillar collagens are predominantly associated with one or other of the major forms.

The collagens of the basement membrane (types IV and VII) provide a mesh, often described as "felt-like," which supports epithelial and endothelial cells, and separates them from the mesenchymal or stromal compartment.

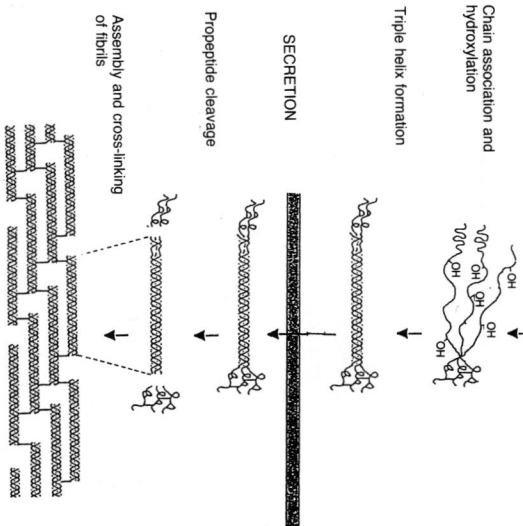

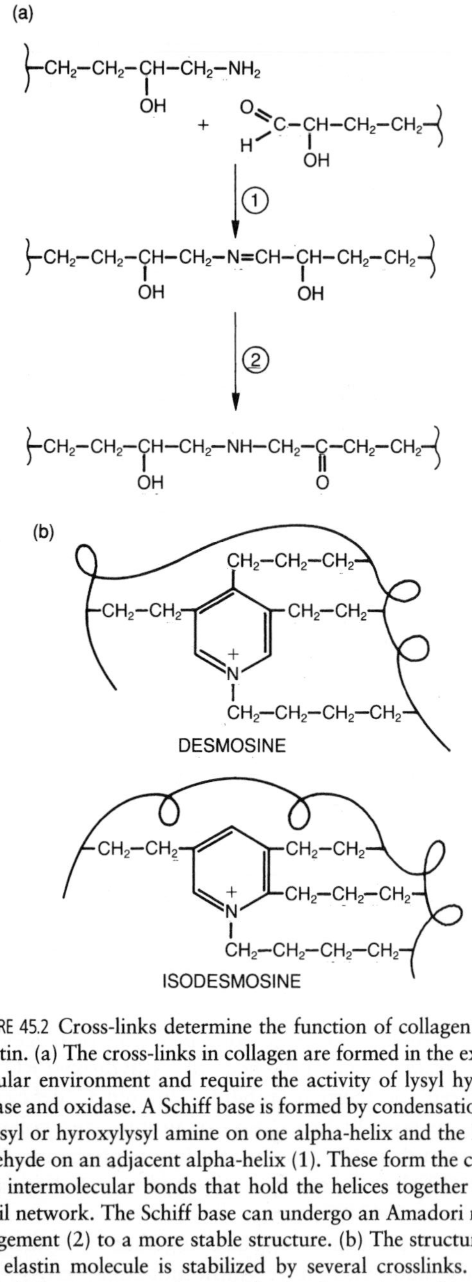

(a)

$\{CH_2-CH_2-CH-CH_2-NH_2$
$\quad\quad\quad\quad OH$
+
$O=C-CH_2-CH_2\}$
$H \quad OH$

①→

$\{CH_2-CH_2-CH-CH_2-N\equiv CH-CH-CH_2-CH_2\}$
$\quad\quad\quad OH \quad\quad\quad\quad OH$

②→

$\{CH_2-CH_2-CH-CH_2-NH-CH_2-C-CH_2-CH_2\}$
$\quad\quad\quad OH \quad\quad\quad\quad\quad O$

(b)

DESMOSINE

ISODESMOSINE

FIGURE 45.2 Cross-links determine the function of collagen and elastin. (a) The cross-links in collagen are formed in the extracellular environment and require the activity of lysyl hydroxylase and oxidase. A Schiff base is formed by condensation of a lysyl or hyroxylysyl amine on one alpha-helix and the lysyl aldehyde on an adjacent alpha-helix (1). These form the covalent intermolecular bonds that hold the helices together in a fibril network. The Schiff base can undergo an Amadori rearrangement (2) to a more stable structure. (b) The structure of the elastin molecule is stabilized by several crosslinks. The cross-link structures unique to elastin, desmosine and isodesmosine, are shown here with their four attachment sites in the coiled, hydrophobic protein. Each of these attachment sites was originally a lysine.

## Elastin

The structural characteristics of elastin (hydrophobic and cross-linked) allow tensile energy to be stored very efficiently, thus ensuring almost perfect recoil properties. Any genetic mutation or pathology compromising this optimum structure has a profound effect on elastin function. The highest concentration of elastin is found in the nuchal ligaments which act as suspensory cords to hold up the head of most four-legged mammals. The elastic cord preserves energy, which is stored in the stretched ligament when the neck muscles pull the head down, as in grazing. The clinical importance of elastin in man is seen in the elastic laminae of arteries and in the recoil properties of elastin in inflated lung and stretched skin.

Tropoelastin is synthesized as a linear protein which contains a high proportion of glycine and hydrophobic amino acids such as valine, the basic amino acid lysine, which is destined to form cross-links, and prolines which will in part (7–16 per cent) become hydroxylated. Many of the lysines in elastin are converted by oxidation and condensation into the unique cross-links desmosine and isodesmosine (Fig. 45.2), which stabilize the coiled hydrophobic structure and ensure its ability to store tensional energy in the stretched state. In lysyl oxidase deficiency or in copper-deficient animals the characteristic dermatosparaxis is seen because the cross-links cannot be formed. In severe forms blood vessels are prone to aneurysm.

The turnover of mature elastin is determined by a balance between proteolytic enzymes (elastases) and inhibitors such as $\alpha_1$-antitrypsin and $\alpha_2$-macroglobulin. In *emphysema*, especially the inherited forms, the inhibitory activity of $\alpha_1$-antitrypsin is absent or compromised, and the tethering of small airways to the connective tissues is eroded due to inadequate inhibition of elastases.

## Fibrillin

Fibrillin (mass 30 kD) is the best characterized protein of the microfibrillar array which is essential, together with elastin, in elastic fibers. It is synthesized as a precursor, glycosylated within the cell and secreted into the extracellular matrix and stabilized by intermolecular disulfide bonds. Two fibrillin classes exist. The gene coding for fibrillin 1 (*FBN1*) is on chromosome 15 (15q21.1). The gene responsible for fibrillin 2 has been mapped to chromosome 5; its gene product is highly homologous to fibrillin 1. A defect in the fibrillin 1 gene results in *Marfan syndrome*. A notable complication of this syndrome is spontaneous arterial rupture. Defects of fibrillin 2 have been linked to *congenital contractural arachnodactyly* (*Beals syndrome*).

## Proteoglycans

The terminology used for proteoglycans and their structures derives from early analytical procedures and can be confusing. The linear, negatively charged carbohydrate chains, or glycosaminoglycans (GAGs), were analyzed as chondroitin sulfates (CS), dermatan sulfates (DS), heparan sulfates (HS), keratan sulfates (KS) and hyaluronan (HA). All, except HA, are usually found attached covalently to protein, known as the proteoglycan core proteins. They are now described and characterized as proteoglycans and their aggregates, as shown in Fig. 45.3.

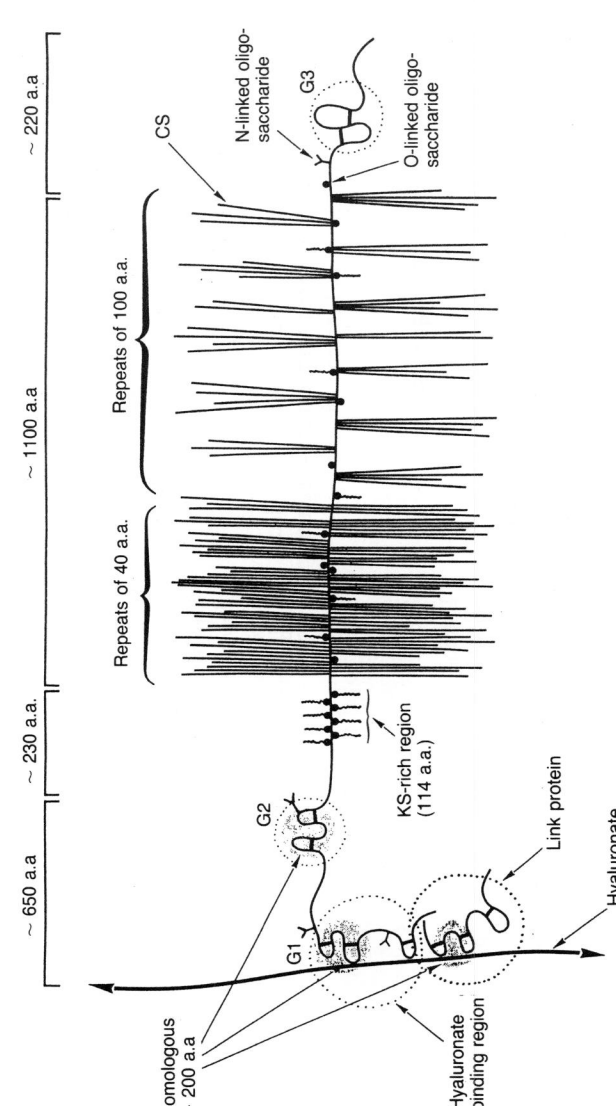

FIGURE 45.3 Proteoglycan structure. The serine hydroxyl groups on the protein core are attached through xylose sugar residues to the GAG side chains. The negatively charged GAG side chains repel one another and acquire counter ions ($Na^+$), thus acquiring the highly hydrated "bottle brush" shape depicted here. The extracellular proteoglycans form complexes with hyaluronan (HA) and the small "link" protein via the basic amino acid clusters in the proteins, which bind specifically to acidic groups in the HA.

There are two major functional classes of proteoglycans. The ECM forms proteoglycans that diffuse freely, depending on their environment, whereas the cell-surface proteoglycans are attached through the cell membrane via transmembrane domains. An example is β-glycan.

There are a bewildering array of proteoglycans which range in size from the large CS-proteoglycan, aggrecan, which forms massive aggregates with HA in cartilage, down to the non-aggregating small PGs found in ovarian follicular fluid.

Their common characteristic is a protein core on which the serine hydroxyl groups are attached through xylose sugar residues to the GAG chains CS, DS, HS, KS. The GAG chains on any proteoglycan often, but not always, are of a similar number of saccharide units. The classic cartilage proteoglycan, aggrecan, forms complexes with the "link protein" and large HA molecules, giving rise to aggregates which are up to $10^8$ Da in mass. The space occupancy of proteoglycans is massive since their high negative charge allows them to sequester counter-ions ($Na^+$) and aqueous fluid. The negative charge allows binding of positively charged amino acid clusters on certain proteins and peptides (see Chapter 17). Aggrecan and link protein also have amino acid motifs which enable specific binding with HA.

Decorin and biglycan appear to have similar functions and are major CS and DS proteoglycans in the extracellular space. They are associated with collagen fibrils in skin and other connective tissues. Biglycan is coded for by a gene on the X chromosome (Xq13qter) and decorin on chromosome 12 (12p12.1). Their function is to interact with type I collagen to affect fibrillogenesis and to alter cell matrix interactions by cell binding to fibronectin.

Aggrecan is the main proteoglycan in cartilage, containing CS and lesser amounts of KS. A common skeletal problem in chickens, nanomelia, has recently been found to be due to mutations in the aggrecan gene. Similarly, a cartilage matrix deficiency seen in mice is caused by an autosomal recessive 7bp deletion in exon 5 of the aggrecan DNA sequence. Apart from skeletal problems, defective aggrecans can cause structural anomalies in the cochlea and thereby *hearing loss*.

## Independent functions for hyaluronan in development

Hyaluronan also acts on cells through specific receptors and stimulates tyrosine kinase activity. One receptor was found to be identical to the lymphocyte cell surface protein, CD44, which also interacts with fibronectin and collagens (see also integrin receptors, the cytoskeleton and FAK, page 69). Later studies have found a group of receptors in human and animal cells (RHAMM – receptors for hyaluronic acid mediated motility) which has the basic amino acid cluster (-B-X₇-B-) as part of its structure. As the name suggests, RHAMM mediates cell locomotion (sperm and T cells), the invasiveness of tumor cells, the outgrowth of neurites from neurons and the tissue penetration of neuronal growth cones (see also netrins and collapsins, page 358). The tracts of hyaluronan in developing tissues have been viewed for many years as highways for migrating cells. That concept now has added validity with the clear description of the hyaluronan receptors which can sense the hyaluronan in the environment and transduce the signal into tyrosine kinase activity.

## BRANCHING MORPHOGENESIS

In the lung, kidney, mammary and salivary glands, the ultimate structure of the organ is determined by the accumulated episodes of branching morphogenesis. These are dependent on epithelial–mesenchymal interactions (see also basic fibroblast growth factor (bFGF) and FGFr, page 280). Interference with proteoglycan or hyaluronan synthesis, or their degradation by enzymes *in vitro*, blocks branching morphogenesis in these organs. In the process of branching, the GAGs and collagen in defined zones of the basement membrane and mesenchyme adjacent to dividing epithelial cells undergo rapid metabolism, but only a few micrometers away, in the clefts where epithelial cells are quiescent, GAGs and collagen are stable and accumulate (Fig. 45.4). Prevention of the synthesis of specific proteoglycans, such as syndecan which has HS and CS chains attached to the core protein, results in a loss of the epithelial phenotype and fibroblastic behavior (complete deprivation of ECM causes epithelial apoptosis or anoikis). Similarly, the condensation of the mesenchyme in the developing limb bud occurs with loss of the hyaluronan-filled spaces between the cells in the chondrogenic and myogenic regions (see also Chapter 44).

Hereditary diseases encompassing abnormalities involving these processes include *mucopolysaccharidoses*, where there is an inability to degrade GAGs which accumulate in lysosomes in sensitive tissues such as the brain.

## MATRIX GLYCOPROTEINS AND THE INTEGRIN RECEPTORS (*see also* Chapter 2)

Laminin is a basement membrane glycoprotein composed of three chains, A (α), B1 (β) and B2 (δ). These are 400kD, 210kD and 200kD, respectively. The three laminin chains combine to form a cruciate structure and can bind a number of other macromolecules (e.g. cell surface proteins, heparin, collagen, nidogen). Laminins play a role in mediating cell adhesion and migration and the structure of the basal lamina. The genes for these chains are located on chromosomes 18p11.3, 7q22, 1q3.1, respectively.

Two related basement membrane (BM) glycoproteins have been identified as functional adhesion com-

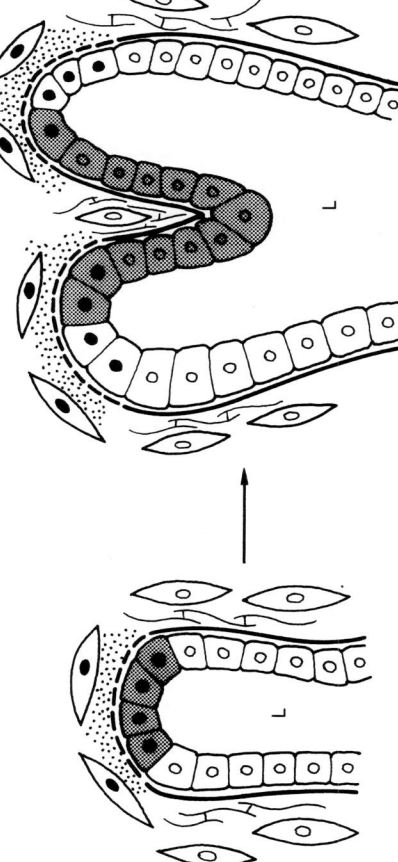

FIGURE 45.4 Matrix and cell biology in branching morphogenesis. The turnover of matrix and basement membrane collagens and proteoglycans (dots) is greatest at the tip of the epithelial bud, allowing plasticity in the matrix for rapid cell growth. The breakdown here is by proteinases, collagenases, and GAGases secreted by the activated mesenchymal cells (dark nuclei). This is also the region of greatest mitotic rate in the epithelia (dark nuclei, shaded) such that the increased cell numbers not only move outward, but also push into the lumen (L), forming a septum or barrier (shaded cells) and increasing the surface area available for secretion or absorption. The septal epithelia derived from the original bud tip (shaded) lose the growth drive. The matrix breakdown in the cleft slows down, and the septal matrix stabilizes, but the epithelia (dark nuclei) now at the tip of the new buds, encounter signals for more growth from the adjacent mesenchymal cells, and the matrix at the tips is again more rapidly degraded. Thus, another cycle of bud formation occurs in the process of branching morphogenesis. Removing the mesenchymal cells, the source of matrix degrading enzymes (and growth factors), or interfering with matrix turnover can block these activities.

ponents of hemidesmosomes. Epiligrin is a BM ligand for basal cell adhesion via integrins $\alpha_3\beta_1$ in focal adhesions and $\alpha_6\beta_4$ in hemidesmosomes. Certain integrin mutations are lethal. An $\alpha_5$-integrin gene null mutation in mice causes defects in mesodermal structures by day E9 and is lethal by day 11 of gestation. Kalinin is an adhesive ligand and is a component of anchoring filaments. Epiligrin, kalinin and nicein have some homology with laminin. Abnormal interactions between these glycoproteins and integrin play a role in the pathogenesis of lethal junctional *epidermolysis bullosa*.

Fibronectin is an ubiquitous adhesive glycoprotein comprising two chains of 250 kD. Fibronectin is involved in cell adhesion, determination of cell morphology and migration. Fibronectin-deficient embryos can implant and gastrulate, but the embryos are shortened with deformed neural tubes and severe defects which are probably caused by disturbed mesodermal activity during development. The serum forms of fibronectin, and the related vitronectin, may have an antithrombolytic function.

There are many other glycoproteins, including nidogen, entactin, versican, biglycan, and a significant proportion of the collagens (up to 25 per cent are glycosylated). Most interact with cell surface receptors such as the integrins and also have specific binding sites (e.g. arg-gly-asp (RGD) sequences) for other matrix molecules.

The behavior of the cells is determined by the matrix, and part of that behavior is the generation of more matrix. Perturbations in matrix or cell behavior caused by trauma or disease, or simply the process of achieving a new differentiation state, can change the relationships which determine the character and quantity of matrix molecules produced.

## SUMMARY

The extracellular matrix molecules provide the three-dimensional structure which is continually regenerated by the cells of the organism. Their magnitude and complexity of interaction are overwhelming. The potential for understanding and applying three-dimensional concepts to human development and pathology, coupled with new information about gene regulation is likely to have increasing application. Many connective tissue disease phenotypes are now defined as the consequence of specific mutations. Further expansion of this knowledge base will provide the means for diagnosis, understanding and therapeutic manipulation of such disorders.

## SELECTED READING

Bateman JF, Lamande SR, Hannagan M *et al.* Chemical cleavage method for the detection of mRNA base changes: experience in the application to collagen mutations in osteogenesis imperfecta. *Am J Med Genet* 1993; **45**: 233.

Byers PH. Molecular genetics of chondrodysplasias, including clues to development, structure and function. *Curr Opin Rheumatol* 1994; **6**: 345.

Hynes RO. Genetic analyses of cell–matrix interactions in development. *Curr Opin Gen Dev* 1993; **4**: 5694.

Turley EA (1992) Hyaluronan and cell locomotion. *Cancer–Metastasis Rev* 1992; **11**: 21.

# 46

# The Skin

Nicholas M. Birchall

The skin is the largest organ of the human body; in the average adult it exceeds 2 m² in area yet in most places it is no more than 2 mm thick. Despite its thinness, its mass exceeds that of all other organs. The skin forms a sheet-like integument contouring and conforming to the movement of the organism within. The skin has several important properties. It provides a physical barrier between the organism and the environment. It contains a vasculature and sweating system adapted to normal regulatory demands. It has a neuroreceptor network to relay environmental information. It is a highly sophisticated component of the peripheral immune system. It has psychosocial and sexual functions.

The skin is a complex, multicellular organ in which the endoderm, neural crest and ectoderm contribute to form a three dimensional unit in a spatially and temporally defined manner. Homeobox genes (*HOX*), which encode information critical for normal embryological development in many organisms (*see page 266*), probably also act as the master genes coordinating the three-dimensional organization of the skin; however their exact role in skin development is still undefined.

Apoptosis, the active, gene directed, pathway of cell self-destruction (see Chapter 2), has been recognized in adult human skin. It would appear logical that it also is involved in fetal skin development and early evidence supports this concept. The idea that programmed cell death occurs during organogenesis is not new, having been recognized for many years. Because cell death was considered a pathological event, the biological significance of physiological cell death previously has been underestimated. It is probable that apoptotic events are involved in development of the epidermis and its appendages, maintenance of homeostasis in the mature epidermis, and in prevention or onset of disease.

## ADULT SKIN

In adult skin the stratum corneum is the outermost layer. It functions to protect the skin from external invasion and prevents the loss of internal fluids. To

date the signals responsible for commitment of basal cells to a particular program of differentiation and the mechanisms involved in establishing tissue shape and size are unknown. Adult keratinocytes are the progeny of basal cells. As keratinocytes proliferate they go through a pattern of differentiation with eventual formation of squamous cells, granular cells, and finally, cells of the stratum corneum as they ascend towards the skin surface. The state of keratinocyte differentiation can be measured by the position of the cell within the epidermal strata, its mitotic potential, surface antigens, enzyme systems, the presence of specific structural proteins and lipids, distinctive cytoplasmic organelles (e.g. keratohyalin granules, lamellar granules) and morphology.

## FETAL SKIN

The establishment of the epidermis and dermis occurs in the first 12 weeks of embryonic life; the dermis lags behind the epidermis in reaching its definitive state. By the end of the second trimester the epidermis is a keratinized, stratified squamous epithelium which includes all of the immigrant cell types and has formed the adnexal structures. The dermis on the other hand at the same stage is less than half its full thickness, lacking certain fibrous components.

## Epidermal growth and regional variation

Epidermal growth, as defined by an increase in thickness and number of cell layers has been found to occur in three stages: a growth spurt between 5–13 weeks' gestation; a plateau between 13–21 weeks; and a second increase in thickness after 21 weeks. The first stage coincides with organogenesis and little growth in the size of the embryo-fetus. During the period of rapid growth of the body (second trimester), the epidermis maintains an approximately constant thickness even though additional cell layers are added. There is considerable regional variation in the rate at which

TABLE 46.1 Comparison of the features of premature newborn, term newborn and adult skin

| | PREMATURE | TERM | ADULT |
|---|---|---|---|
| Full-thickness skin | 0.9 mm | 1.2 mm | 2.1 mm |
| Epidermal surface | Vernix ("gelatinous") | Vernix | Dry |
| Epidermal thickness | 25 µm | ~40–50 µm | ~50 µm |
| Stratum corneum thickness | 5–6 cell layers | 15+ cell layers | 15+ cell layers |
| Spinous cell content | Glycogen | Little glycogen | No glycogen |
| Melanocytes | Few melanosomes | Similar to young adult; low melanin production | Numbers decrease with age; melanin production |
| Dermal–epidermal junction | No significant differences | | |
| Dermis | Changes not marked | | |

HUMAN EPIDERMAL DEVELOPMENT

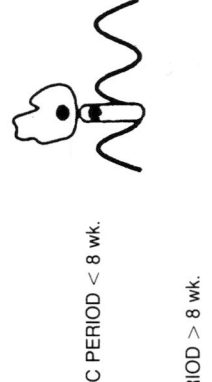

EMBRYONIC PERIOD < 8 wk.

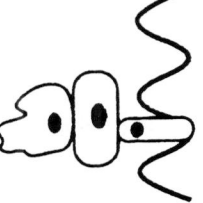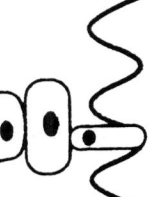

FETAL PERIOD > 8 wk.

EPIDERMAL STRATIFICATION 9–14 wk.

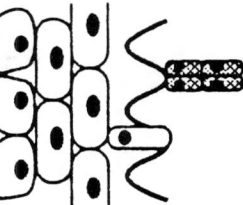

FOLLICULAR KERATINIZATION 14–24 wk.

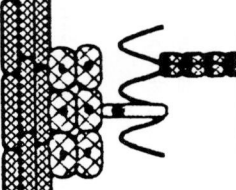

INTERFOLLICULAR KERATINIZATION > 24 wk.

FIGURE 46.1 Schematic diagram of the sequence of human fetal epidermal development. (From Lane AT. Human fetal skin development. *Pediatr Dermatol* 1986; 3: 487. Reproduced with permission.)

these changes occur. During the first trimester, development proceeds simultaneously in all regions except for the palmar and plantar epidermis where it is accelerated; in the second trimester the interfollicular epidermis of both the head and the palmar and plantar surfaces differentiates ahead of that of the remainder of the body. In spite of these regionally specific influences the skin is remarkably similar in ontogenetic pattern and ultimate end product. The differences that do exist reflect primarily the rate or density at which a given structure forms, not the final, fundamental organization of the tissues.

The primitive epidermis is established at 7–8 days when ectoderm and endoderm are defined in the inner cell mass of the implanted blastocyst. At this stage the epidermis is a single-layered "indifferent ectoderm."

Four weeks after conception, human fetal skin is composed of periderm and a basal cell layer. The periderm continues to overlay the fetal epidermis until the period of interfollicular keratinization. With time, an intermediate cell layer develops and begins to stratify between the periderm and basal cells. With continued development, the basal cell layer develops buds, which are the primitive cells of appendage organ development. These buds eventually invaginate into the dermis yielding the peridermal appendages of hair follicles and sebaceous, apocrine, and eccrine glands. Before the time of interfollicular keratinization the epidermis may be less than 70 µm thick. A schema of fetal skin development is shown in Fig. 46.1.

## Periderm

The periderm is the transient, protective covering of the epidermis that is sloughed into the amniotic fluid as soon as differentiation of the underlying epidermal layers is complete. The periderm of the embryo is made up of a pavement epithelium of small polygonal cells, about which little is known, that are modified at the amniotic surface by microvilli and a glycocalyx. The periderm follows a sequence of development with the eventual presence of multiple blebs and microvilli projecting off the surface. The microscopic appearance of the cells suggests a function in secretion or absorption. The source of periderm is not currently known. In the 9-day old developing fetus, the amnio-

this time the cells of the amnion abut the peripheral cells of the epidermis. One week later the epidermis consists of periderm and basal cells. Through the rest of gestation, until it is sloughed off, the periderm remains a solitary layer.

The high glycogen content of fetal epidermis prior to the loss of periderm suggests that the periderm cell may be very important in the early nutrition of the developing fetus. Perhaps absorption of nutrients through the fetal skin is a significant source of nutrition for the early fetus.

### Basement membrane zone

The basement membrane zone (BMZ) that separates the epidermis from the dermis is important in fetal skin development. The BMZ consists of the lower plasma membrane of basal cells, the lamina lucida, and the lamina densa. Biochemically the BMZ is much more complex. Bullous pemphigoid antigen is present in the basal cells and on their periphery in the region of the lamina lucida. Laminin is localized to the lamina lucida, where it crosses with asymmetric arms; Type IV collagen, KF-1 antigen (keratin filament), LDA-1 (lamina densa antigen), and LH 7:2 (London Hospital) are present in fetal region of the lamina densa. Antigens AF-1, AF-2 (anchoring fibrils) and EBA (epidermolysis bullosa acquisita) are present in the sub-lamina densa zone. The sequence of expression of these antigens in the fetus has been mapped out and that in wound healing may be similar. It is interesting to note that the antigens of the basement membrane continue the normal sequence of progression of development in those tissues transplanted in nude mice. Studies further characterizing appendage development, anti-gen development, fetal skin development, wound healing, and basement membrane reformation will help us understand the complexity of the molecular interactions of human BMZ development.

### Keratins

The major structural protein of the keratinocyte is keratin. The sequence of keratin expression in human fetal epidermis has been well characterized (Fig. 46.2). During the embryonic period, keratins associated with simple epithelium, such as the 40, 45 and 50 kD keratins, are expressed. Those associated with mature stratified squamous epithelium, 67 and 56.5 kD keratins, appear during the period of epidermal stratification and follicular keratinization. These keratins initially appear in the developing hair follicle but eventually involve the interfollicular areas after 24 weeks' gestation. In addition, 58 and 50 kD keratins continue to be expressed throughout fetal development in mature neonatal and adult skin. Filaggrin first appears in the hair follicle region around 14 weeks

estimated gestational age (EGA) and slowly increases in quantity until normal amounts are present by 40 weeks.

### Migratory cells

The epidermis is an epithelium of ectodermally derived cells (keratinocytes) which, during the course of development, receives additional cells (immigrant cells) from other germ layers. Three populations of migrant cells exist in the human epidermis, melanocytes, Langerhans cells and Merkel cells. Merkel cells are present in human fetal epidermis before 18 weeks' gestation. Current data do not tell us if these cells are migratory cells or arise *in situ*. The other two cell types are discussed separately below.

### Melanocytes

Cells destined to become melanocytes migrate from the neural crest to the skin early in the second month of embryonic life. The cells often are localized adjacent to nerves and blood vessels. They are evident in the epidermis of embryos and fetuses from 50 days EGA as a population of dendritic cells recognized by the HMB-45 monoclonal antibody that detects a cytoplasmic antigen common to human melanomas and fetal melanocytes. Melanosomes are not evident until approximately 65 days at the earliest. Pigment synthesis in Caucasian fetal skin is thought to begin somewhat later, in the fourth or fifth month. Both the region as well as the race dictates the extent of melanization. The number of melanocytes increases markedly in the late first trimester and early second trimester when the density can reach ~2300 cells/mm².

The number of melanocytes increase in number until around 12–14 weeks EGA. Numbers then gradually decline. Melanocytes are distributed throughout all levels of the epidermis and embryonic

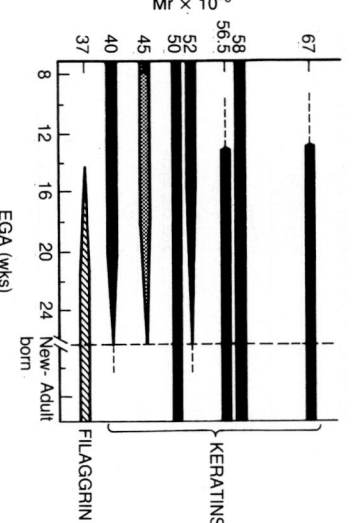

FIGURE 46.2 Diagrammatic representation of the expression of keratin polypeptides and filaggrin in human embryonic and fetal skin. (From Dale BA *et al.* Expression of epidermal keratins and filaggrin during human fetal skin development. J Cell Biol 1985; 101: 1257.)

skin assuming a predominantly basal position at 16–18 weeks. Both the number and the position of melanocytes are constantly changing during early fetal life.

Recent work would suggest that keratinocytes are important in regulating the dynamic interactions of the epidermal–melanin unit. Expression of keratinocyte cell surface adhesion molecules determines the difference between fetal and adult epidermal cells. Interactions between melanocytes and the fibronectin receptors may be one method to control melanocyte adherence and proliferation.

Melanocytes also are under control of a stem cell factor (SCF) otherwise known as melanocyte growth factor (MGF). This cytokine is thought to play a critical role in migration of melanocytes during embryogenesis. Mutations in either the *SCF* gene or its ligand, *c-kit*, result in defects in coat or skin pigmentation both in mice and in humans. SCF regulates expression of integrin receptors and has pleiotrophic effects on melanocyte attachment and migration to extracellular matrix ligands.

## Langerhans cells

Langerhans cells are the antigen-presenting cells of the skin. Like melanocytes, they appear to enter the fetal epidermis very early in development where they are recognized by the expression of human leukocyte antigen-(HLA-DR) on the plasma membrane. Fetal Langerhans cells, but not embryonic ones, also express the T-cell differentiation antigen, CD1a. Langerhans cells change in phenotype during gestation from smaller, truncated cells in embryonic epidermis to larger, more highly dendritic cells in fetal epidermis; the latter cell has a four to five times greater surface area than the embryonic cells. Thus, while the density of cells seems relatively constant throughout the first two trimesters, the fetal Langerhans cells may have a wider field of surveillance and present more surface membrane with immunologically important determinants.

It is uncertain whether Langerhans cells function as antigen-presenting cells or in any other capacity *in utero*. The fetus, however, already has a degree of immunocompetence in the first trimester.

## The dermis

The dermis originates from cells with the superficial dermatome segments of somite mesoderm and from other adjacent mesenchymal areas of the body. The major cell to differentiate from the mesenchyme is the fibroblast. Fibroblasts synthesize and secrete the fibrillar and filamentous collagenous, elastic and glycoprotein components and the non-fibrillar collagens and glycosaminoglycans/proteoglycans that provide mechanical support to the skin. This acts as a scaffolding for other intradermal structures (i.e. it sheaths the epidermal appendages, nerves and vessels). The dermal matrix and cells contain high amounts of glycogen. Hyaluronic acid is the dominant glycosaminoglycan

found in early dermis, but it decreases with age with an associated rise in the amount of dermatin sulfate.

## Hair

The primary hair follicles are the first to form. They appear on the face and scalp. Subsequent follicles develop along a cranio-caudal gradient of differentiation. Developing follicles can be detected at 80 days' gestational age.

Localized proliferations and down growths of basal keratinocytes form the appendages; pilosebaceous structures, eccrine sweat glands, apocrine glands and nails. The hair follicle epidermal cells are under the direct control of a specialized stromal region known as the dermal papilla. Recent evidence indicates that the keratinocyte stem cells are located in specific regions within the skin. It is probable that they lie subadjacent to the stromal cells with which they interact. The exact location of the follicular stem cell is controversial with claims they are either located in the bulge region two-thirds of the way up a hair follicle, or at the base of the follicle (Fig. 46.3). When the epidermal constituent of the hair follicle develops, it penetrates the dermis and partially encloses an undifferentiated ball of fibroblasts which is called the dermal papilla. Once the dermal papilla is formed the adjacent epidermis differentiates and divides to produce the upward growing fiber; dermal papilla cells in culture retain the inductive properties of the intact dermal papilla and are capable of fiber production.

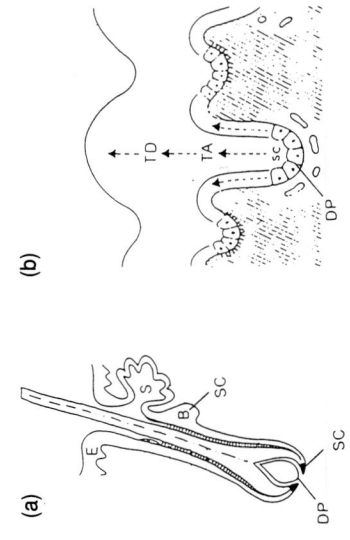

FIGURE 46.3 Location of putative keratinocyte stem cells in (a) the hair follicle and (b) palmar epidermis. B: bulge, DP: dermal papilla, E: epidermis, S: sebaceous gland, SC: stem cells, TA: transiently amplifying cells, TD: terminally differentiated cells. Adapted from Miller SJ, Sun T-T, Lavker RM. Hair follicles, stem cells, and skin cancer. *J Invest Dermatol* 1993; 100: 288S; Cotsarelis G, Cheng S-Z, Dong G, Sun T-T, Lavker RM. Existence of slow-cycling limbal epithelial basal cells that can be preferentially stimulated to proliferate: implications on epithelial stem cells. *Cell* 1989; 57: 201.

## Stem cells

It is generally accepted that there are at least two distinct populations of keratinocyte stem cells in the epidermis. The epidermal stem cells are located in islands evenly dispersed in the basal layer whereas the hair stem cells are thought to be in either the bulge region or at the base of the hair follicle itself (Fig. 46.3). Recently described phenotypic markers for keratinocyte stem cells include the expression of high levels of collagen receptors (β₁-integrin, CD29), and the cells can be partially purified by rapid adherence to collagen.

## Basement membrane zone

Considerable progress has been made in understanding the molecular basis of the cutaneous basement membrane zone (BMZ) with respect to several heritable and acquired diseases of the skin. One of these, *epidermolysis bullosa* (EB) is a heterogeneous group of conditions characterized by the formation of blisters and erosions of the skin and mucous membranes in response to trauma. The clinical and genetic heterogeneity of EB is reflected by the large number of subtypes which in turn, reflect the salient features of the clinical phenotype and the mode of inheritance. In the simplest form of classification, EB can be divided into three major categories on the basis of the level of tissue separation, as demonstrated by diagnostic electron microscopy. In the simplex, non-scarring forms of EB, the blister formation occurs intraepidermally at the level of the basal keratinocytes; in the junctional forms of EB, the tissue separation occurs within the dermal–epidermal basement membrane at the level of the lamina lucida; in the dystrophic, scarring forms of EB the tissue separation occurs below the basement membrane within the upper dermis at the level of the anchoring fibrils. Both autosomal dominant and autosomal recessive patterns of inheritance can be recognized.

Remarkable progress has recently been made in understanding the molecular basis of the non-scarring, simplex forms of EB (EBS), which are inherited in an autosomal dominant manner in the majority of cases. Support for the hypothesis that abnormalities in the keratin genes may underlie EBS was generated by creation of transgenic mice into which truncated constructs of the *keratin 14* gene had been integrated. These animals developed intraepidermal blistering at birth and ultrastructural evidence suggested clumping of tonofilaments. Subsequently, specific mutations have been

demonstrated in patients with EBS, and in two patients with *EBS herpetiformis* (*Dowling–Meara variant*) there was a point mutation in codon 125, which normally encodes an arginine residue.

Previous studies have clearly demonstrated abnormalities in the anchoring fibrils in the dystrophic forms of EB (DEB). In particular, electron microscopy of the skin in patients with the dominantly inherited form of DEB has demonstrated that the anchoring fibrils are reduced in number and/or are morphologically altered. The precise mutations in type VII collagen in DEB are currently under intense investigation. It is probable that there will be a spectrum of mutations.

The potential for genetic manipulation of skin, for example skin grafting of transfected cells to treat such problems, is an exciting advance and indeed the use of gene transfer technology is now just beginning to be applied to these conditions.

CLINICAL PROBLEMS

The preceding information can be used to aid in understanding the clinical patterns of clinical skin problems; a few relevant examples are discussed.

## Pigment cells

Nevus formation may be due to a mistake in migration of melanocytes or to excessive proliferation of melanocytes in the epidermal–dermal region. *Dysplastic nevi* can be regarded as a "continuous trait." This concept implies that acquired or spontaneous mutations cause transitions between ordinary and dysplastic nevi and between dysplastic nevi and *malignant melanoma*. Epidemiological studies and histopathological evidence provide further support for the concept of a continuous transition between pigmented lesions. It is well known that the total number of nevus-cell nevi is an important risk factor for malignant melanoma.

There are three major genetic components involved in the control of dysplastic nevi and malignant melanoma. A gene or set of genes are responsible for pigmentary characteristics, a gene or set of genes control the number of ordinary nevus-cell nevi, and there is a gene or set of anti-oncogenes (tumor repressor genes).

Viral infections during pregnancy can result in genetic changes. Examples of this are *varicella fetopathy* featuring extensive skin defects at birth and *aplasia cutis congenita-like malformations*, which have been reported following herpes simplex type 1 and type 2 infections. It is reasonable to assume that the majority of all nevi are caused by somatic mutations affecting genes involved in early embryogenesis.

A somatic mutation is by definition a postzygotic event. As such it will not affect the entire body but only parts of it. The size and distribution of a nevus will depend on the time and place in embryogenesis when a particular stem cell is affected (i.e. mutates). All cells derived from (or directly influenced by) secretable factors) will form part of the nevus. Clinical experience shows that many nevi are not limited to the skin but can also affect other tissues as is the case, for example, in *hypomelanosis of Ito*.

Supporting the concept of somatic mutations are three lines of evidence. Studies with chimeric mice, the increased risk of persons with epidermolytic epidermal nevi having offspring with bullous ichthyotic erythroderma, and the demonstration of chromosomal mosaicism in a number of patients with hypomelanosis of Ito. Chromosomal mosaicism can be attributed to somatic mutations and various forms of chromosomal mosaicism, as well as chimerism, have been shown to be associated with pigmentary anomalies usually presenting as a hypomelanosis of Ito-like picture.

In his study of epidermal nevi, Blaschko elaborated on the differences between dermatomes which are defined by the area of innervation of spinal ganglia and the lines of Blaschko. These latter are migration routes of pigment cells which are evident as a fountain-like pattern on the back, S-like figures on the flanks and a vertical pattern on the extremities (Fig. 46.4). Interestingly, this pattern of clonal cutaneous growth can also be found in some X-linked dominant skin diseases such as *incontinentia pigmenti* or *focal dermal hypoplasia* and in these situations can be explained as a visible cutaneous mosaic due to X-inactivation.

Few genetic skin diseases with involvement of the entire body have nevoid or segmental variants (e.g. *segmental neurofibromatosis* or *segmental Darier disease*). Interestingly, neurofibromatosis (type 1) has one of the highest mutation rates known in man and this has been related to the enormous size of the gene which spans about 3 million base pairs. It is conceivable that somatic mutations are preferentially seen in genes that are subject to frequent *de novo* mutations.

# Hemangiomas

Hemangiomas are now understood in terms of "hemangiogenesis." Locally produced, angiogenic growth factors act on skin and rarely on visceral endothelial cells to promote their proliferation. Usually the lesions spontaneously involute, presumably due to withdrawal of the previously present angiogenic factors, loss of endothelial receptors for these growth factors, or the influence of an inhibitory message from the surrounding connective tissues.

Smooth muscle cells and pericytes sustain the endothelial cells and interact with them to maintain vascular homeostasis. Basic fibroblast growth factor (bFGF) normally stimulates endothelial cell proliferation and migration. It is a major mediator of hemangiogenesis. bFGF is produced by normal keratinocytes and it is possible that it is produced locally in excess during the growth phase of hemangioma.

Mast cells accumulate in hemangiomas during the proliferative phase, but not during involution. This increased mast cell number may be one of the key factors in growth. Heparin released from mast cells may induce the proliferation of endothelium. The number of mast cells diminishes as the hemangioma enters the regression phase and as the fibro-fatty residuum replaces the cellular component.

Through improved knowledge and understanding of fetal skin development we may be able to benefit neonatal care. The skin of the premature infant is that of the third trimester fetus. It is immature in both structure and function. Infants less than 30 weeks' gestation show extremely fragile, easily injured skin, which makes handling or manipulating them difficult. The quest will be to develop methods to reduce fluid loss and prevent skin sepsis in these premature infants.

In summary, from the above examples it is self-evident that genetic influences play a significant part in the genesis of many cutaneous conditions. The pediatrician or dermatologist would be prudent to conceptualize many of these conditions by combining knowledge of fetal skin development, molecular biology and clinical observation.

## SELECTED READING

Holbrook KA. Structure and function of the developing human skin. In Goldsmith LA ed. *Biochemistry and physiology of the skin*, Vol. 1. New York: Oxford University Press, 1983: 64.

Holbrook KA, Sybert V. Basic science. In Schachner LA, Hansen RC eds. *Pediatric Dermatology.* New York: Churchill Livingstone, 1988: 3.

Lane AT. Human fetal skin development. *Pediatr Dermatol* 1986; 3: 487.

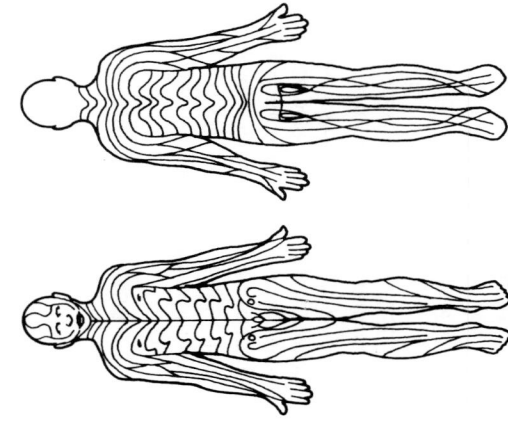

FIGURE 46.4 The lines of Blaschko. These lines are caused by the clonal growth of stem cells during early development. They usually become evident only when a mutation is present in a precursor cell. Linear nevi and dermatoses follow these lines.

# 47

# Wound Healing

## David A. Belford and Rodney D. Cooter

# WOUND HEALING

## INTRODUCTION

Wound healing is a complex series of events that restores tissue integrity. Disruption of tissue and cellular continuity sets in motion a coordinated sequence of biochemical and cellular processes that minimize blood loss, defend against microbial attack, remove damaged tissue, deposit a collagenous extracellular matrix, and seal the wound from the external environment.

## LOCAL INTERCELLULAR MESSENGERS CONTROL THE EVENTS OF WOUND REPAIR

Wound healing is effected by three cell types: skin fibroblasts, endothelial cells, and epidermal cells. These cells change their phenotype in the wound environment to exhibit increased migratory, proliferative and biosynthetic capacities. Attachment and migration of the cells through the extracellular matrix (ECM) is facilitated by expression of specific matrix receptors called integrins, as well as of enzymes that degrade matrix components. Many of these changes are brought about by two classes of intercellular messengers: (1) the leukotrienes and prostaglandins and (2) growth factors and cytokines. Growth factors are polypeptide molecules which act locally in an autocrine or paracrine fashion, by interaction with specific receptors on the surface of target cells, to promote chemotaxis, cell division, and increased biosynthetic activity. Growth factors are delivered to the wound by platelets and macrophages, and also are synthesized in the wound by fibroblast, endothelial and epidermal cells. Although exerting specific effects on several cell types, the biological action of these factors show significant

overlap – most induce new blood vessel formation, are chemotactic for a variety of cells, and stimulate collagen synthesis and fibroblast proliferation.

## PHASES OF WOUND REPAIR

Wound healing can be conveniently described in three phases: (1) hemostasis and inflammation; (2) proliferation and (3) remodeling. It should be emphasized, however, that repair proceeds in an orderly fashion and the transition from one phase to another is indistinct (Fig. 47.1). These phases are common to all soft tissue repair, although as an example, only cutaneous wounds are considered in the following sections.

### Hemostasis and inflammation

Even the cleanest surgical wound will result in some degree of tissue damage and blood loss. Vasoconstriction, initiation of the clotting cascade and the aggregation of platelets combine to achieve hemostasis (see page 886). Provisional wound closure is achieved by a fibrin plug, which serves to protect against bacterial invasion and also provides a scaffolding for the invading inflammatory cells, fibroblasts and endothelial cells.

Wound repair begins with platelet degranulation. Exposure to subendothelial collagen and other mediators including thrombin causes platelet activation and the release of α-granule contents, resulting in a burst of growth factors and cytokines into the wound. These factors both initiate inflammation and the migratory, proliferative and biosynthetic processes of healing (Fig. 47.2).

Inflammation serves to defend against invasion by microorganisms, dispose of injured tissue, and establish a microenvironment that facilitates repair. Activated mast cells and platelets, as well as the

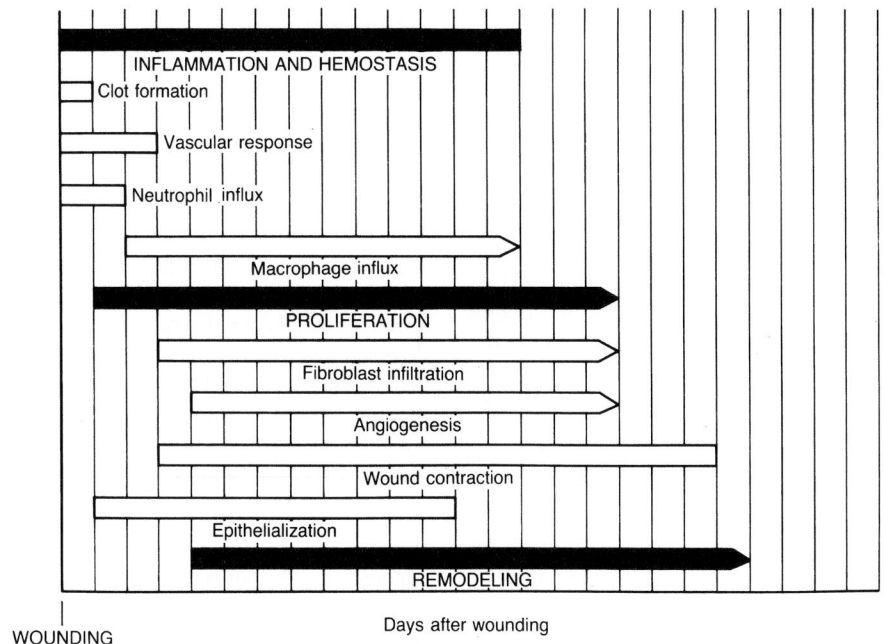

FIGURE 47.1 Events of wound repair.

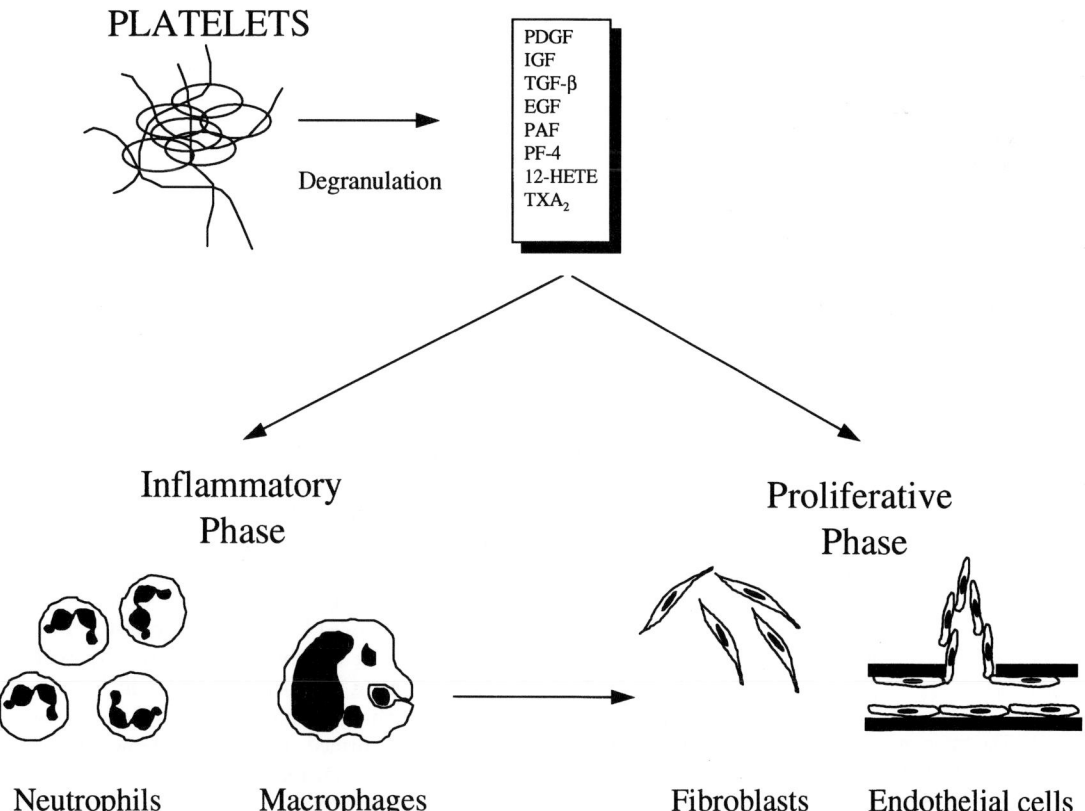

FIGURE 47.2 Platelet activation and degranulation results in release of growth factors, cytokines, prostaglandins and leukotrienes. These mediators help establish the inflammatory response in the wound as well as initiate the proliferative phase of repair. In turn, factors released by the activated macrophage continue to coordinate the migration and proliferation of the repair cells. PDGF, platelet-derived growth factor; IGF, insulin-like growth factor; TGFβ, transforming growth factor β; EGF, epidermal growth factor; PAF, platelet-activating factor; PF-4, platelet factor-4; 12-HETE, 12-hydroxyeicosatetranoic acid; TXA$_2$, thromboxane A$_2$.

damaged tissue itself, release mediators which initiate and establish the inflammatory response in the wound. Subsequent vasodilatation and increased capillary permeability result in extravasation of plasma constituents. Leukocytes adhere to the postcapillary venules and migrate in response to inflammatory mediators such as complement-derived peptide C5a, leukotrienes, bacterial and matrix degradation products, as well as growth factors. Neutrophil numbers peak in the wound at around 24 hours. Their role is mainly defensive, directed at the intra- and extracellular killing of bacteria. They also initiate debridement of damaged tissue through extracellular release of enzymes, such as collagenase and elastase, and the production of oxygen free radicals. However, in uncomplicated wounds, the neutrophil is not essential for ongoing repair.

In contrast, presence of the tissue macrophage is vital. Macrophages appear in the wound after 48–96 hours and continue the wound debriding and antibacterial action initiated by the neutrophil, but their major role is to coordinate the proliferative events of wound repair. They become activated in the wound, releasing a range of mediators, including proinflammatory, chemotactic and fibrogenic cytokines that initiate a cascade of migratory, proliferative and synthetic events that result in the formation of granulation tissue (Fig. 47.3).

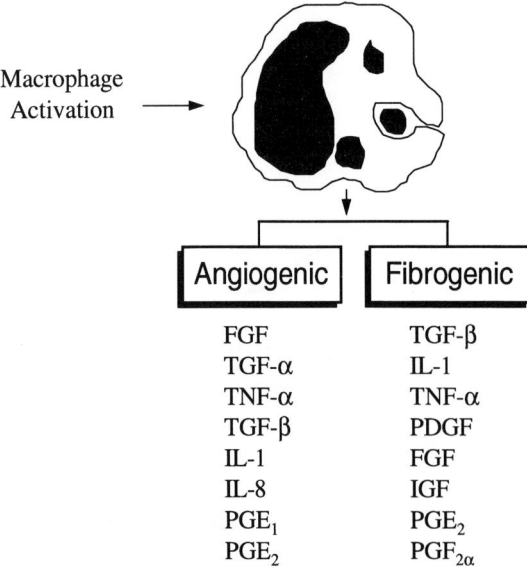

FIGURE 47.3 The tissue macrophage coordinates wound repair. The activated wound macrophage synthesizes and releases a host of mediators that stimulate new blood vessel formation (angiogenic factors), fibroblast proliferation and the synthesis of collagen (fibrogenic factors). FGF, fibroblast growth factor; TGFα transforming growth factor α; TNFα, tumor necrosis factor α; TGFβ, transforming growth factor β; IL-1, interleukin-1; IL-8, interleukin-8; PDGF, platelet-derived growth factor; IGF, insulin-like growth factor; PGE, prostaglandin E; PGF, prostaglandin F.

# Proliferation

The proliferative phase includes the three processes that characterize wound healing in the adult: (1) deposition of connective tissue, (2) wound contraction, and (3) epithelialization. The degree to which each of these processes contributes to repair is dependent on the type, and to some extent, the site of the wound. Close apposition of the dermal edges to allow healing by "primary intention," is achieved mainly by deposition of connective tissue across the wound space. Leaving the wound open to heal by "secondary intention" requires increased connective tissue deposition, wound contraction and prolonged epithelialization. Partial thickness wounds, for example skin graft donor sites, heal primarily by epithelialization alone.

## Deposition of connective tissue

The wound defect is initially filled with granulation tissue, a loose collagen-based matrix containing proteoglycans and other adhesive ligands, along with the invading inflammatory cells, fibroblasts and new capillary buds. A healthy bed of granulation tissue is not only vital to subsequent epithelialization, but also to the ability of a wound to accept a skin graft. Tissue such as bare cortical bone or tendon, which cannot granulate, will not revascularize a graft.

Fibroblast infiltration of the wound is evident at 3–4 days. Fibroblasts migrate in response to proteolytic fragments of matrix components, as well as factors released by activated platelets and macrophages. Platelet-derived growth factor (PDGF) is a potent chemoattractant for fibroblasts. Fibroblast division is controlled by combinations of growth factors that regulate different aspects of the cell cycle. It is likely that factors such as fibroblast growth factor (FGF) and PDGF, both products of the activated macrophage, make the fibroblast competent to respond to systemic factors such as insulin-like growth factor.

New capillary sprouts grow into the wound just behind the migrating front of fibroblasts. Budding of endothelial cells occurs from the postcapillary venules and follows a defined sequence. Degradation of vascular basement membrane on the side of the angiogenic stimulus is followed by endothelial cell migration into the surrounding matrix. Division and differentiation occur to form a number of tubes, which connect to form a branching vascular network. A new basement membrane is formed, followed by remodeling of the new vessels. Several macrophage-derived growth factors have been shown to stimulate angiogenesis (Fig. 47.3).

Collagen synthesis by the fibroblast is modulated by fibrogenic growth factors and cytokines in the wound. The most potent of these is transforming growth factor β (TGFβ), which acts directly on the wound fibroblasts to promote the expression of collagen. Particularly relevant to wound healing is the post-translational processing of the newly synthesized procollagen molecules. Hydroxylation of the proline and lysine residues of procollagen in the endoplasmic reticulum, a step that requires ascorbate (vitamin C) and molecular oxygen, is required to stabilize the triple-helical arrangement. The procollagen chains are then packaged into secretory vesicles and released into the extracellular environment where the propeptides are cleaved off by specific proteinases. Assembly of the collagen molecules into fibrils is stabilized by the formation of intra- and intermolecular bonds, conferring tensile strength to the collagen fiber and, therefore, the healed wound. This process is catalyzed by lysyl oxidase, and continues for many months after wounding as the newly synthesized collagen matrix undergoes remodeling.

## Wound contraction

Wound contraction pulls the margins of the open wound together, such that normal skin is pulled centripetally to reduce the wound defect and volume of the scar. It is to be distinguished from contracture, which occurs within a scar of an epithelialized wound and results in compaction of the scar connective tissue matrix into a tight band. The mechanism of wound contraction remains to be fully elucidated. Early work focused on the contractile ability of granulation tissue, and in particular a fibroblast-derived cell that exhibited characteristics of smooth muscle in the wound environment, the "myofibroblast." As this cell expresses smooth muscle α-actin and possesses actinomyosin stress fibers that connect to the extracellular matrix via a transmembrane complex (a "fibronexus"), wound contraction was thought to be the result of a coordinated ability of myofibroblasts to transmit a contractile force. However, more recently, fibroblasts have been shown to contract a collagenous matrix by cell movement alone, and it is likely that wound myofibroblasts develop in response to tension in the wound, serving to hold the wound margin against the outward force generated by the surrounding tissue.

Wound contraction can be used to clinical advantage in certain circumstances. For example, soft tissue loss from a fingertip of less than $1 \text{cm}^2$, that does not expose bone, will contract substantially such that surrounding glabrous, specialized skin will be drawn into the defect. In this instance, treatment by dressing alone will provide a better reconstruction than a skin graft. In addition, defects in concave areas such as the medial canthal region will contract to an almost imperceptible scar if left to heal by secondary intention.

## Epithelialization

Definitive closure occurs by epithelialization. It is a process largely of cell migration, the epithelium moving as a single layered sheet below the eschar and over the provisional matrix of granulation tissue. Epithelial cells mobilize from both the wound margin and the residual hair follicles and sweat glands by loosening of attachments to both the surrounding cells and the basement membrane. Hemidesmosomal junctions are lost as the migratory cells change shape from a cuboidal to a flattened cell, extend cytoplasmic processes and migrate by lamellipodial crawling. Cells at the leading edge of the migrating front express enzymes, including collagenase, and at the same time become actively phagocytic, removing cellular debris in their path. Receptors for the glycoprotein cell adhesion ligands fibronectin and vitronectin, both components of the provisional wound matrix, are up-regulated. A delayed burst of cell proliferation occurs behind the migrating front of epithelial cells. As the migrating monolayer completes the re-epithelialization process, the cells proliferate and differentiate to re-establish a stratified squamous epithelium. Basement membrane components including type IV collagen, bullous pemphigoid antigen, and laminin are synthesized mainly by the epidermal cells behind the migrating tip, as well as dermal fibroblasts. Ultimately, formation of hemidesmosomes and anchoring filaments link the newly formed epidermis and its basement membrane to the underlying dermal collagen.

# Remodeling

The extracellular environment of the healing wound is in a constant state of flux, representing a balance between the synthesis of ECM components and their degradation by local extracellular proteolysis. In addition to conferring structural integrity to the healed wound, ECM components provide an adhesive scaffolding that regulates cell migration, modulates cell–cell interaction and sequesters growth factors and cytokines in the local environment.

The major structural components of the granulation tissue matrix are fibrin, and later, collagen. The early fibrinous matrix contains components that facilitate cell migration, including the proteoglycan adhesion ligands fibronectin and vitronectin, as well as the glycosaminoglycan hyaluronic acid. The latter maintains a hydrated environment of loosely packed matrix that characterizes many developmental and regenerative processes. Degradation of the proteoglycans and fibrin makes way for the deposition of collagen. Initially, type III collagen is deposited in the wound, although it is replaced by type I collagen fibrils which characterize the mature scar. Remodeling of the collagenous scar by ongoing biosynthesis, degradation and cross-linking, can occur for many years after wounding. Clinical measures aimed at modifying the ultimate scar configuration, including mechanical splintage, strapping, and tailored pressure garments, often require long-term application.

Increasing tensile strength of the wound occurs largely as a result of structural organization of the collagen. The unorganized fibrils that characterize the early repair align in response to mechanical stress and undergo increased cross-linking, such that collagen fiber diameter increases and fibers become more compact. However, the degree of collagen organization in scar tissue never achieves that seen in unwounded dermis, and wound strength always remains less than that of normal skin.

## SELECTED READING

Bennett NT, Schultz GS. Growth factors and wound healing: Part II. Role in normal and chronic wound healing. *Am J Surg* 1993; **166**: 74.

Clark RAF, Henson, PM eds. *The molecular and cellular biology of wound repair*. New York: Plenum Press, 1988.

Cohen IK, Diegelmann RF, Lindblad WJ eds. *Wound healing: biochemical and clinical aspects*. Philadelphia: WB Saunders Co., 1992.

Gailit J, Clark RAF. Wound repair in the context of extracellular matrix. *Curr Opin Cell Biol* 1994; **6**: 717.

Grinnell F. Fibroblasts, myofibroblasts and wound contraction. *J Cell Biol* 1994; **124**: 401.

Hunt TK. The physiology of wound healing. *Ann Emerg Med* 1988; **17**: 1265.

Kovacs EJ, DiPietro LA. Fibrogenic cytokines and connective tissue production. *FASEB J* 1994; **8**: 854.

Martin P, Hopkinson-Woolley J, McClusky, J. Growth factors and cutaneous wound repair. *Prog Growth Factor Res* 1992; **4**: 24.

# PART NINE

# *Thermoregulation*

**Editor: Tania R. Gunn**

# 48

# Thermoregulation

John McIntyre, David Hull, Jan Nedergaard and
Barbara Cannon

As a consequence of the chemical reactions required for growth, activity, maintenance and repair, heat is produced. In most animal species (poikilotherms) this heat is dissipated from the surface of the body, and the body temperature remains similar to that of the surroundings, whether water or air. When mammals developed, they acquired two properties which gave an evolutionary advantage: the ability to breast-feed their young, and the ability to produce extra heat when necessary, i.e. by facultative thermogenesis. The latter allows mammals to defend an elevated and constant body temperature, i.e. they are homeotherms having "a pattern of temperature regulation in which cyclic variation in core temperature, either diurnally or seasonally, is maintained within narrow limits, despite much larger variations in ambient temperature." Their activity is thus independent of ambient temperature; mammals therefore can be active at night when few other predators or competitors are around, and therefore have an evolutionary advantage.

Facultative thermogenesis can be of two types – shivering (in skeletal muscle) and non-shivering. Facultative non-shivering thermogenesis is the distinctive outcome of the metabolism of brown adipose tissue. The earliest mammals were small, and in these small animals brown adipose tissue, and a high thermogenic capacity, probably persisted throughout life. As larger mammals, including man, developed, the need for extra heat production in the adult diminished because loss of heat to the surroundings decreases more rapidly with increasing size than does the resting metabolic rate. However, the smaller size of mammalian neonates still necessitates extra heat production; thus infants rely on brown adipose tissue to remain euthermic.

## PHYSICAL HEAT EXCHANGE

Heat is a form of energy and thus is subject to the laws of thermodynamic conservation which state that "energy cannot be created or destroyed but only converted from one form to another." Heat produced by metabolic processes in the body ($M$) must therefore either be stored in the tissues ($S$) or dissipated to the environment. The channels for dissipating heat are radiation ($R$), convection ($C$), conduction ($K$) and evaporation ($E$). The heat balance can be expressed as

$$M = E + C + K + R + S$$

## Radiation (R)

Energy exchanged by this mode is in the form of electromagnetic waves, ranging from the short wave radiation of the visible spectrum to the long wave infrared radiation. In "natural" environments, solar radiation is the main source of short wave radiation (0.3–3.0 µm). In bright sunlight solar radiation can be the largest single factor in the heat balance equation and the exogenous provision of heat may be as much as 10 times the metabolic heat production. Indirect radiation from scattered sunlight and reflections can increase the net solar radiation flux.

Radiation of a longer wavelength (around 10 µm) is emitted by objects such as people, plants and buildings. At these longer wavelengths energy exchange can result in heat loss or gain depending on the temperature of the body and of the surrounding surfaces. The main factors determining radiant heat exchange are:

- the surface temperature of the two objects, exchange being proportional to the difference to the fourth power of the surface temperatures;
- the respective areas and orientation of the two objects;
- their emissivity and reflectivity.

Normal intact skin has an average emissivity of 0.97–0.98, irrespective of color or pigmentation, and thus for practical purposes the human body can be considered to behave like a black body over most of the thermal spectrum.

## Convection (C)

This describes the transference of heat by the movement of a liquid or gas from a warmer to a cooler region. In still air, free convection occurs in which the air in contact with the body is warmed, becomes lighter and so rises to be replaced with cooler air. The moving air provides an insulation and in the upright position this insulation may be several centimeters thick by the time it reaches the face. The thicker the boundary layer, the lower the convective loss. Large differences in flow patterns and hence insulation can be produced by changes in posture; for example, when lying down the insulating properties of a thick boundary layer are largely lost. When the body is exposed to moving air the natural convective air streams are displaced, disrupting the boundary layer, and heat is lost by forced convection. Prediction of heat loss is difficult; the main determinants of convective heat exchange are the temperature difference between skin and air, air movement across the surfaces and the surface area exposed.

## Conduction (K)

When two bodies are in direct contact, thermal energy can be transferred from molecule to molecule; this is called conduction. The transference of heat will depend on the temperature gradient between the two objects, the area of contact and the heat capacity and conductivity of the materials. In practice the role of conductive heat exchange in humans is small, rarely exceeding 3 per cent of the total.

## Evaporation (E)

When evaporation occurs from the skin or respiratory tract the latent heat of vaporization represents a loss of heat from the body. Evaporative heat exchange is determined by the gradient of absolute humidity. Two processes are involved in evaporative heat loss from the skin. Transepidermal loss is due to the continuous evaporation of water that has been released following passive diffusion through the outer dead layers of the skin. This loss is driven by the difference between the vapor concentration below the epidermis and that in the ambient air. The stratum corneum is the main barrier to diffusion and provided this is intact, transepidermal water loss is a relatively small source of heat loss in the normal indoor environment.

The second process is sweating. In warm environments where non-evaporative heat loss is decreased, large amounts of heat still can be lost by secretion of sweat that evaporates from the skin surface. The heat loss will depend on the rate at which the body can secrete sweat and the environmental humidity. Sweat rate can be adjusted over a wide range of climatic conditions and rates of heat production. It may be as high as 1.5 L/h in unacclimatized adults and up to 4 L/h in someone fully acclimatized.

## Storage (S)

Heat is stored in, or released from, body tissues when their temperature changes. Clearly, over a long period, the mean rate of change of heat storage is zero but it can be an important short-term component of heat balance.

## Developmental aspects

In fetal life there is a continuous exchange of heat between the fetus and its environment. The maternal arterial blood temperature is the single most important determinant of fetal temperature. The heat generated by fetal metabolism is readily transferred to the placenta by the umbilical arteries. Thus, the temperature of the fetus is a little higher than that of the mother, but remains close to it at all times.

The capacity of newborn mammals to control their body temperature varies between species. In newborns of small mammals, the task of maintaining thermal control in the natural environment of their parents would place too great a demand on their energy reserves even if it were biologically possible. The small naked newborn hamster is in many respects immature at birth and lacks obvious thermal control. Thermotaxis appears at around 8 days, behavioral thermoregulation 2 or 3 days later and thermogenesis at around 12–16 days of age. During the first 10 days, the animal is essentially a poikilotherm. For another common laboratory animal, the rat, some thermoregulatory responses are present at birth. However, they develop dramatically during the first week of life. For such mammals, nests, huddling or cuddling are essential for survival and these animals are termed "altricial." In the larger newborn mammals of precocial species, like the lamb, the thermoregulatory capacities are well developed and their responses match, or might even be considered to exceed, those of adults. However, given their smaller size and shorter hair they are still vulnerable to cold conditions that can be weathered by their parents.

The mature newborn human infant has a modest capacity to modulate heat exchange by both behavioral and autonomic responses. Obviously changes in posture and vasomotor control will influence the characteristics of physical heat exchange as well as the characteristics of the environment. Fig. 48.1 illustrates the modes of heat exchange of mature, preterm and very preterm infants nursed in incubators in a thermoneutral environment, that is, at a temperature where the infant need not make any attempt at thermal control. The main external variables are the difference in temperature between the infant's body and the environment, the velocity of air flow, the relative humidity and the area exposed for heat exchange. The size and maturity of the infant are important factors which influence heat flow. In the very preterm infant (<28 weeks' gestation) exchange is powerfully influenced by transepidermal water loss because in the first weeks after birth the skin is only a few cells thick, with a very decreased stratum corneum, and is not watertight. Thus, heat flow is determined by the humidity in the surrounding air. It is difficult to maintain 100 per cent humidity in an incubator though it is important to keep it as high as possible. The use of adhesive semipermeable dressings markedly decreases transepidermal water loss. It is impossible to control the humidity surrounding infants nursed under radiant heaters. This is the main disadvantage of radiant heaters as the heat source for the care of the very preterm infant in temperate climates.

## HEAT PRODUCTION

A relatively constant internal environment allows cellular chemical reactions to proceed at a steady rate. Thus, the homeotherm can maintain a high level of performance despite wide variations in environmental conditions. Such an advantage is, however, expensive in energy terms.

Direct calorimetry measures the heat flux from the subject. Systems have been developed to make such measurements in both children and adults. This approach is technically demanding; it depends on many measurements and requires calculations for which some assumptions have to be made. Indirect calorimetry measures $O_2$ consumption and $CO_2$ production of the subject. Heat production can be calculated by measurements of respiratory gas exchanges, making assumptions about the energy content of nutrients. This is the usual method for measuring energy expenditure and substrate utilization in man.

Heat production varies widely depending on energy expenditure and environmental conditions. Thus to make useful comparisons between individuals the index used is the basal metabolic rate (BMR) which, strictly defined, is "the rate of metabolic free energy production calculated from measurements of heat production or $O_2$ consumption in an organism in a rested, awake, fasting and thermoneutral state." Such a state is often difficult to achieve in children since, if resting, they are usually postprandial and asleep. Thus the measured values are often the resting metabolic rate, which is not a true BMR.

Under similar conditions a larger body will generate more total heat per hour than a smaller one but specific heat production, expressed as watts per kilogram (W/kg), is higher for the smaller individual. This means of expression is appropriate when calculating nutritional requirements. However, as heat loss is determined in part by surface area the metabolic rate is often expressed per unit surface area (W/m²), when considering heat exchange. The data on metabolic rates in infancy and childhood are limited. From birth to sexual maturity there is a steady decline in BMR (in W/kg or W/m²) (Fig. 48.2). The newborn infant has a BMR per unit surface area nearly twice that of an old person. The BMR of males is higher than in comparable sized females. This might be explained by the different amounts of body fat. Body shape affects the BMR; a

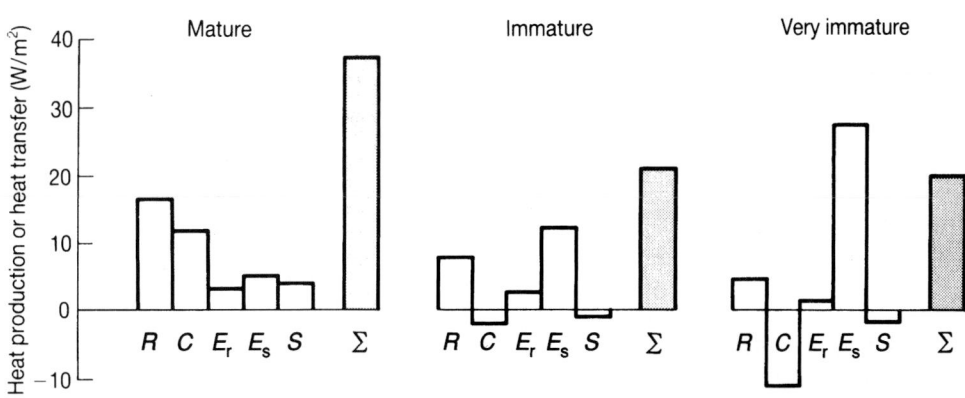

FIGURE 48.1 Physical heat exchange in term and preterm infants. The heat exchange in term, 32-week and < 28-week prematurely born infants nursed in an incubator. $R$, radiation; $C$, convection; $E_r$, evaporation from respiratory tract; $E_s$, evaporation from skin surface; $S$, heat storage; $\Sigma$, net sum of heat exchange.

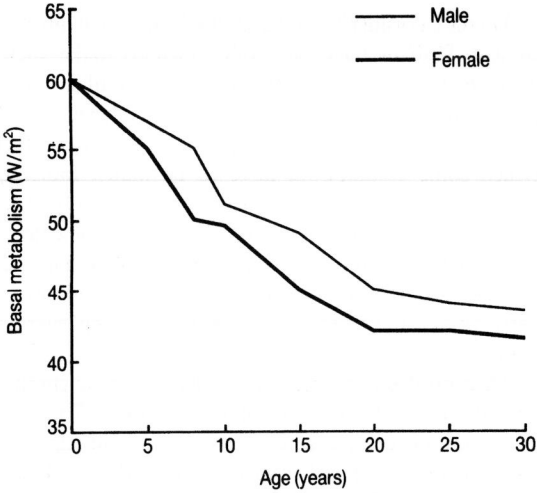

FIGURE 48.2 Basal metabolic rate at different ages. (From Guyton AC. *Textbook of medical physiology*. Philadelphia: WB Saunders, 1986: 847, with permission.)

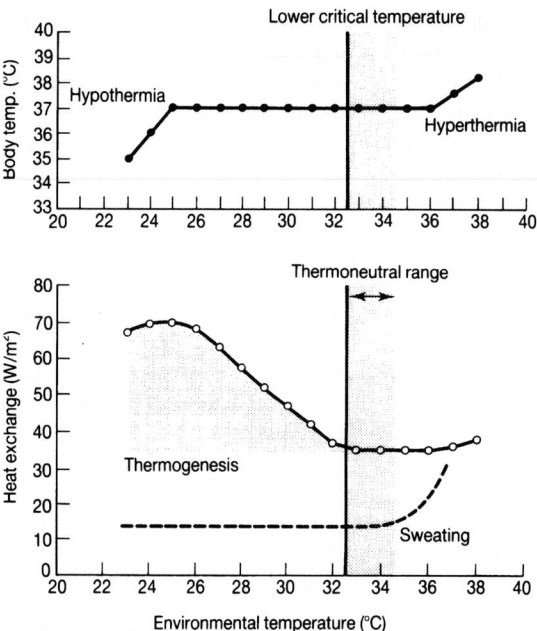

FIGURE 48.3 The relationship between metabolic rate and environmental temperature

lighter individual will have a higher metabolic rate per kilogram body weight than a thicker set person of the same height. This is because BMR depends on active tissue mass and a fat person will have a relatively smaller lean body mass. There are important hormonal influences on BMR. In the *hyperthyroid* state the BMR may increase by 40–80 per cent and in *hypothyroidism* it may fall 40–50 per cent. The BMR also fluctuates over 24 hours. Metabolism and body temperature are greatest during the day and fall during the night. This circadian rhythm appears to develop in the first 4 months of life. Ingestion of food also alters metabolic rate; this so-called specific dynamic action can increase metabolic rate by 6–10 per cent.

Cold conditions and activity have far more impact on energy requirements and heat exchange than the factors that modify basal metabolic rate. The relationship between the metabolic rate and the environmental temperature is illustrated in Fig. 48.3. When the environmental temperature lies in the zone of least thermoregulatory effort, that is the "neutral thermal environment," metabolism is minimal. As environmental temperature falls below this, heat production increases until it reaches a maximum – the cold limit. Cooling beyond this results in a fall in metabolic heat production that, if continued, will cause hypothermia and death. When environmental temperatures exceed the heat dissipating capacity, the hot limit, the metabolic rate will inevitably rise, causing hyperthermia and death unless cooling occurs.

## THE REGULATION OF BODY TEMPERATURE

The central body core temperature is normally maintained within narrow limits. To achieve this, with continuously and rapidly changing rates of heat loss and heat production, requires complex interaction between sensing, integrating and effector units. Thermal sensors are located in the skin, central nervous system and several other locations.

## Thermoreception

Humans can perceive temperature gradations of cold and heat progressing through painful (cold), icy, cold, cool, neutral, lukewarm, warm, hot, painful (hot). Thermoreceptors can be defined in physical terms as nerve endings excited only, or preferentially, by thermal stimuli. This definition holds for any thermosensitive structure irrespective of whether its excitation correlates with temperature sensation. The general properties of specific cutaneous thermoreceptors have been described as follows:

■ they have a static discharge at constant temperature;
■ they show a dynamic response to temperature change with either a positive (warm receptors) or a negative temperature coefficient (cold receptors);
■ they are not excited by mechanical stimuli;
■ activity occurs in the non-painful range.

Cutaneous thermoreceptors have been divided into warm and cold receptors based on these properties. Cold receptors are fairly evenly distributed over the whole body surface. However, the density of warm receptors is more variable with, for example, a high density on the face and hands. The axons of cutaneous thermoreceptors run within the afferent cutaneous nerves to the segmental spinal ganglia and the dorsal root of the spinal cord. Spinal thermosensitive afferents are mainly conveyed in the contralateral spinothalamic tract, giving off collaterals to the midbrain reticular formation and to the hypothalamus.

Much of our current knowledge on central receptors is based on animal studies. Local warming and cooling of the hypothalamus elicits thermoregulatory responses. These thermosensitive neurons are concentrated in the preoptic anterior area of the hypothalamus. There is also evidence for thermosensitive neurons in the midbrain, medulla oblongata and the spinal cord. Thermosensors also are present in deep tissues; for example, in blood vessels, the abdominal cavity, and carotid baroreceptors and chemoreceptors.

Elucidating how thermoregulatory pathways are integrated is difficult. It appears that the brainstem, from the septal preoptic region to the caudal posterior hypothalamus, participates in sensing temperature, integrating the message from different pathways, and organizing efferent pathways. The posterior hypothalamus seems of particular importance and single neurons in this region respond to thermal signals from the anterior hypothalamus and to those arriving from the spinal cord and skin.

# Effector systems

In addition to physiological thermoregulatory mechanisms, homeotherms also regulate body temperature by behavioral means, involving coordinated and voluntary motor activity. Seeking appropriate thermal environments, shelter and clothing are important in maintaining body temperature but this represents modification of thermal environment, not of the subject.

The concept of a "set point" is used to understand how body temperature is maintained in a narrow range. Temperature control mechanisms or effector systems continually attempt to bring back the body temperature to this set point when a deviation is sensed. The temperature-regulated or "controlled variable" was formerly thought to be the deep body temperature best represented by the hypothalamic temperature. However, a more appropriate model may be the multiple input system in which the temperature-regulated variable is a function of several local temperatures; that is, an integrated body temperature. The set point can be thought of as this integrated body temperature that is maintained when output signals from the controller to effector systems are zero. At this point the mechanisms of heat loss and heat production are not being activated. Changes sensed as a deviation from this set point activate thermoregulatory effector systems to return the temperature field towards zero. The short-term control actions of temperature regulation are initiated via nervous pathways. The main effector systems are either behavioral or autonomic. The autonomic systems that respond in sequence from warm to cool are sweating, the vasomotor system, postural adjustments and thermogenesis.

## Sudomotor system (sweat glands)

In conditions where non-evaporative heat loss is limited, sweating becomes the major channel for dissipating heat. Sweat glands are widely distributed over the body. Secretion of sweat is initiated and controlled by the activity of efferent cholinergic sympathetic nerves. It is an eccrine process involving transfer of fluid across the intact cell membrane. The apocrine sweat glands in the axillary and pubic areas are not involved in thermal sweating. The forehead has a particularly high sweating rate. Local skin temperature variations can also appreciably change the rate of eccrine sweat secretion in a small area.

## Vasomotor regulation

A major determinant of heat exchange is the skin temperature and it is the rate of blood flow to the skin that determines its temperature. The blood flow can be altered by changing the diameter of the arterioles, vessels with a thick muscle coat, which can contract or relax in response to nerve impulses. In warm conditions, arterioles dilate, allowing warm blood to flow through the skin capillaries, warming the skin and dissipating heat. This effect is enhanced by returning blood flowing in the superficial veins close to the skin surface. In cold conditions, skin blood flow and hence heat loss is minimized by vasoconstriction, conserving heat to the deeper parts of the body. Furthermore, returning blood flows in the deep veins that lie close to the arteries, a mechanism that helps reduce the temperature gradient across the skin surface. The control of peripheral blood flow varies regionally and three functionally different regions have been identified:

- the extremities, hands, feet, ears, lips, nose;
- trunk and proximal limbs;
- head and brow.

Blood flow through the extremities is under noradrenergic sympathetic control. An increase in sympathetic tone causes vasoconstriction and a decrease in sympathetic tone, vasodilatation. In the trunk and proximal limbs vasodilatation induced by heat is an active process. It is mediated by the release of bradykinin from the sweat glands. Thus cutaneous regions where this active process occurs are the same as those in which pronounced thermal sweating occurs. On the forehead, vasomotor nerves have only a slight effect. With cold exposure there is very little vasoconstriction. In response to heat, however, vasodilatation and sweat production do occur.

## Thermogenesis

Heat production is increased by shivering and non-shivering thermogenesis, both of which are under the control of nervous pathways. In adults the first response to cooling is an increase in muscle tone with muscle units firing out of phase and at different frequencies. This explains the feeling of stiffness on cold exposure. Further cooling causes the discharges to become more synchronized, creating a tremor and eventually frank shivering. The overall heat production can be five to six times the resting rate, but this can only be maintained for a few minutes. Over a period of an hour or more, body heat production may be raised about 50–100 per cent. It is more efficient than voluntary contractions in terms of heat production. Shivering is controlled through the descending tracts of the "shivering pathway" that leave the posterior hypothalamus and run caudally through the midbrain, tegmentum and pons. Here, they contact the supraspinal motor pathways that make synaptic contacts on the motor neurons in the anterior horns of the spinal cord and activate muscles, via the motor nerves.

In the newborn infant heat is generated on cold exposure but shivering does not appear to occur. Over the first year of life the relative contribution of this non-shivering thermogenesis declines to be replaced by shivering thermogenesis (Fig. 48.4). From animal models it is suggested that these two thermogenic effector mechanisms form an interlocked control system. It is thought that under natural conditions shivering will only occur after non-shivering thermogenesis has been evoked to its full extent.

## NON-SHIVERING THERMOGENESIS IN BROWN ADIPOSE TISSUE

Brown adipose tissue is found in several depots in the newborn, but the interscapular and perirenal depots are the most significant (Fig. 48.5). Heat production in brown adipose tissue is a facultative event; heat is only produced when it is needed to maintain the temperature of the newborn. The activity of brown adipose tissue is controlled by centers in the hypothalamus. These include regions around the optic chiasma, responsible for the integration of thermal signals and for the maintenance of body tempera-

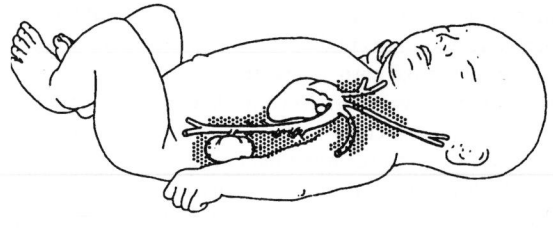

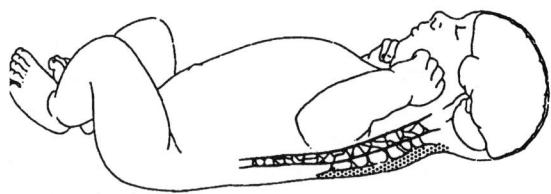

FIGURE 48.5 The distribution of brown adipose tissue as identified by multilocular adipocytes

ture, as well as centers in the ventromedial hypothalamus (VMH) and lateral hypothalamus (LH), responsible for feeding behavior and energetic control.

Physiological stimulation of each of these centers leads to a wide array of effects in the newborn. The temperature centers and the VMH have an inhibitory effect on lower centers which are specifically responsible for stimulating brown fat activity. Thus, when this inhibition is removed the thermogenic function of brown adipose tissue is induced. The signals are transmitted through the sympathetic nervous system. The nerve cell bodies directly responsible for control of brown fat activity are found along the sympathetic chain and especially in the sympathetic ganglia. It is likely that all brown fat depots are activated in parallel. As stimulation of brown adipose tissue occurs via the sympathetic nervous system, the tissue may be stimulated in a stress situation. However, activation of brown adipose tissue should normally be considered a specialized and distinct activation of the tissue through dedicated pathways.

## Adrenergic receptors

Norepinephrine released from the sympathetic fibers within brown adipose tissue interacts with adrenergic receptors on the brown fat cell membrane. The dominant stimulatory pathway proceeds via the recently described $\beta_3$-receptors. These receptors respond to norepinephrine, as do all other $\beta$-receptors, but they have a different pharmacology, e.g. the classical $\beta$-adrenergic inhibitor propranolol is a weaker (10- to 100-fold) antagonist on them than on $\beta_1$- and $\beta_2$-receptors. For thermogenic action $\alpha_1$-receptors are also positively involved, although $\alpha$-stimulation proceeds via

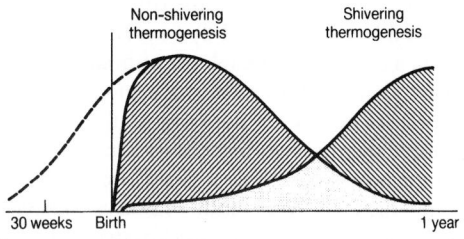

FIGURE 48.4 Shivering and non-shivering thermogenesis

pathways different from those described below and only causes a minor fraction of the heat production. α₂-Adrenergic stimulation inhibits thermogenesis.

## Cytosolic events

The initial intracellular responses in the brown fat cell to β-adrenergic stimulation are not different from those in white adipose tissue (Fig. 48.6). There is first an increase in cAMP which activates intracellular protein kinase, which in turn activates the hormone-sensitive lipase by phosphorylating it on a serine residue. When the lipase is activated, it breaks down the triglycerides in the cytoplasmic fat droplets to fatty acids and glycerol. The released fatty acids have two options: they may be combusted in the brown fat cell itself, as described in more detail below, or they may be exported from the cell and become metabolized in other tissues, e.g. as an energy supply for shivering thermogenesis in muscles.

Continued use of triglycerides for thermogenesis in the newborn rapidly leads to exhaustion of the supply available in the tissue, and therefore ultimately to cessation of thermogenesis. Replenishment of the triglycerides is therefore necessary to ensure thermogenesis. Brown adipose tissue has a comparatively active fatty acid synthesis pathway, but it is doubtful whether this pathway is active during thermogenesis (it is inhibited by norepinephrine and thus is probably mainly active in refilling the triglyceride droplets during periods without thermogenic demand on the tissue). Rather, the major influx of new substrate for thermogenesis comes from the activity of lipoprotein lipase. Lipoprotein lipase is regulated in a unique way in brown adipose tissue; in addition to stimulation by insulin, it also is stimulated by norepinephrine, via a β-adrenergic, cAMP-dependent pathway. The regulation of lipoprotein lipase activity occurs at the transcriptional level. The increased lipoprotein lipase activity in brown adipose tissue is induced via two pathways: when the newborn has an acute need for heat (via the norepinephrine pathway) and also when there is a fresh supply of food, after nursing (via an

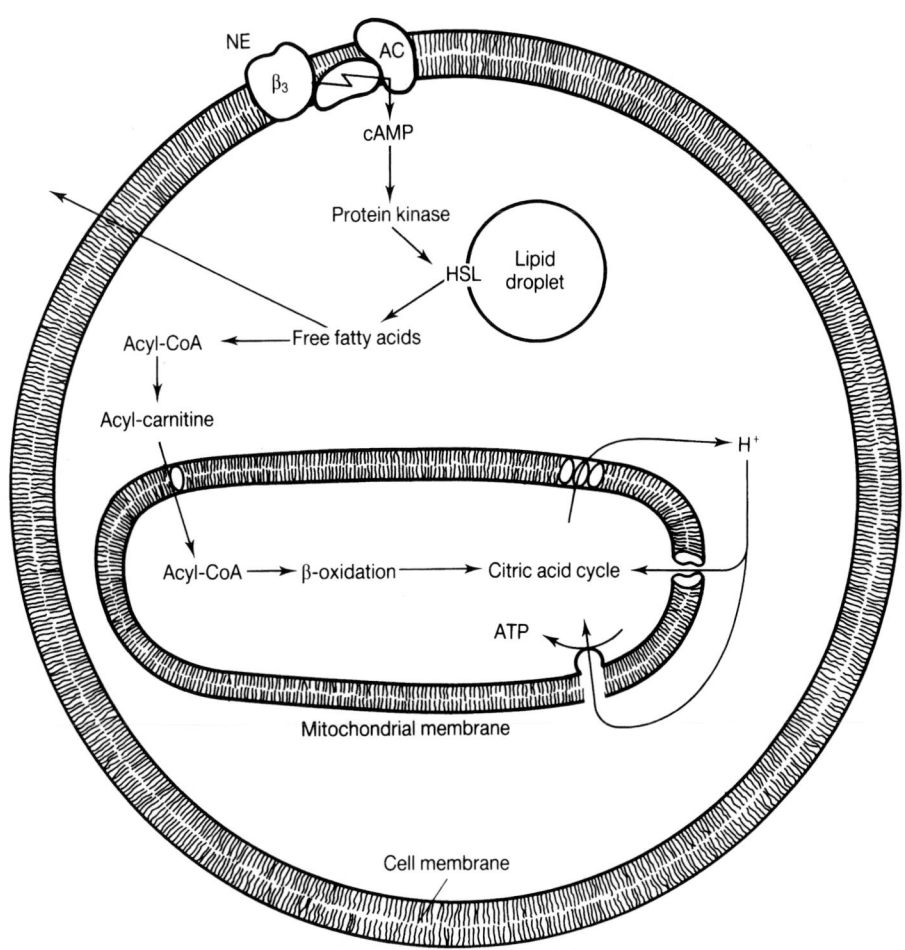

FIGURE 48.6 The cytosolic events in the brown fat cell following β₃-adrenergic stimulation by norepinephrine (NE). AC, adenylyl cyclase; HSL, hormone-sensitive lipase. For details on mitochondrial function, see Fig. 48.7.

insulin pathway similar to that found in white adipose tissue).

## The uncoupling protein, thermogenin and mitochondrial thermogenic events

The combustion of the fatty acids released from the triglycerides takes place in the mitochondria. The fatty acids first are converted on the cytosolic side of the mitochondria to acyl-CoA (acyl-coenzyme A); they then are transported in the form of acylcarnitine derivatives over the mitochondrial membrane, and on the inside, reformed acyl-CoAs are degraded to acetyl-CoA moieties by going through the necessary number of rounds of so called β-oxidation (*see* page 150). The acetyl-CoA formed enters the citric acid cycle, $CO_2$ is released and the electrons from reduced nicotinamide adenine dinucleotide (NADH) and reduced flavine adenine dinucleotide ($FADH_2$) are transported to $O_2$ through the electron transport chain of the mitochondria to form water, all this just as in other fat metabolizing tissues. Here, however, ends the similarity with other mitochondria.

The unique properties of brown fat mitochondria are due to the uncoupling protein, *thermogenin*. As seen in Fig. 48.7, the transport of electrons through the mitochondrial electron transport chain (or

"respiratory chain") is coupled to pumping of $H^+$ out of the mitochondria, into the cytosol. Through this, a proton electrochemical potential is built up; the size of this potential increases, until it is equal to the energy available from electron transport. Then respiration ceases (electrons are no longer transported to $O_2$). In all mitochondria other than those in brown fat, the energy stored in the proton electrochemical potential is primarily utilized when $H^+$ ions re-enter the mitochondrial matrix through the ATP synthetase complex and the energy is captured in the form of ATP.

In brown fat mitochondria, thermogenin (Fig. 48.7) allows protons to re-enter the mitochondrial matrix, without capturing the energy in the form of a chemical bond. The function of this uncoupling protein is thus to short-circuit the protonic circuit, and just as when an electrical circuit is short-circuited, all energy is now released as heat. Thus, the energy which was released when electrons were transported from their high potential in fatty acids via NADH and $FADH_2$ to $O_2$, and which was temporarily stored in the form of the proton electrochemical gradient, now is released in the form of heat. Thus the introduction of this single protein totally changes the purpose of the organized fatty acid degradation pathway to become energy dissipative instead of energy conserving.

Thermogenin is exclusively found in brown adipose tissue, and thus exclusively in mammals. It has a monomeric molecular weight of 32 kD, but probably

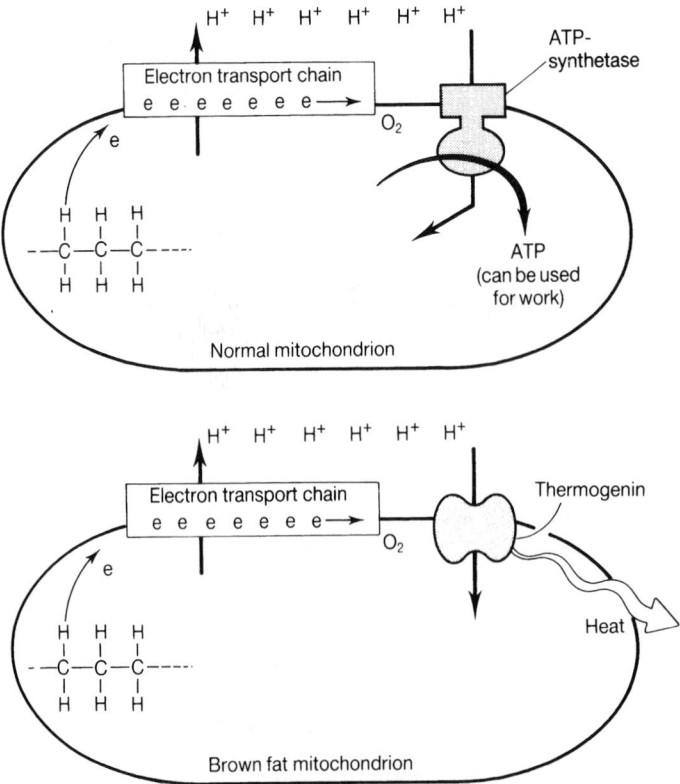

FIGURE 48.7 The mitochondrial events: a comparison of the ATP producing function of "normal" mitochondria (top) with the heat-producing function of brown fat mitochondria (bottom). For structural details of the uncoupling protein thermogenin, see Fig. 48.8.

is active in a homodimeric state. When the sequence of about 300 amino acids is analyzed, it becomes clear that thermogenin has developed from three repeats, each with a length of about 100 amino acids. As thermogenin is a membrane protein, it would be expected that stretches of hydrophobic amino acids should be observed; however, this is not the case. This paradox can be resolved if the structure is analyzed for amphiphilic α-helices. In each 100-amino-acid sequence, two such amphiphilic sequences are found; they are characterized as being α-helices which are hydrophilic on one side and hydrophobic on the other side. It therefore is believed that thermogenin has the structure sketched in Fig. 48.8.

When in an active state, thermogenin transports $H^+$ through the mitochondrial membrane. How this is accomplished molecularly is not known; it is most likely that thermogenin functions as a transporter on which only one $H^+$ can be transported at a time, i.e. not as an open channel with mass flux. Thermogenin is not constantly active, as this would lead to brown fat thermogenesis being permanently switched on, a physiologically unwarranted situation. Rather, thermogenin is endowed with a binding site for purine nucleotides; this binding site can bind ATP, ADP, guanosine triphospate (GTP) and guanosine diphosphate (GDP) with high affinity (this binding site is often referred to as "the GDP-binding site"). Binding of, for example, ATP to this site leads to a conformational change in the thermogenin molecule, including a total inhibition of the $H^+$-transporting activity. Due to the high affinity of the site for ATP and to the high cytosolic concentration of ATP, it is likely that in the resting state, the site is always occupied and thermogenic activity is fully inhibited. Activation of thermogenin thus occurs by overcoming this inhibition, but the mechanism is not yet clear. Based mainly on the fact that free fatty acids added to isolated brown fat cells can elicit thermogenesis without norepinephrine stimulation being necessary, most investigators favor the postlipolytic hypotheses, in which the activation occurs as an effect of fatty acids being released from triglycerides.

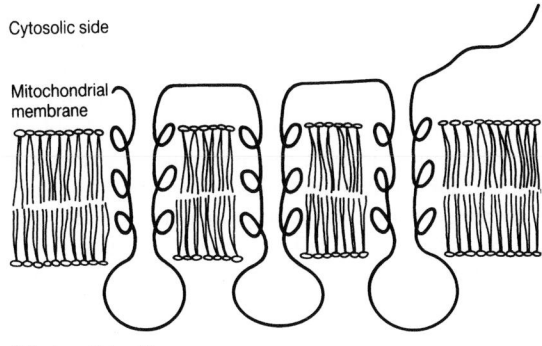

Cytosolic side

Mitochondrial membrane

Mitochondrial matrix

FIGURE 48.8 Some of the accepted structural and functional characteristics of the uncoupling protein thermogenin (see text)

It appears that thermogenin belongs to a family of mitochondrial proteins, which include the oxoglutarate carrier and the ATP/ADP carrier, all of which are found in the mitochondrial inner membrane and all of which function as transporters of specific compounds over the mitochondrial membrane. For thermogenin, the transported species would thus be $H^+$. It can be imagined that these proteins, probably at least 15 different ones, have all developed from an ancestor which developed in free-living bacteria to help take up substrate (food) from the surroundings.

## The recruitment process

Brown adipose tissue is particularly adaptable and responds to an increased demand for its activity by rapidly and extensively increasing its capacity for heat production in two ways: by acquiring more brown fat cells and/or by making "better" cells (cells in a more recruited state with more thermogenin). Mammalian species differ in this respect. The relative importance of these two mechanisms in the human neonate is uncertain.

The number of brown fat cells with which a child is born is probably established early during fetal development. Even in experimental animals it is not known whether there is a postnatal increase in the total number of brown fat cells. However, in adult rats during adaptation to cold the increase in thermogenic capacity mainly corresponds to an increase in the number of brown fat cells. Initiation of division of brown fat cell precursors (brown preadipocytes or stem cells) demands the presence of classical growth factors, but experiments indicate that such growth factors are not physiologically regulatory. Rather it would seem that norepinephrine, released when heat production is needed, can also initiate cell division, but in contrast to thermogenesis, the receptors involved are $\beta_1$-receptors. The undifferentiated cells which can respond in this way do not possess the more specialized $\beta_3$-receptors.

As thermogenin is the rate-limiting step for thermogenesis, an increase in the total amount of thermogenin in brown fat is the only way to increase thermogenic potential. Norepinephrine, working through $\beta_3$-receptors, induces gene expression of thermogenin which can only function if its increased expression is accompanied by an increased amount of mitochondria in the tissue, with an ensuing higher capacity for the combustion of fatty acids. Mitochondrial recruitment has not been shown to be directly under norepinephrine control; rather, the whole differentiation process of the brown fat cells is promoted by norepinephrine, and the lipid metabolizing enzymes are induced as an effect of advanced general differentiation, not as a direct and specified effect.

## Perinatal recruitment

Both the acute thermogenic response and the recruitment process are stimulated by norepinephrine. In many physiological situations this makes good sense, since an increased demand for heat production suggests a requirement for increased total capacity. There are, however, physiological situations in which this relationship does not seem optimal. One of these is found during perinatal recruitment.

The principal patterns of brown fat recruitment in different types of mammalian newborn are shown in Fig. 48.9. The postnatal recruitment in *altricial* species is most easily understood. As noted above, these species, e.g. rats and mice, are born blind and hairless, the pups huddle in the nest and are often warmed by the dam. Recruitment takes place in response to a demand for thermogenesis as the pups are gradually exposed to the cold. In the immature newborn, e.g. hamsters, recruitment does not occur until several weeks after birth due to an initial absence of sympathetic innervation to the brown adipose tissue; once synapses are established, recruitment proceeds. However, many mammalian newborn are *precocial* and are well developed at birth; this is the case for newborn calves and lambs, and indeed for most larger mammals. These newborns not only can walk soon after birth but also have well developed brown adipose tissue at birth, and their acquisition of this represents a regulatory dilemma. *In utero*, there is no demand for thermogenesis, the fetus is warmer than in its later free-living condition. Non-shivering thermogenesis cannot be demonstrated in fetal sheep cooled *in utero*. However, it can be induced following supplemental oxygenation and umbilical cord occlusion. Thus it is likely that physiological inhibitors of fetal cAMP-dependent pathways are present, e.g. in the form of prostaglandins and adenosine produced by the placenta. However, such inhibitors would also inhibit the β-adrenergic pathway which stimulates recruitment, and the fact that recruitment occurs *in utero* thus remains unexplained in such species. After birth, separation from the placenta would remove the placental inhibitors and so allow rapid brown fat thermogenesis to facilitate neonatal adaptation.

The human baby is considered to be "typed" between altricial and precocial at term; newborn babies possess a "basic" amount of active brown adipose tissue, but this can be markedly increased in response to a cooler environment.

# Brown adipose tissue and thyroid hormone

While thyroid hormone stimulates thermogenic processes and the level of basal metabolism of an organism, there also is an interaction between thyroid hormones and non-shivering thermogenesis. Brown adipocytes contain the enzyme type II iodothyronine 5'-monodeiodinase which catalyzes the conversion of thyroxine ($T_4$) to the active form, triiodothyronine ($T_3$). This may lead to local and systemic effects. Increased intracellular $T_3$ levels augment the expression of thermogenin in brown adipocytes. *In vivo*, increases in thermogenin RNA levels seem always to be paralleled or slightly preceded by an increase in the activity of the deiodinase. Brown adipose cells of the newborn have to be in a euthyroid state for norepinephrine to induce thermogenin gene expression. In fetal sheep, thyroidectomy 2 weeks before delivery leads to hypothermia and impaired thermogenesis at delivery, and brown adipocytes from thyroidectomized fetal sheep have reduced tissue respiration in response to norepinephrine stimulation *in vitro*. Thyroidectomized rats have a three-fold reduction in thermogenin levels in brown adipocytes and become hypothermic. Replacement therapy with $T_3$ does not correct the hypothermia or low levels of thermogenin, while replacement with $T_4$ corrects both very rapidly. Thus, optimal thermogenic function of brown adipose tissue seems to require the intracellular conversion of $T_4$ to $T_3$. Circulating $T_4$ as well as intracellular $T_3$ production are essential for neonatal thermogenesis, rather than the circulating $T_3$ surge following delivery.

## DEVELOPMENTAL AND PATHOLOGICAL ASPECTS

At birth the neonate experiences a dramatic change in thermal environment, from a tightly regulated one controlled by the mother to a less predictable one in which the responses of its own thermoregulatory system are essential for survival. Immediately after birth the deep body temperature falls. In the human infant under normal conditions it may fall to below 36°C 3 hours after birth, if care is not optimal, but by 8 hours it usually has returned to the adult range where it remains. The human baby has limited thermal insulation due to a decreased thickness of body shell and a large body surface/volume ratio. As body mass increases to adult size the overall insulation increases by a factor of 1.8. On the first day after birth, control can be exercised

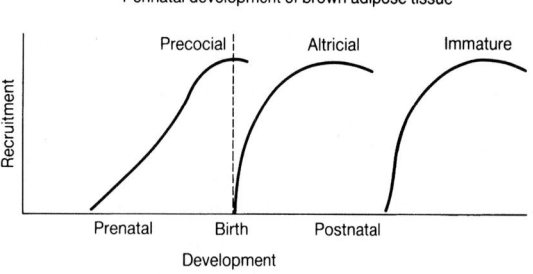

FIGURE 48.9 Perinatal brown fat recruitment in immature, altricial and precocial mammals

over the peripheral vasomotor tone to effect a three-fold change in tissue insulation, although this may still be inadequate insulation. Therefore additional thermal insulation is of great importance. Simply wrapping the baby in a blanket can alter the thermoregulatory range from 36–26°C to 30–10°C. Covering the head is of particular importance as it forms a large proportion of the baby's exposed surface area.

Regulation of temperature by active sweating can occur in babies born at term. About 400 sweat glands per $cm^2$ have been found on the thigh, six times as many as in adults, although each gland produces sweat at only one-third of the rate. With earlier gestation, however, few infants sweat and below 32 weeks' gestation sweating has not been demonstrated.

Soon after birth the newborn is able to respond to a cool environment by an increase in metabolic rate and hence heat production. This takes place without shivering or physical activity, the heat being generated mainly from the brown adipose tissue. The resting metabolic rate of immature infants per kilogram body weight is similar to term infants. Their thermogenic response to cold exposure is more difficult to determine. A breakthrough in the management of preterm infants came with the realization that keeping them in a thermoneutral environment improved survival. While preterm infants have a higher surface/volume ratio, implying more rapid heat loss than term infants, an additional reason for the higher susceptibility to hypothermia is incomplete development of brown adipose tissue, which thus has a limited thermogenic capacity. There is brown adipose tissue present at 28 weeks' gestation; it is unclear whether this can lead to increased heat generation. Further, if nutritional support is inadequate, the brown adipose tissue may encounter a lack of substrate which will hamper the ability of the tissue to produce sufficient heat. Thus, in malnutrition the lack of sufficient food may lead to hypothermia in infants. This problem is not restricted to temperate latitudes; the baby relies on its brown fat thermogenesis to remain warm, even at tropical latitudes.

It has been known for many years that low birth weight infants raised in subthermoneutral conditions grow more slowly than those in thermoneutral conditions, if each group receives identical feeding [120 cal/(kg·day)]. The infants are able to make up this difference when given a caloric supplement sufficient to match the calculated cost of the cold-induced metabolic rise. Using computer-controlled incubator systems, there is an improved caloric efficiency for growth.

The term human baby is born with a large amount of brown adipose tissue, and during early postnatal life the tissue probably becomes further recruited. The tissue remains metabolically important for several years, but with time it tends to become atrophied. It is not known whether this decrease in metabolic significance is an obligatory postnatal event, but extrapolation from other mammals indicates that the decrease does not occur if the young are under constant exposure to comparatively cold conditions. Thus, differences in acute tolerance to lower temperatures may reflect the extent to which the child has been protected from, or exposed to, comparative cold during early years. As brown-fat activity also can be induced via a dietary stimulus, it can be implied that that fraction of the so-called "specific dynamic effect" of food, the increased metabolism seen after a meal, which could derive from brown fat metabolism should be higher in the small child. The lower efficiency (calories gained per calorie eaten) in small children therefore not only may be due to their generally higher rate of metabolism, but also, to some extent, may reflect brown adipose tissue activation.

During anesthesia in infants, body temperature regulation is lost. While central regulation also may be involved, it is clear that commonly used inhalation anesthetics related to halothane dramatically inhibit brown fat metabolism *in vitro* and non-shivering thermogenesis *in vivo*, thereby contributing to the problems of body temperature regulation during anesthesia.

There may be an increased amount of brown adipose tissue in the victims of the *sudden infant death syndrome* (SIDS). This may reflect secondary effects of hypoxic events which have occurred chronically in the prospective victim. This hypoxia would lead to a chronic sympathetic activation which in turn would recruit the tissue. As an alternative hypothesis, it has been suggested that a subgroup of the babies diagnosed as SIDS victims in reality have died of hyperthermia, and that a high brown fat thermogenesis, evoked, e.g. by minor cold, has caused a fatal rise in body temperature in babies who have been too well insulated.

## SELECTED READING

Cannon B, Bengtsson T, Dicker A *et al*. The role of adrenergic stimulation in regulation of heat production and recruitment of brown adipose tissue. In: Zeisberger E, Schönbaum E, Lomax P eds. *Thermal balance in health and disease*. Basel: Birkhäuser Verlag, 1994: 87.

Clark RP, Edholm OG. *Man and his thermal environment*. London: Edward Arnold, 1985.

Gunn TR, Gluckman PD. Perinatal Thermogenesis. *Early Human Develop* 1995, **42**: 169.

Hensel H. *Thermoreception and temperature regulation*. London: Academic Press, 1981.

Nedergaard J, Connolly E, Cannon B. Brown adipose tissue in the mammalian newborn. In: Trayhurn P, Nicholls DG eds. *Brown adipose tissue*. London: Edward Arnold, 1986: 152.

# 49

# Fever and Antipyresis

Eugen Zeisberger

Although body temperature is tightly controlled, the thermoregulatory capacity can be exceeded. At the extremes of climatic conditions, hypothermia or hyperthermia can result. Furthermore, heat production may exceed heat loss, resulting in a rise in body temperature. In *malignant hyperthermia*, for example, there is a state of uncontrolled heat production by peripheral cells. Fever differs from hyperthermia. It can be defined as a body temperature regulated in a resting subject above the range of normal. It is brought about by active thermoregulation and is generally associated with a pathological condition.

Fever is now regarded as part of a complex immunological response to different antigenic stimuli including infections caused by bacteria, viruses and fungi, antigen–antibody complexes, neoplasms, delayed type hypersensitivity reactions and other stimuli inducing inflammation. In homeotherms the thermoregulatory mechanisms behave during fever as if they were adjusted to maintain body temperature at a higher than normal set range. Depending on ambient temperature the heat loss is reduced, and in a cold environment the heat production is additionally increased until the new thermoregulatory set range is reached. Fever is the most universally known symptom of infectious disease and inflammatory responses.

The febrile response may be beneficial, given that it evolved long ago in the phylogeny and persisted as a response to infections. It may facilitate the activation of the immune defense since antibody production and T-cell proliferation are more efficient at higher body temperatures than at normal levels. Moreover, many microorganisms grow best within a relatively narrow temperature range so that a rise in temperature inhibits their growth. Some poikilothermic lizards can resist bacterial infections at elevated ambient temperatures, but will die of the same infection in a cool environment. In humans fevers were artificially induced before the advent of antibiotics for the treatment of *neurosyphilis* and proved to be beneficial. Hyperthermia seems to slow the growth of some tumors and has been found to benefit individuals with some bacterial, viral and fungal diseases.

Very high temperatures are harmful. When the central body temperature exceeds 41°C for prolonged periods, some permanent brain damage may result. At temperatures over 43°C *heat stroke* develops, frequently leading to death. Since the body temperature normally does not exceed 41°C during fever, it has been proposed that the elevation in body temperature is controlled and limited by the actions of endogenous antipyretic substances liberated within the brain during fever. The endogenous antipyresis is thus a normal constituent of the febrile response.

## MEDIATORS OF FEVER

There is increasing evidence that the immune system and the central nervous system (CNS) are functionally connected and interacting. This bilateral communication is mediated by signal substances (Fig. 49.1). Lymphocytes, macrophages and other cells involved in immune responses communicate, in part, by hormone-like chemical messengers called cytokines (*see* page 919). In addition to the immunomodulatory actions, cytokines exert effects on blood vessels, skeletal muscles, the liver and the brain. The effects on the central nervous system include anorexia, increased secretion of corticotrophin-releasing hormone (CRH), increased slow wave sleep and fever. The pyrogenic cytokines are also called endogenous pyrogens and include interleukin-1α (IL-1α), interleukin-1β (IL-1β), interleukin-2 (IL-2), interleukin-6 (IL-6), interferon-β$_2$, tumor necrosis factor (TNF, cachectin), tumor necrosis factor β (TNFβ, lymphotoxin), interferon-α (IFN-α), interferon-γ (IFN-γ) and colony stimulating factors (CSF). The steps in the production of a fever are shown in a simplified form in Fig. 49.2.

The metabolic effects of cytokines, resulting from their actions on liver and muscle, appearing simultaneously with a febrile rise in body temperature are called an acute phase response. They include increased

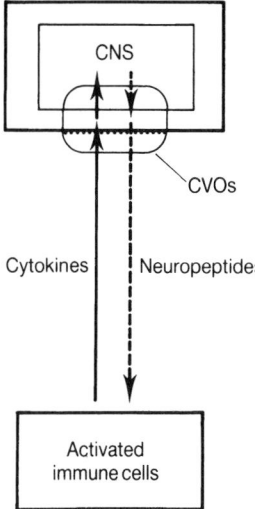

FIGURE 49.1 Bilateral communications between immune and central nervous systems (circumventricular organs, CVOs).

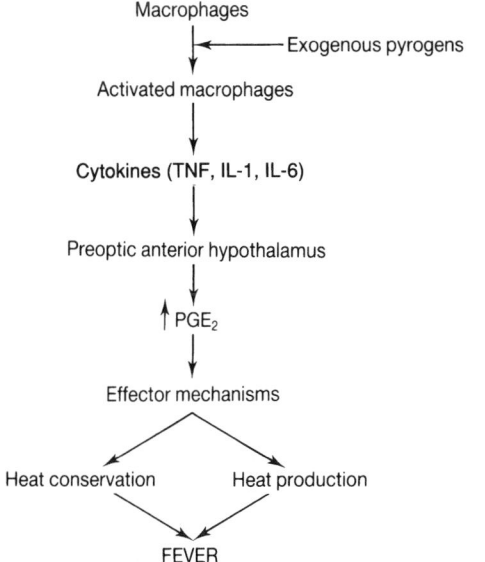

FIGURE 49.2 Steps in production of a fever (simplified)

synthesis of hepatic proteins, increased sodium excretion, increases in ceruloplasmin–copper concentrations, decreases in serum iron and zinc concentrations, negative nitrogen balance, and aminoaciduria. It is accompanied by some hematological effects such as an increased number of circulating neutrophils and decreased number of circulating lymphocytes, increased secretion of colony stimulating factors and by inhibition of lipoprotein lipase.

It is possible to evoke fever by injections of endotoxins which are complex lipopolysaccharides derived from bacterial walls. They are recognized by immune cells as foreign and induce the immune defense reactions resulting in the release of endogenous pyrogens. After intravenous injection of bacterial endotoxin, fever develops after a 30-minute latent period, the time needed by the organism to release endogenous pyrogens like IL-1. In most laboratory animals the normal febrile rise of body temperature peaks about 3 hours after the injection of bacterial endotoxin. At this peak the increase of body temperature amounts to between 1 and 2 °C, and it takes another 3 hours before the temperature returns to the original level. The entire febrile response to an intravenous injection of bacterial endotoxin lasts thus about 6 hours, and after large doses the shape of the fever curve is biphasic. Repeated intravenous injection of endotoxin makes the recipient tolerant, i.e. no response occurs to further injections of endotoxin. There is evidence for both a peripheral immunological component to tolerance and also for central mechanisms (increasing activation of antipyretic systems and septal release of vasopressin). Endogenous pyrogens like IL-1 and TNF evoke fever after 5–15 minutes even in endotoxin tolerant recipients. Originally, it was claimed that endogenous pyrogens do not induce tolerance when administered repeatedly, but recent experiments revealed a partial development of tolerance to peripheral injections of recombinant human cytokines in experimental animals. Repeated injections of cytokines directly into the hypothalamus did not induce tolerance.

The pyrogenic effects of endogenous pyrogens are mediated by local release of prostaglandins. They are released from inflamed tissue. They also are found in the brain and may alter the release or effects of neurotransmitters. Circulatory concentrations increase after injection of pyrogens, probably because IL-1 can stimulate muscle proteolysis during fever by increasing production of prostaglandin $E_2$ ($PGE_2$). Anti-inflammatory steroids, such as cortisol, inhibit the release of arachidonic acid from phospholipid stores and thus block the formation of all eicosanoid products (see page 163). Non-steroidal anti-inflammatory drugs such as aspirin and indomethacin inhibit cyclooxygenase and thus block only the formation of prostaglandins, prostacyclin and thromboxanes, leaving the lipoxygenase pathways intact.

Injections of bacterial endotoxin, endogenous pyrogens or prostaglandins into the brain initiate fevers most promptly from special sites, such as the cluster of neurons in the organum vasculosum laminae terminalis (OVLT), the preoptic region in the limbic system, and the anterior hypothalamus. Also direct mechanical injury or application of chemical substances into the OVLT may release the endogenous $PGE_2$, which results in fever. Neurons and glial cells from these pyrogen-sensitive sites can produce and release $PGE_2$. Some of these cells and others in the hypothalamus can also produce IL-1. Many hypothalamic neurons have receptors for IL-1 and other endogenous pyrogens. In perfusates from these regions increased levels of IL-1, IL-6, TNF and $PGE_2$ can be found during the peripherally induced fever. However, it is very improbable that these increased levels derive from the blood as these molecules are too large to pass the intact blood–brain barrier. How can the peripheral mediators of fever influence the hypothalamic regulatory circuits?

The transduction mechanisms are poorly understood and largely hypothetical. The endogenous pyrogens can enter the perivascular space of circumventricular organs such as OVLT and bind to specific receptors on the surface of the parenchymal microglia and astrocytal end feet. They activate these cells to produce $PGE_2$ and other mediators and release them at the brain side of the barrier. The $PGE_2$ in turn activates neurons in the OVLT which transmit, via their axons, this excitation to neurons and glia at other central sites, e.g. in the preoptic area or anterior hypothalamus. These structures are responsible for simultaneous central release of endogenous pyrogens. They stimulate the local release of $PGE_2$, which can influence the activity of thermosensitive preoptic neurons and thermointegrative hypothalamic neurons, resulting in a change of the thermoregulatory set range with increases of both heat production and heat conservation, and thus a fever.

## DEVELOPMENTAL ASPECTS

Newborn infants can have severe infections, such as meningitis or septicemia, without increasing body temperature. Since the thermoregulatory system is operative at birth, this observation is sometimes ascribed to an immunological defect or inability to form IL-1. However, there is evidence that a febrile response does develop soon after birth and the lack of fever may reflect either a limited thermogenic capacity or the environmental temperature at which they are nursed. Pregnant ewes and guinea-pigs show a progressive loss of fever response to bacterial endotoxins before and after giving birth. Newborn of both species show similarly reduced febrile responses in the first few days of postuterine life in spite of their fully developed abilities to produce endogenous pyrogens and to regulate their body temperature. Such lines of evidence suggest the activation of antipyretic systems. The biological significance of this fever suppression in the near term human and newborn animal is not known.

## ACTIVATION OF ENDOGENOUS ANTIPYRESIS

The febrile signals transduced into the CNS result in a local release of $PGE_2$ in the anterior hypothalamus. This release activates parvocellular neurons in the paraventricular nucleus (PVN) to release mainly corticotrophin-releasing hormone (CRH) from the terminals in the median eminence into the portal hypophyseal blood. CRH stimulates the secretion of adrenocorticotrophic hormone (ACTH) and other pro-opiomelanocorticotrophin derivatives from the corticotropes of the anterior lobe of the pituitary (see page 504). ACTH activates the release of cortisol, which has suppressive effects on the immune system, to inhibit the production of IL-2 by T lymphocytes and thus effectively stop the lymphocyte proliferation. Glucocorticoids have anti-inflammatory and anti-allergic effects and also antipyretic actions because they inhibit phospholipase A, with a consequent reduction in the release of arachidonic acid and all its products including prostaglandins. They also inhibit the release of IL-1 from granulocytes.

Free glucocorticoids inhibit ACTH secretion at both the pituitary and the hypothalamic level. As a consequence the composition of the transmitter cocktail produced by parvocellular neurons in the PVN changes such that instead of CRH they produce arginine vasopressin (AVP). One part of the AVP-immunoreactive neurons does not project to the median eminence but to different areas of the limbic system, including the septum and amygdala. These systems are activated during the fever rise. Exogenous melanocyte-stimulating hormone (MSH) (a metabolite of ACTH) and AVP, microinjected or microinfused into the septum reduce or prevent fevers evoked by bacterial endotoxins, endogenous pyrogens or by intraventricular application of prostaglandins. The antipyretic site can be identified in a small area located ventrally to the lateral septum. The released AVP stimulates the septal neurons via $V_1$ receptors (see Chapter 40). This excitation is then transmitted via septofugal fibers to the hypothalamic thermoregulatory structures, where it cancels the changes induced by pyrogens. Another antipyretic mechanism, also mediated by AVP, has been found in the OVLT.

Thus, endogenous antipyresis can be mediated by at least three mechanisms. The first one is a neuronal pathway from the septum to the hypothalamic thermointegrative neurons which can block the changes induced by pyrogens. The second is the disseminated AVP perivascular system in the OVLT, which is functionally interconnected with the antipyretic septal area. AVP released from this system may influence the permeability or the binding of endogenous pyrogens to their receptors. It can thus change the local production of $PGE_2$, transforming the immune signals into neuronal messages. The third mechanism is peripheral. It is based on the action of some hormones on immune cells. They may act as selective inhibitors of production of endogenous pyrogens and thus reduce the immune signals.

## SELECTED READING

Brück K. Neonatal thermal regulation. In: Polin RA, Fox WW eds. *Fetal and neonatal medicine – physiology and pathophysiology*. Philadelphia: WB Saunders Co., 1991.

Cooper KE. Fever and antipyresis. The role of the nervous system. Cambridge University Press, New York, 1995.

Zeisberger E. The role of septal peptides in thermoregulation and fever. In: Bligh J, Voigt K eds. *Thermoreception and temperature regulation*. Berlin, Heidelberg: Springer-Verlag, 1990.

# PART TEN

# *The Gastrointestinal System and Nutrition*

**Editor: Colin D. Rudolph**

# Introduction

Colin D. Rudolph

## Introduction

Most animal behaviors have evolved primarily for the purpose of efficiently obtaining and selecting food. This process is directed by the central nervous system. An infant cries to signal the mother that it is time to feed. Adults either hunt food, grow food, or earn money to exchange for food. These activities all result in the ingestion of liquid and solid nutrients, which are transported to the stomach where mixing and storage occurs. Complex hormonal and neural feedback mechanisms inform the central nervous system that adequate nutrients have been ingested prior to nutrient absorption. The gastrointestinal system processes complex foodstuffs, providing sustenance to the entire body. Ingested foods are initially lubricated, mechanically ground, and chemically digested into an emulsion in the mouth and stomach. This emulsion, chyme, slowly passes from the stomach to the small intestine, where enzymes and bile secreted by the pancreas and liver further digest complex molecules into simpler carbohydrates, peptides, and fats for absorption into the bloodstream. Subsequent metabolic processing and storage occurs in the liver. Non-absorbed electrolytes, water, and nutrients are salvaged by the colon prior to excretion of waste products as feces.

The initial chapters of this part describe the ontogeny of the structural components of the gastrointestinal tract, including the specialized epithelia, smooth muscle, hormonal, neural and immunologic tissues, and blood vessels. Subsequent sections describe the development of coordinated functions such as propulsion of luminal contents, and the digestion and absorption of fluids, electrolytes, and nutrients. For clarity, liver development and function are discussed separately. Nutrient requirements of the growing human are summarized in the final section.

# 50

# Embryology and Anatomy of the Gastrointestinal tract

Miles L. Epstein and Colin D. Rudolph

The gastrointestinal tract receives tissue contributions from all three germ layers. The primitive gut first forms as a cavity lined by endoderm, which gives rise to the entire epithelial lining of the digestive tube. Most digestive glands, including the liver, gallbladder and pancreas, arise as buds from this endodermal lining. Through lateral folding, the splanchnic mesoderm comes to lie adjacent to, and eventually to surround, the endodermal-lined gut tube, forming the connective tissue and muscular walls. Later, the neural tube derived from the ectoderm gives rise to neural crest cells. These migrate from the neural tube and invade the mesodermal portion of the gut tube, where they form the neurons and glial cells intrinsic to the gastrointestinal tract.

## DEVELOPMENT OF MAJOR STRUCTURES

The timetable of morphologic development of the human gastrointestinal tract is reviewed here briefly (Fig. 50.1). The foregut and hindgut are first identifiable as blind endoderm-lined pouches surrounded by mesoderm. The midgut represents the region opening to the yolk sac and is the last region to be invested with mesoderm. As the gut grows, several key morphological events occur. The respiratory primordium separates from the foregut so that the trachea is distinct from the esophagus. The foregut undergoes differential growth and rotates so that the stomach assumes its adult shape and position. The liver, gallbladder and ventral pancreatic bud develop from an endodermal outgrowth appearing distal to the stomach, while the dorsal pancreatic bud arises from a different outgrowth. Rotation of the duodenum and migration of the ventral pancrea-

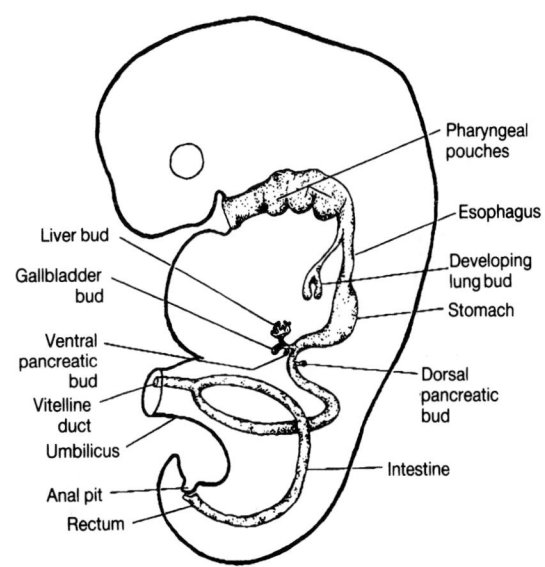

FIGURE 50.1 Schematic representation of the morphologic development of the human gastrointestinal tract at 5 weeks' gestation

tic bud result in juxtaposition, and ultimately fusion, of the pancreatic buds to form a single pancreas, as well as unification of the pancreatic and bile ducts. As the gut elongates, there is insufficient space to accommodate the midgut inside the peritoneal cavity, and the gut expands into the extraembryonic celom within the umbilical cord. During this herniation the gut rotates 90° about the axis of the superior mesenteric artery; an additional 180° counterclockwise rotation occurs upon the return of the midgut to the peritoneal cavity. The net result is to position the cecum in the right lower quadrant of the peritoneal cavity. The mesenteries fuse to the parietal peritoneum, fixing the ascending and descending colon in place. The connection between the yolk sac and the gut is the vitelline duct, which can persist as an outpocketing of the ileum, also called a Meckel diverticulum. The cloaca is divided by the urogenital sinus and eventually separates into the urinary bladder and rectum, which fuses with the overlying ectoderm to form the anus. At the site of the rectum is a depression in the ectoderm called the anal pit; this breaks down to permit continuity between the endodermal lining of the rectum and the ectodermal lining of the anus.

## DEVELOPMENT OF MUCOSA AND MUSCLE

The gastrointestinal wall is composed of external muscle layers, neural plexus, and mucosa throughout the gastrointestinal tract (Fig. 50.2). Differentiation of the epithelial lining, the mucosa, confers specialized functions to each region. Variations in the geometric arrangement of the muscle layers may also confer specialized contractile function. Whereas the esophageal mucosa has the relatively simple function of providing a lubricated conduit for bolus passage and a barrier to infection, the stomach and intestinal mucosa have additional complex secretory, digestive, and absorptive tasks. The maturation of mucosa proceeds in a proximal-to-distal direction. The entire bowel is initially lined with a multilayered epithelium with numerous vacuolizations. In humans, the esophageal epithelium becomes ciliated at 10 weeks' gestation. Replacement by stratified squamous epithelia begins at the fifth month, with patches of ciliated epithelium occasionally persisting until birth. In many mammals, especially those that eat coarse vegetable foods, such as rodents and ruminants, the esophageal mucosa undergoes keratinization.

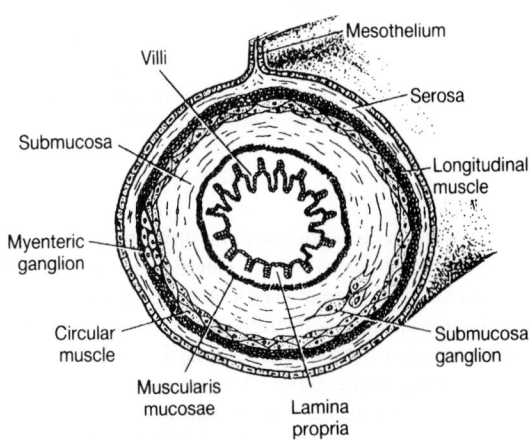

FIGURE 50.2 Schematic representation of a cross-section of the small intestine, demonstrating the layers of the intestinal wall

The mature stomach mucosa is lined with tall columnar cells that have an overlying coat of mucus. Glandular pits contain acid-secreting parietal cells, pepsinogen-secreting chief cells, and goblet-shaped mucus-secreting cells. Slender, flask-shaped cells with slender processes extending to the luminal surface, known as enterochromaffin cells, secrete hormones. Parietal cells are found in the fetal mucosa by 9 weeks' gestation. By 10 weeks enterochromaffin cells can be identified (see Chapter 53), and by 13 weeks cells resembling chief cells are present. By 16 weeks mucus-secreting cells are present. Although peptic activity has been demonstrated in the human stomach by 16 weeks, chief cells cannot be demonstrated to contain pepsinogen until term. Parietal cells contain intrinsic factor by 14 weeks' gestation. The parietal cells do not secrete acid until after birth. The functional development of gastric acid secretion and barrier function are described in Chapter 55.

Finger-like projections, known as villi, project into the lumen of the small bowel, markedly increasing the surface area available for digestion and absorption. Columnar intestinal cells with a microvillus luminal membrane occupy most of the surface of these villi, further increasing surface area. Transport proteins and digestive enzymes are present on the luminal membrane of these cells (see Chapter 56). The various types of villous lining cells are thought to be formed from multipotent stem cells located in the crypts at the villus base. The cells differentiate during migration to the villus tip where they are shed into the bowel lumen. Migration times are longer in the fetus than in the adult. Columnar cells and mucus-secreting goblet cells become recognizable by 8–10 weeks' gestation in the human. By 10–12 weeks villi have appeared and enterochromaffin cells are present. A separate population of pyramid-shaped mucosal cells with prominent secretory granules and little or no turnover, known as Paneth cells, are located at the base of the crypts in humans, monkeys, and ruminants, but not in dogs, cats, or raccoons. These cells appear at 11–12 weeks' gestation. Their functional role is unknown. Aggregations of lymphocytes in the jejunum and ileum called Peyer patches first appear at 5 months' gestation in the human.

Mucosal development of the large intestine follows that of the small intestine. Villi are present at 10–12 weeks' gestation but disappear during later fetal life. The mucosa contains specialized absorptive cells, a large number of mucus-secreting cells, and enterochromaffin cells.

Layers of smooth muscle develop in the mesenchymal layer surrounding the mucosa in a craniocaudal pattern parallel to the rest of the components of the bowel. Circular muscle layers develop in the esophagus and stomach during the fifth week of human gestation and are present in the ileum by 8 weeks. Longitudinal muscle layers are not present until 8 weeks and appear in the ileum by the tenth week. The thin layer of smooth muscle that separates the mucosa and submucosa, the muscularis mucosa, is only fully developed by 20 weeks. The development of smooth muscle has been studied more extensively in the developing chick embryo. In any given region of muscle, the cells develop at approximately the same rate. In the chicken gizzard, actin appears to be expressed on embryonic day (E) 5, whereas myosin is not expressed until E7. The quantity of each contractile protein increases through gestation. The isoforms of the contractile protein also change during development. For instance in rat gut, $\alpha$-vascular smooth muscle actin is expressed first at E14 but is the minor isoform in the adult gut. $\gamma$-Enteric smooth muscle actin is found at E15 in the proximal gut and is the predominant form in the adult. The functional significance of these isoforms is unknown at this time. Gap junctions increase in number and size until they approach mature size by 7 days after hatching. Myoglobin appears only at the time of hatching. In contrast to skeletal muscle, mitoses occur in smooth muscle cells even when the contractile apparatus is mature and cell-to-cell junctions are present.

## DEVELOPMENT OF THE ENTERIC NERVOUS SYSTEM

To study the formation of the enteric nervous system has been difficult in mammal, let alone human preparations. Because the chick embryo can be manipulated and observed readily, studies in this preparation have substantially enhanced our knowledge regarding neural innervation of the intestine. Chickens hatch after 21 days of incubation; the gut is fully operative at hatching. Experiments with avian embryos have permitted elucidation of the source for enteric neuron precursors. These experiments involved either ablation of neural folds or replacement of portions of chick neural tube with comparable portions of quail neural tubes. The quail neural crest cells that migrated into the gut were identified by the unique appearance of quail nucleolar DNA. These experiments indicated that neural crest cells from the hindbrain region (rhombencephalic or vagal neural crest) populate the entire gut. Recent experiments with either localized ablation or injection of retrovirus into somites reveal that the major contribution of crest cells to the gut arises from the neural crest located adjacent to somites 3–6. In addition, a second source of crest cells arising posterior to somite 28, termed sacral crest, give rise to cells that populate the postumbilical gut. These findings have been confirmed in the chicken by injection of cellular tracers such as a fluorescent dye or a replication-deficient retrovirus. After neural crest cells migrate to the bowel, the subsequent increase in neural cell numbers could arise either by migration of late-arriving crest cells or, more likely, by cell division. Cells continue to migrate along the gut and reach the ileocecal junction by embryonic day 5.5 in the chicken, roughly 2 days after entry into the foregut. In the next day the crest cells enter the hindgut.

A large body of indirect evidence from a variety of species supports the idea that neural crest cells enter the gut at both anterior and posterior sites, although in the human fetus a single craniocaudal migration of neuroblasts has been reported. Studies with two neuronal markers, neuron-specific enolase and substance P, indicate that neuronal differentiation is most advanced in the pylorus, less advanced in the colon, and least advanced in the ileum. In the mouse, explant cultures from the embryonic foregut and hindgut reveal that neuronal precursors are present in both the proximal and distal portions of the gut at about the same time. Furthermore, neuronal phenotype markers, reduced nicotinamide adenine dinucleotide phosphate (NADPH) diaphorase and calcitonin gene-related peptide (CGRP) (a peptide neurotransmitter), appear at the ends of the gut before they appear in the middle, an observation consistent with two sources of enteric precursors. More convincing is the finding of fluorescent cells in the fetal mouse hindgut after injection of fluorescent dye into the sacral neural tube.

A number of important questions remain about the sacral contribution to enteric neuroblasts. Although two sources of enteric neuroblasts likely exist in the human, to date they have not been described. In the chick and mouse, where sacral crest cells have been found to enter the hindgut, it is unknown whether the sacral crest cells form neurons. Finally, we need to evaluate the possible role of sacral crest defects in *congenital megacolon*. Does the loss of the sacral crest lead to the absence or reduction in neuron numbers in the terminal hindgut?

## Megacolon and Hirschsprung disease

Megacolon results from the absence of a functional enteric nervous system in the terminal bowel. The region of bowel without functional neurons is chronically contracted, causing obstruction to flow and distension of the normally innervated proximal bowel; hence the name megacolon.

Recent studies of mouse models as well as human patients have yielded insights into the pathogenesis of megacolon and its human counterpart, *Hirschsprung disease*. Two mouse mutants, lethal spotted and piebald lethal, are of special interest because they develop congenital megacolon. Extensive studies with gut cultured from lethal spotted mutants indicate that the defect appears to lie in the terminal bowel because neural crest cells from either normal or mutant mice are unable to colonize the distal colon of this mutant. This inability to enter the bowel may be related to an overabundance of laminin and type IV collagen. Recent work in transgenic mice has identified the defective genes in piebald lethal and lethal spotted mutants. Targeted disruption of the endothelin B receptor ($ET_B$) gene in mice results in aganglionic megacolon. This same receptor gene was found to be deleted in piebald lethal mice. In addition, mapping studies of Hirschsprung disease indicate a locus on human chromosome 13 in the region of the $ET_B$ gene. If expression of the $ET_B$ ligand, endothelin-3 (ET-3), is abolished by gene targeting, the mutant mice also have aganglionic megacolon. A naturally occurring mutation in this gene was found in the lethal spotted mutant. These findings indicate the importance of ET-3 and its receptor to the formation of the enteric nervous system in the terminal bowel. However, more work is necessary to understand how the lack of endothelin receptor activation results in the inability of the hindgut to be colonized by neuroblasts.

A more severe phenotype, the absence of enteric neurons from the entire gastrointestinal tract (not just the terminal bowel), results when the tyrosine kinase domain of the *Ret* gene is disrupted in transgenic mice. Ret is a receptor tyrosine kinase encoded by the c-*ret* proto-oncogene. The human *RET* gene has been cloned and localized to chromosome 10. Mapping studies have found that point mutations of the *RET* gene appear in the DNA of some patients with Hirschsprung disease. Transgenic mice also have provided a number of additional models for megacolon. Megacolon resulted when the homeobox gene *Hox-4* was overexpressed in mice. Expression of this gene is thought to be localized to the smooth muscle in the gut mesenchyme. Electron microscopic examination indicates that the terminal colon contains ganglia. However, these ganglia are abnormal because they have the ultrastructural features found in peripheral nerve but lack the features found in the enteric nervous system. Smooth muscle appeared abnormal, and the basal lamina around the muscularis mucosa was thickened, a condition similar to that observed in lethal spotted mice. It is not clear how overexpression of the Hoxa proteins results in defects in the enteric nervous system.

It is apparent from these studies in transgenic and naturally occurring mutant mice that a number of different genes influence the development of the enteric nervous system in the gut in general, and the hindgut in particular. Hirschsprung disease also appears to be multigenic as mutations on both chromosomes 10 and 13 have been identified. A number of steps contribute to the formation of the enteric nervous system. Neural crest cells enter the gut, proliferate, migrate along the gut, aggregate, and differentiate into neurons (Fig. 50.3). It also is likely that formation relies on interactions between the muscle mesenchyme and the crest cells. Mutations such as those introduced into transgenic mice could block the normal developmental sequence at each step, manifesting with a spectrum of phenotypic patterns with absence of nerves from a segment as in Hirschsprung disease or the entire bowel, or with abnormal differentiation of nerves in the bowel as occurs in various forms of *congenital neuropathic pseudo-obstruction*.

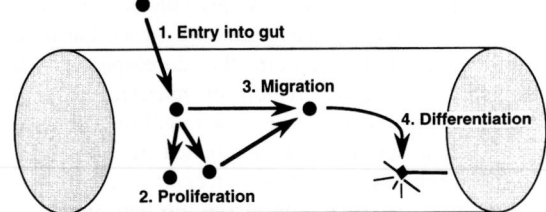

FIGURE 50.3 Schematic diagram showing the steps involved in the formation of the enteric nervous system: (1) neural crest cells enter the gut; (2) crest cells proliferate; (3) crest cells migrate along the gut; (4) crest cells differentiate and form connections with their targets. Cells are also able to migrate and then proliferate so that proliferation does not always precede migration.

# Neuronal differentiation

Mature enteric neurons exhibit a number of transmitter phenotypes including acetylcholine, serotonin, γ-aminobutyric acid (GABA), a large number of neuropeptides, and combinations of these molecules. In the adult gastrointestinal tract groups of chemically-distinguishable neurons are associated with specific functions or targets, a relationship termed neurochemical coding. Neural crest cells migrate off the neural tube and enter the primitive gut. Once within the gut the crest cells appear to migrate, divide and aggregate into small clusters of cells. In the chicken these clusters of cells become connected in a network, increase in size and take on the appearance of nascent ganglia between embryonic days 5 and 10. Within these nascent ganglia, undifferentiated crest-derived cells begin to express the different transmitter phenotypes found in the gut including acetylcholine, vasoactive intestinal peptide (VIP), somatostatin, enkephalin and substance P.

The factors controlling phenotypic differentiation are unknown. However, the appearance of neurotransmitters varies with different regions of gastrointestinal tract and at different times in development. This process has been studied most extensively in the mouse. Choline acetyltransferase activity and serotonin uptake are present on embryonic day 9, before elements with the morphological characteristics of neurons are recognizable. Cells transiently produce catecholamines on E10–12, and then the catecholamines disappear. It is not clear if these transient catecholaminergic (TC) cells die or change their phenotype. TC cells, which have not been found in avian gut, also contain a number of neural markers including neurofilament protein, peripherin, GAP43, and MAP5. The TC cells also proliferate, indicating they are not yet neurons, which are defined as postmitotic cells. However, when day-10 gut explants were grown in culture, many of the TC cells also showed neuron specific enolase, a marker for mature neurons. These results indicate that at least some of the TC cells are able to develop into mature neurons under culture conditions and suggest TC cells may give rise to mature enteric neurons *in situ*. On E12 neuropeptide Y-, on E14 substance P- and VIP-, and on E17 CGRP-immunoreactive neurons are found, while on E18 serotonin is present. Thus, in the mouse there is a pattern of expression of the different transmitter phenotypes in that acetylcholine appears early, followed by peptides and serotonin.

Extrinsic nerves reach the gut at later times. In the developing chick gut, sympathetic neurites reach the duodenum on E12. Sympathetic fibers are functional in the rat small bowel by postnatal day 3, and fibers are found in the myenteric ganglia at that time.

## SELECTED READING

Dow E, Cross S, Wolgemuth DJ *et al*. Second locus for Hirschsprung disease/Waardenburg syndrome in a large Mennonite kindred. *Am J Med Genet* 1994; **53**: 75.

Edery P, Pelet A, Mulligan LM *et al*. Long segment and short segment familial Hirschsprung's disease: variable clinical expression at the RET locus. *J Med Genet* 1994; **31**: 602.

Furness JB, Costa M. *The enteric nervous system*. New York: Churchill Livingstone, Inc, 1987.

Gershon MD, Chalazonitis A, Rothman TP. From neural crest to bowel: development of the enteric nervous system. *J Neurobiol* 1993; **24**: 199.

Hosoda K, Hammer RE, Richardson JA *et al*. Targeted and natural (Piebald-Lethal) mutation of endothelin-B receptor gene produce megacolon associated with spotted coat color in mice. *Cell* 1994; **79**: 1267.

Parikh DH, Tam PK, Van Velzen D, Edgar D. The extracellular matrix components, tenascin and fibronectin, in Hirschsprung's disease: an immunohistochemical study. *J Pediatr Surg* 1994; **29**: 1302.

Puffenberger EG, Hosoda K, Washington SS *et al*. A missense mutation of the endothelin-B receptor gene in multigenic Hirschsprung's disease. *Cell* 1994; **79**: 1257.

# 51

# Development of Primary Dentition and Occlusion

Francisco J. Ramos-Gomez

## DEVELOPMENT AND ERUPTION OF PRIMARY TEETH

Although a child's first 20 teeth are temporary, they serve important and crucial developmental functions: to maintain space and provide guidance for the permanent teeth; to allow for proper speech-pattern development, and, most importantly, to allow children to chew adequately in order to ingest nutrients required for normal growth.

The teeth start forming in the third week of gestation and initially consist of specialized cells of ectodermal and mesodermal origin. There are two broad phases of odontogenesis, or tooth formation, *calcification* and *development*. Odontogenesis is further divided into three histological stages known respectively as the initiation, or bud, the cap, and the bell stages. These are followed by apposition, root formation, and eruption (Fig. 51.1). In general, the mandibular teeth erupt first. Next, the remaining incisors erupt, then the first molars, followed in turn by the canines. The second molars erupt between the ages of 2 to 2.5 years.

Dental development involves many overlapping processes at any one time and is determined by a combination of genetic and environmental factors. In the development of the different histological stages of the tooth there appears to be specific genetic control, and

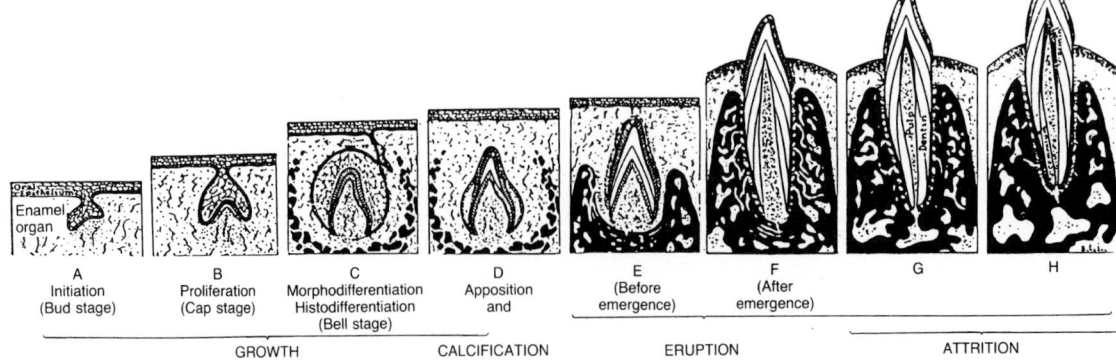

FIGURE 51.1 Representation of the life cycle of a tooth. (From Sharawy M, Bhussry BR. Development and growth of teeth. In Bhaskar SN ed. *Orban's oral histology and embryology,* 10th edn. St Louis: CV Mosby, 1986. Modified from Schour I, Massler M. *J Am Dent Assoc* 1940; **27**: 1785. Reproduced with permission.)

the passage of signals from and between tissues is imperative for proper growth in a systematic fashion. In other words, one specific tissue must develop, and then be able to signal another particular tissue to grow further. This is seen, for example, between mandibular ectomesenchyme and mandibular epithelium. The former is required to interact with the latter to allow the ectomesenchyme to determine incisal and molar form. The types of signaling required for systematic development most likely involve sequential expression of certain genes the proteins of which will regulate the movement and development of the tooth and of craniofacial form. Because the formation of teeth and dentition result from a complex interaction of the various components of orofacial physiognomy, bony as well as muscular structures, the whole developmental process is influenced by the basic developmental mapping, most of which is inherited, as well as environmental factors. Therefore, it is crucial that one be cognizant of the environmental conditions surrounding a child, including nutrition, hygiene and speech patterns; these conditions present not only the possibility of pathogenesis, but also of prevention and intervention.

## Calcification

Calcification of teeth, defined as the process by which organic tissues become hardened by deposits of $Ca^{2+}$ within their substance, occurs *in utero* between 3–6 months' gestation. Primary teeth calcify at different times, beginning with the maxillary central incisor at 14 weeks; first molar at about 15 weeks; lateral incisor at 16 weeks; canine at 17 weeks; and second molar at 18 weeks. The crowns of the teeth continue to grow in width until there is a union of the calcifying cusps. At this stage the chemical structure of the enamel consists of approximately 96 per cent inorganic material and approximately 4 per cent organic material and water. The stages of tooth development are presented in Fig. 51.2.

## Mineralization and root formation

The crowns and roots of primary teeth develop at various times following birth. Enamel formation of primary teeth at birth tends to adhere to the following pattern: enamel of maxillary central teeth is approximately 80 per cent formed; maxillary lateral teeth 70 per cent; mandibular lateral and central teeth 60 per cent; and canines 30 per cent. Enamel formation in all teeth is usually completed by the end of the first year.

The eight incisors, or anterior teeth, erupt within the first year (see below), although the crowns of these teeth are fully developed about 4–6 months before eruption. Crown formation in the remaining 12 primary teeth, which erupt in the second and third years of childhood, requires 6–12 months, during which time the mineralization of hard tissues such as enamel is completed. The crown and root of the earliest erupted tooth tends to mature faster than those of teeth erupting later. Root maturation is completed approximately 1 year after tooth eruption in nearly all primary teeth, so that roots will be completely developed between 18–48 months after birth. A range of 6 months of accelerated or delayed eruption is considered normal. In some mammals the development of pulpal innervation has been linked to nerve growth factor (NGF), although studies in humans have not yet confirmed this.

## Eruption

Eruption is defined as the emergence of the primary dentition from the bony structures of the mandible and the maxilla, resulting in occlusion of each tooth with its opposing tooth. Eruption does not follow the sequence of calcification, and the ages at which eruption occurs may serve as a guide for assessing overall dental development. Eruption patterns, however, have been shown to vary with ethnicity, and African–American children generally display more advanced patterns of primary tooth eruption and development than white children. Mandibular teeth generally erupt before maxillary. The typical eruption sequence (Table 51.1) is as follows: central incisors 6–9 months after birth; lateral incisors next, followed by the first molars, the canines, and finally, the second molars. Usually all teeth have erupted by 2.5 years.

Heredity has been shown to have about an 80 per cent correlation with patterns of primary tooth eruption, whereas environmental factors have proven to have only about a 20 per cent correlation. Primary tooth eruption thus is heavily influenced by genetic disposition.

Eruption also has been shown to vary with hormonal patterns. For example, during night hours eruption is significantly greater than during the day, possibly because of increased metabolic activity associated with circadian hormonal fluctuations. Late eruption of primary molars has been linked to growth hormone deficiency and associated decreased concentrations of circulating growth factors, particularly epidermal growth factor (EGF). There also are gender differences in eruption patterns and until approximately 15 months of age, boys tend to have a greater number of fully erupted teeth than girls. Thereafter, and until primary dentition reaches maturation, girls show full eruption in greater numbers.

The eruption sequence of permanent teeth has significant clinical implications, especially when there is inadequate space in either the maxilla or mandible to accommodate all teeth. Under such circumstances, the last tooth to erupt is displaced in the arch, or may erupt ectopically. The maxillary canine and the man-

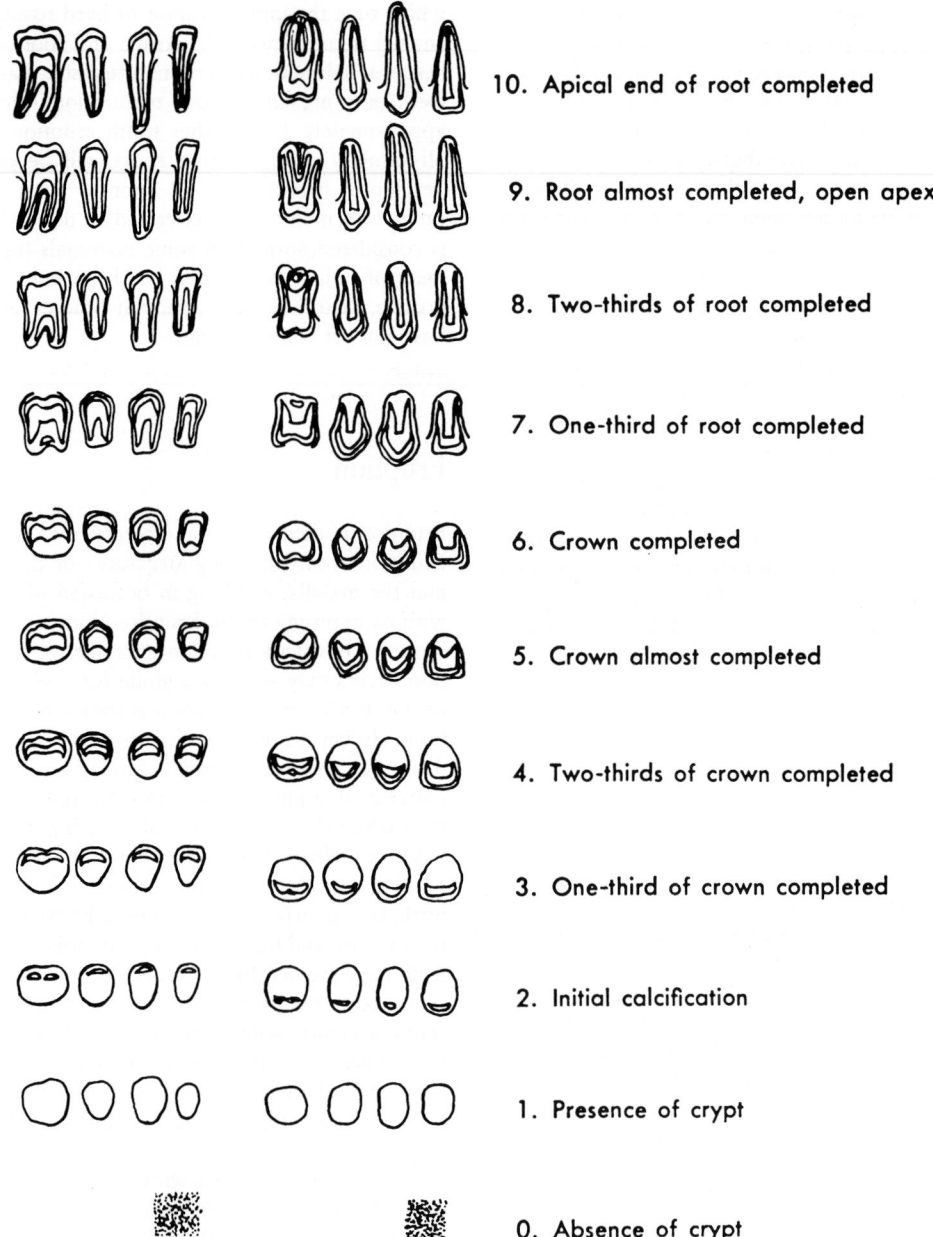

10. Apical end of root completed

9. Root almost completed, open apex

8. Two-thirds of root completed

7. One-third of root completed

6. Crown completed

5. Crown almost completed

4. Two-thirds of crown completed

3. One-third of crown completed

2. Initial calcification

1. Presence of crypt

0. Absence of crypt

FIGURE 51.2 Stages of tooth development. (Based on Nolla CM. Development of permanent teeth. *J Dent Child* 1960; **27**: 254. Reproduced with permission.)

dibular premolar, for example, will erupt ectopically under conditions of inadequate space.

*Exfoliation* occurs approximately 4–6 months before the eruption of permanent teeth (Table 51.1). The central incisors are lost at 6 or 7 years of age, the lateral incisors between 6–8 years, the first molars and mandibular canines between ages 9–12, and, finally, the second molars and maxillary canines between ages 10–12. It is important to understand the implications of premature loss of a primary tooth. The primary teeth are responsible for maintaining space for the corresponding erupting permanent teeth. If a primary tooth in the arch is lost, the rest of the teeth will drift and close the space, and this will lead to impaction or crowding. It is, therefore, important to keep the primary teeth healthy and in place until the appropriate permanent dentition is ready to erupt.

TABLE 51.1 Chronology of the development of primary dentition

| TOOTH | | ERUPTION (months) | EXFOLIATION (years) |
|---|---|---|---|
| Maxillary: | | | |
| Anterior | Central | 7.5 | 6–7 |
| | Lateral | 9 | 7–8 |
| | Canine | 18 | 10–12 |
| Posterior | 1st molar | 14 | 9–11 |
| | 2nd molar | 24 | 10–12 |
| Mandibular: | | | |
| | Central | 6 | 6–7 |
| | Lateral | 7 | 6–8 |
| | Canine | 16 | 9–12 |
| | 1st molar | 12 | 9–11 |
| | 2nd molar | 20 | 10–12 |

## MORPHOLOGY OF PRIMARY TEETH

The primary dentition serves to establish and maintain those patterns of spacing necessary for the eventual eruption of the permanent teeth. This spacing can be noted in the maxillary arch between the laterals and canines, and in the mandibular arch between the canines and first molars (Fig. 51.3). Developmental spacing of the anterior teeth is required for adequate alignment of the permanent incisors.

As in the permanent dentition, there are two subsets of primary teeth: anterior and posterior. Anterior teeth are wider in a mesial–distal direction, while posterior teeth are wider in a buccal–lingual direction. Primary roots tend to be shorter than permanent roots due to resorption. Crown widths of the teeth in all directions will be large by comparison with roots and crevices. Enamel is generally about 1 mm in depth. The dentin which develops between the pulp chambers and the enamel is limited, and the pulp horns tend to be large. Roots are narrow and long when compared to crown dimensions. Molar roots are flared and thinned near the apices.

Genetic disposition correlates significantly with primary tooth size and mineral mass and it may be possible to predict the diameter of permanent teeth based upon existing primary dentition. Recent evidence suggests that the size and morphology of teeth is controlled by genes on the X-chromosome. Primary tooth size also varies among ethnic groups, and given similar socioeconomic conditions and nutritional patterns, primary teeth in African–American children will reach larger sizes at earlier ages than will those of white children. However, information on primary teeth is not as complete as that on permanent teeth, and these differences thus require confirmation.

In addition to effects on eruption, hormonal patterns also influence the morphologic development of primary teeth. Autocrine and paracrine factors affect the development of the primary dentition, from the development of dental lamina to crown and root formation. Primary tooth size tends to vary according to gender, such that boys' teeth generally are larger than those of girls of the same age.

## PRIMARY TOOTH RESORPTION

The eruption of permanent teeth is not the only reason for resorption of primary teeth; in the absence of the corresponding permanent tooth, the resorption process may still occur, although it will be delayed. Factors such as trauma or disease also may affect the resorption process. Furthermore, anomalies in eruption patterns may prevent the resorption of primary teeth – for example, the ectopic eruption of a permanent tooth may result in resorption of only one root of the primary second molar while the second root remains intact. In such a case, when only one root exfoliates, it may be necessary to extract the primary tooth in order to provide adequate space for eruption of the subsequent tooth.

Root resorption occurs bilaterally; if a root is resorbed on one side of the tooth, the root on the other side of the tooth will be resorbed as well. Numerous factors, such as supernumerary primary teeth, may impede resorption and the normal eruption of permanent teeth. Thus, when resorption does not occur bilaterally, an occlusal radiograph is strongly recommended.

## ANOMALIES IN PRIMARY DENTITION

Several anomalies can occur during primary tooth development. Approximately 1 in 2000 to 3000 infants are born with one or more teeth. This condition is described as *natal teeth* (present in the mouth at birth) or *neonatal teeth* (present within 30 days after birth), and there is a higher incidence of these teeth in the mandibular incisor region than in any other region of the mouth. Certain syndromes are associated with this situation. There also is reason to believe that there is a hereditary component to the appearance of these teeth. Neonatal teeth may be supernumeraries or may be part of the primary dentition. They generally have no roots at the time of birth, but in most cases will

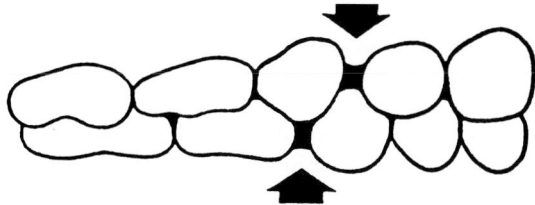

FIGURE 51.3 Primate spaces. Spaces form between the maxillary primary lateral incisor and the primary canine and between the mandibular primary canine and the mandibular first molar. (From Finn SB. *Clinical pedodontics*, 4th edn. Philadelphia: WB Saunders Co, 1973; after Baume LJ. *J Dent Res* 1950; 29: 442. Reproduced with permission.)

develop them shortly thereafter, and subsequently follow the same developmental sequence as normal teeth. It is recommended that neonatal teeth be extracted, for three principal reasons: first, the mother may be injured during breast-feeding; second, the presence of the tooth might cause the child to lacerate his or her soft tissues; and third, the infant might aspirate the tooth, should it become loose, and asphyxiate.

Congenital anomalies such as missing teeth are rare; however, the tooth most frequently missing as a result of congenital factors is the maxillary lateral incisor, followed by the maxillary central incisor and the first primary molar. *Microdontia* and *macrodontia*, defined as teeth appearing disproportionly small or large, respectively, by comparison to the arch or bony base, may occur as single anomalies or in groups of teeth. Peg-shaped teeth, called *"peg laterals,"* are one of the most common anomalies in permanent teeth, but occur with less frequency in the primary dentition. *Dens-in-dente* is "a *tooth-within-a-tooth,"* or an invagination of a lingual pit during morphological differentiation. *Gemination* is the partial cleavage of a tooth bud, or a double crown over a single root with a common root canal, and is largely hereditary. *"Fusion"* refers to two individual crowns joined together; unification may take place at the crowns, at the roots, or at both, and gives the impression that teeth are missing. Gemination and fusion have similar clinical appearances.

Anomalies may also occur in the chronology of tooth eruption. Other conditions include the absence of one or more teeth, known as *hypodontia*; the complete absence of all teeth, called *anodontia*; various defects in tooth enamel, such as *amelogenesis imperfecta*, tetracycline staining, and *fluorosis*; and dentin defects such as *odontogenesis imperfecta*, which appears as a brown or blue discoloration, easily chipped enamel, and missing root canal space and pulp chambers. Recently it has been discovered that the human amelogenin gene is located on both the X and Y chromosomes, so it is likely that a major form of amelogenesis imperfecta is X-linked. In patients with *dentinogenesis imperfecta* and *osteogenesis imperfecta*, it is possible that there is misregulation of expression of the gene(s) responsible for connective tissue formation, causing overabundance of this tissue, which in turn causes pathology. Dentinogenesis has been specifically linked to a defect on chromosome 4. The presence of radiographically visible pulp stones in combination with pulp obliteration and root agenesis is known as *dentin dysplasia*. Developmental defects may result in a variety of tumors, including odontomas and ameloblastomas. Gingival cysts may appear at birth, but these are generally benign, and may be removed or allowed to resorb without intervention.

"Ankylosis," commonly misnamed "submerging," refers to the fusing of primary teeth, particularly molars, to the alveolar process. This condition, which affects lower teeth twice as frequently as uppers, prevents the permanent teeth from erupting. Carious lesions frequently appear secondary to ankylosis, and the resulting loss of space may adversely affect the development of the arch.

## TEETHING

A great deal of misinformation clouds the general perception of teething and its effects on infant health. A full 33 per cent of all infants have no symptoms during teething. Sixty per cent may exhibit a short period of symptoms such as irritability and diarrhea prior to tooth eruption, and severe symptoms such as upper respiratory infections, bronchitis and eczema have at times been attributed to teething. However, there is no scientific evidence to support the association of these symptoms with either teething or tooth eruption.

## DEVELOPMENT OF PRIMARY OCCLUSION

The patterns of occlusal development are strongly related to the growth of the facial musculature and of skeletal structures; both tooth eruption and arch development depend upon the relations that are established during this time of rapid expansion and change. Anomalies in the bone structure or the musculature of either the maxilla or the mandible may have a significant effect on the occlusal patterns of the primary dentition. However, minor disparities and divergence are common even in normal primary occlusal relationships, particularly when compared with occlusal patterns in the permanent dentition. Primary arches, for example, tend to be ovoid, and will display less conformity than do permanent arches. Moreover, there is generalized interdental spacing in the anterior region of the mouth during normal primary occlusion, and this spacing increases continually with age; nevertheless, no spacing pattern will be common to all primary dentition. Common occlusal patterns at 3 years of age will exhibit some shallow cuspal interdigitation, slight overbite and overjet, and some crowding, although very little. "Primate spacing" refers to the spaces between the lower cuspid and the first molar and between the maxillary lateral and cuspid, and is only seen in normal primary dentition (Fig. 51.3). Though it may appear anomalous, primate spacing compensates for the small size of the primary arch and thus establishes the space necessary for emergence of the permanent dentition.

A Class I occlusion is the most common type of occlusal pattern. Growth discrepancies in the mandible and maxilla may occur in a sagittal, vertical, or transverse plane, resulting in a related occlusal disproportion. A mandible that is smaller or more posterior than the maxilla will have an overjet, known as a Class II occlusion. Class III occlusion and anterior cross-bites are related to a maxilla that is smaller or more posteriorly placed than the mandible. A downward and backwardly rotating facial growth is associated with an anterior open-bite, while deep bites are seen in faces with strong forward and upward rotation.

Terminal planes (Fig. 51.4) are imaginary lines placed distally of the second primary molars when viewed from the side. They are used to predict the future occlusion of the first permanent molars and may present in four different ways.

■ Flush terminal plane: allows the first permanent molars to erupt into an end-to-end relationship. Later, when the second primary molars exfoliate, the lower 6-year molar shifts mesially to a greater extent than does the upper 6-year molar. Such a

presentation will eventually develop into a class I occlusion (Angle classification).

■ Slight mesial step terminal plane: allows the 6-year molars to erupt directly into a class I occlusion.
■ Distal step terminal plane: allows the 6-year molars to erupt only into a class II malocclusion.
■ Exaggerated mesial step terminal plane: allows the 6-year molars to be guided only into a class III malocclusion.

Problems seen in primary dentition do have a tendency to self-correct while the child grows. Some problems, however, may get worse and may lead to more serious problems with the permanent dentition and occlusion.

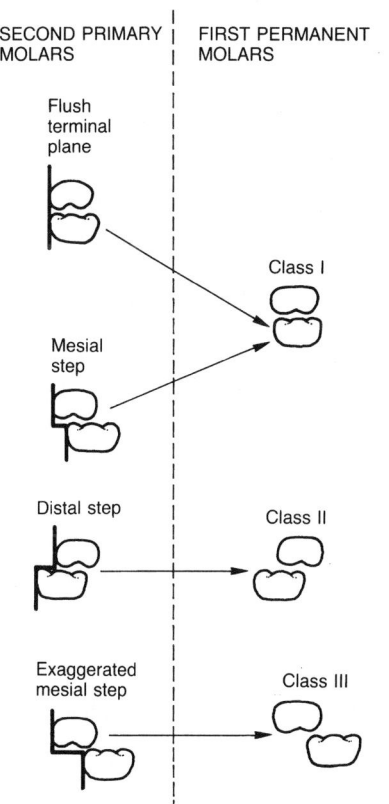

FIGURE 51.4 Representations of the four terminal planes (see text)

## SELECTED READING

Bigeard L, Sommermater J. Dental delay and microdontia in children with somatotropin hormone deficiency. *J Biologie Buccale* 1991; **19**: 291.

Burdi AR, Moyers RE. Development of the dentition and the occlusion. In: RE Moyers, ed. *Handbook of orthodontics*, 4th edn. Chicago: Year Book Medical Publishers Inc, 1988: 99.

Finn SB, ed. *Clinical pedodontics*, 4th edn. Philadelphia: WB Saunders, 1973: 45.

Gartner LP. *Essentials of oral histology and embryology,* 2nd edn. Baltimore: Jen House Publishing Co., 1986: 13.

Lee CF, Profit, WR. The daily rhythm of tooth eruption. *Am J Orthod Dentofacial Orthoped* 1995; **107**: 38.

Naftel JP, Qian XB, Bernanke JM. Effects of postnatal anti-nerve growth factor serum exposure on development of apical nerves of the rat molar. *Brain Res Dev* 1994; **80**: 54.

Nolla CM. Development of permanent teeth. *J Dent Child* 1960; **27**: 254.

Slavkin HC. Molecular determinants during dental morphogenesis and cyodifferentiation: a review. *J Craniofacial Genet Dev Biol* 1991; **11**: 338.

Smith RJ. Identifying normal and abnormal development of dental occlusion. *Pediatr Oral Health* 1991; **38**: 1149.

# 52

# Intestinal Blood Flow and Oxygenation

Karen D. Crissinger

The intestinal circulation provides the substrates and $O_2$ necessary to support the digestive, propulsive, and transport activities of the bowel. It also carries absorbed nutrients, electrolytes, and fluids from the gastrointestinal tract to the tissues of the body. The physiological processes of assimilation of nutrients along with rapid growth of fetal and neonatal intestine increase oxidative demand relative to that of the adult.

## BASIC CONCEPTS

Blood flow to the splanchnic organs is regulated by changes in diameter of muscular arterioles controlled by *extrinsic* and *intrinsic* regulators. Terminal arterioles and precapillary sphincters control the number of capillaries perfused in a specific region, altering the local delivery of $O_2$ and substrates. $O_2$ diffuses from the capillary to the cell, where it is utilized for oxidative metabolism. Thus, intestinal $O_2$ uptake is determined by both intestinal blood flow and $O_2$ extraction:

$$\dot{V}_{O_2} = \dot{Q} \times [A–V]_{O_2}$$

where $\dot{V}_{O_2}$ is $O_2$ uptake, $\dot{Q}$ is blood flow/min, and $[A–V]_{O_2}$ is the arteriovenous $O_2$ content ($Ca_{O_2}$) difference. In adult animals, intestinal $O_2$ uptake remains constant over a wide range of blood flows (Fig. 52.1). $O_2$ uptake is compromised only when blood flow reaches a critically low level, at which point $O_2$ uptake becomes flow-dependent. Modulation of arteriolar tone in small- to medium-sized arterioles changes

blood flow, matching blood flow to the $O_2$ demands of the tissue. Stimulation or inhibition of oxidative metabolism shifts the plateau of the blood flow–$O_2$ uptake curve upward or downward, respectively (Fig. 52.1).

Terminal arterioles and precapillary sphincters modulate the number of capillaries perfused at any given moment, increasing local flow in the face of reduced capillary $P_{O_2}$, thereby increasing $O_2$ delivery. Fig. 52.2 shows the expected influence of capillary density on the relation between blood flow and $O_2$ uptake. If capillary density within an organ is increased, then the level of blood flow required to maintain $O_2$ uptake is reduced (i.e. the curve is shifted to the left) due to an increased capillary surface area and a reduced capillary-to-cell diffusion distance. In adult intestine, changes in flow and numbers of capillaries perfused provide a wide margin of safety against development of tissue hypoxia when metabolic needs increase. In contrast, in newborn intestine, reductions in blood flow in the normal physiological range directly result in reductions in $O_2$ uptake (Fig. 52.3).

The variables that determine cellular $P_{O_2}$ are summarized:

$$P_{O_2\,cell} = P_{O_2\,capillary} - \left(\frac{\dot{V}_{O_2}}{N}\right)$$

where $N$ is the number of perfused capillaries. Normal resting cellular $P_{O_2}$ is above the critical level required to maintain oxidative metabolism, and stepwise reductions in blood flow do not produce concomitant reduc-

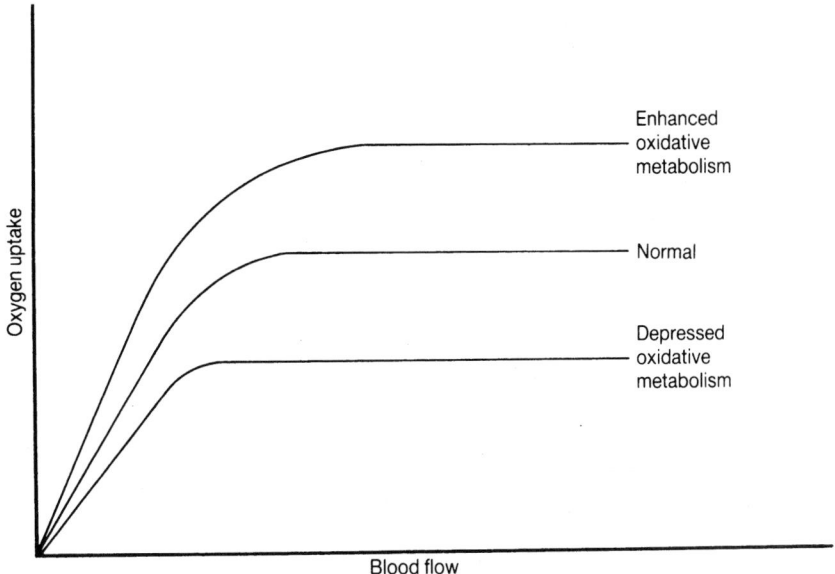

FIGURE 52.1 Relationship between blood flow and $O_2$ uptake under normal conditions and during stimulation or inhibition of oxidative metabolism. (From Kvietys PR *et al*. *Am J Physiol* 1982; **243**: G1, with permission.)

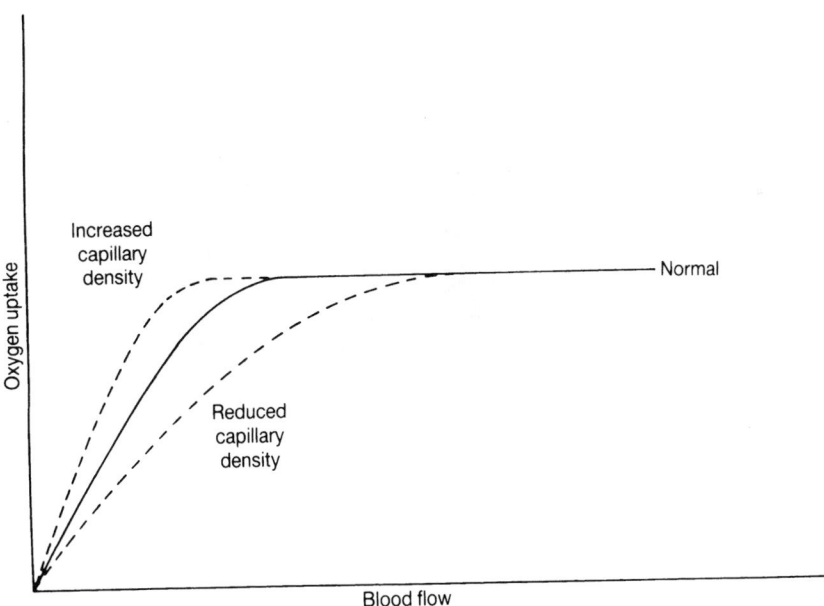

FIGURE 52.2 Relationship between blood flow and $O_2$ uptake under conditions of increased or reduced perfused capillary density. (From Kvietys PR *et al*. *Am J Physiol* 1982: **243**: G1, with permission.)

tions in cellular $Po_2$ until the capacity of the tissue for capillary recruitment is overwhelmed. In contrast, this relationship shows that when the rate of $O_2$ extraction is maximized and blood flow cannot increase, cellular $Po_2$ falls below the critical level required to maintain normal intracellular metabolism. Although the relationship between $O_2$ uptake and cellular $Po_2$ has not been established in developing intestine, studies of postprandial hemodynamics and oxygenation have demonstrated that total wall intestinal blood flow

does not increase in 1-day-old intestine, but $O_2$ extraction increases dramatically so that $O_2$ uptake is maintained (Fig. 52.4). One might speculate that a superimposed cardiovascular stress (e.g. ischemia/ reperfusion) may lead to tissue hypoxia and subsequent mucosal injury in 1-day-old, as compared to older, intestine because it may be unable to increase $O_2$ extraction further to maintain $O_2$ uptake. Information is lacking, however, about the critical cel-

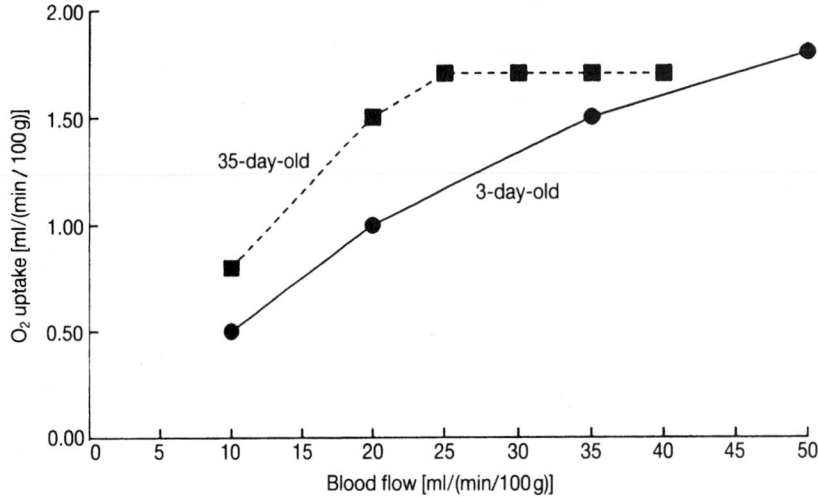

FIGURE 52.3 Relationship between blood flow and $O_2$ uptake in *in vitro* ileal segments from 3- and 35-day-old swine. (Adapted from Nowicki PT *et al. Am J Physiol* 1988; **254**: G189, with permission.)

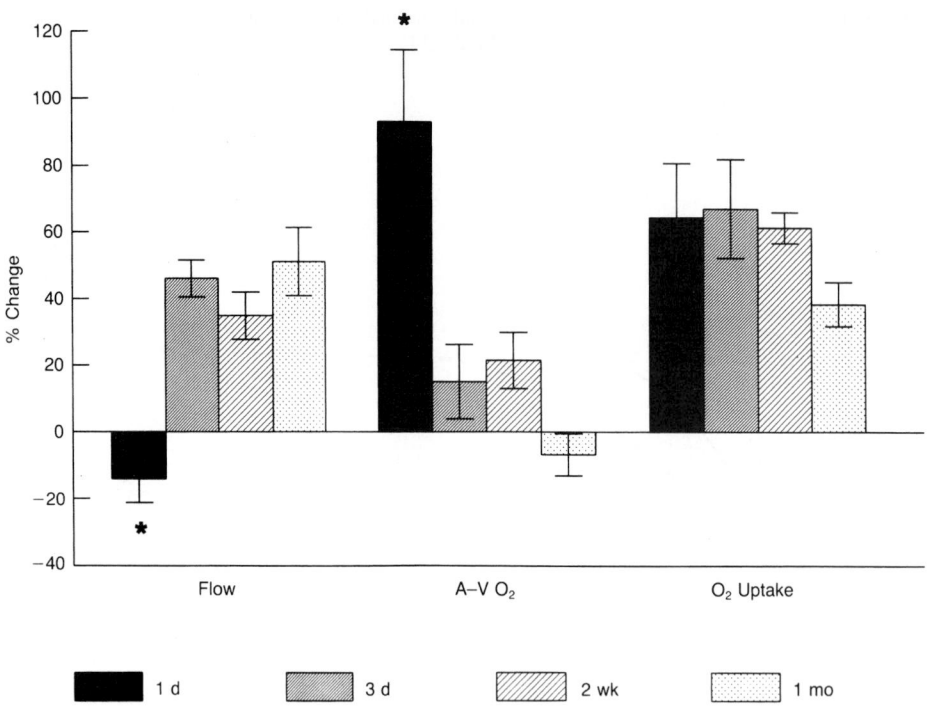

FIGURE 52.4 Percentage change in intestinal blood flow, arteriovenous $O_2$ content difference, and $O_2$ uptake at 30 minutes after luminal instillation of digested and bile acid–solubilized artificial pig milk formula in 1-day-, 3-day-, 2-week-, and 1-month-old piglets. * $P < 0.05$ vs older age groups. (Adapted from Crissinger KD *et al. Am J Physiol* 1991; **260**: G951, with permission.)

lular $Po_2$ at which $O_2$ uptake and oxidative metabolism become compromised.

## EXTRINSIC REGULATION OF INTESTINAL BLOOD FLOW

Neurohumoral (extrinsic) factors are important regulators of blood flow and $O_2$ uptake within the intestine. During reductions in blood pressure due to hypovol-

emia or shock, gastrointestinal flow is markedly reduced in order to redistribute blood flow and $O_2$ to the heart and central nervous system. Extrinsic regulatory mechanisms assure the appropriate response of the intestinal circulation in preserving systemic circulatory homeostasis. Sympathetic noradrenergic nerves play a major role in neural control of intestinal blood flow. α-Adrenergic receptors decrease intestinal flow, whereas β-adrenergic and dopaminergic receptors increase flow.

The net effect of sympathetic stimulation is to decrease intestinal blood flow.

Intestinal blood flow decreases in response to sympathetic stimulation in the ovine fetus. At birth, blood flow to the intestine increases two- to three-fold. The intestinal circulation appears to be under tonic sympathetic vasoconstrictor control. Adrenergic responses of the intestinal circulation are relatively active in newborns and continue to mature postnatally. The immature intestinal circulation appears less capable of vasodilatation, suggesting that neonatal intestine may be at metabolic risk during stresses involving increased sympathetic discharge.

## INTRINSIC REGULATION OF INTESTINAL BLOOD FLOW

Adult intestine has the capacity to regulate its own blood flow after elimination of all nervous and hormonal influences. These local, or intrinsic, microvascular control systems allow the microcirculation to respond to the specific needs of the tissue that it subserves and result in maintenance of the flux of $O_2$ and nutrients to the parenchyma. Several mechanisms of intrinsic vascular regulation probably play a role in this response. The *metabolic hypothesis* suggests that a reduction in blood flow or an increase in parenchymal cell activity causes a decline in tissue $Po_2$ and accumulation of metabolites, dilating arterioles and relaxing precapillary sphincters. The *myogenic hypothesis* proposes that arteriolar tension receptors modulate vascular smooth muscle tone in response to change in microvascular transmural pressure. Resistance vessels dilate when vascular transmural pressure is decreased, while an increase in transmural pressure causes arteriolar vasoconstriction and increased resistance. Endogenous vasodilators (e.g. nitric oxide) may result in increases in intestinal blood flow proportionally to intravascular shear rate or in inverse proportion to vascular transmural pressure.

Intrinsic vascular regulation by the intestine has been studied after altering arterial and venous pressure, after altering arterial $O_2$ concentration, and during periods of increased metabolic activity. In piglets, newborn intestine has a blunted autoregulatory response that does not improve with increased metabolic activity, but does improve with advancing postnatal age (Fig 52.5). Autoregulation of $O_2$ uptake is also compromised in young, compared with older, intestine (Fig. 52.6).

The response of the intestinal vasculature to venous pressure (Pv) elevation is an important criterion for determining whether metabolic or myogenic mechanisms dominate in local vasoregulation. Studies of the stomach, small intestine, and colon in adult animals indicate that vascular resistance rises in response to Pv elevation, findings consistent with a myogenic mechanism. This typical myogenic response can be abolished or reversed by increasing the $O_2$ demands

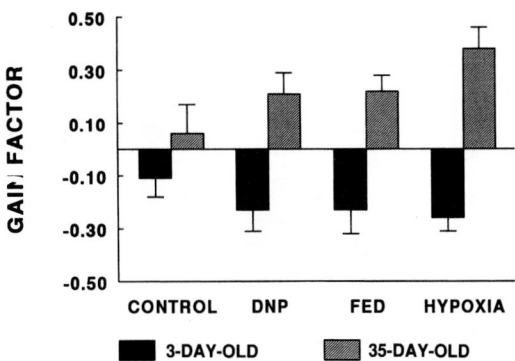

FIGURE 52.5 Autoregulatory capability of intestinal blood flow during control, 2,4-dinitrophenol (DNP) administration (increases metabolic rate), feeding, and hypoxia in 3-day- and 35-day-old swine. A positive gain factor implies that autoregulatory capability is present. (Adapted from Nowicki PT *et al. Am J Physiol* 1991; **261**: G152 and Nowicki PT *et al. Am J Physiol* 1992; **263**: G690, with permission.)

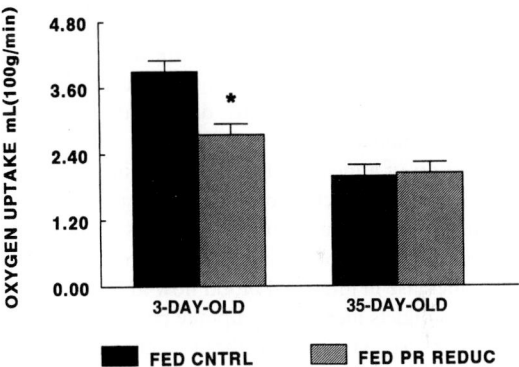

FIGURE 52.6 Autoregulatory capability of $O_2$ uptake during feeding in 3-day- and 35-day-old swine. *$P < 0.05$, pressure reduction fed vs fed control. (Adapted from Nowicki PT *et al. Am J Physiol* 1992; **263**: G690, with permission.)

in adult intestine, suggesting that the response to Pv elevation is also influenced by the metabolic state of the intestine. In newborns, the intestinal circulation dilates, rather than constricts, in response to acute elevation of mesenteric Pv (Fig. 52.7) so that intestinal $O_2$ uptake is not compromised. This indicates that metabolic factors are dominant in the already metabolically active neonatal intestine.

Arterial hypoxemia increases blood flow and elicits capillary recruitment in adult intestine. Decreased vascular resistance and increased capillary density minimize the reduction in $O_2$ uptake induced by limited $O_2$ availability. This response is comparatively reduced in developing intestine. Only a modest vasodilatation can be elicited in response to perfusion with hypoxic blood ($Pao_2$ 35 mmHg; 4.65 kPa), whereas older subjects exhibit a more significant fall in intestinal vascular resistance and rise in blood flow. $O_2$ uptake also falls to a greater extent in developing intestine during arterial hypoxemia than in older animals. These observa-

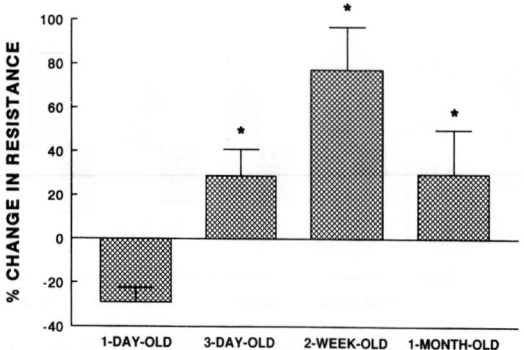

FIGURE 52.7 Percentage change in mesenteric vascular resistance with acute elevation of mesenteric venous pressure (Pv) in 1-day-, 3-day-, 2-week-, and 1-month-old piglets. *$P < 0.05$ vs 1-day-old. (Adapted from Crissinger KD *et al. Am J Physiol* 1988; **254**: G658, with permission.)

tions indicate either that the intrinsic mechanism responsible for hypoxic vasodilatation (i.e. the response to a vasodilator substance) develops postnatally or that the intestinal vessels are already dilated due to increased metabolic activity so that the ability of neonatal intestinal vessels to dilate further during hypoxia is limited.

Ingestion of a meal leads to increases in blood flow to the splanchnic circulation (postprandial hyperemia) in adult intestine. Intraluminal nutrients increase the metabolic demands of the intestinal parenchyma, causing an increase in intestinal blood flow and $O_2$ uptake. Newborn piglets increase $O_2$ uptake postprandially by increasing $O_2$ extraction without a change in total intestinal blood flow (Fig. 52.4). Mucosal blood flow, however, does increase at the expense of muscularis/serosa flow (Fig. 52.8). Thus, $O_2$ extraction and mucosal blood flow may be near maximal during feeding in newborn piglets. This unique response rapidly

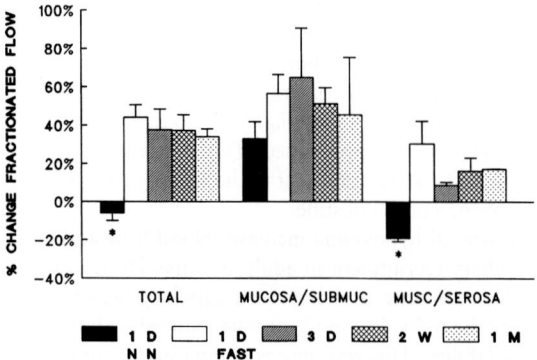

FIGURE 52.8 Percentage change in jejuno-ileal total wall, mucosa/submucosa, and muscularis/serosa blood flow at 30 minutes after luminal instillation of digested and bile acid–solubilized artificial pig milk in 1-day- (never nursed), 1-day- (nursed, fasted), 3-day-, 2-week-, and 1-month-old piglets. *$P < 0.05$ vs all older age groups. (From Crissinger KD *et al. Am J Physiol* 1991; **260**: G951, with permission.)

changes compared to that seen in adult swine intestine within 24 hours of birth.

In summary, the ability to regulate local blood flow and oxygenation in developing intestine appears to improve as a function of postnatal age. The intestine of young animals increases $O_2$ extraction to meet metabolic demands, whereas that of mature animals increases both blood flow and $O_2$ extraction. During periods of decreased $O_2$ delivery due to hypotension or hypoxemia, newborn intestine may be at increased risk for tissue hypoxia and subsequent mucosal injury.

## POSSIBLE RELATIONSHIP OF IMMATURE REGULATORY CAPACITY IN NEWBORN INTESTINE TO NECROTIZING ENTEROCOLITIS

The immature capability to regulate intestinal blood flow may be important in the pathogenesis of *necrotizing enterocolitis*. Mechanical occlusion of groups of vessels in the mesenteric vascular arcades of the distal ileum of piglets causes mucosal injury which is greater in low-birthweight piglets compared to those of normal birthweight. Necrotizing enterocolitis has also been produced in neonatal rats by exposing newborn rats to daily hypoxia, luminal nutrients, and *Klebsiella* bacteria. Another animal model of necrotizing enterocolitis has been produced by the combination of 60 minutes of intestinal ischemia and 60 minutes of reperfusion during luminal perfusion with digested and solubilized preterm infant formula. This combination of insults causes gross and histological mucosal injury in 1-day-old, but not in 1-month-old, piglets and is consistent with the above hemodynamic and oxygenation data, which demonstrate an increased risk for tissue hypoxia/mucosal injury in the youngest intestine during feeding. Efforts directed toward increasing the capacity of developing intestine to meet the oxidative demands of the tissue by increasing $O_2$ delivery while simultaneously minimizing metabolic demand (e.g. by altering the composition of infant formula) may ultimately decrease the incidence of necrotizing enterocolitis.

## SELECTED READING

Crissinger KD. Animal models of necrotizing enterocolitis. *J Pediatr Gastroenterol Nutr* 1995; **20**: 17.

Crissinger KD, Burney DL. Postprandial hemodynamics and oxygenation in developing piglet intestine. *Am J Physiol* 1991; **260**: G951.

Crissinger KD, Granger DN. Gastrointestinal blood flow. In: Yamada T, Alpers DH, Owyang C, Powell DW, Silverstein FE eds. *Textbook of gastroenterology.* Philadelphia: JB Lippincott Co., 1995

Crissinger KD, Burney DL, Velasquez OR, Gonzalez E. An animal model of necrotizing enterocolitis induced by infant formula and ischemia in developing piglets. *Gastroenterology* 1994; **106**: 1215.

Nowicki PT. Neonatal intestinal circulation. In: Schultz SG, Wood JD, Rauner BB eds. *Handbook of physiology. The gastrointestinal system 1.* Bethesda, MD: American Physiological Society, Waverly Press, 1989: 1597.

Nowicki PT, Miller C. Effect of increased tissue oxygen uptake on autoregulation in postnatal intestine. *Am J Physiol* 1992; **263**: G690.

Nowicki PT, Miller CE, Edwards RC. Effects of hypoxia and ischemia on autoregulation in postnatal intestine. *Am J Physiol* 1991; **261**: G152.

Sibbons PD, Spitz L. Necrotizing enterocolitis induced by local circulatory interruption in the ileum of neonatal piglets. *Pediatr Pathol* 1992; **12**: 1.

# 53

# Gastrointestinal
# Hormones

Thomas E. Adrian

Gastrointestinal hormones, such as gastrin and cholecystokinin (CCK), play a key role in the control of alimentary functions. Other regulatory peptides, such as vasoactive intestinal peptide (VIP), substance P, bombesin and the enkephalins, function as neurotransmitters or neuromodulators, not as blood-borne hormones. The integration of these neural and hormonal signals controls the digestion, absorption, and subsequent metabolism of ingested nutrients. Furthermore, some of the gastrointestinal hormones and other peptides, such as epidermal growth factor (EGF), transforming growth factor α (TGFα), and insulin-like growth factor I (IGF-I), appear to play a major role in maintaining the growth and integrity of the alimentary tract.

## BIOCHEMISTRY, PHYSIOLOGY, AND MOLECULAR BIOLOGY

Most gastrointestinal hormones fit into one of three major peptide families: the gastrin/cholecystokinin family, the secretin/glucose-dependent insulinotrophic peptide (GIP)/glucagon/enteroglucagon family, which also includes neurotransmitter relatives such as VIP, pituitary adenylyl cyclase-activating peptide (PACAP), peptide histidine methionine (PHM), and growth hormone-releasing hormone (GRH), and the pancreatic polypeptide (PP)/peptide YY (PYY) family, which has neuropeptide Y (NPY) as its neural cousin. More distant relationships between motilin and gastrin, somatostatin and secretin, and neurotensin and PYY are suggested by some degree of sequence homology.

The receptors for the gastrointestinal hormones have been cloned from several species and sequence similarities have revealed that these are all members of the G-protein-coupled receptor family with seven transmembrane domains (*see* page 55). Multiple receptor subtypes exist for several of these regulatory peptides including CCK, somatostatin and PYY/NPY; it appears likely that this will turn out to be the rule rather than the exception, providing another level of control at the cellular level. Neurotensin and the gastrin family act through the phosphoinositol/$Ca^{2+}$ second messenger pathway. The secretin family utilizes the cAMP system as their second messenger pathway and the PP/PYY family and somatostatin acts, at least in part, by inhibiting adenylyl cyclase. Using the powerful technique of directed mutagenesis, considerable progress has been made in identifying specific amino acid residues within the receptors responsible for ligand binding, G-protein coupling, and internalization. Highly potent, non-peptide receptor antagonists are now available for several of these hormones including gastrin, CCK, and neurotensin; others no doubt will follow soon. Interestingly, these inhibitors appear to bind to sites within the transmembrane domains of the receptors that are distinct from the extracellular binding regions of the peptide ligands. Thus, even though they appear to act as competitive inhibitors, they may stabilize a receptor conformation that has very low affinity for the natural ligand rather than displacing the ligand directly.

The gastrointestinal hormones and their neuropeptide cousins appear to have evolved from common ancestors by the process of gene duplication. Current examples of this evolutionary mechanism include the cosecretion of enteroglucagon and the glucagon-related peptides I and II from the same gene, and neurotensin from the same gene as neuromedin N. Several gastrointestinal hormones exist in multiple molecular forms with differences either in length or side-chain modification, such as sulfation. Many have a C-terminal amide group that renders them resistant to carboxypeptidase activity.

Ten enteric peptides act on the alimentary tract via the circulation. The endocrine cells synthesizing these peptides, with the exception of those producing somatostatin and pancreatic polypeptide, are of the open type, with luminal processes that presumably respond to nutrients and other factors, such as pH within the lumen, to stimulate their secretion. The biochemistry, anatomical localization, and physiological actions of each hormone are discussed below. The site of secretion and major actions are also listed in Table 53.1.

The gastrin family includes members with different chain lengths, all sharing a biologically active C-terminus. The important molecular forms of gastrin have either 17 amino acids (little gastrin) or 34 amino acids (big gastrin). Both are important in the control of gastric acid secretion. About half our gastrin molecules are sulfated, but this modification does not affect biological activity. Gastrin is produced mainly in the gastric antrum, but some is also secreted from the duodenum. The role of gastrin in the control of gastric acid secretion is discussed in Chapter 55. In addition to being an acid secretagogue, gastrin exhibits a potent trophic effect on the gastric mucosa, an action probably of profound importance in the newborn infant.

CCK shares the last five amino acids in the C-terminal end with the gastrins. This property leads to pharmacological overlap in the actions of these peptides. CCK exists in chains of different lengths including 83, 58, 39, 33, 22, 12 and 8 amino acids. All forms of CCK are sulfated, a modification necessary for its biological activity; the larger forms predominate in the

circulation. Biological activity of all forms resides in the common, amidated, C-terminal end of the CCK molecule. CCK is responsible for postprandial pancreatic enzyme secretion, and stimulates gastrointestinal motility, e.g. contracting the gallbladder and slowing gastric emptying. As well as having secretory and motor effects, CCK has been shown to be trophic to the adult pancreas in a number of species and appears to be responsible for the pancreatic growth that accompanies feeding of protease inhibitors and to surgical procedures such as pancreaticobiliary diversion, or small bowel resection. CCK is also a prominent central neuropeptide which appears to be involved in satiety and appetite control. CCK is released from the duodenum and upper jejunum by the presence of fat and protein in the small bowel. Recent evidence suggests a complex mechanism for the release of this peptide involving luminal releasing peptides.

Secretin is a 27-amino-acid peptide with a C-terminal amide group. The whole molecule is required for biological activity. Secretin shares considerable sequence homology with the hormones glucagon and glucose-dependent insulinotrophic peptide, as well as with several neuropeptides as mentioned above. Localized in endocrine cells of the duodenal mucosa, secretin stimulates pancreatic and hepatic bicarbonate secretion. Secretin is released when acid chyme passes through the pylorus into the duodenal bulb. The ensuing bicarbonate secretion rapidly neutralizes the pH of the duodenum. This affords protection to the duodenal

TABLE 53.1 The circulating gastrointestinal hormones and changes in concentrations in the newborn

| HORMONE | LOCALIZATION | MAJOR PHYSIOLOGICAL ACTIONS | OBSERVED CHANGES IN NEONATE |
|---|---|---|---|
| Gastrin | Gastric antrum | Stimulates gastric acid secretion | Hypersecretion at birth, elevated without increased acid secretion |
| Cholecystokinin (CCK) | Duodenum | Stimulates pancreatic enzyme secretion and contracts gallbladder | Marked postnatal surge, concentrations higher than in adult |
| Secretin | Duodenum | Stimulates pancreatic bicarbonate and hepatic bile secretion | Higher than adult in first week after birth, even without enteral feeding |
| Glucose-dependent insulinotropic peptide (GIP) | Upper small intestine | Potentiates glucose-stimulated release of insulin from the pancreas | Low concentrations in first days after birth, then adult pattern develops |
| Motilin | Upper small intestine | Triggers migrating motor complexes (MMCs), speeds gastric emptying | Massive postnatal surge of prefeed concentrations, postfeed fall in concentrations more marked than in adult |
| Neurotensin | Distal ileum | Stimulates mucosal growth, inhibits gastric function | Large postnatal surge, development of marked postfeed response |
| Enteroglucagon | Ileum and colon | Stimulates mucosal growth, inhibits gastric function | Massive postnatal surge, development of marked postfeed response |
| Peptide YY (PYY) | Ileum and colon | Inhibits gastric acid, slows gastric emptying and intestinal transit, enhances absorption | High concentrations at birth, massive postnatal surge |
| Pancreatic polypeptide (PP) | Pancreas | Inhibits exocrine pancreas and relaxes gallbladder | Small postnatal surge of basal concentrations, postfeed response smaller than adult |
| Somatostatin* | Stomach, pancreas, small and large bowel | Inhibits release of all above hormones, inhibits secretions and motor effects | Not reported |

*Note: May act locally (i.e. paracrine peptide). Somatostatin is also found in enteric nerves.

mucosa and provides a neutral environment for the activity of pancreatic enzymes.

Motilin is a straight, 22-amino-acid peptide secreted from the upper small intestine. A larger molecular form of motilin is also found in the circulation in man. The whole sequence of motilin appears important for biological activity. Motilin has powerful motor actions on the gut, including stimulation of the interdigestive migrating motor complexes. Motilin also accelerates gastric emptying and increases colonic motility. Erythromycin and related macrolides are agonists for the motilin receptor, explaining the motor effects of these drugs. Newly developed macrolides, called motilides, have high potency as motilin agonists but no antibiotic activity. These drugs are likely to prove valuable for treating a variety of motility disorders.

Glucose-dependent insulinotrophic peptide (GIP) is a 42-amino-acid member of the secretin family; a larger molecular form exists, but its relative biological potency is unknown. Gastric inhibitory peptide was GIP's original name because of its property of inhibiting acid secretion; however, this effect is only seen at supraphysiological concentrations. GIP releases insulin from the pancreas, although to do this it requires a small (approximately 1 mM) elevation of blood glucose concentrations, like that seen after ingestion of food. Hence, the peptide was renamed glucose-dependent insulinotrophic peptide (retaining the acronym GIP). The secretion of intestinal GIP from the upper small intestine may account in part for the greater insulin response observed after glucose is administered into the bowel as compared with intravenously, previously described as due to a factor, "incretin."

Glucagon-like peptides (enteroglucagon) are produced by the gut, but these differ chemically as well as in biological actions and mechanism of release. Now that the sequence of preproglucagon has been derived from the gene sequence, it is clear that the same gene is transcribed in both gut and pancreas. The post-translational processing of the glucagon precursor differs in these sites, however, giving rise to quite separate products. The glucagon gene encodes for three similar sequences, glucagon and the glucagon-like peptides I and II (GLP-I and II). The glucagon molecule itself is flanked by both C-terminal and N-terminal peptides. In the pancreas, the glucagon sequence is cleaved from these flanking peptides, whereas GLP-I and II are secreted uncleaved as a single peptide. In contrast, in the gut two peptides containing the glucagon sequence are produced, the major one (glicentin) extended by both flanking peptides and the minor one (oxyntomodulin) extended only in the C-terminal end. The glucagon-like peptides are cleaved and secreted separately in the gut (GLP-I, 7-37 amide, and GLP-II). The antibodies used to measure "enteroglucagon" are really N-terminally directed glucagon antibodies that cross-react with enteroglucagon (glicentin and oxyntomodulin). Glucagon concentrations, measured using specific C-terminally directed antisera, are subtracted from those measured using the non-specific antibody, leaving a derived enteroglucagon concentration.

Enteroglucagon is released by carbohydrate and fat in the intestine, whereas these nutrients inhibit the release of glucagon from the pancreas. Although enteroglucagon has not been purified in sufficient quantities to undertake full physiological studies, a mass of circumstantial evidence points to a trophic role for this peptide. A patient with an endocrine tumor producing enteroglucagon had marked villus hypertrophy in the small bowel. Enteroglucagon concentrations are increased, like those of PYY, in any situation associated with *malabsorption*, such as *celiac disease*, or after *small bowel resection*. Enteroglucagon concentrations correlate remarkably with crypt cell hyperplasia in these conditions. In addition, partially purified enteroglucagon stimulates DNA synthesis *in vitro*. Enteroglucagon could, therefore, be considered to be the growth hormone of the intestinal mucosa. It should be emphasized, however, that the evidence linking enteroglucagon and mucosal growth is rather circumstantial. Furthermore, the coreleased glucagon-like peptides might be involved in these trophic effects. Substantial evidence supports an important role for GLP-I in the enteroinsular axis along with GIP.

Peptide YY (PYY) and pancreatic polypeptide (PP) are both 36-amino-acid, tyrosine-rich, straight-chained polypeptides that are amidated at the C-terminal end. Three receptor subtypes exist for PYY and NPY. Structure/activity studies suggest that both ends of these peptides are involved in binding and activity at one receptor subtype (Y1 receptor), whereas C-terminal fragments are sufficient to bind to the other (Y2 receptor). A third receptor subtype is specific for NPY (Y3 receptor). There is also evidence for the endogenous production of a truncated form of PYY (PYY 3–36NH$_2$) that is specific for the Y2 receptor subtype. PP, which is localized to the islets of Langerhans of the pancreas, inhibits pancreatic enzyme secretion and relaxes the gallbladder. As PP concentrations remain high long after concentrations of other hormones, such as CCK, have returned to basal, it has been suggested that PP may play a role in conserving bile and pancreatic enzymes in readiness for ingestion of the next meal. In the adult human PYY is found in the ileum but is more abundant in the colon, with highest levels in the sigmoid colon and rectum. Blood concentrations of PYY increase after ingestion of food, and the magnitude of the response reflects the size of meal ingested. PYY infusion in man, at doses that achieve concentrations within the physiologic range, has potent inhibitory effects on gastric secretion and emptying and causes a marked delay in small bowel transit. These effects appear mediated by inhibition of presynaptic cholinergic transmission. PYY enhances net fluid absorption in the small intestine by inhibition of crypt cell cAMP-mediated chloride secretion. This is a direct effect mediated by receptors linked to the inhibitory G-protein of the adenylyl cyclase complex on the enterocyte. At higher concentrations, PYY infusion in animals also inhibits pancreatic secretion.

Neurotensin is a 13-amino-acid peptide that circulates in low concentrations together with a second peptide, neuromedin N coproduced from the neurotensin gene. The endocrine cells secreting neurotensin are localized to the terminal ileum; release of neurotensin is effected whenever nutrients reach the distal portion of the small bowel. Thus, in normal adult man, meals have little effect on neurotensin release. However, if unabsorbed nutrients pass through the distal small intestine, as in malabsorption due to celiac disease or in patients with postgastrectomy symptoms of dumping, circulating neurotensin concentrations increase. The actions of neurotensin include inhibition of gastric acid secretion and slowing of the rate of gastric emptying. Neurotensin also reduces blood pressure, but this effect is not seen at physiologic concentrations.

Somatostatin (somatotrophin release-inhibiting factor: SRIF) exists in two molecular forms: a 14-amino-acid cyclic peptide (SRIF-14), and a 28-amino-acid peptide, which has the SRIF-14 sequence at its C-terminus. Somatostatin has widespread inhibitory effects on the alimentary tract. It inhibits the secretion of all of the circulating gastrointestinal and pancreatic hormones, inhibits gastric and pancreatic secretion and also has a variety of motor effects. Biological activity resides within the ring, and a potent, long-acting analog (octreotide) is now available for clinical use. Somatostatin is found in endocrine cells of the gastric fundus and antrum, in the islets of Langerhans of the pancreas, and throughout the intestinal tract. Although evidence suggests that somatostatin has some actions through the blood stream, the cells producing this peptide have processes extending to other endocrine and cells, suggesting a paracrine action. Somatostatin is also found in enteric nerves of the myenteric and submucous plexus. The recent cloning of the somatostatin receptor revealed five subtypes which show characteristic specific expression in different tissues. Selective somatostatin analogs are being developed which will be used to selectively target individual receptor subtypes, allowing more specific inhibitory effects than the parent peptide. The commercially available long-acting somatostatin analog, octreotide, is a type 2 somatostatin receptor agonist.

## FETAL DEVELOPMENT OF GASTROINTESTINAL HORMONES

Cells secreting gastrin, somatostatin, motilin and GIP are detectable at 8 weeks' gestation, gastrin and somatostatin cells being most numerous. By 14 weeks, all of the endocrine cell types are present in the intestinal mucosa, although the anatomical distribution is somewhat different from that in the adult. For example, gastrin cells are found in the ileum, neurotensin cells

in the duodenum, PP cells in the colon, and PYY cells in the pancreas early in the second trimester. By the end of the second trimester, however, the cellular distribution resembles that of the adult. Peptidergic nerves are first demonstrable in the myenteric plexus at about 12 weeks' gestation, correlating with the known developmental pattern of enteric nerve plexus. After 3 months, the enteric nerves migrate through to the submucous plexus. By the third trimester all of the regulatory peptide systems appear well developed, although tissue content of some, notably gastrin, rises dramatically just before birth. In early fetal life, large molecular forms of peptides such as GIP and motilin predominate, suggesting that the post-translational enzymatic processing pathways may be immature. At birth, the molecular forms of the gastrointestinal regulatory peptides and their distribution in the gut are similar to those of the adult.

Several alimentary hormones can be detected in umbilical blood, collected at fetoscopy in the second trimester. Moreover, some endocrine cell types are functional, because several hormones such as enteroglucagon, PYY, and GIP are found in higher concentrations in blood from the umbilical artery and vein than in the maternal circulation at 18–21 weeks' gestation. Other peptides, such as gastrin, glucagon, and PP, are also found in the fetal circulation, but at concentrations below those in the maternal blood. Even these hormones show evidence of activity during fetal life as they are found in substantial quantities in amniotic fluid, which is swallowed by the fetus and probably plays a role in gut development. It is tempting to speculate that trophic peptides, such as gastrin, in amniotic fluid play an important role in gastrointestinal development even before luminal nutrition begins at birth.

## NEONATAL DEVELOPMENT OF GASTROINTESTINAL HORMONES

Early neonatal life brings marked functional changes in the alimentary tract, as well as substantial growth, for which surges of gut hormones appear to be responsible. Gastrointestinal hormone secretion changes substantially during this early neonatal period, triggered by the switch from intravenous to enteral feeding. Each of these changes is considered in the following sections. Table 53.1 summarizes the major changes seen in early infant life.

At birth, cord blood concentrations of gastrin are already four or five times higher than those in the adult, and prefeed basal concentrations remain elevated for several weeks. Furthermore, gastrin concentrations increase in response to the first milk feed. Starting 3–4 weeks after birth, basal gastrin concentrations decline, accompanied by development of marked feeding responses. Gastric acid is detectable in the stomach at birth and reaches a peak in the first day or two. Thereafter, acid output decreases for about a month despite the hypergastrinemia and rapid growth of the stomach. It has been suggested that the lack of responsiveness could be due to a lack of receptors in the oxyntic gland mucosa. However, a more likely explanation may be that secretion is suppressed by some inhibitor, such as PYY or neurotensin, thus enabling gastrin to stimulate growth of the gastric mucosa without hyperstimulation of acid secretion.

PYY concentrations are elevated in cord blood and rise postnatally to peak within the first 2 weeks. At their peak, the plasma PYY concentrations are about 50 times higher than fasting concentrations in normal adults. Evidence suggests that gastric emptying and intestinal transit are rapid during the first week after birth, both in term and preterm infants. The triggering mechanism for the ensuing changes is as yet unknown, but factors such as PYY likely play a role. In addition, the very potent inhibitory effect of PYY on gastric secretion may account for the prevention of hypersecretion of acid during the early neonatal period despite the marked hypergastrinemia.

CCK has marked trophic effects on the adult pancreas and appears responsible for regeneration, following resection or acute pancreatitis in the adult. Because of the marked postnatal surge of plasma CCK concentrations, this hormone has been implicated in pancreatic development. However, recent studies failed to show enhanced growth effects of exogenous CCK during this period in neonatal guinea pigs even though secretory responses to the hormone are intact. Furthermore, continuous administration of a CCK receptor antagonist during this period does not affect pancreatic growth or functional development. These findings suggest that some other factor is responsible for the rapid pancreatic growth in the neonatal period. EGF and TGFα, expressed at high levels in the neonatal pancreas, may be responsible as these peptides have potent pancreatotrophic effects during this period.

Basal plasma secretin concentrations are higher at birth than in adults, and during the first 3 weeks a more marked postprandial response develops. As secretin is considered to be a major factor in triggering the neutralization of acid chyme entering the duodenum, the increase in circulating secretin concentrations may be of considerable importance in mucosal protection during this period. Notably, the postnatal surge of secretin, unlike that of the other alimentary hormones, occurs even in the absence of feeding, indicating the importance of this mucosal cytoprotective function.

Basal GIP concentrations are low at birth and increase gradually throughout the first month, along with the development of a marked postfeeding GIP response similar to that seen in the adult after ingestion of a mixed meal. The development of the GIP response to feeding in neonates is mirrored by the postprandial insulin response, which increases through the first month to maintain glucose homeostasis.

Plasma enteroglucagon concentrations show an especially marked postnatal surge that peaks in the first week. This is associated with the development of a marked postprandial enteroglucagon response. As the rate of small intestinal mucosal growth is known to increase during this period, one may speculate that the increase of this trophic hormone is important in neonatal alimentary maturation. The resulting mucosal growth increases the absorptive area for uptake of nutrients from the gut.

Concentrations of PP, which at birth are lower than those of the adult, show a small postnatal surge that is particularly evident in preterm infants. During the first weeks after birth, postprandial PP responses develop, but these are smaller in magnitude than those seen in adults. Overall there is little evidence of a major developmental role for this peptide.

Plasma neurotensin concentrations are higher in the neonate, and an enhanced postprandial response develops in the first month. Both reduced gastric secretion and slowing the rate of gastric emptying decrease the rate at which acid chyme enters the duodenum and, therefore, result in a more steady absorption of nutrients from the gut. Thus, neurotensin may be important in the adaptation of the neonate to enteral nutrition.

Motilin concentrations are low in cord blood, but preprandial basal concentrations show a massive, 10-fold postnatal surge that is particularly evident in preterm neonates. The peak occurs at around 2 weeks. As basal concentrations increase, a fall in motilin concentrations following milk feeding becomes evident, which is more like the pattern seen in the normal adult after a mixed meal. The relationship between maturation of the migrating motor complexes and the late postnatal surge of motilin in the preterm neonates is not clear at present.

## FEEDING AND THE DEVELOPMENT OF GASTROINTESTINAL HORMONAL RESPONSES

Clearly, marked changes in gastrointestinal physiology accompany the introduction of enteral feeding in the infant. It is therefore of considerable interest that the postnatal surges of gut hormones are not seen in infants who have never received enteral feeding. Concentrations of all of these hormones, with the exception of secretin, remain low in babies receiving only parenteral nutrition. The composition of food and its mode of administration are also important in the development of gastrointestinal hormonal responses. This can be demonstrated as early as the first feed in infants, when dextrose elicits a different response than milk. Also, there are differences in hormonal responses between breast- and bottle-fed infants.

## Influence of different feed types on gastrointestinal hormones

The first feed of human milk given 4–6 hours after full-term birth is associated with a marked rise in circulating concentrations of gastrin and enteroglucagon, whereas GIP concentrations are unaffected. The composition of the feed is important, however, as a first feed of glucose has no effect on enteroglucagon although the increment of gastrin is similar to the milk feed.

Substantial differences in gastrointestinal hormone responses are seen between infants fed human breast milk and those fed formula. By day 6, preprandial concentrations of the small intestinal hormones motilin, GIP and neurotensin are much higher in bottle-fed infants, who also have greater postprandial changes in concentrations of insulin, motilin, neurotensin, enteroglucagon and PP. Possible explanations for these alterations include the differences between the composition of human milk and cows'-milk formula (despite attempts to "humanize" it) and the reduced milk intake of breast-fed infants during the first days of life, as lactation is developing. One should note, however, that milk intake was similar in both groups by day 6. The differences in composition include the greater absorbability of fat in human milk and the higher total fat and branched-chain amino acid content of formula. Other factors may include the presence of active lipase and other enzymes as well as hormones in human breast milk. The presence of growth factors, such as EGF, in human milk may also be of profound importance in neonatal gut development.

Several other regulatory peptides have been reported in human milk including gastrin, neurotensin, PYY, VIP, PHM, and bombesin. Of these peptides, bombesin, which has trophic effects in a number of tissues, was present in higher concentrations in breast milk than in plasma.

The differences in hormone responses between breast- and bottle-fed infants may be of considerable practical importance. The enhanced insulin response in bottle-fed infants despite a similar degree of glycemia may result from increased circulating concentrations of branched-chain amino acids or GIP, both of which enhance glucose-stimulated insulin secretion. Because insulin enhances cellular glucose uptake and inhibits lipolysis, the greater insulin release may explain the increased deposition of subcutaneous fat seen in bottle-fed infants. Differences in motilin concentrations may account for the well-known differences in stool frequency between bottle and breast-fed infants. As enteroglucagon is likely to exert a major trophic effect on the small bowel mucosa, changes in concentrations of this hormone may influence postnatal gut development.

## Comparison of continuous infusion feeding with intermittent boluses on gut hormones

Preterm infants receive gastric milk feeds either as continuous feeds or intermittent boluses; however, information is scant concerning the influence of these feeding modes on gastrointestinal hormones and gut development. Both groups show similar increases in plasma motilin, neurotensin, enteroglucagon, and PP concentrations. By 13 days, infusion-fed infants have higher concentrations of insulin, gastrin and GIP. While both methods of feeding result in progressive changes in circulating enteroinsular hormone concentrations, the development of postprandial increases in response to bolus feeding is absent in infusion-fed infants. The absence of meal-stimulated gut hormone responses may have effects on the developing alimentary tract, but does not appear to influence body weight gain, which is similar between the two groups.

## Practical significance of minimal enteral feeding on gut hormones

The relationship between the quantity of milk ingested and the development of postnatal surges of gut hormones has been investigated in infants recovering from hyaline membrane disease. Six-day-old infants exclusively fed parenterally show no postnatal elevation of gastrin, motilin, GIP, neurotensin or enteroglucagon. In contrast, infants who receive restricted enteral feeding over this period have hormone surges similar to those seen in healthy infants on full enteral feeds. Substantial elevations of gastrin, GIP and enteroglucagon are seen after a cumulative enteral feed volume of only 24 mL since birth. By the time infants receive a cumulative intake of 96 mL, the hormone surges have reached maximal concentrations, which are identical to those of enterally fed healthy infants. Greater feed volumes are required to induce the normal surge of motilin and neurotensin, but even these are considerably lower than those required for full enteral feeding. These observations suggest that minimal enteral feeding may have an important therapeutic role in maintaining functional gastrointestinal integrity in infants undergoing prolonged parenteral nutrition.

## SELECTED READING

Adrian TE. Gastrointestinal hormones. In: Wyllie R, Hyams JS eds. *Pediatric gastrointestinal disease: pathophysiology, diagnosis, management*. Philadelphia: WB Saunders, 1992.

Aynsley-Green A. The adaptation of the human neonate to extrauterine nutrition: a prerequisite for postnatal growth. In Cochburn F ed. *Fetal and neonatal growth*. New York: John Wiley and Sons, 1988: 153.

# 54

# Food Ingestion and Gastrointestinal Motility

Colin D. Rudolph

## APPETITE (*see* page 427)

Food intake is regulated by a complex interaction between centers in the hypothalamus, other regions of the central nervous system, and the gastrointestinal system. Although poorly understood, the factors controlling food ingestion and satiation at each meal are better understood than homeostatic regulation of caloric intake over longer periods of time, i.e. weight control. Stimulation of the lateral hypothalamic area results in hunger and food-seeking behavior. Damage to this area results in starvation due to a lack of nutrient ingestion. Stimulation of the ventromedial nucleus of the hypothalamus results in satiety. Gastric distension inhibits continued food ingestion, before nutrients are absorbed into the bloodstream. Distension of the stomach inhibits food intake, whereas when food is allowed to drain from the stomach through a fistula, animals continue eating for long periods of time. The gastrointestinal tract also appears to sense and communicate when an adequate amount of nutrients has been ingested by mechanisms other than gastric distension. The infusion of lipid or glucose into the duodenum or lipid into the ileum results in satiety via neural and/or hormonal feedback to the hypothalamus. Blood-borne nutrients and hormones may also affect satiety. Glucose infusion in the portal vein decreases food intake. Similarly, injection of cholecystokinin (CCK) or gastrin-releasing peptide (GRP) to mimic the pattern of hormone release after feeding decreases food intake, and blockade of CCK receptors augments the satiety response following feeding in dogs.

## TASTE

Taste buds are located on the walls of the tongue with small numbers located throughout the palate, pharynx and proximal larynx, and esophagus. Taste bud response to different stimuli varies with the region of the tongue: sweet and salty at the tip, sour on the sides, and bitter on the soft palate and posterior tongue. Microelectrode recordings indicate that most taste buds respond to two or three different chemical stimuli. Integration of these stimuli occurs in the central nervous system. Taste impulses pass through the chorda tympani of CN VII and CN IX and X to the nuclei of the tractus solitarius. Within the brain, taste stimuli pass through the brainstem to the thalamus and cortex, paralleling the somatic pathways from the tongue.

Taste preferences vary tremendously between individuals and species and with age. For example, humans have a "sweet tooth," whereas cats show no preference for sweets. Interestingly, opioid antagonists reduce the preference for sucrose in humans, suggesting that the pleasurable sensation enjoyed by sweet lovers is mediated by opioid transmitters. Specific taste aversions develop in a wide variety of species when ingestion of a particular taste is linked to an unpleasant experience. Thus, nausea or other discomfort linked to the ingestion of a particular food leads to future avoidance of that particular food. Although taste buds are present in mid-gestation, the number and maturity of taste buds increase postnatally in all species studied. Human infants have taste preferences that change during development. Newborn infants prefer sweet tastes. Infants less than 4 months of age show no salt preference, but between 4 and 24 months children prefer salty solutions. By 30 months children tend to reject saline solutions. Subsequent development of specific taste preferences depends largely on social and cultural factors.

## GASTROINTESTINAL MOTILITY

## Introduction

The muscle coat of the gastrointestinal tract is composed of an inner circular layer and an outer longitudinal layer. Contraction of these muscles results in alterations in the pressure and shape of the lumen, which grinds the food in the stomach and then transports it through the intestine, ensuring adequate mixing and exposure to absorptive surface. The intrinsic gastrointestinal nervous system and extrinsic neural inputs act in concert to alter movement of food by changing the rate and spatial distribution of muscle contractions. In this section, the mechanisms of contraction of smooth muscle are discussed initially. Development of coordinated control of muscular contractile activity in each region of the gastrointestinal tract is then summarized.

## Smooth muscle contraction

A detailed discussion of smooth muscle electrophysiology and mechanics is beyond the scope of this chapter. A resting cell membrane potential is maintained by active extrusion of $Na^+$ in exchange for $K^+$. As in other tissues, the electrochemical gradient generated by the $Na^+$–$K^+$–ATPase pump is directed strongly inward, allowing its use as an energy source for transporting other ions or molecules against their electrochemical gradients. Low intracellular concentrations of $Ca^{2+}$ are maintained by $Ca^{2+}$ extrusion into the extracellular space and sequestration in intracellular organelles by an ATP-dependent pump.

Gastrointestinal smooth muscle undergoes a cyclic variation in basal membrane potential described as "slow waves," "basic electrical rhythms," or "pacesetter potentials." These waves are not associated with smooth muscle contraction, but rather represent changes in the excitability of the muscle cell. During the repolarization phase of the slow wave, the muscle cell is not excitable; thus the slow-wave rate determines a particular smooth muscle's maximal frequency of contraction. Recent data indicate that specialized interstitial cells of Cajal (ICC cells) located on the outer layer of the circular muscle and having gap junction connections to the smooth muscle cells are responsible for the generation of the slow-wave potentials. In transgenic mice with defects in the receptor tyrosine

kinase, c-*Kit*, the ICC cells do not develop and intestinal pacemaker activity is absent. The frequency, plateau, and repolarization rates of slow waves vary in different bowel regions and among species. For example, in the dog the rate decreases from 18/min in the duodenum to 11/min in the ileum, whereas in the human the rate decreases from 12/min in the duodenum to 8/min in the ileum.

Superimposed on the slow wave are action potentials that result in contraction of the smooth muscle (Fig. 54.1). Action potentials can be initiated only during the crest of the slow wave. Depolarization of the membrane opens channels that allow the influx of $Ca^{2+}$, as in skeletal muscle. The membrane is rapidly repolarized due to the outward movement of $K^+$. An increase in the free cytoplasmic $Ca^{2+}$ concentration results in the binding of $Ca^{2+}$ to calmodulin (in skeletal muscle, $Ca^{2+}$ binds troponin), which activates myosin light chain kinase. The myosin and actin then interact, forming an ATPase system leading to mechanical contraction. The slow wave and action potential propagate rapidly around the circumference of the circular muscle, resulting in a synchronized contraction of a ring of smooth muscle. Contraction of this circular muscle ring decreases the diameter and increases the pressure of the bowel lumen that it surrounds. In contrast, action potentials are propagated only for approximately 5 mm longitudinally. Therefore, any coordination of peristalsis requires action potentials to be initiated in each segment of the bowel. If action potentials occur on the peak of every slow wave, a tonic contraction can occur. Some smooth muscles, particularly those associated with sphincters, maintain some contractile activity in the absence of clear action potentials. The electrical events associated with changes in baseline muscle tone are not well described. Patterns of coordination of contractile events in differ-

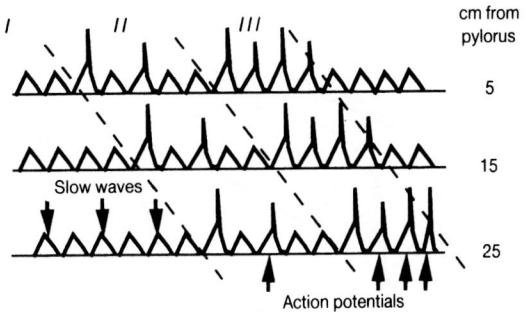

FIGURE 54.1 Electrical activity of smooth muscle in the small intestine. This recording demonstrates the regular cyclic slow wave and overlying action potential. The aboral progression of the phases of the organized migrating motor complexes is also shown. During phase I there are no action potentials. Phase II has irregular action potentials at some of the slow wave peaks. Phase III is characterized by the presence of action potentials superimposed on each slow wave.

ent regions of the gastrointestinal tract are discussed in the following sections.

## Swallowing

Swallowing of secreted saliva occurs constantly during the day. In the adult human, swallowing is composed of four phases (Fig. 54.2). Coordinated contraction of 32 pairs of skeletal muscles is required for the preparatory, oral and pharyngeal phases. During the oral phase food is ground and lubricated to form a bolus. The bolus is then transferred to the pharynx by a sweeping contraction of the tongue against the hard and soft palates. In preparation for bolus passage, the soft palate closes against the posterior pharynx, sealing the nasopharynx; the larynx elevates and the vocal cords close, while the upper esophageal sphincter relaxes. Presence of the food bolus or oral secretions in the upper pharynx initiates a swallow reflex. Peristaltic contractions through the pharynx and esophagus propel the bolus into the stomach. The bolus passes around the airway to enter the esophagus. Sensory feedback via cranial nerves V, IX, and X alters the amplitude and timing of the peristaltic contractions as bolus size and consistency change. Cranial nerves $V_2$, VII, X, and XII control the muscles required for swallowing. Anatomic defects, such as palatal or laryngeal clefts, or neuromuscular disease alter the normal swallow and frequently result in aspiration of food into the lungs.

Infants ingest food only in a liquid form as milk. The infant does not chew food in the oral cavity. The lips are sealed over the nipple and the tongue closes the region between the oral cavity and pharynx.

Lowering the tongue then produces a negative pressure greater than 100 mmHg in the oral cavity, sucking milk from the bottle or breast. Rhythmic bursts of sucks at a rate of 1/second are followed by cessation of breathing and transfer of the liquid bolus into the pharynx, where swallowing proceeds as in the adult. Mature sucking patterns are first noted at about 35 weeks' gestation. Swallowing of pharyngeal contents is seen as early as 11 weeks. The length of the bursts of sucking, the magnitude of the negative pressure produced in the oral cavity, and the coordination of the suck and swallow mechanism gradually improve as the fetus or premature infant approaches term. Non-feeding infants often are comforted by sucking on a thumb or pacifier. "Non-nutritive" sucking is characterized by its rapid rate of approximately 2/second. At 24 weeks the most primitive non-nutritive suck is observed.

As the infant matures the anterior oral cavity enlarges. Between 4 and 6 months of age the tongue begins to transfer soft solids from the oral cavity to the pharynx. Teeth develop over the next year (see Chapter 51), and the tongue and oral muscles develop coordinated movements that transfer solid foods laterally into the buccal pouches for chewing, grinding and lubrication by saliva. This masticated bolus is then transferred into the pharynx and swallowed, as in the adult.

## The esophagus

The esophagus is a conduit between the pharynx and the stomach with muscular sphincters, the upper and lower esophageal sphincters, at either end. In the human the upper quarter of the esophagus is composed of skeletal muscle, and the remainder is smooth muscle. When a food bolus enters the esophagus, rings of circular muscle contract sequentially from the top of the esophagus to the bottom. This "primary peristaltic wave" propels the bolus down into the stomach. The lower esophageal sphincter relaxes to allow bolus passage into the stomach. Stretching of the esophageal wall stimulates a "secondary peristaltic wave," initiated just above the site of distension, which progresses down the esophagus in a similar fashion. Propagation of the peristaltic wave is dependent on the intrinsic myenteric plexus and on vagal afferents. Even in the absence of vagal input, peristaltic waves can be initiated in the smooth muscle portion of the esophagus and transmitted by the intramural myenteric plexus. Abnormal peristalsis results in food impaction and pain. Only limited information regarding the maturation of esophageal peristalsis is available, indicating that peristalsis is poorly coordinated until after 32 weeks' gestation and suggesting that coordinated contractions are not present until several days after birth, even in the term infant.

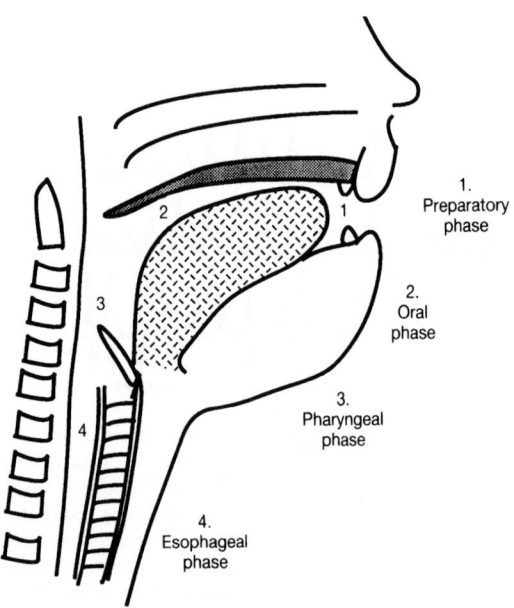

1. Preparatory phase

2. Oral phase

3. Pharyngeal phase

4. Esophageal phase

FIGURE 54.2 The four phases of swallowing in the adult human

The lower esophageal sphincter prevents the acid contents of the stomach from constantly refluxing into the esophagus. Incompetence of the lower esophageal sphincter allows acid to reflux from the stomach, causing inflammation of the mucosal wall and pain. A disorder known as *achalasia* is caused by a lack of relaxation of the lower esophageal sphincter resulting in massive esophageal distension and malnutrition due to an inability to eat. These clinical problems have made the lower esophageal sphincter the focus of a tremendous investigative effort. This sphincter is characterized by its ability to remain tonically contracted. A 2–4 cm zone in the lower esophagus maintains a pressure of approximately 30 mmHg in the adult human. This tonic contraction appears to be a property of the smooth muscle itself. Neural blockade with tetrodotoxin does not affect the tonic pressure. Esophageal or gastric distension or vagal stimulation all cause relaxation of the sphincter muscle. The relaxation of the sphincter elicited by swallowing is mediated by the vagus. The relaxation due to distension is mediated by the intramural neural plexus. Non-cholinergic, non-adrenergic neurons appear to be responsible for these reflex relaxations. A variety of substances including vasoactive intestinal peptide, calcitonin gene-related peptide, peptide histidine isoleucine, and nitric oxide may all play a role in this relaxation response. Although pharmacologic doses of many gastrointestinal hormones have been shown to alter lower esophageal sphincter tone, the physiologic role of these hormones remains controversial.

Recent evidence indicates that the lower esophageal sphincter transiently relaxes in the normal human. Some reflux of acid into the esophagus is a normal event. Secondary peristaltic waves combine with the buffering activity of swallowed saliva to clear the refluxed acid rapidly from the esophagus. Thus, disorders of esophageal clearance may be more important in the pathogenesis of esophageal damage from gastroesophageal reflux than simple incompetence of the sphincter muscle.

Two factors other than the intrinsic smooth muscle tone contribute to competence of the lower esophageal sphincter. In the normal human, a short segment of the esophagus is located below the diaphragm and is constricted when intra-abdominal pressure increases, helping to prevent reflux into the esophagus. In addition, contractions of the crus of the diaphragm, which wraps around the lower esophagus, contribute to the pressure barrier to gastroesophageal reflux during inspiration.

Regurgitation of food is common in infants. The lower esophageal sphincter region of the infant is shorter than in adults. In addition, the anatomic relationship of the stomach and diaphragm is different so that a relatively shorter segment of esophagus lies within the infant's abdominal cavity compared with the adult. At 26 weeks' gestation the lower esophageal sphincter resting pressure is only 4 mmHg, but it increases to 18 mmHg by term. The increased abdominal cavity pressure associated with straining or coughing overcomes this pressure barrier relatively easily, resulting in reflux of gastric contents or regurgitation. Despite an increased tendency toward gastroesophageal reflux, esophageal mucosal damage is rare in infants because refluxed acid is cleared efficiently from the esophagus. Similarly, infants rarely aspirate refluxed material, because inspiration ceases and the airway closes until refluxed material is cleared from the pharynx by swallowing.

## Gastric and small intestinal motility

The stomach grinds and emulsifies food and then serves as a reservoir, gradually emptying nutrients into the intestine for absorption. The fundus and antrum differ in their functional roles. The upper body and fundus of the stomach relax with distension, maintaining a relatively constant intraluminal pressure with variations in volume. This receptive or adaptive relaxation allows the fundus to serve as a reservoir for a large volume of food. The pressure difference between the fundus and duodenum is the most important factor regulating liquid emptying. Adaptive relaxation is mediated by non-cholinergic, non-adrenergic inhibitory vagal neurons. After vagotomy, the reservoir function of the stomach is disturbed and liquids empty rapidly, causing *"dumping" syndrome*.

The tonic contractions of the fundus and body drive liquid and solid food to the antrum. Strong contractions of the antrum mix liquids and grind solid food. Liquid passes easily through the pylorus, whereas solid particles are retropelled back into the body of the stomach. This antral mill grinds the solids into a size small enough to pass through the pylorus, approximately 2 mm. The rate of gastric emptying of solids and liquids is controlled by the central nervous system and by feedback from the intestine. Emotional stress and various central nervous system disorders are associated with a decreased rate of gastric emptying. The presence of acid, fat, carbohydrates, or amino acids (especially tryptophan) in the duodenum decrease gastric emptying. Intramural nerves, vagal pathways, and gastrointestinal hormones, cholecystokinin in particular, all appear to have a role in the feedback regulatory process.

The liquid emulsion that enters the small intestine, chyme, slowly passes from the duodenum to the ileum. In the adult human this occurs over 1–3 hours. Distension of the small intestinal wall results in an aboral peristaltic contraction as in the rest of the bowel. The pattern of constant churning with continual slow movement of the food down the intestinal tract that characterizes the period after feeding is poorly understood. A very complex interaction between the luminal contents and intestinal smooth muscle wall results in this integrated pattern. This process is independent of extrinsic innervation. Recordings of isolated regions of contractile activity in the fed bowel indicate that there are frequent contractions, but a clear, coordinated pattern is difficult to discern. In contrast, in the fasted human there is a cyclic pattern of antral and intestinal contractile activity that migrates from the antrum to ileum called a migrating motor complex (MMC) (see Fig. 54.1). Periods of no contractile activity (Phase I) are interrupted by irregular contractions (Phase II). Then regular contractions occur, at the same rate as the slow wave in the bowel region studied, and the cycle repeats itself every 45–90 minutes. Similar patterns are noted in other species. In the rat cycles recur at intervals of 15–30 minutes. The migrating motor complex functions to remove non-digestible substances, e.g. ingested foreign bodies, from the bowel and sweeps bacteria out of the small intestinal lumen into the large intestine, preventing bacterial overgrowth of the bowel. In most mammals, feeding interrupts the MMC pattern. In weaned ruminants, a MMC pattern persists throughout the day. The movement of intestinal contents occurs during the Phase II portion of the MMC.

The factors controlling gastric emptying appear to be similar in term infants and adults. Although the mechanisms controlling gastric emptying in preterm infants are similar, the rate of emptying may be reduced compared with term infants. Small intestinal contractile patterns are similar in the adult and term infant. In fetal lambs disorganized sporadic contractions are seen from 0.6–0.8 gestation. From 0.8–0.95 gestation clustered rhythmic bursts of activity are noted, which propagate aborally and orally. The MMC pattern appears after 0.95 gestation. In dogs, the clustered burst pattern is present until 15 days after birth, when MMC patterns appear. Therefore, it is evident that food can be adequately propelled and absorbed prior to the development of a mature MMC pattern of fasting small bowel contractile activity. In the human premature infant analogous patterns of intestinal activity are evident. Prior to 30 weeks' gestation contractile patterns are of low pressure, sporadic, and non-propagative. Clusters of rhythmic contractions appear at 30 weeks and then increase in rate of propagation and amplitude over the next several weeks. By approximately 37 weeks the mature MMC pattern is evident.

## Colonic motility and defecation

The smooth muscle wall and innervation of the colon are essentially similar to the small intestine. The longitudinal muscle does not extend around the entire circumference of the colon, and the neuronal phenotypes differ with location and species. In contrast to the small bowel, propulsion of contents through the colon is slow, measured in hours to days, rather than in minutes. The movement of the luminal contents in the colon has only recently been subjected to extensive study. Distension appears to stimulate contractions. Bursts of contractions occur intermittently and are propagated in aboral and oral directions. The proximal and transverse colon have regions of stasis allowing absorption and bacterial fermentation of their contents. The distal colon molds and forms the stool bolus, which is transported into the rectum. The anorectal region temporarily stores the feces until it is convenient to defecate. Like the proximal stomach, the rectum serves as a reservoir, accommodating increased volume with little change in luminal pressure. After meals, the rectal tone increases. Large, high-amplitude, aborally propagated bursts of contraction sweep through the colon, moving a large segment of the luminal contents into the next region. These high-amplitude propagated contractions (HAPCs) are associated with defecation.

Control of defecation is an important skill learned by toddlers during toilet training. Achievement of normal control of defecation is viewed as a major milestone in social development, whereas loss of bowel control results in social censure. Continence of stool is maintained by the anal sphincter, which is composed of a smooth muscle "internal sphincter" and a striated muscle "external sphincter" (Fig. 54.3). The internal sphincter, responsible for anal continence at rest, is not under voluntary control. Passage of stool or gas into the rectum distends the wall of the rectum. An intramural reflex mediated by nitric oxide and vasoactive intestinal polypeptide, the "rectoanal inhibitory reflex," relaxes the internal sphincter when the rectal wall is stretched as stool or gas enters from above. Infants spontaneously pass the stool. Older children and adults sense the need to defecate, but voluntarily contract the external sphincter to prevent passage of stool or gas until a socially acceptable place and time are achieved. The rectum accommodates to the increased volume, and the internal sphincter contracts, allowing relaxation of the external sphincter. During straining to stool, the resting tone of the external anal sphincter decreases, allowing defecation. Passage of flatus alone is achieved when pressure in the rectum increases due to gaseous distension and a small opening in the anal sphincter permits gas, but not feces, to be passed.

Distension of the rectum with a balloon elicits the anorectal inhibitory reflex relaxation of the internal sphincter in normal individuals. In the newborn and premature infant, the magnitude of the resting internal anal sphincter pressure is reduced, but the anorectal inhibitory reflex is intact. In *Hirschsprung disease* the anorectal inhibitory reflex is absent due to the lack of normal intramural neural pathways.

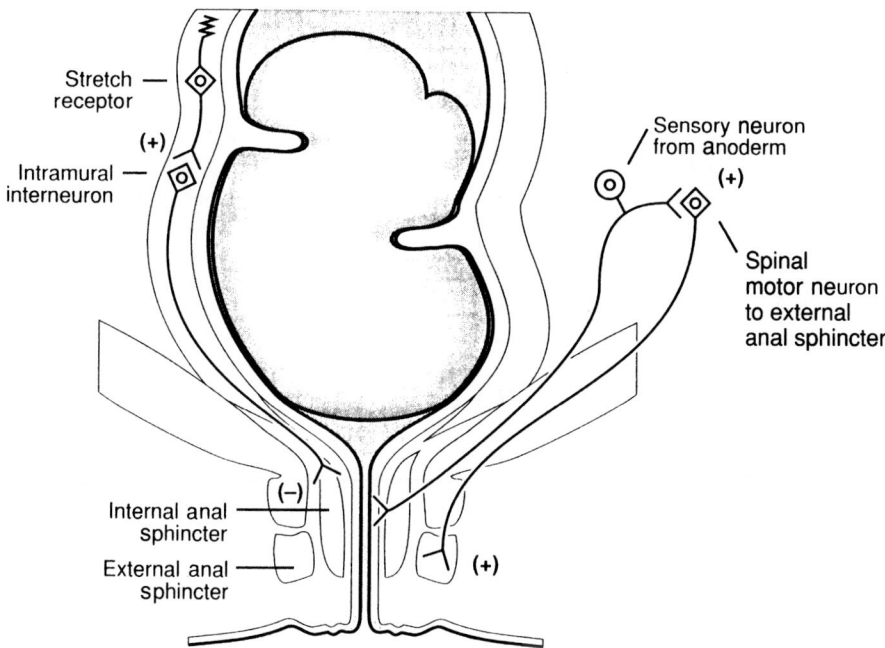

FIGURE 54.3 Diagram of the anorectum. Passage of stool into the rectum activates stretch receptors in the rectal wall, which stimulate intramural interneurons to relax the internal anal sphincter, mediated by nitric oxide. Upon sensation of rectal contents passing onto the epithelium lining the anal sphincter, the anoderm, defecation can ensue, or voluntary contraction of the external anal sphincter prevents stool passage until the rectal wall accommodates and the internal anal sphincter contracts.

## SELECTED READING

Cheng CA, Geoghegan JG, Lawson DC *et al.* Central and peripheral effects of CCK receptor antagonists on satiety in dogs. *Am J Physiol* 1993; **265**: G219.

Dumont RC, Rudolph CD. Development of gastrointestinal motility in the infant and child. *Gastroenterology Clin N Am* 1994; **23**: 655.

Kare MR, Beauchamp K. The role of taste in the infant diet. *Am J Clin Nutrition* 1985; **41**: 418.

Milla PJ ed. *Disorders of gastrointestinal motility in childhood*. Chichester: John Wiley & Sons, Ltd., 1988.

Read NW, French S, Cunningham K. The role of the gut in regulating food intake in man. *Nutr Rev* 1994; **52**: 1.

Rudolph CD. Feeding disorders in infants and children. *J Pediatr* 1994; **125**: S116.

Rudolph C, Benaroch L. Hirschsprung disease. *Pediatr Rev* 1995; **16**: 5.

# 55

# Gastric Acid Secretion and Gastroduodenal Mucosal Defense Mechanisms

Arthur R. Euler

## GASTRIC ACID SECRETION

One of the major physiological functions of the stomach is the secretion of hydrochloric acid by oxyntic gland parietal cells. Gastric acid secretion occurs in three phases: cephalic, gastric, and intestinal. Secretion begins prior to ingestion of food. Simply the smell or thought of food can stimulate gastric acid secretion during the cephalic phase. Entry of food into the stomach or intestine further stimulates secretion.

Gastric glands containing parietal cells are branched, tubular, coiled structures located within the deeper mucosal layers of the gastric fundus and body. In addition to producing hydrochloric acid, which denatures protein, converts pepsinogen to pepsin, and is bacteriostatic or bactericidal for most microbes, these cells also secrete intrinsic factor and small amounts of bicarbonate. The parietal cell contains a network of secretory canaliculi that extend from the luminal surface of the cell through the body of the cell. These canals expand when acid secretion is stimulated.

The synthesis and secretion of hydrochloric acid by parietal cells has been studied intensively. $H^+$ ions are secreted to obtain a pH of 1.0 when intracellular pH is 7.1–7.2, achieving a two-million-fold concentration gradient. The mechanisms by which this is achieved are summarized in Fig. 55.1. Carbonic anhydrase catalyzes the formation of $HCO_3^-$ and $H^+$ ions from $CO_2$ and $H_2O$. $H^+$–$K^+$–ATPase, an enzyme located on the parietal cell luminal surface, secretes $H^+$ ions across the apical membrane in exchange for $K^+$ ions. By a separate pathway, $K^+$ and $Cl^-$ ions are secreted into the canalicular space, down their concentration gradient, with $H_2O$ following. Thus electrochemical and osmotic balance are maintained across the apical membrane. Secretion of this large amount of acid into the lumen requires that an equivalent amount of base be secreted from the basolateral surfaces of the parietal cell to maintain the intracellular pH in the physiological range. $Cl^-$ ions are exchanged for OH ($HCO_3^-$) ions. The $Na^+$–$K^+$–ATPase, located on the basolateral membrane, maintains the higher intracellular $K^+$ concentrations that are necessary to drive $K^+$ ions into the lumen.

Secretion of $H^+$ ions by the parietal cell is stimulated by neurocrine, endocrine, and paracrine pathways through three receptors located on the cell surface membrane: $H_2$-histaminergic, $M_2$-cholinergic, and gastrinergic. The parietal cell also may express receptors for somatostatin and epidermal growth factor (EGF). When histamine from adjacent mast cells occupies $H_2$ receptors on the parietal cell, intracellular cAMP increases. When acetylcholine from the vagus occupies cholinergic receptors, membrane permeability to $Ca^{2+}$ ions increases, allowing an influx of $Ca^{2+}$. Intracellular $Ca^{2+}$ interacts with calmodulin, which probably acts as the second messenger in this pathway. There is conflicting evidence regarding the mechanism of gastrin action on the parietal cell. In some species, gastrin stimulates the mast cell, with histamine secondarily

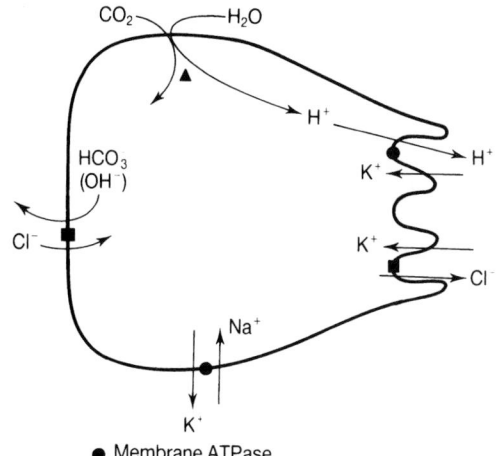

● Membrane ATPase

■ Membrane channel

▲ Carbonic anhydrase

FIGURE 55.1 Schematic representation of the mechanism of $H^+$ ion secretion by the gastric parietal cell. $H_2O$ and $CO_2$ are converted to $H^+$ and $HCO_3^-$ by carbonic anhydrase. $HCO_3^-$ is exchanged for $Cl^-$ across the basal membrane through a membrane channel. $Na^+$ and $K^+$ are exchanged by an energy-requiring ATPase on the basal membrane. $H^+$ is exchanged for $K^+$ on the apical membrane surface. The net effect is to secrete HCl from the apical surface and $NaHCO_3$ from the basal surface.

stimulating the parietal cell. In others, the gastrinergic receptor seems to affect acid secretion in a manner similar to that found after cholinergic stimulation, by increasing $Ca^{2+}$.

## Development of gastric acid secretion

Only the gastric and intestinal phases of gastric acid secretion have been evaluated during the neonatal period. Enterally, or enterally plus parenterally, nourished infants have significantly higher basal and maximal gastric acid secretory rates than those receiving only parenteral nutrition. Enteral feedings, therefore, are necessary for optimal parietal cell function in these infants.

In mammals the upper gastrointestinal mucosa develops early in fetal life, with parietal cells appearing in humans by week 14. Parietal cells have a pink, granular cytoplasm with dark, centrally located nuclei and are usually round or triangular in shape. In the fetal rat, the stomach responds to pentagastrin on day 20. Similar secretory data are not available for the human fetus, although gastrin immunoreactivity has been noted from 18 weeks' gestation onward, with this activity concentrated in the antropyloric area. Parietal cell activity also is noted in the body, antrum, and fundus of human fetuses by the end of the first trimester.

The human newborn has elevated serum gastrin concentrations that are not of maternal origin. These increased gastrin concentrations are not associated with significantly increased gastric acid secretion relative to the older child or adult. This situation is identical to that in the rat, where even 5-day-old pups did not respond to pentagastrin with significant acid secretion. The genes regulating the synthesis of carbonic anhydrase and $H^+$–$K^+$–ATPase appear to be coordinately regulated during acid secretion. The activity of these proteins is diminished in young animals, potentially contributing to the lack of responsiveness to secretagogues in newborns. mRNA coding for these enzymes is present at levels similar to those in the adult rat, suggesting that mRNA translational or post-translational processing is decreased. In addition to gastrin reactivity in the second-trimester human fetus, as well as significant elevations in serum gastrin concentrations in the newborn, somatostatin-like immunoreactivity has been found, in both the plasma and gastric contents of term newborns. The gastrin and somatostatin found in the term newborn are nonsulfated gastrin-34 and somatostatin-14, respectively.

In many mammals, maternal milk prostaglandin $E_2$ ($PGE_2$) content may play a role in regulating acid secretion as PGs are known to suppress gastric acid secretion. Epidermal growth factor (EGF) also is present in mammalian milks and has a number of effects on the gastrointestinal tract, including suppression of gastric acid secretion in a manner similar to $PGE_2$. Solid food intake has the opposite effect and significantly increases acid secretion, doing so to a greater degree than liquids. All of these associations have been documented in animals. One such association also has been confirmed in human neonates: enteral feedings are associated with greater acid secretion than parenteral feedings. This effect may result from specific amino acids contained in the feeds and occurs without a concomitant increase in serum gastrin. This acid secretory response to oral feedings also increases with advancing age, with an approximate two-fold elevation between 1–2 weeks after birth. The role of the central nervous system in gastric acid secretion has been well documented in animals. Vagal stimulation increases gastric acid secretion. In rats, the lateral hypothalamic area has a direct role in gastric acid secretion, and stimulation of this area increases secretory rates. In contrast, enteromedial hypothalamic stimulation decreases secretory rates. L-glutamate and γ-aminobutyric acid likely are the neurotransmitters active within the hypothalamus resulting in gastric acid secretory inhibition and stimulation, respectively. These relationships between the brain and the gut await analysis in the human fetus, newborn, and neonate.

Gastric secretory studies are performed either during fasting conditions (basal acid output: BAO) or after a stimulus (maximal acid output: MAO), e.g. with pentagastrin, histamine, or food. Neither type of secretory study has been reported in the human fetus; however, in the 1-week-old premature infant, BAO was 12 mmol/(kg·h) increasing to 30 mmol/(kg·h) at 4 weeks after birth. MAO after pentagastrin stimulation was 21 mmol/(kg·h) and 44 mmol/(kg·h) at 1 and 4 weeks, respectively. These increases were not associated with elevations in serum gastrin concentrations. In the term newborn, BAO on days 1 and 2 was nearly identical, 0.110 and 0.114 mEq/(kg·h), respectively, while the MAO on the same days, also using pentagastrin as a stimulus, were 0.122 and 0.133 mEq/(kg·h). Serum gastrin concentrations were elevated in these newborns, indicating a relative lack of response by the parietal cells to this supraphysiological stimulus early in life. Betazole, which probably stimulates the histamine $H_2$ receptor on the parietal cell, increases MAO, producing secretory rates approximately 10 times greater 8 weeks after birth than on day 1. This indicates that histamine is a more potent stimulus than gastrin during the neonatal period. When acid secretion is stimulated with a meal (5 per cent glucose plus an elemental formula), newborns respond in a manner similar to older infants (age >6 months), but their response is quantitatively different. Specifically, BAO in the newborn and older infants was 0.038 and 0.067 mmol/(kg·h), respectively, while MAO after the meal was 0.011 and 0.149 mmol/(kg·h), respectively.

Intrinsic factor (IF), a peptide important for absorption of vitamin $B_{12}$, also is secreted by the parietal cell. In rat pups, IF mRNA content changes in parallel with the developmental change in $H^+$–$K^+$–ATPase levels noted above. Similar rates of secretion of IF have been documented in premature and full-term infants (about 11 and 6 ng/(kg·h), respectively). In term infants, IF secretory levels increase from about 7 ng/(kg·h) on day 1 to about 30 ng/(kg·h) by day 28. Normal adult levels (120 ng/(kg·h) are not achieved until 3 months of age. Pepsinogen is secreted by the chief cells in the gastric mucosa. Pepsinogen secretion is reduced in the premature versus full-term infant. The combination of lower acid output and decreased pepsinogen release may place premature infants at considerable disadvantage in gastric proteolysis; thus providing them with amino acids or short-term peptides rather than intact proteins may facilitate nitrogen uptake but this hypothetical advantage has not yet been evaluated. Pepsinogen and gastric proteolysis are discussed in Chapter 56.

## MUCOSAL DEFENSE MECHANISMS

Upper gastrointestinal mucosal damage is believed to result when mucosal destruction by hydrochloric acid, pepsin, or bile salts overcomes the mucosal defense mechanisms. Gastric acid hypersecretion (e.g. due to *Zollinger–Ellison syndrome* or *mastocytosis*) results in mucosal ulceration. More commonly, gastric mucosal destruction is due to inadequate mucosal defense. The protective mechanisms of the gastrointestinal tract have been recognized for over two centuries; however, the importance of mucosal defensive factors was not truly appreciated until Andre Robert described a process he termed *cytoprotection*. Cytoprotection is

defined as the ability of certain substances, especially PGs, to protect the deeper layers of the mucosa, below the surface epithelium, from being injured when exposed to various noxious agents such as strong acids (0.6 M HCl). Cytoprotection occurs with doses of exogenous agents that do not affect gastric acid secretion. This observation has led to an entirely new area of investigation involving the mechanisms of gastrointestinal mucosal protection.

Complex mechanisms underlie the gastroduodenal mucosal defensive barrier. The gastroduodenal mucosa has a well defined layer of mucus overlying the surface epithelial cells. Bicarbonate is secreted into this mucus layer by the surface epithelial cells, forming the *mucobicarbonate barrier*. Mucus is secreted primarily by cells located in the neck segments of gastric glands. These mucus-producing cells have pale foamy cytoplasm, basal nuclei, and large amounts of para-amino-salicylic acid (PAS)-positive mucus. Somatostatin, dopamine, secretin, vasoactive intestinal peptide (VIP), acetylcholine, and particularly $PGE_2$ stimulate mucus secretion, while $PGE_2$, dopamine, VIP, secretin, vagal efferents, and gastric acid stimulate bicarbonate secretion. Neither mucus nor bicarbonate alone is truly an effective defense mechanism, but the two combined form a substantial barrier when the gastric luminal pH is >2–3. When the intraluminal pH is <2 or when noxious agents other than acid are present, the mucosa must enlist other protective mechanisms.

An important alternative mechanism is maintenance of mucosal blood flow and microcirculation. Severe gastroduodenal mucosal damage occurs whenever the vascular supply is compromised because adequate $O_2$ and energy substrates are not available to support intracellular aerobic metabolism. As a result the mechanisms that underlie normal cellular acid–base balance cannot be maintained. These deleterious effects can be avoided by maintaining mucosal blood flow. Endogenous $PGE_2$ increases mucosal blood flow and increases the resistance of the individual mucosal cells to damage. The mechanisms underlying this increased cellular resistance are unknown. EGF, dopamine, and calcitonin gene-related peptide (CGRP) have also been shown to increase mucosal blood flow. These peptide transmitters are contained in the large number of unmyelinated, peptidergic, afferent nerves, called C fibers, within the enteric nervous system. These C fibers probably are the primary splanchnic neurodilatory mechanism; for example, stimulation of these afferents in the stomach will cause vasodilatory peptide release and subsequent increased mucosal blood flow. Surface active phospholipids, which repel water-soluble irritants, also are an important component of mucosal defense. These phospholipids are present as a thin film adhering to the epithelial cells and are stimulated by PGs.

The most important component of the mucosal defensive mechanisms is surface epithelial cellular renewal. It is a slower responding mechanism than those described above, but is essential for maintenance of the epithelium. Soon after injury to an area of the surface epithelium, cells move out of gastric pits onto the surface. Very rapidly they re-establish integrity of the mucosal surface, and an increase in negative potential differences (PDs) is measured. This negativity in PD indicates healing, because during the period when the injury is occurring, the PD rapidly becomes less negative. While repair is underway, subsequent injury is also prevented by secretions from uninjured epithelial cells, which produce a mucoid cap over the area undergoing repair. This mucoid cap is 5–10 times thicker than the normal mucus layer and also is different in composition, consisting primarily of a fibrin gel and necrotic cells. A number of factors previously noted as stimulators of mucus secretion such as PGs and EGF also stimulate these less immediate defense mechanisms.

Although there are fewer studies documenting the relationship between the brain and the gut in the area of mucosal defense in comparison to those documenting the effects of the brain–gut axis on gastric acid secretion, this is a rapidly evolving area in which a number of neurotransmitters have been discovered to play important roles. These neurotransmitters include dopamine agonists that, when given into the mesolimbic tracts of animals, enhance mucosal defenses. Within the stomach, the dopamine 1 ($DA_1$) receptor subtype plays an important cytoprotective role, while CGRP plays a role in maintaining gastric mucosal blood flow and also may be an important neurotransmitter for spinal afferent effects. VIP also is an important neurotransmitter, affecting mucosal defense mechanisms in a number of ways including bicarbonate secretion. As many additional neurotransmitters are discovered, their effects on mucosal defense mechanisms will need to be investigated.

# Development of mucosal protective mechanisms

The limited information on the development of gastroduodenal mucosal defense has not involved human newborns and has been derived from animal studies. In rats, the intrinsic ability of the gastric mucosa to protect itself against acid-induced damage does not develop until 14–21 days after birth. The natural time course of this development seems to depend on endogenous PGs and glucocorticoids. Exogenous hydrocortisone can accelerate this development. Also in rats, surface hydrophobicity, which results from the actions of surface active phospholipids, cannot be consistently induced by exogenous PGs until the third week after birth. This development is not influenced by corticosteroids or thyroxine. Combined, these studies indicate that the gastroduodenal mucosal defensive barrier evolves during the neonatal period and is not fully developed at birth. The exact mechanism(s) underlying the development of the mucosal defense barrier in the human neonate is unknown. It is known that circulating PG concentrations during the first month are greater in both the premature and the fullterm infant than in adults. These concentrations may result from endogenous production by the infant or from PGs in breast milk, where physiologically significant concentrations are present. These PGs are absorbed from the infant's gastrointestinal tract and may have significant influences on many gastrointestinal functions, including the development of various mucosal defensive components.

## SELECTED READING

Allen A, Flemström G, Garner A, Kivilaakso E. Gastroduodenal mucosal protection. *Physiol Rev* 1993; **73**: 823.

Glavin GB, Hall AM. Brain–gut relationships: Gastric mucosal defense is also important. *Acta Physiol Hung* 1992; **80**: 107.

Jacobson ED. Circulatory mechanisms of gastric mucosal damage and protection. *Gastroenterology* 1992; **102**: 1788.

Kelly EJ, Brownlee KG, Newell SJ. Gastric secretory function in the developing human stomach. *Early Hum Dev* 1992; **31**: 163.

Malinowska DH, Sachs G. Cellular mechanisms of acid secretion. *Clin Gastroenterol* 1984; **13**: 309.

Safsten B. Duodenal bicarbonate secretion and mucosal protection. *Acta Physiol Scand Suppl* 1993; **613**: 1.

Schubert ML, Shamburek RD. Control of acid secretion. *Gastroenterol Clin North Am* 1990; **19**: 1.

Shorrock CL, Rees WD. Overview of gastroduodenal mucosal protection. *Am J Med* 1988; **84**: 25.

# 56

# Intraluminal Digestion and Absorption in the Small Intestine

Robert J. Shulman

The primary role of all organs of the gastrointestinal system is to digest complex forms of ingested nutrients into simpler components that are easily absorbed and utilized for energy and growth by the organism. This chapter summarizes the process of digestion and absorption of carbohydrates, fats, proteins, and minerals.

## CARBOHYDRATES

### Digestion of carbohydrates

The primary carbohydrate in the diet of the breast-fed human infant is lactose, which also is the carbohydrate in most infant formulas. Alternative carbohydrates used in infant formulas include sucrose or complex carbohydrates in the form of glucose polymers (molecules of glucose linked almost exclusively by $\alpha$-1,4 bonds in a linear formation). Complex carbohydrates, such as those found in cereals, amylopectins, contain $\alpha$-1,6 bonds as well as $\alpha$-1,4 bonds.

Lactose is digested by the enzyme lactase, which resides in the brush border of the small intestinal mucosa. The $K_m$ for lactase is 18 mM and the optimum pH is 6.0. The products of lactose hydrolysis are glucose and galactose. In adults, the rate of hydrolysis is the rate-limiting step in the absorption of lactose. The rate-limiting step in infants is unknown. Lactase activity is highest in the jejunum and decreases progressively toward the ileum; this gradient is established by the eleventh week of gestation. At the beginning of the third trimester, lactase activity is approximately 25 per cent of that at term. Some lactase activity is demonstrable in the colon in early fetal life, but becomes undetectable by 28 weeks' gestation. The antenatal increase in lactase activity appears to be regulated primarily at the level of transcription and may be in part under glucocorticoid control. In many individuals, lactase activity decreases as age advances. This genetically determined process, begins between 3–5 years of age. The decrease in lactase activity appears to be caused by a reduction in protein synthesis, probably related to changes in transcription, although in some individuals altered post-transcriptional processing seems to play a role. In humans, lactase activity is not inducible by dietary lactose. Despite high lactase activity at birth, most studies suggest that full-term, and especially premature, infants digest and absorb lactose incompletely. In older individuals with low lactase activity, ingestion of lactose may cause diarrhea, flatulence, or cramping (i.e. *lactose intolerance*). Congenital lactase absence has been reported, but is extremely rare.

Digestion of complex carbohydrates is accomplished by a number of enzyme systems (Fig. 56.1), but the quantitative contribution of each remains poorly defined. Salivary and pancreatic amylase (secreted by the salivary glands and pancreas, respectively) have identical actions: hydrolysis of starch at interior $\alpha$-1,4 bonds. They are not active against those bonds located next to $\alpha$-1,6 bonds or those at the reducing end of the starch molecule. The end products of digestion by amylase are maltose, maltotriose, and $\alpha$-limit dextrins. Salivary amylase is present in premature infants, and its activity may increase with increasing gestational age. However, the role of

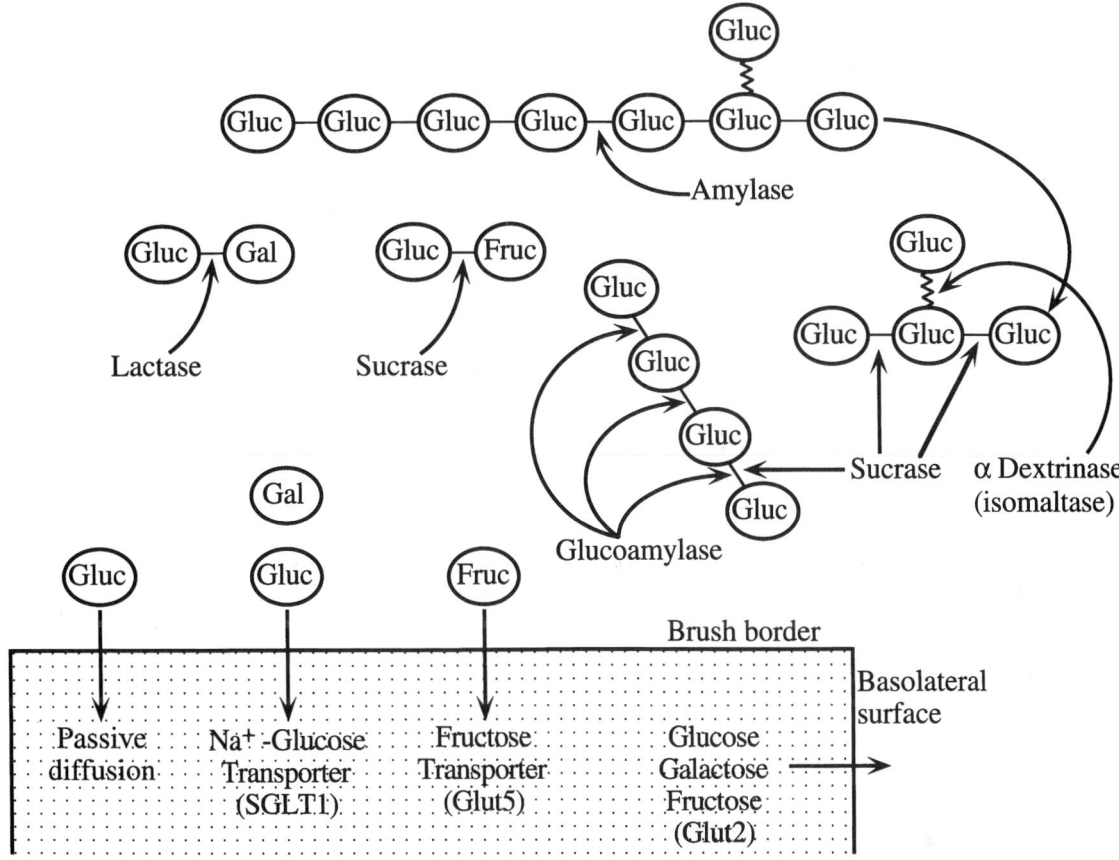

FIGURE 56.1 Small intestinal carbohydrate digestion and absorption. The enzymes lactase, sucrase–isomaltase, and glucoamylase on the small intestinal brush border are responsible for the majority of carbohydrate digestion in the young infant. In older infants and children, pancreatic amylase plays an important role in the digestion of complex carbohydrates (glucose polymers and starches). Gluc, glucose; Gal, galactose; Fruc, fructose (see text for transporter descriptions).

salivary amylase in the digestion of complex carbohydrates remains poorly defined. Although salivary amylase is rapidly inactivated at pH < 4, the inability of some premature infants to generate significant gastric acidity may permit the enzyme to remain active. Additionally, some evidence indicates that complex carbohydrates themselves may offer some protection against destruction of salivary amylase by gastric secretions. Pancreatic amylase activity is extremely low in premature and full-term infants, does not begin to increase until 4–6 months of age, and adult values are not achieved until 1–2 years of age. Pancreatic amylase secretion in newborns does not appear to respond to pancreozymin and secretin stimulation.

The enzyme glucoamylase resides in the brush border of the small intestine. It has activity against complex carbohydrates, primarily those that are non-branched (i.e. only 1–4 bonds), with greatest activity against amylose with a degree of polymerization between 5–9 glucose units. It hydrolyzes α-1,4 bonds from the non-reducing end of the molecule. Thus, the product of glucoamylase activity is glucose. Small intestinal glucoamylase activity is detectable by 20 weeks' gestation, and activity in infants of 28–30 weeks' gestational age is approximately half that at 36–38 weeks. Glucoamylase, like lactase, is present in low levels in the colon only early in fetal life. Glucoamylase activity in the small intestine of young infants is similar to that found in older children and is approximately half that in adults. Because pancreatic amylase activity is low, glucoamylase is the primary determinant of complex carbohydrate digestibility in newborns. Short-chain units of amylose (5–9 glucose units) appear to be digested more easily than longer-chain units. Overall, however, digestion and absorption of complex carbohydrates in the small intestine is incomplete. Rice cereals, for example, contain small amounts of protein, but consist primarily of amylopectin. Recent studies suggest that approximately 30 per cent of rice cereal is not absorbed in the small intestine of infants 1–2 months old.

The disaccharidase sucrase–isomaltase (sucrase-α-dextrinase) is found in the small intestinal brush border; its $K_m$ is 1–4 mM and its pH optimum is ~6. Sucrase–isomaltase is synthesized as a 230-kDa precursor. The molecule is hydrolyzed into sucrase and isomaltase at the brush border by the action of pancreatic proteases, although cleavage is not required for activity. In a pattern similar to that of lactase, a proximo-distal gradient of activity is present by the end of the first trimester. Sucrase–isomaltase activity develops early in gestation under transcriptional control, and by 20 weeks' gestation achieves levels approximately one-half to three-quarters those found in term newborns and adults. Sucrase–isomaltase activity remains high throughout life. Maltase activity is provided mostly by the sucrase–isomaltase complex. A deficiency of sucrase–isomaltase can be transmitted as an autosomal recessive trait.

Not only does sucrase–isomaltase hydrolyze sucrose to its components glucose and fructose, it also is important during the final steps of the hydrolysis of complex carbohydrates. As with glucoamylase, sucrase–isomaltase is capable of hydrolyzing α-1,4 bonds. The hydrolysis of α-1,6 bonds occurs by means of isomaltase activity. Sucrase–isomaltase activity appears to be inducible by sucrose and fructose in the diet. Few data are available on the ability of infants to digest sucrose. Studies in adults suggest that more than 95 per cent of dietary sucrose is digested in the small intestine.

## Absorption of carbohydrates

After hydrolysis, the final step in the assimilation of carbohydrates is the absorption of the component monosaccharides, i.e. glucose and galactose in the case of lactose, glucose and fructose in the case of sucrose, and two molecules of glucose in the case of maltose (Fig. 56.1). Active transport of glucose is demonstrable *in vitro* by 10 weeks' gestation. The maximal absorption rate of glucose increases with age through gestation and after birth to adulthood. Infants less than 37 weeks' gestation have a lower $K_m$ for glucose than full-term infants. Infants who are small for gestational age have a lower apparent $K_m$ than those who are appropriate for gestational age. Recent studies suggest that a *high-affinity transport system* exists throughout the small intestine with a *low-affinity transport system* limited to the proximal small intestine. These systems are present by 17–20 weeks' gestation. The transport of glucose involves movement of the molecule across the brush border and basolateral surfaces (Fig. 56.1); glucose is actively transported by the Na⁺-glucose cotransporter (SGLT1) at the brush border with two molecules of Na⁺. Energy is provided by Na⁺–K⁺–ATPase at the basolateral membrane surface.

Thus, the absorption of glucose facilitates the absorption of Na⁺, which is the rationale for adding glucose to rehydration solutions. On the other hand, Na⁺ is required for the Na⁺–glucose cotransporter to function. Glucose absorption can also occur passively down a chemical gradient. Galactose is believed to be transported by the same system as glucose (SGLT1). In contrast, a separate Na⁺-independent transport system

exists in the brush border for fructose (Glut5), which allows transport down its concentration gradient (Fig. 56.1). The ontogeny of galactose and fructose absorption in the human is unknown. Less than 0.1 per cent of an ingested disaccharide is absorbed intact through passive diffusion. Glucose, galactose, and fructose movement across the basolateral surface out of the cell are by facilitated diffusion, which is Na⁺-independent (Glut2) (Fig. 56.1).

## FATS

## Digestion of fats

Fats not only are a major energy source for newborn infants, but also are integrally involved in normal brain development, are components of cell membranes, and act as vehicles for absorption of fat-soluble vitamins. In contrast to proteins and carbohydrates, fats are water-insoluble molecules that must be solubilized before they can be digested and absorbed.

Most dietary fats (triglycerides) consist of long-chain fatty acids ($\geqslant C_{16}$) and thus are hydrophobic. Digestion of dietary fats primarily involves processes to increase their water solubility. The initial process is *emulsification*, which begins with the mechanical grinding action of the stomach and small intestine. Dietary proteins and the products of fat digestion, fatty acids, monoglycerides, and lecithin, further the emulsification process and stabilize the fat particles. The emulsified particles of fat, which are less than 1.0 mm in size, are further stabilized by bile salts, which are synthesized by the liver and secreted in bile (see Chapter 64). The emulsion is stable at neutral pH. The term *mixed micelles* refers to these spherical particles of bile salts, hydrolysis products, phospholipids, and cholesterol. For micelles to be formed, bile salt concentration must be above the "critical micellar concentration," which is determined by a number of factors including the properties of the individual bile salts. The major enzymes involved in the digestion of fats are the lipases (lingual, gastric, pancreatic). Although pancreatic lipase is the primary enzyme involved in small intestinal fat digestion, it requires the action of pancreatic colipase to anchor lipase to the fat droplet (Fig. 56.2). The products of these actions are mono- and diglycerides, fatty acids, and glycerol. Because medium-chain triglycerides ($C_{10}$–$C_{14}$) are water-soluble, they are absorbed directly through the stomach and the small intestine without the need for emulsification by bile acids.

The lipases undergo dramatic developmental changes. Although lingual lipase is demonstrable at birth, its contribution to lipid digestion is small in contrast to gastric lipase, which is released from the gastric fundus. Lingual and gastric lipases appear before 26 weeks' gestation and have high activities at birth. Newborns can digest 80–90 per cent of ingested fat despite the fact that pancreatic lipase activity is extre-

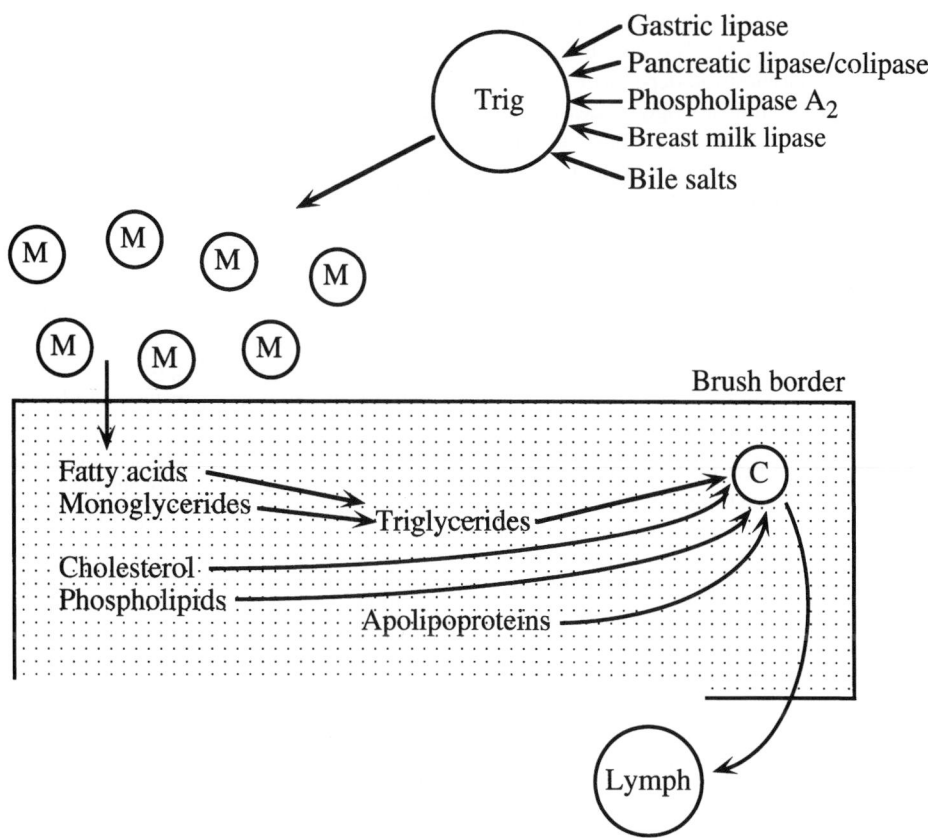

FIGURE 56.2 Small intestinal fat digestion and absorption. In newborn (particularly premature) infants where pancreatic lipase is at low concentrations, gastric lipase probably plays an important role in triglyceride hydrolysis. Trig, triglyceride; M, mixed micelles; C, chylomicrons; Lymph, lymphatic vessels.

mely low at birth. Gastric lipase activity is similar in infants and adults. The underdeveloped gastric acid production of premature and full term newborns provides an optimal milieu for enzyme activity. Approximately 10–30 per cent of dietary fat is hydrolyzed in the stomachs of fullterm infants. Presumably, the relative pancreatic insufficiency of newborn infants results in a lower duodenal pH, which enables lingual and gastric lipases to retain activity and continue fat digestion in the duodenum. Lingual and gastric lipases hydrolyze short- and medium-chain triglycerides more rapidly than long-chain triglycerides. Consequently, the triglyceride profile of the diet fed to newborn infants determines, in part, the digestibility of fat. Pancreatic lipase production is limited even in full-term newborn infants and neither premature nor full-term infants have a lipase secreting response to pancreozymin or secretin either at birth or at 1 month of age. The lipolytic activity of the duodenal contents also is low during the first year. The possible effect of dietary composition on the development of lipase activity and the developmental profiles of the individual lipolytic enzymes, lipase–colipase, phospholipase $A_2$, and cholesterol esterase, remain to be established.

The cholic acid synthesis rate and the cholic acid pool are four-fold less in premature infants 32–36 weeks' gestational age than in full-term infants, who in turn have values approximately half those found in adults (see Chapter 64). Reduced duodenal concentrations of bile salts and pancreatic lipase activity decrease the capacity of infants to digest and absorb lipid. Fat is absorbed more easily from human milk than from formula, which may be the consequence of the presence of a bile salt-sensitive lipase in human milk. Human milk-fed infants 31–36 weeks gestational age do not change fat absorption with increasing postnatal age. Ninety-four per cent of ingested fat is absorbed by the breast-fed infant at 33 days after birth. In contrast, fat absorption in formula-fed infants is correlated with postnatal age and the duodenal concentration of bile acids. In general, the greater the fatty acid chain length and saturation, the poorer the absorption of fat.

## Absorption of fats

Micelles *per se* are not absorbed into the small intestinal epithelial cells (Fig. 56.2). However, because products of lipolysis are fat-soluble, they encounter little difficulty traversing the lipoprotein membrane of the epithelial cells. Uptake of fatty acids occurs by passive diffusion and is concentration-dependent. Most absorption of fatty acids and monoglycerides occurs in the duodenum and upper jejunum. Bile salts are absorbed primarily by active transport in the terminal ileum. Once fat digestion products have entered the cell, they are resynthesized into triglycerides. They are assembled with cholesterol, phospholipids, and apolipoproteins into chylomicrons, which are then discharged into the intercellular space and enter the lymphatic system by exocytosis. The apolipoproteins A-I, B-48, and B-100 are synthesized in the small intestine of the fetus. However, as gestation progresses, the ratio of B-48 to B-100 increases, although overall, the amount of A-I far exceeds that of B-48 and B-100. In the adult, the intestine produces little if any B-100.

Ileal uptake of cholic acid conjugated with taurine (taurocholate), in both premature and full-term infants, is less shortly after birth than at 8 months. When bile acid uptake is reduced, the bile acid pool available for micellar formation presumably is decreased. The duodenal concentrations of bile acids in fullterm infants are roughly one-tenth those found in adults. Premature infants appear to have greater fecal losses of bile acids than older infants, and the loss is greater for infants fed cows'-milk formulas than for those fed human milk.

## PROTEINS

## Digestion of proteins

Protein digestion is a complex process requiring peptidase-mediated hydrolysis of many different peptide bonds (Fig. 56.3). Absorption of the varied products of hydrolysis requires multiple transepithelial transporters. Protein digestion begins in the stomach. Acid denatures proteins, and pepsins I and II begin the process of hydrolysis. The development of gastric acid secretion is covered in Chapter 55. Gastric peptic activity is low in premature infants but increases in proportion to gestational age. Although the stimulated value, corrected for body weight, increases after birth, at 1 month it is still approximately one-third that found in the adult. In 3–4-week-old premature infants (mean age at birth, 31 weeks' gestation), meal-stimulated pepsinogen secretion was 5–10 per cent that found in full-term infants 1–6 months of age. Thus, both pepsin(ogen) production and activity are diminished in premature infants. Activity is low, in part, because gastric pH must be <5 for these enzymes to be

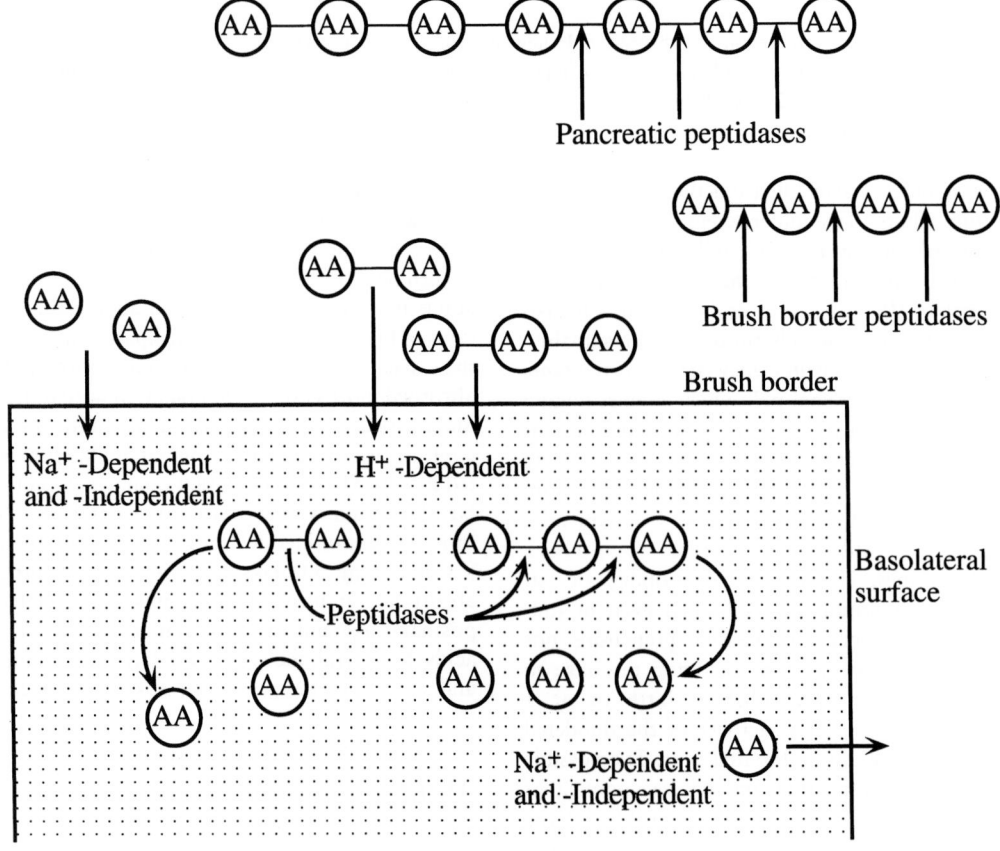

FIGURE 56.3 Small intestinal protein digestion and absorption. Amino acids as well as di- and tripeptides are absorbed across the brush border. AA = amino acids.

activated. Pepsin activity increases approximately two-fold between infancy and adulthood. These studies indirectly support the data suggesting that protein digestion in the stomach of full-term newborns is limited.

The activity of enterokinase, the enzyme responsible for the activation of trypsinogen into trypsin, appears only after 26 weeks' gestation, and its activity at term is approximately 10 per cent of that in adults. However, pancreatic trypsin levels are substantial in both premature and full-term infants. Trypsin in turn activates the other pancreatic proteolytic enzymes.

Trypsin and chymotrypsin activity have been demonstrated *in vitro* at approximately 25 weeks' gestation in the presence of enterokinase. The amount of trypsin secreted in response to pancreozymin and secretin stimulation is similar at birth in premature (32–34 weeks' gestation) and term infants. By 1 week after birth, this response reaches approximately 15–30 per cent of that in children aged 9 months to 13 years. In premature infants (28–34 weeks) trypsin activity (units/mg protein secreted) increases two-fold between birth and 1 month of age. Despite these differences, the trypsin activity level and concentration in duodenal fluid is similar at birth and at 2 years.

Recent studies have focused on the development of other pancreatic peptidases. The responses of chymotrypsin and carboxypeptidase B to pancreozymin and secretin are blunted in the same manner as those of trypsin in newborn and 1-month-old premature infants. Little change in activities occurs over the first month in premature infants of 28–34 weeks' gestation. Activities are approximately one-half those found at 2 years of age. Trypsin, chymotrypsin, and elastase are demonstrable in fetuses at 20 weeks' gestation, with no differences found in histochemical staining compared with full-term infants. The lower activity of pancreatic proteases found in newborn and premature infants compared with full-term infants does not appear to limit protein digestion significantly. Serum albumin is absorbed to a similar extent in premature and full-term newborns during the first month after birth. The ability to digest casein does not appear to be age-related; no apparent change occurs in casein digestion (total proteolytic activity) from 2.5 months of age through adulthood. The action of the luminal proteases produces free amino acids (approximately 30 per cent of ingested protein in adults) and peptides (2–6 amino acid residues in length).

Many proteases are present in the brush border and cytoplasm of the small intestine. The activity of many of these peptidases is detectable between 10–16 weeks' gestation. The activity of dipeptidases is similar in infants, children, and adults. Aminopeptidase activity in infants 28–30 weeks' gestational age is approximately one-half that found at 36–38 weeks. By 22 weeks' gestation, γ-glutamyltranspeptidase, aminopeptidase A, dipeptidylaminopeptidase IV, and carboxypeptidase are detectable, and except for aminopeptidase A, their activities are similar to those in adults. In contrast, γ-glutamyltranspeptidase activity decreases with increasing gestational age. Aminopeptidase activity is also found in the colon of both premature and full-term infants, but at levels approximately half of those found in the small intestine. The contribution of these enzymes to digestion in the premature and full-term infant, however, remains unclear.

## Absorption of protein

*Amino acid transporters* are generally classified on the basis of their Na⁺ dependence, affinity for the amino acid transported, and their possible inhibition by other amino acids. There are at least five different Na⁺-dependent systems for neutral amino acids (Table 56.1). Na⁺-dependent transport is facilitated by the energy derived from Na⁺–K⁺–ATPase at the basolateral cell surface. The movement of Na⁺ across the brush border enables Na⁺-coupled transporters to use the energy for amino acid uptake. A Na⁺-independent (through facilitated diffusion) transport system also exists (Table 56.1). The enzyme γ-glutamyltranspeptidase may also be involved in amino acid transport. After absorption, amino acids (and peptides after hydrolysis) can be converted into other amino acids, converted into proteins, degraded, or transported into blood. Transport of amino acids out of the cell across the basolateral membrane appears to occur through Na⁺-independent and -dependent systems. There is some overlap between the systems for amino acid transport in the small intestine and those in the kidney; the overlap is defined by genetic disorders of amino acid transport common to both organs. (See selected reading for a more complete discussion of the types of amino acid transporters and their specificities.)

Di- and tripeptides can be transported directly into the enterocytes (Fig. 56.3). Peptides larger than three amino acids must be hydrolyzed before they can be absorbed (i.e. by brush border peptidases). Some

TABLE 56.1 Amino acid transporter systems in the small intestinal brush border

| TRANSPORT SYSTEM | SUBSTRATES | Na⁺ GRADIENT REQUIRED |
|---|---|---|
| B | Dipolar α-amino acids | Yes |
| B⁰,⁺ | Dipolar α-amino acids Basic amino acids Cystine | Yes |
| b⁰,⁺ | Dipolar α-amino acids Basic amino acids Cystine | No |
| y⁺ | Basic amino acids | No |
| IMINO | Imino acids | Yes |
| X⁻ₐg | Acidic amino acids | Yes |
| β | β-amino acids | Yes |

amino acids are absorbed more rapidly as di- and tri-peptides than as free amino acids. The absorption of amino acids from a protein hydrolysate is faster than from a mixture of the individual amino acids. The transport systems for peptides are poorly character-ized, but are not those that transport amino acids. Peptide transport probably involves exchange with $H^+$ and is independent of $Na^+$. Most of the peptides within the cell appear to be hydrolyzed by cytoplasmic peptidases, although a small amount of some peptides may be transported intact across the basolateral mem-brane. Little information is available about the trans-port of amino acids and peptides by the developing human small intestine. Amino acid transport appears to have developed by the end of the first trimester. Peptide transport has been demonstrated by the begin-ning of the second trimester. Evidence suggests that absorption of whole proteins can occur but does so with decreasing likelihood as the infant gets older.

## MINERALS

Calcium and phosphorus are the major minerals found in bone. At least 99 per cent of the $Ca^{2+}$ and $PO_4$ in the body are found in bone. Little is known about age-related changes in $Ca^{2+}$ and $PO_4$ absorption in the human.

## Calcium absorption (*see* Chapter 43 for details)

$Ca^{2+}$ absorption is controlled by two processes: active transport and non-saturable diffusion. Active transport of $Ca^{2+}$ occurs through the transcellular route, whereas diffusion occurs through a paracellular pathway. Gastric acidity enhances $Ca^{2+}$ absorption by means of ionization. Most $Ca^{2+}$ absorption occurs in the jeju-num, primarily through active transport, although transport is most efficient in the duodenum. $K_m$ values increase aborally along the small intestine, whereas $V_{max}$ is lowest in the jejunum. Absorption of $Ca^{2+}$ via diffusion occurs throughout the small intestine and decreases aborally with little $Ca^{2+}$ absorption in the colon. Vitamin D ($1,25(OH)_2D$) stimulates active absorption of $Ca^{2+}$ across the brush border, intracel-lular movement of $Ca^{2+}$, and exit of $Ca^{2+}$ across the basolateral membrane (through $Ca^{2+}-Mg^{2+}-ATPase$). In this regard, there is a strong correlation between the concentration of calbindin in the intestine and the rate and efficiency of $Ca^{2+}$ absorption. Calbindin appears to facilitate the intracellular movement of $Ca^{2+}$. Calmodulin, however, may alter the permeability of the cell to $Ca^{2+}$. Calbindin, but not calmodulin, is vita-min D-responsive. At high luminal concentrations, $Ca^{2+}$ is absorbed through vitamin D-independent dif-fusion. Movement of $Ca^{2+}$ out of the enterocyte is mediated through an active $Ca^{2+}-ATPase$ "pump" although there also appears to be a $Na^+-Ca^{2+}$ exchange system facilitated by calmodulin. Some

evidence suggests that $Ca^{2+}$ can also be translocated in vesicles by an energy-dependent mechanism (endocytosis and exocytosis).

$Ca^{2+}$ absorption appears to decrease with age, i.e. absorption in premature infants is approximately 50 per cent, whereas in adults it is closer to 30 per cent. The nature of a diet can affect $Ca^{2+}$ absorption; phy-tates and cellulose decrease $Ca^{2+}$ absorption, whereas carbohydrates that can be digested and absorbed facil-itate $Ca^{2+}$ absorption. *Steatorrhea* also diminishes $Ca^{2+}$ absorption. Active absorption of $Ca^{2+}$ varies inversely with dietary $Ca^{2+}$ intake.

## Phosphorus absorption

$PO_4$ appears to be absorbed both actively and pass-ively. Both absorption routes are more active at pH 6.1 than at pH 7.4. Active transport appears to be the result of a $Na^+$-phosphate co-transport system located at the brush border. The transporter accepts both $H_2PO_4^-$ and $HPO_4^{2-}$. Each phosphate molecule is co-transported with two $Na^+$ ions. As in the case of $Ca^{2+}$, vitamin D ($1,25(OH)_2D$) increases active $PO_4$ transport. Passive diffusion of $PO_4$ occurs predomi-nantly in the duodenum. In contrast to $Ca^{2+}$, thyroid hormone increases $PO_4$ absorption. Studies in animals suggest that $PO_4$ absorption decreases with age. There is disagreement as to whether the movement of $PO_4$ out of the cell is active or passive. Indeed, much regarding $PO_4$ absorption remains to be defined.

## Iron absorption

Absorption of iron is the primary mechanism whereby the content of total body iron is controlled. Most iron absorption occurs in the duodenum and proximal jeju-num. Ferrous iron remains more soluble at the pH of the intestinal lumen and is better absorbed than ferric iron. Iron absorption is also affected by the composi-tion of the diet; absorption is increased by some amino acids and vitamin C and decreased by carbonates and phosphate, which form insoluble precipitates. Hemoglobin iron is absorbed better than non-heme iron. Iron within the cells may come from either the diet or body stores. Because iron is known to bind to receptors on enterocytes, it is believed that when body stores of iron are adequate, the receptors are occupied by the endogenous iron, leaving few receptors available to bind dietary iron. In humans, iron uptake appears to be an active, carrier-mediated process that is mediated, in part, by a membrane protein and free fatty acids. The roles of transferrin and endocytosis in iron uptake by enterocytes have yet to be established.

Iron absorption in animals decreases with age. During iron deficiency, the uptake of other divalent metals (e.g. lead) is increased, presumably because iron and lead share a common transport mechanism. Iron leaves the enterocyte to enter the portal circulation. Iron absorption may be regulated at the brush border as well as at the basolateral membrane.

## SELECTED READING

Argiles JM, Lopez-Soriano FJ. Intestinal amino acid transport: an overview. *Int J Biochem* 1990; **22**: 931.

Cross HS, Debiec H, Peterlik M. Mechanism and regulation of intestinal phosphate absorption. *Min Electrolyte Metab* 1990; **16**: 115.

Flanagan PR. Mechanisms and regulation of intestinal uptake and transfer of iron. *Acta Paediatr Scand* 1989; **S361**: 21.

Grimble GK. The significance of peptides in clinical nutrition. *Annu Rev Nutr* 1994; **14**: 419.

Johnson LR ed. *Physiology of the gastrointestinal tract.* New York: Raven Press, 1994.

Walker WA, Durie PR, Hamilton JR *et al.* eds. *Pediatric gastrointestinal disease.* Philadelphia: BC Decker Inc., 1991.

Wasserman RH, Fullmer CS. On the molecular mechanism of intestinal $Ca^{2+}$ transport. *Adv Exp Med Biol* 1989; **249**: 45.

# 57

# Absorption and Secretion of Electrolytes and Fluid by the Intestine

Mitchell B. Cohen

The intestine is the primary organ of water and nutrient absorption. The intestine also plays an important role in maintaining fluid and electrolyte balance, and intestinal secretory mechanisms aid in food digestion. Disorders of intestinal fluid and electrolyte absorption or of intestinal secretion have a profound impact on health.

## WATER TRANSPORT

In healthy individuals the small intestine absorbs large amounts of water and electrolytes daily. The fluid volume presented to the small intestine is composed of the salivary, gastric, biliary, and pancreatic secretions, which in aggregate significantly exceed the volume of fluid in the diet. Fluid and electrolytes are reabsorbed along the entire length of the gastrointestinal tract; however, the distal segments are more efficient than the proximal segments in their ability to absorb water. The absorptive efficiency of the entire human intestine for water and Na$^+$ is 95–99 per cent. This means that only 1–5 per cent of the water load presented to the upper intestinal tract is actually excreted by the colon. Nonetheless, the human colon is usually not required to absorb fluid to its maximal capacity. In the adult, the human colon can compensate for up to a 50 per cent reduction in small intestinal absorption before stool volume changes.

## SODIUM ABSORPTION

Na$^+$ represents the major driving force for absorption of fluid in the intestine. Furthermore, as fluid progresses to the distal intestine, the ability to absorb Na$^+$ against a high concentration gradient ($\geq$100 mM) increases. The human colon can reduce the intraluminal Na$^+$ concentration to < 15 mM under normal conditions and to 3 mM when required by water and salt deprivation.

Na$^+$ enters the intestinal cell both by diffusion and by active transport. Active transport of Na$^+$ involves two distinct steps. First, there must be carrier- or channel-mediated transport of Na$^+$ across the apical cell membrane. Second, Na$^+$ must traverse the enterocyte and be pumped out by a basolateral membrane Na$^+$ pump. A number of transport mechanisms permit entry of Na$^+$ into the enterocyte through the apical membrane (Fig. 57.1). These include Na$^+$/H$^+$ exchange (HCO$_3^-$-stimulated Na$^+$ absorption), coupled Na$^+$Cl$^-$ absorption, the Na$^+$ channel, which transports Na$^+$ against an electrochemical gradient, and Na$^+$-dependent cotransport with glucose, galactose, amino acids, or volatile fatty acids. Whereas Na$^+$ enters through the apical membrane by several mechanisms, a single active mechanism permits Na$^+$ to exit through the basolateral membrane. The basolateral Na$^+$ pump, Na$^+$-K$^+$-ATPase, is present in sufficient quantity to accommodate the influx of $Na^+$ resulting from the multitude of apical transport systems.

## Bicarbonate-stimulated $Na^+$ transport

The duodenum and jejunum absorb both $Na^+$ and bicarbonate, which results in electrically neutral absorption of both ions. This process begins with the equimolar exchange of $Na^+$ and $H^+$. The $H^+$ liberated into the intestinal lumen is dissipated by combination with bicarbonate. This results in the formation of carbonic acid, which dissociates into $H_2O$ and $CO_2$. $CO_2$ is reabsorbed into the cell and combines with a hydroxyl group to form bicarbonate, which then diffuses across the basolateral membrane.

## Coupled $Na^+$–$Cl^-$ absorption

An important mechanism of $Na^+$ absorption in the ileum and distal colon is that of electrically neutral absorption of $Na^+$ with $Cl^-$. In the ileum, $Cl^-$ is actively exchanged for bicarbonate by the $Cl^-/HCO_3^-$ anion exchanger. The increase in the luminal concentration of bicarbonate drives the intestinal cation exchanger to absorb $Na^+$ in exchange for $H^+$. This double ionic exchange model provides a mechanism

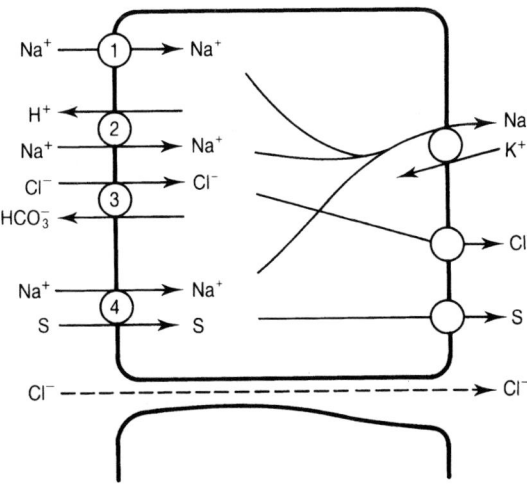

FIGURE 57.1 Major intestinal electrolyte transport systems. $Na^+$ is transported actively across the apical membrane by a number of different processes: (1) through an electrogenic conductance channel, (2) through an intestinal cation exchanger, (3) through an intestinal anion exchanger, and (4) coupled with organic solutes (S) including glucose, galactose, amino acids, and volatile fatty acids. The diagram also shows $Cl^-$ being transported through the paracellular pathway as a result of the electrochemical gradient generated by transport processes 1 and 4. $Na^+$ is excreted through the basolateral membrane via $Na^+$–$K^+$–ATPase. (From Guandalini S, *Drugs* 1988; **36** (Suppl 4): 26, with permission from Adis International.)

whereby volatile fatty acids might also stimulate $Na^+$ and $Cl^-$ transport via fatty acid/bicarbonate exchange.

## Glucose and amino acid-stimulated $Na^+$ transport

Glucose and galactose have a dramatic effect on both $Na^+$ and $H_2O$ absorption via a specific $Na^+$/glucose cotransporter. The maximal stimulatory effect occurs in the range of 50–100 mM glucose. The effects of amino acids on $Na^+$ and $H_2O$ absorption are additive to those of monosaccharides, demonstrating the existence of a separate amino acid/$Na^+$ transporter. These observations have led to the use of glucose-containing oral electrolyte solutions for treatment of dehydration and have also resulted in the preparation of "super" oral rehydration solutions, which contain polymeric monosaccharides (starch) and protein to maximally stimulate $Na^+$ and water absorption.

## Volatile fatty acid-stimulated $Na^+$ transport

Volatile fatty acids are produced by the normal fecal flora as a result of bacterial metabolism of undigested starch and fiber. These volatile fatty acids stimulate colonic $Na^+$ and $H_2O$ absorption (see Chapter 58). Although the mechanism by which these volatile fatty acids exert a stimulatory effect is unclear, there is some evidence for a $Na^+$/fatty acid cotransporter. Alternatively fatty acids may stimulate both $Cl^-$ and $Na^+$ absorption via fatty acid/bicarbonate exchange. Thus, the fatty acids produced by anaerobic fermentation in the colon serve a beneficial role, augmenting $Na^+$ and $H_2O$ salvage in the colon in addition to the role they play in the colon as a useful energy supply. In circumstances where there has not been adequate establishment of the colonic flora (e.g. in the newborn), or where the colonic flora have been drastically reduced (e.g. during antibiotic therapy), there may be inadequate production of volatile fatty acids and an inability to absorb maximally water and electrolytes that have passed through to the colon. In contrast, excess production of volatile fatty acids can result in the clinical phenomena of *cramping* and *osmotic diarrhea*.

## $Na^+$ conductance channel

Several lines of evidence suggest an alternative mechanism of $Na^+$ entry through the apical cell membrane, by way of channels that open and close, primarily in the distal colon. These $Na^+$ conductance channels are inhibited by the diuretic amiloride or its analogs and can be operationally defined as amiloride-sensitive

Na$^+$ channels. During dehydration or states of Na$^+$ depletion, aldosterone increases, which may increase the number and/or sensitivity of the amiloride-sensitive Na$^+$ conductance channels. In addition, mineralocorticoids increase the amount of Na$^+$–K$^+$–ATPase on the basolateral membrane, which may ensure the rapid export of absorbed Na$^+$. Glucocorticoids also increase Na$^+$ absorption by stimulating amiloride-sensitive Na$^+$ transport and Na$^+$–K$^+$–ATPase activity. The response of the colon to aldosterone is not as significant as is the response of the kidney to aldosterone. Nonetheless, aldosterone-stimulated Na$^+$ transport may play an important role in Na$^+$ homeostasis in circumstances of Na$^+$ deprivation or excess loss (e.g. in patients with an ileostomy).

## POTASSIUM ABSORPTION AND SECRETION

The intestine plays an important adjunctive role to the kidney in the maintenance of normal plasma K$^+$ concentrations. K$^+$ is both absorbed and secreted. In the small intestine, K$^+$ is passively absorbed. K$^+$ is normally secreted in the proximal colon, but actively absorbed in the distal colon. However, under the appropriate stimuli, both the proximal and distal colon can be made to secrete K$^+$.

Intestinal K$^+$ secretion results from K$^+$ absorption across the basolateral membrane through the action of Na$^+$–K$^+$–ATPase and subsequent diffusion across the apical membrane through conductance channels. Intestinal K$^+$ absorption results from K$^+$ transport across the apical membrane via K$^+$–H$^+$–ATPase to achieve a net increase in the intracellular K$^+$ concentration. K$^+$ then moves through the basolateral membrane based on an electrochemical equilibrium. Administration of corticosteroids or an elevation in plasma K$^+$ increases basolateral membrane Na$^+$–K$^+$–ATPase. This results in increased K$^+$ secretion. Intestinal diseases that result in inflammation, or in elevated levels of cAMP, also increase intestinal K$^+$ secretion, possibly by increasing apical membrane K$^+$ conductance.

## ACID–BASE HOMEOSTASIS

The intestine complements the primary role of the kidney and the lungs in maintaining acid–base homeostasis.

## Bicarbonate absorption and secretion

The major mechanism of HCO$_3^-$ absorption in the proximal intestine is through HCO$_3^-$-stimulated Na$^+$ transport as described above. HCO$_3^-$ is secreted in the ileum and colon predominately by HCO$_3^-$/Cl$^-$ exchange. Bacterial toxins, such as cholera toxin and *Escherichia coli* heat-labile toxin, as well as

other substances that elevate intracellular cAMP, cause an increase in HCO$_3^-$ secretion in the distal ileum and colon. The increased stool losses of HCO$_3^-$ caused by these agents can result in severe *acidosis*.

## Systemic acid–base balance

Volatile fatty acids which can be absorbed in the colon and metabolized to HCO$_3^-$ make a significant contribution to systemic acid–base balance. Stool electrolyte excretion is altered significantly by conditions of acidosis or alkalosis. Na$^+$ absorption increases during acidosis and decreases during alkalosis. In addition, increased intestinal HCO$_3^-$ secretion occurs during periods of high blood HCO$_3^-$ concentration (metabolic alkalosis and respiratory acidosis) and decreased intestinal HCO$_3^-$ secretion occurs during periods of low blood HCO$_3^-$ concentration (metabolic acidosis and respiratory alkalosis).

## INTESTINAL SECRETION

Intestinal fluid secretion is important to the digestive process. By diluting foodstuffs, the intestine is able to maintain a relatively isotonic environment. In addition, formation of a liquid suspension facilitates mixing and movement of luminal contents. Another important postulated role for intestinal secretion is that of cleansing the intestine of infectious agents and antigens.

A number of agents have been shown to inhibit intestinal water and electrolyte absorption or to stimulate intestinal secretion. These agents include acetylcholine, vasoactive intestinal polypeptide, secretin, bile salts, and bacterial enterotoxins. These agonists presumably bind to an enterocyte receptor, which, when activated, increases the intracellular concentration of a secondary mediator such as cAMP, cyclic guanosine monophosphate (cGMP), or ionized Ca$^{2+}$. These secondary signal transducing agents result in inhibition of coupled Na$^+$ and Cl$^-$ absorption and/or stimulation of Cl$^-$ secretion (Fig. 57.2). Alternatively, these enterocyte-derived secondary messenger molecules may stimulate a neurenteric or enteroendocrine pathway, signaling or amplifying a secretory response in a distant enterocyte(s). In addition, mesenchymal (lamina propria) cells, including mast cells and macrophages, may also elaborate secondary messengers, e.g. histamine, eicosanoids, and platelet activating factor, which stimulate secretomotor enteric neurons and/or directly activate receptors on enterocytes. There is increasing evidence that the enteric nervous system, the mucosal endocrine system (enteroendocrine cells), and inflammatory mediators elaborated by several cell sources strongly influence net intestinal secretion in health and disease.

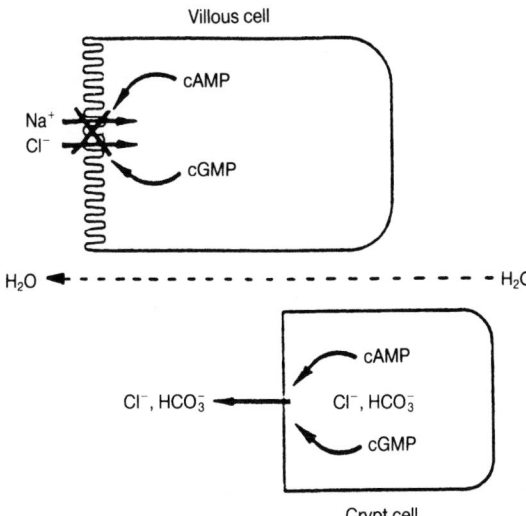

FIGURE 57.2 Scheme of action of cyclic nucleotides on intestinal electrolyte and water transport. cAMP and cGMP inhibit the coupled entry of Na$^+$ and Cl$^-$ into villus cells and stimulate the secretion of Cl$^-$ and bicarbonate from crypt cells. Both of these effects result in net water transport being reversed from absorption to secretion. (From Guandalini S, *Drugs* 1988; **36** (Suppl 4): 26, with permission from Adis International.)

## PARACELLULAR SECRETION AND ABSORPTION

The active transport of Na$^+$ and other ions in the intestine occurs via specific transporters on the apical membrane of the enterocyte. Another mechanism for ion movement is passive diffusion especially through the paracellular space (Fig. 57.3). The paracellular or

intercellular space is marked by the zonula occludens region, which may be viewed as a functional and physical barrier to the passive flow of molecules. However, the zonula occludens may also contain specific ion channels to accommodate the paracellular movement of solutes such as Na$^+$. The paracellular pathway works in cooperation with the active transcellular pathway to effectively couple ion transfer. For example, Na$^+$, which is actively transported across the apical cell membrane, can passively diffuse into the paracellular space. This sets up a transepithelial potential difference across the zonula occludens and drives the passive absorption of Cl$^-$. In fact this particular schema seems to work better in reverse, where paracellular Na$^+$ secretion is coupled to transcellular Cl$^-$ secretion as in the case of *secretory diarrhea*. Recently, a zonula occludens toxin produced by *Vibrio cholerae* has been identified. Thus, disruption of the normal actions of the paracellular pathway may be important in the pathophysiology of some diarrheal diseases.

## SECRETORY DIARRHEA

### Bacterial toxins

Secretory diarrhea is most commonly associated with infections caused by toxin-producing bacteria such as *Vibrio cholerae* and toxigenic *E. coli*. These organisms produce toxins that activate adenylyl cyclase (cholera toxin, *E. coli* heat-labile toxin) or guanylyl cyclase (*E. coli* heat-stable enterotoxin) and increase the intracellular concentrations of the cyclic nucleotides, cAMP or cGMP (Fig. 57.2). This results in increased secretion of Na$^+$ and Cl$^-$ from intestinal crypt cells and/or inhibition of the reabsorption of Cl$^-$ by villus cells. The net result of derangement of the normal absorptive process

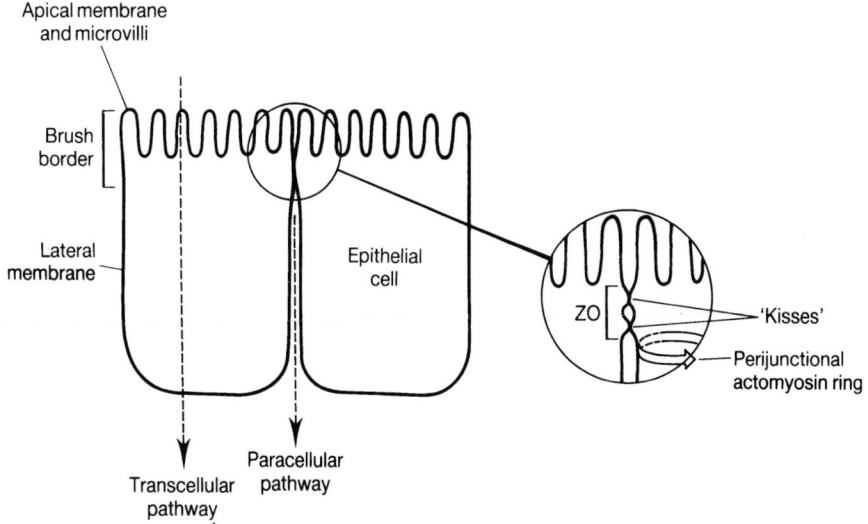

FIGURE 57.3 Schematic representation of intestinal epithelial cells demonstrating transcellular and paracellular pathways. The enlargement of the zonula occludens (ZO) depicts the architecture of this region as it is seen by routine electron microscopy. (From Madara JL, *Cell* 1988; **53**: 497, with permission. © Cell Press.)

is an outpouring of fluid and electrolytes, resulting in secretory diarrhea. The immature intestine may be more sensitive to some of these processes. For example, in immature rats there is an increased response to *E. coli* heat-stable enterotoxin. This may be explained by the presence of an increased receptor number in the immature intestine and/or an inability of the immature intestine to inactivate the toxin. Furthermore, the immature colon may be less able to compensate for increased small intestinal secretion.

## Bile acids

Other examples of secretory diarrhea include *bile acid-induced diarrhea*. Bile acid diarrhea may occur when an increased bile acid load is presented to the colon. Bile acids may alter the net fluid and electrolyte absorption by increasing mucosal cAMP levels, by increasing cytosolic ionized $Ca^{2+}$ levels, and by alterations in prostaglandin metabolism.

## Hormone secreting tumors

Secretory diarrhea can also result from hormone secreting tumors. The term watery diarrhea, hypokalemia, and achlorhydria (WDHA) or *pancreatic cholera* is used to describe a syndrome in which there is massive watery diarrhea related to a *non-islet cell pancreatic adenoma*. This term is now applied to any condition in which there is a tumor producing vasoactive intestinal peptide (VIP). VIP produces net secretion of $Cl^-$ and $Na^+$ by raising intracellular cAMP levels.

## Congenital transport defects

Another mechanism for secretory diarrhea is the presence of a congenital electrolyte transport defect. These defects include *congenital $Cl^-$ diarrhea*, which results from defective $Cl^-$/bicarbonate exchange, and congenital $Na^+$/$H^+$ exchange, which results in *congenital $Na^+$ diarrhea*. Secretory diarrhea can also result from structural abnormalities in the enterocyte, e.g. *microvillus inclusion disease*.

## ORAL REHYDRATION

The laboratory observation that glucose increases intestinal salt and water absorption via the $Na^+$/glucose cotransporter has been directly applied to the care of patients. The addition of glucose to oral rehydration solutions has improved their efficacy, saving millions of children with dehydrating diarrheal disease. Further improvements in this safe, effective and inexpensive therapy may result from future additional understanding of the intestinal mechanisms of absorption of fluid and electrolytes. For example, to maximize further the $Na^+$/glucose cotransporter, as well as to take advantage of the separate amino acid/$Na^+$ cotransporters, recent studies have used hypotonic cereal-based oral rehydration solutions. This approach allows the use of several times as many cotransporting molecules of glucose (as starch) and peptides (as amino acids) while still maintaining a low osmolar solution. Amino acids (L-alanine or glycine) and dipeptides (glycyl-glycine) have also been added to glucose containing solutions to further maximize intestinal absorption of $Na^+$ and water in the treatment of cholera diarrhea.

## SELECTED READING

Cooke HJ. Neuroimmune signaling in regulation of intestinal ion transport. *Am J Physiol* 1994; **266**: G167.

Johnson LR, ed. *Physiology of the gastrointestinal tract,* 3rd edn. New York: Raven Press, 1994.

Lebenthal E, Duffy ME, eds. *Textbook of secretory diarrhea.* New York: Raven Press, 1990.

# 58

# The Nutritional Role of the Colon

Robert D. Murray

The primary functions of the colon are the absorption of electrolytes and water and the storage of fecal material. Recently, a role for the colon in nutrition also has been recognized. Carbohydrates that are not absorbed by the small intestine cross the ileocecal valve. Malabsorbed carbohydrates enter the colon from sloughed cells, secretions, and mucus as well as from exogenous sources including dietary starch, indigestible sugars, and fiber. Bacteria digest these carbohydrates and produce metabolic end products that are readily absorbed (Fig. 58.1), preventing osmotic diarrhea.

In the healthy adult, the colon absorbs 2 L/day of fluid and nearly 275 mmol/day of $Na^+$. Absorption of fluid changes the liquid material in the cecum into formed feces as the luminal contents are moved from the ileocecal valve to the anus. Bacteria are critical to normal colon physiology. Normally bacteria metabolize osmotically active substrates into diffusible anions. When bacteria are prevented from colonizing the large intestine, many morphological and physiological changes occur. The intestinal wall becomes thinner, especially the mucosa. The plasma cells, one of the primary constituents of the lamina propria, become

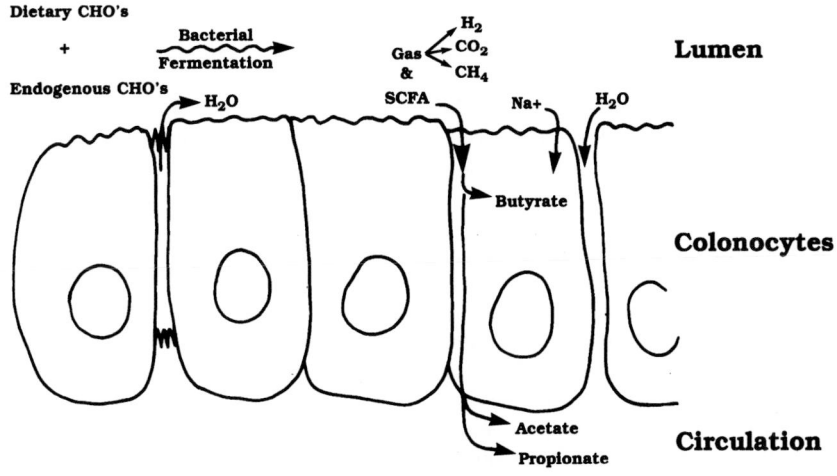

FIGURE 58.1 Carbohydrate that enters the colon is fermented by bacteria to form short-chain fatty acids (SCFA), which are readily absorbed across the colonic epithelium and metabolized by colonocytes or pass into the bloodstream for use as a metabolic substrate.

sparse. The typical cells of the colon change to a cuboidal shape. Cell turnover slows. This results in a drastic reduction in absorption from the germ-free colon. The cecum enlarges and fills with a hypotonic solution that is low in diffusible anions and high in the osmotic particles usually digested by bacteria. As fluid absorption decreases, luminal fluid accumulation increases. In this setting, even minor malabsorption of carbohydrates by the small intestine results in osmotic diarrhea. Clearly, the presence of a healthy bacterial flora fosters the conditions that allow the colon to perform its important absorptive functions.

## BACTERIAL METABOLISM

Normally, daily fecal weight on a Western diet ranges from about 35 g in newborns to 400 g in adults; $10^{11}$ bacteria are present in each gram of feces. Thus, to replenish this massive daily bacterial loss requires substrate, almost exclusively provided by luminal carbohydrates. The solubility of the nonstarch polysaccharides in fiber determine its fermentability in the colon. Under the strict anaerobic conditions of the colon, the flora metabolize carbohydrates to short-chain fatty acids (SCFAs) (i.e. acetate, butyrate, and propionate) and gases (i.e. $CO_2$, $H_2$, and $CH_4$). SCFAs are absorbed by the colonic mucosa, salvaging nutrient energy that otherwise would be lost. In addition, SCFAs stimulate salt and water uptake, increase cell turnover and repair, and serve as substrates for colonocytes. For example, butyrate provides a direct energy source for colonocytes, whereas acetate and propionate enter the systemic circulation and act at distal sites. Recent studies have shown that SCFAs absorbed from the colon can stimulate mucosal proliferation even in an isolated loop of bowel, and a hormonal stimulation of the proliferative crypt region of the isolated mucosa is suggested. In light of these findings, studies are underway to determine whether SCFAs or glutamine, a small bowel energy source, when added to total parenteral nutrition (TPN) might prevent atrophy in patients unable to take enteral feeding.

Given the importance of bacterially derived SCFAs in daily intestinal homeostasis, it is clear that disruptions in bacterial metabolism cause clinical problems. Infections, such as rotavirus, or malabsorption of poorly absorbed carbohydrates, such as lactose, fructose and sorbital, dilute the luminal contents, prevent bacterial fermentation, and result in osmotic diarrhea. Similarly, antibiotics temporarily decrease bacterial number and alter the constituent flora, preventing fermentation. By slowing influx of small bowel fluids, the antidiarrheal agent loperamide may stabilize SCFA production and in turn limit stool losses. One study reported that patients with acute diarrhea had reduced output of watery stool after luminal infusion of SCFAs, supporting the concept that SCFAs are critical to recovery of normal colonic physiology after infection.

## NEONATAL CARBOHYDRATE MALABSORPTION

Lactose is the sole carbohydrate in breast milk and in the most commonly used infant formulas. The newborn infant ingests 12.6 g/(kg·day) of lactose when taking a 120 cal/(kg·day) diet. Studies have shown that intestinal lactase (β-galactosidase) activity is insufficient to digest this daily load of lactose. Although the enzyme lactase is detectable as early as 12 weeks' gestation, it accumulates so slowly that by 34 weeks its activity is only 30 per cent that of a term infant, and by 37–38 weeks, only 70 per cent. Calculation of carbohydrate malabsorption using breath $H^+$ measurements suggests that extensive malabsorption occurs in both the premature and term newborn. Because $H_2$ is a product of bacterial fermentation, its presence in breath can be used as a semiquantitative measure of malabsorbed carbohydrate. Multiple studies on term and premature infants have revealed breath $H_2$ at concentrations of up to 250 ppm, which is well beyond the level observed in physiological malabsorption (<10 ppm). Colonic absorption of $H_2$ is more avid in newborns than adults, partially accounting for higher breath values in infancy. Studies suggest that up to 15–20 per cent of ingested lactose is not absorbed in the small bowel. Doubling the infant's lactose intake doubles pulmonary excretion of $H_2$ but does not increase stool carbohydrate losses, suggesting that increased colonic salvage can occur if necessary.

## BACTERIAL COLONIZATION OF THE COLON

Although the colonic flora is likely to be an important factor for the energy balance of the newborn, its contribution appears limited in the first days of life. The colon is sterile at birth, acquiring an aerobic flora (*E. coli*, streptococci), then a mixed aerobic and facultative anaerobic flora (*Lactobacillus*), and finally a strictly anaerobic flora (*Bifidobacterium*, *Bacteroides*) gradually over the first few weeks. During this time, the SCFA products of bacterial metabolism are modest. Changes in the bacterial flora affect the products of colonic carbohydrate digestion. Lactose infusion into the colonic lumen of piglets during the first postnatal week produces lactate as the primary product of bacterial digestion. After the fourth day, lactate production declines, while SCFA production becomes predominant.

Breast-fed infants appear to have fewer episodes of gastroenteritis than formula-fed babies. Compared with those of bottle-fed infants, feces of breast-fed infants contain a preponderance of bifidobacteria and lactobacilli. Some investigators have postulated that protection is conferred by the unique colonic flora in infants who are breast-fed. However, the degree of protection afforded by the flora during breast feeding is still being debated, and the factors involved have not been delineated. Obviously, sanitation and water-borne infections are avoided by breast feeding. Constituents in breast milk enhance the baby's immune status. Also, psychosocial factors play a role in the choice to breast feed and may affect the infection rate. Recently, the probiotic agent Lactobacillus GG was fed to premature infants in formula in an effort to induce colonization and thereby enhance protection against intestinal infections in formula-fed babies. Colonization was successful. The researchers hypothesized that the metabolic products therefore would also differ, altering colonic physiology and affording an increased level of protection from infection. However, no differences were found in SCFA concentration, lactate concentration, or urinary excretion of metabolites due to anaerobic fermentation, suggesting that the addition of the probiotic had little clinical effect.

The interstitial junction in the small intestine allows ready flux of water and small molecules such as salt and so has been classified as "leaky," whereas that in the colon has been labeled "tight." Thus the colonic luminal bacteria are thought to be prevented from penetrating into the portal and systemic circulation. Yet the colon is not as restrictive as it once seemed. Translocation of luminal bacteria has been found to be common, although it is rarely pathologic in the healthy host. Furthermore, when the epithelial barrier was tested with a molecule that should not cross it (inulin; MW 5000 g/mol), the colon demonstrated permeability in association with water flow. This process is termed "solvent drag." Clearly, not all luminal materials cross the barrier, suggesting that the process is "permselective" for certain substances. A similar phenomenon, but by a different mechanism, has been shown for certain carbohydrates during the neonatal period. Immediately after birth, the colonic mucosa can directly absorb small galactose-containing carbohydrates without bacterial or mucosal enzymatic digestion. Perfusions of the newborn colon show a 20-fold greater absorption of lactose than of its constituent monosaccharides, glucose and galactose. $Na^+$ and water uptake are stimulated by lactose absorption. Thus, in neonates, carbohydrates can substitute for SCFA in stimulating salt and water absorption. The mechanism of lactose absorption was not found to be saturable at concentrations of 15–240 mM. In colonic tissue *in vitro*, lactose, galactose and lactulose, a synthetic disaccharide considered absorbable only after bacterial digestion, traverse the tissue from mucosa to serosa without prior digestion. Glucose-containing sugars and polyethylene glycol (PEG) molecules that are similar in size to lactose did not cross the mucosa, suggesting that simple solvent drag through the tight junctions does not explain this phenomenon. Some molecules may be absorbed from the colonic lumen between the cells by solvent drag or possibly through the cells by the process of endocytosis, a transcellular pathway that is open to the movement of proteins and lipids in the first days of life.

A true symbiosis exists between the human host and the colonic bacterial flora. The colonic flora salvage malabsorbed carbohydrate that would otherwise be lost in feces, preventing both diarrhea and caloric deficit. Yet even in neonates when the flora is attenuated, the colon seems to have a compensatory mechanism for direct carbohydrate assimilation that prevents potentially life-threatening losses of energy and fluids.

## SELECTED READING

Murray RD. Effects of bacterial fermentation end products on intestinal function: implications for intestinal dysfunction. *J Pediatr* 1990; **117**: S59.

Murray RD, Ailabouni AH, Powers PA *et al*. Lactose flux occurs by differing mechanisms in the colon and jejunum of newborn piglets. *Pediatr Res* 1991; **33**: 568.

Potter GD. Development of colonic function. In: Lebanthal E ed. *Human gastrointestinal development*. New York: Raven Press, 1989: 545.

Scheppach W. Effects of short-chain fatty acids on gut morphology and function. *Gut* 1994; **35**: S35.

# 59

# Gastrointestinal Immunology

Barry K. Wershil

The gastrointestinal tract develops in a sterile environment *in utero*, but is exposed to a vast array of foreign antigens immediately after birth. The neonatal gastrointestinal tract adapts to this change in environment by developing mechanisms to limit antigens crossing the intestinal epithelium, the *mucosal barrier*, and mechanisms to control systemic immune responses to foreign antigens, *oral tolerance*.

## THE MUCOSAL BARRIER

The gastrointestinal tract is in continuity with the external environment. A variety of non-immunologic processes act in concert with the mucosal immune system to prevent the attachment and penetration of antigens through the mucosal surface, thus limiting the development of adverse inflammatory reactions (Table 59.1). Thick mucus overlies the epithelial surface and acts as a physical barrier inhibiting antigen attachment. Certain parasitic and microbial infections stimulate additional production and secretion of mucus, increasing the thickness of the layer. Mucus also acts to interfere with bacterial adhesion through direct interaction with specific carbohydrate moieties on bacteria that act like receptors for epithelial cells. The binding of the mucus to these bacterial recognition sites prevents bacterial adhesion and penetration of the intestinal wall.

The composition of the intestinal microvillus membrane is another factor involved in bacterial adhesion. The enterocyte cell membrane changes as the cell migrates from crypt to villus. The composition and functional properties of the enterocyte membrane also change during development. These changes may

TABLE 59.1 Components of the mucosal barrier to antigens

| |
| --- |
| Non-immunological |
|   Intraluminal |
|     Gastric barrier |
|     Proteolysis |
|     Peristalsis |
|   Mucosal surface |
|     Mucosal coat |
|     Microvillus membrane |
| Immunological |
|   Secretory IgA |
|   Secretory IgM |
| Combination of immunological and non-immunological |
|   Immune complex-mediated mucus release of goblet cells |
|   Immune complex-facilitated mucosal surface proteolysis |
|   Kupffer cell phagocytosis of immune complexes |

determine sites of antigen attachment. Microvillus membranes isolated from newborn animals bind certain bacterial enterotoxins and protein antigens more avidly than membranes isolated from adults. This may be due to the lower protein/phospholipid ratio in newborn membranes. These developmental changes in membrane composition may explain the different response to enteric pathogens causing diarrhea.

Secretory immunoglobulin A (sIgA), a major component of the mucosal immune system, plays an important role in barrier function. sIgA constitutes the largest component of the humoral immune system in man. Approximately 3 g sIgA is transported into the adult intestinal tract each day. IgA-secreting plasma cells develop from precursor cells that mature under the influences of accessory cell populations and T cell-derived cytokines, such as interleukin-4, which produce an immunoglobulin isotype switch to predominantly IgA-bearing B cells. These cells deliver polymeric IgA into the submucosa of the intestinal tract, where it is taken up by epithelial cells, covalently linked to secretory component, and secreted into the intestinal lumen. sIgA performs a barrier function by binding to intraluminal microbes and antigens, thereby inhibiting their uptake.

The liver also plays a role in mucosal barrier function through its participation in IgA metabolism. Hepatocytes can remove polymeric IgA from the peripheral circulation and transport it into the bile, thus delivering a significant amount of IgA into the intestinal lumen. In addition, as much as 50 per cent of the IgA in bile is newly synthesized from plasma cells within glands near the large hepatic ducts. The liver can also take up small circulating IgA immune complexes, which may be an important route for elimination of absorbed antigens.

## THE MUCOSAL IMMUNE SYSTEM

The gut-associated lymphoid tissue (GALT) is distinct from the systemic immune system. It is composed of three compartments, organized lymphoid tissues or Peyer patches, diffuse lymphoid tissues of the lamina propria and intraepithelial lymphocytes. In humans, Peyer patches are predominantly found in the ileum and are organized into a germinal center and a parfollicular area composed primarily of B cells and T cells, respectively. These areas underlie specialized epithelium known as M (microfold) cells. M cells appear to function in the uptake and sampling of luminal antigens. Stimulation of GALT occurs when particulate antigens are taken up by M cells and transported into the Peyer patch, as depicted in Fig. 59.1. These antigens are processed and presented to T cells resulting in the activation of lymphoid cells within the Peyer patch. Stimulated T and B cells egress from Peyer patches into the lymph, then pass into the peripheral circulation. These lymphocytes then "home" to the lamina propria of the gut and other exocrine tissues via specific receptors on intestinal vascular endothelium. The B cells mature to plasma cells producing polymeric IgA or IgM. T lymphocytes that reside in the lamina propria are predominantly of the CD4+ (helper) phenotype, while most of the lymphocytes that migrate into the epithelium are CD8+ (cytotoxic/suppressor) cells, known as intraepithelial lymphocytes. In addition to T and B cells, the lamina propria also contains large numbers of macrophages, mast cells and eosinophils.

Intraepithelial lymphocytes (IELs) have several phenotypic characteristics that distinguish them from other T lymphocytes. In mice, 25–50 per cent of IELs express a T cell receptor (TcR) made from γ and δ chains, while the remainder express a TcR pattern of α and β chains as is commonly seen in peripheral T cells. In humans, 2–30 per cent of IELs express γ and δ chains, although the proportion of TcRγδ cells can increase significantly in certain inflammatory conditions such as *celiac disease*. This suggests that TcRγδ-positive T cells either preferentially localize, or mature in the epithelium. The functional significance of these phenotypic variations is not known.

One possible mechanism of IEL activation is presentation of luminal antigens in association with either Class I or Class II molecules of the major histocompatibility (MHC) locus. Macrophages, other accessory cells, and intestinal epithelial cells express Class II antigens and may play a role in antigen presentation to IELs and other cells. Alternatively, certain enterotoxins termed superantigens bind directly to the MHC Class II molecule and can activate many T cells. The function of the intraepithelial lymphocyte is not known, but they may be involved in mucosal immunity in several ways. Some IELs contain cytoplasmic granules and have been shown to have cytotoxic functions that would act to limit microorganism invasion. IELs can secrete a variety of cytokines, which can have protective effects on epithelium and may modulate epithelial cell growth. Finally, it has been suggested that IELs function in the development of oral tolerance.

Oral tolerance, a unique aspect of the mucosal immune system, is a specific immunological state of unresponsiveness induced by prior feeding of an antigen. For example, the single feeding of a soluble protein antigen can suppress systemic IgM, IgG, and IgE antibody production as well as cell-mediated immune responses such as delayed-type hypersensitivity. The mechanisms involved in the development of oral tolerance are complex and have not been defined completely. Oral tolerance has been shown to be due principally to T cell unresponsiveness, while B cells remain potentially active. Animals fed protein antigens develop active immune suppression mediated through T-suppressor cells, but the precise immunoregulatory mechanisms are unclear. It is generally accepted that the development of oral tolerance prevents hypersensitivity reactions to soluble antigens while maintaining active immunity to particulate antigens such as invasive organisms.

## DEVELOPMENT OF THE GASTROINTESTINAL IMMUNE SYSTEM

Immune development occurs in an *antigen-independent stage* prenatally and an *antigen-dependent stage* beginning after birth when luminal antigens are present. During *in utero* human development, columnar epithelium and intestinal villi are present at 9–10 weeks' gestation. Before 11 weeks, only macrophages are found in the lamina propria, but by 11 weeks

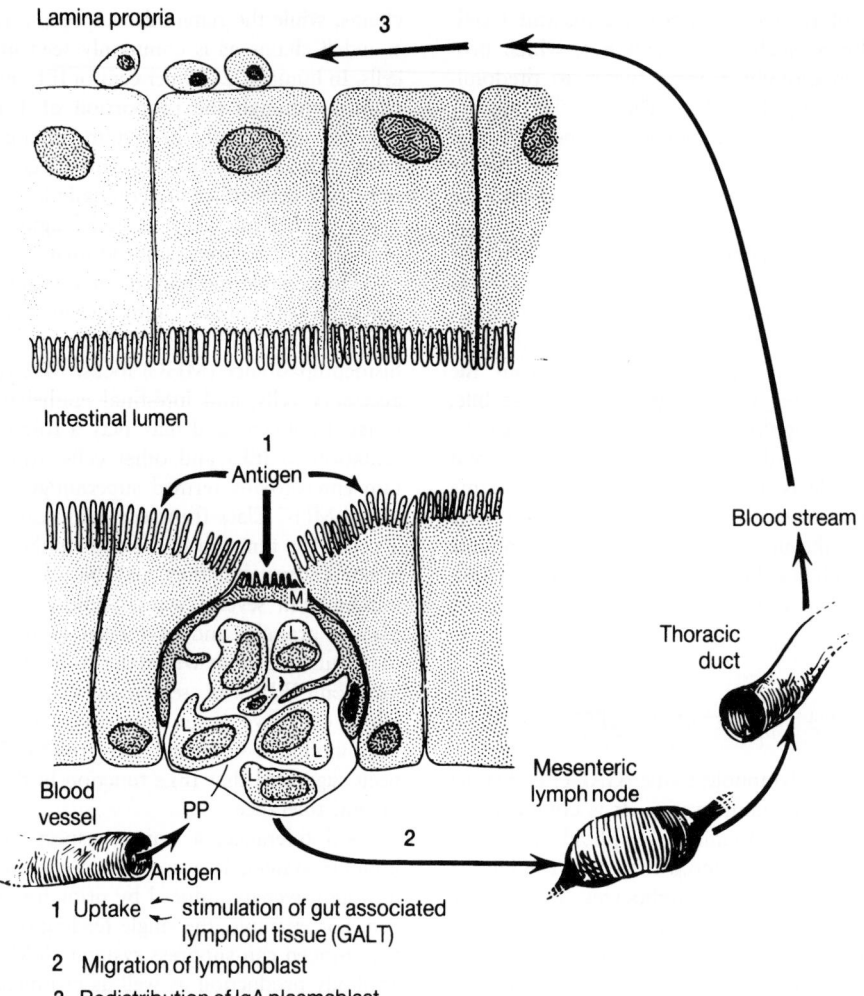

Lamina propria

3

Intestinal lumen

1

Antigen

Blood stream

M

L  L
L  L  L
L
L  L
L

Thoracic
duct

Mesenteric
lymph node

Blood
vessel

PP

Antigen

2

1  Uptake ⇄ stimulation of gut associated
   lymphoid tissue (GALT)
2  Migration of lymphoblast
3  Redistribution of IgA plasmablast

FIGURE 59.1 Lymphocyte migration. Schematic representation of the cell cycle of an IgA-producing plasma cell. Lymphocytes (L) derived from the bone marrow take residence in GALT tissues such as the Peyer patch (PP). Stimulation of lymphoid tissues occurs when antigens are taken up via M cells from the intestinal lumen (1). Lymphoblasts migrate to mesenteric lymph nodes (2) then enter the systemic circulation to redistribute along intestinal mucosal surfaces (3) and produce secretory IgA antibodies in response to absorbed antigens. (From Walker WA, Isselbacher KJ. *N Engl J Med* 1977; **297**: 767, with permission.)

IELs are identifiable. By 17–19 weeks IEL levels increase to about half those seen in postnatal intestines, and approximately half of these are TcRγδ-positive. At 14 weeks, small clusters of CD4+ (helper) phenotype T lymphocytes are present in the lamina propria, but virtually no B cells or plasma cells are seen until after birth. By 16 weeks the secretory component for IgA is detectable, and increases substantially at 20 weeks. Eosinophils are present in the lamina propria at 19 weeks. Peyer patches are not identifiable until 24 weeks' gestation and then increase in size and density until birth. Within Peyer patches, the T cells are mainly CD4+ and the B cells are IgM+, IgD+; there is no cellular zonation, and

almost every cell is Class II MHC-positive. The intestinal epithelium becomes Class II positive between 18 and 22 weeks' gestation.

By birth the mucosal immune system is well developed. Further postnatal development appears to be antigen-driven. Germinal center formation occurs in Peyer patches. The lamina propria is populated by B cells, and the T cell population in the lamina propria expands. The numbers of intraepithelial lymphocytes increase, accompanied by a shift in relative numbers of T cells with γδ and αβ receptors. Ultimately, the fate of the mucosal immune system is directed by the antigens and pathogens present in the gastrointestinal tract.

## SELECTED READING

Brandtzaeg P, Nilssen DE, Rognum TO, Thrane PS. Ontogeny of the mucosal immune system and IgA deficiency. *Gastroenterol Clin North Am* 1991; **20**: 397.

MacDonald TT, Spencer J. Ontogeny of the mucosal immune response. *Semin Immunopathol* 1990; **12**: 129.

Mowat M. The regulation of immune responses to dietary protein antigens. *Immunol Today* 1987; **8**: 93.

Walker WA. Pathophysiology of intestinal uptake and absorption of antigens in food allergy. *Ann Allergy* 1987; **59**: 7.

# 60

# Development and Function of the Exocrine Pancreas

Joel W. Adelson

The exocrine pancreas is the major organ of digestion; its primary task is production of large quantities of alkaline fluid and digestive enzymes, which are secreted into the intestinal lumen. The enzymes function to hydrolyze complex dietary substrates. The fluid neutralizes gastric acid and creates an appropriate alkaline pH milieu for the function of the enzymes.

## MORPHOLOGICAL DEVELOPMENT

The pancreas originates as two separate buds from the differentiating intestine, one dorsal, the other ventral. The dorsal bud is destined to form the greater portion of the gland, including the main body and tail of the organ. The ventral bud originates at the origin of the common bile duct and gallbladder, which explains how the pancreatic–biliary ductular system arises. As pancreatic differentiation and organ enlargement occur, the dorsal bud rotates around the intestinal axis so as to lie directly next to, and cephalad to, the ventral bud. The buds then fuse. The dorsal and ventral buds each contain their own main axial duct; in most cases, these fuse together. Subsequent development of the duct draining the ventral bud results in the formation of the major pancreatic duct, the duct of Wirsung. The dorsal bud's duct will usually drain the head of the pancreas into the ventral or main duct, but not infrequently a separate accessory duct, the duct of Santorini, drains the dorsal pancreatic region into the intestine through its own papillus. This variant is known as *pancreas divisum*, and may contribute to some instances of *pancreatitis*, presumably because of problems in drainage via the accessory duct. Aberrant

fusion of the buds results in an *annular pancreas* in which the intestine is encircled with pancreatic tissue; this can lead to variable degrees of duodenal obstruction, the commonest presentation occurring at birth with complete obstruction. This anomaly occurs sporadically in the general population and relatively commonly with trisomy 21.

Other primary problems with pancreatic development are occasionally reported. These include *hypoplasia* or *complete agenesis of the pancreas*. Excess pancreatic material, known as pancreatic rests, can occur at ectopic locations elsewhere in the gastrointestinal tract, especially the stomach. A complex syndrome, variously named *Schwachman syndrome* or *Schwachman–Diamond syndrome*, is the second commonest cause of pancreatic insufficiency in childhood. This recessively inherited syndrome results in the complete replacement of pancreatic acinar tissue (but not the ductular or endocrine portions) with adipose tissue. These patients present as infants with failure to thrive, steatorrhea, and a normal sweat test. Other accompanying manifestations of the syndrome are noted with varying frequency, including metaphyseal dysostosis – a developmental abnormality of bone, immunodeficiency, short stature, dwarfism, and anemia with cyclic neutropenia.

The histological generation of the pancreas is exemplified by the usual progression from undifferentiated precursor cells without specialized organelles to the highly specialized cells of the mature organ, which can be divided into three functional types: acinar cells, ductular elements, and the endocrine subset comprising the islets of Langerhans. The *acinar cells*, organized into connective tissue-surrounded lobules, constitute the bulk of this relatively homogeneous-appearing gland. Differentiation of the acinar cells proper occurs such that at about 12 weeks' gestation secretory zymogen granules are recognizable. The fully differentiated acinar cell is capable of a great degree of protein synthesis, storage and secretion, nearly all of it devoted to the production of pancreatic enzymes. In fact, the pancreas is so specialized in protein secretion that it was the gland upon which were conducted the original, classical studies on the intracellular route of protein synthesis, processing, storage and secretion. The pyramid-shaped acinar cells are organized into small, round groups or short tubes of cells surrounding a central lumen; the groups are called acini. The secretory granules are located at the apical or luminal pole of the cell. A massive amount of rough endoplasmic reticulum, present in each acinar cell, is primarily devoted to production of the exportable digestive enzymes. The endoplasmic reticulum is located in the basal portion of the cytoplasm, as is the nucleus. The Golgi region lies apical to the endoplasmic reticulum, above the secretory granule-containing region. Near the Golgi, and apparently budding off from it, are immature or condensing vacuoles, which are thought to be the direct precursors of zymogen granules (Fig. 60.1).

During embryogenesis, the digestive enzymes are at first found in extremely low amounts, and then appear in greater and greater quantities in what appears to be a preset sequence, dependent upon the set of genetic instructions with which this organ is endowed. In a singularly revealing experiment in transgenic mice several years ago, the "upstream" or 5′ control region for

mouse chymotrypsinogen was fused with the DNA sequence for human growth hormone and implanted in the transgenic mouse ovum. Following fertilization, implantation, and development, the end result was a mouse that secreted human growth hormone through the pancreatic duct into the digestive lumen! This shows that the placement of a tissue-specific secretory protein into the "right" place at the "proper" time in the differentiation process is due to the information contained in the upstream control region for the structural gene in question.

## FLUID SECRETION

The pancreatic fluid is alkaline in composition due to the presence of a high concentration of bicarbonate ion. The ionic composition of the secretion is rate-dependent with more bicarbonate at higher flow rates and relatively more $Cl^-$ at lower rates. The fluid is secreted by the *ductular system*, which begins at the entrance to the acinar lumen proper. The cells at the acinar opening are centroacinar cells. Ductular secretory cells then continue as a tubular epithelial lining of the pancreatic ducts of increasing caliber, which ultimately drain into the main duct.

One of the main pathophysiological manifestations of *cystic fibrosis* appears to be due to a malfunction of a $Cl^-$ channel present in these ductular cells. The specific $Cl^-$ channel-forming protein is known as CFTR (cystic fibrosis transmembrane conductance regulator). In cystic fibrosis, a relatively common mutation, $\Delta F508$ results in deletion of a phenylalanine residue in position 508 of the 1480 amino acid-long chain. The deletion results in a change in the function of a regulatory portion of CFTR that renders it impossible to open the $Cl^-$ channel. Because $Cl^-$ secretion is necessary for bicarbonate exchange and water flux in the pancreatic gland, the defect results in a failure of fluid and electrolyte secretion, which results in the inability to wash the secreted digestive enzymes from the level of the pancreatic acinus into the intestinal lumen. This ultimately results in a secondary, severe pancreatic enzyme deficit that cripples the digestive process, resulting in loss of fat and other digestive substrates in stool.

## ENDOCRINE PANCREAS

The third element of the differentiated pancreas is the *islets of Langerhans*. These originate from the general exocrine primordium, and not, as previously considered, from the primitive neural crest tissue in the so-called APUD (amine precursor uptake and decarboxylation) system. The embryological and morphological relationships between the endocrine and exocrine pancreas are important. A mini portal system of capillaries leaves the endocrine islets, and enters the peri-insular acinar tissue before finally joining the portal vein drainage. Possibly as a result of hormonal influ-

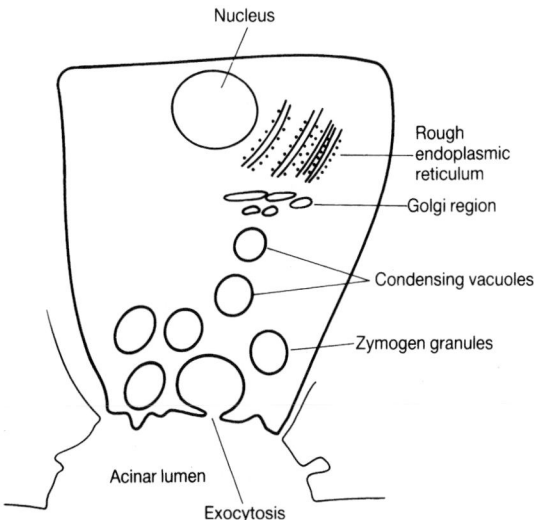

FIGURE 60.1 Generalized schematic of pancreatic acinar cell. Newly synthesized secretory proteins are formed by the rough endoplasmic reticulum, glycosylated in the Golgi region, and packaged in the condensing vacuoles, which mature into zymogen granules. The granule contents are expelled following fusion of the zymogen granule membrane with the plasma membrane.

ences from the "insular–acinar axis," the acinar cells immediately surrounding the islets are distinct from the remaining acinar cells with respect to enzyme composition, cell size, and size of the secretory granules.

## ENZYME SECRETION

Exocrine pancreatic digestive function has been appreciated for several hundred years, and is still an active area of investigation. The gland synthesizes and stores for secretion large quantities of digestive enzymes, making it the body's largest protein secretor with the exception of the lactating mammary gland. The gland produces both exo- and endoproteases, various lipases and phospholipases, nucleases, and amylase; a number of the enzyme species are isoenzymes, alternative enzyme structures differing little from each other in function. Many of the enzymes require activation by various agents prior to reaching full function. All of the proteases are activated by the hydrolysis of a peptide from the proenzyme form; the cleavage is primarily performed by trypsin. Trypsin itself is activated from trypsinogen by enteropeptidase, a proteolytic enzyme secreted by the duodenal mucosa, possibly in response to cholecystokinin (CCK) release, and by autocatalysis by already-activated trypsin. Lipase is activated by another molecule secreted by the gland called colipase.

## Development of pancreatic enzyme secretion

The development of the enzymatic secretory capacity of the pancreas during human gestation is not well studied. The bulk of secretory function is present from birth, and full-term newborns, as well as more developed premature infants, have quite adequate pancreatic function. With respect to the ultimate capacity of the pancreas to handle fats, newborns frequently exhibit a mild steatorrhea. Although a fat absorption coefficient of about 95 per cent is expected in the older child or adult, newborns and young infants are frequently found to absorb less fat; the acceptable norm is 85 per cent or more. Similarly, amylase secretion is not fully developed at birth, and only becomes so after several months. However, there is no indication that infants cannot digest starch polymers, and it may be that the intestinal enzyme glucoamylase is responsible for handling starches in instances where these substances are fed in infancy.

## Stimulus–secretion coupling

The intracellular events leading to enzyme secretion by the acinar cell and fluid secretion by centroacinar and ductular cells have been the subject of much research in recent years. In general, the stimulus–secretion coupling systems found in pancreas resemble those found in most other secretory tissues. The basolateral membranes of acinar cells contain receptors that are highly specific for CCK and cholinergic agonists. Similarly, duct cells have secretin receptors. Numerous other receptors are also found on the cell surfaces. Their roles are not presently clear, but it is thought that the interaction of the receptors with the several ligands that bind to them serves to modulate various aspects of enzyme secretion.

Following binding of a secretagogue to its receptor, a long chain of events ensues, beginning with transmission of information across the cellular membrane by deformation of the receptor itself, which causes activation of a G-protein that exchanges GTP (guanosine triphosphate) for GDP (guanosine diphosphate). This membrane-related event kicks off a further intracellular series of events, depending on the specific G-proteins activated. In the acinar pancreas, both CCK and cholinergic stimuli appear to be connected to the final secretory effectors through the G-proteins by pathways involving metabolism and intracellular production of inositol phosphates and diacylglycerol, as well as via a pathway that leads to mobilization of $Ca^{2+}$ from stores within the acinar cell. Less is known about stimulus–secretion coupling in the ductular cell, but the pathway in that case appears to involve activation of adenylyl cyclase by the secretin receptor with the formation of cAMP. The ultimate activation of the secretory effectors involves phosphorylation of specific proteins involved in the secretory events in the cell membranes leading to fusion of the zymogen granule membrane with the plasma membrane.

## Variations in enzyme secretion

The enzyme composition of the pancreatic zymogen granules and the pancreatic juice can be made to vary with long-term dietary changes so as to match the expensive daily investment in digestive enzymes more closely with the actual substrate upon which these enzymes work. There has been a long-standing controversy as to whether the composition of the digestive enzyme mixture can also be regulated over the short term, i.e. within the digestive time required by the processing of a single meal. Such regulation would be highly economical in terms of saving unnecessary enzymes, but because the zymogen granules were thought to all contain the full mixture of digestive enzymes, the release of their contents by exocytosis must result in a parallel discharge of each enzyme species. However, many examples of non-parallel secretion of digestive enzymes have been reported, and recent work has demonstrated that the exocrine pancreas is a surprisingly heterogeneous organ, secreting digestive proteins from multiple distinct sources containing enzyme mixtures of differing composition.

# Control of secretion

The control of pancreatic secretion, as with other digestive organs, is due to a mixture of hormonal and neural inputs. Neural stimulation is primarily via the vagus nerve, with stimuli originating in the digestive tract or higher centers in the brain, depending on the stage of digestion. Most stimulation, whether neural or hormonal, appears to arise when digestive substrates arrive in the duodenum. The hormone primarily responsible for pancreatic stimulation is CCK, a close relative of the gastric stimulatory hormone gastrin (see Chapter 55). CCK and gastrin share a common sequence at their carboxyl termini, and overlap in actions when the amounts administered are high enough. At physiological concentrations, CCK stimulates pancreatic enzyme release and gallbladder contraction, but the stimulation can be overcome by atropine, which antagonizes the cholinergic nervous system. Thus, it appears that although CCK is classically known as a hormone, its effects may be mediated via the vagus nerve. There now is evidence that pancreatic secretion, at least in the interdigestive period, is cyclic in character with a neurosecretory-like rhythm, akin to the interdigestive migrating motor complex.

Pancreatic enzyme secretion is not only stimulated by the nervous system or by CCK, but also by a CCK-releasing peptide, present in the intestinal lumen, that appears to be derived from intestinal mucosal cells. The peptide is sensitive to proteolytic degradation by pancreatic enzymes, and thereby can act as a signal to the pancreas to secrete more enzyme; when luminal levels of proteolysis fall low enough, the CCK-releasing peptide will survive and signal for further CCK release from the mucosa into the bloodstream. A second peptide called the monitor peptide, secreted in bile, appears to serve a similar function. When food is present in the intestinal lumen, the CCK-releasing peptide is protected from degradation simply by competition with the foodstuffs that serve as a competitive substrate for proteolysis. Thus, during periods when a large amount of undigested protein is present in the lumen, the survival of the CCK-releasing peptide will ensure ongoing stimulation of the pancreas.

Stimulation of pancreatic fluid secretion also depends on neurological and hormonal influences. As with enzyme secretion, the neurological input arises at both the level of the intestine and in higher centers in the brain, depending on the stage of digestion. The major hormone responsible for mediating fluid secretion is known by its elegantly simple name *secretin*, the first hormone ever discovered, by Bayliss and Starling early in this century. Secretin mediates pancreatic fluid secretion independently of the stimulation of enzyme secretion by CCK; however, the two hormones do augment each other's activities when administered together. Because conditions leading to CCK release into the bloodstream – the presence of peptides and proteins in the duodenum – usually overlap directly with the major stimulus for secretin release, acidification of the duodenum, the usual result is simultaneous arrival of both fluid and enzyme in the duodenum. As discussed briefly above, failure of fluid secretion secondarily leads to the insufficiency of pancreatic enzymes seen in cystic fibrosis.

## SELECTED READING

Adelson JW. Pancreatic function in infancy and early childhood. In Heird WC, ed. *Nutritional needs of the six to twelve month old infant,* Carnation Nutrition Education Series, Vol. 2. New York: Raven Press, 1991: 19.

Adelson JW, Clarizio R, Coutu JA. Pancreatic digestive enzyme secretion in the rabbit: rapid cyclic variations in enzyme composition. *Proc Natl Acad Sci USA* 1995; **92:** 2553.

Miyasaka K, Guan D, Liddle RA, Green GM. Feedback regulation by trypsin: evidence for intraluminal CCK-releasing peptide. *Am J Physiol* 1989; **257:** G175.

Owyang C, Williams J. Pancreatic secretion. In: Yamada T, Alpers DH, Owyang C *et al.* eds. *Textbook of gastroenterology.* Philadelphia: JB Lippincott Co., 1991: 294.

# 61

# Embryology and Anatomy of the Liver

Stuart S. Kaufman

The liver of the human embryo begins to differentiate during weeks 3–4 of gestation. A diverticulum of endodermal epithelium extends from the ventral surface of the posterior foregut to meet the adjacent primordial anterior diaphragm, the septum transversum. Primitive hepatocytes (hepatoblasts) mix with and attach to mesodermal mesenchymal cells of the septum. Hepatocytes aggregate into cords up to 10 cells thick, and the cords are separated from one another by small blood vessels or sinusoids, which receive blood from the anterior vitelline vessels from the yolk sac. The vitelline vessels are progressively engulfed by the enlarging liver and ultimately evolve into the portal venous and hepatic venous systems. The primitive hepatocytes mature along two divergent lines. The majority eventually become mature hepatocytes, while the remainder form intrahepatic bile ducts. The functional differentiation of each of these cell types is described below. Pluripotent hematopoietic stem cells are recognizable as clusters between adjacent hepatocytes by the second month of gestation. These cells originate from septal mesenchyma. A discussion of fetal hematopoiesis is included on page 862.

## ACINAR ORGANIZATION

The basic functional unit of the liver is the *acinus* (Fig. 61.1). Acini are organized during the late second and third months of gestation, in concert with formation of constituent cells. The acinus encompasses the region perfused by a terminal portal venule, a branch of the portal vein, and the terminal arteriolar branch of the hepatic artery. Blood flows centrifugally from these vessels through sinusoids emanating radially from each portal area. Drainage from sinusoids is accomplished by terminal hepatic venules positioned at inter-

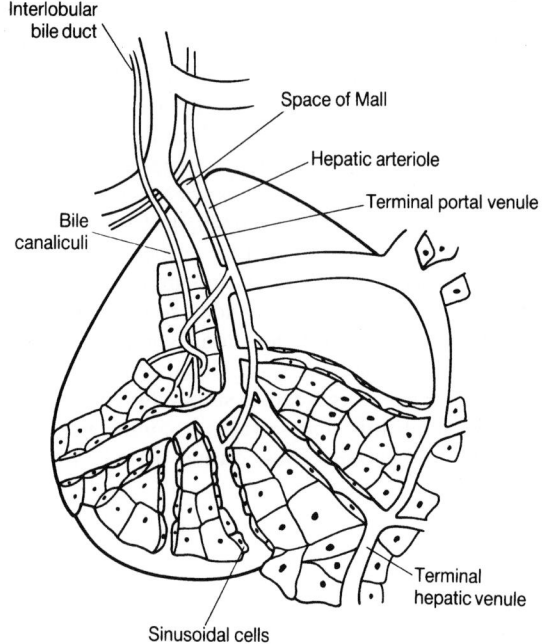

FIGURE 61.1 The liver acinus is supplied with blood from a terminal portal venule and a terminal hepatic arteriole. Blood percolates through the sinusoid to a terminal hepatic venule. The hepatic venules flow into the hepatic veins and drain into the inferior vena cava. Bile is secreted into the bile canaliculus and flows in the opposite direction as blood flow, into the interlobular bile ducts. The interlobular bile ducts receive their blood supply from the hepatic arteries. The space of Mall is an extracellular space through which the hepatic arteriole and portal venule pass. Lautt and Greenway have postulated that the secretion of adenosine into this space plays a role in controlling hepatic arterial blood flow (see Chapter 62).

vals around the border of the acinus. Each hepatic venule receives sinusoidal blood from several adjacent acini.

In mature liver, major functions of hepatocytes vary depending on their position along the sinusoid. This zonal variation in function has been best demonstrated in regard to carbohydrate metabolism. Hepatocytes located closest to portal areas are primarily responsible for gluconeogenesis, containing the key enzymes of gluconeogenesis including phosphoenolpyruvate-carboxykinase (PEPCK), fructose 1,6-biphosphatase, and glucose 6-phosphatase. In contrast, hepatocytes located near the hepatic vein predominantly contain the key enzymes of glycolysis, including glucokinase and pyruvate kinase, and also contain enzymes active in glutamate metabolism. Periportal hepatocytes are primarily responsible for extraction of bile salts from the sinusoidal circulation. Heterogeneity of other liver functions has not been well studied. Some of these regional differences may represent hepatocellular adaptation to regional variations in the $O_2$ or substrate composition of sinusoidal blood because hepatocytes express different phenotypes when cultured in varying $O_2$ or hormone concentrations. Other hormones, growth factors, and innervation patterns may also play a role.

Metabolic zonation is not present until after birth. In newborn rats, zonal heterogeneity of cytosolic PEPCK develops during the first day. The heterogeneous distribution of PEPCK and succinate dehydrogenase is seen by the second week. Changes in hepatic $O_2$ and substrate delivery at birth likely explain the development of zonal heterogeneity.

## HEPATOCYTE DIFFERENTIATION

Small quantities of characteristic hepatocellular proteins including α-fetoprotein, α$_1$-antitrypsin and transferrin are expressed by 4 weeks' gestation. By 5–6 weeks, the rough endoplasmic reticulum and Golgi apparatus enlarge progressively. Selective distribution of proteins to specific regions of the plasma membrane defines the various plasma membrane domains. Each domain is endowed with its own group of receptors, transport enzymes, and other proteins. The canalicular domain borders the canaliculi. The lateral membrane region contains desmosomes and gap junctions between adjacent hepatocytes. The sinusoidal region has a microvillus surface, the increased surface area of which likely promotes exchange with sinusoids.

A basement membrane whose framework is composed of type IV collagen separates hepatocytes and sinusoidal cells. Laminin and another glycoprotein, fibronectin, attach collagen to hepatocytes via specific receptors on the sinusoidal subdomain. Strengthening the interaction of type IV collagen and these attachment glycoproteins are proteoglycans, particularly heparan sulfate, that are embedded within the hepato-

cellular plasma membrane. The composition of the basement membrane and likely that of its adjacent hepatocyte basolateral domain change during development. *In utero*, the relative quantity of heparan sulfate is reduced and laminin increased. The basement membrane, via its interaction with hepatocyte plasma membrane receptors, appears to direct early hepatocellular differentiation during organogenesis. Several extracellular substances including liver cell-adhesion molecule (L-CAM) and the glycoprotein laminin facilitate attachment of hepatocytes to septal cells. Similarly, the basement membrane may maintain hepatocellular differentiation in the mature organ.

The canalicular domain is composed of transport proteins that exteriorize bile constituents to the canalicular lumen. Thus, the canaliculus is the initial site of free bile flow. It is formed by the circular joining of 2–3 canalicular domains of separate hepatocytes, each sealed with a tight junction. Well defined canaliculi appear during the second month of gestation. The canaliculus, like the sinusoidal region of the basolateral domain, has microvilli that increase the surface area available to form bile. Various membrane transport proteins appear at programmed times during development. Development of bile salt secretion (see Chapter 64), bilirubin metabolism (see Chapter 65), and the other metabolic functions of the liver (see Chapters 65 and 66) are discussed elsewhere.

## BILE CELLS AND BILE DUCTS

Bile duct cells first evolve from hepatoblasts at the liver hilum during the second month of gestation. The hilum is the point at which the common bile duct, portal vein, and hepatic artery enter the liver. Just as the affinity of hepatoblasts for septal mesenchymal cells appears mediated by laminin, evolution of hepatoblasts to bile duct cells and the latter's affinity for portal vein branches are also mediated by laminin. At the hilum, hepatoblasts flatten to form a ductal plate of primordial biliary cells. The plate is reorganized into a series of cysts or tubules. Thereafter, tubules fuse into continuous ducts as the tubules progressively extend peripherally into the four partially separated lobes (right, left, caudate, quadrate). These ducts become interlobular bile ducts, remaining in close proximity to terminal portal venules, and are joined by terminal hepatic arteries. Collectively, these groups of three vessels surrounded by scant collagen, define portal areas or triads.

Interlobular bile ducts receive bile from canaliculi via a series of intermediate tributaries penetrating the peripheries of portal areas. These tributaries, the canals of Hering, are also derived from hepatoblasts. Bile is conveyed from canaliculi to canals of Hering to interlobular ducts and then to larger channels, finally reaching the hilum. At the hilum, connection is made with the extrahepatic biliary system. The gallbladder and most proximal portions of the extrahepatic biliary system are derived from the cranial hepatic diverticulum. The remainder of the biliary system comes from the caudal aspect of the hepatic diverticulum. Formation of major biliary vessels is completed by about 10–12 weeks' gestation. Interlobular bile ducts do not completely extend to the hepatic periphery until late in the third trimester.

## SINUSOIDAL CELLS

By 1 month following conception, hepatocytes are organized into multilayered cords. Sinusoids separating the cords have a non-contiguous endothelial lining. However, within a few weeks, hepatocellular cords thin to about three cells deep. Simultaneously, endothelial cells proliferate to become nearly continuous along the length of each sinusoid. Large numbers of vesicles are present within endothelial cytoplasm. This finding suggests that endothelium serves as a structural and functional filter between hepatocytes and the sinusoidal circulation. *In utero*, maturing erythroblasts migrate through perisinusoidal spaces for release into the sinusoidal circulation. During this migration, erythroblasts pass directly through, not between, endothelial cells. In mature liver, gaps in the endothelium known as fenestrae allow large molecules to penetrate the endothelial lining. The time at which endothelial fenestration occurs or the consequences of its early absence are unknown.

In addition to endothelial cells, two additional types of sinusoidal cells, *Kupffer cells* and *Ito cells*, can be identified from the beginning of sinusoidal morphogenesis. Kupffer cells are macrophages that ingest particulate materials passing through the sinusoids. The earliest embryonic Kupffer cells are carried into the liver from the yolk sac by the primordial portal venous system. Later, Kupffer cells are derived from bone marrow macrophages. Kupffer cell density is low through the first half of gestation. Cell densities typical of mature liver can be observed in the neonatal period. Some Kupffer cells are situated within the sinusoidal lumen while others lie on the margins of sinusoids, connecting adjacent endothelial cells. Fetal Kupffer cells are similar, both structurally and functionally, to those present in mature liver. They are large, irregularly shaped, and contain pseudopodial projections. Fetal Kupffer cells also respond to stimuli with production of cytokines that include interleukin-1 and tumor necrosis factor α. In addition, fetal Kupffer cells phagocytose erythrocytes, their extruded nuclei, and other erythrocytic fragments as these cells emerge from the endothelium. Thus, Kupffer cells may be final regulators of hematopoiesis, possibly preventing release of defective blood cells into the circulation.

Ito cells reside in the perisinusoidal space of Disse, where they are attached to inner surfaces of endothelial cells. In mature liver, these cells, also known as fat storage cells or lipocytes, are thought to participate in hepatic vitamin A storage and to produce laminin basement membrane glycoprotein. Along with endothelial cells, they contribute to synthesis of basement membrane type IV collagen. They also may be involved in the control of intrahepatic blood flow resistance (see Chapter 62). Embryonic Ito cells, unlike their mature counterparts, are capable of phagocytosis. Ito cells appear very similar to early fibroblast-like cells in the septum transversum and are thought to originate from those cells.

## WHOLE ORGAN GROWTH PATTERNS

Following formation of the liver during the first trimester, the right lobe enlarges linearly through the remainder of gestation. Left lobar growth slows during the third trimester and, by birth, is about 10 per cent smaller than the right. As with most developing tissues, initial liver growth results primarily from hepatocellular proliferation, i.e. cellular hyperplasia. Hepatocellular proliferation peaks during the second trimester. Hepatocellular levels of so-called proto-oncogenes, sequences that positively modulate mitosis by encoding various stimulatory growth factors, are at maximal concentration at this time. By the third trimester, mitosis slows, coinciding with repression of transcription of enzymes associated with DNA replication, which include thymidine kinase. Subsequently, enlargement of individual hepatocytes, i.e. cell hypertrophy, increasingly contributes to whole organ enlargement. Hematopoiesis peaks by the middle of the second trimester and diminishes through the end of gestation. Following birth, liver growth continues until the end of the second decade. Hepatocellular replication still contributes to postnatal growth. The neonatal liver has less than 20 per cent of the hepatocytes present in the adult organ.

Additional postnatal growth results from hepatocellular hypertrophy associated with attainment of polyploidy. Polyploid hepatocytes are randomly distributed in the acinus. Compared to diploid cells, they are enlarged in direct proportion to their increase in chromosome number. Polyploid hepatocytes are mostly 4N during childhood and 8N by early adulthood. Polyploidy may increase hepatocellular protein synthesis and bile production. However, only remaining diploid hepatocytes are capable of cell division.

Stimulation of hepatocellular hyperplasia is under the combined influence of endocrine, paracrine, and autocrine systems. Placental lactogen, insulin-like growth factors I and II (IGF-I and IGF-II), epidermal growth factor, and transforming growth factor α all may play a role in liver growth.

## SELECTED READING

Andersen B, Zierz S, Jungermann K. Perinatal development of the distributions of phosphoenolpyruvate carboxykinase and succinate dehydrogenase in rat liver parenchyma. *Eur J Cell Biol* 1983; 30: 126.

Enzan H, Hara H, Yamashita Y *et al.* Fine structure of hepatic sinusoids and their development in human embryos and fetuses. *Acta Pathol Jpn* 1983; 33: 447.

Ruebner RH, Blankenberg TA, Burrows DA, SooHoo W, Lund JK. Development and transformation of the ductal plate in the developing human liver. *Pediatr Pathol* 1990; 10: 55.

Sell S. Is there a liver stem cell? *Cancer Res* 1990; 50: 3811.

Traber PG, Chianale J, Gumucio JJ. Physiologic significance and regulation of hepatocellular heterogeneity. *Gastroenterology* 1988; 95: 1130.

# 62

# Fetal and Postnatal Liver Blood Flow

Colin D. Rudolph

Blood from the gastrointestinal tract, pancreas, and spleen drains through the portal vein into the liver before mixing with the systemic circulation. This strategic anatomic arrangement allows the liver to cleanse the portal blood of absorbed toxins, process absorbed nutrients, as well as secrete bile acids in response to gastrointestinal hormonal stimulation. The splanchnic organs that drain into the portal vein utilize $O_2$; thus the $O_2$ content of portal venous blood is reduced. The hepatic artery provides additional $O_2$-rich blood to the liver, assuring that adequate $O_2$ is available to perform the liver's many energy-requiring functions. A similar pattern prevails in the fetus. Nutrients supplied from the placenta pass through the umbilical vein to the liver. However, in many species a portion of this blood bypasses the liver, shunting through the ductus venosus to the systemic circulation.

## LIVER BLOOD FLOW IN THE ADULT

The hepatic artery and portal vein arborize into small terminal vessels in the portal triad (see Fig. 61.1). Both vessels supply blood to the liver parenchyma, emptying into the hepatic sinusoids. The hepatic artery provides the only blood supply to the intrahepatic bile ducts. Sphincters control the flow of portal venous and arterial blood into each liver sinusoid. Blood percolates through the sinusoids to the central vein, into the large hepatic veins, and then into the inferior vena cava. Twenty to 25 per cent of the total cardiac output supplies the liver, providing a total blood flow of about 100 mL/(100 g·min). Approximately 75 per cent of liver blood flow is provided by the portal vein and 25 per cent by the hepatic artery. Hepatic arterial $O_2$ content is high compared with the portal vein; thus, approximately equal portions of the $O_2$ supplied to the liver are derived from each vessel.

Portal blood flow increases after a meal and decreases during fasting. Hepatic arterial blood flow decreases or increases accordingly, maintaining a relatively steady blood flow and $O_2$ delivery to the liver. The intrinsic hepatic mechanisms underlying this "hepatic arterial buffer response" have been elucidated by Lautt and Greenway. The hepatic arterioles and portal venules pass through an extracellular space, the space of Mall (see Fig. 61.1), before entering the sinusoid. Adenosine is produced and released into this space at a constant rate. The concentration of adenosine washed out of the space of Mall varies with portal blood flow; reductions in flow result in the accumulation of adenosine. Adenosine is a potent arteriolar dilator. Thus as portal blood flow decreases, adenosine accumulates and dilates hepatic arterioles, increasing hepatic arterial blood flow. Specific adenosine antagonists suppress this response.

Extrinsic factors also regulate hepatic blood flow. Sympathetic stimulation reduces both portal venous and hepatic arterial blood flow by stimulation of α-adrenergic receptors. β-Adrenergic receptor stimulation reduces hepatic arterial resistance to flow. Other agents released systemically and/or locally may also alter liver blood flow. Tumor necrosis factor (TNF), platelet activating factor (PAF), and prostaglandin $E_2$ ($PGE_2$) all increase the resistance to flow across the liver, possibly by altering sinusoidal diameter. Circulating hormones including angiotensin II and vasopressin also may reduce hepatic blood flow.

The liver is a highly vascular organ, containing about 10 per cent of the total blood volume. During hemorrhage, venoconstriction of hepatic capacitance vessels shifts the blood volume of the liver into the systemic circulation, providing an autotransfusion. This response appears to be mediated by an increase in nitric oxide synthetase activity, at least partially stimulated by endothelin-1, which results in contraction of perisinusoidal lining cells (Ito cells).

## LIVER BLOOD FLOW IN THE FETUS

In the fetus liver blood flow is provided by the umbilical vein, portal vein, and hepatic artery (Fig. 62.1). During fetal development the umbilical–placental circulation receives about 40 per cent of the combined ventricular output. Oxygenated, nutrient-rich blood returns from the placenta to the fetus via the common umbilical vein, which passes toward the liver hilum under the left lobe of the liver. Branches arborize into the left lobe prior to the umbilical vein giving rise to the ductus venosus, which shunts blood across to the inferior vena cava. The umbilical vein then passes into the right lobe of the liver and joins the portal vein. Branches supplying the right lobe of the liver arise in this region. As suggested by the anatomical description, more than 90 per cent of the blood supplying the left lobe of the liver is derived from the umbilical vein. Less than 10 per cent is supplied by the hepatic artery. The right lobe receives 60 per cent of its blood supply from the umbilical vein, 35 per cent from the portal vein, and 5 per cent from the hepatic artery. The percentage of umbilical venous flow shunted through the ductus venosus varies between species and physiologic state. The ductus venosus is absent in several mammalian species, e.g. the horse, pig, and guinea pig.

Total blood flow to the liver is more than four times greater in the fetus compared with the adult, reaching values of approximately 400 ml/(100 g·min). The proportion of umbilical venous blood flow that bypasses the hepatic circulation by shunting to the inferior vena cava through the ductus venosus varies widely, but approximates 50 per cent in the unstressed fetus. This more highly oxygenated blood is then preferentially distributed through the foramen ovale into the

left heart chambers and subsequently to the fetal coronary circulation and to the brain. Most of the blood from the portal vein is distributed to the right lobe of the liver, with less than 10 per cent passing through the ductus venosus.

The fetus responds to various stresses by varying resistance to flow in the umbilical vein, liver, and ductus venosus. These changes in resistance alter the proportion of oxygenated umbilical venous blood shunted through the ductus venosus and may shift the volumes of blood contained in the placenta, liver, and systemic circulations. For example, in response to fetal hypoxemia, vascular resistance in the umbilical veins increases. This increased umbilical venous resistance increases the amount of fetal blood pooled in the placenta, thus distending and recruiting vessels in the placental exchange area and increasing the fetal placental surface area available for blood–gas exchange. This mechanism could compensate for reductions in fetal oxygenation due to placental compression resulting from uterine contraction or altered maternal position, common physiologic causes of fetal hypoxemia.

During hypoxemia, liver blood flow decreases about 20 per cent, with a corresponding increase in shunting of blood across the ductus venosus. It is likely that the volume of blood contained in the liver decreases, with the blood volume shifting to the placenta, but actual changes in liver volume have not been studied. Umbilical cord compression or hypovolemia result in an even more striking increase in the proportion of blood shunted across the ductus venosus with a corresponding large decrease in total hepatic blood flow and a resultant decrease in $O_2$ delivery to approximately 25 per cent of control values. As with hypoxemia, fetal hepatic capacitance is likely markedly reduced during these stresses but has not been studied directly. The volume of blood contained in the liver would be redistributed to the central circulation, an appropriate response to hypovolemic stress.

The proportion of blood flow passing through the ductus venosus versus the liver can be altered by changes in the resistance to flow through the liver or the ductus venosus. There appears to be a sphincter mechanism at the origin of the ductus venosus from the umbilical vein. Neural control of the ductus venosus is unlikely because the administration of atropine to block parasympathetic neural activity, or phentolamine to block α-adrenergic sympathetic neural activity, does not alter ductus venosus flow; however, non-adrenergic, non-cholinergic mechanisms could be operative. Isolated rings of ductus venosus relax when exposed to $PGE_2$ and $PGI_2$ and contract when exposed to indomethacin, an inhibitor or prostaglandin synthesis. The role of these factors in control of ductus venosus sphincter function has not been fully studied *in vivo*. Local autocrine regulators or other hormonal factors may control ductus venosus resistance.

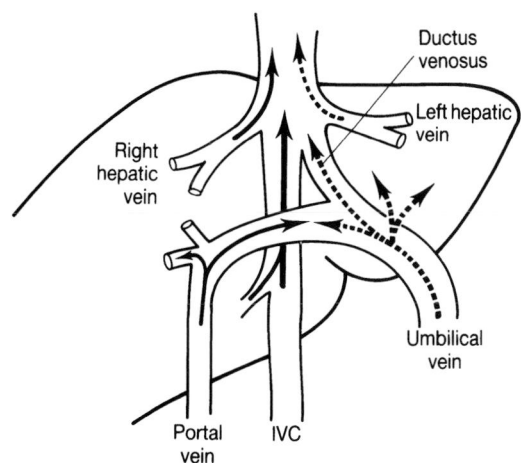

FIGURE 62.1 Schematic representation of liver blood flow in the fetal lamb

## CHANGES IN LIVER BLOOD FLOW AT BIRTH

At birth umbilical blood flow ceases and the liver receives all of its blood supply from the hepatic artery and portal vein, as in the adult. The ductus venosus can remain open for as long as 10 days after birth. Studies in newborn lambs demonstrate that blood flow to the liver abruptly falls to adult rates of approximately 100 mL/(100 g·min) and then rises slowly to approximately 300 mL/(100 g·min) over the first 10 hours after birth. Similar flow rates have been demonstrated in 1-week-old fasted lambs. Changes in total liver blood flow, the proportion of flow provided by the hepatic artery or portal vein, and the intactness of the "hepatic arterial buffer response" have not been well studied in infants or children.

## SELECTED READING

Ballet F. Hepatic circulation: potential for therapeutic intervention. *Pharmacol Ther* 1990; **47**: 281.

Edelstone DI. Regulation of blood flow through the ductus venosus. *J Dev Physiol* 1980; **2**: 219.

Edelstone DI, Rudolph AM, Heymann MA. Effects of hypoxemia and decreasing umbilical blood flow on liver and ductus venosus blood flows in fetal lambs. *Am J Physiol* 1980; **238**: H656.

Lautt WW, Greenway CV. Conceptual review of the hepatic vascular bed. *Hepatology* 1987; **7**: 952.

Paulick RP, Meyers RL, Rudolph CD, Rudolph AM. Venous responses to hypoxemia in the fetal lamb. *J Dev Physiol* 1990; **14**: 81.

Rudolph AM, Rudolph CD. Fetal and postnatal hepatic vasculature and blood flow. In: Polin RA, Fox WW eds. *Fetal and neonatal physiology*, Vol. II. Philadelphia: WB Saunders Co., 1992: 1095.

Zhang JX, Pegoli W Jr, Clemens MG. Endothelin-1 induces direct constriction of hepatic sinusoids. *Am J Physiol* 1994; **266**: G632.

# 63

# Development of Gallbladder Motility

James P. Ryan

Bile salts, which stabilize pancreatic lipolytic enzymes and solubilize the products of lipolysis into micelles, are produced by the liver and are secreted into the biliary ducts. The gallbladder stores and concentrates bile for secretion into the duodenum. Coordination of the motor activities of the gallbladder and the sphincter of Oddi assure that bile salts are released into the intestinal lumen when required for fat digestion. While there is no question that gallbladder emptying involves active contraction of the gallbladder, the dynamics at the sphincter of Oddi are much more controversial. In several species such as the guinea-pig, rabbit and opossum, the sphincter most likely serves the role of a pump and contributes to bile flow into the duodenum by increasing or decreasing the force of its characteristic peristaltic contractions. In other species, such as the human, the sphincter is believed to influence bile flow by serving as a variable resistor, with the magnitude of bile flow being inversely related to sphincter tone.

## EMPTYING PATTERNS IN ADULTS

In adults, gallbladder emptying occurs during both the interdigestive period and after the ingestion of a meal (digestive phase). In adult humans bile flows into the duodenum during the interdigestive period in a cyclical pattern. During this period, water is removed from gallbladder bile because of solvent drag created by active NaCl transport by gallbladder mucosal cells. Mucus and immunoglobulin A (IgA) are also secreted into the gallbladder lumen. The periodic increase in bile delivery into the duodenum correlates closely with Phase II of the migrating motor complex (MMC) discussed in Chapter 54. The periodic increase in bile delivery into the duodenum during the interdigestive period involves cyclical changes in hepatic

secretion of bile and periodic activation of gallbladder emptying involving contraction of the gallbladder and relaxation of the sphincter of Oddi. The physiological role of gallbladder emptying during the interdigestive period remains unsettled. It is proposed that it serves a "housekeeper" function by preventing accumulation of microcrystals or debris in the concentrated bile during fasting. The periodic mixing and emptying of bile may serve to prevent gallbladder stasis during fasting and thus decrease the likelihood of gallstone formation.

The gallbladder empties promptly in response to the ingestion of a meal, generally within 2 minutes. Characteristically, the gallbladder empties 60–70 per cent of its fasting volume and does so with a half-emptying time of 10–20 minutes. The major stimulus for gallbladder emptying occurs during the intestinal phase of digestion and absorption. The gastric emptying of chyme into the duodenum, through activation of neural and hormonal inputs, serves as the primary stimulus for initiation of gallbladder emptying. Preduodenal factors also may contribute to gallbladder emptying during the cephalic and gastric phases of digestion. Excitatory cholinergic vagal fibers, activated by esophageal and gastric distension, input onto the gallbladder and lead to active contraction of the gallbladder smooth muscle.

## REGULATION OF GALLBLADDER EMPTYING

The factors responsible for contraction of the gallbladder during the interdigestive period are unclear. Motilin, when given exogenously during the interdigestive period, increases contractile activity of the stomach, small intestine, and gallbladder. Gallbladder contraction during the interdigestive period closely correlates with increased antral motility during Phase II of the MMC.

Cholecystokinin (CCK) mediates the intestinal phase of gallbladder emptying in a number of animal species (including humans). A close correlation exists between plasma concentrations of CCK and changes in gallbladder volume after ingestion of a meal. Recent evidence indicates that CCK may stimulate gallbladder contraction via activation of excitatory vagal cholinergic fibers. Gallbladder contraction combined with a CCK-mediated decrease in sphincter of Oddi resistance (humans) leads to the prompt delivery of bile into the duodenum.

## DEVELOPMENTAL ASPECTS OF THE GALLBLADDER

The delivery of bile into the duodenum depends not only upon bile acid excretion as determined by hepatic function, but also upon the contractile ability of the gallbladder. Sufficient intraluminal pressure needs to be developed by active contraction of gallbladder smooth muscle to overcome resistances offered by the common bile ducts and the sphincter of Oddi.

The mechanical properties of the gallbladder, assessed by analyzing the pressure–volume relationship of the organ basally and following stimulation with CCK, indicate that the compliance of the unstimulated gallbladder is significantly less in the neonatal pig than in the adult. When stimulated with CCK, gallbladders from adult animals show decreased compliance, whereas gallbladders from newborn animals have no change in compliance. The rise in the intraluminal pressure of the gallbladder in response to CCK stimulation is less in newborn versus adult animals. The reduced gallbladder force generating capacity in the neonate may result from the inability of the gallbladder smooth muscle to generate significant active tension when stimulated with an agonist. The magnitude of the contractile response in adult animals is greater than in preterm and term animals. The differences remain even when the contractile responses are normalized for differences in the cross-sectional area.

The contractile response to $Ca^{2+}$ is concentration-dependent in gallbladder smooth muscle from newborn and adult guinea-pigs; however, at all concentrations examined, the contractile response from newborn animals was significantly less than from adults, supporting the hypothesis that basic differences exist between newborns and adults with respect to the ability of the contractile machinery to generate force in response to an agonist-mediated rise in intracellular $Ca^{2+}$. Recent evidence in vascular and tracheal smooth muscle indicates that postnatal changes in contractile protein content and/or isoforms, as well as changes in the $Ca^{2+}$ concentration and calmodulin sensitivity, might account for the decreased response to $Ca^{2+}$. Perhaps gallbladder smooth muscle exhibits a similar postnatal maturation of the contractile machinery. Other possible explanations for the differences in neonatal versus adult gallbladder contractile activity include age-related differences in the mechanism of action of acetylcholine and CCK, or in the muscle fiber geometric arrangement in the gallbladder.

## SPHINCTER OF ODDI

The delivery of bile into the duodenum involves both gallbladder contraction and the efficient passage of bile through the sphincter of Oddi. The ability of the sphincter of Oddi region to serve as a pump is not fully developed in the newborn guinea-pig. Using an intravital microscopy technique, the contractile activity of the sphincter upon ingestion of a meal is seen to be decreased in newborns, compared with adults. Differences between sphincter smooth muscle or responses to specific agonists in newborns and adults have not been studied.

Limited animal data suggest that the contractile behavior of the gallbladder and the sphincter of Oddi is less in newborns than in adults. Should this also be true for humans, hypomotility of the gallbladder and sphincter may diminish the flow of bile into the duodenum, contributing to physiologic cholestasis in the newborn. Although this is an attractive hypothesis, more data must be obtained before it can be expressed with confidence.

## SELECTED READING

Cox KL, Cheung ATW, Lohse CL *et al*. Biliary motility: postnatal changes in guinea pigs. *Pediatr Res* 1987; **21**: 170.

Denehy CM, Ryan JP. Development of gallbladder contractility in the guinea pig. *Pediatr Res* 1986; **20**: 214.

Lambert R, Ryan JP. Response to calcium of skinned gallbladder smooth muscle from newborn and adult guinea pigs. *Pediatr Res* 1990; **28**: 336.

# 64

# Bile Acid Metabolism and the Enterohepatic Circulation of Bile Acids

James E. Heubi

## NORMAL PHYSIOLOGY

Bile acids serve at least three major functions:

- they stimulate bile flow during secretion across the biliary canaliculus;
- in the upper small intestine they form aggregates called micelles which solubilize the water-insoluble products of lipolysis;
- they are major regulators of sterol metabolism.

In health, the enterohepatic circulation of bile acids is localized to the liver and biliary tract, the intestinal tract, and the portal and peripheral circulations. In the liver, cholesterol is converted to the highly polar bile acids, cholic acid ($3\alpha,7\alpha,12\alpha$-trihydroxy-$5\beta$-cholanoic acid) and chenodeoxycholic acid ($3\alpha,7\alpha$-dihydroxy-$5\beta$-cholanoic acid), which are termed primary bile acids (Fig. 64.1). The initial step of bile acid synthesis involves the $7\alpha$-hydroxylation of the sterol nucleus of cholesterol, which is effected by the rate-limiting enzyme of bile acid synthesis, cholesterol $7\alpha$-hydroxylase. This enzyme is regulated by a mechanism of feedback inhibition based on the quantities of bile acids returning to the liver via the portal vein. After hepatic synthesis, bile acids are conjugated with glycine or taurine as N-acyl conjugates. All but a small fraction of bile acids are conjugated before excretion by the hepatocyte.

Bile is a mixture of organic and inorganic materials. The major organic compounds include conjugated bile acids, phospholipids, cholesterol, and bile pigments. Proteins and hormones are present in low concentrations. Bile acid concentrations in adult bile range from 2–45 mM. Bile acids are amphipathic molecules forming *micelles* (macromolecular aggregates) above a critical micellar concentration (CMC), which in human bile is approximately 2–4 mM. Bile acids in hepatic and gallbladder bile greatly exceed the CMC. Therefore, bile acids in bile and the upper small bowel lumen are present as micelles, with small amounts present as monomers. Bile acids are important in relation to the other organic compounds in bile because hepatocyte secretion of cholesterol and phospholipids is dependent upon bile acid secretion, and the solubility of cholesterol and phospholipids is largely dependent upon bile acids.

Bile acid-dependent bile flow, linked directly to bile acid transport through the hepatocyte and into the canalicular lumen, provides the major impetus for bile flow. The bile acid-independent component accounts for a smaller fraction of bile flow. Uptake of taurocholate into the hepatocyte from portal blood is dependent upon an inwardly directed Na$^+$ gradient, which may be diminished by other bile acids, amino acids, and furosemide. Transcellular passage of bile acids is facilitated by binding to intracellular carrier proteins. Canalicular transport carriers facilitate passage of bile acids into the canalicular lumen. Canalicular transport is via a Na$^+$-independent process driven by a negative transmembrane potential. The osmotic activity of transported bile acids leads to movement of water and other solutes into the canalicular lumen. Choleresis is stimulated by increasing the flux of bile acids across the hepatocyte.

During fasting, most of the bile acid pool is present in the gallbladder; however, some bile acids are always

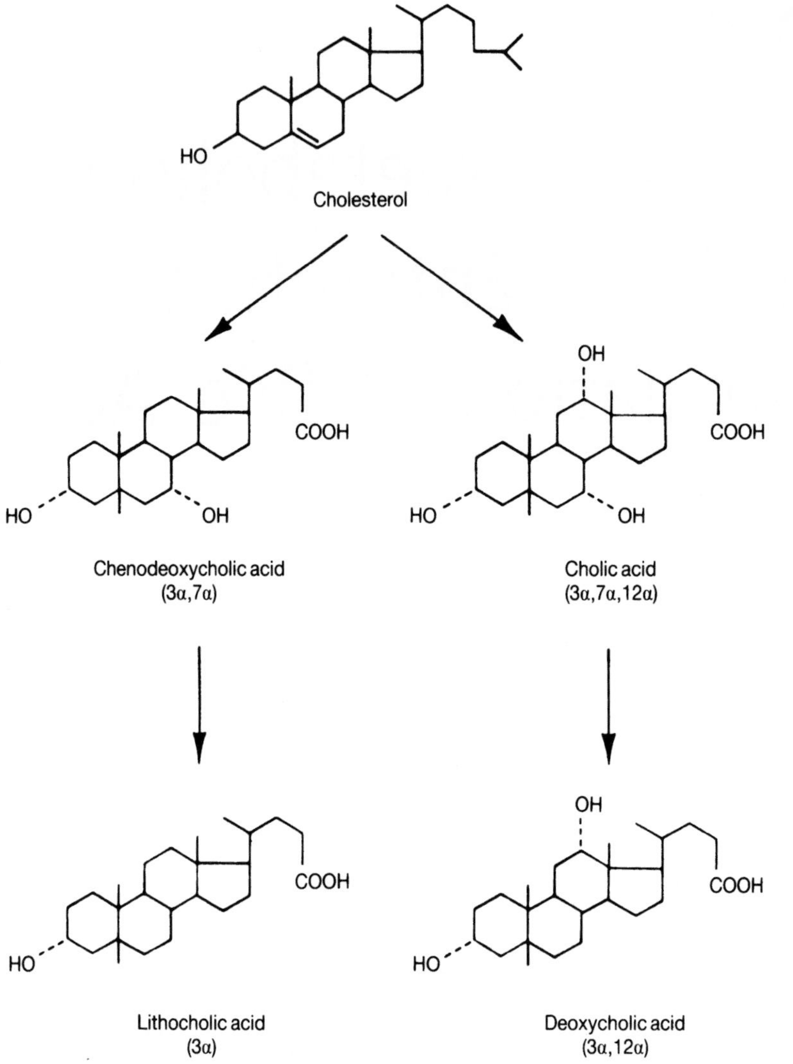

FIGURE 64.1 Primary bile acids synthesized in liver from cholesterol, and the secondary bile acids produced by bacterial $7\alpha$-dehydroxylation

entering the intestinal lumen and produce basal intraluminal concentrations and small but measurable concentrations in the serum because of continuous intestinal absorption with less than complete hepatic extraction from portal blood. When a meal is ingested, the gallbladder contracts at least once, and most of the bile salt pool is emptied into the small intestinal lumen (Fig. 64.2). Within the upper small bowel, bile salts form mixed micelles with the lipolytic products, fatty acids, and monoglycerides. Cholesterol, phospholipids, and fat-soluble vitamins are also solubilized within mixed micelles. The lipolytic products are absorbed and bile acids are thereafter reabsorbed by two mechanisms. A $Na^+$-dependent, active transport system localized to the distal ileum is the principal pathway for reabsorption. Bile acids can competitively inhibit each other for transport across the ileal active transport system. Passive transport by non-ionic diffusion may occur at any location along the length of the small

and large intestine; however, absorption is markedly curtailed for most bile acids because their $pK_a$s are low and they tend to remain ionized at luminal pH. Only unconjugated bile acids and glycine conjugates of dihydroxy bile acids are likely to be non-ionized and in a suitable state for passive absorption. In addition, luminal nutrients tend to inhibit passive uptake of bile acids.

After bile acids are transported out of the enterocyte, they are carried to the liver where transport systems efficiently remove them from the portal blood. A small fraction of the bile acids in portal blood spills over into the systemic circulation leading to a predictable postprandial rise in serum bile acids during each of the 6–10 enterohepatic cycles of bile acids during the day.

Most conjugates of cholic and chenodeoxycholic acid excreted in the bile are reabsorbed without intraluminal bacterial alteration. Approximately one-

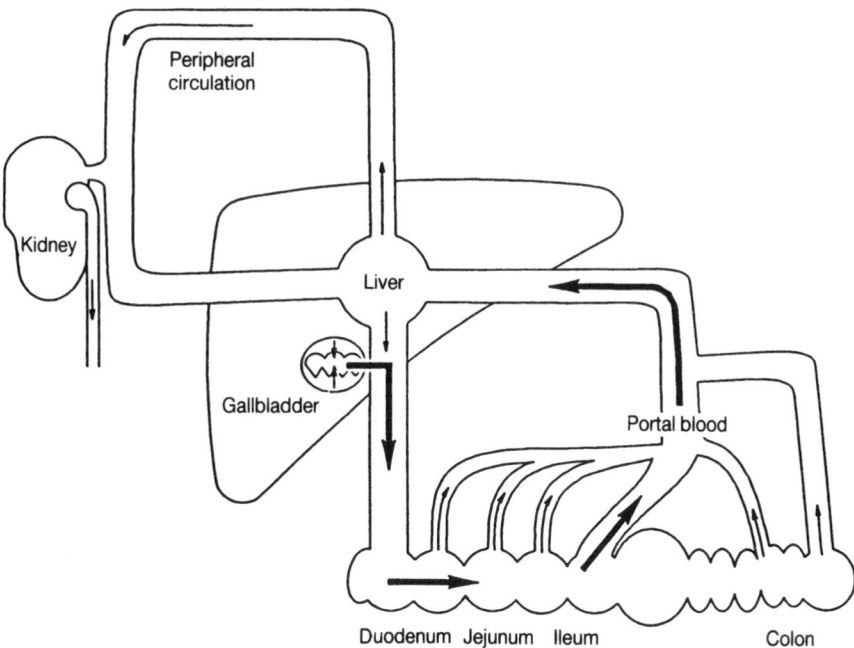

FIGURE 64.2 The enterohepatic circulation of bile acids. With gallbladder contraction, bile acids are expelled into the duodenum. Passive intestinal absorption is depicted by small arrows, and the large arrow in ileum depicts active uptake of bile acids. Bile acids return to the liver via the portal venous system. Despite efficient uptake of bile acids, a small fraction of the bile acids in portal blood spill over into the systemic circulation and may be filtered and excreted by the kidneys. (From Heubi JE, In Banks RO, Sperelakis N eds. *Essentials of basic science: physiology.* Boston: Little, Brown and Company, 1993, with permission.)

quarter of the primary bile acids are deconjugated by bacteria in the terminal ileum and colon. Most of these free bile acids are reabsorbed and reconjugated in the liver with either glycine or taurine. Additional modifications to the steroid nucleus after deconjugation may also be made within the gut lumen. The most common biotransformation made by bacteria is 7α-dehydroxylation with the formation of secondary bile acids (Fig. 64.1). Deoxycholic acid (3α,12α-dihydroxy-5β-cholanoic acid) is formed from cholic acid, and lithocholic acid (3α-hydroxy-5β-cholanoic acid) is formed from chenodeoxycholic acid. The produced deoxycholic acid is absorbed relatively efficiently and reconjugated, whereas lithocholic acid is absorbed poorly. If reabsorbed, lithocholic acid may be conjugated with glycine or taurine; however, the majority of conjugates are sulfated in the three position to form sulfated lithocholate conjugates. Sulfated conjugates are poorly absorbed and are excreted. Fecal bile acids are reflective of major bacterial transformation. The majority of bile acids are unconjugated and lack the 7α-hydroxyl group.

In adults, biliary bile acids are generally cholic (36 per cent), chenodeoxycholic (36 per cent), deoxycholic (24 per cent), and lithocholic (1 per cent) in a glycine:taurine ratio of 3–4:1. Each day about one-quarter to one-third of the cholic acid pool and one-fifth to one-quarter of the chenodeoxycholic acid pool is lost from the adult human enterohepatic circulation. This turnover of bile acids is commonly expressed as the fractional turnover rate (FTR). The bile acid pool is in a steady state in health so that losses of bile acids are replaced by hepatic synthesis by a carefully regulated mechanism of feedback inhibition of the rate-limiting enzyme of bile acid synthesis, cholesterol 7α-hydroxylase.

## DEVELOPMENTAL ASPECTS OF BILE ACID SYNTHESIS AND THE ENTEROHEPATIC CIRCULATION OF BILE ACIDS

The enterohepatic circulation of bile salts is immature at birth. Impairment of hepatic synthesis, secretion, and uptake, intestinal conservation, and gallbladder contractility (see Chapter 63) all contribute to the reduced biliary secretion and intraluminal concentrations encountered in the neonate.

Bile acid biosynthesis is markedly reduced *in utero*; it is first observed near week 12 in the human fetus. A 30-fold increase in the biliary concentrations of cholic and chenodeoxycholic acids is observed between 16–20 weeks' gestation in the human fetus. The bile acids produced (and their metabolic pathways) during gestation are considerably different from those found in the infant, child, and adult. The primary bile acids, cholic and chenodeoxycholic acids, make up less than 50 per cent of the total bile acid pool in the fetus. The ratio of cholic to chenodeoxycholic acid is 0.9 between 16–20 weeks' gestation, in contrast to 2.5 in the neonate and

1.6 in the adult. This suggests that there is immaturity of hepatic 12α-hydroxylation during development. The fetal liver possesses enzymes capable of synthesizing relatively large proportions of bile acids not found in older infants or healthy adults; however, these compounds are found in biological fluids from adults with cholestatic liver disease. These unique bile acids account for 5–15 per cent of the total biliary bile acid of the human fetus. The physiological relevance of almost all of these compounds is unknown; however, they may be directly responsible for the development of cholestasis. Extremely low hepatic bile flow rates secondary to small primary bile acid pool sizes, and the presence of an array of bile acids that are unique to the fetus and may be intrinsically cholestatic, probably exaggerate the immaturity of hepatic excretory function.

The phenomenon of reduced fat absorption in the immediate neonatal period is referred to as *physiologic steatorrhea*. Newborns share two common defects that lead to impaired fat absorption: reduced prandial-related intraluminal bile salt concentrations and diminished pancreatic lipase activity (see Chapter 56). Both are consistently reduced and correlate with gestational and postnatal age. A progressive rise in both occurs in infants in the first few months. Term and preterm infants have markedly reduced primary bile salt pool sizes compared with adults, on a surface-area basis. These reduced pools are accompanied by reduced intraluminal bile salt concentrations (Fig. 64.3). Initial studies suggested that compared with adults, the turnover rate for the primary bile salts might be increased due to impaired intestinal conservation and synthesis rates reduced because of impaired regulation of the rate-limiting enzyme of bile salt synthesis, cholesterol 7α-hydroxylase. Breast-fed preterm infants, when compared with age- and weight-matched infants fed a proprietary formula, have larger bile salt pools and lower turnover rates (both cholic and chenodeoxycholic acids), higher intraluminal concentrations (4.8 versus 2.6 mM compared with the critical micellar con-

centration of 2.00), and better fat absorption efficiency (93 versus 82 per cent) at age 11 days. By 31–38 days, all infants have substantial reductions in the turnover rate for cholate and chenodeoxycholate and increases in cholate and chenodeoxycholate pools; however, synthesis rates for both bile salts remained unchanged. Concurrently, intraluminal bile salt concentrations increase from 5 mM in breast-fed and 3–4 mM in formula-fed infants, while fat absorption increases from 78–83 per cent of dietary intake in both formula- and breast-fed infants. This finding suggests that breast milk may provide a stimulus to maturation of the enterohepatic circulation in the preterm infant.

Because bile acids are the major determinant of bile flow, their synthesis and the development of an adequate pool of bile acids in the neonatal period is essential to biliary excretion. Although unproved in the human neonate, it seems extremely likely that biliary excretory function is impaired in the first weeks after birth. Despite a reduced load of bile acids returned from the intestine in the neonate compared with the adult, elevated serum bile acid concentrations are commonly encountered in preterm and term infants. In term infants, the elevated concentrations decline with postnatal age and normalize at about 6–12 months. This phenomenon has been termed *physiologic cholestasis*. The clearance of additional organic ions, including sulfobromophthalein (BSP), is impaired in term and preterm infants with progressive improvement during the first month after birth. The exact mechanism by which organic ion transport is compromised is unclear, but it likely relates to impaired hepatic uptake at the basolateral membrane, as well as alterations of blood flow and biliary excretion.

Studies on the ontogeny of the enterohepatic circulation in rats have helped to formulate a working model in the mammal that may improve our understanding of developmental physiology in the human. The rat is a particularly good model for comparison to the human premature infant because of its extreme immaturity at birth. In the newborn rat, the bile salt

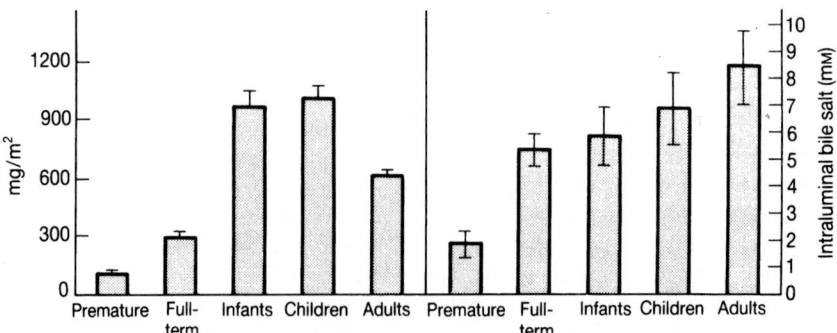

FIGURE 64.3 Left panel: Comparison of cholate pool size (mg/m²) in preterm and term infants (studied by Watkins *et al. N Engl J Med* 1973; **288**: 431; *Gastroenterology* 1975; **69**: 706), infants and children (studied by Heubi *et al. Pediatr Res* 1980; **14**: 943; *J Lab Clin Med* 1982; **100**: 127), and adults (studied by Vlahcevic *et al. Gastroenterology* 1971; **61**: 85). Right panel: Comparison of meal-stimulated intraluminal bile salt concentrations (mM) in preterm and term infants (studied by Watkins *et al. N Engl J Med* 1973; **288**: 431; *Gastroenterology* 1975; **69**: 706), infants and children (studied by Heubi *et al. Pediatr Res* 1980; **14**: 943; *J Lab Clin Med* 1982; **100**: 127), and adults (studied by Porter and Sanders, *Gastroenterology* 1971; **60**: 997).

pool is small at birth and is localized predominantly in the liver and peripheral serum rather than the intestinal lumen, as observed in the adult. Bile acid synthesis begins in the fetal rat on days 15–17. Synthesis rates increase from about 80 pmol/mg dry liver weight on day 18, to about 1000 pmol/mg dry liver weight on day 21. Fetal bile acid synthesis can be enhanced *in vitro* by corticoid treatment. During the first postnatal weeks, hepatocyte bile salt uptake matures. The $K_m$ for hepatic bile salt transport across the basolateral membrane remains unchanged with increasing age; however, the $V_{max}$ increases four-fold between ages 1–8 weeks. This suggests that the transport process is present initially and the number of transport sites increases with postnatal age. Transport across the canalicular membrane appears to be similar in suckling and adult rats. Elevated serum bile acids in the suckling rat decline with increasing postnatal age, suggesting an improvement in the clearance mechanisms. Only passive intestinal bile salt transport is present in the suckling rat; however, during the third postnatal week, ileal active transport first appears with kinetic characteristics that are qualitatively similar to those of older animals. Corticosteroids and thyroxine in pharmacologic doses have been shown to induce precocious development of the active transport mechanism. Concurrently, the pool size, initially located predominately in the liver, increases five-fold between 2 and 8 weeks of age, when it becomes largely localized to the intestinal lumen.

Extrapolating observations made in laboratory animals to humans is difficult; however, fragmentary human data allow inferences regarding postnatal development of the enterohepatic circulation in the human. Hepatic bile acid synthesis is severely reduced, and alternative pathways for synthesis are present in the fetus as well as newborn term and preterm infant. Synthesis of the primary bile acids increases markedly in the first postnatal weeks. Hepatic uptake of bile salts is impaired at birth in term, and especially in preterm infants, with subsequent improvement in the first year, as indicated by high serum concentrations of total serum bile acids and conjugates of cholic and chenodeoxycholate, which decline to levels comparable to older children by 10 months. The turnover rate of bile salts is increased at birth, but declines postnatally. Because the turnover rate reflects biliary secretion rates, intestinal transit, gallbladder contractility and intestinal uptake of bile salts, it is impossible to dissect out exactly which process(es) is compromised at birth and matures with postnatal age. Neither biliary secretion, intestinal transit, nor gallbladder contractility has been directly examined in the human neonate. Results of *in vitro* studies, in which ileal segments were incubated with bile salts, suggest that ileal active bile salt transport is absent in human fetuses, with its first appearance in infants at age 8 months. However, bile salt kinetic studies in preterm and term newborns, infants, and children, strongly suggest that ileal active

bile salt transport is present at birth even in very premature infants.

Intraluminal bile salt concentrations increase postnatally, coincident with pool size enlargement in formula-fed and mixed diet-fed infants and children (Fig. 64.3). Qualitative composition of duodenal bile changes dramatically with age. Although cholic acid and chenodeoxycholic acid predominate in neonatal bile, additional other bile acids have been identified, including 6-hydroxy(OH), 1-OH, and oxo-bile acids. With the appearance of intestinal microflora, secondary bile acids appear in the bile and other less commonly found bile acids disappear. During the first year, cholic acid constitutes 60 per cent of duodenal bile acids, while chenodeoxycholic constitutes 36 per cent. Small quantities of deoxycholic acid are detected between 6–10 months. The glycine:taurine ratio of bile in the preterm neonate is less than 1, but increases to 3.3 during the first year.

Fecal bile acids in the neonate consist of only primary bile acids, with no secondary bile acids detectable. With development of the gut microflora, secondary bile acids appear in the stool. Daily excretion by adults and children are 8–9 times greater than by infants younger than 18 months; however, differences in excretion rates disappear when body surface area differences or weights are taken into account. For all newborns and children, bile acid excretion is relatively consistent when based upon body weight (3–6 mg/(kg·day)), and is similar to that observed in adults.

# CONGENITAL DEFECTS OF BILE ACID BIOSYNTHESIS AND BILE ACID TRANSPORT

Potential inborn errors of primary bile acid synthesis can be identified at each of the multiple enzymatic steps converting cholesterol to bile acids within the hepatic cytosol, mitochondria, microsomes and peroxisomes. The accumulation of toxic metabolites and a small primary bile acid pool may account for the liver injury observed in infants with these metabolic disorders, all of which can be identified, using fast atom bombardment, by the metabolic products that accumulate proximal to the specific enzyme defect. Four inborn errors of bile acid synthesis have been described including *cerebrotendinous xanthomatosis, cerebro–hepato–renal syndrome (Zellweger syndrome), 3β-hydroxysteroid dehydrogenase/isomerase deficiency,* and *Δ⁴-3-oxosteroid 5β-reductase deficiency.* Cerebro–hepato–renal syndrome is characterized by the absence of peroxisomes, causing muscle weakness and central nervous system disease with mental retardation and seizures. Di- and trihydroxycholestanoic acid accumulate, with development of progressive liver damage in infancy. The phenotypic expression of 3β-hydroxysteroid dehydrogenase/isomerase deficiency is quite variable. Most patients present in infancy with jaundice, steatorrhea with fat-soluble vitamin deficiency, normal serum $\gamma$-glutamyl transpeptidase levels, and low serum bile acids. However, some patients present in later childhood or adolescence with chronic liver disease. Bile acid therapy normalizes serum transaminases and serum bilirubin and improves liver histology. $\Delta^4$-3-oxosteroid 5$\beta$-reductase deficiency results in conjugated hyperbilirubinemia with low serum bile acids and neonatal hepatitis. Without bile acid therapy, this condition is uniformly fatal in the first months after birth.

Other defects involving cholesterol synthesis result in reduced bile acid synthesis. *Smith–Lemli–Opitz (SLO) syndrome*, characterized by microcephaly, mental retardation, growth failure, dysmorphic features, cataracts, and cardiac, renal, and endocrine abnormalities purportedly is due to a deficiency of 3$\beta$-hydroxysterol $\Delta^7$-reductase. This leads to an accumulation of 7-dehydrocholesterol in serum with a marked reduction of cholesterol concentrations. Therapy includes supplemental cholesterol and bile acids; however, postnatal therapy cannot correct the *in utero* damage associated with this condition.

In addition to defects of bile acid synthesis, defects of ileal bile acid transport have been described. Two unrelated boys had diarrhea in infancy due to a congenital absence of the ileal active bile salt transport protein. Both had markedly increased fecal bile acid excretion, increased turnover of labeled bile acids, and markedly reduced *in vitro* uptake of bile acids in ileal mucosa. The only therapy available for these children was dietary. Recent cloning of the rat, hamster, and human genes for the ileal bile salt transport protein should allow characterization of the specific molecular defects in these patients. To date, no congenital defects of the hepatic basolateral or canalicular transporters have been described; however, with the cloning of the genes for these transporters, defects may be more readily identified in the future.

## SELECTED READING

Balistreri WF, Heubi JE, Suchy FJ. Immaturity of the enterohepatic circulation in early life: factors predisposing to "physiologic" maldigestion and cholestasis. *J Pediatr Gastroenterol Nutr* 1983; 2: 346.

Hofmann AF. Enterohepatic circulation of bile acids. In: Schultz SG, Forte JG, Rauner BB eds. *Handbook of physiology*. Bethesda, MD: American Physiological Society, 1989: 567.

Setchell KDR, O'Connell NC. Inborn errors of bile acid metabolism. In Suchy FJ ed. *Liver disease in children*. St Louis: Mosby, 1994: 835.

Setchell KDR, Street JM. Inborn errors of bile acid synthesis. *Semin Liver Dis* 1987; 7: 85.

Suchy FJ. Hepatocellular transport of bile acids. *Semin Liver Dis* 1993; 13: 235.

Suchy FJ, Bucuvalas JC, Novak DA. Determinants of bile formation during development: ontogeny of hepatic bile acid metabolism and transport. *Semin Liver Dis* 1987; 7: 77.

Tint SG, Irons M, Elias EF et al. Defective cholesterol biosynthesis associated with Smith–Lemli–Opitz syndrome. *N Engl J Med* 1994; 330: 107.

Wong MH, Oelkers P, Craddock AL, Dawson PA. Expression cloning and characterization of the hamster ileal sodium-dependent bile acid transporter. *J Biol Chem* 1994; 269: 1340.

# 65

# Perinatal Bilirubin Metabolism

Glenn R. Gourley

Bilirubin is formed when the protoporphyrin ring of heme-containing compounds is degraded. Hemoglobin is the largest source for the production of bilirubin, but other heme-containing proteins (e.g. cytochromes, catalases, tryptophane pyrrolase, and muscle myoglobin) are also degraded to bilirubin. The first enzyme system involved in bilirubin formation is microsomal heme oxygenase, located primarily in the reticuloendothelial tissues, and also in tissue macrophages and intestinal epithelium. Heme oxygenase causes cleavage of the tetrapyrrole ring at one of the methine ($=C-$) carbon bridges resulting in equimolar production of the excised carbon (carbon monoxide) and the linear tetrapyrrole, biliverdin. The central (C-10) carbon of biliverdin is then reduced from a methine to a methylene group ($-CH_2-$), by the cytosolic enzyme biliverdin reductase, thus forming bilirubin. Bilirubin is given the IX designation according to Fischer protoporphyrin isomer groups, group IX being the physiological source of bilirubin. Although the tetrapyrrole ring can be cleaved at any of the four ($\alpha$, $\beta$, $\gamma$, and $\delta$) methine bridges, in the fetus, bilirubin IX$\beta$ is first produced and can be found in fetal bile at 14 weeks' gestation. The major human isomer, bilirubin IX$\alpha$, appears in fetal bile at 16 weeks. Bilirubin formation, assessed by carbon monoxide production, indicates that the daily production rate of bilirubin is 6–8 mg/(kg·24 hr) in healthy term infants and 3–4 mg/(kg·24 hr) in healthy adults.

Bilirubin is not linear, but rather contains extensive internal $H^+$ bonding that shields the polar propionic acid groups and makes bilirubin poorly soluble in aqueous media (Fig. 65.1). The carbon–carbon double bonds at positions 4–5 and 15–16 can assume two different configurations depending on whether the higher priority atoms or groups (based on atomic number) are on the same (Z, *zusammen*, German: "together") or opposite (E, *entgegen*: "opposite") sides of the double bond. The naturally occurring form of bilirubin is 4Z,15Z-bilirubin IX$\alpha$. The poor aqueous solubility of bilirubin requires binding to albumin while in the circulation and hepatic transformation to more water-soluble derivatives prior to excretion.

## BINDING AND TRANSPORT

Each albumin molecule possesses a single high-affinity ($7 \times 10^7$ M$^{-1}$) binding site for one molecule of bilirubin. This strong binding results in essentially all bilirubin being transported to the liver bound to albumin, with negligible amounts free to diffuse into other tissues. Secondary binding sites of lesser affinity also exist on albumin. Other substances (e.g. fatty acids, sulfonamides, ceftriaxone, and other drugs) are also bound to bilirubin and can potentially displace bilirubin.

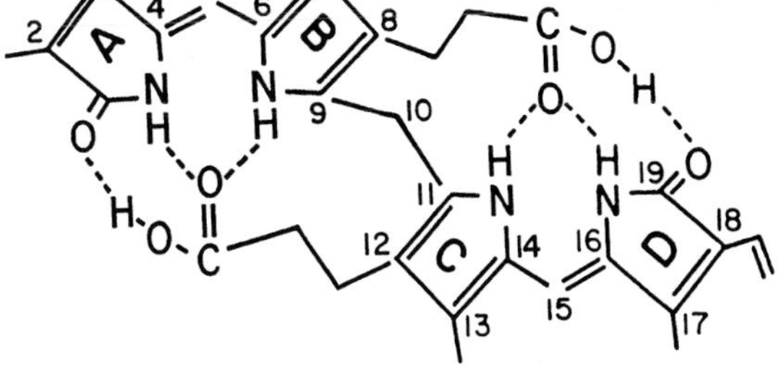

FIGURE 65.1 4Z,15Z-bilirubin IX$\alpha$, the most prominent physiological isomer of bilirubin in humans

## HEPATIC UPTAKE

A receptor in the plasma membrane of the hepatocyte facilitates uptake of bilirubin, and is competitively inhibited by bromsulfophthalein and indocyanin green. Once within the hepatocyte, bilirubin is bound by glutathione $S$-transferase B (GST), traditionally referred to as ligandin. The affinity of purified GST for bilirubin ($K_a = 10^6$) is less than that of albumin, but GST is believed to be of importance in preventing bilirubin and its conjugates from refluxing back into the circulation.

## CONJUGATION

Bilirubin is conjugated with glucuronic acid within the endoplasmic reticulum of the hepatocyte. Bilirubin-UDP-glucuronosyltransferase (BGT) is the enzyme responsible for this conjugation. Uridine diphosphate glucuronic acid (UDPGA) is the glucuronic acid donor. Several different classes of glucuronosyltransferases, with different substrate specificity, have been described. Two BGT isoforms in human liver have been reported to catalyze bilirubin glucuronidation. These BGT isoforms are both expressed by a single complex gene located at the telomeric end of chromosome 2. Bilirubin-UDP-glucuronosyltransferase 1 has been reported to be the only physiologically relevant form of the enzyme. Catalysis of bilirubin by BGT results in both mono- and diglucuronides of bilirubin. BGT activity for bilirubin can be induced by narcotics, anticonvulsants, contraceptive steroids, and bilirubin itself. Alternatively, BGT activity can be decreased by caloric and protein restriction. BGT is present in human fetal liver at levels approximately 0.1 per cent of adult values. At 30 weeks' gestation BGT begins to increase and reaches approximately 1 per cent of adult values by 40 weeks. BGT activity increases postnatally and by 14 weeks plateaus at adult values.

## SECRETION, REABSORPTION, AND EXCRETION

Following bilirubin conjugation, the bilirubin mono- and diglucuronides are secreted into bile via the biliary canaliculi. In normal adult duodenal bile, 70–90 per cent of the bile pigments are bilirubin diglucuronide, and 7–27 per cent are bilirubin monoglucuronides. Smaller amounts of other bilirubin conjugates are also seen. In infants, excretion of bilirubin diglucuronide is decreased with a concomitant increase in mono-glucuronides, consistent with decreased BGT activity. After the first postnatal week secretion of bilirubin conjugates by the hepatocyte is the rate limiting step in bilirubin clearance. Canalicular secretion of bilirubin conjugates can be increased by choleretic agents (e.g. phenobarbital) and decreased by cholestatic agents (e.g. estrogens and anabolic steroids) or pathologic conditions (e.g. liver disease).

Once bilirubin conjugates reach the intestine, several metabolic alternatives arise. In adults and older infants, intestinal bacteria hydrogenate various carbon double bonds in bilirubin to produce urobilinogens. Subsequent oxidation of the C-10 carbon produces the related urobilins. These reduction–oxidation products of bilirubin, known collectively as urobilinoids, are excreted in feces. *Clostridium ramosum* is the most important bacterium for urobilinoid production, and *Escherichia coli* acts synergistically. The conversion of bilirubin conjugates to urobilinoids prevents the intestinal absorption of bilirubin known as the entero-hepatic circulation. Because neonates lack intestinal bacteria, they are more susceptible to bilirubin reabsorption.

Alternatively, intestinal bilirubin conjugates can act as substrate for either bacterial or tissue β-glucuronidase. This ubiquitous enzyme cleaves glucuronic acid from bilirubin glucuronides, producing unconjugated bilirubin, which is more easily absorbed from the intestine. In the fetus, tissue β-glucuronidase, which is detectable by 12 weeks' gestation, is believed to play an important role in facilitating intestinal bilirubin absorption, which enables bilirubin to be cleared via the placenta. Bilirubin glucuronides are present *in utero* by 22 weeks. The effectiveness of bilirubin clearance via the placenta is shown by the fact that almost all infants are born non-icteric, even if they go on to develop severe hyperbilirubinemia in the first days after birth. Lacking placental assistance, the neonate with increased intestinal β-glucuronidase is at risk of experiencing higher serum bilirubin concentrations.

## JAUNDICE

Most, if not all, neonates develop bilirubin concentrations greater than 1.4 mg/dl during the first week. This common observation has led to the term *physiologic jaundice*. Serum concentrations of bilirubin greater than 7 mg/dl result in visible jaundice or icterus, which develops in a cephalopedal manner. Moderate jaundice (bilirubin >12 mg/dl) occurs in at least 12 per cent of breast-fed infants and 4 per cent of formula-fed infants, while severe jaundice (>15 mg/dl) occurs in 2 per cent and 0.3 per cent of these feeding groups, respectively.

Total serum bilirubin includes two fractions: conjugated bilirubin (so-called "direct" reacting because color development takes place directly without the addition of methanol in the van den Bergh test) and unconjugated bilirubin ("indirect" fraction). Traditionally the terms "direct" and "indirect" are used interchangeably with conjugated and unconjugated bilirubin, although it is now recognized that this is not quantitatively correct. Direct bilirubin measurements include delta bilirubin, while specific measurements of conjugated bilirubin do not. Delta bilirubin is the covalently bound bilirubin–protein compound formed spontaneously from bilirubin glucuronides and albumin. Jaundice can result from elevation of either of these fractions. Serum bilirubin measurements are most commonly made with automated laboratory methods. Erroneously elevated direct fractions have been seen with high total bilirubin concentrations.

*Neonatal jaundice* can result if bilirubin is excessively produced or inadequately excreted (see Table 65.1). Recent reviews of this broad subject have been published elsewhere. Pathologic neonatal jaundice is a concern because of the deleterious effects of high unconjugated bilirubin concentrations on the central nervous system known as *kernicterus* or *bilirubin encephalopathy*. Severe neonatal jaundice is an increasing problem today because trends in health care toward very early hospital discharge after birth result in the development of hyperbilirubinemia at home. In this setting parents sometimes do not recognize the severity of the jaundice until potentially toxic bilirubin concentrations have been reached. Therapeutic options to lower serum bilirubin concentrations include phototherapy, exchange transfusion, interruption of the enterohepatic circulation, induction of BGT, interruption of breast-feeding, and inhibition of heme oxygenase. Management of neonatal jaundice has been addressed in a recent practice parameter statement of the American Academy of Pediatrics. Phototherapy is effective because light produces isomers of bilirubin (lumirubin and E isomers), which disrupt the internal $H^+$ bonding and allow direct excretion into bile without conjugation. Recent research has shown that bilirubin has significant antioxidant activity, suggesting the possibility that higher bilirubin concentrations might decrease $O_2$ radical-mediated injury in preterm infants.

TABLE 65.1 Mechanisms of neonatal jaundice

Increased production of bilirubin
   Fetal–maternal blood group incompatibilities
   Extravascular blood in body tissues
   Polycythemia
   Red blood cell abnormalities
Decreased excretion of bilirubin
   Increased enterohepatic circulation of bilirubin
   Breast-feeding
   Inborn errors of metabolism
   Hormones and drugs
   Prematurity
   Hepatic hypoperfusion
   Cholestatic syndromes
   Obstruction of the biliary tree
Combined increased production and decreased excretion of bilirubin
   Sepsis
   Intrauterine infection

## SELECTED READING

American Academy of Pediatrics. Provisional Committee for Quality Improvement and Subcommittee on Hyperbilirubinemia. Practice parameter: management of hyperbilirubinemia in the healthy term newborn. *Pediatrics* 1994; 94: 558.

Gourley GR. Bilirubin metabolism and neonatal jaundice. In: Suchy FJ ed. *Liver disease in children*. St. Louis: Mosby, 1994: 105.

Gourley GR. Disorders of bilirubin metabolism. In: Suchy FJ ed. *Liver disease in children*. St. Louis: Mosby, 1994: 401.

Maisels MJ ed. Neonatal jaundice. *Clin Perinatol* 1990; 17: 245.

McDonagh AF, Lightner DA. "Like a shrivelled blood orange" – bilirubin, jaundice and phototherapy. *Pediatrics* 1985; 75: 443.

Odell GB, Schutta HS. Bilirubin encephalopathy. In: McCandless DW ed. *Cerebral energy metabolism and metabolic encephalopathy*. New York: Plenum Publishing Corp., 1985: 229.

# 66

# Nutritional Requirements

Bonny L. Specker

Nutrient requirements can be considered in three broad categories. First, *macronutrients* including carbohydrates, fats, and proteins, which serve as energy substrates. The proportion of total energy needs provided by each type of macronutrient varies tremendously in different cultures and socioeconomic groups. Second, *minerals,* including $Ca^{2+}$, $PO_4$ and $Mg^{2+}$, are required to synthesize bone. Third, specific components of foods that cannot be synthesized by the human body, *vitamins* or *trace metals*, are required in small amounts for synthesis of other structures, such as iron and hemoglobin, or facilitate specific biochemical reactions. Water and electrolyte requirements are discussed in Chapter 57. Deficiencies due to inadequate intake, malabsorption, or inappropriate losses of these micronutrients result in characteristic patterns of diseases, which are discussed briefly below.

The macronutrient requirements for growth and development have been well established. However, the ideal ratio of carbohydrate, fat, and protein intake remains controversial. The Recommended Dietary Allowances (RDAs), set by the Committee on Dietary Allowances of the Food and Nutrition Board of the National Academy of Sciences, are defined as "the levels of intake of essential nutrients, on the basis of current scientific knowledge, to be adequate to meet the known nutrient needs of practically all healthy persons." These recommended values do not represent optimal or ideal intakes but rather represent amount required for the average American individual of a specific age and gender. Recommended micronutrient amounts are in fact set at a high value to provide a margin of safety, covering the range in the entire population. The values change with illness or other specific defects in absorption of specific nutrients. These nutrient requirements are readily available in several pediatric and nutrition textbooks.

## MACRONUTRIENTS

### Energy requirements

Energy is supplied to the infant and child from protein, carbohydrates, and fat. The distribution of these macronutrients in the diet varies depending upon the food. The energy value of food is typically expressed in terms of heat units or kilocalories (kcal). A kilocalorie is defined as the amount of energy necessary to raise 1 kg of water by 1°C. The *Système International* (SI) unit of measure for energy is the kilojoule (kJ); 1 kJ = 0.24 kcal. During combustion, these sources of energy are oxidized to $CO_2$ and $H_2O$. The ratio of the amount of $CO_2$ produced to $O_2$ consumed is termed the respiratory quotient (RQ):

$$RQ = \frac{CO_2 \text{ produced}}{O_2 \text{ consumed}}$$

The amount of energy produced per liter of $O_2$ consumed is approximately the same for all three nutrients; the amount of energy produced per liter of $CO_2$ produced is higher for fats and lower for carbohydrates.

Indirect calorimetry, used to determine food energy utilization and requirements, involves measurement of

$O_2$ consumption and $CO_2$ production following ingestion of a known quantity of macronutrients. Studies using indirect calorimetry have been used to established energy requirements in infants and children. Energy requirements, which vary throughout infancy and childhood as a result of differing needs, are the sum of basal metabolism (resting energy expenditure: REE), growth of tissues, physical activity, and thermic effect of ingested foods. During the first postnatal year, energy requirement for growth exceeds the energy required for any other use. After the child's weight reaches approximately 15 kg, the growth rate decreases and the REE accounts for 30 per cent of the total energy needs, followed by energy required for physical activity and growth.

## Protein

Protein is essential for the synthesis of enzymes, transport proteins, and other structural components of cells. Proteins supply necessary nitrogen and amino acids. Nitrogen is not stored and must be replaced continuously. Although the body can synthesize and interconvert many of the amino acids, nine cannot be synthesized by the human and therefore must be supplied in the diet. These *essential amino acids* include histidine, isoleucine, leucine, lysine, methionine, phenylalanine, threonine, tryptophan and valine. Taurine, an amino acid present in high concentrations in human milk, appears to have a low endogenous synthesis. Although taurine may be necessary for functional aspects of the brain, retina, heart and liver, a deficiency state has not been identified and its essentiality has not been established.

Serum albumin, transferrin, thyroxine-binding pre-albumin, and retinol-binding protein are often used to assess visceral protein status. However, these proteins are not always specific indicators of protein status; concentrations also are affected by altered metabolism from trauma, stress, sepsis or hypoxia, by specific deficiency of plasma proteins caused by protein-losing enteropathy and liver disease, by capillary permeability changes, or by reduced synthesis from inadequate energy intake, electrolyte deficiency, trace element deficiencies (e.g. iron and zinc) or vitamin deficiency (e.g. vitamin A).

Although results of some studies indicate that a deficiency of protein, rather than energy, is the most common factor limiting growth in infants and children, few objective criteria exist for assessing adequacy of dietary protein and amino acids. The classic features of *kwashiorkor*, the clinical syndrome that results from dietary protein deficiency, include irritability, edema, hypoproteinemia and hypoalbuminemia. Skin abnormalities also occur and include hyperpigmentation, hyperkeratosis, desquamation and ulcerated lesions. Hair becomes sparse and depigmented. Subcutaneous fat stores are preserved and peripheral edema occurs, making it difficult to diagnose kwashiorkor from anthropometric measurements such as weight. *Marasmus*, or non-edematous protein energy malnutrition, is primarily a deficiency of total calories in which there is severe wasting with little edema.

## Carbohydrate

Carbohydrates are needed for the synthesis of nucleic acids and glycoproteins. Twenty-four to 50 per cent of the infant's energy needs are provided by dietary carbohydrates. Glucose, fructose and galactose result from the digestion of dietary carbohydrates. Carbohydrate digestion and absorption are discussed in Chapter 56.

Deficiency of carbohydrates does not occur in healthy human milk-fed or formula-fed infants. Incomplete absorption may occur with rapid transit time, impaired digestion (*disaccharidase deficiency* or *pancreatic insufficiency*), or reduced absorptive surface area (*mucosal atrophy* or *short bowel*). An osmotic diarrhea may occur if excessive amounts of carbohydrates are consumed, overwhelming the absorptive mechanisms.

## Fat

Fats, the main energy source of the infant, are essential to normal development. Fatty acids are necessary for brain development and are an integral part of all cell membranes. Unlike proteins and carbohydrates, fat can be stored in the body in nearly unlimited amounts and is an important source of stored energy.

The major lipid classes consist of glycerides, phospholipids, sterols and fatty acids. *Glycerides* are the result of esterification of glycerol and fatty acids. Three forms occur in nature: monoglycerides, diglycerides and triglycerides. These compounds result from ester links between glycerol and one, two or three fatty acids, respectively. Triglycerides are the most abundant lipid in animal tissue and serve as an important energy source. *Phospholipids* are found in all biologic membranes and are important in oxidative phosphorylation, membrane transport, and electron transport reactions. Phospholipids may be subdivided into three classes: derivatives of glycerol-3-phosphate, sphingosine and glycolipids. *Sterols* are alcohols with a cyclopentanoperhydrophenanthrene skeletal structure. Cholesterol is the principal sterol.

*Fatty acids* are a major energy source and serve as precursors of prostaglandins. Most naturally occurring fatty acids are straight-chained saturated or unsaturated acids containing an even number of carbon atoms. Palmitic acid and stearic acid are by far the most commonly occurring and widely distributed of the saturated fatty acids. The nomenclature of unsaturated fatty acids specifies the total number of carbon atoms and the total number of double bonds that are present. Families of unsaturated fatty acids are defined based on the location of the first double bond, counting from the methyl or ω terminus. Oleic (ω9 family) and linoleic acid (ω6 family) are the most common unsaturated fatty acids. Linolenic (ω3 family) and linoleic acids are considered essential fatty acids and must be supplied in the diet. It has been estimated that 1–4 per cent of total fat intake should consist of polyunsaturated fats from the ω6 family. An elevated triene/tetraene ratio (>0.4) is used as an indicator of essential fatty acid deficiency. The rationale for the use of this ratio is that although the ω9, ω6, and ω3 fatty acids all compete for the same desaturase enzymes in their respective metabolic pathways, ω6 and ω3 fatty acids have a greater affinity for the desaturase that forms tetraene than do ω9 fatty acids. Therefore, when the diet is deficient in linoleic acid (ω6 fatty acid), production of tetraenes is diminished and production of trienes from ω9 fatty acids is increased. Linolenic acid and its longer-chained derivatives (in particular, docosahexaenoic acid) are important to brain development, cell proliferation, myelination, and retinal functions. The developing central nervous system incorporates significant amounts of polyunsaturated fatty acids of 20 carbons or greater; it has been speculated that preterm infants may not be able to desaturate and chain-elongate 18-carbon polyunsaturated fatty acids for several weeks to months following birth.

## WATER-SOLUBLE VITAMINS

## Vitamin C (ascorbic acid)

Ascorbic acid is involved in the synthesis of neurotransmitters, may play an important role as an antioxidant, and is important in enhancing hydroxylation reactions of many biosynthetic reactions, such as *p*-hydroxyphenylpyruvic acid oxidase. Deficiency of ascorbic acid results in petechial hemorrhages and *scurvy*. Infantile scurvy may present with findings of tenderness, swelling, and pseudoparalysis of the lower extremities. Failure to thrive is a common characteristic of preterm infants with scurvy.

Ascorbic acid requirements of preterm infants may be greater than those of term infants due to the hyperoxic environment resulting from mechanical ventilation and transient tyrosinemia and/or relatively high protein intake. Ascorbic acid concentrations of milk are reduced by pasteurization and exposure to iron, copper and $O_2$. High ascorbic acid intake may result in acidosis, decreased vitamin $B_{12}$ absorption, and enhanced iron absorption.

## Vitamin $B_1$ (thiamin)

Thiamin is absorbed by both passive and active transport in the small intestine and is phosphorylated in the intestinal mucosa to form thiamin pyrophosphate and adenylic acid. Thiamin functions as a coenzyme in the metabolism of branched-chain amino acids and of carbohydrates, such as the oxidative decarboxylation of alpha keto acids and pyruvate and transketolase reactions of the pentose pathway.

Deficiency of thiamin during infancy results in *beriberi* and is accompanied by apathy, anorexia, vomiting and restlessness, which can lead to dyspnea, cyanosis and congestive heart failure. Thiamin is inactivated by alkaline solutions, heat, and ionizing radiation. No toxic effects have been noted with high oral doses of thiamin.

## Riboflavin

Riboflavin, as part of the coenzymes flavine adenine dinucleotide (FAD) and flavine mononucleotide (FMN), is involved in metabolism of glucose, fatty acids, and amino acids. Riboflavin deficiency results primarily in abnormalities involving the epithelium (stomatitis, cheilosis, glossitis, seborrheic dermatitis), normocytic anemia, and vascularization of the cornea.

Biochemical riboflavin deficiency, without any clinical signs, has been reported in term infants fed human milk during phototherapy: riboflavin is inactivated by light, particularly that emitted from phototherapy. Toxicity of riboflavin is unlikely in term infants as excess riboflavin can be excreted by the kidney. This may not be the case in preterm infants because renal clearance of riboflavin may be inadequate.

## Vitamin $B_6$ (pyridines)

Pyridoxine (pyridoxol), pyridoxal and pyridoxamine are the three naturally occurring pyridines. Vitamin $B_6$ refers to these three pyridines, in addition to the phosphates of the latter two, pyridoxal-5-phosphate and pyridoxamine-5-phosphate, which are the major forms of vitamin $B_6$ found in blood. Vitamin $B_6$ is important in the biosynthesis of heme and prostaglandins, carbohydrate metabolism, immune development, and conversion of tryptophan to niacin and serotonin.

Vitamin $B_6$ deficiency in infants may result in hypochromic microcytic anemia, vomiting, diarrhea, failure to thrive, listlessness, hyperirritability, and seizures. *Pyridoxine-dependent seizures in the neonate, pyridoxine-responsive hypochromic microcytic anemia, xanthurenic aciduria, cystathioninuria,* and *homocystinuria* are syndromes that require pharmacologic doses of vitamin $B_6$ for adequate function. High dietary protein intakes increase the need for vitamin $B_6$, which is destroyed upon exposure to light. Pyridoxine is used for fortification due to the sensitivity of pyridoxal and pyridoxamine forms to heat. Vitamin $B_6$ deficiency may occur during isoniazid treatment (binding of drug to vitamin) or when an infant is fed human milk from a vitamin $B_6$-deficient mother or exclusively breast-fed for extended periods of time (low vitamin $B_6$ content in milk). Although high doses of pyridoxine do not appear to be toxic, there is a report of sensory neuropathy in adults ingesting megadoses of pyridoxine.

## Vitamin $B_{12}$ (cobalamin)

Vitamin $B_{12}$ is necessary for DNA synthesis and red blood cell formation. The initial release of cobalamin from dietary proteins is facilitated by gastric acid and pepsin. Cobalamin binds to R proteins (haptocorrin) in the stomach, because their affinity for cobalamin is greater than that of intrinsic factor. R proteins are found in saliva, gastric juice and biliary secretions. Whether cobalamin binds to R proteins, however, is dependent upon the oral dose of cobalamin, gastric pH, and the amount of R proteins and intrinsic factor present. Pancreatic proteases degrade R proteins and release cobalamin, which then avidly binds to intrinsic factor and resists digestion by proteases. Intrinsic factor is synthesized by gastric parietal cells and protects cobalamin from bacteria within the intestinal lumen. The cobalamin-intrinsic factor complex binds to specific receptors in the distal small intestine, a process that requires $Ca^{2+}$, but not energy. The complex is believed to be taken up by the enterocyte and split intracellularly, although intrinsic factor is not absorbed into the blood. Cobalamin then binds to transcobalamin II, either within or at the serosal surface and is released into plasma. Release may occur through receptor-mediated endocytosis. When large amounts of cobalamin are ingested, passive diffusion along the length of the small intestine can also occur. Studies in piglets suggest that sows' milk contains a cobalamin-binding protein that promotes cobalamin uptake in newborn piglets more effectively than intrinsic factor.

*Vitamin $B_{12}$ deficiency* may result from congenital defects in absorption and metabolism (lack of intrinsic factor, inborn error of metabolism), surgical resection of terminal ileum (necrotizing enterocolitis, malformations), or bacterial overgrowth in the ileum. Nutritional deficiency may occur in infants fed human milk from strict vegetarian mothers. Manifestations of vitamin $B_{12}$ deficiency include megaloblastic anemia and demyelinization of the spinal cord. In adults, administration of large doses of folic acid may mask vitamin $B_{12}$ deficiency and cause irreversible neurologic damage. Toxicity from vitamin $B_{12}$ has not been reported.

## Niacin

The term niacin refers to nicotinic acid and nicotinamide. Nicotinamide, the predominant form of the vitamin, is a component of the coenzymes nicotinamide adenine dinucleotide (NAD) and nicotinamide adenine dinucleotide phosphate (NADP). Niacin is involved in numerous metabolic processes including fat synthesis, glycolysis, and intracellular respiration. Because of the role of NAD and NADP in the respiratory chain, the allowances for niacin are related to energy expenditure. Approximately 3 per cent of dietary tryptophan is converted to niacin in adults. However, there are no data on this conversion in infants.

Deficiency of niacin results in *pellagra*, which is characterized by a cutaneous inflammation, weakness, inflammation of mucous membranes, diarrhea, vomiting, dysphagia, and in severe cases, dementia. Excessive amounts of niacin may result in cutaneous vasodilatation, reduced serum cholesterol concentrations, arrhythmias, abnormal liver function tests, jaundice, increased gastric acid secretion, and gastrointestinal hypermotility.

## Biotin

Biotin is a coenzyme that is important in fat and carbohydrate metabolism as a component of several carboxylase enzymes. Under normal situations, biotin deficiency is rare. Biotin is produced by intestinal bacteria; the use of antibiotics may decrease biotin synthesis by intestinal flora. There are no reports of toxicity from biotin.

## Folic acid

Folate is a coenzyme necessary for many of the reactions in the synthesis of nucleic acids and in the metabolism of some amino acids. Risk factors for *folate deficiency* are prematurity (rapid growth and decreased hepatic stores), hemolytic disease of the newborn (increased erythropoiesis), anticonvulsant therapy (interference with digestion), prolonged use of antibiotics (decreased production from intestinal bacteria), and any malabsorption syndrome. Manifestations of folate deficiency include, in order of appearance: low serum folate, hypersegmentation of neutrophils, low red cell folate, and macrocytic anemia. Poor growth has been found in some studies. No toxic effects have been reported for folate; however, theoretically, large amounts of folate may partially reverse the anticonvulsant effect of diphenylhydantoin and phenobarbital.

## Pantothenic acid

The primary role of pantothenic acid is its incorporation into coenzyme A, the active factor required for metabolic acetylation processes. Deficiency of pantothenic acid is rare in the human, but may accompany severe malnutrition. Very high doses of pantothenic acid may result in diarrhea.

## FAT-SOLUBLE VITAMINS

Fat malabsorption occurs due to a variety of defects including bile acid deficiencies due to liver disease or bacterial overgrowth of the bowel, pancreatic enzyme deficiencies, and disorders of mucosal function, such as celiac disease. Fat-soluble vitamin deficiencies may occur in any of these clinical settings.

## Vitamin A

Vitamin A exists in several isomeric forms: the basic component of vitamin A is all-*trans* retinol. Retinol is absorbed in the small intestine, incorporated into chylomicrons, and transported to the liver where it is stored and mobilized as a specific complex of retinol-binding protein. Retinol, following isomerization and combination with opsin to form rhodopsin, facilitates visual processing in the rod cells of the retina. Retinol also appears to have a role in regulation and differentiation of epithelial cells. The classic signs of deficiency (night blindness, dry cornea and perifollicular dermatitis) have no practical value in the newborn because overt clinical signs have not been reported. Newborns at risk for *vitamin A deficiency* are those with any form of fat malabsorption (decreased absorption), those born preterm (low hepatic stores), those with bronchopulmonary dysplasia (possible increased requirements due to the healing process), and those on total parenteral nutrition (adherence of vitamin A to plastic intravenous tubings). There is no evidence of dietary deficiency of vitamin A with either formula or human milk feeding of term infants.

Toxicity from vitamin A may occur. Acute toxicity has occurred from single doses of 100 000 IU or more given to infants and includes bulging cranial fontanelles accompanied by nausea, vomiting, fever and neurologic symptoms. Symptoms of chronic toxicity include dry skin, alopecia and headaches. Continued high doses can lead to hepatotoxicity and death.

## Vitamin D (*see also* Chapter 43)

Vitamin D is a fat-soluble vitamin that is necessary for maintaining $Ca^{2+}$ and $PO_4$ homeostasis. Vitamin D is transported to the liver where it is converted to 25-hydroxyvitamin D (25(OH)D), which is often used as an indicator of vitamin D status. 25(OH)D is further converted in the kidney to 1,25-dihydroxyvitamin D (1,25(OH)$_2$D), the most biologically active metabolite of vitamin D. The conversion of 25(OH)D to 1,25(OH)$_2$D is dependent upon the individual's $Ca^{2+}$, $PO_4$, and parathyroid hormone (PTH) status. 1,25(OH)$_2$D increases intestinal absorption and decreases renal excretion of $Ca^{2+}$ and $PO_4$. In conjunction with PTH, 1,25(OH)$_2$D also results in release of $Ca^{2+}$ and $PO_4$ from bone. Deficiency of vitamin D results in disturbances of $Ca^{2+}$ and $PO_4$ homeostasis and ultimately in *rickets*.

Theoretically, vitamin D is not a vitamin because it can be produced endogenously in the skin and is more appropriately considered a hormone. Vitamin D, if not obtained through the diet, is produced endogenously in the epidermis of skin upon exposure to ultraviolet radiation. Unlike other vitamins, vitamin D is not present in significant amounts in naturally occurring food items except oily fish; human milk concentrations of vitamin D also are low. Sunshine exposure results in a significant increase in serum 25(OH) vitamin D concentrations to well within the range where vitamin D deficiency is not observed. Vitamin D supplementation of human milk-fed infants who are not receiving sunshine exposure appears to be necessary to maintain adequate vitamin D status.

Alterations in the metabolism of vitamin D have been proposed as factors in the development of *hypocalcemia* or rickets in preterm infants. The administration of the biologically active vitamin D, both orally and intravenously, for the prevention of hypocalcemia have been investigated. However, only pharmacological doses have been found to be effective and these doses are not recommended until possible long-term or subtle biologic effects are investigated.

## Vitamin E

Vitamin E comprises a group of fat-soluble compounds (tocopherols and tocotrienols) with similar biological roles. α-Tocopherol is the most active of these compounds, and accounts for more than 90 per cent of the vitamin E in human tissues. Due to the different biological activities of the different forms of vitamin E, preparations have been standardized to International Units. The primary role for vitamin E is as an antioxidant. Vitamin E scavenges free radicals that are generated by the reduction of molecular $O_2$ and as normal by-products of oxidative enzymes; thus vitamin E inhibits the naturally occurring peroxidation of polyunsaturated fatty acids in the lipid layers of cell membranes.

Vitamin E status is assessed by measurement of tocopherol in blood. Due to the influence of circulating lipids on tocopherol concentrations, it is preferable to express plasma α-tocopherol as a ratio to cholesterol or total lipid. Vitamin E requirements are increased with high intakes of polyunsaturated fatty acids and, in infants or children, with fat malabsorption. Vitamin E requirements also are increased in preterm infants due to limited tissue stores at birth, poor absorption of fat, and rapid postnatal growth.

Vitamin E is toxic at pharmacological doses. A syndrome of pulmonary deterioration, thrombocytopenia, and liver and renal failure in very-low-birth-weight infants was associated with the use of parenteral α-tocopherol (E-Ferol) in preterm infants. The risk of sepsis and necrotizing enterolitis also may be increased in preterm infants receiving high doses of vitamin E. Thus, extreme caution should be given in treating infants with pharmacologic doses of vitamin E.

## Vitamin K

Vitamin K is necessary for hepatic synthesis of coagulation factors II, VII, IX, X and for the conversion of inactive precursors to the active form of clotting factors. Vitamin $K_1$ (phylloquinone) is synthesized by plants, while vitamin $K_2$ (menaquinone) can be synthesized in animals. In normal adults, up to 50 per cent of the total supply might come from intestinal synthesis by bacterial flora. Because the human infant has a very low storage capacity for vitamin K and the vitamin has a rapid turnover, the time required to reach a deficiency state is deemed to be short.

Vitamin K deficiency is associated with *hemorrhagic disease of the newborn* (HDN), recently subdivided into three categories:

- early HDN, occurring within the first 24 hours after birth and usually associated with maternal anticonvulsant therapy;
- classic HDN occurring between 1 and 7 days after birth;
- late HDN, occurring after 2–4 weeks, which is presently the most common form.

Common factors associated with HDN are a low intake of vitamin K (no supplementation at birth and breast feeding) and, as with all other fat-soluble vitamins, any form of fat malabsorption. There are few data on the toxicity of vitamin K in the human. There does not appear to be any toxicity from phylloquinone since it has become available for use as a prophylaxis.

## MINERALS

## Calcium, phosphorus, magnesium *(see also Chapter 43)*

$Ca^{2+}$, $PO_4$, and $Mg^{2+}$ are essential for tissue structure and function. Mineral absorption is discussed in Chapter 56. Hypocalcemia in the neonatal period may result in seizures; several studies in human infants have shown electroencephalographic seizures during clinically asymptomatic hypocalcemia. Chronic deficiency of $Ca^{2+}$ and $PO_4$ results in bone demineralization or rickets. Toxicity of $Ca^{2+}$ results in high circulating concentrations of these minerals and possible *nephrolithiasis*, *nephrocalcinosis*, bradycardia, and hypertension. Blood concentrations of $Ca^{2+}$, $PO_4$, and $Mg^{2+}$ are maintained within physiological ranges through the combined effects of parathyroid hormone (PTH); 1,25-dihydroxyvitamin D, the biologically active metabolite of vitamin D, and calcitonin. Chronic deficiency of $Mg^{2+}$ may result in an inability to maintain serum $Ca^{2+}$ within physiologic ranges due to the $Mg^{2+}$ requirement of the parathyroid glands for normal functioning.

Cows' milk-based formula feeding during the first postnatal week appears to result in a higher serum $PO_4$ and possibly a lower serum ionized $Ca^{2+}$ concentration than those found in infants fed human milk. Although the clinical significance of these findings is not clear, these studies support the hypothesis that infants fed formula containing high phosphate may be at increased risk for late neonatal hypocalcemia; however, because this disorder is rare, additional risk factors must be present.

Additional $Ca^{2+}$ and $PO_4$ in formula-fed, preterm infants appears to improve net $Ca^{2+}$ retention and bone mineralization, as indicated by increased bone mineral content and lower serum alkaline phosphatase concentrations in those infants receiving high $Ca^{2+}$ and $PO_4$ formula compared with those receiving standard formula.

## Trace elements

Trace elements by definition constitute less than 0.01 per cent of body mass. Those considered essential include iron, zinc, copper, selenium, chromium, manganese, molybdenum, iodine, fluorine and cobalt. Other trace elements may include arsenic, lithium, nickel, silicon, vanadium, bromium, cadmium, lead and tin.

### Iron

Many iron-containing compounds, such as hemoglobin, the cytochromes, and iron–sulfur proteins that are involved in the transport and utilization of $O_2$ for the production of cellular energy. Ferritin and hemosiderin contribute to the maintenance of iron homeostasis. There are marked age-related changes in hemoglobin concentrations following birth; high hemoglobin concentrations at birth resulting from a relative hypoxic environment *in utero* are followed by 4–6 weeks of a marked depression in the rate of red blood cell production and a decline in hemoglobin concentrations. At about 2 months of age, hemoglobin concentrations begin to rise. They plateau at 12.5 g/dl at about 6 months; concentrations then are maintained at this level through age 4 years.

*Iron deficiency*, defined as a lack of iron resulting in a restriction of hemoglobin synthesis, usually is a result of an iron-poor diet and rarely develops prior to 4–6 months of age. Ingesting cows' milk early in infancy also may result in iron deficiency from blood loss in the gastrointestinal tract. Iron stores may be become marginal in unsupplemented human milk-fed infants or in unfortified formula-fed infants around 6 months of age. Because preterm infants have a lower iron store at birth than term infants, iron supplementation or introduction of iron fortified formula should occur at an earlier age in this population.

Measurement of hemoglobin concentrations is one of the most useful laboratory assessments for *iron deficiency anemia*. Red cell indices also are important: mean red cell volume (MCV) decreases with or without a low mean red cell hemoglobin (MCH) in iron deficiency. Confirmatory findings include a low serum ferritin (depressed only in iron deficiency), elevated erythrocyte protoporphyrin (also occurs during infection or lead toxicity), or a low transferrin saturation (serum iron/iron binding capacity which also can occur during infection).

## Zinc

Zinc is an essential cofactor for many enzymes such as DNA and RNA polymerases and alkaline phosphatase. Zinc deficiency results in reduced growth velocity, acro-orificial skin rash, hypoproteinemia, and generalized edema. An autosomal recessive disorder, *acrodermatitis enteropathica*, results from a selective defect in the intestinal absorption of zinc. Long-term exclusively breast-fed infants along with children consuming vegetarian diets may be at a risk of zinc deficiency due to low amounts of this mineral in the diet. *Zinc toxicity* results in copper deficiency and increased cholesterol concentrations.

## Copper

Copper is a coenzyme for many oxidative enzymes involved in collagen and melanin synthesis. In plasma, copper is bound to ceruloplasmin. In the fetus, copper is accumulated mainly in liver during the last trimester of pregnancy. Although preterm infants have smaller copper stores than term infants, their hepatic stores are significant. In the normal infant serum copper concentrations are very low due to limited ceruloplasmin synthesis. Therefore, neither serum copper nor ceuroloplasmin concentrations appear to be good indices of copper status. *Menkes disease* is an inheritable X-linked recessive disorder of copper absorption. Abnormalities include hypopigmentation, bone changes, thrombosis, arterial rupture, progressive cerebral degeneration, and hypothermia. Both serum copper and ceruloplasmin concentrations are very low. *Wilson disease* is a disorder of copper balance. Copper absorption is thought to be normal, but biliary secretion is impaired and high levels of copper accumulate in the body. Abnormalities include hepatitis,

central nervous system impairment, bone demineralization, ophthalmic abnormalities, and hemolytic anemia. Copper toxicity is rare in humans.

## Selenium

Selenium is an important part of the enzyme glutathione peroxidase (GSHPx), which is involved in protecting cells from oxidative damage by destroying cytosolic hydrogen peroxides. Selenium deficiency previously occurred in patients receiving total parenteral nutrition that was not supplemented with selenium and also occurs in free-living populations that reside in areas with low soil selenium concentrations. Clinical symptoms of deficiency include muscle pain and weakness predominantly in the extremities. *Keshan disease*, a selenium-responsive syndrome, has been found to occur in infants, young children, and women of child-bearing age in rural China. The syndrome is characterized by necrosis and fibrosis of the myocardium resulting in acute or chronic heart failure. Erythrocyte fragility associated with low blood selenium concentrations also has been reported in orally-fed preterm infants. Selenium is highly toxic, and blood levels are often monitored during supplementation; a concentration >800 ng/mL is thought to be hazardous to children. Symptoms of toxicity include loss of hair, roughening of nails, nausea and fatigue.

## Chromium

Chromium is important in glucose metabolism because it may potentiate the action of insulin at the cell membrane. Although very rare, chromium deficiency may result after long-term total parenteral nutrition when glucose is utilized as the major energy source. Absorption of chromium is poor, and it is thought to be relatively non-toxic.

## Manganese

Animal studies have indicated that the most vulnerable period for manganese deficiency is during gestation and early infancy. Manganese is important in glycosaminoglycan synthesis, carbohydrate metabolism, lipid metabolism, and central nervous system function. Clinical deficiency of manganese has not been observed in humans. Manganese homeostasis is regulated by the liver, and large doses have been shown to cause mild intrahepatic cholestasis in animals.

## Molybdenum

Molybdenum is involved in sulfur metabolism, where it is incorporated into three known enzymes: sulfite oxidase, xanthine oxidase/dehydrogenase, and aldehyde dehydrogenase. The most important, sulfite oxidase, catalyzes the oxidation of sulfite to sulfate, the terminal step in degradative sulfur metabolism. Molybdenum deficiency is uncommon, although there are several inborn errors of molybdenum metabolism (sulfite oxidase deficiency, xanthine oxidase deficiency, and combined deficiencies of sulfite and xanthine oxidases).

## Iodine

The only known function of iodine is its integral part of the thyroid hormones. Iodine is readily absorbed and taken up by the thyroid gland where it is bound to thyroglobulin, an iodinated glycoprotein from which thyroxine ($T_4$) and triiodothyronine ($T_3$) are formed. The role of iodine in thyroid hormone synthesis is discussed in Chapter 37. Iodine deficiency is rare in regions where supplementation programs (addition to table salt) exist or where soil concentrations are high. Unfortunately, many areas of the world still have a high prevalence of dietary iodine deficiency resulting in goiter and neonatal deficiency. Excessive iodine results in *thyrotoxic goiter*; in the United States, goiter in children is now likely to be associated with higher than normal iodine intakes.

## Fluoride

Fluoride is important in the prevention of dental caries; it strengthens dental enamel by substituting for hydroxyl ions in the hydroxyapatite crystalline mineral matrix of the enamel. Fluoride is incorporated into enamel during the mineralization stage; the resulting fluorapatite is more resistant to both chemical and physical damage. Because the major source of fluoride is water, the need for supplementation will depend on the fluorine exposure of the child from the local water supply. Excessive amounts of fluoride results in *fluorosis* or mottling of the enamel. Acute ingestion of very large amounts of fluoride may cause cardiac and respiratory abnormalities and hypocalcemia.

## SELECTED READING

Farrell PM. Essentials of pediatric nutrition. In: Rudolph AM ed. *Rudolph's pediatrics,* 19th edn. Norwalk, CT: Appleton & Lange, 1991: 215.

Tsang, RC ed. *Vitamin and mineral requirements in preterm infants.* New York: Marcel Dekker, Inc., 1985.

Tsang RC, Nichols BL eds. *Nutrition during infancy.* Philadelphia: Hanley and Belfus, Inc., 1988.

# PART ELEVEN

# *Cardiovascular System*

**Editor: Michael A. Heymann**

# 67

# Vascular Development and Function

## VASCULAR GROWTH AND DEVELOPMENT

The cardiovascular system is the first organ system that forms during embryonic development, beginning to develop when diffusion no longer is able to satisfy the nutritional requirements of the embryo. As morphogenesis of organs begins, vascular channels and capillary plexuses are established throughout stromal tissue, a process essential for continued development of the organ. Numerous studies have begun to elucidate the manner in which various tissues and organs are vascularized. Two separate processes of vascular development, resulting in apparently identical vessels, have been described (Fig. 67.1 schematically illustrates these processes). In the first model, termed *vasculogenesis*, pre-existing endothelial cell precursors or angioblasts are thought to assemble *in situ* to form primitive vascular channels. These channels remodel, giving rise to arteries, veins, and lymphatics. The stimuli and information directing the angioblast to form a particular specialized channel apparently is contained within the surrounding mesenchyme at the site where vascular organization begins. The angioblasts, after organizing into a visible endothelium, either induce the expression of smooth muscle phenotype in the surrounding mesenchyme or recruit existing smooth muscle cells to the forming vessels. In the second model, termed *angiogenesis*, capillaries form by budding or sprouting from pre-existing venules or capillaries. The process of angiogenesis has received a great deal of attention both in embryogenesis as well as in physiological and pathophysiological states. Depending on the tissue studied, vasculogenesis and angiogenesis make greater or lesser contributions to the process of vascularization. There is a consensus that vascularization in the lung, pancreas, and spleen occurs by vasculogenesis, whereas angiogenesis is responsible for development of tissue vasculature in kidney, brain, and retina. As the organ, and thus blood vessels, continue to grow and develop, significant morphological, gene, protein, and functional changes occur in cells of the vessel wall. An understanding of the processes involved in normal vessel wall development is crucial because any external pathophysiological stimulus applied to this changing baseline will have a significant impact on the phenotypic expression of the vascular wall cell. Thus the characteristics of the vascular response to a given stimulus vary with age and state of vascular development at the time of onset of injury.

## NORMAL VASCULAR DEVELOPMENT: STRUCTURE AND FUNCTION

### Structure

Many studies of normal developmental changes in the vasculature have used rat aorta. In the rat embryo (term gestation 21–22 days), the tunica media develops around the endothelial tube at about 12.5 days' gestation when actomyosin filaments are first visible in a cell

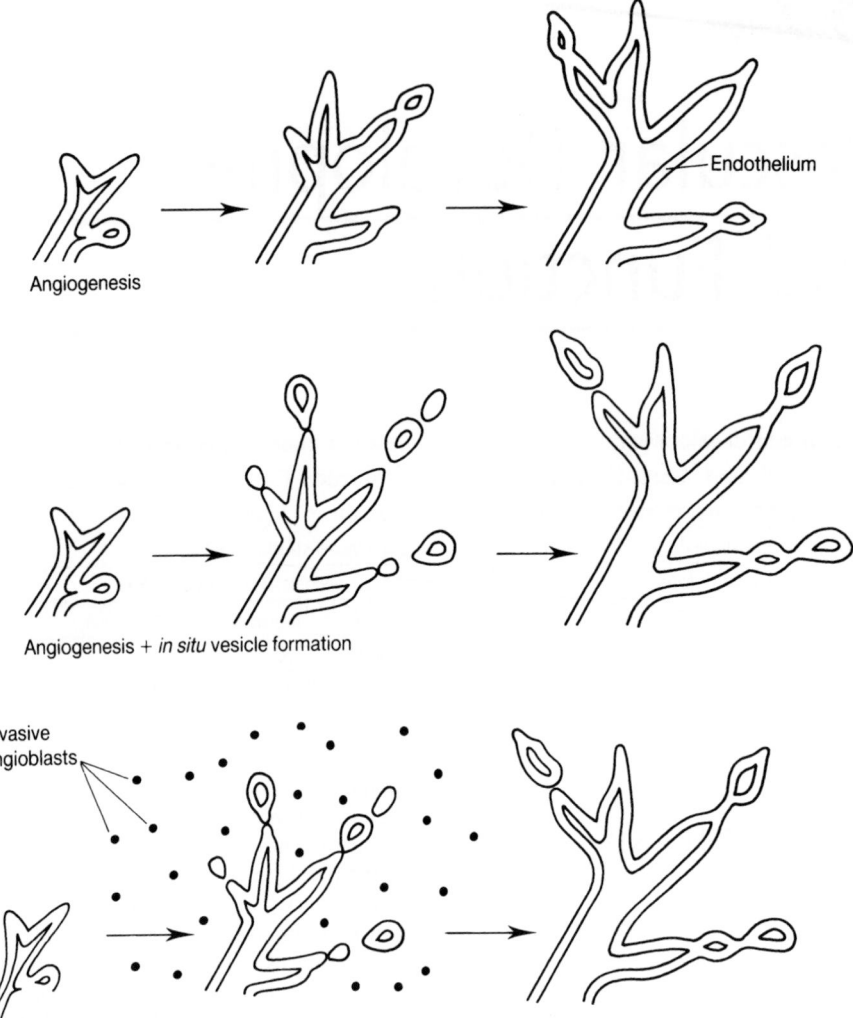

Angiogenesis

Endothelium

Angiogenesis + *in situ* vesicle formation

Invasive angioblasts

Angiogenesis + *in situ* vesicle formation + contributions by invasive angioblasts

FIGURE 67.1 Schematic representation of the processes by which embryonic blood vessels may develop. Angiogenesis results in the formation of sprouts and branches from existing branches. In some instances, endothelial vesicles form independent of existing vessels, and subsequently all endothelial populations coalesce to form new channels. Developing vessels may be formed or receive contributions from invasive angioblasts (shown in black) that move throughout embryonic mesenchyme. (Redrawn from Noden DM. *Am Rev Respir Dis* 1989; **140**: 1097.)

layer surrounding the endothelium. As development proceeds, cell proliferation continues, matrix protein synthesis begins, and lamellar units are established. While the basic structure of the rat aorta is developed by birth, growth of the aorta continues postnatally. Quantitative morphological analysis has indicated that the doubling of wall thickness that occurs in the rat aorta between 1 and 11 days postnatal age is due to the combined effect of a nearly 2-fold increase in muscle cell volume, a 2.6-fold increase in the number of muscle cells, and 8- and 10-fold increases in the amount of elastin and collagen, respectively. The replication index of smooth muscle cells within the aorta during embryonic life (through embryonic day 17) averages 75–80 per cent and slows considerably during the transition to fetal life, averaging 40 per cent for the remainder of fetal life. During postnatal life, the growth of the aorta continues to slow gradually and declines to adult levels by 90 days. In normal adult animals, the replication index of smooth muscle cells in an uninjured vessel is only 0.06 per cent per day. During normal development there is a progressive increase in the DNA ploidy of medial smooth muscle cells and the percentage of tetraploid ($4n$) cells reaches approximately 10 per cent by 12 weeks of age. Virtually nothing is known concerning the significance of this developmental change in smooth muscle cell DNA content. There is a marked heterogeneity between the developmental responses of large and small vessels. Morphometric analysis of arteries less than 250 mm in outer diameter indicates that smooth muscle cell size, but not number, increases during postnatal development.

Extracellular matrix protein production by cells of the vascular wall also changes significantly during the course of normal development. The connective tissue elements of the vascular wall are complex and include molecules from virtually every class of extracellular matrix: elastin, collagens, proteoglycans, and structural and adhesive glycoproteins. The relative proportions of each matrix component appear to reflect either the physical and functional properties expected of a particular vascular segment or the forces to which that vascular segment is exposed. Vascular protein composition therefore changes significantly with development and with type and location of the vessel studied. For example, elastin is the most abundant protein in major arteries subjected to large pulsatile pressures generated by cardiac contraction. Elastogenic progenitor cells giving rise to at least some of the smooth muscle cells that constitute the aorta, and other elastic vessels, arise from mesenchyme adjacent to the myocardium. Elastogenic activity in these cells, at least in developing chick aorta, appears in an orderly, sequential proximal-to-distal deployment, beginning nearest the heart and advancing downstream into all nascent elastic vessels. In the developing rat aorta, peak elastin synthesis occurs during late fetal and early postnatal life and remains high through the first postnatal month. By 2 months, tropoelastin expression is virtually undetectable and no significant tropoelastin is produced by the normal adult vascular smooth muscle cells. As distance from the heart increases, a progressive decrease in the amount of elastin and a progressive increase in the amount of collagen is observed. Mature crosslinked collagen is much stiffer than elastin and thus confers different structural properties to the vessel wall. Collagens are an important family of structural proteins localized in the basement membrane and interstitial spaces of the vascular wall. Many excellent studies have evaluated accumulation of collagen in both systemic and pulmonary vessels during normal development. The amount of collagen in a vessel wall depends on both age and site of the vessel studied. Furthermore, the amount of this fibrous protein, like elastin, can be correlated with differences in vascular wall tension that normally occur in different arteries during growth.

Immunohistochemical studies have evaluated the appearance and distribution of various collagen types in the developing pulmonary artery. The interstitial collagens are deposited in the order of types V, III, and then I during embryonic development. The amount of types I and V collagen in pulmonary arterial media increases with age. Particularly striking is the paucity of type I collagen in resistance-sized pulmonary arteries of the newborn compared with the adult lung. Interesting functional implications can be drawn from these studies. Type I collagen is characterized by a high tensile strength; large quantities of this protein are prominent in tissues that are relatively indistensible. On the other hand, type III collagen is present in distensible connective tissue as is found in the uterus. The relative lack of type I collagen in neonatal pulmonary vessels may explain the plasticity of the pulmonary arteries in early life. As the cells composing the vessel wall change rapidly in shape and position during the first hours of life, and the vessel walls themselves are continually remodeled with growth, these events may be facilitated by the lack of type I collagen. Although present in small amounts, type I collagen appears crucial for the maintenance of vascular integrity during normal development because mutant mice, deficient in type I collagen, die at about 15 days' gestation with ruptured major blood vessels.

Although it has been common to characterize all vascular smooth muscle cells as expressing a common secretory phenotype, the secretory properties of the smooth muscle cell may differ depending on location of the cell within the vessel wall. For instance, secretory properties of smooth muscle cells in small arteries differ from those in conducting vessels or in veins. Recent information suggests a complex heterogeneity of the secretory phenotype of smooth muscle cells at any particular location in the vessel wall. For instance, at certain stages of development in the pulmonary artery, some cells appear actively to produce elastin and collagen and demonstrate very little synthesis of contractile proteins, whereas other cells at the same vessel location express neither collagen nor elastin mRNA, but clearly produce contractile proteins.

Significant changes also occur in expression of contractile and cytoskeletal proteins during normal development. Morphological studies have demonstrated that the volume percentage of myofilaments in the aorta increases from 5 per cent at birth to a maximum of 20 per cent at 8 weeks of age. The non-collagenous, alkaline soluble protein fraction of the vessel wall, which in part represents the contractile proteins, does not change after 10 weeks of age. Thus the net production of contractile protein increases during the first 10 weeks after birth and then remains constant. Concomitant with the increase in actin (a major smooth muscle cell contractile protein) content accompanying smooth muscle cell maturation is a switch from predominant expression of non-muscle β-actin by neonatal aortic smooth muscle cells to predominant expression of smooth muscle (SM)-specific α-actin isoforms by adult smooth muscle cells. In addition to this shift from non-muscle β-actin to the SM-specific form of α-actin during maturation, the cellular content of tropomyosin, vimentin, and desmin in aortic smooth muscle cells increases with age. Recently the SM2 isoform of SM-myosin heavy chain (SM-MHC) was found to be expressed only in adult blood vessels, while the SM1 isoform was found to be expressed earlier in development. Newborn rat aortic smooth muscle cells underexpressing α-actin isoforms exhibit a higher replication rate than α-actin-positive cells, suggesting an inverse correlation between acquisition of the adult phenotype and cell replication.

Studies in the developing human aorta recently have evaluated expression of the regulatory contractile proteins, h-caldesmon and calponin, in conjunction with expression of Sm-specific α-actin and SM-MHC. Actin and myosin are expressed far earlier in development than caldesmon and calponin, suggesting that these proteins, because they are involved in the regulation of contraction, may serve as markers of more highly differentiated smooth muscle cells. In addition, expression of meta-vinculin, a marker of microfilament–membrane association sites, also occurs later in development in more differentiated smooth muscle cells. Interestingly, these investigations have also demonstrated a heterogeneity of smooth muscle phenotype in adult pulmonary and aortic vessel wall. In the subendothelial part of the adult tunica intima, smooth muscle cells express SM-specific α-actin and SM-MHC but lack h-caldesmon, calponin, and meta-vinculin, indicating a much less well differentiated phenotype of these cells. Even the vascular media have now been shown to comprise multiple smooth muscle cell populations with distinct developmental lineages. Neither the reasons for the existence of these multiple smooth muscle cell populations nor the functional implications of their presence are known at present.

Clearly, then, substantial differences exist in the proliferative, secretory, and contractile phenotypes of fetal and adult vascular wall cells. One may reasonably assume that many more such differences exist and that these differences may play pivotal roles in the control of smooth muscle cell replication and gene expression in the adult fully differentiated vascular wall cell.

## Function

Significant changes also occur in the functional responses of the developing vessel to constrictor and dilator stimuli. Many of these changes are due to differences in ability to produce or respond to vasoactive stimuli. For instance, the maximum contractile response of vessel preparations changes significantly during development. Most work to date supports the hypothesis that the maximum contractile response, at least in conduit vessels, increases during early postnatal life and then either declines or remains unchanged at later ages. It has been suggested that in contrast to large vessels, small arteries do not undergo an increase in force generating ability with development, though extensive work in this area has not been performed. Changes in maximum contractile response that occur during development are not due to changes in the active length–tension properties of the muscle. The increase in maximum response early in development might be explained in part by the increasing proportion of actomyosin. However, the decline in this response observed in older animals cannot be explained by a loss of contractile material. Different actin isoforms may interact differently with myosin, which could result in differences in force generating ability. Also, the magnitude of change in maximum

response with development depends on the contractile agent. This observation suggests that developmental changes in excitation–contraction coupling may occur. Changes in the $ED_{50}$ for various contractile agents have been observed during development with large vessels from young animals usually demonstrating a higher sensitivity than adult vessels.

Changes in the ability to contract may be significantly influenced by endogenous activity or locally produced products that control cAMP or cGMP levels in cells within the vessel wall. In ovine pulmonary vascular smooth muscle, for instance, basal adenylyl cyclase activity decreases markedly during the last trimester of fetal development. Further, but lesser, decreases are noted between late gestation and adulthood. Prostacyclin ($PGI_2$) production is three-fold greater in late-gestation pulmonary artery than in the adult. Differences in the coupling of the β-adrenergic receptor to G-proteins ($G_s$ vs $G_i$) in fetal versus adult smooth muscle have been identified. A predominance of $G_i$ activity in fetal tissue, with resultant suppression of cAMP levels, has been observed. The ability of fetal endothelium to produce endothelium-derived relaxing factor (EDRF; i.e. nitric oxide, NO) is significantly less than the adult in response to at least certain agonists (e.g. acetylcholine). Changes in NO activity could account for some of the differences in response to agonists observed between fetal, neonatal, and adult tissues.

## FACTORS INFLUENCING VESSEL GROWTH AND CELL DIFFERENTIATION

Many factors contribute to regulation of new blood vessel growth by influencing cell number, production of extracellular matrix molecules, intracellular contractile proteins, and the state of cell differentiation. Among the factors considered to have the strongest influence are growth factors, vasoactive agents, components of the extracellular matrix, and intercellular interactions.

## Regulation of cell proliferation

As stated above, active cell proliferation occurs during vascular development. For smooth muscle cells, replication slows considerably in early fetal life, continues to decline throughout fetal life, and during early postnatal life, and then virtually ceases under normal conditions. Thus two important concepts and the factors controlling them need to be described. First, the stimuli and factors responsible for cell proliferation must be characterized. Second, and very important for normal growth and development, are investigations of the mechanisms that regulate or suppress endothelial and smooth muscle cell replication once morphogenesis is complete.

Many studies have confirmed roles for various growth factors such as fibroblast growth factors, type β transforming growth factors, the insulin-like growth factors, platelet-derived growth factors, and epidermal growth factors in influencing endothelial and smooth muscle cell proliferation *in vitro*; the *in vivo* roles of these factors during development have not been firmly established to date. However, because some of these growth factors play a role in vascular repair and disease, it is likely that they play a role in the developing vessel. Tables 67.1 and 67.2 list many locally produced and circulating factors known to influence vascular wall cell growth and matrix protein synthesis.

## Fibroblast growth factors (FGFs)

Compelling evidence suggests a role for the FGF family in the control of vascular growth. The FGFs are a family of mitogenic polypeptides of which the prototypic members are the acidic and basic FGFs. There is a 53 per cent sequence homology between basic and acidic FGFs, and both are highly conserved among species. This group of growth factors was characterized and, in fact, initially purified on the basis of their strong affinity for the glycosaminoglycan heparin. A unique characteristic of acidic and basic FGFs is the absence of a consensus signal sequence for secretion; these factors therefore do not appear to be secreted from cells by conventional means. The majority of biologically active proteins in cells known to synthesize

TABLE 67.1 Factors regulating vascular wall cell growth

| FACTORS | ENDOTHELIAL CELL | SMOOTH MUSCLE CELL | FIBROBLAST |
|---|---|---|---|
| bFGF | ↑ | ↑ | ↑ |
| aFGF | ↑ | ↑ | ↑ |
| IGF-I | ↑ | ↑ | ↑ |
| IGF-II | ↑ | ↑ | ↑ |
| Insulin | ↑ | ↑ | ↑ |
| TGFβ[a] | ↑ / ↓ | ↑ / ↓ | ↑ / ↓ |
| TGFα | ↑ | ND | ↑ |
| PDGF | ↔ | ↑ | ↑ |
| EGF | ↑ | ↑ | ↑ |
| HB-EGF | ↔ | ↑ | ND |
| PD-ECGF | ↑ | ↔ | ↔ |
| V-EGF (VPF) | ↑ | ↔ | ↔ |
| Serotonin | ↔ | ↑ | ND |
| Histamine | ↑ | ↑ | ND |
| TNFα | ↔ | ↓ | ↑ |
| IL-1 | ↓ | ↑ / ↓ | ↑ / ↓ |
| Heparan sulfates | ↔ | ↓ | ↓ |
| Interferons | ↓ | ↓ | ↓ |
| Prostaglandins (PGE$_2$, PGI$_2$) | ↔ | ↓ | ↓ |
| Leukotriene C$_4$ (LTC$_4$) | ND | ↑ | ↑ |
| PAF | ND | ↑ | ↑ |

↑, stimulates cell growth; ↓, inhibits cell growth; ↔, no effect on cell growth; ND, effect not determined.
[a] The effects of TGFβ are complex and depend on age of cell and conditions of cell confluency under which experiment was done.

TABLE 67.2 Factors regulating vascular wall matrix protein synthesis

| FACTORS | ELASTIN | TYPE I COLLAGEN |
|---|---|---|
| IGF-I | ↑ | ↑ |
| IGF-II | ↑ | ↑ |
| TGFβ | ↑ | ↑ |
| PDGF | ↑ | ↑ / ↔ |
| Leukotriene C$_4$ (LTC$_4$) | ND | ↑ |
| PAF | ↑ | ND |
| IL-1 | ↓ | ↑ / ↓[a] |
| EGF | ↓ | ↔ |
| PGE$_2$ | ↔ / ↓ | ↓ |
| Interferons | ↓ | ↓ |
| Protein kinase C activation | ↓ | ↓ |

↑, stimulates matrix protein synthesis; ↓, inhibits matrix protein synthesis; ↔, no effect on matrix protein synthesis; ND, effect not determined.
[a] The effects depend on fibroblast type studied.

basic FGF remain cell associated or are deposited into the extracellular matrix. Immunohistochemical analysis has demonstrated the presence of basic FGF in basement membranes in the cornea and skeletal muscle, suggesting that extracellular matrix may serve as a reservoir for basic FGF.

The FGFs have a variety of actions on cells from both mesodermal and neuroectodermal origin. Both acidic and basic FGFs are mitogenic and chemotactic for cells in the vascular wall, including large and small vessel endothelial cells, smooth muscle cells, and pericytes. FGF increases production of proteases by endothelial cells, a function probably important in the formation and remodeling of new blood vessels because movement of cells through the extracellular matrix requires breakdown of that matrix. Furthermore, a number of *in vivo* studies have demonstrated convincingly the ability of these factors to elicit the formation of new blood vessels. Both acidic and basic FGFs are present in high amounts in the major vessels of embryonic rats by day 14 (by immunohistochemical staining) and continue to be expressed by vascular cells into adult life. In a transplanted rat embryo model, antibodies to basic FGF retarded growth of the major vessels. In addition, these factors are important in wound healing and are associated with smooth muscle cell proliferation in atherosclerotic plaque. However, the mechanisms through which FGFs control vascular growth and differentiation remain to be determined.

## Transforming growth factor β (TGFβ)

The TGFβ family contains nearly 20 members; evidence suggests that members of this family play an important role in the control of vascularization. TGFβ stimulates new vessel growth *in vivo*, yet can inhibit smooth muscle cell and endothelial cell proliferation *in vitro*. These two apparently divergent responses to TGFβ demonstrate the importance of the microenvironment in which growth factors act in determining the ultimate effect they have on cells. The angiogenic effect of TGFβ may be due to its extremely potent chemoattraction for monocytic cells that may mediate neovascularization by the release of other angiogenic factors. Thus *in vivo* TGFβ may induce new vessel growth through either a direct or indirect action on endothelial cells. Further evidence suggests that TGFβ is probably important during normal vascular wall development. These peptides are capable of controlling the proliferation, biosynthetic phenotype, and differentiation of a variety of cell types. The effects of TGFβ on vascular smooth muscle cells, for instance, are diverse and include control over gene expression, organizational behavior, connective tissue synthesis, cell hypertrophy, and cell proliferation. TGFβ is a bifunctional, density-dependent regulator of smooth muscle proliferation, the actions of which may be mediated through distinct receptor subtypes. In adult cells, TGFβ causes inhibition of growth in sparsely plated cells and stimulates growth in confluent cells. However, preliminary work suggests that TGFβ always causes inhibition of growth in neonatal cells.

## Insulin-like growth factors (IGFs)

IGFs may play a role in vascular remodeling and, by analogy, in normal development of the blood vessel wall. IGF-I has mitogenic effects on aortic smooth muscle cells and significantly increases collagen and elastin production by smooth muscle cells as well as fibroblasts. Localization of IGF-I in the media by immunostaining varies with vascular load, suggesting that IGF-I expression is modulated by hemodynamic forces. IGF-I mRNA has been localized by *in situ* hybridization to adventitial areas of human fetal pulmonary arteries. Both porcine fibroblasts and aortic smooth muscle cells produce IGF-I *in vitro* and production by porcine aortic smooth muscle cells is stimulated by platelet-derived growth factor. In addition to local production within the vessel wall, IGF-I is present in serum in concentrations up to 1000 ng/mL, and serum-derived IGF-I could have increased access to the vascular media in the presence of an altered endothelial barrier function. Importantly, vascular smooth muscle cells have receptors for IGF-I and IGF-II (type I and type II receptors), and receptor expression appears to vary during vessel development. Less is known regarding the role of IGF-II and blood vessel development. IGF-II expression precedes that of IGF-I in the developing vessel, and IGF-II recently has been shown to have significant effects on the proliferation of neonatal smooth muscle cells and fibroblasts, in addition to increasing elastin and collagen synthesis. The effects of IGF-II on vascular wall cells, however, appear to be mediated through the type I IGF receptor.

## Platelet-derived growth factor (PDGF)

PDGF, an extremely potent mitogen for vascular smooth muscle cells and fibroblasts, is a 30-kD dimeric protein consisting of homodimers or heterodimers of two distinct polypeptide chains (the A and B chains). Three isoforms, AA, AB, and BB, and two receptor subtypes have been described. The A chain recognizes the α-receptor, and the B chain, in contrast, binds to either the α- or β-receptor. The receptor protein is a glycoprotein with tyrosine kinase activity. The receptor kinase activity is believed to generate a mitogenic signal leading to DNA synthesis. PDGF is stored in platelets (α-granules), and PDGF-like molecules are known to be synthesized by endothelial cells, smooth muscle cells, and activated macrophages. Growth factors, such as PDGF, produced locally in the vascular wall can act through separate receptors and signaling pathways to additively or synergistically effect cell proliferation. Fig. 67.2 schematically illustrates the multiple pathways through which various stimuli can initiate cell proliferation.

A role for PDGF in regulation of vascular wall development is suggested by experiments documenting its effects on cultured smooth muscle cells. In addition to its potent mitogenic effects on mesenchymal cells, PDGF is chemotactic for a variety of cells including neutrophils, monocytes, smooth muscle cells, and fibroblasts. These actions are not thought to be mediated through the tyrosine kinase receptor pathway. Furthermore a subtype of smooth muscle cells derived from neonatal rats express increased amounts of a PDGF-like mitogen. This neonatal smooth muscle cell subtype demonstrates autocrine growth characteristics, in contrast to the adult smooth muscle cells, suggesting a possible role for PDGF. Early mouse embryos express PDGF-AA and α-receptor mRNA. The appearance of the β-receptor lags two days behind, and the PDGF-BB product still later in development. Therefore, there is evidence that PDGF is developmentally regulated and may play a role in the proliferative response of smooth muscle cells *in vivo* during normal and abnormal vascular growth.

# Negative growth control mechanisms

Cells in mature vessel walls normally exhibit a very low index of replication. In addition, smooth muscle cells in the vessel wall are highly resistant to tumor formation, suggesting that at least in these cells, potent growth suppressive activities exist. This suggests that strict growth control mechanisms exist for smooth muscle cells of the adult vessel wall and that these mechanisms are largely absent in fetal (i.e. replicating) vessels or in neointima responding to atherosclerotic or other injurious mechanisms.

A variety of potential mechanisms (discussed below) may contribute to the establishment and/or

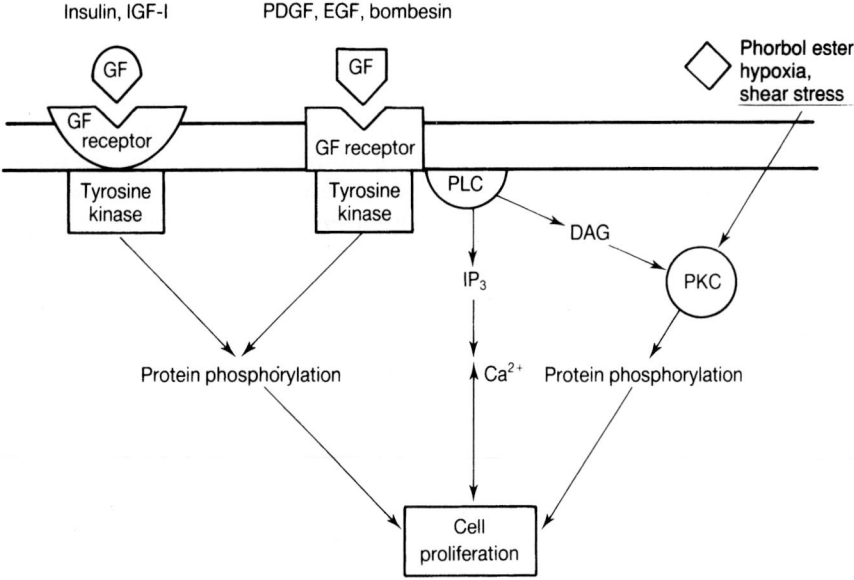

FIGURE 67.2 Schematic representation of the multiple pathways through which growth factors and other stimuli can act to stimulate cell proliferation. For instance, IGF-I appears to stimulate cell proliferation through a protein kinase C (PKC)-independent pathway. When agents are present that activate PKC, marked enhancement of the IGF-I effects occurs.

maintenance of smooth muscle cell quiescence following development. Active growth arrest could occur in response to inhibitors of smooth muscle cell replication such as heparin-like glycosaminoglycans, tumor necrosis factor α (TNFα), interferon-γ, or TGFβ. Further specific proteins from "tumor suppressor" genes (e.g. p53 or the retinoblastoma gene) may be responsible for suppression of cell proliferation in adult cells. While smooth muscle cells are capable of expressing each of these factors, the timing and expression of these potential active growth inhibitors during development and the contribution of these factors to growth inhibition *in vivo* are not known. It is also clear that novel, as yet unidentified growth inhibitors, operative in the vessel wall, may also exist. Should growth arrest in the developing vessel wall be dependent on the induced synthesis of an active growth inhibitor, much further work will be required to determine the physical or biochemical signals (such as $O_2$ environment) underlying the induction of this factor.

Passive growth arrest might result from absence of growth stimulatory cytokines, growth factors, or their receptors. Little is known about the expression of growth factors, cytokines, or receptors during smooth muscle cell development and maturation. As mentioned above, cultured neonatal rat smooth muscle cells secrete a PDGF-like mitogen that is not secreted by cultured adult cells; however, the mRNAs for both chains of PDGF are not significantly different in neonatal versus adult vessels *in vivo*. As suggested above, IGF-II expression has been demonstrated in fetal, but not in adult arteries. Fetal smooth muscle cells have been suggested to grow in an autocrine fashion in culture. If early arterial development is characterized by autocrine smooth muscle growth mechanisms, factors

responsible for turning off expression of the autocrine factor must be identified.

Extracellular matrix-mediated growth arrest might occur indirectly as the result of alterations in the extracellular matrix, which collectively might constitute a growth restrictive environment. Various studies have shown that the extracellular matrix can exert significant effects on the replication of cells in culture. Of particular relevance for the smooth muscle cells are thrombospondin (a growth factor-inducible matrix protein known to facilitate smooth muscle cell replication), heparin-like glycosaminoglycans (potent inhibitors of smooth muscle cell replication both *in vivo* and *in vitro*), and an uncharacterized heparin-inducible collagen, the synthesis of which correlates with heparin-regulated growth inhibition. In addition, immunolocalization studies have demonstrated that a heparan sulfate proteoglycan, potentially capable of inhibiting smooth muscle growth, is present in the endothelial basement membrane, thus placing this molecule in a strategic location to mediate endothelial–smooth muscle interactions during arterial morphogenesis.

Extracellular matrix-mediated growth arrest might also occur directly. Smooth muscle cells cultured on the basement membrane components laminin or type IV collagen, or in the presence of heparin-like molecules, exhibit reduced replicative capabilities. In addition, smooth muscle cells cultured on intact basement membranes do not replicate and appear to exhibit a more differentiated phenotype compared to smooth muscle cells cultured on plastic. These data suggest that smooth muscle cells may acquire a growth-suppressive basement membrane during development that largely prevents mitogenic responses *in vivo*.

Differentiation-mediated growth control might also play a role in the regulation of vessel wall growth. In many cell systems (e.g. skeletal muscle), terminal differentiation is accompanied by a complete loss of replicative ability. This does not seem to be true for vascular smooth muscle cells: following experimental arterial injury *in vivo*, fully "differentiated" smooth muscle cells enter $G_1$ and S phase with kinetics comparable to cultured cells. $G_1$ and S are the first two stages of the cell cycle; thus "differentiated" smooth muscle cells, in contrast to "differentiated" skeletal muscle cells, can easily be induced to proliferate in response to many agonists. No consensus has yet emerged as to what constitutes a differentiated smooth muscle cell. Smooth muscle cells exist along a continuum from a relatively immature fetal state to a more mature adult state, but the functional significance of smooth muscle cell maturation in terms of growth control is not known. Interestingly, recent work has demonstrated that smooth muscle cells near the lumen even in adult vessels retain certain characteristics of fetal cells. It has been suggested that this may allow these cells to migrate more easily and replicate in response to injury. Possibly, maturation of the smooth muscle cell to an adult phenotype occurs concomitant with the acquisition of certain growth restrictive characteristics conferred by the tunica media environment.

# Regulation of connective tissue production

## Elastin

In most mammalian tissues, the bulk of elastin production occurs during the fetal and neonatal periods and is essentially complete by the first decade of life. The temporal sequence of elastogenesis is unique in that elastic fibers are deposited during a defined developmental window, whereas many other extracellular matrix proteins are made and turned over continually. A number of factors have been demonstrated to participate in the normal regulation of tropoelastin expression. However, none has been definitively implicated in controlling elastin gene expression during normal vascular wall development.

The limited developmental expression of elastin indicates that a finely tuned and complex regulatory system controls production of this extracellular matrix protein. The microenvironment within which the elastin-producing cell exists certainly influences differentiation to the elastin phenotype, and this induction involves signals that traverse to the cell surface. For instance, it has been shown that the developing elastogenic cell may have the capacity to create a microenvironment conducive to its own phenotypic differentiation by the production of an extracellular matrix which autocatalyzes the induction of elastogenesis. In addition, it has been shown that the mature elastic matrix can also stimulate tropoelastin synthesis by cells already producing elastin and can elevate the very low levels of elastin production noted in adult cells. Thus the tissue milieu influences both the start and maintenance of elastin production. In addition, cell–matrix contact is required for complete differentiation, suggesting strongly that a cell surface molecule is involved as the instructive signal for elastogenesis.

Numerous other factors are able to modulate elastin synthesis in vascular wall cells. IGF-I stimulates tropoelastin synthesis and mRNA levels in neonatal arterial smooth muscle cells. Circulating concentrations of IGF-I and hepatic mRNA levels for IGF-I correlate with tropoelastin synthesis in the developing chick aorta suggesting that IGF-I may be involved in embryonic production of elastin. In addition, IGF-I mRNA levels in the embryonic chick aorta have been correlated with the onset of tropoelastin expression in this tissue. $TGF\beta_1$ also enhances tropoelastin expression in cultured neonatal arterial smooth muscle cells. However, there is no evidence from *in vivo* experiments to confirm the role of $TGF\beta_1$ in normal vascular wall development, nor to demonstrate convincingly that $TGF\beta_1$ is required for the increased elastin deposition seen during vascular remodeling. During periods of elevated elastin deposition, increased expression of tropoelastin may be controlled by a soluble cytokine-like factor that may act in both an autocrine and paracrine fashion. This factor, called smooth muscle elastogenic factor (SMEF), is secreted by smooth muscle cells derived from the pulmonary arteries of calves with severe pulmonary hypertension. SMEF stimulates tropoelastin synthesis in actively producing cells and induces expression in pre-elastogenic cells. The biochemical properties of SMEF have not been characterized, although it is not thought to be one of the known cytokines capable of regulating elastin synthesis. Glucocorticoids have also been shown to increase elastin production and, notably, these compounds seem to be acting through age-specific mechanisms. Elastin-producing cells from the fetus or neonate demonstrate increased production of tropoelastin upon exposure to glucocorticoids. Glucocorticoids do not induce tropoelastin expression in pre-elastogenic cells or in fully differentiated adult cells.

Many factors have also been shown to down-regulate tropoelastin gene expression. Marked inhibition of tropoelastin synthesis and mRNA levels and elastin deposition in various cultured cells is mediated by epidermal growth factor, recombinant interleukin-1β (rIL-1β), TNFα, interferon-γ, 1,25-dihydroxyvitamin $D_3$ ($1,25(OH)_2D_3$) and the phorbol esters.

Thus, although both stimulators and repressors of tropoelastin production have been identified, the actual physiological action of these modulators is not known. Conditions such as the developmental stage, the composition of the extracellular matrix with which the cell interacts, the proliferative potential of the elastin-producing cells, the presence of migratory cells, and physical forces add to and complicate the influences affecting extracellular matrix gene activity.

## Collagens

Factors controlling collagen formation during normal growth and development remain unclear. However, studies on cultured cells have provided some insights into factors that may be important in modulating at least type I collagen formation. TGFβ and insulin-related peptides are two substances that clearly can induce large increases in collagen formation by smooth muscle cells and fibroblasts in culture. Recent studies have also demonstrated that the potent inflammatory mediator leukotriene C$_4$ (LTC$_4$) can increase type I collagen formation. Many other molecules such as prostaglandin E$_2$ (PGE$_2$) and interferon-γ inhibit collagen accumulation. Thus the net accumulation of collagen, at least as it is controlled by cytokines, depends on the interaction of these and, of course, many other factors. Collagen accumulation and incorporation in the matrix is also limited by intracellular and extracellular degradation of intact collagen fiber by enzymes. Newly synthesized collagen can be degraded intracellularly. Furthermore, although the assembly of collagen fibers involves the formation of crosslinks that render the collagen molecule relatively resistant to protease digestion, mature extracellular collagen can be degraded by several mammalian collagenases. TGFβ$_1$, which stimulates the type I collagen gene, inhibits the expression of collagenase and transin/stromelysin, members of a family of matrix-degrading metalloproteinases. Also, TGFβ$_1$ stimulates production of an inhibitor of the metalloproteinases (TIMP-1). The regulation of connective tissue synthesis and degradation within the vessel wall therefore appears to be well coordinated and controlled by a balance of stimulators, inhibitors, and degradation pathways of the collagen molecules.

## STRUCTURAL REMODELING IN VASCULAR DISEASE

Abnormal cell proliferation and connective tissue deposition by vascular smooth muscle cells characterizes both *atherosclerosis* and *hypertension*. Atherosclerotic lesions consist of a proliferation of smooth muscle cells in the intima of large vessels with concomitant lipid and connective tissue accumulation, producing enlargement of the atherosclerotic plaque and focal narrowing of the vascular lumen. In hypertension (pulmonary or systemic), cell proliferation and an increased connective tissue deposition can occur in any of the three vessel compartments (intima, media, or adventitia). The resulting increase in wall mass produces a diffusely narrowed lumen and a vessel with altered mechanical and functional properties. Common to both atherosclerosis and hypertension is a phenotypically altered smooth muscle cell that appears to escape from its normal, tightly controlled state of quiescence to undergo high rates of replication. These cells also exhibit altered patterns of expression of connective tissue components compared to cells in normal, uninjured vessels.

Multiple changes in the phenotype of smooth muscle cells within the atherosclerotic plaque have been observed. These cells escape normal growth control mechanisms, migrate into the intima and proliferate abnormally. Both immunohistochemical and *in situ* hybridization studies have shown increases in elastin, collagen, and fibronectin synthesis. Changes in the cytoskeletal and contractile phenotype of the smooth muscle cells within the atherosclerotic lesion have also been reported, with cells characterized as having "fetal-like" characteristics.

A number of changes in the phenotype of the smooth muscle cell have also been documented during the development of *pulmonary hypertension* (Fig. 67.3). A newborn calf model of severe neonatal pulmonary hypertension induced by hypobaric hypoxia has demonstrated severe pulmonary vascular changes that mimic those found in forms of severe human neonatal pulmonary hypertension. A significant increase in smooth muscle cell and fibroblast proliferation occurs almost immediately after exposure of the newborn animal to hypoxia as opposed to cells in the normal developing pulmonary artery, which in the neonatal period have a low replication index. This marked hyperplastic response is seen in both large and small vessels of the hypertensive pulmonary vascular bed. Moreover, when examined by *in situ* hybridization techniques, pulmonary arterial tissue from hypertensive calves

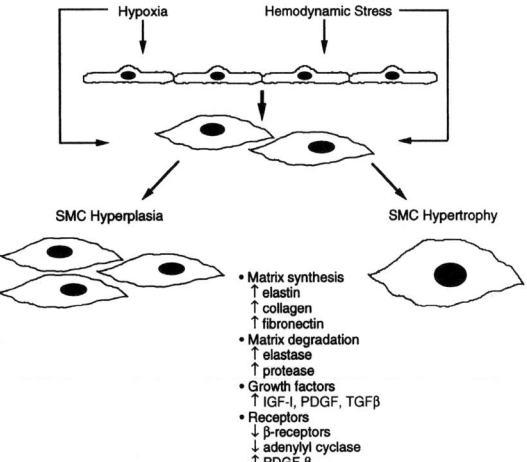

FIGURE 67.3 Schematic representation of the phenotypic changes which occur in the pulmonary vascular smooth muscle cell (SMC) during the development of chronic hypoxic pulmonary hypertension. Hypoxia and/or hemodynamic forces act through the endothelial cell, or directly, to cause a "transformation" of the smooth muscle cell. This cell exhibits several characteristics that are very different from the smooth muscle cell in the normal pulmonary artery.

exhibits a very different pattern of matrix protein gene expression than tissue from age-matched normal calves. In large vessels a marked decrease in tropoelastin mRNA expression occurs immediately after birth; this decrease in mRNA occurs in a radial fashion, progressing from the outer to the inner wall. In contrast the fetal and neonatal pattern of tropoelastin gene expression persists in neonatal animals with severe pulmonary hypertension. This could have significant functional implications for the vessel wall and could also imply that other genes in the hypoxic pulmonary hypertensive animal may not undergo the same postnatal transition in gene expression that occurs during normal development. Animals developing severe neonatal pulmonary hypertension rapidly exhibit marked increases of type I collagen gene expression in the media and adventitia of the small pulmonary artery walls. As stated above, these rapid changes in collagen gene expression and collagen accumulation could have marked functional implications during this critical period of transition. A marked increase in wall stiffness would be expected, as well as an inability to adapt rapidly to the changes taking place in neonatal life. Interruption of the normal postnatal adaptation process by early injury may have long-lasting implications. Although on removal of the stimulus the newborn vessels appear to return to a morphologically and functionally "normal" state, upon re-exposure to the injurious stimulus (i.e. hypoxia) 6 weeks after apparent full recovery, animals that had been exposed to hypoxia in the neonatal period show greater vascular remodeling and higher pulmonary arterial pressures than animals that had adapted normally to extrauterine life.

The primary stimuli responsible for vascular remodeling remain unclear. Mechanical forces (increased wall tension and shear stress) and hypoxia have received considerable attention with regard to their effects on cell phenotype. Various models including vessel coarctation, venous to arterial autologous grafts, and in vitro preparations of stretched vessel segments or isolated vascular smooth muscle cells have been employed to evaluate the effects of increased load on vascular wall cells. In general, these studies have shown that increased tension or load stimulates an almost immediate increase in net protein production. Expression of connective tissue proteins increases before that of contractile proteins, and the amounts of specific proteins within individual classes can change independently. The effects of elevated strain on cellular hyperplasia are unclear and may depend on the age and type of vessel examined. However, some studies suggest that direct mechanical stretch of the vascular wall is sufficient to induce cell replication. Significant differences between the responses of veins and arteries have been observed, again suggesting a heterogeneous response to vascular load. Recent studies have documented both stretch-activated and stretch-inactivated ion channels within various cell types, including muscle. These voltage-dependent channels can lead to electrical polarization changes within the cell, perhaps directly activating second messenger systems necessary for protein synthesis or cell proliferation. Changes in $Na^+$ can also stimulate protein production, and $Na^+$-channel blockers have been demonstrated to ameliorate the response to increased load. Cells may also sense deformation of the membrane directly via filaments connecting the cell surface to the nucleus. Complex cell–cell interactions are certainly important in this response as endothelial cells have been shown to modulate the responses of smooth muscle cells to hemodynamic forces.

The effects of chronic hypoxia on vascular wall cells are especially important in the pulmonary circulation. Chronic hypoxic exposure is associated with significant pulmonary hypertension in most species, as well as changes in the vessel wall that include cell proliferation (predominantly in the adventitial fibroblast) and significant increases in the production and deposition of elastin and collagen. The direct effect of hypoxia on these changes, however, is uncertain. Hypoxia alone has been demonstrated to decrease smooth muscle cell proliferation and elastin and collagen production in cultured neonatal smooth muscle cells. On the other hand, hypoxia has been shown to stimulate fibroblast proliferation. In addition, in certain cell types (including the endothelium), hypoxia has been demonstrated to enhance growth factor production and responsiveness. One possible hypothesis is that hypoxia induces cellular changes that make cells more responsive to mechanical and hormonal stimuli.

Recent studies have begun to evaluate some of the locally produced factors that may be involved in mediating the vascular remodeling process. Basic FGF seems to be involved in the proliferation of cells observed in the atherosclerotic plaque and in the initial smooth muscle cell replication observed during restenosis of vessels following induced endothelial injury such as occurs with angioplasty procedures. In addition, PDGF-BB, angiotensin II, $TGF\beta_1$, and thrombin have been implicated in this process. In models of pulmonary hypertension, $TGF\beta$, IGF-I, IGF-II, and PDGF have been correlated in a temporal fashion with the changes in cell proliferation and matrix production that are observed. $TGF\beta$, for instance, was found to be temporally and specifically related to areas in the vessel wall that were undergoing intense remodeling. Importantly, it also is known that endogenous vascular elastases and proteinases are activated in vascular disease states. It is clear that changes in the activity of these proteins contribute to smooth muscle cell proliferation and increased matrix synthesis through as yet undescribed mechanisms.

Characterization of the signals involved in initiating the vascular response to injury as well as of the mediators generated by endothelial, smooth muscle, and fibroblast cells during the vascular remodeling response require intense investigation. In addition, evaluation of the mechanisms responsible for cell activation and protein synthesis will be an important new direction for further research into the molecular and cellular mechanisms responsible for regulating cell proliferation and connective tissue synthesis in normal and diseased vessels.

## SELECTED READING

Carey DJ. Control of growth and differentiation of vascular cells by extracellular matrix proteins. *Annu Rev Physiol* 1991; 53: 161.

Cook C, Weiser M, Schwartz P *et al.* Developmentally timed expression of an embryonic growth phenotype in vascular smooth muscle cells. *Circ Res* 1994; 74: 189.

D'Amore PA. Developmental aspects of vascular disease. In Bernfield M, Cole FS, eds: *Developmental mechanisms of disease in the newborn. Report of the 101st Ross Conference on Pediatric Research.* Columbus, Ohio: Ross Laboratories, 1991: 95.

Durmowicz AG, Parks WC, Hyde DM *et al.* Persistence, re-expression, and induction of pulmonary arterial fibronectin, tropoelastin, and type I procollagen mRNA expression in neonatal hypoxic pulmonary hypertension. *Am J Pathol* 1994; 145: 1411.

Feinburg RN, Sheser GK, Auerbach R, eds. *The development of the vascular system.* Basel, Switzerland: Karger, 1991.

Mitchell JJ, Reynolds SE, Leslie KO *et al.* Smooth muscle cell markers in developing rat lung. *Am J Respir Cell Mol Biol* 1990; 3: 515.

Noden DM. Embryonic origins and assembly of blood vessels. *Am Rev Respir Dis* 1989; 140: 1097.

Stenmark KR, Majack RA. Response of the developing pulmonary circulation to injury. In Bernfield M, Cole FS, eds: *Developmental mechanisms of disease in the newborn. Report of the 101st Ross Conference on Pediatric Research.* Columbus, Ohio: Ross Laboratories, 1991: 102.

Stenmark KR, Durmowicz AG, Roby J *et al.* Persistence of the fetal pattern of tropoelastin expression in hypoxic pulmonary hypertension. *J Clin Invest* 1994; 93: 1234.

Zhu L, Wigle D, Hinek A *et al.* The endogenous vascular elastase that governs development and progression of monocrotaline-induced pulmonary hypertension in rats is a novel enzyme related to the serine proteinase adipsin. *J Clin Invest* 1994; 94: 1163.

# Vascular endothelium and smooth muscle function

## BLOOD VESSEL STRUCTURE

Blood vessel walls consist of three tissue layers called the tunica intima, tunica media and tunica adventitia. The tunica intima is subdivided into endothelium, subendothelium and internal elastic or basal lamina. The endothelium is a single layer of polygonal, flattened squamous epithelium, lining the interior of blood vessels. The luminal side of the endothelial cell membrane is coated with proteoglycans forming the endo-endothelial coat. The subendothelium consists of loose connective tissue and elastic fibers with a few longitudinally oriented smooth muscle cells. The endothelial cells rest on a basal lamina that contains a fenestrated layer of elastic fibers. The basal lamina is more prominent in large arteries, is very thin in veins, and is absent in arterioles, venules and capillaries.

The tunica media contains smooth muscle cells distributed in concentric and helical layers, varying in number from 3 to 40 layers, depending on the size and type of artery. The smooth muscle cells are surrounded by basal laminae and communicate with each other via gap junctions. The tunica media also contains proteoglycans, collagen (type III) and reticular and elastic fibers, all secreted by the smooth muscle cells. The elastic fibers are more abundant in conduit arteries. At the junction with the tunica adventitia of muscular distributing arteries, the elastic tissue forms the external elastic lamina. In capillaries, the media consists of pericytes, which contain myosin, actin and tropomyosin, indicating a contractile function for these cells.

The tunica adventitia contains collagen (type I) and elastic fibers, longitudinally oriented, fibroblasts, a few mast cells and smooth muscle cells. In large vessels, vasa vasorum (blood vessels of blood vessels) are present in the adventitia and outer media, to provide metabolites for the outer layers of the media. The adventitia also contains a network of unmyelinated sympathetic or parasympathetic fibers, that release neurotransmitters. Gap junctions between the smooth muscle cells propagate the response to the inner cell layers.

## VASCULAR ENDOTHELIAL CELL FUNCTION

The vascular endothelium is a monolayer of squamous epithelial cells situated at the interface between the flowing blood and the vascular wall, in a unique location for interaction with the soluble and cellular elements of the blood on one side, and with the subendothelium and the smooth muscle cells on the other. The endothelium is a metabolically active tissue that functions to maintain vascular homeostasis and integrity, to produce and inactivate various substances, to regulate the growth and function of the surrounding vascular components as well as that of the cellular elements in the blood. Endothelial cell function is regulated by physical and chemical forces occurring in the blood and in the vascular wall.

The following sections, will present briefly the various components synthesized by the endothelial cells and discuss their physiological contribution.

### Extracellular matrix components

Extracellular matrix components are a chemically diverse group of molecules (Table 67.3), that form an

TABLE 67.3 Factors released from endothelium (see text for abbreviations)

---

*Extracellular matrix components*

Collagen, elastin, fibronectin, laminin, thrombospondin, vitronectin, vWF, glycosaminoglycans (dermatan sulfate, heparan sulfate, chondroitin sulfate)

*Growth factors*
Growth stimulants
   PDGF, bFGF, IGF-I, ET, AII, $O_2^-$, thrombospondin
Growth inhibitors
   NO, $PGI_2$, heparin, heparan sulfate, TGFβ, collagen type V, glycoproteins, glycosaminoglycans

*Proteases*
Metalloproteases, collagenases, elastases, gelatinases, serine proteases, plasminogen activators (t-PA, u-PA)

*Proteinase inhibitors*
Inhibitors of: metalloproteases, collagenases, elastases, gelatinases, serine proteases, PAI-1 and PAI-2

*Adhesion factors/chemoattractants*
Vascular endothelial growth factor (VEGF)/vascular permeability factor, PDGF, bFGF, macrophage colony stimulating factor, monocyte chemoattractant factor, granulocyte-macrophage colony stimulating factor (GM-CSF), PAF, TGFβ, selectins, ICAMs, VCAM-1, sialomucins, major histocompatability complex (MHC) class I and II antigens, IL-8

*Vasoactive factors*
Relaxants
   NO, endothelium-derived hyperpolarizing factor (EDHF), aceytlcholine, substance P, ATP, $PGI_2$, $PGE_2$
Constrictors
   ET, $TXA_2$, $PGH_2$, $PGF_{2\alpha}$ LTs, $O_2^-$, AI, AII, endothelium-derived constricting factors

*Cytoprotective factors*
NO, $PGI_2$

*Cytotoxic factors*
NO, $O_2^-$, IL-1, IL-6, IL-8

*Coagulation cascade factors*
Procoagulants
   Tissue factor, PAF, vWF, coagulation cascade factors V and X, factor V and XII activators, HMWK, fibronectin, binding sites on the endothelium for factors VIII, IX, IXa, X, Xa
Anticoagulants
   NO, $PGI_2$, t-PA, u-PA, glycosaminoglycans, thrombomodulin, proteins S and C. Endothelium constitutes a functional barrier between factor VII and tissue factor, and between platelets and vWF
Fibrinolytic factors
   t-PA and u-PA, PAI-1 and PAI-2
Thomboregulatory factors
   $PGI_2$, $TXA_2$, EDRF/NO, ADPase

---

insoluble three-dimensional mesh, providing strength, elasticity and structural integrity to the vascular wall. These components interact strongly with one another, as well as with the molecules released by the endothelium and by the blood. For example, some of the endothelial collagens, and also laminin, fibronectin, vitronectin and glycosaminoglycans, provide support for endothelial cell attachment and detachment, modulating their movement, growth, proliferation and the ability of endothelial cells to participate in angiogenesis and mechanotransduction. In addition, heparan sulfate, von Willebrand factor (vWF) and vitronectin

convey anticoagulant and procoagulant function, respectively, to endothelial cells. The extracellular matrix contains various other molecules such as proteases, proteinase inhibitors (Table 67.3) and growth factors.

## Growth factors

Endothelial cells produce a number of chemically diverse substances that are able to stimulate or inhibit the growth of vascular wall components (Table 67.3). In normal quiescent blood vessels, the growth inhibitory factors dominate. In pathological alterations of endothelial cell function, there is an increased production of growth stimulators, generated by the adhering and aggregating monocytes and platelets, and by the endothelium, leading to increased smooth muscle proliferation and migration, fibrin deposition and growth and maturation of the connective tissue cells. The secretion of growth stimulants by endothelial cells is of particular importance in blood vessel formation during embryogenesis, and also in the development of collateral vasculature and wound repair in adults.

## Adhesion factors

A key step in the inflammatory response is the ability of circulating leukocytes, which are subjected to strong shear forces by the blood flow, to slow down and become attached to the vascular endothelium at the site of injury (*see* also p. 863). These highly selective and transient interactions are mediated by several families of cell adhesion molecules (CAMs) (Tables 67.3 and 67.4, Fig. 67.4): (1) selectins, which include L-, E- and P-selectins (Table 67.4A); (2) $\beta_2$ integrins, that include LFA-1, Mac-1 and p150,95. Some $\beta_1$, $\beta_3$, and $\beta_7$ integrins also play an important role in leukocyte–endothelial cell interactions (Table 67.4B); (3) intercellular adhesion molecules (ICAMs), belong to the immunoglobulin superfamily and include ICAM-1, ICAM-2, ICAM-3, as well as other CAMs (Table 67.4C); (4) sialomucins and carbohydrates (Table 67.4D) complete the constantly increasing list of CAMs.

The leukocyte–endothelial cell interactions, referred to as the adhesion cascade (Fig. 67.4), ensure a rapid self-limiting response to isolate and destroy invading microorganisms, with minimum damage to healthy tissue. First, the P-selectin and then E-selectin, expressed on activated endothelial cells, initiate the slowing down and rolling of leukocytes, through $Ca^{2+}$-dependent recognition sites of leukocyte cell surface carbohydrates such as sialyl Lewis X ($SLe^X$). Second, endothelium-generated chemoattractants, such as leukotriene $B_4$, interleukin (IL)-1, IL-8, platelet activating factor (PAF) and granulocyte-macrophage colony stimulating factor (GM-CSF), activate the rolling leuko-

TABLE 67.4 Cellular adhesion molecules (CAMs)

| NAME | CD-NAME | PREVIOUS NAME | EXPRESSED BY: | TARGET CELL/LIGAND | FUNCTION |
|---|---|---|---|---|---|
| *A. Selectins (LEC-CAMs)* | | | | | |
| L-selectin (constitutive) | CD62L | LAM-1, LECAM-1, MEL-14 | Leukocytes, (neutrophils, monocytes, lymphocytes) | Cytokine-activated ECs, peripheral lymph nodes, mesenteric lymphoid tissue, high endothelial venule (HEV)/GlyCAM-1, CD34, MAdCAM-1, sialyl Lewis X (SLe$^X$), sialyl Lewis A (SLe$^A$), peripheral node addressins (PNAd), heparin, E-selectin | Lymphocyte homing receptor, neutrophil adhesion to activated ECs |
| E-selectin (inducible) | CD62E | ELAM-1 | Cytokine activated ECs | Neutrophils, monocytes, eosinophils, granulocytes, T-lymphocyte subsets, some tumor cells/SLe$^X$, SLe$^A$, Le$^X$, lymphocyte antigen (CLA), P-selectin-glycoprotein ligand-1 (PSGL-1), L-selectin, CD66, $\beta_2$ integrins | Leukocyte rolling and adhesion |
| P-selectin (constitutive and inducible) | CD62P | GMP-140, PADGEM | Thrombin-activated platelets and ECs (Weibel–Palade bodies), histamine and cytokine-activated ECs | Neutrophils, monocytes, eosinophils, granulocytes, lymphocyte subsets, some tumor cells/Le$^X$, SLe$^X$, SLe$^A$, PSGL-1, L-selectin, heparin | Leukocyte rolling and adhesion, platelet adhesion to myeloid cells |
| *B. Integrins* | | | | | |
| $\beta_1$: VLA-4 (very late activation antigen) (LPAM-2) | CD49d/CD29 | | Lymphocytes, monocytes, basophils, B-cells and T-cells | Cytokine-activated ECs, leukocytes, Peyer patch on HEV/VCAM-1, fibronectin, thrombospondin and other ligands on leukoyctes | Cell–cell adhesion receptor, cell–matrix binding, T-cell homing |
| $\beta_2$: | | | | | |
| LFA-1 | CD11a/CD18 | | All leukocytes | ECs/ICAM-1, ICAM-2 | Leukocyte adhesion |
| Mac-1 (CR3) | CD11b/CD18 | | Granulocytes, monocytes, macrophages, some activated lymphocytes, large granular lymphocytes | ECs/ICAM-1, factor X, fibrinogen, certain carbohydrates, iC3b, LPS, *Leishmania* | Leukocyte adhesion, complement receptor 3 (CR3) |
| p150,95 (CR4) | CD11c/CD18 | | Granulocytes, monocytes, macrophages, some activated lymphocytes, large granular lymphocytes | ECs/fibrinogen, iC3b | Leukocyte adhesion, CR4, neutrophil adhesion to serum-coated surfaces, monocyte adhesion to ECs |
| $\beta_3$: vitronectin receptor (VNR) | CD51/CD61 | | Neutrophils, tumor cells | ECs/vitronectin, fibrinogen, thrombospondin, wWF, C5b-7 | Neutrophil–EC adhesion |
| $\beta_7$: $\alpha_4\beta_7$ | | | Leukocytes | Lymphoid HEV/MAdCAM-1, VCAM-1 on activated ECs, fibronectin | Leukocyte mucosal homing receptor |
| *C. Immunoglobulin (Ig) superfamily* | | | | | |
| ICAM-1 (constitutive and inducible) | CD54 | | ECs, lymphocytes, monocytes, synovial cells, epithelial cells, fibroblasts, hepatocytes, keratinocytes | Malaria-infected RBCs, rhinovirus, lymphocytes, monocytes, granulocytes/LFA-1, Mac-1, CD43 (syalophorin) | ECs–leukocyte interactions, cell-mediated cytolysis, Ag presentation |
| ICAM-2 (constitutive) | CD102 | | ECs, lymphocytes (activated) | Lymphocytes, monocytes, granulocytes/LFA-1 | Leukocyte adhesion |
| MAdCAM-1 (mucosal addressin) | | | HEV in mucosal lymph nodes (Peyer patch) | Leukocytes/$\alpha_4\beta_7$ integrin, L-selectin | Lymphocyte emigration |
| PECAM-1 (constitutive) | CD31 | | ECs, platelets, monocytes, neutrophils, some peripheral lymphocytes | Leukocytes/PECAM-1 | Leukocyte homophilic adhesion to ECs, and transmigration |

*(contd)*

TABLE 67.4 Cellular adhesion molecules (CAMs) (*contd*)

| NAME | CD-NAME | PREVIOUS NAME | EXPRESSED BY: | TARGET CELL/LIGAND | FUNCTION |
|---|---|---|---|---|---|
| VCAM-1 (inducible) (vascular CAM) | CD106 | INCAM-1 | ECs, epithelial cells, dendritic cells | Lymphocytes, basophils, monocytes, eosinophils/ VLA-4 | Leukocyte adhesion |
| *D. Other CAMs* Sialomucins: (addressins) MAdCAM-1 | | | HEV in mucosal lymph nodes (Peyer patch), mammary gland venules | Leukocytes/$\alpha_4\beta_7$ integrin, L-selectin | Bind subsets of lymphocytes that express homing receptors |
| PNAd PSGL-1, GlyCAM-1 CD34, CD44 | | | HEV in peripheral lymph nodes | Leukocytes/L-selectin | All bind subsets of lymphocytes that express homing receptors |
| VAP-1 | | | HEV in mucosal peripheral lymph nodes, synovium | Lymphocytes | ? |
| L-VAP-2 (constitutive) | | | Human umbilical vein endothelium, B-cells, CD8$^+$ T-cells | Lymphocytes | ? |
| CD14 | | | Monocytes, neutrophils | Cytokine activated ECs | |
| Carbohydrates: Lewis X (Le$^X$) | CD15 | | Neutrophils | P-selectin | Leukocyte adhesion |
| Sialyl Lewis X (SLe$^X$) | CD15s | | Neutrophils | E-selectin, P-selectin | Leukocyte adhesion |
| Lewis A (Le$^A$) | | | Tumor cells | E-selectin, P-selectin | Tumor metastases |

cytes to express the $\beta_2$ integrins, LFA-1 and Mac-1, which bind to another group of adhesion molecules expressed by the endothelial cells, the ICAMs (ICAM-1, ICAM-2, VCAM-1 and MAdCAM-1). ICAM-1, as a receptor for Mac-1 integrin, brings the leukocytes to a complete stop. The leukocytes then undergo morphological changes and migrate between the endothelial cell junctions. By releasing elastase, which digests the basement membrane, the leukocytes proceed through it by diapedesis to the site of injury or infection. This process, known as transendothelial migration or extravasation, is mediated by the $\beta_1$, $\beta_2$ and $\beta_7$ integrins and PECAM-1 on the leukocyte cell surface and by ICAM-1, VCAM-1 and PECAM-1 on the endothelium. The subendothelial migration of leukocytes to the injury site is mediated by $\beta_1$ and $\beta_2$ integrins on the leukocytes and by different extracellular matrix components and chemoattractants released in the subendothelium.

Regulation of the expression and function of adhesion molecules that lead to the recruitment of different subtypes of leukocytes to the site of tissue injury is a normal process in the inflammatory response and follows a temporal sequence. For example, an intradermal injection of lipopolysaccharide first induces an influx of neutrophils which is followed by accumulation of mononuclear macrophages for the next 48 hours. However, deficiencies in this series of events and the ability of the cells involved to generate highly reactive oxidants, nitric oxide, proteinases and proin-

flammatory agents can contribute to the pathogenesis of pediatric inflammatory diseases such as ischemia–reperfusion injury (manifested in newborns as necrotizing enterocolitis, postasphyxial central nervous system injury and acute tubular necrosis). Other disorders involving adhesion cascade abnormalities include pulmonary oxygen injury, intraventricular hemorrhage, retinopathy of prematurity, hemolytic uremic syndrome in newborns, and rheumatoid arthritis, inflammatory skin disease, and respiratory distress syndrome in adults. In allergic inflammations such as asthma, a selective accumulation of eosinophils occurs as a response to PAF released from the cytokine-activated endothelial cells. Eosinophil adhesion occurs in a similar manner to that of neutrophils, involving the selectins, integrins and ICAM-1. The only difference is the expression of VLA-4 ($\beta_1$) integrins, which can bind VCAM-1 on cytokine-activated endothelial cells. A new generation of drugs that use antagonists of selectin- or integrin-mediated adhesion may be therapeutically useful in a variety of inflammatory diseases as well as in some genetic disorders such as leukocyte adhesion deficiency (LAD).

## Vasoactive factors

The endothelium contributes to the modulation of vasomotor tone by secreting both vasodilator and vasoconstrictor factors (Table 67.3).

| Adhesion Steps / Cell Type | Slowing down + rolling | Aggregation + adhesion | Transendothelial migration | Chemotactic subendothelial migration |
|---|---|---|---|---|
| **Leukocytes** | SLe$^X$, L-selectin | $\beta_1$, $\beta_2$, $\beta_7$ integrins | $\beta_1$, $\beta_2$, $\beta_7$ integrins PECAM-1 | $\beta_1$, $\beta_2$ integrins |
| **Endothelium** | P-selectin, E-selectin | ICAM-1, VCAM-1, MAdCAM-1 | ICAM-1, VCAM-1, PECAM-1 | Extracellular matrix components, Chemoattractants |

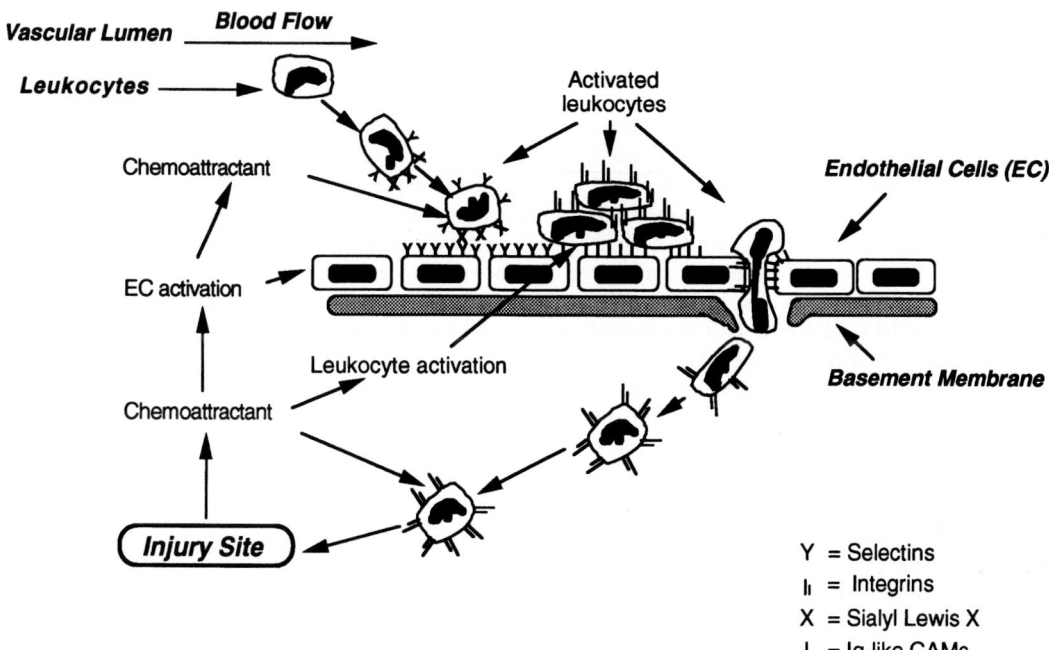

FIGURE 67.4 The leukocyte–endothelial cell (EC) adhesion cascade requires multiple interactions between different adhesion molecules expressed on their cell surfaces. First, the chemoattractants produced at the injury site activate both ECs and circulating leukocytes, which slow down and start rolling on the endothelium. This step is mediated by P-selectin and E-selectin on the activated ECs and by sialyl Lewis X (SLe$^X$) or L-selectin on the leukocytes. Secondly, the activated leukocytes develop an increase in avidity of the $\beta_1$ integrin (VLA-4) and $\beta_2$ integrins (LFA-1 and Mac-1) for their respective immunoglobulin-like (Ig-like) ligands (ICAM-1, VCAM-1 and MAdCAM-1) on the activated endothelium, which results in the aggregation and firm adhesion of leukocytes to the ECs. The third step, transendothelial migration, is mediated by ICAM-1, VCAM-1 and PECAM-1 on the ECs and by $\beta_1$, $\beta_2$ and $\beta_7$ integrins and PECAM-1 on the leukocytes. The final step, the chemotactic subendothelial migration to the injury site, is mediated by the leukocyte $\beta_1$ and $\beta_2$ integrins and the extracellular matrix components and the chemoattractants from the subendothelial tissue.

## Endothelium-derived relaxing factors (EDRFs)

Despite the knowledge that vascular endothelial cells displayed various synthetic, degradative, and secretory functions, the modulatory role of the endothelium on vascular tone remained unrecognized until 1980, when Furchgott and Zawadzki discovered EDRF. In this original study, acetylcholine-elicited relaxation of isolated rabbit aorta preparations was shown to be endothelium-dependent and due to the release of an endothelium-derived relaxing factor that was chemically unstable. An attractive hypothesis was offered that this relaxing substance might be a lipoxygenase product of arachidonic acid. Furchgott and coworkers went on to propose that EDRF is also responsible for the arterial relaxant responses to bradykinin, histamine, ATP, ADP and Ca$^{2+}$ ionophores. Over 16 years ago, our laboratory discovered that bubbling nitric oxide (NO) gas into Krebs bicarbonate solution containing isolated strips of bovine coronary artery caused a rapid and marked, yet transient, relaxation that was antagonized by hemoproteins and methylene blue. NO activated soluble guanylyl cyclase in coronary artery preparations, and this was inhibited by hemoproteins and methylene blue. These observations were made before the discovery of EDRF. Shortly after the discovery of EDRF, we found that NO activated human platelet guanylyl cyclase, elevated platelet cyclic

GMP (cGMP) levels, and produced a profound inhibition of platelet aggregation. When we started to study the pharmacological properties of EDRF, we did not envision that EDRF could be NO, although we found that endothelium-dependent vascular smooth muscle relaxation was associated with marked tissue formation of cGMP, both of which were inhibited by the soluble guanylyl cyclase inhibitor methylene blue. Further studies revealed the remarkable similarities in biological properties between EDRF and NO and in 1986 we proposed that EDRF is NO or a labile nitroso precursor. The following year, we and others provided chemical evidence for the identity of EDRF as NO.

Many studies reported the similarities between EDRF and authentic NO. As had been shown for NO, EDRF activated purified soluble guanylyl cyclase by heme-dependent mechanisms and inhibited platelet aggregation and adhesion by mechanisms involving cGMP. Several inconsistencies were reported in which EDRF was suggested to be a labile nitroso precursor, rather than NO. Definitive evidence has not been provided, however, to refute the well-accepted concept that EDRF is NO. EDRF or NO is released from artery and vein and appears to be involved intimately in the regulation of vascular smooth muscle tone. NO is responsible, at least in part, for the endothelium-dependent vasodilator action of acetylcholine, bradykinin, histamine, serotonin, ATP, ADP, substance P, and thrombin (Fig. 67.5). These endogenous substances interact with selective receptors located on the extracellular surface of the vascular endothelial cell. Agonist–receptor interaction is coupled to the intracellular formation of NO via a $Ca^{2+}$-dependent process. Receptor occupancy by agonist results in the influx of $Ca^{2+}$, which combines with calmodulin to activate NO synthase (NOS), thereby stimulating NO production (Fig. 67.5) (see also Chapter 10).

The vascular endothelium is capable of modulating the tone of the underlying smooth muscle in arteries in response to local changes in shear stress, pressure, and other mechanical factors. The purpose of endothelial regulation is to adapt blood vessel diameter to sudden changes in tissue perfusion demands. Studies using isolated arterial segments and cultured arterial endothelial cells have shown that endothelium-derived NO is likely responsible for shear stress-induced or flow-dependent vasodilatation, perhaps through a potassium channel-mediated mechanism (discussed on page 703). Thus, NO likely plays an important physiological role in the regulation or modulation of blood flow. Endothelium-derived NO plays a role in modulating the systemic blood pressure. In vitro studies have shown that inhibitors of NO synthesis (discussed below) cause endothelium-dependent contractions of isolated arterial preparations. In vivo studies have shown that the same inhibitors of NO synthesis cause a marked increase in peripheral vascular resistance and systemic blood pressure. Endothelium-derived NO also plays a role in modulating platelet adhesion and aggregation, thereby endowing the vas-

cular endothelium with the capacity to provide a thrombogenic-free surface. Local damage to the vascular endothelium can promote local vasoconstriction and blood clot formation. Fig. 67.5 illustrates some of the important influences of the endothelium on vascular smooth muscle tone.

NO is synthesized from L-arginine through a multistep oxidation reaction catalyzed by NOS (see also Chapter 10). The second byproduct of this reaction is L-citrulline (Fig. 67.6). In mammalian cells NOS exists as three basic isoforms. Neuronal NO synthase (ncNOS) and endothelial NO synthase (ecNOS) are constitutively present in their respective cell types, whereas inflammatory NO synthase (iNOS) can be induced on demand by a variety of cytokines. The iNOS can be induced not only in macrophages but also in vascular smooth muscle and endothelial cells as well as other cell types. Endothelium-dependent vasorelaxants such as acetylcholine and bradykinin interact with selective receptors on the endothelial cell surface to trigger the opening of receptor-operated $Ca^{2+}$ channels, thereby promoting $Ca^{2+}$ influx. Increased intracellular free $Ca^{2+}$ results in the activation of ecNOS and subsequent production of NO (Fig. 67.5). Lipopolysaccharide and cytokines including interferon-$\gamma$ and tumor necrosis factor $\alpha$ promote the transcriptional expression (increased mRNA) of relatively large quantities of iNOS, resulting in the production of large amounts of NO. The NO generated by iNOS in vascular smooth muscle causes a profound vasorelaxation that is difficult to reverse with vasoconstrictor agents. The much smaller amounts of NO generated in vascular endothelial cells by ecNOS serve a physiological role in regulating the systemic vascular resistance.

$Ca^{2+}$ activates ecNOS by promoting the binding of calmodulin to the enzyme protein. Calmodulin facilitates the transfer of NADPH-derived electrons from the flavin domain of ecNOS to the heme iron prosthetic group. Electron transfer results in the reduction of heme iron to the ferrous state so that it can bind and activate oxygen. The $O_2$ is incorporated into the L-arginine substrate to yield NO plus L-citrulline. Tetrahydrobiopterin, another required factor, appears to function not as a stoichiometric reactant but rather to stabilize the NOS protein during catalysis. NO also acts as a negative feedback modulator of ecNOS, ncNOS and iNOS, and tetrahydrobiopterin can prevent this inhibitory action of NO.

Like ecNOS, ncNOS is activated by $Ca^{2+}$/calmodulin, whereas iNOS appears to be independent of $Ca^{2+}$/calmodulin. Calmodulin is already tightly bound to iNOS as a subunit and, therefore, $Ca^{2+}$ is not required to promote calmodulin binding. $N^{\omega}$-substituted analogs of L-arginine including the methyl, nitro and amino derivatives are competitive inhibitors of NOS, and inhibition can be overcome by addition of excess L-arginine. These inhibitory analogs of L-arginine have been shown to cause vasoconstriction, hypertension and thrombosis, and have been used extensively to assess the physiological and pathophysiological roles

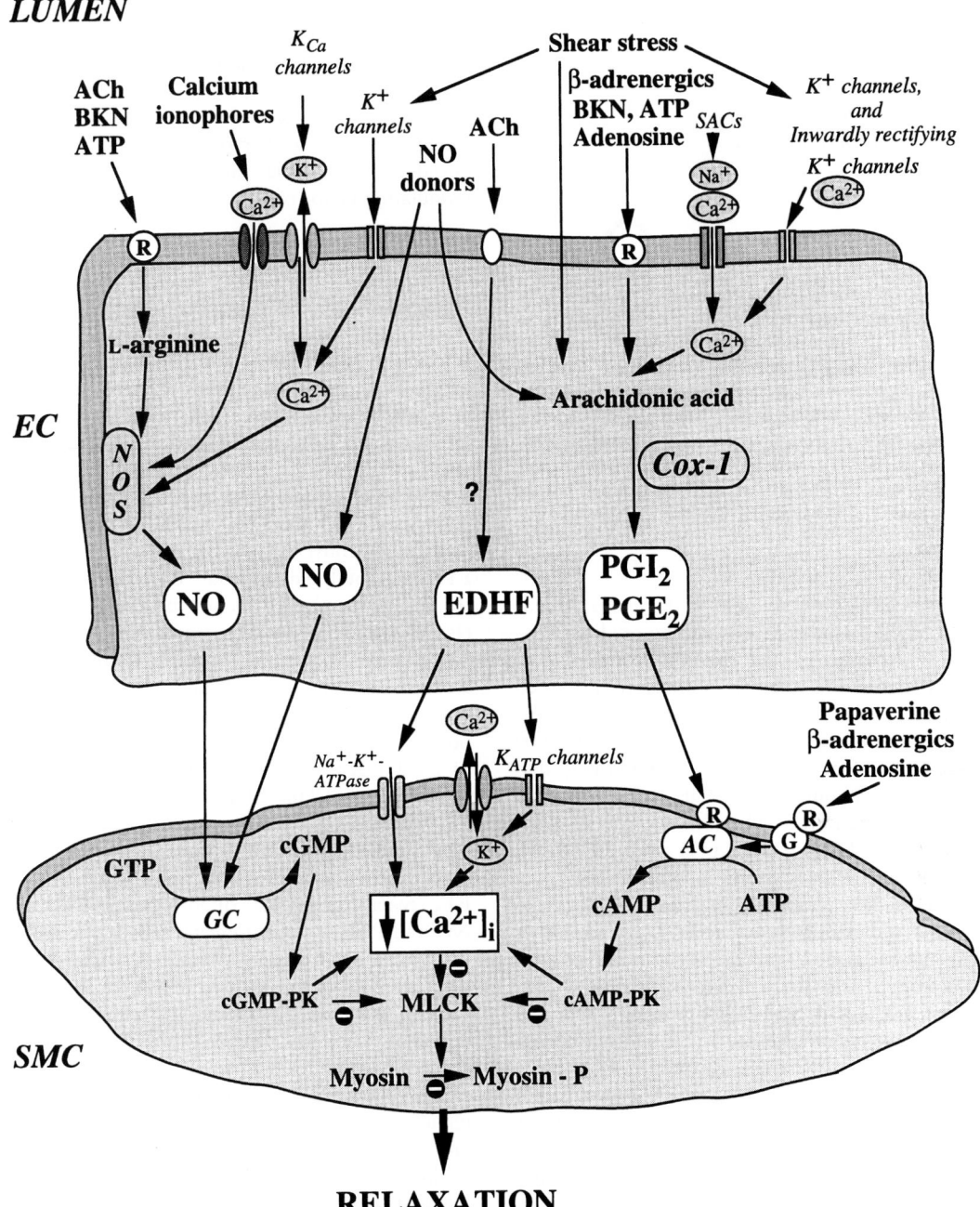

FIGURE 67.5 Vasorelaxation occurs via chemical or mechanical stimulation of endothelial cells (EC), resulting in the generation and release of nitric oxide (NO), vasodilatory prostaglandins (prostacyclin ($PGI_2$) and prostaglandin $E_2$ ($PGE_2$)) and endothelium-derived hyperpolarizing factor (EDHF). NO diffuses into the smooth muscle cell (SMC) and activates guanylyl cyclase (GC), causing an elevation in cyclic GMP (cGMP) which leads to a reduction in free intracellular $Ca^{2+}$ ($[Ca^{2+}]_i$) levels and produces SMC relaxation via activation of cGMP-dependent protein kinase (cGMP-PK) or via modulation of cAMP signal transduction system. Abluminally released $PGI_2$ and $PGE_2$ from EC activate the adenylyl cyclase (AC) in the SMC, resulting in elevation of cyclic AMP (cAMP), reduction in $[Ca^{2+}]_i$ and SMC relaxation. EDHF released by acetylcholine (ACh) and other transmitters hyperpolarizes the SMC membrane either by activating the ATP-sensitive potassium channels ($K_{ATP}$) or by activating the $Na^+$-$K^+$-ATPase. ( ●, decreased activity.)

of endogenous NO formed in many different cell types. Endothelial cell physiology is disrupted in hypercholesterolemia, where the acetylcholine-induced relaxation is diminished, suggesting an impaired production and/or rapid degradation of NO. However, the vasodilator response to organic nitrates and other endothelium-independent relaxants is not affected in hypercholesterolemia. In *atherosclerosis*, in addition to the impaired responses to endothelium-dependent relaxants, the response to NO is also affected as a result of increased

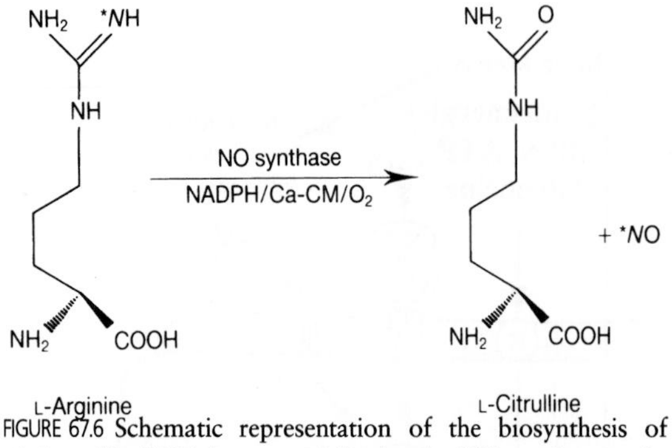

L-Arginine                    L-Citrulline

FIGURE 67.6 Schematic representation of the biosynthesis of nitric oxide (NO) from L-arginine by the NO synthase pathway. Ca-CM signifies the $Ca^{2+}$-calmodulin complex. Although a single arrow depicting the reaction is shown, the enzymatic conversion of L-arginine to NO plus L-citrulline is a complicated, multistep oxidation process. NO synthase activity also requires tetrahydrobiopterin, FAD (flavin adenine dinucleotide) and FMN (flavin mononucleotide), all of which are bound to NO synthase.

superoxide generation in the inflammatory cells attached to the endothelial cells and by oxidized low-density lipoprotein in the atherosclerotic plaque. Abnormal vasomotor regulation leads to increased production of vasoconstrictors and to vasospasm, elicited by acetylcholine and serotonin, which in normal vasculature produce relaxation. Hypertension, diabetes mellitus and homocystinuria also cause abnormal vascular reactivity in the NO pathway.

Prostacyclin ($PGI_2$) (Table 67.3 and Fig. 67.5), synthesized and released from endothelial cells, is a potent vasodilator, platelet aggregation inhibitor, profibrinolytic and cytoprotective agent. $PGI_2$, like other prostaglandins, is a 20-carbon (eicosanoid) unsaturated carboxylic acid with a cyclopentane ring, synthesized from arachidonic acid via the sequential action of the constitutive cyclooxygenase 1 (COX-1) peroxidase and prostacyclin synthase (see Chapter 8). $PGI_2$ has a half-life of about 3 min and, like NO, has mostly a local action. In smooth muscle cells, $PGI_2$ activates the membrane-bound adenylyl cyclase, and the elevated cyclic AMP (cAMP) activates intracellular kinases to produce relaxation. $PGI_2$-induced increases in cAMP in platelets inhibit the release of proaggregatory agents such as thromboxane $A_2$ ($TXA_2$), ADP and serotonin. $PGI_2$ synthesis can be stimulated by a number of agents that elevate intracellular $Ca^{2+}$ levels, such as kinins, catecholamines, ATP, $Ca^{2+}$ antagonists, angiotensin-converting enzyme (ACE) inhibitors and NO donors. Decreased synthesis of $PGI_2$ in maternal vessels may lead to pregnancy-induced hypertension, diabetic pregnancy or intrauterine growth retardation, and subsequent abnormalities in the development of fetal vasculature.

Prostaglandin $E_2$ ($PGE_2$) (Table 67.3 and Fig. 67.5), another vasodilator prostanoid synthesized from arachidonic acid, is released into the microcirculation, but not the macrocirculation. Endothelium-derived hyper-polarizing factors (EDHFs) (Table 67.3 and Fig. 67.5) are vasodilator compounds of as yet undetermined chemical composition that depolarize the smooth muscle cell membrane, by opening ATP-sensitive $K^+$ channels ($K^+_{ATP}$), or by activating the $Na^+$-$K^+$-ATPase. The recently discovered C-type natriuretic peptide produced by the vascular endothelium may be another modulating factor of vascular tone.

## Endothelium-derived constricting factors (EDCFs)

Endothelin (ET) (Table 67.3 and Fig. 67.7) is a 21-amino acid peptide that exists in three isoforms: ET-1, produced by endothelial cells, ET-2, produced in the intestine, and ET-3, synthesized in the brain. mRNA translation produces the preproendothelin (203 amino acids), which is converted to proendothelin by endopeptidases, and then to big endothelin (39 amino acids). The conversion of big endothelin (big ET) to ET-1 is catalyzed by the ET-converting enzyme (ECE), a membrane-bound metalloproteinase that cleaves the bond between tryptophan and valine of big ET to produce ET-1. ET-1 is about 100-fold more potent than big ET and 10-fold more potent than angiotensin II (AII), being considered the most potent vasoconstrictor yet identified. Two subtypes of ET-1 receptors, named $ET_A$ and $ET_B$, have been characterized. All three ET isoforms bind to $ET_B$ receptor, whereas ET-1 binds specifically to the $ET_A$ subtype. Both receptors are G-protein linked. ET-1 causes vasoconstriction and hypertension when it binds to the $ET_A$ receptor of vascular smooth muscle. ET-1 releases NO and $PGI_2$ from endothelial cells when it binds to the $ET_B$ receptor causing a transient fall in blood pressure prior to its hypertensive effect. In some circumstances, such as the pulmonary circulation in the perinatal period (see page 751), this vasodilating effect predominates.

Physiologically, ET-1 may serve in local and systemic hemostasis, in the event of blood vessel injury and hemorrhage. Locally, ET acts by eliciting a long-lasting vasoconstriction, along with the serotonin released from activated platelets. Systemically, in synergism with AII, ET-1 increases the peripheral vascular resistance and enhances fluid retention via its indirect antinatriuretic effects. In the perinatal period, ET may play an important role in regulation of amniotic fluid volume, in parturition and in closure of the ductus arteriosus and umbilical vessels at birth. During parturition, ET may have a direct action on the myometrium as well as an indirect action in stimulating myometrial prostaglandin production. Overproduction or overreaction to ET may result in reduction of fetoplacental blood flow and intrauterine growth retardation. High levels of ET-1 have also been found in myocardial infarction, cardiogenic shock, hypertension and pregnancy-induced hypertension and also in heart and renal failure.

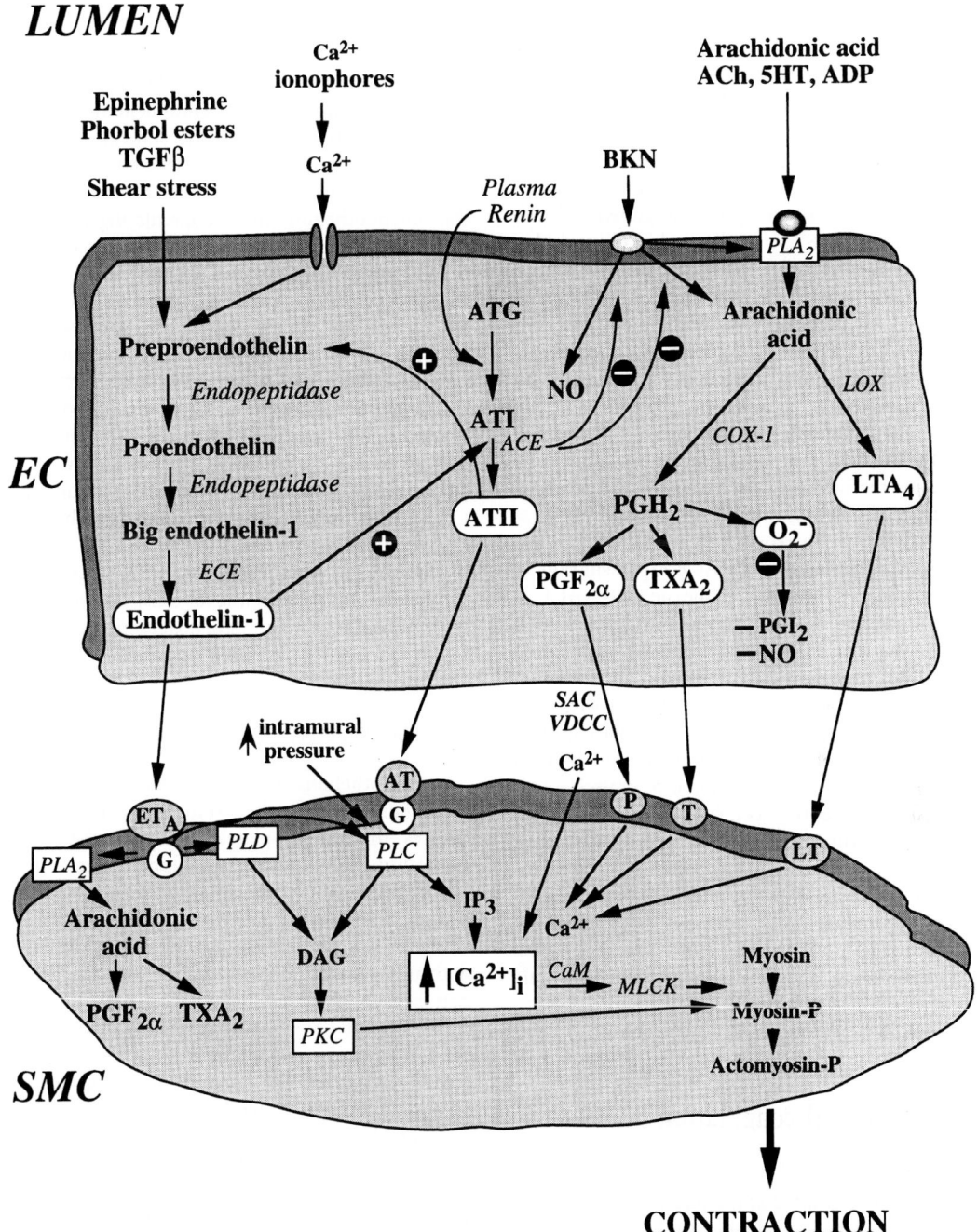

FIGURE 67.7 Vasoconstriction occurs by chemical or mechanical stimulation of endothelial cells (EC), resulting in the synthesis and release of contractile substances such as endothelin-1 (ET-1), angiotensin II (AII), thromboxane $A_2$ (TXA$_2$) and prostaglandin $F_{2\alpha}$ (PGF$_{2\alpha}$). These compounds interact with their receptor-operated $Ca^{2+}$ channels to cause $Ca^{2+}$ influx and elicit the smooth muscle cell (SMC) contraction via myosin light chain kinase (MLCK) activation, myosin phosphorylation and actomyosin-P formation. Superoxide radical ($O_2^-$), generated by cyclooxygenase-1 (COX-1) produces vasoconstriction indirectly by inhibiting the synthesis or the action of vasodilatory compounds such as prostacyclin (PGI$_2$) or nitric oxide (NO). Involvement of phospholipase $A_2$ (PLA$_2$), phospholipase C (PLC) and phospholipase D (PLD) as a result of ET-1 and AII action on the SMC specific receptors causes formation of contractile metabolites of arachidonic acid (PGF$_{2\alpha}$ and TXA$_2$) and protein kinase C (PKC) activation, respectively, which also lead to SMC contraction. ( ⊕, increased activity; ⊖, decreased activity.)

The COX-1 pathway (Fig. 67.7 and Table 67.3) generates proaggregating vasoconstrictors such as $TXA_2$, endoperoxides ($PGH_2$) and also superoxide anion ($O_2^-$). The net effect of free radical production in the endothelium is vasoconstriction, as a result of NO destruction and $PGI_2$ synthesis inhibition. There is no significant effect on $TXA_2$ synthesis. A number of other compounds generated by the cyclooxygenase, lipoxygenase and cytochrome $P_{450}$-dependent monooxygenase pathways also produce vasomotor effects.

In the renin–angiotensin system, angiotensin I (AI) (Fig. 67.7 and Table 67.3) synthesized in the endothelial cells, is converted to AII by endothelial ACE, which also inactivates bradykinin, a stimulator of NO and $PGI_2$ release. AII is the second most potent vasoconstrictor after ET-1. These two potent vasoconstrictors have an enhancing effect on each other. ET-1, by stimulating ACE activity, increases the production of AII. Similarly, AII potentiates ET-1 synthesis from preproendothelin. Both peptides also act synergistically by increasing the vascular tone and the blood pressure, as well as in stimulating smooth muscle cell proliferation and aldosterone secretion from the adrenal cortex.

In normal adult vasculature, ACE is present only in the endothelium. However, in the neonate, ACE is highly expressed in the tunica media and it has been suggested that AII may exert a growth-stimulating effect on the smooth muscle cells, via induction of platelet-derived growth factor (PDGF), transforming growth factor β (TGFβ) and basic fibroblast growth factor (bFGF). In adult vessels injured after balloon angioplasty, the neointimal smooth muscle cells express ACE. This represents a reversal of the contractile phenotype, which characterizes the normal adult smooth muscle, to the neonatal secretory form. This increased local AII synthesis results in neointimal proliferation. There are three subtypes of angiotensin receptors: AT1A and AT1B, expressed in normal adult blood vessels, and AT2 receptors, present only in the developing vessels and in adult injured neointimal smooth muscle cells.

# Endothelium and coagulation (see also Chapter 82)

The endothelium, situated at the interface between the circulating blood and vascular tissue, plays a central role in modulation of hemostasis and blood fluidity by participating in the procoagulant and anticoagulant pathways, in the regulation of fibrinolysis and in thrombus formation.

## Procoagulant action (Table 67.3)

The endothelium may directly stimulate the coagulation cascade by secreting PAF, factors V, X, tissue factor, vWF, fibronectin and high-molecular-weight kininogen (HMWK). Endothelial cells also secrete activators for factors V and XII and display binding sites for factors VIII, IX, IXa, X, Xa, and HMWK.

## Anticoagulant action (Table 67.3)

The main effect of endothelial cells on the coagulation cascade is inhibitory. The endothelium constitutes a functional barrier between the subendothelial procoagulant, tissue factor, and intraluminal factor VIIa, and between the proaggregating collagen and vWF in the subendothelium and the circulating platelets. The endothelial cells express cell surface glycosaminoglycans, such as heparan sulfate and dermatan sulfate. Heparan sulfate stimulates antithrombin II (which inactivates thrombin), coagulation factors IXa, Xa, XIa, XIIa, and lipoprotein-associated coagulation inhibitor (LACI), a potent factor Xa inhibitor. Dermatan sulfate has an inhibitory action on thrombin, by stimulating heparin cofactor II. The anticoagulant action is also evident in the autoregulatory pathway of the coagulation cascade, involving thrombomodulin, protein C and protein S, which inactivate thrombin and coagulation factors Va and VIIIa. Thrombin is also inactivated by protease nexin I, a protease inhibitor synthesized by the endothelial cells. Recently, an inhibitor of contact activation of coagulation via Hageman factor inactivation has been described.

## Thromboregulatory action (Table 67.3)

The endothelium modulates the early phases of thrombus formation by producing a number of substances that affect platelet function. NO activates platelet guanylyl cyclase and inhibits platelet degranulation, aggregation and adhesion to endothelial cells. The eicosanoids released from endothelial cells have either an antiaggregating action, such as $PGI_2$, which activates platelet adenylyl cyclase and has synergistic action with NO, or have a proaggregating action as in the case of $TXA_2$. vWF secreted by endothelial cells binds to platelet membrane glycoproteins and stimulates aggregation. The endothelial cell surface ectonucleotidase (ADPase) metabolizes ADP to adenosine to prevent platelet recruitment. Adenosine then elevates cAMP in platelets and further inhibits their aggregation. Endothelial cells, in turn, respond to platelet-derived products that may cause negative feedback modulation of the platelet function. Histamine, serotonin and ADP released during platelet activation stimulate the formation of NO and $PGI_2$ in endothelial cells, which inhibit aggregation. Platelet-derived TGFβ, histamine and serotonin stimulate secretion of vWF, a proaggregatory compound, from endothelial cells.

## Fibrinolytic action (Table 67.3)

The endothelium modulates clot dissolution, or fibrinolysis, by synthesizing plasminogen activators (PAs) and plasminogen activator inhibitors (PAIs). Fibrin is degraded by plasmin, a serine protease, originating in the proenzyme plasminogen. The PAs are serine proteases of urokinase type (u-PA) that activate plasminogen in the fluid phase, or tissue type (t-PA) which are active only when they are bound to fibrin. Endothelial cells also secrete two PAIs, PAI-1 and PAI-2. In pathological disruption of endothelial cell function such as in atherosclerosis, diabetes mellitus and homocystinuria, the altered extracellular matrix secreted by endothelial cells leads to reduced anticoagulant action and loss of inhibitory effects on smooth muscle cell proliferation, causing increased platelet aggregation and adherence, and reduced fibrinolytic ability.

## Endothelial control of vascular permeability

The endothelium constitutes a selective permeability barrier modulating the passage of plasma components from the lumen to the tissue. Transport of water, solutes and macromolecules across the endothelial monolayer occurs either through a small and large pore system or via transcytotic vesicles formed in the endothelial plasmalemma. During an acute inflammatory response, endothelial permeability increases to both solutes and macromolecules, leading to edema formation, also known as plasma protein leakage. Several stimuli, such as bradykinin, histamine, thrombin, oxygen radicals and PAF, elevate intracellular $Ca^{2+}$ ($[Ca^{2+}]_i$) and protein kinase C (PKC) activity, leading to alterations in the endothelial cell cytoskeleton and increased plasma leakage. Vascular permeability can be regulated by substances released from the endothelium that increase (ET-1) or decrease ($PGE_1$) the permeability of the endothelial monolayer to plasma components. Neutrophil adhesion and transendothelial migration also increase vascular permeability.

## Endothelium and blood flow

Blood vessels are continually exposed to hemodynamic forces that are the result of interacting physical, chemical and electrical events within the vascular wall. Physical forces, such as transmural pressure and luminal shear stress provide opposing mechanical stimuli that control the vasomotor activity. The endothelial monolayer, situated at the interface between vessel wall and the blood flowing through the lumen, responds to both acute and chronic changes in transmural pressure and shear stress by converting the physical force into a cellular response, a process known as mechanotransduction.

Acute increases in intramural pressure lead to contraction in smooth muscle cells via the myogenic response or by activating signal transduction pathways such as stretch-activated ion channels or phospholipase C (PLC), resulting in release of endothelial vasoconstrictors.

Acute increases in shear stress cause hyperpolarization of the endothelial cell membrane by activating $Ca^{2+}$-sensitive $K^+$ channels ($K^+_{Ca^{2+}}$). This change in membrane potential is transmitted via myoendothelial gap junctions, inducing relaxation in the smooth muscle cells. Simultaneous $[Ca^{2+}]_i$ elevation via GTP-binding protein activation by inositol phosphate (IP) and cyclic nucleotide generation trigger the release of endothelium-derived compounds such as acetylcholine, substance P, ATP, NO and $PGI_2$, causing further vascular relaxation.

Chronic shear elevation activates the nuclear factor κB (NF-κB) transcription complex (which may play a regulatory role in gene responses to flow), induces some early response genes (c-myc, c-fos, c-jun), and also induces a number of other genes such as those for PDGF-β, TGFβ, iNOS, t-PA, E-selectin, ICAM-1, VCAM-1, tissue factor and monocyte chemotactic protein-1. A putative positive shear stress response element (+SSRE) containing a GAGACC motif is required for the increased transcription of these genes. Renin and histamine release also is stimulated, whereas the production of ET-1, erythropoietin and fibronectin is inhibited. Down-regulation of ET-1 by shear stress, through a decrease in gene transcription rate without changes in ET-1 mRNA stability, occurs via an as yet unidentified negative shear stress response element (−SSRE). This process is dependent on intracellular $Ca^{2+}$, tyrosine kinase activity, and intact microtubules and is inhibited by cycloheximide. Shear stress acts first on the endothelial cell membrane, then is transmitted across to the cytoskeleton, and to the focal adhesion points at the sites of attachment, where the actin stress fibers are anchored to the cell membrane. Therefore, mechanotransduction occurs at both luminal and abluminal sites, and the dynamic cellular response to stress transmission leads to changes in cell signaling, adhesion, differentiation and morphology, resulting ultimately in vascular wall remodeling via smooth muscle cell hypertrophy or hyperplasia. Also, shear stress increases endothelial cell permeability, endocytosis, and decreases vascular thromboresistance and accelerates thrombus formation. In high-shear areas there is increased platelet interaction with the tumor cells and endothelium, enhancing metastatic dissemination. High shear stress also causes an increase in selectin-mediated rolling of leukocytes on the endothelium, whereas their adhesion to endothelial cells decreases.

## Ion channels in endothelial cell membrane

Endothelial cells do not produce action potentials and, therefore, are non-excitable. In these cells $Ca^{2+}$ plays a critical physiological role, and there are a number of mechanisms that regulate $Ca^{2+}$ influx, via either voltage-independent $Ca^{2+}$ channels (VICCs) or other types of channels. Depending on their regulatory mechanism, the VICCs can be subdivided into three groups: (1) receptor-operated $Ca^{2+}$ channels (ROCCs) are tightly coupled to the receptor and are G-protein regulated; (2) second messenger-operated $Ca^{2+}$ channels (SMOCCs) are regulated by intracellular $Ca^{2+}$ increases resulting from receptor stimulation, and by $IP_3$, $IP_4$ and other second messengers; (3) depletion-operated $Ca^{2+}$ channels (DOCCs) are regulated by the depletion of $Ca^{2+}$ pools in sarcoplasmic reticulum and their function is to refill the intracellular $Ca^{2+}$ stores.

The other ion channels that participate in endothelial cell function can also be divided into three categories: (1) channels activated in unstimulated cells; (2) channels activated in chemically stimulated cells; (3) channels activated in mechanically stimulated cells.

In unstimulated cells the most frequently activated are inwardly rectifying and other potassium ($K^+$) channels which upon activation cause membrane hyperpolarization. There are also cation channels that cause depolarization upon activation, as well as chloride ($Cl^-$) channels, which hyperpolarize the plasma membrane.

Endothelial cells chemically stimulated by acetylcholine, bradykinin, thrombin and ATP, via specific membrane receptors, respond by activating $K^+$ and non-selective cation channels (NSCCs). Many of the $K^+$ channels are activated by $Ca^{2+}$ [$Ca^{2+}$-activated potassium channels ($K^+_{Ca^{2+}}$)]. Thus, $Ca^{2+}$-activated $K^+$ currents increase the inward $Ca^{2+}$ conductance and $K^+$ efflux, which can stimulate NOS in endothelial cells to produce NO and induce vasodilatation. Depolarizing cation currents increase $Ca^{2+}$ efflux, thus diminishing the formation of NO and causing vasoconstriction. The inflammatory mediators such as bradykinin and histamine activate $K^+_{Ca^{2+}}$ channels, which by increasing $[Ca^{2+}]_i$ stimulate the contraction of endothelial cell actin and myosin, leading to increased transendothelial permeability.

Mechanical deformation of endothelial cells produced by elevated shear stress activates the inward rectifying $K^+$ channels, causing membrane hyperpolarization. Increased intraluminal pressure activates the *NSCCs* (also known as stretch-activated cation channels or *SACs*) that increase $Ca^{2+}$ permeability. The myogenic contraction of vascular smooth muscle cells in response to stretch is thus limited by the increased NO release in endothelial cells, resulting in autoregulation of vascular diameter and appropriate changes in blood flow.

## VASCULAR SMOOTH MUSCLE CELL FUNCTION

Smooth muscle cells are elongated, non-striated, and range in size from 10 to 200 μm (pregnant uterus) in length, and from 2 to 5 μm in width. Each cell is surrounded by a basement membrane consisting of collagen type IV, laminin, entactin and heparan sulfate. The role of the basement membrane is to maintain vascular smooth muscle cell homeostasis, regulate intercellular transport and function as a link with the extracellular matrix. The extracellular matrix, which limits the distention of cell lengths near the optimum for force development, contains elastic laminae, fibrils of collagen types I and III, chondroitin sulfate and dermatan sulfate.

The contractile elements form bundles consisting of thin actin and tropomyosin filaments, thick myosin filaments, and intermediate desmin (skeletin) and vimentin filaments. Both thin and intermediate filaments are attached to membrane-associated and cytosolic *dense bodies*, containing α-*actinin*, that transmit the contractile force to adjacent cells and their surrounding matrix. The sliding filament–crossbridge mechanism, characteristic of skeletal muscle contraction, also underlies smooth muscle cell contraction. Contraction velocities are much slower in vascular smooth muscle than in skeletal muscle, this being attributed to a myosin isoform with low ATPase activity. Smooth muscle cells contract tonically (sustained partial activation) and this is characterized by reduced rates of crossbridge cycling. Smooth muscle contraction is activated by $Ca^{2+}$, which stimulates myosin phosphorylation by myosin light chain kinase (MLCK) and the actin-activated myosin $Mg^{2+}$-ATPase. MLCK is $Ca^{2+}$ and calmodulin-dependent (Fig. 67.8). Troponin, the $Ca^{2+}$ regulatory protein in the thin filaments of skeletal and cardiac muscle, is absent from the vascular smooth muscle. Although vascular smooth muscle cells contain sarcoplasmic reticulum, most neurotransmitters, hormones and drugs that cause contraction are largely dependent on extracellular $Ca^{2+}$ influx for maximal responses. $Ca^{2+}$ influx depends either on a slow voltage-operated $Ca^{2+}$ channel (VOCC) that responds to changes in the membrane potential and leads to depolarization, or via NSCC. Smooth muscle cell membranes do not possess fast channels. Many neurotransmitters, hormones, and drugs interact with selective ROCCs to cause $Ca^{2+}$ influx and thus elicit contractile responses, often without changing the membrane potential (Fig. 67.8). $[Ca^{2+}]_i$ mobilization from the sarcoplasmic reticulum, via either $IP_3$ or ryanodine receptor $Ca^{2+}$ release channels, can also be involved.

Pharmacomechanical coupling represents the chain of events that takes place in the smooth muscle cell leading to contraction, and proceeds as follows: the elevated $[Ca^{2+}]_i$ binds to calmodulin producing a conformational change that promotes binding with MLCK. This $Ca^{2+}$–calmodulin–MLCK complex, representing the active form of MLCK, catalyzes the phosphorylation of light chain myosin. This process initiates the cycling of myosin crossbridges along the thin actin filaments, and as a result causes vascular smooth muscle cell contraction.

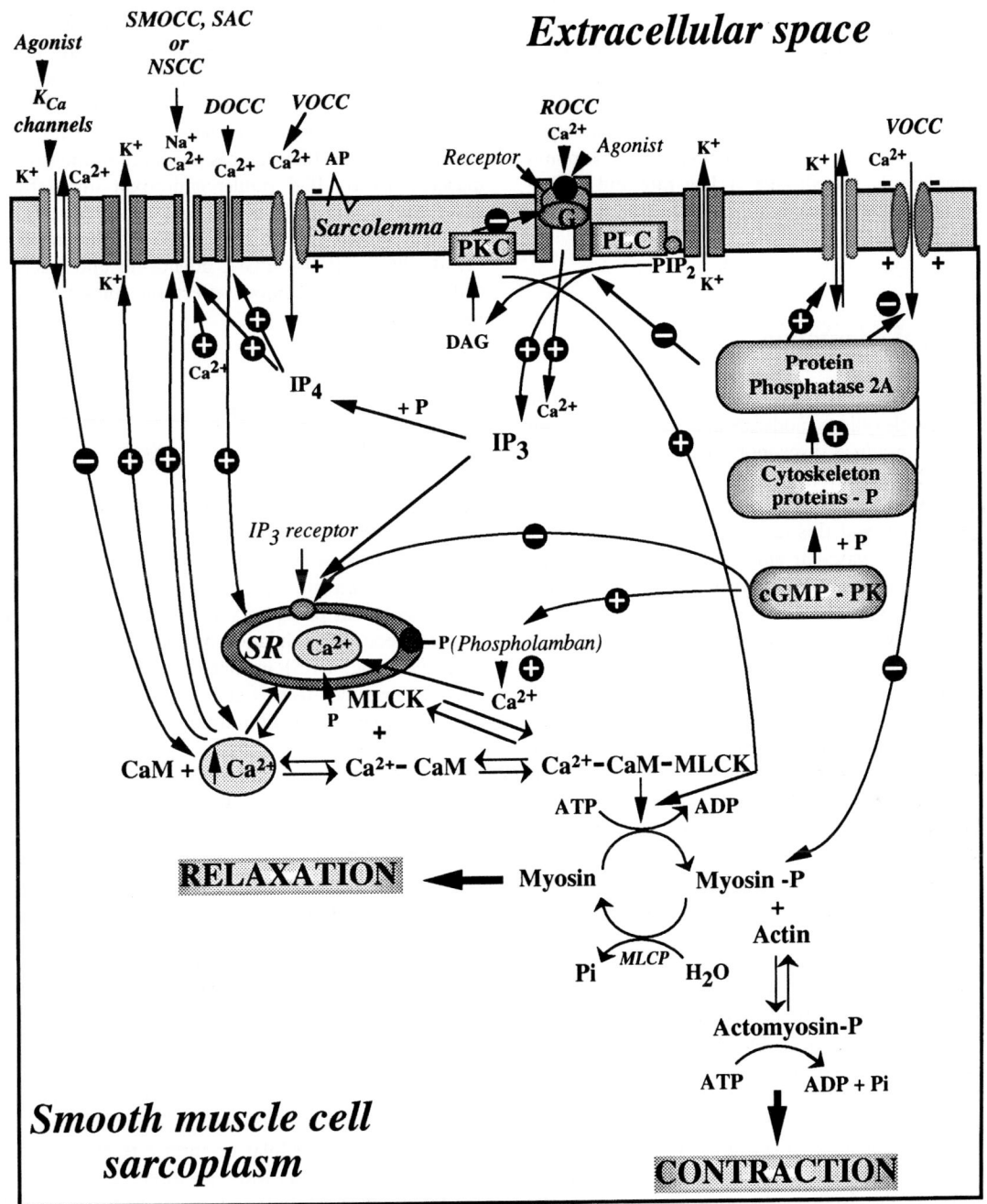

FIGURE 67.8 Schematic illustration of the role of $Ca^{2+}$ and cGMP-dependent protein kinase (cGMP-PK) in regulation of smooth muscle cell function. Agonists may act through receptor-operated $Ca^{2+}$ channels (ROCC), G protein-linked (G) to phospholipase C (PLC), which hydrolyzes the substrate phosphatidylinositol 4, 5-bisphosphate ($PIP_2$), producing inositol 1,4,5-trisphosphate ($IP_3$) and diacylglycerol (DAG). $IP_3$ formation activates the $IP_3$ receptor (calciosome) on the sarcoplasmic reticulum (SR) and causes the release of stored $Ca^{2+}$ into the cytoplasm. Inositol tetrakisphosphate ($IP_4$) formed from $IP_3$ activates the membrane non-selective cation channels (NSCC) and the depletion-operated $Ca^{2+}$ channels (DOCC) resulting in extracellular $Ca^{2+}$ influx. Activation of other ion channels such as $Ca^{2+}$-activated potassium channels ($K_{Ca}$), stretch-activated cation channels (SAC) and slow voltage-operated $Ca^{2+}$ channels (VOCC) also increase extracellular $Ca^{2+}$ influx. Elevated intracellular $Ca^{2+}$ binds to calmodulin (CaM) and to myosin light chain kinase (MLCK). This complex phosphorylates the myosin and initiates the cycling of myosin crossbridges along the actin filaments, resulting in smooth muscle cell contraction. Relaxation occurs from increased $Ca^{2+}$ efflux and/or sequestration into the SR, which leads to MLCK inactivation and myosin dephosphorylation. Cyclic GMP-dependent protein kinase (cGMP-PK) reduces the cytosolic $Ca^{2+}$ levels either by inhibiting $IP_3$ formation via PLC inactivation, by inhibiting the $IP_3$ receptor on the SR, by activating the $Ca^{2+}$-ATPase via its regulatory protein phospholamban, or by membrane hyperpolarization via $K_{Ca}$ channel activation. ( ⊕ , increased activity; ⊖ , decreased activity.)

Relaxation results from increased $Ca^{2+}$ efflux and/ or intracellular sequestration, that restores the resting $[Ca^{2+}]_i$ levels. MLCK is inactivated by the dissociation of calmodulin and myosin is dephosphorylated by myosin light chain phosphatases. Two potential regulatory proteins associated with actin filaments, calponin and caldesmon, have been identified. Calponin may regulate the crossbridge cycling rate and caldesmon may modulate the crosslinking of actin and myosin filaments.

## Functional adaptation

Because of the structural arrangement of vascular smooth muscle cells, a moderate shortening of smooth muscle can produce disproportionately large volume changes. The overall volume reduction is 30–40-fold for an arterial segment that undergoes a 50 per cent cell shortening, and this can stop blood flow. Unlike skeletal muscle, vascular smooth muscle shows little dependence on extrinsic innervation for maintaining contractile activity.

During development and growth smooth muscle cells are involved in the migration, proliferation and synthesis of extracellular matrix components, processes that confer a distinct "synthetic" phenotype (abundant endoplasmic reticulum and few contractile elements) to neonatal smooth muscle cells. Adult smooth muscle cells exhibit a "contractile" phenotype represented by a reduced rough endoplasmic reticulum and a well-developed contractile system. Other differences involve the extracellular matrix proteins, where fibronectin, osteopontin, tropoelastin and procollagen are expressed abundantly in the neonate and are absent in the adult vasculature. Similarly contractile elements and growth factors are expressed differently in the neonatal compared with the adult vessel. In adults, the tissue mass increases if the smooth muscle is subjected to a sustained increase in mechanical work (compensatory hypertrophy). A striking example of this principle is the thickening of the tunica media of arterioles in patients with essential hypertension. This may actually be attributed to cellular hypertrophy and hyperplasia. The response of adult smooth muscle cells to injury involves the re-expression of neonatal genes and the formation of neointima, either via dedifferentiation of adult smooth muscle cells or from an undifferentiated cell that, in response to injury, undergoes proliferation and migration. The growth factors and their receptors that are expressed in neonatal smooth muscle cells are present only in the adult injured tissue.

Vascular smooth muscle cell proliferation can be stimulated by exogenous mitogens such as PDGF, epidermal growth factor (EGF), insulin-like growth factor-I (IGF-I), FGF, IL-1 and IL-6, and TGFβ (which has both inhibitory and stimulatory effects). Also, vasoactive mediators such as catecholamines, serotonin, substance P, substance K (neurokinin A), ET, $PGE_2$, $PGI_2$, and $PGF_{2\alpha}$ and leukotrienes stimulate smooth muscle proliferation. Smooth muscle cells produce mitogens of their own (endogenous mitogens) that include PDGF (B chain in newborns and A chain in adults), smooth muscle cell-derived growth factor (SMCGF), IGF-I (in response to the inhibitory effects of PDGF), and heparan sulfate. Other factors produced in the smooth muscle cells are IL-1 (under endotoxin stimulation), bFGF and acidic FGF (aFGF) and ET or prostaglandins that inhibit growth by modulating the effects of PDGF. $PGE_1$, $PGE_2$, $PGI_2$, adenosine and heparan sulfate have an inhibitory effect on smooth muscle proliferation.

## Second messenger functions of cGMP and cAMP

Relaxation of vascular smooth muscle is caused by a variety of hormones and drugs that stimulate the intracellular formation of cAMP or cGMP. These second messengers activate specific protein kinases (PK), which results in phosphorylation of various enzymes with consequent modulation of their activities.

cGMP (Fig. 67.5) mediates the vascular smooth muscle relaxant effect of endogenous NO as well as that of exogenously administered NO donors, such as nitroglycerin and nitroprusside. Vascular smooth muscle contains two isoforms of guanylyl cyclase. The cytosolic isoform contains heme and is activated markedly by NO and EDRF. NO donors are converted in vascular smooth muscle cells to NO, which then activates guanylyl cyclase. The membrane-bound isoform is not influenced by NO but is activated by atrial natriuretic peptides or atriopeptins. Activation of either isoform of guanylyl cyclase results in intracellular cGMP formation and vascular smooth muscle relaxation.

cAMP (Fig. 67.5) mediated relaxation is caused by β-adrenergic agonists, certain prostaglandins, adenosine, and other activators of adenylyl cyclase. Adenylyl cyclase is a membrane-bound enzyme that is coupled to extracellular or surface receptors via G-proteins. Interaction with $β_2$-adrenergic receptors, prostaglandin receptors, and receptors for other substances results in adenylyl cyclase activation, intracellular cAMP formation, and vascular smooth muscle relaxation. Both cyclic nucleotides lower the intracellular concentration of $Ca^{2+}$ in vascular smooth muscle, thereby causing a decrease in tone.

cGMP-dependent protein kinase (cGMP-PK) has been shown to regulate several pathways that control cytosolic $Ca^{2+}$ levels in vascular smooth muscle (Fig. 67.8), such as $IP_3$ production and activity as well as activation of $Ca^{2+}$-ATPase, and the $K^+_{Ca^{2+}}$ channels. $IP_3$ production and activity is inhibited by cGMP-PK via phosphorylation of cytoskeleton proteins such as the actin-binding vasodilator-stimulated phosphoprotein (VASP) which inhibits PLC activation by removing it from the substrate, phosphatidylinositol 4,5-bisphosphate ($PIP_2$). $IP_3$ receptor (calciosome) function on the sarcoplasmic reticulum may also be inhibited by cGMP-PK. Another modulatory action of cGMP-PK on $[Ca^{2+}]_i$ levels occurs by phosphorylation of the sarcoplasmic reticulum, $Ca^{2+}$-ATPase regulatory protein, phospholamban, resulting in $Ca^{2+}$-ATPase activation and reduction of the $[Ca^{2+}]_i$ level, by increasing its sequestration into the sarcoplasmic reticulum. cGMP-PK also phosphorylates okadaik acid-sensitive protein phosphatases, which activate $K^+_{Ca^{2+}}$ channels and lead to membrane hyperpolarization and decreased cytosolic $Ca^{2+}$ entry through VOCCs. Thus by regulating $[Ca^{2+}]_i$, cGMP-PK modulates vascular smooth muscle tone.

# Control of vascular smooth muscle function

The vascular smooth muscle is the tissue responsible for the control of peripheral vascular resistance, arterial and venous tone, and distribution of blood throughout the body. Contractile activity is elicited by either neuronal or humoral stimuli. Some blood vessels show spontaneous contractions; this is termed electrical–mechanical coupling. Most of the arteries and veins are innervated by sympathetic adrenergic fibers, which release norepinephrine as the neurotransmitter. Therefore, the predominant autonomic tone output to blood vessels is sympathetic, and vasoconstriction or increased smooth muscle tone is the prevailing effect.

## Extrinsic control of vascular smooth muscle tone

The sympathetic division of the autonomic nervous system exerts its influence on arteries and veins via the action of norepinephrine on postsynaptic $\alpha_1$-adrenergic receptors. Inhibition of the sympathetic nerves, either centrally or peripherally, causes passive vascular smooth muscle relaxation and vasodilatation. Although the major neuronal control of the peripheral blood vessels is provided by sympathetic adrenergic vasoconstrictor fibers, sympathetic cholinergic fibers innervate primarily the resistance arteries in the skeletal muscle. These fibers release acetylcholine and cause vasodilatation, but the physiological role of these cholinergic fibers in the regulation of local blood flow is unknown. The cholinergic efferent fibers of the parasympathetic division innervate some blood vessels in the head and viscera, and their stimulation causes vascular smooth muscle relaxation and vasodilatation. The mechanism by which acetylcholine causes relaxation is thought to be attributed to an endothelium-dependent interaction resulting in the formation and release of EDRF/NO. Studies indicate that non-adrenergic non-cholinergic (NANC) neurons innervate some, but not all, arteries; the smooth muscle in the gastrointestinal tract and corpus cavernosum are two such examples. Electrical stimulation of NANC neurons causes vascular smooth muscle relaxation by releasing NO. Humoral factors such as circulating epinephrine, released from the adrenal medulla, affect vascular smooth muscle tone. Contraction or relaxation can occur depending on the tissue distribution of $\alpha_1$- and $\beta_2$-adrenergic receptors. Locally synthesized bradykinin, histamine, and serotonin in certain species, can cause local vasodilatation that is endothelium-dependent and attributed to the generation of EDRF/NO. The direct action of these endogenous substances on vascular smooth muscle is contraction, but this generally is not observed in normal, healthy blood vessels *in vivo*. Locally synthesized eicosanoids (prostaglandins, thromboxanes, leukotrienes) can cause contraction or relaxation depending on the blood vessel, species, and eicosanoid. Other chemical substances, such as the potent vasoconstrictors ET-1 and AII, serve a physiological role in regulating blood pressure and circulating blood volume.

## Intrinsic control of vascular smooth muscle tone

In a variety of tissues, local blood flow is modulated or adjusted to the existing metabolic activity or functional state of the smooth muscle. For example, changes in local blood flow or perfusion pressure can result in changes in vascular resistance or vascular smooth muscle tone that tend to maintain a constant blood flow. The mechanism of this autoregulation of local blood flow is not well understood and multiple mechanisms likely exist.

The myogenic hypothesis states that vascular smooth muscle contracts in response to stretch (sudden increase in local blood flow). Thus, the initial increase in flow is followed by a return of flow to prior control levels. The myogenic hypothesis may explain the vasoconstriction that occurs in the lower extremities when one changes position from reclining to standing.

The metabolic hypothesis requires that local blood flow is regulated by the metabolic activity of the smooth muscle or a decrease in oxygen supply to the smooth muscle. This appears to occur in many tissues including the heart and skeletal muscle, where blood flow closely parallels metabolic activity. The metabolic hypothesis may explain the increase in local blood flow that occurs during exercise. Numerous chemical substances have been proposed as mediators of metabolic vasodilatation including adenosine, certain prostaglandins ($PGE_2$ and $PGI_2$), and EDRF/NO.

The flow hypothesis is based on the observations that if arterial inflow to a vascular bed is stopped for a few seconds or longer, the local blood flow increases immediately on release of the occlusion (Fig. 67.9). The mechanism of this reactive hyperemia is unknown but may be attributed to the increased local formation of EDRF that is triggered by an increase in intracellular

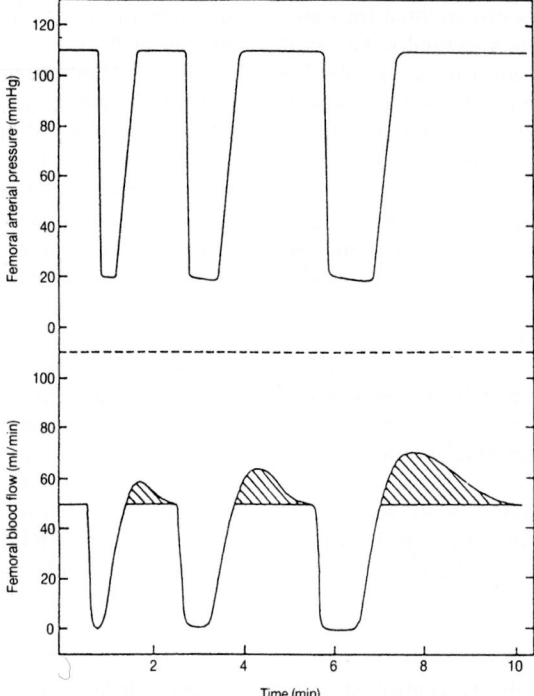

FIGURE 67.9 Schematic of experimental tracings illustrating reactive hyperemia in the hind limb of the dog after 15-, 30- and 45-second occlusions of the femoral artery. The hatched areas in the lower tracing represent the reactive hyperemia.

$Ca^{2+}$ levels in the affected smooth muscle. This situation may be analogous to the concept of flow-dependent vasodilatation, where a sudden local increase in blood flow causes a downstream vasodilatation to accommodate the increase in blood flow. Flow-dependent vasodilatation is an endothelium-dependent phenomenon. The stimulus for flow-dependent vasodilatation is increased shear forces or tangential forces imposed on the vascular endothelial cells by the increase in blood flow. The chemical agent that mediates the vascular smooth muscle relaxation appears to be EDRF/NO, as the response can be abolished by inhibitors of EDRF/NO synthesis (*see also* page 697).

Clearly, the direct changes in vascular smooth muscle tone brought about by neuronal influences are modified by the concomitant changes in the flow and pressure of the blood. Nevertheless, the control of vascular smooth muscle tone by both intrinsic and extrinsic mechanisms allows for vascular adjustments to provide changes in local blood flow as required under the prevailing conditions of metabolic organ function. Intrinsic flow-regulating mechanisms predominate in vital organs such as the heart and brain, and sympathetic nervous system activation during severe hemorrhage or shock has negligible effects on the arterioles within these areas, whereas marked vasoconstriction occurs in the skin, renal and splanchnic regions. Extrinsic flow-regulating mechanisms predo-

minate in the skin, especially through reflex hypothalamic pathways, to contribute to the regulation of body temperature. In skeletal muscle there appears to be more of a balance between extrinsic and intrinsic flow-regulating mechanisms. For example, neuronal control (vasoconstriction) predominates in resting muscle, whereas intrinsic control (vasodilatation) predominates in exercising muscle. Moreover, mere anticipation of impending skeletal muscle activity results in a predominance of intrinsic over extrinsic mechanisms.

## CONCLUSIONS

The vascular endothelium functions as a general endocrine gland by secreting a multitude of biologically active chemical substances that serve to regulate or modulate vascular smooth muscle function. Vascular smooth muscle receives its signal input not only from various innervations, but also from chemical agents generated in the adjacent endothelial cells. Thus, vascular smooth muscle function is critically dependent on normal endothelial cell function.

Endothelial cell pathology contributes to conditions such as atherosclerosis, hypertension, vasospasm, tissue inflammation, thrombosis, acute respiratory distress syndrome, and also diabetes and tumor growth. Pathophysiological alterations in endothelial cell function during the perinatal period can lead to a number of disorders such as intracerebral hemorrhage in the fetus and newborn, and altered fetoplacental circulation, persistent pulmonary hypertension, and preeclampsia, hypertension, thrombosis and other related diseases in the pregnant mother. Abnormalities in endothelial cell function that affect hemostasis during the perinatal period can result in inflammation of the placental vasculature (vasculitis) such as in chronic placental insufficiency. Interruption of the large placental vessels that occurs during complications of abruptio placenta and placenta previa are frequently followed by vessel rupture and hemorrhage. Abnormally developed blood vessels due to either congenital or metabolic disorders, such as in abnormal synthesis of collagen or of extracellular matrix components, are also accompanied by excessive hemorrhaging.

Given the life-threatening implications of the above-described disorders, the understanding of the complexity of cellular interactions that take place in the vascular wall, and how these interactions may be altered in pathological states, is of crucial importance.

## SELECTED READING

Allen BG, Walsh MP. The biochemical basis of the regulation of smooth-muscle contraction. *Trends Biochem Sci* 1994; **19**: 362.

D'Angelo G, Meininger GA. Transduction mechanisms involved in the regulation of myogenic activity. *Hypertension* 1994; **23**: 1096.

Davies MG, Hagen PO. The vascular endothelium. A new horizon. *Ann Surg* 1993; **218**: 593.

Davies PF, Barbee KA. Endothelial cell surface imaging: insights into hemodynamic force transduction. *News Physiol Sci* 1994; **9**: 153.

Feldman PL, Griffith OW, Stuehr DJ. The surprising life of nitric oxide. *Chem Eng News* 1993: **71**: 26.

Ignarro LJ. Nitric oxide-mediated vasorelaxation. *Thromb Haemost* 1993; **70**: 148.

Inagami T, Naruse M, Hoover R. Endothelium as an endocrine organ. *Annu Rev Physiol* 1995; **57**: 171.

Lincoln TM, Komalavilas P, Cornwell TL. Pleiotropic regulation of vascular smooth muscle tone by cyclic GMP-dependent protein kinase. *Hypertension* 1994; **23**: 1141.

Luscher TF. The endothelium as a target and mediator of cardiovascular disease. *Eur J Clin Invest* 1993; **23**: 670.

Masters BSS. Nitric oxide synthases: why so complex? *Annu Rev Nutr* 1994; **14**: 131.

Meidell RS. Southwestern internal medicine conference: endothelial dysfunction and vascular disease. *Am J Med Sci* 1994; **307**: 378.

Reinhart WH. Shear-dependence of endothelial functions. *Experientia* 1994; **50**: 87.

Rubanyi GM, Parker Botelho LH. Endothelins. *FASEB J* 1991; **5**: 2713.

Springer TA. Traffic signals on endothelium for lymphocyte recirculation and leukocyte emigration. *Annu Rev Physiol* 1995; **57**: 827.

# 68

# Cardiac and Myocardial Structure and Myocardial Cellular and Molecular Function

James D. Bristow

## ANATOMICAL DEVELOPMENT

The familiar four-chambered heart of mammals has its beginnings in the early embryo as two amorphous collections of cells. Not surprisingly, an extraordinary series of transformations is required to produce the configuration of the mature heart, and the complexity of this process has long fascinated embryologists. Driven by the wide spectrum of congenital heart defects occurring in children, an extremely detailed anatomical account of cardiac development has now been produced which provides a very useful framework for the categorization and understanding of many human congenital heart defects.

### Normal development

The earliest heart cells can be recognized as a collection of cardiac progenitor cells located on opposite sides of the lateral plate of the presomite embryo (approximately 17 days after conception in the human). These cells form bilateral tubular structures that migrate to the midline and fuse to form the primitive cardiac tube by day 21 of gestation. Shortly after its formation, the cardiac tube commences beating. Although the regions of the early heart tube are not morphologically distinct, each portion of the tube is named according to the structure that will arise from it. Hence, the caudal portion of this tube is called the sinus venosus, followed sequentially as one moves cephalad by the primitive atrium, ventricle, and bulbis cordis (Fig. 68.1a). At about 25 days' gestation, the cardiac tube bends and elongates, forming a loop anteriorly and to the right, the so called D-loop (Fig. 68.1b). This process positions the atrial portion of the tube posteriorly, the proximal portion of the ventricular segment, which will form the left ventricle, leftward, and the distal portion, which will form the right ventricle, rightward. At this stage, a frontal section through the heart demonstrates division of the tube's lumen into the primordial cardiac chambers (Fig. 68.1c). The inlet from the posterior atrium into the left portion of the primitive ventricle is through the atrioventricular (AV) canal. Outlet is superiorly, from the right portion of the ventricle into the conus cordis, which will form the outflow tracts of both ventricles. The transverse portion of the loop between halves of the primitive ventricle contains a slight swelling, which marks the beginning of the interventricular septum that will eventually close this communication. Finally, the conus cordis is in continuity with the truncus arteriosus, which will give rise to pulmonary artery and the aorta.

In the 3 weeks following completion of looping, the atria, AV canal, ventricles, conus cordis, and truncus arteriosus must all be septated. Beginning at 38 days' gestation, the atrial septum is closed, first by upward growth of the primum septum from the endocardial cushions, then by downward growth from the roof

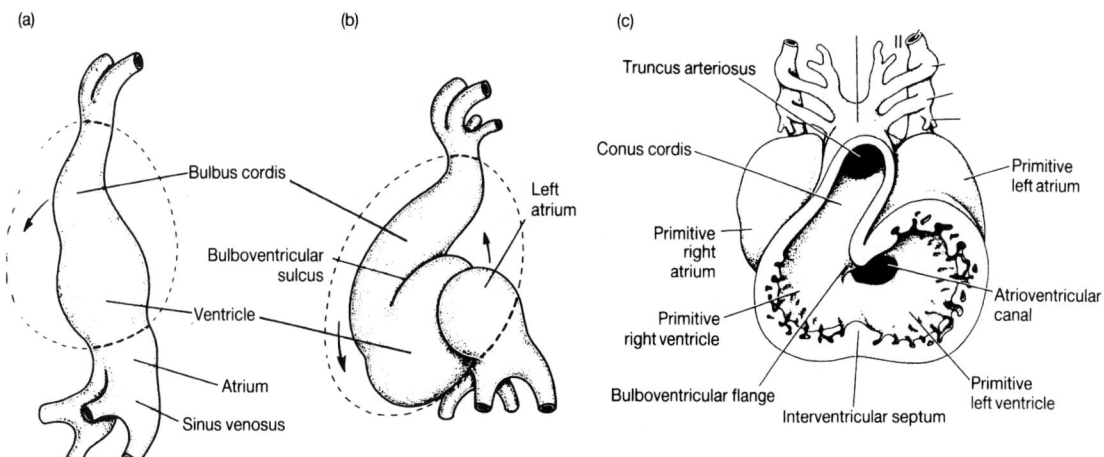

FIGURE 68.1 Looping of the cardiac tube. (a) Regions of the cardiac tube before looping. (b) The cardiac tube after looping viewed from the left. (c) Frontal section of the heart shown in (b). Note inlet is to the primitive left ventricle and outlet is from the primitive right ventricle. (From Langman J. *Medical embryology: human development – normal and abnormal,* 3rd edn. Baltimore: Williams and Wilkins, 1975, with permission.)

of the atrium (Fig. 68.2a). A portion of this septum is then resorbed, and the hole thus produced is closed by growth of the secundum septum just to the right of the primum septum. The secundum septum does not completely close, but leaves a centrally placed hole, the foramen ovale, which is covered by a flap valve consisting of primum septum. At the same time as the atria

are being septated, the AV canal must be divided into the tricuspid and mitral orifices. This occurs by upward and downward growth of the endocardial cushions located at the superior and inferior margins of the AV canal (Fig. 68.2b). This same process provides tissue to close the inlet portion of the ventricular septum. The remainder of the ventricular septum in

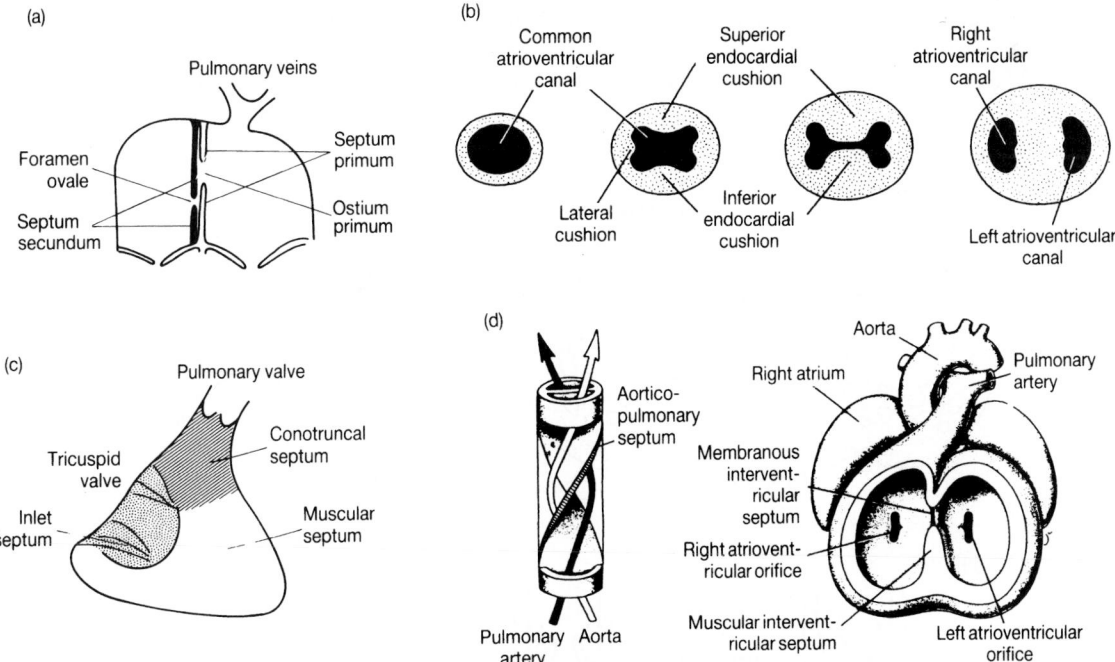

FIGURE 68.2 Formation of cardiac septa. (a) Apposition of the primum and secundum septa closes the atrial septum, but leaves a communication, the foramen ovale. (b) Division of the AV canal into left and right atrioventricular orifices. The valve leaflets will form later. (c) View of the mature ventricular septum from the right ventricle showing the origin of its three parts. (d) Schematic view of the conotruncal septum, showing that the septum rotates within the conus cordis and truncus, leading to the mature configuration of the great vessels. (From Langman J. *Medical embryology: human development – normal and abnormal,* 3rd edn. Baltimore: Williams and Wilkins, 1975, with permission.)

turn is closed by tissues from two other regions (Fig. 68.2c). First, the muscular septum is formed by upward growth of ventricular muscle from the inferior margin of the primitive ventricle. Second, within the conus cordis a spiraling septum divides it into right and left ventricular outflow tracts. The inferior margin of this septum comes in contact and fuses with the muscular septum. Fig. 68.1c demonstrates that if the conus cordis is to supply the outlet from both ventricles, it must move substantially to the left. This is accomplished by resorption of the bulboventricular flange (Fig. 68.1c). The truncus arteriosus is septated in concert with the conus cordis so that the anterior pulmonary artery is ultimately in continuity with the right ventricle and the posterior aorta is in continuity with the left ventricle (Fig. 68.2d).

Formation of the cardiac valves occurs immediately after septation of the AV canal and the truncus arteriosus (Fig. 68.3). Formation of the mitral and tricuspid valves begins with proliferation of undifferentiated cells surrounding both orifices, accompanied initially by growth of ventricular muscle below. Gradually the ventricular muscle below becomes hollowed out, leaving the tips of the nascent valve attached to the ventricular wall by muscular strands or chordae tendineae. The tissue in the chordae and the valve leaflets is eventually replaced by dense connective tissue, and the valves are complete. The semilunar valves are produced in similar fashion.

After septation, three outpouchings grow from the wall of the aorta and pulmonary artery. In this case resorption of tissue above the valve and at the commissures between valve leaflets, combined with continued growth of the central portion, produces elongation and

thinning of the valve leaflets. Resorption above the valve is complete so that the valve leaflets are attached to the vessel wall only at the hinge points.

By 55 days' human gestation the basic form of the heart has been attained and the remaining 80 per cent of gestation is used for growth and maturation of cardiac structures. Myocardial cells proliferate in tandem with the dramatic accumulation of contractile proteins and metabolic machinery required to meet the circulatory needs of the rapidly growing fetus.

## Abnormal development

Not surprisingly, abnormalities in each of the morphogenetic transformations described above occur and give rise to characteristic congenital heart lesions. Many of these defects are best understood as arrested development producing abnormal mature configurations that closely resemble normal stages in cardiac development. Several common examples, beginning with cardiac looping, are illustrated in Fig. 68.4 and serve to illustrate this point. If the primitive cardiac tube loops to the left rather than to the right, the primitive ventricles will be right–left reversed. If the remainder of cardiac morphogenesis proceeds normally but also right–left reversed, a functionally normal, mirror image heart will be produced, as is commonly seen in complete situs inversus. A functionally normal heart can also result after looping to the left if malrotation of the conus cordis establishes continuity between the left-sided "right" ventricle and the aorta, and between the right-sided "left" ventricle and

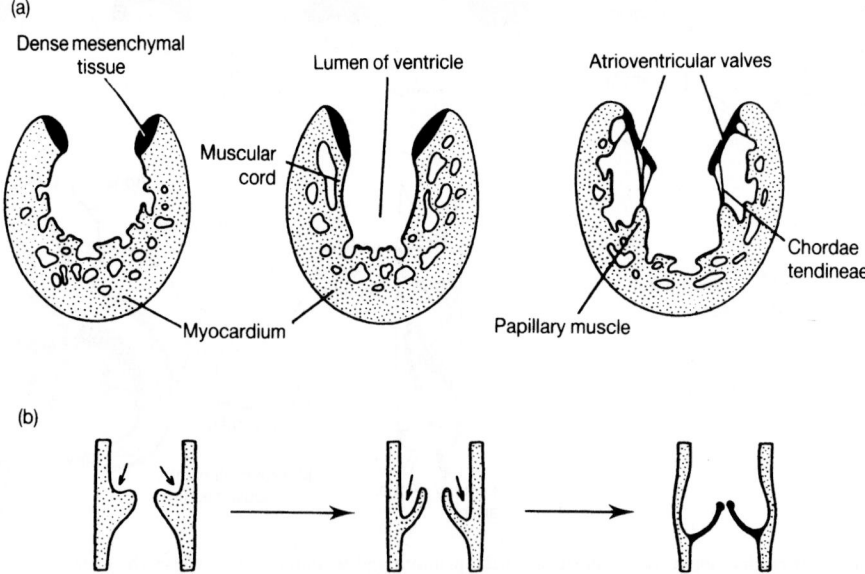

FIGURE 68.3 Formation of cardiac valves. (a) The atrioventricular valves are formed by incomplete resorption of underlying myocardium, leaving papillary muscles and chordae tendineae attached. (b) The semilunar valves are formed by more complete regression of tissue from above the valve. (From Langman J. *Medical embryology: human development – normal and abnormal*, 3rd edn. Baltimore: Williams and Wilkins, 1975, with permission.)

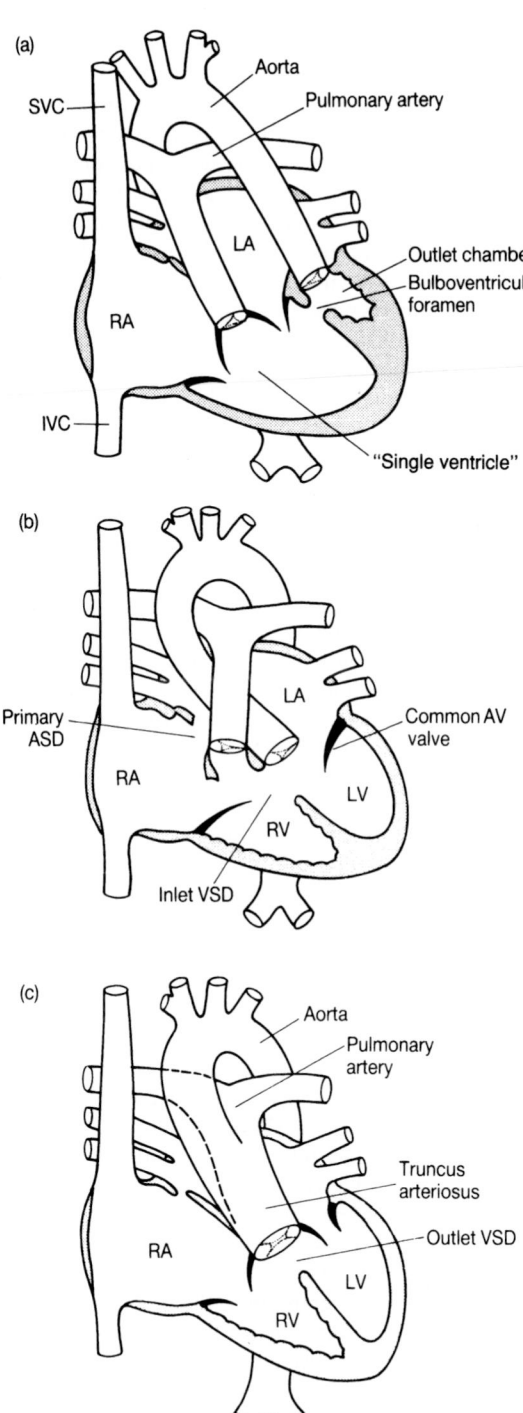

FIGURE 68.4 Congenital heart defects arising from arrested maturation. (a) Single ventricle and L-transposition. Atrioventricular connection is to the left ventricle, which connects to an outlet chamber derived from conus cordis. (b) Complete AV canal defect. The AV canal was not septated, leaving a single atrioventricular orifice. Septal defects are present both above and below this orifice. (c) Persistent truncus arteriosus. Failure of conotruncal septation leaves a single outlet from the ventricles and leaves a defect in the outlet portion of the ventricular septum.

the pulmonary artery. This rare malformation is called congenitally corrected transposition of the great arteries or *L-transposition* because the malrotation of the conus cordis corrects the abnormality in cardiac looping. More frequently, looping to the left is accompanied by arrest of ventricular septation giving rise to a *double inlet single ventricle* (Fig. 68.4a). In this case the conotruncal septum forms but is malrotated so that the single ventricle gives rise to a posterior pulmonary artery while the aorta arises from the persistent bulbis cordis. Not surprisingly, septation of the AV canal may also fail. In this circumstance the atrial and ventricular anatomy is strikingly similar to that in Fig. 68.1c.

The most common cardiac defects arise from incomplete septation of the atria or ventricles and are termed *atrial septal defect* (ASD) and *ventricular septal defect* (VSD), respectively. Predictably, defects in both the primum and secundum atrial septum and defects in each of the three components of the ventricular septum also occur. Occasionally, development of the endocardial cushions is abnormal, causing failure of septation of the AV canal as well as the inferior portion of the atrial septum and inlet portion of the ventricular septum. Clinically this is termed a *complete AV canal defect* (Fig. 68.4b) and is common in children with *Down syndrome*.

Abnormalities of conus cordis and truncus arteriosus development are commonly seen, and are usually grouped together as conotruncal malformations (Fig. 68.4c). If the conotruncal septum fails to form, one would predict the finding of *persistent truncus arteriosus*. This lesion is always found with a defect in the outlet portion of the ventricular septum because this portion of the ventricular septum is actually derived from the conotruncal septum. In each of these circumstances, the defect of the mature heart arises by persistence of normal embryological configurations. Not all congenital heart disease arises from arrested maturation, but analyses like that above have provided considerable information about the genesis of congenital heart lesions, and have suggested avenues for experimental inquiry.

## GENETICS OF CONGENITAL HEART DISEASE

Based on the high frequency of heart defects that accompanies human chromosomal aberrations, especially trisomy syndromes, it has been suspected for many years that certain congenital heart defects have a hereditable component. However, because these syndromes account for only a small fraction of congenital heart defects, another model needed to be constructed to account for the bulk of these lesions. The primary problem with defining the genetic basis of human congenital heart disease was (and is) how to explain the less than 25 per cent recurrence risk in all but a very few families, and the phenotypic variability of defects found in the families with more than one affected member. The most widely applied model of causation of congenital heart disease is the multifactorial threshold model proposed by Nora in 1968 (Fig. 68.5). The basic premise of this model is that each family carries a unique set of susceptibility genes that together define the family's risk. On this genetic background, environmental factors act to produce the actual risk observed.

This model has been useful for counseling of families as it predicts that environmental factors may play a major role in causation of congenital heart disease. Clearly this can be the case, as the association of heart defects with drugs (alcohol, lithium, and thalidomide), infectious agents (rubella), and fetal environment (phenylketonuria) or maternal environment (diabetes) has been shown. The major problem with this prediction is that these conditions explain only a small fraction of heart defects. Moreover, the incidence of heart defects appears to have been remarkably stable over the past 60 years, showing little variation with time or region across the globe, as might be expected if environmental factors were of major importance.

Recently, studies on the etiology of congenital heart disease have shifted emphasis to attempt to identify single genes capable of causing heart defects. Remarkable progress has been made in the course of a very few years. Evidence now supports the concept that single congenital heart disease genes can be identified and may ultimately explain the bulk of congenital heart diseases. The congenital heart defects shown in Fig. 68.4 will serve as examples of this approach.

As noted in the previous section, heart defects frequently accompany abnormal looping. Our understanding of this process has been aided greatly by the availability of an inbred mouse model (*iv*) that displays abnormal cardiac looping as an autosomal recessive trait. In *iv/iv* animals, situs is established randomly, and defects in laterality are frequently found in other viscera as well, as is the case in humans. The gene

defect has been mapped to the telomeric region of mouse chromosome 12, but the specific gene is not yet identified. The major importance of this model is in the incidence and variability of the heart defects. Depending on the strain, the incidence of heart defects may be substantially less than predicted by simple Mendelian genetics, and affected mice display a broad range of defects from simple ASD to the complex defects shown in Fig. 68.4a. Hence mice with identical genotypes and maternal environments may display the same phenotypic variability that is characteristic of human congenital heart defects.

With the information that a single gene might cause defects in laterality in hand, it has recently been shown that some patients with abnormal laterality and severe congenital heart defects have mutations in the *connexin43* gene, encoding a gap junction protein that may play a role in intercellular signaling during cardiac development. Whether all patients with abnormal laterality will have defects in this, or related genes, is not yet known.

We next turn to the example of *AV canal defects*. These defects are common in children with *Down syndrome* who have an extra copy of chromosome 21. However, not all children with features of Down syndrome carry complete extra copies of this chromosome. As a result of unbalanced translocations, some patients have triplication of portions of chromosome 21. Analysis of a number of such patients has shown that the phenotype of these patients is correlated with the portion of chromosome 21 that is triplicated. It now appears that AV canal defects are seen in patients who are trisomic for a region of about 6 million bp of chromosome 21; an intensive hunt is underway for genes within this region that might be responsible for the cardiac phenotype.

It is reasonable to ask what such a gene or genes might be doing. To begin thinking about the problem, first it is important to understand how the endocardial cushions develop. The cushions develop as acellular collections of extracellular matrix that lie between the endothelial lining of the heart (the endocardium) and the myocardial muscle cell layer that lies beneath. By a process known as endothelial–mesenchymal transformation, endothelial cells bud off from the endothelium and migrate into the cushion matrix. Because these cells ultimately form the valve leaflets and contribute to the primum atrial septum and inlet ventricular septum, this process has been the focus of ongoing experiments in several laboratories analyzing endocardial cushion development in the chick. Our present understanding of endothelial–mesenchymal transformation is depicted in Fig. 68.6.

This process also has played a central role in the thinking about phenotypic variability in congenital heart disease. Kurnitt in 1987 developed a computer model that simulated endothelial–mesenchymal transformation and subsequent cell migration and aggregation. He demonstrated that no matter how he varied the parameters of his model, a random variation in final

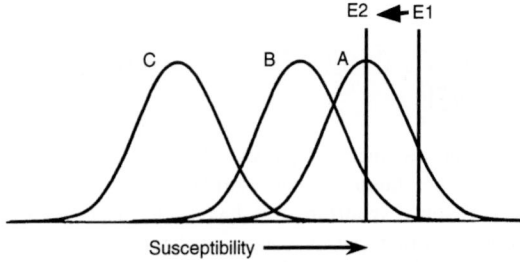

FIGURE 68.5 The multifactorial threshold model. Three families, each with a unique set of susceptibility genes, are represented by the bell-shaped curves labeled A, B, and C. Given a standard exposure to environmental teratogens, each will have a given incidence of congenital heart disease. If exposure to an environmental teratogen occurs (E2) the threshold for congenital heart disease is reduced, and the incidence of disease increases for high- (A) and moderate-risk (B) families, but not appreciably for the low-risk family (C).

pattern was achieved. This is not surprising, but it leads directly to the conclusion that randomness in heart development must be acknowledged, and that phenotypic variability in congenital heart defects may reflect this randomness more than genetic heterogeneity.

The final example, *persistent truncus arteriosus*, is an uncommon congenital heart defect, but 50 per cent of patients with this lesion also have defects in development of the thymus gland (producing T lymphocyte deficiency) and parathyroid gland (producing hypocalcemia), as well as characteristic abnormal facies (*DiGeorge syndrome*). All of the organs affected in DiGeorge syndrome require the presence of neural crest cells for normal morphogenesis. These cells migrate from the cranial neuro-ectoderm, and in the heart they can be demonstrated experimentally in the conotruncal portion of the ventricular septum. Although the precise mechanism responsible for deficient neural crest migration or subsequent function is not known, it seems reasonable to speculate that a single gene defect might be responsible for DiGeorge

syndrome and perhaps sporadic truncus arteriosus as well.

This hypothesis has been boosted by the recent demonstration that most patients with *DiGeorge syndrome* have a deletion on chromosome 22q11. Most of these patients have a *de novo* deletion, but a few have inherited the deletion from a parent without heart disease, suggesting that phenotypic variability should be expected. Several genes have now been identified within the deleted segment, and it is not yet clear whether the developmental defects arise from loss of a single or multiple genes within the region. Surprisingly, the same deletion is found in another genetic syndrome, the *velo-cardio-facial syndrome*, which has distinct features including *cleft palate*, *tetralogy of Fallot*, and characteristic facies. Clearly these two syndromes constitute a spectrum with a single etiology. The next surprise was the finding that 15–30 per cent of children with sporadic tetralogy of Fallot will also carry the deletion. The final piece of the puzzle is the identification of the gene or genes responsible for these several phenotypes and correlation of phenotypes with genotypes.

Given the clinical experience with congenital heart defects, it might be predicted that single gene defects will be found to explain the bulk of patients with the heart defects discussed here, but that phenotypes and genotypes will not be tightly correlated. In other words, a single genetic defect may give rise to a spectrum of related defects or, at times, no defect at all. This probably occurs because the gene defects producing congenital heart disease act early in heart development, producing abnormalities that have secondary effects which influence subsequent development. The challenge is first to identify the molecular pathology and then to characterize the secondary effects at both the molecular and anatomical/functional level.

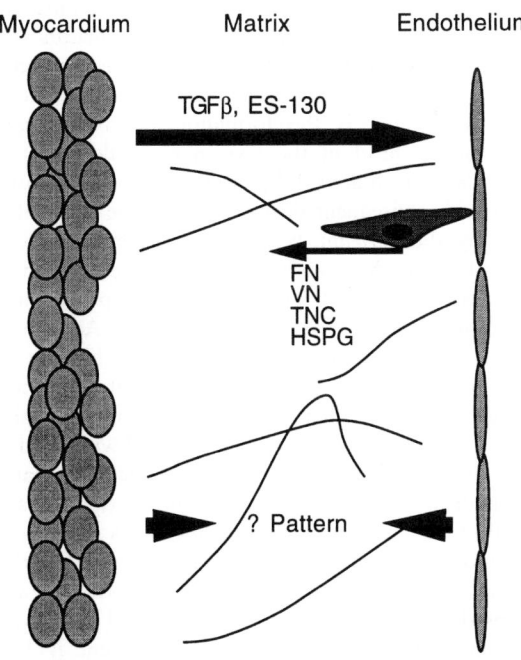

FIGURE 68.6 Cellular interactions in the atrioventricular endocardial cushions. A schematic longitudinal section of the post-looped heart shows the myocardial and endocardial cell layers, and the extracellular matrix between them. The myocardial layer secretes transforming growth factor β (TGFβ) and ES-130 (a novel matrix element) that induce an endothelial–mesenchymal transformation. Such a transformed endothelial cell can be seen budding from the endothelial lining where it migrates on a substrate rich in fibronectin (FN), vitronectin (VN), tenascin-C (TNC), and heparan sulfate proteoglycan (HSPG). The migration and maturation of these cells results in the formation of the fibrous crux of the heart. The signals responsible for patterning of these cells (arrowheads) may arise from the myocardium, endocardium or both, but the nature of these signals is completely unknown.

## MICROSCOPIC ORGANIZATION AND FUNCTION OF THE HEART

The developing heart, like the mature heart, is made up of several different cell types, including myocytes, specialized conducting cells, fibroblasts, neural cells, and vascular elements. During the process of cardiac morphogenesis, the heart also contains numerous undifferentiated cells, termed mesenchymal cells, that ultimately differentiate into mature cardiac cells or may die (as in the formation of the cardiac valves). The predominant cell type in the mature heart is the myocyte, which can be identified by the numerous myofibrils that contain the contractile apparatus. Within each myocyte the myofibrils are arranged in parallel along the cell's long axis, giving the myocyte its characteristic striated appearance. In the embryonic heart the first myocytes appear in the primitive cardiac tube; however, these contain relatively few myofibrils, the arrangement of which is somewhat more random than in the mature heart. After the developing heart reaches the four-chambered adult configuration, cardiac mass increases rapidly by myocyte division (hyperplasia). The myofibrillar content of myocytes increases steadily through gestation (hypertrophy). After birth, most species, including humans, have relatively little capacity for hyperplasia, but myocyte hypertrophy continues.

The cardiac myocyte, a relatively large and highly specialized cell, has a subcellular structure uniquely organized to carry out its contractile function. Myocytes are packed with myofibrils, each containing numerous sarcomeres, the fundamental contractile unit, linked end to end. Each myofibril is surrounded by a complex network of membranes called the sarcoplasmic reticulum (SR), which supplies $Ca^{2+}$ to activate the contractile apparatus for each contraction and removes $Ca^{2+}$ during cardiac relaxation. Also nearby are vast numbers of mitochondria, the site of oxidative phosphorylation, which supply the high-energy phosphates necessary for cellular contraction and maintenance of cellular integrity. The transmission of tension from the contractile apparatus to the whole ventricle requires a series of links from the sarcomere to the fibrous supporting matrix. This function is assumed by the cytoskeleton and the extracellular matrix. Each of these several cellular components will be examined in detail.

# The sarcomere

As noted above, the myocyte contains many myofibrils arranged in parallel, each in turn composed of many sarcomeres arranged in series. As seen in Fig. 68.7, the sarcomere consists of an array of partially overlapping thick filaments composed of myosin as well as thin filaments composed primarily of actin. The sarcomere has been divided into various regions according to its microscopic appearance, and the content of each region is now known with some precision. Hence the dark Z line is the fibrous end of the sarcomere to which the actin filaments are anchored. The I band corresponds to the proximal portion of the actin filament not overlapping with myosin, while the A band corresponds to the length of the myosin filament. A great deal is now known about the several components of the sarcomere, the precise mechanism of sarcomere shortening, and the expression of contractile proteins during development.

The thick filament is approximately 1.6 μm in length and about 10 nm in diameter at the center, but tapers toward each end. It is composed of overlapping double-stranded myosin heavy chain molecules, each of which contains a rod-like portion and a globular head. The myosin heads are radially oriented, and attached to each is a myosin light chain molecule. The head of the heavy chain contains the contractile ATPase. The thin filament is composed of a double-stranded helix of actin, through the center of which

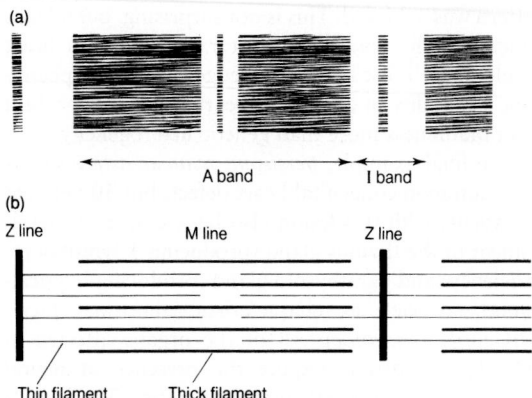

FIGURE 68.7 The sarcomere is the fundamental contractile unit. Its appearance under the electron microscope (a) is produced by overlapping of thick filaments composed of myosin and thin filaments composed primarily of actin (b).

runs a third protein called tropomyosin. At regular intervals (0.3 μm), the troponin complex is found. Troponin comprises three proteins: troponin C, which binds $Ca^{2+}$; troponin I, which inhibits intrinsic ATPase activity; and troponin T, which anchors the complex to the actin/tropomyosin chain. It is now generally accepted that the fundamental event in sarcomere shortening is the formation of crossbridges between the head of the myosin molecule and the thin filament, followed by rotation of the myosin head with consequent displacement of the actin filament by about 10 nm. Following displacement of the thin filament, the myosin head is released, and the cycle can be repeated. The details of this process are diagrammatically represented in Fig. 68.8. According to this model, the process is begun by the binding of $Ca^{2+}$ to troponin C. This produces a conformational change in the thin filament that allows binding of the myosin heads, which are already charged with adenosine-5'-diphosphate (ADP) and inorganic phosphate, the hydrolysis products of adenosine-5'-triphosphate (ATP). Once the myosin head is bound, its rotation is induced and the thin filament is displaced. After the stroke is completed, the ATP hydrolysis products are released and a new ATP molecule is bound before the myosin head is released from the thin filament. ATP is finally hydrolyzed in the process of restoring the activated conformation of the myosin heavy chain. One immediate consequence of this cycle arises from the observation that ATP must bind to the myosin head before the latter is released from the thin filament. In circumstances that deplete ATP, myosin remains attached to the thin filament. In skeletal muscle this gives rise to rigor mortis, and in cardiac muscle is a potential mechanism for impaired relaxation during periods of metabolic failure.

This model of sarcomere function has been greeted with enthusiasm because it provides an ultrastructural basis for several important physiological properties of the heart, the most important of which is the Starling

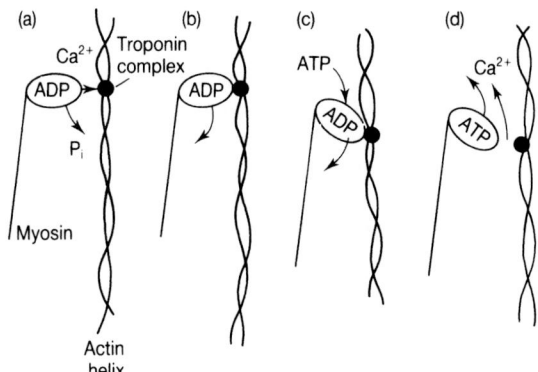

FIGURE 68.8 The contractile cycle. (a) In response to increased Ca$^{2+}$, the myosin heads form crossbridges with actin thin filaments. (b) The myosin head rotates, thereby displacing the thin filament. (c) ADP and inorganic phosphate (P$_i$) are released and ATP is bound by the myosin head before the crossbridge is broken. (d) Ca$^{2+}$ is removed and the crossbridge is broken. ATP is hydrolyzed, and the energy is stored as a change in conformation of the myosin head.

law of the heart (*see* page 739). Most simply stated, this law suggests that the heart is able to change the force of contraction as its initial size (or length) is changed. As seen in Fig. 68.9, this phenomenon can be explained based on the overlapping of thick and thin filaments. At a sarcomere length of 3.6 μm, there is essentially no force generation, because there is no overlap between thick and thin filaments. As the sarcomere is shortened, force generation increases due to increasing overlap of thick and thin filaments. At a sarcomere length of 2 μm, overlap and force generation are maximal. With further shortening, thin filaments begin to overlap each other, interfering with myosin crossbridge formation and force generation. The minimum sarcomere length corresponds to the length of the thick filament at which time the I band can be seen to disappear.

Over the past several years, intense interest has centered on the molecular biology of contractile proteins, the best studied of which are the myosin heavy chains. As has long been known, myosin heavy chains exist in

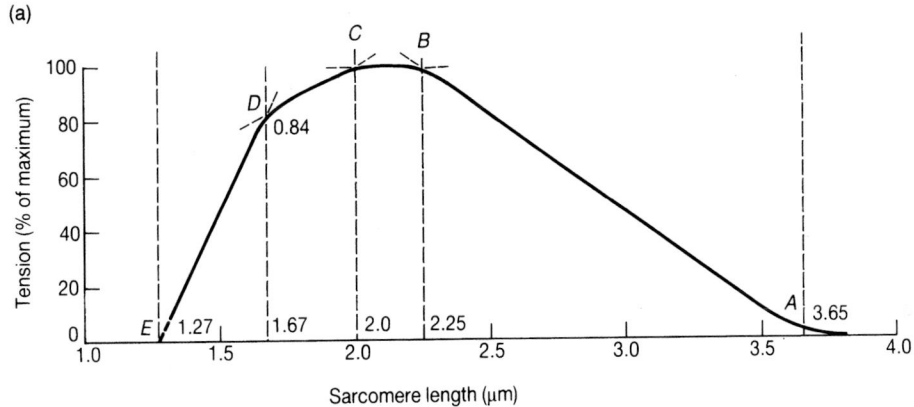

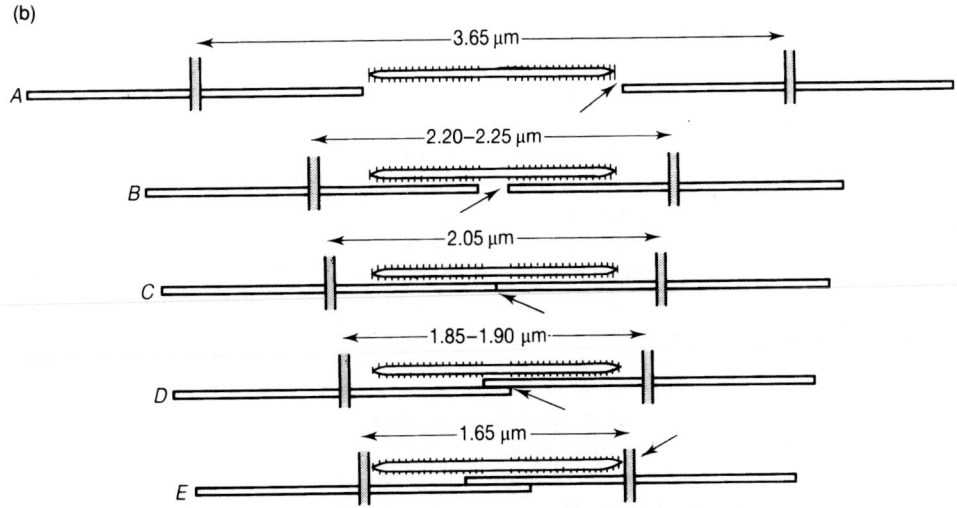

FIGURE 68.9 The ultrastructural basis for Starling's law of the heart. (a) Developed tension as a function of sarcomere length. (b) Force generation is dependent upon initial sarcomere length which determines overlap between thick and thin filaments. Maximal tension occurs with optimum overlap (about 2 μm). (From Braunwald E, ed. *Heart disease, a textbook of cardiovascular medicine*. Philadelphia: Saunders, 1980, p. 427, with permission.)

three forms, denoted V1, V2, and V3, which differ in their relative rates of ATP hydrolysis. We now know that two myosin heavy-chain genes give rise to distinct isoforms called $\alpha$ and $\beta$. Dimerization of these isoforms yields the three V isoforms: V1 and V3 are $\alpha$ and $\beta$ homodimers, respectively, while V2 is an $\alpha\beta$ heterodimer. It is also known that in most mature mammals, ventricular muscle contains the V1 isoform with the highest ATPase activity. However, before birth the V3 isoform predominates. In human heart, ventricular muscle does not switch from V3 expression after birth, but whether contractile protein expression may be altered in some disease states is not known.

Switching of myosin heavy chain genes occurs in many other muscles throughout the body, but not all switch from V1 to V3. This raised an interesting molecular question: why under the influence of thyroid hormone does one muscle switch from V1 to V3, while another will switch from V3 to V1 or V2? The basis of neonatal myosin heavy chain switching is now known to be due to the neonatal increase in thyroid hormone concentrations, and the answer to this question comes from knowledge of thyroid hormone receptors. This ever-expanding family of receptors binds thyroid hormone, and the complex can then bind to the regulatory regions of responsive genes either to enhance or to repress transcription of specific genes. The myosin heavy chain genes contain several sequences upstream (5' in DNA language) of the coding sequences that are capable of binding the thyroid hormone receptor complex. Hence tissue-specific expression of myosin heavy chain genes depends on the thyroid hormone receptor(s) being expressed by each muscle at a particular time. This observation was very important in developmental biology because it demonstrated one way in which expression of a single gene can be independently regulated by the several tissues that must express the gene at one time or another.

The genetics of contractile proteins has recently achieved clinical importance with the demonstration that point mutations in three contractile proteins, the $\beta$ myosin heavy chain, troponin T, and $\alpha$ tropomyosin, are responsible for the human disease *familial hypertrophic cardiomyopathy*. This disease is an autosomal dominant disorder, which produces gradually increasing ventricular mass beginning in the second or third decade. Histologically, the hypertrophic muscle is characterized by disorganization of myofibrils and fibrosis (presumably due to myocyte death). The hypertrophy causes symptoms by producing left ventricular outlet obstruction in some patients, and sudden cardiac death in others. A benign course is also seen in many of these patients. The first mutations identified were in the $\beta$ myosin heavy-chain gene, which, remarkably, became a candidate gene only after it was shown by a positional cloning strategy to be tightly linked in one large kindred. Many mutations in the $\beta$ myosin heavy-chain gene have been detected, and many of them involve replacement of charged residues with neutral amino acids in the head region.

Although this makes molecular diagnosis somewhat difficult, researchers have been rewarded by finding that some mutations carry a much higher risk for sudden death than others. This is important because it allows identification of affected individuals before hypertrophy is documented. Early therapy and close surveillance are clearly warranted for such individuals.

Another issue raised by this disease is how the molecular defects lead to hypertrophy. It is attractive to speculate that myocytes containing both normal and abnormal contractile proteins initially have a mild defect in tension development, and that this leads to increased synthesis of contractile proteins. This is plausible because the normal response to increased wall tension is synthesis of contractile proteins and myocyte hypertrophy. Hence a mechanism must exist that transduces tension into synthesis of contractile proteins. As abnormal contractile proteins accumulate, more myofibrils are affected and tension generation worsens, leading to further hypertrophy. Recently, mutant human $\beta$ myosin heavy-chain genes have been inserted in mice which then develop hypertrophy. It is hoped that a better understanding of the mechanism of abnormal tension generation and its transduction into gene expression will be gained from these animals. Armed with this information, new strategies to intervene in this and other forms of cardiac hypertrophy may be developed.

## SR and excitation–contraction coupling

For the myocyte to contract and relax as frequently as three or four times per second, an extremely rapid mechanism must activate and deactivate myofibrillar contraction. The SR is now well known to play the central role in this process. The SR is a membrane-limited intracellular organelle that surrounds each sarcomere with longitudinal tubules. The SR alternately releases and sequesters intracellular $Ca^{2+}$ ions that ultimately are responsible for myofibrillar contraction. The cell membrane of the myocyte contains invaginations localized over the Z line of each sarcomere, and from these, further extensions called T tubules penetrate the myocyte. At some points the SR and T tubule lie very close (10 nm), and in these regions the SR flattens into sac-like structures called cisternae. One should remember that although the T-tubule system and the SR are both membrane systems, they do not communicate directly. The T-tubule system is in communication with the extracellular space, while the SR is an intracellular organelle. They are, however, closely coupled, as depolarization of the cell membrane is channeled through the T tubules, leading to a small increase in intracellular $Ca^{2+}$ concentration during the plateau phase of the action potential. This increase in $Ca^{2+}$ is not sufficient to activate contraction, but does activate release of $Ca^{2+}$ from the SR, which raises intracellular $Ca^{2+}$ by 100-fold, which in turn activates myofibrillar contraction. This integrated process is termed *excitation–contraction coupling*.

In mature myocytes the primary site of $Ca^{2+}$ release and storage is the cisternae of the SR, where $Ca^{2+}$ is sequestered by a binding protein called calsequestrin. Because of its central role in excitation–contraction coupling, $Ca^{2+}$ concentration in the cisternae of the SR is believed to play an important role in determining the inotropic state of the myocyte. During relaxation, $Ca^{2+}$ is actively transported into the SR by a $Ca^{2+}$-dependent ATPase and bound by a second $Ca^{2+}$-binding protein, phospholamban. Both the $Ca^{2+}$-dependent ATPase and phospholamban are confined to the longitudinal tubules. Because the sites of systolic and diastolic $Ca^{2+}$ flux are different, it is not surprising that abnormalities of systolic and diastolic function are frequently separable.

Present evidence suggests that $Ca^{2+}$ handling by the sarcolemma of immature myocytes is relatively well developed. Conversely, $Ca^{2+}$ transport by the SR is less well developed. There are fewer cisternae in the SR, and $Ca^{2+}$ uptake by the SR has been shown to be decreased due to a lower rate of ATP hydrolysis and a lower coupling ratio (mol $Ca^{2+}$ pumped/mol ATP hydrolyzed). The first implication of these findings is that extracellular $Ca^{2+}$ may be quantitatively more important for activation of the contractile apparatus in immature myocardium, which may explain its more pronounced $Ca^{2+}$ sensitivity when compared with mature myocardium. Furthermore, the impaired $Ca^{2+}$ uptake by SR may be responsible for altered diastolic function in the fetus. Finally, in mature myocardium, the availability of intracellular $Ca^{2+}$ to the contractile proteins obviously is a major determinant of inotropic state. This is true for increases in inotropy due to increased heart rate, following both a premature extrasystole and administration of cardiac glycosides (digoxin). Because both release and uptake of $Ca^{2+}$ by SR are reduced in the immature heart, it has been postulated that fetal cardiac function is impaired relative to the adult. Whether this speculation will be borne out in intact animals remains an open question.

## Extracellular matrix (ECM) and cytoskeleton

During each systole, individual myocytes obviously must shorten. It is equally true that for this to occur there must be a link between the myofibril and the cell wall and between the cell wall and the ECM. Individual myofibrils are linked together and to the cell wall through a complex network of microtubules and microfilaments. In recent years interest has grown in the connections of the cell with the ECM. For many years it was believed that the ECM was a static collection of structural elements that merely provided support for the cellular elements. While the ECM certainly fills this function, it is now known to be a dynamic mix of adhesive, structural proteins such as collagens, fibronectin, and laminin, antiadhesive proteins such as tenascin, Secreted Protein Acidic Rich in Cysteine (SPARC), and thrombospondin, as well as a host of other regulatory molecules including growth factors and proteases. This is especially true during cardiac development. Indeed much of the interest in cardiac ECM has been stimulated by observations suggesting that the ECM plays important roles in cell migration, proliferation, and maturation during organogenesis in organisms as diverse as *Drosophila* and humans, and in organs as diverse as skin and brain.

Cell migration is an integral part of cardiac morphogenesis, and the ECM plays a critical role in cell migration throughout cardiac development. The earliest cardiac progenitor cells appear to migrate along a fibronectin gradient on their way to forming the primitive cardiac tube. Experimental perturbations that disrupt the interaction between these cells and ECM components (especially fibronectin) completely prevent heart formation at this stage. Once formed, the primitive cardiac tube consists of a thick layer of ECM sandwiched between an epithelial layer of cardiac progenitor cells above and an endothelial layer below. It has long been suspected that the process of looping depends upon the presence and composition of the ECM. The ECM also plays a crucial role in the closure of the endocardial cushions. The endocardial cushions begin as acellular masses of ECM, into which mesenchymal cells must migrate, followed by proliferation and subsequent maturation. Alteration of the ECM has been shown to interfere with this process, leading to the hypothesis that the primary error leading to endocardial cushion defects is an augmentation of cell adhesion to ECM. Finally, closure of the conotruncal septum has been shown to require the influx of migrating cranial neural crest cells. Although not shown directly for migration into developing heart, the migration of neural crest cells is known to require both adhesive and antiadhesive matrix interactions.

The precise mechanism of ECM interaction with cells is known for very few matrix elements; however, the interaction of fibronectin with cells is prototypic in this respect (Fig. 68.10). Fibronectin appears to bind to cells through a specific receptor or integrin. The fibronectin receptor is one of a large family of related receptors with overlapping affinities for ECM components. Fibronectin is a large molecule containing three different types of protein domains, each repeated several times. The different domains have affinities for cells or other matrix components. The primary binding of fibronectin to its receptor involves a very short amino acid sequence (Arg-Gly-Asp-Ser), and several other matrix proteins appear to bind to integrin receptors using this short sequence. As one might expect from the discussion above, occupancy of the receptor may do more than anchor the cell to the ECM. The integrin receptor is coupled to the cytoskeleton through the protein talin, and in this way can dramatically affect cell shape. Remarkably, occupancy of the receptor can

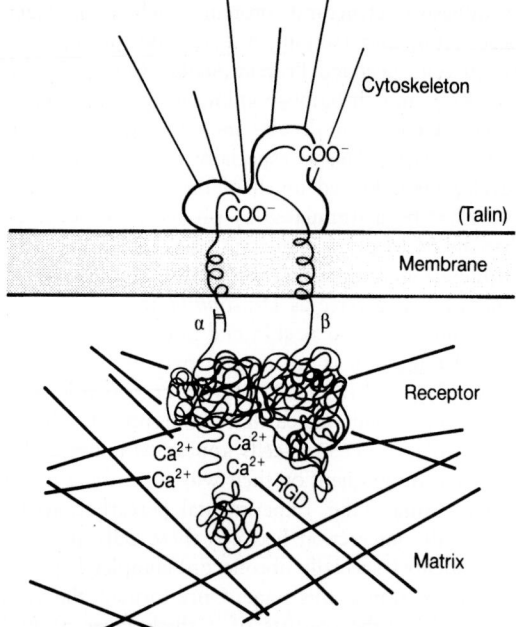

FIGURE 68.10 Integrins establish a physical link between the cytoskeleton and extracellular matrix. The integrin receptor is composed of one α and one β chain. Binding of the sequence Arg-Gly-Asp (RGD) by the globular extracellular domain requires extracellular $Ca^{2+}$. Both integrin chains span the cell membrane and contact the cytoskeleton through the membrane-associated protein talin. This mechanism allows cells to flatten themselves by pulling on a rigid matrix or to deform the matrix if it is weak. (From Ruoslahti E, Pierschbacher MD. *Science* 1987; **238**: 496, with permission.)

also lead to changes in gene expression, which in turn could stimulate or repress cellular proliferation or lead to the production of new proteins associated with the maturing myocyte phenotype. The mechanism(s) by which the ECM can turn on gene expression is unknown, but an intriguing hypothesis is that a change in cell shape also produces a change in nuclear shape, which alters expression of certain genes in some unknown fashion.

Evidence is accumulating that other ECM proteins also interact with cells through specific receptors, and one can easily envision that interaction with different receptors may produce quite different cellular behaviors. A useful model, although clearly oversimplified, defines cellular interactions with ECM as either adhesive or antiadhesive. How these interactions might be important in morphogenesis is best demonstrated by two relevant but hypothetical examples. The first is the case of cardiac progenitor cells migrating to form the primitive cardiac tube (Fig. 68.11). It is considered axiomatic that to migrate, cells must adhere to ECM. As mentioned above, cardiac progenitor cells migrate along a path rich in fibronectin, the prototypic adhesive molecule. One can easily envision the cells sticking to such a matrix, but what allows them actually to move? One possibility is that the leading edge of migrating cells is firmly attached to the ECM, while the trailing edge is freed by competing antiadhesive forces. This may entail elaboration at the trailing edge of antiadhesive proteins (like tenascin) by the cell or weakening of the interaction of cell with matrix by proteolysis of the matrix. In some cell types, occupancy of certain integrin receptors with fibronectin fragments can induce expression of proteases that break down ECM proteins, including fibronectin. Hence a feed-forward loop is established that could rapidly free the trailing edge of the migrating cell. What then signals migrating cells to stop? Again at least two possibilities exist. Perhaps as the cells encounter a greater concentration of adhesive matrix components, the antiadhesive forces are simply overwhelmed. More likely, some new signal turns off the elaboration of antiadhesive proteins or proteases.

The interaction of adhesive and antiadhesive forces can also be invoked to explain changes in organ shape. The most energetically favorable cell shape is round, the shape assumed by myocytes when in solution rather than attached to ECM. The primitive cardiac tube is composed of a cardiac epithelium resting on a layer of ECM. When the tube is straight, the epithelial cells are flattened onto the matrix. If the matrix is

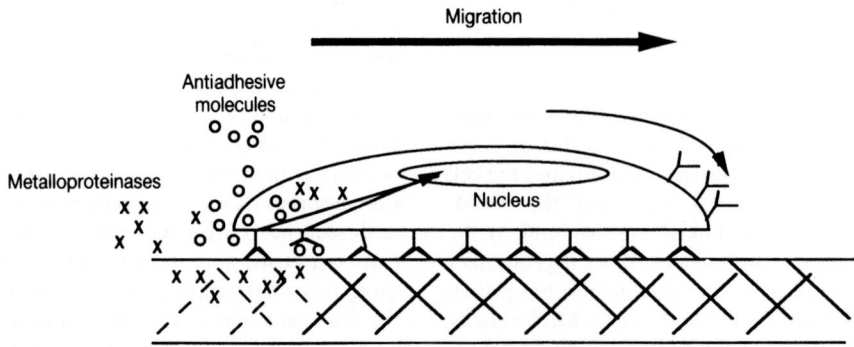

FIGURE 68.11 Adhesive and antiadhesive effects are required for cell migration. During migration the leading edge of the cell is anchored while the trailing edge is freed by elaboration of antiadhesive factors. Migration ceases when the antiadhesive signal is interrupted.

weakened, e.g. by proteolysis, cells will seek a more energetically favorable conformation and will begin to deform the matrix as shown in Fig. 68.12. If the weakening of the matrix is radially asymmetric, the tube will begin to bend, with the weak matrix on the convex side. Cells on the convex side may need their interaction with the matrix to be weakened by antiadhesive proteins that allow the matrix to be deformed without undue strain on the myocytes. Some experimental evidence supports this hypothesis: incubation of cardiac tubes with colchicine, which disrupts microtubules that are critical for maintenance of cell shape, prevents looping. This observation suggests that the energy to deform the tube is supplied by the cardiac cells rather than by deforming forces within the ECM.

## MITOCHONDRIA AND MYOCARDIAL O₂ AND ENERGY METABOLISM

Heart muscle is unique among the body's tissues because of the frequency with which it must perform mechanical work. Mechanical work uses much more energy than metabolic interconversions or transport processes. This is demonstrated by the observation that the $O_2$ consumption of the resting heart is less

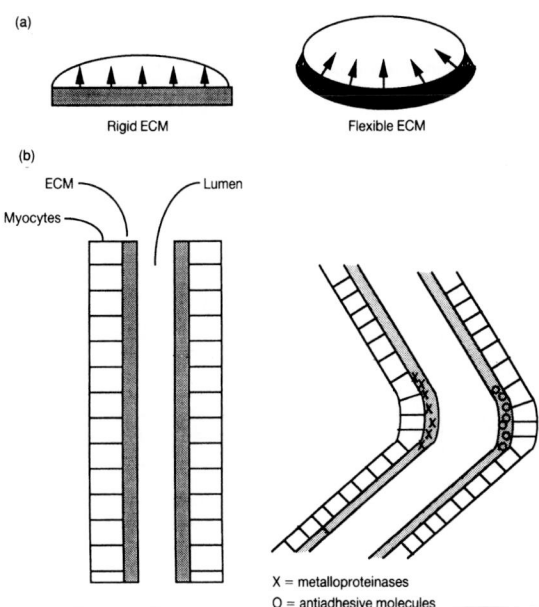

FIGURE 68.12 Deformation of the cardiac tube. (a) When adherent to a rigid matrix, myocytes are flattened. When the matrix is weakened, tension from the myocyte is transmitted across the sarcolemma to the extracellular matrix (ECM) at points of attachment and the matrix is pulled up around the myocytes. Bending of the ECM allows myocytes to assume an energetically more favorable configuration. (b) Radially asymmetric weakening of the ECM, by the action of matrix-degrading enzymes, will lead to bending of the tube.

than 20 per cent that of the contracting heart. The primary determinant of myocardial $O_2$ consumption is wall tension or stress, although heart rate, contractility, and stroke volume are also important. The $O_2$ consumption of the fetal and adult heart are similar. However, because fetal blood $O_2$ content is substantially less than that of the adult, and because both fetal and adult hearts extract nearly all of the available $O_2$ from blood, fetal myocardial blood flow is roughly twice that of the adult. This is probably accomplished by a greater capillary density in the fetus than in the adult. For the first few months of postnatal life in most mammalian species, muscular growth of the ventricles (hypertrophy) is accompanied by growth of new blood vessels. The mechanism(s) responsible for new vessel growth during hypertrophy and its cessation with time are presently unknown.

As pointed out above, $O_2$ extraction by the heart is maximal under basal conditions, and therefore increased $O_2$ demands must be met with increases in blood flow. Normally, $O_2$ demand and coronary blood flow are closely coupled and both increase approximately four-fold with maximal exertion (see page 733). The difference between basal and maximal coronary blood flow is termed coronary flow reserve, and because it is so large in infants and children imbalances between myocardial $O_2$ demand and delivery are unusual. However, such an imbalance can occur in response to severe aortic stenosis. In this setting, left ventricular outlet obstruction causes muscular hypertrophy. During the first few months of life, this is accompanied by new blood vessel growth. Eventually, new vessel growth stops; at this point, blood flow to new muscle reduces coronary reserve. If hypertrophy becomes massive, or if additional stresses of hypoxemia, anemia, exercise, or tachycardia are added, $O_2$ demand eventually may outstrip coronary flow reserve, and ischemia results, especially in the subendocardium, the deepest layer of the myocardium. During ischemia, myocardial concentrations of high-energy phosphates fall, interfering with contraction and eventually leading to myocyte death. It is not at all unusual to see patchy areas of fibrosis or necrosis in hearts of children with severe aortic stenosis, especially in the subendocardium, although this rarely produces a macroscopic myocardial infarction. With surgical relief of obstruction, hypertrophy gradually regresses and coronary reserve is returned to normal.

Although $O_2$ consumption is similar in adult and fetal myocardium, the fuels used by the two are dramatically different. The adult heart preferentially uses fatty acids, while the fetal heart is an obligatory user of carbohydrates – the fetal lamb heart metabolizes about 35 per cent glucose, 60 per cent lactate, and 5 per cent pyruvate. This observation is of some clinical importance; severe hypoglycemia can precipitate metabolic failure and seriously depress cardiac function in neonates, but is quite unlikely to do so in older children or adults.

The perinatal difference in myocardial fuel preference was initially felt simply to reflect substrate availability, i.e. comparatively low fatty acid concentrations in the fetus, and low lactate concentrations in the adult. However, it is now known that exogenous free fatty acids are not utilized by the fetal heart *in vitro* or *in vivo*. In fact, they are actually detrimental to fetal cardiac function. To gain insight into how myocardial fuel preference is regulated in the fetus and the adult, we must first understand something about the metabolism of energy substrates and the process of high-energy phosphate production in the heart.

Within the cell, the site of $O_2$ consumption and ATP production is the mitochondrion. Consistent with its role as the primary source of the high-energy phosphates required for contraction, cardiac mitochondria are tightly packed between adjacent myofibrils. They are also numerous, occupying as much as 30 per cent of total myocyte volume. Mitochondria are bounded by an outer membrane and an inner membrane. Associated with the inner membrane are the enzymes of the citric acid cycle, which oxidizes two carbon fragments to $CO_2$ and supplies NADH and $FADH_2$ to the respiratory chain for generation of ATP (Fig. 68.13).

The inner membrane is folded into numerous cristae, which greatly increase the surface area available for these reactions. ATP is not freely diffusible out of mitochondria. ATP is transported across the mitochondrial membrane in exchange for ADP by the adenine nucleotide antiporter. Once outside mitochondria, ATP is still not freely diffusible as it quickly transfers its high-energy phosphate to creatine using the enzyme mitochondrial creatine kinase. Creatine phosphate then diffuses to sites of ATP hydrolysis (such as the contractile apparatus) where the high-energy phosphate is transferred back to ADP by other creatine kinase isoforms. Regardless of the fuel used, these reactions represent the pathway for ATP production, so regulation of fuel preference clearly must be proximal to the citric acid cycle.

The counterregulation of fuel substrates in mature myocardium is illustrated in Fig. 68.14. Fatty acids entering the cardiac cell are quickly esterified to coenzyme A, forming acyl-CoA. This is necessary because unesterified fatty acids can associate with and injure many of the cell's membranes. However, acyl-CoA is unable to cross the mitochondrial membranes for subsequent metabolism, so a specific transport mechanism is required. For transport, acyl-CoA is transesterified

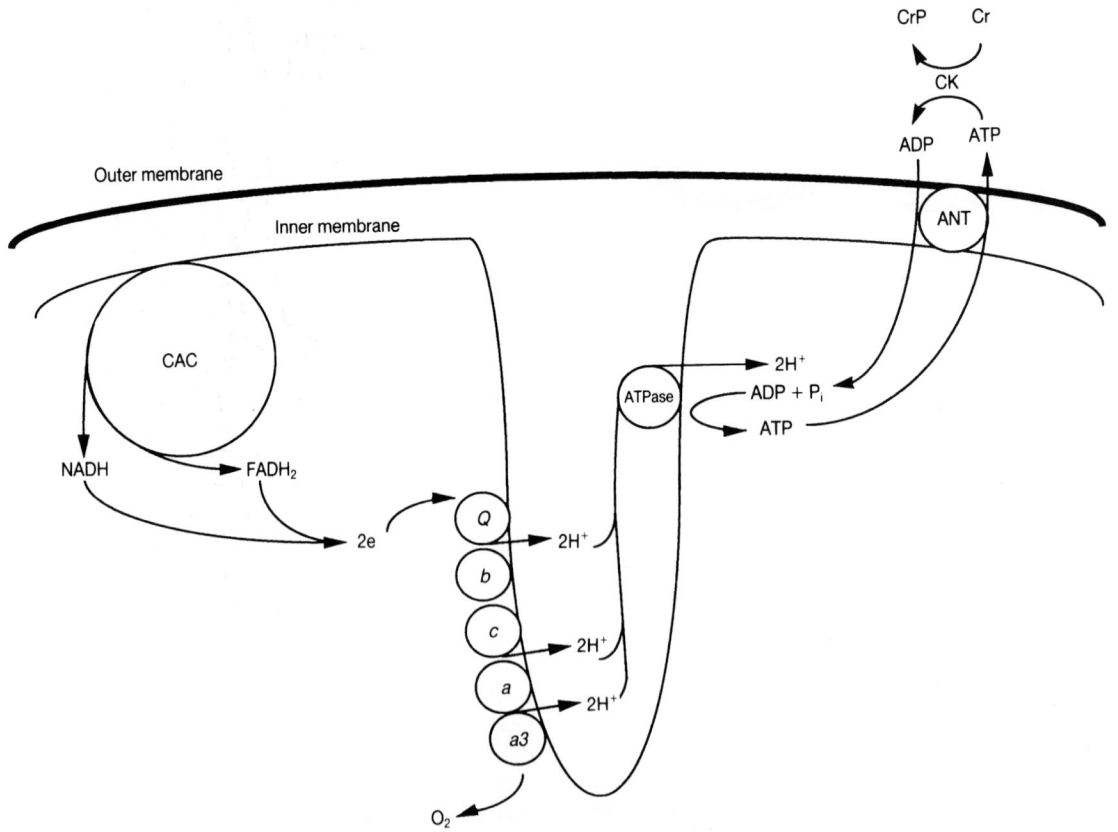

FIGURE 68.13 Mitochondrial generation of ATP. The enzymes of the citric acid cycle (CAC) oxidize acetyl-CoA to $CO_2$, reducing NAD and FAD in the process. NADH and FADH, transfer their electrons (2e) to the respiratory chain where electron transport causes $H^+$ to be transported across the inner membrane. This creates a pH gradient. Movement of $H^+$ back across the inner membrane is coupled with phosphorylation of ADP to ATP. Finally, high-energy phosphate from ATP is transferred to creatine (Cr) via the adenine nucleotide transporter (ANT) and creatine kinase (CK). CrP, creatine phosphate; $P_i$, inorganic phosphate; $Q$, $b$, $c$, $a$, $a3$, cytochromes.

with carnitine to form acylcarnitine and free coenzyme A. A specific transport protein called carnitine-palmitoyl transferase 1 (or CPT1) mediates this transfer. A second enzyme termed CPT2 mediates transfer across the inner mitochondrial membrane and conversion back to acyl-CoA. The fatty acid then undergoes β-oxidation, liberating acetyl-CoA for entry into the citric acid cycle. The primary site of regulation in this pathway appears to be the entry of fatty acids into mitochondria, and this is accomplished through inhibition of CPT1 by malonyl-CoA, the first committed intermediate in fatty acid synthesis. Concentrations of malonyl-CoA are lower in muscle than in liver (where fat synthesis is active), but muscle CPT is far more sensitive to malonyl-CoA inhibition than is liver CPT. Malonyl-CoA concentrations in turn are regulated by circulating concentrations of glucagon. After birth, glucagon concentrations surge, removing malo-

nyl-CoA inhibition of CPT1 and allowing fatty acid oxidation to begin.

The next question is how fatty acid oxidation feeds back to inhibit glucose utilization. In contrast to fatty acids, primary regulation of glucose metabolism occurs in the cytosol. As shown in Fig. 68.14, the glycolytic pathway splits glucose into two molecules of pyruvate. This initial phase of glucose metabolism nets only a small amount of ATP and is quantitatively unimportant for both fetal and mature myocardium. A much larger yield of ATP is produced when pyruvate enters the mitochondrion where acetyl-CoA is generated and oxidized by the citric acid cycle. It has been known for many years that when fatty acids are being oxidized, glucose utilization is limited by inhibition of the glycolytic enzyme phosphofructokinase (PFK$_1$), which catalyzes the phosphorylation of fructose 6-phosphate (F-6-P) to fructose 1,6-bisphosphate (F-1,6-P) in an ATP-requiring reaction. This highly regulated enzyme has

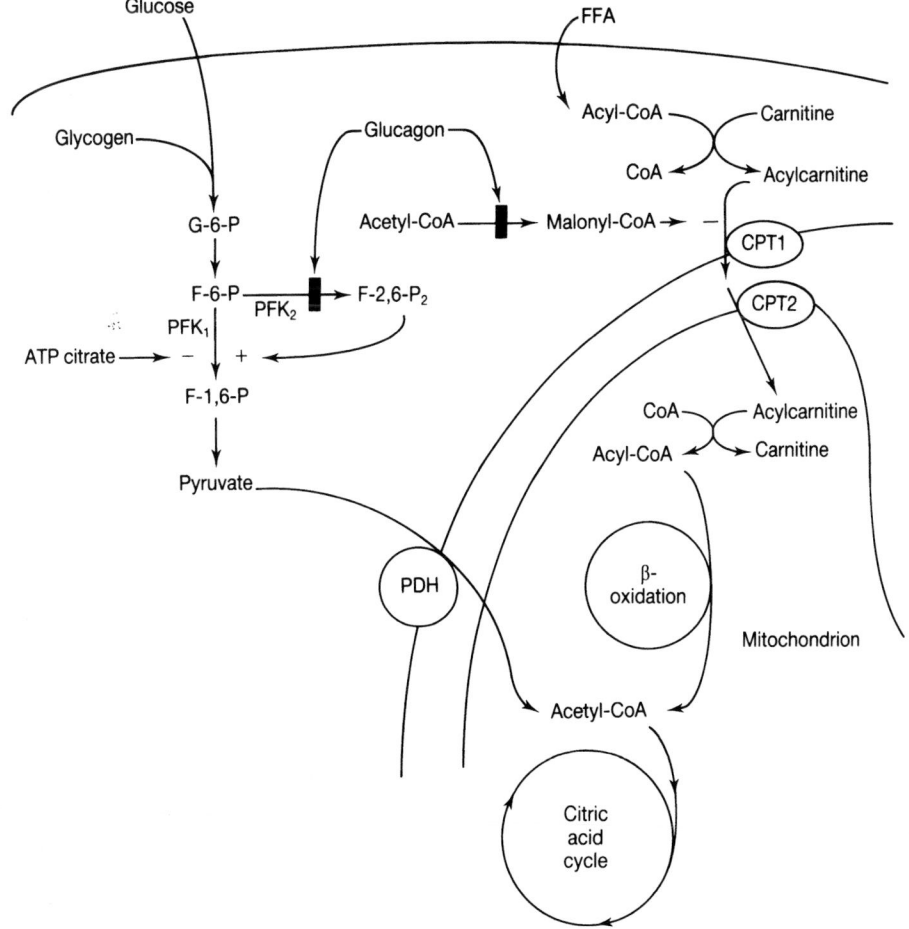

FIGURE 68.14 The probable role of glucagon in the regulation of fatty acid and glucose utilization. The glycolytic pathway leading from glucose to pyruvate is regulated at the PFK$_1$ reaction. This reaction is potently inhibited by ATP and citrate and activated by F-2,6-P$_2$. The latter is formed by PFK$_2$, the activity of which is decreased by glucagon in a cAMP-dependent mechanism. Fatty acid oxidation is regulated at the level of acylcarnitine transport across the outer mitochondrial membrane, mediated by CPT1. CPT1 is inhibited by malonyl-CoA, which is synthesized from acetyl-CoA and HCO$_3^-$ in the cytosol. Malonyl-CoA levels are also decreased by glucagon. The postnatal glucagon surge will decrease both F-2,6-P$_2$ and malonyl-CoA, allowing fatty acid oxidation while inhibiting glycolysis. PDH, pyruvate dehydrogenase; see text for remaining abbreviations.

been the focus of many investigations through which more than a dozen different metabolites have been found to affect the activity of the purified enzyme *in vitro*. The most potent inhibitors of PFK activity are ATP and citrate. In isolated perfused hearts, the rise in cytosolic citrate accompanying fatty acid oxidation probably is primarily responsible for inhibition of PFK. Indeed, citrate and ATP inhibition are so powerful that in the presence of physiological concentrations of its substrates and its numerous positive and negative effectors, there is no demonstrable PFK activity *in vitro*. How then does the cardiac cell metabolize glucose *in vivo*? Only recently a powerful new positive effector was discovered, capable of overcoming the inhibition produced by ATP and citrate. Its identity is fructose 2,6-bisphosphate (F-2,6-$P_2$), and it is formed by a second PFK enzyme (PFK$_2$ ), so named because it phosphorylates the 2 position of F-6-P and because it was the second PFK enzyme discovered. F-2,6-$P_2$ is present in both fetal and mature hearts at concentrations that activate PFK$_1$ sufficiently to account for glycolytic fluxes observed *in vivo*.

It seems likely that in heart, as in liver, glucose and fatty acid oxidation are regulated in parallel. In liver, both malonyl-CoA and F-2,6-$P_2$ concentrations are regulated by the circulating glucagon:insulin ratio, and it is likely that the same is true in the heart. In the fetus the insulin:glucagon ratio is high, malonyl-CoA and F-2,6-$P_2$ concentrations are both high, and CPT is inhibited, while PFK$_1$ is stimulated. After birth, the glucagon surge dissipates malonyl-CoA and F-2,6-$P_2$, releasing CPT inhibition and allowing fatty acid oxidation to proceed, while allowing citrate and ATP to inhibit PFK and glycolytic flux. The extent to which the hormonal milieu may influence myocardial fuel preference of adult hearts on a day-to-day basis is largely unexplored.

## SELECTED READING

Anderson PAW. Immature myocardium. In: Moller J, Neal WA, eds. *Fetal, neonatal and infant cardiac disease.* Norwalk, CT: Appleton & Lange, 1990: 35.

Bristow J. The search for genetic mechanisms of congenital heart disease. *Cell Mol Biol Res* 1995; **41**: 307.

Clark EB, Markwald RR, Takao A, eds. *Developmental mechanisms of heart disease.* Armonk, NY: Futura Publishing, 1995.

Damsky CH, Bernfield M. Cell-to-cell contact and extracellular matrix. *Curr Opin Cell Biol* 1991; **3**: 777.

Icardo JM. The growing heart: an anatomical perspective. In: Zak R, ed. *Growth of the heart in health and disease.* New York: Raven Press, 1984: 41.

Van Mierop LH. Morphological development of the heart. In: Berne RM, ed. *Handbook of physiology, Section 2: The cardiovascular system, Vol. 1: Circulation.* Bethesda, MD: American Physiologic Society, 1979: 1.

# 69

# Myocardial Receptors

Einat Birk

## MYOCARDIAL RECEPTORS AND GUANINE NUCLEOTIDE-BINDING PROTEINS

Receptors can be defined as cellular macromolecules that, when bound to a discrete group of compounds, lead to a cascade of intracellular events. Many receptors reside in the plasma membrane and, when bound to an appropriate ligand, propagate its signal into the cell. The formation of a receptor–ligand complex leads to a cellular effect either directly or by inducing the release or synthesis of another regulatory molecule (the latter known as a second messenger). This chain of events eventually leads to biochemical and physiological responses.

Mammalian myocardium contains a variety of receptors. These receptors can be activated by neurotransmitters released from autonomic efferent nerve fibers, by hormones secreted from distant organs, or by autacoids produced locally by cardiac tissue.

Receptors elicit a cellular response through a series of steps. The activated receptor couples to a membrane-associated signal transducer, which in turn stimulates a response element (Fig. 69.1). A common succession of such a pathway (Fig. 69.2) begins with the coupling of a guanine nucleotide (GTP)-binding protein (G-protein) to an activated receptor. The G-protein is then coupled to a cellular response element, which is either an enzyme or an ion channel. Coupling to an enzyme produces a second messenger, which in turn leads to a physiological event either directly or via activation of other cellular enzymes.

G-proteins are a family of proteins; each one is formed by heterotrimers, consisting of α-, β-, and γ-subunits. The α-subunit is thought to be the actual signal transducer of the G-protein, interacting with the effector. It also serves as the activation–deactiva-

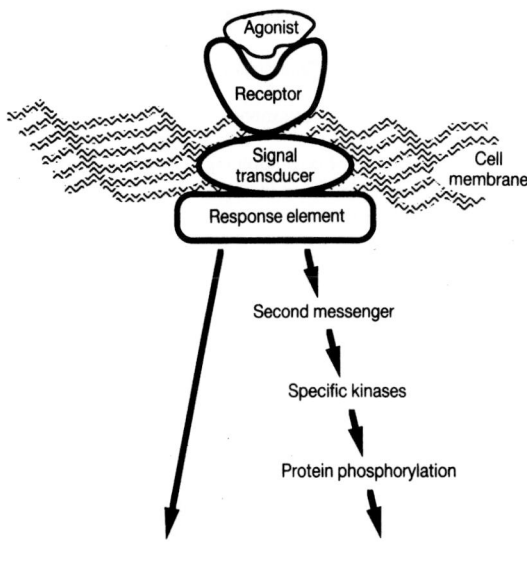

FIGURE 69.1 Description of transmembrane signal transduction: an agonist activates a receptor, which in turn stimulates a signal transducer (e.g. G-protein). Once activated, the signal transducer stimulates a response element (e.g. ion channels, enzymes) that, either directly or via additional steps, results in a physiological response.

tion element of the G-protein by binding and hydrolyzing GTP, respectively. Once activated by a stimulated receptor, the α-subunit releases a GDP molecule and binds GTP instead; at the same time, the affinity of the α-subunit to βγ-subunits is decreased, and a βγ complex is released. Deactivation of the G-protein occurs by GTPase activity of the α-subunit (releasing a free phosphate from the α-subunit-bound GTP) and by reassociation with the βγ complex.

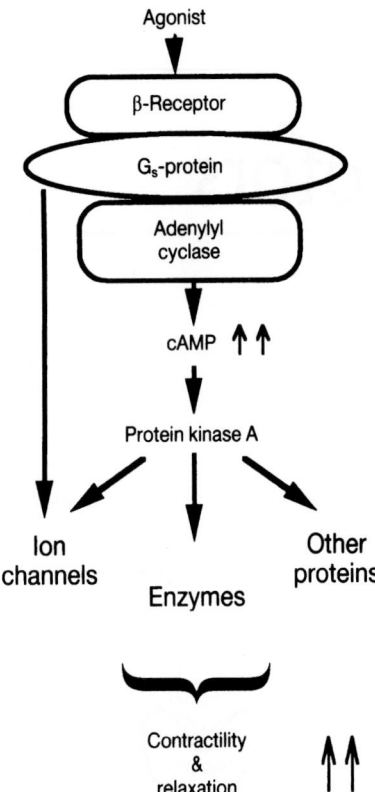

FIGURE 69.2 Activation of a β-adrenergic receptor leads to a chain of events resulting in an increase in myocardial contractility and relaxation rate

G-proteins can have a stimulatory ($G_s$-protein) or an inhibitory ($G_i$-protein) effect on cellular response elements.

Several G-proteins may regulate myocardial function. Some appear able to interact with more than one receptor and with more than one cellular response element. Therefore, activation of different receptors may cause the same cellular response; on the other hand, activation of a single receptor group can stimulate various cellular responses.

Little information exists regarding developmental changes in the expression and function of cardiac G-proteins. There is an increase in the G-protein that mediates $α_1$-adrenergic responses in developing neonatal rat myocytes. This increase is associated with developing myocardial innervation, and changes the chronotropic effect of $α_1$-adrenergic stimulation from a positive to a negative one. Ventricular $G_{iα}$ decreases during development and aging in rat myocardium. However, the regulatory consequences of this process are not clear.

The G-proteins transmit the signals generated by hormone–receptor interactions to a diverse group of effectors, including adenylyl cyclase, phospholipase C, and ion channels.

## SPECIFIC RECEPTORS AND THEIR SIGNAL TRANSDUCTION PATHWAYS

### β-Adrenergic receptors

β-Adrenergic receptor activation provides a major means of regulating myocardial contractility: adrenergic agonists potentiate myocardial contraction and enhance the rate of relaxation.

β-Adrenergic receptors are glycoproteins located in the membrane bilayer. β-Adrenergic receptors are not uniform, and can be classified into two major groups: the $β_1$ subtype, which provides a major cardiac signaling pathway, and the $β_2$ subtype, which mediates signal transduction in smooth muscle cells. Most mammalian ventricular myocardium contains the $β_1$-receptor subtype almost exclusively; in humans, the $β_1$ subtype constitutes approximately 80 per cent of the myocardial β-receptor population. Both subtypes are coupled to adenylyl cyclase and a positive inotropic response.

β-Adrenergic receptors utilize G-proteins in translating receptor occupancy into a biochemical response. The receptor interacts with $G_{sα}$ to stimulate adenylyl cyclase-mediated production of the second messenger cAMP. Next, cAMP activates its protein kinase. The activated enzyme, in turn, phosphorylates several key regulatory proteins of the cardiac muscle, including phospholamban and troponin 1. $G_{sα}$ can also stimulate mammalian cardiac $Ca^{2+}$ channels and inhibit $Na^+$ channels in neonatal ventricular myocytes, both directly and via cAMP production (Fig. 69.2).

Maturation of β-adrenergic receptors, in terms of their ability to respond to an agonist with the production of a second messenger and their ability to elicit a physiological response, has been shown to occur early during fetal myocardial development. The pharmacological characteristics and function of the β-adrenergic receptors are similar in fetal, newborn, and adult myocardium. Changes in receptor concentration and adenylyl cyclase activity occur with aging as well as with myocardial disease.

The β-adrenergic receptor cascade appears to play a substantial role in compensatory mechanisms during fetal stress as well as in increasing heart rate and cardiac output during labor and delivery. Such an adrenergic effect can be modulated by changes in β-receptor agonist concentration, e.g. catecholamines, as well as by a change in receptor availability and function. Indeed, it appears that more than one mechanism regulates the β-adrenergic pathway.

Circulating catecholamine concentrations increase significantly during fetal stress (e.g. hypoxemia), as well as during birth and shortly thereafter; the latter has been shown both in humans and sheep. Moreover, the density of myocardial receptors is higher in neonates than in adults. Changes in myocardial adrenergic responsiveness during fetal and neonatal development are modulated by thyroid hormones. An increase, or decrease, in hormone concentrations results in a significant increase, or decrease, in β-adrenergic receptor number, respectively. In other systems, steroids modulate receptor number. In the failing heart, β-adrenergic receptor concentrations and the contractile response to stimulation by β-adrenergic receptor agonists declines. A gradual decline also occurs with aging.

## $\alpha_1$-Adrenergic receptors

$\alpha_1$-Adrenergic receptors, found in mammalian and human myocardium, have both a chronotropic and an inotropic effect. However, their density is significantly lower than that of the β-adrenergic receptors, and their physiological role is not clearly understood. $\alpha_1$-Adrenergic stimulation results in a negative chronotropic effect in the adult. Reports regarding myocardial mechanical responses to $\alpha_1$-adrenergic stimulation have been conflicting; some have indicated a positive inotropic effect, while others have shown no effect on cardiac contraction.

Three $\alpha_1$-adrenergic receptor subtypes are present in humans. The distribution of the subtypes is tissue selective, and also varies between species. In the heart $\alpha_1$-adrenergic receptors are coupled to hydrolysis of phosphatidylinositol to produce two second messengers: inositol trisphosphate (IP$_3$) and diacylglycerol (DAG). IP$_3$ is linked to Ca$^{2+}$ metabolism, and DAG is linked to the activation of protein kinase C, which has several myocardial substrates.

The ontogeny of α-adrenergic receptors and their role in myocardial development are not clear. One study describes a reduction in myocardial receptor concentration with advancing gestational age during the third trimester in fetal sheep. During early postnatal development, the chronotropic response to $\alpha_1$-adrenergic stimulation changes from positive to negative in the rat and dog heart. As mentioned above, this change is associated with myocardial innervation, and with an increase in the G-protein that mediates $\alpha_1$-adrenergic responses. α-Adrenergic mechanisms appear to play an essential role in regulating cardiovascular responses during stress in growth-retarded fetal lambs, because α-blockade during acute hypoxic stress results in death. However, the relative role of the myocardium in this process is not well established.

Another potential role for α-adrenergic mechanisms during growth and development may stem from their ability to induce myocyte hypertrophy in neonatal rats. Again, the importance of this mechanism in myocardial development remains to be elucidated.

## Muscarinic receptors

Muscarinic receptor activation has been associated with negative chronotropic and inotropic effects in adult hearts. Muscarinic receptors are not structurally and functionally uniform, and at least five different receptor genes (M$_1$–M$_5$) have been cloned and pharmacologically characterized. They are expressed in a tissue-specific manner, and their affinity to cellular response elements varies. In most mammalian hearts, including human, the muscarinic subtype identified is M$_2$.

The presently known biochemical responses to muscarinic stimulation in the heart include a reduction in cAMP concentration, an increase in the hydrolysis of phosphoinositides, activation of K$^+$ channels, and interaction with Na$^+$ channels.

The inhibitory myocardial effects of muscarinic stimulation may be executed through coupling with G$_i$ leading to inhibition of adenylyl cyclase activity. Receptor interaction with a different G-protein, G$_p$, stimulates phospholipase C to cause phosphoinositide hydrolysis. The effect of the latter response is not clear; as stated above, the products of phosphoinositol hydrolysis are the two second messengers, IP$_3$ and DAG. IP$_3$ is linked to Ca$^{2+}$ metabolism, and DAG is linked to the activation of protein kinase C, which has several myocardial substrates. Several recent studies have associated phosphoinositol hydrolysis with a positive inotropic effect (Fig. 69.3).

The ontogeny of myocardial muscarinic receptors and their physiological importance during myocardial growth and development are not clear. Prior to vagal innervation, the response of embryonic chick heart to muscarinic stimulation is low; following vagal ingrowth, this response increases, while no change in receptor density is detected. Later in gestation,

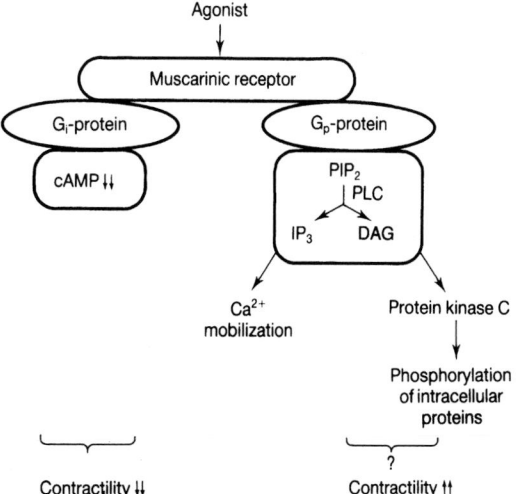

FIGURE 69.3 Activation of a muscarinic receptor leads to a G$_i$-mediated reduction in cAMP and reduced contractility. G$_p$-mediated phospholipase C (PLC) activation leads to the hydrolysis of phosphatidylinositol 4,5-bisphosphate (PIP$_2$). The latter reaction produces the two second messengers, inositol trisphosphate (IP$_3$) and diacylglycerol (DAG), leading to a cascade of intracellular events that may increase contractility.

myocardial muscarinic receptor concentrations in fetal myocardium appear to be significantly higher than in adults. The receptor signal transduction pathway in the fetus is intact, and is capable of mediating a cellular response. The physiological significance of this pathway in cardiac development is not clear.

## SELECTED READING

Brodde OE. Beta-adrenoceptors in cardiac disease. *Pharmacol Ther* 1993; **60**: 405.

Chen FM, Yamamura Hl, Roeske WR. Ontogeny of mammalian myocardial β-adrenergic receptors. *Eur J Pharmacol* 1979; **58**: 255.

Cheng BC, Cornett LE, Goldfien A. Decreased concentration of myocardial α-adrenoceptors with increasing age in foetal lambs. *Br J Pharmacol* 1980; **70**: 515.

Cheng JB, Goldfien A, Cornett LE, Roberts JM. Identification of β-adrenergic receptors using [³H]dihydroalprenolol in fetal sheep heart: direct evidence of qualitative similarity to the receptors in adult sheep heart. *Pediatr Res* 1981; **15**: 1083.

Galper JB, Klein W, Catterall WA. Muscarinic acetylcholine receptors in developing chick heart. *J Biol Chem* 1977; **252**: 8692.

Gupta RC, Neumann J, Watanabe AM. Comparison of adenosine and muscarinic receptor-mediated effects on protein phosphatase inhibitor-1 activity in the heart. *J Pharmacol Exp Ther* 1993; **266**: 16.

Nedoma J, Slavikova J, Tucek S. Muscarinic acetylcholine receptors in the heart of rats before and after birth. *Pflugers Arch* 1986; **406**: 45.

Price DT, Lefkowitz RJ, Caron MG *et al*. Localization of mRNA for three distinct α₁-adrenergic receptor subtypes in human tissues: implications for human α-adrenergic physiology. *Mol Pharmacol* 1994; **45**: 171.

Robishaw JD, Foster KA. Role of G proteins in the regulation of the cardiovascular system. *Annu Rev Physiol* 1989; **51**: 229.

Simpson P. Stimulation of hypertrophy of cultured neonatal rat heart cells through an α-adrenergic receptor and induction of beating through an α₁- and β₁-adrenergic receptor interaction. Evidence for independent regulation of growth and beating. *Circ Res* 1985; **56**: 884.

Tobise K, Ishikawa Y, Holmer SR *et al*. Changes in type-VI adenylyl cyclase isoform expression correlate with a decreased capacity for cAMP generation in the aging ventricle. *Circ Res* 1994; **74**: 596.

Whitsett JA, Pollinger J, Matz S. β-Adrenergic receptors and catecholamine sensitive adenylate cyclase in developing rat ventricular myocardium: effect of thyroid status. *Pediatr Res* 1982; **16**: 463.

# 70

# Myocardial Nervous Innervation and Regulation

David F. Teitel and Julien I.E. Hoffman

## DEVELOPMENTAL ASPECTS

Adrenergic, muscarinic, and other receptors appear early and function before autonomic innervation occurs; parasympathetic precedes sympathetic innervation in all species. The earliest viable human premature infants have rudimentary autonomic innervation. Innervation is most advanced in those species that are independent immediately after birth.

## ANATOMY AND PHYSIOLOGY

Cardiac sympathetic nerves arise from cervical sympathetic ganglia and stellate ganglia, and the upper four thoracic sympathetic ganglia. Right sympathetic nerves innervate the right and anterior portions of the heart, and left sympathetic nerves innervate the left and posterior portions of the heart. The efferent sympathetic nerve endings produce and store dopamine, norepinephrine and neuropeptide Y; the latter two are coreleased with nerve stimulation. Vagal nerves from the medullary centers supply both atria and ventricles, and the proximal part of the bundle of His; the distal part of the bundle of His has only sympathetic nerve supply. Vagal nerve endings contain not only acetylcholine but also vasoactive intestinal peptide (VIP) and somatostatin. Sympathetic and vagal afferents leave the heart, carrying information from baroreceptors that are stimulated by high pressures in the ventricles and lower pressures in the atria, cavae, and pulmonary veins, and from chemoreceptors that can be stimulated by exogenous (e.g. veratridine) and endogenous (e.g. bradykinin and eicosanoids) substances. Bradykinin released during ischemia is a candidate for the source of pain in myocardial ischemia. The cell bodies of the afferent sympathetic nerves produce the vasodilator peptides substance P, neurokinin A, and CGRP (calcitonin gene-related peptide), which are transported down the axon to the nerve endings and are coreleased on stimulation of the nerves.

The heart can function without cardiac nerves; cardiac function is normal after cardiac transplantation. However, the response to exercise in denervated hearts is slower than normal, being mediated by increases in circulating catecholamines and the rise in body temperature. In innervated animals and humans, β-adrenergic receptor blockade blunts the heart rate increase with exercise and abolishes the inotropic response, as judged by an increase in $dP/dt_{max}$ (the maximal rate of change of pressure). Consequently, acceleration of blood leaving the left ventricle is reduced, an effect used to attempt to prevent dissection of the aorta in patients with *Marfan syndrome*.

## SYMPATHETIC–VAGAL INTERACTION

Neurogenic cardiac control varies with the state of consciousness and the basal level of sympathetic and parasympathetic tone. In conscious animals, resting sympathetic tone is low, and parasympathetic tone is high. Therefore, sympathetic blockade changes heart rate and myocardial contractility minimally, but vagal blockade causes significant tachycardia. By contrast, many anesthetics depress the sympathetic nervous system further, and lead to impaired contractility. After surgery, patients often have high circulating catecholamine concentrations, and their myocardial function depends on the balance of catecholamine concentrations, stimulation of the sympathetic nervous system by pain, and the degree of myocardial depression by the drugs used for sedation.

## PATTERNS OF STIMULATION

With exercise and hemorrhage, plasma catecholamines and heart rate increase greatly, but inotropic responses differ. $dP/dt_{max}$ increases up to 400 per cent with exercise, but by only 30–50 per cent with hemorrhage. The peripheral vascular bed dilates and cardiac output increases with exercise, whereas cardiac output falls and most vascular beds vasoconstrict with hemorrhage. Thus, the pattern of sympathetic neural stimulation, rather than the circulating catecholamine concentrations, determines how the heart responds to these stimuli.

## VAGAL EFFECTS

Vagal stimulation decreases heart rate, but may also depress myocardial contractility that depends on existing sympathetic tone. Vagal stimulation has little effect on myocardial contractility when there is little sympathetic tone, but markedly reduces the inotropic effects of increases in circulating catecholamines or sympathetic nerve stimulation. Conversely, blockade of muscarinic receptors can intensify the myocardial contractile response to sympathetic stimulation. Vagal stimulation slows conduction through the atrioventricular node, an effect used in treating supraventricular tachycardias.

## BARORECEPTORS

Carotid and aortic baroreceptors respond to changes in arterial blood pressure. With normal low basal sympathetic tone, inhibiting sympathetic tone by raising aortic pressure has little effect on myocardial contractility. However, lowering arterial pressure reflexly increases sympathetic tone, and increases heart rate and contractility. Baroreceptor sensitivity increases

throughout gestation in fetal lambs, but may decrease after birth. In fetal lambs, denervation of the baroreceptors does not alter mean arterial blood pressure or heart rate, but increases their variability; in adult sheep denervation increases variability of pressures, but not of heart rate.

Ventricular mechanoreceptors are also involved in the response to postural changes. Normally, decreased ventricular filling, as occurs immediately after standing up, stimulates sympathetic output and causes vasoconstriction, thereby preventing hypotension. Sometimes, however, decreased ventricular filling paradoxically activates ventricular mechanoreceptors, increases afferent traffic to the brain stem and inhibits sympathetic output; therefore, heart rate slows and blood pressure falls and if the changes are marked, the individual faints (neurocardiogenic syncope). Other mechanisms must also occur, however, because syncope can occur with a transplanted denervated heart.

## CHEMORECEPTORS (see also p.834)

Carotid and aortic chemoreceptors are stimulated by decreases of $P_{O_2}$ and pH, and marked increases of $P_{CO_2}$, but the increase in myocardial contractility is modest; the fetus is less sensitive than the adult to chemoreceptor stimulation, and responds with bradycardia rather than tachycardia. The bradycardia seen postnatally with severe hypoxemia is due to vagal stimulation plus direct depression of the sino-atrial (SA) node.

## VASCULAR INNERVATION

The autonomic nerves innervate coronary vessels, and interact with circulating and local hormones to regulate coronary vascular tone. Because of the major effect of metabolic regulators on coronary vascular tone, it is difficult to ascribe specific actions to the autonomic nerves, but α-adrenergic vasoconstriction is well recognized. It may play a part in the onset of angina pectoris in patients with coronary arterial disease.

## SELECTED READING

Randall WC, ed. Nervous control of cardiovascular function. Oxford: Oxford University Press, 1984.

Shepherd JT. Cardiac mechanoreceptors. In: Fozzard HA, Haber E, Jennings RB, Katz AM, Morgan HE, eds. The heart and cardiovascular system. Scientific foundations. New York: Raven Press, 1991: 1481.

Vatner SF. Sympathetic mechanisms regulating myocardial contractility in conscious animals. In: Fozzard HA, Haber E, Jennings RB, Katz AM, Morgan HE, eds. The heart and cardiovascular system. Scientific foundations. New York: Raven Press, 1991: 1709.

# 71

# Coronary Circulation and Myocardial Oxygen Consumption

David F. Teitel and Julien I.E. Hoffman

## DETERMINANTS OF MYOCARDIAL $O_2$ CONSUMPTION

### Pressure work

Pressure work by the heart consumes more $O_2$ than does volume work, and Sarnoff and colleagues found a good correlation between the area under the left ventricular pressure curve in systole (the tension time index) and left ventricular $O_2$ consumption ($LV\dot{V}O_2$). Later work showed that peak wall tension (or stress) was a better predictor of left ventricular $O_2$ consumption. Therefore, wall thickness and ventricular dimensions must be used in estimating myocardial $O_2$ consumption ($M\dot{V}O_2$); this explains why the tension time index, which ignores wall stress, is not a good predictor of myocardial $O_2$ consumption, particularly in abnormal hearts. Increased contractility or heart rate also increases myocardial $O_2$ consumption, but they decrease ventricular size, and thus wall stress, so that the increased $O_2$ consumption is not as great as would be expected from studies in muscle strips.

### Volume work

Stroke volume is an added predictor that must be considered. Suga and colleagues found that the best predictor of left ventricular $O_2$ consumption was the area in the pressure–volume loop plus the area representing end-systolic pressure energy (Fig. 71.1a,b); the total area was termed the pressure–volume area (PVA). Note that the line relating myocardial $O_2$ consumption to PVA (Fig. 71.1b) intercepts the $\dot{V}O_2$ axis at a positive value, because some of the $O_2$ consumption is independent of the PVA; this $O_2$ consumption is due to excitation–contraction (E–C) coupling and basal metabolism. The slope of the line is the reciprocal of contractile efficiency. An increase in contractility (defined by $E_{max}$) is linearly related to the PVA-independent $\dot{V}O_2$ (Fig. 71.1c,d). Furthermore, certain interventions, e.g. acidosis, make the slope of this relation between PVA-independent $\dot{V}O_2$ and $E_{max}$ steeper, i.e. they decrease the efficiency of the system (Fig. 71.1d).

### Substrate effects

Because more $O_2$ is used oxidizing fats than carbohydrates, there should be more $O_2$ used per unit of work when metabolizing fatty acids. This has sometimes been found, but has not been carefully studied. Because fetal myocardium uses mainly carbohydrate as a substrate, rather than fatty acids as in the adult, this difference could be considered a mechanism for conserving $O_2$ in the fetus.

## STRUCTURE AND DEVELOPMENT OF THE CORONARY CIRCULATION

### Embryology

In the early embryo, the primitive cardiac tube has an inner wall that is heavily trabeculated and derived from endothelium, whereas the myocardium is derived from

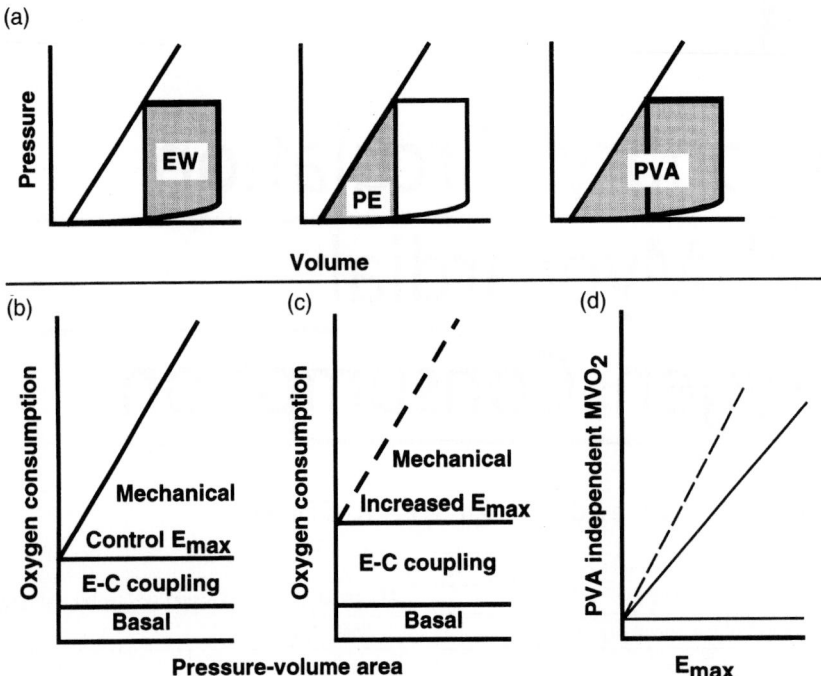

FIGURE 71.1 Determinants of myocardial $O_2$ consumption. (a) Pressure–volume diagrams to show the component of external work (EW) on the left, of potential energy (PE) in the middle, and on the right the combination of both to make up the pressure–volume area (PVA). The PVA is closely related to myocardial $O_2$ consumption ($M\dot{V}O_2$). (b,c) Relation between myocardial $O_2$ consumption (vertical axis) and pressure–volume area (horizontal axis) at normal (b) and increased contractility (defined by $E_{max}$) (c). Increased contractility increases the component of myocardial $O_2$ consumption related to excitation–contraction coupling (E–C coupling) but not the other two, so that myocardial $O_2$ consumption and mechanical work remain proportional. (d) Relation of contractility (defined by $E_{max}$) and PVA-independent myocardial $O_2$ consumption. The dashed, more steeply sloping line shows that during hypercapnic acidosis the $O_2$ cost of contractility increases, i.e. the system becomes less efficient. (Adapted from the publications of Suga and his colleagues.)

mesoderm. Connective tissue grows out from the base of the truncus arteriosus to enter the muscle and form its connective tissue, and from this tissue the coronary arteries are formed. Initially, the inner myocardial layer is supplied with $O_2$ and substrates by diffusion from the cavity, but as the heart grows and its metabolic needs increase, the coronary arteries take over the role of supplying the actively growing and working muscle.

## Anatomy

In the human heart there are two major extramural coronary arteries. The right coronary artery comes off the right anterior sinus of Valsalva. It is dominant in two-thirds of people, i.e. it reaches the crux of the heart and gives off the posterior descending coronary artery which supplies the posterior third of the ventricular septum and part of the adjacent left ventricular wall. The left coronary artery comes off the left sinus of Valsalva. In about 15 per cent of people it is dominant, i.e. it reaches the crux of the heart and gives off the posterior descending coronary artery, so that the left coronary artery supplies all the left ventricle and a small part of the right ventricle. In the remaining 18

per cent of people, neither artery is dominant; they are said to have a balanced circulation. The right coronary artery usually gives off the artery to the sino-atrial (SA) node, and the posterior descending artery supplies the atrioventricular (AV) node.

## Microcirculation

The arteries penetrate the muscle and course towards the endocardium, giving off branches as they go and forming a subendocardial plexus. The major control of coronary vascular resistance lies in arterioles <400 μm in diameter. The myocardium of the left ventricle has a relatively large blood volume of about 15 per cent of wall volume, and this can change substantially during contraction. In systole, blood is squeezed out of the left ventricular subendocardium and midmyocardium; some of this blood passes retrogradely into the extramural coronary arteries, some into the coronary veins, and some actually passes into the subepicardial vessels, which therefore receive a dual blood supply: in systole from the subendocardium and in diastole from the extramural coronary arteries.

# MYOCARDIAL O$_2$ DEMAND–SUPPLY RELATIONSHIP AND CORONARY BLOOD FLOW

## Basic features

The left ventricle extracts about 60–75 per cent of the O$_2$ from the blood passing through the myocardium. Therefore, because it is impossible to remove the residual O$_2$ from hemoglobin without producing dangerously low O$_2$ tensions, increased myocardial O$_2$ demand must be met by increased myocardial blood flow. Normally, with maximal exertion, left ventricular O$_2$ consumption increases four-fold, and so does left ventricular blood flow. If coronary perfusion pressure does not change during exertion, the increased flow has to be achieved by a decrease in coronary vascular resistance.

Coronary vascular resistance has three components: a basal low resistance in the arrested heart with maximally dilated vessels, an added resistance when vessels have tone, and a phasic resistance added whenever the ventricle contracts. The second of these resistances can be abolished with vasodilator drugs, and then perfusion of the left ventricular myocardium will produce a steep pressure–flow relation that is linear at higher flows but usually curvilinear at low pressures and flows (Fig. 71.2a). Because the vessels are maximally dilated, flow is uncoupled from metabolism and depends only on driving pressure and resistance. If heart rate is increased, the maximal flow at any perfusion pressure will decrease because the heart is in a relaxed state for a smaller proportion of each cardiac cycle.

## Autoregulation

If coronary vessels have tone, then the pressure–flow relationship can be assessed at different perfusion pressures after cannulating the left coronary artery. Cannulation is necessary because when cardiac metabolism and blood flow are coupled, increasing aortic blood pressure will increase coronary flow by increasing myocardial O$_2$ demand. If perfusion pressure is raised or lowered from its control value, flow changes transiently in the direction of the change of pressure and then tends to return towards the previous steady-state. There is a range over which there is almost no change in steady-state flow; a rise in pressure has caused vasoconstriction, and a fall in pressure has caused vasodilatation. This response, in which for a constant myocardial O$_2$ consumption flow remains almost constant despite changes in perfusion pressure, is termed autoregulation. At perfusion pressures above the upper end of the range, flow increases, probably because the pressure overcomes the constriction. At pressures below about 40 mmHg (5.3 kPa) (but varying: see below) flow decreases (Fig. 71.2a), indicating

that some vessels are maximally dilated and can no longer decrease resistance to compensate for the decreased perfusion pressure. Animal studies have shown that at these low pressures flows are decreased in some small pieces of myocardium, particularly in the subendocardium, although adjacent small pieces of muscle may have normal flows. As pressures are lowered still further, more and more pieces of muscle develop low flows and become ischemic, and the majority of the hypoperfused and ischemic pieces are in the subendocardium. Similar changes occur if the perfusion pressure is kept constant and the pressure in the left ventricle, systolic or diastolic, is greatly elevated, or the heart rate is greatly increased, or the O$_2$ content of coronary arterial blood is decreased. In each of these circumstances, an imbalance between myocardial O$_2$ consumption and myocardial blood (and O$_2$) supply develops. These changes have their counterparts in human disease; for example, subendocardial ischemia and patchy subendocardial necrosis occur in *critical aortic stenosis, cyanotic heart disease, severe anemia* (especially if chronic), carbon monoxide poisoning, extreme tachycardia, *dilated cardiomyopathy,* or *coronary artery atheroma.*

## Role of vasoactive peptides and other vasoregulators

Although control of tissue O$_2$ tensions seems to be the aim of the autoregulatory and other metabolic control systems, the mechanisms by which tissue O$_2$ is kept fairly constant are poorly understood. Adenosine, a powerful coronary vasodilator, is a prime candidate for a control mechanism. More cardiac work or decreased coronary perfusion results in increased breakdown of ATP to adenosine monophosphate; this is broken down by 5′ nucleotidase to adenosine which could then dilate the vessels. On the other hand, less cardiac work or increased perfusion decrease the amount of adenosine produced and so might lead to some vasoconstriction. Adenosine is not essential for coronary regulation, because a great decrease in its concentration produced by infusing adenosine deaminase does not affect autoregulation, and also because certain dynamic considerations do not fit the adenosine model. Nevertheless, it could play a role during ischemia.

Several powerful vasoactive peptides are known to affect the coronary circulation. Cardiac sympathetic afferent nerves can be stimulated by ischemia, perhaps by release of local bradykinin or eicosanoids. On stimulation, these nerves release substance P and calcitonin gene-related peptide (CGRP) from their nerve endings, and these are powerful coronary vasodilators. Once coronary flow is increased, the coronary endothelium is stimulated (probably by increased shear stress) to release nitric oxide (NO), and this helps to maintain the vasodilatation (*see* page 697 for further details). Coronary vasodilators like acetyl-

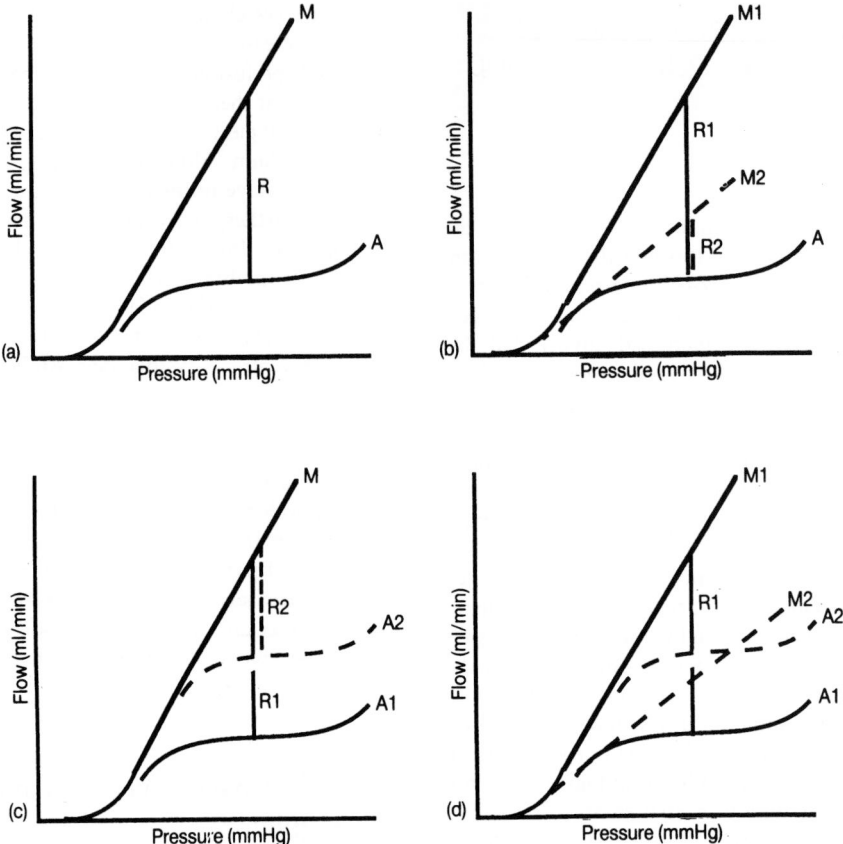

FIGURE 71.2 Coronary flow reserve diagrams. (a) Coronary flow reserve diagram with autoregulation curve (A), pressure–flow line of maximal vasodilatation (M), and coronary flow reserve (R) at normal perfusion pressure. (b) Normal coronary flow reserve diagram which shows in addition to the normal maximal pressure–flow line (M1) the dashed line of reduced maximal pressure–flow relation. The normal flow reserve (R1) is reduced to R2 (short dashed line). (c) Normal coronary flow reserve diagram which shows in addition to the normal autoregulation curve (A1) a curve showing autoregulation at an increased level of flow (A2). Once again, flow reserve is reduced from the normal value of R1 to a lower value of R2 (short dashed line). (d) Normal coronary flow reserve diagram with an abnormally high autoregulation curve (A2) and an abnormally low maximal pressure–flow line (M2). As can be seen, at a normal perfusion pressure there is no reserve left. This combination can occur with hypertrophy, polycythemia and hypoxemia, as well as with other combinations of factors.

choline and substance P act entirely through the release of NO. Endothelial damage from air embolism or atheroma decreases or prevents NO release, and the absence of this potent vasodilator (and platelet antiaggregatory agent) may explain some instances of coronary spasm. Finally, atrial natriuretic peptide (ANP) is released from atria (and to some extent from ventricles) when these are distended. ANP dilates renal vessels and aids diuresis, and also inhibits sympathetic tone. What part it plays in coronary vasomotion is not clear. Finally, recent studies have shown that ATP-dependent potassium channels are important in the coronary bed and cause vasodilatation (possibly through NO production). Ischemia has been shown to activate these channels, and reactive hyperemia can be reduced by about 60 per cent when these channels are inhibited.

There are also potent coronary vasoconstrictors. Norepinephrine released from sympathetic nerve endings activates α-adrenergic receptors and produces vasoconstriction, and so does neuropeptide Y, which is coreleased with norepinephrine. The endothelium also produces endothelins, a family of powerful vasoconstrictors. These are released by ischemia and appear in high concentration in patients with congestive heart failure, but their role in pathophysiology is not yet defined. Another vasoconstrictor hormone is vasopressin, which may also rise in concentration during congestive heart failure. Finally, there are potent eicosanoids that are vasoconstrictors, notably some of the leukotrienes and thromboxane $A_2$. The latter is released from platelets that are activated during aggregation; the vasoconstriction and the platelet plug help to prevent hemorrhage from any break in the vascular wall. Coronary endothelial damage, by reducing local endothelial production of prostacyclin ($PGI_2$) and NO, encourages platelet aggregation which may play a role in coronary spasm.

# Coronary blood flow reserve

## General principles

At any pressure, the difference between autoregulated and maximal flows is termed coronary flow reserve; this has the same units as the original flows, but a dimensionless ratio with similar implications can be obtained by dividing maximal by resting flow. Flow reserve depends greatly on perfusion pressure because of the steepness of the pressure–flow relation in maximally dilated vessels. Coronary flow reserve indicates how much added flow the myocardium can receive at a given pressure to meet increased demands for O$_2$; if reserve is much reduced, then flow cannot increase sufficiently to meet demands, and myocardial ischemia occurs. Decreases in coronary flow reserve are always more profound in the subendocardium than in the subepicardium, so that myocardial supply–demand imbalance and ischemia will occur in the subendocardium before the subepicardium.

## Decreased maximal blood flow

If autoregulated flow is normal but maximal flow is decreased (Fig. 71.2b), then coronary flow reserve will be reduced. Such a change can occur with marked tachycardia; a decrease in the number of coronary vessels due to small vessel disease, as in some collagen vascular diseases, especially systemic lupus erythematosus; increased resistance to flow in one or more large coronary vessels because of embolism, thrombosis, atheroma, or spasm; impaired myocardial relaxation due to ischemia or hypothermia; myocardial edema; a marked increase in left ventricular diastolic pressure; a marked increase in left ventricular systolic pressure if coronary perfusion pressure is not also increased, as in aortic stenosis or incompetence; and an increase in blood viscosity, most commonly seen with an hematocrit over 65 per cent but also occurring with macroglobulinemia or very high white blood cell counts in leukemia.

## Increased control (autoregulated) blood flows

Coronary flow reserve will also be reduced if maximal flows are normal but autoregulated flows increase (Fig. 71.2c). Myocardial flows increase above normal values with exercise, tachycardia, anemia, hypoxemia, carbon monoxide poisoning, leftward shift of the hemoglobin O$_2$ dissociation curve as in infants with a high proportion of fetal hemoglobin or certain abnormal hemoglobins (hemoglobinopathies), thyrotoxicosis, acute ventricular dilatation (because of increased wall stress), inotropic stimulation by catecholamines, and acquired ventricular hypertrophy.

## Effects of ventricular hypertrophy

When hypertrophy occurs after about 4–6 months of age in lambs and swine, ventricular muscle mass increases without a concomitant increase in conducting coronary blood vessels. Ventricular hypertrophy returns wall stress to normal, and myocardial flow per minute per gram of muscle remains approximately normal. Total left ventricular flow is increased in proportion to ventricular mass, but because maximal flow per ventricle is usually unchanged, the coronary flow reserve is diminished. Often autoregulated flow is increased and maximal flows are reduced at the same time; for example, with severe tachycardia or cyanotic heart disease with hypoxemia, ventricular hypertrophy, and polycythemia. Under these circumstances, coronary flow reserve can be drastically reduced or even absent at normal perfusion pressures (Fig. 71.2d).

## Hypertrophy and angiogenic potential

Hypertrophy occurring in fetal life, or very soon after birth, has in experimental animals been associated with an increased total number of conducting coronary vessels and no loss of coronary flow reserve. This angiogenic potential disappears within the first few months after birth.

## Myocardial wall stress, O$_2$ consumption, and coronary blood flow reserve

Myocardial wall stress is regulated within a fairly narrow range, with or without myocardial hypertrophy. Consequently, myocardial blood flow per unit mass is fairly constant at about 1 mL/(min·g) of left ventricle at rest. There is a close relationship between left ventricular mass-to-volume ratio and peak wall stress in systole, as shown by Strauer. If the heart dilates acutely, then the mass-to-volume ratio decreases, wall stress and myocardial O$_2$ consumption increase, and coronary flow reserve falls. This is particularly serious when there is hypertrophy in which coronary flow reserve is already reduced. Decreasing ventricular dilatation by afterload and preload reduction reverses these unfavorable events and is another reason for the value of this therapy.

Note from Fig. 71.2a–d that because the line of maximal pressure–flow relations slopes up and to the right, any decrease in that slope (Fig. 71.2b) or any increase in autoregulated flow (Fig. 71.2c) causes autoregulation to fail at pressures much higher than usually occurs.

# Right ventricular myocardial blood flow

Right ventricular myocardial blood flow is governed by the principles described above, but there are differences due to the low right ventricular systolic pressure and because right ventricular pressure work is not changed by alterations in aortic and coronary artery blood pressures. Acute right ventricular hypertension, e.g. from pulmonary embolism or severe pulmonary vasoconstriction, will, if severe, cause right ventricular failure; the increased wall stress increases right ventricular $O_2$ consumption but the increased systolic pressure reduces the coronary flow, and right ventricular myocardial ischemia occurs because supply cannot match demand. Under these circumstances, if aortic perfusion pressure is increased mechanically or with $\alpha$-adrenergic agonists, right ventricular myocardial blood flow will increase and restore right ventricular function to normal.

With chronic right ventricular hypertension and hypertrophy, as in severe pulmonic stenosis, many forms of cyanotic congenital heart disease, and some chronic lung disease, then right ventricular myocardial blood flow behaves in the same way as left ventricular blood flow. If aortic pressure is lowered, however, left ventricular pressure decreases, as does left ventricular work and $O_2$ consumption, but in the right ventricle the workload may not be reduced, so that imbalance between myocardial $O_2$ supply and demand may occur. The greatest imbalance occurs when right ventricular systolic pressure is maintained but coronary perfusion pressure decreases, as can happen in a child with *tetralogy of Fallot* who has an excessively large aorto-pulmonary anastomosis. The right ventricular systolic pressure will be raised because of the systemic aortic and left ventricular systolic pressures, but the low diastolic aortic pressure due to the shunt lowers coronary perfusion pressure in diastole and can cause both left and right ventricular ischemia and failure. A similar imbalance occurs when there is severe pulmonary hypertension without a connection between the two sides of the heart. A fall in systemic pressure then causes right ventricular underperfusion and may lead to sudden death.

# Reperfusion injury

When a heart is ischemic for 15–20 min and is then reperfused, there is a transient period of impaired function that may last for hours but recovers completely; this phenomenon is known as stunning and is due to unknown biochemical processes. Periods of ischemia longer than 40–60 min lead to regions of cell death, predominantly in the subendocardium of the left ventricle. It seems that it is the reperfusion rather than the ischemia that causes much of the damage, because the use of certain experimental reperfusates may allow up to 6 hours of normothermic ischemia without any cell death. Cell death is preceded by overload of $Ca^{2+}$ in the mitochondria and by loss of nucleotides from the cytosol, both of these being in part due to profound membrane damage. Some of this damage may be due to free radicals like superoxide and hydroxyl radicals, and recently investigators have shown that NO released during reperfusion may generate peroxynitrite anions which produce hydroxyl radicals. It is possible that $O_2$ free radical injury plays a particularly important role in the reperfusion after cardiac surgery of hearts of children with cyanotic heart disease.

## SELECTED READING

Hata K, Takasago T, Saeki A, Nishioka T, Goto Y. Stunned myocardium after rapid correction of acidosis. Increased $O_2$ cost of contractility and the role of the $Na^+$-$H^+$ exchange system. *Circ Res* 1994; **74**: 794.

Hata K, Goto Y, Kawaguchi O *et al.* Hypercapnic acidosis increases $O_2$ cost of contractility in the dog left ventricle. *Am J Physiol* 1994; **H266**: 730.

Hoffman JIE. Maximal coronary flow and the concept of coronary vascular reserve. *Circulation* 1984; **70**: 153.

Hoffman JIE. Transmural myocardial perfusion. *Prog Cardiovasc Dis* 1987; **29**: 429.

Hoffman JIE. Coronary artery physiology. In: Garfein OB, ed. *Current concepts in cardiovascular physiology*. New York: Academic Press, 1990: 289.

Strauer BE. Myocardial oxygen consumption in chronic heart disease: role of wall stress, hypertrophy and coronary reserve. *Am J Cardiol* 1979; **44**: 730.

# 72

# Ventricular Function

David F. Teitel and Julien I.E. Hoffman

## ISOLATED MUSCLE

### General considerations

In addition to the components of individual myocytes, factors that affect the interaction between myocytes determine the force developed by a muscle strip. Relative concentration and organization of myocytes within a region affect force generation, as do the extracellular matrix and connective and vascular tissues. Developmental changes occur at all these levels. Contractile elements increase as a proportion of total volume throughout gestation, increasing the force generated per gram of tissue. Collagen, the major protein responsible for the complex network which connects myocytes and allows maximal force generation, changes greatly throughout development, from initially showing only small quantities of very disorganized material to a well-developed and structured framework to which the myocytes attach. Collagen type also changes over development, although the functional significance of the different types is not known. Other extracellular components, including fibronectin and growth factors, may have important effects on cardiac growth and development.

If a muscle is stimulated to contract, it develops force. Isometric contractions occur at infinite afterload so that no shortening occurs; the function of the isometrically contracting muscle can be described entirely by the extent and rate of force generation. If the muscle is allowed to shorten, the amount and rate of shortening are also parameters of function. In the extreme, a fully unloaded muscle reaches maximal velocity of shortening with no force generation. Thus indices of force generation and shortening have been applied to the study of isolated muscle strips in a variety of conditions and at different developmental stages.

### Length–tension relationships in muscle strips

A basic property of cardiac muscle is defined by the *Frank–Starling relationship*: the greater the initial stretch (preload) of that muscle the greater the force it generates on contraction. At a sarcomere level, this phenomenon can be understood in terms of crossbridge units: the greater the length of a sarcomere prior to contraction, the more crossbridges are available for the myosin heads to shorten the sarcomere, and the greater the sensitivity of the crossbridge complex to $Ca^{2+}$ (length-dependent activation).

To study the Frank–Starling relationship in cardiac muscle strips, investigators have isolated small pieces of tissue, usually in papillary muscle with its nearly parallel fibers, but also in portions of the ventricular walls. The muscle strip is placed in a water bath. One end is tied to a pivoted lever, and the other is attached to a force transducer (Fig. 72.1). Weights attached to the other end of the lever extend the muscle to any desired length before contraction (preload); excessive stretching is prevented by a stop. Other weights added to the lever after initial length has been set affect the muscle only after contraction has begun, and are therefore termed the afterload. Muscle length and force can be measured before and during contraction. The muscle is stimulated to contract by an electrical impulse. Instruments to measure sarcomere length, $Ca^{2+}$ entry, and many other functions can be added.

Active contraction is studied in two ways (Fig. 72.2). If cardiac muscle is stimulated to contract at different initial muscle lengths, but is not allowed to shorten (isometric contraction), no force is generated at the shortest lengths; the muscle remains slack. Then as sarcomere lengths increase, force is generated, and this force increases to reach a maximum at sarcomere

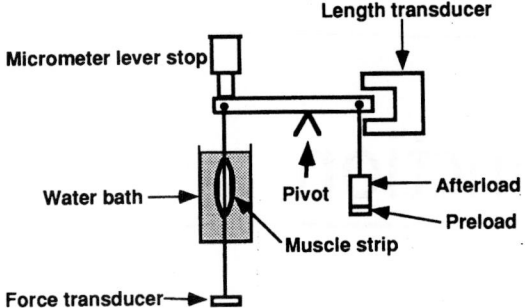

FIGURE 72.1 Diagram of muscle bath. The muscle is in a water bath. One end is suspended from a pivoted lever, and the other is attached to a force transducer. The other end of the lever is attached to a length transducer. A weight (preload) attached to the lever stretches the muscle to an extent determined by the stop. Then another weight (afterload) is added, and the muscle is stimulated to contract by electrodes (not shown) in the bath.

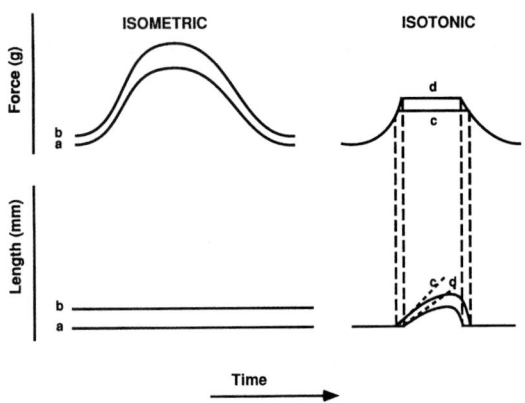

FIGURE 72.2 Length–tension curves during isometric (left) and isotonic (right) contractions. Left panels: the isometric curves are made at two different initial muscle lengths (a and b) and show no shortening (below). The maximum force generated from the longer initial length (b) is greater than that generated by the shorter length (above). Right panels: isotonic curves are made at two different afterloads. As shown in the upper diagram, force rises until the afterload is reached, and then it remains constant at the afterloads of c and d, as shown by the intervals between the two sets of dashed lines, until relaxation begins. The corresponding shortening curves (below) show an initial rapid shortening; tangents to this initial rapid upstroke (dotted lines) are used to calculate the initial velocity of shortening. Note that for the higher afterload (d), it takes longer before shortening begins, the initial velocity of shortening is less, and relaxation begins earlier.

lengths of about 2.2 μm. At longer sarcomere lengths, there may even be a decrease in force, because the sarcomere is overstretched so that the actin filaments are separated from the myosin filaments and efficient crossbridging cannot be achieved. (This cannot occur in the intact heart, because the stiffness of the extramyocytic components – part of the parallel elastic element – limits the extent to which the sarcomere can be

stretched.) If at any muscle or sarcomere length passive tension is subtracted from the tension generated during isometric contraction, the resulting curve demonstrates active tension as a function of length. If afterload is small, the contracting muscle generates an appropriate force, and then shortens while force remains constant (isotonic contraction). The rate of shortening is fastest at the onset of shortening, and from it the velocity of shortening is measured (Fig. 72.2, right panels). The shortening velocity will range from zero when the load is so heavy that it prevents shortening to a maximum when the external load is zero; because of internal viscosity and elastic forces, however, true zero loading is impossible. Increases in cytosolic $Ca^{2+}$ increase the force generated during contraction, but have little effect on the maximal velocity of shortening.

Conceptually the sarcomeres can be considered to have at least three functional components: an inelastic contractile element (CE) and two elastic elements, one in series with the contractile element (SE) and one in parallel with it (PE). These elastic elements were needed to explain the results of stretching the muscle passively, and of releasing it suddenly during contraction. The exact arrangement of these elements is still debated; in one popular model (Maxwell model), the PE is parallel to both the CE and SE which are in series, whereas in the other popular model (Voigt model) the PE is parallel only to the CE, and both are in series with the SE. In addition, there is internal viscosity that affects some of the changes noted in these experiments.

## Force–frequency relationship

Another basic property of cardiac muscle is that force generation is altered by the frequency of contraction. If intrinsic contractility of a muscle is defined as the alterations in force generation or shortening caused by changes in either $Ca^{2+}$ availability to or $Ca^{2+}$ sensitivity of the sarcomere, then the force–frequency relationship can be considered a product of beat-to-beat changes in contractility. If the frequency of contraction changes suddenly from one steady rate to a higher frequency, there is an increase in contractility over several contractions until some maximum is attained. This increase is due to a greater influx of $Ca^{2+}$ into the cells because of the greater duration of membrane depolarization per minute and a lesser reuptake by the sarcoplasmic reticulum because of a shorter duration of diastole. Eventually $Ca^{2+}$ influx and efflux equilibrate, but with a greater level of (releasable) intracellular $Ca^{2+}$ that is responsible for the increase in contractile force. Transient analyses are based on the phenomenon of post-extrasystolic potentiation, namely that force is reduced during a premature beat but is supernormal after the compensatory pause. This phenomenon can be tested formally in muscle strips to obtain the force–frequency or the force–interval relationship. The muscle is stimulated to beat at a regular rate, and then every eighth stimulus is applied prematurely; this procedure is repeated with varying intervals between the last regular stimulus and the premature stimulus. In the second stage, a second premature stimulus is applied at varying intervals after the first premature stimulus. The maximal force achieved in each contraction is plotted against the interval between the last normal beat and the first or second premature beat. The force achieved is low at short interstimulus intervals, and rises to a maximum at an interval of about 1 s. The force is about twice as high after two premature stimuli as after one. The interpretation of this relationship is that when the muscle is excited to contract, $Ca^{2+}$ enters the cytosol from outside and also from the sarcoplasmic reticulum. In diastole, $Ca^{2+}$ is taken up by the sarcoplasmic reticulum, but is not available for release until some time has passed. Therefore, after a premature beat, a subnormal amount of $Ca^{2+}$ is available to generate force, which is submaximal. After the compensatory pause, however, more releasable $Ca^{2+}$ is in the storage sites, and when released produces a supramaximal contraction. Thus, post-extrasystolic potentiation requires a well-functioning sarcoplasmic reticulum and a condition in which $Ca^{2+}$ availability is not maximal, i.e. a low initial contractile state.

## Developmental aspects

Active tension per square millimeter cross-sectional myocyte area at any given afterload is below adult values, but is proportional to the reduced number of myofibrils present; about 60 per cent of adult cardiac muscle consists of contractile material, whereas this amounts to only 30 per cent in the fetus. The extent and velocity of shortening are also reduced in fetal heart muscle, but correction for the amount of contractile machinery suggests that the intrinsic performance of fetal and adult actin–myosin filaments is similar. Some of the differences between fetal and adult cardiac muscle may be due to differences in collagen and cytoskeletal composition. The change from fetal to adult performance seems to occur fairly soon after birth, when myofibrillar array becomes regular and when the T tubules and the sarcoplasmic reticulum develop into their adult form. For this reason, prematurely born infants (and, to a lesser extent, full-term infants) have a reduced ability to tolerate an increase in afterload, and are also unduly sensitive to reductions in serum $Ca^{2+}$ concentrations. Early in fetal development, post-extrasystolic potentiation is limited because of immaturity of the sarcoplasmic reticulum. Post-extrasystolic potentiation increases in late fetal life in the sheep, but then after birth decreases again because of the high resting β-adrenergic state that exists following birth. With the increased catecholamine stimulation necessary to drive the increased $O_2$ demands of respiration and thermoregulation, $Ca^{2+}$ influx to the cytosol is

near maximal with each beat, so that the sarcoplasmic reticulum is limited in its ability to increase this further.

Most of these developmental differences have been observed in animals, not humans. Because in humans the distances from $Ca^{2+}$ release sites to myofilaments are much shorter in fetuses than in adults, the availability of $Ca^{2+}$ to the myofilaments may not be very different at different ages.

## INTEGRATED MUSCLE FUNCTION: INTACT VENTRICLE

### Systolic function

There are factors that determine heart function *in vivo* beyond those which determine the function of the isolated muscle, but nevertheless there are close correlations between what is found in muscle strips and in the whole ventricle. If one defines the contractile performance of the isolated muscle in terms of force developed and length, one can define the global systolic performance of the intact ventricle in terms of pressure and volume. The amount and rate of pressure developed and the amount and rate of blood volume ejected per beat can fully describe the performance of the heart as a pump. Thus evaluation of systolic performance is best made in the pressure–volume plane, which has been the primary direction of studies over the past 20 years.

In the adult heart, the four major determinants of systolic performance are preload, afterload, contractility and heart rate. It is important to define these determinants clearly, because in many studies the definitions have not been appropriately used.

### Frank–Starling mechanism (preload effects)

The preload that stretches a muscle strip is equivalent to end-diastolic fiber length of the intact ventricle. This length can be measured readily by various devices in animals, but in the intact human ventricle is best related to end-diastolic diameter or volume. Frequently, end-diastolic pressure has been used interchangeably with end-diastolic volume as an index of preload, but this can be misleading if the distensibility of the ventricle changes or if pressure outside the heart (pericardial or intrathoracic) rises. Furthermore, there is normally little rise in tension for a fairly considerable change of fiber length, so that similar end-diastolic pressures might coexist with very different fiber lengths. Now that ventricular volumes can be measured fairly accurately by modern imaging methods, there is no reason for not using length or volume to assess preload.

The Frank–Starling relationship is active in the intact ventricle as well as in isolated muscle. Increasing preload increases the pressure generated by an isolated ventricle that is not allowed to eject, as described over 100 years ago by Otto Frank. If the ventricle is allowed to eject, then increased preload allows the heart to eject the same stroke volume against an increased afterload, or else to eject a greater stroke volume against a constant afterload; this is what Ernest Starling showed. The Frank–Starling mechanism has been shown in fetal sheep as well as in the embryonic chick heart. The reserve to increase output, and the plateau pressure at which output is maximal, are significantly lower in fetal as compared with postnatal sheep. Thus, although intact, the Frank–Starling mechanism cannot be invoked to a great extent prior to birth to increase output in times of increased demand (see below).

## Afterload effects

Afterload is more complicated in the intact ventricle than in isolated muscle strips. Frequently, aortic systolic pressure is equated with afterload. However, in the muscle strip, afterload represents the force exerted by the muscle during contraction, and pressure and force are not the same. The afterload against which the intact ventricle ejects includes the peripheral resistance of the systemic vascular bed, the impedance of the central vasculature, and the inertia of blood and the ventricular wall. Because the stress in the wall of the ventricle is equal to the force or afterload against which it is contracting, stress is the most accurate estimate of afterload. It is preferable to calculate circumferential or meridional wall stress, which, at the mid wall, is a function of ventricular pressure, diameter, and wall thickness. Both peak systolic and end-systolic wall stress can be used in assessing ventricular function. Calculations of wall stress are based on the LaPlace relationship:

$$\text{wall stress} = \frac{Pr}{2h}$$

where $P$ is pressure, $r$ is radius of curvature, and $h$ is wall thickness. Because the left ventricle is not a regular sphere, particularly in systole, the LaPlace formula is an oversimplification. A fairly simple and accurate formula for meridional wall stress that incorporates the important variables was developed by Grossman and others:

$$\text{wall stress} = \frac{1.35Pd}{4h(1 + h/d)}$$

where $P$ is pressure, $d$ is left ventricular minor axis dimension, and $h$ is wall thickness at the level of the minor axis.

## Heart rate effects

Heart rate as a determinant of performance in the intact heart is more complex than in isolated muscle. The force–frequency relationship has been demonstrated in intact hearts, measuring ventricular minor axis diameter with ultrasonic crystals, and using the two-stage extra stimulus procedure described above. The maximal rate of change of pressure ($dP/dt_{max}$) in the ventricles was similar to that found previously in muscle strips. In cats and dogs, after steady pacing, an optimal $dP/dt_{max}$ occurred 720 ms after the last normal beat; this was shortened to 560 ms during epinephrine infusion, and $dP/dt_{max}$ increased if the control pacing rate was elevated. These findings can be explained by the effects of these maneuvers on $Ca^{2+}$ stores and their release. Applying this technique to humans with normal or abnormal left ventricular function, the optimal R–R interval was 800 ms. If two beats were given at optimal intervals after the premature stimulus, $dP/dt_{max}$ of the first normal beat after the premature beat was potentiated because the extra $Ca^{2+}$ introduced into the cytosol by the premature beat was available to potentiate the first beat after the premature stimulus. The second post-premature beat was also potentiated, but less so; the ratio of the potentiation of these two beats can be used to calculate the fraction of $Ca^{2+}$ recirculating from one beat to the next. This amount is constant in any one individual, but much less in those with left ventricular dysfunction.

In addition to the force–frequency relationship, heart rate affects systolic performance by the Frank–Starling relationship by virtue of its effects on diastolic filling. At normal rates, the ventricle fills and ejects a normal stroke volume. As heart rate increases, stroke volume falls slightly at first because there is a decrease in filling time; however, the increase in contraction frequency may more than offset the decrease in stroke volume so that cardiac output is maintained or may increase. When heart rate increases further, diastolic filling is impaired enough that cardiac output falls. Similarly, as heart rate decreases, cardiac output is maintained through a certain range because of an increase in preload and thus stroke volume. When heart rate decreases further, the increase in preload is insufficient to maintain cardiac output. The range over which cardiac output is maintained is an index of the heart rate sensitivity; the wider the range, the lesser the sensitivity. The newborn and adult heart are relatively insensitive to changes in heart rate over a wide range. The fetal heart, however, is quite rate-sensitive, and heart rate may be the major determinant of cardiac output under normal conditions. This is partly because the fetal ventricles are relatively less compliant than are the ventricles postnatally, so that increasing diastolic filling time is not associated with compensatory increases in preload, and partly because the fetal heart is exposed to positive rather than negative extracardiac pressures. In addition to rate sensitivity, the filling of the ventricles is exquisitely sensitive to venous flow patterns, because the right atrial return is the main source of left ventricular filling as well. Thus, a change in the site of the pacemaker (left versus right atrium) has significant effects on relative right and left ventricular output as well as combined ventricular output.

## Contractility

The last major determinant of systolic performance is contractility. This is the most difficult determinant of performance to define and yet it is the one most studied. Contractility can perhaps best be defined as the alterations in cardiac function that occur secondary to changes in cytosolic $Ca^{2+}$ availability or sarcomere sensitivity to $Ca^{2+}$. Thus, β-adrenergic agonists or phosphodiesterase inhibitors, which increase cytosolic $Ca^{2+}$, and thyroxine, which alters myosin ATPase sensitivity to $Ca^{2+}$ in some species by altering the dominant isoform, are positive inotropic agents. However, to quantify contractility in the intact heart or to assess the contractile effects of an intervention is very difficult. This is because all presumed indices of contractility are in fact indices of overall performance. Insofar as the indices change with changes in the other determinants of performance (loading conditions and heart rate), they are not entirely specific for changes in contractility. For example, cardiac output is an excellent index of the systolic performance of the intact ventricle, but it is so sensitive to preload, afterload and heart rate that it is not useful as an index of contractility.

This has led many investigators to search for indices of performance that are load-insensitive and thus specific for changes in contractility. Unfortunately, it is increasingly clear that such a search is fruitless and in fact misdirected, because contractility is itself not independent of the other determinants of performance. For example, changes in contractility are not independent of changes in heart rate; as described above, the force–frequency relationship describes increases in contractility secondary to increases in heart rate. It is now apparent that changes in both preload and afterload also directly alter contractility. Direct preload effects on contractility have been clearly shown in the intact heart and at the sarcomere level by demonstrating length-dependent changes in contractility likely secondary to increased $Ca^{2+}$ sensitivity of the sarcomere at longer initial lengths. Afterload dependence has also been demonstrated; recent studies in the intact circulation have shown that acute increases in afterload acutely increase contractility independent of indirect effects of β-adrenergic stimulation. Some of this afterload dependence has been thought to be on the basis of beat-to-beat changes in $Ca^{2+}$ flux related to shortening deactivation. Recently it has also been shown that ejecting beats actually can generate greater rather than lesser pressures than isovolumic beats, so that there appear to be subcellular processes which act in

a direction opposite to shortening deactivation. It is likely that these as yet poorly defined processes which lead to pressure deficits and excesses in ejecting beats will be based on beat-to-beat alterations in $Ca^{2+}$ flux and sensitivity.

## Developmental aspects

In the immature heart, and particularly in the fetal environment, factors other than those described above may be important determinants as well. Most importantly, the right ventricle fills to a greater extent and under a higher pressure than the left, and it ejects more blood under the same pressure and against a greater impedance. Thus, the effects of the right ventricle on left ventricular performance (termed *ventricular interaction*) may well be another major determinant of left ventricular performance in the fetus, and must be considered. In addition, it is possible that the constraining effects of the pericardium and the uninflated lungs have a greater effect in the fetus than they will have postnatally. Lastly it is important to realize that the fetal circulatory environment is very different to that of the postnatal environment. Most importantly, the ventricles do not function strictly in series and the left ventricle is in physical continuity with a high pressure right ventricle. Thus the right ventricle may have a far more significant direct effect on left ventricular filling and ejection in the fetus than in the postnatal state.

After birth, as pulmonary arterial resistance and pressure progressively decrease, the right ventricle becomes thinner and more distensible than the left ventricle. The ventricular septum now bulges into the right ventricular cavity, so that the left ventricle is more circular on cross-section, the septum contracts in concert with the rest of the left ventricular wall, and left ventricular systolic function becomes more efficient. Left ventricular function at this stage is relatively unaffected by big changes in right ventricular volume or modest changes in right ventricular pressure. On the other hand, ventricular interaction can be more important than in the fetus if there is a marked increase in pulmonary vascular resistance; not only is it more difficult for right ventricular output to reach the left ventricle, but the distended high-pressure right ventricle compresses the septum and the left ventricle and can interfere with left ventricular function. Such a significant effect of the right ventricle on left ventricular performance has been demonstrated in the setting of pulmonary hypertension in the adult dog, and large increases in maximal left ventricular output shown in fetal sheep during *in utero* ventilation supports this hypothesis. Thus it is likely that ventricular interaction, although only a minor determinant of left ventricular output postnatally, may be a major determinant prior to birth.

In summary, the major determinants of fetal cardiac output may be quite different from those of postnatal cardiac output. Heart rate may normally be the major determinant of output; fetal bradycardia has a very detrimental effect on blood flow and $O_2$ delivery. The fetal heart can respond to increased preload (Frank–Starling law) with increased stroke volume, but this response is limited, perhaps because of a concomitant increase in afterload and the interactive effects of the right ventricle on left ventricular filling and ejection. The importance of inotropic stimulation in the fetus also appears limited. Conversely, whereas direct ventricular interaction appears to be a minor determinant in the postnatal state, it may be a major determinant of output in the fetus and, more importantly, alterations in ventricular interaction at birth may substantially contribute to the ability of the left ventricle to more than double its output after birth.

# Indices of performance and contractility

If it is clear that one cannot evaluate myocardial contractility specifically because it is intricately dependent upon loading conditions and heart rate, it becomes important to rethink all the indices of systolic performance which in the past have been used to separate the effects of contractility from those of preload and afterload. It seems more appropriate to accept that all indices are reflections of global performance and, rather than try to dissect out the independent contributions of various determinants, to determine the nature and magnitude of their interaction (equivalent to the interaction of sarcomere length, $Ca^{2+}$ dynamics and frequency of contraction in the isolated myofibrils). Prior to discussing indices of performance, it is worth making two general statements. First, because different determinants of performance are more important at different phases of systole (for example, preload during the isovolumic phase and afterload during ejection) it is worthwhile dividing the indices of systolic performance by the phase or phases of systole during which they occur. Second, because contractility is intricately related to load, any single beat index of performance is by necessity very load-sensitive and thus of limited usefulness in evaluating the contractile state of the heart. Thus any acceptable index of the contractile state of the heart should be obtained over a range of loading conditions. That is, a relationship of systolic performance over different loads would best describe the intrinsic ability of that heart to contract and eject blood.

## Pressure–volume loops: ventricular elastance

Because the systolic function of the intact heart is to generate pressure and eject blood, many recent investigators have studied performance in the pressure–volume plane. If left ventricular pressure and volume are measured simultaneously, the resulting pressure–volume loop gives information about ventricular function and can be used to assess myocardial contractility

in the intact heart. The modern approach to analyzing these loops is based on the elastance concept of Suga and Sagawa; by definition, elastance is the ratio of pressure change to volume change. Consider first an isolated ventricle containing a balloon that can be inflated to different volumes. At each volume the ventricle is stimulated to contract and generates a peak systolic pressure (Fig. 72.3a); as volumes increase, so do the peak systolic pressures generated, and the relationship is relatively linear. The line joining the peak pressures intercepts the volume axis at a positive value, termed $V_0$, that indicates the unstressed volume of the ventricle. The equation for this line is:

$$P_{es} = E_{es}(V_{es} - V_0)$$

where $P_{es}$ is end-systolic pressure, $E_{es}$ is the slope of the line, $V_{es}$ is the end-systolic volume, and $V_0$ is the unstressed volume (the ventricular volume when the transmural ventricular pressure is zero). If contractility increases (more $Ca^{2+}$ enters the cells), the ventricle can generate greater pressures at any given volume, thereby generating a steeper pressure–volume line (higher value of $E_{es}$), as shown by the dashed line $C^+$ in Fig. 72.3a. If contractility decreases, the ventricle generates lower pressures at any given volume, and the pressure–volume line is less steep (lower value of $E_{es}$).

If the ventricle ejects in the intact circulation, the typical pressure–volume loops shown in Fig. 72.3b are seen. During diastolic filling, volume increases and there is a slight rise in diastolic pressure due to the increase in passive tension. At the end of diastole, isovolumic systole occurs and ventricular pressure rises with no change in volume. When ventricular pressure exceeds aortic diastolic pressure, the aortic valve opens, blood is ejected, and ventricular volume decreases. Then ejection ends and pressure falls to diastolic levels as isovolumic relaxation occurs. The pressure and volume reached at the end of systole are those that would have been reached by the isolated ventricle at that same end-systolic volume; in other words, at a given volume, no higher pressure can be generated (loop 1, Fig. 72.3b). The decrease in volume during ejection is the stroke volume, which divided by the end-diastolic volume gives the ejection fraction; normally, ejection fraction is over 65 per cent.

To evaluate contractility in the intact circulation, one needs to evaluate the index (here, end-systolic elastance) over changing load, as discussed above. This has been done with pressure–volume loops with increases (volume infusion) and decreases (inferior vena caval occlusion) in preload or increases (aortic occlusion) in afterload. For example, if afterload is increased by raising aortic pressure, the normal heart responds as shown in Fig. 72.3b, loops 2 and 3. In the first beat after the increase, the ventricle has to generate a higher pressure before the valve opens. Then it ejects, but cannot eject a normal stroke volume because of the higher pressure that is required from the same end-diastolic length (preload). In fact, the end-systolic

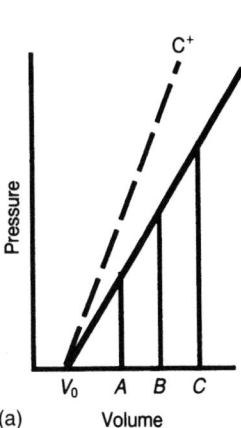

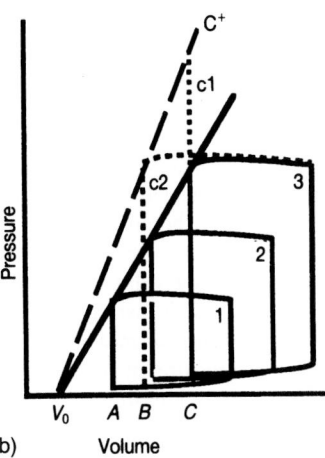

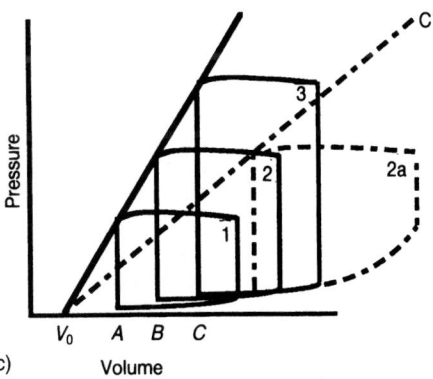

FIGURE 72.3 Ventricular pressure–volume relations. (a) Pressure–volume characteristics of non-ejecting (isometric) ventricle. $A$, $B$, and $C$ are three arbitrary ventricular volumes, and $V_0$ is the unstressed volume. The solid diagonal line is the pressure–volume relation of the normal ventricle, and the diagonal dashed line $C^+$ is the corresponding relation when contractility is increased. (b) Pressure–volume characteristics of ejecting ventricles. Loops 1, 2, and 3 in solid lines represent three ejecting beats at three different aortic pressures. The diagonal solid line is the elastance line obtained at end-systole; it is usually the line of maximal elastance when afterload is measured accurately. The end-systolic volumes for loops 1, 2, and 3 are the same volumes $A$, $B$, and $C$ as appeared in (a). When contractility is increased, as shown by the diagonal dashed line $C^+$, the ventricle with pressure–volume loop 3 can either generate a higher pressure at the same stroke volume (extension c1) or expel a greater stroke volume at the same aortic pressure (extension c2). (c) Pressure–volume characteristics when contractility is greatly impaired (as shown by the diagonal dashed line $C^-$). Loops 1, 2, and 3 are as in (b). Loop 2a indicates the pressure–volume loop during impaired contractility. Note that if the ventricle cannot dilate, as in restrictive cardiomyopathy, it can eject only a small stroke volume as shown by the vertical dashed line at end-systole for loop 2. If the ventricle can increase its end-diastolic volume, as in loop 2a, then it can eject a normal stroke volume, but at the expense of a very elevated end-diastolic pressure.

volume is that which is appropriate for the higher pressure. Because the ventricle has emptied incompletely, the next normal diastolic inflow increases end-diastolic volume, and this increase of end-diastolic volume continues until the ventricle ejects a normal stroke volume, but now at a higher end-diastolic volume (compare loops 1 and 2, and loops 2 and 3). The ventricle has adapted to the higher afterload by increasing end-diastolic fiber length, a phenomenon described by Starling and also discussed by Ross under the term "preload reserve." If different afterloads are used, the end-systolic pressure–volume points define a sloping line that is predicted to have the same slope as the line obtained

in the isolated heart at those same volumes, the line of maximal ventricular elastance. This end-systolic pressure–volume relationship can then be described by its slope ($E_{max}$) and intercept ($V_0$); these indices have been used separately and together to describe changes in contractility in the intact animal and human. However, this theoretical relationship does not hold exactly in the intact circulation. First, there is no theoretical reason for the relationship to be linear. Second, ejecting beats, probably through beat-to-beat changes in contractility, can achieve either higher or lower pressures than isovolumic beats. For these reasons, both curvilinearity and load dependence have been demonstrated in the adult and young heart, particularly when studied over a wide range of loads or at very high or very low contractile states. In the physiological range of measurements, however, and particularly in the young animal, the relationship appears to be linear enough to ignore the adjustments of curvilinearity, and $E_{max}$ appears to be reasonably sensitive to changes in contractility. However, because of curvilinearity in the far ranges of load, extrapolation to unstressed volumes probably is not valid. Thus, the positional index of the relationship generally used is a volume at a pressure in the range of measurement, such as $V_{100}$ (volume at a pressure of 100 mmHg [13.25 kPa]) rather than $V_0$. It is important to note that the end-systolic pressure–volume relationship can be generated over load using a variety of techniques, and afterload increases are not necessarily the best, because of rapid baroreflex responses. Typically, the relationship is generated during inferior vena caval occlusion. This alters preload over an adequate range to be able to define the slope and position of the relationship, but without producing large changes that would induce major and rapid neural responses to those changes.

## Increased contractility and elastance

If ventricular contractility increases, then the ventricle can attain higher ejection pressures at any given volume, and the end-systolic pressure–volume points are on a steeper line that lies above and to the left of the normal line, as shown by dashed line $C^+$ in Fig. 72.3b. Therefore, as shown by the dotted lines extending from loop 3, the ventricle can eject a higher stroke volume (see extension c2) at the same end-diastolic pressure (which is what happens during exercise) or can eject the same stroke volume at a higher pressure (see extension c1).

## Decreased contractility and elastance

If ventricular contractility decreases, then the ventricle cannot generate normal pressures at any given end-diastolic volume, and the end-systolic pressure–volume line lies below and to the right of the normal line, as shown by the dashed line $C^-$ in Fig. 72.3c. Note from Fig. 72.3c that the ventricle with impaired contractility can either eject a normal stroke volume at much increased end-diastolic volumes and pressures (loop 2a), or can eject at a normal end-diastolic volume and pressure only by reducing its stroke volume drastically (loop 2). Any increase in afterload causes a further increase in end-diastolic volume, and this increase causes diastolic pressures to rise rapidly to high values that cause pulmonary congestion. The normal preload reserve has been used up in attempting to eject a reasonable stroke volume against a modestly increased afterload. In hearts that are even more depressed, even normal afterloads cannot be handled by the ventricle without getting a pathologically raised diastolic pressure in the ventricles or a drastic decrease in stroke volume. Note that in these hearts, because of the relatively flat slope of the maximal ventricular elastance line, a slight reduction of afterload produces a relatively large increase in stroke volume and a relatively large decrease in ventricular end-diastolic volume and pressure. This is one of the mechanisms for cardiac improvement with afterload reduction.

# Ventricular function curves

## Ejection phase indices

More classical evaluation of systolic performance during ejection uses ventricular function curves. Sarnoff and colleagues first measured left ventricular diastolic pressure and stroke work, then infused fluids and examined the relationship between these two variables. A pressure–stroke work curve (N) is shown in Fig. 72.4. If contractility increased (I), the curve shifted up and to the left; i.e. at any end-diastolic pressure, a greater stroke work was achieved. If contractility decreased (D), the curve shifted down and to the right. Sarnoff recognized a major problem with this technique, namely that curvilinearity of the diastolic length–pressure relationship produced an S-shaped curve when relating stroke work to end-diastolic pressure, and at that time techniques for measuring fiber

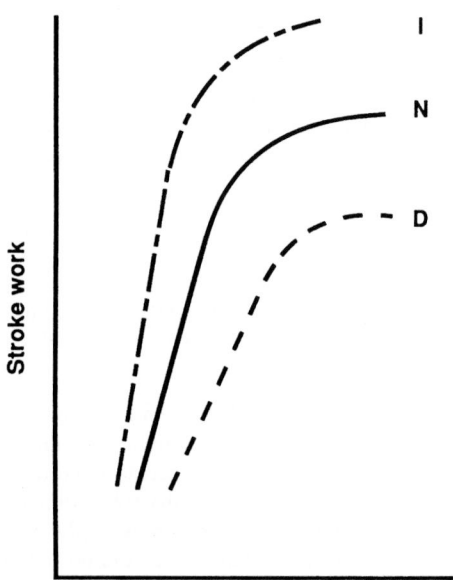

FIGURE 72.4 Curves to illustrate the ventricular function curves introduced by Sarnoff and colleagues. Curve N is the normal relation which can be moved up and to the left by increased contractility (I) or down and to the right by decreased contractility (D).

length or ventricular volume were inadequate. In addition, using pressure instead of fiber length or volume may lead to misinterpretations if there are substantial changes of pericardial or pleural pressures. Subsequent groups of investigators used similar function curves to examine the stroke volume–end-diastolic pressure relationship; this is even less satisfactory because stroke volume is affected by increases of afterload.

In conscious dogs with autonomic blockade the relationship of stroke work to end-diastolic fiber length or ventricular volume, termed preload recruitable stroke work, is linear and independent of changes in afterload. The line intercepts the length or volume axis at values close to the unstressed length or volume. $Ca^{2+}$ infusion increases the slope of the line without changing the intercept on the length axis. In ischemic ventricles, depression of ventricular function shifts the stroke work–end-diastolic segment length relationship to the right (increases the intercept on the horizontal axis) and decreases the slope. These two effects can be evaluated simultaneously by calculating the area under the curve, termed the preload recruitable stroke work area. These concepts and the ventricular elastance concept have much in common, and both give acceptable approaches to assessing myocardial function independent of changes in preload and afterload provided it is possible to measure wall force, stroke work, ventricular volume, or minor axis diameter and to change these over a range so that the lines or areas defining these indices can be obtained.

In addition to ejection phase analyses, it is possible and useful to evaluate performance during other phases of systole, and in other planes. The force–velocity relationship is another well-described attribute of cardiac muscle, and can be evaluated prior to ejection (during isovolumic contraction). The concept of the maximal velocity of contraction against zero load ($V_{max}$) was once popular; this value in muscle strips was independent of muscle length but varied in the right way with inotropic changes. The principle, based on studies of skeletal muscle by A.V. Hill, was reasonable, but the complexity of the mechanics of cardiac muscle, with its mixture of contractile, series elastic, and parallel elastic elements as well as viscosity made it difficult to assess what would have been the true index, namely the $V_{max}$ of the contractile element alone. In practice, too, it is not possible to abolish internal loading of the muscle fiber. Applying this concept to the intact heart was even more difficult.

As a substitute for $V_{max}$, investigators began to use $dP/dt_{max}$ (the maximal rate of change of ventricular pressure). However, this index is affected markedly by changes in afterload, and so must be used with care when afterloads are very different. A variant of this method is to measure $dP/dt$ at a developed ventricular pressure of 40 mmHg (5.3 kPa), because this virtually guarantees that the aortic valve will still be closed when the measurement is made. Little has recently described an index of ventricular performance by varying load while measuring the change in $dP/$ $dt_{max}$. The $dP/dt_{max}$–end-diastolic volume relation is similar to the end-systolic pressure–volume relation and to the preload recruitable stroke work index, is relatively linear, and varies with changes in contractility, but is less sensitive than are the other two indices.

## Combined ejection and isovolumic phase indices

Combining ejection and isovolumic phase indices may be the best way to evaluate systolic performance. Such an index has been created in both adults and children by providing normal data for the relationship between end-systolic wall stress and velocity of shortening. As contractility increases, the relationship shifts upward. Unfortunately, the effect of decreasing afterload beyond the range of the normal data has not been carefully explored, and from early studies it appears that, just as would be predicted from the force–velocity relationship, such decreases in afterload also appear to increase the stress-corrected velocity of shortening.

# Arterial and venous coupling

## Arterial coupling

Because the heart is a mechanical pump that ejects blood into the arterial system and in turn is supplied with blood by the venous system, these three components interact. One way to evaluate this is to consider what would happen if the heart were disconnected (uncoupled) from the rest of the circulation and each component considered separately. The heart's pumping ability can be tested by finding out how much it can eject against different afterloads; similarly, how much force a muscle strip can exert can be tested by increasing the afterload. As the load against which the left ventricle pumps increases, the output decreases until, at some high load, the heart cannot eject. The relationship of load to output is approximately linear (Fig. 72.5a). Then a pump is connected to the aorta and the amount of blood that can be pumped through the system at different perfusion pressures is determined; the higher the pressure, the more the flow through the system. For simplicity, this relationship is shown in Fig. 72.5b as linear, although the actual shape of the curve depends on many variables. In the intact circulation, there is an afterload for the ventricle and a perfusion pressure that pushes blood around the body; both of these are in equilibrium, and cardiac output and peripheral flow will be equal and occur where the two pressure–flow lines intersect (Fig. 72.5c). With decreased contractility, the heart can pump less blood at any given pressure, which produces the dashed line shown in Fig. 72.5d; where this crosses the (normal) peripheral resistance line gives the new equilibrium, and shows that both pressure and cardiac output will be reduced. If peripheral resistance is elevated without a change in contractility, then cardiac

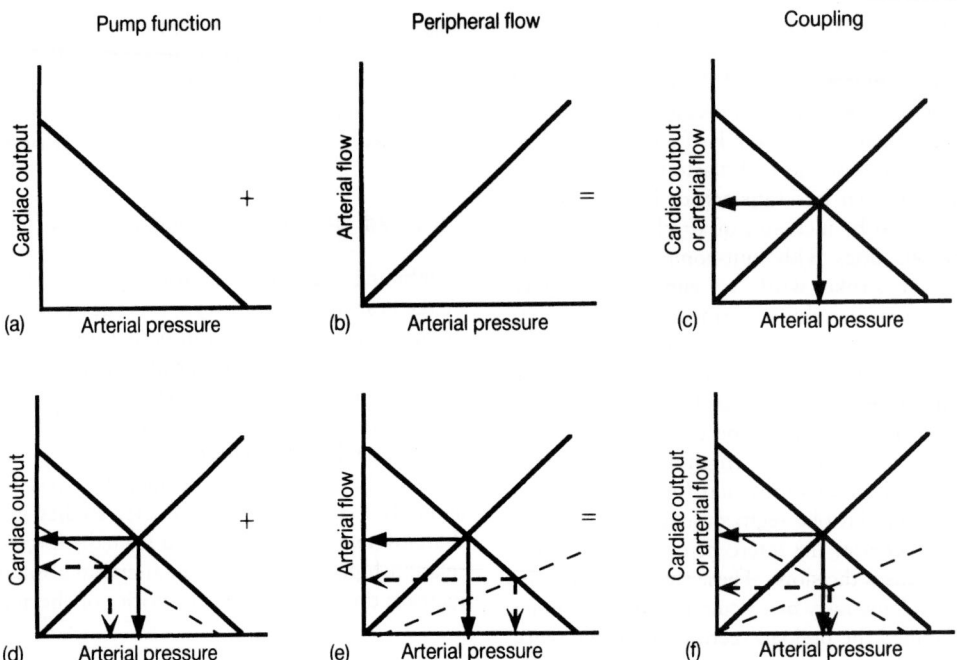

FIGURE 72.5 Arterial coupling. (a) Pump function of heart shown by plotting pump (cardiac) output at increasing peripheral (arterial) pressures. As the afterload increases, the output decreases. (b) Arterial function shown by how much flow is obtained at different perfusion pressures. The slope of the line is the resistance. (c) Normally cardiac output and arterial flow are equal, and the values for these flows occur where the two function lines cross. The solid arrows show the normal operating flow and pressure. (d) With decreased pump function, the cardiac output–afterload line is depressed (dashed line), and if peripheral resistance is normal both output and arterial pressure will be low, as shown by the dashed arrows. (e) With normal pump function but an increased peripheral resistance (as shown by the decreased slope of the dashed pressure–flow line) cardiac output is also decreased, but arterial pressure may be increased, as shown by the dashed arrows. (f) With heart failure, both a decrease in pump function and an increase in peripheral resistance will occur (dashed lines). Therefore, both cardiac output and arterial pressure will be reduced, the former more than the latter (dashed arrows).

output will be low but arterial pressure can be normal (dashed lines and arrows in Fig. 72.5e). However, with severe heart disease, there is an increase in peripheral resistance as well as a decrease in contractility, so that the two function lines cross at a markedly reduced stroke volume, even though the arterial pressure may be fairly normal (Fig. 72.5f). Therefore, treatment by agents that reduce afterload or increase inotropy, or both, will raise the crossover point and increase stroke volume by raising the equilibrium point at which the two function lines cross.

## Venous coupling

To study venous coupling, first the relationship between ventricular output and atrial pressure is examined (Fig. 72.6a). Increases in pressure cause a large increase in output at first (preload effect); then at increasing atrial pressures, output rises less markedly because preload reserve is used up, i.e. sarcomeres have reached their optimal lengths. On the other hand, if the effects of changing atrial pressures on venous return are examined (Fig. 72.6b), the venous return does not change for small increases in atrial pressure, but **above** atrial pressures of about 10–12 mmHg (1.3–

1.6 kPa) the venous return decreases more or less linearly as atrial pressures increase. The point at which these two curves cross is the operating point for the normal circulation (Fig. 72.6c); this is normally on the plateau of the venous return curve. In the normal heart, decreasing venous return decreases cardiac output (Fig. 72.6d), as is seen transiently in the brief hypotension that occurs when suddenly standing up from a sitting position. In other words, cardiac output is normally limited by venous return and not by cardiac performance. In *congestive heart failure*, however, the venous system is overfilled and at high pressure. The crossover point occurs on the sloping portion of the venous return curve because cardiac output is now determined by the depressed cardiac function and is low, and because venous pressure is high, cardiac function is not limited by venous return (Fig. 72.6e). What happens to the circulation when sodium nitroprusside is given? Systemic venous capacity increases, and causes a shift of blood from the pulmonary to the systemic circuits. Left ventricular filling pressure is decreased, thus reducing left ventricular preload with resulting improvement in left ventricular function, partly by improving subendocardial blood flow. Therefore, cardiac output increases and the patient improves. Increased cardiac output from vasodilators

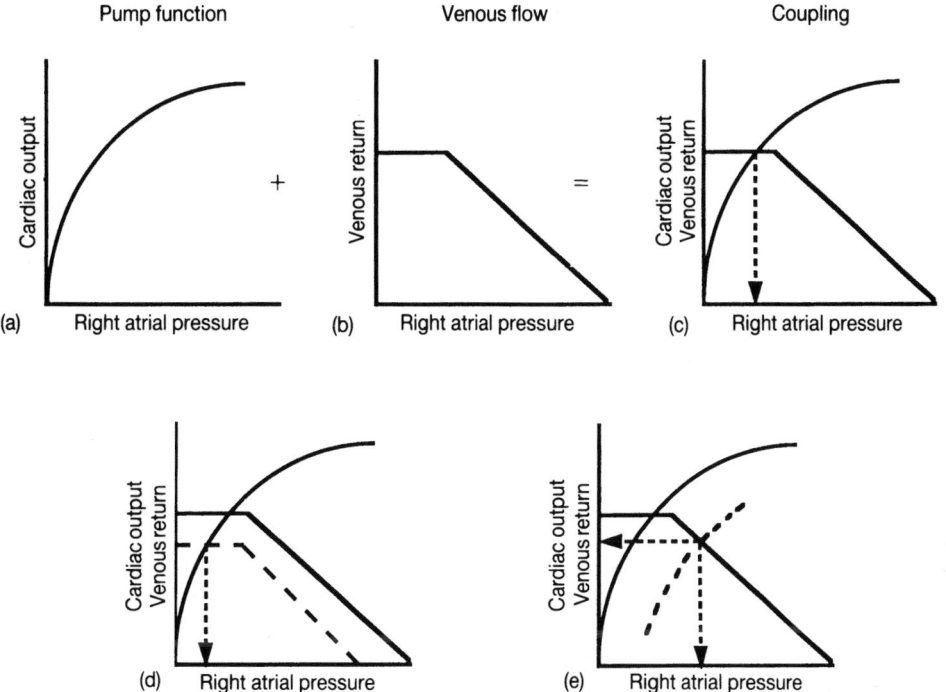

FIGURE 72.6 Venous coupling. (a) Typical preload–flow relation of an atrium. (b) Typical normal venous return–right atrial relation. As right atrial pressure is increased from very low values, the venous return does not change because of the systemic venous waterfall. At higher pressures, raising right atrial pressure will lower venous return. (c) Where the right atrial pressure–cardiac output and the right atrial pressure–venous return curves cross will determine the venous return and right atrial pressure for that subject. As shown by the dotted arrow, this is usually on the plateau of the venous return–atrial pressure curve. (d) A sudden decrease in venous return, as occurs with standing up, decreases right atrial pressure and cardiac output. (e) With decreased cardiac contractility, right atrial pressure rises until it impedes venous return.

also tends to lower venous pressure and increase venous return.

## Diastolic function

Systolic function affects the force and rate of ventricular contraction, and the amount of blood ejected with each beat; diastolic function concerns the rate and extent of ventricular relaxation. Many forms of heart disease manifest abnormalities of both systolic and diastolic function, but dysfunction of one or the other may predominate and determine the type of therapy needed.

Diastolic dysfunction is indicated by an increased ventricular diastolic pressure at normal ventricular volumes. It is thus determined by active processes (crossbridge dissociation or myofilament deactivation) and passive processes (the distensibility or compliance of the fully relaxed ventricle). Dysfunction may be caused by increased passive stiffness (decreased compliance) of the ventricles due to chronic infiltrates (e.g. amyloid), myocardial scars (e.g. after ischemia), constrictive pericarditis, or diffuse myocardial fibrosis. It also can be due to impaired relaxation. Normally, ventricular muscle relaxes rapidly in diastole, the primary

mechanism being the rapid release of $Ca^{2+}$ bound to troponin and its uptake by the sarcoplasmic reticulum. Removing $Ca^{2+}$ allows actin–myosin crossbridges to dissociate and the sarcomeres to lengthen, so that the ventricle can dilate. Decreased $Ca^{2+}$ removal because of abnormalities in major contractile proteins or transport processes decreases the rate and extent of relaxation. Ischemia is one major factor that impairs $Ca^{2+}$ metabolism and diastolic ventricular function, but many other forms of heart disease have similar effects. Clinically, the passive component of diastolic function is assessed by relating end-diastolic pressure and volume. The active component is assessed by observing the rate of ventricular filling by angiography or by Doppler studies of the mitral valve inflow, by measuring the peak rate of fall of ventricular pressure (negative $dP/dt_{max}$), or by calculating the time constant of the fall in ventricular pressure.

## Role of the pericardium

The parietal pericardium is a stiff membrane that surrounds the heart, separated from it only by a small amount of pericardial fluid. Normally, the pressure in the pericardial cavity is negative, due to the negative intrapleural pressure. Therefore, normally, transmural diastolic pressure across the wall of the left ventricle is slightly greater than diastolic ventricular pressure. Pericardial pressure can become positive and may restrict dilatation of the left ventricle if there is a tense *pericardial effusion (tamponade)* or if the ventricles dilate acutely because of a sudden volume load or sudden myocardial depression. In some patients with *acute myocardial ischemia*, left ventricular diastolic pressure can be greatly increased without much change in ventricular volume because of tension in the pericardium. This mechanism makes it difficult to interpret changes in diastolic pressure–volume relations only in terms of myocardial stiffness.

It is important to realize that the pericardium can restrict ventricular dilatation even when pericardial cavity pressure is not positive. Imagine replacing the pericardium with a loose mesh of fibers resembling a tennis net. These fibers can press against the surface of the heart and exert a surface force that restrains the heart, but there can be no positive liquid pressure in the cavity because it is very leaky. The difference between surface and liquid pressures explains some of the discrepancies previously reported in the literature. Some investigators believe that the right atrial pressure is the closest approximation to pericardial surface pressure, so that it could be used when calculating transmural ventricular pressure, but caution is advised when doing this because there is not yet clear evidence that the surface pressures are identical at every part of the external cardiac surface.

## Pericardial tamponade

The positive pericardial pressure of pericardial tamponade is the major cause of pulsus paradoxus (a fall in systemic arterial blood pressure of more than 6–8 mmHg [0.8–1.06 kPa] with inspiration). It acts via two main mechanisms. One of them is that with inspiration the intrathoracic pressure decreases, and so do pressures in the pulmonary veins. Normally, left atrial pressure decreases to a similar extent with inspiration, and left atrial filling is changed little by inspiration. However, when pericardial pressure is positive, left atrial pressure remains high during inspiration and there may even be a pressure gradient from left atrium to pulmonary veins that produces retrograde flow. Consequently, left ventricular filling is impaired and arterial blood pressure decreases. The second major mechanism is discussed below.

# Ventricular interaction

Because the left and right ventricles share the ventricular septum, distension of the right ventricle, e.g. in acute pulmonary embolism, pushes the septum to the left, thereby decreasing left ventricular volume and preload. The resulting decrease in cardiac output should not be taken to indicate left ventricular dysfunction. In fact, a lesser degree of this shift occurs with each inspiration, and is one of the mechanisms responsible for the slight fall of systemic arterial pressure that takes place with each inspiration. This mechanism is accentuated when there is pericardial tamponade, because the stiff pericardium does not allow the total intrapericardial volume to increase. Therefore, when the right ventricle dilates during the inspiratory increase in venous return, the left ventricular volume is much reduced and arterial pressure falls significantly. This is one of the major mechanisms responsible for the pulsus paradoxus that is the primary method of diagnosing pericardial tamponade.

## SELECTED READING

Friedman WF. The intrinsic physiologic properties of the developing heart. In: Friedman WF, Lesch M, Sonnenblick EH, eds. *Neonatal heart disease*. New York: Grune & Stratton, 1973: 21.

Hori M, Suga H, Baan J, Yellin EL, eds. *Cardiac mechanics and function in the normal and diseased heart*. Tokyo: Springer-Verlag, 1989.

Kass D, Maughan WL. From "$E_{max}$" to pressure–volume relations: a broader perspective. *Circulation* 1988; 77: 1203.

Mahony L. Development of myocardial structure and function. In: Emmanouilides GC, Allen HD, Riemenschneider TA, Gutgesell HP, eds. *Moss and Adams heart disease in infants, children and adolescents: Including the fetus and young adult*, 5th edn. Baltimore: Williams & Wilkins, 1995: 17.

Ross J Jr. Mechanisms of cardiac contraction. What roles for preload, afterload and inotropic state in heart failure? *Eur Heart J* 1983; 4 (Suppl A): 19.

Smith V-E, Zile MR. Relaxation and diastolic properties of the heart. In: Fozzard HA, Haber E, Jennings RB, Katz AM, Morgan HE, eds. *The heart and cardiovascular system. Scientific foundations*. New York: Raven Press, 1991: 1353.

Teitel DF, Sidi D, Chin T *et al*. Developmental changes in myocardial contractile reserve in the lamb. *Pediatr Res* 1985; 19: 948.

# 73

# Specific Circulations

## PULMONARY CIRCULATION

### MORPHOLOGICAL DEVELOPMENT

The morphological development of the pulmonary circulation affects the physiological changes that occur in the perinatal period. In the fetus and newborn, pulmonary arteries (regardless of their size) have a thicker medial smooth muscle coat relative to the external diameter of the artery than do similar size (external diameter) pulmonary arteries in the adult. This greater muscularity accounts, in part, for the higher pulmonary vascular resistance (PVR) and greater pulmonary vascular reactivity in the near-term fetus than in the adult. In the fetus, pulmonary arteries 20–50 μm in external diameter have the thickest medial smooth muscle coat. These are the resistance vessels. After birth and for the first few months, the medial smooth muscle coat of the arteries thins. These morphological changes account, in part, for the gradual decrease in PVR and pulmonary vascular reactivity over the first few months of life.

Small pulmonary arteries (20–50 μm in external diameter) can be identified by their relationship to airways (Fig. 73.1). Preacinar pulmonary arteries are proximal to, or course with, the terminal bronchioli, while intraacinar pulmonary arteries course with the respiratory bronchioli and alveolar ducts, or are within the alveolar walls. In the late-gestation fetus, only about 50 per cent of the pulmonary arteries associated with respiratory bronchioli are muscularized (either partially or completely). The pulmonary arteries within the alveolar wall are non-muscularized. The partially muscularized and non-muscularized pulmonary

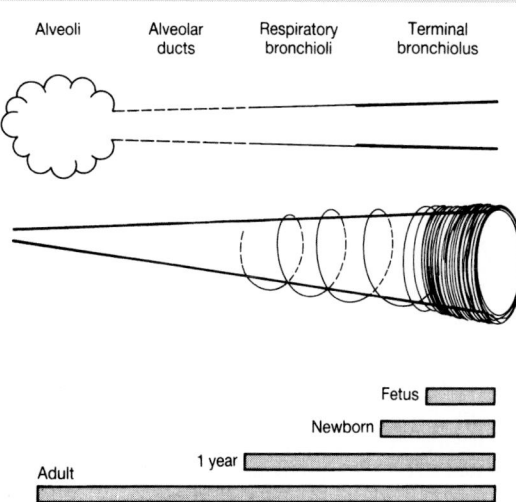

FIGURE 73.1 Diagrammatic representation of smooth muscle distribution in normal human pulmonary vessels. (Adapted from Reid LM, *Chest* 1986; **89**: 279, with permission.)

arteries contain pericytes and intermediate cells (intermediate in position and structure between pericytes and smooth muscle cells), which are the precursors of smooth muscle cells. With advancing age after birth, these cells differentiate into smooth muscle cells, completely muscularizing the majority of the small pulmonary arteries within alveolar walls in the adult.

### PHYSIOLOGY

#### Fetal pulmonary circulation

In the fetus, because gas exchange occurs in the placenta, pulmonary blood flow is low, supplying only nutritional requirements for lung growth and performing some metabolic functions. In the mid-gestation fetal lamb (term is approximately 142–145 days), pulmonary blood flow is approximately 3–4 per cent of the total combined left and right ventricular outputs of the heart (fetal cardiac output), while in the near-term fetal lamb pulmonary blood flow is approximately 100 mL/100 g of lung weight per minute), or 8–10 per cent of the fetal cardiac output [400–450 mL/(kg · min)]. Fetal pulmonary arterial pressure increases with advancing gestation. At term, mean pulmonary arterial pressure is about 50 mmHg (6.6 kPa), generally exceeding mean descending aortic pressure by 1–2 mmHg.

## Determinants of pulmonary vascular resistance

PVR changes throughout gestation and after birth. PVR is related to several factors and can be estimated by applying the resistance equation and the Poiseuille–Hagen relationship. The resistance equation (the hydraulic equivalent of the Ohm law) states that the resistance to flow between two points along a tube equals the decrease in pressure between the two points divided by the flow. For the pulmonary vascular bed, where $R_p$ is the pulmonary vascular resistance and $\dot{Q}_p$ the pulmonary blood flow per minute, the decrease in mean pressure is from the pulmonary artery ($P_{pa}$) to the pulmonary vein ($P_{pv}$):

$$R_p = \frac{(P_{pa} - P_{pv})}{\dot{Q}_p}$$

PVR increases when pulmonary arterial or pulmonary venous pressure increase. The latter also causes an increase in pulmonary arterial pressure to maintain the driving pressure across the lungs. Similarly, PVR also increases when pulmonary blood flow decreases.

Other factors that affect PVR can be defined by applying a modification of the Poiseuille–Hagen relationship, which describes the resistance ($R$) to flow of a Newtonian fluid through a system of round, straight glass tubes of constant cross-sectional area:

$$R_p = \frac{8l\eta}{\pi r^4}$$

where $l$ is length of the system of vessels, $r$ is the internal radius of the system of vessels, and $\eta$ is the viscosity of the fluid. The assumption is that each pulmonary artery is a round, straight glass tube, and that the pulmonary circulation consists of many of these tubes. Changes in viscosity or radius affect PVR; increasing the viscosity of blood perfusing the lungs or decreasing the radius or cross-sectional area ($\pi r^4$) of the pulmonary vascular bed increases PVR. Early in gestation, PVR is much higher than in the newborn or the adult because there are fewer pulmonary arteries in the fetal lung, and therefore a decreased cross-sectional area. Secondary to the growth of new pulmonary

arteries and the increase in cross-sectional area of the pulmonary vascular bed, PVR decreases during fetal life. However, near term, PVR is still much higher than after birth.

Differences between physical and biological systems may make these relationships inaccurate. First, blood is not a Newtonian fluid. The viscosity of blood is related to red cell number, fibrinogen concentration, and red cell deformability. An increased hematocrit (secondary to fetal hypoxemia, twin-to-twin blood transfusion or maternal-to-fetal blood transfusion, or delayed clamping of the umbilical cord) will increase viscosity. PVR increases logarithmically (not linearly) when the hematocrit increases (Fig. 73.2). Second, blood flow through the pulmonary circulation is pulsatile, not laminar, and the small pulmonary arteries are branched, curved, and tapered, not smooth. In addition, the small pulmonary arteries are in parallel, and the radii of these arteries may differ in different lung zones. Although these factors tend to increase PVR, their actual effects on fetal PVR are minimal.

## Regulation of fetal pulmonary vascular resistance

Many factors, including mechanical effects, state of oxygenation, and the production of vasoactive substances, regulate the tone of the fetal pulmonary circulation (Fig. 73.3). In unventilated fetal lungs, fluid filling the alveolar space compresses the small pulmonary arteries, increasing the PVR. In addition, the high PVR is associated with the normally low $O_2$ tension in pulmonary and systemic arterial blood. In fetal lambs, the pulmonary arterial blood $P_{O_2}$ is 17–20 mmHg (2.6 kPa) and the femoral arterial $P_{O_2}$ is 20–24 mmHg (3.2 kPa). Reducing $P_{O_2}$ to similar values in newborn lambs after birth increases PVR. The mechanism of this hypoxia-induced pulmonary vasoconstriction is unknown. Similarly, fetal PVR is increased by decreasing fetal $P_{O_2}$ either by maternal hypoxia or by compression of the umbilical cord,

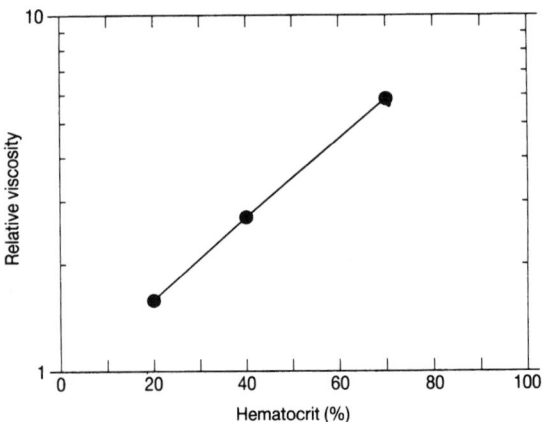

FIGURE 73.2 Relationship of relative viscosity (blood viscosity relative to plasma viscosity) and hematocrit at a shear rate likely to be found in the pulmonary circulation

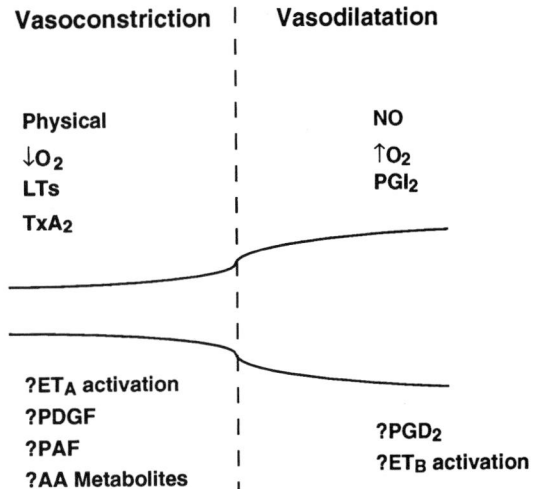

FIGURE 73.3 Factors considered to be involved in the control of pulmonary vascular resistance and pulmonary blood flow during fetal life. AA, arachidonic acid; ET, endothelin; LTs, leukotrienes; NO, nitric oxide; PAF, platelet activating factor; PDGF, platelet-derived growth factor; $TXA_2$, thromboxane $A_2$; $ET_A$, ET A receptor; $ET_B$, ET B receptor.

and is decreased by increasing $Po_2$ by maternal hyperoxia. Whether the low fetal $Po_2$ acts directly to constrict pulmonary vascular smooth muscle and increase PVR or indirectly through the release of vasoactive substances is not known. $O_2$-related changes in PVR are affected by pH: acidemia increases PVR and also accentuates hypoxic vasoconstrictor responses.

Metabolites of arachidonic acid may be actively involved in the control of fetal PVR either directly or as mediators of "hypoxia-induced" pulmonary vasoconstriction. Leukotrienes (LTs) are synthesized from arachidonic acid by a 5'-lipoxygenase enzyme in pulmonary arterial tissue. $LTC_4$ and $LTD_4$ produce pulmonary vasoconstriction in newborn and adult animals. Inhibition of LT synthesis or action prevents hypoxia-induced pulmonary hypertension in older animals, and markedly decreases fetal PVR and increases fetal pulmonary blood flow similarly to ventilation at birth (see below). LTs have been isolated from tracheal fluid of near-term fetal lambs and from lung lavage fluid of newborns with the syndrome of persistent pulmonary hypertension. This suggests that LTs may contribute to maintaining the high PVR in the fetus. The pulmonary vasoconstriction produced by LTs is not mediated through secondary production of constrictor prostaglandins.

Other vasoactive substances may also play a role in maintaining the high PVR in the fetus. Thromboxane $A_2$, synthesized from arachidonic acid by the cyclooxygenase enzymes, is a vasoconstrictor, as is platelet activating factor. Both produce potent pulmonary vasoconstriction in newborn and adult animals. Several growth factors, particularly platelet-derived growth factor (PDGF), which are involved in vascular smooth muscle growth and proliferation (see page

688), also have vasoconstrictor effects. Whether any of these, or other compounds yet to be defined, contribute to maintaining the high PVR in the fetus is unknown.

In addition to the production of vasoconstrictors, the fetal pulmonary circulation actively and continuously produces vasodilating substances that modulate the degree of vasoconstriction under normal conditions and may play a more active role during periods of fetal stress. These substances are mainly endothelial-derived and include prostacyclin ($PGI_2$) and nitric oxide (NO; formerly called endothelial-derived relaxing factor (EDRF) or endothelial-derived nitric oxide (EDNO)) (see below and also page 697).

$PGI_2$ is synthesized from arachidonic acid (by cyclooxygenase enzymes) primarily in vascular endothelial cells, and produces vasodilatation by activating adenylyl cyclase via receptor–G protein coupled mechanisms. Activation of adenylyl cyclase results in increased cyclic adenosine monophosphate (cAMP) concentrations, thus initiating a cascade that results in smooth muscle relaxation. There is a maturational increase in $PGI_2$ production throughout gestation that parallels the decrease in PVR in the fetal third trimester. However, in vivo, prostaglandin inhibition does not significantly change resting PVR, questioning the importance of basal $PGI_2$ activity in mediating resting fetal pulmonary vascular tone.

NO is synthesized by the oxidation of the quanidino nitrogen moiety of L-arginine (see page 698). Once synthesized in the endothelial cell, NO diffuses into vascular smooth muscle cells, stimulates guanylyl cyclase, and increases the concentration of cyclic guanosine monophosphate (cGMP), which initiates a cascade that results in smooth muscle relaxation and vasodilatation (Fig. 73.4). In fetal lambs, inhibition of NO synthesis by $N^{\omega}$-nitro-L-arginine, a competitive inhibitor of L-arginine, increases PVR which suggests that basal NO production, in part, mediates pulmonary vascular tone. In the fetus, NO is synthesized and released by activation of nitric oxide synthase both by receptor-mediated mechanisms (via endothelium-dependent vasodilators) and by stretch or increased shear forces acting on the pulmonary vascular endothelium (via activation of ATP-dependent $K^+$ channels). $PGI_2$ production by endothelial cells can also be stimulated by increasing shear forces.

Endothelin-1 (ET-1) is a 21-amino-acid polypeptide also produced by vascular endothelial cells that has potent vasoactive properties (see also page 700). The hemodynamic effects of ET-1 are mediated by at least two distinctive receptor populations, $ET_A$ and $ET_B$. $ET_A$ receptors are located on vascular smooth muscle cells, and are likely responsible for the vasoconstricting effects of ET-1, whereas the $ET_B$ receptors may be located on endothelial cells, and are likely responsible for the vasodilating effects of ET-1 via NO production (Fig. 73.4). In the pulmonary circulation, exogenous ET-1 produces vasoconstriction in adult animals, but produces pulmonary vasodilatation in both fetal and

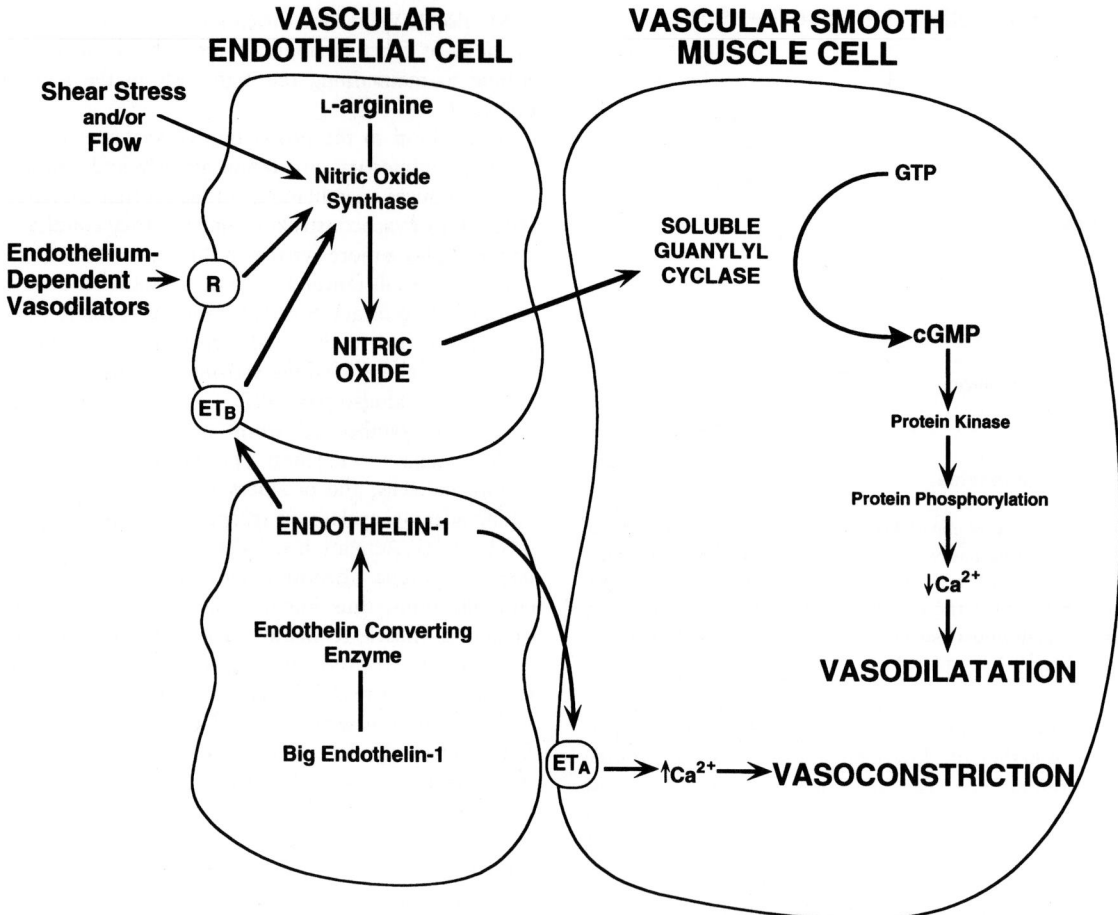

FIGURE 73.4 Schematic representation of the interactions, in vascular endothelial and smooth muscle cells, between the NO–cGMP cascade and ET-1 and its receptors in modulating pulmonary vascular tone

neonatal lambs. In fetal lambs, selective $ET_A$ receptor blockade slightly decreases resting fetal PVR, as does selective $ET_B$ stimulation. This suggests a potential role for $ET_A$ stimulation in maintaining the high fetal PVR and $ET_B$ stimulation in producing pulmonary vasodilatation after birth (see below).

## Changes in the pulmonary circulation at birth

After birth, with initiation of ventilation by the lungs, and the subsequent increase in pulmonary and systemic arterial blood $O_2$ tensions, PVR decreases and pulmonary blood flow increases by eight- to ten-fold to match systemic blood flow (300–400 mL/(kg·min)). This large increase in pulmonary blood flow increases pulmonary venous return to the left atrium, increasing left atrial pressure. Then the valve of the foramen ovale closes, preventing any significant atrial right-to-left shunting of blood. In addition, the ductus arteriosus constricts and closes functionally within several hours after birth (see page 755) effectively separating the pulmonary and systemic circulations. Mean pulmonary arterial pressure decreases, and by 24 hours of age is

approximately 50 per cent of mean systemic arterial pressure. Adult values are reached 2–6 weeks after birth.

## Regulation of postnatal pulmonary vascular resistance

Many factors cause the decrease in PVR with ventilation and oxygenation at birth (Fig. 73.5). Physical expansion or ventilation of the fetal lung without increasing $O_2$ tension increases fetal pulmonary blood flow and decreases PVR, but not to newborn values. A very small proportion of this decrease relates to replacement of fluid in the alveoli with gas, which allows unkinking of the small pulmonary arteries, and to the changes in alveolar surface tension, which exert a negative dilating pressure on the small pulmonary arteries, maintaining their patency. Physical expansion of the lungs also releases vasoactive substances such as $PGI_2$, which increases pulmonary blood flow and decreases PVR in the fetal goat and lamb. There is a net production of $PGI_2$ by the lung with the initiation of ventilation at birth. In addition, inhibitors of prostaglandin synthesis (such as indomethacin) not only

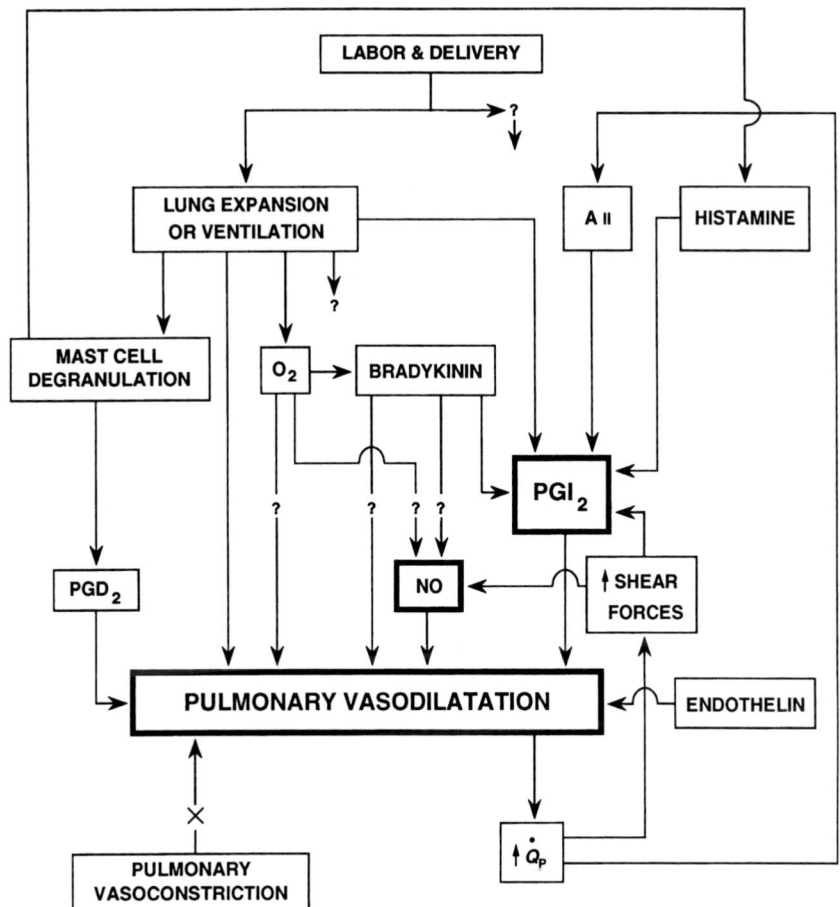

FIGURE 73.5 Factors likely to be responsible for the changes of pulmonary vascular resistance and pulmonary blood flow with ventilation and oxygenation at birth.

block $PGI_2$ production, but also attenuate the increase in pulmonary blood flow and decrease in PVR that occur with physical expansion of the fetal lung, although not the changes that occur with oxygenation. Therefore, $PGI_2$, or perhaps, but less likely, another metabolite of arachidonic acid, plays an important role in the increase in pulmonary blood flow and decrease in PVR that occur in association with the mechanical component (stretch) of ventilation at birth.

Other prostaglandins may also play a role in these circulatory changes. $PGE_2$, produced in the fetal vasculature and the placenta, not only maintains patency of the ductus arteriosus, but also decreases PVR in fetal lambs and goats. The effects are non-specific. $PGD_2$, produced and released by lung mast cells that are located near the small pulmonary arteries, is a selective pulmonary vasodilator in fetal and newborn goats and lambs, and a pulmonary vasoconstrictor in older animals. Because there is mast cell degranulation at birth, $PGD_2$ may play a role in the postnatal pulmonary circulatory changes.

Ventilation of fetal lungs with air or $O_2$ to increase $O_2$ tension increases pulmonary blood flow and decreases PVR to newborn levels. As described

above, ventilation of the fetus without oxygenation produces partial pulmonary vasodilatation, while ventilation with oxygenation produces complete pulmonary vasodilatation. The increase in alveolar or arterial $O_2$ tension may decrease PVR either directly by dilating the small pulmonary arteries, or indirectly by stimulating the production of vasodilator substances. Bradykinin, a potent pulmonary vasodilator, is produced by the fetal lung during $O_2$ ventilation and during exposure of pregnant ewes to hyperbaric oxygenation. Bradykinin stimulates $PGI_2$ production, which would enhance vasodilatation. Increased oxygenation is also a direct stimulus for $PGI_2$ production, as is angiotensin II (AII), which increases markedly in concentration at birth, indicating a complex interaction between various vasodilating stimuli. In addition, bradykinin stimulates ($B_1$-receptor-mediated) the production of NO by endothelial cells. However, selective bradykinin receptor blockade does not prevent the increase in pulmonary blood flow and decrease in PVR that occur during $O_2$ ventilation. NO has been implicated as an important mediator of the decrease in PVR at birth. In fetal lambs, inhibition of NO synthesis attenuates the increase in pulmonary blood flow and decrease in PVR produced during $O_2$ ventilation and during exposure of pregnant ewes to hyperbaric oxygenation. Therefore, there are at least two components to the decrease in PVR with the initiation of ventilation and oxygenation. First, there is partial pulmonary vasodilatation caused by physical expansion of the lung and the production of prostaglandins ($PGI_2$ and $PGD_2$). This is probably independent of fetal oxygenation, and results in a modest increase in pulmonary blood flow and decrease in PVR. Next, there is a further maximal pulmonary vasodilatation associated with fetal oxygenation, which is not necessarily dependent on prostaglandin production. This results in an increase in pulmonary blood flow and decrease in PVR to newborn values. This latter pulmonary vasodilatation is likely caused by the synthesis of NO, although the exact stimulus or stimuli for NO production are not yet defined. Both components are necessary for the successful transition to extrauterine life. Pulmonary vasodilatation may also occur when the initial increase in pulmonary blood flow increases shear forces on endothelial cells increasing the production of both NO and $PGI_2$. It is possible that after the initial fall in PVR, due to another mechanism, this particular mechanism acts to maintain pulmonary vasodilatation.

Control of the perinatal pulmonary circulation, therefore, probably reflects a balance between factors producing pulmonary vasoconstriction (low $O_2$, LTs, and other vasoconstricting substances and those producing pulmonary vasodilatation (high $O_2$, $PGI_2$, NO, and other vasodilating substances such as perhaps calcitonin gene-related peptide [CGRP] or the related peptide, adrenomedullin). The dramatic increase in pulmonary blood flow with the initiation of ventilation and oxygenation at birth reflects a shift from active pulmonary vasoconstriction in the fetus to active pulmonary vasodilatation in the newborn.

## Metabolic function

Pulmonary vascular endothelium is capable of producing (e.g. $PGI_2$, NO, bradykinin, AII) and removing from the circulation (e.g. catecholamines, bradykinin, $PGE_2$) many different substances. This activity is present in the fetus and changes at the time of transition to air breathing.

Concomitant with the increasing metabolic activity of the fetal lung (particularly increasing antioxidant enzyme and surfactant phospholipid synthesis) in the latter weeks of gestation, resting pulmonary blood flow increases (from about 4 per cent of combined ventricular output to about 8 per cent). After birth, and associated with the dramatic increase in pulmonary blood flow, pulmonary vascular metabolic capacity also increases markedly, to a large extent due to a significant increase in pulmonary vascular endothelial functional surface area. AI conversion to AII, by the endothelial enzyme, angiotensin converting enzyme (ACE), increases, and the same enzyme is responsible

for the metabolic breakdown of the vasoactive peptide bradykinin. Metabolic removal of $PGE_2$ also increases, and this is an important component of the transition as $PGE_2$ is responsible for ductus arteriosus patency (*see* page 755).

## FAILURE OF PULMONARY VASCULAR RESISTANCE TO DECREASE AT BIRTH

In a number of clinical conditions (e.g. *respiratory distress syndrome, meconium aspiration*, or *sepsis*), PVR does not decrease normally at birth, which may result in *persistent pulmonary hypertension*, right-to-left shunting of blood through the foramen ovale, and/or patent ductus arteriosus and hypoxemia. The syndrome of persistent pulmonary hypertension of the newborn accounts for approximately 1 per cent of all admissions to newborn intensive care units. Treatment is supportive, consisting of administration of supplemental $O_2$, mechanical hyperventilation, correction of metabolic abnormalities, infusion of non-specific vasodilators to lower pulmonary arterial pressure, and infusion of cardiotonic drugs to improve cardiac function. Extracorporeal membrane oxygenation (ECMO) has been used. More recently, inhaled NO has improved oxygenation in some but not all newborns with persistent pulmonary hypertension. The clinical course is variable, though the mortality rate is decreasing.

The pathophysiological mechanisms preventing the normal pulmonary vasodilatation and fall in PVR with ventilation and oxygenation at birth are not fully known. Morphological abnormalities are present: extracellular matrix protein changes are found (*see* pages 685, 691), the thickness of the medial smooth muscle coat of the small pulmonary arteries is increased, and this muscle extends to normally nonmuscularized arteries in infants who die with persistent pulmonary hypertension syndrome. The underlying mechanisms (such as alterations in smooth muscle growth-stimulating or growth-inhibiting factors) producing these changes are unknown. These structural changes take time to develop, indicating that, in some instances, prolonged *in utero* events may have altered the pulmonary circulation. One such phenomenon that is considered a possible mechanism is chronic partial constriction of the ductus arteriosus *in utero*. In addition to structural changes there may be functional alterations as well. There may be increased concentrations of, or responsiveness to, vasoconstricting substances (e.g. $LTC_4$, $LTD_4$, thromboxane $A_2$ and $ET_A$ receptor activation) or decreased concentrations of, or responsiveness to, vasodilating substances ($PGI_2$, $PGD_2$, NO, $ET_B$ receptor activation, and increased $O_2$ tension). A better understanding of the mechanisms that control PVR in the perinatal period will lead to improved treatment of these infants.

## SELECTED READING

Abman SH, Chatfield BA, Hall SL, McMurtry IF. Role of endothelium-derived relaxing factor during transition of pulmonary circulation at birth. *Am J Physiol* 1990; **259**: H1921.

Fineman JR, Wong J, Morin FC *et al.* Chronic nitric oxide inhibition *in utero* produces persistent pulmonary hypertension in newborn lambs. *J Clin Invest* 1994; **93**: 2675.

Fineman JR, Soifer SJ, Heymann MA. Regulation of pulmonary vascular tone in the perinatal period. *Annu Rev Physiol* 1995; **57**: 115.

Iwamoto HS, Teitel D, Rudolph AM. Effects of birth related events on blood flow distribution. *Pediatr Res* 1987; **22**: 634.

Kinsella JP, Neish SR, Shaffer E, Abman SH. Low-dose inhalational nitric oxide in persistent pulmonary hypertension of the newborn. *Lancet* 1992; **340**: 819.

Leffler CW, Hessler JR, Green RS. The onset of breathing at birth stimulates pulmonary vascular prostacyclin synthesis. *Pediatr Res* 1984; **18**: 938.

Moore P, Velvis H, Fineman JR *et al.* EDRF inhibition attenuates the increase in pulmonary blood flow due to oxygen ventilation in fetal lambs. *J Appl Physiol* 1992; **73**: 2151.

Roberts JD Jr, Polaner DM, Lang P *et al.* Inhaled nitric oxide in persistent pulmonary hypertension of the newborn. *Lancet* 1992; **340**: 818.

Roberts JD, Schaul PW. Advances in the treatment of persistent pulmonary hypertension of the newborn. *Pediatr Clin North Am* 1993; **40**: 983.

Shaul PW, Farrar MA, Zellers TM. Oxygen modulates endothelium-derived relaxing factor production in fetal pulmonary arteries. *Am J Physiol* 1992; **262**: H355.

Velvis H, Moore P, Heymann MA. Prostaglandin inhibition prevents the fall in pulmonary vascular resistance due to rhythmic distension of the lungs in fetal lambs. *Pediatr Res* 1991; **30**: 62.

Wong J, Fineman JR, Heymann MA. The role of endothelin and endothelin receptor subtypes in regulation of fetal pulmonary vascular tone. *Pediatr Res* 1994; **35**: 664.

Wong J, Vanderford PA, Fineman JR *et al.* Endothelin-1 produces pulmonary vasodilation in the intact newborn lamb. *Am J Physiol* 1992; **265**: H1318.

# DUCTUS ARTERIOSUS

## REGULATION OF DUCTUS ARTERIOSUS PATENCY

The ductus arteriosus represents a persistence of the terminal portion of the left pulmonary or sixth branchial arch. More muscular than the elastic pulmonary artery and aorta at either end, the ductus arteriosus also has a looser structure with increased amounts of hyaluronic acid in the muscle media. During fetal life, it serves to divert blood away from the fluid-filled, non-ventilating lungs towards the descending aorta and placenta.

## Fetal regulation

Although it was commonly believed that the ductus arteriosus was a relatively passive structure in the fetus, it is now obvious that the relative patency of the ductus arteriosus, even during fetal life, is regulated by both dilating and contracting factors (Fig. 73.6). Vasodilator *prostaglandins*, especially PGE$_2$, play a significant role in maintaining ductus patency during fetal life. Inhibitors of prostaglandin synthesis (e.g. indomethacin) constrict the fetal ductus arteriosus both *in vitro* and *in vivo*. Conversely, PGE$_2$ will dilate the constricted fetal ductus both *in vitro* and *in vivo*. The response of the ductus to PGE$_2$ is unique among blood vessels in that it is extraordinarily sensitive to this vasodilating substance.

The factors that oppose prostaglandin dilatation and constrict the vessel *in utero* have not been fully evaluated. In contrast with other vessels, the ductus appears to be unresponsive to the vasoconstrictor thromboxane A$_2$. *Endothelin-1 (ET-1)* appears to be a prime candidate for maintaining fetal vessel tone as it is the most potent vasoconstrictor of the ductus that is currently known. At fetal O$_2$ tension (P$_{O2}$) levels, ET-1 is made by both ductus arteriosus luminal endothelial cells and the muscle media. When tested at these O$_2$ tensions, phosphoramidon, an inhibitor of ET-1 synthesis, relaxes basal tone in both intact and endothelium-denuded strips of ductus arteriosus. Other factors that play a role in fetal ductus arteriosus patency and constriction have yet to be discovered.

## Neonatal regulation

Since the initial studies of Kennedy and Clark in 1942, many investigators have demonstrated that O$_2$ is responsible for constricting the ductus arteriosus after birth. However, the biochemical basis for the O$_2$ response has never been fully explained. Associated with a rise in intracellular Ca$^{2+}$, O$_2$ causes membrane depolarization in smooth muscle cells of the ductus arteriosus. This increase in intracellular Ca$^{2+}$ stems from voltage-dependent Ca$^{2+}$ channels in the sarcolemma of the smooth muscle cells and inhibitors of these channels block the O$_2$-induced contraction of the ductus arteriosus. The sarcoplasmic reticulum does not appear to be a major source of the O$_2$-induced rise in cytosolic Ca$^{2+}$. The cause of this O$_2$-induced membrane depolarization is currently unknown.

During the last decade, members of the *cytochrome P$_{450}$ family* have been examined as potential receptors for the O$_2$-induced events in the ductus arteriosus. Carbon monoxide (CO), an inhibitor of cytochrome P$_{450}$, inhibits the O$_2$-induced constriction; this CO

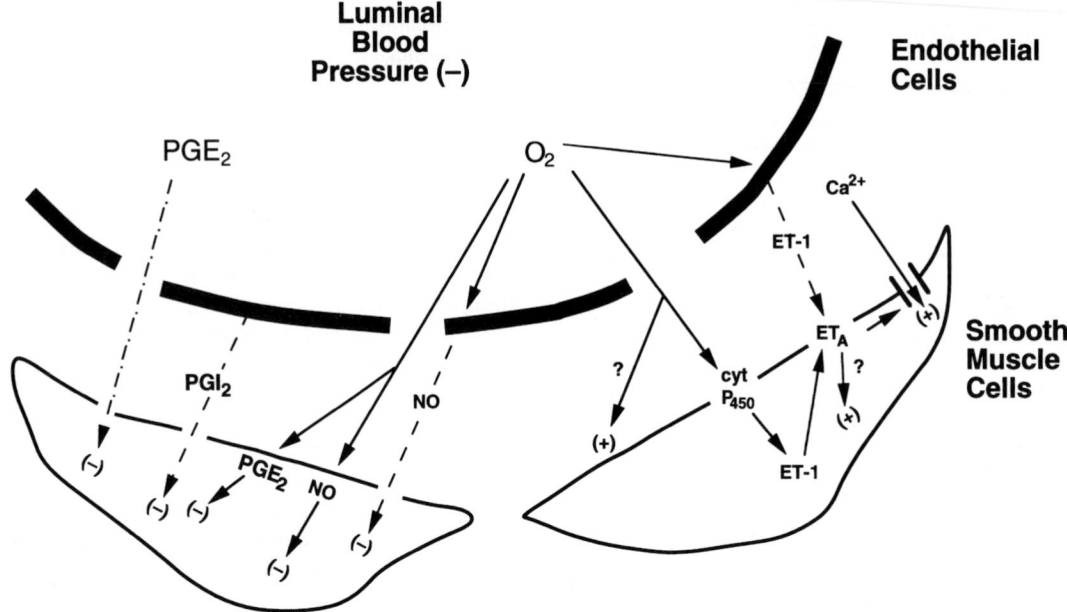

FIGURE 73.6 Mediators of ductus arteriosus contraction and relaxation. cyt $P_{450}$, cytochrome $P_{450}$; ET-1, endothelin 1; $ET_A$, endothelin A receptor; NO, nitric oxide; $O_2$, oxygen; $PGE_2$, prostaglandin $E_2$; $PGI_2$, prostacyclin; (+), constricts; (−), dilates

relaxation can be reversed by light with a wavelength of 450 nm. Both $O_2$ and CO require an intact sarcolemma to exert their effects, and immunostaining of cultured smooth muscle cells from the ductus arteriosus demonstrates the presence of a glucocorticoid-inducible cytochrome $P_{450}$ in the sarcolemma of these cells. However, no cytochrome $P_{450}$-monooxygenase activity has been found in the fetal or neonatal ductus arteriosus, and none of the known monooxygenase metabolites have been shown to constrict the ductus arteriosus. Future studies will determine whether this cytochrome $P_{450}$ transducer works through a yet to be defined monooxygenase reaction or through some other conformational change not associated with catalytic activity.

ET-1 appears to be a downstream mediator of the $O_2$/cytochrome $P_{450}$ interaction. ET-1 is formed in both ductus arteriosus endothelial and muscle cells and is the most potent vasoconstrictor of the vessel. ET-1 synthesis by the ductus arteriosus increases with increasing $O_2$ tensions. CO, which inhibits cytochrome $P_{450}$, inhibits ET-1 release from both the endothelium and muscle media. Blockade of ET-1 synthesis with phosphoramidon or blockade of $ET_A$-receptor activation with BQ123 inhibits the contraction of the ductus to $O_2$; however, ET-1 can still contract the ductus arteriosus even when the ability of $O_2$ to do so is inhibited by CO. Thus there appear to be two successive events in the process of ductus arteriosus closure: initial interaction of $O_2$ with a cytochrome $P_{450}$ hemoprotein that is located in the plasma membrane of muscle cells, and the subsequent formation of a constrictor ET-1.

Following delivery, the ductus arteriosus produces several vasodilator substances that inhibit the ability of $O_2$ to constrict the ductus arteriosus. The postnatal increase in $Po_2$ stimulates the release of $PGE_2$ from cells in the muscle media and adventitia of the ductus arteriosus, and this rise in $Po_2$ does not alter the extreme sensitivity of the ductus to $PGE_2$.

In addition to prostaglandins, an increase in $Po_2$ stimulates the release of a *nitric oxide (NO)*-like vasodilator from isolated muscle strips of ductus arteriosus. There are both endothelial and non-endothelial sources of NO in the ductus arteriosus. The endothelial-derived NO can be stimulated by agents like bradykinin and the $Ca^{2+}$ ionophore A23187, whereas the non-endothelial-derived NO is not stimulated by these agents. Similar to the heightened sensitivity to $PGE_2$, the ductus arteriosus is more sensitive than adjacent vessels, like the aorta, to the vasodilating effects of NO. Exogenous NO donors (such as sodium nitroprusside) dilate the ductus arteriosus at both fetal and neonatal $Po_2$ levels. In contrast, inhibitors of NO synthesis (e.g. $N^\omega$-nitro-L-arginine methyl ester, L-NAME) constrict the ductus arteriosus when it is incubated at neonatal $O_2$ tensions, but not at fetal $O_2$ tensions. As a result, NO appears to be released in significant amounts only when the environmental $Po_2$ rises into the neonatal range; basal NO release appears to be negligible at fetal $Po_2$ levels. This is consistent with studies performed *in vivo* in fetal lambs that found no spontaneous generation of NO within the fetal ductus arteriosus.

Therefore, closure of the ductus arteriosus at birth occurs through a process that alters the balance between dilating and contracting factors. The postnatal increase in $Po_2$ increases the local formation of the constrictor ET-1. This overwhelms the vasodilating effects of $PGE_2$ and NO, and leads to ductus arteriosus closure. This process can be modulated by other events. The vascular pressure within the ductus arteriosus lumen opposes the rate of ductus constriction. In the fetus, pulmonary vascular resistance is high and intravascular pressure at the pulmonary end of the ductus is 2–3 mmHg greater than at the aortic end. With the onset of air breathing, pulmonary vascular resistance and pressure drop precipitously. This produces a drop in the mean intravascular pressure opposing ductus arteriosus constriction, thereby facilitating closure. Conversely, the persistently elevated pulmonary vascular pressures that occur in *pulmonary hypertension syndromes of the newborn* inhibit ductus closure and are associated with an increased incidence of *persistent patency of the ductus arteriosus (PDA)*.

The relative importance of the two vasodilators, PGE$_2$ and NO, can also change after birth. In the case of incomplete closure of the ductus arteriosus lumen, one can envision an increased role for NO in maintaining patency. The flow of oxygenated arterial blood through the narrowed ductus lumen, in association with increased shear stress, may stimulate increased NO and prostaglandin synthesis. Mechanical injury to the vessel wall, resulting from transient ductus closure, also may stimulate the inducible NO system through the release of cytokines within the vessel wall. These mechanisms may play a role in persistent PDA after birth.

## PERSISTENT PATENCY OF THE DUCTUS ARTERIOSUS IN PRETERM INFANTS

O$_2$ has been shown to have a greater constrictor effect on the ductus arteriosus from near-term compared with immature fetuses. The increased effectiveness of O$_2$ late in gestation, compared with 0.7 gestation (70 per cent of full term), is *not* due to increased muscle development in the vessel wall. Rather, the increased contractile response of the mature ductus arteriosus to O$_2$ is due to a developmental alteration in the sensitivity of the vessel to locally produced vasodilators. Isolated ductus arteriosus, from preterm animals, are much more sensitive to the dilating action of PGE$_2$ and NO than those from animals near term. The ductus arteriosus from animals younger than 0.7 gestation have decreased muscle development and decreased contractile capacity in addition to being much more sensitive to the vasodilators PGE$_2$ and NO. These factors probably account for the higher incidence of persistent PDA in preterm infants. Inhibitors of prostaglandin production like indomethacin, ibuprofen, and mefenamic acid have proved to be effective agents in promoting ductus arteriosus closure. It follows that drugs interfering with NO synthesis or function also could become a useful adjunct, especially in situations where indomethacin has proved ineffective.

The factors that alter the sensitivity of the ductus arteriosus to locally produced PGE$_2$ or NO are unknown. Elevated cortisol concentrations in the fetus have been found to decrease the sensitivity of the ductus arteriosus to PGE$_2$; consistent with these findings, prenatal administration of glucocorticoids causes a significant reduction in the incidence of PDA in premature human infants and animals. During normal fetal development, there is an increase in circulating cortisol, which occurs near the end of gestation; this probably influences ductus arteriosus development in a manner similar to the experiments that used exogenously administered steroids.

## Sites of production of PGE$_2$

The exact source of the PGE$_2$ responsible for regulation of the ductus arteriosus *in vivo* is unclear. Isolated rings of ductus arteriosus produce very little PGE$_2$ at the low ambient O$_2$ tensions found in the fetus. What, then, is the source of the prostaglandins in the fetus? Circulating PGE$_2$ concentrations in the fetus are markedly elevated when compared with the newborn or adult, and this probably controls ductus arteriosus patency in the fetus. Removal of the placenta, an important source of the circulating PGE$_2$ in the fetus, and expansion of the pulmonary circulation, which is the major site of PGE$_2$ removal, contribute to the decrease in circulating concentrations that facilitates ductus arteriosus closure after delivery. In preterm animals, the ability of the lungs to clear circulating PGE$_2$ is decreased compared with full-term animals; this leads to elevated circulating PGE$_2$ concentrations, and this may play a significant role in maintaining ductus arteriosus patency during the first days after premature birth. In addition, during episodes of necrotizing enterocolitis, circulating concentrations of PGE$_2$ reach the pharmacological range and are often associated with reopening of the ductus arteriosus. However, after birth, when arterial blood $P_{O_2}$ rises, the cells of the ductus arteriosus are capable of producing large quantities of PGE$_2$. It appears that after birth the ductus itself is the primary source of the PGE$_2$ responsible for maintaining its patency. There is some evidence to suggest that after delivery PGE$_2$ production in the ductus arteriosus may be stimulated by reactive O$_2$ metabolites.

## LOSS OF DUCTUS ARTERIOSUS REACTIVITY AND REOPENING OF THE VESSEL

In normal, full-term animals, loss of responsiveness to PGE$_2$ shortly after birth prevents the ductus arteriosus from reopening once it has constricted. Loss of ductus arteriosus responsiveness is directly related to the degree of prior ductus arteriosus constriction because constriction causes loss of luminal blood flow and ischemia of the inner vessel wall. This appears to be the first step in permanent closure of the ductus. In contrast to full-term infants, premature infants are more likely to have a ductus arteriosus that continues to dilate in response to PGE$_2$. This occurs even after complete obliteration of ductus luminal blood flow. Consequently, once the ductus arteriosus has closed in the premature infant (either spontaneously or as a result of indomethacin), it may reopen at a later date, with recurrence of the left-to-right shunt. The incidence of ductus arteriosus reopening is inversely related to birth weight: 33 per cent of infants with birthweights <1000 g exhibited ductus arteriosus reopening after initial closure while only 8 per cent of infants with birthweights >1500 g exhibited ductus arteriosus reopening.

When the ductus arteriosus reopens after initial successful closure, it is most frequently due to the effects of endogenous PGE$_2$. As a result, 70 per cent of those ductus that reopen can be closed again with a second treatment course of indomethacin. The factors that maintain ductus arteriosus responsiveness to PGE$_2$ after postnatal constriction in immature newborns are unknown. The O$_2$ consumption of the near-term ductus arteriosus is normally greater than that of other vascular structures containing smooth muscle. In contrast, the O$_2$ consumption of the premature ductus arteriosus appears to be much lower than that obtained near term. This might be due to the low circulating concentrations of thyroid hormones in immature fetuses and neonates. Since O$_2$ consumption is reduced in the preterm ductus arteriosus, the preterm vessel is more resistant to ischemic damage during postnatal constriction. Consistent with this hypothesis is the observation that premature infants with low concentrations of thyroid hormones have an increased incidence of PDA compared with those with normal concentrations. Conversely, when fetal lambs are infused with triiodothyronine (T$_3$) for 48 hours *in utero* and then delivered prematurely, there is a generalized loss of ductus arteriosus responsiveness following constriction of the ductus arteriosus after birth. The loss of ductus arteriosus responsiveness during postnatal constriction in T$_3$-infused premature lambs is similar to that found in full-term lambs. In contrast, the ductus arteriosus of premature lambs that are not infused with T$_3$ are still responsive to vasoactive agonists, even after postnatal constriction. Therefore, increases in thyroid hormone concentrations, which occur with advancing gestation, may play a role in preventing ductus arteriosus reopening once the vessel has constricted after birth.

## ANATOMICAL CLOSURE

In full-term infants, once the ductus arteriosus constricts, rapid histological changes ultimately lead to obliteration of the vessel's lumen and prevent reopening at a later date. As the fetus approaches term, there is intimal thickening and fragmentation of the internal elastic lamina. After birth, the intima continues to increase in size, forming mounds that ultimately occlude the lumen. The rapid increase in intimal thickening that occurs after birth is due to extensive constriction and shortening of the vessel, in addition to migration of smooth muscle cells from the muscle media into the intima.

Once ductus arteriosus luminal blood flow has been obliterated, by the combination of postnatal constriction and intimal mound formation, cells in the inner part of the muscle media begin to disintegrate. Over the next number of weeks, the muscle fibers of the media ultimately atrophy and are replaced by connective tissue. Anatomical closure is complete one to several months after birth.

Preterm infants who experience ductus arteriosus reopening following a successful, initial spontaneous or indomethacin-induced closure fail to develop the anatomical changes seen in full-term neonates. The ductus in these preterm infants remain essentially fetal in appearance with diminished intimal mounds, an intact internal elastic lamina, and absence of cytolytic necrosis.

In the late-gestation fetus, the process of intimal cushion formation starts with the accumulation of hyaluronan (HA) below the luminal endothelial cells. This is accompanied by the loss of laminin and collagen IV from the basement membrane of the endothelial cells and their subsequent separation from the internal elastic lamina. Laminin and collagen IV ultimately re-form under the detached endothelial cells, but HA continues to accumulate in the subendothelial space. The hygroscopic properties of HA cause an influx of water and widening of the subendothelial space; this creates an environment well suited for cell migration. Accompanying the increase in HA is an increase in fibronectin and chondroitin sulfate in the neointimal space (Fig. 73.7).

The endothelial cells and smooth muscle cells (SMCs) of the ductus arteriosus differ from those of adjacent vessels in their ability to form neointimal cushions. Isolated endothelial cells of the ductus arteriosus have an increased rate of HA accumulation compared with those of the aorta or pulmonary artery; this increase appears to be regulated by transforming growth factor β (TGFβ). Following delivery, there is a marked increase in ductus arteriosus TGFβ expression, which accentuates the accumulation of HA within the neointima.

HA makes ductus arteriosus SMCs migrate faster than aortic SMCs. The potentiating effect of HA on ductus SMCs is mediated through a hyaluronan-binding protein (RHAMM). Ductus SMCs synthesize more RHAMM than aortic SMCs and concentrate it at the leading edges of the cells. Antibodies against RHAMM will reduce the migration of ductus SMCs to the level found in aortic SMCs.

Ductus arteriosus SMCs also secrete more fibronectin and chondroitin sulfate than those of the aorta or pulmonary artery. This does not appear to be regulated by TGFβ. Fibronectin plays an important role in facilitating ductus SMC migration, but has no effect on the

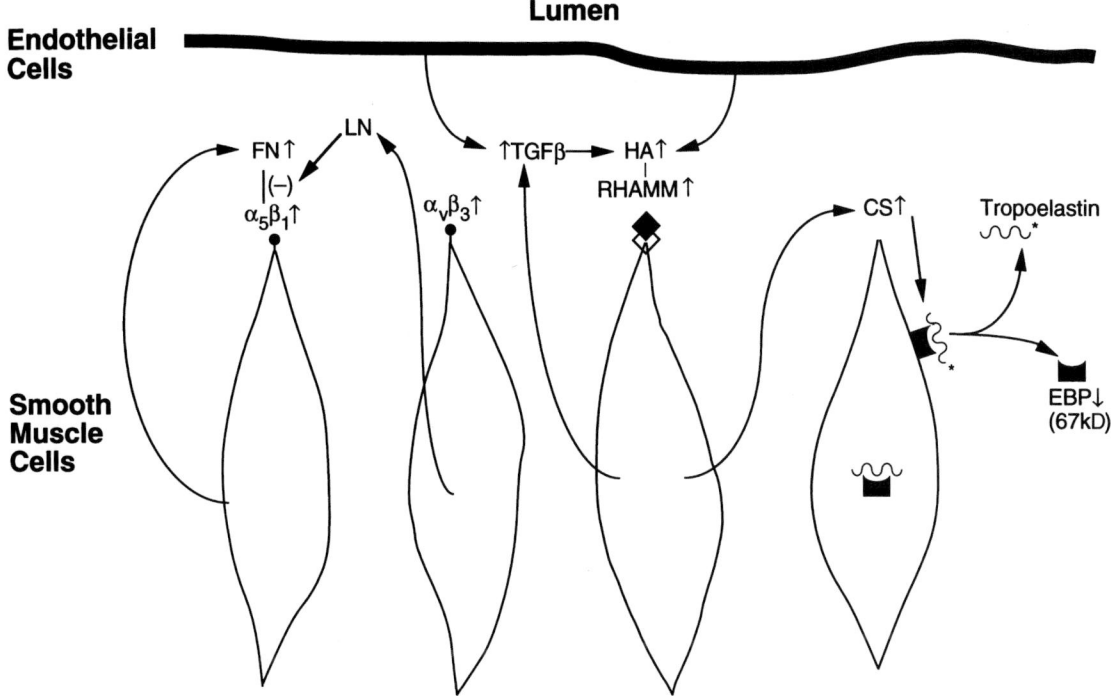

FIGURE 73.7 Factors promoting ductus arteriosus neointima formation. $\alpha_5\beta_1$, integrin receptor $\alpha_5\beta_1$ (for fibronectin); $\alpha_V\beta_3$, integrin receptor $\alpha_V\beta_3$; CS, chondroitin sulfate; EBP, 67-kD elastin-binding protein; FN, fibronectin; HA, hyaluronan; LN, laminin; RHAMM, hyaluronan-binding protein; TGFβ, transforming growth factor β.

migration of aortic SMCs. The increased production of chondroitin sulfate, on the other hand, appears to have no direct effect on either ductus or aortic SMC migration.

Ductus arteriosus SMCs use a family of cell surface receptors, called integrins, to interact with, adhere to, and migrate through the extracellular matrix that surrounds them. When SMCs of the ductus are in a quiescent, contractile state, they express the same integrins on their cell surface as SMCs of the aorta. However, when ductus SMCs of the inner muscle media begin to migrate into the subendothelial space, two new integrin complexes appear on their cell surface: the $\alpha_V\beta_3$ and $\alpha_5\beta_1$ receptors. The $\alpha_V\beta_3$ integrin is a promiscuous receptor that interacts with most extracellular matrix glycoproteins and is essential for migration of ductus SMCs *in vitro*. The $\alpha_5\beta_1$ integrin binds exclusively to fibronectin and mediates the potentiating effects of fibronectin on ductus SMC migration. During the process of migration, ductus SMCs secrete laminin, which also has an important promigratory role. Laminin facilitates SMC migration by destabilizing the interactions of the cells' integrin receptors with other matrix glycoproteins. Because strong adhesion between a cell and its surrounding matrix makes a cell ill suited for migration, this antiadhesive property of laminin allows the cell to make and break contacts with the surrounding matrix rapidly, thus promoting locomotion. Antibodies against laminin will inhibit ductus SMC migration.

Intimal cushion formation in the ductus arteriosus is also associated with striking alterations in elastin fiber assembly. In contrast to the aorta, where formation of well-developed elastic laminae is seen between layers of muscle cells, SMCs of the ductus muscle media are surrounded only by thin and fragmented elastin fibers. SMCs in the ductus neointima are surrounded by even fewer elastin fibers than those in the muscle media. The disruption of normal elastin fiber assembly in the ductus does not appear to be due to increased elastase activity or decreased tropoelastin production. Rather, it appears to be due to a developmental mechanism that reduces insolubilization of elastin and prevents formation of intact elastic laminae.

Vascular SMCs synthesize a 67-kD elastin binding protein (EBP) that is central to the assembly of soluble tropoelastin molecules into a mature matrix of insoluble elastic fibers. The 67-kD EBP appears to be an alternatively spliced, catalytically inactive variant of β-galactosidase. It has three separate binding sites: one for the VGVAPG hydrophobic region of tropoelastin, one for the cell membrane, and one for galactosugars, respectively. The 67-kD EBP binds the hydrophobic tropoelastin molecule intracellularly and escorts it through the SMC's secretory pathways, protecting it from premature self-aggregation and premature proteolytic degradation. Tropoelastin is secreted, with the 67-kD EBP, as a complex. The 67-kD EBP attaches the tropoelastin molecule to the cell's surface. When galactosugars come in contract with the lectin-binding site of the 67-kD EBP, the affinity for both tropoelastin and the cell-binding site is lowered. As a result, bound tropoelastin is released and the 67-kD EBP dissociates from the cell membrane. Coordinated presentation of galactosugars, contained within the growing elastin microfibrillar scaffold, may regulate the orientation and proper alignment of tropoelastin for crosslinking during normal elastin fiber assembly. On the other hand, excess galactosugars, from other matrix elements, may compete with this process and lead to abnormal assembly.

Ductus arteriosus SMCs have less 67-kD EBP on their cell surface when compared with aortic SMCs. As a result, ductus SMCs deposit little insoluble elastin compared with aortic SMCs. They also secrete large amounts of a truncated form of tropoelastin, which appears to be due to proteolytic intracellular degradation caused by the 67-kD EBP deficiency. This truncated tropoelastin lacks the C-terminus of the molecule and is impaired in its ability to align on microfibrils and crosslink. Ductus SMCs also secrete increased amounts of chondroitin sulfate, an N-galactosamine-containing glycosaminoglycan, compared with aortic SMCs. Chondroitin sulfate, through its galactosugar side chains, removes the 67-kD EBP from SMC surfaces, thereby interfering with elastin fiber assembly.

The exact relationship between impaired elastin assembly and SMC migration into the neointima is still open for speculation. Impaired assembly of thick elastic laminae would seem to facilitate SMC migration by removing a physical barrier to which they might attach. Ductus SMCs are able to migrate through elastin membranes that restrain aortic SMC migration. Treatment of aortic SMCs with chondroitin sulfate causes the release of the 67-kD EBP from the aortic cells' surface and enables them to migrate through elastin membranes at the same rate as ductus SMCs. Finally, the accumulation of a relatively stable, soluble, truncated tropoelastin may act as a chemoattractant for SMCs. Thus, there appear to be mechanisms that link elastin fragmentation and formation of ductus arteriosus intimal cushions. Conversely, when intimal cushions fail to develop, as occurs in the genetic form of PDA, the elastic laminae of the ductus appear abnormally well developed and similar to those in the aorta.

## HEMODYNAMIC AND PULMONARY ALTERATIONS

The pathophysiological consequences of a PDA depend both on the magnitude of left-to-right shunt through the ductus arteriosus and on cardiac and pulmonary responses to the shunt. There are important differences between immature and mature infants in the heart's ability to handle a volume load (see p. 741). Immature infants have less cardiac sympathetic innervation. Before term, the myocardium has more water and less contractile mass. Therefore, in the

immature fetus the ventricles are less distensible than at term and also generate less force per gram of myocardium (even though they generate the same force per sarcomere as those in more mature infants). The relative lack of left ventricular distensibility in immature infants is more a function of the ventricle's tissue constituents than of poor muscle function. As a result, in immature infants, left ventricular distension secondary to large left-to-right PDA shunts may produce higher left ventricular end-diastolic pressures at smaller ventricular volumes. The increase in left ventricular end-diastolic pressure increases pulmonary venous pressure and causes pulmonary congestion.

Studies in preterm lambs with a PDA have shown that despite these limitations, the lambs are able to increase their left ventricular output to maintain "effective" systemic blood flow, even with left-to-right shunts equal to 50 per cent of left ventricular output. With shunts greater than 50 per cent of left ventricular output, "effective" systemic blood flow falls despite a continued increase in left ventricular output. The increase in left ventricular output is accomplished not by an increase in heart rate, but by an increase in stroke volume. Stroke volume increases primarily as a result of the simultaneous decrease in afterload resistance on the heart and the increase in left ventricular preload. Despite the ability of the left ventricle to increase its output in the face of a left-to-right ductus arteriosus shunt, blood flow distribution is significantly rearranged. This redistribution of systemic blood flow occurs even with small shunts. Blood flow to the skin, bone, and skeletal muscle is most likely to be affected by left-to-right ductal shunts; the next most likely organs to be affected are the gastrointestinal tract and the kidneys. These organs receive decreased blood flow due to a combination of decreased perfusion pressure (related to a drop in diastolic pressure) and localized vasoconstriction. These organs may experience significant hypoperfusion before there are any signs of left ventricular compromise.

Very-low-birthweight infants with a PDA have been found to have increased flow in the ascending aorta and decreased flow in the descending aorta. Such alterations in cardiac output distribution have been implicated in the high incidence of *intracranial hemorrhage* and *necrotizing enterocolitis* associated with PDA. Significant aortic backflow has been observed over large distances in some infants with PDA, consistent with a "diastolic steal" of blood from the aorta and abdominal organs to the pulmonary artery. The continuous distension of the pulmonary vessels during diastole may be important in the production of pulmonary vascular disease and *bronchopulmonary dysplasia*.

The decreased ability of the preterm infant to maintain active pulmonary vasoconstriction may be responsible in part for the earlier presentation of a "large" left-to-right PDA shunt in the most immature infants. Therapeutic maneuvers (e.g. surfactant replacement) that lead to a more rapid drop in postnatal pulmonary vascular resistance can exacerbate the amount of ductus arteriosus left-to-right shunt in preterm infants with respiratory distress syndrome. Two separate recent meta-analyses have demonstrated an increase both in the incidence of PDA and in the incidence of pulmonary hemorrhage when infants are treated with synthetic surfactant prophylactically.

The factors responsible for preventing fluid and protein movement from the plasma to the lung interstitium (microvascular barrier) and from the interstitium to the air spaces (alveolar barrier) have been described elsewhere (see pages 818 and 821). With a wide open PDA, the pulmonary vasculature is exposed to systemic blood pressure and increased pulmonary blood flow. Because the premature infant, with respiratory distress syndrome, frequently has low plasma oncotic pressure and increased capillary permeability, increases in microvascular perfusion pressure that result from PDA may increase interstitial and alveolar lung fluid. Leakage of plasma proteins into the alveolar space would inhibit surfactant function and increase surface tension in the immature air sacs, which are already compromised by surfactant deficiency. The increased $F_IO_2$ and mean airway pressures required to overcome these early changes in compliance may be important factors in the association of PDA with chronic lung disease. However, these changes in pulmonary mechanics appear to occur only after several days of exposure to a PDA. While it is true that preterm animals with a PDA have increased fluid and protein clearance into the lung interstitium, due to an increase in pulmonary microvascular filtration pressure, a simultaneous increase in lung lymph flow appears to eliminate the excess fluid and protein from the lung. This compensatory increase in lung lymph flow acts as an "edema safety factor," inhibiting fluid accumulation in the lungs. As a result, there is no net increase in water or protein accumulation in the lung, or change in pulmonary mechanics. This delicate balance between PDA-induced fluid filtration and lymphatic reabsorption is consistent with the observation, made in human infants, that ligation of the ductus arteriosus, within the first 24 hours after birth, has no effect on the course of the newborn's respiratory disease. However, if lung lymphatic drainage is impaired, as it is in the presence of pulmonary interstitial emphysema or fibrosis, the likelihood of edema increases dramatically. After several days of lung disease and mechanical ventilation, the residual functioning lymphatics are more easily overwhelmed by the same size PDA shunt that could be accommodated on the first day after delivery. As a result, it is most common for infants with a persistent PDA to develop a "hemodynamically significant shunt" with pulmonary edema and alterations in pulmonary mechanics at 7–10 days after birth. In these infants, improvement in lung compliance occurs following ligation of the PDA.

Not all of the changes associated with a PDA are necessarily detrimental to the immature infant with respiratory distress syndrome. In fact, decreases in systemic arterial $O_2$ content have been observed following PDA closure, despite the absence of any alterations in pulmonary mechanics. This phenomenon is due to recirculation of oxygenated arterial blood through partially expanded lungs. Therefore, continued patency of the ductus arteriosus after birth may serve a temporary but useful function in infants whose lungs are not fully expanded. However, the interpretation of arterial blood $Po_2$ values, which are commonly, but mistakenly, assumed to reflect only changes in pulmonary function, may be confounded when there are changes in the amount of left-to-right ductus shunt (due to either ductus closure or alterations in pulmonary vascular resistance).

## SELECTED READING

Boudreau N. Turley E, Rabinovitch M. Fibronectin, hyaluron and a hyaluron binding protein contribute to increased ductus arteriosus smooth muscle cell migration. *Dev Biol* 1991; 143: 235.

Coceani F, Kelsey L, Ackerley C et al. Cytochrome P450 during ontogenic development: occurrence in the ductus arteriosus and other tissues. *Can J Physiol Pharmacol* 1994; 72: 217.

Coceani F, Kelsey L. Seidlitz E. Evidence for an effector role of endothelin in closure of the ductus arteriosus at birth. *Can J Physiol Pharmacol* 1992; 70: 1061.

de Reeder EG, Girard N, Poelmann RE et al. Hydaluronic acid accumulation and entothelial cell detachment in intimal thickening of the vessel wall. The normal and genetically defective ductus arteriosus. *Am J Pathol* 1988; 132: 574.

Hinek A. Boyle J, Rabinovitch M. Vascular smooth muscle cell detachment from elastin and migration through elastic laminae is promoted by chondroitin sulfate-induced "shedding" of the 67-kDa cell surface elastin binding protein. *Exp Cell Res* 1992; 203: 344.

Hinek A, Rabinovitch M. The ductus arteriosus migratory smooth muscle cell phenotype processes tropoelastin to a 52-kDa product associated with impaired assembly of elastic laminae. *J Biol Chem* 1993; 268: 1405.

Nakanishi T, Gu H, Hagiwara N, Momma K. Mechanisms of oxygen-induced contraction of ductus arteriosus isolated from the fetal rabbit. *Circ Res* 1993; 72: 1218.

Slomp J, van Munsteren JC, Poelmann RE et al. Formation of intimal cushions in the ductus arteriosus as a model for vascular intimal thickening. An immunohistochemical study of changes in extracellular matrix components. *Atherosclersosis* 1992; 93: 25.

Zhu L, Dagher E, Johnson DJ et al. A developmentally regulated program restricting insolubilization of elastin and formation of laminae in the fetal lamb arteriosus. *Lab Invest* 1993; 68: 321.

# 74

# Circulatory Changes During Gestation

## MATERNAL CARDIOVASCULAR ALTERATIONS DURING PREGNANCY

### UTEROPLACENTAL VASCULAR CHANGES IN PREGNANCY

This chapter presents an overview of maternal uteroplacental and systemic cardiovascular changes that normally occur in pregnancy. The uteroplacental vascular bed demonstrates dramatic and unique changes in pregnancy, providing essentially the only direct link between the maternal and fetal blood compartments. In this review we define the "peripheral or systemic cardiovascular system" collectively to include all vascular beds other than the uteroplacental.

The changes that occur in the uterine vascular bed during gestation must be evaluated with regard to the uterus as a single unique vascular bed, as well as to its component vascular beds, the endometrium, myometrium, and maternal placenta. Because accurate quantitation of individual tissue blood flow and vascular distribution are invasive and cannot be performed in humans, most studies have centered around ovine models. However, much of the ovine data correlates with human pregnancy, especially when adjusted to relative gestational age. For comparison purposes, term pregnancy in the ewe is 145 days, with the second and third trimesters commencing at around 50 and 100 days, respectively.

## Total uteroplacental perfusion

Total uterine blood flow increases 50- to 70-fold above non-pregnant levels during the course of normal gestation in women and sheep. Moreover, because of additional metabolic demands, the flow increases in multifetal gestations are directly related to the number of fetuses, i.e. single < twins < triplets. The rise in uteroplacental perfusion accounts for 7–25 per cent of cardiac output at term in the sheep, dog, guinea pig, rhesus monkey, rabbit, and human. Because blood flow to any organ is controlled acutely by relative changes in both vascular resistance and perfusion pressure, the latter estimated from mean arterial blood pressure, this dramatic increase in blood flow occurs while perfusion pressure falls, although slightly (see below). Thus there are substantial decreases in uterine vascular resistance, which can be estimated using the following equation:

$$\text{Uterine vascular resistance} = \frac{\text{Mean arterial pressure}}{\text{Uterine blood flow}}$$

In sheep, uterine vascular resistance decreases around 25-fold by 60–100 days' gestation (from about 5 mmHg/[mL · min] during the non-pregnant state to about 0.2 mmHg/[mL · min]) and around 70-fold (to 0.07 mmHg/[mL · min]) by 130–140 days' gestation, providing what has been interpreted as direct evidence of profound vasodilatation. The increase in total uterine perfusion during normal pregnancy may be explained by two important phenomena: first, growth of existing myoendometrial vascular beds and the development of the placental vascular bed and, second, the subsequent vasodilatation of each of these vascular beds. The vascular growth component also is associated with an increase in total organ blood flow, but not flow per gram of tissue and is likely controlled by the expression of placental and/or uterine angiogenic factors which induce neovascularization. In contrast, the vasodilatation component is reflected by increases in total perfusion per gram of tissue without a change in perfusion pressure. The patterns of change in total uterine weight, uterine blood flow, and uterine blood

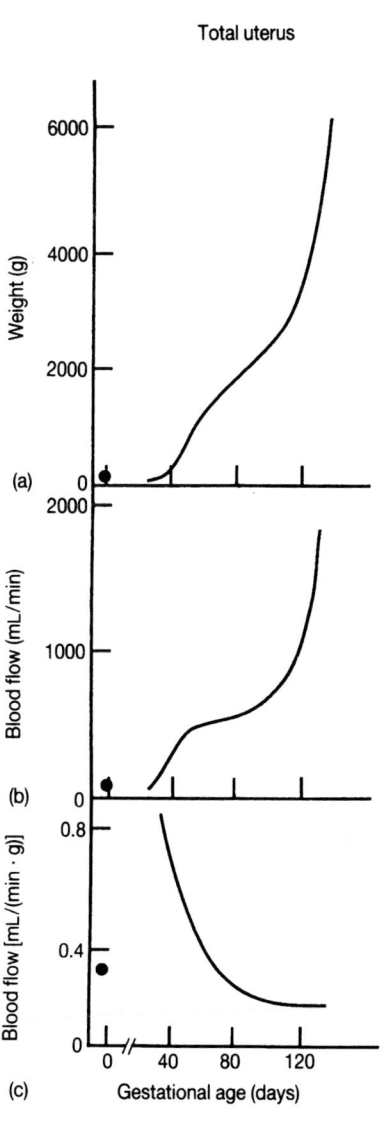

**Total uterus**

FIGURE 74.1 Changes in uterine weight (a), blood flow (b), and blood flow per gram of total uterine weight (c) during ovine gestation. Total uterine weight is defined as the sum of the metabolically active tissues, i.e. endometrium, myometrium, placentomes, fetal membranes, and fetus. ● = Non-pregnant. (From Rosenfeld CR, *et al. Gynecol Invest* 1974; 5: 252, with permission from Karger, Basel.)

flow per gram of tissue during ovine pregnancy are illustrated in Fig. 74.1. Total uterine weight was considered as the sum of the metabolically active tissues, i.e. endometrium, myometrium, placentomes (caruncles and cotyledons), fetal membranes, and fetus. Prior to 50–60 days' gestation (first trimester) uterine weight increases relatively little (Fig. 74.1a). Thereafter weight increases rapidly, continuing in a logarithmic manner throughout gestation. This weight increase during the last two trimesters reflects growth and development not only of uterine tissues and the placenta, but also of the fetus, and is accompanied by rather large increases in absolute blood flow (Fig. 74.1b). The pattern of gestational increase in uterine blood flow suggests two periods of rapid absolute blood flow (mL/min) increase, the first between 50 and 80 days, during the second trimester and the second from 110 days' gestation until term (i.e. during the third trimester). The former is associated with placentation and will be discussed in detail later. The latter is temporally related to rapid fetal growth in the third trimester. When these changes in blood flow are expressed per gram of tissue (Fig. 74.1c), thereby taking into account both metabolically active (consuming) tissue mass and growth, an inverse pattern is observed, i.e. there are extremely high blood flows in the first 50 days (early implantation/attachment and initiation of placentation), followed by a gradual fall until 90–100 days, after which blood flow remains relatively unchanged or may increase slightly. These data indicate that during the first two trimesters of pregnancy the increase in uterine weight is substantially greater than the increase in total uterine blood flow, while thereafter increases in tissue weight and blood flow are proportional. The third trimester modifications can also be interpreted as demonstrating vasodilatation of this vascular bed at a time when the greatest fetal metabolic demand for growth occurs. The high uterine perfusion early in gestation likely reflects high metabolic needs of the uterine tissues and the early embryo, as well as increases in the production of steroid hormones (estrogen and/or progesterone) necessary for maintenance of pregnancy, or a combination of these factors. Therefore these blood flow patterns likely reflect the need for increased uterine $O_2$ and other nutrient substrate delivery.

## Distribution of uterine blood flow throughout pregnancy

Changes in the pattern of total uteroplacental blood flow represents the sum of the patterns of the individual uterine tissues receiving flow. Using radiolabeled microspheres, changes in distribution of total blood flow to individual uteroplacental tissues that occur during ovine pregnancy can be measured (Fig. 74.2). In non-pregnant sheep, uterine blood flow is evenly distributed among the endometrium, myometrium, and caruncles.

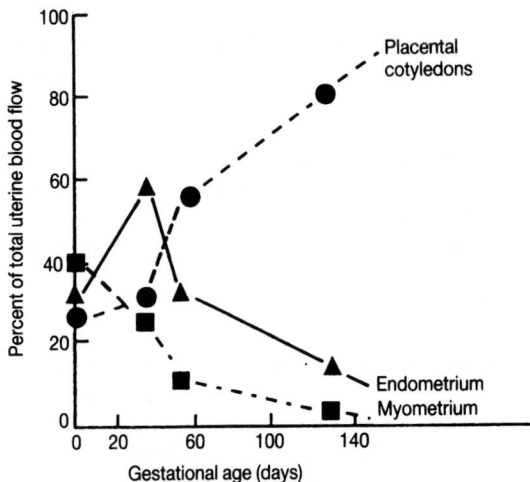

FIGURE 74.2 Distribution of uterine blood flow during ovine pregnancy; term is 145 days. Placental cotyledonary flow is maternal (caruncular) blood flow. (From Rosenfeld CR. *Semin Perinatol* 1984; 8: 42, with permission from W.B. Saunders Co.)

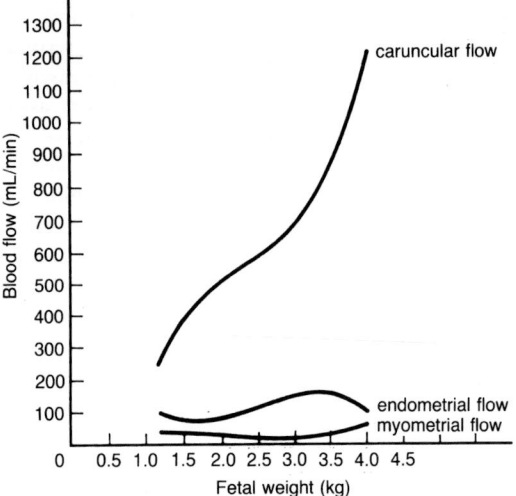

FIGURE 74.3 Regional absolute blood flows (mL/min) to the maternal placental "cotyledon" (caruncle), endometrium, and myometrium in the third trimester gravid sheep uterus plotted against fetal weight. (From Makowski EL, *et al. Am J Obstet Gynecol* 1968; **101**: 409, with permission.)

The latter are specialized sites for implantation/placentation in the sheep and will develop into the maternal compartment of the placentome, in direct apposition to the fetal cotyledonary portion of the placentome. At 40–50 days' gestation, i.e. before placentation is complete, the endometrium receives nearly 60 per cent of total uterine blood flow, while the remaining blood flow is evenly distributed between the myometrium and the enlarged caruncles, which exhibit both hypertrophy and hyperplasia. This suggests that significant functional and metabolic alterations occur in the endometrium and the caruncles early in gestation, and that these are important for maintenance of early pregnancy. This early time in ovine gestation lies between about days 12 and 45 when "maternal recognition of pregnancy" first ensues and the attachment/implantation phases occur, respectively. It therefore sets the stage for maternal placental development. Between 60 and 80 days' gestation, when ovine placental development is being completed, there is a redistribution of uterine blood flow and by 80 days maternal placental (caruncular) blood flow accounts for 60 per cent, endometrial flow 30 per cent, and myometrial flow 10 per cent. Thereafter, the proportion of uterine blood flow to the maternal component of the placentome continues to increase, with commensurate decreases in the proportions perfusing the endometrium and myometrium. This redistribution toward maternal placental blood flow reflects the metabolic needs of placental and fetal growth and demonstrates that, anatomically and physiologically, the placenta is the key link between the maternal and fetal circulations. These relationships between the changes in blood flow to the maternal placenta, endometrium and myometrium relative to fetal weight are shown in Fig. 74.3. The increase in fetal weight during the third trimester is related primarily to increases in

maternal placental blood flow and not endometrial or myometrial perfusion.

By term maternal placental blood flow accounts for 80–85 per cent of total uterine blood flow, while the endometrium receives 10 per cent and the myometrium 5 per cent, suggesting that the changes in total uterine blood flow late in gestation (Fig. 74.1) primarily reflect alterations in the placental vascular bed. Therefore, studies that measure only total uteroplacental blood flow may not determine vascular responses to the individual tissues which comprise the gravid uterus, especially the caruncular portion of the placentome in early and mid versus late gestation. Therefore we will describe the changes in each of these vascular beds during gestation.

## Endometrial and myometrial blood flow throughout gestation

The patterns of change in endometrial (Fig. 74.4) and myometrial (Fig. 74.5) tissues during advancing gestation differ for absolute blood flow, but are similar for weight and blood flow per gram of tissue. Both tissues have biphasic increases in weight, the first by about 60 days and the second from around 120 days until term. These phases likely reflect both placental development as well as expression of maternal and/or fetoplacental factors, necessary for the observed increases in tissue weight and blood flow. Blood flow per gram of tissue decreases substantially in both tissues as pregnancy progresses until the end of gestation when a relatively small increase is seen. The extremely high endometrial blood flow prior to 40–50 days' gestation (Fig. 74.4c) most likely reflects the need to highly perfuse this tissue

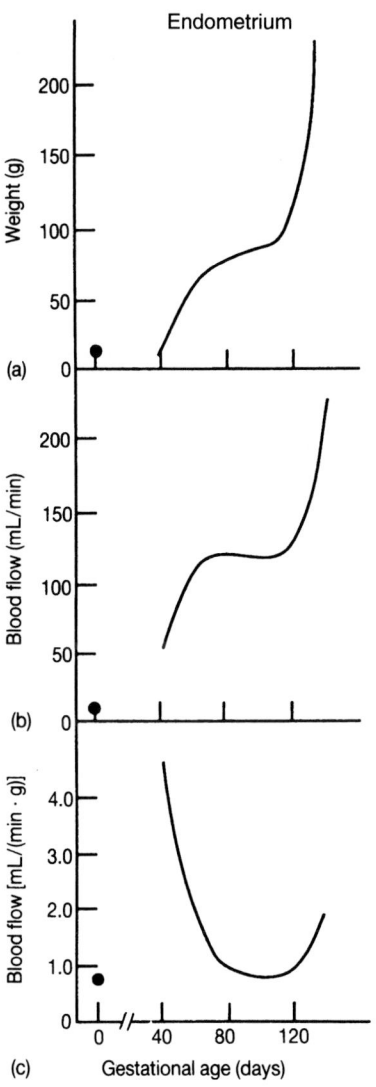

FIGURE 74.4 Changes in endometrial weight (a), blood flow (b), and blood flow per gram of endometrium (c) during ovine gestation. •, Non-pregnant. (From Rosenfeld CR, *et al. Gynecol Invest* 1974; 5: 252, with permission from Karger, Basel.)

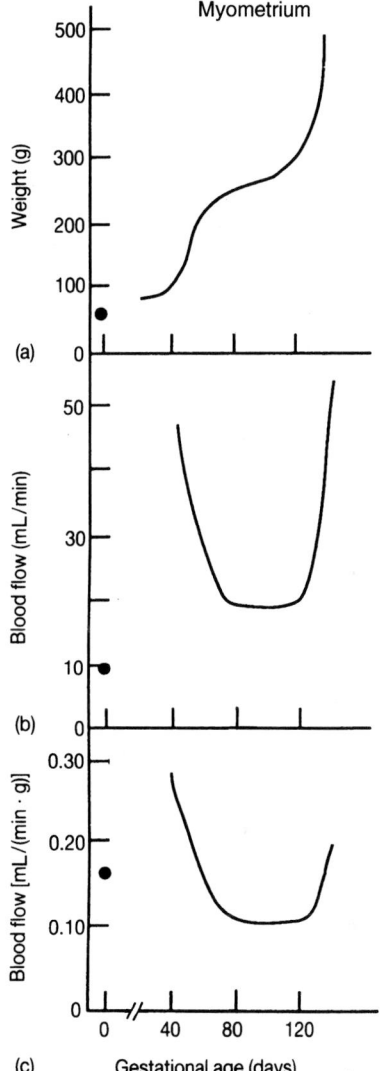

FIGURE 74.5 Changes in myometrial weight (a), blood flow (b), and blood flow per gram of myometrium (c) during ovine gestation. •, Non-pregnant. (From Rosenfeld CR, *et al. Gynecol Invest* 1974; 5: 252, with permission from Karger, Basel.)

so that implantation and placentation can occur. It also is thought to be regulated by embryonic and/or ovarian steroid hormones.

## Maternal placental blood flow throughout gestation

Patterns of change in weight and blood flow differ in the placentomes (Fig. 74.6). Placental growth begins around 60 days and is completed by 80–90 days' gestation; thereafter placental weight remains relatively unchanged or even decreases slightly in the last 1–2 weeks of gestation. Similar patterns occur

for placental DNA content and numerical density of nuclei in the maternal placental stroma. The biphasic pattern of change for placental blood flow (Fig. 74.6b) is similar to that observed for the uterus as a whole. When placental growth and blood flow to the maternal component of the placentome are combined and expressed in terms of blood flow per gram of tissue (Fig. 74.6c), the pattern is different from that for the total uterus, endometrium or myometrium. Rather than the decrease in myoendometrial blood flow with only a minor rise at term, there is a dramatic rise in maternal placental blood flow after about 110 days that continues until term. Thus the first phase of increase in absolute maternal placental blood flow between 50 and 90 days represents the

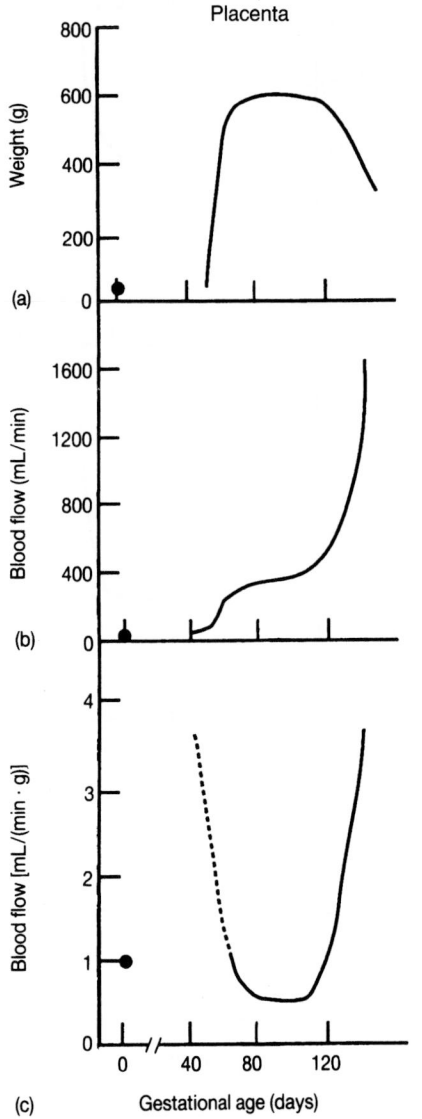

(a)
(b)
(c)

FIGURE 74.6 Changes in placental weight (a), blood flow (b), and blood flow per gram of placenta (c). Observations on the non-pregnant animals (●) represent the caruncles or future sites of implantation. (From Rosenfeld CR, *et al. Gynecol Invest* 1974; 5: 252, with permission from Karger, Basel.)

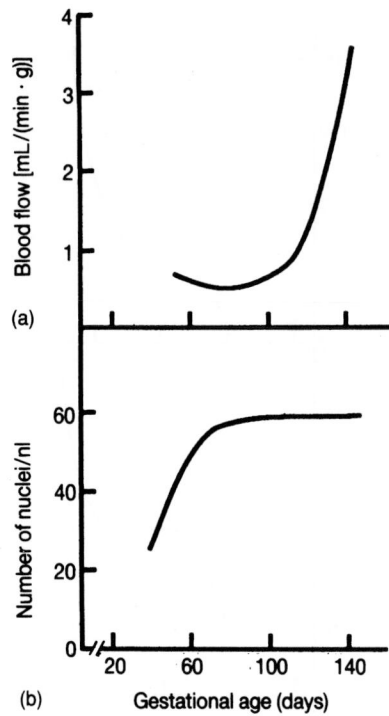

(a)
(b)

FIGURE 74.7 Comparison of maternal placental blood flow per gram of placenta (a) with the numerical density of nuclei of the maternal placental stroma (b). (From Teasdale F. *Anat Rec* 1976; **185**: 187. Copyright © 1976. Reprinted with permission from John Wiley and Sons, Inc.)

namic changes are similar, and occur at relatively similar times in gestation.

## Angiogenesis and uteroplacental blood flow

During pregnancy, formation of new placental blood vessels from pre-existing vessels (angiogenesis) has been well characterized. The placenta, uterus and corpus luteum, tissues undergoing periodic growth and development, are normal adult reproductive tissues exhibiting angiogenesis. Angiogenesis also occurs in pathological conditions such as tumors, or the healing of wounds or fractures, and vascular growth generally reflects the high metabolic demands of the tissues, normal or abnormal.

Placental angiogenesis occurs in many species including the human and sheep. In sheep, angiogenesis occurs throughout gestation, but the origin of the growth factors stimulating angiogenic activity differs during gestation (Fig. 74.8), suggesting important temporal developmental regulation, as seen with uteroplacental growth and blood flow. During the early first trimester, angiogenic activity, evaluated as endothelial cell proliferation, occurs primarily in the maternal, but

development and growth of the placental vascular bed, whereas the secondary rise in placental blood flow after 100–110 days must represent the vasodilatation of the placental vascular bed because there were: (1) no alterations in overall uteroplacental perfusion pressure (arterial pressure), (2) no alterations in placental weight so that blood flow per gram of tissue increased, and (3) no changes in total numbers of maternal stromal cells (Fig. 74.7). Changes in placental blood flow observed in sheep correspond to patterns reported in women. Although the human and ovine placentas are anatomically different, the overall local and systemic (described below) hemody-

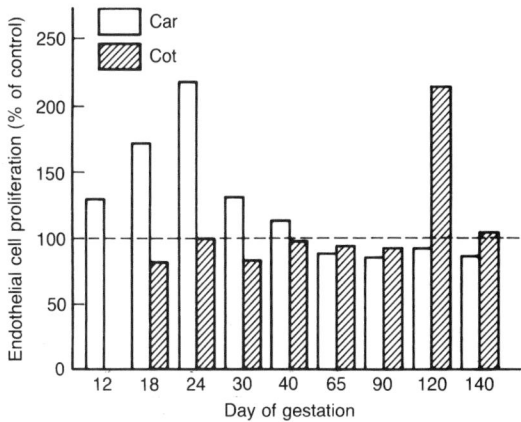

FIGURE 74.8 Angiogenic activity in media conditioned by ovine maternal (Car) and fetal (Cot) compartments of the placenta throughout gestation. Angiogenic activity was evaluated as the proliferation of bovine aortic endothelial cells above that observed using control (unconditioned media) which represents 100%. (From Reynolds LP, Redmer DA. *J Anim Sci* 1995; **73**: 1839, with permission.)

not fetal, portion of the placenta. Angiogenesis in the placentome remains relatively unchanged during the second trimester, the time when blood flow per gram of tissue is expected to fall and then plateau (Fig. 74.6). During the last trimester, however, angiogenic activity is found primarily in the fetal, but not maternal, placenta. These angiogenic patterns likely account for the differences in vascular growth patterns in individual placental tissues during gestation since they correlate with the increased vascular density in the maternal placenta (caruncle) during the first trimester and in the fetal placenta (cotyledon) during the last trimester.

Although not yet fully characterized, this angiogenic activity may relate to at least two well-known families of growth factors, fibroblast growth factors (FGFs) and vascular endothelial growth factors (VEGFs), both of which are implicated in the processes regulating placental vascular growth. These growth factors also are involved in other physiological, endocrine and metabolic functions in the placenta. For example, in addition to the very important properties of direct and specific stimulation of proliferation and migration of endothelial cells, VEGFs, which are highly expressed in the fetal placenta, also increase microvascular permeability. The angiogenic effects may be important in modulating placental perfusion, especially during the last trimester and the increased expression of VEGFs and/or FGFs in the ovine placenta likely correlates with the increase in placental perfusion during this period.

Formation of new blood vessels is a critical component of growth and development of all tissues. However, in contrast to most tissues, in which vascular development is proportional to the growth of the other cellular components of the tissue, the ovine placenta exhibits a substantial increase in vascular density relative to cross-sectional area/tissue mass (Fig. 74.9). At

the beginning of placentation, caruncular (maternal placentome) vascular density increases by day 24 and is associated with a four- to six-fold increase in uterine blood flow as well as a nearly two-fold elevation in angiogenic activity (Fig. 74.8). From day 40 to 80, caruncular vascular density continues to increase (approximately two-fold) and remains relatively unchanged thereafter. This vascular growth is directly correlated with changes in the density of nuclei of the maternal caruncular stroma during the last trimester of gestation (Fig. 74.7) and with placental blood flow (Fig. 74.6). The variation in maternal placental (caruncular) vascular density until approximately 80 days also is concomitant with the changes in absolute maternal placental blood flow (mL/min) and total placentome weight (Fig. 74.6). Unlike maternal placental vascular growth, however, the cotyledonary (fetal placenta) vascular density remains relatively constant until around 80–90 days' gestation, and then increases dramatically (Fig. 74.9). This cotyledonary vascular growth correlates with the increase in both absolute and relative uteroplacental blood flow (ml/[min · g]; Fig. 74.6), and in fetoplacental blood flow and with fetal growth during the third trimester.

Although placental vascular growth is important to placental blood flow, it may account for only part of the increase in placentome blood flow during gestation. For example, even though caruncular vascular density remains relatively unchanged from 80–90

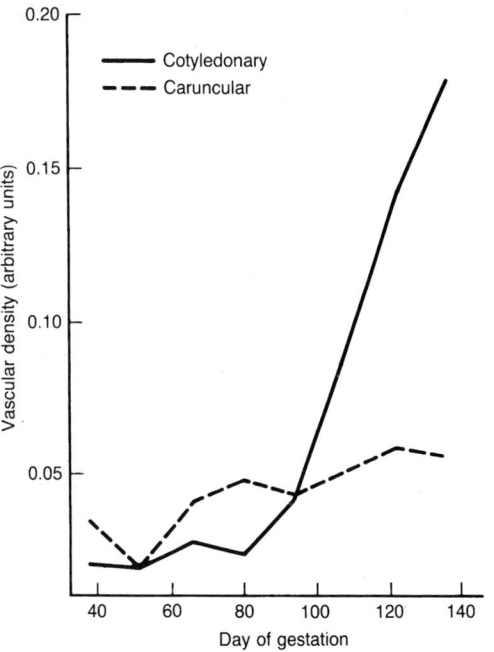

FIGURE 74.9 Microvascular density of the maternal (caruncular) and fetal (cotyledonary) compartments of the ovine placentome during gestation. (From Reynolds LP, Redmer DA. *J Anim Sci* 1995; **73**, 1839, with permission; derived from original data published by Stegeman, JHJ. *Bijdragen Tot de dierkunde (Contrib Zool)* 1974; **44**: 3.)

days' gestation until term, uteroplacental blood flow per gram of tissue increases about five-fold. Similarly, during the same period, cotyledonary vascular density increases only around seven-fold, but fetal placental blood flow increases nearly 20-fold. Therefore, factors other than vascular growth alone, e.g. vasodilators, also must play a role in regulating placental blood flow changes (see below). This may have clinical significance since both fetoplacental and uteroplacental blood flows continue to increase until term and fetal weight is highly correlated with blood flow to both sides of the placenta (Fig. 74.3).

Thus during the third trimester when fetal growth is the greatest, the increase in fetal placental (cotyledonary) blood flow may be dependent upon both angiogenic processes and vasodilatation whereas the increase in uteroplacental blood flow is related primarily to vasodilatation of the maternal placental but not endometrial and myometrial vascular beds. The increase in maternal placental blood flow is thought to be in response to the metabolic demands of the rapidly growing fetus as well as those of the fetal membranes and uterine tissues.

## PERIPHERAL VASCULAR CHANGES IN HUMAN AND OVINE PREGNANCY

In addition to the changes described for the uteroplacental vascular bed, there are also numerous changes in the maternal peripheral vascular bed. For example, although there is a relatively minor decrease in arterial blood pressure, there is a gradual, but more substantial, increase in cardiac output (Fig. 74.10) associated with a proportional fall in systemic vascular resistance. Thus pregnancy is a state of both uterine and systemic vasodilatation. Maternal blood and plasma volumes, body weight and interstitial fluid volume also increase and there is relative refractoriness to the pressor effects of infused angiotensin II, α-adrenergic agonists, and several other vasoconstrictors. Moreover, cardiac output is redistributed, primarily reflecting the growth and development of the uteroplacental vascular bed and, later in pregnancy, the growth of the mammary gland vascular bed (Fig. 74.11). All of these cardiovascular alterations return to non-pregnant levels within 2–5 weeks of delivery.

In normal pregnant women in the second trimester (12–20 weeks), cardiac output is increased approximately 25–40 per cent in singleton and 50–60 per cent in multifetal pregnancies. It then plateaus and remains unchanged or falls slightly during the third trimester. However data on cardiac output in humans after the second trimester are inconsistent as the increasing size of the gravid uterus often compresses, and partially occludes, both the inferior vena cava and the aorta causing transient falls in cardiac output as venous return decreases (cardiac preload). For example, cardiac output is 22 per cent lower in the same patients in the supine versus lateral recumbent

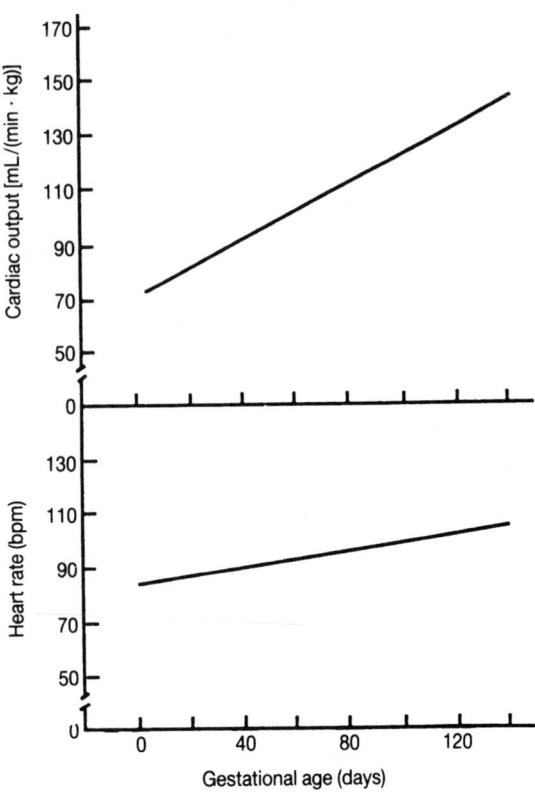

FIGURE 74.10 Changes in cardiac output and heart rate during ovine pregnancy. (From Rosenfeld CR. *Am J Physiol* 1977; **232**: H231, with permission.)

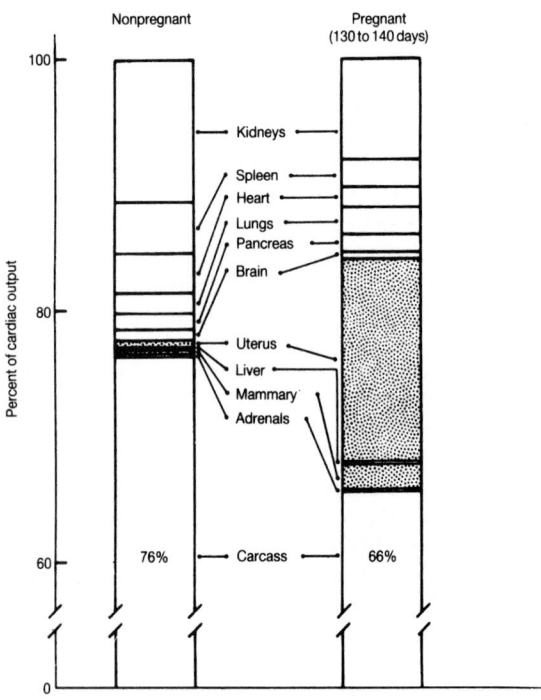

FIGURE 74.11 Distribution of cardiac output in non-pregnant and pregnant ewes at 130–140 days of gestation. Stippled areas represent mammary gland and uterine mass. (From Rosenfeld CR. *Am J Physiol* 1977; **232**: H231, with permission.)

positions. More definitive data have been obtained in sheep in which the uterus does not rest upon the great vessels; cardiac output progressively rises (Fig. 74.10), increasing from non-pregnant values of about 75 mL/(min·kg) to about 150 ml/(min·kg) by the end of gestation. This has been confirmed in several species using different techniques, e.g. dye-dilution, thermal dilution, radiolabeled microspheres, two-dimensional echocardiography and electromagnetic flow transducers.

Cardiac output is expressed by the mathematical equation:

$$\text{Cardiac output} = \text{Heart rate} \times \text{Stroke volume}$$

Therefore, it is important to determine which component is responsible for the observed increase in cardiac output. In humans and sheep, heart rate increases similarly, i.e. 20–30 per cent (Fig. 74.10). In women, heart rate increases gradually from about 8 weeks' gestation and plateaus around 28–32 weeks. This rise is attributed both to changes in the autonomic nervous system and to increases in placental steroids; however, their specific roles remain unproven. Because the rise in heart rate is proportionately less than the rise in cardiac output, the increase in cardiac output must also reflect an increase in stroke volume. As measured by echocardiography during normal singleton pregnancy, both left ventricular wall mass and end-diastolic dimensions increase and the increase in stroke volume is directly proportional to end-diastolic volume, implying little change in myocardial inotropic state. However, in multifetal gestations the additional 20–30 per cent rise in cardiac output occurs predominantly by increased inotropy demonstrated by an increased fractional shortening of the ventricular diameter. Taken together these changes suggest a decrease in cardiac reserve in normal pregnancy. In addition, the aorta has been noted to be larger and more compliant in pregnant women, which may contribute to the decreased afterload on the heart seen in pregnancy.

The rise in cardiac output also correlates directly with an increase in blood volume. This important relationship follows from the direct proportionality between stroke volume, end-diastolic volume and blood volume as described by the Starling law of the heart (see Chapter 72). The magnitude of increase in blood volume in pregnancy depends on the presence of a singleton or multifetal pregnancy and varies from 30 to 50 per cent. During normal human pregnancy, increases in plasma volume begin around 6 weeks and plateau around 30–34 weeks. There is enhanced erythropoiesis, and thus total red blood cell mass also increases; however, the rise in plasma volume in women, but not sheep, generally exceeds the increase in red cell mass which explains the development of the "physiological anemia of pregnancy." The following equation defines this relationship:

$$\text{Blood volume} - \text{Plasma volume} = \text{Red blood cell mass}$$

In addition to increases in cardiac output and blood volume, pregnant women exhibit a 10–15 per cent decrease in systemic arterial blood pressure and a 50–75 per cent decrease in systemic vascular resistance near the end of the first trimester. This normal systemic vasodilatation appears to be absent, or reversed, in pregnancies complicated by proteinuric hypertension (pre-eclampsia). The hypotensive effect of pregnancy commences at 8 weeks' gestation and becomes significant by 12 weeks at which time some pregnant women suffer from dizziness or even syncope with postural changes. The nadir occurs around 20 weeks, blood pressure remains low until 30–32 weeks and then slowly returns to near non-pregnant levels by term (38–40 weeks). The greater decreases in diastolic than systolic blood pressures suggest that significant decreases in vascular tone also are involved in these cardiovascular alterations. In pregnancies destined to develop pregnancy-induced hypertension or pre-eclampsia, the small, but significant, fall in mean arterial blood pressure that occurs early in the second trimester in normal pregnancy may not occur. In ovine pregnancy, the decrease in mean arterial pressure is noted as early as the first trimester and persists throughout gestation. Nevertheless, the best index of systemic vasodilatation is not blood pressure, but rather peripheral or systemic vascular resistance, which takes into consideration changes in both blood pressure and cardiac output during pregnancy, i.e. the increases in total systemic flow. Systemic vascular resistance is calculated by the equation:

$$\text{Systemic vascular resistance} = \frac{\text{Central arterial pressure} - \text{Central venous pressure}}{\text{Cardiac output}}$$

Because central venous pressure is generally very low (1–3 mmHg), this calculation can be estimated more easily as:

$$\text{Systemic vascular resistance} = \frac{\text{Mean arterial pressure}}{\text{Cardiac output}}$$

The combination of reduced blood pressure and increased cardiac output early in pregnancy indicate substantial decreases in systemic vascular resistance beginning well before the uterine vascular bed enlarges, placentation occurs, or uterine vascular resistance has changed to any great extent. Therefore, these changes reflect peripheral vasodilatation at a time when changes in the uteroplacental vascular bed cannot account for the observed systemic vasodilatation and rise in cardiac output. These data therefore dispel the theory that the systemic alterations merely reflect the formation of a "uterine arteriovenous shunt." Moreover, because blood and plasma volume expansion are not proportional in human pregnancy and hematocrit falls, blood viscosity will decrease. Since viscosity is inversely proportional to vascular resistance (*see* page 750), this may be one more mechanism contributing to the rise in systemic flow in pregnancy.

In view of the 40–80 per cent fall in systemic vascular resistance, surprisingly little attention has been paid to why substantial hypotension does not occur during normal pregnancy. If the above equation is reversed to evaluate pressure as the dependent variable, i.e.

> Mean arterial pressure
> = Systemic vascular resistance × Cardiac output

then as resistance falls, a rise in cardiac output will in part maintain blood pressure. Increases in blood volume as well as activation of both the renin–angiotensin–aldosterone system and the sympathetic division of the autonomic nervous system play key roles not only in maintaining blood pressure during this state of substantial vasodilatation, but also in the positive chronotropism of pregnancy. These systems function peripherally by vasoconstricting vascular smooth muscle of various resistance vascular beds. Determining the role of the integrative reflex functions of these systems on blood pressure and cardiac output control are quite invasive and thus have not been critically evaluated in human pregnancy.

Another important issue to consider is the redistribution of the increased cardiac output, which presently cannot be determined in pregnant women. In pregnant ewes, cardiac output increases by as much as 3.5 L/min (100 per cent) at term. Using radiolabeled microspheres (Fig. 74.11), the greatest increase in organ or tissue blood flow occurs in the uteroplacental vascular bed, from about 0.06 per cent of cardiac output in non-pregnant ewes to about 8 and 16 per cent at 60–100 and 130–140 days' gestation, respectively. Increases in mammary gland blood flow also occur, increasing 10-fold, from about 0.2 per cent of cardiac output in the non-pregnant ewe to about 2 per cent at term. It is unclear how much of the increase in uteroplacental blood flow late in gestation results in relative systemic "underfilling," thereby stimulating a further increase in cardiac output and blood volume via activation of the renin–angiotensin–aldosterone system, each of which is increased in pregnancy. However, when increases in blood flow to the gravid uterus and mammary gland are summed, only 1.5–2.0 L/min or 40–55 per cent of the observed increase in cardiac output can be accounted for. Therefore, 45–60 per cent of the increase in cardiac output is directed towards other systemic tissues and organs. Even though the proportion of cardiac output to non-reproductive tissues falls from 76 to 66 per cent, this actually reflects a 73 per cent increase in absolute blood flow to these tissues. In the skin, the largest organ in the body, blood flow per gram of tissue increases nearly 100 per cent. Studies in women also have suggested rather substantial increases in blood flow through the extremities as pregnancy progresses, supporting the hypothesis that blood flow to the skin may account for a substantial portion of the observed rise in cardiac output; however, this has not been critically evaluated. The percentage of cardiac output to other major organs falls, but there is little or no significant change in their absolute blood flows or blood flow per gram of tissue compared with uterine and mammary tissues, demonstrating that pregnancy is characterized by a substantial redistribution of cardiac output towards important reproductive tissues.

## FACTORS CONTROLLING THE UTERINE AND SYSTEMIC VASCULATURE IN PREGNANCY

Proposed factors involved in controlling the uteroplacental and systemic vascular changes that occur in normal pregnancy include estrogen, progesterone, prostaglandins, sympathetic and parasympathetic mediators of the autonomic nervous system, endothelial-derived relaxing factor (nitric oxide, NO), histamine, growth factors, and even $Ca^{2+}$ channel blockade. A conclusive direct cause-and-effect relationship has not been established between any of these substances or pathways and the pregnancy-associated alterations described.

Endogenous estrogen production by the fetoplacental unit is increased during gestation. The uterine and systemic vasodilatation found in normal pregnancy can be mimicked, in part, by exogenous estrogen (estradiol-17$\beta$, E$_2\beta$) administration to non-pregnant castrated sheep (Figs 74.12 and 74.13); these responses also are similar to the systemic responses of postmenopausal women treated with conjugated estrogens. In sheep, estrogen increases uterine blood flow, cardiac output, and blood volume while decreasing uterine and systemic vascular resistance. The uterine and systemic vascular beds vasodilate independently in response to estrogen, and furthermore, the uterine vascular bed is substantially more responsive than the systemic vascular bed (Fig. 74.12). The gradual rise in cardiac output with exogenous estrogen mirrors the pattern of increase in uterine blood flow, suggesting that they occur by similar mechanisms. However, the rise in cardiac output (systemic blood flow) could not be accounted for by the observed increase in uterine blood flow.

A somewhat different pattern of circulatory changes emerges when "pregnancy-like" concentrations of estradiol-17$\beta$ are achieved by infusion into non-pregnant sheep (Fig. 74.13). These include decreases in mean arterial blood pressure (8–10 per cent), systemic vascular resistance (40–50 per cent) and angiotensin II pressor responses, in association with increases in cardiac output, due to increases initially in heart rate but subsequently stroke volume, blood volume, plasma volume and red blood cell mass. The rise in stroke

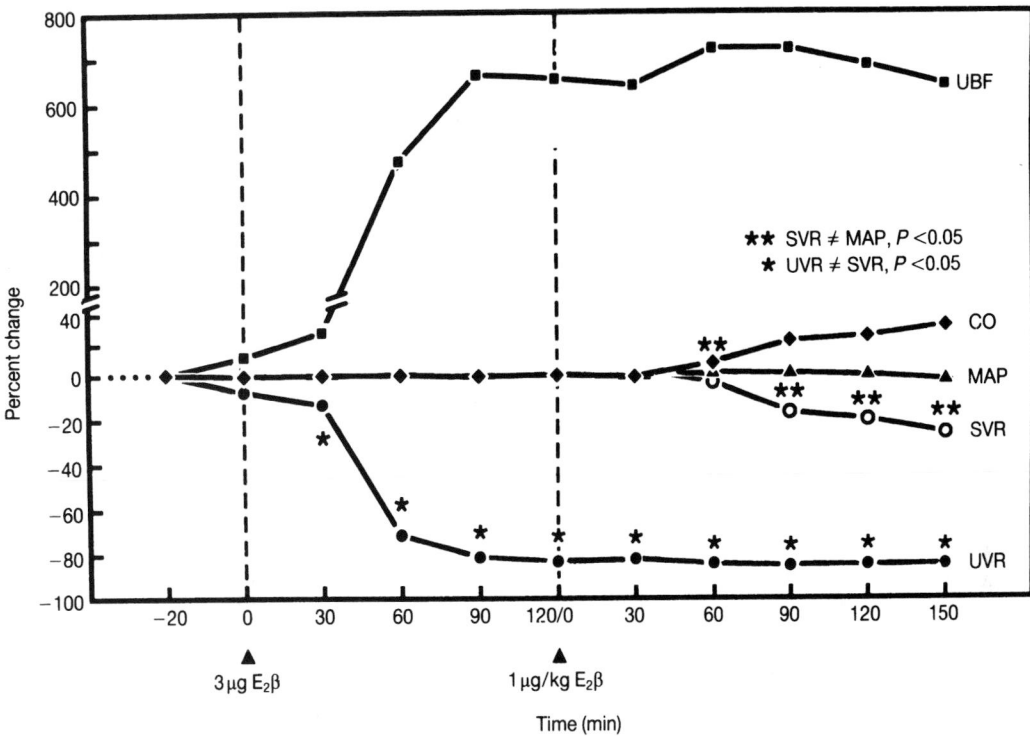

FIGURE 74.12 Effects of local and systemic estradiol-17β (E₂β) on relative responses of uterine blood flow (UBF), cardiac output (CO), mean arterial pressure (MAP), systemic vascular resistance (SVR), and uterine vascular resistance (UVR) in non-pregnant oophorectomized sheep. (From Magness RR, Rosenfeld CR. *Am J Physiol* 1989; **256**: E536, with permission.)

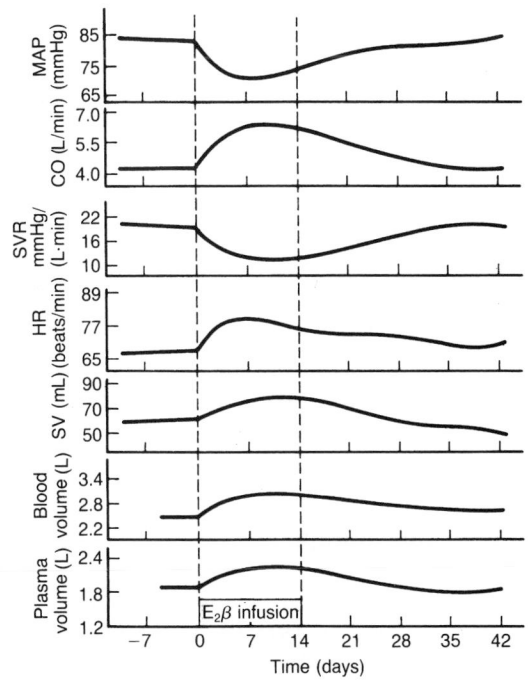

FIGURE 74.13 Effects of prolonged systemic (i.v.) estradiol-17β (E₂β) administration on daily responses of mean arterial pressure (MAP), cardiac output (CO), systemic vascular resistance (SVR), heart rate (HR), stroke volume (SV), blood volume, and plasma volume in non-pregnant oophorectomized sheep. (From Magness RR, *et al. Am J Physiol* 1993; **265**: E690, with permission.)

volume, but not heart rate, correlates with the estradiol-17β-induced increase in blood and plasma volume. Uterine blood flow initially increases but with time tachyphylaxis is observed. Thus for continued uterine vasodilatation, repetitive relatively high systemic concentrations of estradiol-17β or lower continuous local concentrations of estradiol-17β may be needed to increase, and then maintain elevated, uterine blood flow. It is unknown if progesterone also is needed to sustain the estrogen vasodilatory response in the uterine vascular bed as was observed in the systemic vasculature. In pregnancy the ovine uteroplacental vascular bed is not maximally vasodilated and has the capacity to further vasodilate after systemic administration of either estradiol-17β or its C₁₉-androgen precursor, dehydroepiandrosterone. Together these observations suggest that estrogen may be important in modulating and maintaining uteroplacental blood flow during pregnancy; however, cause-and-effect relationships have yet to be established fully. As with pregnancy, it also is not known whether estradiol-17β has a direct action on the vasculature to cause these uterine and/or systemic changes, or if an intermediary vasodilator is produced (e.g. prostacyclin or NO).

Although several investigators have suggested that the increase in prostaglandin production normally seen in pregnancy is necessary for the pregnancy-associated vasodilatation in both the systemic and uteroplacental vascular beds, data are available to question this conclusion. Decreases in prostaglandins of 40–70 per cent after systemic and local indomethacin infusion have no effect on basal blood flows or other cardiovascular parameters. Other mechanisms that need to be critically evaluated in this manner include NO production, growth factors and even progesterone. Thus the mechanisms responsible for the systemic and/or uteroplacental vasodilatation seen in pregnancy remain unclear.

## SELECTED READING

Cunningham FG, MacDonald PC, Gant NF. Maternal adaptations to pregnancy. In: Patterson L, ed. *Williams obstetrics*, Vol 18. Norwalk: Appleton and Lange, 1989.

Magness RR. Ovarian secretion and vascular function. In: Naftolin F, Sarrel PM, Gutmann JN, DeCherney AH, eds. *Cardiovascular and neurological function and ovarian secretions*, Vol 80. Norwell: Raven Press, 1990: 93.

Magness RR, Rosenfeld CR. Eicosanoids and the regulation of uteroplacental hemodynamics. In: Mitchell MD, ed. *Eicosanoids in reproduction*. Boca Raton: CRC Press, 1990: 139.

Magness RR, Rosenfeld CR. The role of steroid hormones in the control of uterine blood flow. In: Rosenfeld CR, ed. *The uterine circulation*, Vol 10. New York: Perinatology Press, 1989: 239.

Magness RR, Rosenfeld CR. Local and systemic estradiol-17β: effects on uterine and systemic vasodilatation. *Am J Physiol* 1989; **256**: E536.

Magness RR, Parker CR Jr, Rosenfeld CR. Systemic and uterine responses to chronic infusion of estradiol-17β . *Am J Physiol* 1993; **265**: E690.

Reynolds LP, Redmer DA. Studies of utero-placental growth and vascular development. *J Anim Sci* 1995; **73**: 1839.

Rosenfeld CR. Changes in uterine blood flow during pregnancy. In: Rosenfeld CR, ed. *The uterine circulation*, Vol 10. New York: Perinatology Press, 1989: 135.

# UMBILICAL–PLACENTAL AND UTERINE CIRCULATIONS

Development of an adequate, and increasing, blood flow to both maternal and fetal sides of the placenta is necessary for the increasing nutrient and respiratory demands of the fetus as it develops and grows throughout gestation. In both circulations of the placenta, this is achieved by a combination of remodeling or growth of vessels, the direct influence of vasoactive agents, and by systemic cardiovascular changes.

## UMBILICAL–PLACENTAL CIRCULATION

### Anatomy

The human fetal extracorporeal circulation is established by 6 weeks' gestation and adapts to continuous fetal growth and increasing demand throughout gestation so that at term about 40 per cent of fetal cardiac output (combined ventricular output) reaches the umbilical–placental circulation. The umbilical arteries branch from the internal iliac arteries and then run 30–60 cm within the cord without branching. The paired arteries and veins are embedded in a loose connective tissue, Wharton jelly, consisting of fibroblast-like stellate cells, dispersed in an extracellular matrix. A single layer of amnion cells lines the cord. The three vessels run parallel and are twisted an equal, though highly variable number of times, the twisting protecting the vessels from torsional forces. The vessels have the normal three layers, intima, muscular, and adventitia, each enclosed by a thin connective tissue sheath. Collagen fibers from the adventitia extend between the smooth muscle cells of the muscular layer and also into the Wharton jelly. The muscle fibers have a defined outer circular and inner layer, which in arteries contains small amounts of elastin and collagen, whereas the vein is richly endowed with connective tissue elements.

Endothelial cells, their basement membrane, and connective tissue constitute the intima. The vein, but not the artery, has an internal elastic lamina. The *in vivo* luminal diameter of the umbilical vein is 6–8 mm, and that of the arteries 3–4 mm. Hoboken nodules give the cord a segmental appearance, although the nodules do not appear to function as valves. The umbilical vessels are unusual in that they lack a nerve supply and do not have vasa vasorum, and therefore derive their nutrition by diffusion from the lumen or the amniotic fluid. The umbilical cord is inserted centrally or slightly off center on the chorionic plate of the placenta. The umbilical arteries each divide into two chorionic arteries, which then divide successively as they move towards the periphery to give first-, second-, third-, and sometimes fourth-order chorionic plate arteries. Each of these terminal umbilical arterial branches then penetrates the chorionic plate to become the stem artery of a cotyledon. Within the cotyledon, the arteries divide to give second, third, and fourth vessels, and finally villous vessels enter the chorionic villi. The previllous arterioles are the major resistance vessels of the placenta. The veins follow the arteries and all drain into the one umbilical vein.

## General physiology

Umbilical–placental blood flow increases throughout gestation; however, it decreases as a proportion of fetal cardiac output until at term it is 100–150 mL/(min · kg) (fetal weight) measured by Doppler flow. The flow in the two arteries presumably is equally distributed, but may be unequal in pathological pregnancies. The pressure in the umbilical artery is 40–50 mmHg (5.3–6.6 kPa) and 10 mmHg (1.3 kPa) in the vein. The corresponding blood $P_{O_2}$ and pH are 25 mmHg (3.3 kPa) and 7.30–7.35 and 45 mmHg

(6.0 kPa) and 7.37–7.40 for artery and vein, respectively. To accommodate the increasing flow, resistance in the umbilical–placental circulation normally decreases throughout gestation and can be characterized by an increase in end-diastolic flow velocity relative to peak systolic velocity when umbilical arterial flow velocity waveforms are examined by Doppler ultrasound. Such measurements in the umbilical vessels are indicative of downstream impedance in the villous tree. In pre-eclampsia and intrauterine growth retardation (IUGR), the normal gestational increase in end-diastolic velocity is not seen on ultrasound studies suggesting reduced flow. This correlates with a reduced number of vessels and a narrowing of the lumen and thickening of vessel walls in the villous vascular tree, which increases impedance. Blood flow in the umbilical–placental circulation may also be profoundly affected by changes in the fetal cardiovascular system that alter fetal systemic arterial pressure, and hence alter umbilical–placental perfusion pressure.

# Regulatory mechanisms

## General mechanisms

Changes in blood $Po_2$, $Pco_2$, and pH may affect umbilical blood flow. Decreases in $Po_2$ do not affect umbilical–placental flow in the sheep fetus, whereas flow is increased to the coronary, cerebral, and adrenal circulations. Hypoxemia and acidemia appear to favor the placenta, brain, and heart by redistribution of flow. Very high $Pco_2$ levels give small decreases in umbilical vascular resistance. Increasing maternal blood pressure in the intervillous space has been suggested to increase fetal–placental vascular resistance and, hence, reduce flow. However, this hypothesis has not been supported. Alterations in the hydrostatic pressure difference across the placenta, e.g. by reducing fetal arterial pressure, is suggested to increase maternal-to-fetal water flow, which would increase fetal venous backflow and cardiac output and restore umbilical pressure and flow. Maternal and fetal flows in the placenta may be matched as are ventilation/perfusion ratios in the lung. This would optimize $O_2$, nutrient, $CO_2$, and waste product exchange and requires an agent that easily crosses the placenta and has opposing (vasoconstrictor/vasodilator) effects on either side of the placenta. While prostaglandins have been considered as filling this role, conclusive experimental proof is lacking. Indeed, *in vitro* in human placenta, only 6 per cent of the $PGE_2$ and $PGF_{2\alpha}$ present in one placental circulation will cross to the other circulation, and the majority of that which crosses ends up as an inactive metabolite. Angiotensin II has also been considered as a possible mediator of perfusion matching. Vascular reactivity and the ability to produce vasoactive agents vary along the length of the umbilical–placental circulation with the umbilical veins responding

differently under certain conditions. The villous vascular tree is responsive to vasoactive agents and is the major determinant of resistance in the umbilical–placental circulation, accounting for about 90 per cent of the total resistance (umbilical veins account for the remainder). Vasoactive substances (autacoids) affect umbilical blood flow in two ways: (1) by altering perfusion pressure and/or fetal heart rate with no change in umbilical–placental vascular resistance, or (2) by directly altering umbilical–placental vascular resistance. The families of autacoids that may affect umbilical–placental vascular resistance include the renin–angiotensin system, the eicosanoids (arachidonic acid metabolites), catecholamines, and the endothelial-derived vasoactive factors, nitric oxide (NO) and endothelin.

## Adrenergic and cholinergic control

In isolated vessels, extremely high concentrations of adrenergic or cholinergic agents are necessary to affect vessel tone, suggesting no or slight physiological effects. Fetal cholinergic blockade increases umbilical blood flow secondary to increasing systemic pressure and heart rate. β-Adrenergic agonists given to the fetus increase umbilical blood flow and lower vascular resistance, whereas β-antagonists have opposite effects. α-Adrenergic agonists or antagonists do not alter umbilical blood flow. Although circulating catecholamines do not affect arteriolar tone, they do increase umbilical venous tone and almost certainly are responsible for the constriction of those vessels associated with hypoxemia. By increasing umbilical–placental outflow impedance, and thereby distending the veins and recruiting placental exchange area, this may improve gas exchange.

## Renin–angiotensin system

Both the umbilical vessels and the villous vascular tree are constricted by angiotensins I (AI) and II (AII) and also, surprisingly, by AIII, all of which act via the AII receptor and can be inhibited by receptor antagonists such as saralasin. AI acts following its conversion to AII by angiotensin converting enzyme (ACE), which is present in high concentrations in the vascular endothelium. ACE inhibitors should be used with great caution in pregnancy as they cross the placenta and may have detrimental effects on the fetus.

## Eicosanoids

Of the eicosanoids, thromboxane $A_2$ is a potent vasoconstrictor throughout the umbilical–placental circulation. The vasodilator prostaglandins, $PGD_2$, $PGE_1$, and $PGI_2$ (prostacyclin) cannot affect resting tone *in vitro*, suggesting that the umbilical–placental circulation is maximally vasodilated. However, all three of these eicosanoids will relax the preconstricted umbilical–placental circulation. The rank order of their potency suggests they all act via a PGI$_2$ receptor. Increased synthesis of PGI$_2$ and PGE is found when the umbilical–placental circulation is constricted, for example by AII, suggesting these eicosanoids act as compensatory vasodilators to attenuate the actions of vasoconstrictors. However, prevention of prostaglandin synthesis by cyclooxygenase inhibitors does not affect resting tone, suggesting that prostaglandins are not major determinants of resting tone in the umbilical–placental circulation. The responsiveness of the umbilical–placental circulation to these autacoids appears to be greatest at the placental end of the circulation, i.e. in the villous resistance vessels. Increased synthesis and release of thromboxane and decreased synthesis and release of PGI$_2$ by maternal and fetal vessels purportedly is characteristic of placental insufficiency syndromes, including pre-eclampsia and IUGR and may contribute to the altered indices of fetal–placental vascular resistance measured by Doppler ultrasound in vivo. Low-dose aspirin therapy (80 mg/day), which selectively inhibits thromboxane synthesis while leaving PGI$_2$ synthesis relatively unchanged, is reported to increase fetal–placental blood flow and to improve outcome in some patients thought to be at risk of IUGR on the evidence of altered umbilical blood flow velocity waveform indices. The peptidyl leukotrienes C$_4$, D$_4$ and E$_4$ are also vasoconstrictors of the umbilical–placental circulation in vitro.

## Endothelin (ET) and other vasoactive peptides (see pages 700 and 751 for further details)

The endothelins are a family of 21 amino acid peptides (ET-1, ET-2, and ET-3) coded for by three separate genes. They are potent, long-acting (45–60 min) vasoconstrictors and usually have greater potency on veins than on arteries. The genes for ET-1 and ET-3 are expressed in human placenta. Both ET-1 and ET-3 are potent vasoconstrictors of the human fetal–placental circulation in vitro. The precursor 39-amino-acid peptide big ET-1 is also a vasoconstrictor in vitro, but is less potent than ET-1. The action of big ET-1 appears to be indirect following its conversion to ET-1 by a converting enzyme (ECE, a neutral metalloprotease) in the fetal–placental circulation.

Receptors for ET-1 have been demonstrated in the smooth muscle of the umbilical, chorionic plate and villous vasculatures and also in the syncytiotrophoblast. The selective ET$_A$ receptor subtype (ET-1 and ET-2 > ET-3) predominates in the chorionic plate vessels, whereas the non-selective ET$_B$ receptor (ET-1 = ET-2 = ET-3) is found in the veins of stem villi and blood vessels of distal regions of the villous tree. In pre-eclampsia, which is associated with increased fetal–placental vascular resistance, increased or unaltered umbilical plasma ET-1 concentrations have been reported in comparison with normotensive pregnancies. No differences in ET receptors have been reported in pre-eclamptic pregnancies.

Other peptide hormones that are vasoactive in the umbilical–placental circulation include calcitonin gene-related peptide (CGRP), corticotropin releasing hormone (CRH), parathyroid hormone (PTH), PTH-related peptide (PTHrP) and the natriuretic peptides, atrial natriuretic peptide (ANP) and brain natriuretic peptide (BNP), all of which are vasodilators in vitro, and vasoactive intestinal peptide (VIP), a vasoconstrictor (see below). ANP is a much weaker vasodilator than BNP and also than NO or PGI$_2$ in this vasculature. Receptors for ANP have been described in the human fetal–placental vasculature. ANP and BNP are synthesized and released by the fetal cardiac atria and ventricles and may act as circulating stress hormones in the fetus. Increased concentrations of BNP have been measured in cord blood of distressed fetuses.

## Endothelial-derived relaxing factor/NO (see pages 697 and 751 for further details)

Endothelial-derived relaxing factors (EDRFs) are found in the umbilical–placental circulation. Umbilical cord and chorionic plate vessels appear to produce very little of these but will relax in response to them if the vessels are preconstricted. One major EDRF appears to be NO, which acts as a vasodilator via stimulation of vascular smooth muscle cGMP production to cause relaxation. Agents that generate NO will vasodilate the villous vascular tree preconstricted in vitro with either thromboxane mimetics, ET, bradykinin, serotonin, or AII. By using competitive substrate inhibitors of the NO synthase (NOS) enzyme, which forms NO and L-citrulline from the basic amino acid L-arginine, it has been shown that endogenous NO synthesis contributes to maintenance of the low resting tone of the fetal–placental circulation and that it attenuates the actions of vasoconstrictors in vitro. The major stimulus to NO synthesis in placental vessels may be hydrodynamic, possibly shear stress related. The small resistance vessels of the villous vascular tree appear to have a greater capacity to produce NO than the larger umbilical or chorionic plate vessels. In pre-eclampsia, the ability of umbilical cord arteries and veins to produce NO in vitro is significantly reduced compared with vessels from normotensive pregnancies, suggesting that, like PGI$_2$, a deficiency of NO synthesis may be associated with increased vascular resistance and reduced flow. Synthesis of NO is greater in arteries than veins and may account for the lower potency of ET in arteries than in veins.

NOS exists in at least three distinct isoforms. The endothelial isoform, ecNOS, has been localized to the endothelium of umbilical, chorionic plate and stem villous vessels, but is not seen in the capillary endothelium of the terminal villi where there is no underlying smooth muscle. Further, ecNOS is also found in syncytiotrophoblast, but not the underlying progenitor cytotrophoblast cell layer. The function of syncytiotrophoblast-derived NO is probably to prevent platelet adhesion to the syncytiotrophoblast surface and platelet aggregation in the intervillous space. There are no conclusive reports of altered placental NOS activity in pre-eclampsia. Immunohistochemical ecNOS distribution and intensity appear similar in normotensive, pre-eclamptic and intrauterine growth restricted pregnancies. However, in pre-eclampsia, vessels in the terminal villous region which have thickened walls and narrow lumens show ecNOS immunostaining in their endothelium in contrast to the absence in terminal villous capillary endothelium of normotensive pregnancy. This may be an adaptive response to the altered vascular tone and blood flow seen in the pre-eclamptic placenta.

## UTEROPLACENTAL CIRCULATION

### Anatomy

Uterine blood flow must increase during pregnancy both to the myometrium and to the decidua and intervillous space of the placenta. The uterine artery arises from the hypogastric or internal iliac artery, descends to the broad ligament and crosses towards the uterus, then divides into the cervicovaginal artery and the ascending uterine artery. The latter vessel runs along the uterus and gives a major branch to the upper portion of the cervix and 8–24 arcuate branches to the uterus. The arcuate arteries are usually paired, traversing the uterus anteriorly and posteriorly within the outer one-third of the myometrium and anastomozing with the vessels from the other side. The radial arteries branch from the arcuate arteries to supply the inner two-thirds of the myometrium and terminate in the spiral arteries, which supply endometrium, decidua, and placenta. The ascending branch of the uterine artery ends as it reaches the fallopian tube, where it trifurcates to the fundal, tubal, and ovarian branch. The ovarian branch anastomoses with the uterine artery. The spiral arteries supply the endometrium in the non-pregnant uterus and undergo a physiological adaptation to accommodate the increased flow of pregnancy. In the first trimester of pregnancy, extravillous trophoblast migrates in a retrograde manner down the spiral arteries and removes the endothelial and musculoelastic layers of the artery and replaces them with fibrinoid. In the second trimester, the adaptation continues into the myometrial portion of the spiral arteries, the net result being conversion of the tortuous narrow spiral arteries to flaccid, distended vessels with no musculoelastic elements. This implies that the response of these resistance vessels to neural or humoral agents is lost. In pre-eclampsia and IUGR, the secondary wave of trophoblast invasion is absent and some spiral arteries within the placental bed do not appear to be invaded at all, the net result being an increase in vascular resistance and reduction in flow

of up to 50 per cent, which can be estimated *in vivo* by Doppler ultrasound measurements in the arcuate arteries. The known uteroplacental pathology associated with these conditions makes it likely that the increased impedance is due to the lack of structural alteration of the spiral arteries rather than an alteration in vascular reactivity.

## Physiology

As fetal demands increase, uterine blood flow increases 20–80-fold during pregnancy by virtue of vasodilatation and growth of the vascular bed. At term, human uterine blood flow may be up to 800 mL/min or 10–20 per cent of cardiac output. The majority of this flow (80 per cent) is diverted through the spiral arteries to the intervillous space of the placenta.

## Regulatory mechanisms

The vasoactive agents to which the uteroplacental circulation is likely to respond include the same families of autacoids that act on the fetal–placental circulation. The unique features of the uteroplacental circulation include the flaccid distended spiral arteries and the intervillous space that will not respond to neural or humoral agents. Blood flow through these vessels is thus determined by the reactivity of the larger uterine, arcuate, and radial arteries and by systemic cardiovascular changes. What effect the absence of the secondary wave or the total lack of trophoblast invasion of spiral arteries in pre-eclampsia or IUGR have on uterine vascular reactivity remains to be determined. Overall uterine blood flow has two components: to the myometrium and to the placental intervillous space. Vascular reactivity studies in species such as sheep in which the maternal placenta has a resistance bed obviously bear no relationship to the hemomonochorial human placenta with invaded spiral arteries and an intervillous space with no vascular response elements.

### Innervation

The uterus is richly supplied with sympathetic and parasympathetic fibers. There is a reduction in transmitter substances and neural elements in the uterus during pregnancy; this accounts for the reduced response to autonomic agonists in pregnancy. The maximal vasodilatation of the uterine circulation makes it difficult to demonstrate vasodilatation to local β-adrenergic stimulation. There are very few or no data for autoregulation, i.e. alteration of resistance to maintain constant flow when perfusion is altered, in the human uterine circulation.

## Steroid hormones, uterine blood flow, and NO

The large increases in estrogen and progesterone synthesis in pregnancy and the correlation with changes in blood flow in pregnancy make the steroid hormones potential candidates for regulating blood flow. Estradiol infusion in non-pregnant animals significantly increases uterine blood flow by a mechanism that is dependent on RNA and protein synthesis with a time delay of 20–30 min. Progesterone alone has no effect on uterine blood flow, but will attenuate the estradiol effect. The search for the mediator of this estrogen-induced hyperemia has proved elusive. Recent data suggest that NO may mediate a large proportion of the estrogen-induced increase in uterine blood flow as competitive substrate inhibitors of NO synthesis appear to antagonize the effect in experimental animals. In pregnant animals, increases in uterine NOS activity have been measured and NOS inhibitors decrease uterine blood flow suggesting that increased NOS activity mediates the increased uterine blood flow of pregnancy. Estrogen has been shown to stimulate ecNOS activity in some tissues. As indicated above, there are at least three isoforms of NOS and blood vessels appear to possess both the "constitutive" and "inducible" forms. The latter form appears to be stimulated by cytokines and inhibited by glucocorticoids, which also inhibit estrogen-induced hyperemia.

Chronic administration of NOS inhibitors in pregnant rats produces a pre-eclampsia-like syndrome with increased mean arterial pressure, loss of refractoriness to pressors such as AII, decreased fetal weight, and placental necrosis and infarction and renal glomerular swelling. While this evidence has been suggested to define a role for NO deficiency in the etiology of pre-eclampsia, it more likely highlights the major role that NO plays as an active vasodilator agent in normal physiological circumstances.

## Endothelin

ET-1 is also a vasoconstrictor of the uterine circulation in animals. The contribution of circulating ET in humans is unclear as concentrations are below the threshold necessary to activate ET receptors. Subthreshold concentrations of ET may, however, increase the sensitivity of vessels to other vasoconstrictors. In pre-eclampsia, disparate findings of either unaltered or increased maternal and fetal ET-1 concentrations have been reported.

## Renin–angiotensin system

The ovine uteroplacental circulation is vasoconstricted by AII; however, the responsiveness is less than that of the systemic vasculature. The greater increase in systemic resistance with AII sometimes indirectly increases uterine blood flow, falsely suggesting that AII is a uterine vasodilator. Such observations serve to illustrate the interaction between perfusion pressure, vascular resistance, and blood flow in the uterine circulation and the potential dangers of systemic vasodilatation during pregnancy. The reduced reactivity of the uteroplacental circulation to AII, concentrations of which are increased during pregnancy, has been associated with an increase in $PGI_2$ production by this vasculature in pregnancy. Of course, increased NO synthesis also must now be considered. Blockade of prostaglandin synthesis with indomethacin does not affect resting uterine blood flow in late-gestation pregnant sheep but potentiates the response to AII, suggesting that as in the fetal placental circulation vasodilator prostaglandins attenuate the actions of vasoconstrictors. Indeed, AII acting via its receptors increases $PGI_2$ production in isolated uterine vessels.

## Eicosanoids

Whole-body and uterine vessel synthesis of $PGI_2$ is increased during pregnancy, this perhaps being hormonally regulated, but also possibly arising from increasing flow and/or shear stress over endothelial cells in the vasculature. In pre-eclampsia and IUGR, there is a generalized deficiency of $PGI_2$ synthesis relative to thromboxane when compared with normotensive pregnancy, and reactivity to AII is increased. This deficiency of $PGI_2$ is associated with the increased vascular resistance of these conditions. This may be more important in the uteroplacental circulation, where $PGI_2$ plays a greater role in attenuating the action of vasoconstrictors.

## Peptide hormones

The presence of unidentified factors that mediate non-adrenergic non-cholinergic nervous control of uterine function has been recognized for a long time. These could include the peptides such as VIP, neuropeptide Y, CGRP, and also radicals such as NO. VIP, a 28-amino-acid peptide present in female genital nerves, can produce a dose-related increase in myometrial and total uterine blood flow in non-pregnant animals, an effect not mediated via α- or β-adrenergic receptors. Neuropeptide Y, a 36-amino-acid peptide with both N- and C-terminal tyrosines and structural homology to other peptides of the pancreatic polypeptide family, is a potent vasoconstrictor in the myometrial circulation *in vitro*. CGRP, a 37-amino-acid peptide derived from alternative tissue-specific RNA splicing and transcription of the calcitonin gene, has no structural similarity to calcitonin. CGRP may be distributed in the same nerve fibers as substance P, and CGRP-immunoreactive nerve fibers are found adjacent to blood vessels. CGRP is a potent inhibitor of smooth muscle activity.

## Calcium channel blockers

An increase in intracellular $Ca^{2+}$ is a common denominator in smooth muscle contraction. A vast array of agents have the ability to block $Ca^{2+}$ influx and have dramatic effects on both uterine vascular and myometrial tissue. The $Ca^{2+}$ channel blockers do appear to cross the placenta. In addition to any direct effect on the uteroplacental vasculature, the systemic cardiovascular effects of $Ca^{2+}$ channel blockers will influence uterine perfusion. In pregnant ewes, the dihydropyridine, nifedipine, infused at $10 \, \mu g/(min \cdot kg)$ gives a 22-per cent reduction in maternal peripheral resistance, a slight but significant decrease in maternal arterial pressure, an increase in heart rate, and a 21-per cent reduction in uterine blood flow despite no change in uterine vascular resistance. The decrease in uterine blood flow therefore is due to the maternal systemic hypotensive effect. A significant decline in fetal arterial blood hemoglobin $O_2$ saturation and a tendency to fetal hypoxemia and acidemia is seen. Similar effects are seen in the primate, where transfer of dihydropyridines to the fetus is low, suggesting rather that changes in fetal oxygenation are secondary to decreases in maternal systemic arterial blood pressure. The limited number of human studies at present using dihydropyridines as tocolytics show no apparent deleterious effects on neonatal outcome. In human chorionic plate vessels, the dihydropyridines, nifedipine and nitrendipine, give concentration-dependent inhibition of agonist-induced contractile activity, suggesting that $Ca^{2+}$ channel blockers would increase placental perfusion, although this has not been confirmed in vivo.

## Smoking, recreational drugs, and exercise

Nicotine from cigarette smoking produces a systemic sympathomimetic effect of elevated heart rate and blood pressure. Smoking in pregnancy results in lower-birthweight babies due either to lower prenatal weight gain in the mother or to direct fetal effects of nicotine or carbon monoxide. In pregnant sheep, nicotine or simulated cigarette smoking do not have an acute effect on uterine blood flow, although constant infusion of nicotine may chronically reduce uterine blood flow. Human intervillous blood flow is reported to decrease acutely about 20 per cent by smoking a single cigarette. Cocaine stimulates the central nervous system, producing sympathetic stimulation, increased heart rate and blood pressure, and vasoconstriction. An increased incidence of cerebrovascular accidents and placental abruption is associated with cocaine use. The response to cocaine appears to be heightened during pregnancy in sheep and somehow is related to

increased circulating progesterone concentrations. Low doses of intravenous cocaine are reported to increase uterine vascular resistance by up to 52 per cent in the pregnant sheep. There is no evidence that heroin affects uteroplacental perfusion. Exercise during pregnancy decreased uterine blood flow in animal models in direct relationship to the intensity of exercise, probably by redistribution of cardiac output and by increasing catecholamines. Women who exercise vigorously in pregnancy have lighter infants than do sedentary women.

## Local anesthetics

Local anesthetics, bupivacaine, lidocaine, and chloroprocaine can decrease uterine blood flow and uterine activity in the pregnant ewe in vivo, but only at concentrations exceeding those seen during epidural block for labor and delivery. Epidural or spinal anesthesia that results in maternal hypotension can produce a decrease in uterine blood flow and affect fetal well-being as a consequence of decreasing uterine perfusion pressure. In part, these effects may be related to placing the patient in the supine position. Well-conducted regional anesthesia without hypotension and supine positioning do not have a detrimental effect on uterine blood flow or fetal well-being. In some studies, an increase in uterine blood flow is seen in patients with epidural analgesia, especially those with pregnancy-induced hypertension, probably by reduction of blood epinephrine and norepinephrine concentrations.

## SELECTED READING

Battaglia FC, Meschia G. *An introduction to fetal physiology.* Orlando: Academic Press, 1986.

Brinkman CR III. Circulation in the pregnant uterus. In: Carsten ME, Miller JD, eds. *Uterine function, molecular and cellular aspects.* New York: Plenum Press, 1990: 519.

Kaufmann P. Basic morphology of the fetal and maternal circuits in the human placenta. In: Schneider H, Dancis J, eds. In vitro *perfusion of human placental tissue. Contributions to Gynecology and Obstetrics, Vol 13.* Basel: Karger, 1985: 5.

Magness RR, Rosenfeld CR. Eicosanoids and the regulation of uteroplacental hemodynamics. In: Mitchell MD, ed. *Eicosanoids in reproduction.* Boca Raton: CRC Press, 1990: 139.

Myatt L. Current Topic: Control of vascular resistance in the human placenta. *Placenta* 1992; **13**: 329.

Myatt L, Brockman DE, Eis ALW, Pollock JS. Immunohistochemical localization of nitric oxide synthase in the human placenta. *Placenta* 1993; **14**: 487.

Page K. *The physiology of the human placenta.* London: UCL Press, 1993.

# 75

# Oyxgen Transport and Consumption

George Lister

## RELATION BETWEEN OXYGEN TRANSPORT AND OXYGEN CONSUMPTION

Transport of oxygen ($O_2$) from the environment to the tissues requires the integration of three organ systems: the lungs, the circulation, and the blood. The pressure gradient for $O_2$ drives the diffusion from atmosphere to the blood in the lungs and from the blood to the tissues in the periphery, whereas convection is responsible for transport of $O_2$ from the lungs to the periphery. At rest transport of $O_2$ to the tissues is in great excess of metabolic rate or $O_2$ consumption. This buffer between transport and consumption of $O_2$ permits modest reductions in $O_2$ transport to be tolerated without any change in $O_2$ consumption. With stress such as exercise or fever, $O_2$ consumption increases abruptly, as does $O_2$ transport. These observations are used as evidence that metabolic rate usually dictates the level of $O_2$ transport rather than the converse. However, little $O_2$ is stored in the body. Therefore, severe reductions in $O_2$ transport or marked increases in metabolic demands can quickly exhaust the usual reserve and cause hypoxia, a mismatch between $O_2$ supply and demand, unless these organ systems can respond to restore the balance. These integrated responses, which are central adaptations to virtually all forms of cardiorespiratory disturbances, are the focus of this chapter.

The rate of $O_2$ transport to the tissues (Fig. 75.1) can be quantified as the systemic $O_2$ transport (SOT or $\dot{Q}_{O_2}$), the product of cardiac output or systemic blood flow ($\dot{Q}$) and arterial blood $O_2$ concentration ($C_a O_2$)

$$SOT = \dot{Q} \times C_a O_2$$

SOT here is expressed in vol of $O_2/t$, $\dot{Q}$ is in vol blood/$t$, and $C_a O_2$ is in vol $O_2$/vol blood. $C_a O_2$ is a function of hemoglobin concentration (Hb), arterial blood hemoglobin $O_2$ saturation ($S_a O_2$), and arterial blood $O_2$ pressure or tension ($P_a O_2$) as follows:

$$C_a O_2 = (Hb \times S_a O_2 \times 1.34) + (P_a O_2 \times 0.003)$$

where Hb is in g/dL blood; $S_a O_2$ is a fraction; $P_a O_2$ is in mmHg; the $O_2$-carrying capacity of hemoglobin, 1.34, is in mL $O_2$/g Hb; and 0.003, the solubility of $O_2$ in blood, is in mL $O_2$/(dL blood·mmHg). These equations demonstrate that $O_2$ transport may be decreased by reductions in cardiac output (stagnant hypoxia), hemoglobin concentration (anemic hypoxia), or $P_a O_2$ or $S_a O_2$ (hypoxic hypoxia).

As $O_2$ is consumed from the blood by the tissues in the periphery it must be taken up in the lung at an equal rate. Therefore $O_2$ consumption ($\dot{V}_{O_2}$) can be quantified from either of two methods: (1) measurements of respiratory gas concentrations and volumes or (2) measurements of arterial and mixed venous blood $O_2$ contents ($C_a O_2$ and $C_{\bar{v}} O_2$, respectively) and blood flow ($\dot{Q}$). Each approach has its merits and unique problems.

## Method 1

Measurement of the net $O_2$ flow entering and leaving the respiratory system can be obtained quite precisely and non-invasively according to the following mass balance (Fig. 75.1):

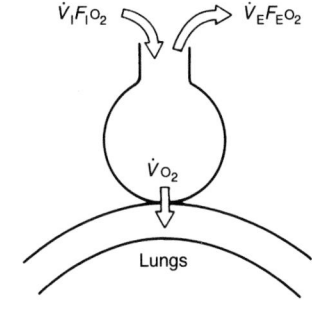

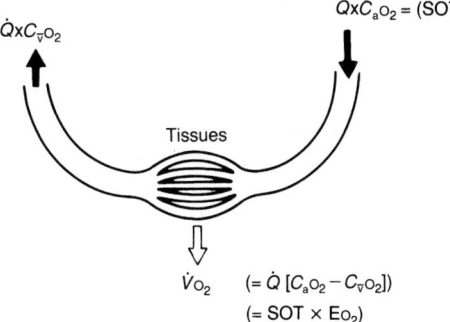

FIGURE 75.1 Mass balance for $O_2$ showing $O_2$ consumption ($\dot{V}_{O_2}$) at the lungs and at the tissues. The schema demonstrates the principle for two methods of measuring $O_2$ consumption, from respiratory gases or from blood flow and blood $O_2$ contents. The schema also shows that the product of systemic blood flow ($\dot{Q}$) and arterial $O_2$ content ($C_aO_2$) is systemic $O_2$ transport, which can be related to $O_2$ consumption by the fractional $O_2$ extraction ($E_{O_2}$).

$$\dot{V}_{O_2} = [\dot{V}_I \times F_IO_2] - [\dot{V}_E \times F_EO_2]$$

where $F_IO_2$ and $F_EO_2$ are the fractional concentrations of $O_2$ in inspired and expired gas, respectively, and $\dot{V}_I$ and $\dot{V}_E$ are the volumes of inspired and expired gas, respectively (corrected to STPD conditions). Even though gas concentrations can be measured in inspired gas, it is usually difficult or cumbersome to quantify inspired gas volume accurately; therefore, it is common to collect only expired gas and to determine inspired volume from expired volume by correcting for changes in nitrogen ($N_2$) concentration because there is no net consumption or production of $N_2$ in the steady state. Therefore,

$$\dot{V}_I \times F_IN_2 = \dot{V}_E \times F_EN_2$$

or

$$\dot{V}_I = \dot{V}_E \frac{1 - F_EO_2 - F_ECO_2}{1 - F_IO_2 - F_ICO_2}$$

because ($F_{N_2} + F_{O_2} + F_{CO_2} = 1$). Finally, when there is no $CO_2$ in inspired gas, $\dot{V}_{O_2}$ is most easily calculated from the following equation:

$$\dot{V}_{O_2} = \dot{V}_E \frac{F_IO_2[1 - F_EO_2 - F_ECO_2]}{[1 - F_IO_2] - F_EO_2}$$

It may be technically difficult to measure $O_2$ consumption in children whose trachea is intubated with an uncuffed tube owing to potential air leaks around the tube (loss of $\dot{V}_E$). It also is apparent from the above equation that there is potential for inaccuracy when the inspired $O_2$ concentration is high because $(1 - F_IO_2)$ approaches 0 and small measurement errors are magnified; therefore, when inspired $O_2$ concentration is 100 per cent, inspired and expired gas volumes must be known, or other approaches must be used. Variations on the above equations can be used to measure $\dot{V}_{O_2}$ by a flow-through technique in which air is drawn by the face of a subject at a constant rate and mixed expired gas is sampled for $O_2$ and $CO_2$ concentrations. This has the advantage that it neither requires a sealed system nor cooperation by the subject, so it is particularly useful in infants.

## Method 2

Alternatively, by rearranging the Fick equation for cardiac output $\dot{V}_{O_2}$ can be determined by invasive means using a mass balance (Fig. 75.1) without concern for the inspired gas concentrations or sources of air leak.

$$\dot{V}_{O_2} = \dot{Q}(C_aO_2 - C_{\bar{v}}O_2)$$

However, this approach is less precise owing to difficulties in measuring blood flow.

From these concepts it is apparent that SOT and $\dot{V}_{O_2}$ can be related to each other by multiplying the above equation by $C_aO_2/C_aO_2$ and regrouping terms, which yields:

$$\dot{V}_{O_2} = \dot{Q} \times C_aO_2 \times \frac{C_aO_2 - C_{\bar{v}}O_2}{C_aO_2}$$

or

$$\dot{V}_{O_2} = SOT \times E_{O_2}$$

where $(C_aO_2 - C_{\bar{v}}O_2)/C_aO_2$ is the fractional $O_2$ extraction, $E_{O_2}$. This equation shows clearly that any decrease in SOT must be attended by a comparable increase in $O_2$ extraction if $\dot{V}_{O_2}$ is to be maintained constant. Furthermore, because the fractional $O_2$ extraction is generally in the range of 0.25–0.30 under normal conditions, this equation also emphasizes the usual abundance of $O_2$ transport even though $\dot{V}_{O_2}$ and $O_2$ transport undergo substantial changes from birth to maturity.

# $O_2$ UPTAKE IN THE LUNGS

## Normal gas exchange

Before considering the developmental changes in $O_2$ transport and the adaptive responses to specific disturbances, it is important to understand the factors that influence the components of $O_2$ transport, cardiac output and arterial blood $O_2$ content. The focus here will be on pulmonary gas exchange and its effect on arterial oxygenation.

As $O_2$ is taken up in the lung $CO_2$ is eliminated, and the ratio of $O_2$ consumption to $CO_2$ production is the respiratory gas exchange ratio, $R$, which is dictated by the metabolic fuels being utilized. $O_2$ uptake and $CO_2$ elimination occur because mixed venous blood normally comes into close proximity with inspired air across the alveolar–capillary membrane where complete equilibrium of pressure between the blood and gas phase is attained for both respiratory gases. The resultant $Po_2$ (or $Pco_2$) in pulmonary capillary blood is determined by that equilibrium.

For any given metabolic rate, the arterial blood $Pco_2$ ($P_aco_2$) is normally controlled by changes in alveolar ventilation.

In contrast to the regulation of $P_aco_2$, factors other than overall alveolar ventilation influence the arterial blood $Po_2$ ($P_ao_2$) during both physiological and pathological conditions. To understand these it is useful first to consider an alveolar–capillary unit under static conditions; the equilibrium $Po_2$ would be a function of the volume of $O_2$ in the gas phase (inspired air) relative to that in the blood phase (mixed venous blood) and the movement of $O_2$ from one phase to the other would result from the $Po_2$ gradient. During dynamic conditions, the equilibrium $Po_2$ depends on the respective volume flow of $O_2$ in inspired gas (which is a function of the inspired $Po_2$ and the alveolar ventilation) and in mixed venous blood (which is a function of mixed venous blood $O_2$ content and pulmonary capillary blood flow). In any alveolar–capillary unit, capillary blood $Po_2$ will be closer to inspired $Po_2$ when the ratio of alveolar ventilation to capillary perfusion ($\dot{V}_A/\dot{Q}_c$ or $\dot{V}/\dot{Q}$) is high, and conversely capillary blood $Po_2$ will be lower if $\dot{V}/\dot{Q}$ is low. Normally $\dot{V}/\dot{Q}$ varies throughout the lung within a narrow range (mean = 0.8 with most units between 0.5 and 2.0); $\dot{V}/\dot{Q}$ is relatively high in the apices and lower at the bases in the upright individual, owing primarily to the effect of gravity on blood flow distribution. The mean (weighted by volume of blood) pulmonary capillary blood $O_2$ content from all of the alveolar–capillary units determines the arterial blood $O_2$ content (which thereby determines the arterial blood $Po_2$). Without detailed knowledge of ventilation and perfusion in all regions of the lung, it is not possible to predict the (volume-weighted) mean pulmonary capillary blood $O_2$ content (or pulmonary capillary blood $Po_2$). However, if the entire lung were assumed to be uni-

form with respect to $\dot{V}/\dot{Q}$, an ideal alveolar $Po_2$ ($P_Ao_2$) or ideal pulmonary capillary blood $Po_2$ ($P_{c'}o_2$) can be estimated and this represents the highest value possible for arterial blood $Po_2$ ($P_ao_2$), so it is a useful first-order estimate of an expected $P_ao_2$ with normal gas exchange (Fig. 75.2). The ideal alveolar $Po_2$ is the pressure of $O_2$ in the alveolar gas after equilibrium is reached; it can be derived conceptually for the whole lung from knowledge of: (1) the inspired $Po_2$ (where $P_Io_2 = [P_B - P_{H_2O}]F_Io_2$; $P_B$ is barometric pressure, $P_{H_2O}$ is water vapor pressure at body temperature, and $F_Io_2$ is the fraction of $O_2$ in inspired gas), (2) the decrease in $Po_2$ that occurs when $O_2$ moves from gas into blood and (3) the overall $R$. Since the $O_2$ leaving the alveolus is replaced by $CO_2$ in a ratio, $R$, and the $CO_2$ pressure in the alveolus can be approximated from arterial blood $Pco_2$ ($P_aco_2$) then:

$$P_Ao_2 \approx P_Io_2 - \frac{P_aCO_2}{R}$$

## Causes and quantitation of hypoxemia

Two common pathological processes cause arterial blood $Po_2$ ($P_ao_2$) to be decreased relative to ideal alveolar $Po_2$ ($P_Ao_2$) and result in an increased alveolar-arterial $Po_2$ difference (AaDo$_2$) (Table 75.1).

■ When mixed venous blood bypasses ventilated alveoli there is true right-to-left shunt and this produces venous admixture and arterial hypoxemia. Right-to-left shunting can occur within the lung from alveolar consolidation or collapse, within the heart associated with certain congenital cardiac malformations, or through vascular connections, e.g. patent ductus arteriosus in the presence of pulmonary hypertension. The normal child has an AaDo$_2$ of about 5–10 mmHg in room air owing to shunting through the bronchial and thebesian circulations.

■ When there is marked $\dot{V}/\dot{Q}$ heterogeneity (Fig. 75.3), hypoxemia is produced even though each alveolar–capillary unit may achieve $Po_2$ equilibrium (i.e. $P_Ao_2 = P_{c'}o_2$). The hypoxemia occurs when the subject breathes room air or a relatively low $F_Io_2$ because the reduced $Po_2$ of capillary blood from the low $\dot{V}/\dot{Q}$ areas does more to depress the overall $O_2$ content than the blood from the high $\dot{V}/\dot{Q}$ does to increase it; this, in turn, is caused by the curvilinear shape of the hemoglobin–$O_2$ dissociation curve and the increased contribution of the low $\dot{V}/\dot{Q}$ (i.e. relatively high $\dot{Q}$ ) areas to the overall weighted mean for blood flow.

Diffusion impairment is another reason often cited as a cause for hypoxemia and an increased AaDo$_2$; however, it is unclear whether this is an important consideration except under very unusual circumstances in children. Although hypoxemia can also be caused by

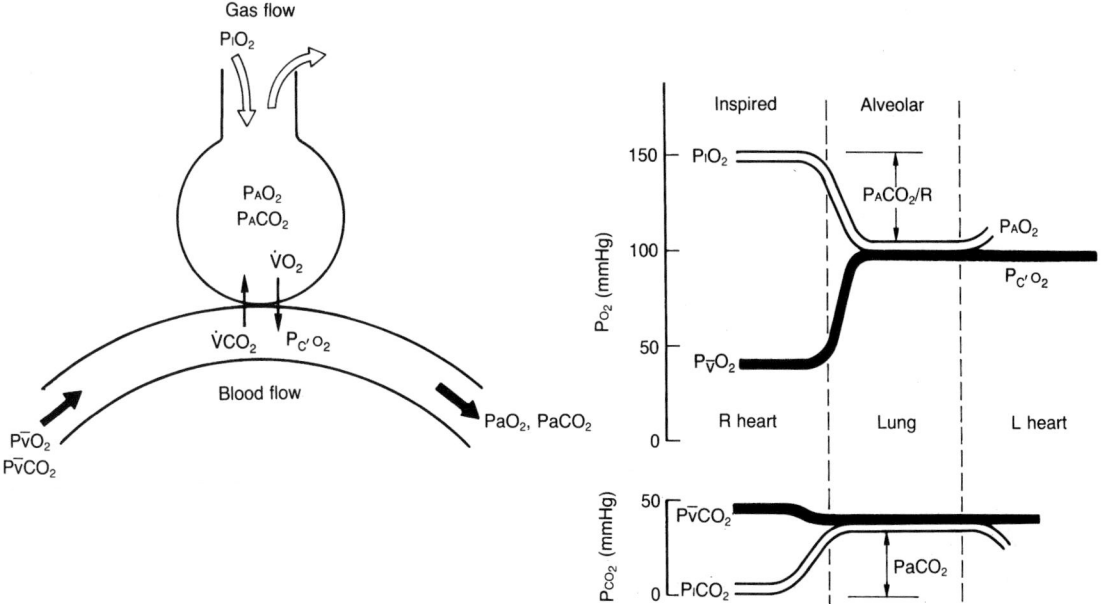

FIGURE 75.2 The determination of alveolar $P_{O_2}$ ($P_{A}O_2$). On the left is a schema demonstrating that inspired gas and venous blood attain equilibrium for $O_2$ and $CO_2$ across the alveolar–capillary membrane. As $O_2$ is taken up ($\dot{V}O_2$) and $CO_2$ is produced in the alveolus ($\dot{V}CO_2$) the blood increases its $P_{O_2}$ from the mixed venous ($P_{\bar{v}}O_2$) level towards the alveolar ($P_{A}O_2$) level and decreases its $P_{CO_2}$ from mixed venous ($P_{\bar{v}}CO_2$) towards alveolar ($P_{A}CO_2$) or arterial ($P_{a}CO_2$) levels. At the same time the gas $P_{O_2}$ decreases from the inspired ($P_{I}O_2$) to the alveolar level and gas $P_{CO_2}$ increases from 0 towards $P_{A}CO_2$ levels. Thus, at equilibrium the alveolar $P_{O_2}$ is equivalent to the pulmonary capillary $P_{O_2}$ ($P_{c'}O_2$). On the right, the schema shows that the streams of inspired gas (open lines) and mixed venous blood (dark lines) interface in the lung and that the decrease in $P_{O_2}$ from inspired to alveolar level is approximately equivalent to the increase in alveolar $P_{CO_2}/R$, where $R$ is the ratio of $\dot{V}CO_2$ to $\dot{V}O_2$.

TABLE 75.1. Responses to $O_2$ breathing

| CAUSE OF HYPOXEMIA | $AaD_{O_2}$ | $\dot{Q}_s/\dot{Q}_t$ | EFFECT OF BREATHING 100% $O_2$ | ARTERIAL $P_{CO_2}$ ($P_{a}CO_2$) |
|---|---|---|---|---|
| True shunt | ↑ | ↑ | $\dot{Q}_s/\dot{Q}_t$ unchanged; $P_{a}O_2$ ↑ (change depends on initial $P_{a}O_2$) | usually ↓ |
| $\dot{V}/\dot{Q}$ heterogeneity | ↑ | ↑ | $\dot{Q}_s/\dot{Q}_t$ ↓; $P_{a}O_2$ ↑ to normal | usually ↓ |
| Global hypoventilation | No change | No change | $\dot{Q}_s/\dot{Q}_t$ unchanged; $P_{a}O_2$ ↑ to normal | ↓ |

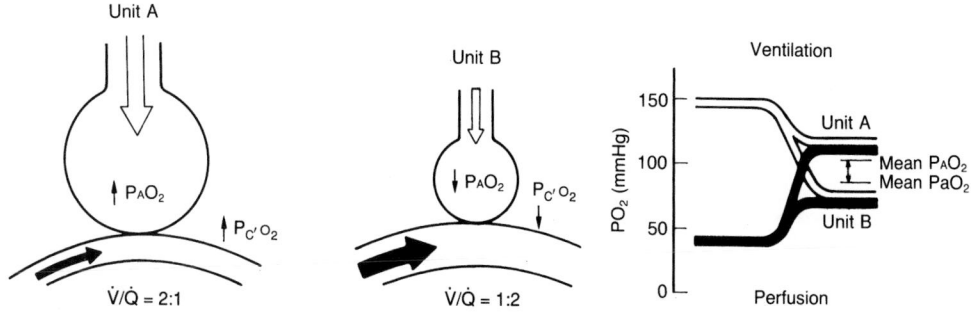

FIGURE 75.3 The development of an alveolar–arterial $P_{O_2}$ difference from heterogeneity of ventilation to perfusion ratios. In this schema an extreme example of ventilation ($\dot{V}$) to perfusion ($\dot{Q}$) mismatching is shown. On the left alveolar–capillary Unit A has a $\dot{V}/\dot{Q}$ of 2:1, producing a high $P_{A}O_2$ and $P_{c'}O_2$. In contrast, Unit B with low $\dot{V}/\dot{Q}$ produces a low $P_{A}O_2$ and $P_{c'}O_2$. When the gas from the high and low $\dot{V}/\dot{Q}$ units mix, the mean gas $O_2$ tension ($P_{A}O_2$) is weighted towards the higher $\dot{V}/\dot{Q}$ owing to a larger gas volume from Unit A (i.e. two parts gas from Unit A mix with one part gas from Unit B). Three factors influence mean arterial blood $O_2$ tension ($P_{a}O_2$): the blood mixture is a function of $O_2$ content ($C_{O_2}$) rather than $P_{O_2}$, the content from the low $\dot{V}/\dot{Q}$ is disproportionately low because of the curvilinear shape of the hemoglobin–$O_2$ dissociation curve, and the mean value is weighted towards lower $\dot{V}/\dot{Q}$ owing to a larger blood volume from Unit B (one part from Unit A with two parts from Unit B). Thus, $\dot{V}/\dot{Q}$ heterogeneity produces a difference between alveolar and arterial $P_{O_2}$.

global hypoventilation, there is no increase in $AaDO_2$ because the decrease in arterial $PO_2$ is proportional to the increase in $P_aCO_2$ (see calculation of $P_{AO_2}$) (see Table 75.1). Although determination of the $AaDO_2$ is a useful means for detecting aberrations in gas exchange, this value varies with many conditions including a change in $F_IO_2$.

Another way to describe the magnitude of derangement in gas exchange is to calculate the per cent venous admixture (also commonly referred to as net shunt or shunt fraction, $\dot{Q}_s/\dot{Q}_t$). The circulation is viewed as comprising two streams, one with perfect gas exchange in which the capillary blood $PO_2$ is equivalent to the ideal $P_{AO_2}$ and the other with no gas exchange (the shunt) and, hence, a $PO_2$ equivalent to that of mixed venous blood (Fig. 75.4). The shunt fraction is the ratio of the volume flow through the shunt divided by the total flow, and it can be calculated as follows:

$$\frac{\dot{Q}_s}{\dot{Q}_t} = \frac{C_{c'}O_2 - C_aO_2}{C_{c'}O_2 - C_{\bar{v}}O_2}$$

where $C_{c'}O_2$ is the $O_2$ content of ideal pulmonary capillary blood, which is calculated by assuming that the $PO_2$ of capillary blood is equivalent to ideal alveolar $PO_2$, and that the arterial and mixed venous $O_2$ contents are measured directly or are estimated from blood $PO_2$ using the hemoglobin–$O_2$ dissociation curve. In calculating the $\dot{Q}_s/\dot{Q}_t$ it does not matter whether the shunts are intrapulmonary, intracardiac or both.

Computation of either the $AaDO_2$ or the $\dot{Q}_s/\dot{Q}_t$ is helpful in detecting and quantifying the disruption in gas exchange causing hypoxemia; however, it is essen-

tial to recognize that these values will change depending on a variety of conditions. One of the most important considerations is the effect of $O_2$ breathing on both of these, because $O_2$ is frequently used in treatment of hypoxemia and the response can be used to determine the cause(s) of the gas exchange disturbance as illustrated in Fig. 75.5.

It also is important to stress that arterial blood $O_2$ content ($C_aO_2$), $PO_2$, and $O_2$ saturation ($S_aO_2$) increase with $O_2$ breathing even when there is a fixed right-to-left shunt. In fact, the best initial estimate of how much the $O_2$ content will increase can be derived from the projected change in $C_{c'}O_2$, which will increase because alveolar $PO_2$ rises. This can be best appreciated by rearranging the equation for $\dot{Q}_s/\dot{Q}_t$ to show the factors determining $C_aO_2$:

$$C_aO_2 = C_{c'}O_2 - \frac{\dot{Q}_s}{\dot{Q}_t}[C_{c'}O_2 - C_{\bar{v}}O_2]$$

If $\dot{Q}_s/\dot{Q}_t$ is constant and cardiac output does not change (i.e. $C_{\bar{v}}O_2$ increases the same amount as $C_aO_2$) when changing from room air to 100 per cent $O_2$ breathing, then $C_{c'}O_2$ and $C_aO_2$ increase by the same amount (approximately 2–3 mL $O_2$/dL or about a 10–15 per cent increase in $S_aO_2$ if initially there is hypoxemia). For any given change in $C_aO_2$, the change in $P_aO_2$ will depend on the initial value. When the initial $P_aO_2$ is very low, the change in $PO_2$ will be relatively small owing to the steep part of the hemoglobin–$O_2$ dissociation curve, and when the initial $S_aO_2$ and $P_aO_2$ are high, as $S_aO_2$ approaches 100 per cent the increase in $PO_2$ can be quite dramatic. Accordingly, subjects with venous admixture from an intracardiac shunt often have very little change in $P_aO_2$ when breathing $O_2$, because the shunts are relatively large, and there-

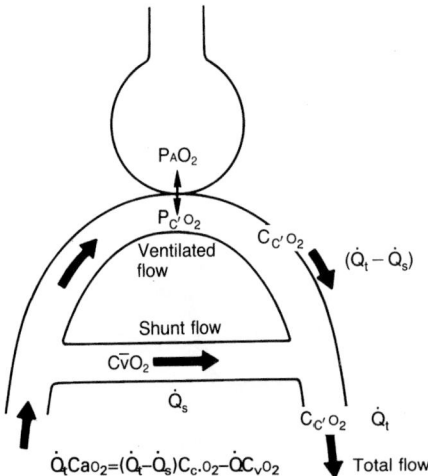

FIGURE 75.4 The concept of net shunt. In this schema, total systemic venous return splits into two streams of blood: (1) shunt flow ($\dot{Q}_s$) which has an $O_2$ content of mixed venous blood ($C_{\bar{v}}O_2$) and (2) ventilated flow (equivalent to $[\dot{Q}_t - \dot{Q}_s]$) which attains complete equilibrium with alveolar gas such that $P_{AO_2}$ = $P_{c'}O_2$, and pulmonary capillary $O_2$ content ($C_{c'}O_2$) can be derived from $P_{c'}O_2$. Therefore, the systemic $O_2$ transport (SOT) is the sum of these two streams of $O_2$ flow as shown.

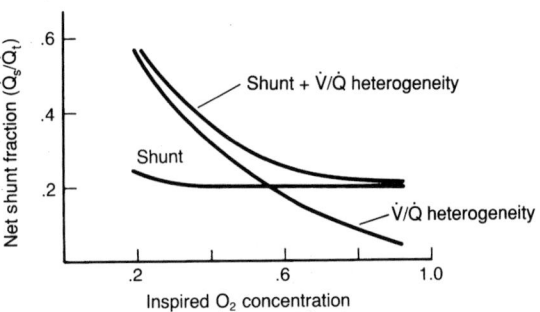

FIGURE 75.5 The effect of increasing inspired $O_2$ concentration on the net shunt fraction. In the presence of true shunt, the $\dot{Q}_s/\dot{Q}_t$ is virtually constant except for a slight initial decrease owing to the normal small amount of $\dot{V}/\dot{Q}$ heterogeneity which produces venous admixture at low $O_2$ inspired concentrations. In the presence of $\dot{V}/\dot{Q}$ heterogeneity, $\dot{Q}_s/\dot{Q}_t$ progressively decreases as the effect of low $\dot{V}/\dot{Q}$ regions on venous admixture is diminished. Finally, in the presence of shunt and $\dot{V}/\dot{Q}$ heterogeneity, $\dot{Q}_s/\dot{Q}_t$ decreases towards an asymptote which defines the true shunt fraction. Thus, the patterns of changing $\dot{Q}_s/\dot{Q}_t$ help define the type of disturbance of gas exchange present.

fore the initial $P_aO_2$ is low. In contrast, some subjects with intrapulmonary causes for venous admixture can have a large change in $P_aO_2$ when breathing $O_2$ because some of the hypoxemia is caused by $\dot{V}/\dot{Q}$ heterogeneity and the net shunt decreases (Fig. 75.5).

Factors other than $O_2$ breathing can also affect $C_aO_2$ in the absence of any change in net shunt. Again, this can be appreciated from the above equation. If cardiac output increases, then $C_{\bar{v}}O_2$ rises, thereby increasing $C_aO_2$; this effect is particularly prominent when cardiac output is low or the shunt is large (Fig. 75.6). If hemoglobin concentration increases $C_aO_2$ also rises just as it does with $O_2$ breathing even if the relationship between arterial, mixed venous and pulmonary capillary blood $O_2$ contents is constant. Finally, if $\dot{V}O_2$ decreases, less $O_2$ is extracted so that $C_{\bar{v}}O_2$ can increase. In practice, these changes rarely produce the predicted change in $C_aO_2$ because usually there are secondary responses which blunt the effect. For example, either an increase in hemoglobin concentration or decrease in $\dot{V}O_2$ may cause cardiac output to decrease in response. However, it is useful to recognize these factors when trying to dissect the causes for hypoxemia or when attempting to maximize oxygenation in a subject with critical hypoxemia.

## POSTNATAL CHANGES IN $O_2$ TRANSPORT AND $O_2$ CONSUMPTION

### $O_2$ consumption ($\dot{V}O_2$)

$\dot{V}O_2$ per mass in newborns is relatively high compared with adults or fetuses (Fig. 75.7). $\dot{V}O_2$ increases tran-

siently after birth, then progressively declines to adult values, which are approximately one-half those of the neonate. When $\dot{V}O_2$ is normalized to body surface area, much of this age-related difference disappears, suggesting that the high newborn rate is in large part related to dissipation of heat from a high surface area:mass ratio. In addition, a higher fraction of metabolism is devoted to growth in the newborn than in the more mature subject. These age-related differences are even more accentuated in rapidly growing mammals, such as the premature child. Other factors such as postnatal increases in thyroid hormone ($T_3$ and $T_4$) concentrations also contribute to the higher metabolic rate of the neonate.

Some caution must be used when interpreting values of $\dot{V}O_2$ in infants under widely different conditions. Environmental factors have a marked effect on metabolic rate. For example, $\dot{V}O_2$ increases by nearly 50 per cent when newborns are placed in an environment only 6°C below thermoneutral temperature. Moreover, because activity and sleep state markedly alter $\dot{V}O_2$, these need to be specified before comparing data.

## Cardiac output

Cardiac output normalized to mass is also much higher in the newborn than in the fetus or in the mature subject. Combined ventricular output of the fetus is about 500 mL/(kg · min), of which 30 mL/(kg · min) contributes to systemic tissues other than the placenta. After birth blood flow from each ventricle is about

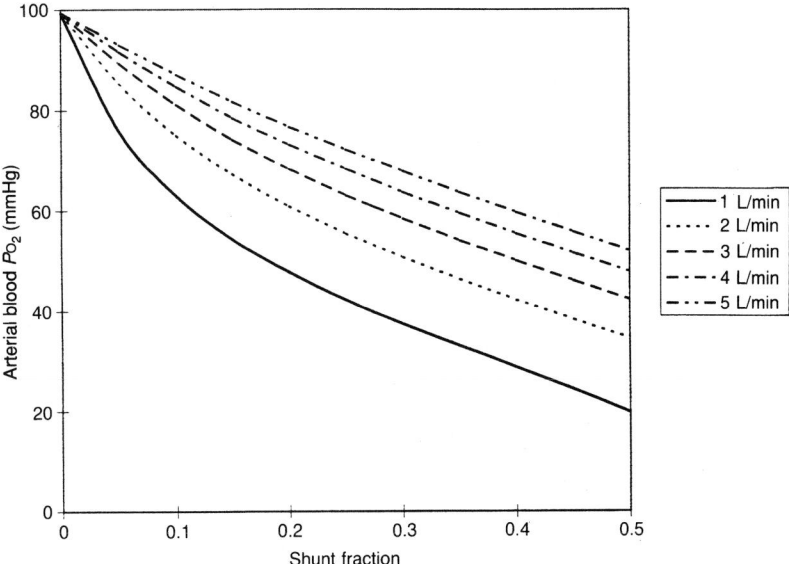

FIGURE 75.6 The effect of a change in cardiac output on oxygenation in the presence of a right-to-left shunt. The arterial blood $P_{O_2}$ achieved while breathing room air is shown as a function of shunt fraction. Isopleths demonstrate the effect of altering cardiac output at any given shunt fraction. Note that cardiac output has a more significant effect on oxygenation when shunt fraction is large. For this figure $O_2$ consumption is assumed to be 120 mL/min and hemoglobin concentration to be 14 g/dL.

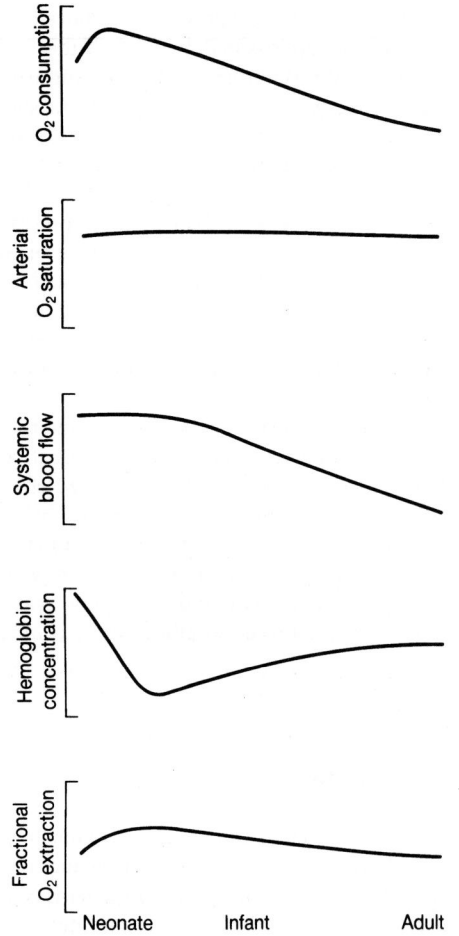

FIGURE 75.7 Stylized schema demonstrating postnatal changes in the factors contributing to the changes in $O_2$ transport. The relationships shown are not precise for humans, but are inferred from data in humans and experimental animals.

400 mL/(kg · min); this decreases progressively to the adult value, which is closer to 80 mL/(kg · min). Because of the high resting cardiac output of the neonate, there may be limited reserve for augmenting blood flow further under conditions of stress. This may be a factor reducing the capacity to respond if $O_2$ transport must increase suddenly to meet changing metabolic demands. In the mature subject cardiac output can increase by a factor of 3–4 (or as much as 6 with training) because stroke volume can increase by a factor of 1.5 and heart rate by 2–4 times. It is doubtful that the infant can sustain such high levels of cardiac output.

## Hemoglobin concentration

After birth there is a progressive fall in hemoglobin concentration and hematocrit, with a consequent decrease in $O_2$-carrying capacity of blood. Hematocrit usually decreases from approximately 55

per cent at birth to 33 per cent by 2 months and then gradually increases to about 45 per cent by adolescence. This decline in hemoglobin concentration is referred to as *physiological anemia* because it is unresponsive to transfusion or to hematemic agents and it occurs in healthy infants with no recognized nutritional deficiency. The anemia is accentuated in premature infants and even occurs in chronically hypoxemic infants, although the decrease in hemoglobin concentration is less marked than in normal infants. Furthermore, the postnatal anemia occurs in infants with left-to-right shunts and can increase shunting. With the decline in viscosity when hematocrit decreases systemic and pulmonary vascular resistance decrease (roughly in proportion to each other, *see* page 750), pulmonary and systemic blood flows increase (also in proportion) in response, and the left-to-right shunt thereby increases. Thus, postnatal changes in hemoglobin concentration may worsen or provoke circulatory failure and not be "physiological" in the presence of cardiopulmonary pathology.

## $P_aO_2$ and $S_aO_2$

Normally, $S_aO_2$ does not change much with postnatal development even though $P_aO_2$ increases from approximately 50–60 mmHg (6.6–8.0 kPa) shortly after birth to approximately 100 mmHg (13.3 kPa) in childhood. Based on changes in $P_aO_2$, breathing 100 per cent $O_2$, the low $P_aO_2$ of the neonate has been attributed to both ventilation/perfusion inequalities and fixed intrapulmonary right-to-left shunting (see above). As a result, healthy newborn infants breathing 100 per cent $O_2$ usually have a $P_aO_2$ of about 300 mmHg, which may represent a right-to-left shunt of approximately 20 per cent caused by anatomical shunts (via bronchial and thebesian circulations), atelectasis, and airway closure during expiration. However, owing to the high hemoglobin $O_2$ affinity (see below) $S_aO_2$ at birth is in the range of 95 per cent even with the relatively low $P_aO_2$, and it does not change with postnatal development. Thus, except under unusual circumstances, changes in arterial oxygenation do not contribute to the marked alterations in $O_2$ transport with postnatal development. Moreover, if hemoglobin concentration or cardiac output are reduced, increases in $S_aO_2$ provide little compensation for the reduced $O_2$ transport.

## $O_2$ extraction

Simultaneous with the decrease in hemoglobin concentration after birth, there is a progressive rightward shift of the hemoglobin–$O_2$ dissociation curve (Fig. 75.8). If $P_aO_2$ is normal and mixed systemic venous blood $PO_2$ ($P_{\bar{v}}O_2$) is constant, this rightward shift would permit progressively more $O_2$ to be unloaded from oxygenated hemoglobin, increasing arteriovenous blood $O_2$

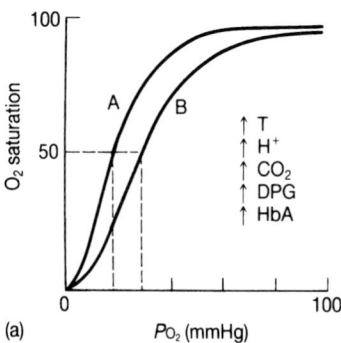 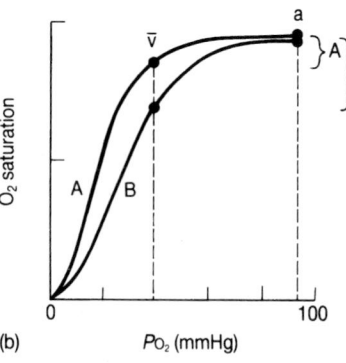 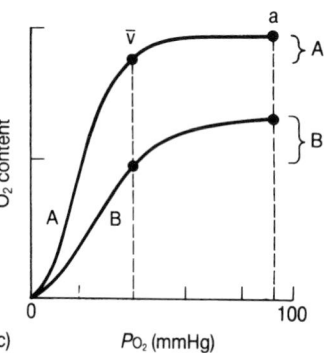

FIGURE 75.8 Effect of changes in hemoglobin (Hb) $O_2$ affinity on $O_2$ unloading. (a) With increases in temperature (T), serum $H^+$ concentration, $CO_2$, concentration, or DPG content in the red cell, the relationship between Hb $O_2$ saturation and $Po_2$ shifts to the right (curve A to curve B). This shift reduces Hb $O_2$ affinity and increases $P_{50}$, the $Po_2$ at 50 per cent Hb $O_2$ saturation. Similarly, when the fraction of adult hemoglobin (HbA) increases during postnatal development, $P_{50}$ also increases because HbA binds to DPG more avidly than does fetal Hb, and this binding to DPG decreases the affinity of Hb for $O_2$ (see text). Curve A is typical for a newborn, and curve B for an adult. (b) As shown by the brackets, a rightward shift of the dissociation curve (A → B) causes a larger arteriovenous $O_2$ saturation difference when arterial (a) $Po_2$ and mixed venous (v̄) $Po_2$ are normal and fixed. (c) In the presence of postnatal anemia, a rightward shift in the curve permits more $O_2$ to be unloaded for the same arterial (a) and mixed venous (v̄) $Po_2$. When anemia occurs, the relationship between $O_2$ saturation and $Po_2$ does not fully characterize the effects on $O_2$ transport; therefore, in this figure $O_2$ content has replaced $O_2$ saturation on the y axis to demonstrate the effect of anemia. Curve A represents the neonate with a low $P_{50}$ (similar to curve A in other panels) and high Hb concentration. Curve B shows the combined effects of an increase in $P_{50}$ and a decrease in Hb concentration. Despite the marked decrease in a total $O_2$ capacity of blood, curve B permits a larger arteriovenous $O_2$ content difference, as shown by the brackets.

content difference, an important mechanism for compensation during postnatal anemia. Thus there is a slight increase in fractional $O_2$ extraction particularly during the nadir of the anemia. Remarkably, however, despite large differences in $O_2$ transport, $\dot{V}o_2$, and hemoglobin $O_2$ affinity during development, there is apparent constancy of $P_{\bar{v}}o_2$, which is in the range of 39–40 mmHg (5.2–5.3 kPa) in normal resting subjects. Therefore, there is reasonable basis for estimates of the capacity to extract $O_2$ using the position of the $O_2$ dissociation curve, the hemoglobin concentration, and an assumed $P_{\bar{v}}o_2$.

The postnatal decrease in hemoglobin $O_2$ affinity (or increase in $P_{50}$, the $Po_2$ at which hemoglobin is 50 per cent saturated with $O_2$) is caused by an increase in the proportion of adult relative to fetal hemoglobin and an increase in the concentration of 2,3-diphosphoglycerate (DPG) (or 2,3-bisphosphoglycerate) as follows. There is a gradual decline in fetal hemoglobin from about 77 per cent at birth to less than 2 per cent by 8 months. DPG, a product of the Rapaport–Leubering shunt present in red cells, decreases the affinity for $O_2$ (increases $P_{50}$) through its allosteric interaction with the hemoglobin molecule. Because DPG does not bind to fetal hemoglobin as avidly as it does to adult hemoglobin, hemoglobin $O_2$ affinity is high immediately after birth ($P_{50}$ approximately 20 mmHg [2.7 kPa]). In contrast, by 8 months $P_{50}$ increases to about 30 mmHg (4.0 kPa); after adolescence, $P_{50}$ reaches adult values (about 27 mmHg [3.6 kPa]). Therefore, in early infancy when the concentration of fetal hemoglobin is high, change in DPG has little effect

on $P_{50}$, whereas modulation of hemoglobin $O_2$ affinity is an important compensatory mechanism in the older subject in response to hypoxemia, anemia, or low cardiac output.

Capillary density and surface area also influence $O_2$ extraction (see below), but no data describe developmental differences in these important factors. Based on observations, when $O_2$ extraction must increase with acute stress there seems to be no limitation in the young subject, suggesting that there are no large differences in the microcirculation of newborn and mature subjects.

## PHYSIOLOGICAL O₂-SUPPLY DEPENDENCY

When $O_2$ transport has been reduced progressively under experimental conditions in which demands are kept relatively constant, the response in whole body $\dot{V}o_2$ appears to be biphasic (Fig. 75.9). Initially $\dot{V}o_2$ is constant and independent of $O_2$ transport. With further reductions in $O_2$ transport, $\dot{V}o_2$ becomes dependent on $O_2$ transport and declines in proportion, a relationship described as physiological supply dependency. Experimental studies comparing the effects of hypoxic hypoxia, anemic hypoxia, and stagnant hypoxia suggest a single, critical $O_2$ transport above which $\dot{V}o_2$ is independent of transport. This in turn suggests that resting $\dot{V}o_2$ is equivalent to metabolic demand, whereas the depressed $\dot{V}o_2$ (below the critical transport) underestimates true demand. Therefore,

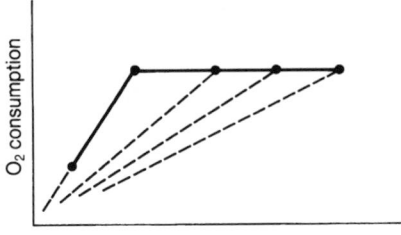

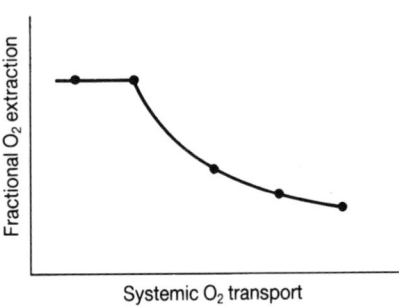

FIGURE 75.9 Stylized schema showing the change in $O_2$ consumption and fractional $O_2$ extraction as $O_2$ transport is reduced. Note that $O_2$ consumption initially remains constant owing to increases in $O_2$ extraction. $O_2$ extraction is the instantaneous slope of each point on the top figure, as shown by the dashed lines emanating from the origin. This is typical of the relationships seen in controlled experiments using anesthetized animals during graded reductions in $O_2$ transport.

when $O_2$ transport is reduced below the critical level, some tissues become hypoxic of necessity. At this point metabolism must be maintained by anaerobiosis (and lactate concentrations may increase in arterial blood) or the tissues must decrease metabolic rate, or both. Such a biphasic relationship between $O_2$ transport and consumption has been demonstrated in intact experimental animals as well as in isolated organs and tissues. Much less evidence is available in intact humans. Although there is no reason to believe that the relationship described in animals is substantially different in humans, this issue has been called into question and is difficult to resolve experimentally in normal subjects.

## Effects on metabolic demands

An implicit assumption in studying the effects of changing $O_2$ transport on $\dot{V}O_2$ is the maintenance of constant metabolic demands, a condition difficult to ensure in clinical studies. Decreases in $O_2$ transport may provoke ventilation or cardiac output to increase, raising cardiorespiratory work. Even though this work can be quantified, responding changes in $\dot{V}O_2$ are not always predictable because the efficiency ([work/$t$]/[energy consumption/$t$]) of these systems can vary

widely. When $O_2$ transport is reduced, other factors increase metabolic demands in a less predictable manner. The release of catecholamines into the circulation or infusion of related drugs with β-adrenergic action can increase $\dot{V}O_2$ by stimulating thermogenesis. Other drugs may stimulate catecholamines indirectly and produce a similar effect. Finally, if an increase in ventilation (e.g. with hypoxemia) causes alkalemia, this raises whole body $\dot{V}O_2$ (as much as 15–20 per cent), an effect not related to respiratory work because it occurs with mechanical as well as spontaneous breathing.

On the other hand, some factors decrease metabolic demands when $O_2$ transport is reduced. For example, if renal blood flow decreases, so does metabolic work of the kidney, because sodium transport (which accounts for 75 per cent of renal $\dot{V}O_2$ at rest) declines. Similarly, metabolic work of the liver, which depends on substrate delivery, decreases if hepatic blood flow is reduced. Thus, for experimental purposes, keeping metabolic demands constant in intact, non-anesthetized subjects as $O_2$ transport is decreased or increased may be quite difficult.

## Matching of flow and metabolism

Fractional $O_2$ extraction must increase progressively as $O_2$ transport is reduced if $O_2$ consumption is to remain constant. The mechanisms by which $O_2$ extraction increases to maintain $\dot{V}O_2$ when $O_2$ transport is disturbed involve regulation of blood flow at both the organ level and in the microcirculation. In general, blood and $O_2$ flow are distributed to match nutritional demands of the tissue. Such distribution of blood flow occurs both at rest and when metabolic demands are altered. For example, muscle blood flow increases with exercise, and gut blood flow increases following feeding. However, there are important exceptions. Tissues that perform specialized tasks may demand relatively high blood flow. The skin has a high rate of blood flow relative to metabolism because of its importance in heat exchange. The kidney, which is responsible for filtration, also has a very high blood flow rate relative to its metabolism. Accordingly, both of these organs have relatively low fractional $O_2$ extraction at rest. The heart and the brain, on the other hand, have low blood flow rates relative to their metabolic demands and have high fractional extraction at rest. The fractional extraction for the whole body is the flow-weighted average of each organ. When $O_2$ transport is reduced or metabolic demands are increased, whole body fractional $O_2$ extraction is expected to increase in response, as this is a measure of the distribution of $O_2$ flow relative to demands. Accordingly, in states of limited $O_2$ supply, a failure of $O_2$ extraction to increase in response provides strong presumptive evidence of a defect in peripheral $O_2$ uptake, which could be caused by $\dot{V}O_2$–blood flow mismatch (analogous to ventilation/perfusion mismatch in the lung), peripheral arteriovenous shunting, or interference with cellular utilization of O$_2$.

When O$_2$ transport is disturbed, overall organ perfusion results from the balance between factors that permit vasodilatation and those that promote vasocon-striction (Fig. 75.10). Three important factors influence organ vascular resistance: the capacity of the organ for autoregulation, the response to neural stimulation, and the response to humoral stimulation. When perfusion pressure to an organ is reduced there can be autoregulation, a simultaneous decrease in vascular

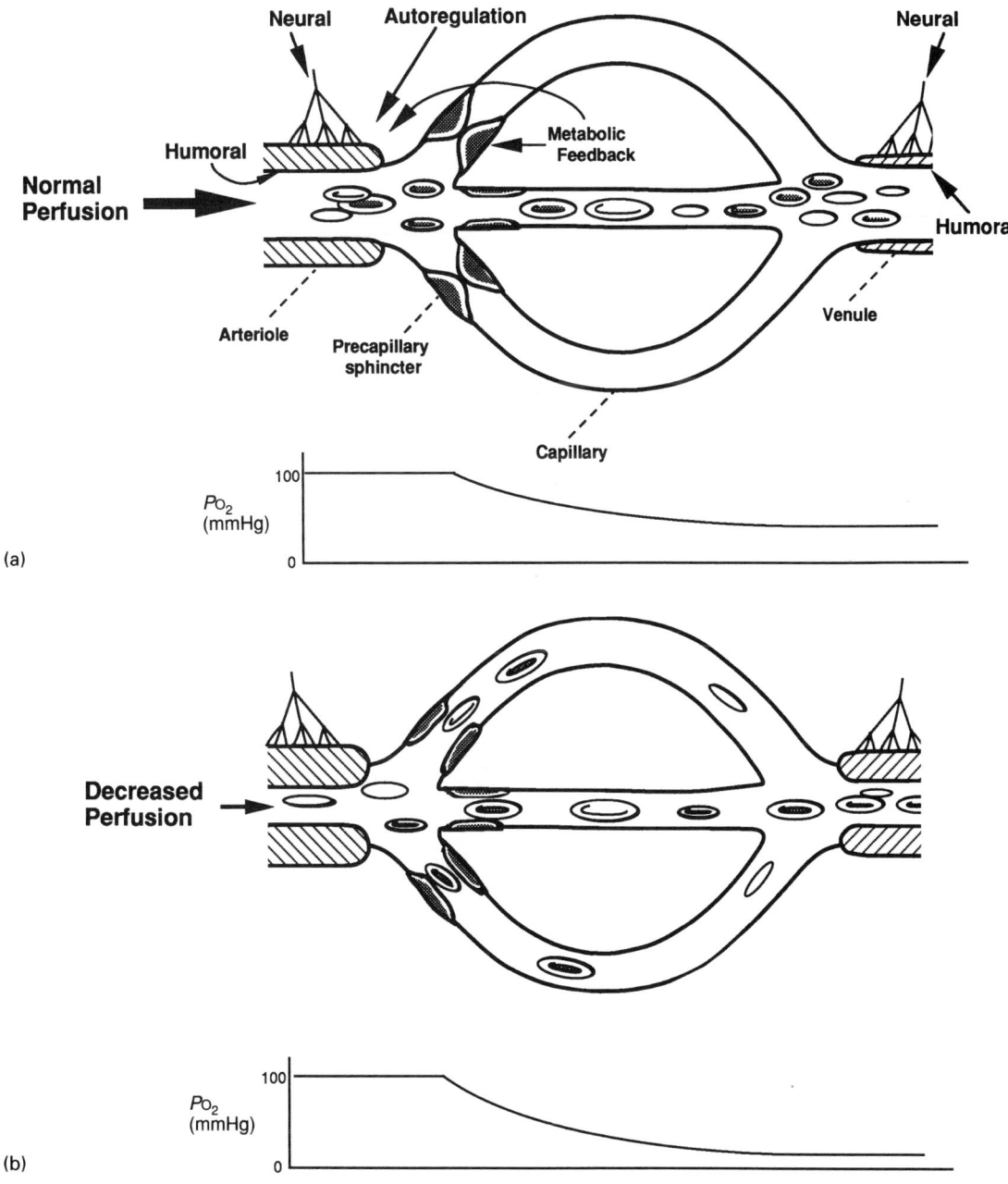

FIGURE 75.10 Schematic diagram of the microcirculation during conditions of (a) normal perfusion to metabolism and (b) decreased perfusion to metabolism. As shown, arteriolar resistance controls perfusion of the microcirculation, and precapillary sphincters control the distribution of microcirculatory blood flow. Arteriolar tone is controlled by neural and humoral influences, autoregulation, and, to some extent, feedback from local metabolic factors. Venular tone is also under the influence of neural and humoral control. (a) When perfusion is normal, not all of the capillaries are open. O$_2$ extraction by the tissues is shown by the decline in O$_2$ pressure as a function of distance through the microcirculation (diagram immediately below the vascular bed). (b) When perfusion is markedly decreased by arteriolar and venular constriction, O$_2$ extraction is increased by the opening of previously closed capillaries, which increases surface area for diffusion, shortens diffusion distance, and increases transit time. The higher extraction is shown by the lower venous O$_2$ pressure.

resistance that serves to maintain blood flow at its previous level. This vasodilatation and ability to sustain organ perfusion (probably mediated by metabolic feedback) is particularly prominent in the heart, brain, and kidney, but less important in other organs.

In the intact subject, blood flow is also influenced by an organ's responses to humoral and nervous input that cause vasoconstriction when $O_2$ transport is limited. Whenever $O_2$ supply is limited, catecholamines increase, stimulating cardiac contractility and rate and causing peripheral vasoconstriction. In most tissues low cardiac output is accompanied by a local neural release of norepinephrine in response to activation of arterial baroreceptors and cardiopulmonary receptors. In addition, circulating catecholamine concentrations increase in response to chemoreceptor (with anemia and hypoxemia) and baroreceptor (with low cardiac output) activation, which causes the release of epinephrine and norepinephrine from the adrenal medulla. Circulating concentrations of other vasoconstricting hormones also increase. With low cardiac output, renin is released in response to reduced renal blood flow and increased sympathetic stimulation. Renin catalyzes conversion of angiotensinogen to angiotensin I and angiotensin I is hydrolyzed to angiotensin II by angiotensin converting enzyme. Angiotensin II stimulates the release of aldosterone from the adrenal cortex and vasopressin from the pituitary gland. Vasopressin is also stimulated directly by decreased aortic or atrial pressure. Vasopressin, aldosterone, and angiotensin II are all potent vasoconstrictors. These nervous and humoral responses generally increase regional vascular resistance and divert blood flow away from organs that respond.

Perfusion to a given organ during a reduction in $O_2$ transport thereby depends on the relative importance of autoregulation, which serves to sustain flow, and the neural and humoral factors, which serve to reduce it. The brain and heart have little sympathetic innervation and are relatively resistant to sympathetic control, whereas the kidney is quite sensitive. Thus, in contrast to the kidney or to other organs that are richly innervated with sympathetic fibers, the brain and heart maintain blood flow during conditions in which $O_2$ supply is limited. Organs with relatively low resting $O_2$ extraction (gut, skin, kidney) reduce blood (and $O_2$) flow relative to demand and increase their fractional extraction as well as that of the whole body when $O_2$ supply decreases, a response that helps to sustain oxidative metabolism.

## Adjustments in the microcirculation

In addition to the alterations in vascular resistance that control organ blood flow, adjustments in the microcirculation enhance $O_2$ extraction and serve to preserve organ metabolism. These adaptations include the opening of previously closed capillaries and changes in hemoglobin $O_2$ affinity. Some tissues have precapillary sphincters, which are located at the arterial end of each capillary and maintain the capillary either open or closed. The exact control of these sphincters is not fully understood, although both local metabolic factors and local $P_{O_2}$ play a role. Whenever the number of perfused capillaries increases, tissues can extract more of the available $O_2$ via three mechanisms: (1) the increase in capillary density decreases the distance for diffusion between blood and the site of $O_2$ utilization; (2) the increased number of capillaries increases the lateral surface area for diffusion; and (3) the increase in cross-sectional area of the capillaries reduces the linear velocity of blood and increases transit time for diffusion. These mechanisms permit very high levels of $O_2$ extraction when $O_2$ demand is increased or when $O_2$ supply is curtailed.

In addition to the changes in diffusion as perfusion is altered acutely, $H^+$ concentration can increase locally, which causes a rightward shift of the $O_2$ dissociation curve (Fig. 75.8) and permits more unloading of $O_2$ from hemoglobin (for any given venous blood $P_{O_2}$, venous $O_2$ saturation is lower). However, because arterial blood pH is more alkaline than venous blood pH and $P_{a}O_2$ is on the flat part of the $O_2$ dissociation curve, $O_2$ loading usually is not compromised by acidemia. Normally hemoglobin $O_2$ affinity differs between arterial and venous blood because of the differences in $H^+$ and $CO_2$ concentrations in the two circulations. In a state of low $O_2$ transport this difference is exaggerated, which generally enhances $O_2$ extraction at the periphery as an acute adaptation. With the marked intraorgan differences in flow relative to metabolism, the shift in the dissociation curve may vary widely.

In addition to this acute shift in hemoglobin $O_2$ affinity, the $O_2$ dissociation curve may be affected by changes in the concentration of DPG if the disturbance in $O_2$ transport is sustained. The concentration of DPG is regulated primarily by the red cell $H^+$ concentration because the rate-limiting enzyme is pH-sensitive. A high pH stimulates DPG synthesis. Because deoxyhemoglobin provides better buffering than oxyhemoglobin and thereby raises red cell pH relative to plasma pH, the low venous $O_2$ concentration in any form of chronic hypoxia can promote DPG synthesis. However, this adaptive mechanism is less prominent in young infants with fetal hemoglobin, which binds DPG poorly, because synthesis is inhibited by unbound DPG.

## SPECIFIC DISTURBANCES IN $O_2$ TRANSPORT

## Low cardiac output

When cardiac output is reduced abruptly, systemic $O_2$ transport decreases in parallel because there is little or no change in hemoglobin concentration. Therefore, an increase in $O_2$ extraction (decrease in $P_{\bar{v}}O_2$) provides the only acute mechanism for sustaining oxidative metabolism. Under some circumstances a reduction in blood flow may even be more disruptive to metabolism than anemia or hypoxemia because it limits the supply of substrates other than $O_2$ and there may be accumulation of metabolites, which can alter substrate utilization. In experimental animals, cardiac output can be reduced acutely by about 50 per cent before there are signs of tissue hypoxia, but this tolerance depends on the hemoglobin concentration; with anemia, the tolerance is less than when the hemoglobin concentration is higher.

When cardiac output is reduced chronically, DPG can increase, which will increase $P_{50}$ and $O_2$ extraction and restore $P_{\bar{v}}O_2$ towards normal. However, if systemic acidemia persists, this can decrease red cell pH, inhibit DPG synthesis, and interfere with this important hematological adaptation. There is no evidence that a low cardiac output stimulates hemoglobin synthesis even though erythropoietin production is presumably stimulated by low renal venous blood $P_{O_2}$. It has been suggested that reduced renal blood flow decreases renal $O_2$ consumption, thereby restoring renal venous blood $P_{O_2}$ towards normal.

## Anemia

When hemoglobin concentration is reduced acutely, cardiac output and $O_2$ extraction increase. Therefore, $O_2$ transport does not decrease in proportion to the decline in hemoglobin. In intact animals an isovolemic decrease in hematocrit to about 15 per cent is tolerated without signs of tissue hypoxia as long as the augmentation of cardiac output can occur. Cardiac output increases with anemia because cardiac contractility and heart rate are stimulated by catecholamines and the decrease in blood viscosity reduces vascular resistance. Thus, cardiac output may increase quite significantly at low hematocrit concentrations.

When anemia is sustained, the $O_2$ dissociation curve shifts to the right, which permits venous $O_2$ saturation to be quite low and $O_2$ extraction to be quite high even though $P_{\bar{v}}O_2$ returns towards normal. With anemia there may also be an increase in plasma volume, which helps to increase cardiac output further by increasing stroke volume. Despite these adaptations, the problems of decreased $O_2$-carrying capacity may be compounded if red cell deformability is abnormal as with iron deficiency and sickle cell disease, both of which interfere with microcirculatory flow and have been implicated as causes of vascular occlusion and strokes.

## Hypoxemia

The response to hypoxemia depends in part on the method used to produce the disturbance. With alveolar hypoxia, $O_2$ extraction increases and cardiac output increases somewhat, although less so than with a comparable decline in $C_aO_2$ produced by anemia. Part of the contrast relates to the reduced viscosity with anemia and the limitation of systemic blood flow with alveolar hypoxia owing to the increase in pulmonary vascular resistance, which restricts right ventricular output. The concentration of inspired $O_2$ that is tolerated before there is evidence of tissue hypoxia varies widely with age, species, size, and ambient environment, but in young subjects $O_2$ consumption usually decreases when inspired $O_2$ concentration is near 10 per cent. However, when neonates are placed in a cool environment (stimulating metabolic demands), even mild alveolar hypoxia can decrease $\dot{V}_{O_2}$, which is in contrast to observations in neutral thermal environment.

When hypoxemia is sustained chronically, two important hematological adjustments occur: hemoglobin synthesis increases, and the $O_2$ dissociation curve shifts. In the presence of hypoxemia from either alveolar hypoxia or from intracardiac shunt, there is an inverse relationship between the hemoglobin concentration and the $S_aO_2$, which keeps $C_aO_2$ nearly constant. However, the polycythemia may limit the anticipated augmentation in cardiac output and, when severe, can cause SOT to decrease.

The utility of a change in $P_{50}$ to enhance extraction of $O_2$ from venous blood depends on the degree to which $O_2$ loading of arterial blood is affected simultaneously (Fig. 75.11). With anemia or low cardiac output, arterial and pulmonary capillary blood $P_{O_2}$ are high and $O_2$ loading occurs on the flat part of the $O_2$ dissociation curve; thus, there is a large increase in extraction with a rightward shift of the dissociation curve (little decrease in $S_aO_2$ but a marked decrease in $S_{\bar{v}}O_2$). With arterial hypoxemia the effects of the shift in the curve are more complex. If there is alveolar hypoxia, then a rightward shift of the dissociation curve may interfere with $O_2$ loading; whether a rightward or leftward curve is beneficial depends on the severity of the alveolar hypoxia. In general, rightward shift in the dissociation curve enhances $O_2$ unloading with mild alveolar hypoxia, and leftward shift enhances unloading with severe alveolar hypoxia. In contrast, with shunt hypoxemia, as occurs with cardiac disease, pulmonary capillary blood $P_{O_2}$ remains relatively high, and a rightward shift to the dissociation curve interferes minimally with $O_2$ loading and increases $O_2$ unloading at the periphery. Accordingly, patients with congenital cardiac disease causing hypoxemia usually have an increase in $P_{50}$ except shortly after birth, whereas the response in subjects with alveolar hypoxia varies.

## Metabolic responses

In all subjects the final evidence of impairment of $O_2$ transport is a disturbance in cellular energy

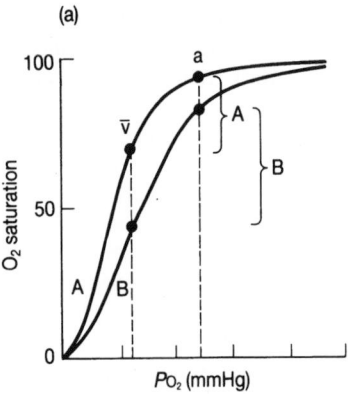
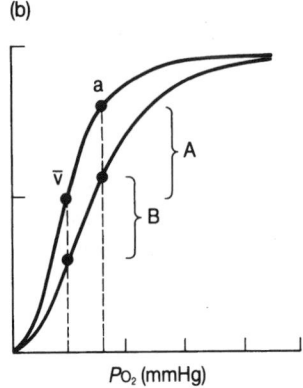

FIGURE 75.11 The effect of a shift in the $O_2$ dissociation curve on $O_2$ unloading with alveolar hypoxia. The height of the brackets indicates the quantity of $O_2$ unloaded by hemoglobin. (a) With mild alveolar hypoxia, a shift to the right enhances $O_2$ unloading while it produces less impairment of $O_2$ loading. The reason is that the $P_aO_2$ is fixed by the alveolar $Po_2$, which is on a less steep part of the curve than the mixed venous point (v̄). Therefore, the arteriovenous $O_2$ saturation difference is greater with curve B than curve A. (b) With more severe alveolar hypoxia, both alveolar and arterial $Po_2$ are very low and both the arterial and mixed venous points are on a steep part of the curve. Hence, in this case the arteriovenous venous $O_2$ saturation difference is smaller with the right-shifted curve.

metabolism. When $O_2$ transport is inadequate, insufficient $O_2$ is available for oxidative phosphorylation. The electron transport chain slows, the rate of phosphorylation of adenosine diphosphate (ADP) to adenosine triphosphate (ATP) is decreased, and cytochromes remain in the reduced state. There is also an increase in the concentration of adenosine monophosphate (AMP), which is rapidly catabolized to inosine and hypoxanthine during hypoxia. Thus, the state of phosphorylation of the nucleotides, the presence of products of catabolism, and the redox state of one or more of the cytochromes provide inferential information about the state of tissue oxygenation. The tissues of some organs, particularly skeletal muscle, and to some extent brain and heart, can synthesize ATP for brief periods by transferring a high-energy phosphate to ATP. In the presence of the enzyme creatine kinase, creatine phosphate serves as an energy reservoir during hypoxic stress, but such a resource is rapidly depleted.

ADP can also be phosphorylated anaerobically during hypoxia when $O_2$ supply is reduced, but this is considerably less efficient than aerobic metabolism in terms of moles of ATP per mole glucose. Furthermore, with anaerobic metabolism, lactic acid accumulates in tissues and in venous blood, thereby decreasing serum as well as tissue pH. Each of the metabolic changes has been used as a sign of inadequate tissue oxygenation, although the utility of any one measure depends on experimental conditions and the specific tissue.

More subtle signs of tissue hypoxia are difficult to quantify, but one clear finding in the child with chronic hypoxia is failure to thrive. Thus, growth failure of the fetus or the infant is a common consequence of chronic hypoxia, whether produced by hypoxemia, anemia, or limited cardiac output. This finding is strong evidence that adaptation has failed.

## SUMMARY

The aim here has been to demonstrate the functioning of a highly integrated system that readily tolerates acute and chronic changes in metabolic demands by adjusting the rate of $O_2$ transport and extraction. As has been emphasized, disruption in any component of $O_2$ transport demands quick adaptive changes in other parts of the system. However, any reserve may be exhausted rapidly when such adaptations are disturbed. An infant with cyanotic congenital cardiac disease may maintain sufficient $O_2$ transport to grow and be active because of an increased cardiac output, increased $O_2$ extraction, and increased hemoglobin concentration. However, tissue hypoxia may rapidly ensue when cardiac output is compromised, metabolic demands increase, or there is even a mild reduction in hematocrit.

## SELECTED READING

Cain SM. Peripheral oxygen uptake and delivery in health and disease. *Clin Chest Med* 1983; 4: 139.

Dantzker DR. Pulmonary gas exchange. In: Dantzker DR, ed. *Cardiopulmonary critical care.* Philadelphia: WB Saunders, 1986: 25.

Finch CA, Lenfant C. Oxygen transport in man. *N Engl J Med* 1972; 286: 407.

Lister G, Fahey JT. Oxygen transport. In: Chernick V, Mellins RB, eds. *Mechanisms of pediatric respiratory disease: cellular and integrative.* Philadelphia: BC Decker, 1991: 129.

Lister G, Moreau G, Moss M, Talner NS. Effects of alterations of oxygen transport on the neonate. *Semin Perinatol* 1984; 8: 192.

Schumacker PT, Samsel RW. Oxygen supply and consumption in the adult respiratory distress syndrome. *Clin Chest Med* 1990; 11: 715.

# 76

# Electrophysiology

George F. Van Hare

## IMPULSE FORMATION

Cardiac impulses are formed by cardiac cells that exhibit "pacemaker activity," or spontaneous automaticity. In adults, such cells are found primarily in the sinus and atrioventricular nodes, and to a lesser extent in atrial muscle and the His–Purkinje (distal conducting) system. Action potentials recorded from these cells by micropuncture techniques differ from action potentials recorded from cells in other parts of the heart in several respects (Fig. 76.1). They have a slower rate of rise (phase 0) than action potentials recorded elsewhere, as well as a shorter plateau phase (phase 3). They are known as "slow-response" potentials, in con-

trast to "fast-response" potentials recorded elsewhere. When they are not being overdriven by another source of repetitive stimulation, slow-response cells exhibit a gradual rise in transmembrane potential during electrical diastole (phase 4) until the threshold potential is reached, giving rise to an action potential. This spontaneous diastolic depolarization is mediated by various ionic mechanisms depending on the location of the cell, and is the origin of normal pacemaker activity in the heart.

Spontaneous cardiac electrical activity begins very early in embryological development, by 35 hours in the chick embryo. Rhythmic contractions are first observed in the embryonic ventricle, and pacemaker potentials may be recorded in nearly all ventricular cells early in gestation. Very quickly, however, these cells lose their capability for normal automaticity, and the site of cardiac activation shifts to the developing atrium.

The sinus node develops quite early as a well-demarcated structure at the junction of the right atrium and superior vena cava. This cluster of cardiac cells becomes progressively more compact with further fetal development. It is made up of normal working atrial myocardial cells, a second cell type termed "typical nodal cells" or "P cells," and finally "transitional cells," which are found mainly at the margins of the sinus node. P cells are thought to be primarily responsible for sinus node automaticity, and transitional cells may be important in providing excellent contact with the working atrial myocardium. In addition, the sinus node is well invested with a collagenous matrix that separates cells from one another. While fibrosis of the sinus node has been reported with age, this probably represents loss of sinus node cells rather than the formation of new fibrous tissue.

While sinus node automaticity is mainly responsible for the heart rate, automaticity (at lower rates) may occur in cells lower in the cardiac conduction system, if allowed to "escape" from overdrive suppression by the sinus node. This may occur in individuals with sinus node disease in response to increased vagal

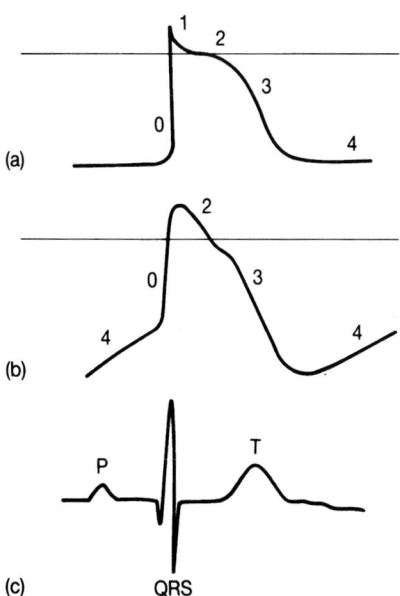

FIGURE 76.1 Cardiac action potential. Numbers correspond to the phases of the action potential. (a) Fast-response cells (atrial and ventricular myocardium). (b) Slow-response cells (sinus and atrioventricular nodes). (c) Surface electrocardiogram.

tone or certain drugs, or because of congenital or acquired atrioventricular block (Table 76.1). This escape automaticity is normal and adaptive. In the presence of diseases such as myocarditis or following surgery, abnormal automaticity may develop in any part of the heart, and this produces rates that are greater than the escape rates found higher in the conducting system. These sites of abnormal automaticity overdrive other foci.

## IMPULSE PROPAGATION

Cardiac muscle cells have the ability to pass electrical impulses to adjacent cells via gap junctions, specialized structures that make the cytosol of adjacent cardiac cells electrically continuous. Cardiac muscle is not a syncytium; the cells maintain their cell membranes. However, these specialized cell-to-cell connections allow cardiac muscle to function electrically as a syncytium. An action potential that spreads down one cardiac cell will be passed easily to adjacent cardiac cells, leading to propagation throughout the heart. While cardiac muscle may be viewed as an electrical syncytium, recent evidence suggests this view is overly simplistic. Instead of homogeneous conduction in all directions, as one would expect with a syncytial model, in fact propagation is known to be more rapid along the long axis of cardiac cells than along the transverse axis. This property, known as "anisotropic conduction," reflects greater axial than longitudinal resistivity. Collagenous septa, oriented longitudinally and acting as insulators, may be largely responsible for this difference, along with other factors. These characteristics may lead to discontinuous and heterogeneous conduction, and anisotropic conduction has been hypothesized as an important factor in the genesis of lethal ventricular arrhythmias.

Micropuncture studies in fetal and newborn preparations have shown age-related changes in action potential characteristics in several species, including chicks, rats, and canines. There is a gradual increase in negativity of the resting potential from the time the heart beat is first established; in many species, this increase continues into adulthood. The increasing negativity of the resting potential is thought to be due to increasing permeability to $K^+$ with development, as well as to increasing activity of $Na^+$-$K^+$-ATPase.

The velocity of impulse propagation in cardiac muscle depends on a number of factors, including fiber orientation, passive properties of cardiac muscle such as membrane excitability threshold, resistance and capacitance, and active properties related to the action potential. The most important of these factors is the rate of rise of phase 0 of the action potential, also known as $dV/dt$ or $\dot{V}_{max}$. Conduction velocity is directly related to the magnitude of $\dot{V}_{max}$, and factors that affect $\dot{V}_{max}$ also affect conduction velocity.

Phase 0 of the action potential occurs when the transmembrane potential is increased from its resting negative value to its excitability threshold. In fast-response cells, this results in the opening of voltage-sensitive $Na^+$ channels and the rapid entry of positively charged $Na^+$ ions, and the further increase in the membrane potential toward 0 potential. The $Na^+$ channel is time-dependent and inactivates, allowing other ionic mechanisms eventually to return the membrane potential to its resting potential. Phase 0 corresponds to the QRS complex on the surface electrocardiogram. Phase 1 (early repolarization) is due to $Na^+$ channel inactivation, but also to a transient outward $K^+$ current. This is not well seen in slow-response cells. During phase 2 (plateau), membrane conductance is low with respect to all ions, but $Na^+$-$K^+$-ATPase and an inward $Ca^{2+}$ current are active. Rapid repolarization occurs during phase 3 and is quite complex. Both time-dependent and voltage-dependent outward $K^+$ currents are active, and the inward $Ca^{2+}$ current is inactivated, returning the cell to a negative resting potential. In addition, other $K^+$ channels important in repolarization have been described; they are sensitive to acetylcholine, adenosine triphosphate, and $Na^+$. The end of phase 3 roughly corresponds to the refractory period of the cell as well as the occurrence of the T wave on the surface electrocardiogram. Finally, in pacemaker cells, phase 4 depolarization occurs. In the sinus node, it is mediated by the inactivation of a repolarizing outward $K^+$ current, as well as the slow recovery of the inward $Ca^{2+}$ current.

Fast $Na^+$ channels may be studied using micropuncture techniques, and may be blocked using tetrodotoxin. Antiarrhythmic agents with class 1 antiarrhythmic activity, such as procainamide and quinidine, are thought to exert their effects by blocking fast $Na^+$ channels, therefore slowing the rate of rise of phase 0 and consequently decreasing conduction velocity.

Studies using tetrodotoxin in embryonic chick hearts have shown that these fast $Na^+$ channels are not present initially. Before they appear, phase 0 of the action potential is mediated by an inward $Na^+$ current carried by slow-response tetrodotoxin-insensitive $Na^+$ channels. $\dot{V}_{max}$ is much lower, and the amplitude of the action potential is lower as well. Tetrodotoxin-sensitive $Na^+$ channels appear at about 5 days' gestation in the chick heart, and there is a transitional period when both slow and fast $Na^+$ channels are present. By 8 days' gestation, all $Na^+$ channels are tetrodotoxin-sensitive. It is not clear whether the same phenomenon exists in other species; tetrodotoxin-insensitive slow $Na^+$ channels have not been found in

TABLE 76.1 Escape rates for intrinsic cardiac pacemaker foci

|  | 0–1 MONTH | 1 YEAR | 5 YEARS | ADULT |
|---|---|---|---|---|
| Sinus node | 90–180 | 90–150 | 65–135 | 60–120 |
| Atrioventricular node | 80–90 |  |  | 40–70 |
| Ventricle | 30–70 |  |  | 25–50 |

canines studied at an early gestational age, nor in human fetuses at 7 weeks.

In slow-response cells like those found in the sinus and atrioventricular node, the upstroke of the action potential, and therefore the velocity of conduction, is much lower than in fast-response cells found elsewhere. Phase 0 of the action potential is not mediated by the opening of fast $Na^+$ channels, but instead by the slow inward $Ca^{2+}$ current.

In normal sinus rhythm, the spread of cardiac excitation proceeds from the sinus node through the atrial muscle to excite both right and left atria (Fig. 76.2). Excitation reaches the atrioventricular node by way of cell-to-cell intraatrial conduction. Three specialized internodal tracts were once thought to be responsible for conduction directly from sinus to atrioventricular node. However, careful histological studies have failed to find evidence of specialized conduction tissue. The previously described internodal tracts currently are thought instead to be simply preferred routes for intraatrial conduction, made up of normal atrial myocardial cells.

The atrioventricular node is an atrial structure lying at the apex of the triangle of Koch and delineated by three landmarks: the tendon of Todaro (continuous with the eustachian valve), the mouth of the coronary sinus, and the tricuspid valve annulus. The atrioventricular node gives rise to a bundle (bundle of His) that penetrates the central fibrous body, then divides to form the left and right bundle branches, made up of Purkinje cells. The atrioventricular node is made up of slow-response cells that are histologically similar to those found in the sinus node. The slower upstroke of the action potential in the atrioventricular node is associated with a lower conduction velocity than elsewhere in the heart, and the atrioventricular node is responsible for introducing a significant delay between atrial and ventricular contraction.

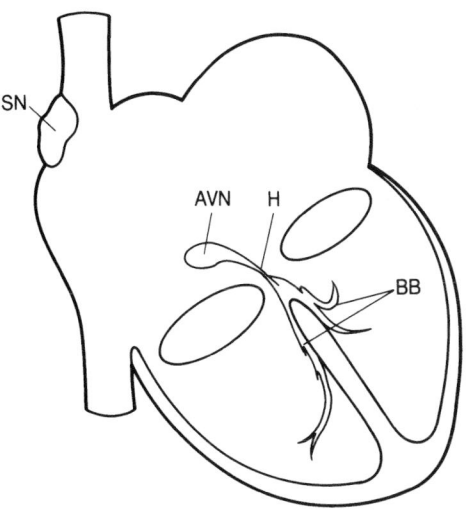

FIGURE 76.2 Cardiac conduction system. AVN, atrioventricular node; BB, bundle branches; H, bundle of His; SN, sinus node.

Nodal conduction time is age related. Little is known about conduction time in the node in fetal life. However, nodal conduction time may be measured clinically by recording the atrial electrogram at the approaches to the atrioventricular node, and the His electrogram. The atrial–His bundle (AH) interval is a measure of atrioventricular nodal conduction. Normally quite short at birth (20–40 ms), the AH interval increases progressively with age to as long as 200 ms in adulthood. Conduction in the distal conducting system (His bundle and bundle branches) may also be measured by timing the HV interval, i.e. the time from His bundle activation to earliest ventricular activation on the surface electrocardiogram. The HV interval, normally 20 ms at birth, increases to 40–50 ms in adulthood.

In addition to introducing a delay, the atrioventricular node also limits the number of atrial impulses that may conduct to the ventricles. This function is adaptive; arrhythmias such as atrial flutter or atrial fibrillation occur with atrial rates as high as 500–600 beats per minute. Refractoriness in the atrioventricular node limits the resulting ventricular rate. Refractoriness is also age-dependent. In late fetal life and in the newborn period, the atrioventricular node may conduct atrial rates as high as 300 beats per minute without block; however, with increasing age, atrioventricular block occurs at progressively slower atrial rates. Atrioventricular node refractoriness is also quite sensitive to autonomic influences.

## REGULATION OF IMPULSE FORMATION AND PROPAGATION

While both cardiac automaticity and conduction are under autonomic control, various other mechanisms may affect heart rate and conduction velocity. For example, both automaticity and conduction velocity increase with increasing temperature, acidity, and $CO_2$, and with decreasing $O_2$.

The adult heart is well invested with nerve fibers, and both the sympathetic and parasympathetic nervous systems influence cardiac automaticity and conduction. While sympathetic fibers reach the sinus node, atrioventricular node, bundle branches, and atrial and ventricular myocardium, vagal fibers are more limited in distribution, affecting mainly the atrial myocardium and the sinus and atrioventricular nodes. However, innervation of the ventricles by the vagus is limited, and vagal stimulation can lead to mild decreases in ventricular contractility.

Sympathetic fibers, when stimulated, release norepinephrine, which acts on local β-adrenergic receptors, enhancing the activity of adenylyl cyclase and converting ATP to cAMP, the "second messenger." Most norepinephrine is then taken up by the sympathetic terminals to be released again, and a small amount is metabolized. Sympathetic stimulation leads to increased automaticity of both the sinus and atrioventricular nodes, shortening of refractory periods and conduction times through the atrioventricular node, and shortening of refractory periods in both atrial and ventricular myocardium. Fast $Na^+$ channels do not appear to be regulated by autonomic influences or catecholamines. $Ca^{2+}$ channels, on the other hand, are under β-adrenergic control, mediated by a cAMP-dependent protein kinase. Sympathetic stimulation, of course, may have a host of other effects on the circulation, including increased contractility, changes in blood pressure, and effects on the coronary circulation.

Parasympathetic fibers innervating the heart release acetylcholine when stimulated. Cardiac cholinergic receptors are muscarinic in type. Activation of these receptors produces effects that, in general, are the opposite of effects produced by sympathetic stimulation. Therefore, decreases in sinus and atrioventricular node automaticity and increases in atrioventricular node conduction time are demonstrable.

Sympathetic and parasympathetic effects on the heart are age related, and change during fetal and post-natal development. The two opposing influences may develop at different rates during fetal life, but the results of investigations in this area are quite species specific. In sheep, sympathetic effects on the circulation probably appear before parasympathetic effects, but development of both is probably complete by 12 weeks' gestation. In contrast, sympathetic development is not complete at birth in canines, rats, and primates including humans. In these species, heart rate is thought to be primarily under vagal control at the time of birth. Differences in responsiveness to nerve stimulation are not thought to be due to lack of adrenergic or cholinergic receptor activity in the heart. In fact, compared with adults, fetuses appear supersensitive to the effects of infused norepinephrine, isoproterenol, and acetylcholine.

In species that exhibit incomplete sympathetic innervation of the heart at birth, postnatal maturation takes place. Such maturation may be non-uniform and may follow an irregular pattern of progression, as shown by experimental nerve stimulation in puppies. Adrenergic stimulation has been demonstrated to shorten ventricular action potential duration and refractory periods dramatically. Left stellate ganglion stimulation, or right stellate ganglion removal, is known to lower the threshold for ventricular fibrillation and to prolong the QT interval, and right stellate stimulation, or left stellate removal, raises the threshold. Conceivably, a developmental heterogeneity of sympathetic innervation may create a period of electrical instability due to dispersion of refractoriness, when stress and increased sympathetic activity may lead to ventricular arrhythmias. Schwartz was the first to propose the idea that autonomic instability could lead to ventricular arrhythmias and subsequently to sudden infant death syndrome (SIDS). There is evidence that abnormalities in the relationship between the QT interval and heart rate changes are detectable in at least some infants who later developed SIDS.

## SELECTED READING

Klitzner TS. Maturational changes in excitation–contraction coupling in mammalian myocardium. *J Am Coll Cardiol* 1991; **17**: 218.

Kralios FA, Millar CK. Functional development of cardiac sympathetic nerves in newborn dogs: evidence for asymmetrical development. *Cardiovasc Res* 1978; **12**: 547.

Kralios FA, Millar CK, Kralios AC. Developmental changes of ventricular fibrillation threshold and spontaneous defibrillation in young dogs. *J Dev Physiol* 1992; **17**: 163.

Malfatto G, Steinberg SF, Rosen TS *et al.* Experimental QT interval prolongation. *Ann NY Acad Sci* 1992; **644**: 74.

Mizeres NJ. The anatomy of the autonomic nervous system in the dog. *Am J Anat* 1955; **96**: 285.

Moak JP. Developmental cellular electrophysiologic effects of *d*-sotalol on canine cardiac Purkinje fibers. *Pediatr Res* 1991; **29**: 104.

Reder RF, Miura DS, Danilo P, Rosen MR. The electrophysiological properties of normal neonatal and adult canine cardiac fibers. *Circ Res* 1981; **48**: 658.

Schwartz PJ. Cardiac sympathetic innervation and the sudden infant death syndrome. *Am J Med* 1976; **6**: 167.

Schwartz PJ, Snebold NG, Brown AM. Effects of unilateral cardiac sympathetic denervation on the ventricular fibrillation threshold. *Am J Cardiol* 1976; **37**: 1034.

Yanowitz F, Preston JB, Abildskov AJ. Functional distribution of right and left stellate innervation to the ventricles. *Circ Res* 1966; **18**: 416.

# PART TWELVE

# *Respiratory System*

**Editor: Samuel Hawgood**

# 77

# Pulmonary Structure and Function

## LUNG DEVELOPMENT

### EMBRYOGENESIS

Lung development can be subdivided into five stages: (1) embryonic period – development of major airways; (2) pseudoglandular period – development of airways to terminal bronchioles; (3) canalicular period – development of the acinus and vascularization; (4) terminal sac (saccular) period – subdivision of saccules by secondary crests; and (5) alveolar period – the appearance of alveoli.

## Airways and alveoli

### Embryonic period

The lung originates from a diverticulum of the ventral wall of the caudal end of the laryngotracheal tube, which divides into two knob-like bronchial buds at 3–4 weeks' gestation. Outgrowth of these buds into the splanchnic mesenchyme produces the left and right primary bronchi. Each primary bronchial bud divides monopodially to give rise to a lateral diverticulum or bud; subsequently, the right lung bud gives rise on its craniodorsal side to a second monopodial diverticulum. Each secondary bronchus is a stem bronchus that will be a lobar bronchus. These stem bronchi are destined to branch and rebranch and, with the surrounding pulmonary mesenchyme, which will provide the elastic tissue, smooth muscles, cartilage, vascular system and other connective tissues, will give rise to the definitive pulmonary lobes that characterize adult lung organization.

## Pseudoglandular period

In the pseudoglandular period (6–16 weeks' gestation), the tracheobronchial tree of the fetal lung resembles a system of branching tubules that terminate in exocrine gland-like structures. These tubules are lined by distinct epithelium composed of columnar or approximately cuboidal cells, and are surrounded by mesenchyme.

## Canalicular period

During this period (16–28 weeks' gestation), the gas-exchanging portion of the lung becomes delineated with the appearance of new tubular branches, the respiratory bronchioles. Each respiratory bronchiole terminates in two or three thin-walled dilatations called terminal sacs or primitive alveoli.

## Terminal sac period

The terminal sac period (28–36 weeks' gestation) is characterized by further differentiation of the respiratory portion of the lung; respiratory bronchioles rapidly subdivide into an array of thin-walled primitive alveolar ducts and primitive alveoli. The saccules contain both cuboidal and flat types of alveolar epithelial cells, type II and type I epithelial cells, respectively. By the end of the terminal sac period, the organizational pattern of the respiratory portion of the lung is complete.

## Alveolar period

This period (32 weeks to term and postnatally in humans) is marked by the appearance of the alveoli, lined with extremely thin squamous type I cells. These type I cells become so thin that the underlying capillaries bulge into the space of each terminal sac. By the late fetal period, the lungs are capable of respiration because the alveolar capillary membrane is sufficiently thin to allow gas exchange.

# Vasculature

During the first month of gestation, a vascular plexus (originating from the splanchnic plexus) forms within the lung bud, which receives its blood supply from primitive pulmonary arteries as well as from a pair of branches from the dorsal aorta. Subsequently, numerous paired dorsal intersegmental arteries supply the vascular plexus, but by the end of the fifth week of gestation, as the true pulmonary arteries form and unite with the vascular plexus, the "primitive" pulmonary arteries become incorporated into the sixth aortic arch and the intersegmental arteries involute. The bronchial arteries develop only after the ninth week of gestation; they supply the bronchi down to a level several generations proximal to the terminal bronchioli.

Differentiation of true intrapulmonary arteries within the vascular plexus occurs at the same time as the airways develop so that by the sixteenth week of gestation all preacinar branches are present: both the conventional arteries that run alongside the airways and the supernumerary arteries that provide additional blood supply to the alveolar region. After the sixteenth week of gestation the preacinar arteries increase mainly in diameter and length, and the intraacinar arteries begin to form along the developing acinus (i.e. the primitive alveolar ducts and alveoli).

The pulmonary veins develop from an outgrowth of the left atrium. These structures start as a blind chamber that grows posteriorly to contact the lung buds; it bifurcates, and by the eleventh week of gestation, four separate veins enter the left atrial chamber. The veins within the lung develop at the same time as the arteries so that all preacinar veins are also present halfway through gestation. The conventional veins branch at right angles to the arteries, and there are many supernumerary veins as well. At 20 weeks' gestation, all the veins are non-muscular, but by 28 weeks scattered muscle bundles appear.

# Tissue interactions

In the embryonic lung, branching of the epithelium is controlled by epithelial–mesenchymal tissue interactions. The mesenchymal component dictates the branching pattern of the epithelium, and the inductive capacity of the mesenchyme is organ and species specific. Forces within the epithelial cells alter cell and tissue shape to produce branch points. Extracellular matrix proteins at the epithelial–mesenchymal interface, such as proteoglycans, fibronectin, laminin, and collagen, may act as morphogenetic factors controlling the organ- and species-specific pattern of lung branching. Growth factors have also been implicated in regulating branching morphogenesis. Platelet-derived growth factor (PDGF-AA), keratinocyte growth factor (KGF), and epidermal growth factor (EGF), have characteristics compatible with transferring information between adjacent tissue layers.

## PRENATAL GROWTH

As is evident from the preceding section, fetal lung morphogenesis involves major structural changes that are associated with cell proliferation as well as with cell differentiation (*see* Chapter 17). The following section summarizes current knowledge of prenatal lung growth.

## Physical factors

Increasing evidence suggests that a variety of physical factors influence normal fetal lung growth. These include the amount of amniotic and lung fluid, available space for lung in the thorax, and fetal respiration. How these factors affect lung growth remains to be defined, but the available evidence strongly supports the concept that strain is an important stimulus for fetal lung growth.

## Hormonal factors

Hormones such as glucocorticoids, androgen, thyroid hormone, and insulin affect lung differentiation. Current data, however, suggest that they play no important role in normal fetal lung growth.

## Growth factors

Growth factors are a group of small molecular mass (8–40 kD) polypeptides that regulate the proliferation of cells by inducing DNA synthesis and cell division. Such growth factors have been isolated from a variety of sources including tissue, serum, plasma and conditioned medium from cell cultures. Growth factors function as autocrine or paracrine messengers. Once synthesized, they are released and act on target cells via specific cell-surface receptors. A number of intracellular metabolic pathways are activated after receptor stimulation, which may lead to DNA synthesis and cell replication. Not all growth factors are stimulatory; some inhibit cell proliferation. Many growth factors have been identified in the fetal lung, where they apparently mediate the effects of physical forces on cellular proliferation.

## Lung cell growth

Lung cell proliferation is confined mainly to morphogenetically active regions, which shift from central to peripheral tubules during development. The rate of proliferation of both epithelial and mesenchymal cells decreases during development, but the decline is unequal. The proportion of dividing cells that are epithelial increases initially during fetal development but declines dramatically near term. The decline in epithelial mitotic activity is associated with an increase in cellular differentiation that occurs in the course of

lung morphogenesis. Unlike epithelial cells, the proportion of dividing cells that are mesenchymal decreases in the earlier stages of development, but mesenchymal proliferation increases sharply at the canalicular phase of development because of capillary growth. Capillary formation continues at a rapid rate during late fetal life and, consequently, mesenchymal cells are the predominant dividing cell type near term. The period of alveolarization is accompanied by a phase of rapid cellular proliferation in both epithelial and mesenchymal lung populations. Interstitial fibroblasts proliferate actively early in the period but then slow down, whereas endothelial cell growth is brisk throughout this period. The dividing endothelial and interstitial cells are primarily located in septal crests. Epithelial cell division in this period occurs on septal buds and walls. Both alveolar epithelial cell populations, type II and type I cells, increase during this growth period. However, only alveolar epithelial type II cells proliferate actively, indicating that alveolar type I cells arise from type II cells.

## Mesenchymal–epithelial interactions

As mentioned above, the mechanism(s) controlling the ontogenic pattern of lung cell proliferation remains to be elucidated. However, it is well known that bronchial epithelial growth is stimulated by bronchial mesenchyme. Embryonic bronchial mesenchyme seems to have the ability to maintain most or all of the epithelial cells at the branching points in the cell cycle, thereby stimulating epithelial budding. Growth factors, synthesized and released by mesenchymal cells, are most likely responsible for this local effect on epithelial cell growth. However, growth inhibitory factors may also be involved in controlling this process.

## DIFFERENTIATION

## Epithelium

### Type II cells

The commitment of apparently undifferentiated respiratory epithelium to subsequent expression of the type II cell phenotype occurs prior to 13 days' gestation in the fetal rat lung and is dependent upon epithelial–mesenchymal interactions (Fig. 77.1a).

Once the future type II cell is committed to its phenotypic pathway, glycogen deposition precedes lamellar body formation. At the appropriate developmental stage, the synthesis of glycogen in the alveolar epithelium is regulated by corticosteroids, which requires the presence of mesenchyme. Later, the onset of lamellar body formation is associated with glycogen breakdown. Significant quantities of surfactant are not synthesized until close to term. The fine regulation of this quantitative progression in expression of

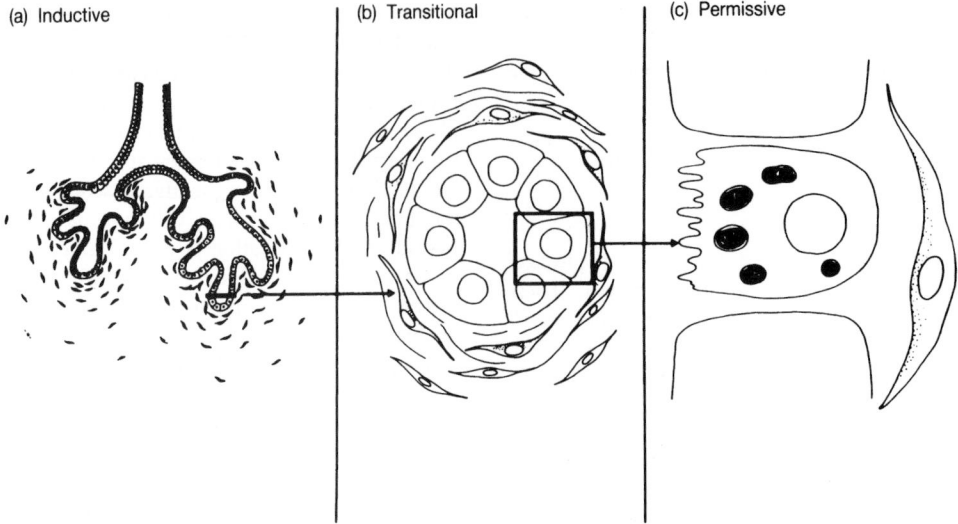

(a) Inductive    (b) Transitional    (c) Permissive

FIGURE 77.1 Schematic representation of the time and nature of mesenchymal–epithelial interactions during the organogenesis and differentiation of lung parenchyma. (a) Role of mesenchyme in directing the branching of epithelium and in establishing the future phenotype of the alveolar type II cell. As these involve expression of new gene products, these represent inductive influences. (b) Acquisition of glucocorticoid receptors by mesenchymal cells closest to differentiating epithelium. These influences may involve either new gene expression or quantitative increase in expression of genes, and are termed transitional. (c) Role of fibroblast-derived fibroblast-pneumonocyte factor in enhancing surfactant phospholipid production by the type II cell in anticipation of birth and the need for air breathing. As no new gene products are expressed, but quantitative increases occur, this is termed permissive induction.

phenotype is under multihormonal control, yet local cell and tissue interactions continue to modulate the endocrine signals.

## Hormonal factors

A central role in epithelial type II cell maturation is played by endogenous fetal glucocorticoids. They are largely in the inactive form (cortisone), but in the fetal lung fibroblast are "activated" by reduction of cortisone at the eleventh carbon to produce cortisol. Once activated, the glucocorticoid also acts directly within the fibroblast to induce the production of fibroblast-pneumonocyte factor (FPF) (Figs. 77.1c and 77.2), which in turn acts upon the adjacent type II cell to induce surfactant phospholipid synthesis. The elaboration of FPF in response to glucocorticoid is inhibited in the presence of insulin and androgen. Thyroid hormones increase the responsiveness of fetal type II cells for FPF (Fig. 77.2).

## Alveolar type I cells

The alveolar epithelial type I cell is the attenuated alveolar lining cell across which gas exchange takes place. This phenotype appears quite late in development, in keeping with its terminally differentiated state. Its embryonic precursor is the alveolar type II cell. As the appearance of the type I cell occurs at the time that the mesenchyme is regressing and the vascu-

lar cells are coming to lie in closer approximation to the alveolar epithelium, it is tempting to speculate that the phenotypic conversion from type II cell to type I cell could be induced by endothelial interactions (or withdrawal of fibroblast interactions).

# Vascular cells

The development of blood vessels in the lung (angiogenesis) most likely depends on a coordinated set of stimulatory and inhibitory signals from a variety of interstitial and blood-borne cell types (see Chapter 67). The vascular cells themselves contribute. The signals include insulin-like growth factors, interferon-γ, proteins with a high affinity for heparin such as acidic and basic fibroblast growth factors, and the transforming growth factors α and β. The growth and angiogenic factors induce proteolytic activity, which alters basement membrane and other connective tissue proteins. This stimulates not only cell migration and proliferation, but also the elaboration of a different matrix, which may then have an inhibitory or "stop" action on the proliferating cells and induce proliferation or differentiation of another cell type. Subtle changes in the extracellular protein milieu probably contribute to specialization of vascular cells, and flow patterns ultimately determine whether a vessel is destined to be a capillary, an artery, or a vein. The whole process, while very active in the developing lung, must be held in check after it is completed.

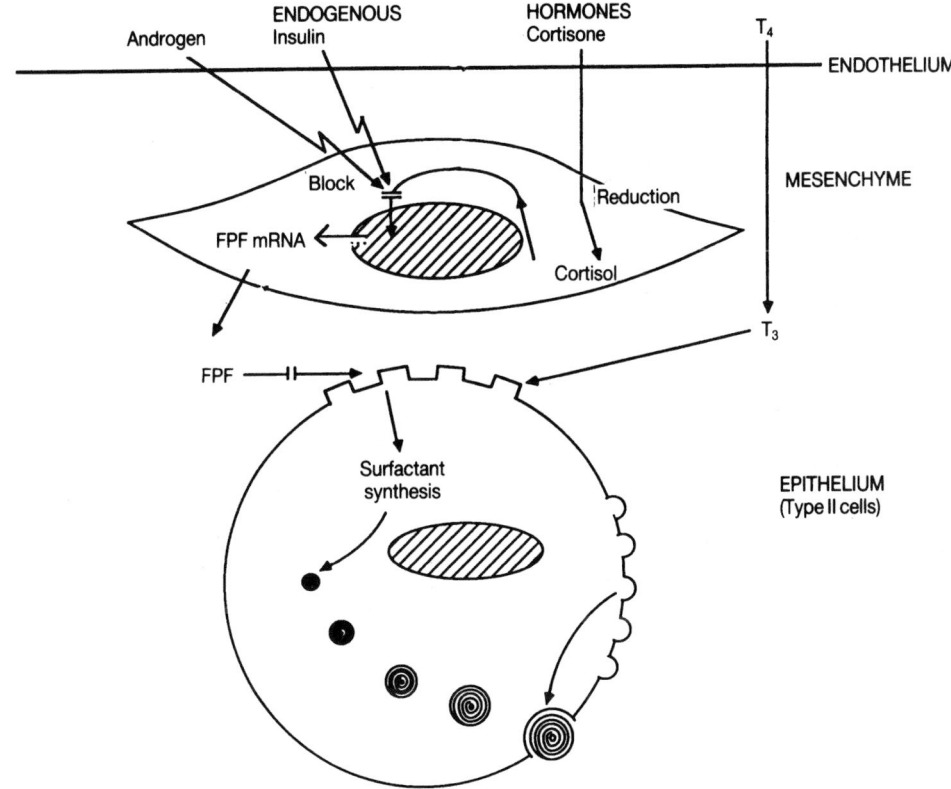

FIGURE 77.2 Schematic representation of hormonal influences on epithelial type II cell differentiation. FPF, fibroblast-pneumonocyte factor

## SELECTED READING

Adams JC, Watt FM. Regulation of development and differentiation by the extracellular matrix. *Development* 1993; 117: 1183.

Minoo P, King RJ. Epithelial–mesenchymal interactions in lung development. *Annu Rev Physiol* 1994; 56: 13.

Post M, Smith BT. Hormonal control of surfactant metabolism. In: Robertson B, Van Golde LMG, Batenburg JJ, eds. *Pulmonary surfactant: from molecular biology to clinical practice*. New York: Elsevier, 1992: 379.

Smith BT, Post M. Tissue interactions. In: Crystal RG, West J, eds. *The lung*. New York, Raven Press, 1991: 671.

# UPPER AND CONDUCTING AIRWAYS

The upper airway and the tracheobronchial tree are a continuous system of tubes that connect the gas-exchange regions of the lung to ambient air. The upper airway extends from the nasal choanae to the larynx, and may be divided into three parts based on functional anatomy: the nasal passage, the pharynx, and the larynx. It is important to note that the oral cavity can also contribute to respiration under normal and pathological conditions, but its role will not be covered in depth. The tracheobronchial tree begins at the larynx and may be divided into three major sections based on anatomy: the cartilaginous airways, including the extrapulmonary airways and the bronchi down to 1 mm in diameter; the membranous bronchioles, comprising the last four to five generations of airways leading to the gas-exchange areas of the lung; and the respiratory bronchioles. The conducting airways include the first two sections and, together with the upper airway, constitute the anatomical dead space. Although the principal function of the upper and conducting airways is to act as a conduit for gas flow, they also have important non-respiratory functions, e.g. humidifying, warming, and filtering inspired air. They play an important role in defense against microorganisms, particles, and noxious agents in inspired air. The upper airway has separate but important functions in speech, swallowing, digestion, smell, and taste. The rigid conducting airways have the additional function of providing a supporting framework for the surrounding lung parenchyma.

## UPPER AIRWAY

### Upper airway structure

The upper airway is composed of both fleshy, collapsible segments and rigid, bony segments. Collapsible segments include the nasal valve, the muscular pharynx, and the cartilaginous larynx. Rigid segments include the nasal cavity from the nasal valve to the choanae, the paranasal sinuses, and upper portions of the nasopharynx.

Collapsible segments of the upper airway are organized in three layers: mucosa, submucosa, and musculomembranous. The mucosa is composed of a ciliated pseudostratified columnar epithelium superiorly, and a non-cornified stratified squamous epithelium inferiorly, overlying a lamina propria of variable thickness, depending on the site. The transition between typical respiratory epithelium and squamous epithelium, high in the nasopharynx, is indistinct. At the nasal opening, the mucosa is normal skin with a ring of coarse hairs protruding into the nasal vestibule. The submucosal layer contains blood vessels, adipose cells, lymphoid tissue, nerves, and glands. In the wall of the pharynx, a layer of striated muscles surrounded by fascia underlies the submucosa. These muscles extend from the skull, hyoid, cervical cartilage, and mandible to visceral layers of fascia that connect muscle groups. These muscles are an important structural element of collapsible segments of the upper airway and are controlled by neural input from the motor nuclei in the brainstem through cranial nerves VII, IX, X, and XII and spinal nerves C1–2. The motor nuclei of the brainstem receive input from the respiratory control centers and multiple sensory afferent nerves.

In rigid segments of the upper airway, the mucosa is tightly attached to underlying periostium and composed of a ciliated pseudostratified columnar epithelium resting on a basal lamina. Epithelial cell types include ciliated and non-ciliated columnar cells, basal cells, intermediate cells, and mucus-secreting goblet cells interspersed in the epithelium. Cilia are more numerous in the nasal epithelium and at the openings of the sinuses. Within the sinuses, the epithelium is more cuboidal with fewer cilia. The underlying submucosa is highly vascular and has numerous submucosal glands, densely distributed throughout the nasal cavity. The superficial submucosa has numerous arterioles, capillaries, veins, venous plexi, and venous lakes that can become engorged with blood, resulting in thickening of the submucosa. Deep in the submucosa, fenestrated capillaries allow vascular fluid to move quickly into the submucosa resulting in edema. Sensory innervation from this area to the brain is via branches of the trigeminal nerve. Efferent innervation is directed to submucosal glands and blood vessels via postganglionic parasympathetic fibers from the sphenopalatine ganglion and postganglionic sympathetic fibers from the superior cervical ganglion.

## Development

Fetal development of the oral, nasal, and pharyngeal structures is crucial to overall development of the face, and is structurally complete by 10 weeks' gestation. The anterior structures (mouth and nose) derive from ectoderm, and the posterior structures (pharynx and larynx) derive from endoderm. Muscular components of the mouth, pharynx, and larynx develop from ill-defined collections of mesenchyme along the lateral aspects of the developing airway.

The oral cavity (stomodeum) is seen in the first weeks of gestation and fuses with the caudal end of the developing pharynx (primitive foregut) by disintegration of the buccopharyngeal membrane (fourth week). The nasal cavity begins as ectodermal thickenings called placodes (fourth week) that develop into sacs (sixth week) and fuse with the developing pharynx forming the nasal choanae (seventh week). Failure of this fusion or retention of epithelial plugs can result in choanal atresia or stenosis. The palate develops medially from the sides of the maxillary process and fuse with the nasal septum anteriorly (seventh week). Fusion proceeds posteriorly towards the nasal choanae, completing palate development by the twelfth week. Failure of this fusion results in a cleft palate. Ossification of the palate also begins anteriorly and proceeds posteriorly, terminating at the posterior edge of the nasal septum. The remaining palate becomes a muscular flap, the soft palate. The anterior nasal passage and the oral cavity become lined with stratified squamous epithelium, whereas the posterior nasal passage develops ciliated epithelium. Goblet cells are first seen in the anterior nasal cavity (thirteenth week) and migrate posteriorly along the floor of the nose and then superiorly, completing their migration by the thirtieth week. Submucosal glands are first seen anteriorly in the eleventh week and migrate in a fashion similar to goblet cells, covering the nasal cavity by the eighteenth week.

The pharyngeal cavity develops from the caudal end of the primitive foregut in association with derivatives of deep clefts of surface ectoderm (branchial arches). The primitive pharynx has four pairs of pouches that extend laterally between the aortic arches and make direct contact with the branchial arches. Structures such as the eustachian tubes, middle ears, tonsilar fossae, and parathyroid glands are formed from the pharyngeal pouches. Supporting structures such as the mandible, hyoid, thyroid cartilage, and cricoid cartilage are derived from the associated branchial arches. The pharyngeal cavity becomes lined with stratified squamous epithelium up to the level of the dissolved buccopharyngeal membrane.

The larynx develops from a midline groove in the anterior pharyngeal cavity, first seen in the fourth week of gestation. As this laryngotracheal groove becomes a tube, the upper part forms the larynx and the lower part becomes the trachea and developing lung buds. By the sixth week, the larynx is a T-shaped opening in the laryngotracheal groove and the surrounding structures of the arytenoids and epiglottis become evident. The epithelium of the larynx is derived from the pharynx and transiently grows over the laryngeal opening. Failure of complete dissolution of this epithelium can result in congenital obstruction of the larynx. The cartilage of the arytenoid and the epiglottis develop from the branchial arches and the muscles of the larynx arise from mesenchymal collections associated with the third and fourth arches.

## Control of upper airway patency

Even though the upper airway has multiple functions, its role in respiration is primary. The upper airway makes up a significant portion of the anatomical dead space and contributes a predominant portion of the total resistance to breathing. Airflow through the upper airway is complex and controlled by multiple interrelated factors including airflow rate, transmural pressure, airway size, airway muscle tone, head position, and sleep state. Moreover, because regions of the upper airway have fleshy collapsible segments, important dynamic changes in airflow resistance can occur under different conditions. These factors can be variably effective at different sites in the upper airway. Control of upper airway patency is achieved by a balance of collapsing and dilating forces that are generated by airflow properties and structural elements of the airway wall (Fig. 77.3).

### Airflow through collapsible segments

The structure of the upper airway results in turbulent airflow, which has important and distinctive features. Because of turbulence, resistance to airflow through the upper airway is non-linear, increasing geometrically as airflow rate increases (Fig. 77.4). During turbulent flow, resistance is directly proportional to the density of gas and inversely proportional to the fifth power of the radius. Thus, the resistance offered by the upper airway varies significantly with the rate at which air is moved through it and is exquisitely sensitive to airway caliber. Use of less dense gases, such as helium, can be effective in altering resistance and have clinical usefulness in patients with *upper airway obstruction.*

Much of the upper airway is collapsible and, therefore, the pressure difference across the airway wall (transmural pressure) must be considered (Fig. 77.5). During inspiration, the pressure within the airway lumen becomes less than the pressure in surrounding tissues (atmospheric). As a result, the transmural pressure difference acts as a collapsing force on the upper airway wall. Higher transmural pressures lead to more collapse of the airway, potentially to the point of complete obstruction. During exhalation, the transmural pressure difference provides a distending force on the

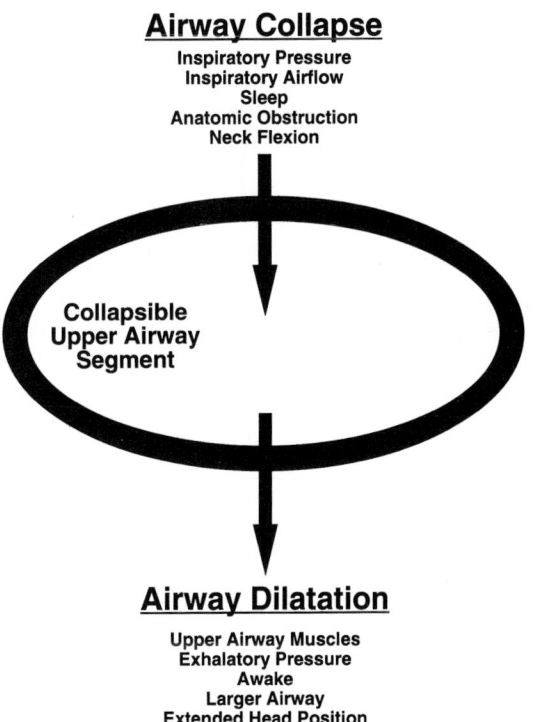

**Airway Collapse**

**Inspiratory Pressure**
**Inspiratory Airflow**
**Sleep**
**Anatomic Obstruction**
**Neck Flexion**

**Collapsible**
**Upper Airway**
**Segment**

**Airway Dilatation**

**Upper Airway Muscles**
**Exhalatory Pressure**
**Awake**
**Larger Airway**
**Extended Head Position**

FIGURE 77.3 Balance of forces controlling upper airway patency. The major collapsing forces (inspiratory transmural pressure and flow) are balanced against the dilating forces (action of the upper airway muscles). Excess inspiratory flow or negative intraluminal pressure result in airway closure, whereas increased tension or contraction of upper airway muscles can open the airway. Sleep state, airway size, and head position can alter the effect of these forces, affecting the balance.

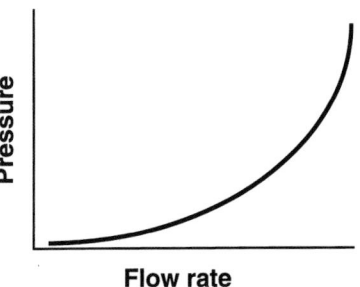

FIGURE 77.4 Turbulent flow. The pressure–flow relationship is non-linear during turbulent flow. Resistance is the slope of this relationship, and increases as pressure or flow rate increase.

airway wall, explaining why dynamic obstruction of the upper airway is usually apparent during inspiration. The combined effects of transmural pressure on the collapsible airway and airway caliber on resistance make the upper airway most vulnerable to collapse during inspiration. The lowest transmural pressures required to collapse the airway of newborn infants and, hence, the greatest vulnerability to collapse are found in the oropharynx and nasopharynx. This is the region of the upper airway where snoring and

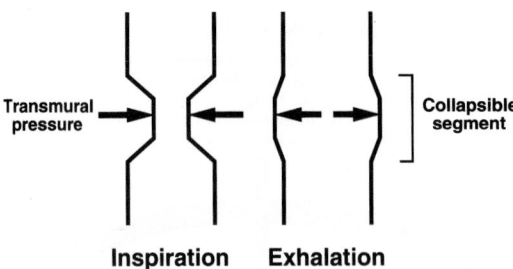

**Inspiration    Exhalation**

FIGURE 77.5 Effect of transmural pressure on collapsible segments of the upper airway. During inspiration, the intraluminal pressure is less than the pressure in the surrounding tissues and transmural pressure tends to collapse the airway. During exhalation, intraluminal pressure is greater than in the surrounding tissue and the airway is slightly distended.

*obstructive apneas* occur. Evidence for a relationship between collapsing pressures and airway size is seen in patients with increased dynamic obstruction due to anatomical narrowing of the airway (hypertrophy of lymphoid tissues, nasal obstruction due to inflammation, enlargement of the tongue, and craniofacial abnormalities) or positional narrowing due to flexion of the neck. This relationship is clarified by the relief of obstruction seen after slight extension of the head, surgical correction of anatomical airway narrowing, and application of continuous positive airway pressure.

In the collapsible segments of the upper airway, muscles in the airway wall provide the dilating force that maintains airway patency. As many as 39 muscles assist in maintaining upper airway patency. Their action is coordinated by neural input from motor nuclei in the brainstem that receive input from the respiratory centers, afferent nerves responding to stretch, airflow, pressure changes and temperature, peripheral and central chemoreceptors, and neural centers controlling state. In general, contraction of these upper airway muscles results in dilatation or increased tension in the airway wall. Muscles of the upper airway are structurally adapted to provide rapid contraction and resistance to fatigue. Some muscles are continuously active; many muscles contract phasically during inspiration, providing dynamic stability in the airway; a small number of muscles are active primarily during exhalation; and some muscles are variably active, remaining inactive during rest and increasingly active as ventilatory effort increases. The contraction of these muscles is coordinated such that contraction of upper airway muscles precedes the action of inspiratory muscles. This timing is affected by central respiratory centers; peripheral afferent nerves from the lungs, lower airways, and the upper airway muscles themselves; and sleep state. The importance of proper function and timing of muscle contraction is illustrated by common uncoordinated breaths such as snoring and hiccoughs, and pathological conditions such as *obstructive sleep apnea* (Fig. 77.3), upper airway obstruction in premature newborns, airway obstruc-

tion in patients with cerebral palsy or depressed mental states (anesthesia, intoxications, or brain injury), and obstruction during phrenic nerve pacing. State of arousal has an important effect on upper airway muscles. During sleep, the timing of respiratory muscle contraction is altered and activity in dilating muscles is decreased, promoting upper airway obstruction. The activity of upper airway muscles can be stimulated by hypercapnia, mild degrees of hypoxia, and arousal.

## Airflow through rigid segments

Resistance offered by the rigid nasal passage makes the single greatest contribution to the overall resistance of the upper airway. In adults, 40–60 per cent of the total airway resistance during quiet breathing is contributed by the nose. Like the collapsible segments, resistance to airflow through the nose is variable. The previously described features of resistance to turbulent flow also apply to the nose. There is a non-linear relationship between airflow rate and pressure drop through the nose, and resistance is very sensitive to small changes in airway caliber. As a result, it becomes very difficult to sustain nasal breathing as airflow increases. During exercise, when airflow is high, people naturally change to mouth breathing, decreasing the work of breathing by about 30 per cent. Absolute nasal resistance is higher in infants than adults, but the relative contribution of nasal resistance to the total resistance is less. In addition, the larynx is positioned higher in newborns, bringing the epiglottis close to the soft palate and the oral portion of the tongue is apposed to the soft palate. These features make nasal breathing easier in infants. In young infants, who do not easily change to mouth breathing, increases in nasal resistance, resulting from changes in flow or airway size, can result in significant respiratory distress.

Airflow through the nose is directed along the floor of the nasal cavity, between the nasal turbinates and the septum, such that resistance is also regulated by the mucosa over the turbinates and septum. The nasal mucosa acts as an erectile tissue that can swell and shrink causing large alterations in nasal resistance. In adolescents and adults, these changes can be cyclical (nasal cycle), causing the nasal resistance to increase and decrease in an alternating fashion between the two sides of the nose and the total nasal resistance to remain relatively constant. In younger children, the nasal cycle occurs simultaneously on both sides of the nose, resulting in cyclical variation in total nasal resistance. The nasal cycle is not well understood but may be regulated by autonomic neural input. Non-cyclical variation in nasal resistance is generated by autonomic neural input, hormones (estrogen, testosterone, epinephrine, and thyroid), body and head position, lung volume, ambient temperature and humidity, inflammatory mediators (histamine, prostaglandins), emotions, and sexual activity.

## CONDUCTING AIRWAYS

### Airway structure

The conducting airways are organized into three concentric layers: mucosa, submucosa, and adventitia. The innermost layer, the mucosa, is composed of a continuous layer of epithelial cells covered by a thin layer of liquid and mucus. The submucosa is separated from the mucosa by the lamina propria and contains glands, smooth muscle, nerves, cartilage, and blood vessels. The outermost layer, the adventitiá, is a collection of loose connective tissue that contains nerves, ganglia, and bronchial vessels. This loose connective tissue layer provides a sump for collection of excess lung liquid, and contains lymphatics that are an important route for clearance of excess liquid from the gas-exchange regions of the lung. The structure of these layers changes as the airways branch out toward the periphery of the lung.

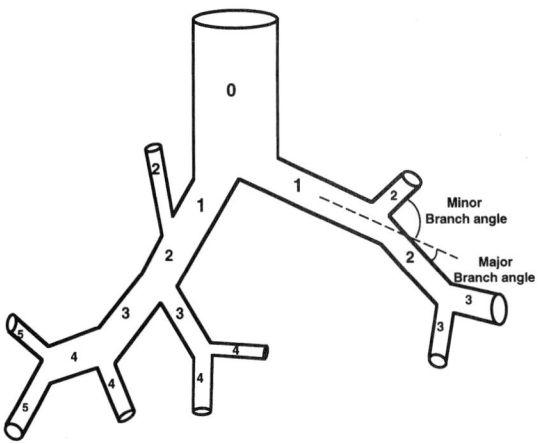

FIGURE 77.6 Irregular dichotomous branching of the conducting airways. Airway generation is labeled from the trachea to successive daughter branches which may be different in length and diameter. The larger branch has a smaller angle (major angle) and the smaller branch has a larger angle (minor angle) to the line of the parent branch.

### Airway development

Airway development is important in determining the ultimate shape of the mature lung. As the primitive airways grow, a balance between proliferation and migration of epithelial cells as well as specific interactions between the epithelium and the surrounding mesenchyme govern airway branching. Each parent branch gives rise to two smaller daughter branches that differ in length and diameter. This pattern of branching is called irregular dichotomous branching, an important feature of mature airways. After branching, airways become encased in dense mesenchymal tissue that ultimately develops into smooth muscle, connective tissue, and cartilage. The structural development of the airways is complete well before birth. After birth, several terminal generations of airways are lost by development of terminal bronchioles into respiratory bronchioles. This process is complete by about 3 years of age. Thereafter, growth in airway length and diameter continues until growth of the chest cavity stops. During postnatal development, the rate of growth in both length and diameter of the larger airways exceeds that in the smaller airways.

### Airway morphology

Airway morphology in the mature lung is well suited for efficient transport of gas to an expansive gas-exchange surface. The irregular dichotomous branching system results in progressive reduction in length and diameter of the branches as they approach the gas-exchange region (Fig. 77.6). The diameter of a given branch is proportional to the volume of gas-exchange region that it ventilates. The angles between branches vary according to the diameter of the airway. There is considerable heterogeneity in the distance and number of branches required to reach gas-exchange sites. In the mature lung, the total number of divisions between the trachea and the respiratory bronchioles averages about 15 but can vary between 8 and 25. The distance from the carina to the distal bronchioles can vary from 8 to 22 cm.

### Functional consequences of airway morphology

Transport of gas in the lung involves bulk movement of gas through the conducting airways and diffusion of gas in the distal lung. The physical characteristics of these two processes are very different and place complex and seemingly contradictory requirements on airway structure. Efficient diffusion requires short diffusion distances and large total cross-sectional areas. Efficient bulk movement of gas requires increased airway volume in order to decrease airflow resistance. However, increasing airway volume increases wasted ventilation by taking volume away from gas-exchange regions, and increases airway tissue mass.

These opposing requirements are well balanced by the morphological features of conducting airways. As the number of branches increases, the cumulative volume and total cross-sectional area of the airways increases. Airflow velocity decreases as the airway branching increases. Thus, as air moves from the proximal airways to the distal airways, the total cross-sectional area increases and the airflow velocity decreases, allowing for efficient diffusion of gas in terminal respiratory regions (Fig. 77.7). The irregular branching

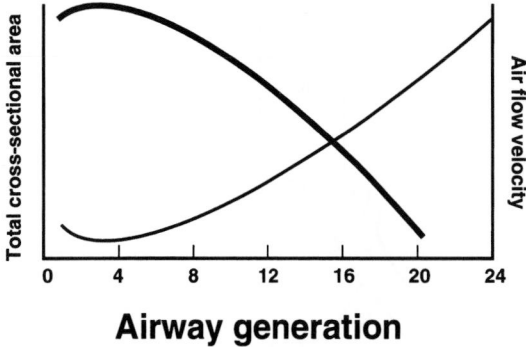

**Airway generation**

FIGURE 77.7 Relationship of cross-sectional area and airflow velocity as the airways branch. As the airways branch toward the periphery, airflow velocity (bold line) decreases to near zero at the level of the gas-exchange units. Total cross-sectional area (thin line) increases toward the alveoli.

branch angles causing higher resistances in airways to proximal gas-exchange sites. Thus, the balance of structural features that determine airflow in the airways acts to minimize potential differences in ventilation between proximal and distal gas-exchange units.

## Structural elements of the airways (Table 77.1)

### Surface epithelium

Cells that line airways and secretory glands are derived from endodermal cells in the primitive foregut. Ciliated and basal cells are seen early in gestation, followed later by secretory cells. Differentiation of the epithelium starts centrally and extends peripherally during development. In the mature lung the mucosal epithelium of the trachea and larger bronchi is a pseudostratified columnar ciliated epithelium. As the airways narrow and branch out toward the lung periphery, the epithelium becomes thinner and more cuboidal. Ciliated cells are the most common cells in the surface epithelium of larger airways; however, they are less numerous in bronchioles. Intermediate cells are relatively undifferentiated cells found submerged within the pseudostratified columnar epithelium. Basal cells form a row of flattened cells along the basement membrane. Brush cells are relatively rare cells located throughout the airways. Goblet cells are mucus-secreting cells seen primarily in the larger airways, and are relatively uncommon in bronchioles under normal conditions. Serous cells are seen in the surface epithelium during fetal life but are rare after birth. Clara cells

system also enhances bulk flow by minimizing the energy required for gas transport, optimizing airflow that is intermediate between laminar and turbulent, and by minimizing the distance from the airway entrance to each point in the gas-exchange region.

Variability in airway length, airway diameters, and the number of branches required to reach different alveoli would be expected to result in higher airflow resistance to more distal gas-exchange sites. Differences in airflow resistances, transit times, and airway lengths may further contribute to variability in the time it takes for air to reach different alveoli and inhomogeneity of ventilation within the lung. While longer airway lengths and more branch points may lead to higher resistances and longer times for air to reach more distal alveoli, this is balanced by wider

TABLE 77.1 Structural elements of the conducting airways

| STRUCTURE | LOCATION | | | FUNCTION |
|---|---|---|---|---|
| | LAYER | CARTILAGINOUS AIRWAYS | MEMBRANOUS BRONCHIOLES | |
| Surface epithelium | | | | |
| Ciliated cell | Mucosa | ++ | + | Clearance, ion transport, barrier |
| Intermediate cell | Mucosa | + | + | Undifferentiated, ? repair |
| Basal cell | Mucosa | ++ | + | Epithelial adhesion |
| Mucous (goblet) cells | Mucosa | + | + | Secretion |
| Clara cells | Mucosa | − | ++ | Barrier, ion transport, secretion, repair and regeneration |
| Submucosal glands | Submucosa | ++ | − | Secretion, defense |
| Smooth muscle | Submucosa | + | + | Control of airway caliber |
| Neural elements | | | | |
| Motor nerves | Submucosa, adventitia | + | + | Airway caliber, secretion, ion transport |
| Sensory nerves | Mucosa, submucosa, adventitia | + | + | Airway caliber, secretion |
| Neuroepithelial | Mucosa | ++ | + | Neuroregulatory |
| Immunological cells | Submucosa | + | + | Defense, airway caliber, secretion, ion transport |
| Connective tissue | | | | |
| Cartilage | Submucosa | ++ | − | Structural support |
| Elastin and collagen | Submucosa | + | ++ | Structural support |

are non-ciliated cuboidal secretory cells that are common in bronchioles of the mature lung.

The surface epithelium has several important functions. The airway epithelium forms a barrier against foreign material entering the lung tissue and leakage of interstitial liquid into the air spaces. Surface epithelial cells maintain the thin liquid layer that lines airways by transporting ions and water across the epithelial barrier. Secretory epithelial cells provide a variety of substances that contribute to lung defense and clearance mechanisms. Ciliated cells help propel these secretions up the airways. Serous and intermediate cells contribute to repair and regeneration of the epithelium while basal cells help other epithelial cells adhere to the basement membrane. Clara cells appear to serve regenerative and secretory functions in the bronchioles. Surface epithelial cells also play a regulatory role through interactions with other airway cells.

## Submucosal glands

Submucosal glands are acinar structures with tubular ducts that pierce the lamina propria and open into the surface epithelium. They first appear in the central airways as clumps of undifferentiated cells, which then migrate into the submucosa. After migration, gland cells differentiate into mucous and serous cells and proliferate to form cystic structures. Ducts form by separation and canalization of cells leading to the surface epithelium. Later in development, primitive glands extend peripherally into the bronchi. Gland formation is largely complete before birth. The glands continue to increase in size and complexity until adolescence and early adulthood. In the mature lung, submucosal glands are seen primarily in the proximal airways. They become smaller and less numerous in more distal airways, and are normally absent in small bronchi and bronchioles.

Submucosal glands are important to lung defense by secreting a complex mixture of mucins and proteins that entrap debris, microorganisms, inflammatory cells, and inhaled foreign particles. The density of glands within the submucosa parallels the deposition of inhaled particles, and increases in chronic inflammatory conditions.

## Airway smooth muscle

Smooth muscle cells, elongated contractile cells found in the airway submucosa, are joined by gap junctions and are grouped in muscle bundles. The location and orientation of these bundles in the airway wall varies according to the location in the tracheobronchial tree. In the trachea and larger bronchi, they form bands of muscle that connect the ends of incomplete cartilage rings. Further down the airway, they form a separate layer of muscle between the surface epithelium and the cartilage. Smooth muscle spirals around smaller airways in a helical fashion.

During development, smooth muscle forms from dense condensations of mesenchyme around proximal airways, and later develops more peripherally in parallel with developing nerves. Although the amount of smooth muscle in the proximal airways increases substantially after birth, very little increase occurs normally in peripheral airways.

Airway smooth muscle controls airflow within the lung by regulating local airflow resistance through changes in airway caliber. In response to stimulation, the muscles contract slowly, resulting in a gradual increase in tension followed by slow relaxation. The effect of airway smooth muscle contraction depends on the size of the airway. Muscle contraction in the larger cartilaginous airways pulls the ends of the cartilage rings together, diminishing airway caliber. In smaller bronchi, muscle contraction decreases airway diameter and length, and increases wall stiffness.

## Neural elements

The conducting airways have a generous supply of afferent and efferent nerves as well as receptors that are stimulated by local or humoral substances. These neural elements interact with epithelium, submucosal glands, smooth muscle, and airway vasculature to regulate numerous airway functions. Development of neural elements in the airways begins early in gestation and continues after birth. Ganglion cells and nerves are seen in the proximal airways early in gestation and extend peripherally along with target structures. Cholinergic nerves are found in airways earlier in gestation than adrenergic nerves. A mature pattern of innervation is achieved by the end of the first year of life.

The airways receive both parasympathetic and sympathetic efferent (motor) nerves. Preganglionic parasympathetic fibers start in the central nervous system, travel to the lung in the vagus nerve, and end in ganglia located around the airway wall. Postganglionic fibers then penetrate into the submucosa to innervate smooth muscle, epithelium, and glands. Parasympathetic innervation is mediated by acetylcholine binding to postsynaptic muscarinic receptors. Preganglionic sympathetic nerves start in the central nervous system and end in the upper thoracic sympathetic ganglia. Postganglionic sympathetic fibers are less numerous than cholinergic fibers. They terminate on glands, airway ganglia, and blood vessels with very little direct input to airway smooth muscle. Despite the sparse sympathetic innervation, adrenergic receptors are found on smooth muscle, glands, epithelial cells, and mast cells and adrenergic agonists have important effects on these target structures. The physiological agonist for these receptors may be circulating epinephrine released from the adrenal gland.

In addition to the input from the parasympathetic and sympathetic nervous systems, there is a third system that is important in the conducting airways. This system, which does not utilize catecholamines or acetylcholine, has been called the non-adrenergic, non-cholinergic nervous system. Mediators in this system include substance P, neurokinin A, vasoactive intestinal peptide, peptide histidine methionine, calcitonin gene-related peptide, neuropeptide Y, and galanin. These mediators have competing effects on smooth muscle, submucosal glands, and airway vasculature.

Three types of afferent (sensory) nerves are found within the airways. They travel in the vagus nerve and contribute to reflexes that alter bronchial caliber, vascular resistance, and control of breathing. Sensory nerves of the first type, slowly adapting sensory nerves or stretch receptors, are concentrated in the smooth muscle of central airways and decrease in number peripherally. These receptors respond to increases in bronchial wall tension and transpulmonary pressure. Response is diminished in newborns due to higher thresholds of stimulation, lower discharge rates, decreased myelination, and differences in mechanics of the newborn lung. Stimulation of slowly adapting receptors results in laryngeal and bronchial dilatation, increased heart rate, decreased vascular resistance, and apnea during the Hering–Breuer inflation reflex. Sensory nerves of the second type, rapidly adapting nerves or irritant receptors, have nerve endings in the epithelium of the extrapulmonary airways. They respond to a variety of stimuli including inhaled irritants, inflammatory mediators, prostaglandins, and mechanical deformation of the airways. Response of these receptors is decreased in newborns due to reduced numbers of fibers. Stimulation of these receptors results in reflex bronchoconstriction, cough, increased mucus secretion, and laryngeal constriction. Sensory nerves of the third type, bronchial C-fibers, have nerve endings in the epithelium of the intrapulmonary bronchi. They are very sensitive to chemical stimuli and less sensitive to mechanical stimuli. Stimulation causes reflex bronchoconstriction, mucus secretion, cough, and rapid, shallow breathing. The stimuli and the reflex events caused by sensory nerves overlap; together they play an important regulatory role in cough, control of airway caliber, and airway secretion.

Neuroendocrine cells are granular cells similar to amine precursor uptake and decarboxylation (APUD) cells seen in the gastrointestinal tract. They occur as single cells within the airway epithelium or as clumps (neuroepithelial bodies) associated with bifurcations in the intrapulmonary airways. They are well positioned to respond to chemical changes in the airway lumen and may serve a sensory function. They also receive external nerve input and may have regulatory effects on lung growth and differentiation, response to hypoxemia, and hypersensitivity immune responses.

## Immunological cells

Immunological cells are found predominantly in the larger airways, concentrated where the greatest deposition of inhaled particles and antigens occurs. They include local resident cells such as mast cells, lymphocytes, and macrophages as well as migratory cells derived from the blood. Lymphocytes form lymphoid aggregates, called bronchial-associated lymphoid tissue, that increase during development in response to stimulation by foreign antigen. Mast cells, found predominantly in the submucosa of the proximal airway, release a variety of mediators that cause edema, smooth muscle contraction, and altered function of the epithelium. Resident macrophages within the airspace lumen are phagocytic cells that sequester foreign particles, kill microorganisms, and present digested foreign antigens to other immunological cells.

## Connective tissue

Connective tissue elements such as cartilage, elastin, and collagen are important structural components of the airway walls. In the trachea and extrapulmonary bronchi, cartilage forms incomplete rings connected by a muscular membrane. Beyond the main stem bronchi, rings of airway cartilage are irregularly shaped and helical in configuration. Elastin and collagen are present beneath the cartilage in larger airways but become more prominent in small bronchi and bronchioles where cartilage is absent. Elastin is composed of amorphous and microfibrillar components that are closely associated and impart the distinctive springiness to lung tissues. Elastin is most prominent in the parenchyma and contributes to tethering of the airways by lung parenchyma. Loss of parenchymal elastin in emphysema results in small airway obstruction. Collagen, a large protein with a complex structure that is found in different forms in the lung, contributes to structural rigidity of airways; excess collagen, as seen in fibrotic diseases, decreases compliance of the airway wall.

# Control of airway caliber

Airway caliber and resistance to airflow result from a balance of opposing forces produced by the airway structure, elasticity of the airway wall, mechanical interaction between the airway wall and surrounding parenchyma, contraction of airway smooth muscle, fluid balance within the airway wall, and mucus secretion (Fig. 77.8). During inspiration, the pressure gradient across the airway wall (transmural pressure) and traction on the airway by the expanding parenchyma distend the airway. During exhalation, the transmural pressure difference is reversed and airway distension by the surrounding parenchyma is decreased, resulting in a tendency toward airway collapse.

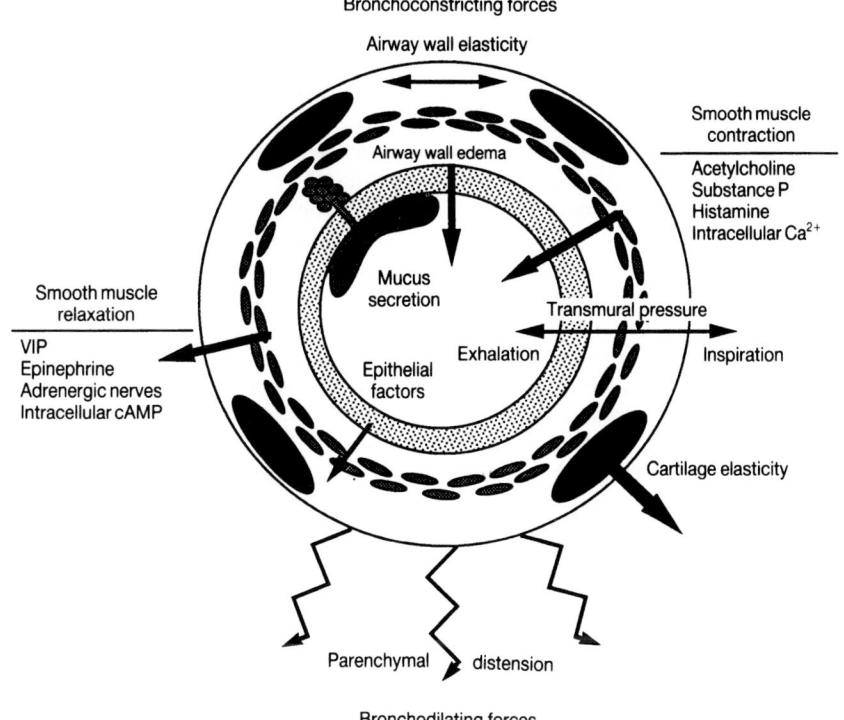

FIGURE 77.8 Forces controlling conducting airway caliber. Schematic diagram of an intrapulmonary bronchus demonstrates the forces that determine airway caliber. The caliber of the airway results from the balance of these competing forces.

The degree to which these forces result in dynamic changes in airway caliber is determined by the structural rigidity of the airway wall, the size of the airway, and the elasticity of the airway wall. In the larger airways, cartilage provides structural rigidity to the airway wall that limits these dynamic changes in caliber. Cartilage also limits the reduction in airway caliber that results from smooth muscle contraction. The abnormal shape and laxity of airway cartilage seen in patients with *tracheomalacia* results in excessive dynamic collapse during exhalation. In small bronchi and bronchioles, dynamic changes and contraction of smooth muscle are opposed by traction on the airway wall from surrounding lung parenchyma and the elasticity of the bronchial wall. Smooth muscle contraction has a more direct effect in decreasing airway caliber in the distal airways. The force generated per muscle mass and length is greatest in the peripheral airways. In addition, smaller airways require less increase in wall tension to produce the same percentage decrease in airway caliber. Therefore, equivalent contraction of smooth muscle leads to a relatively greater decrease in airway diameter. All these factors suggest that control of small airway caliber is more dynamic and sensitive to altered smooth muscle tone than that in larger airways. Therefore, smooth muscle contraction within the membranous bronchioles may be important in determining distribution of ventilation to gas-exchange regions.

Contraction of airway smooth muscle is controlled by complex and often competing local interactions between smooth muscle, nerves, epithelium, and inflammatory cells as well as interactions between smooth muscle and neurohumoral input from outside the lung. Smooth muscle tone is determined by the balance of these multiple inputs. Response of smooth muscle to these extracellular stimuli is controlled by a complex biochemical process within the smooth muscle cell. Activation of receptors on the surface of smooth muscle cells stimulates contraction through the production of second messengers that cause phosphorylation of myosin. Phosphorylation causes a conformational change that allows myosin to interact with actin, and resultant hydrolysis of ATP provides the energy needed for shortening of the muscle. The magnitude of the response to receptor stimulation depends on the balance of intracellular enzymes that phosphorylate and dephosphorylate myosin. Thus, phosphorylation of myosin is a major regulatory site in the biochemical coupling of receptor stimulation to muscle contraction.

Intracellular $Ca^{2+}$ concentration is highly regulated and also important to stimulus–contraction coupling. Polyphosphoinositides and their metabolites are important second messengers that increase intracellular $Ca^{2+}$ concentration. Release of intracellular $Ca^{2+}$ results in formation of a $Ca^{2+}$–calmodulin complex that activates an enzyme which phosphorylates myosin. The $Ca^{2+}$–calmodulin complex may also regulate enzymes that inactivate myosin. Intracellular concentrations of cAMP have an inhibitory effect on myosin phosphorylation through the activation of a cAMP-dependent kinase. This kinase might decrease the affinity of the myosin phosphorylating enzyme for the $Ca^{2+}$–calmodulin complex. Alternatively, cAMP might inhibit contraction by causing a decrease in intracellular $Ca^{2+}$ concentration. Selective phosphodiesterase inhibitors, an important class of drugs used for treatment of asthma, act to prevent the breakdown of cAMP in smooth muscle cells, resulting in bronchodilatation.

The myoneural junction is a major extracellular site for regulating smooth muscle tone. Binding of acetylcholine to muscarinic receptors on the surface of smooth muscle cells stimulates contraction through the release of intracellular $Ca^{2+}$. Cholinergic nerves participate in bronchoconstricting reflexes that are regulated, at the ganglion, by both local and systemic mediators. Adrenergic input to the smooth muscle is sparse and may not be important in regulating smooth muscle tone under normal conditions. However, when tone is increased, adrenergic input may cause relaxation by inhibition of vagally mediated contraction. Bronchodilatation results from stimulation of β-adrenergic receptors that are found with increased density on smooth muscle of the distal airways. Epinephrine can decrease bronchial tone through interaction with these receptors; however, the physiological role of circulating catecholamines in regulating bronchial tone is unclear. These receptors are important pharmacological sites of action for medications commonly used in the treatment of asthma.

Non-adrenergic, non-cholinergic nerves containing vasoactive intestinal peptide and peptide histidine isomethionine are found with greater density in larger airways than peripheral airways and may provide direct inhibitory neural input to airway smooth muscle. These substances cause bronchodilatation by stimulating receptors that activate adenylyl cyclase, increasing cAMP levels inside smooth muscle cells. Non-adrenergic, non-cholinergic nerves containing substance P, neurokinin A, and calcitonin gene-related peptide are potent bronchoconstrictors. These neuropeptides are released by local axon reflexes in bronchial C-fiber nerve endings.

Non-neural regulation also plays an important role in regulation of bronchial smooth muscle tone. Resident mast cells found in the submucosa of the airways can be stimulated to release a variety of mediators that cause smooth muscle contraction. Binding of foreign antigen to IgE antibody on the mast cell surface results in release of histamine, eosinophilic chemotactic factor, leukotrienes, and cyclooxygenase products. Release of mediators by mast cells is regulated by cyclic nucleotides, prostaglandins, respiratory heat loss, β-adrenergic agonists, and histamine. The airway epithelium also plays an important role in regulation of airway smooth muscle tone. The integrity of the epithelial barrier affects access of mast cells and sensory nerve endings to foreign antigens and noxious irritants. Epithelial cells release $PGE_2$ and epithelium-derived relaxing factor that act directly on smooth muscle to

decrease tone. Epithelial cells also possess neutral endopeptidases that metabolize bronchoconstricting neuropeptides.

*Asthma*, an important disease in children, is characterized by intermittent and reversible airway obstruction due to bronchial hyperresponsiveness, edema of the airway wall, and excessive mucus secretion. Bronchial hyperresponsiveness may result from an imbalance between endogenous bronchoconstricting and bronchodilating factors. Inflammation plays a critical role in asthma and airway hyperresponsiveness. Inflammatory cells and their mediators can result in many of the pathological and pathophysiological abnormalities seen in asthmatic patients. How inflammation upsets the normal balance of factors regulating bronchial tone is presently the subject of intense research interest. Abnormalities in the β-adrenergic receptor have been proposed but probably do not play a major role in the pathogenesis of asthma. Recent evidence also suggests that deficiencies in vasoactive intestinal peptide, excesses in bronchoconstricting neuropeptides, and abnormalities in enzymes responsible for degradation of these mediators are possible explanations for hyperresponsiveness. Loss of epithelial integrity may play a role in hyperresponsive states associated with epithelial damage through loss of endopeptidase activity, decreased production of smooth muscle relaxing factors, increased exposure of irritant receptors to noxious substances, and increased access of mast cells to foreign antigen. Abnormalities in smooth muscle have also received considerable attention. Increased mass, altered distribution, increased force generation, and increased responsiveness to stimulatory mediators have been proposed to explain the role of smooth muscle in hyperresponsiveness. Morphological features of asthmatic airways may also be potential factors in hyperresponsiveness. The thickness of airway walls is increased in asthmatic patients due to smooth muscle hypertrophy and edema. In the presence of thickening, the amount of smooth muscle shortening required to narrow the airway is decreased so that a normal amount of smooth muscle contraction causes increased obstruction. Edema in the airway wall has been postulated to decrease the tethering of airways by the surrounding lung parenchyma. Thus, asthma and bronchial hyperresponsiveness can be considered the final common pathway for any of a variety of abnormalities that upset the normal balance of factors determining airway caliber.

## INTERACTION WITH THE EXTERNAL ENVIRONMENT

### Air conditioning

The upper and conducting airways play an important role in humidifying, warming, and cleaning the inspired air before it reaches the fluid-lined gas-exchange regions. Most humidification of inspired air is provided by the nasal mucosa. This appears to be accomplished by engorgement and fluid displacement into the nasal mucosa from its vasculature. The nasal mucosa also plays an important role in temperature regulation by a similar mechanism. This results in minimal change in the temperature of inspired air at the opening to the conducting airways even with large variation in ambient temperature. The remaining conditioning of inspired air is accomplished in the conducting airways. The relative contribution of the proximal conducting airways to this process may increase under certain conditions such as exercise or mechanical bypassing of the upper airway.

# Host defense mechanisms

The upper and conducting airways possess a variety of non-specific and specific mechanisms that contribute to pulmonary defenses. Non-specific mechanisms include morphological features that result in deposition of inhaled particles and absorption of inhaled gases, airway secretions, ciliary clearance, epithelial barrier function, phagocytic cells, mechanical mechanisms such as cough or sneeze, and biochemical defenses. Specific mechanisms involve both local and systemic, humoral and cellular immunological reactions.

## Cleansing of inspired air

The upper and conducting airways remove particles and noxious vapors from inhaled air by deposition of particles along the airway wall and absorption of vapor by the airway epithelium. Factors that govern clearance of inhaled substances may be important in determining airway damage from inhalation injuries and the efficacy of therapeutic aerosols.

### Deposition of particles

Deposition of particles along the airway mucosa is determined by the physical characteristics of the particle, airflow properties, and airway anatomy. Particles are deposited by filtering, impaction, sedimentation, and diffusion. The nasal passage is efficient at trapping and clearing the majority of larger particles (including microorganisms) in inspired air. The hairs in the nasal vestibule trap the largest particles by bulk filtering. Deposition of the remaining large particles by impaction is the result of inertia and is determined by particle mass, airflow velocities, and turbulent flow. Impaction is greatest in the upper airway and proximal large conducting airways. Deposition of particles by sedimentation results from settling of particles by gravity and is determined by the density and size of the particles. Sedimentation occurs primarily in more distal airways where airflow velocity and turbulence are decreased. Deposition of particles by diffusion occurs only with very small particles and in the absence of airflow.

Diffusion occurs primarily in the terminal airways and alveoli. Smaller airways, higher respiratory rates, smaller tidal volumes, and increased turbulent flow result in greater impaction of particles. For these reasons, deposition of particles is greater in the proximal airways of children compared with adults.

### Absorption of vapors

Absorption of vapors by the airway mucosa differs slightly from deposition of particles and is dependent on the physical properties of the gas, gas concentration, tidal volume, and respiratory rate. In general, gases that are highly soluble in water, e.g. sulfur dioxide and ammonia, are readily absorbed by the liquid layer lining the airway and are cleared in the upper and larger conducting airways. Higher concentrations of these gases or deep breathing are required for them to reach the distal lung. In contrast, gases with low solubility in water, e.g. nitrogen dioxide and chlorine, are not readily absorbed by the large airways and are more likely to penetrate deep into the lung.

## Mucociliary clearance

Clearance of particles deposited along the airway depends on the production of respiratory secretions by mucosal cells and submucosal glands, the action of cilia on mucus, and the exchange of electrolytes and liquid across the epithelium (Fig. 77.9). Particles that are deposited along the airway wall are trapped in the mucus or gel layer overlying the mucosa and propelled, by cilia, toward the mouth where they are cleared from the airway by swallowing. Cilia beat within a liquid or sol layer that contributes to humidification of inspired air and proper hydration of the mucus layer. The volume and composition of this sol layer is maintained by epithelial transport of ions and water. These three processes are regulated by similar mechanisms, constituting a coordinated and integrated system. Abnormalities in any of these processes can result in abnormal airway function and clinical disease.

### Airway secretions

Airway mucus is a complex mixture of water, electrolytes, mucins, proteoglycans, and proline-rich proteins produced by secretory cells in the surface epithelium and submucosal glands. The physical properties of mucus are largely determined by complex interactions between these elements. Mucins, the major mucoid component of airway secretions, are produced by goblet cells in the surface epithelium and mucous cells in the submucosal glands. Proteoglycans play an important role in hydration of mucins. Proline-rich proteins appear to affect the physical properties of mucus by interaction with mucins. Proteoglycans and proline-rich proteins are secreted by serous cells in submucosal glands. These macromolecules are stored in secretory cells as compact granules that are secreted by exocytosis. After secretion, mucus droplets rapidly

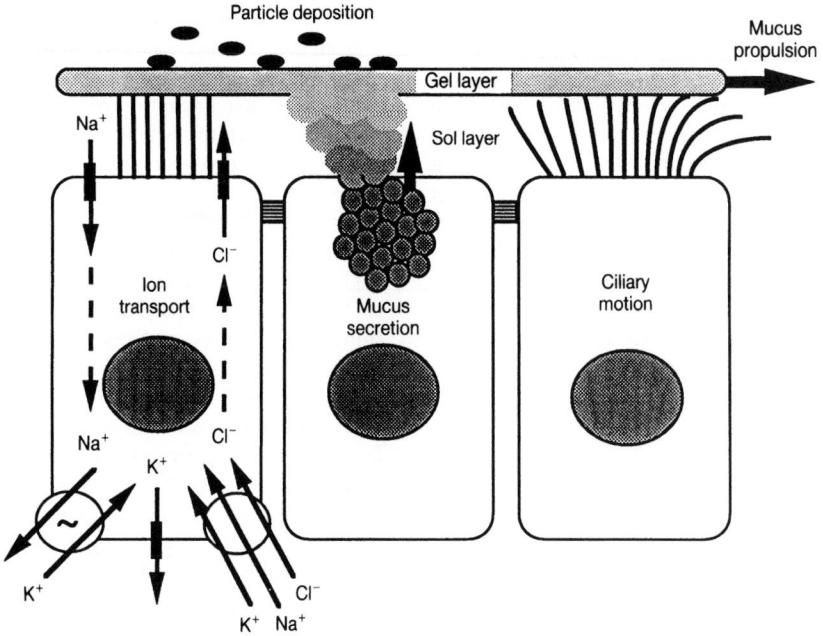

FIGURE 77.9 Mucociliary clearance, showing the major components of normal clearance. Particles deposited along the airway adhere to the gel layer and are propelled up the airways by the action of cilia on mucus. Dense granules of mucus are released by secretory cells and quickly expand as the gel is hydrated by the sol layer. The sol layer is maintained by epithelial ion transport. $Cl^-$ enters surface epithelial cells through a $Na^+$-$K^+$-$Cl^-$ cotransporter that is driven by the $Na^+$ concentration gradient. $Cl^-$ that builds up in the cell exits through apical $Cl^-$ channels. $Na^+$ moves down its concentration gradient into the cell through apical $Na^+$ channels and is subsequently removed by the basolateral $Na^+$-$K^+$-ATPase. $K^+$ is recycled across the basolateral membrane in order to maintain the electrical driving force for apical $Cl^-$ movement and to prevent cell swelling.

swell by absorption of water. Normal hydration appears to be very important in determining the chemical and physical properties of mucus.

In addition to mucus, secretory cells produce a variety of substances that have antimicrobial properties and assist in defense of the lung. Submucosal gland serous cells secrete lysozyme, an enzyme that acts on bacterial cell walls and has antimicrobial activity against Gram-positive organisms. Serous cells also secrete lactoferrin, an iron-binding protein with bacteriostatic properties. Epithelial mucous cells secrete peroxidase, which is active against a variety of microorganisms.

The volume and physical properties of respiratory mucus are regulated by neural input, inflammatory mediators, chemical irritants, and mechanical stimulation of the airway mucosa. In the nose, mucus clearance is affected by temperature, humidity, inflammation, infection, histamine, and adrenergic agents. In the conducting airways, cholinergic neural input does not change the physical properties of mucus but increases secretion rate by stimulating both mucous and serous cells. Stimulation of submucosal glands by α-adrenergic input increases the volume of secretions and lowers the viscosity by selectively stimulating serous cells. In contrast, β-adrenergic stimulation has questionable effects on the volume of secretions but increases the viscosity through the relatively selective stimulation of mucus cells.

Neuropeptides also act to stimulate mucus secretion. Chemical irritation of the mucosa stimulates goblet cells to increase in number and secretion rate. A variety of humoral and inflammatory mediators including histamine, bradykinin, and arachidonate metabolites can stimulate mucus secretion by both direct and reflex mechanisms.

## Cilia

The action of cilia is crucial to normal mucociliary clearance. Cilia beat in waves, and their motion can be divided into three distinct phases. The first or preparatory stroke phase involves slow backward and clockwise motion of the cilia. At the end of this phase, the cilia are extended and point upstream. They proceed immediately into the propulsive stroke phase, during which they remain extended and rapidly move forward. After the propulsive phase, the cilia enter a rest phase in which they await the next cycle. Ciliary motion results from mechanical stimulation and is initiated by the preparatory stroke. Waves of ciliary motion, called metachronal waves, can propagate across an area of mucosa by the movement of one cilium mechanically stimulating neighboring cilia. Once the preparatory phase is initiated, the cilia will proceed through a complete cycle and return to the resting position. The ciliary beat frequency varies according to the location within the airway, the mechanical load, temperature, and regulatory input.

Cilia are more dense and beat more rapidly in the proximal airways than in the distal airways. Cilia also beat faster as the strength of the mechanical stimulus increases. These features of cilia may help prevent excessive accumulation of mucus as it converges on proximal airways from more distal airways. Ciliary beat frequency may also be increased by cholinergic and β-adrenergic stimulation.

Ciliary movement results from interaction between microtubules that are organized in a distinctive longitudinal array within the shaft of the cilia. This organization consists of nine microtubular doublets arranged around a central pair. Doublets are connected to each other by nexin links and to the central pair by radial linkages. One microtubule of each doublet has two dynein arms that contain ATPase. Hydrolysis of ATP by the dynein arms results in sliding of microtubules along each other. Linkages between microtubules direct this sliding so that it results in bending of the ciliary shaft. Defects in this basic structure and the biochemical processes causing ciliary motion have been identified that result in abnormal ciliary motion. This group of primary ciliary dyskinesias result in similar clinical consequences and have been grouped together as the *immotile cilia syndrome*.

## Mucus and ciliary interactions

Cilia propel mucus using small, claw-like projections that are anchored in the tip of the cilia shaft. These projections allow force to be transmitted from the internal structures that produce ciliary movement to the overlying mucus. The physical properties of mucus are very important to the action of cilia on mucus. The viscosity of mucus tends to decrease in proportion to force that is applied to it, i.e. the harder cilia beat, the less viscous mucus becomes. In addition, the elasticity of mucus allows transmission of applied force; a large sheet of mucus may be moved by acting on only one portion of the sheet. Because the recoil or relaxation time of mucus is relatively slow, ciliary action results in forward propulsion rather than oscillation back and forth as cilia attach and release the mucus sheet. Thus, the physical properties of mucus enhance the action of cilia by allowing mucus to help pull itself along the airway.

## Ion transport

Epithelial ion transport plays a role in controlling the physical properties of mucus and affects ciliary motion by regulating the volume and composition of the sol layer. Complex intercellular junctions allow epithelial cells to segregate ion-transporting proteins into either the apical or basolateral cell membrane. Segregation of ion-transporting proteins and expenditure of energy to generate ion concentration differences between the inside and outside of the cell allow the epithelium to transport ions across the mucosa. Transepithelial movement of ions generates osmotic differences that draw water back and forth across the epithelium according to the net movement of ions. The airway epithelium can simultaneously secrete $Cl^-$ and absorb $Na^+$. Secretion of $Cl^-$ into the airway results in liquid production by the airway epithelium. Absorption of $Na^+$ results in removal of liquid from the airway lumen. $Na^+$ and $Cl^-$ movement accounts for nearly all the transepithelial ion and water movement. Therefore, the balance of these two ion transport processes regulates the charge, composition, volume, and net production of airway liquid by the airway epithelium.

The importance of the balance between these two ion transport processes to fluid balance across the respiratory epithelium is illustrated by dramatic developmental changes in ion transport. During fetal life the lung is filled with liquid that plays an important role in normal lung development. This liquid is produced by the active secretion of $Cl^-$ and water by the respiratory epithelium. Absorption of $Na^+$ plays little or no role in fluid balance at this point. In the days immediately preceding birth, the volume of liquid and the rate of liquid secretion slows. During labor, stimulation of $Na^+$ absorption results in removal of liquid from the lung lumen. This clearance of liquid plays an important role in the preparation for air breathing at birth. After birth, $Na^+$ absorption increases and $Cl^-$ secretion decreases. In the mature airways, $Na^+$ absorption is the dominant ion transport process with $Cl^-$ and bicarbonate moving across the epithelium as counterions.

The importance of a proper balance between secretory and absorptive ion transport processes in the airway epithelium is also illustrated by genetic abnormalities in epithelial ion transport. The mature airway epithelium retains the capacity for $Cl^-$ and water secretion under certain circumstances. $Cl^-$ secretion can be stimulated by a variety of humoral, neural, and inflammatory mediators. These mediators may stimulate $Cl^-$ secretion by increasing intracellular cAMP concentrations. Increased cAMP results in increased intracellular $Ca^{2+}$ concentrations and activation of cAMP-dependent protein kinase which, in turn, activates $Cl^-$ transport pathways within the apical membrane of the epithelial cell. $Cl^-$ secretion can be stimulated by β-adrenergic agonists, prostaglandins, vasoactive intestinal peptide, leukotrienes, adenosine, bradykinin, eosinophil myelin basic protein, and neurokinins. Activation of $Cl^-$ transport by cAMP is abnormal in individuals with cystic fibrosis. This abnormality results in deficient liquid secretion and excessive water absorption by the airway epithelium. In cystic fibrosis, this abnormal balance alters the volume of airway liquid and hydration of mucus, resulting in tenacious mucus that obstructs airways.

## Immunological defenses

Immunological responses in the airways are similar to responses elsewhere in the body and include both humoral and cellular components of the immune system. In the upper airway, the nasal mucosa contains immunological cells such as mast cells, neutrophils, and eosinophils and secretes lysozyme, interferon, and immunoglobulin (IgG, IgE, and IgA). Collections of lymphoid tissue in the pharynx (Waldeyer ring) and larynx presumably play a role in immunological defense against infection, although this role is not well defined.

Immune responses in the conducting airways are largely produced locally and are mediated by immunological cells within the airway. Secretory IgA is the predominant immunoglobulin in airway secretions; it assists in viral neutralization, agglutinates microorganisms, and prevents attachment of bacteria to epithelial surfaces. Secretory IgA is derived from local aggregations of lymphoid cells in the submucosa of the large airways. The concentration of IgA decreases toward the periphery of the lung in association with decreases in the size and organization of these lymphoid aggregates. IgG is present in much lower concentrations in the airways. IgE antibody plays an important role in immediate hypersensitivity reactions within the lung. Interferon is produced by macrophages and serves antiviral and immunoregulatory roles within the lung. Complement is normally found in very small amounts in airway secretions but can be increased in inflammatory states, where it serves an immunoregulatory role in controlling vascular permeability and in chemotaxis. The cellular component of immune responses in the lung involves both local and migratory phagocytic cells and lymphocytes. When circulating leukocytes are activated they adhere to the vascular endothelium and migrate from the vascular space under the influence of chemotaxins to the site of an immune response. Resident macrophages predominantly serve a local phagocytic role and to a lesser extent an immunoregulatory function. Both local and circulating lymphocytes play a role in the production of immunoglobulin and cell-mediated immunity within the airways. Local T-lymphocytes are important to the defense against viruses and have extensive interactions with macrophages that result in the production of lymphokines.

## SELECTED READING

### Upper airway

Crelin E. Development of the upper respiratory system. *Clin Symposium (CIBA)* 1976; **28**: 1.

Mathew O. Maintenance of upper airway patency. *J Pediatr* 1985; **106**: 863.

Nunn JF. Resistance to gas flow and airway closure. In: *Applied respiratory physiology* 3rd edn. London: Butterworths, 1987: 46.

Proctor D. Form and function of the upper airways and larynx. In: Fishman AP, Macklem PT, Mead J, eds. *Handbook of physiology, Section 3, The respiratory system, Vol III Mechanics of breathing, Part I*. Bethesda: American Physiological Society, 1986: 63.

Reed W, Roberts J, Thach B. Factors influencing regional patency and configuration of the human infant upper airway. *J Appl Physiol* 1985; **58**: 635.

Thach BT. Neuromuscular control of the upper airway. In: Beckerman RC, Brouillette RT, Hunt CE, eds. *Respiratory control disorders in infants and children*. Baltimore: Williams and Wilkins, 1992: 47.

van Lunteren E. Upper airway effects on breathing. In: Crystal RG, West JB, eds. *The lung: scientific foundations*. New York, Raven Press, 1991: 1631.

### Conducting airways

Horsfield K, Cumming G. Morphology of the bronchial tree. *J Appl Physiol* 1968; **24**: 373.

Horsfield K, Cumming G. Functional consequences of airway morphology. *J Appl Physiol* 1968; **24**: 384.

Leff AR. Endogenous regulation of bronchomotor tone. *Am Rev Respir Dis* 1988; **137**: 1198.

Murray JF. Defense mechanisms. In: *The normal lung*. Philadelphia: WB Saunders, 1986, 313.

Sleigh MA, Blake JR, Liron N. The propulsion of mucus by cilia. *Am Rev Respir Dis* 1988; **137**: 726.

Weibel ER. Lung cell biology. In: Fishman AP, Fisher AB, eds. *Handbook of physiology, Section 3, The respiratory system, Vol 1 Circulation and non-respiratory functions*. Bethesda: American Physiological Society, 1985: 47.

Widdicombe JH. Ion transport by airway epithelia. In: Crystal RG, West JB, eds. *The lung: scientific foundations*. New York, Raven Press, 1991: 263.

# ALVEOLAR REGION

## ORGANIZATION OF THE ALVEOLAR REGION

The alveolar region of the lung lies distal to the smallest of the conducting airways, the respiratory bronchiole. The primary function of the alveolar region is the exchange of $O_2$ and $CO_2$ between the inspired air and the blood. The alveolus is the basic anatomical unit of gas exchange; the human lung contains about 500 million alveoli. The average alveolar diameter in the human lung is approximately 200 µm; at birth, alveolar diameter is about 50–100 µm. When the adult lung is 60 per cent inflated, the alveolar surface area available for gas exchange is approximately $140 \, m^2$. Thousands of individual, cup-shaped alveoli, separated by septa and interconnected by alveolar ducts, make up a respiratory acinus. The acinus constitutes the basic unit of ventilation in the lung. Each acinus is connected to a single respiratory bronchiole. The basic perfusion unit, the capillary bed between each pulmonary arteriole and the corresponding pulmonary venule, is less easy to define anatomically but clearly extends over several alveoli because paired arterioles and venules are separated by 0.5–1.0 mm. The pulmonary microvasculature has a large capillary surface area that almost matches the alveolar surface area available for gas exchange. The total estimated volume of the pulmonary microcirculation is approximately 200 mL.

## ALVEOLAR STRUCTURE

The structure of the alveolar region promotes efficient gas exchange between alveolar gases and blood in the microvasculature by keeping the tissue space between the two to a minimum. Adjacent alveoli share a very thin common wall, or alveolar septum, only 5–8 µm thick. Over most of their length the septa are covered by the very attenuated cytoplasmic extensions of specialized epithelial cells (type I cells), which rest on a basement membrane shared with the underlying endothelial cells of the pulmonary capillary in the septum. Throughout more than half of the enormous gas-exchange area in the lung there is little or no interstitial space. This fragile architecture creates special problems of maintaining structural stability while allowing for the distensibility necessary during ventilation. As the luminal surface of the alveolar epithelium is lined by a thin but continuous liquid layer, surface forces also potentially compromise alveolar structural stability.

The alveolar region of the lung is supported, in part, by a system of interstitial fibers, collagen and elastin, that follow the branching of the airways and run through the alveolar ducts to connect with the strands of connective tissue that support the alveolar septa. Additional mechanical support is provided by a fibrous network that extends in from the visceral pleura along the interlobular septa. These three fibrous systems are interconnected and between them provide a supportive scaffolding for the alveolar region. Fibroblasts and other cells are found in the proximity of the fibrous bundles in the interstitial space. The surface forces present in the liquid layer that lines the alveolar epithelium are reduced to low levels by a unique surfactant secreted by a second, specialized epithelial cell of the alveolar lining, the type II cell. Absence or dysfunction of this surfactant leads to volume loss in the gas-exchange region and respiratory failure. These basic elements of the alveolar region will be discussed in greater detail below.

## ALVEOLAR EPITHELIUM

Because the alveolar region has such an enormous surface area and a generally thin interstitial space, the epithelial cells lining the alveolus constitute more than 20 per cent of the total number of cells in the lung. The alveolar epithelium consists of just two cell types, known as type I and type II cells. Each human alveolus is lined by approximately 40 type I cells and 70 type II cells. The specialized design of the alveolar epithelium creates a tight barrier between the interstitial space and the alveolar lumen. This barrier regulates the accumulation and composition of fluid in the alveolus while imposing a minimal resistance to respiratory gas diffusion. The alveolar epithelium, particularly the type II cell, secretes many biologically active substances, including pulmonary surfactant, into the alveolar lumen. Other major cells of the alveolar region, including interstitial fibroblasts and endothelial cells, are discussed in other parts of this section.

## Type I cells

Type I cells cover about 95 per cent of the alveolar surface area. Type I cells are very large and extremely thin cells with complex branched cytoplasmic extensions. A single type I cell covers an area of approximately 5000 µm², but its average thickness over most of this enormous area is only 0.2 µm. This extreme cytoplasmic attenuation presumably facilitates gas exchange by limiting the total tissue space across which gas exchange must occur to less than 0.5 µm in much of the alveolar region. No functions other than this important barrier role have been ascribed to the type I cell. The cells have relatively few mitochondria and a small endoplasmic reticulum and Golgi apparatus, suggesting limited metabolic capacity; however, because of difficulties in isolation and culture, type I cells have not been directly studied *in vitro*. Type I cells do contain a relatively large number of pinocytic vesicles and therefore may have an important role in the bidirectional traffic of small solutes and proteins between the alveolar lining liquid and the interstitial space. The water channel, Chip28, is abundant in the alveolar epithelium.

The basement membrane beneath the type I cell appears to be fused or intermingled with the basement membrane of the closely apposed capillary endothelial cell. Along much of the alveolar septum there is almost no discernible interstitial space between type I cells and the underlying capillaries. The contact between type I cells and other type I or type II cells is formed by tight junctions, making the alveolar epithelium a relatively tight or impermeable barrier for solutes and proteins in the interstitial space. Type I cells appear in the fetal lung in the early third trimester. Whether type I cells differentiate directly from the progenitor columnar epithelium or transdifferentiate from type II cells is uncertain. Type I cells are acutely susceptible to a wide variety of lung injury including that caused by oxidants, barotrauma, and infection. Injured type I cells readily detach from the basement membrane. In the adult lung, epithelial integrity apparently is restored after injury by division and subsequent transdifferentiation of type II cells. Adult type I cells are thought to be terminally differentiated and to lack the capacity for mitosis. The signals regulating the mitogenic responsiveness and differentiated state of alveolar epithelial cells are unknown, but may include soluble factors secreted by mesenchymal cells and alveolar macrophages as well as molecules in the extracellular matrix.

## Type II cells

The relatively small, cuboidal type II cells are approximately twice as abundant as type I cells but cover only about 5–10 per cent of the alveolar surface area. Type II cells are frequently but not exclusively situated in the corners of the alveoli. Ultrastructurally, type II cells are distinguished by numerous short microvilli on the luminal surface and unique secretion granules known as lamellar bodies. The lamellar bodies store surfactant and other molecules including lysosomal enzymes. Type II cells each contain about 150 lamellar bodies. Type II cells contribute to the barrier functions of the alveolar epithelium by forming tight junctions with neighboring type I cells. Type II cells have the following additional known functions: synthesis, storage, secretion, and clearance of surfactant; active transport of solutes and possibly proteins between the alveolar and interstitial spaces; and progenitor cells for alveolar epithelial repopulation after injury. Type II cells also appear to synthesize and secrete many other bioactive molecules such as components of the complement cascade, coagulation factors, lysozyme, lysosomal enzymes, growth factors, and cytokines. The biological role of most of these products in the alveolar space is unknown.

Morphologically recognizable type II cells appear in the human fetal lung early in the third trimester of pregnancy. In culture, morphological maturation of the columnar epithelium lining the developing air spaces can be synchronized and induced by a number of factors, including cAMP, prostaglandins, and glucocorticoids, but the precise sequence of signals regulating type II cell differentiation *in vivo* is unknown.

## SURFACTANT

### Surface forces and lung mechanics

The presence of the large air–liquid interface in the alveolus (approximately $140 \, m^2$ in the adult lung) leads to a tension in the interface or a surface force that promotes retraction of the interface (lung collapse) and accumulation of fluid in the alveolar lumen (pulmonary edema). Pulmonary surfactant accumulates at the alveolar air–liquid interface and reduces the tension in the interface. Surfactant therefore stabilizes the alveolus against collapse, or atelectasis, on expiration (helps maintain residual volume), promotes expansion on inspiration (reduces compliance and work of breathing), and helps to keep the alveolar space relatively dry. A surfactant-deficient lung has a reduced lung volume and is stiff or has a decreased

compliance. If the alveolus is considered as a spherical structure the relationships between alveolar size ($r$), surface tension ($\sigma$) and transsurface or transpulmonary pressure ($P$) can be modeled using the law of Laplace for thin-walled spheres:

$$P = 2\sigma/r$$

If the surface tension $\sigma$ is high (70 dynes/cm, as in the absence of any surfactant) a transsurface pressure ($P$) of approximately $28 \, cm \, H_2O$ would be required to maintain a radius ($r$) of $50 \, \mu m$. Simplistically, a similar calculation in the context of the lung infers that a positive end-expiratory pressure (PEEP) of $28 \, cm \, H_2O$ would be required to maintain a reasonable functional residual volume (FRC) in the absence of any surfactant. Surfactant lowers the surface tension to very low values by accumulating at the air–liquid interface. The transpulmonary pressure required to maintain FRC in the normal lung is therefore very low. The complex geometry of the alveolar region is clearly not adequately modeled as a simple collection of non-interacting, thin-walled spheres. The Laplace law cannot therefore be strictly applied, but it does serve to highlight the importance of surface forces to volume stability.

### Surfactant composition

Pulmonary surfactant is predominantly lipid consisting of approximately 45 per cent dipalmitoylphosphatidylcholine (DPPC), 25 per cent unsaturated phosphatidylcholines, 15 per cent phosphatidylglycerol, and lesser amounts of several other lipids. DPPC is the component that accumulates at the air–liquid interface and reduces surface tension. At least three specific apolipoproteins are associated with surfactant. SP-A is a large complex, oligomeric, collagen-like lectin that binds to surfactant lipids and modifies their structure and surface properties. SP-A also may have roles in regulating the alveolar surfactant pool size and possibly immunoregulatory functions in the alveolus. SP-B is a smaller (79 amino acids), hydrophobic, cationic protein with a detergent-like effect on lipid membranes that probably destabilizes surfactant so that it can spread rapidly at the air–liquid interface. SP-B may also have a central role in lamellar body formation. Congenital SP-B deficiency, secondary to one of several point mutations in the *SP-B* gene, is a rare autosomal recessive cause of fatal *respiratory distress syndrome* in term infants. SP-C is a very small (35 amino acids), covalently palmitoylated, hydrophobic protein that has similar but not identical properties to SP-B. All three surfactant apolipoproteins likely act as a cooperative unit to facilitate the delivery of DPPC from the type II cell to the air–liquid interface. The proteins may also have other roles related to the clearance of used surfactant from the alveolar space.

## Surfactant metabolism

Surfactant is synthesized in type II epithelial cells (Fig. 77.10). The phospholipids and apolipoproteins are synthesized from blood-borne precursors in the endoplasmic reticulum and are transported through the Golgi apparatus to the lamellar body. These organelles are the intracellular storage site for surfactant. Roughly half the total pool of lung surfactant is stored in lamellar bodies, and half is in the alveolar lumen. In the newborn, the luminal surfactant pool size is several times larger than in the adult. Lamellar bodies are released from the type II cell in a regulated manner in response to a number of pharmacological stimuli including β-adrenergic agonists. Circulating catecholamines may therefore play a role in the secretion of surfactant. Expansion of the lung towards total lung capacity and the hyperventilation of exercise also stimulate surfactant release. Periodic sighs therefore may be an important mechanism to maintain adequate alveolar surfactant levels. Conversely, prolonged ventilation at a fixed tidal volume without intermittent sighs may lead to a deficiency of surfactant in the alveolar lumen with a loss of compliance and atelectasis. Approximately 10 per cent of the intracellular surfactant pool is secreted into the alveolar space each hour at rest. The secretion rate can increase four-fold during exercise.

The lamellar body contents are secreted into the alveolar lining liquid and transform into an unusual morphological form called tubular myelin. This form of surfactant, containing the apolipoproteins and lipids, appears to be specialized for the transport of phospholipids, particularly DPPC, to the interface. At the air–liquid interface, DPPC forms a surface layer and surface tension falls. Like all phospholipids, DPPC is an amphipathic molecule with a polar head group (choline) and apolar tails (palmitate). This amphipathicity allows DPPC to accumulate in the surface layer. Additionally, the straight acyl chains of DPPC and the high melting point of this lipid allow it to pack very tightly in the surface film, exclude water, and therefore reduce surface tension to very low values. With ventilation some DPPC is lost from the surface layer and must be replaced by new material. Therefore, a continuous and balanced cycle of surfactant secretion and clearance occurs in the alveolus. The pathways of clearance are not well understood but include active reuptake into type II cells (conservation and reuse of surfactant) and clearance by alveolar macrophages (degradation of surfactant). The total amount of surfactant in the alveolar space at rest is about 10 mg/kg body weight but only about half this amount is actually in the surface layer. The concentration of surfactant in the alveolar space is more difficult to establish, but is probably about 15 mg/mL.

## Surfactant ontogeny

Active synthesis of surfactant components begins early in the third trimester of fetal life. Adult pool sizes are not attained until 35–36 weeks in most fetuses, but noticeable disease from surfactant deficiency is rare after 34–35 weeks. The hyperinsulinemia in infants of diabetic mothers delays some aspects of lung maturation and may cause respiratory distress in more mature infants. At term, about 10 per cent of the normal alveolar luminal surfactant pool is present in lung liquid, which fills the fetal alveoli. A dramatic burst of secretion occurs with lung inflation at birth.

The regulation of surfactant synthesis during fetal life is complicated. Several hormones, cytokines, and growth factors interact with combinations of transcription factors to bring about the orderly maturation of the surfactant system. Glucocorticoids contribute to the normal maturation of the surfactant system and can be used to prematurely stimulate surfactant production from very early in fetal life. Glucocorticoids also stimulate morphological maturation of the alveolar epithelium and pulmonary interstitium. Other hormones, including thyroxine, prolactin, and cAMP and growth factors such as epidermal growth factor may act synergistically with glucocorticoids in the induction of surfactant synthesis. *In vitro*, insulin and transforming growth factor β down-regulate the expression of some of the surfactant apolipoprotein genes, but the biological significance of these findings has not been clarified. Maturation of the surfactant system in male fetuses is delayed by 1–2 weeks relative to female fetuses. This has been attributed to the higher circulating levels of androgens in the male fetus.

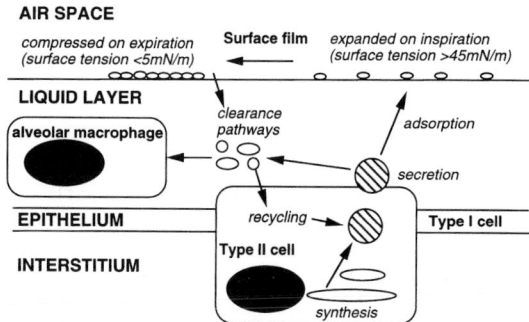

FIGURE 77.10 Hypothesized pathways of surfactant metabolism in the alveolus. The alveolar epithelium consists of two cell types, the type I and type II cell. A thin liquid layer separates the epithelium and the air space. Surfactant is synthesized in type II cells and stored in lamellar bodies. After secretion surfactant spontaneously forms a surface film at the air–liquid interface and reduces the surface tension at this interface. Surfactant is continuously recycled requiring regulated synthesis, secretion, and clearance.

# Surfactant deficiency: *respiratory distress syndrome (RDS)*

The relationship between surfactant deficiency or dysfunction and acute respiratory failure is clearly established. Infants born before the surfactant system fully matures develop RDS manifested by widespread atelectasis, poor lung compliance, intrapulmonary shunts and pulmonary edema. Following the logic of the Laplace relationship, treatment is directed towards restoring lung volume by the application of PEEP. Infants breathing spontaneously try to achieve the same result by expiring through a partially closed glottis. This pattern of breathing often is accompanied by a characteristic expiratory grunt.

Therapeutic surfactant, derived from animal surfactant or assembled from synthetic components, can also be administered via the trachea. The formulations of the exogenous surfactants vary, but all contain high concentrations of DPPC and an agent included to promote spreading of the DPPC at the air–liquid interface. Exogenous surfactant therapy approximately halves the mortality from RDS. In several diseases where acute respiratory failure with stiff lungs and low lung volumes is a final common end point (*adult respiratory distress syndrome* or *ARDS*), surfactant may be present in normal amounts but be inactivated by the presence of soluble inhibitory agents present in the edema fluid in the alveolar space. The specific pathway of inhibition is unclear, but the surfactant dysfunction that results undoubtedly contributes to the morbidity of these conditions. The role of surfactant therapy in ARDS has not been clarified.

## ALVEOLAR FLUID BALANCE

The enormous capillary surface area of the pulmonary microvasculature allows for a large solute, protein and fluid flux between the vascular space and the interstitium. A number of physical forces, classically described by the Starling law of capillary fluid exchange, determine the flux of fluid between these compartments. The lymphatics of the pulmonary interstitium control fluid accumulation in the interstitial space and the relatively tight epithelial barrier limits alveolar flooding and frank pulmonary edema. In the normal lung the alveolar epithelium is covered with a thin but continuous fluid layer. The volume and ionic composition of this alveolar lining fluid appears to be primarily regulated by active epithelial processes including ion pumps and transcytotic vesicular pathways.

## Capillary fluid exchange

Transcapillary fluid movement in the pulmonary microcirculation is discussed on page 821.

## Epithelial barrier

Fluid and protein entering the interstitial space generally do not spill over into the alveolar lumen. This is because under normal circumstances the alveolar epithelium forms a tight barrier restricting passive fluid, solute, and protein movement. Alveolar epithelial cells are linked by morphologically recognizable tight junctions. Some passive diffusion of water and small solutes occurs across the normal epithelial barrier, but the actual anatomical sites (paracellular or transcellular) through which this flux occurs are not known. Epithelial injury, hyperventilation, and surfactant deficiency increase epithelial permeability.

Active epithelial transport processes appear to be very important in maintaining a dry alveolar lumen. Type I and type II cells have vesicular pathways that may contribute to the selective bidirectional movement of proteins, including albumin and immunoglobulins, between the interstitial space and alveolar lumen. The alveolar epithelium also has active ion transport potential. In the fetal lung the predominant process is cAMP-dependent $Cl^-$ secretion by the epithelium lining the developing potential air spaces. The mature alveolar epithelium actively transports $Na^+$ from the luminal to interstitial spaces. This transport is regulated by cAMP and β-adrenergic agonists *in vitro* and *in vivo*. In the mature epithelium, active $Na^+$ resorption followed by passive $Cl^-$ and $H_2O$ resorption likely is primarily responsible for keeping the normal alveolar space relatively dry and for clearing fluid that accumulates during pulmonary edema. The factors that control the transition from a predominantly $Cl^-$-secreting state before birth to a $Na^+$-resorbing state after birth are not fully defined, but circulating hormones including catecholamines and vasopressin are thought to play a major role. Although all cells can be expected to express ion pumps on their surface, pulmonary type II epithelial cells appear to be particularly rich in basolateral $Na^+$-$K^+$-ATPase and may therefore play a primary role in regulating alveolar liquid homeostasis.

## Alveolar liquid lining layer

The alveolus in the mature lung is not completely dry. The epithelial layer is lined by a thin but probably continuous layer of fluid. The interface between this fluid layer and the respiratory gases imposes the problem of special surface forces with regard to the volume stability of the lung. The volume of the liquid layer is difficult to assess but is probably in the order of 35–70 mL in the adult human lung. The average depth of this layer, sometimes referred to as the alveolar subphase or hypophase, is about 1 μm, but in large areas over the type I cells the subphase is very thin, covering little more than the cell's glycocalyx. The alveolar subphase (pH 6.9) is more acidic than plasma (pH 7.4). In the fetal lung, the free $Ca^{2+}$ concentration of the lung liquid is 0.5 mmol/L.

The subphase $Ca^{2+}$ concentration rises after birth and rapidly reaches a level (2 mmol/L) similar to the plasma concentration. The importance of these values and their changes with birth is unknown, but $Ca^{2+}$ may regulate certain important aspects of surfactant function such as the rate of surface layer formation. Major derangements in alveolar subphase protein and ion concentration, as may occur in states of pulmonary edema, could interfere with surfactant function.

## Pulmonary edema

The normal lung does not become edematous, even though fluid filtration increases, until pressure in the microvasculature rises to very high levels. As fluid filtration increases, compensatory decreases in interstitial oncotic pressure and increases in interstitial pressure slow the rate of fluid filtration (see Starling equation, page 821). The flow through the pulmonary lymphatics can also increase dramatically, limiting accumulation of fluid in the interstitium. In the injured lung, the fluid filtration rate increases at much lower microvascular pressures. Eventually, with a sufficiently high rate of fluid filtration, the capacitance of the interstitial space is exceeded; alveolar flooding occurs when the interstitial volume has increased by approximately 50 per cent. Epithelial injury from barotrauma, oxidant injury, surfactant deficiency, infection, etc. allows earlier alveolar flooding. Gas exchange deteriorates markedly with alveolar flooding.

The mechanisms involved in the clearance of liquid and protein from the alveolar space after alveolar flooding are not fully understood. Active $Na^+$ resorption with passive water resorption by the alveolar epithelium, particularly the type II cells, is probably a central mechanism of edema clearance. In diseases with a major component of epithelial injury and permeability edema (high protein concentration in the edema fluid), the subphase protein concentration may rise to very high levels as the water is cleared from the alveolar lumen. The mechanisms of protein clearance from the alveolar space during the recovery phase of pulmonary edema are not known, but probably include alveolar macrophage phagocytosis and degradation and asymmetric epithelial transcytosis.

## IMMUNE EFFECTOR CELLS IN THE ALVEOLUS

In the normal lung the major immune effector cells in the alveolar region are alveolar macrophages and T-lymphocytes. Macrophages are by far the most numerous, but both cell types are found scattered throughout the alveolar interstitium and in the alveolar space. The functional characteristics of the cells in the interstitium of the lung appear to be similar to those of the luminal cells. In lavage fluid from the distal lung, 80–85 per cent of the cells are alveolar macrophages and 10–15 per cent are activated or memory T-lymphocytes. Less than 5 per cent of the cells in normal lavage fluid are neutrophils or eosinophils, but the number of these cells can increase dramatically in disease states. A variety of other alveolar cells can act as antigen-presenting accessory immune cells, including cells of the dendritic lineage, which are scattered throughout the alveolar interstitium. The responses of all these alveolar immune effector cells to foreign antigens, particulates, and pathogens are similar to the responses of immune cells elsewhere in the body. The details of the general immune response are described in detail elsewhere (Chapters 83–87); only the rather specialized alveolar macrophage will be briefly discussed here.

## Alveolar macrophages

Fetal lung liquid is virtually acellular. The number of alveolar macrophages increases steadily after birth. The average adult alveolus contains 10–50 macrophages closely associated with the alveolar epithelium in the subphase fluid. Both tissue macrophages and intravascular macrophages are also found in the alveolar region. Alveolar macrophages are predominantly derived from blood monocytes and are quite long lived in the alveolus. Alveolar macrophages also have some limited potential to proliferate in the alveolar space. Alveolar macrophages are multifunctional cells with beneficial roles in antigen presentation to T-lymphocytes, phagocytosis of particulates and microorganisms, recruitment and functional regulation of other immune cells, and stimulation of repair processes in the injured alveolus. A broad array of receptors, including those for complement components and immunoglobulins, have been localized to the surface of the alveolar macrophage. Subpopulations of alveolar macrophages with possibly different functions have been described. The ability of the alveolar macrophage to produce and secrete many bioactive compounds including prostanoids, cytokines, growth factors, proteases, and other enzymes has led to the belief that products of the alveolar macrophage may also play harmful roles in many diseases.

## SELECTED READING

Avery ME, Mead J. Surface properties in relation to atelectasis and hyaline membrane disease. *Am J Dis Child* 1959; **97**: 517.

Clements JA, Hustead RF, Johnson RP, Gribetz I. Pulmonary surface tension and alveolar stability. *J Appl Physiol* 1961; **16**: 444.

Fels A, Cohn Z. The alveolar macrophage. *J Appl Physiol* 1986; **60**: 353.

Taylor AE, Barnard JW, Barman SC, Adkins WK. Fluid balance. In: Crystal RG, West JB, eds. *The lung: scientific foundations*, Vol 1. New York: Raven Press, 1991: 1147.

Weibel ER. Morphological basis of alveolar–capillary gas exchange. *Physiol Rev* 1973; **53**: 419.

# PULMONARY VASCULATURE

The pulmonary vasculature plays a central role in normal and abnormal lung function. A critical and obvious role of the pulmonary vasculature is to provide a conduit through the lungs for the oxygenation of systemic venous blood. While providing this pathway is essential, the pulmonary vasculature is not simply a system of inert tubes. It regulates its own blood flow and distribution and is intimately involved with multiple circulating components in the blood.

## INTEGRATIVE PHYSIOLOGY

The pulmonary circulation serves the indispensable function of delivering deoxygenated blood to the distal air spaces where $O_2$ and $CO_2$ are exchanged.

## Blood volume

The fetal lungs contain relatively less blood than they do postnatally. After birth, the blood volume of the lung increases approximately 40 per cent. If estimates for adults are applicable to children, then approximately 10–15 per cent of the total blood volume is contained in the lungs. Because of this, the lungs can act as a reservoir of volume for the maintenance of cardiac output; this reservoir may be needed during postural changes.

## Blood flow

### Developmental considerations

In the fetus only about 8 per cent of the combined ventricular output of the heart traverses the pulmonary circulation, a result of the high pulmonary vascular resistance, which shunts blood from the pulmonary artery to the descending aorta through the ductus arteriosus. Within the first day after birth, pulmonary arterial pressure, which is slightly greater than aortic pressure in the fetus, falls to roughly 50 per cent of the *in utero* value while systemic arterial pressure remains relatively constant. The regulation of this fall in pulmonary vascular resistance, and vasomotor tone in general, are discussed in Chapters 67 and 73.

### Effect of gravity

Because the postnatal pulmonary circulation is a low pressure circuit that is influenced by alveolar and interstitial pressure, the distribution of blood within the lungs is not uniform; rather, blood flow depends on the interplay of lung position and gravity.

By convention, physiologists divide the lung into several different zones; blood flow through each is determined by the interrelationship of pulmonary arterial pressure, alveolar pressure, and pulmonary venous pressure. Zone 1 is the uppermost section of lung, and the remaining zones follow one below the other. Furthermore, physiologists label vessels in the lung as either alveolar or extraalveolar. The alveolar vessels are subject to the pressure in the alveolar space and are compressed by lung inflation, while extraalveolar vessels are not affected by alveolar pressure and expand with lung inflation. The concepts of lung zones and alveolar and extraalveolar vessels are functional, and not anatomically based. They are most useful in terms of understanding and explaining the results of experimental manipulations of the lung.

*Zone 1* is that area of the lung in which alveolar pressure is greater than pulmonary arterial and pulmonary venous pressures. Consequently there is no blood flow through alveolar vessels because alveolar pressure exceeds pulmonary arterial pressure; alveolar pressure acts, in effect, as a clamp on the alveolar vessels in this zone. Blood flow does occur in extraalveolar vessels in zone 1. In an upright patient, zone 1 comprises the area of the lung near the apices.

In *zone 2*, which begins just below zone 1, pulmonary arterial pressure exceeds alveolar pressure, but alveolar pressure exceeds pulmonary venous pressure. Blood flow in zone 2 increases with distance down zone 2 because pulmonary arterial pressure increases with distance down zone 2.

*Zone 3* begins at the point where alveolar pressure equals pulmonary venous pressure. Although in this area of the lung blood flow is determined by the difference between pulmonary arterial and pulmonary venous pressures, blood flow increases with distance down zone 3 just as in zone 2. This is rather unexpected because the difference in driving pressure for fluid movement (the difference between pulmonary arterial and pulmonary venous pressures) remains constant in zone 3. The increase in observed blood flow is thought to be secondary to vessel recruitment and distension.

The most dependent area of the lung is sometimes referred to as *zone 4*. Determinants of blood flow are more complicated in this zone and, as a result, blood flow is influenced to a greater extent by flow in vessels other than those in close approximation to alveoli. Blood flow often decreases with distance down zone 4 as blood vessels are compressed by gravity.

### Sites of vascular resistance

In the pulmonary circulation, the total cross-sectional area in the pulmonary vasculature decreases as vessels branch distally. Direct microvascular pressure measurements have shown that as a result of this, the pressure drop across the microcirculation is substantial. This contrasts with the situation in the systemic circulation, where the greatest site of resistance is in the small arterioles, upstream from the microcirculation.

## Effect of vascular pressure and lung volume

The pulmonary circulation can accommodate substantial changes in blood volume and flow. For instance, an increase in pulmonary arterial pressure or left atrial pressure decreases pulmonary vascular resistance as a result of vascular distension and vessel recruitment. Likewise, an increase in pulmonary blood volume also causes vascular distension and recruitment and results in a decrease in pulmonary vascular resistance. Thus, during exercise, even though cardiac output may increase substantially, pulmonary arterial pressure does not rise dramatically because pulmonary vascular resistance decreases.

When the lung is at functional residual capacity (FRC), pulmonary vascular resistance is lowest. During inspiration, which increases lung volume above FRC, or during a forced expiration at the end of a tidal breath, which lowers lung volume below FRC, pulmonary vascular resistance increases.

Although commonly believed, the concept that interstitial pulmonary edema *per se* increases pulmonary vascular resistance (by "filling up" the interstitial space) is not supported by experimental evidence at present. There is evidence, however, that alveolar edema results in a local increase in pulmonary vascular resistance secondary to vasoconstriction. This results in redistribution of blood flow to areas of the lung with well-ventilated alveoli.

## Liquid and solute transport

The pulmonary vasculature is the first barrier to liquid and solute movement into the parenchyma of the lung, and as such is the first line of defense against pulmonary edema. Although edema in peripheral tissues is cosmetically unappealing, edema in the lungs can be life-threatening. Conditions that increase the rate of transport of liquid into the lungs are common but, fortunately, the pathways for liquid removal can accommodate excess fluid under most circumstances. Pulmonary edema results when the mechanisms for liquid removal are overwhelmed.

Water probably crosses the endothelial barrier directly through the endothelial cell or through interendothelial cell junctions. Macromolecules probably cross the endothelial barrier through interendothelial cell junctions, which do not restrict small particles but do restrict large proteins. There is some evidence for vesicular transport across the endothelial cell itself, but how much this type of solute transport contributes to overall liquid and protein movement is unclear.

In general, fluid transport across a semipermeable membrane can be described conceptually by the Starling equation:

$$Q = Kf[(P_{mv} - P_{pmv}) - \sigma(\pi_{mv} - \pi_{pmv})]$$

where $Q$ is the net liquid flow across the membrane, $Kf$ represents the conductance of the membrane, $P$ is the hydrostatic pressure term, $\sigma$ represents the reflection coefficient, and $\pi$ represents the protein osmotic pressure; the subscripts mv and pmv represent the microvascular and perimicrovascular sites of measurement, respectively. The major portion of the fluid exchange occurs in the vicinity of the alveolar walls in the small vessels, collectively termed the microvasculature (Fig. 77.11).

## Permeability

The conductance of the vascular barrier, $Kf$, is a function of both the permeability to water and the surface area available for fluid exchange. From the above equation, if permeability increases, $Kf$ would increase, resulting in more fluid transport across the pulmonary vasculature. Likewise, if the surface area for fluid exchange increases, $Kf$ would increase, and fluid flow across the endothelial barrier would increase.

The other term in the equation that affects permeability is $\sigma$, the osmotic reflection coefficient. The reflection coefficient indicates the relative resistance of a barrier to solute movement. In limiting cases, impermeant molecules have a reflection coefficient of 1 and

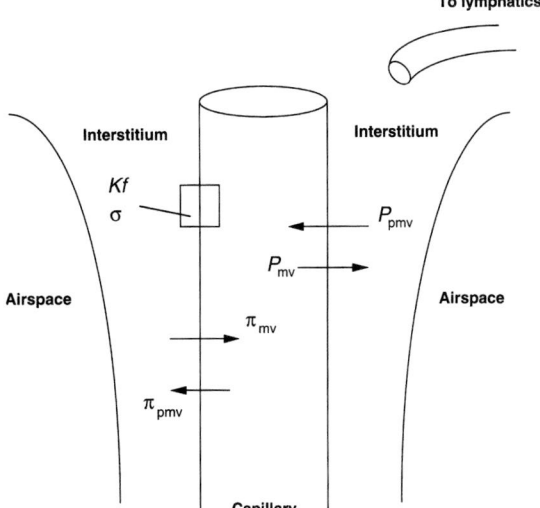

FIGURE 77.11 Characterization of fluid exchange across the microcirculation in the lung. Under normal circumstances, hydrostatic pressure in the microvasculature ($P_{mv}$) and protein osmotic pressure in the perimicrovascular space ($\pi_{pmv}$) act to move fluid into the interstitium. Hydrostatic pressure in the perimicrovascular space ($P_{pmv}$) and protein osmotic pressure in the microcirculation ($\pi_{mv}$) oppose fluid entry into the interstitium. Fluid leaves the interstitium at least in part by lymphatic drainage. $Kf$ and $\sigma$ are properties of the vascular barrier. The airway and alveolar epithelium prevents interstitial fluid from entering the air spaces.

molecules with no restriction to movement, such as serum electrolytes, have a value of 0. The term $\sigma$ represents the sum of the permeability characteristics for all the plasma solute components. The relevant solutes in plasma generally are proteins. As a practical matter, any condition that increases the water conductance of the barrier also increases the protein permeability and results in an increase in $Kf$ and a decrease in $\sigma$.

The adult respiratory distress syndrome affects not only adults but many pediatric patients as well. The pulmonary endothelium is more permeable than normal ($Kf$ is increased and $\sigma$ is decreased), which results in an exaggerated filtration of fluid across the vascular barrier and resultant pulmonary edema. In the respiratory distress syndrome of prematurity, a condition initiated by insufficient pulmonary surfactant, the pulmonary endothelium is also abnormally permeable.

## Vascular and osmotic pressure

From the Starling relationship, it is clear that a rise in microvascular hydrostatic pressure will increase fluid filtration. The difference between the microvascular and perimicrovasular pressures actually determines whether a change in hydrostatic pressure will change fluid transport. For the most part, however, increases in microvascular pressure are not accompanied by equivalent increases in interstitial pressure; therefore, excess fluid is filtered across the circulation.

Likewise, the protein osmotic pressure terms must be considered together. That is, the difference between the microvascular and perivascular protein osmotic pressures determines the effect on fluid filtration.

Equilibration between protein concentrations in the intravascular and interstitial spaces of the lung is more rapid than is generally appreciated. In normal lungs, for instance, the albumin concentration in interstitial fluid is approximately 80–90 per cent that of plasma. It rapidly reaches a new equilibrium when plasma albumin concentration changes. In conditions where the permeability of the endothelial barrier is compromised, the concentration of albumin in the interstitium is even closer to that of plasma. Infusions of albumin to increase plasma oncotic pressure in patients with increased vascular permeability are unlikely to result in any substantial benefit to the patient as the albumin will equilibrate rapidly between the plasma and interstitium. Such an infusion may increase pulmonary vascular pressures and enhance fluid filtration into the lung

## ENDOTHELIAL CELL BIOLOGY (see also Chapter 67)

# Metabolic functions

The pulmonary endothelium is not an inert cell lining; it is metabolically active and sensitive to a number of components that come in contact with its surface. After birth the entire cardiac output passes through the pulmonary circulation; therefore, the lung is in a unique position to respond to mediators present in the circulation.

## Prostaglandins

Prostaglandins are a class of arachidonic acid metabolites synthesized by virtually all cell types (see Chapter 8). Pulmonary endothelium is no exception and makes predominantly $PGI_2$ which affects vasomotor tone (see page 700). $PGI_2$ is not metabolized in the lung. In contrast, $PGE_2$, $PGE_1$, and $PGF_{2\alpha}$ are all inactivated in the lung. $PGE_2$ inactivation is gestationally dependent in the perinatal period with less circulating $PGE_2$ being cleared in a single passage through lungs from immature fetuses. Pulmonary inactivation of circulating $PGE_2$ is important in functional closure of the ductus arteriosus at birth.

## Endothelial-derived relaxing factor (EDRF)

Now known to be nitric oxide (NO) and also termed endothelial-derived nitric oxide (EDNO), this substance is released in response to various stimuli. It too plays a major role in pulmonary vasoregulation (see pages 697 and 751).

## Inactivation of biogenic amines

Catecholamines, histamine, and serotonin are potent vasogenic bioamines. The pulmonary circulation plays a major role in the inactivation of two of these substances, serotonin and norepinephrine. The pulmonary circulation plays little or no role in the inactivation of epinephrine, dopamine, or histamine.

### Serotonin

Serotonin (5-hydroxytryptamine), a potent vasoconstrictor, is found in a variety of tissues. The pulmonary endothelium contains a specific uptake mechanism for the removal of serotonin. This extraction process is carrier mediated, driven by the $Na^+$ gradient produced by $Na^+$-$K^+$-ATPase and it is saturable and temperature-dependent. Once inside the cell, serotonin is metabolized by a monoamine oxidase. The uptake system is quite efficient, clearing over 90 per cent of plasma serotonin during a single pass through the lung. It is inhibited by cocaine and tricyclic antidepressants.

### Norepinephrine

Norepinephrine is also a potent vasoconstrictor. Like serotonin, norepinephrine is taken up and inactivated by the pulmonary endothelium; 25–50 per cent of circulating norepinephrine is cleared during a single pass through the lungs.

The uptake of norepinephrine by endothelial cells is biochemically similar to the uptake of serotonin, although the carriers responsible for transport are distinct. Once inside the cell, norepinephrine is metabolized by either a monoamine oxidase or catechol-O-methyltransferase. Uptake inhibitors are similar to those for serotonin.

## Vasoactive peptides

### Bradykinin

Bradykinin is a nine-amino-acid peptide formed in plasma by the kininogen–kinin system. It is a potent hypotensive substance, inactivated by angiotensin converting enzyme (ACE), an endothelial cell-surface dipeptidylcarboxypeptidase. Roughly 80 per cent of circulating bradykinin is removed during one pass through the lungs.

### Angiotensin I

Angiotensin I is a 10-amino-acid peptide formed in plasma from angiotensinogen. As angiotensin I passes through the lungs, it is converted by ACE to angiotensin II, an eight amino acid peptide that causes hypertension. Although other endothelial cells possess ACE activity, the lung is the most important site for converting angiotensin I to angiotensin II. Angiotensin II is not metabolized by the lung, but is metabolized by other vascular beds.

# Pulmonary circulation and hemostasis

The pulmonary endothelium, like other endothelial beds, normally maintains a non-thrombogenic surface. However, a number of lung diseases are associated with disordered hemostasis in the pulmonary circulation. Often it is unclear whether the abnormal hemostasis causes or aggravates the lung disorder or whether it is secondary to a primary endothelial cell abnormality.

## Anticoagulant characteristics (see also Chapters 67 and 82)

### Prostaglandins

PGI$_2$ is not only a potent vasodilator but also inhibits platelet aggregation. Platelet aggregation occurs early in response to vascular injury, promoting conversion of prothrombin to thrombin, and releasing thromboxane A$_2$, a powerful vasoconstrictor. PGI$_2$ released by endothelial cells serves to counteract these responses.

### Endothelial-derived nitric oxide

NO, much as PGI$_2$, is not only a potent vasodilator but also inhibits platelet aggregation.

### Heparan sulfate

In addition to synthesizing PGI$_2$ and NO, endothelial cells express cell-surface-associated molecules involved in anticoagulation. One such molecule is heparan sulfate, a proteoglycan that has heparin-like characteristics. Heparin, and similarly heparan sulfate on the cell surface, act as anticoagulants because they bind to circulating antithrombin III, which enhances thrombin inactivation. In addition to inactivating thrombin, antithrombin III also inactivates factors IXa, Xa, XIa, and XIIa. Antithrombin III acts by blocking a serine residue necessary for coagulant enzyme activity. If endothelial cells are damaged in such a manner as to block or destroy the heparan sulfate molecules on the cell surface, their antithrombin III-mediated anticoagulant property is lost.

### Thrombomodulin

Endothelial cells express a thrombin-binding protein called thrombomodulin. This protein avidly binds thrombin to form a complex that dramatically enhances thrombin catalyzed activation of protein C. The endothelial cell provides a surface for activated protein C to interact with protein S, a circulating glycoprotein. When the activated protein C–protein S complex is formed, activated protein C blocks the function of factors Va and VIIIa, inhibiting the coagulation process.

There is also evidence that after thrombin binds to thrombomodulin, this ligand–receptor complex is internalized. This process tends to promote anticoagulation because thrombin bound to thrombomodulin can still convert fibrinogen to fibrin.

## Procoagulant characteristics

The major procoagulant property of endothelial cells is the cell-surface expression of tissue factor, a glycoprotein with a molecular mass of 40–50 kD. Tissue factor acts as a cofactor with factor VII to enhance the activation of factors IX and X. Normal endothelium does not express tissue factor, but certain molecules known to be associated with pulmonary vascular injury are stimulants for tissue factor expression by endothelial cells. These include thrombin, endotoxin, interleukin-1 (IL-1), and tumor necrosis factor (TNF).

## Fibrinolysis

The endothelium plays a balancing act in fibrinolysis, producing molecules that promote and inhibit clot lysis. Like every other aspect of the coagulation cascade, regulated production of these factors is the critical element.

Endothelial cells produce two plasminogen activators, urokinase plasminogen activator (u-PA) and tissue plasminogen activator (t-PA). t-PA binds to fibrin and plasminogen, forming a complex that accelerates the formation of plasmin from plasminogen. Plasmin then cleaves fibrin and fibrinogen to begin clot lysis.

Endothelial cells also produce plasminogen activator inhibitor. This molecule inhibits both t-PA and u-PA. Thus the endothelial cell participates intimately in the regulation of clot formation and dissolution. Factors like endotoxin and TNF disturb this balance and promote endothelial procoagulant activity.

## Non-hemostatic effects

Some of the molecules formed during hemostasis have additional effects on the pulmonary vasculature. For instance, thrombin is a crucial clotting enzyme, but also appears to increase pulmonary vascular permeability, pulmonary vascular resistance, and pulmonary arterial pressure. Thrombin also causes neutrophils to adhere and accumulate in the lung and stimulates platelet aggregation and adherence of platelets to endothelial cells. In addition, heparan sulfate produced by endothelial cells acts as a growth inhibitor for pulmonary vascular smooth muscle.

# Neutrophil–endothelial cell interaction

Although the interaction of endothelial cells and circulating neutrophils is essential for normal host defense, when this interaction occurs in an unregulated fashion, neutrophils can initiate or enhance tissue damage.

Neutrophils play a role in lung injury and the subsequent development of pulmonary edema.

The requisite step in neutrophil migration into the interstitium is adhesion to the vascular wall (Fig 77.12). This adhesion is modulated, at least in part, by neutrophil-dependent and endothelial cell-dependent mechanisms (see also page 694). The extent to which each of these mechanisms contributes to neutrophil-mediated lung injury is not completely certain.

## Neutrophil-dependent adhesion

Two general classes of adhesion molecules, present on neutrophils, mediate their binding to endothelial cells, the $\beta_2$ integrins and L-selectin.

### $\beta_2$ Integrins

The three $\beta_2$ integrins are more commonly recognized by their CD classifications: CD11a/CD18, CD11b/CD18, and CD11c/CD18. All three integrins normally are present on the neutrophil plasma membrane.

A number of diverse agonists induce neutrophil-dependent, integrin-mediated adhesion to endothelial cells, including f-Met-Leu-Phe, fragments of complement activation, platelet activating factor (PAF), interleukin-8 (IL-8), and leukotriene $B_4$. Adhesion appears to be dependent on a conformational change in the $\beta_2$ integrins present on the surface at the time of stimulation. Although new $\beta_2$ integrins may translocate to the cell surface after agonist stimulation, neutrophil

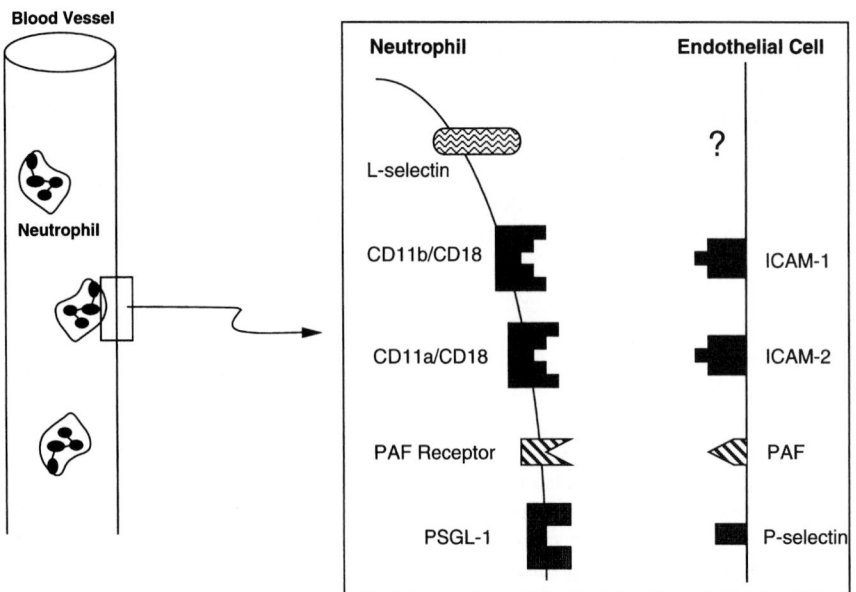

FIGURE 77.12 Cell adhesion molecules that are potentially important in neutrophil–endothelial cell interactions in the lung. Following stimulation, P-selectin binds to P-selectin glycoprotein ligand-1 (PSGL-1) on the neutrophil. At the same time, platelet activating factor (PAF) binds to its receptor on the neutrophil, which increases $\beta_2$ integrin (CD11/CD18) binding. CD11a/CD18 binds to intercellular adhesion molecule-2 (ICAM-2); CD11a/CD18 and CD11b/CD18 bind to ICAM-1. The counter receptor for neutrophil-bound L-selectin is uncertain.

adhesion occurs even in the absence of additional integrin expression.

The $\beta_2$ integrins bind to the intercellular adhesion molecules 1 and 2 (ICAM-1, ICAM-2) on the endothelial surface. The $\beta_2$ integrins may also bind to other uncharacterized ligands.

### L-selectin

L-selectin (also known as LAM-1, MEL-14 and LECAM-1) is one of three molecules in the selectin family, the others being E-selectin and P-selectin. L-selectin is the only one, however, known to be present on neutrophils. The adhesion molecule on endothelial cells to which L-selectin binds is uncertain.

The binding characteristics of neutrophil adhesion to endothelial cells mediated by L-selectin have not been explored as extensively as those of the $\beta_2$ integrins. It is interesting that under certain conditions there may be cooperation between L-selectin and $\beta_2$ integrins since reagents that interfere with either $\beta_2$ integrins or L-selectin inhibit neutrophil adhesion to cytokine-stimulated endothelial cells.

## Endothelial cell-dependent adhesion

### Platelet activating factor

PAF is a phospholipid that is rapidly synthesized in endothelial cells in response to a number of agonists including leukotriene $C_4$, histamine, and thrombin. After it is synthesized, PAF is not released but remains cell-associated. PAF binds to a receptor on the neutrophil surface, a process that results in an increase in neutrophil adhesiveness, further anchoring the neutrophil to the endothelial cell. The enhanced neutrophil binding triggered by PAF is mediated by the $\beta_2$ integrins CD11a/CD18 and CD11b/CD18. PAF can also prime the neutrophil to respond in an exaggerated fashion to chemotactic factors.

### Interleukin-8

Another molecule, IL-8, is synthesized by endothelial cells and participates in neutrophil binding and subsequent neutrophil migration. After endothelial cells are stimulated by TNF, IL-1, or lipopolysaccharide (LPS), transcription of IL-8 mRNA begins, ultimately resulting in maximal IL-8 expression 4–24 hours later. IL-8 is secreted by the endothelial cell and exerts its effect by binding to a receptor on the neutrophil. In response to IL-8 stimulation, neutrophil adhesion is mediated through the integrin complex.

### P-selectin

When endothelial cells are activated by histamine or thrombin, P-selectin moves rapidly from storage granules in the endothelial cell to the plasma membrane. Cell-associated P-selectin binds a receptor on the neutrophil surface that is distinct from the $\beta_2$ integrin family. The time course for expression of P-selectin activity is similar to expression of PAF activity. Thus,

P-selectin may initially bind the neutrophil, allowing PAF to activate the neutrophil. This would result in enhanced neutrophil adhesion secondary to $\beta_2$ integrin binding and enhanced responsiveness to chemotactic factors. The receptor for P-selectin on the neutrophil is the P-selectin glycoprotein ligand-1.

### E-selectin

E-selectin (also known as endothelial–leukocyte adhesion molecule 1, or ELAM-1) is a molecule expressed and retained on the endothelial cell plasma membrane in response to stimulation with TNF, IL-1, or LPS. Expression requires protein synthesis and is maximal at 4–8 hours. $\beta_2$ Integrins are not required for E-selectin-mediated neutrophil binding, nor is neutrophil activation required. The receptor on the neutrophil for E-selectin is unknown.

## Mediators of neutrophil-induced damage

There is abundant evidence that oxidants released from stimulated neutrophils are responsible in part for damage caused by these cells. Antioxidants like superoxide dismutase and catalase ameliorate neutrophil-mediated damage in vivo and in vitro. Likewise, reduced amounts of natural antioxidants like glutathione increase the susceptibility of endothelial cells to neutrophil-mediated damage. The exact mechanism of injury under these circumstances is unclear, but oxidants may alter cell phospholipids and thereby impair membrane function.

Neutrophils also cause damage by releasing proteases in response to activation. These proteases may disturb endothelial cell–matrix attachments and may alter molecules expressed on the endothelial cell surface such as heparan sulfate. Oxidants may also inactivate naturally occurring antiproteases.

## SELECTED READING

Albelda SM, Smith CW, Ward PA. Adhesion molecules and inflammatory injury. *FASEB J* 1994; 8: 504.

Bland RD, Carlton DP. Neonatal lung edema. In: Said SI, ed. *The pulmonary circulation and acute lung injury*, 2nd edn. Mount Kisco, NY: Futura Publishing Company, Inc., 1991: 10.

Carlos TM, Harlan JM. Membrane proteins involved in phagocyte adherence to endothelium. *Immunol Rev* 1990; **114**: 5.

Fishman AP. Pulmonary circulation. In: Fishman AP, Fisher AB, eds. *Handbook of physiology, Vol 1, Section 3.* Baltimore: Waverly Press, 1985: 93.

Godin C, Caprani A, Dufaux J, Flaud P. Interactions between neutrophils and endothelial cells. *J Cell Sci* 1993; **106**: 441.

Hughes JMB. Distribution of pulmonary blood flow. In: Crystal RG, West JB, eds. *The lung: scientific foundations*, Vol 1. New York: Raven Press, 1991: 523.

Staub NC. Pulmonary edema. *Physiol Rev* 1974; **54**: 678.

Stern DM, Kaiser E, Naworth PP. Regulation of the coagulation system by vascular endothelial cells. *Haemostasis* 1988; **18**: 202.

# PULMONARY INTERSTITIUM

Anatomically, the pulmonary interstitium is considered to encompass the area between the alveolar epithelium and capillary endothelium. This space is contiguous with the loose connective tissue that surrounds the airways and larger blood vessels; thus this entire region is in series. The interstitium contains a number of different cells and molecules necessary for maintenance of normal lung function, and is also the area through which water and solutes travel after they have filtered across the vascular endothelium or have been reabsorbed from the alveolar air space.

## STRUCTURAL DESIGN

The interstitial area throughout the lung contains an organized connective tissue framework that gives the lung its characteristic shape. The elements of this framework are predominantly collagen and elastin. The framework is divided into three components. The first component, the peripheral fiber system, begins in the interstitium of the visceral pleura. These fibers surround the lung in the pleural interstitium and also travel centrally, subdividing the lung into segments as they move towards the hilum. The second component, the central fiber system, begins at the hilum and moves peripherally, surrounding and supporting airways and vessels. The third component, the septal fiber system, is composed of small connective tissue fibers that provide support for the alveoli. This design gives the lung its strength and its elastic characteristics.

## LIQUID MOVEMENT

The fibrous network of the interstitium permits efficient liquid movement away from the alveoli to a more central location, thus minimizing interference with gas exchange. Normally, fluid is removed by lymphatics as it moves out of the alveolar septal area, and the volume of lymphatic drainage is considered to be equal to transvascular fluid filtration. There is always a net movement of liquid from the circulation into the interstitial space. The lymphatics do not begin in the alveolar septal area, but rather in the peribronchovascular space around terminal airways and vessels. Lymphatics are lined by continuous endothelium and contain numerous valves, similar in function to those in the systemic veins, which results in unidirectional lymphatic flow centrally. Smooth muscle cells that surround larger lymphatic vessels are responsible for the pulsatile movement of lymph towards the hilum. The

lymph eventually drains into regional lymph nodes, and ultimately the systemic circulation.

The alveolar septal connective tissue space is in series with the peribronchovascular space, the loose connective tissue that surrounds the larger airways and blood vessels. When abnormal amounts of fluid are filtered from the circulation and overwhelm the lymphatic system, this excess fluid moves to fill the peribronchovascular space. Again this minimizes the volume of liquid filling the alveolar septal space. The driving force for this movement is an increasingly negative pressure gradient from periphery to hilum.

## EXTRACELLULAR MATRIX (*see also* pages 71 and 693)

Together, collagen and elastin in the interstitium are estimated to constitute most of the total protein in the lung, well over 95 per cent of the connective tissue, and 15–20 per cent of dry lung weight. Of the two, collagen is the most abundant. Together they give the lung its structural integrity, expansive limit, and elastic recoil.

## Collagen

Collagen collectively consists of about 25 different proteins. Their chemical properties give them great tensile strength. Types I and III collagen are the most abundant forms found in the lung, accounting for over 75 per cent of the connective tissue. All collagen molecules share relatively unique amino acid sequences of repeating trimers containing glycine. In addition to the large amount of glycine, proline and hydroxyproline are also abundant. The latter is an uncommon amino acid and, in fact, is often used as a marker of collagen as virtually no other protein contains hydroxyproline. The other unique molecular characteristic of collagen is that it is composed of three subunits that form a triple helix. Depending on the collagen type, the subunits may be the same or different.

Collagen synthesis is not restricted to one cell type in the lung. Fibroblasts, epithelial cells, and endothelial cells all synthesize collagen, but the fibroblast is considered to be the model cell for collagen production. Collagen is initially translated as procollagen. While still inside the cell, the appropriate proline, and sometimes lysine, residues are hydroxylated. Three individual procollagen subunits then associate and form a more mature procollagen, which then undergoes helix formation. Before secretion, the hydroxylysine residues are glycosylated. The extra peptides present on the procollagen molecules are thought to have several functions, one of which is to keep the collagen precursor soluble in the cell until secretion. After secretion, C- and N-terminal regions of the procollagen subunits are cleaved to form mature collagen. Mature collagen is known to bind to fibronectin and to certain cells, but the biological significance of these findings is unclear. Collagen synthesized in response to injury is predominantly type I. This is a result of enhanced fibroblast production and an overall increase in fibroblast number.

Collagens are degraded by metalloproteinases referred to as collagenases, but what role collagenases play in the turnover of lung collagen is unclear. Neutrophils, macrophages, and fibroblasts each secrete collagenases, but their specificity for a particular collagen type is different. A number of cells, including fibroblasts, macrophages, and neutrophils, produce enzymes capable of destroying collagen, which is undoubtedly important in lung diseases where destruction of the delicate interstitial elements occurs.

## Elastin

Elastin is the other major component of the connective tissue in the lung. Although not as prominent as collagen, it is extremely important, giving the lung its "elastic" quality and aiding in normal alveolarization (Fig. 77.13). Although elastin can be found relatively early in gestation, the majority of elastin production takes place during the latter part of gestation, temporally associated with alveolarization; after this portion of lung development is complete, new elastin formation is minimal.

Elastin is first secreted in a soluble form, tropoelastin. Tropoelastin then associates with microfibrils, after which lysyl oxidase links tropoelastin molecules together to form mature elastin; chemically, mature

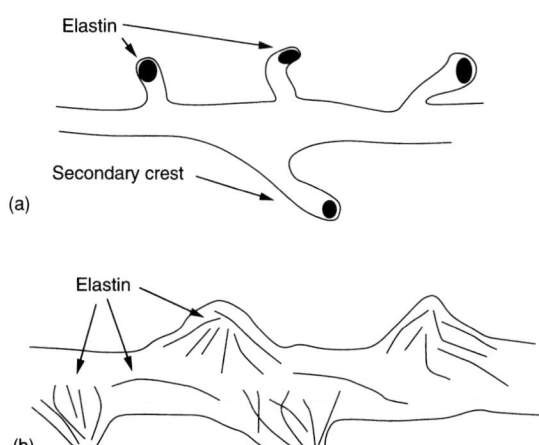

FIGURE 77.13 Appearance of elastin in alveolar septa. Normal alveolarization is associated with collections of elastin at the leading tip of secondary crests, the finger-like structures that begin future alveoli (a). After injury (b), elastin fails to aggregate and instead appears as disorganized strands throughout the interstitium. Under these circumstances, secondary crests are abnormal, alveoli are immature and air-space formation is delayed.

elastin is quite insoluble. A variety of cells, including smooth muscle cells, endothelial cells, myofibroblasts, and some types of fibroblasts, are believed to be capable of producing elastin. The normal turnover rate for elastin is extraordinarily slow. Mature elastin that does turn over is degraded by elastases. These enzymes are promiscuous and degrade not only elastin but also proteoglycans, collagen, and fibronectin. The normal site in the lung for elastase production is unknown.

## Fibronectins

The role of fibronectins in the extracellular matrix of the lung is unclear. They are large glycoproteins with molecular mass of approximately 500 kD, and at least 20 isoforms have been identified. Although plasma fibronectin is produced by hepatocytes, a "cellular" fibronectin produced locally by lung cells is considered important in normal lung development. Pulmonary endothelial cells, epithelial cells, fibroblasts, alveolar macrophages, and smooth muscle cells all are capable of producing fibronectin in vitro. Although at this time it is uncertain whether fibronectin detected in the lung is derived from plasma or is produced in the lung, the balance weighs in favor of plasma deposition.

Fibronectins contain an RGD (Arg-Gly-Asp) sequence that acts as a binding site for lung fibroblasts, which possess a fibronectin receptor complex. Fibronectin–fibroblast interactions allow the fibroblasts to migrate and spread. Other cell types, including endothelial and epithelial cells, also bind to fibronectin, but whether this binding is mediated in the same fashion as fibroblasts is unclear.

The role of fibronectin in lung development is deduced from experiments showing increased fibronectin content associated with cell differentiation. This role for fibronectin in a general biological sense is strengthened because of similar associations in other organs during development. Furthermore, experiments with antibodies that interfere with fibronectin–receptor binding in vitro disturb normal lung development.

Although normal adult lungs have very little cellular fibronectin, injured lungs show a dramatic increase in cellular fibronectin production. The importance of this finding is unknown, but probably reflects the role of fibronectin in cell migration.

## BASEMENT MEMBRANE

Basement membranes consist of molecules assembled to form a matrix that supports and surrounds the endothelium and epithelium. Basement membranes are also associated with smooth muscle cells and nerves. The basement membrane serves as a somewhat selective barrier for macromolecules and inhibits cell movement, unless the cells possess specific proteases that dissolve the matrix (e.g. inflammatory cells).

## Collagen

Type IV collagen is a major constituent of basement membranes. It is similar in basic constitution to other collagens and has a molecular mass of approximately 500 kD. The C-terminal globular domains are joined together, which allows the N-terminal ends from four collagen molecules to interact. This interaction results in a lattice or meshwork of collagen.

## Laminin

Laminin, another major component of basement membranes, is a large glycoprotein with a molecular mass of around 850 kD. Fully assembled, laminin exists as a four-armed "cross"-like structure composed of three distinct chains. Laminin is not one molecule but, like fibronectin, exists as several different isoforms. Also like fibronectin, laminin has several sites of attachment that permit binding of cells and other constituents of the extracellular matrix. Laminin probably plays a role in cell migration and lung development (Fig. 77.14).

## Entactin

Entactin, also known as nidogen, is a glycoprotein of molecular mass 150 kD. It apparently exists in basement membrane only, and is closely associated with laminin. The entactin molecule has binding sites for type IV collagen; therefore, entactin may serve to link laminin and collagen.

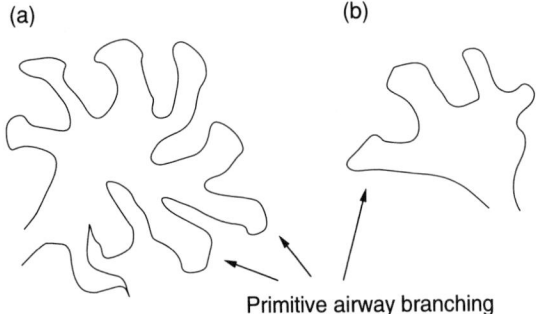

(a)             (b)

Primitive airway branching

FIGURE 77.14 The importance of laminin in lung development. If laminin binding is prevented experimentally, airways do not form properly in the developing lung and maturation is disturbed. (a) Normal airway branching pattern. (b) Airway branching pattern if laminin binding is prevented (adapted from Schuger L *et al. Dev Biol* 1989; **137**: 26). Although results like these demonstrate the importance of one component of extracellular matrix in lung formation, a number of other extracellular matrix components, adhesion molecules and growth factors are likely critical for lung development under normal conditions and following injury.

## Heparan sulfate proteoglycans

These molecules are proteins bound to heparan sulfate chains. Because of their negative charge, they may serve to restrict movement of negatively charged molecules. There are a number of different heparan sulfate proteoglycans. Some are known to bind laminin, type IV collagen, and fibronectin.

## INTERSTITIAL CELLS

## Fibroblasts

These cells constitute the major cell type of the lung interstitium. Although sometimes presented as distinctly different cells, fibroblasts, myofibroblasts, and pericytes probably represent different forms of a similar cell type.

Fibroblasts contain many mitochondria, a large amount of endoplasmic reticulum, and an obvious Golgi complex. These findings are consistent with the synthetic capabilities of the fibroblast to produce collagen, fibronectin, and proteoglycans. Fibroblasts possess cell-surface receptors capable of binding a number of interstitial elements including fibronectin, laminin, and collagen. The fibroblast–connective tissue interactions may serve to arrange the interstitial components during development and repair.

## Pericytes

Pericytes are associated with the capillaries in the alveolar system. They are partially surrounded by a basement membrane, and cytoplasmic extensions are often found in direct contact with the endothelial cells. Their function is uncertain but they are considered by some to be smooth muscle cell precursors.

## Myofibroblasts

Myofibroblasts are present in the alveolar septum. They possess contractile characteristics, but their biological significance is unknown. They are abundant, perhaps constituting 40 per cent of the volume of the interstitial space.

Certain diseases resulting in pulmonary fibrosis are associated with alterations in fibroblasts and extracellular matrix. For instance, bleomycin induces pulmonary fibrosis and is associated with diminished fibroblast growth, but enhanced collagen production.

## SELECTED READING

Bienkowski RS, Gotkin MG. Control of collagen deposition in mammalian lung. *Proc Soc Exp Biol Med* 1995; **209**: 118.

Foster IA, Curtiss SW. The regulation of lung elastin synthesis. *Am J Physiol* 1990; **259**: L13.

Goldstein RH. Control of type I collagen formation in the lung. *Am J Physiol* 1991; **261**: L29.

Hilfer SR, Rayner RM, Brown JW. Mesenchymal control of branching pattern in the fetal mouse lung. *Tissue Cell* 1985; **17**: 523.

McDonald JA. Extracellular matrix assembly. *Annu Rev Cell Biol* 1988; **4**: 183.

McGowan SE. Extracellular matrix and the regulation of lung development and repair. *FASEB J* 1992; **6**: 2895.

Minoo P, King RJ. Epithelial–mesenchymal interactions in lung development. *Annu Rev Physiol* 1994; **56**: 13.

Yurchenco PD, Schittny JC. Molecular architecture of basement membranes. *FASEB J* 1990; **4**: 1577.

# LUNG INJURY

Aerobic organisms are continually exposed to the risk of *oxidant injury* caused by partially reduced, reactive oxygen metabolites (ROM). ROM can cause injury by reacting with cellular proteins, lipids, and nucleic acids. To protect against oxidant injury, aerobic cells have evolved a multilayered, interdependent antioxidant system that includes enzymatic and non-enzymatic components. This antioxidant system exists in the mature lung of all air-breathing organisms. In human diseases, an imbalance between oxidants and antioxidants is involved in the pathogenesis of diverse pulmonary and non-pulmonary disorders. This section characterizes the nature and source of ROM and describes the function of key antioxidant compounds.

## PULMONARY OXIDANT INJURY

An imbalance between pulmonary oxidants and antioxidants often results from exposure to excess oxidants. In the lung, oxidants arise from three major sources.

- Increased production of endogenous oxidants which can arise intracellularly from mitochondrial or cellular oxidizing enzyme systems, or from activated inflammatory cells.
- By exposure to inhaled oxidants including hyperoxia, ozone, and particulates like silica and asbestos. Hyperoxia increases mitochondrial production of ROM and ozone is metabolized to reactive oxygen and lipid peroxide compounds. An additional source of inhaled oxidant stress is tobacco smoke which contains several compounds that generate ROM in respiratory epithelium.
- Many drugs and environmental xenobiotics can generate pulmonary ROM. Atmospheric pollutants and antineoplastic agents such as bleomycin can cause oxidant lung injury. Ionizing radiation also causes lung injury, presumably by increasing pulmonary ROM production.

Reactive oxygen species include the partially reduced oxygen metabolites superoxide anion ($O_2^-$), hydrogen peroxide ($H_2O_2$), hydroxyl radical ($OH^\bullet$), and singlet oxygen ($O^-$) (see Chapter 9). The initial reaction of oxygen radicals with cellular constituents can also generate a secondary cascade of lipid and protein "radicals" that further propagate oxidant injury. Three key features of oxidant injury should be recognized. First, oxidants are produced at specific subcellular sites, which vary depending on the oxidant stress. Second, because of their reactivity, ROM are diffusion-limited and oxidant injury tends to occur near the site of ROM production. For example, mitochondrial damage is a central feature of hyperoxia-induced injury because oxygen increases mitochondrial production of ROM. Hydrogen peroxide, which is able to cross membranes, may provide a way to export ROM. Third, because of the specificity of ROM production and injury, protective antioxidants must be located either at the site of ROM production or at the oxidant target. Therefore, increased mitochondrial antioxidants would be expected to protect mitochondria from locally produced ROM during hyperoxia, while an increase in extracellular or cytoplasmic antioxidants might not.

## Nitric oxide

Nitric oxide (NO) was recently discovered to be a potent vasodilator. Its discovery ended the search for the endothelial-derived relaxing factor, which had begun several years previously (see Chapter 67). Since the original description of NO as a physiological messenger, it has been shown to be a major regulator of cardiovascular, immune, and nervous systems. More recently it has been implicated in disease states including septic shock and adult respiratory distress syndrome (ARDS). NO is a prooxidant, and its adverse effects may in part be due to its ability to react with cellular constituents. NO also combines with $O_2^-$ to form another oxidant, peroxynitrite, which may mediate the neurological, mitochondrial, and cardiovascular toxicities of NO. In experimental animal models, inhaled NO causes an increase in peroxynitrite and reactive nitrotyrosine species. Future work may demonstrate that inhaled NO is a useful pulmonary vasodilator. However, care must be taken to explore the potential adverse, oxidant, effects of NO.

## PULMONARY ANTIOXIDANT ENZYMES

The cascade of oxidizing radicals requires a matched system of substrate-specific antioxidant enzymes. $O_2^-$, the initial radical formed by one electron reduction of molecular oxygen, is eliminated by the superoxide dismutases (SODs). Eukaryotic organisms contain at least three SODs: a cytosolic CuZn-SOD, a mitochondrial Mn-SOD, and an extracellular SOD. All three SODs efficiently catalyze the reaction:

$$2O_2^- + 2H^+ \rightarrow H_2O_2 + O_2$$

Eukaryotic cells are well protected against $H_2O_2$ by catalase and glutathione peroxidase, which eliminate $H_2O_2$. The subcellular distributions of catalase and glutathione peroxidase are different: catalase is present in peroxisomes, and glutathione peroxidase in cytosol and in the mitochondria. Their affinity for $H_2O_2$ also differs: glutathione peroxidase has a $K_m$ of $10^{-6}$ mol/L; catalase has a $K_m$ of $10^{-3}$ mol/L. Although glutathione peroxidase has a greater affinity for $H_2O_2$, it has a smaller capacity than catalase. Glutathione peroxidase may, therefore, be important at times of low $H_2O_2$ production, with catalase assuming greater importance during times of high $H_2O_2$ production. It is imperative that $O_2^-$ and $H_2O_2$ be rapidly eliminated because they can combine to generate a cascade of more reactive species. In the presence of iron, which is ubiquitous in mammalian systems, $O_2^-$ and $H_2O_2$ react to produce hydroxyl radical ($OH^\bullet$), an extraordinarily reactive species capable of oxidizing most cellular constituents:

$$Fe^{3+} + O_2^- \rightarrow Fe^{2+} + O_2$$

$$Fe^{2+} + H_2O_2 \rightarrow Fe^3 + OH^\bullet + OH^-$$

Eukaryotic cells have no specific enzymatic protection against $OH^\bullet$, other than "suicide" reactions in which sulfhydryl groups or unsaturated fatty acids react nonspecifically with $OH^\bullet$. These reactions irreversibly oxidize the SH groups on cellular proteins, or lipids, frequently producing other reactive compounds.

Inherent in the eukaryotic cellular antioxidant system is the interdependence of the components. Augmentation of one antioxidant, without commensurate changes in other components, may not be beneficial. For example, when SOD is increased in cultured mammalian cells, oxidant cytotoxicity increases. Presumably, the increased toxicity results from an inability to cope with the increased $H_2O_2$ generated by SOD.

## NON-ENZYMATIC ANTIOXIDANTS

Several important antioxidants are non-enzymatic. Vitamin E (more precisely α-tocopherol) is a membrane antioxidant that detoxifies oxygen and lipid radicals to protect membrane fatty acids. When there is vitamin E deficiency, membrane polyunsaturated fatty acids (PUFA) are more sensitive to reactive species that are formed in normal metabolism, and to any oxidative stress (hyperoxia, radiation, ozone, oxidant drugs). Peroxidation of membrane PUFA changes the physical and functional characteristics of the membrane.

Although not strictly an antioxidant, glutathione (GSH), a peptide thiol, is an important component of the antioxidant system. GSH, a required cofactor in

detoxification pathways of xenobiotics, is used by glutathione peroxidase in metabolism of $H_2O_2$ and lipid peroxides, and is necessary for regeneration of several antioxidants including ascorbate and α-tocopherol. When cellular GSH is insufficient, eukaryotic cells are more sensitive to reactive species generated during normal metabolism, and to exogenous oxidant stress. Manifestations of GSH deficiency are diverse, but include profound mitochondrial damage, presumably due to oxidant damage by mitochondrially produced ROM.

Vitamin A (retinoic acid) is often classified as an antioxidant. Although vitamin A may have antioxidant properties, it is more important as a regulator of cell growth and differentiation. Repair and regeneration of damaged epithelia requires adequate vitamin A. *Vitamin A deficiency* is associated with dysplastic epithelial changes that are reminiscent of the chronic lung changes that develop after pulmonary oxygen injury. There is strong evidence that inadequate vitamin A worsens the chronic lung sequelae that result from *neonatal pulmonary oxygen injury*.

## DEVELOPMENTAL ASPECTS OF PULMONARY ANTIOXIDANTS

The developmental patterns of antioxidants have an important impact on neonatal pulmonary oxygen injury. The ontogeny of the pulmonary antioxidants mirrors the development of the surfactant system; maturation of the surfactant and antioxidant systems is part of a generalized preparation of the lung for birth. Lung antioxidant enzyme activities are low until immediately prior to term, when they are strongly induced. Activities peak in the immediate postnatal period and then decline to normal adult levels. The genetic and cellular mechanisms involved in regulation of lung antioxidant activities involve complex interactions between hormones, growth factors, and local substances. Less is known about the ontogeny of non-enzymatic lung antioxidants. Several are nutritionally regulated, and vitamin E and A levels in the lung require adequate liver stores. For most nutritional factors, lung levels are low throughout gestation, and normal postnatal increases require adequate enteral intake.

The preterm infant is ill prepared for an increase in oxidant stress because of low enzymatic and non-enzymatic antioxidant capabilities. Many preterm infants require supplemental oxygen because of pulmonary immaturity. The combination of increased oxidant stress and low antioxidants places important biological components at risk of oxidant damage. Although life-saving, hyperoxia causes significant morbidities that are mediated by reactive oxidant metabolites.

Despite normal levels of antioxidants, *pulmonary oxidant injury* occurs as part of other common pediatric diseases. Chronic infection and inflammation in children with *cystic fibrosis* or *asthma* results in lung injury that is partly mediated by oxidants. Iatrogenic oxidant injury develops in the lungs of children receiving chemotherapy or ionizing radiation.

## LUNG PROTEASES AND ANTIPROTEASES

Proteolytic lung injury can be either primary, caused by a deficiency of protective antiproteases, or secondary. Secondary proteolytic lung damage occurs as a result of a pulmonary inflammation. Lung injury or infection elicits an influx of inflammatory cells which release proteolytic compounds and activated oxygen species. This causes further lung injury.

The human lung is normally protected from proteases capable of attacking the extracellular matrix by a group of proteins, the antiproteases. The extracellular antiproteases in lung include $\alpha_1$-antitrypsin ($\alpha_1$AT), secretory leukoprotease inhibitor (SLPI), $\alpha_1$-antichymotrypsin ($\alpha_1$ACT), tissue inhibitor of metalloproteases (TIMP) and $\alpha_2$-macroglobulin ($\alpha_2$M). Antiproteases functionally inactivate proteases by specific binding, usually at the active proteolytic site. The binding is either irreversible or slowly reversible. Thus, the antiproteases act as a "substrate" with a greater affinity for the protease than other substrates. The kinetics of protease inhibition involve both the time of inhibition (association rate constant) and the concentration of antiprotease required for inhibition (equilibrium constant), again emphasizing the concept of balance between protease and antiprotease. None of the lung antiproteases is protease-specific; however, most are class-specific. For example, $\alpha_1$AT and SLPI inhibit all serine proteases, while TIMP inhibits metalloproteases.

$\alpha_1$AT, the most abundant pulmonary extracellular antiprotease, provides most of the protection against neutrophil elastase in the lower respiratory tract. The major site of $\alpha_1$AT production is the liver, although other cells make small amounts. Pulmonary levels of $\alpha_1$AT ultimately are controlled by hepatocyte synthesis and secretion. The critical importance of $\alpha_1$AT is demonstrated by the genetic condition $\alpha_1$-antitrypsin deficiency. In these patients, plasma $\alpha_1$AT levels are less than 35 per cent of normal, and the patients develop severe emphysema in young adulthood. Relative $\alpha_1$AT deficiency probably is involved in other conditions. Premature infants who later developed *bronchopulmonary dysplasia* were reported to have inactive $\alpha_1$AT in their airways. Chronic inhalation of tobacco smoke appears to inactivate pulmonary antiproteases, perhaps explaining the higher incidence of *emphysema* in cigarette smokers.

SLPI, a serine antiprotease, is produced in the lung by mucosal cells in large and small airways. In distal respiratory tract, SLPI is made in non-ciliated (Clara) epithelial cells. The major role of SLPI appears to be to protect the upper respiratory tract from neutrophil elastase. TIMP, a specific inhibitor of metalloproteases, such as collagenase, gelatinase, and the stromolysins, is produced within the lung by fibroblasts and alveolar macrophages. Although the exact role of TIMP in the

lung is unclear, it is induced by pulmonary oxygen injury, perhaps as an adaptive protective response.

## PROTEASES AND LUNG INJURY

The balance between proteases and antiproteases appears to be heavily weighted towards excess antiprotease protection in the healthy lung. Disturbance of this balance, with unlimited proteolysis, results in damage to and loss of the extracellular matrix. Without the support of their underlying connective tissue, alveoli are lost, resulting clinically in emphysema. Extensive work with animal models has demonstrated that administration of exogenous proteases, or stimulation of endogenous proteases, causes lung injury. Imbalance between proteases and antiproteases can occur as a primary pathophysiology in human lung; the best evidence for this mechanism is $\alpha_1AT$ *deficiency, cigarette smoke toxicity,* and *idiopathic pulmonary fibrosis.* More commonly, increased proteolytic injury occurs subsequent to lung inflammation with release of proteolytic enzymes from neutrophils and alveolar macrophages. The influx of inflammatory cells can occur in response to a variety of stimuli, including infection, acute lung injury, or complement activation. The acutely injured lung produces many substances that are chemotactic for neutrophils. These activated inflammatory cells release proteases and reactive oxygen species that cause further lung injury. Reactive oxygen species may also oxidize the active site of $\alpha_1$AT, rendering it inactive, further tipping the balance towards proteolysis and lung injury. Because pulmonary inflammation is an almost universal response to lung injury, the major role of proteolysis in human lung disease may be to amplify and prolong acute lung injuries incited by diverse causes. In the future, it may be possible to augment the antiprotease defenses of the lower airway in order to prevent proteolytic injury.

## SELECTED READING

Crystal RG, West JB, eds. *The lung, scientific foundations*, Vol 2. New York: Raven Press, 1991: 1763, 1803.

Fridovich I. Antioxidant defenses in the lung. *Annu Rev Physiol* 1986; **48**: 693.

Halliwell B, Gutteridge JMC. Oxygen toxicity, oxygen radicals, transition metals and disease. *Biochem J* 1984; **219**: 1.

Hubbard RC, Ogushi F, Fells GA *et al.* Oxidants spontaneously released by alveolar macrophages of cigarette smokers can inactivate the active site of $\alpha_1$-antitrypsin, rendering it ineffective as an inhibitor of neutrophil elastase. *J Clin Invest* 1987; **80**: 1289.

Merritt AT, Cochrane CG, Holcomb K *et al.* Elastase and $\alpha_1$-proteinase inhibitor activity in tracheal aspirates during respiratory distress syndrome. *J Clin Invest* 1983; **72**: 656.

Proteases and antiproteases. Proceedings of the 9th Transatlantic Airway Conference. Lucerne, Switzerland, January 1994. *Am J Respir Crit Care Med* 1994; **150**: S107.

Wispé JR, Roberts RJ. Molecular basis of pulmonary oxygen toxicity. *Clin Perinatol* 1987; **14**: 651.

# 78

# Control of Breathing

## PHYSIOLOGICAL CONTROL OF RESPIRATION

The respiratory system has both metabolic and behavioral functions. To survive for more than a few minutes, the organism must absorb $O_2$ and excrete $CO_2$ through the lungs. The metabolic function must always be fulfilled and, at times, exclusively determines the magnitude of ventilation and the timing of respiratory muscle contraction. However, during certain activities, such as exercise and phonation, behavioral control of breathing takes precedence. For instance, during swimming, the pattern of breathing must be closely matched to the locomotor rhythm while metabolic needs for $O_2$ and $CO_2$ are met. The metabolic and behavioral functions have separate but related control systems in the central nervous system.

The metabolic and behavioral control systems converge on brainstem and spinal lower motor neurons that innervate the respiratory muscles (Fig. 78.1). Spontaneous respiration occurs as a result of the rhythmic and coordinated discharge of inspiratory and expiratory neurons innervating respiratory muscles. During inspiration, the diaphragm and external intercostal muscles contract expanding the thoracic cavity and drawing fresh air into the lungs. These muscles are innervated by the phrenic (cervical segments 3–5) and thoracic lower motor neurons. Other inspiratory muscles, which maintain patency of the pharynx and larynx, are innervated by cranial nerves, especially the glossopharyngeal (IX), vagus (X), and hypoglossal

(XII) nerves. Expiratory muscles, the internal intercostals and abdominals, are less active during resting, unloaded breathing. Expiration is largely driven by the elastic recoil forces accumulated during inspiration.

The behavioral, or voluntary, control system results from cerebral cortical activity stimulating respiratory lower motor neurons via the corticospinal and corticobulbar tracts. The metabolic, or automatic, control system centers on activity of upper motor neurons in the medulla. The medullary respiratory centers comprise a spontaneously active neural oscillator, or central pattern generator, that maintains a characteristic discharge pattern even if it is disconnected from the pons above and the spinal cord below. The central pattern generator is arranged as a self-sustaining, oscillating neural network distributed fairly widely in the brainstem. Activity of the medullary neurons is modulated by numerous excitatory and inhibitory inputs, e.g. chemoreceptors, mechanoreceptors, forebrain, pontine, and hypothalamic inputs. The numerous neurotransmitters and neuromodulators involved include acetylcholine, dopamine, $\gamma$-aminobutyric acid (GABA), substance P, and opioid peptides. An understanding of the respiratory control system will help the clinician understand disorders of breathing (Table 78.1).

## ORGANIZATION OF CENTRAL RESPIRATORY NEURONS

Many medullary respiratory neurons project downwards to phrenic or intercostal neurons. During quiet breathing, expiration is passive and most expiratory

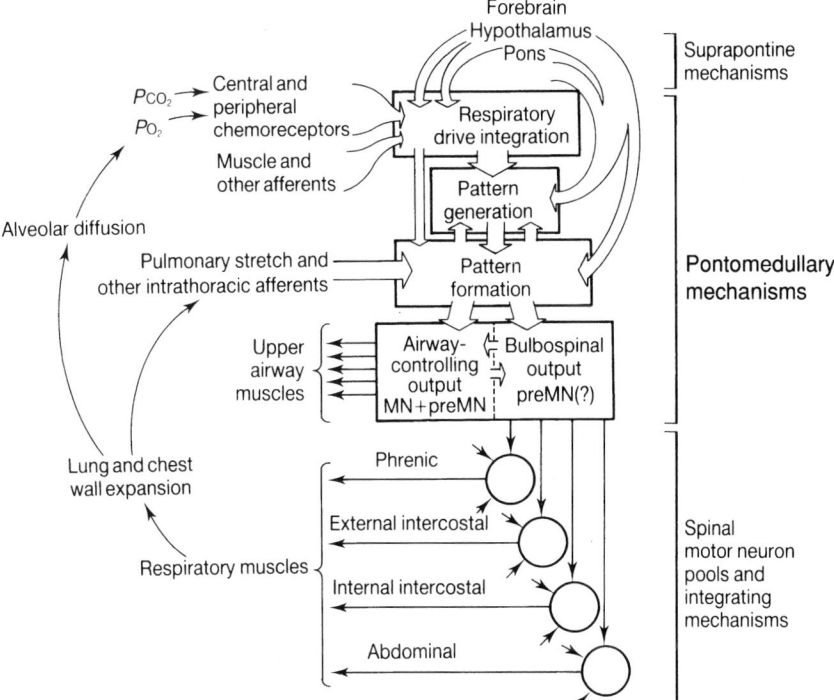

FIGURE 78.1 Organization of the metabolic, or automatic, control of breathing. Emphasis is placed on the mechanisms for respiratory drive integration, respiratory pattern generation and formation and their influences on the two main output systems which control the upper airway and respiratory muscles. The behavioral control system with direct connections between cerebral cortex and lower motor neurons is not shown. (From Euler CV. Breathing behaviour. In: Euler CV, Lagercrantz H, eds. *Neurobiology of the control of breathing*. New York: Raven Press, 1987: 4. Reproduced with permission of Raven Press.)

TABLE 78.1 Structures involved in respiratory control, examples of disorders, and breathing patterns

| STRUCTURE | DISORDER (EXAMPLE) | BREATHING PATTERN |
|---|---|---|
| Forebrain | Convulsion | Apnea; irregular breathing |
| Medulla | Arnold–Chiari malformation | Low respiratory rates; hypoventilation |
| Cervical spinal cord | High cord transection | Respiratory muscle paralysis |
| Phrenic nerve | Brachial plexus birth injury | Diaphragmatic paralysis |
| Diaphragm | Eventration | Increased work by accessory muscles |
| Lung | Bronchopulmonary dysplasia | Tachypnea; increased work of breathing |
| Upper airway | Adenotonsillar hypertrophy | Obstructive sleep apnea |

neurons are active only when ventilation is increased. Medullary respiratory neurons are grouped into two main areas. First, the predominantly inspiratory, dorsal respiratory group (DRG) located in the dorsal medulla in the nucleus tractus solitarius (NTS) near the fourth ventricle and the hypoglossal (XII) nucleus. Most DRG neurons have bulbospinal connections to phrenic or inspiratory intercostal neurons. Second, the ventral respiratory group (VRG) contains both inspiratory and expiratory neurons. Located ventral and lat-

eral to the DRG, the VRG extends from the caudal border of the pons in the retroambiguous, paraambiguous and retrofacial nuclei to the caudal medulla.

The pontine respiratory group (PRG) (also called the pneumotaxic center) consists of neurons in the Kölliker–Fuse and parabrachial nuclei of the rostral pons. These cells are thought to be important in terminating inspiration because PRG lesions, especially when combined with vagotomy, result in prolonged inspiration (apneusis). A similar pattern is seen when the brainstem is transected between the pons and medulla.

The mechanism(s) causing the periodic alternation of inspiration and expiration remain uncertain but must involve the membrane properties of individual respiratory neurons and the connections between them. Intracellular recordings have suggested that there are at least three patterns of brainstem neuronal discharge: inspiratory, postinspiratory (early expiratory), and expiratory. Investigators now have identified in the pre-Bötzinger complex, just rostral to the VRG, neurons with intrinsic oscillatory properties. Others have tried to identify a neural network characterized by reciprocal inhibition of inspiratory and expiratory activity. It seems likely that different mechanisms initiate inspiration, terminate inspiration, and control the rate of inspiratory discharge. Progress in defining the membrane, synaptic, neurotransmitter, and neuromodulator characteristics of respiratory neurons will undoubtedly result in a deeper understanding of the control of breathing.

## EFFECTS OF SLEEP/WAKE STATE ON RESPIRATORY CONTROL

Sleep/wake state profoundly influences the pattern of breathing. Sleep, particularly rapid eye movement (REM) sleep, depresses ventilatory and arousal responses and many respiratory reflexes. During quiet wakefulness the rate and depth of breathing are primarily set by the metabolic control system. During exercise, phonation and other states of active wakefulness, the behavioral control system assumes primary control; corticospinal and corticobulbar impulses drive respiratory lower motor neurons. Of course, metabolic needs to absorb $O_2$ and to excrete $CO_2$ must still be met. Specific wakeful behaviors can markedly affect breathing. In infants during sucking, breathing may be interrupted to the point that hemoglobin desaturation and bradycardia occur.

As state changes from quiet wakefulness to quiet sleep, respiration becomes remarkably regular in rate and depth, the level of ventilation then being determined solely by metabolic rate and the chemical ($Po_2$, $Pco_2$, pH) drive to breathe. A slight increase in arterial blood $CO_2$ and decrease in ventilation, compared to quiet wakefulness, occur. The higher level of ventilation in wakefulness compared to quiet sleep is thought to be due to the wakefulness drive to breathe, tonic excitatory inputs from the reticular activating (arousal) system to the metabolic respiratory control system. Two examples will highlight the importance of the wakefulness drive to breathing. In a normal infant or child, hyperventilation, which withdraws the chemostimulatory drive to breathe, results in apnea during quiet sleep but not during wakefulness. In children with *congenital central hypoventilation syndrome*, because of a defect in the metabolic control system,

each time they enter quiet sleep they hypoventilate and become severely hypoxemic. Breathing may be normal during wakefulness.

REM sleep is characterized by marked variability in the rate and depth of breathing and by loss of muscle activity in intercostal and airway-maintaining musculature. Periods of hyperpnea can alternate with apnea. As in states of active wakefulness, breathing is primarily controlled by the behavioral system. Most brain activity is increased during REM sleep, but brainstem and spinal lower motor neurons are inhibited and brain activity is, by and large, not translated into motoric activity. Diaphragmatic activity, however, is not inhibited. In infants, REM sleep inhibition of intercostal muscle activity causes inspiratory chest wall collapse, and puts an increased load on the diaphragm because of the very compliant chest wall. In children predisposed to airway obstruction, REM sleep inhibition of upper airway-maintaining musculature increases upper airway resistance and may lead to *obstructive sleep apnea* and hypoxemia (Fig. 78.2).

## CHEMICAL REGULATION OF BREATHING

Respiratory depth and rate are regulated by chemical feedback mechanisms that monitor arterial blood $Po_2$ ($P_aO_2$) and $Pco_2$ ($P_aCO_2$), adjusting ventilation so that blood gases and pH are kept within normal limits. A rise in $P_aCO_2$ and/or a fall in $P_aO_2$ increases afferent input to the central pattern generator that then increases inspiratory muscle activity and ventilation to facilitate excretion of $CO_2$ and absorption of $O_2$. Conversely, blood gas changes in the opposite direction depress breathing. These effects on respiration are mediated by chemoreceptors responsive to changes in arterial blood $Po_2$ and $Pco_2$ and/or hydrogen ion concentration. Under normoxic conditions the central chemoreceptors are predominant and $P_aCO_2$ is more precisely regulated than $P_aO_2$.

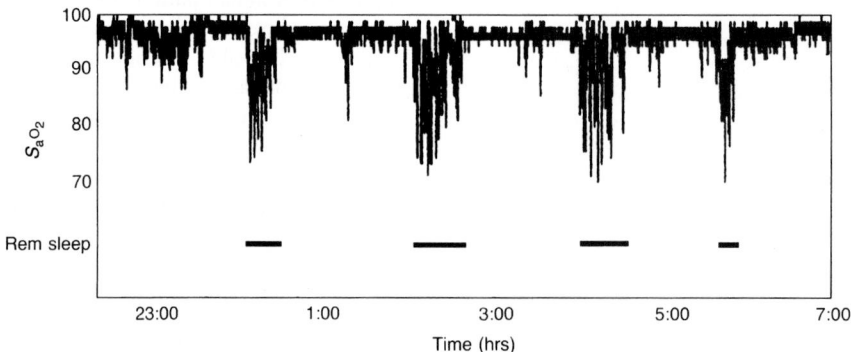

FIGURE 78.2 The important influence of sleep state on breathing. Recurrent obstructive apnea and drops in hemoglobin oxygen saturation ($S_aO_2$) occur during each of four epochs of REM sleep in this 20-month-old child with enlarged tonsils and adenoids. During periods of quiet sleep there is much less obstructive apnea and hypoxemia. REM sleep mechanisms decrease pharyngeal, airway-maintaining, muscular activity. This pharyngeal hypotonia allows the pharynx to collapse when the diaphragm generates negative pressure during inspiration. Brief arousals, required to reestablish airway patency, do not usually result in a change of sleep state.

## Inputs from central chemoreceptors: $CO_2$ drive (*see also* page 840)

An increase in $P_aCO_2$ causes a proportional (linear) increase in ventilation. The sensors for $CO_2$ level are primarily the central chemoreceptors located on the ventral surface of the medulla. However, the peripheral chemoreceptors are also $CO_2$ responsive and account for some ventilatory stimulation. Cooling or anesthesia of the ventral medullary surface causes apnea while perfusion with an acidotic mock cerebrospinal fluid stimulates breathing. The central chemoreceptors affect output of the VRG and the DRG, possibly through connections to pontine respiratory neurons. The biochemical mechanism by which increased $CO_2$ stimulates the central chemoreceptors involves the transfer of $CO_2$ across the blood–brain barrier, hydration to carbonic acid, and release of hydrogen ion into the brainstem interstitial space and/or cerebrospinal fluid. The time course of ventilatory changes to changes in $P_aCO_2$ is measured in minutes. The linear $CO_2$ ventilatory response, the relatively slow response time of the central chemoreceptors, and the large body stores of $CO_2$ tend to stabilize the rate and depth of breathing.

## Inputs from peripheral chemoreceptors: hypoxemic drive

A fall in $P_aO_2$ results in an exponential ventilatory response mediated by the peripheral chemoreceptors located in the carotid and aortic bodies. The carotid bodies are innervated by a branch of the IX nerve and are situated at the junction of the internal and common carotid arteries. The aortic chemoreceptors, situated in the aortic arch, are innervated by the vagus nerve. The peripheral chemoreceptors project afferents to the nucleus tractus solitarius in the medulla. Afferent discharge increases when $P_aO_2$ falls and is silenced by inhalation of oxygen. The exact mechanism by which carotid and aortic chemoreceptors sense changes in $P_aO_2$ is still a subject of debate. Removal or denervation of the carotid bodies has little effect on resting ventilation but results in loss of the ventilatory responses to hypoxia and a diminished response to hypercapnia. The peripheral chemoreceptors respond within a few seconds to changing $O_2$ status. The exponential shape and the rapid time course of the peripheral chemoreceptor response and the small body stores of $O_2$ promote periodic breathing but allow the organism to respond quickly to an asphyxiating environment. Hypoxia, when severe, also has a direct depressant effect on ventilation that is most marked in the neonate. Whether this decrease in ventilation is due to down-regulation of metabolism and/or a depression of central respiratory control is the subject of active research.

## PULMONARY MECHANORECEPTORS

Inflation of the lungs inhibits inspiratory discharge by a reflex mechanism known as the Hering–Breuer inflation inhibition reflex. The reflex is more pronounced in infants and in anesthetized animals than in adult humans. Lung stretch receptors, whose afferents run in the vagus nerve to the nucleus tractus solitarius, are stimulated by lung inflation and terminate inspiration. Larger volume changes are required to halt inspiration early in inspiration than later on in inspiration.

In contrast to the slowly adapting pulmonary stretch receptors, other vagally innervated pulmonary receptors, the irritant receptors, are rapidly adapting. They can be stimulated both chemically (e.g. by cigarette smoke, noxious gases, histamine, bradykinin, antigens) and mechanically (e.g. by particulate matter or increases in airflow). These receptors are spread throughout the epithelial cells of the trachea and bronchi but most are in the larger airways. Stimulation of these receptors augments inspiratory activity, but can also constrict the airway and cause coughing or rapid, shallow breathing. Irritant receptor stimulation may also initiate the augmented breaths or sighs that occur periodically during normal breathing and that maintain lung expansion. Irritant receptor stimulation by histamine and other substances released in response to allergens may increase ventilation during asthma attacks by augmenting inspiration. Rapid, forceful inspiration, as may occur with mechanical ventilation, particularly in infants, may also augment inspiration and promote lung inflation.

## PROPRIOCEPTOR AFFERENTS

Afferents from chest wall proprioceptors convey information about chest wall movement and the forces exerted by respiratory muscles. Such information can help coordinate breathing during speech or postural changes and may also assist ribcage stabilization when breathing is impeded by increased airway resistance or decreased lung compliance. Joint and tendon afferents also stimulate the respiratory centers and may increase ventilation during exercise.

## LARYNGEAL CHEMOREFLEX

The larynx contains chemoreceptors that are sensitive to various stimuli, especially milk, water, and other hyposmolar solutions. Afferent information is carried in the superior laryngeal nerve. Behavioral responses include cough, expiratory efforts, and swallowing. However, in neonates the response is characterized by apnea followed by swallowing before resumption of breathing. This response pattern is most marked in the premature infant. *Gastroesophageal reflux* may stimulate laryngeal receptors inducing *apnea* or *apparent life-threatening events*. Some evidence suggests that *pertussis* and/or *respiratory syncytial virus* infection induces apnea in young children by stimulating laryngeal receptors. In older infants these infections/inflammation stimulate cough.

## SELECTED READING

Beckerman RC, Brouillette RT, Hunt CE, eds. *Respiratory control disorders in infants and children.* Baltimore: Williams & Wilkins, 1992.

Bryan AC, Bowes G, Maloney JE. Control of breathing in the fetus and newborn. In: Cherniack NS, Widdicombe JG, eds. *Handbook of physiology. Section 2: The respiratory system.* Bethesda, MD: American Physiological Society, 1986: 621.

Feldman JL. Neurophysiology of breathing in mammals. In: Mountcastle VB, ed. *Handbook of physiology. Section 1: The nervous system.* Bethesda, MD: American Physiological Society, 1986: 463.

Johnson SM, Smith JC, Funk GD, Feldman JL. Pacemaker behavior of respiratory neurons in medullary slices from neonatal rat. *J Neurophysiol* 1994; 72: 2598.

Mortola JP, Matsuoka T. Interaction between $CO_2$ production and ventilation in the hypoxic kitten. *J Appl Physiol* 1993; 74: 905.

Phillipson EA, Bowes G. Control of breathing during sleep. In: Cherniack NS, Widdicombe JG, eds. *Handbook of physiology. Section 2: The respiratory system.* Bethesda, MD: American Physiological Society, 1986: 649.

# NEONATAL, PERINATAL, AND DEVELOPMENTAL ASPECTS OF RESPIRATORY CONTROL

## INTRODUCTION

To the lay person, breathing is probably the best-known vital sign, and its presence and pattern in neonatal life are anxiously observed, e.g. by parents or siblings. There is good reason for this concern, as disturbances of respiratory control are major causes of morbidity and mortality in the newborn. The processes by which breathing is controlled in perinatal life are poorly understood. It is a common misconception that breathing starts at birth, despite the first observations of fetal breathing movements (FBM) more than 100 years ago. Although lay persons usually can enumerate factors that affect breathing in the adult (exercise, emotional states, lack of oxygen, sleep, etc.), these processes do not affect FBM in the same way. Despite these differences, the control of fetal and postnatal breathing has some similarities, and the neural circuitry employed is similar. The responses that appear qualitatively different are, in fact, largely due to quantitative differences, e.g. altering the balance of excitatory and inhibitory mechanisms. This section discusses

this concept in relation to the development of respiratory control.

## FETAL BREATHING MOVEMENTS

### Ontogeny and incidence

FBM are present from early gestation, e.g. from 10 weeks in humans. Initially, they occur more or less continuously, although their amplitude is irregular (Fig. 78.3). As gestation proceeds, FBM become clustered into episodes and are related to behavioral state. Although the classification of states may not be the same in humans and sheep, in late-gestation sheep FBM occur about 40 per cent of the time in association with the low-voltage (LV) electrocortical (ECoG) state (Table 78.2). There is also a circadian rhythm in the incidence of FBM, determined largely by maternal influences (the rise in blood glucose after meals increases the incidence of FBM in humans and sheep). Maternal corticosteroids play a major role in determining FBM incidence, and there is usually a peak in FBM during the evening (Fig. 78.4). FBM cease 24–36 hours before birth. Again this is likely to be due to the associated endocrine changes; in sheep, the fall in

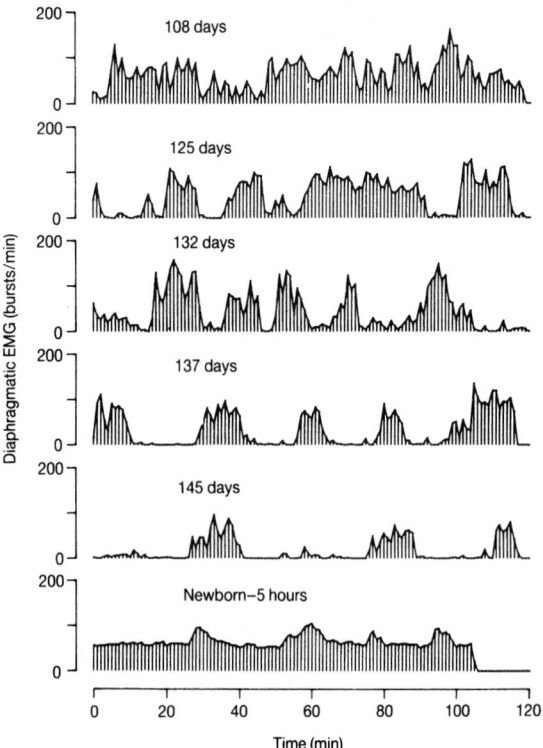

FIGURE 78.3 Analysis of diaphragmatic EMG of a fetus at five gestational ages (108–145 days) and as a 5-hour-old newborn. Each graph displays time in minutes on abscissa and diaphragmatic electromyogram (EMG) activity in bursts/min on ordinate. (Reproduced with permission from Bowes G *et al. J Appl Physiol* 1981; 50: 693.)

TABLE 78.2 Association of fetal breathing movements with behavioral variables

|  | ECoG LV | ECoG HV |
|---|---|---|
| Fetal breathing movements | + | − |
| Rapid eye movements | + | − |
| Postural muscle tone | − | + |

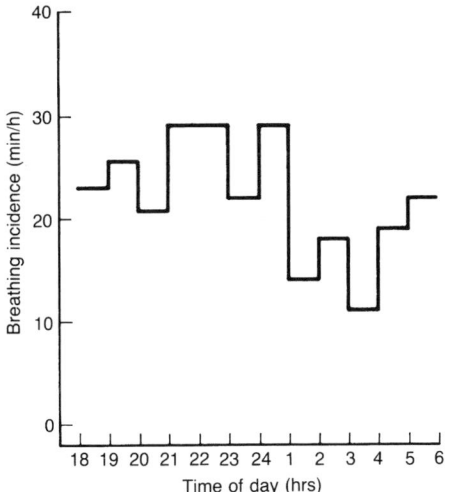

FIGURE 78.4 Changes in the incidence of fetal breathing movements measured overnight in fetal sheep in late gestation. Highest circadian incidence occurs in late evening. (From Koos BJ *et al. J Dev Physiol* 1988; **10**: 161.)

plasma concentrations of progesterone and the rise in $PGE_2$ are involved.

## Importance for lung development

The secretion of liquid by the fetal lungs (*see* page 239) produces a net efflux of liquid, which is greater during FBM due to the reduction of laryngeal resistance accompanying the breathing. FBM are necessary for normal lung development. Prevention of FBM by section of the spinal cord above the level of the phrenic outflow produces pulmonary hypoplasia. Congenital defects such as diaphragmatic hernia, which permit FBM but prevent them from producing mechanical distortions of the developing lungs, similarly produce pulmonary hypoplasia. However, in view of the episodic nature of FBM and their return during the adaptation to prolonged fetal hypoxemia (see below), it is not safe to predict that a lack of observed FBM in the human fetus on ultrasound will be associated with pulmonary hypoplasia.

## Peripheral control

FBM are less under reflex control than are postnatal breathing movements. Hypocapnia stimulates FBM, but the effect is overridden by the high-voltage electrocortical state (HV ECoG) when FBM cease (Table 78.2). The stimulation is due to increased activity of both peripheral and central chemoreceptors via the rise in arterial and brain tissue $P_{CO_2}$, respectively. Hypoxia also stimulates the fetal arterial chemoreceptors (Fig. 78.5), but this does not produce an increase in FBM: in fact, FBM cease initially in hypoxia and, in sheep, the ECoG switches to HV. Peripheral chemoreceptor and mechanoreceptor inputs are not important in determining the incidence of FBM, as this incidence is not altered (or only transiently affected) by bilateral division of the carotid sinus nerves and/or vagi, after several days are allowed for postoperative recovery.

Cooling the fetus, either with a coil in the amniotic cavity or via an extracorporeal circuit, stimulates FBM. The effect can persist even in HV ECoG, but the duration is not known. Clearly the powerful effect of cooling in the establishment of continuous breathing after birth can be elicited at least partially *in utero*.

## Central control

FBM are produced by contractions of the diaphragm initiated by synchronous discharge of phrenic motor neurons. In this respect, they are similar to unstimulated postnatal breathing. Apart from occurring in episodes, FBM also differ from postnatal breathing in being more irregular in amplitude and faster (up to 4 Hz). It is not known whether these differences are predominantly due to differences in central control, or whether they arise from the mechanical condition of the fluid-filled lung. However, centrally acting drugs

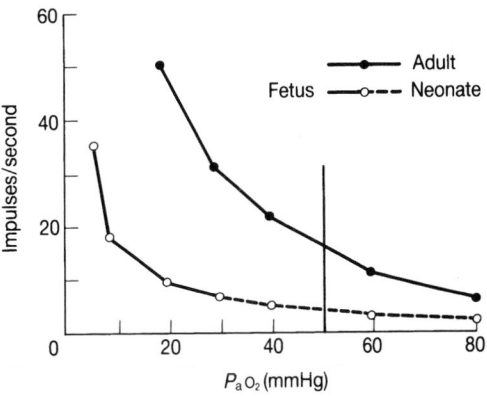

FIGURE 78.5 Arterial chemoreceptor response curves to changing arterial blood $P_{O_2}$ ($P_aO_2$) in sheep. The fetal curve (open symbols, continuous line) lies to the left of the adult curve (solid symbols, continuous line). In the neonate (open symbols, interrupted line) the $P_aO_2$ has risen well above the fetal range and discharge is quiescent. Resetting then shifts the response curve up and to the right to its adult position. At any $P_aO_2$ (e.g. 50 mmHg [6.66 kPa] shown by vertical line) both mean discharge and slope of the response line to changes in $P_aO_2$ are greater.

can alter the characteristics of FBM (Table 78.3). The inhibition of FBM in hypoxia involves descending processes in the brainstem. Transection through the upper pons (Fig. 78.6), but not higher at the level of the caudal hypothalamus, abolishes the effect: after such pontine transection, breathing becomes continuous and is stimulated by hypoxia. More detailed studies have involved placing lesions bilaterally in the rostral pons. Once again, FBM are stimulated in hypoxia, but this stimulation is removed by subsequent denervation of the peripheral chemoreceptors. Thus there are two opposing processes in the intact fetus: stimulation from the peripheral chemoreceptors, and inhibition mediated by the upper pons or lower mesencephalon (Fig. 78.6). The neurophysiology of this brainstem mechanism is currently under investigation.

FBM do not cease when hypoxia is induced in the ewe and the maternal side of the placenta while the fetus is maintained normoxic by an extracorporeal oxygenation circuit; thus the mechanisms detecting the fall in $P_{O_2}$ appear to be fetal. FBM are triggered by low $P_{O_2}$ in the fetal brain as they also occur in anemia and with carboxyhemoglobinemia. This rules out the possibility that FBM are due to low arterial blood $P_{O_2}$ ($P_{a}O_2$), e.g. detected by the peripheral chemoreceptors. The drug almitrine, which mimics hypoxia at the peripheral chemoreceptors, also causes FBM to cease; adenosine, which is released in the fetal brain in hypoxia, reduces FBM. Both agents mediate

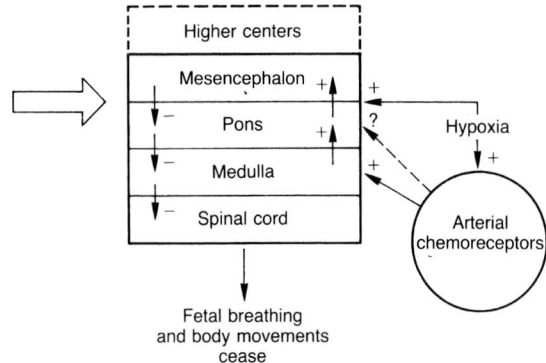

FIGURE 78.6 Diagram of brain stem processes involved in effects of hypoxia on fetal breathing and body movements. The excitatory input (+) from the arterial chemoreceptors to the medulla may be relayed rostrally and it is likely that hypoxia also excites neurons in the mesencephalon/pons. Descending inhibitory influences (−) are mediated at this level, as revealed by the removal of the inhibitory effects of hypoxia on fetal breathing movements by transection or lesioning at the level shown by the large arrow (but not by more rostral damage). Thus, after such lesions hypoxia can stimulate fetal breathing, an effect abolished by destruction of the arterial input.

their actions via the upper pons – transection or lesions at this level abolish their effects, but denervation of the peripheral chemoreceptors does not. The only pharmacological antagonist drugs that reduce inhibition of FBM in hypoxia are theophylline and the α-adrenergic blocker phentolamine. Many other drugs, with agonist actions, affect the incidence of FBM (Table 78.3), but their effects are overridden by hypoxia, and the significance of their actions is not clear.

## Transition at birth

A remarkable aspect of perinatal respiratory control is of course the transition at birth when, after a period of quiescence just before delivery, breathing becomes continuous and persists postnatally regardless of changes in sleep/wake state. The processes involved in the initiation of continuous breathing are distinct from those that contribute to its maintenance. The former must act rapidly to produce breathing that is independent of sleep state (unlike the fetus, where HV ECoG inhibits breathing), and the initial effect must be independent of oxygenation. In fact, the inhibitory effects of hypoxia persist during birth, as a fall in $P_{a}O_2$ delays the onset of postnatal breathing. Cooling is an important stimulus to continuous postnatal breathing; fetal lambs delivered by cesarean section into a warm saline bath with the umbilical circulation intact continue to show periodic episodes of breathing associated with LV ECoG. The level of $P_{a}CO_2$ is also an important determinant of the onset of postnatal breathing (Fig. 78.7); this may provide a link whereby the increased

TABLE 78.3 Pharmacological and other stimuli affecting fetal breathing movements

| STIMULUS | EFFECT |
|---|---|
| High-voltage ECoG | ↓ |
| Fetal hypoxia (fetal distress) | ↓ |
| Labor | ↓ |
| Prostaglandins (PGE₁, PGE₂) | ↓ |
| Starvation (hypoglycemia) | ↓ |
| Barbiturates | ↓ |
| Ethanol | ↓ |
| Diazepam | ↓ |
| Meperidine/pethidine (Demerol) | ↓ |
| Adenosine | ↓ |
| Norepinephrine | ↓ |
| Adrenocorticotropic hormone | ↓ |
| Clonidine | ↓ |
| Almitrine | ↓ |
| | |
| Low-voltage ECoG | ↑ |
| Hypercapnia (only during low voltage) | ↑ |
| Glucose | ↑ |
| Prostaglandin synthetase inhibitors (e.g. indomethacin) | ↑ |
| Isoproterenol | ↑ |
| Epinephrine | ↑ |
| Morphine | ↑ |
| Theophylline/caffeine | ↑ |
| Thyrotropin releasing hormone | ↑ |
| Corticotropin releasing hormone | ↑ |
| Corticotropin releasing factor | ↑ |
| α-Adrenergic blockade | ↑ |

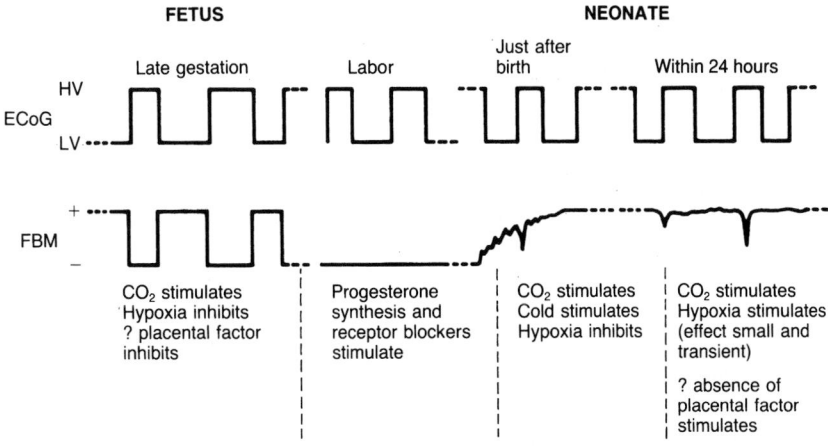

FIGURE 78.7 Relation of fetal breathing movements (FBM) to sleep state (ECoG) and the effects of stimuli and inhibitors in the perinatal period

metabolic rate at this time stimulates breathing. Metabolism increases about four-fold after birth; this is accomplished by switching on brown adipose tissue thermogenesis, by shivering, and by a generalized increase in the metabolic rate of many organs (see Chapter 48). Endocrine changes are important in these effects, mainly the rise in catecholamines that occurs especially with vaginal delivery, and thyroid hormones. It has also been proposed that occlusion of the umbilical cord removes from the fetus a thermogenic inhibitory factor of placental origin, possibly adenosine or $PGE_2$. The changes at birth involve the onset of the first clear signs of arousal, with LV ECoG being associated with postural muscle tone, breathing, variable heart rate, and apparent wakefulness with a lowered threshold of response to stimuli. This arousal involves the brainstem reticular formation and also locus coeruleus. In part the mechanisms involve the γ-aminobutyric acid (GABA)-mediated inhibitory processes.

The processes that initiate breathing at birth are complemented, over a longer time frame, with those that maintain continuous respiration. The metabolic drive to breathe remains important; evidence supports the notion that declining fetal plasma concentrations of endocrine factors of placental origin which inhibit breathing may play a role. The nature of these factors is uncertain, but adenosine and $PGE_2$ are candidates. They both inhibit fetal and postnatal breathing, and are cleared from the plasma over several hours postnatally.

## NEONATAL BREATHING

The changing balance of processes involved in respiratory control provides a good example of neonatal adaptation to a new environment. As indicated earlier, this shift has the effect of making some neonatal responses appear qualitatively different from fetal responses, although there is no evidence that different components are involved. Moreover, the balance changes further during neonatal life, as respiratory control mechanisms mature to become similar to those of the adult (Fig 78.8).

## Metabolism

Oxidative metabolism increases several-fold after birth caused by the increasing activity of a range of systems, e.g. cardiac and skeletal muscle, gut, kidneys, etc., to meet the increased demands placed on them, and by shivering and non-shivering thermogenesis needed to maintain body temperature. This produces a greater "feed-forward" drive to breathe in terms of $O_2$ demand and $CO_2$ excretion. Combined with air breathing it produces oscillations in blood $P_{O_2}$, $P_{CO_2}$,

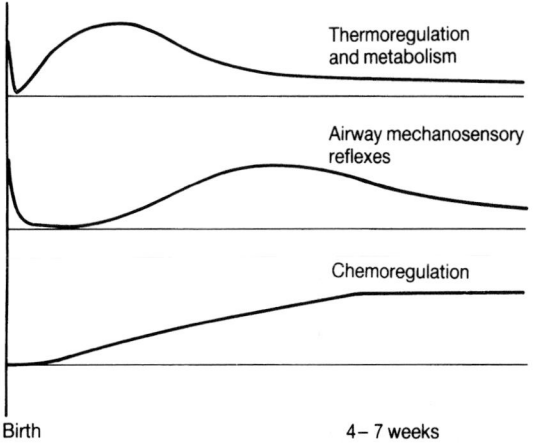

FIGURE 78.8 Diagrammatic representation of the phases of postnatal respiratory control. (Modified from Johnson P. In: *Respiratory control and lung development in the fetus and newborn*. Ithaca, NY: Perinatology Press, 1986: 384.)

and pH that provide an important stimulus to breathe. Reduction of metabolic $CO_2$ delivery to the lungs, using an extracorporeal gas exchanger, reduces ventilation despite a constant mean $P_aCO_2$.

# Thermal drive

This is an important drive to continuous breathing at birth. As far as is known, cutaneous and hypothalamic thermoreceptors are functional in late fetal life (see Chapter 48). The neonatal reduction in thermoneutral range and the widening difference between upper and lower critical temperatures affect respiratory control. Moreover, the ability to thermoregulate, by changes in metabolism and control of cutaneous blood flow, develops postnatally, even though the metabolic role of brown adipose tissue declines. Human infants also show development of a diurnal rhythm in body temperature within about 2 months. In animals, and possibly in human neonates, increasing environmental temperature reduces the gain of respiratory responses. Combined with the reduced metabolic drive to breathe at warmer temperatures, this can predispose to apnea. The mechanisms are not known.

# Mechanoreceptors

The pulmonary mechanics of the neonate differ from the adult because the chest wall in newborn, especially preterm, neonates is very compliant. If ventilatory drive increases, this can result in inward movements of the ribs as the diaphragm descends during inspiration. This is countered to some extent by the use of external intercostal muscles, even during relatively quiet breathing, to "splint" the chest wall, and by abdominal muscles (usually expiratory muscles) during inspiration, to make the abdominal wall less compliant. Even so, "paradoxical" breathing is often observed to a greater or lesser degree in many newborn babies; the chest wall and abdominal wall appear to move in opposite directions both during inspiration and expiration. Measurement of respiratory volumes, e.g. by inductance plethysmography, necessitates placement of measuring bands around both the mid-thorax and the abdomen; tidal volume is derived from the sum of the excursions of each.

The compliant thorax of the neonate also tends to make the functional residual capacity (FRC) low. This is countered by contraction of the adductor muscles of the larynx during "braking" of expiratory airflow and, in extreme cases, by giving an expiratory "grunt."

Patency of the upper airway during inspiration is also vital for maintaining adequate pulmonary ventilation. This is achieved by the abductors of the larynx and the hypoglossal muscles, which protrude the tongue. The force of contraction of these muscles is under reflex control; e.g. subatmospheric pressure

and collapse of the upper airway potentiates hypoglossal activity to reduce the obstruction. Enhanced respiratory drive, e.g. associated with increased $P_{CO_2}$, can augment this effect; however, it can be inhibited during hypoxia (see below).

The pharyngeal and laryngeal sensory receptors are extremely sensitive to mechanical or osmotic stimulation. For example, instillation of water (but not physiological saline) into the larynx produces an immediate apnea, even in a tracheotomized animal under general anesthesia. This is therefore a powerful reflex. Similarly, application of water to the face can evoke apnea, as in the initial phase of the adult diving response. Stimulation of such receptors is associated with a pronounced bradycardia, which is exacerbated if accompanied by apnea. This is because apnea removes the central respiratory drive and volume-related feedback from the lungs, which normally produce a rise in heart rate. Moreover, if the apnea produces hypoxia, chemoreceptor stimulation augments the bradycardia.

# Chemoreceptors

The peripheral arterial chemoreceptors are the body's first line of defense against hypoxia or asphyxia; they respond rapidly to changes in $P_aO_2$ or $P_aCO_2$, and changes in their discharge can affect ongoing respiratory patterns. For example, a sudden increase in chemoreceptor firing during expiration prolongs the duration of that expiration.

Carotid chemoreceptor afferent fibers have their cell bodies in the petrosal ganglion and project to the nucleus tractus solitarius. As noted above, increasing chemoreceptor discharge is prevented from affecting respiratory output after a few minutes of hypoxia in the neonate. Hence a shift in the balance of excitatory and inhibitory influences favors the latter, and ventilation falls.

A change in the hypoxia sensitivity of the peripheral arterial chemoreceptors occurs during the first few days of postnatal life, shifting their hypoxia response curves up and to the right (see Fig. 78.5). This has a two-fold effect. First, chemoreceptor discharge at any $P_aO_2$ is increased. Second, resetting increases chemoreceptor sensitivity to small changes in $P_{O_2}$ that occur about any mean $P_{O_2}$.

Similar resetting of hypoxia sensitivity occurs in the aortic chemoreceptors. The mechanism of chemoreceptor resetting is not known, but is initiated by the rise in $P_{O_2}$ at birth and probably involves a change in the cellular transduction mechanisms by which chemoreceptors detect hypoxia. Raising fetal $P_aO_2$ artificially *in utero* initiates the resetting before birth; conversely, chronic hypoxia postnatally delays or reduces it. This may explain in part the weak chemoreflexes in hypoxemic infants.

Resetting of hypoxia sensitivity is necessary because of the increase in $P_aO_2$ at birth. However, only small changes in $P_aCO_2$ occur at this time; therefore, the peripheral arterial chemoreceptor sensitivity to $CO_2$ does not need to change. Sensitivity to $CO_2$, which is present in the fetus and immediately after birth, is important in the initiation of breathing at birth and in matching ventilation to metabolism in the neonate. Because hypoxia and $CO_2$ interact as stimuli to the chemoreceptors, the situation is complex: the net result is that steady-state $CO_2$ sensitivity increases as hypoxia sensitivity resets, but the dynamic response to rapid changes in $CO_2$ remains unaltered.

## Neural mechanisms

Much research is now directed to elucidating the CNS mechanisms involved in breathing control in the neonate. While there is no evidence at present that the fundamental neural circuitry that produces breathing differs in the neonate and the adult, respiratory responses to stimuli differ. The differences are best considered in terms of an altered balance of peripheral and central influences impinging on the respiratory neurons in the brainstem. Thus the respiratory response to hypoxia in the neonate is "biphasic": an initial increase in ventilation over the first 1–2 min of hypoxia followed by a decline to, or below, control (Fig. 78.9). The first phase is due to stimulation of the peripheral arterial chemoreceptors. The magnitude of this increase in ventilation becomes larger over the first few days/weeks after birth, as the sensitivity of the chemoreceptors to hypoxia increases (see above). The second phase, decline in ventilation, is due to descending inhibitory processes that reduce respiratory output and prevent the sustained stimulation of the arterial chemoreceptors from stimulating ventilation. In fact, a decline in respiratory output in hypoxia also occurs in the adult; thus similar processes may operate throughout life, being strongest in the fetus (when hypoxia produces a cessation of FBM) and least potent

in the adult. As the neonate is at a transitional stage, the shifting balance of opposing forces is most clear at this stage.

As in the fetus, the descending inhibitory processes are mediated by the upper pons or lower mesencephalon. Transections through the pons at the level of the colliculi abolish the response, and hypoxia then produces a sustained increase in breathing (Fig. 78.10). Destruction of neural tissue more rostrally (by supra-collicular decerebration) does not prevent the secondary fall in ventilation. Similar effects are produced by cooling the dorsal rostral pons in the region of the locus coeruleus in newborn lambs; this technique has the advantage of a reversible effect. This effect is not seen in older lambs, which also do not exhibit a biphasic respiratory response. Electrical stimulation in the region of the locus coeruleus reduces respiratory output in normoxia in the neonate, which may be important in view of its role at birth (see below). However, stimulation in the pontine reticular nuclei or raphe nuclei and in parts of the parabrachial complex also reduces respiratory output. Due to the interconnections among these pontine structures and respiratory neurons, it is not yet possible to state the site of origin

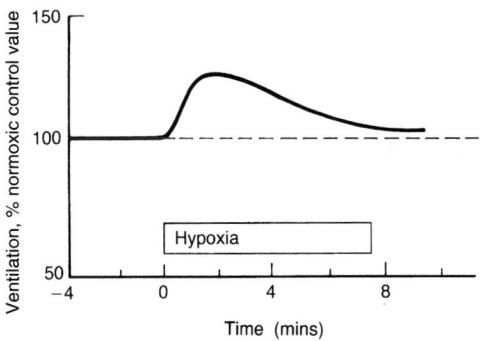

FIGURE 78.9 Neonatal ventilatory response to isocapnic hypoxia shows an initial stimulation of breathing over 1–2 min, followed by a fall towards prehypoxic levels by the 5–6 min period

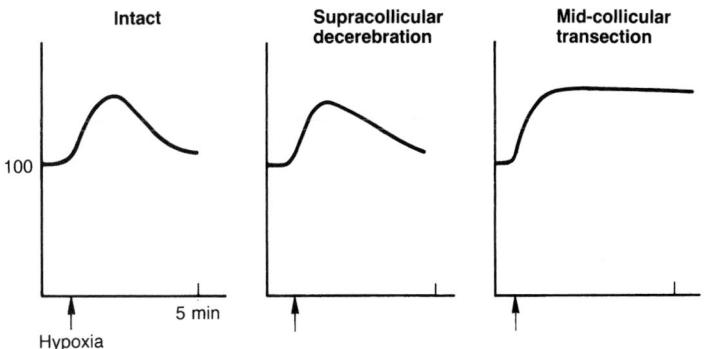

FIGURE 78.10 Ventilatory responses of neonatal rat pups to hypoxia when intact, after decerebration and then after transection of the brainstem through the pons. (Reproduced with permission from Hanson MA, Williams BA. *J Physiol* 1989; **414**: 24P.)

of the descending inhibition, or whether electrical stimulation at any locus excites cell bodies or merely axons passing through the region. As in the fetus, however, the descending inhibition is believed to be mediated by structures rostral to the pons. Direct evidence for this has been gained only recently, when it was shown that electrical or chemical stimulation in the red nucleus (RN) inhibits respiratory output, and that bilateral RN lesions abolish the secondary decline in ventilation with hypoxia. Unilateral lesions in the RN, or lesions at adjacent sites in the mesencephalon, do not alter the biphasic response. The role of the RN in fetal and neonatal life is not known; however, as it is involved in motor control in the adult, it may form an important part of the brainstem mechanisms that inhibit fetal breathing and body movements and reduce neonatal ventilation in hypoxia.

As in the fetus, neuromodulators released in the CNS during hypoxia may play an important role in the neonatal responses. Adenosine administration reduces neonatal breathing, and the effect is reduced by cooling in the rostral pons. Furthermore, adenosine antagonists reduce the fall in ventilation in hypoxia.

## Behavior and arousal

Neonatal breathing control is considerably affected by sleep state. Breathing is more regular during quiet sleep than in active sleep; it is also thought to be more under chemical control during quiet sleep. Thus during upper airway obstruction, arterial blood $O_2$ saturation ($S_aO_2$) falls to lower levels in active sleep than in quiet sleep before arousal and respiratory stimulation occurs. This may be of great importance in the etiology of apnea (see below). The role of the brainstem, e.g. the locus coeruleus, in arousal has been mentioned above. Naturally, the effects of sleep state on ventilation are clearly demonstrable in small animals only after the postnatal development of clearly defined electroencephalographic states, e.g. at about 1 month in the kitten.

## Effects of anesthetics and drugs

Inhalation anesthetics, such as halothane, depress resting chemoreceptor discharge in animals (Fig. 78.11). This effect is independent of the accompanying hypotension, which would be expected to increase chemoreceptor discharge. Halothane also impairs the reflex ventilatory response to hypoxemia, and its effects may be long-lasting (at least several hours). It has been implicated in *respiratory failure after general anesthesia*, especially in preterm babies. Metabolic inhibitors, such as cyanide, stimulate chemoreceptors, mimicking hypoxia at the carotid body. Doxapram and almitrine are stimulants of chemoreceptors that may also act at the hypoxia-sensing mechanisms. The former has been used clinically as a respiratory stimulant in the neonate.

Narcotics and general anesthetics also depress respiratory output centrally. Their site of action varies. Some reduce the level of arousal from higher centers via the reticular activating system; in addition, the effects of some (e.g. barbiturates) may be mediated via the brainstem. By altering the balance of tonic excitatory and inhibitory mechanisms, these drugs may increase the activity of the descending inhibitory processes that reduce respiratory output in the neonate. Thus they may interact positively with central effects of mild hypoxia.

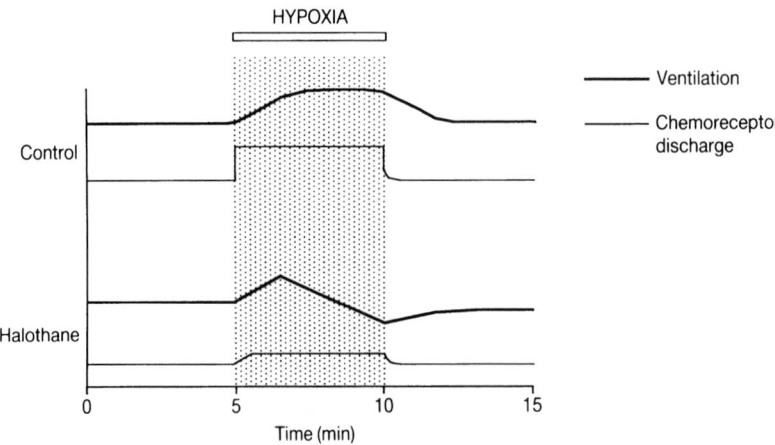

FIGURE 78.11 Effects of inspired halothane (0.5–1.0 per cent) on the ventilatory and carotid chemoreceptor responses to a brief period of hypoxia. Chemoreceptor discharge in normoxia and in hypoxia is reduced by halothane. With halothane, stimulation of ventilation during hypoxia is not maintained.

# APNEA

## Classification

In *central apnea*, respiratory output is interrupted; thus there is failure of contraction of the diaphragm, intercostal muscles, and some upper airway muscles. In contrast, in *obstructive apnea*, the diaphragm and intercostal muscles contract, but patency of the upper airway is not maintained. In fact, many apneas fall under a third heading, that of *mixed apnea*, when an initial central component is followed by an obstructive element at the time when vigorous contractions of the diaphragm and intercostal muscles resume. Alternatively, an initial obstruction can produce hypoxemia, which triggers a fall in respiratory output by CNS mechanisms.

Apneas are usually detected from measurements of surface diaphragm electromyogram (EMG), by intrathoracic pressure monitoring (e.g. with an esophageal balloon), or from monitoring abdominal and chest-wall movements (e.g. with strain gauge inductance or impedance pneumography). Airflow is measured with a pneumotachometer attached to a facial or nasal mask, by monitoring air temperature changes with thermal prongs, $P_{CO_2}$ changes at the nares, or even the sounds of respiratory movement with a microphone. Hence, central apneas are characterized by cessation of muscle EMG or intrathoracic pressure changes along with cessation of airflow. Obstructive apneas are characterized by persistence of EMG and large intrathoracic pressure changes, with absence of airflow at the nares.

Brief pauses in breathing (< 15 s) are common during both waking and sleep, especially in newborns. In waking the pauses are associated with voluntary acts such as speech; in rapid eye movement (REM) sleep they tend to be associated with rapid eye movements; and in non-REM sleep they may follow augmented breaths (sighs). Such spontaneous apneas should be distinguished from cyanotic breath-holding spells in which some children, when frustrated, angry, or frightened, expire actively, reducing FRC and holding lung volume below the normal end-expiratory point. The rapid fall in $O_2$ saturation during such episodes has been ascribed to alveolar collapse and pulmonary arterial–venous shunting. The rapid desaturation can result in loss of consciousness, which usually restores respiratory rhythm. The spells can occur as early as 2–3 months of age, but are most common between 6 months and 4 years.

## Causes

*Hypoventilation* and *central apnea* can result from the reduced respiratory output associated with diffuse encephalopathies, focal brainstem lesions in the region of the respiratory control neurons, and the action of respiratory depressants, e.g. barbiturates, benzodiazepines, narcotics, ethanol. Apnea is also associated with prematurity; preterm infants frequently experience recurrent 15–20 s pauses in respiration, sometimes with desaturation and bradycardia. Most infants less than 32 weeks' gestation have such apneas. Although such apneas generally are not considered pathological, if they are recurrent they may be the first sign of septicemia, hypoglycemia, hydrocephalus, or intraventricular hemorrhage. The chain of cause and effect in such apneas has not clearly been established, but a relatively common sequence would be one in which hypoventilation (associated with sleep state) produces mild hypoxemia, which reduces the output of motor neurons that normally maintain upper airway patency, e.g. the hypoglossal motor neurons (see above). Thus, even relatively mild hypoxemia can produce a fall in $P_{O_2}$ sufficient to be associated with obstructive apnea. This sequence is relatively similar to obstructive sleep apnea. In the neonate the neural mechanisms are probably akin to those involved in controlling FBM, in which hypoxemia stops respiratory output completely (see above). The operation of such mechanisms may persist into adult life, but this has not been established. As in the adult, the use of a small level of continuous positive airway pressure may be adequate to ensure patency of the airway in the neonate.

Apart from the prevention of marked hypoxemia, some treatment strategies involve the use of mild respiratory stimulants such as theophylline or caffeine. Their mechanism of action is unknown: they stimulate peripheral chemoreceptors but, as discussed above, this may not be beneficial in the face of powerful central nervous inhibitory processes. The drugs may play a role by reducing the depressant effects of centrally released adenosine (see above).

*Congenital central hypoventilation syndrome (Ondine curse)* is associated with loss of respiratory output during Stage 2 non-REM sleep. In this regard, it is similar to the adult condition and may involve disorders of the systems that regulate the peripheral chemoreceptor input similar to those operating in the neonatal biphasic response (see above).

Infants who experience isolated or recurrent episodes of apnea, pallor, and cyanosis with hypotonia and difficulty in arousing from sleep are said to suffer from *apparent life-threatening events (ALTEs)*. At one extreme such infants may have anatomical anomalies of the upper airway, e.g. *Pierre Robin syndrome*. There may also be upper airway dysfunction related to changes in oropharyngeal dimensions over the first 6 months of neonatal life. At the other extreme, ALTEs may result from enhanced central depressive mechanisms (e.g. excessive persistence of those operating in the fetus) or an exaggerated obstructive component of mixed apnea. As chronic hypoxemia reduces ventilatory responses, and as ALTEs produce severe episodes of hypoxemia, a vicious circle can result in which recurrent ALTEs are more likely to precipitate such cyanotic periods.

## Chronic hypoxemia

Because the normal arterial chemoreceptor resetting process depends on the rise in $P_aO_2$ at birth, limiting this increase reduces the extent of resetting. Infants born at high altitude and animals reared in 15 per cent $O_2$ have a blunted chemoreflex response to hypoxia (Fig. 78.12). Chronic hypoxemia due to *bronchopulmonary dysplasia* or repeated acute hypoxemia from recurrent apnea has similar effects. The blunting seems to be in part at the carotid body, but the precise mechanism of the resetting is not known. The carotid body hypertrophies by an unknown mechanism in high-altitude natives and adults suffering from chronic hypoxemia. It should also be noted that chronic hypoxemia may alter the brainstem inhibitory processes operating in the neonate (see above) and may thus reduce the gain of reflex responses to superimposed episodes of acute hypoxia. This may result in exacerbation of the failure of respiratory control and in gradual neuronal damage. Such processes have been suggested to operate in adult disorders such as *Pickwickian syndrome*.

## SUDDEN INFANT DEATH SYNDROME (SIDS)

It is now widely believed that the etiology of *SIDS* is multifactorial. Whatever the combination of factors, it is clear that some failure of respiratory control must almost invariably be involved; mature chemoreflex

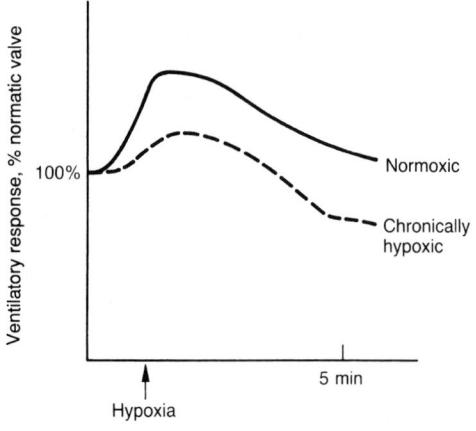

FIGURE 78.12 Ventilatory responses to hypoxia are blunted in chronically hypoxic neonates. The initial increase in ventilation is smaller, and the secondary fall in ventilation is greater.

mechanisms, which produce cardiorespiratory responses and arousal in hypoxemia/asphyxia, would not permit death to occur quietly during sleep, as is common in SIDS. If respiratory control is immature, due to reduced resetting of peripheral chemoreceptor sensitivity or an imbalance favoring the operation of central nervous inhibitory processes, such chemoreflex failure can be explained. Additionally, genetic influences or pathological processes may play a role, e.g. hypoxemia *in utero* or postnatally.

Poor chemoreflexes have been reported in some groups of infants at high risk for SIDS, i.e. those with a recurrent apnea or bronchopulmonary dysplasia. This may represent a genetic or environmental difference, or could be a pathophysiological change resulting from hypoxemia. There are reports that the carotid-body dopamine levels of some SIDS victims are higher than those of infants dying of other causes. The significance of this is unknown.

*ALTEs* confer a higher risk of SIDS; it may be that the positively interacting components of the phenomenon take some months to develop, explaining the peak incidence of SIDS between 2 and 5 months after birth. Further research is necessary before the contribution of perturbation of perinatal respiratory control mechanisms to pathological conditions over the long term can be defined.

## SELECTED READING

Adamson SL. Regulation of breathing. *J Dev Physiol* 1991; **15**: 45.

Bentele KHP, Albani M. Are there tests predictive for prolonged apnea and SIDS? A review of epidemiological and functional studies. *Acta Paediatr Scand* 1988; **342**: 1.

Dawes GS. The central control of fetal breathing and skeletal muscle movements. *J Physiol* 1984; **346**: 1.

Haidmayer R, Kerschaggl P, Kerbl R, Pfeiffer KP, Kurz R, Kenner T. Investigations of respiratory control in infants to assess possible risk for SIDS. In: Rolfe P, ed. *Neonatal physiological measurements*. London: Butterworths, 1986; 335.

Hanson MA, ed. *The fetal and neonatal brainstem*. Cambridge: Cambridge University Press, 1991.

Hanson MA, Spencer JAD, Rodeck CH, Walters DV. *The fetus and neonate, Vol II, Breathing*. Cambridge: Cambridge University Press, 1994.

Lagercrantz H. What does the preterm infant breathe for? Controversies on apnea of prematurity. *Acta Paediatr Scand* 1992; **81**: 733.

Nijhuis JG. Breathing movements in the human fetus in normoxia and hypoxia. In: Kunzel W, Kirschbaum M, eds. *Oxygen: basis of the regulation of vital functions in the fetus*. Berlin: Springer-Verlag, 1992: 117.

Richardson BS. Fetal adaptive responses to asphyxia. *Clin Perinatol* 1989; **16**: 595.

# 79

# Mechanics of Breathing

J. Julio Pérez Fontán

As aquatic animals adapted to life on land, their gas-exchange systems needed to maintain a large contact surface with air without losing large amounts of water to evaporation. Therefore, the lungs of most terrestrial species evolved as invaginated structures. An invaginated lung, however, required a mechanism to force air in and out of the gas-exchanging spaces. In mammals and other higher vertebrates, this mechanism resembles a bellows pump, in which a group of respiratory muscles apply force on the passive elements of the chest wall (rib cage and abdomen) to inflate and deflate the lungs. The function of the pump is regulated by a complex network of sensors, which relay both mechanical information from the pump's components and chemical information from blood to a control center in the brainstem. Despite the relative simplicity of the pump and the obvious complexity of the regulatory network, the respiratory system is more vulnerable to mechanical than to control dysfunctions. In fact, the increase in energy demand imposed by various types of mechanical breakdown usually causes most of the signs and symptoms of respiratory disease and ultimately leads to respiratory failure.

From a mechanical point of view, the function of the respiratory system is best analyzed in terms of work and energy. Above, the mammalian respiratory system is compared to a bellows pump. Basic physics indicates that the amount of work ($\Delta W$) done by such a pump in order to produce a certain volume change ($V_0$ to $V_1$) with a pressure change $P$ can be computed as (equation 1):

$$\Delta W = \int_{V_0}^{V_1} P \, dV$$

For the respiratory system, the total amount of work done by the respiratory muscles during a single breath depends on the mechanical characteristics of the lungs and chest wall (which define the magnitude of $P$) and on the needs for gas exchange (which define the limits of the volume change, $V_1 - V_0$).

However, work alone is not a direct measure of the energy that the muscles must extract from the metabolic fuels provided by the circulation. The reason is that the respiratory muscles transform energy ($\Delta Q$) into work with variable efficiency ($\varepsilon$) (equation 2).

$$\Delta Q = \Delta W / \varepsilon$$

In this regard, the relationship between the work needed to ventilate the lungs and the work done by the respiratory muscles can be envisioned as a see-saw resting on a sliding fulcrum, the position of which defines the efficiency of the system (Fig. 79.1). Excluding extreme conditions (e.g. shock), the circulation provides the respiratory muscles with abundant substrates, and small increases in work or decreases in efficiency caused by mild or even moderate mechanical dysfunction can be easily compensated by extracting more energy from these substrates. With more severe mechanical dysfunction, however, substrates either may not be available or, more commonly, may not be processed fast enough into work by the muscles' metabolic and contractile machinery. If so, the balance is tipped beyond the limits of compensation, leading to the gas-exchange abnormalities that characterize respiratory failure.

To keep with this view of the respiratory system, I first analyze the factors that determine the work of breathing; then examine the conditions that modify the efficiency with which the energy used by the respiratory muscles is applied to do this work; and, finally, discuss the ability and limitations of the respiratory muscles to respond to the increased demands imposed by disease. When appropriate, I will highlight any unique characteristics that may render the developing respiratory system more vulnerable to both mechanical dysfunction and failure.

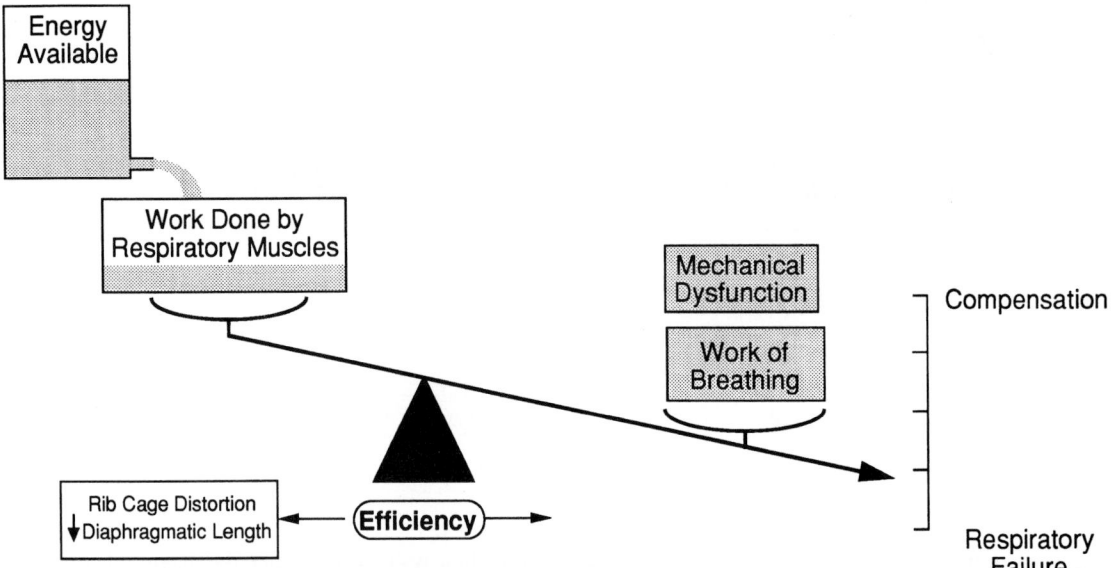

FIGURE 79.1. Relationship between the work needed to ventilate the lungs and the work done by the respiratory muscles. The relationship is represented as a see-saw resting on a fulcrum that can slide to the right or left, depending on whether the efficiency of the respiratory system increases or decreases. Lung mechanical dysfunction increases the workload that must be performed to maintain adequate gas exchange, forcing the respiratory muscles to use more energy. If the added workload exceeds the amount of energy that can be transformed by the muscles into work for a given time, then the mechanical dysfunction cannot be compensated and respiratory failure ensues. Alterations such as rib-cage distortion and decreased diaphragmatic length, which are frequently associated with respiratory mechanical dysfunction, decrease the efficiency with which energy is transformed into work and cause respiratory failure to occur at lower levels of workload.

## DETERMINANTS OF VOLUME–PRESSURE WORK

As shown by equation 1, the volume–pressure relationships of the respiratory system are the only determinants of how much work the respiratory muscles must do during breathing. These relationships summarize the mechanical behaviors of the lungs and the chest wall. Because lungs and chest wall are linked by a non-compressible boundary (the pleural space), their volumes cannot change independently of each other or of the respiratory system as a whole, and therefore (equation 3):

$$\Delta V_L = \Delta V_W = \Delta V_{RS}$$

where $\Delta V_L$, $\Delta V_W$, and $\Delta V_{RS}$ represent the volume changes that the lungs, chest wall, and respiratory system, respectively, undergo during breathing.

In contrast, the pressures that the respiratory muscles need to generate in order to inflate the lungs ($P_L$), chest wall ($P_W$), and respiratory system ($P_{RS}$) depend on the pressure difference across each component, and consequently they are all different (equations 4–6):

$$P_L = P_{ao} - P_{pl}$$
$$P_W = P_{pl} - P_B$$
$$P_{RS} = P_{ao} - P_B$$

where $P_{ao}$ is the pressure at the airway opening (the nares or the mouth, during normal breathing), $P_{pl}$ is the representative pressure in the pleural space, and $P_B$ is atmospheric pressure. These equations can be easily reworked into the following expression (equation 7):

$$P_{RS} = P_L + P_W$$

which indicates that, at any time during breathing, the total pressure needed to produce a certain volume change in the respiratory system is equal to the sum of the pressures needed to produce the same change individually in the lungs and the chest wall.

## Pressures acting on the respiratory system

To move both air and respiratory tissues during breathing, the respiratory muscles must overcome several types of forces, which when applied on tissue surfaces are translated into pressures. Depending on whether the energy consumed in the effort leaves the system as heat or simply remains stored to be recovered later, the pressures acting on the respiratory system can be classified into non-dissipative and dissipative. Non-dissipative pressures include elastic or volume-dependent pressures that arise from the tendency of the lung and chest wall to recover their original shape upon deformation, inertial or acceleration-dependent pressures produced by the changes in velocity experienced by gas and tissues during breathing movements, and gravitational or mass-dependent pressures related to the weight of the tissues. Dissipative pressures are commonly grouped together as resistive pressures, and include flow-dependent pressures generated primarily by the friction of the gas against the airway walls, and viscoelastic or time-dependent pressures created by the molecular movements that occur in the tissues and in the gas–liquid interface as the respiratory system changes volume.

## Non-dissipative pressures

Inertial and gravitational pressures are small during normal breathing in children and can be neglected. Elastic pressures, in contrast, can be quite large. Their magnitude depends on the volume of the respiratory system, much as the tension developed by a rubber band depends on the extent to which it is stretched. Elastic pressures are best characterized when there are no other pressures operating in the respiratory system. For this to happen, respiratory system volume must be maintained constant for at least a few seconds (e.g. by breath-holding at a given level). Under such circumstances, gas ceases to flow in the airways, and pressures at the airway opening and in the alveoli ($P_A$) become the same. Equations 4–6 can then be rewritten (equations 8–10):

$$P_{L,el} = P_A - P_{pl}$$
$$P_{W,el} = P_{pl} - P_B$$
$$P_{RS,el} = P_A - P_B$$

where $P_{L,el}$, $P_{W,el}$, and $P_{RS,el}$ represent the elastic pressures generated by the lungs, the chest wall, and the whole respiratory system, respectively.

The relationships between volume changes and elastic pressures in the respiratory system and its components are quite complex. Graphically, their shape can be described by a sigmoid curve: volume increases much less for a given pressure change at low and high volumes than at intermediate volumes, when the volume–pressure relationship is steeper (Fig. 79.2). From a mathematical point of view, the description is more difficult. Like any other continuous function, each volume–pressure relationship has a well-specified slope at each volume ($\Delta V/\Delta P$). This slope defines the *compliance* of the lungs, chest wall, or respiratory system for that volume depending on whether $\Delta P_{L,el}$, $\Delta P_{W,el}$ or $\Delta P_{RS,el}$ is substituted for $\Delta P$. Unfortunately, no single slope or compliance can accurately describe the totality of the volume–pressure relationship. Only for the intermediate range of volumes is the relationship relatively linear, and $\Delta V/\Delta P$ can be considered constant.

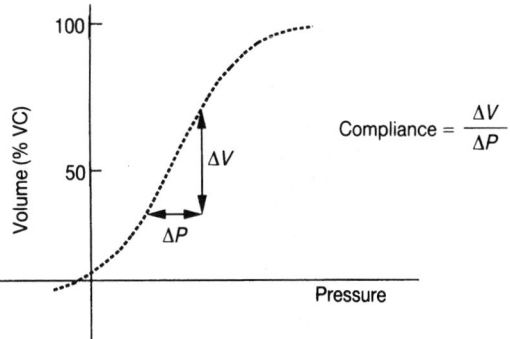

FIGURE 79.2 Idealized relationship between volume and elastic pressure in the lungs. Volume is represented as a proportion of the vital capacity of the lungs (VC, the maximal volume that can be inhaled after a complete exhalation). The relationship is relatively flat at high and low lung volumes and steeper at intermediate volumes, where breathing normally takes place. At these intermediate volumes, the slope is relatively constant, and the relationship can be described with a single compliance.

If equations 8–10 are rearranged in a way similar to equation 7, it would be apparent that, just like the total pressure, the elastic pressure developed by the respiratory system is the sum of the elastic pressures developed by the lungs and the chest wall. A graphic analysis demonstrates how this additive interaction of the lungs and the chest wall shapes the volume–pressure behavior of the entire respiratory system (Fig. 79.3). For instance, at the points at which the volume–pressure curves intersect the volume axis, the respiratory system and each of its components (lungs and chest wall) are at their respective relaxation volumes (i.e. the volumes at which the elastic elements generate no recoil). Lungs and chest wall have different relaxation volumes. The relaxation volume of the lungs is rather small; if allowed to collapse freely, the lungs would end up containing a gas volume smaller than the normal residual volume (the gas volume of the lungs after a forced expiration). The relaxation volume of the chest wall, on the other hand, is considerably larger; in the adult, it exceeds 50 per cent of the vital capacity (the gas volume of the lungs after a maximal inspiratory effort). The discrepancy between the relaxation volumes of the lungs and the chest wall has three important mechanical consequences. First, it causes the relaxation volume of the respiratory system to occupy a position intermediate between that of the lungs and the chest wall; beyond the newborn period, the relaxation volume of the respiratory system coincides with the functional residual capacity of the lungs (the gas volume of the lungs at the end of a tidal breath). Second, the opposing recoils of the lungs and chest wall create a negative pressure in the pleural space at the end of a normal breath. This negative pressure attaches the lungs to the chest wall and promotes venous return into the heart. Finally, for at least a portion of the volume range, the passive outward recoil of the chest wall contributes to the work of expanding the lungs, thereby reducing the energetic demands on the respiratory muscles (Fig. 79.3).

The elastic recoil generated per unit of lung volume is relatively constant during development. In contrast, the recoil of the chest wall increases substantially after the perinatal period, when a high chest wall compliance is essential to facilitate passage through the birth canal. As a result of this high chest wall compliance, the inward recoil of the newborn's lungs is partially unopposed, and the relaxation volume of the respiratory system is proportionally smaller than that of the adult (Fig. 79.3). Because a small lung volume represents a disadvantage in terms of both alveolar stability and oxygenation, newborns of most mammalian species have developed strategies to maintain the functional residual capacity of their lungs above the relaxation volume of their respiratory system. These strategies combine mechanisms directed at prolonging

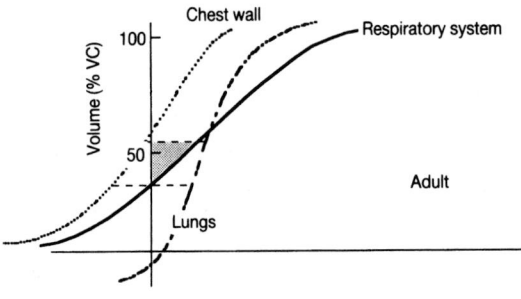

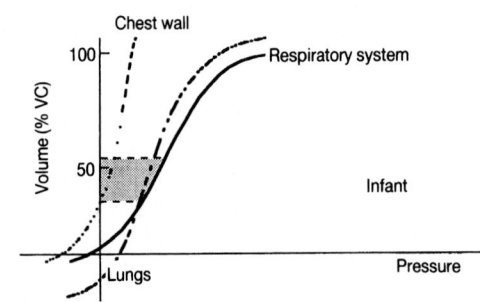

FIGURE 79.3 Elastic volume–pressure relationships of the lungs, chest wall, and respiratory system for the range of vital capacity (VC) in an adult and an infant. These relationships show that the pressure needed to inflate the respiratory system to any given volume is the sum of the pressures that would be needed to inflate the lungs and the chest wall individually to the same volume. The intersection of each relationship with the ordinate represents the relaxation volume of each component. The volume–pressure relationships of the lungs are similar in the adult and in the infant; the volume–pressure relationship of the chest wall, however, is much steeper in the infant, causing both the relaxation volumes of the chest wall and the respiratory system to be lower as well. The stippled area represents the elastic work done by the respiratory muscles for a typical tidal volume. Note that this work tends to be greater in the infant because, at normal breathing volumes, the recoil of the chest wall does not contribute to inflating the lungs as it does in the adult.

expiratory flow (such as sustaining the tonic activity of the inspiratory muscles during expiration or contracting the adductor muscles of the larynx) with a relatively high breathing rate, which reduces the time available for expiration. The resultant dependence of lung volume on neural control renders the functional residual capacity of newborn and small infants' lungs very vulnerable to changes in muscle coordination and tone. Concurrent decreases in intercostal and upper airway muscle tone during rapid eye movement (REM) sleep, for example, prevent expiratory flow prolongation and may decrease lung volume substantially, particularly in the premature infant. Likewise, muscle weakness, deep sedation, and central nervous system depression all can reduce the functional residual capacity of the lungs, increasing the work of breathing and impairing gas exchange.

## Dissipative pressures

A pressure is characterized as dissipative when the energy that is used to overcome it leaves the system (usually as heat) and cannot be used again. In the respiratory system, most dissipative energy losses result from friction between the gas and the internal surface of the air passages. A measurable amount of energy, however, is also lost in reshaping the structure of the lungs and the chest wall, either by producing reversible molecular rearrangements in the tissue or the alveolar gas–liquid interface (e.g. incorporation of surfactant molecules to the surface of the alveolar liquid as the lungs expand) or by causing alterations in the gross architecture of the lung (e.g. recruitment of previously collapsed alveoli). Although difficult to separate in practice, the processes responsible for these non-frictional energy losses are frequently described as viscoelastic or plastoelastic depending on whether the pressure changes that they cause depend primarily on the rate or the amplitude of the lung volume change (many materials present in the lungs, like pulmonary surfactant or smooth muscle, exhibit both viscoelasticity and plastoelasticity when studied in isolation).

Regardless of whether the final pathway is frictional, viscoelastic, or plastoelastic, the energy dissipated during inspiration can no longer contribute to work performed during expiration. Thus, whenever present, dissipative losses cause the volume–pressure behavior of the respiratory system to vary depending on the direction, inspiratory or expiratory, of the volume changes. This property, known as *hysteresis*, is responsible for the formation of loops when the volume–pressure relationships of the respiratory system are plotted during breathing (Fig. 79.4). In such graphic representation, the dissipative pressures can be identified at any volume as the distance between the point in the loop and the point that the elastic volume–pressure relationship would occupy at a similar volume ($\Delta P$ in Fig. 79.4). The area enclosed by the loop provides a measure of the total amount of work done

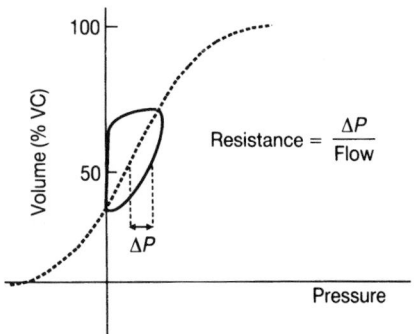

FIGURE 79.4 Dynamic volume–pressure relationship showing hysteresis (loop) caused by dissipative energy losses. The magnitude of the dissipative pressure losses can be estimated at any point as the distance between the hysteretic loop and the elastic volume–pressure relationship ($\Delta P$). The resistance of the respiratory system is usually calculated by dividing the dissipative pressure losses calculated in this fashion by the gas flow.

against dissipative pressures (Fig. 79.5). Under normal circumstances, however, only the inspiratory portion of the work is performed by the respiratory muscles. The dissipative work done during expiration is performed at the expense of the energy accumulated in the elastic elements of the lungs and the chest wall during inspiration.

Similar to the elastic pressures, the dissipative pressures in the respiratory system cannot be accurately predicted with a simple mathematical expression. This is in part because viscoelastic and plastoelastic pressures are complex, non-linear functions of gas flow and respiratory system volume. Frictional pressures, in contrast, are generally considered to relate linearly to the gas flow present in the airways ($\dot{V}$).

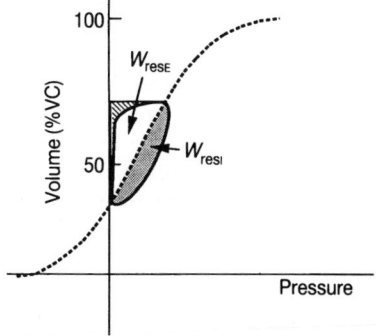

FIGURE 79.5 Work performed during a typical tidal breath. The area enclosed by the loop is a measure of the work done against dissipative forces. However, only the inspiratory portion of this work ($W_{\text{resI}}$, stippling) needs to be performed by the respiratory muscles; the expiratory portion of the dissipative work ($W_{\text{resE}}$, no stippling) is done by the energy accumulated in the elastic elements of the system during inspiration. A small portion of this elastic energy is used to overcome the tone left in the inspiratory muscles during expiration (cross-hatched area).

Because friction is the main mechanism of pressure loss in the airways, the pressure difference between the airway opening ($P_{\text{ao}}$) and the alveoli ($P_{\text{A}}$) are often described with equation 11:

$$P_{\text{ao}} - P_{\text{A}} = R_{\text{aw}}\dot{V}$$

where the constant $R_{\text{aw}}$ represents the flow resistance of the airways. However, even if only referred to frictional pressure losses, this formulation involves an oversimplification: volume-dependent variations in airway caliber as well as turbulence and other flow perturbations common at points of airway narrowing and bifurcation cause substantial departures from flow–pressure linearity that cannot be accounted for by a constant $R_{\text{aw}}$.

## Airway dynamics

An understanding of the relationship between airway caliber and lung volume is essential for the recognition and diagnosis of airway obstruction. Central to this understanding is the idea that the airways are elastic tubes, whose caliber is determined by the coupling of airway wall compliance and airway transmural pressure. Airway wall compliance depends on the state of health and maturity of the airways and on the tone of the airway muscle. The latter is regulated by a complex network of central nervous system neurons, which influences the output of the somatic motor neurons that innervate the upper airway skeletal muscles and the general visceral motor neurons that innervate the tracheal and bronchial smooth muscle. In all appearance, the main function of this regulatory network is to stiffen the airways and thus limit airway distortion (collapse and distension) during breathing. Accordingly, the neural output to the airway muscles varies depending on the intensity of the respiratory drive: it increases in the presence of ventilatory stimuli such as hypoxia and hypercarbia and disappears during *neural apnea*.

Airway transmural pressure, defined as the difference between the pressures of the gas column inside the airway and the tissue outside the airway, changes during the breathing cycle in a fashion that depends on whether the airway is extrathoracic or intrathoracic. Extrathoracic airways (nose, pharynx, larynx, and trachea between the cricoid cartilage and the thoracic inlet) are exposed to atmospheric pressure on the outside. Because the pressure inside is subatmospheric during inspiration and supraatmospheric during expiration, the transmural pressure of these airways is always negative (promoting airway collapse) during inspiration and always positive (promoting airway distension) during expiration. The outside surface of the intrathoracic airways (trachea and bronchi) is exposed to a pressure similar to pleural pressure (independent of whether they are embedded in the lung tissue or the mediastinum). Because inspiratory flow requires the pressure inside the airways to be greater than alveolar pressure, and alveolar pressure must in turn be greater than pleural pressure (the difference being equivalent to the elastic recoil of the lungs – $P_{L,el}$ in equation 8), the transmural pressure of the intrathoracic airways becomes increasingly positive (causing the airways to become distended) during inspiration. Expiratory flow, in contrast, requires the pressure inside the airways to be lower than alveolar pressure. Whether the pressure at a specific point inside an airway ($P_{aw}$) is higher or lower than the outside pleural pressure ($P_{pl}$), however, depends on the balance between the frictional pressure losses that occur upstream from the airway ($P_A - P_{aw}$) and the elastic recoil of the lungs ($P_{L,el}$). If, at a certain point, friction causes ($P_A - P_{aw}$) > $P_{L,el}$, then it follows that (equation 12):

$$P_A - P_{L,el} > P_{aw}$$

or, from equation 8 (equation 13):

$$P_{pl} > P_{aw}$$

which means that from this critical point all the way to the thoracic inlet, the transmural pressure is negative and the airway tends to collapse. Obviously, diseases that increase the frictional resistance of the airways (e.g. *asthma*) or decrease the elastic recoil of the lungs (e.g. *emphysema*) will move the critical point closer to the alveoli, causing airway collapse and further increasing airway resistance during expiration.

Depending on the airway wall compliance and caliber, airway collapse during expiration can lead to flow limitation, a situation in which expiratory gas flow does not increase regardless of the effort made by the subject to raise alveolar pressure. Flow limitation can be caused by both the increase in frictional pressure losses (viscous flow limitation) and the formation of areas of critical velocity above which pressure disturbances cannot travel upstream (wave speed flow limitation) as airway flow increases. Regardless of which of these two mechanisms is operative, the flow rate at which flow limitation occurs at a given lung volume depends only on the caliber and collapsibility of the airways and is highly reproducible. Determinations of maximal expiratory flow during respiratory function testing take advantage of this reproducibility to assess and follow the functional state of the intrathoracic airways over time or in response to therapeutic interventions.

## Airway obstruction

Airway obstruction can result from space-occupying lesions that impinge on the airway lumen (e.g. edema of the airway mucosa in *croup* or compression of the trachea by a *vascular ring*) or from failure of airway muscle control (e.g. pharyngeal collapse in *sleep apnea*). In either case, the clinical manifestations typically reflect an exaggeration of the normal cyclic changes of the airway caliber described above (Fig. 79.6). When the obstruction is extrathoracic (e.g. croup), the pressure inside the airway segment downstream from the narrow point must become more negative during inspiration in order to overcome the increased frictional resistance of the narrowing. The segment therefore tends to collapse, producing both an inspiratory exacerbation of the obstruction and a characteristic turbulent noise (*inspiratory stridor*). The obstruction is somewhat relieved during expiration, as the pressure inside the airways must become more positive, again to overcome the narrowing's increased resistance. When the obstruction is intrathoracic (e.g. *asthma* or *tracheobronchomalacia*), very negative pleural pressures tend to dilate the airways during inspiration. During expiration, however, increased frictional pressure losses create a marked pressure gradient from the alveoli toward the airway opening. As a result, the pressure inside the airways is rapidly exceeded by pleural pressure as the lungs deflate, causing an expiratory exacerbation of the obstruction and a distinctive mid- to end-expiratory wheeze on auscultation.

## Restrictive and obstructive respiratory disease

The total amount of work that the respiratory muscles must do during breathing is the sum of the work done to overcome the non-dissipative and dissipative pressures. Depending on which of these two work components predominates, the mechanical dysfunctions of the respiratory system can be classified as restrictive or obstructive.

Restrictive disease is caused by processes that increase the elastic recoil of the lungs (e.g. *pulmonary edema, respiratory distress syndrome of the newborn*) or the chest wall (e.g. abdominal distension, *scoliosis*). The increased recoil has two major consequences. First, it increases the amount of work that the respiratory muscles must do during inspiration (expiration continues to be passive). Second, by lowering the relaxation volume of the respiratory system, the increased recoil also decreases the functional residual capacity of the lungs, promoting alveolar collapse and increased venous admixture. In an attempt to counteract the effects of restrictive disease on lung volume, infants and children often close their glottis toward the end of expiration, generating a grunt, which is a helpful diagnostic sign. Positive end-expiratory pressure and continuous airway pressure are therapeutic modalities both directed at preserving alveolar stability.

The small caliber and high compliance of the developing airways renders them particularly vulnerable to obstruction. During normal breathing, small airways represent no particular disadvantage for the child because gas flows are low and dissipative pressure losses also remain small. When obstruction occurs,

Inspiration                    Expiration

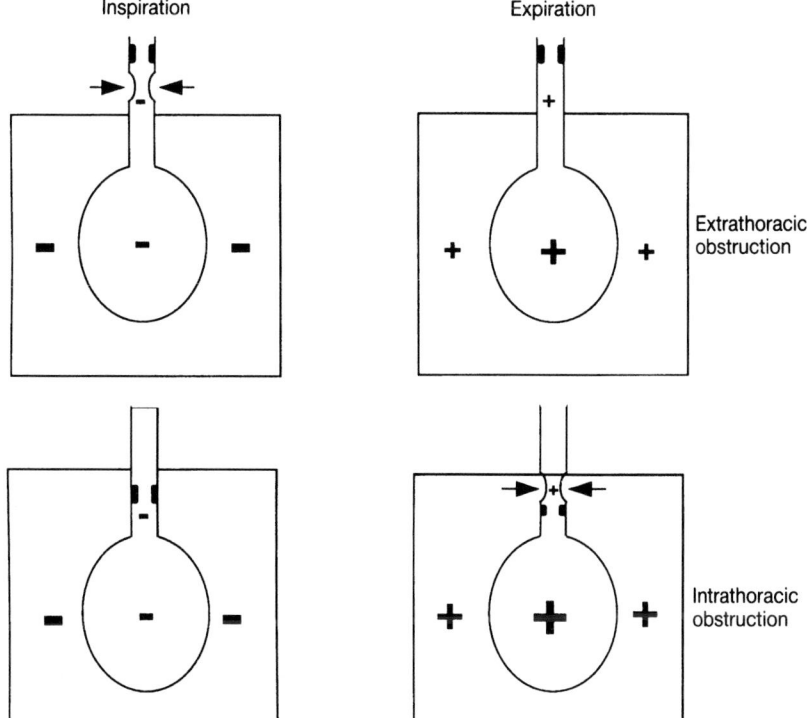

FIGURE 79.6 Effects of airway obstruction on airway caliber during inspiration and expiration. Extrathoracic obstruction is exacerbated during inspiration because the highly negative pressure inside the airways is unopposed by the atmospheric pressure outside, causing the airway to collapse (arrows). Intrathoracic obstruction, in contrast, worsens during expiration because, as gas starts to flow towards the mouth, the pressure outside the airways (which is similar to pleural pressure) rapidly exceeds the pressure inside, causing the airways downstream from the obstruction point to collapse (arrows). (From Pérez Fontán JJ, Lister G. In: Touloukian RJ, ed. *Pediatric trauma*, 2nd edn. St Louis: Mosby-Year Book Inc., 1990: 46, with permission.)

however, frictional pressure losses increase exponentially with the reduction in airway diameter, an increase that is compounded by the tendency of flow to develop into turbulent patterns in low-caliber tubes. Consequently, the same degree of obstruction has much more dire consequences in the small infant and child than in the adult.

## DETERMINANTS OF BREATHING EFFICIENCY

In a thermodynamic system, efficiency can be defined as the proportion of free energy that is transformed into external work. In the case of the respiratory system, for any given period of time (equation 14):

$$\varepsilon = \frac{\text{Work}}{\text{Respiratory muscle energy consumption}}$$

The numerator of this expression (which is a direct application of equation 1) represents the amount of work done by the respiratory muscles to inflate and deflate the lungs during that time. The denominator is the amount of energy consumed by the respiratory muscles to do this work. In practice, the calculated

efficiency is always an underestimate of the true efficiency of the respiratory system for two reasons. First, the volume–pressure work done on themselves by the respiratory muscles (which are part of the chest wall) cannot be measured. Second, the muscles consume a substantial amount of energy to perform postural or isometric tasks, which, in a physical sense, do not constitute work and therefore are included in the denominator but not in the numerator. Accordingly, the problem of analyzing the transformation of energy into work during breathing is usually approached with an operative definition of efficiency in which the numerator represents strictly the work done on the lungs (thereby excluding the chest wall) and the respiratory muscle energy consumption is estimated from the difference between the whole-body oxygen consumption measured while the subject breathes spontaneously and while ventilation is fully supported by a mechanical ventilator. Accepting its evident limitations, this approach has the advantage of identifying inefficient activities which, like chest wall distortion, are a source of real work for the respiratory muscles, but do not contribute to the inflation of the lungs or gas exchange. Considered in these terms, the respiratory system is an extremely inefficient machine. Efficiency values as low as 8–25 per cent occur in adult humans at rest; even lower ones in healthy premature infants (4 per cent) and in patients with respiratory disease (1–3 per cent). Because of these low starting values, very small changes in efficiency have a large effect on the energy required for breathing. A clear understanding of the factors that influence respiratory system efficiency is important for both the diagnosis and the treatment of most breathing disturbances. Among these factors are breathing pattern, diaphragmatic configuration, chest wall distortion, and the contractile state of the respiratory muscles.

## Breathing pattern

The amount of work that the respiratory muscles must do to generate a given alveolar ventilation (and thus maintain a certain $P_aCO_2$) depends on the breathing pattern (Fig. 79.7). Each individual has a well-defined optimal breathing frequency, above and below which the work of breathing increases hyperbolically. This theoretical frequency is linked to the volume–pressure relationships of the respiratory system: it increases when the elastic recoil of the lungs or the chest wall increases (e.g. with pulmonary edema) and decreases when the dissipative pressures of the respiratory system increase (e.g. with airway obstruction). In practice, most subjects, including those with respiratory mechanical disturbances, adopt breathing frequencies that approach their predicted optimal frequency. As a result, one can usually categorize respiratory disease as primarily restrictive or obstructive depending on whether the patient breathes rapidly or slowly. However, the breathing pattern is regulated through neural pathways that respond more to mechanical and irritant stimuli from the respiratory system or to cortical influences than to energetic convenience. Therefore, it is not uncommon for children with respiratory disease to

breathe transiently at frequencies that depart substantially from the optimal frequency. In this manner, airway irritation, stretch receptor stimulation, crying, and agitation can reduce the energetic efficiency of the respiratory system and precipitate respiratory failure.

## Diaphragmatic length and configuration

Just like any other muscle, the diaphragm develops its maximal contractile force at a certain optimal length (see below), which happens to be attained when the lungs approximate their functional residual capacity. At this volume, the diaphragm is configured as a dome-capped cylinder, an arrangement that has several advantages. First, a cylindrical shape allows a much greater volume displacement for a given fiber shortening than a simple dome shape. Second, as the sides of the cylinder shorten during inspiration, making the dome descend toward the abdomen in a piston-like motion, the area of contact between the internal surface of the rib cage and the lungs increases. This increase provides a way to accommodate without distortion the inevitable increase in lung surface that occurs as the lungs expand. Finally, for most of the tidal volume range, the sides of the diaphragmatic cylinder are apposed to the internal surface of the rib cage. By transmitting to the ribs and the sternum the increase in intraabdominal pressure that occurs as the diaphragm descends into the abdomen, this area of apposition establishes a mechanical link between the abdomen and the rib cage, helping to stabilize the chest wall and facilitating inspiration.

The developing diaphragm may lack some of these advantages. Particularly in the newborn and small infant, the lower portion of the rib cage has proportionally wider diameters than in the adult. As a result,

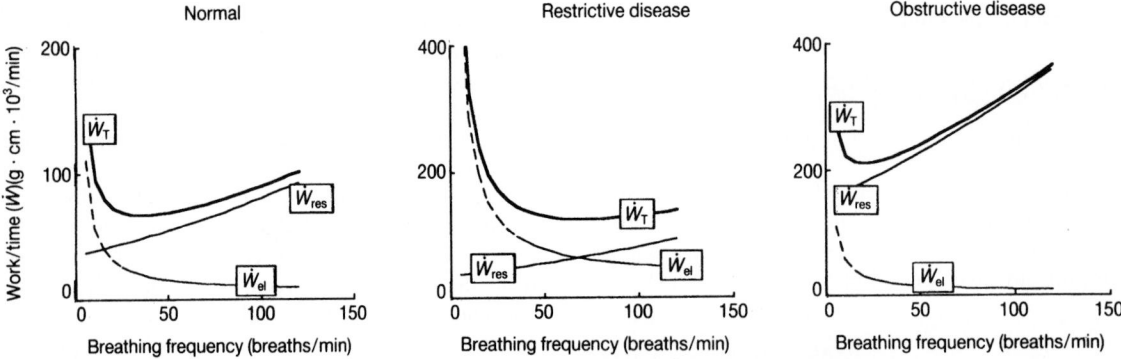

FIGURE 79.7 Calculated effect of breathing frequency on the energy expended per unit of time (breathing power, $\dot{W}$) to overcome elastic forces ($\dot{W}_{el}$), resistive forces ($\dot{W}_{res}$), and their sum ($\dot{W}_T$) in a normal infant and in two infants with respiratory disease, one restrictive and the other obstructive. Calculations are based on assumptions that minute alveolar ventilation is constant, breathing pattern is sinusoidal, and volume– and flow–pressure relationships are linear. Elastic and resistive power decrease and increase with frequency, respectively. As a result, total power follows a bimodal course, decreasing at low frequencies and increasing at high frequencies. The point at which total power reaches a minimum is the optimal frequency in terms of energy expenditure. The figure shows that the predominance of elastic and resistive power shifts this optimal frequency to higher frequencies in restrictive disease and to lower frequencies in obstructive disease. Note different scales used to accommodate the increase in breathing power caused by restrictive and obstructive disease.

the muscle's insertions are spread out, and the sides of the diaphragmatic cylinder are short (Fig. 79.8). Under such conditions, fiber contraction can only increase the radius of the dome; therefore, the volume displaced (and the work done) by a given fiber shortening (or for a certain energy expenditure) is limited. In addition, the shortness of the area of apposition lessens the stabilizing and inspiratory effects of intraabdominal pressure, further reducing the work-to-energy ratio and the efficiency of the respiratory system.

## Chest-wall distortion

Until this point, it has been assumed that every portion of the chest wall undergoes a similar displacement during breathing, regardless of its location. In reality, not only can different portions of the rib cage and abdomen change volume independently of each other, but they often do it in opposite directions.

Chest-wall distortion is primarily the consequence of regional variations in chest wall compliance. In the case of the rib cage, areas without bony support (intercostal, suprasternal, and subcostal spaces) are particularly prone to move inward as pleural pressure decreases during inspiration. When pleural pressure becomes very negative to overcome an increased elastic recoil or an airway obstruction, this inward movement of the rib cage becomes more pronounced, causing visible retractions.

The chest walls of newborns and infants are very susceptible to distortion. As discussed above, the limited ossification of ribs and sternum increases markedly the passive compliance of the rib cage during early life. In addition, the developing intercostal muscles, the main function of which is to stabilize the chest by contracting simultaneously with the diaphragm, appear to have decreased tone, especially during REM sleep. Finally, the lack of a substantial area of apposition between the diaphragm and the rib cage eliminates the additional stabilizing effect of intraabdominal pressure on the lower ribs and subcostal area at these ages.

Chest wall distortion can be quantified as a change in volume caused by a change in pressure. Therefore, it represents a form of work and has a measurable energy cost. Unfortunately, the work done to produce the distortion is not applied to lung inflation, and therefore distortion can be considered a source of inefficiency (see above). This point of view is well illustrated by a simple analysis of the work done by the diaphragm in the presence of rib-cage retractions (Fig. 79.9). Regardless of whether such retractions are present or not, the tidal volume of the lungs ($\Delta V_L$) has to be equivalent to the sum of the volume changes undergone by the rib cage ($\Delta V_{rc}$) and abdomen ($\Delta V_{ab}$) (equation 15):

$$\Delta V_L = \Delta V_{rc} + \Delta V_{ab}$$

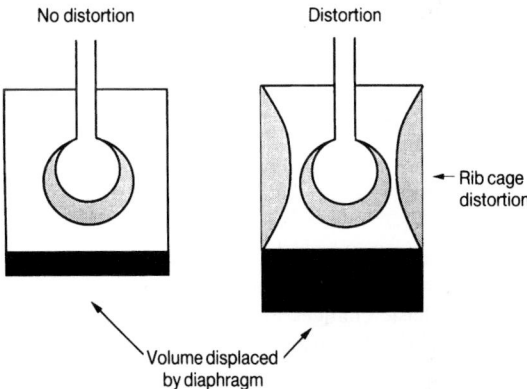

FIGURE 79.9 Effects of rib-cage retractions on the volume displaced by the diaphragm during inspiration. During a nondistorted inflation, both rib cage and abdomen expand. During a distorted inflation, however, the diaphragm must increase its volume displacement (and therefore do more work) to offset the inward movement of the rib cage and maintain the tidal volume of the lungs constant. (From Pérez Fontán JJ. Mechanical dysfunction of the respiratory system. In: Fuhrman BP, Zimmerman JJ, eds. *Pediatric critical care*. St Louis: Mosby-Year Book Inc., 1992: 399, with permission.)

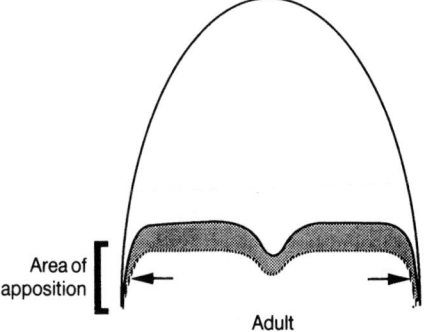
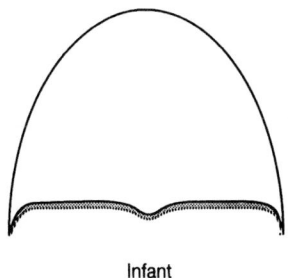

FIGURE 79.8 Configuration of the diaphragm in the adult and the infant. In the adult, the diaphragm has the shape of a cylinder with a dome cap. The sides of the cylinder adhere to the internal surface of the rib cage, forming an area of apposition that is used by intraabdominal pressure to push the ribs and the sternum during inspiration. In the infant, the diaphragmatic insertions are more spread out and both the sides of the cylinder and the area of apposition are smaller. As a result, the volume displaced by the muscle's contraction (stippling) is smaller, and the abdomen and rib cage are linked in a less efficient manner.

Consequently, decreases in $\Delta V_{rc}$ caused by rib-cage retractions during inspiration must be accompanied by a commensurate increase in $\Delta V_{ab}$, if $\Delta V_L$ is to remain constant. In extreme cases, $\Delta V_{ab}$ can in fact be greater than $\Delta V_L$ if $\Delta V_{rc}$ becomes negative. Because $\Delta V_{ab}$ approximates the volume displaced by the diaphragm, the work performed by the muscle is increased markedly by rib-cage distortion without a parallel change in the work done on the lungs. The resultant energy waste may contribute to the poor weight gain and easy diaphragmatic fatigability of small infants suffering from respiratory distress.

## Contractile state of the respiratory muscles

Muscle fatigue (the decrease in contractile force that follows excessive muscle activity) appears to increase the energy needed by respiratory muscles to perform a certain amount of work on the lungs, thereby reducing their efficiency. *Metabolic disturbances* and simple *malnutrition* may have similar effects.

## RESPIRATORY MUSCLE FUNCTION

The respiratory muscles form a heterogeneous group of skeletal muscles the primary function of which is to generate phasic changes in lung volume. Frequently, they are classified as inspiratory or expiratory, depending on whether their contraction results in lung inflation or deflation. The diaphragm is, for instance, a purely inspiratory muscle because, under physiological conditions, it can only generate inspiratory flow. The abdominal wall muscles are, on the other hand, expiratory muscles because their contraction forces air out of the lungs. In humans, only the diaphragm and the intercostal muscles participate regularly in breathing. Other muscles, the primary function of which is not respiratory, are incorporated into the breathing effort when the ventilatory output increases to meet the demands of exercise or fever and when the respiratory drive is stimulated by gas-exchange abnormalities. The most important of these so-called accessory muscles are the scaleni, the sternocleidomastoid, and the abdominal muscles (external and internal obliques, transversus abdominis, and rectus abdominis).

## Actions of the respiratory muscles during normal breathing

Each respiratory muscle, and even different fiber groups within a muscle, makes highly specialized contributions to the motion of the chest wall during breathing. The diaphragm can, in this regard, be considered as composed of two muscles: a costal muscle, composed of the fibers that originate from the inner surfaces of the lower six ribs; and a crural muscle encompassing all the fibers which arise from the first three lumbar vertebrae and the medial and lateral arcuate ligaments. Even in the absence of a significant area of apposition (see above), contraction of the costal fibers expands the rib cage anteriorly and laterally; in contrast, contraction of the crural fibers has no direct expanding effect on the rib cage (in fact, it decreases the antero-posterior diameter of the chest) and serves only to displace the abdominal contents downward.

The chief function of the intercostal muscles is to stiffen the rib cage during inspiration, thereby limiting the inward movement of the soft intercostal tissues in the presence of subatmospheric intrathoracic pressures. When this function is absent (as happens during REM sleep in premature infants), the work that the diaphragm must do to inflate the lungs increases and breathing becomes inefficient (see above). Considered individually, the external intercostal muscles raise the ribs and thus increase lung volume, and, at least for their interosseous portion, the internal intercostal muscles lower the ribs and decrease lung volume.

The abdominal muscles are the main muscles of expiration. Because expiration is normally driven by the recoil accumulated in the lungs and chest wall during inspiration, these muscles do not have a substantial participation in breathing at rest. They become active, however, during coughing, when ventilatory demands are raised, and whenever lung emptying needs to be shortened to limit increases in functional residual capacity during intrathoracic airway obstruction. By virtue of their insertions, the abdominal muscles (particularly the rectus abdominis) pull down the lower ribs and decrease the diameter of the rib cage. At the same time, they raise abdominal pressure and, if the diaphragm is relaxed, pleural pressure. As a result, expiration is accelerated. Paradoxically, abdominal muscle contraction is frequently detected during inspiration in children and adults with respiratory distress. Under such circumstances, the abdominal muscles may act as accessory inspiratory muscles by enhancing the effects of intraabdominal pressure on the diameter of the lower rib cage.

## Transformation of energy into work by the respiratory muscles

Similar to other skeletal muscles, respiratory muscles can obtain energy from both oxidative and glycolytic processes. This is reflected in their heterogeneous fiber composition, which includes fast-twitch glycolytic fibers suitable for short-term actions, oxidative fast-twitch red fibers designed to maintain long-term phasic activities, and slow-twitch oxidative fibers adapted for sustained tonic activity. The relative proportions of these fiber types vary depending on the respiratory muscle in question, the species, and the stage of development. In the human adult, 55 per cent of the diaphragmatic fibers are slow-twitch fibers, the remainder being distributed equally between fast-twitch glycolytic and oxidative fibers. In many species, the proportion of slow fibers is increased during the early postnatal period, a feature that slows down the speed of the muscle's contraction, but may also render it fatigue-resistant. Premature infants, on the other hand, appear to have a decreased number of slow oxidative fibers in their diaphragm and intercostal muscles, and therefore may be more susceptible to respiratory muscle fatigue. Although the exact functional correlation of these histochemical changes remains controversial, there is little doubt that these changes are part of a differentiation process that involves variations in the gene expression of the contractile proteins, sarcoplasmic reticulum, and transverse tubular system.

Despite their glycolytic abilities, respiratory muscles rely primarily on aerobic metabolism for their most important repetitive functions. They are therefore highly dependent on the vascular supply of oxygen and nutrients. Although breathing only accounts for 1–5 per cent of the human body's energy expenditures at rest, the oxygen consumption of the respiratory muscles increases out of proportion with minute ventilation. Moderate ventilatory demands can be met easily by extracting more oxygen from the blood or by increasing diaphragmatic blood flow. More stringent demands, such as those imposed by severe restrictive lung disease or airway obstruction, may exceed the diaphragm's maximum vascular supply. Then the ability of the muscle to rise to the challenge becomes impaired. In situations such as shock and congestive heart failure in which perfusion is limited, even physiological levels of spontaneous ventilation cannot be supported, and respiratory failure ensues.

## Response of the respiratory muscles to mechanical dysfunction: fatigue

The respiratory system responds to the development of mechanical dysfunction by increasing the contraction force of the regular muscles of respiration (diaphragm and intercostal muscles) and, if the dysfunction is severe enough, by recruiting accessory muscles. This process is similar to the one leading to ventilation increases during exercise and is triggered by a combination of chemoreceptor and mechanoreceptor stimuli and supramedullary influences acting on a network of premotor neurons in the medulla. The final result is an increase in the firing rate of already active spinal motor neurons and the activation of previously quiescent spinal motor neurons. Particularly in the presence of substantial workloads, neural activation of the respiratory muscles frequently follows an alternating pattern, which allows fiber or muscle groups periods of rest while other muscles carry the load. It has been proposed that neural apnea in infants represents a similar resting strategy directed at

breaking prolonged periods of increased muscle activity and preventing respiratory muscle fatigue.

In this context, respiratory muscle fatigue can be defined as the situation in which the respiratory muscles become unable to generate sufficient force to support adequate alveolar ventilation. The site of the responsible limiting step or steps remains controversial. Decreases in neural output during loaded breathing have been observed experimentally, but they may represent an adaptive response designed to protect the motor units. Neuromuscular transmission failure, presynaptic or postsynaptic, impaired excitation–contraction coupling, and simple exhaustion of cellular energy resources all probably play a role in the progressive decrease in contraction force observed in patients with prolonged respiratory difficulty.

The detection of respiratory muscle fatigue in infants and children requires a high degree of awareness. A decrease in the frequency of the diaphragmatic electromyogram appears to correlate with the development of decreased contraction force in children and adults, but electromyographic recordings are difficult to perform and interpret. The clinical signs are sometimes subtle and cannot be distinguished from the normal response to a mechanical dysfunction. However, the findings of increased tachypnea with reduced tidal volumes, irregular breathing, and inward movement of the abdominal wall during inspiration are usually an ominous indication. Decreased perfusion, hypoxemia and hypercapnia, malnutrition, and suboptimal configurations of the respiratory muscles (e.g. pulmonary hyperinflation) accelerate the development of fatigue and should therefore raise the clinician's level of concern in the presence of respiratory distress in an infant or child.

## SUMMARY

As the previous discussion establishes, the developing respiratory system has some mechanical disadvantages. The reader, however, should not be left with the impression that infants and children are constantly on the brink of respiratory failure. On the contrary, they have a remarkable capability to compensate for most mechanical disturbances. This capability is based on the maintenance of a large functional reserve. Recognizing when this reserve becomes threatened is perhaps the most important point in the rational management of children with respiratory disease.

## SELECTED READING

Mead J. Mechanical properties of the lungs. *Physiol Rev* 1961; **41**: 281.

Mortola JP. Dynamics of breathing in newborn mammals. *Physiol Rev* 1987; **67**: 187.

Roussos C, Campbell EJM. Respiratory muscle energetics. In: Macklem PT, Mead J, eds. *Handbook of physiology: The respiratory system*. Vol III, Part 2. Bethesda: American Physiological Society, 1986: 481.

# PART THIRTEEN

# *Blood*

**Editors: Charles A.J. Wardrop and Barbara M. Holland**

# 80

# Hematopoiesis and the Lymphoid System

Robert D. Christensen and Kurt R. Schibler

## HEMATOPOIESIS

Each of the cellular elements of blood has a finite life-span and consequently must be continually replaced. The collective process by which new blood cells are generated is termed hematopoiesis. In the "steady state," hematopoiesis proceeds at a relatively fixed pace, constantly maintaining the circulating concentration of each cell type within remarkably narrow limits. Despite this usual stability, the hematopoietic system is highly responsive, with the capacity to markedly up-regulate production of any of the various cell types on demand.

The processes regulating hematopoiesis are necessarily complex. This intricacy is needed not only to maintain equilibrium between cellular production and utilization and to assure the necessary responsiveness to rapidly changing demands for cells, but also to accommodate the unique spans of the various cellular elements. For instance, in adults erythrocytes circulate for about 120 days, platelets for about 10 days, and neutrophils only for hours (steady state $t_{\frac{1}{2}} = 6.5$ hours). Empirically, independent mechanisms would be needed to regulate the production of each variety of blood cell. Indeed, a large and constantly increasing list of hematopoietic growth factors now can be assembled, each with a unique set of actions on clonal development of the various mature blood cell types from hematopoietic progenitors.

## Hematopoietic progenitor cells

A schematized hierarchy of the hematopoietic progenitors is shown in Fig. 80.1. Although the progenitors can be categorized as existing at the various develop-mental stages shown, progress from pluripotent progenitors to mature hemic cells undoubtedly occurs as a continuous process, proceeding through numerous intermediate stages.

Bradley and Metcalf first established the existence of pluripotent, self-renewing, hematopoietic stem cells by showing that transfusion of irradiated mice with marrow cells obtained from normal mice repopulated their entire hematopoietic system. Subsequently, the capacity to culture hematopoietic progenitors in semi-solid media, beginning with the work of Pluznick and Sachs, permitted the categorization, functional analysis, and definition of growth factor requirements of the various hematopoietic progenitors.

Progenitor cells that develop into clones containing neutrophils, macrophages, erythrocytes, and megakaryocytes (and sometimes eosinophils and mast cells) are termed CFU-GEMM (colony forming unit-granulocyte, erythrocyte, macrophage, megakaryocyte). These progenitor cells are categorized as "primitive" on the basis of their pluripotentiality. They appear to have a limited capacity for self-renewal, however, and therefore are not true "stem cells." In contrast to pluripotent progenitors, committed progenitors are those that give rise to colonies containing cells of only one (or sometimes two) types. Examples include BFU-E (burst forming unit-erythrocyte), CFU-E, CFU-GM, CFU-Eo, CFU-Baso, and CFU-Meg.

The more primitive variety of erythroid progenitors, BFU-E, appears to be derived from pluripotent progenitors. BFU-E subsequently differentiate into clones of mature erythroid progenitors, CFU-E (colony forming unit-erythrocyte). Subsequently, under the influence of erythropoietin, CFU-E generate clones of normoblasts. Although BFU-E and CFU-E appear to be two stages in a continuum, they differ in important ways. For instance, BFU-E require factors

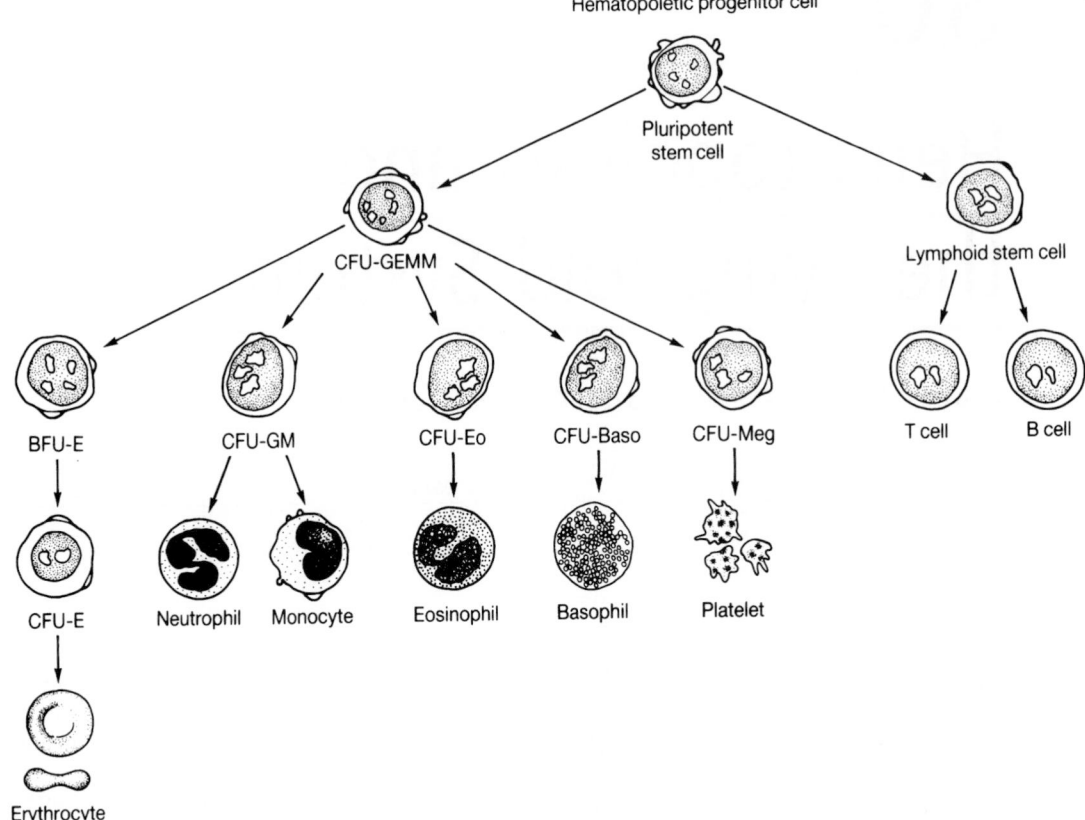

FIGURE 80.1 Pluripotent hematopoietic progenitors (see text) differentiate into either myeloid multipotent progenitors (CFU-GEMM) or lymphoid multipotent progenitors that further clonally differentiate into mature hematopoietic cells. Stages of intermediate progenitors are recognized by the colonies formed from them *in vitro*, as well as their unique sensitivities to recombinant hematopoietic growth factors.

with "burst-promoting" activity (detailed in the next section) in order to develop into CFU-E, while CFU-E do not require such factors to differentiate into clones of normoblasts. BFU-E are found in the blood as well as in the bone marrow, but CFU-E are scarce in blood. (Fetal blood is an exception, particularly blood of extremely preterm infants, which is rich in CFU-E.) Other differences between BFU-E and CFU-E include the large number of normoblasts per mature BFU-E colony (often as many as 10 000 normoblasts/colony) compared with the small number per CFU-E colony (64 to 200–300). Another difference is the length of time required in culture to produce a mature clone of normoblasts from BFU-E (14 days) compared with CFU-E (7 days). Of note, both BFU-E and CFU-E of fetal origin mature into clones of normoblasts in culture more rapidly than do those of adult origin.

Granulocyte-macrophage progenitors (CFU-GM) also appear to be differentiated from pluripotent progenitors, having been restricted in their capacity to produce only granulocytes and macrophages. CFU-GM can differentiate further into cells capable of generating clones of macrophages only (CFU-M) or neutrophils only (CFU-G).

Progenitors with features that are intermediate between those shown in Fig. 80.1 are identified frequently. For instance, colonies are seen that contain neutrophils, macrophages, and normoblasts, but not megakaryocytes. Others contain neutrophils and normoblasts. Any colony that contains a mixture of normoblasts with another variety of cells is referred to as a MIX colony, and thus derived from a progenitor termed CFU-MIX. Such a progenitor might be thought of as intermediate between a CFU-GEMM and a committed progenitor.

The proliferative state of hematopoietic progenitors can be categorized as either quiescent (in the $G_0$ phase of the cell cycle) or as actively cycling (*see* Chapter 2). Further categorization of cycling cells can be accomplished by assessing, during a "flash label" (a 20-min exposure to tritiated thymidine of high specific activity), the proportion of progenitors that are in S phase. The proliferative state, as well as clonogenic maturation, of hematopoietic progenitors appears to be regulated by hematopoietic growth factors.

Pluripotent progenitors (CFU-GEMM and CFU-MIX) obtained from the bone marrow of healthy adults are generally relatively quiescent. In contrast, at least 10–30 per cent of the committed progenitors (such as CFU-E and CFU-GM) are generally in S phase. On this basis it has been proposed that "steady-state" demands are met by the committed progenitors. During a period of increased demand for cells, a greater percentage of committed progenitors will usually be in S phase, and pluripotent progenitors might also be cycling. For instance, during bacterial infection cycling of CFU-MIX as well as CFU-GM increases, and following acute blood loss cycling of BFU-E as well as CFU-E increases.

Unlike the situation in adult marrow, pluripotent progenitors in fetal blood and marrow (and in animals, progenitors in the liver and spleen as well) are actively cycling. For instance, generally less than 5 per cent of CFU-MIX cultured from adult bone marrow are in S phase, compared with 20–30 per cent from fetal blood or marrow. Similarly, as many as 40–60 per cent of CFU-GM from fetal blood or marrow are generally in S phase, compared with 10–30 per cent from adult marrow. This high rate of progenitor cell cycling is consistent with the rapid myeloid (and somatic) growth of the fetus. Rapid cycling of CFU-GM in the uninfected fetus has been interpreted as a potential limitation in capacity to further up-regulate neutrophil production during an infectious challenge. Indeed, in infected newborn rats the percentage of CFU-GM in S phase does not appear to increase substantially from the already high baseline rate. Whether human neonates have a similar limitation is not known. An argument against a limitation as severe as that observed in neonatal rats is that the baseline CFU-GM cycling rate

in uninfected human neonates, although high, is not maximal.

## Hematopoietic growth factors

Recent advances in molecular biology have permitted the production, purification, and characterization of factors that support hematopoiesis *in vitro*. Experiments using such factors have allowed a more sophisticated scrutiny of hematopoietic regulation. Moreover, production of relatively large amounts of these factors has permitted clinical trials in which their *in vivo* actions have been assessed.

Table 80.1 lists the factors known to influence hematopoietic growth and differentiation, their molecular mass, chromosomal location, and the principal varieties of cells that they influence.

One approach to defining the physiological roles of the various hematopoietic growth factors has been to produce mice that are genetically deficient in a specific factor. The technique of homologous recombination in embryonal stem cells has been particularly useful in these "knock-out" endeavors. Using these techniques, murine models for deficiencies of granulocyte colony stimulating factor (G-CSF), granulocyte-macrophage colony stimulating factor (GM-CSF), and macrophage colony stimulating factor (M-CSF) have been reported.

G-CSF-deficient mice are viable, fertile, and superficially healthy, but have chronic neutropenia. They also have a marked reduction in granulocyte, macro-

TABLE 80.1 Hematopoietic growth factors

| FACTOR | MOLECULAR MASS (kD) | CHROMOSOMAL LOCATION | TARGET CELL |
|---|---|---|---|
| Interleukin-1 | 17 | (beta) 2q13–21 | Hepatocyte, endothelial cell |
| | | (alpha) 2q13 | Osteoclast, neutrophil, macrophage, TH2 lymphocyte |
| Interleukin-2 | 15.5 | 4q26–27 | T lymphocyte, cytotoxic lymphocyte |
| Interleukin-3 | 15–30 | 5q23–31 | CFU-GEMM, CFU-MIX, CFU-MEG, CFU-GM, BFU-E, cytotoxic lymphocyte, macrophage |
| Interleukin-4 | 16–20 | 5q31 | T lymphocyte, B lymphocyte |
| Interleukin-5 | 46 (dimer) | 5q31 | CFU-Eo, B lymphocyte |
| Interleukin-6 | 19–21 | 7p15 | CFU-GEMM, CFU-MIX, B lymphocyte, T lymphocyte, fetal CFU-GM, fetal BFU-E, macrophage, hepatocyte, neural cell |
| Interleukin-7 | 25 | 8q12–13 | B lymphocyte |
| Interleukin-8 | 8–10 | 4 | Neutrophil, endothelial cell, T lymphocyte |
| Interleukin-9 | 16 | 5q31–32 | BFU-E, CFU-GEMM, CFU-MIX, fetal CFU-GM |
| Interleukin-10 | 35–40 | 1 | T lymphocyte, B lymphocyte, mast cell |
| Interleukin-11 | 20 | 19q13.3–13.4 | CFU-GEMM, CFU-MIX, fetal BFU-E, T lymphocyte |
| Interleukin-12 | 70–75 (dimer) | – | T lymphocyte |
| Interleukin-13 | 9 | 5q23–31 | Pre-B lymphocyte, macrophage |
| Interleukin-14 | 53 | – | B lymphocyte |
| Interleukin-15 | 14–15 | – | B lymphocyte, T lymphocyte, cytotoxic lymphocyte |
| GM-CSF | 18–30 | 5q23–31 | CFU-GM, CFU-MIX, BFU-E, CFU-GEMM, macrophage, neutrophil |
| G-CSF | 20 | 17q11.2–21 | CFU-G, neutrophil, CFU-MIX, BFU-E, CFU-GEMM |
| M-CSF | 70–90 (dimer) | 5q33.1 | CFU-M, CFU-GM, macrophage, placenta |
| Stem cell factor | 28–35 | 12q4.3–12 | All hematopoietic progenitors |
| Erythropoietin | 34–39 | 7q11–22 | CFU-E, mature BFU-E, fetal BFU-E |
| Thrombopoietin | 35 | 3q26–27 | CFU-MEG, megakaryocytes |

phage, and blast-cell progenitors, a small marrow neutrophil reserve, and a marked impairment in controlling infection. Treatment of the animals with recombinant G-CSF (rG-CSF) completely restores these defects. These observations indicate that G-CSF is indispensable for maintaining the normal balance of neutrophil production during the "steady state," and also for increasing neutrophil production in times of acute need.

The significant overlap in function of certain hematopoietic growth factors is illustrated by the GM-CSF and M-CSF "knock-out" studies. Neither GM-CSF deficiency nor M-CSF deficiency produces animals with markedly abnormal hematopoiesis or impaired survival, but the combination does. GM-CSF-deficient mice have relatively unperturbed baseline hematopoiesis, in terms of the number of circulating hemic cells and the concentrations of hematopoietic progenitors in the various hematopoietic organs. However, they display a non-fatal lung disease characterized by alveolar proteinosis, and a vulnerability for pulmonary infections with a range of bacterial and fungal organisms. M-CSF-deficient mice develop osteopetrosis, are toothless, and have an age-dependent macrophage deficiency. By inbreeding GM-CSF-deficient and M-CSF-deficient mice, animals deficient in both factors have been produced. These mice have reduced survival, repeated bronchopneumonia and lobar pneumonia, severe often fatal alveolar proteinosis, and a marked susceptibility to bacterial infections. Interestingly, mice deficient in GM-CSF and M-CSF maintain normal monocyte/macrophage production and function, indicating that other factors can be used for these functions. Congenital deficiencies of hematopoietic growth factors in humans have not yet been reported.

# Cell-surface receptors for hematopoietic growth factors

All of the hematopoietic growth factors appear to interact with target cells by way of specific cell-surface receptors. Although not all have been identified, the receptors appear, in general, to be members of the superfamily of receptors that couple to guanine nucleotide-binding proteins (G-proteins) (*see* Chapter 2). Little information is available concerning the signal transduction mechanisms resulting from interaction of hematopoietic growth factors with their receptors. Certain inherited and acquired disorders of hematopoiesis likely will be identified eventually as due to defects in hematopoietic growth factor receptors or the subsequent signal transduction mechanisms.

Specific receptors for hematopoietic growth factors were thought to be lineage restricted. For instance, erythropoietin receptors (EPO-R) were thought to be expressed only on cells of the erythroid lineage or on their progenitors. However, EPO-R have been detected on human umbilical vein endothelial cells, human

macrophages, murine liver stromal cells, two rodent cell lines of neural origin, and monocytes obtained from human fetal blood. In general the density of EPO-R on these non-erythroid cells appears to be lower than on erythroid cells. The physiological role of EPO-R on non-erythroid cells is not known.

# Developmental/clinical aspects

Human and animal studies indicate that, compared with adults, neonates have an increased susceptibility to acquiring certain infections and, when infected, have an increased likelihood of developing a severe resultant illness. This susceptibility is considerably more marked in neonates delivered prematurely. Multiple factors appear to contribute to this reduced host defense status of neonates, including hyporesponsiveness of B cells, T cells, and granulocytes, and reduced quantities of granulocytes and their progenitors per kilogram of body weight. Specific defects include delayed maturation of B cells into antibody-producing cells, deficient stimulation of T-cell maturation, and delayed induction of hematopoietic progenitor cell cycling.

Actions of several hematopoietic growth factors, including G-CSF, GM-CSF, interleukin (IL)-6 and IL-8, closely parallel these areas of diminished host defense. For example, the actions of G-CSF include stimulation of myeloid progenitor cycling, clonal development of neutrophils, and enhancement of neutrophil functions such as phagocytosis, superoxide production, and bactericidal activity. Similarly, IL-6 acts to induce antigen-specific antibody production, T-cell maturation, and hematopoietic progenitor cell cycling. Thus, one possible mechanism accounting for a number of the host defense defects in neonates is defective production or action of certain of the hematopoietic growth factors.

## Generation of hematopoietic growth factors by the fetus and neonate

Studies of explanted human fetal cells support the hypothesis that preterm neonates produce certain hematopoietic growth factors poorly. Normal term newborns exhibit diminished production of interferon-γ by leukocytes, decreased GM-CSF production by mononuclear cells, and diminished IL-6 production and decreased *IL-6* gene transcription by explanted monocytes. Preterm neonates exhibit much more severe decreases in IL-6 production by monocytes. Studies of hematopoietic growth factor production *in vivo* during bacterial infection are incomplete, but such studies will be needed to determine the clinical significance of the *in vitro* observations.

In order to interpret the significance of the reduced production of certain hematopoietic growth factors by preterm neonates, information must be obtained regarding the actions of such factors on fetal and neo-natal target cells. For instance, reduced production of G-CSF by fetal marrow stroma during bacterial infection might be completely counterbalanced by a heightened responsiveness of fetal CFU-G to the actions of G-CSF. If diminished production of certain hematopoietic growth factors by fetal cells is a clinically relevant limitation, the mechanism that results in this limitation will also be an important topic for investigation. Such a mechanism might include either "programming" of otherwise fully functional fetal cells by extrinsic factors to produce certain products efficiently and others poorly, or a "developmental defect," such that fetal cells lack a specific capacity to respond to an inflammatory agonist. Potential examples of this include a reduced density of cell-surface receptors capable of interacting with a particular ligand critical to hematopoietic growth factor generation, reduced signal transduction specific for that ligand, a limitation relating to specific gene transcription for that growth factor, diminished message stability, and diminished stability of that protein. Understanding the biology responsible for the diminution in production of certain hematopoietic growth factors by fetal cells is a critical step toward the clinical testing of cytokine-based therapy for infected neonatal subjects.

## Neutrophil production in the fetus and neonate

During bacterial sepsis, newborn mice, rats, dogs, and humans are much more susceptible than adults to developing neutropenia, exhaustion of the marrow neutrophil reserves, and death. The basis for this susceptibility appears to include: (1) lack of rapid up-regulation of neutrophil production during infection, (2) a small neutrophil storage pool per kilogram body weight, and (3) specific defects in neutrophil function, permitting greater bacterial growth and, subsequently, the requirement for more neutrophils than would be needed if the infection was sterilized rapidly.

Whether the development of neutropenia and marrow neutrophil reserve exhaustion could be prevented or treated by administration of hematopoietic growth factors is not known. In part, this depends on such factors as the extent to which neutrophil production can be further increased in infected neonates, the sensitivity of hematopoietic progenitors from infected neonates to recombinant hematopoietic growth factors, and the likelihood of adverse reactions to administration of cytokines. Indeed, studies aimed at assessing the benefits versus risks of administration of recombinant hematopoietic growth factors to infected infants should probably await a better definition of precisely which hematopoietic growth factors are produced poorly by infected preterm neonates. Also, the actions of those specific recombinant growth factors on target cells of neonates should probably be assessed *in vitro* before such trials begin.

## Neutrophil function in the fetus and neonate

Among the many explanations for the unique susceptibility of neonates to overwhelming infection are biochemical, structural, and functional abnormalities of neutrophils. Developmental defects in signal transduction, cell-surface receptor up-regulation and mobility, cytoskeletal rigidity, microfilament contraction, $O_2$ metabolism, and intracellular antioxidant generation have all been described.

Neutrophil–endothelial cell interactions, which form the basis of neutrophil adhesion, are mediated by interacting sets of adhesion molecules and chemoattractants (*see also* page 694). As the inflammatory process begins, neutrophils flowing in postcapillary venules undergo a slowing, mediated by substances termed selectins. Adhesion of neutrophils to the vessel wall then occurs by way of interaction of the CD11/CD18 integrins on neutrophils to ligands such as intercellular adhesion molecule 1 (ICAM-1) located on endothelial cells. Finally, transmigration of neutrophils into the tissues occurs, a process which requires a chemotactic stimulus and engagement of platelet endothelial cell adhesion molecule 1 (PECAM-1). The sequence of maturation of this system during human gestation, and the results of incomplete development on neutrophil function of preterm infants, remain areas of investigation. Future therapeutic approaches to control unwanted inflammation might include targeted interruption of one or more of these processes.

## Transplacental passage of hematopoietic growth factors

Studies in sheep suggest that no placental transfer of erythropoietin occurs. However, two groups recently observed that after administration of large doses of recombinant erythropoietin (rEPO) to pregnant rats at term increased erythropoietin activity was present in the fetal blood. No studies have been published that address the issue of transplacental transfer of erythropoietin in humans.

Scanty evidence in mice and humans suggests that G-CSF, at least in small amounts, can cross from the maternal to the fetal circulations. Recombinant G-CSF given to pregnant rats subsequently is detected in the fetal circulation. Although the transplacental transfer is relatively poor, in one animal study it was sufficient to increase fetal neutrophil function and production and to increase the survival of pups subsequently exposed to group B streptococci. The mechanism and physiological relevance of transplacental passage of rEPO and rG-CSF in human parturients are topics of current investigation.

## Clinical use of recombinant hematopoietic growth factors in perinatal medicine

Large clinical trials on three continents have shown that treatment with rEPO can reduce transfusion requirements in very low birth weight infants (*see* page 869). Some studies have administered rEPO during the first days after birth, in order to determine whether this reduces transfusion requirements that result predominantly from phlebotomy losses. Other studies have administered rEPO after 2–4 weeks of age, to determine whether this would reduce the transfusion requirements that result from the hyporegenerative anemia of prematurity. Both approaches have been effective; however, no long-term evaluations have been published.

Animal and clinical studies indicate that, during bacterial infection, neonates do not generate G-CSF and GM-CSF as efficiently as adults. Similarly, *in vitro* studies of G-CSF generation by macrophages show relatively poor G-CSF production by cells obtained from preterm neonates, generation of higher quantities and in a more prompt fashion by macrophages obtained from term neonates, and rapid and prompt production of G-CSF by macrophages obtained from adults. Neutrophils from newborn infants appear to express functional G-CSF and GM-CSF receptors, and have about the same density and binding characteristics as neutrophils from adults. Recombinant G-CSF and rGM-CSF have been administered to preterm neonates in a limited number of published trials. From those studies, it appears that preterm neonates respond to rG-CSF and rGM-CSF administration in a manner similar to adults, i.e. with a dose-dependent increase in neutrophil (G-CSF) and neutrophil and monocyte (GM-CSF) production and function. Whether either of these potential treatments will have any clinical utility in preventing or treating infections in neonates is not yet clear. The risks, benefits, and long-term effects of rG-CSF and rGM-CSF administration to neonates have not been defined. Neither is it clear whether combinations of immunotherapy, such as hematopoietic growth factors and preformed antibody, will be of clinical value.

## LYMPHOID SYSTEM

The goals of lymphopoiesis are to produce cells that possess the capacity to: (1) distinguish between foreign and self antigens, (2) facilitate elimination of antigens determined to be foreign, and (3) maintain a memory of previous foreign antigen exposures. To accomplish these tasks, lymphoid development proceeds along two pathways, culminating in the formation of B lymphocytes involved in antibody-mediated immunity, and T lymphocytes responsible predominantly for cell-mediated immunity.

## T lymphocytes (*see* also Chapter 85)

### Ontogeny

Differentiation of T-cell precursors into functional T lymphocytes involves interaction between non-lymphoid and lymphoid elements of the thymus. The thymus develops relatively early in humans. Morphologically, the primitive thymic rudiment formed from the ectoderm of the third branchial cleft and the endoderm of the third branchial pouch is evident at approximately 4 weeks' gestation. These structures move caudally, and at week 8 fuse in the midline. Distinct cortical and medullary regions are identified at 14 weeks, and by 16 weeks Hassall bodies are present and the thymus assumes the histological configuration seen postnatally.

Before week 7, T-cell precursors, identified by monoclonal antibodies to early T-cell markers CD7 and CD45, are present in the yolk sac, neck, upper thorax, and liver. Between 7 and 8.5 weeks' gestation they migrate to the thymic rudiment, an event that appears to be regulated by chemotactic factors elaborated from the thymic epithelium. These cells colonizing the thymus differentiate into T-cell colonies expressing markers of T-cell lineage (CD2, CD4, CD8, and WT31) if cultured *in vitro* with T-cell-conditioned medium and IL-2. However, they retain the capacity to differentiate into cells of myeloid lineage if provided with an appropriate environment.

Lymphoid cells from the thymus at 8.5 weeks react with antibodies to CD2 (sheep erythrocyte rosette receptor). Arrest of T-lymphocyte maturation at this stage is identified in some cases of severe combined immunodeficiency disease. At 8.5 weeks thymocytes fail to react with monoclonal antibodies directed against CD3, CD5, CD4, CD8, and A1G3-p80; however, at 10 weeks these antigens are present. Thus, between 8.5 and 10 weeks' gestation, thymocytes develop from stage I ($CD7^+$, $CD2^+$) to stage II ($CD4^+$, $CD8^+$, and $CD3^+$).

### Generation of diversity

During maturation, T cells are programmed to recognize antigenic determinants in the context of the self major histocompatibility (MHC) antigens. T lymphocytes of the CD4 population recognize antigens in conjunction with MHC class II molecules, while CD8 T cells recognize antigens in conjunction with MHC class I molecules. To acquire these capacities, prothymocytes migrate to the thymus and undergo rapid division and rearrangement in the T-cell receptor gene. There are two sets of the receptor gene, $\gamma\delta$ and $\alpha\beta$, which encode different receptors. Each gene comprises multiple components that rearrange; these are designated as diversity (D) sequences, variable (V) sequences, joining (J) sequences, and constant (C) sequences of DNA. Successful rearrangement of genes encoding $\gamma\delta$ stops rearrangement of $\alpha\beta$ genes. Likewise, $\alpha\beta$ rearrangement precludes further $\gamma\delta$ rearrangement. The tremendous diversity of T-cell receptors is generated through rearrangement and joining of these gene elements. The most common T-cell receptor lineage is the $\alpha\beta$ heterodimer pair. Following successful rearrangement of these genes, thymocytes stop proliferating.

Peripheral T-cell maturation and proliferation is influenced by exposure to antigens and soluble factors. Exogenous antigen encountered by antigen-presenting cells is processed and presented to T cells expressing the appropriate MHC determinants. The signal thereby delivered induces IL-2 secretion by T cells, which initiates a cascade of events leading to proliferation. A second signal initiating activation of T cells is IL-1.

Recognition of a foreign antigen by accessory cells such as macrophages initiates the following chain of events culminating in T-cell activation. The macrophage processes the antigen and re-expresses this modified antigen on its surface. Additionally, the macrophage secretes IL-1 in response to the antigenic stimulus. The T cells recognize the foreign antigen in the context of their appropriate MHC antigen.

Soluble factors influencing T-cell function include the interleukins and interferons. IL-1, which is produced by monocytes and thymic epithelial cells, has varied effects on T cells, B cells, monocytes, neutrophils, fibroblasts, and a host of other cells. Its chief effect on T cells is to induce IL-2 production. IL-2, also called T-cell growth factor, induces proliferation and maturation of T cells, B cells, and natural killer (NK) cells. The interferons are a group of glycoproteins produced in response to viral infection and by other immune stimulatory events. Three classes of interferons have been characterized. Interferon-$\alpha$ and interferon-$\beta$ are produced by leukocytes and by fibroblasts in response to viral infection. Interferon-$\gamma$ is synthesized by T cells in response to antigenic stimulation. Interferons induce a number of cell membrane effects including augmentation of MHC I and II expression, and up-regulation of IgG receptors. Interferons stimulate increased macrophage cytotoxicity, increase cytotoxic activity of NK cells, and increase the reactivity of cytotoxic T cells. Paradoxical effects of interferon have been reported with respect to its effect on lymphocyte proliferation and immunoglobulin production.

## Alterations in T-cell function

Congenital T-cell defects are relatively rare, e.g. *DiGeorge syndrome* (congenital thymic aplasia). More commonly, T-cell defects are combined with defects in humoral immunity. This category includes *severe combined immunodeficiency (SCID)*, *Wiskott–Aldrich syndrome*, *ataxia telangiectasia*, and *adenosine deaminase deficiency*. These diseases generally become clinically apparent during infancy due to repeated infections with a wide variety of microorganisms.

Acquired abnormalities in T-cell function are relatively common, occurring in conjunction with *viral infections*, *malignancy*, *immunosuppressive drug administration*, *renal failure*, *autoimmune diseases*, *human immunodeficiency virus (HIV) infection*, and *malnutrition*. Transient T-cell dysfunction often accompanies infections such as *measles*, *rubella*, and *Mycoplasma*. Quantitative and functional abnormalities in the suppresser T-cell population are observed in a variety of autoimmune disorders.

Infection with HIV causes profound derangements in T-cell-associated immunity. Marked reduction in CD4 (helper/inducer) T-cell numbers and in T-cell function render these patients susceptible to a variety of microorganisms and to malignancy.

## T-cell function in the fetus and neonate

Mitogen-responsive T cells are identifiable in the peripheral blood and spleen by week 12 of gestation and increase in number until approximately 20 weeks, at which time they approach numbers seen at term. While the proportion of T cells in the blood at term has been reported to be low in some studies and normal in others, their absolute numbers generally exceed adult levels due to a relative lymphocytosis. Response to the mitogens phytohemagglutinin and concanavalin A is diminished in very low birth weight infants, but is normal or increased in term infants.

While T-cell numbers and mitogen sensitivity are relatively normal in term neonates, a number of functions are deficient, including cytotoxic effector functions of T cells and NK cells, lymphokine production, and regulation of B-cell function. T-cell-mediated cytotoxicity requires sensitization followed by cell lysis. Cell-mediated lympholysis has been detected as early as 18 weeks' gestation. However, in term infants it is only 50 per cent of adult levels. Similarly, NK cell function has been demonstrated early in gestation (9 weeks); however, NK activity and cell numbers are decreased at birth.

Production of some lymphokines by fetal and neonatal T cells appears to be normal, while others are diminished. Normal production of IL-2 and IL-2 receptor have been reported, but production of other lymphokines is defective. Among these are interferon-$\gamma$, lymphocyte-derived chemotactic factor, and macrophage-activating factor.

Immunoregulatory functions of neonatal T cells have been studied, particularly with regard to interaction with B cells. The impaired capacity of human newborns to produce specific immunoglobulins despite normal numbers of B cells in peripheral lymphoid organs and in the blood is at least in part due to interaction between T cells and B cells. Experiments in which neonatal T cells were cultured with adult B cells demonstrated suppression of B-cell proliferation and immunoglobulin secretion. Conversely, when adult T cells were coincubated with neonatal B cells, the B cells were transformed into plasma cells capable of producing immunoglobulins including IgA and IgG, although at lesser quantities than similar studies involving adult B cells. Although a number of investigators have identified increased suppressor activity in neonatal cord blood, controversy remains as to the cellular or humoral nature of this suppression.

## B lymphocytes (*see* also chapter 84)

### Ontogeny

Pluripotent stem cells in the fetal liver and bone marrow give rise to pre-B cells identified by intracytoplasmic IgM. These B-cell precursors appear first in the fetal liver at 8 weeks' gestation. By 10 weeks' gestation IgM surface receptors are detectable. Between 10 and 12 weeks, clones of immature B cells segregate and develop isotype specificity (i.e. IgE, IgG, IgM, etc.). By 15–18 weeks the absolute number and proportion of B cells expressing each of the different immunoglobulin isotypes reaches adult numbers; however, immunoglobulin secretion remains limited.

### Generation of diversity

The molecular basis for generation of antibody diversity results from extensive rearrangement of genetic information encoding heavy-chain variable ($V_H$), diversity ($D_H$), and joining ($J_H$) regions and light chain variable ($V_L$) and joining ($J_L$) regions. Heavy-chain variable and constant genes are located on chromosome 14 in humans. Genes encoding $\lambda$ light chains are located on chromosome 2, and those encoding $\kappa$ light chains are on chromosome 22. There are approximately 1000 heavy-chain variable regions, 20 diversity regions, and six joining segments. Heavy-chain diversity generated by DNA excision and splicing of these elements would account for one million antigenic determinants. Light-chain diversity occurring in a similar manner also accounts for about one million combinations. Thus, combinatorial joining of heavy and light chain products of these genetic rearrangements forms a repertoire of complete immunoglobulin molecules capable of recognizing approximately one billion antigenic specificities. Somatic mutations occurring during the rearrangement of these elements further expand this array of antibody determinants.

### B-cell development

During the pre-B cell stage, DNA rearrangements, i.e. joining of $V_H D_H J_H$ elements, occur that culminate in assembly of a complete heavy-chain variable gene, termed the $\mu$ gene. Expression of this gene produces $\mu$ chains evident in the cytoplasm of pre-B cells. The absence of light-chain production at this stage precludes formation of complete immunoglobulin molecules. The next stage of maturation, the early B cell, is marked by assembly and expression of light-chain genes. The $\mu$ and light chains are assembled into complete IgM molecules, which are expressed on the cell surface. The final stage of B-cell maturation is distinguished by secretion of immunoglobulin molecules. Interaction with T cells and exposure to antigens are integral in maturation of B cells into activated B cells or plasma cells. This transition requires RNA splicing to express secretory exons preferentially. Switching of heavy-chain isotypes, regulated by the T cell, also occurs at this stage of development.

### Antibody response

Following initial exposure to an antigen there is a 10–14 day delay before appearance of specific antibody in the circulation. During this primary response to an antigen, the predominant immunoglobulin class is IgM. Upon subsequent exposure to the same antigen, an antibody response of far greater magnitude and consisting predominantly of IgG isotype occurs within 4 days. This secondary response is initiated by binding of the foreign antigen to long-lived memory B cells expressing specific antigen receptors on their surface.

The antibody response is a regulated process involving interaction between macrophages, T cells, and B cells. During the initial phase of this response the antigen is contacted by cells of the monocyte/macrophage system within the spleen and lymph nodes. The antigen is processed by these antigen-presenting cells and displayed on the cell surface in conjunction with MHC antigens to facilitate recognition by T cells. The dual signal, antigen plus MHC determinants, is required for T-cell interaction but not B-cell interaction with an antigen. The second phase (proliferative phase) of the antibody response involves both cellular interaction and response to lymphokines. Direct interaction between T cells and B cells enables the B cell: (1) to differentiate into an antibody-producing plasma cell, (2) to become a long-term memory B cell, or (3) to proliferate, forming clones of antigen-sensitive cells. In addition to direct cellular interactions, B cells are influenced by exposure to lymphokines elaborated by T cells. Activated T cells release IL-4, which induces proliferation of antigen-specific B cells and up-regulates the expression of IL-6 receptors on B cells. In addition, T cells secrete IL-6, which induces B cells to differentiate into antibody-producing plasma cells. The final stage of the antibody response involves production and secretion of specific antibodies.

### Developmental aspects of B-cell function

Immunoglobulin synthesis by the fetus is limited, constituting primarily IgM. The fetus acquires circulating levels of maternal IgG through placental transport.

This transplacental acquisition begins at approximately 12 weeks. Maternal IgG renders the infant relatively protected from many viral and bacterial diseases during the first 4–6 months of postnatal life. However, infants born prematurely, particularly those delivered before 30 weeks' gestation, generally do not receive sufficient quantities of maternal IgG to provide the same level of protection.

Following birth, serum concentrations of IgG fall gradually, due to catabolism of maternal IgG, to 300–500 mg/dL by 4 months of age. This *physiological hypogammaglobulinemia* is more protracted in infants born prematurely. Significant IgG production generally begins at 4 months of age and increases gradually over the first 10 years. By 1 year of age the infant's serum IgG concentrations are approximately 60 per cent of adult levels.

The capacity for IgM production is intact *in utero*. In fact, during congenital infection the fetus produces IgM at levels usually exceeding 20 mg/dL. After birth, production of IgM precedes that of IgG. The majority of antibodies to enteric Gram-negative bacteria are of IgM isotype, and production of IgM accelerates during the first week of life as colonization of the gastrointestinal tract occurs. IgM synthesis reaches 80 per cent of adult levels by 1 year of age. IgA, IgD, and IgE are not transplacentally acquired. Synthesis of these immunoglobulins increases slowly, approaching adult levels by about 15 years of age.

## SELECTED READING

Albelda SM, Smith CW, Ward PA. Adhesion molecules and inflammatory injury. *FASEB J* 1994; **8**: 504.

Cairo MS. Therapeutic implications of dysregulated colony-stimulating factor expression in neonates. *Blood* 1993; **82**: 2269.

Christensen RD. Hematopoiesis in the fetus and neonate. *Pediatr Res* 1989; **26**: 531.

Demetri GD, Griffin JD. Granulocyte colony-stimulating factor and its receptor. *Blood* 1991; **78**: 2791.

Gillan ER, Christensen RD, Suen Y *et al*. A randomized, placebo-controlled trial of recombinant human granulocyte colony-stimulating factor administration in newborn infants with presumed sepsis: significant induction of peripheral and bone marrow neutrophilia. *Blood* 1994; **84**: 1427.

Lieschke GL, Grail D, Hodgson G *et al*. Mice lacking granulocyte colony-stimulating factor have chronic neutropenia, granulocyte and macrophage progenitor cell deficiencies, and impaired neutrophil mobilization. *Blood* 1994; **84**: 1737.

Maier RF, Oblanden M, Scigalla P *et al*. The effect of epoietin beta (recombinant human erythropoietin) on the need for transfusion in very-low-birth-weight infants. *N Engl J Med* 1994; **330**: 1173.

Metcalf D. Review: Hematopoietic regulators: redundance or subtlety? *Blood* 1993; **82**: 3515.

Nathan DG. Regulation of hematopoiesis. *Pediatr Res* 1990; **27**: 423.

Schibler KR, Liechty KW, White WW, Christensen RD. Production of granulocyte colony-stimulating factor *in vitro* by monocytes from preterm and term neonates. *Blood* 1993; **82**: 2478.

Shannon KM, Keith JF, Mentzer WC *et al*. Recombinant human erythropoietin stimulates erythropoiesis and reduces erythrocyte transfusion in very low birth weight preterm infants. *Pediatrics* 1995; **95**: 1.

Sieff CA. Hematopoietic growth factors. *J Clin Invest* 1987; **79**: 1549.

Strauss RG. Erythropoietin and neonatal anemia. *N Engl J Med* 1994; **330**: 1227.

# 81

# Red-Cell Physiology

## Charles A.J. Wardrop, Barbara M. Holland and J.G. Jones

Oxygen is transported as a complex with hemoglobin (*see* also Chapter 75), which is contained within a flexible red blood cell – the erythrocyte. Adequate production of healthy erythrocytes is essential for proper tissue oxygenation as these cells determine the concentration of hemoglobin, control hemoglobin–$O_2$ affinity, and contribute to both blood volume and viscosity.

## ERYTHROPOIESIS

Erythrocytes develop from pluripotent stem cells, which are capable of both replication and differentiation to a wide spectrum of blood cells including red cells, granulocytes, monocytes, and megakaryocytes/platelets (*see* Fig. 80.1). The earliest recognizable red blood cell is the normoblast, which matures, without further replication, to a reticulocyte, and finally becomes an erythrocyte. The normoblast is preceded by other cell lines that, although committed to becoming red cells, are still capable of replication. These are represented *ex vivo* by the burst forming unit-erythrocyte (BFU-E) and colony forming unit-erythrocyte (CFU-E). *In utero*, erythropoiesis begins in the yolk sac, but this function migrates to the liver at about 6 weeks' gestation and ultimately to the bone marrow at about 20 weeks' gestation. Blood serves as the intermediary medium for this transfer, and blood from premature neonates still contains measurable numbers of hematopoietic progenitor cells (Table 81.1).

### Erythropoietin

The maturation of these red cell precursors, in neonates and adults, is controlled by the hormone erythropoietin (EPO), which binds to specific receptor sites in the membrane. If the receptor sites are not complexed with EPO, then the progenitor cells do not survive. In general the responsiveness to EPO is inversely related to the ability of the progenitor cells to replicate. Hence

TABLE 81.1 Numbers of stem cells in cord blood from preterm and term infants.

| GESTATIONAL AGE (weeks) | CFU-GM | | CFU-E | |
|---|---|---|---|---|
| | (per $10^5$ LDNAs) | (per mL) | (per $10^5$ LDNAs) | (per mL) |
| 25–31 | 175 | 10 000 | 4200 | 21 000 |
| 32–36 | 75 | 4 000 | 100 | 6500 |
| 38–41 | 35 | 3 000 | 125 | 11 000 |

LDNAs, low-density non-adherent cells.
(Adapted from Clapp DW, Baley JE, Gerson SL. *J Lab Clin Med* 1989; **113**: 422, with permission.)

BFU-E are very proliferative cells but are not very responsive to EPO; in contrast, CFU-E are less able to replicate but are entirely dependent on EPO for further maturation to normoblasts. EPO, a glycoprotein containing about 30 per cent carbohydrate, is produced in fetal liver but largely in adult kidney, although adults retain some potential for hepatic synthesis. EPO synthesis is regulated by blood $P_{O_2}$, and the sensor in adults is believed to be a heme protein synthesized largely, but not exclusively, in the kidney. Like hemoglobin, this protein is thought to be an allosteric molecule that exists in two separate conformations, corresponding to oxygenated and deoxygenated forms, the latter postulated to stimulate EPO synthesis. EPO concentrations peak about 24 hours following acute blood loss. The kinetics of EPO synthesis are insensitive to the degree of hypoxia, suggesting that the sensor "flips" from low to high saturation with $O_2$ over a narrow range of concentration of the gas. This behavior is entirely consistent with the view that the sensor is an allosteric protein with a sigmoidal binding curve for $O_2$. The deoxygenated form of the sensor is believed to enhance EPO synthesis by stimulating the *EPO* gene, and it may also stabilize the resulting mRNA. The consequence of this sensitive control is an inverse relationship between hematocrit and the mean plasma concentration of EPO (Table 81.2), but there can be a 10-fold difference in measured EPO at any hematocrit. This individual variability stems from the complex relationships between plasma $Po_2$ and a variety of interrelated physiological processes. Hence, in addition to red cell numbers, the tissue $Po_2$ depends on other factors such as cardiopulmonary function, blood volume, hemoglobin concentration, hemoglobin–$O_2$ affinity, and $O_2$ consumption. In response to anemic hypoxia, cardiac output is increased, and there are compensatory changes in hemoglobin–$O_2$ affinity and interorgan distribution of blood (see below). Each of these physiological functions has a separate $O_2$ sensor with its own unique response time. Although these different control mechanisms are interrelated, it is not surprising that there is considerable individual variation in the relationship between EPO concentration and hematocrit, which is just one hematological variable measured at a single moment in time.

The *EPO* gene has been isolated, copied, cloned, and expressed in a biologically active form in Chinese hamster ovarian cells. This recombinant human EPO (rhEPO) has been used therapeutically, at doses of 50–150 U/kg three times per week, with spectacular success as replacement therapy in patients with *anemia associated with renal failure*. Larger doses of 600 U/kg three times per week have been used to facilitate therapeutic venesection in iron overload and to provide blood for later autologous transfusion. Such pharmacological doses can also promote red cell production in patients with mild to severe anemia, but the response is variable and the proper dosage requires further investigation.

## EPO after term and preterm birth

The increase in plasma $Po_2$ after birth switches off EPO production and concentrations decline, with a half-life of about 4 hours. In term infants, red blood cell numbers then decline more gradually, from a mean count of $5.4 \times 10^{12}$/L of blood at birth to a nadir of $3.4 \times 10^{12}$/L at 7 weeks, rising again to $3.7 \times 10^{12}$/L at 12 weeks; this is then maintained by renewed and balanced EPO synthesis. The timing of these maturational processes is not affected by preterm delivery.

Anemia, associated with low EPO, is seen in children with renal failure and in preterm infants. The former reflects failure of synthesis due to renal damage and can be treated with recombinant EPO (rEPO).

The *anemia of the preterm infant* represents "immaturity" of the hormonal response, but evidence is growing that this may also respond to higher pharmacological doses of rEPO. In this context, it is pertinent to note that an infant growing from 1 kg to 3 kg requires at least a further 90 mL of red blood cells, and this degree of synthesis demands adequate nutritional and hematinic support. A reserve capacity, a supranormal rate of erythropoiesis, is seen in experimental animals but not in preterm infants treated with rEPO, e.g. from birth to 6 weeks of age. In untreated infants, erythropoiesis has ceased and its rate can be stimulated by thrice-weekly administration of subcutaneous rEPO to about normal values but not beyond. The effectiveness of rEPO is insufficient to offset the need for donor blood transfusions during intensive clinical management in the first 4–6 weeks after birth when phlebotomy losses are heaviest. Thereafter, refractory early anemia of prematurity is alleviated by rEPO but the overall effect, with present schedules, is estimated to reduce transfusion needs by 10–20 per cent. Limitations of the efficacy of rEPO in this clinical situation are associated with inordinate phlebotomy losses and the inhibitory effect of infections and other inflammatory problems on rEPO stimulation of erythropoiesis. Losses of hematopoietic stem cells and progenitors with the circulating blood will also reduce the efficacy of rEPO therapy. Again nutritional support, particularly with iron and proteins, is essential for effective erythropoiesis and nutrition is difficult to optimize in sick infants. Further work is needed to define better the indications for rEPO in preterm infants but those of less than 32 weeks' gestational age may benefit from a reduced need for donor blood transfusion for signs of the early anemia of prematurity. Allowing placental transfusion at birth, in addition to present management with surfactant when needed, represents the best opportunity for avoiding blood transfusion after preterm delivery (see below). This practice will ameliorate respiratory distress syndrome and hence the need for respiratory support and concomitant phlebotomy losses.

## HEMOGLOBIN AND O₂ TRANSPORT

## Genetics of hemoglobin synthesis

The decline in hemoglobin (Hb, Hgb) concentration after birth is accompanied by a change in the type of circulating hemoglobin. During human development, six genetic variants of hemoglobin are produced. Each complete protein is a tetramer made from two pairs of identical dimers, and each dimer contains one α-like subunit (ζ or α) combined with one β-like subunit (ε or γ or β or δ). The α-like globins are coded

TABLE 81.2 Erythropoietin concentrations and hematocrit

| HEMATOCRIT | EPO CONCENTRATION (mU/mL) |
|---|---|
| 45 | 10–20 |
| 30–45 | 20–200 |
| 20–30 | 200–2000 |
| Transfusion-dependent | 2000–20000 |

Adapted from Erslev AJ. *Semin Hematol* 1991; **28**: 2, with permission.

by genes on chromosome 16, while β-like globins are coded by genes on chromosome 11. Adult hemoglobin (HbA) is composed of two α–β dimers with a minor form (HbA$_2$, < 5 per cent of total circulating hemoglobin) containing ε globins in place of β. The major fetal form of hemoglobin (HbF) is composed of two α–γ dimers and is first produced at about 6 weeks' gestation; prior to that, three separate embryonic proteins are produced from dimers of ζ–ε (hemoglobin Gower 1), ζ–γ (hemoglobin Portland), or α–ε (hemoglobin Gower 2). HbF is itself heterogeneous with 75 per cent of the γ globin (G-γ) having glycine in position 136, while the remainder (A-γ) contains alanine in this position. In functional terms, both forms of HbF are identical and are usually considered as one. The switching from HbF to HbA synthesis begins *in utero* at 34 weeks' gestation and proceeds with a half-life of about 6 weeks. This is not altered by preterm delivery but can be delayed by maternal hypoxia or by *diabetes* and in *infants who are small for gestational age*. In term infants at birth, 60 per cent of hemoglobin is HbF; this declines to below 1 per cent over the first year of life. The switching from HbF to HbA synthesis changes the affinity of the hemoglobin for O$_2$ with important consequences in terms of O$_2$ delivery. An understanding of these changes in O$_2$ affinity requires a brief description of the quaternary molecular structure of human hemoglobin.

## Structure and function of hemoglobin

All hemoglobins exist in two different quaternary structures (tense or *T-state* and relaxed or *R-state*) that are linked by a reversible equilibrium. The R-state has an affinity for O$_2$ 100-fold higher than that of the T-state and, in the absence of O$_2$, the ratio of T/R is $1 \times 10^5$. Thus, as O$_2$ binds to hemoglobin, the equilibrium shifts to give a higher concentration of the high-affinity R-state, and this accounts for the sigmoidal hemoglobin–O$_2$ binding curve. The affinity of hemoglobin for O$_2$ can be modified by altering the equilibrium between the T and R states of the protein.

It is instructive to examine the bonds that stabilize both the R-state and T-state of hemoglobin and pay particular attention to those that are present in one state but not the other.

The subunits of the R-state are held together by hydrophobic interactions between unlike subunits. There are no α–α nor β–β links. The major interactions involve some 35 amino acids and link α to β subunits. They are termed α$_1$/β$_1$ interactions and are identical with α$_2$/β$_2$ contact areas. These bonds stabilize the basic α/β dimer that is duplicated to form the intact tetramer. These dimers are linked by smaller, but significant, hydrophobic interactions between α and β subunits that involve some 19 amino acids and are commonly referred to as the α$_1$/β$_2$ contact (α$_2$/β$_1$ is identical). The same α$_1$/β$_1$ contacts are found in the

T-state as they are not significantly altered by O$_2$ binding. However, the α$_1$/β$_2$ contact is altered in the T-state, being shifted in position and slightly reduced in magnitude. This relative movement of the two dimers is primarily stabilized by eight extra electrostatic bonds that are only found in the T-state (Fig. 81.1).

Since the binding of O$_2$ favors the R-state of hemoglobin, it follows that this process involves the breaking of these bonds and they are worthy of more detailed attention. All eight electrostatic bonds involve the C-terminal amino acid residues of each globin chain. These amino acids are arginine (α) or histidine (β), which have positive side-chains and contribute one negative and one positive charge to separate electrostatic bonds. The penultimate amino acid in each subunit is the hydrophobic tyrosine, which is sandwiched between two helical segments of the same subunit and serves to anchor the C-terminal residue in a favorable position to form two new electrostatic bonds with other charged groups in the protein. Hence, in total, each globin chain contributes one extra hydrophobic interaction and two new electrostatic bonds that stabilize the T-state of hemoglobin. As these bonds are not apparent in the R-state, and this form predominates in the presence of excess O$_2$, they must be broken when O$_2$ is bound to the protein. There are three important questions to answer.

- What is the trigger that causes the C-terminal region to move and breaks the extra bonds that stabilize the T-state?
- Why does the binding of O$_2$ improve with increasing saturation of hemoglobin with O$_2$, i.e. why is the binding curve sigmoidal?
- Why is the affinity of the R-state for O$_2$ higher than that of the T-state?

First, in the T-state of hemoglobin, the Fe(II) lies out of the plane of the porphyrin ring because of the large

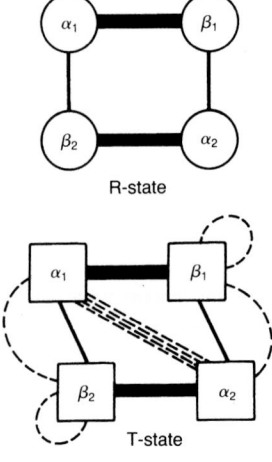

FIGURE 81.1 Schematic structure for R-state and T-state hemoglobin. Solid lines represent hydrophobic interactions. Dotted lines represent electrostatic interactions.

radius of the iron atom that exists in the high spin state when coordinated with four nitrogens of the porphyrin ring and one nitrogen of the proximal histidine in the globin subunit. When the sixth coordination position is occupied by $O_2$, the Fe(II) converts to a low-spin state and contracts in size. This allows the $O_2$ to "pull" the Fe into the plane of the porphyrin ring (Fig. 81.2). This movement involves the attached histidine and hence the remainder of the polypeptide chain. This initiates the conformational change of T-state to R-state.

Second, the conformational change results in a closing of the gap between the helical regions that "anchor" the penultimate tyrosine. The tyrosine is therefore expelled along with the C-terminal basic amino acid – this weakens two of the electrostatic bonds that served to stabilize the T-state. The equilibrium between the two conformational states then shifts towards the R-state. As each $O_2$ binds, two new electrostatic bonds and one hydrophobic interaction are weakened and there is a further shift in the T–R equilibrium. Each new $O_2$ molecule "sees" more of the hemoglobin in the R-state, which has a higher affinity for $O_2$ than the T-state. Thus the affinity of the equilibrium mixture of T and R states for $O_2$ increases with increasing saturation.

Third, the binding of $O_2$ to the T-state of hemoglobin involves large conformational changes as outlined above and is therefore energetically unfavorable. In contrast, binding to the R-state requires no such investment of energy and is therefore easier. There is also a change in the orientation of the heme in the R-state that makes it easier for the $O_2$ to approach the Fe(II).

Compounds that bind to the T-state will inhibit $O_2$ binding and there are three important physiological inhibitors. $H^+$ ions and $CO_2$ are important extra-erythrocytic modulators of binding, and both decrease $O_2$ affinity when blood moves from the lungs to the tissues, thereby enhancing $O_2$ release. An increase in pH results in an increase in $O_2$ affinity by weakening the electrostatic bonds that stabilize the T-state (alkaline Bohr effect). A more long-term modulator of hemoglobin–$O_2$ affinity is provided by the intraerythrocytic metabolite 2,3-bisphosphoglycerate (BPG) (2,3-diphosphoglycerate, 2,3DPG). Hypoxic or anemic hypoxia is often compensated for by an increase in BPG with a resulting decrease in hemoglobin–$O_2$ affi-

nity. In contrast, a decrease in plasma pH decreases the rate of BPG production and increases the affinity of hemoglobin for $O_2$. This effect is seen in *diabetic ketoacidosis* or in bank blood stored at low pH. Fetal blood has a higher affinity for $O_2$ than adult blood, again related to the physiological function of BPG. HbF has a lower affinity for BPG than HbA and hence, at a given concentration of BPG, a higher affinity for $O_2$. The $O_2$ tension required to half-saturate blood ($P_{50}$) at pH 7.4 and $P_{CO_2}$ of 40 mmHg (5.33 kPa) is 27 mmHg (3.6 kPa) in adults and 20 mmHg (2.67 kPa) in preterm infants with 90 per cent HbF. These various differences in hemoglobin–$O_2$ affinity are generally too small to affect $O_2$ loading in the lungs but make a significant contribution to $O_2$ release in the tissues (see below).

Compounds that bind to the R-state enhance $O_2$ binding and include carbon monoxide (CO) and nitric oxide (NO). CO therefore reduces $O_2$ delivery by reducing the $O_2$-carrying capacity of hemoglobin and by increasing the affinity of remaining binding sites for $O_2$. The result is a secondary polycythemia. CO also inhibits $O_2$ utilization by competing for binding sites on enzymes with heme prosthetic groups. The reduced form of cytochrome oxidase is particularly sensitive and CO poisoning produces similar effects to *cyanide poisoning*. NO will exert a similar effect by combining with deoxygenated hemoglobin to produce nitrosylhemoglobin Hb-NO. However, unlike CO, NO binds reversibly with methemoglobin and reacts irreversibly with oxygenated sites of native hemoglobin:

$$Hb\text{-}Fe(II)O_2 + NO \Rightarrow Hb\text{-}Fe(III) + NO_3^-$$

This reaction probably accounts for the attenuation by hemoglobin of the biological actions of nitrovasodilators and endothelium-derived relaxing factor (NO) (*see* Chapters 10, 67 and 73). Hence the vasodilatatory effects of nitroprusside, mediated through NO production, may be prolonged but that of NO itself will be curtailed to the site of production or administration.

## Hemoglobinopathies

Hemoglobinopathies arise from a single base substitution in one of the globin genes giving rise to a single amino acid substitution in the corresponding globin chain. Over 400 mutant hemoglobins have been described and whether the abnormal hemoglobin is reflected in a clinical disorder depends on the location of the affected site. In general, amino acids on the periphery of the folded protein do not play an important role in the function of the protein. Hence about 50 per cent of mutant hemoglobins are clinically benign. However, modifications in other sites can lead to predictable changes in the allosteric properties of the hemoglobin. The important sites are discussed below.

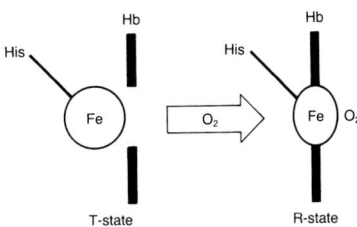

FIGURE 81.2 Trigger for transition from T to R states of hemoglobin (Hb) when $O_2$ binds. His, histidine.

## C-terminal region

This region stabilizes the T-state of hemoglobin and modifications here (e.g. hemoglobin Rainier) are likely to diminish this stability and produce a high-affinity hemoglobin.

## $\alpha_1/\beta_2$ contact

This contact area changes during the T to R transition and modifications here will alter the equilibrium between the two conformational states. A shift to the R-state is more common and produces a high-affinity hemoglobin (e.g. hemoglobin Chesapeake). A shift to the T-state will produce a low-affinity hemoglobin (e.g. hemoglobin Kansas).

## BPG-binding site

The binding of BPG stabilizes the T-state and modifications here diminish this stability and produce a hemoglobin with a high affinity for $O_2$ when in the normal environment of an erythrocyte (e.g. hemoglobin Syracuse). High-affinity hemoglobin is associated with a lower $Po_2$ for a given level of $O_2$ consumption (see Chapter 75). The physiological response is an increased production of erythropoietin by the kidney, with a concomitant polycythemia. Conversely, a low-affinity hemoglobin reduces the stimulation of erythropoietin production and is often, but not invariably, associated with anemia.

## $\alpha_1/\beta_1$ contact

Amino acid substitutions in this area lead to a weakened tetrameric structure and precipitation of hemoglobin as Heinz bodies.

## The heme binding pocket

Each heme group is tightly wedged in a hydrophobic pocket in an orientation that allows free access of $O_2$ to and from its binding site – the Fe(II). Changes in the amino acids that bind the periphery of the heme molecule will change its orientation and alter the affinity of that subunit for $O_2$. The environment of the heme is also designed to minimize, but cannot prevent, the oxidation of Fe(II) to Fe(III) (methemoglobin) when $O_2$ is bound. This end is achieved partly by the positive charge of the histidine that binds the Fe(II) (the proximal histidine) and another histidine that is nearby (the distal histidine). The presence of these groups favors the Fe in the divalent rather than trivalent state and their replacement with an electronegative group is likely to alter this balance and produce an excess of methemoglobin that cannot be reduced fast enough by the NADH-dependent methemoglobin reductases,

which are cytochromes and responsible normally for 95 per cent of the reduction of methemoglobin. The clinical consequence is methemoglobinemia (e.g. hemoglobin Iwate, hemoglobin Hyde Park, hemoglobin Boston, hemoglobin Saskatoon). Inherited deficiencies of these reducing enzymes can also result in a *methemoglobinemia* as can the administration of a wide variety of oxidant drugs. Neonates can be susceptible to methemoglobinemia due to a transient deficiency of cytochrome $b_5$ reductase activity.

## Peripheral amino acids

Substitution of amino acid residues on the surface of the protein are normally without physiological/clinical consequences. There are few exceptions to this rule but notable examples include HbS (sickle cell hemoglobin), HbC and HbE and they are also the most common of all hemoglobinopathies. About 10 per cent of American Blacks and 25 per cent of African Blacks are thought to be heterozygous HbS carriers. In HbS a hydrophobic valine replaces a hydrophilic glutamate ($\beta$-6) and creates a hydrophobic area that allows polymerization of HbS into long fibers that precipitate within the erythrocyte, which then appears to be sickle-shaped. This process is termed *sickling* and the altered cells block capillaries *in vivo* and cause extreme ischemic pain. Sickling is common in homozygous HbS patients but is absent in the heterozygous carriers. The polymerization is only possible with the T-state of hemoglobin and therefore can be minimized by avoiding excessive $O_2$ consumption as in exercise or hypothermia. The prevalence of HbS results from the protection it affords to heterozygotes against malaria. The global distribution of HbC and HbE also coincides with that of the malarial parasite.

# Available $O_2$

The predicted physiological consequence of simultaneous changes in hemoglobin concentration and $O_2$ affinity is provided by the derived "available $O_2$" (AO). It is the calculated difference in $O_2$ content of blood at arterial $Po_2$ and at an assumed mixed venous $Po_2$ of 20 mmHg and represents the amount of $O_2$ that can be extracted from blood before the need arises for an increase in cardiac output. AO can be calculated from the measured $O_2$ affinity of the blood or, for untransfused preterm infants up to 10 weeks' postnatal age, can be estimated from the total postconceptual age:

$$AO\,(mL/g\,Hgb) = 0.54 + 0.005 \times age\,(weeks)$$

This predicts age-dependent increases in AO reflecting the decreasing affinity of hemoglobin for $O_2$, which compensates for the decline in circulating hemoglobin in term infants. The compensatory value of a decrease in $O_2$ affinity in anemia is often illustrated with another calculation analogous to, but different from, AO. This is the $O_2$ release capacity, which uses an assumed mixed venous $P_{O_2}$ of 40 mmHg, chosen to reflect *in vivo* conditions at rest rather than in a period of high $O_2$ demand. This difference appears trivial but is highly significant; changes in $P_{50}$ that restore $O_2$ release capacity to normal, after preterm delivery, may leave the AO suboptimal. In these circumstances, the infant will not cope with $O_2$ demands above those required at, or near to, resting conditions. Symptoms of anemic hypoxia can arise in preterm infants born at less than 30 weeks' gestation, when the nadir of hemoglobin occurs before there is significant switching to HbA synthesis, and this tips the balance to clinical signs of anemia. This is likely to occur when AO drops to 6.0 mL/dL of blood. In healthy adults the normal AO is 12.2 mL/dL. Similar problems will be relevant in older infants with abnormal hemoglobin or with metabolic disturbances that alter the hemoglobin–$O_2$ affinity. An abnormal, high-affinity hemoglobin will result in chronic hypoxia, which may stimulate EPO synthesis and an elevated production of red cells. The resulting polycythemia will be associated with abnormal blood flow due to the increase in blood viscosity (see below).

## BLOOD VOLUME AND $O_2$ TRANSPORT
(*see* also Chapter 75)

In addition to the concentration of hemoglobin, the total volume of circulating red cells (RCV) is also an important hematological variable that influences tissue oxygenation. When considering blood volume variables, it is useful to consider hemoglobin concentration as the proportion of blood occupied by the red blood cells, which for a sample of peripheral blood is defined as hematocrit (Hct). The relationship between Hct and hemoglobin concentration will, of course, vary with the amount of hemoglobin contained within each cell, the mean corpuscular hemoglobin (MCH). The whole body hematocrit (HctB) is defined by equation (1):

$$HctB = \frac{RCV}{(RCV + PV)}$$

where RCV is the total volume of circulating red cells, PV is the volume of plasma within which these cells are circulating, and the sum of RCV and PV is blood volume (BV). In neonates and adults, a plot of peripheral Hct versus RCV is hyperbolic with a large degree of individual scatter attributed to inequality in maintenance of plasma volume between individuals. Importantly, there is little evidence of compensatory changes in PV to maintain circulating BV at low

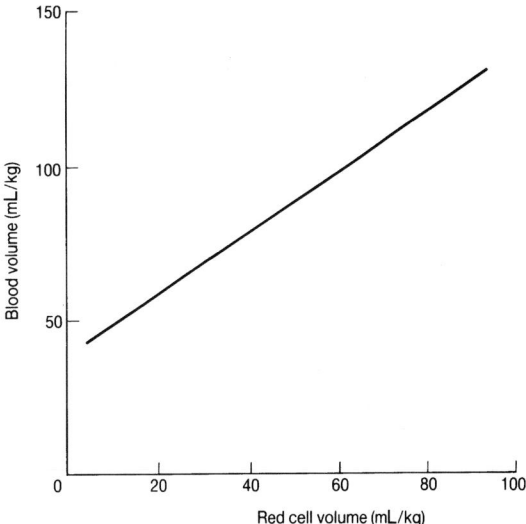

FIGURE 81.3 Relationship between red cell volume and blood volume. (From Jones JG, Holland BM, Hudson · IR, Wardrop CA. *Br J Haematol* 1990; **76**: 288, with permission.)

RCV. The corollary to this is a linear relationship between BV and RCV, and a low RCV is likely to be associated with oligovolemia as well as anemia (Fig. 81.3).

Average values for RCV and BV in healthy male adults are quoted at about 30 and 75 mL/kg, respectively. The corresponding figures for healthy young females are 25 and 70 mL/kg. These figures are only crude guides and vary with the method of measurement and the height of individuals at the same weight. RCV and BV for infants weighing between 10 and 30 kg are the same as those for adults. The normal neonate has a higher BV, which is attributed entirely to an increased RCV and hence HctB. The quoted range is very wide and depends on the extent of placental–fetal transfusion at birth. Placental vessels contain about 150 mL of blood and the amount of blood transferred to the infant will depend on the timing of cord clamping, gravity, uterine contractions and lung expansion. About 25 per cent of placental transfusion occurs in the first 15 s with 80 per cent within 5 min. Typical values for RCV and BV in neonates, from one study, illustrate these points and are collected in Table 81.3. These data also illustrate that, during the first 2 hours, a 17 per cent decrease in BV is seen in infants receiving the extra transfusion. This reduction represents a diminution of PV with plasma extravasation and a resulting increase in Hct. Thereafter an increase in PV, particularly after early cord clamping, leads to a similar BV in both groups by 120 hours after birth.

There seems to be general agreement on this point although this similarity in BV, in the first few days, varies according to the extent of transfusion and the difference can remain as large as 10 mL/kg. This extra blood is crucial because a large part of placental blood (about 45 mL) is needed to fill the pulmonary circula-

TABLE 81.3 Red-cell volume (RCV) and blood volume (BV) in term neonates delivered vaginally

| | IMMEDIATE CLAMPING | | CLAMPING DELAYED BY 3 MIN | |
|---|---|---|---|---|
| | BV (mL/kg) | RCV (mL/kg) | BV (mL/kg) | RCV (mL/kg) |
| At birth | 70 | 31 | 90 | 39 |
| 2 hours after birth | 71 | 31 | 75 | 39 |
| 120 hours after birth | 78 | 31 | 80 | 39 |

From Nelle M, Zilow EP, Kraus M *et al. Am J Obstet Gynecol* 1993; **169**: 189, with permission.

tion. A delay in cord clamping of just 30 s, with appropriate juxtaposition of fetus and placenta, may reduce respiratory complications in preterm infants. BV in normal fetuses is believed to be about 110 mL/kg and present evidence is consistent with that being relatively constant during fetal development. A higher BV per kilogram, reported for preterm infants, probably reflects a lower amount of fatty tissue which is generally more poorly supplied with blood. In summary a healthy neonate, with adequate placental transfusion, would be expected to have BV and RCV values of about 90 and 45 mL/kg, respectively. Higher values will lead to hypervolemia, polycythemia and hyperviscosity (*see* below and also *see* Chapter 73) while lower values lead to hypovolemic anemia.

A reduction in blood volume decreases venous compliance and capacity, which occurs unevenly, leading to redistribution of blood flow through organs such as the heart and brain to protect them from $O_2$ deprivation. This circulatory adaptation delays major physiological responses, such as an increase in cardiac output at rest, until anemia becomes severe. Theory predicts a biological response will occur when RCV in neonates falls to about 15–20 mL/kg. The biological responses could be normal physiological compensatory mechanisms as well as signals of the need for clinical intervention in severely affected individuals. Clinical data from

preterm neonates support these conclusions and identify 25 mL/kg as the critical RCV below which cardiac output at rest and the level of clinical attention increases (Fig. 81.4). From the early stages of anemia, however, a more immediate but equally undesirable result of uneven redistribution of blood in oligovolemia is chronic underperfusion and possible hypoxia in some tissues. The liver and bowel are particularly vulnerable to decreasing blood $O_2$ content, and the bowel is a major source of lactic acid in endotoxic shock. It is therefore important to address problems associated with reduced RCV early before the situation is serious enough to invoke an increase in cardiac output at rest. The increased cardiac output, which is stimulated by, and correlated with, a low RCV, is not related to Hct alone but is correlated with both Hct and BV as independent predictors. Hct predicts $O_2$-carrying capacity of the blood, and BV is a measure of the effective proportion of the total tissue vasculature that is perfused. RCV has been used in some investigations as the single measurement reflecting both of these important variables and has been considered the logical target and monitor in red-cell-transfusion regimens. However, the best hematological guide to possible tissue hypoxia is a combination of Hct and BV, and methods for measuring BV are becoming increasingly important. Apart from indirect methods such as hydrostatic pressure in major blood vessels, there are two ways of obtaining this measurement: (1) independent measures of RCV and PV; or (2) from equation (1) using measured Hct and either RCV or PV.

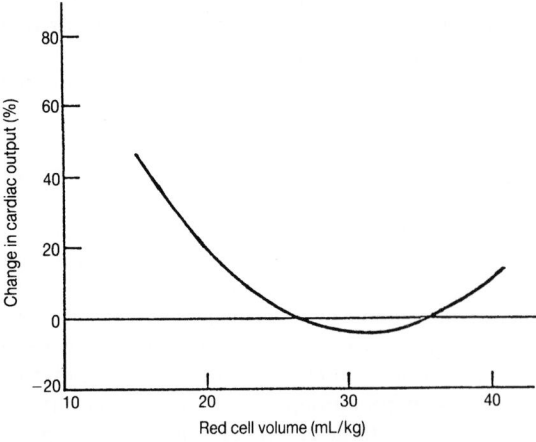

FIGURE 81.4 Association between red cell volume and changes in cardiac output after altering red cell volume with blood transfusion in preterm neonates. (From Hudson I, Cooke A, Holland B *et al. Arch Dis Child* 1990; **65**: 672, with permission.)

## Measurement of RCV

In general, measurements of RCV depend on labeling autologous cells with radioisotopes or biotin and measuring the degree of dilution after retransfusion of the labeled cells into the original donor. Radioisotopes are invasive, and biotin involves lengthy and labor-intensive procedures. However, neonatologists often transfuse neonates with adult red cells as part of clinical therapy, and the administered cells are diluted with those of the infant receiving the transfusion. In these circumstances, dilution of autologous HbF by donor HbA forms the basis of a simple, rapid, and proven graphical method for RCV measurement, although it does become less sensitive with multiple transfusions as the proportion of HbA in the circulation increases.

RCV measurement is also relevant in the clinical management of *polycythemia*, presently recognized as an elevated Hct or hemoglobin concentration. The distinction between true erythrocytosis and contracted PV, an essential part of hematological diagnosis in adults, is less appreciated in infants. In these patients, the estimation of RCV must depend on more traditional dilution techniques, and the biotin method, proven effective in neonates as well as adults, may be a possibility in an environment with the appropriately trained staff and technology. The need is growing for easier methods of RCV estimation.

## Measurement of PV

PV, the volume of fluid within which the red cells are distributed, is estimated in practice as the volume of distribution of macromolecules believed to be confined to the vascular space. The usual molecule is albumin, labeled with a suitable radioactive isotope or chromophoric dye. The volume of distribution of albumin is probably greater than that of the larger erythrocyte; this difference is likely to be exaggerated in sick infants with compromised capillary permeability. This method of estimating PV is therefore unsatisfactory, and an alternative is required. In neonatology, the immunoglobulin IgM is emerging as a useful molecule in this context as it is reduced or absent from neonatal blood and is administered clinically during plasma transfusion. In these circumstances, the volume of distribution of IgM is easily calculated and has been used as a measure of PV. From studies of neonatal blood, it is now clear that the volume of distribution of red blood cells is closer to that of IgM than to that of albumin.

## Measurement of BV

The use of equation (1) for estimating BV from Hct and either RCV or PV has been questioned because of the reported variable relationship between measured peripheral Hct and HctB. The ratio HctB/Hct varies from 0.75 to 0.97 and two possible reasons have been postulated.

∎ The distribution of flowing blood cells and plasma in the microvasculature varies with the diameter of the vessel, and the Hct of blood from a peripheral vein or artery is not the same as that found in narrow capillaries or venules. A dynamic decrease in the Hct of flowing blood begins to appear in vessels of about 300 μm diameter and is maximal at about 10 μm (the Fåhraeus effect). However, less than 10 per cent of blood is found in systemic capillaries and any difference in Hct here will have to be unrealistically large to produce the observed difference between peripheral Hct and HctB.

∎ HctB is calculated from independent measures of RCV and PV and the latter is accepted as the volume of distribution of labeled albumin, which is not confined to circulating blood. The volume of distribution of macromolecules is inversely related to their molecular size and, with molecules as large as IgM, the ratio of HctB/Hct in human neonates is about 0.96. Traditional measurements of PV therefore provide an overestimate of true circulating plasma and this error is exaggerated in sick individuals with impaired capillary integrity. Until a suitable plasma marker is found, the use of PV to predict BV is likely to be unsatisfactory and should be avoided.

For the present, and provided care is taken to standardize the drawing of blood samples, to estimate BV from the peripheral Hct and RCV should be acceptable. The BV, calculated in this way, and the peripheral Hct are the primary determinants of whole body tissue oxygenation.

## BLOOD VISCOSITY

The oxygenation of tissues also depends on blood flow, which is sensitive to changes in blood viscosity that affect vascular resistance to flow (*see* page 750). Hyperviscosity has been reported in about 5 per cent of infants at birth, and 2 per cent of those may present with clinical problems. The viscosity of blood is determined by plasma viscosity, the number of red cells, and the rheological properties and aggregability of those cells. Except in extreme leukocytosis, the white cells do not influence blood viscosity but have profound effects on flow through the microcirculation. Plasma viscosity reflects the concentration of high molecular weight proteins such as fibrinogen. The concentration of fibrinogen increases from about 25 g/L in term infants to about 35 g/L in adults with a concomitant increase in plasma viscosity from 1.25 to 1.46 mPa. The viscosity of blood at a high shear rate is typically

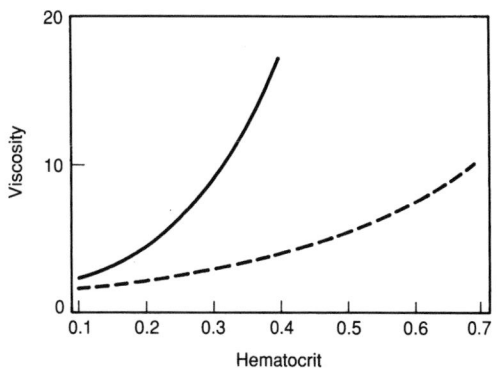

FIGURE 81.5 Hematocrit and blood viscosity at low (——) and high (- - - -) shear rates

five-fold higher than that of plasma due to the red blood cells. This difference is exaggerated at low shear rate due to the aggregation of the red cells (Fig. 81.5). The viscosity of blood is therefore very sensitive to Hct but, at any Hct, is lower in neonates than adults due to the lower concentration of plasma fibrinogen and the larger size of the red cells. Increasing the Hct produces a linear increase in $O_2$-carrying capacity and a logarithmic increase in viscosity. In terms of $O_2$ delivery to tissues therefore there is a theoretical optimum Hct, but quoted values lie within a broad range from 0.3 to 0.56. These disparate values have been derived by various theoretical predictions, measurements *in vitro* and *in vivo* and a variety of clinical management and assessment procedures and are worthy of comment.

Theoretical predictions and measurements *in vitro* do not allow for the oligovolemia which is often associated with a low Hct, is corrected by transfusion and is crucial *in vivo*. Thus blood transfusion to preterm infants causes the expected increase in BV, Hct and viscosity but the latter effect is offset by a decrease in peripheral resistance. This effect can be assumed to reflect the reversal of the vasoconstriction apparent in hypovolemic infants before transfusion.

An optimum Hct derived from clinical studies relates to one particular end-point and results cannot be extrapolated to all others. For example, normovolemic hemodilution is found to aid recovery in adults who have suffered a stroke. It is important to emphasize that the adherence to normovolemia is an essential part of this treatment. Conversely an induced short-term polycythemia is considered to improve physical performance in endurance athletes – hence the forbidden practice of blood doping. However polycythemia is recognized as a high-risk factor for coronary disease in adults and reduces pulmonary blood flow in children with high-flow congenital heart disease (e.g. ventricular septal defect). Clinical evidence now shows that increased Hct and BV, after delayed cord clamping in preterm infants, increases the ratio of arterial/alveolar $Po_2$ in the first day and reduces the subsequent need for supplemental $O_2$. The beneficial effect here is believed to reflect better filling of pulmonary vessels by the larger BV.

Hence an overemphasis on the importance of an optimum Hct is mistaken; a chronic anemia in neonates, children, and adults is hypovolemic and probably associated with hypoperfusion of some tissues in order to protect others. Hence an Hct below the normal value will not correct the oligovolemia, will leave an impaired total tissue oxygenation, and is the wrong target in blood transfusion therapy.

## SELECTED READING

Brace RA. Fluid distribution in the fetus and neonate. In: Polin RA, Fox WW, eds. *Fetal and neonatal physiology*. Philadelphia: WB Saunders, 1992: 1288.

Christensen RD. Hematopoiesis in the fetus and neonate. *Pediatr Res* 1989; 26: 531.

Jones JG, Holland BM, Hudson IRB, Wardrop CAJ. Total circulating red cells versus haematocrit as the primary descriptor of $O_2$ transport by the blood. *Br J Haematol* 1991; 76: 288.

Jones JG, Holland BM, Wardrop CAJ. Disorders of red cells 3: red cells and $O_2$ transport. In: Lilleyman JS, Hann IM, eds. *Paediatric haematology*, 2nd edn. Edinburgh: Churchill Livingstone, 1992: 257.

Kinmond S, Aitchison TC, Holland BM *et al*. Umbilical cord clamping and preterm infants: A randomised trial. *Br Med J* 1993; 306: 172.

Lipton JM, Nathan DG. The anatomy and physiology of hematopoiesis. In: Nathan DG, Oski F, eds. *Hematology in infancy and childhood*, Vol I. Philadelphia: WB Saunders, 1987: 128.

Maier RF, Obladen M, Scigalla P *et al*. The effect of Epoetin Beta (recombinant human erythropoietin) on the need for transfusion in very-low-birth-weight infants. *N Engl J Med* 1994; 330: 1173.

Wardrop CAJ, Jones JG, Holland BM. Detection, correction and ultimate prevention of anaemias in the preterm infant. *Transfusion Sci* 1991; 12: 257.

Weatherall DJ. Haemoglobin and its disorders. In: Kendrew J, ed. *The encyclopedia of molecular biology*. Oxford: Blackwell Science, 1994: 472.

# 82

# Hemostasis

Maureen Andrew and M. Patricia Massicotte

## DEVELOPMENTAL HEMOSTASIS

The discovery of individual components of the hemo-static system over the past century has been accompanied by the realization that in infants and children this system is profoundly different from that in adults, and throughout childhood is a dynamic, evolving system that exists in many unique forms. Although hemostasis in the young can be considered immature, this also must be considered physiological because it provides protection from hemorrhagic and thrombotic complications in healthy children. Indeed, the hemostatic system of children has some significant advantages over the adult system. For example, thrombotic complications rarely occur during childhood but occur frequently enough in adults to warrant prophylactic anticoagulant therapy in many conditions. However, the immaturity of the hemostatic system in the very young does leave them vulnerable to some disorders, such as *hemorrhagic disease of the newborn* secondary to vitamin K deficiency. These examples illustrate the need to fully understand the ontogeny of hemostasis, and the effects of aging on hemostasis. An understanding of developmental hemostasis in the broadest sense will optimize the prevention, diagnosis and treatment of hemostatic problems during childhood and will undoubtedly provide new insights into the pathophysiology of hemorrhagic and thrombotic complications at all ages. In this chapter, coagulation, fibrinolysis and platelet function are reviewed in general and in the context of developmental hemostasis.

## COAGULATION

### Thrombin generation: general

Under physiological conditions, blood is maintained in a fluid phase. In response to damage to the vessel wall, platelets, plasma coagulation proteins and the vessel orchestrate the formation of a hemostatic plug. A schematic outline of blood coagulation is shown in Fig. 82.1. The amino acid and nucleic acid sequences of the corresponding gene are known for virtually all coagulation proteins (Table 82.1). The central purpose of these proteins is to generate thrombin from

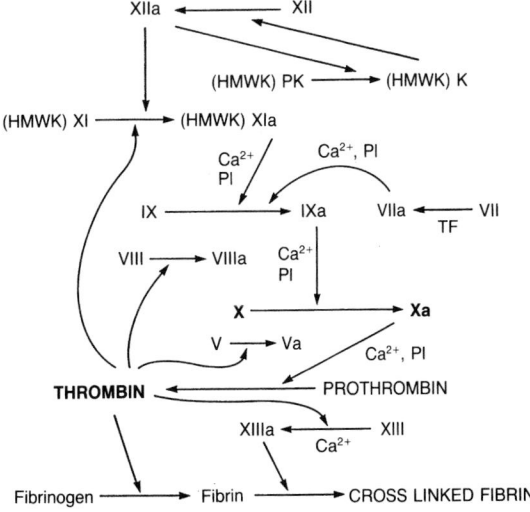

FIGURE 82.1 The coagulation system. HMWK, high-molecular-weight kininogen; PK, prekallikrein; K, kallikrein; TF, tissue factor; Pl, phospholipid.

TABLE 82.1 Properties of components of the coagulation and fibrinolytic systems

| | SITE OF SYNTHESIS | PROTEIN CHARACTERISTICS | MOLECULAR MASS (kD) | PLASMA CONCENTRATION | CHROMOSOMAL LOCATION | GENE ORGANIZATION |
|---|---|---|---|---|---|---|
| *Blood coagulant proteins* | | | | | | |
| Fibrinogen (factor I) | Hepatocyte | Dimeric, three subchains/ monomer | 333 | 200–400 mg/dL | 4 | Separate genes for α, β and γ |
| Prothrombin (factor II) | Hepatocyte | Vitamin K-dependent | 72 | 100 µg/mL | 11 | 14 exons |
| Factor V | Hepatocyte | Vitamin K-dependent | 330 | 10 µg/mL | 1 | Similar to FVIII |
| Factor VII | Hepatocyte | Vitamin K-dependent | 55 | 0.5 µg/mL | 13 | 9 exons; adjacent to FX gene |
| Factor VIII | Hepatocyte | Cofactor to FIXa | 330 | 0.1 µg/mL | X | 26 exons |
| Factor IX | Hepatocyte | Vitamin K-dependent | 55 | 5 µg/mL | X | 8 exons |
| Factor X | Hepatocyte | Vitamin K-dependent | 55 | 10 µg/mL | 13 | 8 exons; adjacent to the FVII gene |
| Factor XI | Hepatocyte | Homodimeric | 160 | 5 µg/mL | 4 | 15 exons |
| Factor XIII | Hepatocyte | Tetrameric ($a_2b_2$) | 320 | 10 µg/mL | 1(b) 1(a) | a and b genes on different chromosomes |
| Tissue factor | Many cell types | Transmembrane protein | 37 | 0 | 1 | 5 exons |
| *Inhibitors of coagulation* | | | | | | |
| Antithrombin | Hepatocyte | Protease inhibitor | 50 | 140 µg/mL | 1 | 6 exons |
| Heparin cofactor II | Hepatocyte | Protease inhibitor | 65.6 | 40 µg/mL | 22 | – |
| $\alpha_2$-Macroglobulin | Hepatocyte | Protease inhibitor | 725 | 2500 µg/mL | – | – |
| Protein C | Hepatocyte | Vitamin K-dependent | 62 | 4 µg/mL | 2 | 9 exons |
| Protein S | hepatocyte | Vitamin K-dependent | 69 | 25 µg/mL | 3 | 15 exons |
| *Fibrinolytic system* | | | | | | |
| Plasminogen | Hepatocyte | Protease zymogen | 92 | 200 mg/mL | 6 | 19 exons |
| $\alpha_2$-Antiplasmin | Hepatocyte | Inhibitor | 70 | 70 mg/L | 18 | – |
| Tissue plasminogen activator | Endothelium Monocyte | Protease zymogen | 68 | 0.005 mg/L | 8 | 14 exons |
| Plasminogen activator inhibitor 1 | Endothelium | Inhibitor | 52 | 10 µg/mL | 7 | – |
| Plasminogen activator inhibitor 2 | Placenta Monocyte | Inhibitor | 40 non-glycosylated 60 glycosylated | Not detectable | 18 | – |
| Histidine-rich glycoprotein | Endothelium | Inhibitor | 75 | 100 mg/L | – | – |
| Tissue factor pathway inhibitor | Endothelium | – | 40 | 115 µg/mL | 2 | 9 exons |
| Thrombomodulin | Endothelium | Glycoprotein | 75 | 0 | 20 | No introns |

prothrombin. Although blood coagulation theoretically can be initiated both by the contact system or by exposure of blood to tissue factor (TF), the latter is the physiologically important activation pathway.

## Initiation of coagulation

Factor VIIa (FVIIa) binding to TF, in the presence of $Ca^{2+}$ and a phospholipid surface, initiates coagulation as FVIIa–TF activates both FX and FIX. FVII is a vitamin K-dependent protein with 10 γ-carboxy glutamic acid (Gla) residues at the amino-terminal region. The latter are critical for the $Ca^{2+}$-mediated binding of vitamin K-dependent proteins to coagulant surfaces where thrombin production occurs. Whether or not the

zymogen form of FVII displays some intrinsic enzymatic activity in its native form is still unclear. FVII is cleaved to a two-chain serine protease by several coagulation enzymes including FXa, FXIIa, FIXa, and thrombin. Patients with no measurable FVII activity have severe bleeding problems, in keeping with the importance of FVIIa–TF activation and coagulation. TF is a transmembrane protein with an extended surface domain, a small transmembrane domain, and a short cytoplasmic domain. TF is produced by several cell types and is present in almost all tissues. Endothelial cells in culture have minimal TF activity, but can be induced to synthesize and express TF on their surfaces.

FXI is one of four factors comprising the contact system (FXII, prekallikrein, and high-molecular-weight kininogen (HMWK)). Although FXI can be activated by FXIIa, the physiological activator of FXI likely is small amounts of thrombin generated by the TF pathway. FXIa, in the presence of $Ca^{2+}$ and a phospholipid surface, activates FIX to FIXa. Of the contact factors, only inherited deficiency of FXI is associated with a bleeding risk.

FIX is a vitamin K-dependent protein with 12 Gla residues. FIX is converted to FIXa by limited proteolytic cleavage by either FVIIa or FXIa. FIXa, in the presence of FVIIIa, $Ca^{2+}$, and a phospholipid surface activates FX to FXa. Inherited deficiencies of FIX constitute hemophilia B, a serious bleeding disorder. FVIII is converted to FVIIIa by limited cleavage by thrombin and to a lesser extent by FXa. FVIIIa functions as the cofactor when FIXa activates FX. The importance of FVIII is evidenced by the severe bleeding disorders in FVIII deficient patients (*hemophilia A*).

## The prothrombinase complex

The final reaction of the coagulation pathway is catalyzed by the prothrombinase complex which consists of FVa (cofactor), FXa (enzyme), $Ca^{2+}$ and a phospholipid surface. The prothrombinase complex converts prothrombin to thrombin by two peptide bond cleavages in the zymogen, giving rise to prothrombin fragment 1.2 (F1.2) and α-thrombin. Both FX and prothrombin are vitamin K-dependent serine proteases that also bind to negatively charged phospholipids through their Gla residues. The activated form of FV, FVa, is the cofactor necessary for prothrombin activation by FXa to proceed at a physiologically relevant rate. FVa functions as a receptor in platelet membranes binding both prothrombin and FX in close proximity. Thus, FX and prothrombin bind to surfaces by two separate but complementary mechanisms (FVa and $Ca^{2+}$ mediated by the Gla regions).

Human α-thrombin consists of an A chain linked by a disulfide bond to a B chain. Three principal functional domains of α-thrombin have been described and consist of the catalytic center where substrates are cleaved, a substrate-recognition exosite necessary for initial interaction, and an anion-binding exosite(s) where polyanions (e.g. heparin) bind. Thrombin is also a serine protease with many coagulant functions including: cleavage of fibrinopeptides A and B from fibrinogen resulting in fibrin formation; activation of FXI, FVIII, and FV to enhance its own generation; activation of FXIII which promotes covalent crosslinking of fibrin; and activation of platelets.

Fibrinogen consists of two symmetrical half-molecules, each of which has three polypeptide chains termed Aα, Bβ, and γ. The two halves are joined by three disulfide bridges between γ(2) and Aα(1) chains in the central amino-terminal domain (E domain). Cleavage of fribrinopeptide A (Aα 1–16, FPA) and fibrinopeptide B (Bβ 1–14, FPB) in the E domain by thrombin initiates fibrin assembly. Fibrin monomers can be considered as tridominal structures with a central E domain and two outer D domains which assemble in an antiparallel, staggered, overlapping manner with non-covalent interactions between E and D domains to form two-stranded fibrils. At the same time, the fibrils undergo non-covalent lateral associations to form thicker fibers.

## Crosslinking of fibrin

In the presence of FXIIIa, assembled fibrin undergoes covalent crosslinking by formation of ε-γ-Glu-Lys isopeptide bonds, initially between γ chains and more slowly between α chains. Crosslinking provides structural stability and integrity to an otherwise easily deformable fibrin clot. Several plasma proteins (including α2-antiplasmin (α2AP)) also become crosslinked to α chains by FXIIIa. A secondary binding site for thrombin is also present on the E domain and is dependent on the Bβ 15–42 sequence. This secondary site serves to protect thrombin from its natural inhibitors (*see* p. 881) and permit the ongoing conversion of other fibrinogen molecules to fibrin. During fibrinolysis, the peptides connecting the D and E domains are cleaved with the generation of E and/or D-containing fragments. The D products in these fragments contain crosslinked γ chains (i.e. D-dimer, etc.).

## Laboratory testing of the coagulation system

An overall assessment of the coagulation system can be made with two general screening tests, the prothrombin time (PT) and activated partial thromboplastin time (APTT). The PT measures thrombin generation following activation of FX by FVIIa and the APTT measures thrombin generation following activation of the contact system. Expression of the PT as an International Normalized Ratio (INR) is encouraged because it standardizes for different thromboplastin reagents. Plasma concentrations of individual coagulation proteins also can be measured directly with functional or immunological assays. These assays provide an important means of assessing the coagulation system; however, they do not provide sensitive indices of *in vivo* activation of the coagulation system. Sensitive laboratory tests that reflect *in vivo* generation of thrombin include measurement of: a fragment formed following proteolytic cleavage of prothrombin, F1.2; a peptide released by thrombin cleavage of fibrinogen, FPA; the remaining portion of the fibrinogen molecule called fibrin monomer; or thrombin complexed to its natural inhibitor antithrombin forming thrombin–antithrombin (TAT) complexes. Together these tests provide an effective means to evaluate hemostasis under physiological and pathological conditions.

# Thrombin generation: infancy and childhood

Components of the coagulation system do not cross the placenta; rather they are synthesized by the fetus, initially appearing by approximately 10 weeks' gestation. Samples obtained at fetoscopy provide the best representative assessment of the coagulation system for the very immature infant (Table 82.2). Studies of hemostasis following birth and during infancy and early childhood have been hindered by problems in obtaining adequate samples from healthy infants, by greater variability in plasma concentrations of coagulation proteins, and by the need for microassays to measure coagulation proteins in small volumes of plasma. Despite these problems, normal ranges for the coagulant proteins in premature and full-term infants are available during the first 6 months after birth, and throughout childhood.

At birth, plasma concentrations of most coagulant proteins differ significantly from adults (Fig. 82.2); however, the patterns of change in plasma concentrations of coagulant proteins from the fetus to the adult are not all similar. At birth plasma concentrations of the vitamin K-dependent coagulant proteins and contact factors are half of adult values, whereas plasma concentrations of fibrinogen, FVIII, von Willebrand factor (vWF), and FV are not decreased at birth (Table 82.2) nor during early childhood (Fig. 82.2). By 6 months of age, the coagulation system evolves

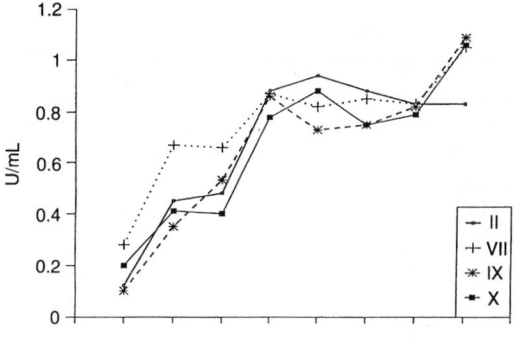

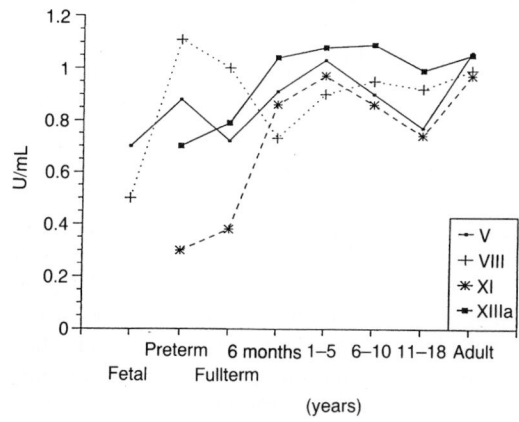

FIGURE 82.2 Plasma concentrations of the vitamin K-dependent coagulation factors (II, VII, IX, and X) and other coagulation factors (V, VIII, XI, XIIIa) at different ages

TABLE 82.2 Reference values for components of the coagulation system in healthy fetuses (19–27 weeks' gestation) and premature infants at birth (28–31 weeks' gestation)

| TEST | GESTATIONAL AGE | |
|---|---|---|
| | 19–27 Weeks | 28–31 Weeks |
| PT (s) | – | 15.4 (14.6–16.9) |
| APTT (s) | – | 108.0 (80–168) |
| Fibrinogen (g/L) | 1.00 (±0.43) | 2.56 (1.60–5.50) |
| II (U/mL) | 0.12 (±0.02) | 0.31 (0.19–0.54) |
| V (U/mL) | 0.41 (±0.10) | 0.65 (0.43–0.80) |
| VII (U/mL) | 0.28 (±0.04) | 0.37 (0.24–0.76) |
| VIII (U/mL) | 0.39 (±0.14) | 0.79 (0.37–1.26) |
| vWF (U/mL) | 0.64 (±0.13) | 1.41 (0.83–2.23) |
| IX (U/mL) | 0.10 (±0.01) | 0.18 (0.17–0.20) |
| X (U/mL) | 0.21 (±0.03) | 0.36 (0.25–0.64) |
| XI (U/mL) | – | 0.23 (0.11–0.33) |
| XII (U/mL) | 0.22 (±0.03) | 0.25 (0.05–0.35) |
| Prekallikrein (U/mL) | – | 0.26 (0.15–0.32) |
| High molecular weight kininogen (U/mL) | – | 0.32 (0.19–0.52) |
| Antithrombin (U/mL) | 0.24 (±0.03) | 0.28 (0.20–0.38) |
| Heparin cofactor II (U/mL) | 0.27 (±0.05) | – |
| Protein C (U/mL) | 0.11 (±0.03) | – |

PT, prothrombin time; APTT, activated partial thromboplastin time; VIII, factor VIII pro-coagulant; vWF, von Willebrand factor. All factors except fibrinogen are expressed as units per milliliter (U/mL) where pooled plasma contains 1.0 U/mL. Values are expressed as a mean followed by the lower and upper boundary.

to one with many similarities to the adult (Fig. 82.2); however, important differences still remain. Plasma concentrations of the vitamin K-dependent factors and contact factors are 10–20 per cent lower than adult values and the lower limits of normal are also decreased compared with adults.

## Thrombin generation

The first clue that the capacity to generate thrombin is reduced in the neonatal coagulation system is provided by the presence of prolonged PT and APTT during infancy (Table 82.2). More sensitive assays of thrombin generation in newborn plasma show that thrombin generation is both delayed and decreased compared with adult plasma. The degree of impairment reflects the low plasma concentrations of prothrombin, which are similar to those found in plasma from adults receiving therapeutic amounts of coumadin or heparin. Following infancy, the capacity to generate thrombin increases but remains approximately 20 per cent less than that in adults.

## Fibrinogen

At birth, fibrinogen has an increased sialic acid content compared with adult fibrinogen. The thrombin clotting time (TCT), if performed without $Ca^{2+}$ in the system, is prolonged in newborns, reflecting the "fetal" fibrinogen. If the sialic acid is removed, fetal fibrinogen appears indistinguishable from adult fibrinogen. The physiological significance of fetal fibrinogen is unknown. Fetal fibrinogen disappears during early infancy and plasma concentrations during childhood remain similar to those in adults.

## Physiological significance

The physiological significance of the age dependency of hemostasis is still unknown. However, some of the subtle differences in plasma concentrations of certain coagulation proteins may contribute to observed differences for the risk of thromboembolic disease during childhood. Prospective studies in adults have shown a significant relationship between plasma concentrations of FVII and the occurrence of ischemic cardiovascular events. Plasma concentrations of prothrombin are directly related to the amounts of thrombin generated. That lower plasma concentrations of FVII and prothrombin during childhood are in part responsible for the lower risk of thrombotic complications is plausible, but remains unproved.

# Thrombin regulation: general

## Direct inhibitors of thrombin

Thrombin generation and activity are regulated by plasma inhibitors, endothelial cells, and fibrin. The direct inhibitors of thrombin in plasma include antithrombin (AT, formerly ATIII), $\alpha_2$-macroglobulin ($\alpha_2$M), and heparin cofactor II (HCII). AT is a single-chain polypeptide chain belonging to the serine proteinase family of inhibitors (serpins). AT inactivates serine proteases, including thrombin, by forming a 1:1 covalent bond with the active site. AT-mediated inhibition of thrombin is potentiated by the glycosaminoglycans, heparan sulfate and heparin. Physiologically, endothelial cell surface-associated heparan sulfate potentiates AT-dependent inhibition of thrombin. Therapeutically, heparin and its low-molecular-weight derivatives are the most commonly used anticoagulants for the prevention and initial treatment of venous thrombosis. $\alpha_2$M, like AT, binds to several serine proteases of blood coagulation, including thrombin. However, $\alpha_2$M inhibits a smaller fraction of thrombin than AT in adult plasma, and inhibition of thrombin by $\alpha_2$M is not enhanced by glycosaminoglycans. When $\alpha_2$M binds to thrombin, it inhibits the ability of thrombin to cleave protein substrates such as fibrinogen, but not small molecules such as chromogenic substrates.

HCII, like AT, inactivates thrombin forming a 1:1 covalent bond that completely neutralizes thrombin's activity. However, HCII inhibits only a small fraction of thrombin added to plasma. Inhibition of thrombin by HCII can be potentiated by dermatan sulfate, which is present in the subendothelium and, to a lesser degree, on the surface of endothelial cells. *In vivo*, the potentiation of HCII inhibition of thrombin by the glycosaminoglycan, dermatan sulfate, may increase the importance of this inhibitor. The safety and effectiveness of dermatan sulfate is currently being evaluated in animal models and in humans.

## Protein C/protein S system

A second mechanism for inhibiting thrombin coagulant activity is the protein C/protein S system. When it binds to the endothelial cell surface receptor, thrombomodulin (TM), thrombin no longer functions as a coagulant. TM is a protein integrated into endothelial cell membranes through a membrane-spanning domain. TM binds to thrombin through an epidermal growth factor (EGF)-like region on TM and at a site on thrombin distant from the active site. Thrombin bound to TM no longer cleaves fibrinogen or FV and FVIII, nor activates platelets. However, it can activate the vitamin K-dependent inhibitor protein C to its activated form. Protein C consists of a heavy chain, which contains the active site, and a light chain. Activated protein C (APC) is a serine protease that inactivates FVa and FVIIIa by limited proteolysis. APC activity is enhanced by another vitamin K-dependent inhibitor, protein S, that functions as a cofactor. Protein S is a single-chain glycoprotein present in two forms: a free active form and an inactive form that circulates bound to $C_4B$-binding protein. APC is inhibited by at least two plasma inhibitors: protein C inhibitor (PCI) and $\alpha_1$-antitrypsin inhibitor. Patients with *inherited deficiencies of protein C and protein S* are at risk for thrombotic complications as adults. In addition, patients who are resistant to APC activity due to a single-point mutation in FV are also at risk for thrombotic complications.

## Tissue factor pathway inhibitor

A third mechanism for regulating the generation of thrombin is by an inhibitor of the FVIIa–TF pathway, tissue factor pathway inhibitor (TFPI). TFPI is a Kunitz-type serine proteinase inhibitor synthesized by endothelial cells. The inhibition of FVIIa–TF by TFPI occurs after the generation of FXa. FXa binds to TFPI in a $Ca^{2+}$-independent reaction requiring the active site of FXa. The TFPI–FXa complex binds to FVIIa–TF in a $Ca^{2+}$-dependent reaction resulting in the inhibition of FVIIa. Following the generation of small amounts of thrombin, TFPI prevents further generation of thrombin via FVIIa–TF. The small amount of thrombin generated activates FXI which results in a burst of thrombin generation independent of FVIIa–TF.

## Regulation of thrombin by fibrin

A fourth mechanism for regulating thrombin activity is fibrin itself. Thrombin binds to fibrin and is relatively protected from inactivation by plasma antiproteases. Thrombin bound to fibrin functions as a procoagulant by activating FV, FVIII, FXI and potentially converting fibrinogen to fibrin but at a considerably slower rate.

# Thrombin regulation: infancy and childhood

There are several important physiological differences in thrombin regulation that likely partly explain the lower risk of thrombotic complications in children.

## Direct inhibitors of thrombin

Plasma concentrations of AT and HCII during the first weeks of life are approximately 50 per cent of those in adults (Table 82.1, Fig. 82.3). One anticipates that low concentrations of these inhibitors would markedly impair the inhibition of thrombin and place infants at greater risk of thrombotic complications. However, when measured directly, the inhibition of thrombin is slower but the total capacity to inhibit thrombin is similar in plasma from newborns and adults. In contrast to AT and HCII, plasma concentrations of $\alpha_2 M$ in newborns are increased compared with adult values and are approximately twice adult values by 6 months of age (Fig. 82.3). Increased plasma concentrations of $\alpha_2 M$ likely compensate, at least in part, for the low plasma concentrations of AT in newborns.

In addition to the increased binding of thrombin to $\alpha_2 M$ in newborn plasma, the amount of thrombin complexing to HCII is disproportionately increased due to the presence of a circulating dermatan sulfate proteoglycan (DSPG) that catalyzes thrombin inhibition by HCII. The plasma concentration of DSPG is 0.29 $\mu g/mL$ and its molecular mass is 150 kD. DSPG also is present in plasma from pregnant women, is produced by the placenta and disappears within days of delivery. The length of time that DSPG circulates in newborns is not known, except that it is still present during the first week of life in sick premature infants with *respiratory distress syndrome*.

Postnatally average values for plasma concentrations of AT increase to adult values by approximately 3 months of age (Fig. 82.3). In contrast, plasma concentrations of $\alpha_2 M$ remain increased throughout childhood and do not decrease to adult concentrations until the third decade of life (Fig. 82.3). The capacity of $\alpha_2 M$ to complex with thrombin remains increased during childhood, likely contributing to both the decreased

thrombotic risk in healthy children as well as in children with heterozygous AT deficiency.

## Protein C/protein S system

Similar to adults, thrombin generation in the young is also controlled by the protein C/protein S inhibitor system. Plasma concentrations of protein C and protein S are significantly reduced in early childhood (Table 82.1, Fig. 82.3). In the newborn, protein C circulates in a fetal form that differs from the adult by a two-fold increase in single-chain protein C. The physiological significance of fetal protein C is unknown. Protein S circulates completely in the free, active form because $C_4B$-binding protein is absent in newborn plasma. The latter likely compensates for the low plasma concentrations of total protein S (Table 82.1, Fig. 82.3). The lower limits of normal for protein C and protein S remain decreased throughout early childhood and are important to consider when assessing children for inherited deficiencies of these inhibitors (Fig. 82.3). In contrast to protein C and protein S, plasma concentrations of TM are increased during infancy and early childhood, decreasing to adult values during the teenage years.

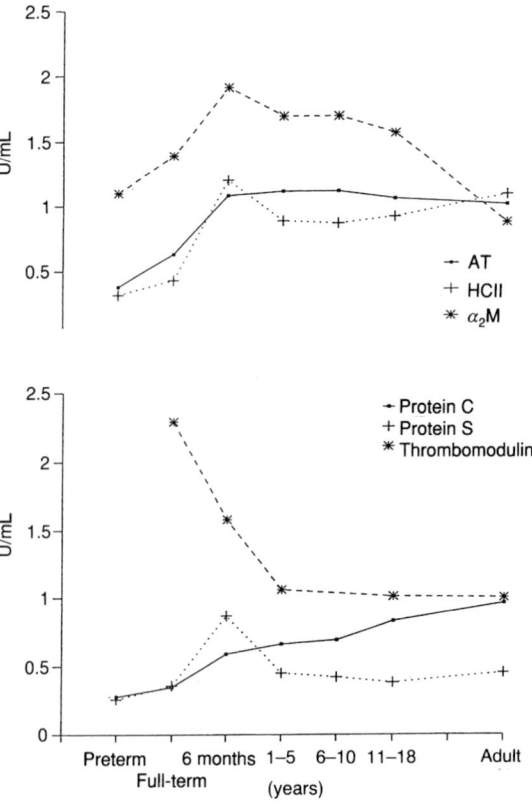

FIGURE 82.3 Plasma concentrations of the inhibitors of coagulation at different ages. AT, antithrombin III; HCII, heparin cofactor II; $\alpha_2 M$, $\alpha_2$-macroglobulin.

## Tissue factor pathway inhibitor

There is limited information on the influence of age on TFPI. Cord plasma concentrations of TFPI are decreased to 64 per cent of adult values.

## Regulation of thrombin by fibrin

The capacity of newborn fibrin clots to bind thrombin has been assessed by measuring FPA production by fibrin clots prepared from adult and cord plasmas. Cord plasma clots generated significantly less FPA compared with adult plasma clots. Decreased plasma concentrations of prothrombin in cord plasma resulted in decreased thrombin bound to cord clots. Increasing cord plasma concentrations of prothrombin similarly increased FPA production by cord clots. These observations suggest that thrombi in newborns may not have the same propensity to propagate compared with thrombi in adult patients.

## The influence of age on endogenous regulation of thrombin

Activation of coagulation *in vivo* with the generation of thrombin can be quantitated by specific activation peptides such as F1.2, FPA, and protein C activation peptide; and by enzyme–inhibitor complexes, such as TAT, protein C–PCI, and protein C–$\alpha_1$AT. Increased cord plasma concentrations of FPA and TAT suggest that coagulation is activated at birth. However, this process seems to be well controlled and self-limited. Indeed, activation of coagulation during the birth process does not result in significant consumption of circulating plasma coagulation proteins nor clinical morbidity. Plasma concentrations of F1.2 and TAT complexes are similar in children and young adults (ages 20–40 years). However, with increasing age (over 40 years), plasma concentrations of F1.2 increase along with age-dependent increases in the plasma concentrations of FPA and protein C activation peptide. This *ex vivo* evidence of impaired thrombin regulation in older adults, in combination with *in vitro* evidence of enhanced regulation of thrombin during childhood, strongly suggests that the regulation of thrombin deteriorates with age, paralleling an increased risk of thrombotic complications.

## Potential mechanisms: ontogeny and thrombin regulation

Potential mechanisms responsible for differences in plasma concentrations of coagulation components include decreased synthesis, increased clearance or consumption, and presence of proteins with decreased activity. mRNA levels have been measured for FVII, FVIII, FIX, FX, fibrinogen, AT, and protein C in hepatocytes from 5–10-week-old human embryos and fetuses, and from adults. The embryonic–fetal transcripts and adult mRNAs were similar in size; and the nucleotide sequences of embryonic, fetal and adult FIX and FX mRNA were identical. However, the expression of mRNA was variable, with adult values for some coagulation proteins and decreased expression for others. Similar concentrations of prothrombin mRNA are found in newborn and adult rabbit livers; one study has reported lower prothrombin mRNA concentrations in sheep.

At least some coagulation proteins are cleared more rapidly in newborns compared with adults. The half-life of fibrinogen is significantly shorter in newborn animals and in infants with respiratory distress syndrome than that in corresponding adults. The half-life of AT is shorter in infants requiring an exchange transfusion for hyperbilirubinemia than that in healthy adults. Reasons for the faster clearance of these proteins in newborns are incompletely understood but in part may be due to an increased basal metabolic rate in newborns.

Activation of coagulation during the birth process does occur but does not provide an explanation for low concentrations of coagulation proteins in newborns. Similarly there is no evidence that fetal proteins significantly affect functional measurements of coagulation proteins, thereby contributing to low plasma activities of the protein involved.

# FIBRINOLYSIS

## Plasmin regulation: general

Once a fibrin clot has formed *in vivo*, it is modified by the fibrinolytic system (Fig. 82.4). Analogous to thrombin, plasmin is the critical enzyme in fibrinolysis. Plasminogen circulates in two forms, one with an

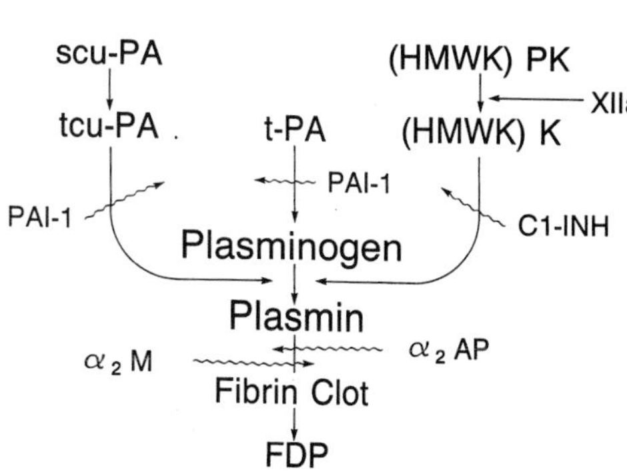

FIGURE 82.4 The fibrinolytic system. t-PA, tissue plasminogen activator; PAI-1, plasminogen activator inhibitor-1; HMWK, high-molecular-weight kininogen; PK, prekallikrein; K, kallikrein; $\alpha_2$M, $\alpha_2$-macroglobulin; $\alpha_2$AP, $\alpha_2$-antiplasmin; scu-PA, single-chain urokinase plasminogen activator; tcu-PA, two-chain urokinase plasminogen activator; C1-INH, C1-inhibitor; FDP, fibrin degradation products.

NH$_2$-terminal glutamic acid residue (glu-plasminogen) and a second form with NH$_2$-terminal lysine, valine, or methionine residues (lys-plasminogen). Glu-plasminogen can be converted to lys-plasminogen by limited proteolytic degradation. Lys-plasminogen has both a higher affinity for fibrin and an increased fibrinolytic activity than glu-plasminogen. Both forms of plasminogen bind to fibrin through specific lysine-binding sites that also mediate the interaction of plasminogen with its inhibitor, α$_2$-antiplasmin (α$_2$AP). Plasminogen is converted to its enzymatically active form, plasmin, by several activators. Tissue plasminogen activator (t-PA) is the most important physiological activator of plasminogen. t-PA is a serine protease that also binds to fibrin through lysine-binding sites. t-PA is a relatively poor enzyme in the absence of fibrin; however, fibrin greatly enhances the rate of plasminogen activation by t-PA. Urokinase (u-PA) is a second physiological activator of plasminogen. Single-chain urokinase (scu-PA) has relatively low thrombolytic activity until it is activated to its two-chain form (tcu-PA) by limited cleavage by plasmin or kallikrein. Plasminogen also is activated by components of the contact system; however, this does not appear to be of physiological importance. The plasmin molecule is a two-chain trypsin-like serine proteinase. Once formed on the fibrin clot, plasmin cleaves fibrin in sequential steps resulting in fibrin degradation products.

When bound to the fibrin surface, plasmin is relatively protected from inhibition by its major inhibitor α$_2$AP. α$_2$AP belongs to the serpin family of inhibitors and binds to the active site of plasmin forming a 1:1 stoichiometric complex that has no further activity against fibrin. α$_2$M is a less important inhibitor of plasmin than α$_2$AP in adults. Plasmin bound to α$_2$M retains some fibrinolytic activity. The fibrinolytic system is also regulated by inhibitors of t-PA and u-PA. There are three plasminogen activator inhibitors: PAI-1, PAI-2, and PAI-3. PAI-1 is the major inhibitor of t-PA and tcu-PA in adults. PAI-2 is present in plasma during pregnancy and is produced by the placenta. PAI-2 is likely the physiological mechanism by which fibrinolysis is suppressed during pregnancy. Recently it was shown that PAI-3 is identical to PCI.

## Plasmin regulation: infancy and childhood

During infancy and childhood, plasmin is generated and inhibited in a fashion similar to that in adults; however, as with thrombin regulation, there are important differences when compared with the adult fibrinolytic system (Table 82.3, Fig. 82.5). Plasma concentrations of fibrinolytic proteins differ significantly (Table 82.3). In newborns, plasma plasminogen concentrations are 50 per cent of adult values, α$_2$AP concentrations 80 per cent, and plasma concentrations of PAI-1 and t-PA are significantly increased over adult values. The increased plasma concentrations of t-PA and PAI-1 in newborns on day 1 are in marked contrast to values from cord blood, in which concentrations of these two proteins are significantly lower than in adults. The discrepancy between newborn and cord plasma concentrations of t-PA and PAI-1 can be explained by enhanced release of t-PA and PAI-1 from the endothelium shortly following birth. PAI-2 is detectable in cord blood but at significantly lower concentrations than in pregnant women. PAI-2 has not been measured in newborns. Plasminogen, like fibrinogen, has a fetal form. Fetal plasminogen exists in two glycoforms, but with increased amounts of mannose

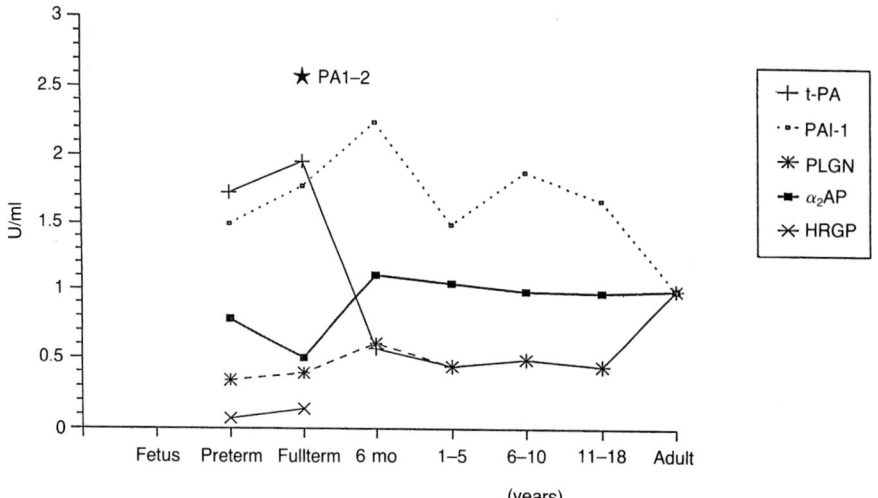

FIGURE 82.5 Plasma concentrations of the components of the fibrinolytic system. t-PA, tissue plasminogen activator; PAI-1, plasminogen activator inhibitor 1; PAI-2, plasminogen activator inhibitor 2; PLGN, plasminogen; α$_2$AP, α$_2$-antiplasmin; HRGP, histidine-rich glycoprotein.

TABLE 82.3 Reference values for infants and children for the coagulation and fibrinolytic systems

| | FULL-TERM MEAN (BOUNDARY) | CHILDREN 6–10 YEARS MEAN (BOUNDARY) | ADULT MEAN (BOUNDARY) |
|---|---|---|---|
| Fibrinogen (g/L) | 2.83 (1.67–3.99) | 2.79 (1.57–4.0) | 2.78 (1.56–4.0) |
| II (U/mL) | 0.48 (0.26–0.70) | 0.88 (0.67–1.07) | 1.08 (0.70–1.46) |
| V (U/mL) | 0.72 (0.34–1.08) | 0.90 (0.63–1.16) | 1.06 (0.62–1.50) |
| VII (U/mL) | 0.66 (0.28–1.04) | 0.85 (0.52–1.20) | 1.05 (0.67–1.43) |
| VIII (U/mL) | 1.00 (0.50–1.78) | 0.95 (0.58–1.32) | 0.99 (0.50–1.49) |
| vWF (U/mL) | 1.53 (0.50–2.87) | 0.95 (0.44–1.44) | 0.92 (0.50–1.58) |
| IX (U/mL) | 0.53 (0.15–0.91) | 0.75 (0.63–0.89) | 1.09 (0.55–1.63) |
| X (U/mL) | 0.40 (0.12–0.68) | 0.75 (0.55–1.01) | 1.06 (0.70–1.52) |
| XI (U/mL) | 0.38 (0.10–0.66) | 0.86 (0.52–1.20) | 0.97 (0.67–1.27) |
| XII (U/mL) | 0.53 (0.13–0.93) | 0.92 (0.60–1.40) | 1.08 (0.52–1.64) |
| Prekallikrein (U/mL) | 0.37 (0.18–0.69) | 0.99 (0.66–1.31) | 1.12 (0.62–1.62) |
| High molecular weight kininogen (U/mL) | 0.54 (0.06–1.02) | 0.93 (0.60–1.30) | 0.92 (0.50–1.36) |
| XIIIa (U/mL) | 0.79 (0.27–1.31) | 1.09 (0.65–1.51) | 1.05 (0.55–1.55) |
| XIIIb (U/mL) | 0.76 (0.30–1.22) | 1.16 (0.77–1.54) | 0.97 (0.57–1.37) |
| Antithrombin (U/mL) | 0.63 (0.39–0.87) | 1.11 (0.90–1.31) | 1.0 (0.74–1.26) |
| $\alpha_2$-Macroglobulin (U/mL) | 1.39 (0.95–1.83) | 1.69 (1.28–2.09) | 0.86 (0.52–1.20) |
| $C_1$-esterase inhibitor (U/mL) | 0.72 (0.36–1.08) | 1.14 (0.88–1.54) | 1.0 (0.71–1.31) |
| $\alpha_1$-Antitrypsin (U/mL) | 0.93 (0.49–1.37) | 1.00 (0.69–1.30) | 0.93 (0.55–1.30) |
| Heporin cofactor II (U/mL) | 0.43 (0.10–0.93) | 0.86 (0.40–1.32) | 1.08 (0.66–1.26) |
| Protein C (U/mL) | 0.35 (0.17–0.53) | 0.69 (0.45–0.93) | 0.96 (0.64–1.28) |
| Protein S (U/mL) | | | |
| Total | 0.36 (0.12–0.60) | 0.78 (0.41–1.14) | 0.81 (0.60–1.13) |
| Free | – | 0.42 (0.22–0.62) | 0.45 (0.27–0.61) |
| Plasminogen (U/mL) | 0.54 (0.35–0.74) | 0.92 (0.75–1.08) | 0.99 (0.77–1.22) |
| Tissue plasminogen activator (ng/mL) | 9.6 (5.0–18.9) | 2.42 (1.0–5.0) | 4.90 (1.40–8.40) |
| $\alpha_2$-Antiplasmin (U/mL) | 0.85 (0.55–1.15) | 0.99 (0.89–1.10) | 1.02 (0.68–1.36) |
| Plasminogen activator inhibitor (U/mL) | 6.4 (2.0–15.1) | 6.79 (2.0–12.0) | 3.60 (0–11.0) |

VIII, factor VIII procoagulant; vWF, von Willebrand factor; PK, prekallikrein; HMWK, high-molecular-weight kininogen; AT, antithrombin; $\alpha_2$M, $\alpha_2$-Macroglobulin; $C_1$E-INH, $C_1$-esterase inhibitor; $\alpha_1$AT, $\alpha_1$-antitrypsin; HCII, heparin cofactor II; t-PA, tissue plasminogen activator; $\alpha_2$AP, $\alpha_2$-antiplasmin; PAI, plasminogen activator inhibitor. All factors, except fibrinogen, are expressed as units per milliliter (U/mL), where pooled plasma contains 1.0 U/mL. All values are expressed as the mean, followed by the lower and upper boundary encompassing 95 per cent of the population. Between 40 and 77 samples were assayed for each value for the newborn. Some measurements were skewed due to a disproportionate number of high values. The lower limit, which excludes the lower 2.5 per cent of the population, has been given.

and sialic acid. There probably is decreased enzymatic activity of "fetal plasmin" as well as decreased binding to cellular receptors for fetal plasminogen.

By early childhood, plasma concentrations of plasminogen and $\alpha_2$AP are similar to adult values while physiological plasma concentrations of t-PA are decreased and PAI-1 increased (Fig. 82.5).

## The influence of age on endogenous regulation of fibrinolysis

Short whole-blood clotting times, short euglobulin lysis times and increased plasma concentrations of the Bβ 15–42 fibrin-related peptides all suggest that the fibrinolytic system is activated at birth. At the same time, the capacity of the fetal fibrinolytic system to generate plasmin in response to stimulation with a thrombolytic agent is decreased compared with adults. The latter reflects low plasma concentrations of plasminogen in newborns. The reduced capacity to generate plasmin impairs the overall ability of cord plasma to lyse fibrin clots. Increasing plasma concentrations of plasminogen, either with purified plasminogen or with plasma supplementation, enhances the fibrinolytic capacity of

cord plasma. During childhood, the increased t-PA and decreased PAI-1 concentrations result in a decreased fibrinolytic capacity, as assessed by venous occlusion. Thus, the fibrinolytic system does not appear to provide a mechanism for lowering the risk of thromboembolic complications in children. Furthermore, the suppressed fibrinolytic system in the young may impair endogenous lysis of thrombi. The latter will be important to determine in long-term follow-up studies of children with large vessel thrombotic complications.

## PLATELETS

## General information

The cell surface properties and internal constituents of platelets both contribute to the central role of platelets in hemostasis. Platelets, disc-shaped cells produced by megakaryocytes in the bone marrow, are released into the circulation. Platelet counts in adults range between 150 and 400 × $10^9$/L with mean platelet volumes of 7–9 fL. Platelet counts and mean platelet volumes in newborns are not different from adult values, although the average count in premature infants is slightly lower than in full-term infants. Platelet counts in fetal blood (18–30 weeks' gestation) also fall within the adult range with a mean of $250 \times 10^9$/L. Platelet lifespan is approximately 7–10 days in adults at which time platelets are removed from the circulation by macrophages in the reticuloendothelial system. Platelet survival has not been measured in healthy infants. However, as measured with indium oxide-labeled adult rabbit platelets, platelet survival is similar for adult and newborn rabbits. Platelet survival in thrombocytopenic infants is shorter than that in adults, with platelets from the least thrombocytopenic infants having the longest survival, some in the normal adult range. Together these studies suggest that platelet survival in newborns does not differ significantly from that in adults.

Because of the sample volume required to evaluate platelet function, most studies of newborn platelet function in fact have been performed on cord platelets, not platelets obtained directly from newborns. Cord and newborn platelets may have some differences in function and thus are designated separately in this section. Although studies agree that cord and adult platelets function differently, there is not uniform agreement on the details of the differences. Differences in the timing and method of collection, different sources (newborn vs cord), and differing methods of measuring platelet function all contribute to apparently conflicting information.

## Platelet structure

### Adult platelets

The outer surface of platelets contains several adhesive glycoproteins that bind specific adhesive proteins to facilitate platelet–surface interactions, and platelet to platelet aggregation. Under the glycocalyx, there is a phospholipid bilayer that provides a procoagulant surface after platelets are activated for thrombin generation, and an internal membrane system that participates in platelet secretion of granular contents. Platelets contain two types of granules: dense bodies and α-granules. Dense bodies contain substances that promote platelet aggregation such as ADP, serotonin and $Ca^{2+}$. The α-granules contain several substances that have a wide variety of functions: thrombospondin, an adhesive protein; growth factors such as platelet-derived growth factor, transforming growth factor β, and fibroblast growth factor; platelet factor 4 (PF-4), a substance that interferes with heparin–AT interaction; several coagulation proteins and β-thromboglobulin, a marker of platelet activation.

### Cord platelets

Cord platelets have been examined for the presence of secretory granules and defects in release mechanisms.

Electron microscopy studies have demonstrated normal numbers of granules; however, serotonin and ADP, which are stored in dense granules, are present at concentrations less than 50 per cent of those in adults.

## Adhesion, activation, aggregation

### Adhesion: adult platelets (Fig. 82.6) (*see* also page 702)

Under normal circumstances, circulating platelets do not adhere to vessel walls or to other cells. When the vascular endothelial lining is damaged or removed, platelets adhere to subendothelial layers, undergo shape change, spread over the surface and bind to each other. Adhesion initiates the secretion of platelet granule contents that include ADP and adhesive proteins such as vWF and fibrinogen. These substances promote both adhesion and formation of aggregates. The process of platelet adhesion is mediated by a specific component of the platelet membrane, glycoprotein Ib (GPIb) and an adhesive protein, vWF. GPIb, an integral membrane protein bound to the actin skeleton of the platelet, is a sialoglycoprotein composed of two disulfide-linked subunits (Ibα, 143 kD, and Ibβ, 22 kD). There are approximately 25 000 molecules of GPIb per platelet and these serve as binding sites for vWF. The extracellular component of the Ibα chain is carbohydrate rich and is called glycocalicin. vWF is secreted by both endothelial cells and platelets, and is present in both the subendothelium and plasma.

### Adhesion: cord platelets

*In vitro* measurement of cord platelet adhesion has not produced consistent results. GPIb is present on fetal platelet membranes in adult amounts. Both the plasma concentration of vWF and the proportion of high molecular weight multimers of vWF are increased in newborns, and these achieve adult levels within the first weeks after birth. The abnormal multimeric forms appear similar to the forms released by endothelial cells suggesting that mechanisms for processing the multimeric structure may not be fully developed at birth. The increase in high-molecular-weight multimers may be responsible for the enhanced cord platelet agglutination to low concentrations of ristocetin and may contribute to the short bleeding time found in newborns.

### Platelet aggregation: adult platelets (Fig. 82.6)

Following activation of platelets, glycoproteins IIb (GPIIb) and IIIa (GPIIIa) come together on the platelet surface to form a 1:1 complex that forms a binding site for fibrinogen and, to a lesser extent, vWF and fibronectin. Platelet to platelet adherence or aggregation is mediated by fibrinogen bound to GPIIb/IIIa. GPIIb and

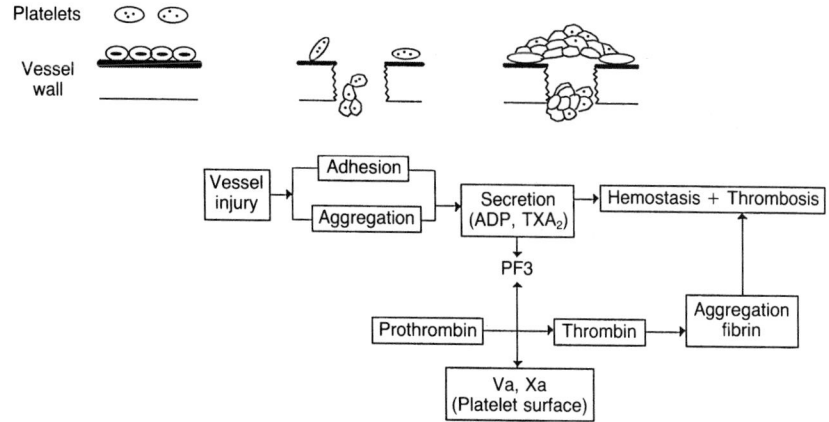

FIGURE 82.6 Platelet aggregation and adhesion. ADP, adenosine diphosphate; TXA$_2$, thromboxane A$_2$; PF3, platelet factor 3.

GPIIIa are the most abundant platelet surface glycoproteins with approximately 50 000 copies of each per platelet. GPIIb is composed of two disulfide-linked subunits (GPIIbα, 125 kD and GPIIbβ, 25 kD, while GPIIIa is a single polypeptide chain (105 kD). GPIIb/IIIa are the site of some platelet-specific alloantigens such as Bak$^a$ on GPIIb and P1$^{A1}$ antigen on GPIIIa.

## Platelet aggregation: cord platelets

The IIb/IIIa platelet glycoproteins are present on fetal platelet membranes from early gestation. The capacity of cord platelets to aggregate following exposure to a variety of agonists including ADP, epinephrine, collagen, thrombin and arachidonic acid has been variable with some observations, more consistent with others. Cord platelet aggregation in response to epinephrine is markedly impaired due to decreased numbers of α-adrenergic receptors. This may be due to delayed maturation of these receptors or to occupation by catecholamines that are released during the birth process. Of the other agonists, decreased cord platelet aggregation to collagen is the most consistent defect.

## Activation and secretion: adult platelets (Fig. 82.7)

Regulation of platelets is a dynamic process initiated when specific platelet surface receptors are occupied by a wide variety of extracellular molecules that result in excitatory and/or inhibitory signals. These signals can be grouped as strong agonists (thrombin, collagen, prostaglandin endoperoxides (PGG$_2$, PGH$_2$), thromboxane A$_2$, platelet-activating factor; weak agonists (ADP, epinephrine, vasopressin and serotonin) and antagonists (PGI$_2$, PGD$_2$, endothelium-derived relaxing factor (nitric oxide, NO). Receptor occupation activates membrane-associated enzymes through receptor-linked changes in signal-transducing GTP-binding regulatory proteins (G-proteins). These in turn generate intracellular second messengers, phospholipase C, which promotes platelet activation in a wide variety of ways, and adenylyl cyclase, which

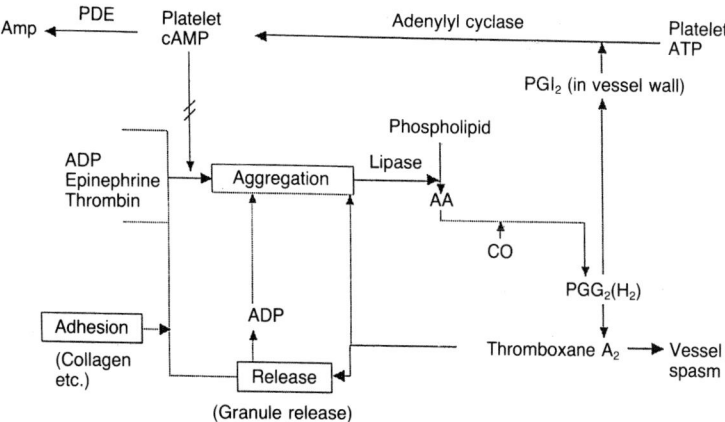

FIGURE 82.7 Platelet activation. ATP, adenosine 5'-triphosphate; ADP, adenosine 5'-diphosphate; AMP, adenosine 5'-monophosphate; cAMP, cyclic 3',5'-adenosine monophosphate; PDE, phosphodiesterase; AA, arachidonic acid; PGI$_2$, prostacyclin; PGG$_2$, PGH$_2$, prostaglandin endoperoxides; CO, cyclooxygenase.

promotes platelet inhibition by converting intracellular ATP into cAMP, a molecule that antagonizes all $Ca^{2+}$-dependent activation events.

Platelet secretion is a process whereby platelet granules form a cluster, and then fuse with the membranes of other granules or the open connected canalicular system. The clustering of granules depends on the interaction of actin and myosin filaments, which in turn is dependent on $Ca^{2+}$–calmodulin activation of myosin light-chain kinase. The fusion of granules depends on protein kinase C.

## Activation and secretion: cord platelets

Studies of activation pathways leading to release have not identified specific abnormalities in cord platelets. Inositol phosphate production and protein phosphorylation are normal, as is production of arachidonic acid and its metabolites. In fact, in response to thrombin stimulation, cord platelets release more arachidonic acid than adult platelets. This may be due to platelet membranes made more reactive by low levels of vitamin E. Agonist receptors, with the exception of α-adrenergic receptors discussed previously, do not appear to be decreased in number. Despite a poor response to collagen stimulation, cord platelets have normal amounts of the collagen receptor GPIa/IIa present on platelet membranes. Coupling of agonist receptors to phospholipases may be the site of this transient activation defect in response to collagen.

## Studies of platelets from newborns

A few studies have assessed platelet aggregation using newborn platelets obtained during the first few days after birth; others have evaluated older neonates. In one study, abnormal platelet aggregation to ADP (decreased primary wave and absent secondary wave) was observed in platelet-rich cord plasma. However, improved platelet aggregation was seen in newborn platelets drawn 2 hours after birth, with normalization of platelet aggregation by 48 hours.

## Bleeding time

Currently, the bleeding time is the best *in vivo* test of platelet interaction with the vessel wall. This is particularly true for newborns, in whom platelet aggregation studies frequently are not feasible. Recently, automated devices modified for newborns and children have become available and the methodology for performing bleeding times standardized. Bleeding times in infants during the first week after birth are significantly shorter than adult values. Several mechanisms probably contribute to this enhanced platelet–vessel wall interaction: higher plasma concentrations of vWF in newborns; enhanced function of vWF due to increased amounts of high-molecular-weight, active

multimers; large red cells; and high hematocrits. The significance of mild platelet aggregation defects in cord platelets compared with adult platelets is uncertain when bleeding times in newborns are even shorter than those in adults. Throughout the rest of childhood, bleeding times are prolonged compared with adult values for reasons that are not apparent. Platelet aggregation studies are similar in children compared with adults.

## Activation during the birth process

There is strong evidence that platelets are activated during the birth process. Cord plasma concentrations of thromboxane $B_2$, β-thromboglobulin and PF-4 are increased. Consistent with these observations, the granular content of cord platelets is decreased and epinephrine receptor availability on platelets is reduced, perhaps secondary to occupation. The mechanisms of activation are likely multifactorial and include thermal changes, hypoxia, acidosis, adrenergic stimulation and thrombogenic effects of amniotic fluid.

## AGE AND THE VESSEL WALL

The last decade has established that the endothelium plays a complex role in hemostasis, preventing thrombotic complications under physiological conditions and promoting fibrin formation when injured. The following is a brief summary of endothelial anticoagulant properties, which can be grouped under the headings of eicosanoids, proteoglycans, NO, protein C/protein S system, and fibrinolysis (see also Chapter 67).

### Eicosanoids

One of the anticoagulant properties of endothelial cell surfaces is mediated by lipoxygenase and cyclooxygenase metabolites of unsaturated fatty acids synthesized by the endothelium. Prostacyclin ($PGI_2$) is a potent vasodilator that inhibits platelet aggregation and release, as well as enhancing fibrinolysis. $PGI_2$ regulates the extent of *in vivo* platelet plug formation in response to injury. 13-Hydroxyoctadecadienoic acid, produced by the lipoxygenase pathway, inhibits the adhesion of platelets to endothelial surfaces.

### Endothelial cell surface proteoglycans

Endothelial cell surface heparan sulfate proteoglycans promote AT neutralization of thrombin as well as other serine proteases that promote thrombin generation (see above).

## Nitric oxide

NO is a labile agent that modulates vascular tone in the fetal and postnatal lung, as well as in other organs, and contributes significantly to the normal decline in pulmonary vascular resistance at birth (see Chapter 73). Like $PGI_2$, NO is a potent inhibitor of platelet activation and adhesion to the damaged vessel wall.

## Protein C/protein S system

The endothelial cell receptor TM binds thrombin, which accelerates protein C activation to APC. APC in the presence of protein S proteolytically inactivates FVa and FVIIIa (see page 881).

## Fibrinolysis

Endothelial cells produce many components of the fibrinolytic system including t-PA, PAI-1, and urokinase. In addition, there are binding sites for components of the fibrinolytic system on endothelial cell surfaces.

## Age and anticoagulant properties of the vessel wall

The process of vessel wall aging is likely a continuum with important developmental changes already occurring during early infancy and childhood. However, there is little information on anticoagulant properties of the vessel wall during infancy and childhood. Structurally, there is some evidence that vessel wall glycosaminoglycans differ in the young. Very crude parameters of capillary bed fragility suggest that the capillary system is more fragile in newborns compared with adults. Metabolically, cord vessel production of $PGI_2$ exceeds that of vessels from adults. Thrombin generation in cord plasma is decreased in the presence of human umbilical endothelial cells compared with plastic. However, increasing cord plasma concentration of AT further enhances the anticoagulant properties of human umbilical vein endothelial cells (HUVEC).

## CONCLUSIONS

Developmental aspects of hemostasis are important because they influence the clinical presentation of hemostatic problems and the effectiveness of therapeutic options for pediatric patients. The physiological development of hemostasis in humans is a dynamic process that assumes many forms depending on the age of the subject. Hemostasis evolves from a relatively immature form in early fetal life to a mature adult form. In healthy fetuses, infants and children appropriate hemostasis is achieved and neither hemorrhagic nor thrombotic complications occur. Thus the hemostatic system at these times of life must be considered physiological, not pathological, variations of the adult system. However, the age-related differences in hemostasis alter the risk of hemorrhagic and thrombotic complications compared with adults. For example, the low stores of vitamin K and markedly reduced capacity to generate thrombin in the first days after birth leave newborns more vulnerable than adults for hemorrhagic complications secondary to vitamin K deficiency. In contrast, enhanced thrombin regulation in plasma by the vessel wall likely contributes to the low incidence of thromboembolic events in children. Further research on age-dependent variations in hemostasis will likely provide further insight into hemostatic problems in children and adults.

## SELECTED READING

Andrew M, Paes B, Johnston M et al. Development of the human coagulation system in the full-term infant. Blood 1987; 70: 165.

Andrew M, Paes B, Johnston M. Development of the hemostatic system in the neonate and young infant. Am J Pediatr Hematol Oncol 1990; 12: 95.

Andrew M, Paes B, Milner R et al. Development of the human coagulation system in the healthy premature infant. Blood 1988; 72: 1651.

Andrew M, Vegh P, Johnston M et al. Maturation of the hemostatic system during childhood. Blood 1992; 80: 1998.

Hassan H, Leonardi C, Chelucci C et al. Blood coagulation factors in human embryonic–fetal development: Preferential expression of the FVII/tissue factor pathway. Blood 1990; 76: 1158.

Michelson AD. Neonatal thrombosis and hemorrhage. In: Loscalzo J, Schafer AI, eds. Thrombosis and hemorrhage. Cambridge: Blackwell, 1994: 999.

Yamamoto N, Greco NJ, Barnard MR, et al. Glycoprotein Ib (GPIb)-dependent and GPIb-independent pathways of thrombin-induced platelet activation. Blood 1991; 77: 1740.

# PART FOURTEEN

# *Immune System*

**Editor: Melissa E. Elder**

# 83

# Ontogeny of the Immune System

Hans D. Ochs

Studies of the ontogeny of the immune system are key to understanding the complex machinery that ensures recognition of self and non-self and effective elimination of infectious agents. Furthermore, awareness of normal lymphocyte differentiation aids understanding of the physiological immune deficiency of newborns and young infants, and of primary immunodeficiency syndromes.

## LYMPHOCYTE ONTOGENY

The cells involved in the immune response are part of the hematopoietic system derived from stem cells originating in the yolk sac. In humans, the function of the yolk sac is replaced by that of the fetal liver and bone marrow at 5 weeks' gestation. Natural killer (NK) cells and T- and B-lymphocyte precursors are detectable in the fetal liver at 6 weeks and 7–8 weeks, respectively. The fetal thymus is subsequently colonized by T-cell precursors at 8–9 weeks, and pre-B cells are found in the bone marrow by 13 weeks. These lymphocytes and their progeny are identified by the expression of cell surface cluster of differentiation (CD) molecules. Mature T and B lymphocytes are detectable by the onset of the second trimester of pregnancy. Some complement components can be detected between 6 and 14 weeks' gestation; all are present at birth, although at lower levels than in adults.

## B CELLS

### Antibody structure (see also page 900)

Immunoglobulins or antibodies, which consist of paired identical heavy and light chains, are highly vari-able in sequence at the antigen-binding (Fab) portion and constant at the Fc region of the molecule. Antibody diversity is determined by the structure of the Fab portion and is generated during B-lymphocyte differentiation in the pre-B and B-cell stages. The ability to bind most antigens encountered by humans is accomplished by B-lineage cells through the utilization of a complex recombinase system in which multiple gene segments encoding immunoglobulin heavy and light chains are assembled by sequential rearrangement. This process occurs for heavy-chain gene segments prior to that for light chains. The heavy-chain locus consists of multiple copies of $V_H$ (variable), $D_H$ (diversity), and $J_H$ (joining) gene segments. The VDJ region is linked to a cluster of constant gene sequences that encode the different heavy-chain classes ($\mu$, $\delta$, $\gamma3$, $\gamma1$, $\alpha1$, $\gamma2$, $\gamma4$, $\epsilon$, $\alpha2$; see Chapter 84, Fig. 84.2). Each heavy-chain class defines an immunoglobulin isotype with distinct biological functions, such as half-life, passage across the placenta, and complement fixation. The system of VDJ rearrangement, together with somatic hypermutation (addition or loss of nucleotides at the VDJ junctions) permit an antibody repertoire of more than $10^{11}$ specificities to be generated from a relatively small number of somatic gene segments.

Once membrane-bound, immunoglobulins act as antigen receptors, providing specific antigen recognition and initiating a cascade of events that lead to B-lymphocyte activation (see Chapter 84, Fig. 84.1). Membrane-associated immunoglobulins have very short intracytoplasmic sequences that are unsuitable for signal transduction. Instead, surface IgM forms a complex with a heterodimer consisting of two glycoproteins designated Ig-$\alpha$ and Ig-$\beta$ (CD79). These constitutively expressed components of the antigen receptor complex have long cytoplasmic tails that provide binding sites to one, or more, non-receptor protein tyrosine kinase involved in transmitting signals to the nuclei of B lymphocytes.

# B-cell development

## B-cell progenitors

B lymphocytes are derived from pluripotent hematopoietic stem cells. Commitment to the B-cell lineage is achieved before the formation of progenitor B lymphocytes. Proliferation and differentiation of progenitor B lymphocytes occur in close contact with a marrow microenvironment containing diverse cells referred to as stromal cells. At this stage, progenitor B-lymphocyte development is dependent on cell–cell contact and on multiple cytokines (messenger molecules that can affect cellular responses without requiring direct cell–cell contact) secreted by stromal cells. Progenitor B lymphocytes do not express B lineage-specific markers and have not begun to rearrange their immunoglobulin genes (Fig. 83.1).

## Pre-B cells

Pre-B cells can be detected in the human fetal liver by 8 weeks' gestation, and in the fetal bone marrow by 13 weeks. Pre-B cells are distinguished by the presence of μ heavy chains in the cytoplasm. Cell-surface expression of immunoglobulins is not seen because light-chain gene segments have not yet rearranged.

## Immature B cells

Immature IgM⁺IgD⁻ B cells have been observed at 10 weeks' gestation. These may develop anergy if exposed to antigen; clonal anergy and physical deletion of autoreactive B lymphocytes may guarantee B-cell tolerance to self antigens throughout life. IgM⁺IgD⁺ B cells develop between 10 and 12 weeks' gestation; thereafter, they increase rapidly in numbers and can be found in the spleen, bone marrow, and circulation.

## Mature B cells

The subsequent differentiation of IgM⁺IgD⁺ B cells into mature B cells expressing other immunoglobulin isotypes, as well as the development of memory B cells and antibody-secreting plasma cells, requires antigen exposure and the cooperation of CD4⁺ helper T ($T_H$) cells. Antigenic stimulation of IgM⁺IgD⁺ B cells results in loss of expression of IgD and initiation of isotype or class switch whereby IgG, IgA, or IgE is expressed on the B-cell membrane. These antigen receptors will have different effector functions as specified by the Fc region, but the Fab regions and antigen specificity will be identical with that of the initially expressed IgM and IgD molecules. Isotype switch requires physical contact of the B cell with CD4⁺ $T_H$ cells through binding of CD40 and CD40 ligand (CD40L or gp39).

IgG⁺ and IgA⁺ B cells are abundant in lymph nodes, spleen, tonsil, appendix, and Peyer patches, and circulate in the peripheral blood. Following exposure to antigen, positive selection of antigen-specific B lym-

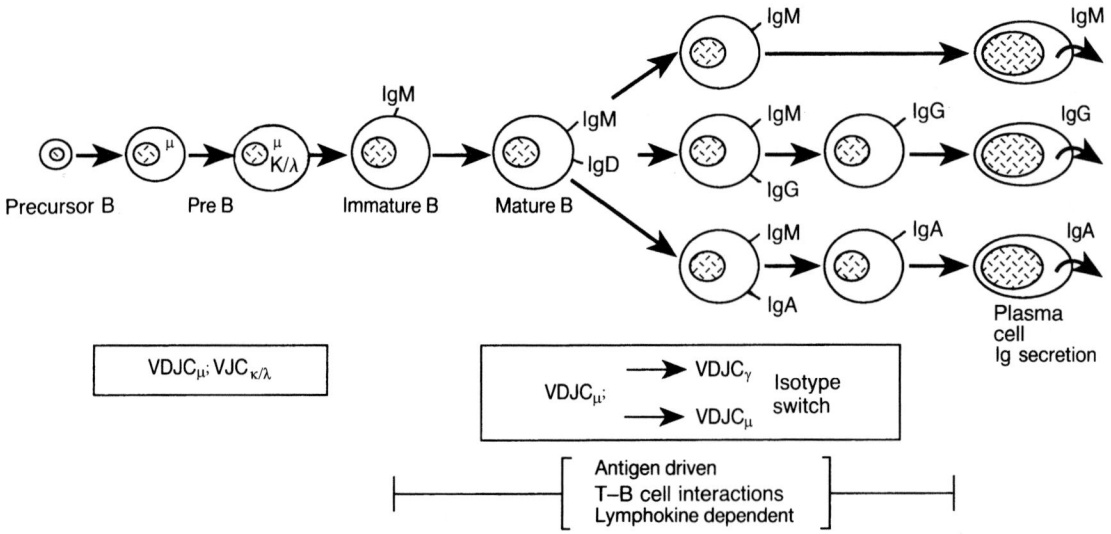

FIGURE 83.1 B-cell ontogeny. Early (antigen-independent) and late (antigen-dependent) stages of B-cell development can be identified by immunoglobulin isotype expression. B-cell precursors have not rearranged their immunoglobulin genes, and pre-B cells are identified by the presence of cytoplasmic μ chains. After light-chain rearrangement (κ or λ) is completed, IgM is expressed on the surface of immature B cells, which are tolerized if exposed to antigen. Subsequent B-cell stages also require T-cell help via exposure to lymphokines such as IL-4 and IL-6 and cell–cell contact through interactions of CD40 and CD40 ligand. VDJCμ (VDJCγ and VDJCα), rearranged variable-diversity-joining-constant segments of μ (γ and α) heavy-chain gene segments; VJCκ/λ, rearranged variable-joining-constant segments of κ or λ light-chain gene segments.

phocytes is initiated and further diversity generated by somatic hypermutation. Germinal center formation in lymph nodes and spleen plays a central role in T cell-dependent and T cell-independent antigenic challenge. A major role in T cell–B cell interactions within germinal centers is played by the ligand–receptor pairs, CD40L and CD40, and CD28/CTLA4 and B7. Interactions of these molecules and production of lymphokines (cytokines produced by lymphocytes), such as interleukin (IL)-2, by CD4$^+$ T$_H$ cells are necessary for development of humoral immunity.

## B-cell function

The CD40-dependent and lymphokine-modified pathways, which are crucial for B-lymphocyte proliferation and differentiation as well as secretion of antigen-specific antibodies of various isotypes and subclasses, are poorly developed during the fetal and newborn periods. Furthermore, memory B cells and plasma cells are rarely detected in the non-infected neonate. The infant is largely protected from infections in the first few months after birth by the presence of maternal IgG, which is actively transported across the placenta during the third trimester of pregnancy.

## T CELLS

## Thymus

The thymus is derived from primitive germ layers: the thymic cortex is formed from endoderm of the third branchial pouch; the thymic medulla is derived from third branchial cleft ectoderm; and mesenchymal elements contribute to formation of the fibrous capsule, stroma, and vessels. A structurally normal thymus is necessary for T-cell ontogeny to occur correctly. *DiGeorge syndrome* is a developmental field defect resulting in facial dysmorphism, hypoparathyroidism, cardiac outflow tract abnormalities, and cellular immunodeficiency as a consequence of thymic hypoplasia. Many affected children have an associated monosomy of 22q11. The T-cell defects found in DiGeorge syndrome include variably decreased numbers of T cells and/or depressed T-cell proliferative responses; these abnormalities often improve with age, suggesting that the thymus continues to develop postnatally.

## T-cell development

Thymocyte differentiation begins when immature CD34$^+$CD7$^+$ prothymocytes enter the fetal thymus from the bone marrow between 8 and 9 weeks' gestation (*see* Chapter 85, Fig. 85.4). At the type I thymocyte stage, T-cell receptor (TCR) genes have not begun to rearrange, and the cells lack expression of CD3,

CD4 and CD8 (triple-negative thymocytes). The thymic microenvironment triggers further thymocyte maturation by initiating VDJ rearrangement events that encode the TCRβ chain or VJ rearrangements that encode the TCRα chain. This recombination process is analogous to that of immunoglobulin genes in pre-B cells and similarly depends on the activities of recombination-activating genes (*RAG-1* and *RAG-2*) (*see* also pages 900 and 905). More than 95 per cent of thymocytes become TCRαβ$^+$. The remaining thymocytes will alternatively express a TCR composed of γ and δ chains; the roles of these TCRγδ$^+$ cells in ontogeny and in immune responses are not well understood.

After successful TCR rearrangement, type II thymocytes, found mainly in the thymic cortex, express TCRαβ-CD3 and both CD4 and CD8 (double-positive thymocytes). At this stage, thymocytes undergo vigorous positive and/or negative selection depending on their TCRαβ specificity. During positive selection, T cells expressing TCRαβ that recognize peptides bound to self major histocompatibility complex (MHC) class I or II molecules are stimulated to continue differentiation. If this signal fails to develop, the thymocyte undergoes apoptosis (programmed cell death) and is eliminated. Negative selection occurs when the TCRαβ recognizes self peptide–MHC complexes. This may be the most important process during ontogeny to eliminate autoreactive T lymphocytes. Failure to express a functional TCRαβ and the processes of positive and negative selection result in the elimination of most thymic precursors. Type III thymocytes, the most mature cell population in the thymus, are found primarily in the thymic medulla. These cells express TCRαβ-CD3 and either CD4 or CD8 alone (single-positive thymocytes). These complex intrathymic selection processes ensure that the resulting mature T lymphocytes demonstrate diversity in recognizing antigen and can discriminate between self and non-self.

## T-cell subsets

Peripheral T cells express either CD4 or CD8 alone. In the majority of lymphocytes, these molecules are associated with specific T-cell functions: CD4$^+$ cells primarily produce helper effects, and CD8$^+$ cells are usually cytotoxic T (T$_C$) cells. T$_H$ cells secrete lymphokines and provide other signals required for normal B cell and T$_C$ functions; T$_C$ cells kill target cells that are expressing non-self antigens. CD4 or CD8 expression is thought to be dependent on the TCR expressed by the developing double-positive thymocyte and its interactions with the thymic microenvironment. For example, thymocytes expressing a TCRαβ that binds MHC class I molecules will differentiate into CD8$^+$ T cells; in contrast, a TCRαβ that binds MHC class II antigens will be expressed by T cells destined to be CD4$^+$.

## Helper T cells

CD4$^+$ T$_H$ cells constitute the majority of T cells in the peripheral blood and function by amplifying or down-regulating immune responses. Functionally, three CD4$^+$ T$_H$ cell subsets can be differentiated by their pattern of cytokine secretion: (1) T$_H$1 cells produce predominantly interferon (IFN)-γ, tumor necrosis factor (TNF) β, granulocyte-monocyte colony-stimulating factor (GM-CSF), and IL-2; (2) T$_H$2 cells preferentially produce IL-4, IL-5, IL-6, and IL-10; and (3) a T$_H$0 subset may be a precursor population. Following initial encounter with antigen, mature T$_H$ cells acquire memory function, which is defined by rapid proliferation to previously administered antigens. In adults, approximately 40 per cent of TCRαβ$^+$CD4$^+$ T cells are memory T cells and express the low-molecular-weight isoform of CD45 (CD45RO) and high levels of CD29 (CD29$^{hi}$); the remaining CD4$^+$ T cells express the high-molecular-weight isoform of CD45 (CD45RA), but not CD45RO, and low levels of CD29 (CD29$^{lo}$). Memory CD4$^+$ T cells have enhanced capacity to produce IL-4 and IFN-γ, but not IL-2, and proliferate vigorously in response to anti-CD3 antibodies. Circulating neonatal CD4$^+$ T cells are predominantly naive T cells (CD45RA$^+$, CD45RO$^-$, and CD29$^{lo}$), consistent with limited exposure to antigens. The proportion of memory CD4$^+$ T cells increases with age, presumably as a result of antigen exposure.

## Helper T-cell function

*In vitro* tests of T-cell function include proliferative responses to stimulation by mitogens and non-self MHC antigens in mixed lymphocyte cultures (MLC). Proliferation of fetal T cells to stimulation by various mitogens can be seen as early as 10–12 weeks' gestation and in MLC by 14 weeks; however, responses do not reach that of adult T cells until approximately 18 weeks' gestation. Activated neonatal CD4$^+$ T cells synthesize normal amounts of IL-2, but markedly depressed amounts of IL-3, IL-4, IL-5, IFN-γ, and GM-CSF, and lack ability to express CD40L, when compared with adult T lymphocytes. This defect can be corrected by exposing neonatal T cells to an *in vitro* preactivation process, suggesting that the apparent immune deficiency of neonatal T cells reflects immunological naiveté rather than an intrinsic defect.

## Cytotoxic T cells

CD8$^+$ T$_C$ cells recognize non-self antigens presented by MHC class I molecules on the surfaces of target cells. These endogenous antigens are often proteins produced by viruses, parasites, or other intracellular organisms, or are tumor-associated molecules. Induction and amplification of cell-mediated cytotoxic reactions are dependent on the production of IL-2 by T$_H$1 cells.

## Cytotoxic T-cell function

The ability of T$_C$ cells to kill target cells in *in vitro* cell-mediated lympholysis assays is not seen until 15–22 weeks' gestation and is not comparable to that of adult CD8$^+$ T cells until birth.

## NATURAL KILLER CELLS

NK cells originally were defined by their ability to lyse target cells without presensitization or restriction by MHC antigens. NK cells are considered a lymphocyte subset and can be identified by their expression of CD16 and/or CD56 and absence of CD3. Some NK cells are CD8$^+$ and most are CD2$^+$ and CD7$^+$, markers expressed by all T lymphocytes. However, NK cells develop normally in the absence of a thymus, do not rearrange TCR or immunoglobulin genes, and are present in patients with *severe combined immunodeficiency*. In contrast to T cells, which recognize foreign antigens in association with self MHC molecules, NK cells appear to recognize the absence of self MHC expression. NK antigen receptors are not well characterized, but may be associated with CD3ζ, which forms a complex with the IgE Fc receptor (FcεRIγ) and the IgG Fc receptor (CD16). The cytotoxic activity of NK cells is initiated by engagement of antigen and IgG with CD16, which is known as antibody-dependent cell-mediated cytotoxicity, or is initiated through contact with target cells lacking expression of self MHC antigens (natural killing). NK cells have roles in defense against intracellular pathogens; absence of NK cells has been associated with *recurrent severe infections due to herpes viruses*.

Cells with an NK phenotype have been detected as early as 6 weeks' gestation and are present in normal numbers throughout the second half of gestation. However, neonatal NK cells have diminished cytotoxic activity, which can be improved *in vitro* by incubation with IL-2 or IFN-γ.

## COMPLEMENT PATHWAYS

The complement system consists of the classical and the alternative pathways (Fig. 83.2). These sequential reactions converge on the late or common pathway, which generates the membrane attack complex (C5b6789). The components of these pathways interact in a cascade fashion, forming complexes and releasing fragments that are important for cell lysis, opsonization, and chemotaxis.

The classical pathway is activated by antigen–antibody complexes that bind the three components of the C1 system (C1q, C1r, and C1s). Bound C1 cleaves and binds C4 and C2, which then cleaves C3, forming the

## Classic pathway

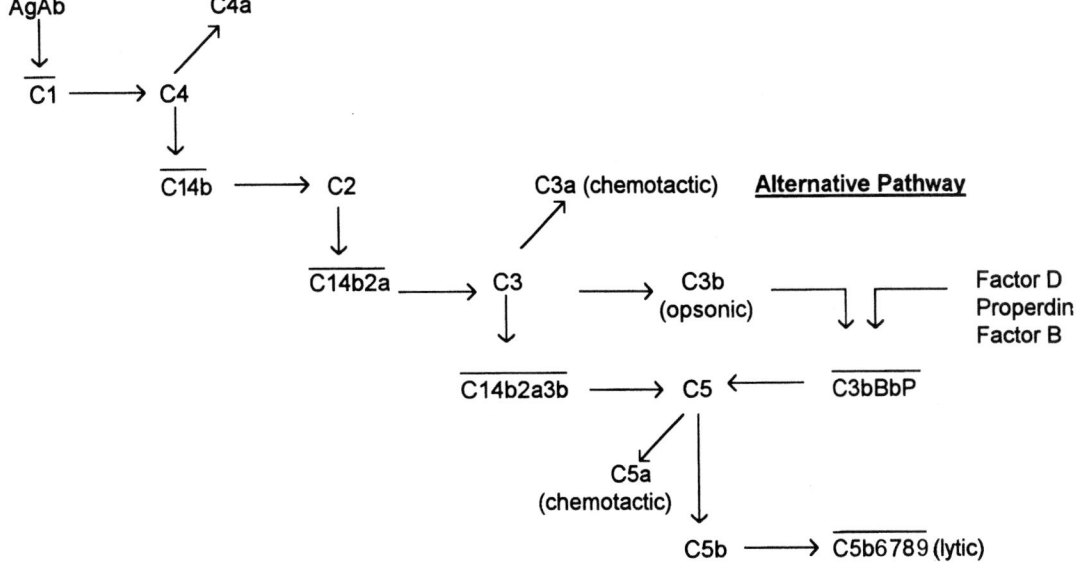

FIGURE 83.2 The complement system. The classical and alternative pathways activate C3, followed by activation of the common pathway, which forms the membrane attack complex (C5b6789). Enzymatically active proteases (indicated by a horizontal bar) cleave subsequent components, generating new proteases.

complex C4b2a3b, which cleaves C5. The larger C5b fragment binds the terminal complement components that form the membrane attack complex on the cell membrane, resulting in cytolysis.

Activation of the phylogenetically older alternative pathway is not dependent on antigen–antibody complexes, but occurs with exposure to polysaccharides, endotoxin, and other structures. If sufficient C3b is generated through the alternative pathway, C5 is cleaved and the common pathway is activated. Complement components are produced principally by hepatocytes and to a lesser extent by macrophages. Because complement components are not actively transferred across the placenta, the fetus is dependent on its own synthesis of these proteins. Some complement components can be detected between 6 and 14 weeks' gestation. In newborns, in comparison with adult levels, classical pathway components and activity are nearly normal. In contrast, the activity and components of the alternative pathway are moderately reduced, and the components of the late attack phase are less than 20 per cent. The effect of this relative complement deficiency on defense against microorganisms in the newborn is unknown.

## SELECTED READING

Colten HR, Rosen FS. Complement deficiencies. *Annu Rev Immunol* 1992; **10**: 809.

Hollenbaugh D, Ochs HD, Noelle RJ, *et al.* The role of CD40 and its ligand in the regulation of the immune response. *Immunol Rev* 1994; **138**: 23.

Lanier LL, Spits H, Phillips JH. The relationship between NK and T cells. *Immunol Today* 1992; **13**: 392.

Lewis DB, Wilson CB. Developmental immunology and role of host defenses in neonatal susceptibility to infection. In: Remington JS, Klein JO, eds. *Infectious diseases of the fetus and newborn infant*. Philadelphia: WB Saunders, 1995: 20.

Ochs HD, Winkelstein J. Disorders of the B cell system. In: Stiehm ER, ed. *Immunologic disorders in infants and children*, 4th edn. Philadelphia: WB Saunders, 1996: 296.

Rolink A, Melchers F. Molecular and cellular origins of B lymphocyte diversity. *Cell* 1991; **66**: 1081.

# 84

# B Cells

Kathleen E. Sullivan

The primary function of a B lymphocyte is to produce neutralizing antibodies. Various lymphoid tissues may produce antibodies of different classes or isotypes (IgM, IgD, IgG$_1$, IgG$_2$, IgG$_3$, IgG$_4$, IgA$_1$, IgA$_2$, and IgE), each of which has specialized biological functions. Control of antibody production involves several levels of regulation: T cells and cytokines regulate the proliferation and differentiation of B cells, and B cells themselves have the capacity to fine-tune antibody affinity. Regulation of antibody production is crucial, because the production of antipathogen antibodies is an important effector arm of the immune response, while production of aberrant or pathological antibodies is the basis of many autoimmune disorders.

## B CELL-SURFACE MOLECULES

The B lymphocyte is distinguished from other cell types by the expression of membrane-bound immunoglobulin molecules, which are utilized as high-affinity antigen receptors. Other B cell-surface proteins include those involved in cell trafficking, in responses to proliferative signals, and in antigen presentation (Fig. 84.1). Many of these molecules have been given a cluster of differentiation (CD) designation, although immunoglobulin molecules, cytokine receptors, and proteins of the major histocompatibility complex (MHC) retain their own nomenclature.

Three cell-surface proteins play particularly important roles in interactions between B cells and T cells. CD40 is expressed on mature B cells, and the ligand for CD40 (CD40L or gp39) is present on T cells. The binding of CD40L by CD40 provides signals necessary for the production of antibody isotypes other than IgM. Patients with defective expression of CD40L on their T cells develop *X-linked hyper-IgM syndrome*, a disease in which only IgM is produced because immunoglobulin class switching does not occur. This disease is characterized by recurrent sinopulmonary infections characteristic of patients who fail to make functional antibodies, as well as neutropenia and opportunistic infections. The occurrence of opportunistic infections in these children implies that T-cell function is also aberrant in this disorder, although clinical assays for T-cell function typically are normal. CD40L may have costimulatory functions for T cells as well, and it may be on this basis that T-cell function is abnormal in X-linked hyper-IgM syndrome. CD11a/18, an integrin molecule expressed by T cells, binds intercellular adhesion molecule 1 (ICAM-1, CD54) expressed by B cells, providing signals necessary for B-lymphocyte activation. Defective expression of CD11a/18 on T cells occurs as part of leukocyte adhesion deficiency, which primarily results in a failure of neutrophil chemotaxis, but also is associated with impaired antibody production. Interactions between the B cell-surface molecules B7.1 (CD80) and B7.2 (CD86) and the T cell-surface molecule CD28/CTLA4 are also crucial for feedback stimulation and function of B cells. Other membrane proteins that have been implicated in B-cell signaling and function include CD19, CD21, CD22, CD45, and CD81.

B cells express interleukin (IL) receptors at various stages during ontogeny. Disease states in which one or more of these cytokines are over- or under-produced can profoundly affect B-cell development and antibody production. Many chronic infections such as *human immunodeficiency virus (HIV)* are associated with increased levels of IL-1 and IL-6 in the circulation, which induce polyclonal B-cell activation and, consequently, hypergammaglobulinemia.

Another cell-surface protein, CD5, designates a clinically important subset of B cells. CD5 is also expressed on T cells, but within the B-cell compartment CD5 identifies those B cells in which the immunoglobulin repertoire is skewed toward production of autoantibodies. These cells appear to differentiate along a distinct pathway and have the capacity for self-renewal in the absence of antigenic stimulation. Most *B-cell chronic lymphocytic leukemias* express CD5.

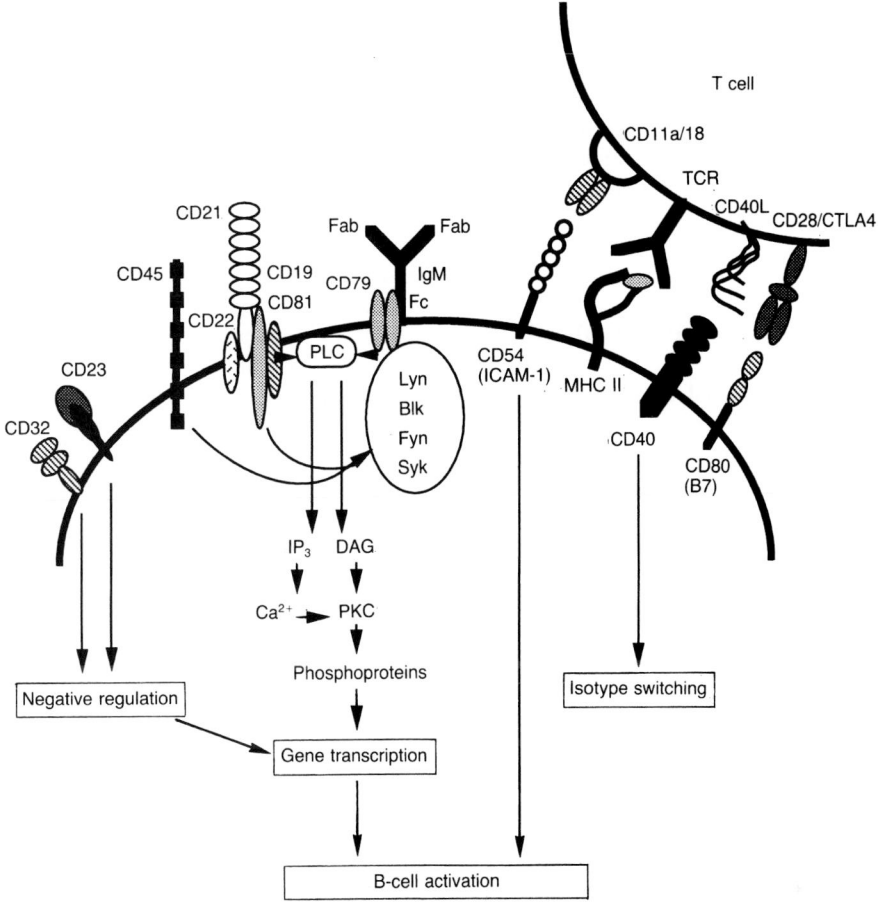

FIGURE 84.1 B cell-surface proteins. These molecules have roles in adhesion, trafficking, signaling, and interactions with T cells. Many of the functions are interrelated and share intracellular signaling pathways. In this figure, the IgM molecule is shown associated with accessory molecules that interact through cytoplasmic protein tyrosine kinases such as Lyn, Blk, Fyn, and Syk. The association of CD54, CD80, CD40, and MHC class II molecules is shown along with their T-cell ligands. PLC, phospholipase Cγ; DAG, diacylglycerol; PKC, protein kinase C; IP₃, inositol trisphosphate; TCR, T-cell receptor; MHC, major histocompatibility complex; ICAM-1, intercellular adhesion molecule 1.

In addition to molecules that participate in cell activation, signal transduction, and cell adhesion, proteins are expressed that belong to the MHC (or the human leukocyte antigen system; HLA) class II loci. These molecules, which include HLA-DR, -DQ, and -DP, function to bind and "present" antigen to CD4⁺ helper T (T$_H$) cells, which in turn secrete lymphokines that augment B-cell responses and antibody production. For proper antigen presentation, protein antigens bound to surface immunoglobulins are first internalized and processed in the cytoplasm, then re-expressed on the B-cell surface as peptide fragments within a protein cleft of the MHC class II molecule. MHC class II proteins are extremely polymorphic, and each molecule favors the presentation of peptides with certain physical characteristics. Interference with antigen presentation by B cells is a strategy used in the treatment of certain autoimmune diseases and is the basis for chloroquine therapy in *systemic lupus erythematosus*.

## IMMUNOGLOBULIN STRUCTURE

B lymphocytes must differentiate into plasma cells in order to secrete antibodies. Immunoglobulin molecules comprise two identical light chains and two identical heavy chains. In contrast to other isotypes, IgA and IgM exist as dimers and pentamers, respectively, of this basic immunoglobulin unit. Each heavy chain comprises an isotype-specific Fc region and a Fab region that is physically involved in antigen binding. The light chains contribute to Fab structure and are either of the λ or κ isotype.

The Fc regions of antibody molecules mediate different effector functions depending on heavy-chain isotype. Both IgG and IgM undergo conformational changes after binding antigen such that the capacity to activate the complement cascade is acquired. There are also isotype-specific Fc functions that rely on cell- and organ-specific expression of certain Fc receptors. For example, Fc receptors for IgE and IgA on eosinophils function to direct these cells to parasites, and IgE Fc receptors present on mast cells and basophils mediate most allergic responses. Gut epithelial Fc receptors are involved in the transport of IgA produced in mucosal lymphoid tissues across epithelial surfaces. Another organ-specific Fc function is the transplacental transport of maternal IgG during the third trimester of pregnancy.

## Immunoglobulin gene rearrangement

Antigen specificity is generated through the random use and the sequential rearrangement of multiple gene segments encoding immunoglobulin heavy and light chains (combinatorial joining; Fig. 84.2). Immunoglobulin genes are dispersed as multiple coding segments along the chromosome and include 100–200 variable (V) region segments, five to six joining (J) segments, and a constant (C) region segment for each isotype. Heavy-chain genes also have diversity (D) segments located between the V and J segments. The V, D, and J gene segments encode the Fab portion, and the C segments encode the structural and Fc regions of the antibody molecule. Immunoglobulin genes and T cell-receptor genes share a sophisticated VDJ recombinase

system of proteins that brings V, D, and J coding segments into close proximity on the chromosome through somatic recombination such that transcription can occur. The recombinase machinery is activated by the recombination-activating genes (*RAG-1*) and (*RAG-2*), which are developmentally regulated and are expressed only in pre-B cells and early cortical thymocytes. Infants with defects in *RAG-1* and *RAG-2* expression fail to produce mature T cells and B cells and have severe combined immunodeficiency syndrome. The recombinase is targeted to unrearranged V, D, and J segments by specific DNA-recognition sequences consisting of conserved heptamer and nonamer sequences separated by non-conserved spacers of 12 or 23 bp. Gene rearrangement is initiated in an orderly and sequential fashion; initial heavy-chain VDJ joining subsequently stimulates light-chain recombination. Allelic exclusion (productive rearrangement on one chromosome prevents a subsequent rearrangement of the other allele) and isotypic exclusion (successful κ-chain rearrangement precludes λ-chain rearrangement) ensure that a given B cell and its progeny will produce antibodies of only one antigen specificity and light-chain type (clonal restriction). Heavy-chain isotype switching also utilizes the recombinase machinery, but the recognition sequences and the stimuli are different.

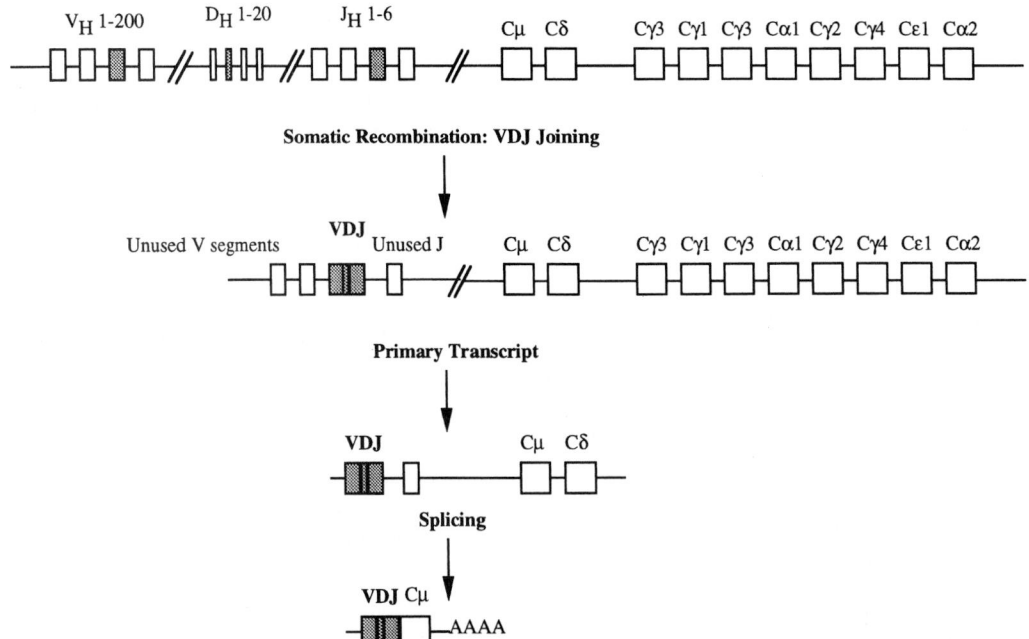

FIGURE 84.2 Immunoglobulin heavy-chain gene rearrangement. Antibodies are capable of recognizing over $10^{11}$ antigen epitopes. This molecular diversity is accomplished through the use of random combinations of multiple gene segments, frameshifts, nucleotide additions, and somatic hypermutation. Multiple gene segments are combined by somatic recombination, a phenomenon that is unique to lymphocytes. Heavy-chain genes recombine initially, followed by κ and then λ genes. This figure demonstrates the sequence of events for heavy-chain recombination, although light-chain events use a similar mechanism. At the B-cell progenitor stage, diversity (D) and joining (J) segments rearrange initially, followed by variable (V) segments. If a functional VDJ recombination occurs, the other chromosome will remain in its germline configuration. The primary transcript is quite long and can be spliced to include either the IgM constant (C) region or the IgD constant region. Further recombination associated with isotype switching requires T-cell interaction via CD40.

Random combinations of V, D, and J segments result in antibody diversity. Such diversity is also increased by other cellular mechanisms: (1) the joints between segments are imprecise, resulting in changes in the DNA reading frame; (2) random nucleotides are inserted at segment ends during VJ or VDJ joining by terminal deoxynucleotidyltransferase; (3) various combinations of heavy and light chains occur during antibody formation; and (4) increased mutation rates are seen in rearranged VJ and VDJ sequences (somatic hypermutation). Somatic hypermutation occurs mainly in memory B cells and participates in affinity maturation, a phenomenon in which higher affinity antibodies are produced with time during an immune response. Ultimately, more than $10^{11}$ antigen epitopes can be recognized by every individual.

## IMMUNOGLOBULIN CLASSES

IgG constitutes approximately 75 per cent of total serum antibodies in adults. Newborns have predominantly maternal IgG in their serum, but after 3 months most serum IgG is produced by the infant. IgG is divided into four subclasses that differ somewhat in their function. The serum concentrations of the four subclasses are not evenly distributed, with $IgG_1 > IgG_2 > IgG_3 > IgG_4$. $IgG_1$ and $IgG_3$ activate the complement cascade more efficiently than the other two IgG subclasses and also bind Fc receptors more avidly. Serum $IgG_2$ and $IgG_4$ concentrations do not rise to appreciable levels until the second year of life.

IgA is secreted as dimers in association with J chain and secretory component peptide. IgA is abundant in tears, saliva, intestinal secretions, and bronchial mucus, and blocks access of microbes to the blood by neutralizing organisms at mucosal surfaces. Because IgA does not activate the complement cascade, antigen binding does not result in mucosal inflammation. In the serum, IgA circulates as a monomer and represents a small portion of total immunoglobulins.

IgM is produced during primary immune responses and responses to polysaccharide antigens. IgM typically represents about 10 per cent of total serum immunoglobulins; however, during acute infections, total IgM may rise dramatically. IgM usually circulates as pentamers stabilized by disulfide bonds and the same J chain utilized by secretory IgA.

Membrane-bound IgD functions in B-cell signaling and activation. It is present in serum in only trace amounts. The structure of IgD is very similar to IgG, although it is more susceptible to proteolysis.

IgE resembles IgG structurally and is normally detected in the blood at very low concentrations. However, markedly elevated concentrations of IgE may be seen in *atopic conditions*. The Fc region of IgE molecules triggers mast-cell release of mediators responsible for *allergic reactions*. When skin testing is performed, the intradermal antigen binds to tiny amounts of IgE present in the skin and triggers mast-cell release, resulting in a wheal and flare reaction.

## B-CELL ONTOGENY

In the developing fetus, islands of B-cell hematopoiesis are found in the liver and bone marrow after 8 weeks' gestation. In older children and adults, production of B cells is confined to the bone marrow, and maturation into plasma cells occurs in lymph nodes and other lymphoid tissues. Naive B cells circulate continuously between the peripheral blood and lymphoid tissues, where they percolate through T cell-dense regions and briefly rest in B-cell follicles before recirculating. B cells that display self-reactive immunoglobulin receptors are eliminated through apoptosis or competition for the follicular microenvironment, or may persist but become functionally inert (anergy). This is the basis for B-cell tolerance to self antigens. B-cell subsets include immature B-cell precursors, mature resting B cells, memory B cells, activated B cells, and terminally differentiated antibody-producing plasma cells (Fig. 84.3).

### Pre-B cells

Pre-B cells undergo μ heavy chain re-arrangement and express μ chains in the cytoplasm. Mutations in a cytoplasmic protein tyrosine kinase encoded by the Bruton tyrosine kinase (*BTK*) gene cause the disorder *X-linked agammaglobulinemia*, which is associated with arrested B-cell development at the pre-B-cell stage and failure of antibody production. This disorder is characterized by recurrent infections with pyogenic organisms. The patient's T cells are normal, and replacement therapy with monthly intravenous immunoglobulin provides effective prophylaxis against infections.

### Immature B cells

To be transported to the cell surface in the absence of rearranged κ or λ light chains, the cytoplasmic μ heavy chains must first associate with surrogate (non-κ and non-λ) light chains. The resulting complexes are transported to the plasma membrane, and the surrogate light chains are subsequently replaced by κ or λ chains after appropriate developmental signals have triggered light-chain gene rearrangement. Consequently, the next identifiable subset of B cells is the immature $IgM^+IgD^-$ B cell. In spite of membrane-bound IgM, these cells are unable to proliferate in response to antigen. It is at this stage that cells begin to be released into the periphery and self-reac-

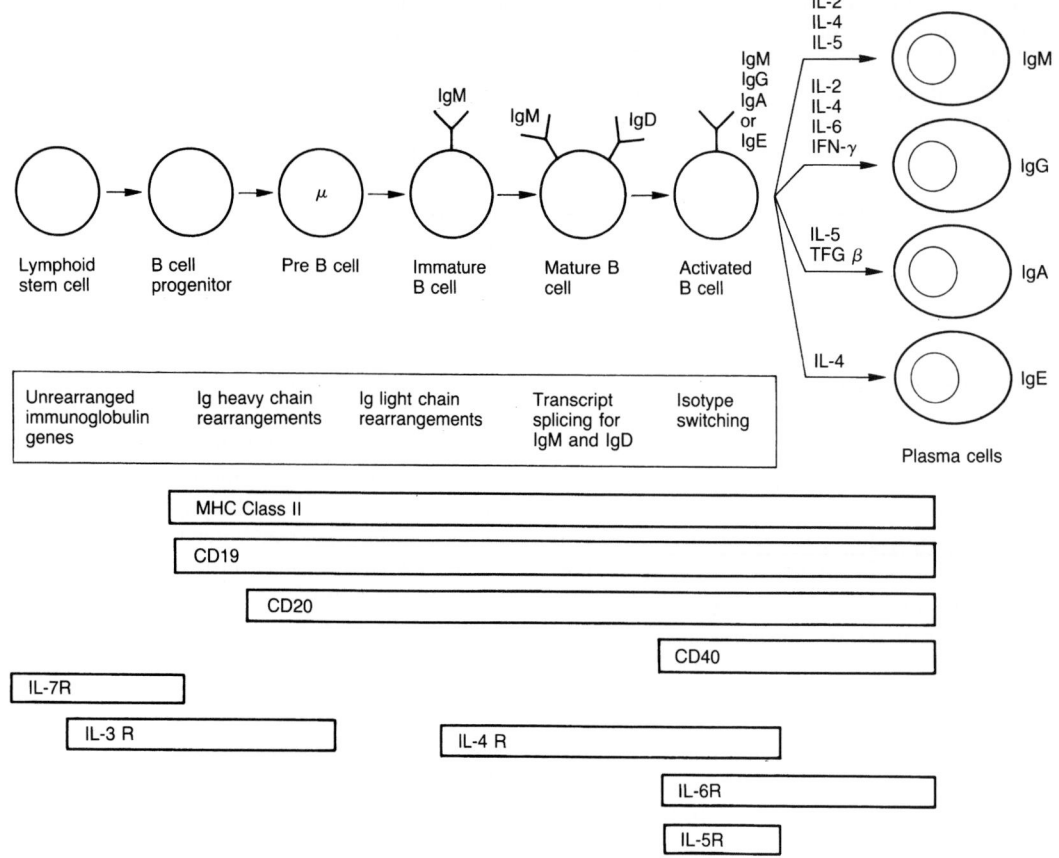

FIGURE 84.3 B-cell ontogeny. B-cell maturation is divided into discrete stages; events prior to the development of mature B cells do not require antigenic stimulation. During these early stages, the B cell resides in the bone marrow and is stimulated to proceed through development by cytokines and microenvironmental clues. At the immature B-cell stage, IgM is expressed on the cell surface, and any cells capable of recognizing self antigen are eliminated before reaching the peripheral blood. The course of immunoglobulin gene rearrangement is shown along with the sequential expression of interleukin (IL) receptors (R) and other pertinent cell-surface proteins. Plasma cells are produced as the final step in this developmental pathway. The immunoglobulin isotype produced by an individual plasma cell is regulated by the cytokines shown in the figure.

tive B cells are eliminated. In contrast, non-self-reactive B cells begin to express IgD in addition to IgM and are allowed to survive. All isotypes expressed by a B cell and its progeny will have the same antigen specificity, such that both IgD and IgM receptors on the B-cell surface will recognize the same antigen epitopes.

## Mature B cells

Subsequent exposure to protein antigens induces the proliferation and differentiation of these immature IgM⁺ IgD⁺ B cells into mature B lymphocytes expressing immunoglobulin receptors of the IgG, IgA, or IgE isotype. These B cells require "help" (CD40–CD40L interaction and lymphokine production by CD4⁺ T_H cells) in order to undergo isotype or class switch, and then to proliferate and differentiate into memory B cells and plasma cells.

## Plasma cells

With appropriate antigen exposure and T-cell help, mature B cells differentiate into plasma cells capable of secreting large amounts of antibody. These cells are principally found in lymphoid tissues, such as tonsils, lymph nodes, intestinal Peyer patches, and bone marrow, and are not normally found in the blood. Plasma cells have short lifespans of a few weeks and must be replenished from the mature B-cell pool in order to maintain serum immunoglobulin levels.

Although infants are born with functional B cells, plasma cells are not present at birth unless exposure to foreign antigens has occurred *in utero*, as is seen in toxoplasmosis, rubella or syphilis infections. Instead, Fc receptor-bound maternal IgG is actively transported across the placenta after 32 weeks' gestation, providing full-term infants with maternal antibodies to common pathogens. After birth, infants begin to produce their own IgM and IgG while maternal IgG levels fall, such that by about 4 months the concentration of maternal IgG in the infant's serum is about 10 per cent of that at delivery. As a consequence of maternal antibody protection, most children with *congenital B-cell defects* rarely become ill until after 6 months of age. In contrast, premature infants are relatively immunodeficient due to lack of protective maternal IgG.

## ANTIBODY PRODUCTION

Primary antibody responses to protein antigens are characterized by low-affinity IgM production after approximately 5–10 days. During initial antigen exposure, a cascade of signal transduction events is initiated, stimulating resting B cells to enter the cell cycle and increase cell-surface expression of MHC class II proteins, adhesion molecules, and costimulatory proteins. Memory B cells are produced so that subsequent exposure to the same antigen will result in a secondary or anamnestic response. Anamnestic antibody responses are characterized by the production of high-affinity antibodies in 1–3 days that are predominantly IgG (or IgA in the mucosa).

As stated previously, B cells internalize protein antigens and re-express the processed peptides on their surface bound to MHC class II molecules to be recognized by CD4+ $T_H$ cells. Simultaneous CD40–CD40L interaction and lymphokine production amplify the immune response and dictate the antibody isotype that plasma cells will secrete. This contact-based regulation of antibody production ensures that B cells specific for the presented antigen will preferentially proliferate. IL-2, IL-4, and IL-5 augment the proliferative effects, while other cytokine combinations specify the antibody isotype.

Early B-cell proliferative responses occur at the edges of the T cell-dependent areas of lymphoid tissues. Subsequently, B cells migrate to the lymphoid germinal centers and proliferate rapidly. Additional stimuli are required for the differentiation of mature B cells into plasma cells, which generally occurs in lymphoid tissues where the architecture facilitates cell–cell interactions. The humoral immune response is augmented by activation of the complement cascade; immune complexes containing the complement C3b component are actively bound by follicular dendritic cells. These bound antigen–antibody–C3b complexes serve as reservoirs for restimulation and provide a milieu for the continuous development of memory B lymphocytes and plasma cells.

Important differences exist in humoral responses to polysaccharide antigens. Complex polysaccharide antigens can stimulate B cells without T-cell help. Examples of polysaccharide antigens are blood group antigens and the coat proteins of encapsulated organisms. Responses to polysaccharide antigens are characterized by production of IgM and $IgG_2$. Neither memory B cells nor secondary antibody responses

develop. Furthermore, the ability to respond to polysaccharide antigens is developmentally regulated. In humans, $IgG_2$ production to polysaccharide antigens is not seen until 2 years of age, which partially explains why *Haemophilus influenzae* and *Streptococcus pneumoniae* infections are most common in young children. The vaccine for *H. influenzae* utilizes polysaccharide antigen conjugated to a protein carrier that stimulates a T cell-dependent humoral response, production of $IgG_1$ antibodies, and acquisition of immunity to *H. influenzae* that otherwise would not be possible in infants.

*Common variable immunodeficiency* is a disorder in which B cells fail to produce functional antibodies. In contrast to *X-linked agammaglobulinemia*, B cells usually are present and the age at onset is typically later. The etiology is not understood, although most patients have a defect in T-cell regulation of antibody production. B cells from these patients can be induced to secrete immunoglobulins *in vitro*. This disorder highlights T cell–B cell interactions and the dependence of normal B-cell function on T-cell regulation.

The cell-surface events that drive B-cell developmental changes and the production of antibodies are not completely understood. Resting B cells express IgM and IgD in association with Igα/β (CD79), linking antigen-binding events to activation of cytoplasmic protein tyrosine kinases. Activation of this signaling cascade results in the phosphorylation of target proteins, some of which are direct transcriptional regulators of B-cell activation genes. Other cell-surface molecules, such as CD22 and CD45, also participate in B-cell signal transduction. Ultimately, these biochemical events result in entry into the $G_1$ stage of the cell cycle, increased expression of adhesion and costimulatory molecules, cellular differentiation, and antibody production.

## SELECTED READING

Abbas AK, Lichtman AH, Pober JS. Maturation of B lymphocytes and expression of immunoglobulin genes. In: *Cellular and molecular immunology*. Philadelphia: WB Saunders, 1994: 65.
Clark EA, Ledbetter JA. How B and T cells talk to each other. *Nature* 1994; 367: 425.
Cooper MD. B lymphocytes normal development and function. *N Engl J Med* 1987; 317: 1452.
Feldman M. Cell cooperation in the antibody response. In: Roitt I, Brostoff J, Male D, eds. Immmunology, 3rd edn. London: Mosby Press, 1993: 7.1.
Hollenbaugh D, Ochs HD, Noelle RJ *et al*. The role of CD40 and its ligand in the regulation of the immune response. *Immunol Rev* 1994; 138: 23.
Pleiman CM, D'Ambrosio D, Cambier JC. The B cell antigen receptor complex: structure and signal transduction. *Immunol Today* 1994; 15: 93.

# 85

# T Cells

Terry O. Harville

## T CELL-SURFACE PROTEINS

### Cluster of differentiation (CD) designations

Cells derived from the thymus (T lymphocytes) have important roles in both the development and the function of the immune system. T lymphocytes have been shown to (1) "help" B lymphocytes differentiate into antibody-secreting plasma cells; (2) recognize and "kill" cells that are infected with viruses or intracellular organisms; and (3) recognize and "kill" cells from other individuals (allogeneic graft rejection). Depending on their functions, T cells have been categorized as either helper T ($T_H$) or cytotoxic/suppressor T ($T_C$) cells. By using monoclonal antibodies (mAbs) against various lymphocyte cell-surface proteins, subpopulations of T and B lymphocytes have been identified and specific developmental stages and functional properties ascribed to each. Membrane proteins identified by groups of similarly reactive mAbs are assigned the same CD designation or number (Tables 85.1 and 85.2). This has facilitated lymphocyte characterization; e.g. $T_H$ cells are primarily CD4$^+$ and $T_C$ cells are usually CD8$^+$.

TABLE 85.1 Markers of human T-lineage cells

| CD | OTHER DESIGNATION | T-CELL SUBPOPULATION | FUNCTION |
|---|---|---|---|
| CD1 | T6 | Cortical thymocyte | Role in antigen presentation? |
| CD2 | T11, LFA-2 | Pan-T lineage | Binds CD58, costimulation signal transduction |
| CD3 | T3 | Thymocyte, T cell | TCR signal transduction |
| CD4 | T4 | Thymocyte, $T_H$ cell | Binds MHC class II, signaling |
| CD5 | T1, Lyt-1 | Pan-T lineage | Binds CD72 |
| CD6 | T12 | Thymocyte, T cell | Signal transduction? |
| CD7 | gp40 | Earliest T-cell marker, pan-T lineage | IgM Fc receptor?, costimulation in TCRγδ$^+$ T cells |
| CD8 | T8, Lyt-2 | Thymocyte, $T_C$ cell | Binds MHC class I, signaling |
| CD25 | Tac | Activated T cell | IL-2R α chain, IL-2 signaling |
| CD26 | DPP IV | T cell | Cleaves N-terminal proline dipeptides |
| CD27 | – | Medullary thymocyte, T cell | Disappears from cell surface with memory acquisition |
| CD28 | Tp44 | Thymocyte, >75% CD4$^+$ and 50% CD8$^+$ T cells | Binds B7 (CD80, CD86), costimulation signal transduction |
| CDw90 | Thy-1 | Some thymocyte | Costimulation |
| CD122 | – | Activated T cell | IL-2R β chain, IL-2 signaling |
| – | IL-γc | Activated T cell | Common γ chain of receptors for IL-2, IL-4, IL-7, IL-9, IL-13, IL-15, signaling |
| – | TCRαβ | Thymocyte, T cell | Recognition of antigen presented by MHC class I or MHC class II |
| – | TCRγδ | 5% T cell (TCRαβ not coexpressed) | Antigen recognition, not presented via classic MHC |
| – | gp39, CD40L | T cell | Stimulates B cells via CD40 for Ig production and isotype switch |

CD, cluster of differentiation; TCR, T-cell antigen receptor; IL, interleukin; R, receptor; $T_H$, helper T cell; $T_C$, cytotoxic T cell; MHC, major histocompatibility complex; Ig, immunoglobulin.

TABLE 85.2 Other T-cell markers

| CD | OTHER DESIGNATION | LYMPHOCYTE SUBPOPULATION | FUNCTION |
|---|---|---|---|
| CD11a | LFA-1 | Pan-lymphocyte | Dimer with CD18, binds CD54 and CD102, cell adhesion |
| CD11b | MAC-1, Mo-1 | NK cell, low on T cell | Dimer with CD18, binds CD54 and CD102, cell adhesion |
| CD18 | gp95 | Pan-lymphocyte | Integrin β2, dimer with CD11, binds CD54 and CD102, cell adhesion |
| CD29 | 4B4 | Memory T cell | Integrin β1, dimer with CD49, cell adhesion |
| CD30 | Ki-1 | Activated T and B cell | T cell activation? |
| CD34 | My-10 | Earliest lymphocyte progenitor | ? |
| CD35 | CR1 | B cell, some T cell | Binds complement C3b and C4b |
| CD38 | T10 | Early T and B lineage, activated T and B cell | ? |
| CD43 | Sialophorin | Pan-T lineage, B cell | Interacts with CD54, costimulation |
| CD44 | PgP-1 | Thymocyte, T cell | Cell adhesion |
| CD45RO | | Activated T cell, B cell | Phosphotyrosine phosphatase, signaling |
| CD45RA | T200 | Naive T cell, B cell | Phosphotyrosine phosphatase, signaling |
| CD49 (a–f) | VLA-(1–6) | Memory T cell, B cell | Integrin α chains, dimer with CD29, cell adhesion |
| CD54 | ICAM-1 | Activated lymphocyte | Binds CD11/CD18, cell adhesion |
| CD58 | LFA-3 | Medullary thymocyte, memory T cell | Binds CD2, cell adhesion, costimulation |
| CD69 | Leu-23 | Thymocyte, activated T and B cell | Early activation marker, ? role |
| CD71 | T9 | Thymocyte, activated T and B cell | Transferrin receptor, costimulatory |
| CD73 | Ecto-5'-nucleosidase | Thymocyte, T cell, B cell | 5' dephosphorylation of nucleotides to nucleosides, costimulatory |
| CD102 | ICAM-2 | Lymphocytes | Binds CD11/CD18, cell adhesion |
| – | MHC class I | Pan-lymphocyte | HLA-A, -B, -C; presents endogenous antigen |
| – | MHC class I | B cell, activated T cell | HLA-DR, -DP, -DQ; presents exogenous antigen |

CD, cluster of designation; HLA, human leukocyte antigen; MHC, major histocompatibility complex.

# T-cell antigen receptor

## T-cell receptor (TCR) gene rearrangement

The human genome is not large enough to encode all of the antigen specificities that are recognizable by TCRs. Analogous to antibody formation, the process of rearrangement of individual variable (V), diversity (D), and joining (J) gene segments into VDJ recombinants allows new sequences that encode the vast repertoire of TCR specificities to be generated (Fig. 85.1). TCR heterodimers of $\alpha$ and $\beta$ chains provide the antigen-recognition component found on 90–95 per cent of circulating T lymphocytes, with TCR $\gamma\delta$ heterodimers expressed on the remaining cells. There are approximately 100 V$\alpha$, 100 J$\alpha$, 100 V$\beta$, 2 D$\beta$, 13 J$\beta$, 14 V$\gamma$, 5 J$\gamma$, 6 V$\delta$, 3 D$\delta$, and 3 J$\delta$ coding segments dispersed along the chromosome. As with immunoglobulin rearrangements, TCR recombination events proceed sequentially, with DJ rearrangements occurring before VDJ formation. At each junctional site (D–J and V–DJ), further sequence diversity is created by exonuclease removal of bases and terminal deoxynucleotidyl transferase (TdT) addition of bases in a non-template-dependent manner (a process termed N-diversification). TCR VDJ recombination occurs in immature CD4$^-$CD8$^-$ cortical thymocytes that subsequently express TCR only in association with CD3. TCR$\alpha\beta^+$ thymocytes then undergo intrathymic positive and negative selection processes and complete differentiation before release into the peripheral circulation.

VDJ recombination is brought about by proteins that are common to both T-cell and B-cell lineages. An individual protein has not been identified as the "recombinase"; recombinase system activity instead is found in a collection of enzymes and DNA-binding proteins, some of which are normal constituents of nucleated cells involved in DNA replication and repair. Others are lymphocyte-lineage-specific proteins that provide the specificity necessary for VDJ recombination, such as TdT, recognition signal sequence (RSS)-binding proteins, and molecules encoded by the recombination-activating genes 1 and 2 (RAG-1, RAG-2). RSS-binding proteins bind to and align RSS sites (consensus sequences of 7 and 9 bases separated by non-consensus sequence spacers of 12 or 23 bases), which flank each V, D, and J gene segment so that proper recombination can occur. VDJ rearrangement is controlled by RAG-1 and RAG-2. Expression of RAG-1 and RAG-2 are cell type and tissue specific, occurring in pre-B lymphocytes in the bone marrow and in cortical thymocytes (Fig. 85.2). Interleukin (IL)-7 appears to be an important cofactor for inducing RAG-1 and RAG-2 expression. During thymocyte and pre-B lymphocyte ontogeny, there is a window of time during which RAG-1 and RAG-2 are expressed and recombination of the respective TCR and immunoglobulin gene segments can occur. Failure to undergo successful VDJ rearrangement during this interval results in cell death.

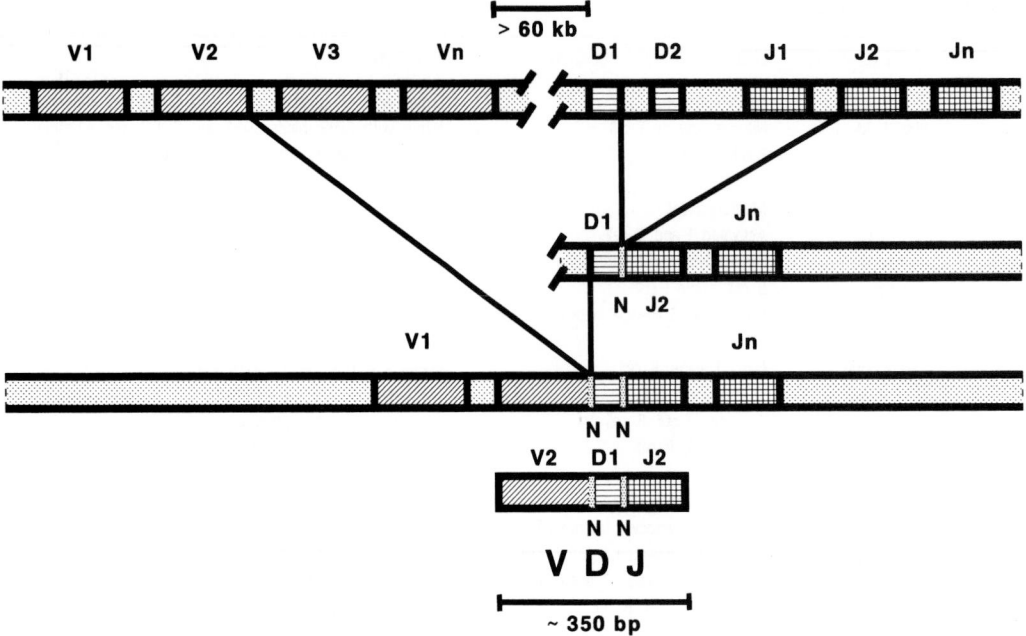

FIGURE 85.1 T-cell antigen receptor (TCR) gene rearrangement events. Somatic recombination of variable (V), diversity (D), and joining (J) gene segments generates DNA sequences encoding antigen specificities of TCR. DJ joining proceeds first, followed by V–DJ joining. Intervening nucleotides are excised during recombination. To further increase TCR diversity, an exonuclease cleaves nucleotides at the joining sites, followed by random insertion of new bases by terminal deoxynucleotidyltransferase prior to ligation of the joins. From DNA segments spanning 60–800 kb, VDJ recombinants of approximately 350 bp are generated.

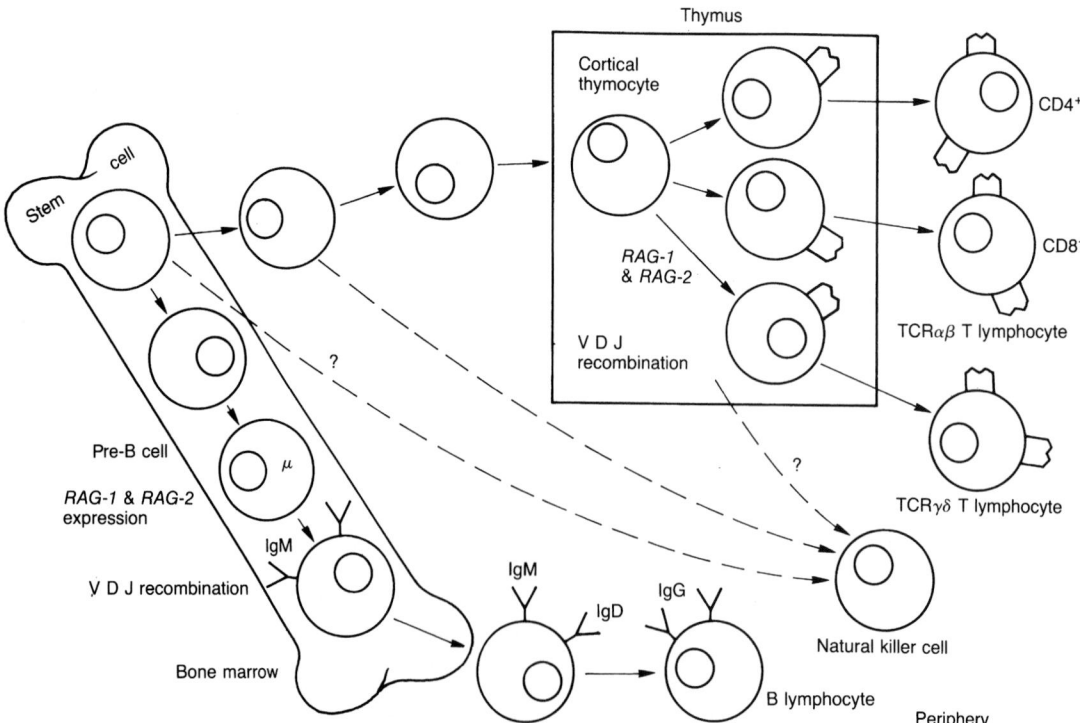

FIGURE 85.2 Recombinase activity in T- and B-lymphocyte development. Immunoglobulin VDJ rearrangement occurs in the bone marrow and is controlled by the products of the recombination-activating genes (RAG-1, RAG-2). Early cortical thymocytes express RAG-1 and RAG-2 and initiate T-cell receptor (TCR) gene rearrangement. After productive rearrangement and expression of TCRαβ in association with cluster of differentiation (CD) 3 on the cell surface, the developing thymocytes undergo positive and negative selection and exit the thymus as mature T cells expressing CD4 or CD8 alone. T cells expressing TCRγδ do not require thymic education for differentiation into mature lymphocytes. V, variable; D, diversity; J, joining.

## TCR structure and function

The TCR is composed of eight proteins expressed on the T-lymphocyte membrane (Fig. 85.3). The TCR α and β chains are analogous to the immunoglobulin light and heavy chains, respectively, and are only expressed on the cell surface in association with CD3. Both TCR α and β chains contain variable domains created by VJ and VDJ recombination, and constant domains that allow interactions with the cell membrane and CD3. The TCRαβ heterodimer is required for antigen binding and recognition, and the coexpressed CD3 proteins are pivotally involved in signal transduction. CD3 is a complex composed of εγ, εδ, and ζζ dimers that interact directly with TCRαβ and couple antigen-binding signals to intracellular biochemical pathways, resulting in T-cell activation. Specifically, these signals activate cytoplasmic protein tyrosine kinases (PTKs), such as Lck, Fyn, and ZAP-70, which in turn phosphorylate other cytosolic proteins and ultimately lead to T-cell activation, differentiation, and proliferation. Activation of one such intracellular substrate, calcineurin, results in the increased expression of IL-2 and IL-2 receptor. The drugs cyclosporin A and FK506, which are used to prevent *transplant rejection* and *graft-versus-host disease (GVHD)*, bind calcineurin and consequently prevent T-cell activation and T cell-mediated immune responses.

## Major histocompatibility complex

The process of rejection or acceptance of allogeneic grafts (transplantation compatibility) is dictated by cell-surface proteins called histocompatibility antigens that are recognizable by T and B cells. Mapping of these antigens reveals that most are encoded by genes inherited together as the major histocompatibility complex (MHC), or the human leukocyte antigen (HLA) locus. The primary function of MHC is not to provide a means of host recognition and rejection of cells from another individual, but to "present" antigen to T lymphocytes so that a specific immune response can be generated. MHC class I proteins and MHC class II molecules are required to bind and "present" endogenous and exogenous antigens, respectively. Subpopulations of T lymphocytes are selected within the thymus to recognize antigens presented by either MHC class I or MHC class II molecules; CD8[+] $T_C$ cells recognize antigens presented by MHC class I proteins, and CD4[+] $T_H$ lymphocytes respond to antigens bound to MHC class II molecules. MHC class I antigens are found on the surfaces of all nucleated cells and present peptides derived during intracellular processing to $T_C$ lymphocytes. In this manner, cells that have been infected with viruses, intracellular organisms or parasites, or transformed due to cancer can be detected by the presentation of viral, parasitic, or tumor antigens, respectively, in the binding groove of MHC class I proteins. Specialized antigen-presenting cells (APCs) express MHC class II molecules on their surface membranes for the presentation of internally processed foreign antigens phagocytosed by APC. CD4[+] $T_H$ lymphocytes then provide signals (lymphokine secretion and via CD40–CD40L interaction) for the selection of B cells capable of secreting antibodies directed against the same antigen. APCs include B lymphocytes, monocytes, macrophages, dendritic cells, histiocytes, and microglial cells.

MHC class I molecules are composed of two protein chains: invariant β2-microglobulin and a variable

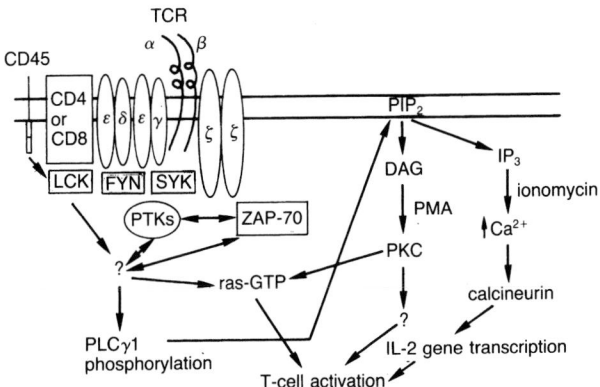

FIGURE 85.3 T-cell signal transduction pathway. Numerous membrane-bound and cytosolic proteins are involved in T-cell activation. The T-cell receptor (TCRαβ) is depicted in association with the ε, δ, and ζ chains of the cluster of differentiation (CD) 3 complex. CD45 and either the CD4 or CD8 coreceptor are also expressed. Associated with these molecules are protein tyrosine kinases (PTKs), including Lck, Fyn, Syk, and ZAP-70. Activation of these PTKs results in the phosphorylation of phospholipase Cγ1 (PLCγ1) and other target proteins, culminating in the production of second messengers, interleukin (IL)-2 gene transcription, and T-cell activation. PIP2, phosphatidylinositides; DAG, diacylglycerol; IP3, inositol trisphosphate; PMA, phorbol myristic acetate; PKC, protein kinase C; Ca$^{2+}$, intracellular free calcium.

α chain that is involved in antigen binding. The α chains can be subdivided by sequence homologies into HLA-A, -B, and -C families that are detectable by mAbs. Polymorphisms of the α chain allow for diversity in the types of antigens presented and presumably add to the immunological vigor of the species.

MHC class II molecules are composed of a heterodimeric complex of structurally similar α and β chains. Three main families exist: HLA-DR, -DP, and -DQ. Serological techniques can detect HLA-A, -B, -C, -DR, and -DQ, but not HLA-DP. Based on serological testing, there are 30 different HLA-A, 60 HLA-B, 10 HLA-C, 20 HLA-DR, and 9 HLA-DQ antigens. MHC class II specificities were initially determined by *in vitro* mixed lymphocyte proliferative responses, and at least 25 "HLA-D types" have been detected, including 6 HLA-DP members. Although serological testing is highly standardized, lack of detection of minor amino acid differences and cross-reactivities between closely related proteins occur. With the availability of molecular biological techniques such as polymerase chain reaction, HLA typing via DNA sequence analysis is allowing more precise definition of HLA antigens.

# T-CELL SUBSETS

## CD4+ T cells

Mature TCRαβ+ T lymphocytes are divided into two subpopulations based on the cell-surface expression of CD4 and CD8. In the majority of cases, after binding of antigen presented by MHC class II molecules on APCs, CD4+ T$_H$ lymphocytes secrete lymphokines such as IL-4 and IL-6 that stimulate antigen-specific B lymphocytes to proliferate, undergo class switch, differentiate into plasma cells, and produce memory B lymphocytes for subsequent encounters with the same antigen. This helper-cell function requires physical interactions between B cells and CD4+ T$_H$ cells via membrane-bound CD40 and CD40L. Subsequently, stimulated CD4+ T$_H$ lymphocytes proliferate and memory T lymphocytes are generated. In addition, CD4+ T$_H$ cells secrete IL-2, interferon (IFN)-γ, and other lymphokines that are involved in stimulation of T$_C$ cells and in induction of cytotoxicity.

## CD8+ T cells

CD8+ T$_C$ lymphocytes recognize endogenous antigens presented by MHC class I proteins. Non-self antigens related to intracellular infection (such as by virus) are recognized and killed by the release of toxic substances from stimulated CD8+ T$_C$ lymphocytes. Similarly, self proteins that have been altered or are not usually presented by MHC class I molecules except as a result of malignant transformation are recognized by CD8+ T$_C$

cells. While these associations between cellular phenotype and function have been useful in the understanding of cellular immunity, in rare instances cytotoxic CD4+ T cells and helper CD8+ T lymphocytes have been detected.

# Thymic selection

The thymus acts as a "school" for educating thymocytes to recognize foreign (non-self) antigens presented by self MHC proteins. The education process accomplishes three goals: (1) selection of thymocytes that can interact with self MHC class I or MHC class II proteins (this leads to positive selection of potentially useful T lymphocytes); (2) non-selection of thymocytes that have poor ability to bind to self MHC antigens (resulting in apoptosis or programmed cell death); and (3) active elimination of any thymocytes with too great an affinity for self MHC antigens or that recognize self proteins (negative selection to eliminate potentially autoreactive thymocytes). The process of positive selection occurs in cortical thymocytes that have undergone TCR gene rearrangement and express TCRαβ-CD3 on their cell membranes (Fig. 85.4). These double-positive thymocytes coexpress both CD4 and CD8 and through interactions with the thymic cortical epithelium and APCs are "selected" for further differentiation into single-positive thymocytes that express either CD4 or CD8 alone. If immature CD4+CD8+ thymocytes express TCRαβ that interact with MHC class I proteins, then CD4 expression is subsequently lost. In contrast, if TCRαβ interaction with MHC class II proteins is favored, then only CD4 expression is maintained. Thymocytes failing to interact with self MHC molecules are thought to apoptose from the absence of signals necessary for further cell differentiation and proliferation. During negative selection, interactions between thymocytes and dendritic cells in the thymic medulla allow for identification and subsequent death of thymocytes whose TCRαβ recognize self antigens or interact so avidly with MHC proteins that stimulatory signals would be generated even if the TCR-binding site is not occupied by antigen. As a consequence of positive and negative selection, potentially useful T lymphocytes capable of recognizing foreign antigens are produced and most autoreactive T lymphocytes are eliminated. Less than 10 per cent of all thymocytes survive selection and exit the thymus as mature T cells.

# T-CELL FUNCTIONS

## Helper T cells

### Cytokine patterns

T$_H$ lymphocytes primarily express CD4, but not all CD4+ T lymphocytes are capable of providing B-cell

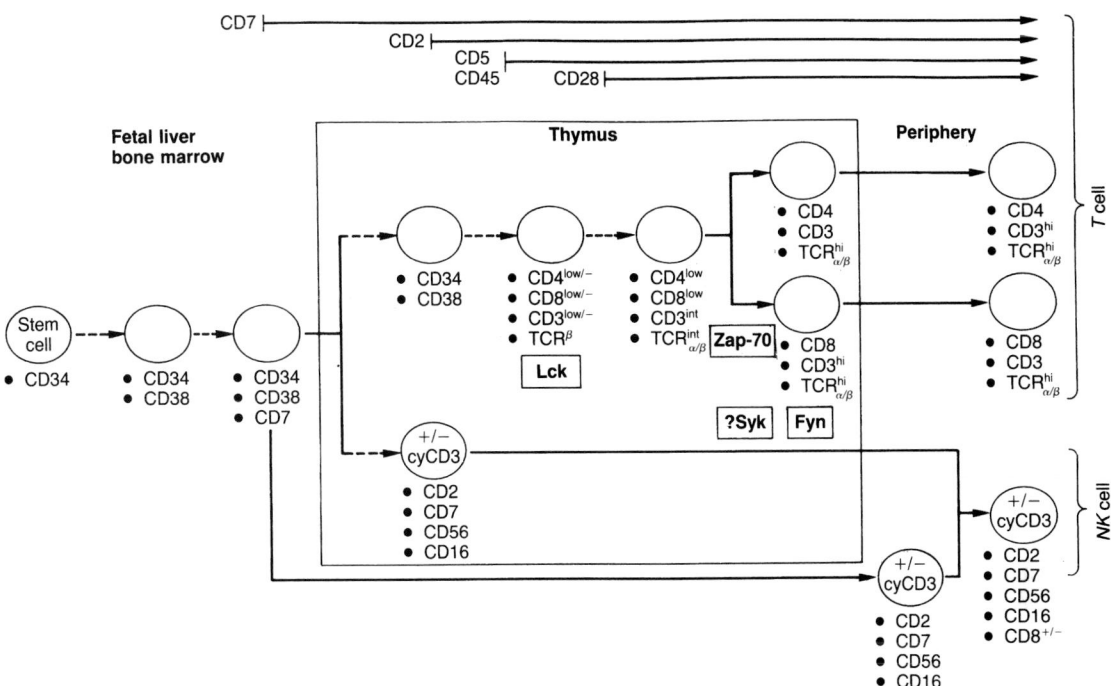

FIGURE 85.4 T-cell ontogeny. Cells of the T-lymphocyte lineage may be identified by flow cytometry analysis. Lymphoid progenitor stem cells express cluster of differentiation (CD) 34; the acquisition of additional CD molecules identifies cells of the T lymphocyte or natural killer (NK) cell lineage. CD38+CD7+ cells enter the thymus, rearrange their T-cell receptor (TCR) genes and undergo selection. Surviving thymocytes express TCRαβ in association with CD3 and either CD4 or CD8 alone. Also shown are additional cell surface markers expressed by differentiating T cells and developmental stages at which activities of certain protein tyrosine kinases (Lck, Fyn, ZAP-70, Syk) are critical. TCRγδ+ T-cell ontogeny is not depicted. Although cytoplasmic CD3 (cyCD3) can be demonstrated, cells destined to become NK cells neither express TCR or CD3 on the cell surface nor undergo thymic selection.

help or eliciting a *type IV delayed hypersensitivity (DTH) response.* Three subpopulations of $T_H$ cells have been distinguished by their predominant cytokine secretion profile (Fig. 85.5): (1) $T_H1$ lymphocytes are responsible for DTH reactions and secrete IL-2, IL-3, IFN-γ, tumor necrosis factor (TNF) β, and granulocyte-monocyte colony-stimulating factor (GM-CSF); (2) $T_H2$ lymphocytes are involved in B-lymphocyte proliferation and differentiation and isotype switching, and secrete IL-4, IL-5, IL-6, IL-9, IL-10, and IL-13; and (3) $T_H0$ cells secrete a mixed pattern of cytokines and are probably precursors of both $T_H1$ and $T_H2$ cells. IL-12 may participate in the conversion of $T_H0$ cells to $T_H1$ lymphocytes. These $T_H1$ and $T_H2$ lymphocyte subsets are thought to have counter-regulatory roles in the modulation of immune responses. Despite difficulties in identifying $T_H$ subpopulations in normal people, abnormal cytokine production and dysfunctional $T_H$ subsets are thought to occur in certain disease states.

## B-cell help

In addition to lymphokine secretion, B cells require direct contact with CD4+ $T_H$ lymphocytes in order to proliferate, differentiate into plasma cells, and secrete antibodies. $T_H2$ lymphocytes provide help via cognate interactions of T-cell and B-cell surface proteins (CD2–CD58, CD28/CTLA4–B7, CD40L–CD40, TCRαβ-CD3–MHC class II, CD4–MHC class II, CD5–CD72, CD11a/CD18–ICAM-1). IL-6 secretion induces B-lymphocyte proliferation, and IL-4 is important for B-cell differentiation into plasma cells and isotype switching from IgM to IgG, IgA, or IgE. Other lymphokines required by B cells include IL-2, IL-9, and IL-13.

## Cytotoxic T-cell help

CD8+ $T_C$ lymphocytes mediate cell-mediated cytotoxicity and respond to endogenous antigens that have been processed to peptides of approximately 7–15 amino acids in length and presented in the antigen-binding cleft of MHC class I molecules. IL-2 drives $T_C$ responses and IFN-γ enhances activities of $T_C$ cells; these lymphokines are produced by $T_H1$ cells that have recognized the same antigen as $T_C$ cells, but in association with MHC class II proteins. This requirement for both CD4+ and CD8+ T cells to

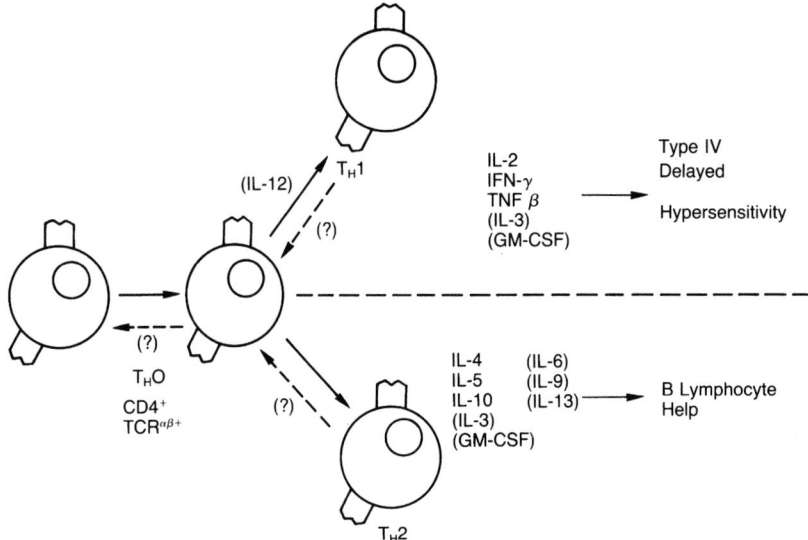

FIGURE 85.5 Helper T-cell subpopulations. Subpopulations of mature cluster of differentiation (CD) 4⁺ T cells can be distinguished by their lymphokine secretion patterns and the types of "help" provided. T_H0 cells are thought to be a precursor population that can give rise to both T_H1 and T_H2 cells. T_H1 lymphocytes secrete interleukin (IL)-2, interferon (IFN)-γ, tumor necrosis factor (TNF) β and granulocyte-monocyte colony-stimulating factor (GM-CSF) and are involved in type IV delayed hypersensitivity responses. T_H2 lymphocytes secrete IL-4, IL-5, IL-6, IL-10 as well as other lymphokines, and are required for B-cell development, antibody production and isotype switching.

mount cell-mediated cytotoxic responses has been well demonstrated in *GVHD* and *transplant rejection*.

## Cytotoxic T cells

### Mechanism of killing

CD8⁺ T_C lymphocytes physically contact potential target cells through accessory and adhesion molecules, such as CD2–CD58, CD8–MHC class I, and CD11a/CD18–ICAM-1. Recognition of peptides presented by MHC class I molecules on the plasma membranes of target cells initiates activation of naive T_C cells. CD4⁺ T_H1 lymphocytes provide help by secreting IL-2. Previously activated T_C cells can mediate cytolysis of target cells immediately after antigen binding and do not require further CD4⁺ T-cell help to kill target cells or to maintain the activated killer state. However, T_C lymphocytes may require T_H1-cell help to reinitiate active killing if sufficient time has passed since initial stimulation.

Direct cell–cell contact is required for cell-mediated cytotoxicity. Once a target cell is recognized and cell–cell adherence occurs, perforin, granzymes, lymphotoxin (TNFβ), and acidic chondroitin sulfate proteoglycans from T_C cytoplasmic vesicles are released into the cell membrane of the target cell. This process has been termed "the tight embrace with the kiss of death." Perforin has sequence homology with the membrane attack complex of the complement cascade and is thought to act in a similar fashion by creating pores

in the target cell membrane. Granzymes are serine proteases that initiate proteolytic digestion of cytosolic enzymes, and TNFβ initiates DNA fragmentation. T_C cells secrete IFN-γ and TNFα that potentiate the inflammatory response.

## Immunological memory

T lymphocytes exist as both naive and antigen-specific memory cells. The ability to respond to previously seen antigen is called antigenic recall. Memory T lymphocytes have been demonstrated to be long-lived and may survive the entire lifespan of an individual. Conversion of T cells from the naive to the memory state is associated with changes in the expression patterns of certain T cell-membrane proteins; memory CD4⁺ T_H lymphocytes express CD45RO, CD26, CD29, and increased levels of the adhesion molecules CD2, CD11a/CD18, CD54, and CD58. This may help T cells adhere to vascular endothelial cells and transmigrate to areas of inflammation. In contrast, naive T lymphocytes express CD45RA and lower levels of adhesion molecules. In general, greater concentrations and/or more potent forms of stimulants are required to activate naive T lymphocytes.

DTH is a memory T cell-mediated response, and characteristic clinical findings of DTH occur in some contact allergies. With initial antigen contact (such as poison ivy), APCs in the skin capture the antigen and migrate to local lymph nodes where naive T_H1 lymphocytes are stimulated and converted to memory T cells. These T cells subsequently remigrate to the skin and with subsequent antigenic exposure produce DTH reactions within 24–72 hours. Each antigen reexposure further potentiates the DTH response so that worsening clinical symptoms may develop.

## SEVERE COMBINED IMMUNODEFICIENCY

Severe combined immunodeficiency (SCID) comprises a heterogeneous group of genetically determined disorders affecting approximately 1 per 100 000 live births with a 4:1 male predominance. These infants characteristically have a paucity or complete absence of mature functional T lymphocytes. There is concomitant B-lymphocyte dysfunction, which may result from lack of T-cell help or from intrinsic defects shared by both cell types. Natural killer cells are present in variable numbers in different SCID forms; this occurs as a consequence of both heterogeneity of inheritance and heterogeneity of underlying molecular defects. Approximately 20 per cent of patients with SCID have autosomal recessively inherited adenosine deaminase deficiency; these children present with severe lymphopenia that involves all cell lineages. Approximately 40 per cent of affected children have X-linked SCID with the lesion resulting from mutations in the IL-2 receptor γ chain; the γ chain subsequently has been shown to be a subunit of the receptors for IL-4, IL-7, IL-9, and IL-15 as well. These male infants generally present with a relative increase in B-lymphocyte numbers. A similar phenotype of absent T cells and normal to increased B-cell numbers is seen in SCID patients with a deficiency of Jak 3, a tryosine kinase also involved in IL-2 signaling. Lesions underlying many of the remaining cases of SCID are unknown. Defects in CD3, HLA molecules, ZAP-70, and other signaling proteins have been reported in isolated patients and consanguineous families. Defects in DNA repair (as observed in *scid* mice) have not yet been detected in humans. Currently, the only effective long-term therapy is bone marrow transplantation (BMT). Transplantation with histocompatible or HLA-identical bone marrow from a related donor (usually a sibling) is successful in reconstituting immunity and providing long-term survival in more than 80 per cent of patients, but is only available for about 15 per cent of infants with SCID. Removal of mature T lymphocytes from HLA non-identical donor bone marrow by lectin agglutination and other methods has allowed successful haplocompatible (one HLA allele match) BMT for most infants with SCID. Haplocompatible BMT usually uses a parent as the donor, and worldwide success with haploidentical BMT is greater than 60 per cent. Affected infants generally present by 3 months of age, but may not become ill for several months, delaying diagnosis. Viral, fungal, bacterial, and parasitic infections are problematic. In particular, *Pneumocystis carinii*, parainfluenza type 3, cytomegalovirus, Epstein–Barr virus, adenovirus, and *Candida albicans* have caused much of the morbidity and mortality associated with SCID. Additional morbidity may be due to *in utero* engraftment of maternal T cells, which can cause GVHD and complicate treatment in these patients. Suspicion and prompt evaluation are imperative for successful outcomes in these children.

## PEDIATRIC ACQUIRED IMMUNODEFICIENCY SYNDROME

Pediatric acquired immunodeficiency syndrome (PAIDS) is a profound T-cell immunodeficiency that results from infection with the human immunodeficiency virus (HIV), a member of the retroviral subgroup termed lentivirus. HIV preferentially infects CD4$^+$ T$_H$ cells, monocytes/macrophages and microglial cells of the brain; this cell preference is explained by the fact that the CD4 molecule functions as the specific HIV receptor to allow virus inside target cells. HIV binds CD4 via its viral envelope glycoprotein gp120. An unidentified cell surface molecule that binds the V3 loop of gp120 is thought to exist and acts exclusively to restrict HIV entry to human cells.

Although only a minority of CD4$^+$ T lymphocytes are actually infected with HIV, concomitant loss of uninfected T cells occurs. Mechanisms to explain this depletion of all T cells are not well understood, but include "bystander" cell killing from HIV-induced syncytium formation and profound deleterious effects on lymphocyte proliferation as a result of abnormal antigen presentation and cytokine production by HIV-infected APCs. Antibody-bound HIV virions are efficiently trapped by Fc receptor-bearing follicular dendritic cells (FDCs) within lymphoid follicles. With time, FDCs and lymphoid follicles are destroyed, leading to the loss of memory B and T lymphocytes and an inability to mount anamnestic immune responses. T$_H$1 cells tend to be preferentially depleted by HIV, resulting in more severe effects on cell-mediated immunity than on B-cell proliferation and immunoglobulin production. However, compromised B-cell responses are eventually seen, reflecting B-cell dependence on normal T-cell function.

More than 95 per cent of children with PAIDS are infected perinatally. Potential factors affecting maternal–fetal transmission of HIV include viral genotype, prematurity, multiple pregnancy (first twin is more likely to acquire HIV), maternal–fetal blood transfusion and stage of maternal disease (advanced AIDS or primary HIV infection with viremia). The clinical course of PAIDS is bimodal; approximately 20 per cent of children develop PAIDS within a few months of birth, while the remainder may be asymptomatic for several years. This bimodal pattern may reflect timing of HIV transmission from mother to child. *In utero* HIV infection is suggested by virus detection in cord blood, presentation in infancy and rapid disease progression. In contrast, intrapartum HIV transmission is suggested by discordance of infection in twins, absence of HIV in early infant blood samples, indolent course and delayed presentation, often for more than 6 years. Recently, antiretroviral therapy with zidovudine has been demonstrated to significantly decrease intra-partum maternal–fetal transmission of HIV.

PAIDS is characterized clinically by recurrent bac-terial infections, non-central nervous system (CNS) opportunistic infections (*P. carinii*, cytomegalovirus), early onset encephalopathy, lymphocytic interstitial pneumonitis (LIP), parotitis, chronic mucocutaneous candidiasis, and failure to thrive secondary to chronic diarrhea and gastrointestinal infections. In contrast to adults with AIDS, children rarely develop CNS oppor-tunistic infections or neoplasms, although lymphoid hyperplasia is common. Guidelines have been devel-oped for the use of antiretroviral therapies, intravenous gammaglobulin and *P. carinii* prophylaxis in infants and children with HIV and PAIDS.

## SELECTED READING

Baeuerle PA, Henkel T. Function and activation of NF-κB in the immune system. *Annu Rev Immunol* 1994; **12**: 141.

Berke G. The binding and lysis of target cells by cytotoxic lymphocytes: molecular and cellular aspects. *Annu Rev Immunol* 1994; **12**: 735.

Chan AC, Desai DM, Weiss A. The role of protein tyrosine kinases and protein tyrosine phosphatases in T cell antigen receptor signal transduction. *Annu Rev Immunol* 1994; **12**: 555.

Gibb D, Wara D. Pediatric HIV infection. *AIDS* 1994; **8**: S275.

Gray D. Immunological memory. *Annu Rev Immunol* 1993; **11**: 49.

Harding CV, Song R, Griffin J *et al.* Processing of bacterial antigens for presentation to class I and II MHC-restricted T lymphocytes. *Infect Agents Dis* 1995; **4**: 1.

Leiden JM. Transcriptional regulation of T cell receptor genes. *Annu Rev Immunol* 1993; **11**: 539.

Levy JA. Pathogenesis of human immunodeficiency virus infection. *Microbiol Rev* 1993; **57**: 183.

Morimoto C, Schlossman SF. P. Rambotti Lecture. Human naive and memory cells revisited; new markers (CD31 and CD27) that help define CD4+ T cell subsets. *Clin Exp Rheumatol* 1993; **11**: 241.

Pannetier C, Even J, Kourilsky P. T cell repertoire diversity and clonal expansions in normal and clinical samples. *Immunol Today* 1995; **16**: 176.

Pantaleo G, Graziosi C, Fauci AS. The immunopathogenesis of human immunodeficiency virus infection. *N Engl J Med* 1993; **328**: 327.

Robey E, Fowlkes BJ. Selective events in T cell development. *Annu Rev Immunol* 1994; **12**: 675.

Romagnani S. Lymphokine production by human T cells in disease states. *Annu Rev Immunol* 1994; **12**: 227.

Seder RA, Paul WE. Acquisition of lymphokine-producing phenotype by CD4+ T cells. *Annu Rev Immunol* 1994; **12**: 635.

Trowbridge IS, Thomas ML. CD45: an emerging role as a protein tyrosine phosphatase required for lymphocyte acti-vation and development. *Annu Rev Immunol* 1994; **12**: 85.

Weiss RA. How does HIV cause AIDS? *Science* 1993; **260**: 1273.

# 86

# Hypersensitivity Immune Responses

Richard S. Shames

The function of the immune system is to protect the individual from invasion by foreign antigens by distinguishing self from non-self. A normal immune response relies on the careful coordination of a complex network of specialized cells, organs, and biological factors necessary for the recognition and subsequent elimination of foreign antigens. An exaggerated immune response can result in hypersensitivity to foreign antigens with resultant tissue injury and the expression of a variety of clinical syndromes.

The Gel and Coombs classification scheme defines four basic immunopathological mechanisms of hypersensitivity (types I–IV; Table 86.1); two other mechanisms (types V, VI) have also been proposed. Types I–III are antibody-mediated (humoral immune responses), while type IV results from the actions of sensitized T lymphocytes (cell-mediated immune response). These mechanisms require an initial exposure to antigen (sensitizing dose), which induces a primary immune response (sensitization). Subsequent exposure to the same antigen (challenge dose) following a lag period of at least 1 week evokes the hypersensitivity response.

Antigen elimination by cellular or humoral processes is integrally linked to the inflammatory response in which cellular messengers (cytokines) and antibodies trigger the recruitment of additional cells and the release of endogenous vasoactive and proinflammatory substances (inflammatory mediators). Inflammation

TABLE 86.1.   Hypersensitivity reactions

| TYPE | IMMUNE MECHANISM | CLINICAL DISEASES | DIAGNOSTIC TESTS |
|---|---|---|---|
| Type I: Immediate hypersensitivity | IgE; mast cell and basophil mediators | Local: allergic rhinitis, asthma, atopic dermatitis, urticaria/angioedema, gastrointestinal food allergies Systemic: anaphylaxis | Immediate skin testing (20 min) RAST (*in vitro* IgE) |
| Type II: Antibody-mediated cytotoxicity | IgG or IgM against cell-surface antigens; complement activation | Transfusion and drug reactions Graves disease Myasthenia gravis | Demonstration of antibody *in vitro* |
| Type III: Immune complex | Antigen–antibody complexes; complement activation | Arthus-type reaction: hypersensitivity pneumonitis Serum sickness SLE Autoimmune vasculitis | Late (Arthus) skin test (6–8 hours) Demonstration of tissue-fixed or circulating immune complexes Demonstration of specific antibody |
| Type IV: Delayed hypersensitivity | Lymphocytes | Contact dermatitis Granulomatous disease: sarcoidosis, *M. tuberculosis* Allograft rejection | Delayed skin test (24–48 hours) *In vitro* proliferation |

RAST, radioallergosorbent test; SLE, systemic lupus erythematosus.

has both positive and deleterious effects. Tight control of inflammatory mechanisms promotes efficient elimination of foreign substances and prevents uncontrolled lymphocyte activation and antibody production. However, inappropriate activation or dysregulation can perpetuate inflammatory processes that lead to tissue damage and organ dysfunction. Inflammation is responsible for hypersensitivity reactions and for many of the clinical effects of autoimmunity.

## TYPE I HYPERSENSITIVITY

*Anaphylactic* or *immediate hypersensitivity reactions* represent an inflammatory response mediated by the interaction of antigen with IgE-bound mast cells and basophils, and subsequent release of inflammatory mediators that leads to tissue damage in specific target organs. Examples of type I-mediated reactions include *allergic rhinitis, allergic asthma, acute drug reactions,* and *systemic anaphylaxis.*

## Mechanisms

Initial antigen exposure in a genetically predisposed host results in synthesis of antigen-specific IgE constituting the atopic state. Induction of IgE synthesis requires two signals that are primarily elaborated by cluster of differentiation (CD) $4^+$ helper T ($T_H$) lymphocytes: one influences IgE expression, and the other activates B cells. Secretion of interleukin (IL)-4 by $T_H$ cells is critical for IgE isotype switching; additional B-lymphocyte activation and differentiation factors, triggered through the B-cell-membrane receptor CD40, are required for IgE synthesis. In contrast, interferon-$\gamma$ (IFN-$\gamma$) inhibits IL-4-dependent IgE synthesis; therefore, an imbalance favoring IL-4 over IFN-$\gamma$ may induce IgE production.

Three subsets of $T_H$ lymphocytes have been identified by their patterns of cytokine synthesis: (1) $T_H$1 cells elaborate IL-2, IFN-$\gamma$, IL-3, and granulocyte-monocyte colony-stimulating factor (GM-CSF), and participate in type IV-delayed hypersensitivity (DTH) reactions; (2) $T_H$2 cells secrete GM-CSF, IL-4, IL-5, IL-6, and IL-10, and have been implicated in type I allergic responses; and (3) $T_H$0 cells probably represent precursor cells. IL-3 induces mast cell differentiation and proliferation, IL-5 promotes activation and chemotaxis of eosinophils, and GM-CSF stimulates proliferation and differentiation of phagocytic cells. Activated $T_H$2 lymphocytes have been demonstrated at sites of inflammation in allergic airway disease and are believed to direct the immune response toward allergic inflammation.

Antigen-specific IgE binds to Fc receptors on tissue mast cells, basophils, macrophages, eosinophils, and platelets, thus sensitizing these cells to future allergen encounters. Upon re-exposure to allergen, the sensitized individual mounts a secondary or anamnestic

immune response. $IgE^+$ mast cells bind and crosslink allergen, which triggers a sequence of biochemical events that results in mast cell and basophil activation and degranulation (Fig. 86.1a). These events include both the release of preformed mediators from cytoplasmic granules (histamine, chemotactic factors, and enzymes), and the synthesis and release of newly generated mediators (prostaglandins, leukotrienes, and platelet-activating factor (PAF)).

Interactions of inflammatory mediators with specific target organs and cells frequently induces a biphasic response: (1) an early effect on blood vessels, smooth muscle, and secretory glands marked by vascular leakiness and smooth muscle constriction; and (2) a late response characterized by tissue edema and influx of inflammatory cells. Early-phase events are primarily mediated by histamine, while late-phase events are induced by cytokines, preformed chemotactic mediators, leukotrienes, and PAF.

The early-phase response occurs within minutes of antigen exposure with the release of histamine, leukotrienes, $PGD_2$, kinins, and other mediators from mast cells and basophils. The late phase may either follow the early-phase response (dual response) or occur as an isolated event (isolated late-phase response). Late-phase reactions begin 2–4 hours following initial antigen exposure, reach maximal activity at 6–12 hours, and usually resolve within 12–24 hours. Mediators of the early-phase response, except for $PGD_2$, reappear during the late-phase response in the absence of antigen rechallenge; absence of $PGD_2$, an exclusive product of mast-cell release, suggests that basophils are the predominant source of mediators during late-phase events. The late-phase response is characterized histologically by an influx of, primarily, eosinophils and mononuclear cells. Eosinophils and products of activated eosinophils, such as major basic protein and eosinophilic cationic protein, are destructive to epithelial tissues and predispose to persistent tissue reactivity. Inflammatory cells infiltrating target tissues (bronchi, skin, or nasal mucosa) during the late phase also release chemical mediators and thus precipitate a sustained inflammatory response resulting in localized edema, epithelial disruption, and further influx of polymorphonuclear cells and mononuclear cells.

## Clinical manifestations

Pathophysiological events of the late-phase response characterize a persistent inflammatory state thought closely to mimic clinical allergic diseases, including *allergic rhinitis, asthma, food-sensitive atopic dermatitis,* and *systemic anaphylaxis.* Therefore, therapeutic interventions that prevent or reverse inflammatory processes are most effective in the control of chronic and severe allergic disease. Evidence of local type I clinical syndromes may be confirmed by the finding of antigen-specific IgE bound to skin mast cells (positive immediate hypersensitivity skin testing) or by the presence of antigen-specific IgE in serum (*in vitro* radioallergosorbent test [RAST]).

## TYPE II HYPERSENSITIVITY

Cytotoxic reactions involve antigen–antibody reactions on the surfaces of cells that result in cellular destruction or dysfunction. Clinical manifestations vary with the cells and tissues involved and include erythrocyte, neutrophil, and platelet disorders and Goodpasture syndrome.

## Mechanisms

Cell-bound antigen stimulates production of IgM and IgG, resulting in destruction of cells to which the antigen is bound by several mechanisms (*see* Fig. 86.1b): (1) activation of the complement cascade and binding of the membrane attack complex (C5b6789); (2) phagocytosis by Fc or C3b receptor-bearing macrophages that attach to the cell-bound antigen–antibody complexes (opsonization); and (3) antibody-dependent cell-mediated cytotoxicity (ADCC) in which cell-bound antigen–antibody complexes are recognized by natural killer cells. ADCC is sometimes described as type VI hypersensitivity. Additionally, cell-bound antigen may induce the formation of antibodies that do not cause outright cell destruction but may alter cell function instead; this type of mechanism has also been called type V hypersensitivity.

## Clinical disorders

The spectrum of injury by type II hypersensitivity depends on the cell types affected. Immunopathologic red-cell destruction may result in *blood transfusion reactions*, *hemolytic disease* of the newborn, and drug- or infection-induced hemolytic disease. Blood transfusion reactions constitute normal immune responses against foreign erythrocyte antigens, but are classified as hypersensitivity disorders because of the adverse clinical effects. Acute reactions are due to ABO incompatibility, which induces complement-mediated intravascular hemolysis. Delayed hemolytic reactions result from sensitization to foreign non-ABO erythrocyte antigens, which induce clinical hemolysis 3–10 days after transfusion and result from immune phagocytosis by splenic macrophages. Hemolytic disease of the newborn occurs when maternal IgG anti-fetal Rh antibodies cross the placenta. Drug-induced hemolytic disease is due to the formation of immunogenic drug–hapten complexes; typical drugs behaving as small-molecular-weight haptens are penicillin and phenacetin. Type II reactions also involve neutrophils, platelets, or basement membrane antigens

and induce *neonatal leukopenias*, neonatal or *idiopathic thrombocytopenia*, and *Goodpasture syndrome*, respectively. Although type II hypersensitivity generally results in cell destruction, antigen–antibody interactions may also cause only a disruption of cellular function, such as seen in *autoimmune primary hyperthyroidism (Graves disease)* and *myasthenia gravis*.

## TYPE III HYPERSENSITIVITY

Immune complex-mediated reactions occur when immune (antibody–antigen) complexes escape phagocytosis by the reticuloendothelial system and deposit in tissues or vascular endothelium, inducing complement activation, anaphylatoxin generation, polymorphonuclear leukocyte migration, and tissue injury (*see* Fig. 86.1c). *Serum sickness* and *lupus nephritis* are examples of type III-mediated diseases.

## Mechanisms

Immune complexes may deposit locally in various organs or remain in the circulation. Arthus-type reactions and serum sickness are due to type III hypersensitivity. Arthus reactions result from tissue necrosis at the site of antigen entry, with the severity of the reaction generally proportionate to the antigen dose. Precipitating antibodies in the serum formed with repeated antigen exposure lead to the development of large antigen–antibody complexes that deposit in small blood vessels, activating the complement cascade and causing hemorrhage and tissue necrosis. Serum sickness defines a more common manifestation of type III reactions in which large antigen doses (foreign serum proteins, drugs, viral or microbial antigens) induce the formation of immune complexes in the serum. Large multivalent protein antigens and IgG or IgM antibodies favor formation of immune complexes by facilitating interactions with complement. Antigen–antibody complexes formed at either moderate antigen or antibody excess tend to persist in the circulation and deposit in the walls of small blood vessels. The deposited immune complexes activate complement, which leads to necrotizing vasculitis.

## Clinical manifestations

Circulating immune complexes are found in many diseases, such as *serum sickness*, *systemic lupus erythematosus*, *poststreptococcal glomerulonephritis*, and *hepatitis B viral infections*. Arthus-type reactions occur in *hypersensitivity pneumonitis*, which are a group of interstitial and/or alveolar-filling granulomatous diseases resulting from inhalation of organic dusts. The occurrence of serum sickness syndromes

## (a) TYPE I

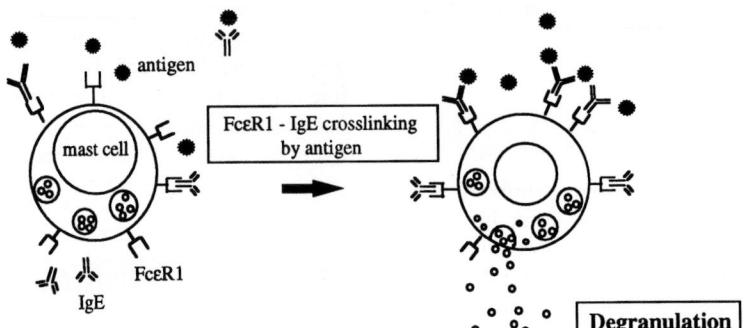

## (b) TYPE II

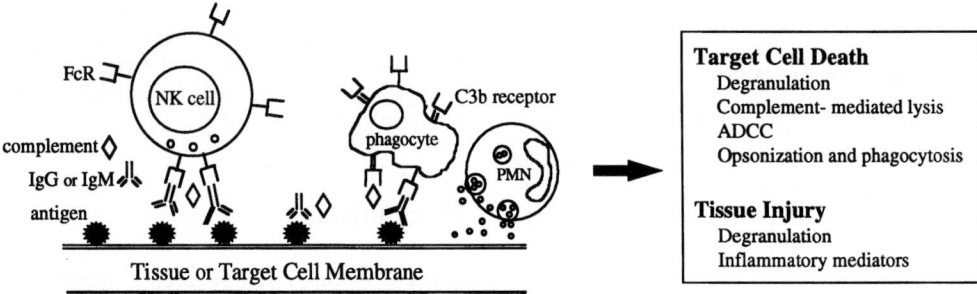

## (c) TYPE III

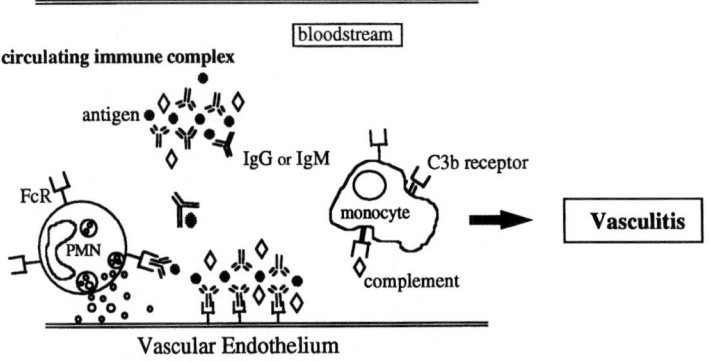

## (d) TYPE IV

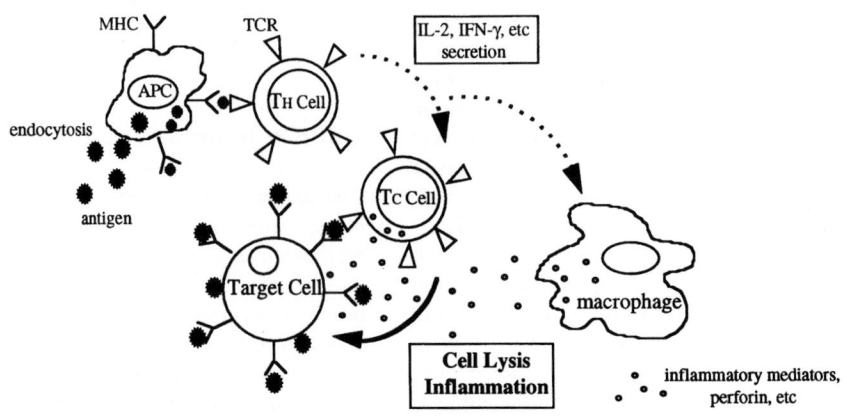

has declined with the decreased use of heterologous serum. Currently, penicillin is the most common cause of serum sickness, but the exact immunopathogenesis is not well understood. Clinical manifestations usually require a latent period following initial antigen exposure of 8–12 days to allow for antibody formation; both the antigen dose and the timing of antigen re-exposure influence the severity of the reaction.

## TYPE IV HYPERSENSITIVITY

Type IV DTH reactions are mediated primarily by T lymphocytes and in contrast to type I reactions, which often occur within minutes of antigen challenge, this immune injury does not manifest for 24–72 hours. Classic examples of type IV immunopathology are the *tuberculin skin test reaction, sarcoidosis,* and *contact dermatitis.*

## Mechanisms

Inappropriate activation or dysregulation of cell-mediated cytotoxicity results in type IV DTH (*see* Fig. 86.1d). Killing of target cells by cytotoxic T ($T_C$) lymphocytes requires cell–cell contact in order for activated $T_C$ cells to inject perforin and other lytic products into targets expressing non-self proteins bound to MHC class I molecules. Target cell lysis ensues with changes in cell membrane permeability and apoptosis (programmed cell death). The histological appearance of cell-mediated cytotoxicity is characterized by marked lymphocytic infiltration and necrosis of affected tissues. Cell-mediated immunity also involves secretion of IFN-γ and other lymphokines by activated $T_H$ cells that promote migration of mononuclear phagocytes into sites of antigen deposition. Type IV DTH may result from the uncontrolled activation of tissue macrophages.

## Clinical manifestations

Clinical examples of type IV DTH include *contact dermatitis*, sarcoidosis, *Mycobacterium tuberculosis* infections, and *allograft rejection*. Cutaneous DTH is the basis for skin tests used in the diagnosis of *M. tuberculosis*, histoplasmosis, and coccidiomycosis. Intradermal injection of inactivated antigen that appears as an indurated nodule signifies antigen re-exposure and likely is the result of either previous infection or specific immunization. Histological appearance of the site at 24–48 hours demonstrates deposition of fibrin, tissue edema, and marked infiltration by primarily $CD4^+$ T cells and mononuclear cells. The pathogenesis of cutaneous DTH involves antigen presentation to $CD4^+$ memory T cells in the skin, local lymphokine release, and activation of tissue macrophages. Contact sensitivity is seen following application of antigen to the skin of previously sensitized individuals. Antigens that commonly induce contact dermatitis include nickel, drugs, dyes, and plants such as poison ivy and poison oak. Skin biopsy demonstrates a characteristic cell-mediated inflammatory response with marked dermal perivascular infiltration of lymphocytes and macrophages, tissue edema, and fibrin deposition. Diagnosis is confirmed by a positive patch test, which appears as a vesicular or eczematous patch 24–72 hours after direct application of the suspected antigen to the skin. Granulomatous inflammation is defined by chronic persistent antigenic stimulation of T cells, which induce morphological changes in macrophages and a characteristic inflammatory response. Aggregates of macrophages, lymphocytes, plasma cells, and palisading fibroblasts are characteristically observed in affected tissue sites. Antigens that induce granulomatous inflammation include microorganisms that persist in phagocytic cells such as *Mycobacterium,* sarcoidosis, metals and inert foreign bodies.

FIGURE 86.1 Hypersensitivity immune responses. (a) Type I reaction. Mast cells and basophils bind IgE via high-affinity Fc receptors (FcεR1). Antigen binding and crosslinking of FcεR1–IgE complexes induce cellular degranulation and release of inflammatory mediators. (b) Type II reaction. IgG or IgM antibodies against tissue or cellular antigens induces complement activation, which results in cell death and tissue injury by several mechanisms. These include complement-mediated lysis, opsonization and phagocytosis of target cells via FcR and complement (C3b) receptors on polymorphonuclear cells (PMN) and other phagocytes, and neutrophil degranulation. Antibody-dependent cell-mediated cytotoxicity (ADCC) by natural killer (NK) cells is also triggered by the binding of antibodies to target cell antigens. (c) Type III reaction. Circulating immune complexes composed of soluble antigen and IgG or IgM eventually deposit on vascular endothelium of various tissues, which activates the complement cascade. PMN and other phagocytes are attracted to these sites of immune complex deposition via their Fc and C3b receptors and are induced to degranulate and phagocytose the complexes, resulting in local tissue injury and vasculitis. (d) Type IV reaction. Via their T-cell receptors (TCR), helper T ($T_H$) cells recognize target cell antigenic peptides bound to self major histocompatibility complex (MHC) class II molecules on antigen-presenting cells (APC). This T-cell recognition results in the secretion of interleukin (IL)-2, interferon (IFN)-γ and other lymphokines that are required for the activation of tissue macrophages and cytotoxic T ($T_C$) cells. $T_C$ cells recognize the same antigen bound to MHC class I molecules on the target cell, inducing target cell lysis by perforin and other molecules secreted by $T_C$ cells. Macrophage activation results in mediator release and inflammation.

## SELECTED READING

Barnes PJ. Pathophysiology of allergic inflammation. In: Middleton E, Reed CE, Ellis EF, Adkinson NF, Yuninger JW, Busse WW, eds. *Allergy principles and practice*, Vol I. St Louis: Mosby-Year Book, 1993: 243.

Barnett EV. Circulating immune complexes: their biologic and clinical significance. *J Allergy Clin Immunol* 1986; **78**: 1089.

Dannenberg AMPR. Immune mechanisms in the pathogenesis of pulmonary tuberculosis. *Rev Infect Dis* 1989; **11**: S369.

Engelfrie CP, Overbeeke MAM, von dern Borne AEG. Autoimmune hemolytic anemia. *Semin Hematol* 1992; **29**: 3.

Geha RS. Regulation of IgE synthesis in humans. *J Allergy Clin Immunol* 1992; **90**: 143.

Kaliner M. Asthma and mast cell activation. *J Allergy Clin Immunol* 1989; **83**: 510.

Lawley TJ. Immune complexes. In: Frank MM, Austen KF, Claman HF, Unanue ER, eds. *Samter's immunologic diseases*. Boston: Little, Brown and Company, 1994: 321.

Maibach HI, Dannaker CJ. Contact skin allergy. In: Middleton E, Reed CE, Ellis EF, Adkinson NF, Yuninger JW, Busse WW, eds. *Allergy principles and practice*, Vol II. St Louis: Mosby-Year Book, 1993: 1605.

Romagnani S. Lymphokine production by human T cells in disease states. *Annu Rev Immunol* 1994; **12**: 227.

Shames RS, Adelman DC. The immune system. In: McPhee S, Lingappa V, eds. *Pathophysiology of disease: an introduction to clinical medicine*. Norwalk: Appleton and Lange, 1995.

Waters AH. Autoimmune thrombocytopenia: clinical aspects. *Semin Hematol* 1992; **29**: 18.

# 87

# Structure and Function of Cytokines

## James D. Watson

## INTRODUCTION

Cytokines are soluble proteins produced by many cell types that act as chemical communicators between cells. Most are secreted, but some can exert activity as membrane-bound ligands. Cytokines bind to specific receptors on the surface of target cells that are coupled to intracellular signal transduction and second messenger pathways. Most cytokines are growth or differentiation factors. Cytokine nomenclature is a reflection of the different historical approaches to naming new factors that were based either on cell of origin or initial defining bioassay. The colony-stimulating factors were first identified by the type of blood cell colony that emerged in soft-agar culture from the stimulation of bone marrow cells. The interleukin (IL) nomenclature assigns a sequential number to new factors, but has not been universally applied to new factors. This has created anomalies such as IL-8 which is clearly a member of a chemokine family. Tumor necrosis factor (TNF) is another. TNF was originally defined as causing necrosis of solid tumors, but is now thought to be primarily an inflammatory cytokine.

The major cytokines are discussed here in three general groups. The divisions are based on current nomenclature, effector function and protein structure. The groups are: (1) the hematopoietic growth factors, including colony-stimulating factors; (2) the interleukins (IL-1 to IL-15); and (3) the TNF receptor family.

## CYTOKINE RECEPTOR FAMILIES

The receptors for most known cytokines have been cloned. The analysis of primary structures has led to the grouping of these receptors into superfamilies. The main cytokine receptor superfamilies (see also page 53) are detailed below:

- The hematopoietin receptor superfamily is characterized by cytokine and fibronectin type III domains in the extracellular regions and a Trp-Ser-X-Trp-Ser (WSXWS) motif.
- The immunoglobulin receptor superfamily is made up of membrane polypeptides with immunoglobulin domains in their extracellular regions. These domains are made up of a structural unit of about 100 amino acids with a folding pattern known as the immunoglobulin fold.
- The protein tyrosine kinase receptor superfamily all have a large glycosylated, extracellular ligand-binding domain, a single transmembrane domain and an intracellular catalytic domain.
- The TNF receptor superfamily (also known as the nerve growth factor receptor superfamily) have three or four cysteine-rich repeats of about 40 amino acids in the extracellular region of the receptor.

## CYTOKINES THAT REGULATE HEMATOPOIESIS (Table 87.1) (see also Chapters 80 and 81)

The earliest members of this family of growth factors were identified by the stimulation of hematopoietic cell colonies in soft-agar medium, hence the name colony-stimulating factors. The blood system is in constant renewal. From early in fetal development and throughout adult life, hematopoietic stem cells found in bone marrow constantly give rise to the mature cell types found in blood – erythrocytes, granulocytes, macrophages, dendritic cells, megakaryocytes and platelets, mast cells, eosinophils, B lymphocytes and T lympho-

TABLE 87.1 Hematopoietic growth factors

| NAME | MOLECULAR MASS (kD) | PROTEIN STRUCTURE | BIOLOGICAL ACTION | RECEPTOR FAMILY |
|---|---|---|---|---|
| SCF | 30 | Short chain 4α helical bundle, homodimer type 1 transmembrane protein | Stimulates proliferation, differentiation and function of mast cells; stimulates proliferation and differentiation of HSC; synergizes with other growth factors in regulating growth of hemopoietic progenitor cells | Tyrosine kinase |
| Flt-3 ligand (Flk-2) | 30 | Short chain 4α helical bundle, homodimer type 1 transmembrane protein | Synergizes with other regulators in stimulating the proliferation and differentiation of HSC and dendritic cells | Tyrosine kinase |
| GM-CSF | 18–32 | Short chain 4α helical bundle, monomer | Stimulates proliferation, differentiation, activation and survival of myeloid cells and their progenitors | Hematopoietin, shared β chain with IL-3 and IL-5 |
| G-CSF | 18–25 | Long chain 4α helical bundle, monomer | Stimulates proliferation, differentiation, functional activation of HSC, granulocytes and macrophages | Hematopoietin |
| M-CSF | 45–90 | Short chain 4α helical bundle, homopolymer, type I transmembrane protein | Stimulates proliferation, differentiation, activation and survival of macrophages and osteoclasts and their progenitors; weak stimulus of granulocytes | Tyrosine kinase |
| TPO | 38 | 4α helical bundle | Stimulates proliferation, differentiation, functional activation and survival of megakaryocytes | Hematopoietin |
| EPO | 30 | Long chain 4α helical bundle, monomer | Stimulates proliferation, differentiation, functional activation and survival of erythrocytes and megakaryocytes | Hematopoietin |

HSC, hematopoietic stem cells. For other abbreviations, see text.

cytes. Seven cytokines with predominantly hematopoietic cell targets are summarized below and in Table 87.1.

## Stem cell factor (c-kit ligand)

Stem cell factor (SCF) stimulates the development of hematopoietic and pigment cell lineages. It has a wide range of activities on myeloid and lymphoid cell development and synergistic effects with other growth factors such as granulocyte-macrophage colony stimulating factor (GM-CSF) and IL-7. SCF is encoded by the *steel* locus of the mouse and is the ligand for the c-*kit* protooncogene. Alternative mRNA splicing gives rise to two forms of SCF, both of which have a transmembrane domain and are inserted into the cell membrane. The larger form contains a peptide cleavage site that is processed to yield secreted SCF. Both membrane-bound and soluble forms are biologically active. The SCF receptor (*c-kit*) belongs to the tyrosine kinase receptor family.

## Flt-3 ligand (Flk-2)

Flt-3 ligand, like SCF, is involved in the early development of hematopoietic cells. It has a wide range of activities on myeloid, dendritic, and lymphoid progenitors, and shows synergistic effects with other hematopoietic growth factors. Flt-3 also belongs to the tyrosine kinase receptor family, and is also known as Flk-2.

## Granulocyte-macrophage colony-stimulating factor

GM-CSF is a growth factor for hematopoietic progenitor cells, and a differentiation and activating factor for granulocytic and monocytic cells.

The high-affinity GM-CSF receptor is a complex of a low-affinity α-chain with a second affinity-converting β-chain that is also shared with the IL-3 and IL-5 receptor β-chains. Both the α- and β-chains of the GM-CSF receptor are members of the hematopoietin family of receptors. The intracytoplasmic domain of the β-chain is not required to form a high-affinity receptor.

## Granulocyte colony-stimulating factor (G-CSF)

G-CSF is a growth, differentiation and activating factor for neutrophils and their precursors. It also synergizes with IL-3 to stimulate growth of hemato-poietic progenitors, and also can cause proliferation of endothelial cells.

The G-CSF receptor is a hybrid structure containing an immunoglobulin domain and a hematopoietin domain. The human receptor exists as two forms varying in their intracytoplasmic domains. A soluble form of the human receptor has the transmembrane region deleted. The G-CSF receptor shares 46 per cent sequence homology to the gp130 chain of the IL-6 receptor.

## Macrophage colony-stimulating factor (M-CSF)

M-CSF is a growth, differentiation and activating factor for macrophages and their progenitor cells. M-CSF can be produced as membrane-bound or secreted protein variants.

The M-CSF receptor is identical to the product of the c-*fms* protooncogene and is related to *c-kit* (the SCF receptor). These receptors are all autophosphory-lating tyrosine kinases. The M-CSF receptor exists in a single affinity form.

## Megakaryocyte colony-stimulating factor (thrombopoietin, TPO)

TPO is a megakaryocytic lineage-specific growth and differentiation factor. It acts as a regulator of platelet numbers. The TPO receptor, also known as *c-mpl*, is a member of the hematopoietic receptor family. A soluble form of the receptor is also found. A portion of the *c-mpl* (TPO receptor) gene has been found fused to viral sequences encoding the envelope protein of a strain of Friend leukemia virus called myelo-proliferative leukemia virus (MPLV). The viral oncogene v-*mpl* includes the entire cytoplasmic and transmembrane domains of the *c-mpl* gene and 40 amino acids of the extracellular domain. The remainder of the extracellular domain is replaced by viral envelope sequences.

## Erythropoietin (EPO)

EPO is produced by kidney and liver. Its major function is stimulating erythroid precursors to generate red blood cells, but also can stimulate platelet generation. The EPO receptor also belongs to the hematopoietin receptor family.

## INTERLEUKINS: CYTOKINE SECRETION PROFILES OF T LYMPHOCYTES (Table 87.2)

Most cloned lines of murine CD4+ T cells can be classified into two groups, $T_H1$ and $T_H2$, based on the cytokines they produce and their related functional activities. $T_H1$ cells are defined by their production of IL-2, interferon γ (IFN-γ) and TNFβ; $T_H2$ cells are defined by their production of IL-4, IL-5, IL-6, IL-10 and IL-13. Both cell types produce IL-3, TNFα and GM-CSF. There are T-cell clones that coexpress $T_H1$ and $T_H2$ cytokines in various combinations. Clones of this phenotype have been classified as a third subset, $T_H0$, and are proposed to be precursors of $T_H1$ and $T_H2$ clones. However, it remains an open question as to whether cells must pass through a $T_H0$ stage of unrestricted cytokine gene expression before expressing a more restricted cytokine profile.

The reciprocal relationship often observed between inflammatory and humoral responses is now attributed to the preferential activation of $T_H1$ and $T_H2$ cells, respectively. A number of human and murine immune reactions *in vivo* and *in vitro* display patterns of cytokine gene expression that are predominantly of $T_H1$ or $T_H2$ type.

## $T_H$ subsets and disease

$T_H1$ and $T_H2$ cells are involved in the pathogenesis of immunological disorders. $T_H2$ cells play a prominent role in the induction of antibody synthesis and immediate-type hypersensitivity, as IL-4 is the critical stimulus inducing a switch to IgE antibody production. Conversely, $T_H1$ cells are considered to be involved in the induction of inflammatory responses and a range of experimental autoimmune diseases. Evidence for this is based on adoptive transfer experiments demonstrating that CD4+ cells producing $T_H1$-type cytokines can transfer disease, in models of experimental allergic encephalomyelitis (EAE) and insulin-dependent diabetes mellitus (IDDM). However, cytokine regulation is complex; for example, in EAE, IFN-γ also can mediate a protective effect. In addition, TNFα and IL-10 have opposite effects on IDDM, depending on the developmental stage of the immune system.

$T_H1$ cells also appear to be involved in human, organ-specific, *autoimmune diseases*. CD4+ T-cell clones isolated from lymphocytic infiltrates of *Hashimoto thyroiditis* or *Graves disease* exhibit a clear-cut $T_H1$ phenotype. In addition, most T-cell clones derived from peripheral blood or cerebrospinal fluid of multiple sclerosis patients show a $T_H1$-type cytokine profile. The situation is less clear in systemic autoimmune disorders. In general, heterogeneous cytokine profiles are found in the serum or target organs of patients with systemic autoimmunity, such as *systemic*

TABLE 87.2 The interleukins

| NAME | MOLECULAR MASS (kD) | PROTEIN STRUCTURE | BIOLOGICAL ACTION | RECEPTOR FAMILY |
|------|---------------------|-------------------|-------------------|-----------------|
| IL-1α | 17 | β-trefoil tetrahedral monomer | Synergizes with GM-CSF to stimulate proliferation of myeloid cells; stimulates differentiation and sIgM expression in B cells, proliferation of $T_H2$ cells, secretion of cytokines by macrophages, and survival of granulocytes | Immunoglobulin |
| IL-1β | 17.5 | β-trefoil tetrahedral monomer | Same as for IL-1α | Immunoglobulin |
| IL-1Ra | 17–25 | β-trefoil tetrahedral monomer | Same as for IL-1α, inhibits actions of IL-1α and IL-1β by non-productive receptor binding | Immunoglobulin |
| IL-2 | 15–20 | Short chain 4α helical bundle, monomer | Stimulates proliferation, differentiation, and functional activation of T, B, and NK cells; stimulates macrophage function | Hematopoietin, shared γ-chain with IL-4, IL-7, IL-9, IL-13, IL-15 |
| IL-3 | 14–30 | Short chain 4α helical bundle, monomer | Stimulates proliferation, differentiation, activation, and survival of HSC, erythrocytes, myeloid, and B cells | Hematopoietin, shared β chain with GM-CSF and IL-5 |
| IL-4 | 18–20 | Short chain 4α helical bundle, monomer | Stimulates proliferation, differentiation, and functional activation of T and B cells; suppresses proliferation and function of macrophages; suppresses proliferation of erythrocytes | Hematopoietin, shared γ-chain with IL-2, IL-7, IL-9, IL-13, IL-15 |
| IL-5 | 2 × 21.5 | Short chain 4α helical bundle, homodimer | Stimulates proliferation, differentiation, activation and survival of eosinophils and basophils; and B cells (mouse only) | Hematopoietin, shared β chain with GM-CSF and IL-3 |
| IL-6 | 21–26 | Long chain 4α helical bundle, monomer | Stimulates proliferation, differentiation, functional activation and survival of HSC, T cells, B cells, megakaryocytes, granulocytes and macrophages | Hematopoietin, shared gp130 with IL-11, IL-12α |
| IL-7 | 22–28 | Short chain 4α helical bundle, monomer | Stimulates proliferation, differentiation, and functional activation of pre-B cells, B cells, thymocytes and T cells; stimulates macrophage function | Hematopoietin, shared γ-chain with IL-2, IL-4, IL-9, IL-13, IL-15 |
| IL-8 | 8 | Three antiparallel β-strands and one α helix, $H^+$ bonded dimer | Chemotactic for granulocytes, T cells and basophils; stimulates functional activation in granulocytes and macrophages; stimulates histamine and leukotriene release in basophils; suppresses proliferation of myeloid progenitors | Rhodopsin (chemokine receptor family) |
| IL-9 | 32–39 | Short chain 4α helical bundle, monomer | Stimulates proliferation of T cells and mast cells; erythrocyte differentiation; and enhances IgE and IgG production by B cells | Hematopoietin, shared γ-chain with IL-2, IL-4, IL-7, IL-13, IL-15 |
| IL-10 | 18 | Long chain 4α helical bundle, monomer | Inhibits cytokine synthesis by T cells, NK cells and macrophages; costimulates T cells in the presence of IL-2, IL-4 and IL-7 | Interferon |
| IL-11 | 19–21 | Long chain 4α helical bundle, monomer | Stimulates proliferation, differentiation, functional activation and survival of HSC, B cells, erythrocytes, megakaryocytes and macrophages | Hematopoietin, shared gp130 with IL-6 |
| Il-12 | 35–40 (heterodimer) | Long chain 4α helical bundle, monomer | Induces IFN-γ production and stimulates cytolytic activity in T and NK cells, suppresses IgE synthesis, inhibits the action of IL-2 on γδ+ T cells | Hematopoietin, homology to gp130 |
| IL-13 | 14–40 | Short chain 4α helical bundle, monomer | Stimulates proliferation, differentiation and functional activation of B cells, suppresses proliferation and activation of macrophages | Hematopoietin, shared γ-chain with IL-2, IL-4, IL-7, IL-9, IL-15 |

TABLE 87.2 The interleukins (*contd.*)

| NAME | MOLECULAR MASS (kD) | PROTEIN STRUCTURE | BIOLOGICAL ACTION | RECEPTOR FAMILY |
|------|---------------------|-------------------|-------------------|-----------------|
| IL-14 | 50–60 | Monomer | Enhances proliferation of activated B cells, inhibits immunoglobulin secretion | ? |
| IL-15 | 14–15 | 4α helical bundle | Promotes clonogenic growth of pre-B cells; stimulates differentiation of more mature B cells and pre-T cells | Hematopoietin, shared γ-chain with IL-4, IL-7, IL-9, IL-13, IL-15 |

HSC, hematopoietic stem cells. For other abbreviations, see text.

*lupus erythematosus*, *Sjögren syndrome* and *primary vasculitis*. However, screening of synovial tissues from patients with *rheumatoid arthritis* for cytokine expression has revealed a $T_H1$-type pattern in most samples.

# Interleukin-1

IL-1 has a range of biological activities on many different target cell types, including B cells, T cells, monocytes. It induces hypotension, fever, weight loss, and the acute phase response. There are two molecular forms of IL-1 (IL-1α and IL-1β) derived from two different genes. Amino acid sequence homology between human IL-1α and IL-1β is 20 per cent. These molecules bind to the same receptor and have very similar biological properties. IL-1α is mostly cell associated and IL-1β is mostly released. An IL-1 receptor antagonist (IL-1Ra) has been described that is structurally related to IL-1β. The antagonist is made by the same cells that secrete IL-1. A cysteine protease releases mature IL-1β. A cowpox virus inhibitor (CRMA) of the IL-1 converting enzyme inhibits the host inflammatory response. IL-1 is secreted from most cell types.

There are two IL-1 receptors. The type I receptor is a transmembrane glycoprotein with a molecular mass of 80 kD. It is a member of the immunoglobulin superfamily. The receptor binds IL-1α and IL-1β and IL-1Ra mature proteins. This appears to be the major IL-1 receptor. The type II receptor is a glycoprotein with a molecular mass of 60 kD. The type II receptor can bind IL-1α, IL-1β and IL-1Ra. Its function is unclear.

# Interleukin-2

IL-2 is a T-cell-derived cytokine also known as a T-cell growth factor. It stimulates growth and differentiation of T cells, B cells, natural killer (NK) cells, lymphokine-activated killer (LAK) cells, monocytes and macrophages.

The IL-2 receptor is a complex of three distinct polypeptide chains. The α-chain binds IL-2 with low affinity while the β-chain binds IL-2 with a higher affinity. The high-affinity receptor complex is an α/β/γ heterotrimer. The IL-2 receptor β- and γ-chains are both members of the hematopoietin receptor superfamily. The γ-chain is also a functional component of the IL-4, IL-7, IL-9, IL-13 and IL-15 receptors. Mutations in the IL-2 receptor γ-chain are responsible for *X-linked severe combined immunodeficiency (X-SCID)* in humans. This is a lethal disease characterized by normal B-cell numbers, absent or greatly reduced T cells, and severely depressed cell-mediated and humoral immunity.

# Interleukin-3

IL-3 is a growth factor that stimulates colony formation of erythroid, megakaryocyte, neutrophil, eosinophil, basophil, mast cell and monocytic lineages. IL-3 also stimulates multipotential progenitor cells. Many of the activities of IL-3 are enhanced or are dependent upon costimulation with other cytokines. IL-3 is a growth factor for B lymphocytes and activates monocytes. IL-3 has been used clinically to expand hematopoietic precursors after *bone marrow transplantation, aplastic anemia and chemotherapy*.

The high-affinity IL-3 receptor is formed by association of a low-affinity IL-3 binding α-subunit with a second β-subunit. In humans, the β-subunit is common to the IL-3, IL-5 and GM-CSF receptors, but does not itself bind any of these cytokines. The IL-3 receptor α-subunit is a member of the hematopoietin receptor family, with homology to sequences in the α-subunits of the IL-5 and GM-CSF receptors. It has a short cytoplasmic domain, and is unable to signal. The β-subunit has a much longer cytoplasmic domain with regions in common with the IL-2 receptor β-chain and the IL-4 receptor.

# Interleukin-4

IL-4 is derived from T cells and mast cells with multiple biological effects on B cells, T cells and non-lymphoid cells including monocytes, endothelial cells and fibroblasts. It also induces secretion of $IgG_4$ and IgE by human B cells. The IL-4-dependent production of IgE is due to IL-4-induced isotype switching.

The IL-4 receptor is a complex consisting of at least two chains: a high-affinity IL-4 binding (α-chain) chain and the IL-2 receptor γ-chain. The high-affinity IL-4 binding chain belongs to the hematopoietin receptor family. The IL-2 receptor γ-chain is a functional component of the IL-4 receptor.

## Interleukin-5

IL-5 is a T-cell-derived disulfide-linked homodimer that stimulates eosinophil differentiation in humans.

The IL-5 receptor consists of a low-affinity binding α-chain and a non-binding β-chain shared with the IL-3 and GM-CSF receptors. Both chains belong to the hematopoietin receptor family.

## Interleukin-6

IL-6 is secreted by both lymphoid and non-lymphoid cells that regulates B and T cell function and acute phase reactions.

High-affinity IL-6 receptors are formed by the non-covalent association of two subunits. The IL-6 receptor α-chain binds IL-6 with low affinity but does not signal. The β-chain (gp 130) does not itself bind IL-6, but associates with the α-chain–IL-6 complex and is responsible for signal transduction.

## Interleukin-7

IL-7 is a stromal cell-derived growth factor for progenitor B and T cells. The main population in the thymus responsive to IL-7 is CD4$^-$CD8$^-$. IL-7 also stimulates proliferation and differentiation of mature T cells, similar to IL-2.

The IL-7 receptor is a complex consisting of an IL-7 binding chain and the IL-2 receptor γ-chain, which augments IL-7 binding.

## Interleukin-8

IL-8 is an inflammatory cytokine, produced by many cell types, and functions mainly as a neutrophil chemoattractant. It also attracts basophils and a sub-population of lymphocytes.

There are two IL-8 receptors, one high affinity and another of lower affinity. Both receptors possess seven transmembrane spanning domains and are G-protein-linked receptors of the rhodospin superfamily. The high-affinity receptor is 77 per cent identical to the low-affinity receptor. The low-affinity receptor has an unglycosylated molecular mass of 32 kD. The

high-affinity receptor has an unglycosylated molecular mass of 40 kD and only binds IL-8, whereas the low-affinity receptor binds other chemokines.

## Interleukin-9

IL-9 enhances the proliferation of T lymphocytes, mast cell, megakaryoblastic leukemia cell lines and erythroid precursors. IL-9 is produced by IL-2-activated T$_H$2 lymphocytes and Hodgkin lymphoma cells. The single IL-9 receptor belongs to the hematopoietin receptor family. Both membrane-bound and soluble forms of the IL-9 receptor exist. The IL-2 receptor γ-chain is also part of the IL-9 receptor.

## Interleukin-10

IL-10, secreted by T$_H$0 and T$_H$2 subsets of CD4$^+$ T lymphocytes, inhibits activation of cytokine synthesis by T$_H$1 cells, activated monocytes and NK cells. IL-10 also stimulates proliferation of B cells, thymocytes and mast cells. There is 70 per cent homology between IL-10 and an open reading frame (BCRF1) in the Epstein–Barr virus genome. The protein encoded by BCRF1 exhibits some of the activities of IL-10 and has been designated vIL-10. The IL-10 receptor belongs to the hematopoietin receptor family.

## Interleukin-11

IL-11 is a growth factor for plasmacytomas, multi-potential and committed megakaryocytic and macrophage progenitor cells. IL-11 is distantly related to IL-6. A single IL-11 receptor has been identified that belongs to the hematopoietin receptor family. The IL-6 signal transducer gp130 also functions as part of the IL-11 receptor.

## Interleukin-12

IL-12 is a heterodimeric cytokine made up of two chains. It induces IFN-γ production by T and NK cells, enhances NK activity, and costimulates peripheral blood lymphocyte proliferation. IL-12 also stimulates proliferation and differentiation of the T$_H$1 subset of T lymphocytes. The receptor for IL-12 is found on T cells and NK cells and is a member of the hematopoietin receptor family with homology to gp130 of the IL-6 receptor.

...

## Interleukin-13

IL-13 is produced by activated T cells and inhibits the production of inflammatory cytokines (IL-1β, IL-6, TNFα, IL-8) by lipopolysaccharide-stimulated monocytes. Human IL-13 promotes B-cell proliferation in combination with other stimuli and stimulates secretion of IgM, IgE and IgG₄. Human and mouse IL-13 have no known activity on mouse B cells. The receptor for IL-13 is a member of the hematopoietin receptor superfamily and shares a γ-chain with the IL-2, IL-4, IL-7, IL-9 and IL-15 receptors.

## Interleukin-14

IL-14 is produced by T cells enhances the proliferation of activated B cells, and inhibits immunoglobulin synthesis. IL-14 is unrelated to other cytokines, but shares homology with complement factor Bb. A single receptor type is detected on B cells and B-cell leukemias. IL-14 causes up-regulation of its receptor on B cells. IL-14 receptors also bind complement fragment Bb.

## Interleukin-15

IL-15 shares many of the biological properties of IL-2, including stimulation of T-cell proliferation, *in vitro* generation of cytotoxic T cells and non-antigen-specific LAK cells. The IL-2 receptor β- and γ-chains are both components of the IL-15 receptor, but the IL-2 receptor α-chain is not.

## TNF RECEPTOR FAMILY

Mechanisms that regulate cell death are essential for normal development and homeostasis. Cell death can be developmentally controlled, by the expression of novel genes that induce the death signal at a specific stage of differentiation in response to defined physiological stimuli. The most common morphological expression of such programmed cell death is apoptosis (*see* page 99), characterized by cell shrinkage, blebbing of the plasma membrane, and nuclear collapse and fragmentation of the nuclear chromatin at internucleosomal sites due to activation of an endogenous nuclease.

Three structurally-related cell surface receptors have been associated with the transduction of death signals in a broad range of cell types. They are the Fas antigen (APO-1), and two distinct TNF receptor chains, p55 and p75. All three receptors belong to a family of cell surface glycoproteins that includes nerve growth factor receptor, the T-cell antigen CD27, the B-cell receptor CD40, and the T cell-associated receptors CD30 and 4-1BB.

TNF receptors are broadly distributed in both normal and tumor cells and bind two related TNF molecules, TNFα and TNFβ. TNFα is one of the principal mediators of inflammation, and interaction between TNF and TNF receptors produces a range of effects that depend on the nature of the target cell.

Fas is a cell surface glycoprotein that is constitutively and inducibly expressed in a variety of normal tissues and tumor cell lines. Administration of anti-Fas antibody triggers apoptosis of Fas-expressing cells. Mutations that inactivate Fas have been shown to be associated with the lymphoproliferative disorder of *Lpr/Lpr* mice, and Fas is also involved in cytotoxic T lymphocyte-mediated target cell death.

Although Fas and TNF receptors are currently grouped together as the principal cell death receptors, it is unclear whether they trigger the death signal along the same or distinct pathways. A conserved death domain is found in the intracellular region of these receptors.

CD40 is structurally related to the TNF receptor and Fas but has no known cytotoxic function. Stimulation of CD40 by CD40 ligand (CD40L) induces B-cell activation and immunoglobulin class switching. Mutations that inactivate CD40L are associated with *X-linked hyper-IgM syndrome*.

## Tumor necrosis factor (TNF) and TNF receptors

TNFα is a potent mediator of inflammatory and immune functions. It also regulates growth and differentiation of a wide variety of cell types. TNFα is selectively cytotoxic for many transformed cells, especially in combination with IFN-γ. *In vivo*, it leads to necrosis of some murine sarcomas. Many of the actions of TNFα occur in combination with other cytokines. TNFα is expressed as a type II membrane protein attached by a signal anchor transmembrane domain and is processed by a metalloproteinase.

TNFβ has 35 per cent homology with TNFα. Like TNFα, it has a wide range of biological activities. It is also an important mediator of inflammation and immune function. Whereas TNFα can be expressed as a membrane protein TNFβ is secreted.

There are two receptors for TNF that both bind TNFα and TNFβ. The type I receptor has a molecular mass of 55kD and the type II receptor has a molecular mass of 75 kD. Both receptors have four Cys-rich repeats in the extracellular domain. The two receptors have no more homology to each other than to other members of the TNF receptor family. There is no significant homology between the intracellular domains of the two TNF receptors, indicating different signaling mechanisms. Soluble forms of both the human p55 and p75 TNF receptors have been found in serum and urine of cancer patients. The soluble TNF receptors are derived from the extracellular domain of each

TABLE 87.3 TNF family of ligands

| NAME | MOLECULAR MASS (kD) | PROTEIN STRUCTURE | BIOLOGICAL ACTION | RECEPTOR FAMILY |
|---|---|---|---|---|
| TNFα | 3 × 17 | β-jellyroll non-covalent trimer | Inhibits proliferation of erythrocytes and myeloid progenitors; stimulates functional activation of macrophages and granulocytes; stimulates proliferation of B and T cells | TNF/NGF |
| TNFβ | 20–25 | β-jellyroll non-covalent trimer | Suppresses proliferation of certain hematopoietic progenitor cells, stimulates B and T cell growth, stimulates macrophage differentiation | TNF/NGF |
| Fas ligand | 43 | β-jellyroll | Costimulator for T cell activation. Induces apoptosis in B and T cells, and macrophages | TNF/NGF |
| CD40 ligand | 39 | β-jellyroll | Stimulates proliferation and function of B cells, stimulates functional activation of macrophages | TNF/NGF |

NGF, nerve growth factor. For other abbreviations, see text.

membrane-bound receptor and are thought to act as inhibitors of TNF action. Myxoma virus encodes a soluble protein related to the TNF receptor.

## Fas and Fas ligand

Fas ligand is a type II membrane protein of the TNF receptor family. Some 150 amino acids in the extracellular domain have significant homology with other ligands of the TNF receptor family. The expression of Fas ligand is induced on most T cells, and can act as a costimulator in the activated cells and tumor cell lines. The Fas ligand binds to Fas, which is a type I membrane protein belonging to the TNF receptor family. Both Fas ligand and Fas appear to exist as trimeric structures in the plasma membrane.

## CD40 ligand (CD40L)

CD40L is a type II integral membrane glycoprotein expressed on activated T cells. It has significant sequence homology with TNFα and a predicted tertiary structure very similar to the TNF trimer. CD40L binds to CD40 on B cells, and in combination with IL-4 induces isotype switching to IgE. CD40 is a type I integral membrane glycoprotein also belonging to the TNF receptor family. Activation of cells expressing CD40 with CD40L also appears to have an anti-apoptotic effect when these target cells are exposed to agents that normally induce apoptosis.

The structure and biological actions of these TNF ligands are summarized in Table 87.3

# SELECTED READING

Callard RE, Armitage RJ, Fanslow WC, Spriggs MK. CD40 ligand and its role in X-linked hyper-IgM syndrome. *Immunol Today* 1994; **14**: 559.

Callard RE, Gearing AJH. *The cytokine facts book*. London: Academic Press, 1994.

Gruss H-J, Dower SK. Tumor necrosis factor ligand superfamily: involvement in the pathology of malignant lymphoma. *Blood* 1995; **85**: 3378.

Lyman SD, James L, Johnson L *et al.* Cloning of the human homologue of the murine flt3 ligand. *Blood* 1994; **83**: 2795.

Metcalf D. Haematopoietic regulators: redundancy or subtlety? *Blood* 1983; **82**: 3513.

Mosmann TR, Coffman RL. Th1 and Th2 cells: different patterns of lymphokine secretion lead to different functional properties. *Annu Rev Immunol* 1990; **7**: 145.

Nagata S, Suda T. Fas and Fas ligand: *lpr* and *gld* mutations. *Immunol Today* 1995; **39**: 39.

Williams DE, de Vries P, Namen AE *et al.* The *steel* factor. *Dev Biol* 1992; **151**: 368.

# PART FIFTEEN

# *Renal Function, Fluid and Electrolyte Balance*

**Editor: Jean E. Robillard**

# 88

# Anatomical Development of the Kidney

Jean E. Robillard

The development of the human kidney proceeds from a simple system of aglomerular tubules, the pronephros, through simple glomerulonephrons, the mesonephros, to culminate in the elaboration of the final complex glomerulonephron units found in the mature kidney, the metanephros (Figs 88.1–88.3).

The *pronephros*, sometimes referred to as the "cervical kidney," is the first evidence of a renal excretory system in the human embryo. It appears about the middle of the third week of gestation and gives rise to about seven paired tubules, which undergo regression by degeneration by the fifth week (Figs 88.1 and 88.2). The pronephric structures do not differentiate into recognizable nephrons and are of no significance as a functioning excretory organ. The main role of the pronephros is that it gives rise to the pronephric duct, which persists after the pronephric tubules regress. The pronephric duct extends into the cloaca and is important in the development of the mesonephros.

The *mesonephros* (Figs 88.1 and 88.2), which corresponds to the mature kidney of fish and amphibians, appears immediately caudal to the last of the pronephric tubules. The first mesonephric nephrons are seen around 24–25 days' gestation (middle of the fourth week). As with the pronephros, the earliest mesonephric nephrons (the more cephalic) start to degenerate during the fifth week of gestation while the more caudal nephrons are still differentiating. The formation of the mesonephric nephrons differs from the pronephric tubules in that the mesonephric nephrons arise by induction of differentiating vesicles within the solid cell mass of the nephrogenic cord. The mesonephric glomerulus is vascularized and the tubules differentiate into a definite proximal tubule with convolutions and brush border, but they have no loop of Henle or distal tubule. Collectively, the mesonephros constitutes the

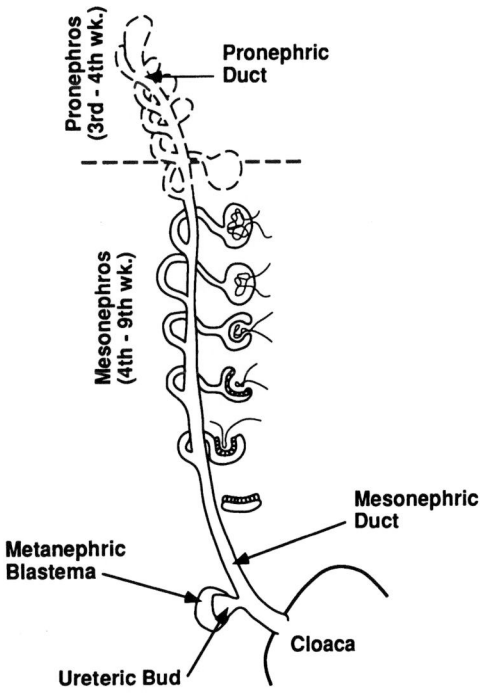

FIGURE 88.1 Schematic representation of the development of the mammalian kidney during intrauterine life. The pronephros, which contains no glomeruli, and the mesonephros, which possesses glomeruli and tubules, are only present during embryonic life and regress *in utero*. The mesonephros gives rise to the mesonephric duct, which induces the ureteric bud that is required for the formation of the metanephros.

first true functional glomerulonephron unit formed during renal embryogenesis. The mesonephros remains actively functional during early development of the metanephros so that for a time nephrons in both struc-

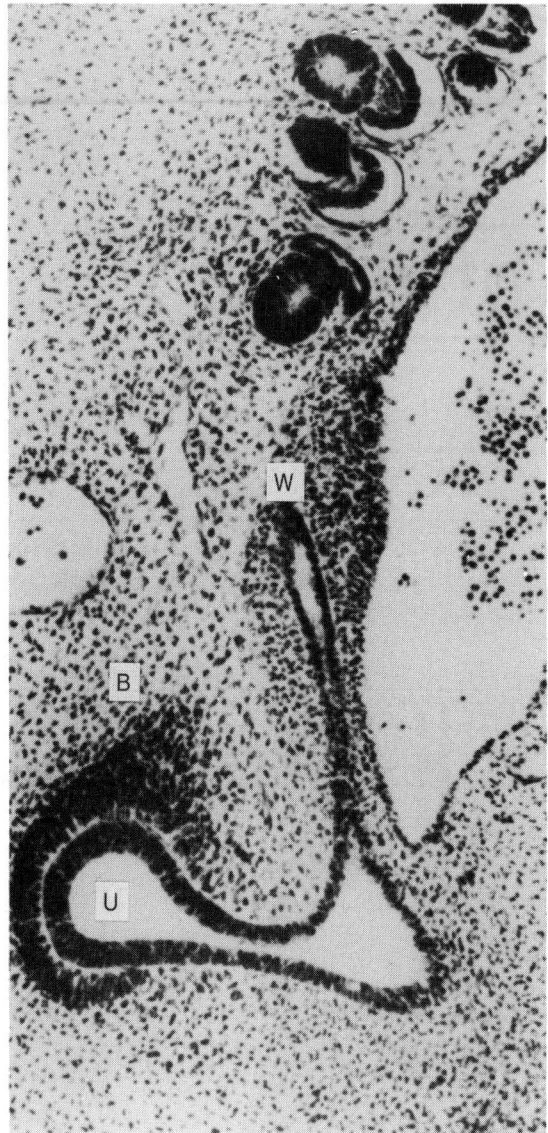

FIGURE 88.2 Caudal extremity of the mesonephros from a 38-day human embryo (7 mm). U, ureteric bud; B, nephrogenic blastema; W, Wolffian duct. Magnification: ×98. (From DuBois, 1969 (*see* Selected Reading), with permission.)

The main contribution of the mesonephros during embryogenesis is that it gives rise to the mesonephric duct, which induces the ureteric bud that is required for the formation of the metanephros. The ureteric bud, which arises during the fourth week of gestation, is essential for the formation of the urinary collecting system, beginning with the ureter and terminating with the collecting tubules, and for initiating nephron formation by inducing the metanephric blastema (Figs 88.1 and 88.2).

The *metanephros* or "hind kidney" begins to develop in the human fetus early during the fifth week of gestation and starts to function by the eighth week. As the ureteric buds extend dorsocranially into the nephrogenic ridges, it begins to divide and to form calyces and early divisions of the collecting ducts. The induction of nephron element formation starts shortly after the ureteric bud begins dividing (Fig. 88.3). Mesenchymal cells condense in a spherical mass (vesicle) located adjacent to an ampulla originating from dividing collecting ducts (ureteric bud). This spherical mass of mesenchymal cells forms an S-shaped body. Cells from one side of the S-shaped body become glomerular epithelium and cells from the other side become proximal tubules. Capillary endothelium and mesangium also arise from undifferentiated mesenchymal cells and invade the S-shaped body to form glomerular capillaries and glomerular mesangial cells. The development of new nephron units proceeds in a centrifugal fashion from the center toward the periphery of the kidney until 32–34 weeks' gestation, when the formation of new nephrons is completed and approximately 800 000 nephrons have appeared in each kidney. The inner portion of the cortex, near the corticomedullary junction, contains the older glomeruli. The peripheral cortex contains the more recently formed glomeruli, the tubules of which are more shallowly placed and may remain in the cortex. This pattern of development results in a high degree of structural heterogeneity with nephron populations and nephron segments developing at different times.

Before the metanephric blastema develops into a fully developed kidney, certain conditions need to be met. First, the undifferentiated cells of the metanephric blastema have to be committed to become nephrons well before the earliest evidence of differentiation. This process of "nephric determination" is unique to this phase of development and never recurs in the adult animal, where all growth and regeneration involves committed epithelial cells. The second step in the development of the metanephric blastema is the progression of committed mesenchymal cells into differentiated epithelial cells under the influence of the ureteric bud, which acts as an inducer.

This conversion of metanephric mesenchymal cells into epithelial cells is regulated by developmental changes in the expression of genes and proteins encoding extracellular matrix components, cell adhesion molecules, structural proteins, and growth factors and receptors. The molecular interactions forming

tures function simultaneously. However, the functional contribution of the mesonephros during fetal development is minimal because it degenerates as the metanephros begins functioning.

The size and functional importance of the mesonephros in various species is directly related to that of the allantois. The mesonephros and allantois are largest in species with a simple appositioned type of placenta, and are short-lived in primates, in which the placenta is highly permeable and the allantois is rudimentary. In species with a large allantoic cavity, such as the pig, rabbit and sheep, the mesonephros has an excretory function early during development.

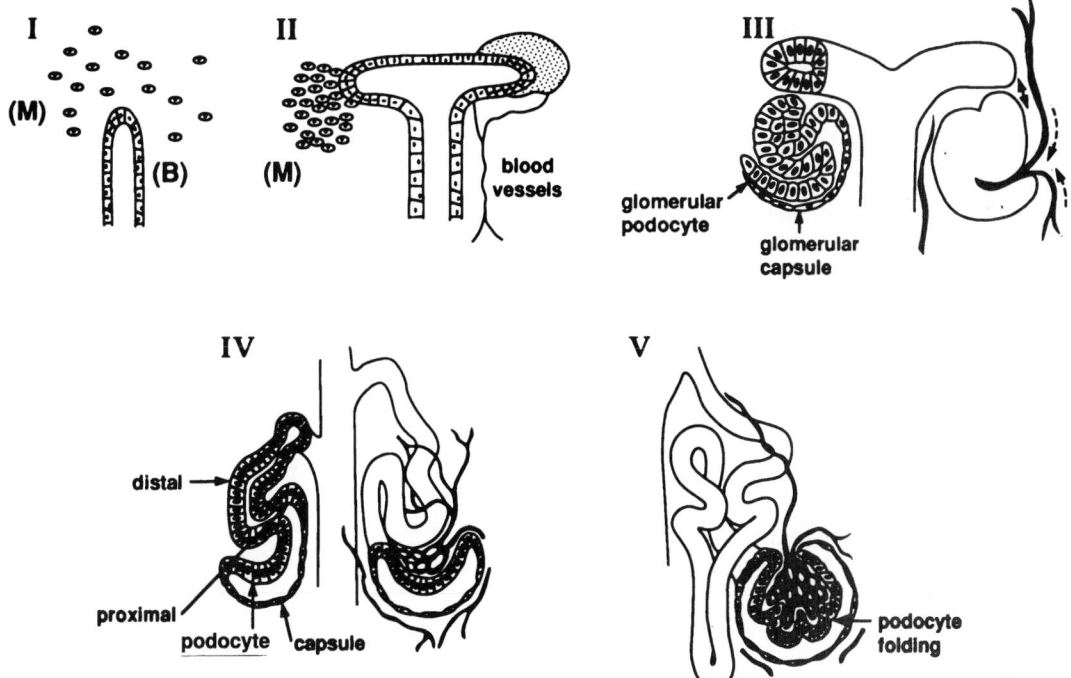

FIGURE 88.3 Schematic representation of the development of the metanephros or permanent kidney. Panels I and II show the mesenchymal cells (M) condensing around the ureteric bud (B). Panel III is a representation of mesenchymal cells differentiating into epithelial cells and forming the S-shaped body. Panel IV shows the fusion of the S-shaped body with the terminal end of the ureteric bud. Panel V is a representation of tubular elongation and folding of the podocytes.

the basis of this set of events are complex. Among the transcription factors involved in early epithelial differentiation, oncogenes, homeobox (*Hox*) and paired-box (*Pax*) genes and products of the Wilms tumor suppressor gene (*WT1*) appear to play an important role (Fig. 88.4). For example Pax-2 proteins are present in the ureteric bud, the nuclei of condensed mesenchymal cells, comma-shaped bodied and early collecting duct epithelium. After the formation of the S-shaped bodies, the expression of *Pax-2* decreases and is not observed in mature glomeruli and tubules suggesting that the early expression and subsequent down-regulation of *Pax-2* may be important components of the events leading to the formation of S-shaped bodies.

Multiple lines of evidence also suggest that *WT1* plays an important role during nephrogenesis. *WT1* is expressed in condensed mesenchyme, S-shaped bodies and glomerular epithelial cells. Mutations of the *WT1* gene are associated with renal developmental abnormalities while *Wt1* homozygous knockout mice fail to develop metanephri and have no ureteric bud.

Different oncogenes also play an important role in the regulation of early nephrogenesis. Among these, the protooncogene c-*myc* is widely expressed during early renal embryogenesis, being detected in uninduced mesenchyme and in early epithelial structures (Fig. 88.4). In contrast, n-*myc* is not expressed in uninduced mesenchyme, but is rapidly up-regulated during early

epithelial differentiation and decreases after formation of S-shaped bodies (Fig. 88.4).

In addition to the transcription factors, a number of growth factors probably act synergistically in kidney cell differentiation and play a critical role in modulating the different kidney developmental programs. Polypeptide growth factors such as transforming growth factors α and β, platelet-derived growth factor,

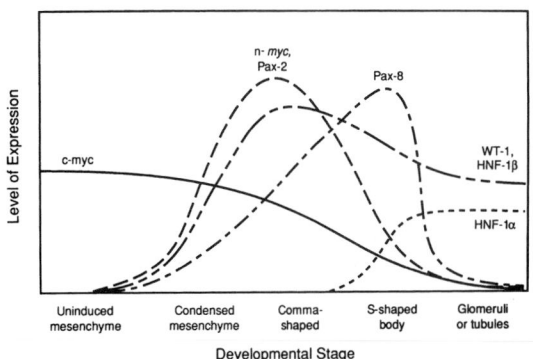

FIGURE 88.4 Temporal expression of selected transcription factors during early nephrogenesis. HNF, hepatocyte nuclear factor; WT-1, Wilms tumor suppression gene; Pax, paired-box gene. (From Igarashi P. *Curr Opin Nephrol* 1994; **3**: 308, with permission.)

epidermal growth factor, insulin-like growth factor, acidic and basic fibroblast growth factors and nerve growth factors have been shown to influence renal organogenesis.

## SELECTED READING

Bacallao R, Fine FG. Molecular events in the organization of renal tubular epithelium: from nephrogenesis to regeneration. *Am J Physiol* 1989; **257**: F913.

DuBois AM. The embryonic kidney. In: Rouiller C, Muller AF, eds. *The kidney: morphology, biochemistry, physiology*, Vol 1. New York: Academic Press, 1969: 1.

Igarashi P. Transcription factors and apoptosis in kidney development. *Curr Opin Nephrol Hypertens* 1994; **3**: 308.

McCrory WW. Embryologic development of the kidney. In: McCrory WW, ed. *Developmental nephrology*. Cambridge, MA: Harvard University Press, 1972: 1.

Potter EL. Development of the kidney. In: *Normal and abnormal development of the kidney*. Chicago: Year Book Medical Publishers, 1972: 3.

Reeves WH, Kanwar YS, Farguhar MG. Assembly of the glomerular filtration surface. Differentiation of anionic sites in glomerular capillaries of newborn rat kidney. *J Cell Biol* 1980; **85**: 735.

# 89

# Renal Hemodynamics

Jean E. Robillard

## DISTRIBUTION OF BLOOD FLOW

The fetal kidneys receive only 2–4 per cent of the combined ventricular output during the last trimester of gestation. The proportion of cardiac output distributed to the kidneys increases to about 6 per cent in the first week after birth, and to approximately 15–18 per cent during the first month. In adults, the kidneys receive 20–25 per cent of the cardiac output. In the fetus, renal blood flow (RBF) is in the order of 1.5–2.0 mL/(g kidney weight · min). This relatively low rate of RBF is associated with high renal vascular resistance and a low filtration fraction when compared with newborn animals (Fig. 89.1). In human subjects, the clearance of para-aminohippurate (PAH), traditionally used to measure effective renal plasma flow, increases from $20 \, mL/(1.73 \, m^2 \cdot min)$ at 30 weeks gestation to $45 \, mL/(1.73 \, m^2 \cdot min)$ at 35 weeks, $83 \, mL/(1.73 \, m^2 \cdot min)$ at term, $300 \, mL/(1.73 \, m^2 \cdot min)$ at 3 months, and $650 \, mL/(1.73 \, m^2 \cdot min)$ in adults.

During fetal life, the intrarenal blood flow distribution is quantitatively different from that observed postnatally. Concordant with the morphological development of the kidney, which occurs from the center toward the periphery of the cortex, intrarenal blood

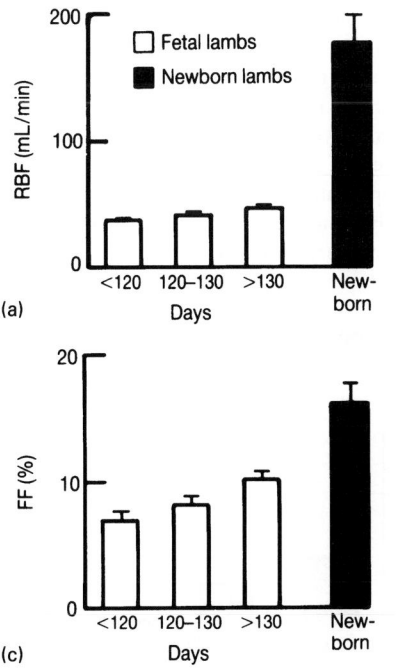

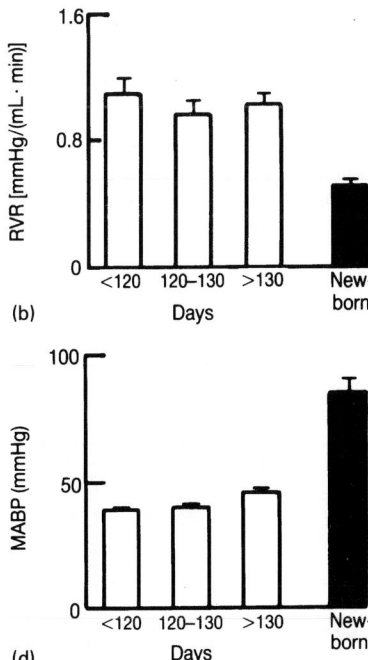

FIGURE 89.1 Renal hemodynamic values in fetal and newborn sheep. The duration of gestation in sheep is 145 days. Newborn lambs were studied between 3 and 19 days postnatally. (a) RBF, renal blood flow; (b) RVR, renal vascular resistance; (c) FF, filtration fraction; (d) MABP, mean arterial blood pressure. (Adapted from Robillard JE, Nakamura KT. *Am J Physiol* 1988; **254**: F771, with permission)

flow distribution progresses in a centrifugal pattern (Fig. 89.2). Intrarenal distribution of glomerular perfusion, used as an index of intrarenal blood flow distribution, remains the same across the cortex during the last third of gestation, but the quotient between outer and inner glomerular blood flow increases significantly at birth, reflecting a shift of blood flow toward the superficial cortex. This shift in intrarenal blood flow distribution at birth is not accompanied by immediate changes in RBF or vascular resistance. Only in the days following birth are significant increases in RBF observed (Fig. 89.1). This intrarenal redistribution of blood flow toward the outer zone of the renal cortex may contribute to changes in glomerular and tubular function observed postnatally.

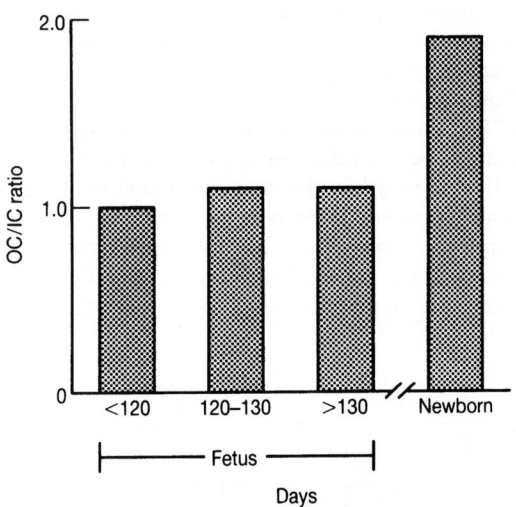

FIGURE 89.2 Intrarenal blood flow distribution in fetal and newborn sheep. Newborn lambs were studied between 3 and 19 days postnatally. OC, outer cortex; IC, inner cortex. (Adapted from Robillard JE *et al. Pediatr Res* 1981; **15**: 1248, with permission.)

## REGULATION OF BLOOD FLOW

The mechanisms involved in the age-related increase and redistribution of RBF involve both anatomical and hemodynamic factors. Increase in the diameter of resistance vessels, formation and/or development of new glomeruli, and changes in the intrarenal vascular system are important anatomical factors that contribute to the increase in RBF during fetal and postnatal development. In addition to these anatomical changes, hemodynamic factors play an important role in the rise in RBF postnatally. The two main hemodynamic determinants involved in the age-related increase in RBF during development are the rise in renal perfusion pressure (2.5-fold) and the decrease in renal vascular resistance (2.9-fold). The decrease in renal vascular resistance during development is due to either myogenic or neurohormonal mechanisms. Several vasoactive systems play a role in the regulation of RBF during development; these include the adrenergic nervous system, the renin–angiotensin system, the kallikrein–kinin system, eicosanoids, endothelin and atrial natriuretic peptide (ANP).

## Sympathetic nervous system

The influence of the adrenergic nervous system on RBF during development is both maturation and species dependent. For example, the renal circulation in the pig is under tonic neural vasoconstrictor influence, whereas that of the sheep is not. As such, surgical or pharmacological renal denervation is not associated with significant changes in RBF in fetal lambs, but does result in increased RBF in piglets. On the other hand, renal nerves play an important role in modulating fetal RBF during stressful conditions such as hypoxemia or hemorrhage. The fetal and postnatal developmental differences in the regulation of renal hemodynamic responses to increased efferent renal nerve activity have been investigated in sheep (Fig.

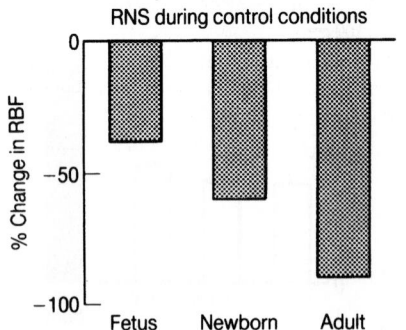

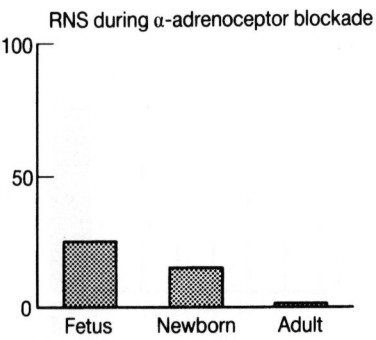

FIGURE 89.3 Effect of renal nerve stimulation (RNS) on renal blood flow (RBF) during development. The effect of stimulation at 8 Hz on renal blood flow is smaller in fetuses than in newborn lambs or adult sheep (left panel). Renal nerve stimulation during α-adrenoreceptor blockade with phentolamine increases renal blood flow in fetal and newborn sheep, but not in adult sheep (right panel). (Adapted from Robillard JE, Nakamura KT. *Am J Physiol* 1988; **254**: F771, with permission.)

89.3). Renal nerve stimulation decreases RBF and increases renal vascular resistance at all stages but the overall vasoconstrictor response is smaller in fetuses than in newborn and adult animals (Fig. 89.3).

In addition to renal vasoconstriction, renal nerve stimulation can also produce renal vasodilatation during α-adrenergic receptor blockade in fetal and newborn animals (Fig. 89.3). The ability of renal nerve stimulation to induce renal vasodilatation is particular to this developmental period, because it does not occur in adults. This renal vasodilatation, which is of greater magnitude in fetal than in newborn sheep, is independent of activation of cholinergic or dopaminergic receptors but is completely blocked by selective β2-adrenergic receptor antagonists. These results are of interest in several respects. First, they suggest that renal nerve fibers activated during renal nerve stimulation are essentially noradrenergic. Second, they provide evidence of an age-dependent neural renal vasodilator mechanism in mammals. Third, the observation that the renal vasodilatation observed during renal nerve stimulation decreases postnatally suggests that maturation of the adrenergic system is associated with a down-regulation of β-adrenergic receptors in renal vessels. In favor of this hypothesis is the observation in different vascular beds that β-adrenergic receptor relaxation declines with advancing age. Furthermore, the renal β2-adrenergic receptor is the main β-adrenergic receptor subtype in the fetal kidney.

After the immediate newborn period, the neonatal renal circulation is more sensitive to α-adrenergic stimulation in dogs, pigs, and guinea pigs, but not in sheep. Factors contributing to the increased sensitivity of the neonatal renal vasculature to catecholamines have been studied. First, the newborn kidney shows increased expression of the α1B-adrenergic receptor gene and α1B-adrenergic receptor protein. Second, the renal vasodilator effect of dopamine is decreased in the newborn in spite of "mature" levels of receptors. In this instance, decreased formation of vasodilating second messengers (e.g. cAMP) may be involved.

In sheep, the intrarenal infusion of dopamine produces renal vasoconstriction during both fetal and postnatal life. The absence of renal vasodilatation with low dopamine doses in fetal and newborn sheep confirms results from other species demonstrating that "α-adrenergic receptor" effects of dopamine are predominant in immature animals. During α- and β-adrenergic receptor blockade, dopamine did not increase RBF in 1–2-week-old puppies, but did increase RBF and glomerular filtration rate (GFR) in older puppies. Similar results were observed following intravenous dopamine administration in young piglets. Intrarenal dopamine infusions during renal α- and β-adrenergic receptor blockade produce similar renal vasodilator responses in fetal, newborn and adult sheep, suggesting that in sheep dopamine has no age-related vasodilator effect as previously observed in dogs and piglets.

## Renin–angiotensin system

Studies of the role of the renin–angiotensin system in controlling renal hemodynamics during development have shown that the vasopressor response and the renal vasoconstrictor response to infusion of angiotensin II (AII) are less during fetal life than after birth, possibly due to a high receptor occupancy by endogenous AII early in life. However, administration of AII to fetal sheep increases arterial blood pressure and decreases umbilical and renal blood flow. GFR remains unchanged, suggesting that AII acts primarily by increasing the tone of the efferent arteriole, as previously shown in adults.

Intrarenal localization of AII-specific binding has shown that AII receptors are present in the afferent and efferent arterioles early during glomerular development, and in mesangial cells and in peritubular vessels just before birth. Immunolocalization of AII also has been found in the proximal tubule and in the thick ascending limb of Henle in fetal rats. Intravenous administration of the AII subtype 1 (AT1) receptor antagonist losartan to third-trimester fetal sheep reduces fetal arterial blood pressure and causes a fall in renal vascular resistance and a rise in RBF. This rise in RBF is associated with a significant decrease in glomerular filtration.

## Atrial natriuretic factor (atrial natriuretic peptide)

Atrial natriuretic factor comprises a class of peptides with potent natriuretic, diuretic, and vasodilator effects. The renal hemodynamic responses to systemic infusion of ANP differs in fetal, newborn, and adult animals. Whereas no significant changes occur in adults, systemic infusion of ANP in fetal and newborn animals decreases RBF and increases renal vascular resistance. This decrease in RBF may be secondary to a decrease in cardiac output, as shown in adults, an increase in renal sympathetic tone and circulating catecholamines, a direct vasoconstrictor action of ANP on the fetal and neonatal vasculature, or a combination of these. However, intrarenal infusion of ANP causes a direct renal vasodilatation in fetal and newborn animals, suggesting that the renal vasoconstriction observed during systemic infusion of ANP is secondary to activation of compensatory mechanisms.

## Eicosanoids

Prostaglandins produced by the kidney may be involved in the regulation of renal hemodynamics and function during development. In fetal and newborn animals a transient reduction in fetal RBF occurs following administration of the prostaglandin inhibitors meclofenamate or indomethacin. Interestingly, administration of prostaglandin synthetase inhibitors to stop *preterm labor* in humans is associated with oligohydramnios in as many as 50 per cent of cases. This oligohydramnios probably results from a decrease in fetal urinary output secondary to a decrease in fetal RBF. Observations made in pregnant women given a short course of indomethacin suggest that the inhibition of prostaglandin synthesis leads to a significant decrease in GFR combined with low urine output in their offspring immediately after exposure. Although the alterations in renal function may be transient, one should consider prolonged treatment with prostaglandin synthetase inhibitors during pregnancy to be an important risk factor for the developing fetus.

## Nitric oxide (NO)

In fetal sheep and newborn piglets the endothelium-derived relaxing factor, NO, is produced by the renal vascular endothelium early during development and modulates renal vascular resistance. For example, inhibition of NO synthesis in third trimester fetal sheep is associated with an increase in renal vascular resistance, a decrease in GFR and a decline in urinary excretion of $Na^+$. Similar changes in renal hemodynamics have been observed in newborn piglets following inhibition of NO formation.

## Endothelins

Endothelins produced by endothelial cells are potent vasoconstrictors and mitogens, and are involved in the regulation of renal hemodynamics in the adult. In the human fetal kidney, specific binding sites for endothelins have been found in the cortex, medulla, and renal vessels. The presence of endothelin-binding sites in the developing kidney and the high endothelin-1 concentrations in the first 5 days after birth in humans may indicate a role for endothelin in modulating renal hemodynamics early in life and in influencing renal development. However, the renal vasoconstrictor effect of endothelin appears to be less during early development than later in life.

## Autoregulation

The mature kidney is capable of maintaining RBF relatively constant when major changes in perfusion pressure occur, a phenomenon known as autoregulation. It has been suggested that RBF autoregulation is negligible at birth, but increases with postnatal development. Limited data are available on the renal autoregulatory phenomenon in the fetus. During infusion of vasopressin or AII to fetal sheep RBF is unchanged despite a moderate increase in arterial blood pressure suggesting that the fetus may autoregulate RBF during modest increases in renal perfusion pressure. In the newborn, autoregulation of RBF is present but is set at a lower perfusion pressure set point than in the adult. Autoregulation of RBF also is less efficient in the young than in the adult. This reduced autoregulatory efficiency in the neonate is apparently due to prostaglandin-dependent renin release, which causes vasoconstriction at lower levels of perfusion pressure.

## SELECTED READING

Guillery EN, Porter CC, Page WV, *et al.* Developmental regulation of the $\alpha_{1B}$-adrenoceptor in the sheep kidney. *Pediatr Res* 1993; 34: 124.

Jose PA, Haramati A, Fildes RD. Postnatal maturation of renal blood flow. In: Polin RA, Fox WW, eds. *Fetal and neonatal physiology*. Philadelphia: WB Saunders, 1992: 1196.

Segar JL, Smith FG, Guillery EN *et al.* Ontogeny of the renal response to specific dopamine receptor stimulation in sheep. *Am J Physiol* 1992; 263: R868.

Seikaly MG, Arant BS Jr. Development of renal hemodynamics: glomerular filtration and renal blood flow. *Clin Perinatol* 1992; 19: 1.

Semana DS, Thonney M, Guignard J-P *et al.* Effects of endothelin on renal function in newborn rabbits. *Pediatr Res* 1993; 34: 120.

# 90

# Glomerular Filtration

Jean E. Robillard

In all vertebrate classes, the specialized filtration structure formed by the endothelium of the glomerular capillaries, the glomerular epithelial cells, and the basement membrane serves as an ultrafilter. The rate at which the glomerular filtrate is formed, or glomerular filtration rate (GFR), is determined by measuring the clearance of inulin ($C_{in}$). $C_{in}$ is defined as the virtual volume of plasma that is completely cleared of inulin by the kidney per unit time and is expressed as

$$C_{in} = \frac{UV}{P}$$

where $U$ is the concentration of inulin in the urine, $V$ is the rate of urine flow, and $P$ is the concentration of inulin in plasma. Inulin, a starch-like polymer of fructose, is considered the best marker of GFR since it is freely filterable through the glomerular capillary, is biologically inert and is neither reabsorbed nor secreted by the renal tubule.

Glomerular filtration begins between 9 and 12 weeks' gestation in the human fetus and contributes to the formation of urine and the accumulation of amniotic fluid. During nephrogenesis, the first developed glomeruli, which appear in the juxtamedullary cortex, have higher filtration rates than the most recently formed glomeruli in the superficial cortex. As the embryonic development of the kidney proceeds in a centrifugal fashion, most of the increase in GFR during fetal life is due to an increase in the number of filtering nephron units. In fetal sheep, GFR increases about 2.5-fold during the last trimester of gestation (from 1.24 mL/min at 100 days' gestation to 3.25 mL/min at term) (Fig. 90.1). The rise in GFR during fetal life increases in parallel with the rise in kidney mass and in fetal body weight. In newborn infants delivered between 27 and 43 weeks' gestation GFR

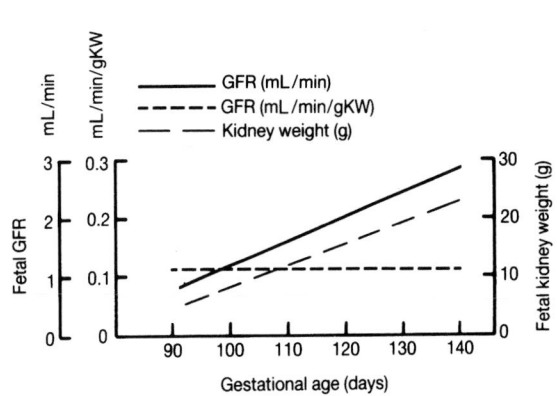
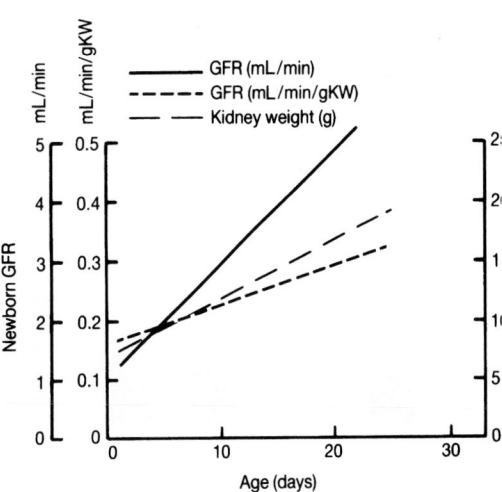

FIGURE 90.1 Maturation of glomerular filtration rate (GFR) during fetal (left panel) and postnatal (right panel) life. (From Robillard JE, *et al. Am J Obstet Gynecol* 1977; **128**: 727; and Kleinman LI, Lubbe RJ. *J Physiol* 1972; **223**: 395, with permission)

(mL/min) measured in the first 24 hours after birth correlates with gestational age.

The transition from fetal to newborn life brings a sudden surge in GFR. In sheep, GFR increases three-fold during the first 24 hours following birth (Fig. 90.2). This rise in GFR is not associated with significant changes in total renal blood flow, but appears to be due to an increase in the number of functional nephrons in the outer portion of the renal cortex. Following the newborn period, GFR continues to increase. In the human, GFR corrected for body surface area doubles from birth to 2 weeks of age, increases to 50 per cent of adult levels by 2 months of age, and reaches adult levels by about 2 years.

## REGULATION BY VASOACTIVE SUBSTANCES

Vasoactive substances such as vasopressin, angiotensin II (AII), prostaglandins, catecholamines, bradykinin, parathyroid hormone, nitric oxide, endothelin and acetylcholine can alter not only distribution of blood flow within the cortex, but also the perfusion of individual nephrons within a cortical region. For example, the renin–angiotensin system may influence changes in GFR during the transition from fetal to newborn life. In support of this, during early fetal life the expression of renin mRNA and protein extend to the arcuate and interlobular arteries, whereas in the newborn renal renin distribution shifts to a more classic juxtaglomerular location (Fig. 90.3). In addition, inhibition of AII synthesis with captopril tends to decrease renal blood flow and GFR during the first 24 hours after birth.

Renal prostaglandins also may contribute to the regulation of GFR in special conditions during development. Inhibition of prostaglandin synthesis in unstressed fetal and newborn animals does not appear to decrease GFR. On the other hand, inhibition of prostaglandin synthesis with indomethacin, in premature infants with patent ductus arteriosus, has resulted in transient renal failure that could be attenuated by the administration of furosemide, a diuretic that stimulates prostaglandin production. Thus during development, prostaglandins may not play an important role in modulating GFR during normal conditions, but may

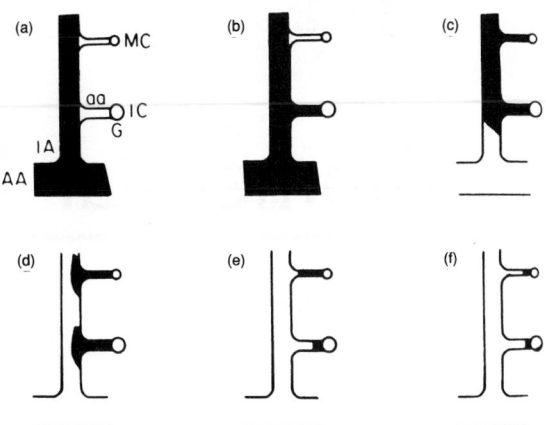

FIGURE 90.3 Schematic representation of changes in intrarenal renin distribution during maturation in rats. Dark areas represent arterial segments expressing renin at different stages of renal maturation. AA, arcuate artery; IA, interlobular artery; aa, afferent arteriole; G, glomerulus; IC, inner (juxtamedullary) cortex; MC, middle cortex. (a) 19-day-old fetus; (b) 20-day-old fetus; (c) 5-day-old newborn; (e) 20 days postnatal; (f) adult. (From Gomez et al. J Hypertens 1986; 4: S31, with permission.)

be important in controlling the effects of stress-induced vasoconstriction such as by catecholamines or AII.

Because plasma catecholamine concentrations are elevated in human infants delivered vaginally, the changes in plasma catecholamines may play an important role in the regulation of GFR during the transition from fetal to newborn life. However, renal denervation prior to birth in fetal sheep does not appear to alter the postnatal rise in GFR.

## REGULATION BY PHYSICAL FACTORS

Changes in physical factors known to affect single nephron glomerular filtration rate (SNGFR) in the adult may also regulate the changes in SNGFR during development. Changes in the effective area used for filtration, the glomerular surface area ($S$), effective filtration pressure ($P_{UF}$) [$P_{UF} = P_{GC} - (P_T + \mu_{GC})$ where $P_{GC}$ is the mean glomerular capillary pressure, $P_T$ is the proximal tubule pressure, and $\mu_{GC}$ is the mean colloid osmotic pressure in the glomerular capillary] and effective hydraulic permeability ($k$) are all known to affect SNGFR during the newborn period. These interrelationships are expressed by the equation:

$$GFR = k \cdot S \cdot P_{UF}$$

These factors have not been quantified during fetal life. It appears, however, that low $S$, low $k$, and low $P_{UF}$ may contribute to the low GFR in the fetus. In the newborn, it has been shown that the large increase in GFR (25 times) during development depends predominantly on an increase in the glomer-

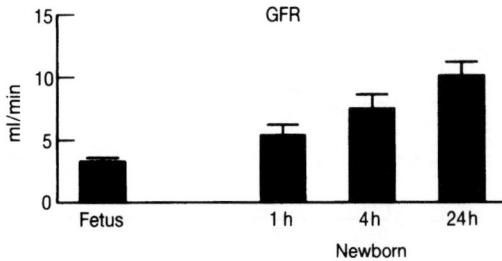

FIGURE 90.2 Changes in glomerular filtration rate (GFR) during the transition from fetal to newborn life. (From Nakamura KT et al. Pediatr Res 1987; 21: 229, with permission.)

### Newborn

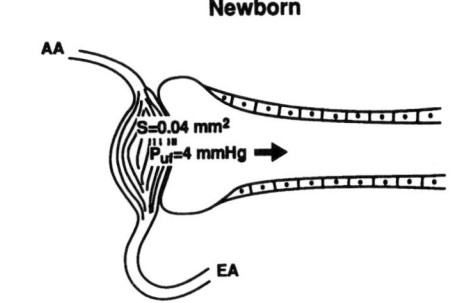

### Adult

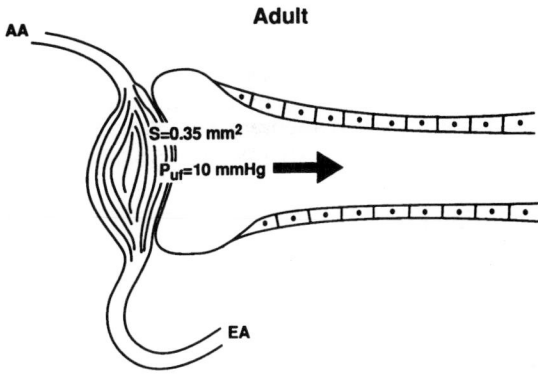

FIGURE 90.4 Determinants of single nephron glomerular filtration rate (SNGFR) during kidney development. $SNGFR = k \cdot S \cdot P_{UF}$ (see text). From newborn to adult life $S$ increases 8-fold, $P_{UF}$ increases 2.5-fold and $k$ about 1.3-fold. Developmental changes in these variables allow superficial nephron SNGFR to increase from 0.9 nl/min at birth to 19 nl/min in adult guinea pigs. AA, arcuate artery; EA, efferent arteriole.

ular surface area (8 times) and, to a lesser extent, on a rise in $P_{UF}$ (2.5 times) (Fig. 90.4). Changes in the hydraulic permeability of the glomerular capillary (1.3 times) contribute only minimally to the postnatal rise in GFR.

## SELECTED READING

Corey HE, Spitzer A. Renal blood flow and glomerular filtration rate during development. In: Edelmann CM Jr, ed. *Pediatric kidney disease*. Boston: Little, Brown and Company, 1992: 49.

Gibson KJ, Lumbers ER. Changes in renal function and blood volume in the newborn lamb delivered by cesarean section. *Pediatr Res* 1994; **36**: 506.

Nakamura KT, Matherne GP, McWeeny OJ *et al.* Renal hemodynamics and functional changes during the transition from fetal to newborn life in sheep. *Pediatr Res* 1987; **21**: 229.

Robillard JE, Smith FG, Segar JL *et al.* Functional role of renal sympathetic innervation during fetal and postnatal development. *News Physiol Sci* 1992; **7**: 130.

Robillard JE, Smith FG, Smith FG Jr. Developmental aspects of renal function during fetal life. In Edelmann CM, ed. *Pediatric kidney disease*, Boston: Little, Brown and Company, 1992: 3.

Seikaly MG, Arant BS Jr. Development of renal hemodynamics: glomerular filtration and renal blood flow. *Clin Perinatol* 1992; **19**: 1.

# 91

# Tubular Function

## SODIUM HOMEOSTASIS

### REGULATION OF Na$^+$ HOMEOSTASIS

It is essential for the mammalian organism to maintain both arterial blood pressure and intracellular electrolyte composition within normal limits. In healthy adults, this process is so efficient and sensitive that, despite wide daily variations in salt and water intake, blood volume, blood pressure, and intracellular electrolyte composition generally are well maintained, and only large pathological losses offset this balance.

The kidney plays an important role in this regulation. Both short- and long-term adjustments of salt and water balance are accomplished by variations in the rate of tubular reabsorption. Tubular reabsorption is under the control of renal nerves, catecholamines, and both peptide and steroid hormones. It is also regulated by hydrostatic and oncotic pressures. These physical forces in turn influence tubular and glomerular function because the glomerular filtration rate and the filtration fraction have an important influence on the hydrostatic and oncotic pressures in the peritubular capillaries and in the tubular lumen.

### ION TRANSPORTERS

Na$^+$ crosses the cell membrane via specific transporting proteins. Located in the basolateral membrane of all tubular cells, Na$^+$-K$^+$-ATPase, by transferring the energy from ATP hydrolysis to a vectorial transport of Na$^+$ and K$^+$ with a coupling ratio of 3:2, creates an electrochemical gradient across the cell membrane. Na$^+$-K$^+$-ATPase uses approximately 80 per cent of all O$_2$ that is consumed by the kidney. The Na$^+$-K$^+$-ATPase-mediated gradient allows for a downhill transport of Na$^+$ from the tubular lumen into the cell via cotransporters and countertransporters and channels. Na$^+$-K$^+$-ATPase is a ubiquitous protein, but most of the in-transporters are selectively distributed. Some examples of Na$^+$ in-transporters are the Na$^+$-glucose and Na$^+$-amino acid cotransporters, which are only expressed in proximal tubular cells, and the furosemide-sensitive Na$^+$-K$^+$-Cl$^-$ cotransporter, which is expressed in the thick ascending limb of Henle. The important Na$^+$-H$^+$ exchanger is most abundant in the proximal tubule.

As many of the Na$^+$-transporting proteins are cloned, information about the transcriptional and translational regulation of these proteins is starting to emerge. Because these proteins are differentially distributed to the basolateral or apical membrane, the means by which they are directed to the appropriate side of the cell is an important developmental question.

## Paracellular transport

Tubular reabsorption of salt and fluid is both transcellular and paracellular. In the proximal tubule, which is a relatively leaky epithelium, a large fraction of salt and water reabsorption occurs via the paracellular pathway. Paracellular fluxes depend on the establishment of osmotic and chemical gradients across the epithelium, which are generated by the active transcellular transport of solute. The paracellular fluxes also depend on the hydraulic conductivity of the cell junctions.

## NEUROTRANSMITTERS AND HORMONES MODULATING Na$^+$ BALANCE

Regulation of Na$^+$ excretion is bidirectional. Some of the best known salt-regulating factors are atrial natriuretic peptide (ANP) and dopamine, which act natriuretically, and aldosterone, angiotensin, and norepinephrine, which act antinatriuretically. Many other hormones, such as prostaglandins, bradykinin, and endothelin, also have a modulating effect on Na$^+$ transport in various parts of the nephron, but the mechanism(s) of action of these hormones are less well known. Both aldosterone and ANP are circulating factors. Aldosterone is released in response to changes in electrolyte balance. Increased circulating concentrations of aldosterone generally are an early sign of salt depletion. ANP is released from the heart in response to changes in blood volume. Recent evidence suggests that ANP is also locally produced in the kidney. Angiotensin and dopamine are formed in the kidney and act as both paracrine and autocrine factors. Dopamine is synthesized in the proximal tubular cells; the rate of synthesis is sensitive to changes in salt balance. Norepinephrine is released from nerve endings. Renal nerve activity can be influenced by many physiological factors (e.g. volume expansion will decrease renal nerve activity).

Aldosterone is a steroid hormone with an intracellular receptor that, when activated by the hormone, crosses the nuclear membrane and acts as a transcriptional factor. Several lines of evidence suggest that both aldosterone and glucocorticoid hormones can regulate the transcription of Na$^+$-K$^+$-ATPase. The effects of aldosterone differ from those of glucocorticoid hormones: aldosterone is more specific (aldosterone receptors are selectively distributed in the distal parts of the nephron), and is age-independent and present in the mature kidney. The age-dependent effects of glucocorticoid hormones are described below.

Both peptide hormones and catecholamines act on membrane receptors that, following activation, initiate a signal that is forwarded by second messengers such as cAMP, Ca$^{2+}$, and diacylglycerol to third messengers such as protein kinases. Eventually the activity of the Na$^+$-transporting protein will be altered by phosphorylation/dephosphorylation, the most common form of covalent modification of a protein. Although the physiological responses are entirely different, the principles for regulation of ion transporters via protein phosphorylation are similar in the brain and kidney.

The balance between the effect of protein kinases and the effect of phosphatases determines the basal activity of ion transporters. Hormones that act natriuretically drive the reaction in one direction, resulting in inactivation of the ion transporter, while hormones that act antinatriuretically drive the reaction in the other direction, resulting in activation of the ion transporter. Antinatriuretic hormones often stimulate both the Na$^+$ in-transporters and Na$^+$-K$^+$-ATPase, while natriuretic hormones often inhibit both in-transporters and Na$^+$-K$^+$-ATPase.

## DEVELOPMENTAL ASPECTS

The infant mammalian kidney is not as efficient as the adult kidney in maintaining body fluid volume and composition. Low salt intake results in negative salt balance more rapidly in the infant than in the adult. Because the newborn kidney also has a lower capacity to excrete a Na$^+$ load, the risk for salt and water accumulation following high salt intake is greater in the infant than in the adult.

The low capacity of the infant to vary Na$^+$ excretion rapidly in response to changes in salt intake does not seem to be due to a lack of regulatory factors. Most of the hormones known to be important for the regulation of Na$^+$ balance are appropriately released in the neonate and also in the near-term fetus.

In many infants renal tubular cells seem to have an altered sensitivity to hormones regulating Na$^+$ transport. Renal sympathetic nerves already can influence salt excretion during fetal life. In fact, high renal nerve activity might contribute to the infant's low capacity to excrete a salt load. Renal tubular cells in preterm infants and in rat pups are relatively insensitive to aldosterone due to low availability of aldosterone receptors. A blunted natriuretic response to ANP also has been reported in infants of many species, and a blunted response to dopamine occurs in rat and dog pups. There is a natriuretic response to dopamine in the human infant and in rabbit pups, but the magnitude of the response in infants and adults has not been compared. Apparently the ontogeny of signal transduction systems in the renal tubular cells is quite complex. Most developmental studies on signal transduction in the kidney so far have been performed on signal pathways that are coupled to dopamine receptors. The ontogeny of the cellular response to dopamine differs in different parts of the nephrons. In the proximal tubule, the coupling of the dopamine 1 receptor to the adenylyl cyclase unit increases during ontogeny. The reverse appears to be the case in the medullary thick ascending limb of Henle. Protein kinase C, which might also be a third messenger of dopamine in the kidney, can phosphorylate and inactivate Na$^+$-K$^+$-ATPase. This response is blunted in the infant kidney. Yet protein kinase C activity is higher in the infant than in the adult renal cortex. From the relatively few studies conducted so far in this interesting field, one can conclude that the effect of a particular hormone on natriuresis in the infant cannot be predicted from that hormone's effect in the adult. It is tempting to speculate that in the developing kidney, signal transduction pathways also are used for growth and differentiation and that they might therefore be occupied when $Na^+$-regulating factors try to forward a signal.

The $Na^+$-transporting capacity of the infant kidney also is limited by a low number of transporting proteins. So far most determinations of available transporters are indirect and are based on studies of the activity of the transporter when it is saturated with regard to substrates. In rat pups, the activities of the $Na^+$-$K^+$-ATPase/$Na^+$-$H^+$ exchanger and the $Na^+$-glucose transporter have been shown to increase significantly after birth. The most rapid increase generally occurs during or just before the weanling period. This coincides with an upsurge in plasma concentrations of glucocorticoid hormone. Several lines of evidence suggest that glucocorticoid hormones can act as an inducer of $Na^+$-transporting proteins and that, at least in the case of $Na^+$-$K^+$-ATPase, this is mediated by a direct transcriptional effect on the genes of the two subunits of the enzyme. Of interest for the understanding of renal differentiation, this effect is transient and appears to be lost or attenuated in the adult kidney.

The increase in the number of transporting proteins is paralleled by an increase in the reabsorptive capacity of the tubule and also by an increase in the size of the membrane where the protein is located. If the ion transporters are prematurely induced by administration of glucocorticoid hormones, this will be followed by an increase in the functional capacity of the kidney. Observations from experimental studies indicate that the infant proximal convoluted tubule has a large hydraulic conductance and suggest that the transepithelial shunt pathway may contribute to reabsorption to a larger extent in the early postnatal period than in later life.

## CLINICAL ASPECTS

During the first weeks after birth, the preterm infant has a very low capacity to vary salt excretion and is therefore extremely sensitive to large variations in salt intake. Because the capacity to regulate body fluid tonicity is also low (*see* Chapter 93), disturbances in serum $Na^+$ concentration are common. All infants have difficulties in rapidly excreting a salt load. This capacity develops gradually during the first year. Disturbances in salt and water balance have many adverse effects. High $Na^+$ and fluid intake results in blood volume expansion, which may delay closure of the ductus arteriosus and might compromise the circulation to the gut and the lungs, contributing to necrotizing enterocolitis and bronchopulmonary dysplasia. Salt deficiency retards growth. Both hyponatremia and hypernatremia can lead to brain damage. The low capacity of the $Na^+$-$H^+$ exchanger predisposes to acidosis.

Healthy full-term infants generally maintain $Na^+$ balance well, provided they receive breast milk or a formula with corresponding electrolyte composition. If the infant has kidney disease that has led to a mod-

erate decrease in renal function, the risk for disturbances in $Na^+$ balance is high. Hyponatremia and acidosis (low capacity of the $Na^+$-$H^+$ exchanger) are common in infants with moderate renal insufficiency. Like salt deficiency, acidosis will retard growth; therefore, even mild acidosis must be corrected in infants with renal insufficiency.

## SELECTED READING

Aperia A, Celsi G. Ontogenic processes in nephron epithelia. Structure, enzymes, and function. In: Seldin DW, Giebisch G, eds. *The kidney: physiology and pathophysiology*, Vol 11, 2nd edn. New York: Raven Press, 1992: 803.

Celsi G, Nishi A, Akusjarvi G, Aperia A. Abundance of $Na^+$-$K^+$-ATPase mRNA is regulated by glucocorticoid hormones in infant rat kidneys. *Am J Physiol* 1991; **260**: F192.

Haycock GB, Aperia A. Salt and the newborn kidney. *Pediatr Nephrol* 1991; **5**: 65.

Robillard JE, Smith FG, Segar JL *et al*. Mechanisms regulating renal sodium excretion during development. *Pediatr Nephrol* 1992; **6**: 205.

Seldin DW, Giebisch G, eds. *The kidney: physiology and pathophysiology*, Vol 11, 2nd edn. Section 111: Renal regulation of sodium and chloride: normal. New York: Raven Press, 1992: 1807.

# RENAL REGULATION OF POTASSIUM HOMEOSTASIS

The kidney, the major route for elimination of potassium ($K^+$) from the body, is responsible for excretion of approximately 90 per cent of the average 100 mmol $K^+$ ingested daily by adults. Small obligatory extrarenal losses of $K^+$ occur in sweat (1–2 mmol/day) and stool (7–15 mmol/day).

In general, the rate of urinary $K^+$ excretion parallels dietary intake, thereby maintaining serum $K^+$ concentration within a narrow range of 3.5–5.0 mmol/L. However, extreme adjustments in the $K^+$ excretory rate cannot be achieved as rapidly as for $Na^+$, nor are they as complete. Whereas urinary $Na^+$ virtually disappears from the urine within 3–4 days of $Na^+$ restriction, a minimum urinary $K^+$ loss of approximately 5 mmol/day persists in the $K^+$-restricted adult. In response to an abrupt increase in $K^+$ intake (oral, parenteral), urinary $K^+$ promptly increases, yet maximal excretory rates may not become apparent for 1–2 days.

## SITES OF POTASSIUM TRANSPORT IN THE KIDNEY

Most of the information available regarding the renal handling of $K^+$ has been derived from *in vivo* micropuncture studies of segments exposed to the cortical surface (superficial nephrons) or papillary tip (juxtamedullary nephrons); segments inaccessible to micropuncture have been examined by *in vitro* microperfusion. The transport characteristics of individual nephron segments are summarized in Fig. 91.1. Filtered $K^+$ is reabsorbed almost entirely in proximal segments of the nephron, urinary $K^+$ being derived predominantly from distal $K^+$ secretion. Thus $K^+$ balance, at least in the adult, is maintained by renal secretion rather than reabsorption (as in the case of $Na^+$).

## Superficial nephron

$K^+$ is freely filtered at the glomerulus. Approximately 50 per cent of the filtered load of $K^+$ is reabsorbed along the initial two-thirds of the superficial proximal tubule. Reabsorption in this segment is passive, closely following the reabsorption of water and $Na^+$; thus, the concentration of $K^+$ in the proximal tubular fluid remains similar to that of plasma.

In the adult, 5–15 per cent of the filtered load of $K^+$ reaches the superficial early distal tubule, indicating that significant net reabsorption of $K^+$ occurs in the intervening nephron segments. A major site of avid $K^+$ reabsorption therein is the thick ascending limb of the loop of Henle, which possesses a luminal electroneutral cotransporter that translocates one $Na^+$ and one $K^+$ with two $Cl^-$ ions into the cell (Fig. 91.2a); the powerful *loop diuretics* (e.g. furosemide, ethacrynic acid) inhibit this cotransporter, resulting in $Na^+$ and $K^+$ escape into the distal tubular fluid.

Comparison of the fractional delivery of $K^+$ to the early distal tubule with that present in the final urine indicates that the rate of $K^+$ secretion along the intervening segments (late distal tubule, collecting duct) is highly variable, depending on the metabolic state and $K^+$ balance, but can approach 20–50 per cent of the filtered load.

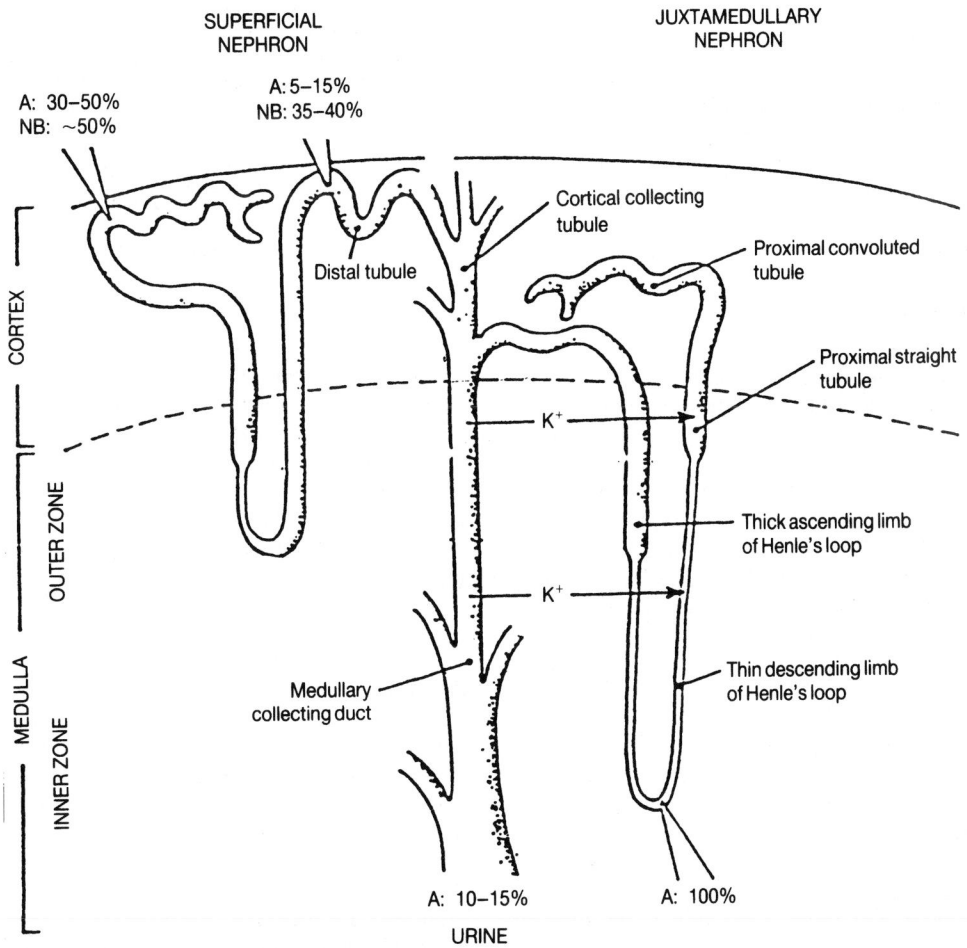

FIGURE 91.1 Segmental handling of $K^+$ in superficial and juxtamedullary nephrons of the rat. The percentage of filtered $K^+$ remaining at each site is provided for the adult (A) and, when known, the newborn (NB) animal. Arrows show the direction of net $K^+$ transport, either reabsorption or secretion. (Modified from Giebisch G *et al.* Renal transport and control of potassium excretion. In: Brenner BM, Rector FC Jr, eds. *The Kidney*. Philadelphia: WB Saunders, 1991: 291, with permission.)

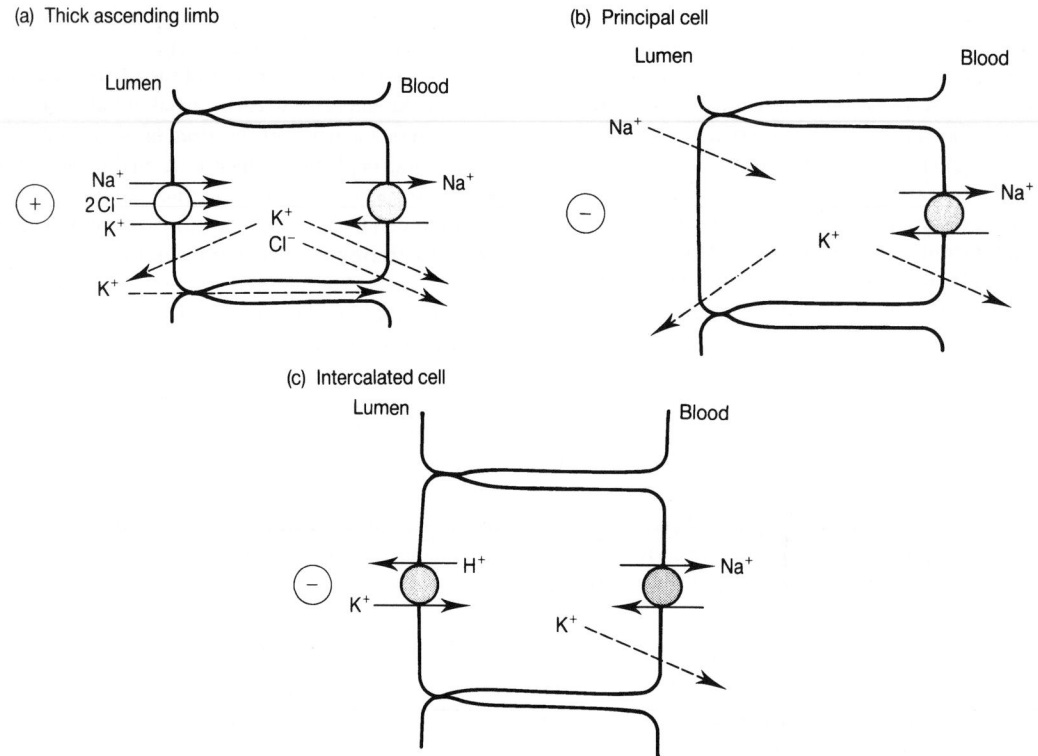

FIGURE 91.2 Pathways of transepithelial K$^+$ transport in (a) thick ascending limb and cortical collecting duct, (b) principal cell and (c) intercalated cell. Broken arrows denote passive pathways whereas solid arrows depict active transport mechanisms. (Modified from Wright FS, Giebisch G. Regulation of K$^+$ excretion. In: Seldin DW, Giebisch G, eds. *The Kidney*. New York: Raven Press, 1985: 1223, with permission.)

## Juxtamedullary nephron

Analysis of the tubular fluid collected by micropuncture at the tip of the adult rat papilla indicates that the rate of K$^+$ delivery to the end of the descending limb of the loop of Henle may exceed the filtered load. Presumably, K$^+$ diffuses passively from the medullary interstitium down its concentration gradient into the proximal straight tubule and thin descending limb of the loop of Henle. The high concentration of K$^+$ in the medullary interstitial fluid is derived from reabsorption by the thick ascending limb and the outer medullary collecting duct. K$^+$ reabsorption by the latter segment is primarily passive, following a favorable electrochemical gradient generated by the high tubular fluid K$^+$ concentration leaving the cortical collecting duct and the lumen positive voltage.

The physiological role of medullary K$^+$ recycling (reabsorption by the thick ascending limb and medullary collecting duct; secretion into the proximal straight tubule and descending limb of the loop of Henle) remains unclear. However, it may serve to amplify the fraction of K$^+$ being delivered to distal segments of the juxtamedullary nephron and may account for an increase in K$^+$ excretion under conditions of K$^+$ loading.

## Distal nephron

The cortical collecting duct is the main regulatory site of K$^+$ secretion, capable of generating K$^+$ concentrations in excess of 100 mmol/L in the luminal fluid. This segment is composed of two major cell types. The majority cell type, the principal cell, secretes K$^+$ and absorbs Na$^+$. The less numerous intercalated cells, primarily responsible for transepithelial acid–base transport, may play a role in K$^+$ reabsorption.

### Principal cell

The model for transcellular K$^+$ secretion in the principal cell (Fig. 91.2b) requires the active cellular uptake of two K$^+$ ions against a large concentration gradient in exchange for the extrusion of three Na$^+$ ions at the basolateral membrane, a process driven by Na$^+$-K$^+$-ATPase; the unequal exchange ratio is responsible, in large part, for the negative voltage within the cell. Cell K$^+$ then diffuses passively into the lumen through apical K$^+$-selective channels. In the presence of an adequate number of channels, the magnitude of K$^+$ secretion is determined by the cell-to-lumen electrochemical gradient. The lumen-negative potential difference across the cortical collecting duct, generated by apical Na⁺ entry and electrogenic basolateral extrusion (via Na⁺-K⁺-ATPase), and high cell K⁺ provide a favorable driving force for cell K⁺ exit into the luminal fluid.

## Intercalated cell

Intercalated cells, specialized for proton secretion in the medullary collecting duct, may actively absorb K⁺ (Fig. 91.2c). K⁺ deficiency is associated with selective hypertrophy of the apical surfaces of medullary intercalated cells and appearance of an ATP-coupled H⁺-K⁺ pump (which secretes protons into the urine in exchange for K⁺ reabsorption) in the apical membrane of these cells.

## REGULATION OF K⁺ BALANCE BY THE DISTAL NEPHRON

K⁺ secretion by the cortical collecting duct depends on the interaction of various cellular, luminal, and circulating factors capable of influencing K⁺ transport (Table 91.1). Factors that enhance the electrochemical driving force or apical membrane permeability to K⁺ of the principal cell facilitate secretion of this cation.

## Cell K⁺ concentration

The chemical concentration of K⁺ in the intracellular fluid ranges between 100 and 150 mmol/L. K⁺ activity, the effective concentration that is ionically active, appears to be substantially lower, reflecting intracellular binding of K⁺ to proteins or compartmentalization of this ion within cells.

The intracellular concentration of K⁺ can be altered by numerous factors, including K⁺ intake. An increase in dietary K⁺ results in a transient rise in plasma K⁺ concentration, which in turn stimulates renal K⁺ excretion and adrenal release of aldosterone. At the level of the principal cell, hyperkalemia reduces the concentration gradient across the basolateral membrane against which the Na⁺-K⁺ pump must function, thereby stimulating basolateral uptake of K⁺. This, in combination with an increase in transepithelial voltage, augments K⁺ secretion.

TABLE 91.1 Factors that influence K⁺ transport

Cellular
  Cell K⁺ concentration
Luminal
  Tubular fluid flow rate
  Luminal Na⁺ and K⁺ concentrations
  Transepithelial voltage
Circulating
  Acid–base balance
  Aldosterone activity

Chronic K⁺ loading leads to "K⁺ tolerance" in the distal nephron, an adaptation that enables the animal to survive an otherwise lethal acute K⁺ load. The cellular mechanisms underlying this adaptation include increases in Na⁺-K⁺-ATPase activity and permeability of the apical membrane of the principal cell, modifications that together create a more favorable driving force for K⁺ diffusion from cell to lumen. A similar adaptive response is seen in chronic renal insufficiency.

## Rate of tubular fluid flow

K⁺ secretion is strongly influenced by the rate of tubular fluid flow (Fig. 91.3) and the concentration of K⁺ in the tubular fluid. At low flow rates, distal K⁺ secretion results in a gradual increase in the tubular fluid K⁺ concentration that opposes further K⁺ secretion. As flow rate increases, the tubular fluid K⁺ concentration remains constant or falls, thereby preserving or enhancing the favorable chemical gradient for the secretion of K⁺. Thus volume expansion and diuretics, which increase urinary flow rate, facilitate K⁺ secretion in the distal nephron.

## Distal Na⁺ delivery

Extracellular volume expansion and administration of diuretics (osmotic or those acting on proximal tubule or loop) promote an increase in K⁺ excretion. Whereas the kaliuresis is due in part to the increase in tubular flow rate, the increased luminal Na⁺ concentration reaching the cortical collecting duct can, in itself, enhance K⁺ secretion. Specifically, stimulation of electrogenic Na⁺ reabsorption increases the intraluminal

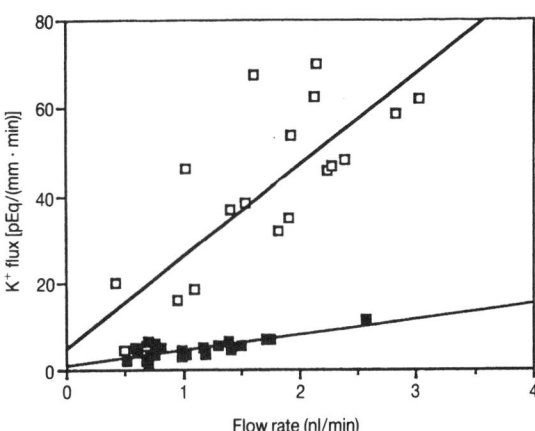

FIGURE 91.3 Effect of tubular fluid flow rate on K⁺ secretion (K⁺ flux) in isolated perfused rabbit cortical collecting ducts. Solid squares, data from animals fed a control diet. Open squares, animals fed diet to elevate plasma aldosterone concentrations and thereby enhance K⁺ secretion. (From Engbretson BG, Stoner LC. *Am J Physiol* 1987; **253**: F898, with permission.)

negativity, further enhancing the electrochemical gradient favoring passive diffusion of K$^+$ from cell to lumen.

Luminal Na$^+$ concentrations exceeding 35 mmol/L do not further influence the K$^+$ secretory rate; however, K$^+$ secretion is markedly suppressed when the tubular fluid Na$^+$ concentration falls below 10 mmol/L, as might occur under conditions of maximal Na$^+$ retention. *In vivo* measurements of distal tubular Na$^+$ concentration in both adult and suckling rats generally exceed 35 mmol/L, indicating that luminal Na$^+$ concentration does not regulate distal K$^+$ secretion under physiological conditions.

## Transepithelial voltage

Because the transepithelial voltage is generated by apical Na$^+$ entry and electrogenic basolateral extrusion, any agent that decreases active Na$^+$ transport (e.g. basolateral ouabain, luminal amiloride) will reduce the lumen-negative potential difference and thereby reduce K$^+$ secretion. A small increase in luminal electronegativity in the cortical collecting duct occurs when Na$^+$ delivered to that segment is accompanied by a poorly reabsorbable anion (e.g. β-hydroxybutyrate in diabetic ketoacidosis, bicarbonate, or carbenicillin) instead of Cl$^-$.

## Acid–base balance

For both respiratory and metabolic derangements, acute alkalosis increases whereas acute acidosis reduces urinary K$^+$ excretion (Fig. 91.4). Although alkalosis shifts K$^+$ into cells and acidosis causes cells to lose K$^+$, principal cell K$^+$ concentration changes little in response to perturbations in acid–base balance. Presumably, enhanced uptake is accompanied by accelerated exit through apical pH-sensitive K$^+$ channels, which open in response to cell alkalinization and close with acidosis.

The effect of chronic acid–base disturbances on K$^+$ secretion is more complex and may be influenced by the rate of delivery of fluid to the distal nephron, modification of the glomerular filtrate (replacement of Cl$^-$ with bicarbonate), and circulating aldosterone concentrations.

## Mineralocorticoid effects

Mineralocorticoids stimulate net Na$^+$ reabsorption and K$^+$ secretion in the cortical collecting duct (Figs 91.3 and 91.5). Aldosterone action requires its initial binding to receptors on principal cells, followed by translocation of the hormone–receptor complex to the nucleus, where specific genes are stimulated to code for physiologically active proteins (e.g. Na$^+$-K$^+$-ATPase). Cellular effects include increases in the apical membrane permeability to Na$^+$ and K$^+$ and enhancement of basolateral Na$^+$-K$^+$-ATPase activity, the latter promoting active uptake of K$^+$. Stimulation of Na$^+$ reabsorption additionally leads to an increase in lumen-negative transepithelial voltage. In sum, mineralocorticoids modulate both the electrochemical gradient and luminal membrane permeability across the distal nephron, stimulating K$^+$ secretion.

Prolonged administration of mineralocorticoids results in a persistent kaliuresis but only a transient phase of Na$^+$ retention. "Escape" from the Na$^+$-retaining effects presumably follows extracellular volume expansion to a new steady state with subsequent depression in proximal or loop Na$^+$ reabsorption.

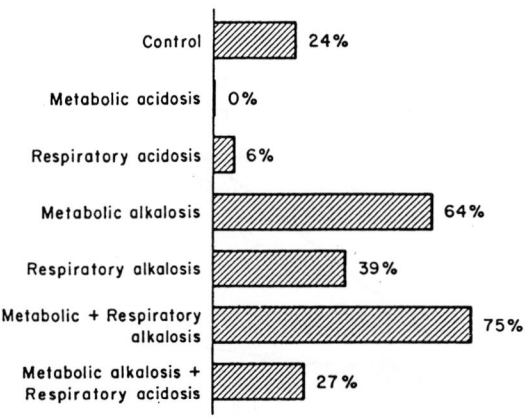

FIGURE 91.4 Effect of acid–base disturbances on distal tubule K$^+$ secretion. Bars indicate the percentage of the amount of K$^+$ in glomerular filtrate present under the designated condition. (From Giebisch G *et al.* Renal transport and control of K$^+$ excretion. In: Brenner BM, Rector FC Jr, eds. *The Kidney*, Vol I. Philadelphia: WB Saunders, 1991: 305 with permission.)

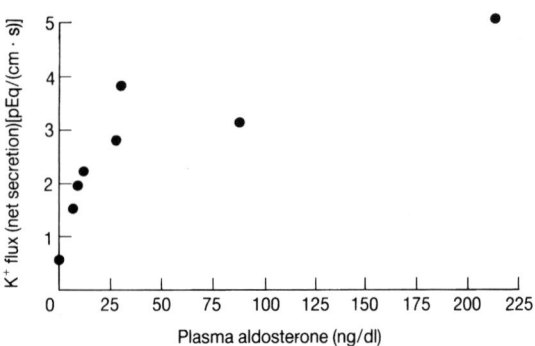

FIGURE 91.5 Relationship between circulating concentrations of aldosterone and K$^+$ secretion (K$^+$ flux) in isolated perfused rabbit cortical collecting ducts. (From Schwartz GJ, Burg MB. *Am J Physiol* 1978; **235**: F583, with permission.)

# DEVELOPMENTAL ASPECTS

## Overview of the renal contribution to K⁺ homeostasis

Unlike adults, who are in zero balance, growing infants maintain a state of positive K⁺ balance. The relative conservation of K⁺ early in life is generally associated with higher plasma K⁺ concentrations than those in the adult (Table 91.2). The renal clearance of K⁺ ($C_K^+$) in the infant is less than that in the older child, even when corrected for glomerular filtration rate ($C_{cr}$) (Table 91.2). Children and adults ingesting a regular diet containing Na⁺ in excess of K⁺ excrete urine with a Na⁺-to-K⁺ ratio greater than 1. Although the Na⁺-to-K⁺ ratio of breast milk and commercial infant formulas averages 0.5, the urinary Na⁺-to-K⁺ ratio of the newborn is also greater than 1, consistent with significant K⁺ retention.

Infants, like adults, can excrete K⁺ at a rate that exceeds its filtration when given a K⁺ load, indicating the capacity for net tubular secretion; however, the rate of K⁺ excretion per unit body weight in response to exogenous K⁺ loading is less in newborn compared with older animals.

The limited K⁺ secretory capacity of the immature kidney becomes clinically relevant only under conditions of K⁺ excess. Under normal circumstances, K⁺ retention by the newborn kidney is appropriate and a requirement for growth.

## Sites of K⁺ transport in the kidney

Micropuncture studies indicate that approximately 50 per cent of the filtered load of K⁺ is reabsorbed along the initial two-thirds of the superficial proximal tubule of the suckling rat (Fig. 91.1). In contrast to the situation in the adult, up to 40 per cent of the filtered load of K⁺ reaches the superficial distal tubule of the newborn (Fig. 91.1), providing evidence for functional immaturity of the loop of Henle. Estimates of the mass flow of K⁺ entering the tubular fluid between the late distal tubule and final urine suggest that the

rate of K⁺ secretion along the intervening nephron segments, i.e. the collecting ducts, is less in the newborn compared with that in the adult. Recent studies of cortical collecting ducts microperfused *in vitro* confirm that segments isolated from neonatal animals show negligible K⁺ secretion into the tubular fluid (Fig. 91.6).

## Regulation of K⁺ transport in the neonate

Net K⁺ secretion in the cortical collecting duct reflects the sum of the opposing processes of K⁺ secretion by principal cells and K⁺ absorption by intercalated cells. The limited capacity of the immature principal cell for K⁺ secretion may be due to a low electrochemical gradient across the luminal membrane, a limited apical permeability to K⁺ and/or Na⁺ or a low activity of the Na⁺-K⁺ pump. Both a high rate of K⁺ absorption by intercalated cells possessing apical H⁺-K⁺-ATPase and

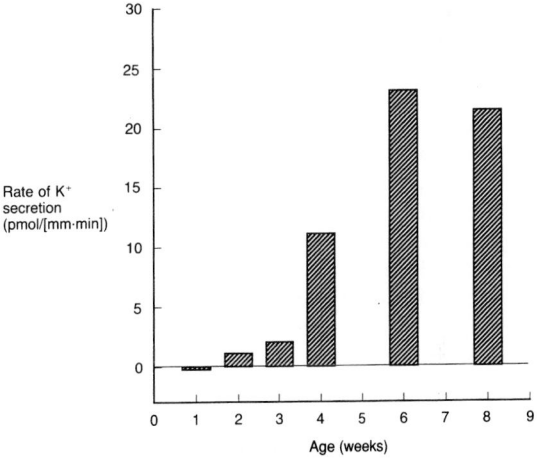

FIGURE 91.6 Relationship between postnatal age and net K⁺ secretion in microperfused cortical collecting ducts isolated from maturing rabbits. No net K⁺ secretion is observed until the fourth week of postnatal life; 8-week-old rabbits are considered to be adults. (Modified from Satlin LM. *Am J Physiol* 1994; **266**: F59, with permission.)

TABLE 91.2 Mean plasma concentrations and renal clearance of K⁺ for infants and children without significant renal disease on regular diet

| AGE (years) | $P_{K^+}$ (mEq/L) | $C_{cr}$ (mL/[1.73 m² · min]) | $C_{K^+}$ (mL/[1.73 m² · min]) | FEK⁺ (%) | $U_{Na^+/K^+}$ |
|---|---|---|---|---|---|
| 0–4 months | 5.2†‡ | 62†‡§ | 4.8†‡§ | 8.5†‡ | 1.1 |
| 5 months–1 year | 4.9†‡ | 99†‡ | 13.5† | 14.6 | 0.8 |
| 3–10 | 4.2 | 141 | 19.6 | 14.5 | 1.5 |
| 11–20 | 4.3 | 137 | 21.2 | 16.2 | 1.4 |

$P_{K^+}$, plasma K⁺ concentration; $C_{cr}$, glomerular filtration rate (calculated as renal excretion/plasma level); $C_{K^+}$, renal clearance of K⁺ (calculated as renal excretion/plasma level); FEK⁺, fractional excretion of K⁺; $U_{Na^+/K^+}$, urinary Na⁺/K⁺ ratio.
†$P < 0.05$ vs 11–20 years. ‡$P < 0.05$ vs 3–10 years. §$P < 0.05$ vs 5 months–1 year.
From Satlin LM, Schwartz GJ. Metabolism of potassium. In: Ichikawa I, ed. *Pediatric textbook of fluids and electrolytes*. Baltimore, Williams & Wilkins, 1990: 90, with permission.

substantial paracellular backleak, if present in the neonatal tubule, may further reduce net urinary K+ loss.

Assuming that K+ activity bears a constant relationship to concentration throughout postnatal life, cell K+ content in the neonatal cortical collecting duct is similar to that measured in the mature segment, averaging 120 mmol/L intracellular water. Yet Na+-K+-ATPase activity in neonatal segments is only 50 per cent of that measured in the mature nephron. Taken together, these findings suggest that a low apical membrane permeability to K+, possibly due to a paucity of conducting channels, restricts K+ exit from principal cells; such a situation would both maintain cell K+ concentration and limit K+ movement from cell to lumen. Whereas the "chemical" component of the electrochemical gradient driving K+ secretion appears to remain constant during postnatal life, the "electrical" component has not been rigorously examined.

The rate of distal tubular flow is presumed to be low early in postnatal life due to the prevailing low single nephron glomerular filtration rate. In the adult, K+ secretion in the cortical collecting duct is profoundly influenced by the rate of tubular flow (Fig. 91.3); thus, a low urinary flow rate could theoretically limit K+ secretion in the neonatal distal nephron. However, microperfused cortical collecting ducts isolated from newborn animals show only a negligible rise in net K+ secretion in response to an increase in tubular fluid flow rate. These results suggest that low distal tubular flow rates *in vivo* do not limit urinary K+ excretion in the neonate.

Electrogenic Na+ transport generates the lumen-negative potential difference across the cortical collecting duct, which in turn influences the magnitude of K+ secretion. Studies of microperfused rabbit cortical collecting ducts indicate that the capacity for Na+ reabsorption appears earlier in postnatal life than that for K+ secretion. The contribution of a maturational increase in Na+ entry into the principal cell towards activation of K+ secretion remains to be examined.

Plasma aldosterone concentrations in the newborn are higher than those in the adult, yet clearance studies demonstrate a relative insensitivity of the immature kidney to this hormone. The density of aldosterone-binding sites and receptor affinity are similar in mature and immature rats, suggesting that the early hyposensitivity to aldosterone represents a postreceptor phenomenon.

Thus, the neonatal cortical collecting duct is well adapted to retain K+, a necessary condition for growth. The postnatal onset of K+ secretion in the distal nephron may reflect activation of principal cell secretory pathways and/or modification of absorptive and paracellular transport pathways.

## SELECTED READING

Giebisch G, Malnic G, Berliner RW. Renal transport and control of K+ excretion. In: Brenner BM, Rector FC Jr, eds. *The kidney*, Vol I. Philadelphia: WB Saunders, 1991: 283.

Lelievre-Pegorier M, Merlet-Benichou C, Roinel N, de Rouffignac C. Developmental pattern of water and electrolyte transport in rat superficial nephrons. *Am J Physiol* 1983; 245: F15.

Satlin LM. Maturation of renal K+ transport. *Pediatr Nephrol* 1991; 5: 260.

Satlin LM. Postnatal maturation of potassium transport in rabbit cortical collecting duct. *Am J Physiol* 1994; 266: F57.

Satlin LM, Schwartz GJ. Renal regulation of K+ homeostasis. In: Edelmann CM Jr, ed. *Pediatric kidney diseases*. Boston: Little, Brown and Company, 1992: 127.

# RENAL CALCIUM AND PHOSPHORUS HOMEOSTASIS

## CALCIUM (see also Chapter 43)

Urinary Ca2+ excretion is low in the first few months of life in both preterm and term infants, and rises progressively over the next several weeks. By 3 months of age, urinary Ca2+ excretion, normalized by body surface area, is comparable to that in adults. Other than providing a general description of Ca2+ handling by the infant, few studies have specifically examined the renal regulation of Ca2+ homeostasis during development. Therefore, the basic principles described below are largely derived from studies in adults. Nevertheless, it is clear that the regulation of Ca2+ homeostasis involves two important elements: first, maintenance of positive Ca2+ balance, meaning that Ca2+ output (excretion) is less than Ca2+ input (dietary intake) so that sufficient Ca2+ is provided for the growing tissues; and second, maintenance of plasma Ca2+ concentration within a narrow range, which serves to minimize changes in the electrochemical Ca2+ gradient across the cell membranes that could greatly affect cell function. These processes occur through the coordinated action of several hormonal systems, principally parathyroid hormone (PTH), calcitonin, and vitamin D, acting on bone, gastrointestinal tract, and the kidney.

More than 98 per cent of total body Ca2+ is contained in the skeleton, one-third of which is readily exchangeable with the extracellular fluid. Of the Ca2+ circulating in plasma, approximately one-half exists in the free, ionized form, another 10 per cent is complexed to various anions such as phosphate, bicarbonate, citrate, and sulfate, and the rest represents Ca2+ that is bound to protein (primarily albumin).

The homeostatic regulation of Ca2+ balance occurs largely at the level of the intestine, where adjustments in the rate of Ca2+ absorption control the influx of Ca2+ into the extracellular pool. The role of the kidneys in Ca2+ homeostasis is to reabsorb essentially all

(98 per cent) of the filtered $Ca^{2+}$ and to limit urinary $Ca^{2+}$ losses. Consequently, the kidney functions as an important contributor, rather than a primary regulator of $Ca^{2+}$ balance.

## Tubular handling of calcium

Approximately 60 per cent of the total plasma $Ca^{2+}$ (representing the ionized and complexed forms) is filtered at the glomerulus. However, only 2 per cent of the filtered $Ca^{2+}$ load is normally excreted in the urine. The bulk of $Ca^{2+}$ reabsorption (50–60 per cent) occurs in the proximal tubule (both proximal convoluted and proximal straight segments) by a process that is linked to $Na^+$ reabsorption (Fig. 91.7). This involves mostly passive $Ca^{2+}$ diffusion, occurring via the paracellular pathway, although there is evidence for a small active transport component as well (Fig. 91.8).

In the loop of Henle, the thin descending and ascending limbs are reportedly impermeable to $Ca^{2+}$. The thick ascending limb, however, is a significant site where about 20 per cent of the filtered $Ca^{2+}$ load is reabsorbed. The transport of $Na^+$, $K^+$, and $Cl^-$ in this segment, via a $Na^+$-$K^+$-$Cl^-$ carrier, results in a lumen-positive transepithelial potential difference. This, together with thehigh permeability of this segment to $Ca^{2+}$, drives the passive, paracellular reabsorption of $Ca^{2+}$. In addition, $Ca^{2+}$ is reabsorbed actively, particularly in the cortical thick ascending limb, by a transport system that is stimulated by PTH.

The distal convoluted tubule and the cortical collecting tubule are nephron segments that actively transport $Ca^{2+}$ and are PTH-dependent. These sites combine to reabsorb efficiently 10–15 per cent of the filtered $Ca^{2+}$, and serve to minimize loss of $Ca^{2+}$ in the urine.

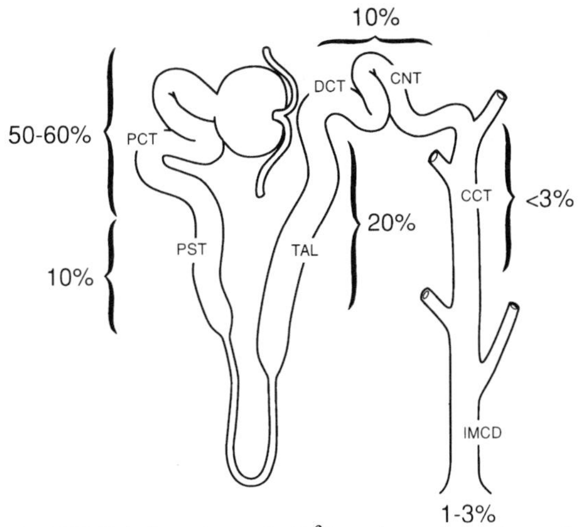

## Cellular mechanisms of renal calcium transport

Renal $Ca^{2+}$ transport occurs through several mechanisms, involving both transcellular and paracellular pathways. $Ca^{2+}$ enters the tubular cells by passive diffusion down its electrochemical gradient, as well as by facilitated diffusion via $Ca^{2+}$-binding protein carriers. The translocation of intracellular $Ca^{2+}$ ions to the basolateral membrane is not well defined, but appears to involve cytosolic $Ca^{2+}$-binding proteins and the action of mitochondria and other organelles, which "shuttle" $Ca^{2+}$ from the luminal to the basolateral membrane. Because of the low intracellular $Ca^{2+}$ concentration, exit across the basolateral membrane into the extracellular fluid occurs against an electrochemical gradient and is energy-dependent, primarily through $Na^+$-$Ca^{2+}$ countertransporters, and $Ca^{2+}$-activated ATPases (Fig. 91.8).

The movement of $Ca^{2+}$ between renal epithelial cells occurs passively by diffusion, and depends upon the transepithelial electrochemical gradient and permeability characteristics of the cell membranes and tight junctions in the various nephron segments.

## Factors regulating renal calcium reabsorption

PTH decreases the urinary excretion of $Ca^{2+}$, an action consistent with its overall function to protect against large declines in the plasma $Ca^{2+}$ concentration. PTH stimulates bone resorption, which releases $Ca^{2+}$ and

FIGURE 91.7 Tubular sites of $Ca^{2+}$ reabsorption along the nephron. The percentage of filtered $Ca^{2+}$ reabsorbed in the various segments is indicated. The numbers at the end of the IMCD segment represent the fraction of filtered $Ca^{2+}$ excretion. PCT, proximal convoluted tubule; PST, proximal straight tubule; TAL, thick ascending limb of the loop of Henle; DCT, distal convoluted tubule; CNT, connecting tubule; CCT, cortical collecting tubule; IMCD, inner medullary collecting duct.

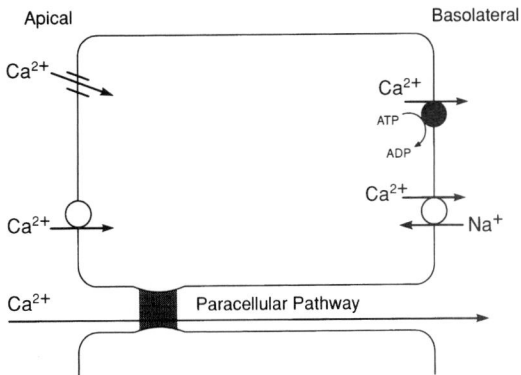

FIGURE 91.8 Model of transepithelial $Ca^{2+}$ transport in renal tubules. The amount of $Ca^{2+}$ transport which passes through the paracellular pathways varies from 90 per cent (of the total) in proximal tubules to 50 per cent in the loop of Henle. No paracellular $Ca^{2+}$ transport is thought to occur in the distal convoluted tubules.

PO$_4$ to the extracellular fluid. However, the effects of PTH to decrease renal Ca$^{2+}$ excretion and increase PO$_4$ excretion assure that plasma Ca$^{2+}$, and not plasma PO$_4$, is elevated. At the tubular level, the action of PTH to increase Ca$^{2+}$ reabsorption in the loop of Henle and distal nephron segments is mediated by membrane receptors coupled to adenylyl cyclase and the subsequent generation of cAMP as a second messenger. The PTH receptor–adenylyl cyclase–cAMP pathway is active in the fetal and postnatal kidney, but is not as responsive as in the adult kidney.

Vitamin D plays a key role in raising the plasma Ca$^{2+}$ concentration through stimulation of intestinal Ca$^{2+}$ absorption. This role is particularly important in the period between weaning and puberty, when there is an increase in the activity of the renal 1-hydroxylase, which converts 25(OH) vitamin D to its active form of 1,25(OH)$_2$ vitamin D. Indeed, the renal production of 1,25(OH)$_2$ vitamin D increases rapidly during this period of growth, provided sufficient amounts of the substrate (25(OH) vitamin D) are available. Whether vitamin D also contributes directly to enhancing renal Ca$^{2+}$ reabsorption in the neonate is unknown.

Because of the dependence of Ca$^{2+}$ reabsorption on NaCl transport in the proximal tubule and the Na$^+$-K$^+$-Cl$^-$ cotransporter in the loop of Henle, factors that increase NaCl excretion, such as administration of diuretics that act at those sites, or expansion of the extracellular volume, also cause parallel increases in Ca$^{2+}$ excretion. However, thiazide diuretics reduce urinary Ca$^{2+}$ excretion. This decrease results from a direct effect of the thiazide diuretics to enhance distal tubule Ca$^{2+}$ reabsorption and not from a secondary effect of volume contraction.

Several other factors have been associated with altered urinary Ca$^{2+}$ excretion. For example, *hypercalciuria* occurs during reduced PO$_4$ uptake and in metabolic acidosis. Should these conditions continue for a prolonged period of time, the impairment in Ca$^{2+}$ balance will likely affect growth adversely.

## PHOSPHORUS (see also Chapter 43)

In the neonatal and prepubertal period, the regulation of PO$_4$ homeostasis is crucial to proper growth and development. As with Ca$^{2+}$, the neonate maintains positive balance for PO$_4$. This is a consequence of a relatively high intake of PO$_4$, efficient intestinal absorption, and reduced urinary PO$_4$ excretion, all of which involve the integrated action of several hormonal systems. Unlike Ca$^{2+}$, the primary regulation of PO$_4$ homeostasis is at the level of the kidney, where adjustments in the rate of renal PO$_4$ reabsorption control the plasma PO$_4$ concentration and PO$_4$ balance.

The majority (80 per cent) of total body phosphorus is present in the skeleton, the rest being in soft tissues, muscle, and extracellular fluids. Two-thirds of the phosphorus in plasma is in the form of

organic phosphates (esters and phospholipids) and one-third is inorganic PO$_4$ (mostly orthophosphates). Most of the orthophosphates circulate as free phosphate in a 4:1 ratio of the dibasic (HPO$_4^{2-}$) to monobasic (H$_2$PO$_4^-$) form; these together with the small amounts of phosphate complexed with Ca$^{2+}$ and Mg$^{2+}$ or protein-bound are reported as the plasma PO$_4$ concentration. The plasma PO$_4$ concentration in infants and children is 50 per cent higher than that observed in adults, which is a consequence of the relatively high rate of PO$_4$ reabsorption by the neonatal kidney.

## Tubular handling of phosphate

Approximately 90 per cent of the plasma PO$_4$ is freely filtered at the glomerulus. Under normal conditions, adult kidneys reabsorb 75–80 per cent of the filtered PO$_4$ load and excrete the rest. The bulk (60–70 per cent) of the filtered PO$_4$ is reabsorbed in the proximal convoluted tubule, and the remainder (10–15 per cent) is reabsorbed in the proximal straight tubule, distal convoluted tubule, and cortical collecting tubules (Fig. 91.9). The latter sites become most significant during states of PO$_4$ conservation such as hypoparathyroidism and dietary phosphate deprivation, where complete reabsorption of the filtered PO$_4$ load can occur.

The neonate, with a rapid growth rate and large PO$_4$ requirement, normally reabsorbs about 90 per

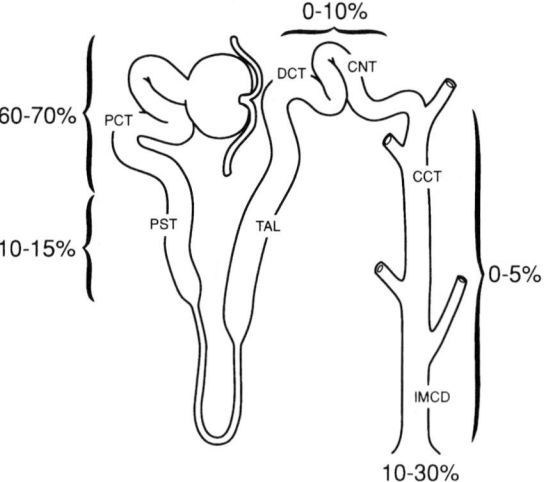

FIGURE 91.9 Tubular sites of PO$_4$ reabsorption along the nephron. The percentage of filtered PO$_4$ reabsorbed in the various segments is indicated. The numbers at the end of the IMCD segment represent the fraction of filtered PO$_4$ excreted. PCT, proximal convoluted tubule; PST, proximal straight tubule; TAL, thick ascending limb of the loop of Henle; DCT, distal convoluted tubule; CNT, connecting tubule; CCT, cortical collecting tubule; IMCD, inner medullary collecting duct.

cent of the filtered $PO_4$. The proportionately greater conservation of $PO_4$ involves enhanced reabsorption in the proximal convoluted tubule and in more distal segments. However, the precise sites and mechanisms of increased $PO_4$ transport are not known.

Another important element that may explain the renal retention of $PO_4$ in the neonate is nephron heterogeneity. The capacity to transport $PO_4$ is greater in deep (juxtamedullary) nephrons compared with superficial (cortical) nephrons. Because nephrogenesis begins in the corticomedullary region and proceeds toward the outer cortex, the relative preponderance of functioning deep nephrons in the juxtamedullary area of the immature kidney may contribute to its overall enhanced capacity for tubular $PO_4$ reabsorption.

## Cellular mechanisms of renal phosphate transport

Transcellular $PO_4$ transport is a $Na^+$-coupled, electroneutral, secondary active process, which depends on an electrochemical gradient for $Na^+$ entry into the cell, generated by the $Na^+$-$K^+$-ATPase pump on the basolateral membrane of the proximal tubule cell. $PO_4$ enters the cell via specific $Na^+$-$PO_4$ carrier proteins on the proximal tubule brush border membrane. In the cell, $PO_4$ can be incorporated into various organic compounds through one of several biosynthetic pathways, or it can simply pass through the cell. The amount of $PO_4$ exiting the cell can vary depending on the metabolic needs of the cell. When the intracellular $PO_4$ pool increases, $PO_4$ leaves the cell passively down its electrochemical gradient and crosses the basolateral membrane via both $Na^+$-dependent and $Na^+$-independent carriers (Fig. 91.10).

Evidence from animal studies indicates that proximal tubule brush-border $PO_4$ uptake is higher in neo-

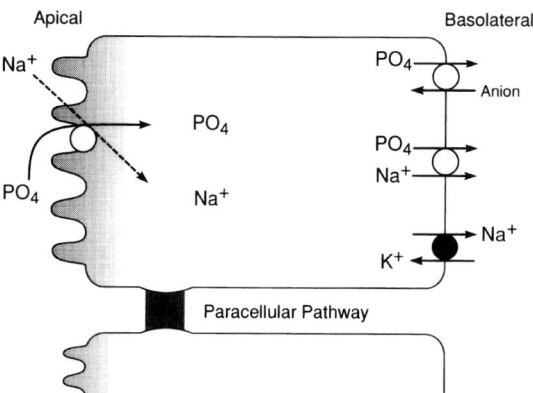

FIGURE 91.10 Model of transepithelial $PO_4$ transport in renal proximal tubules. $PO_4$ enters the cells via a $Na^+$–$PO_4$ cotransporter located on the apical brush border membrane (shaded area). $PO_4$ exits cells via $Na^+$-dependent and $Na^+$-independent carriers. (At pH 7.4, $PO_4$ will be in a 4:1 ratio of the dibasic ($HPO_4^{2-}$) to monobasic ($H_2PO_4^-$) form.)

nates compared with adults as a result of an increased velocity of $PO_4$ transport ($V_{max}$). This could occur from either an increased turnover rate or an increased number of $Na^+$-$PO_4$ cotransporters in the neonatal kidney. Interestingly, studies examining renal intracellular $PO_4$ concentrations have shown lower levels in kidneys of neonates compared with adults, despite the higher rate of $PO_4$ entry into the tubular cells. This suggests that the rate of basolateral $PO_4$ efflux must also be higher in newborns. With the recent cloning of several different $Na^+$-$PO_4$ cotransporters, ideal tools are now in hand to address some of the unanswered questions regarding the cellular mechanisms of renal $PO_4$ transport during growth and development.

## Factors regulating renal phosphate reabsorption

Because the rate-limiting step in transepithelial $PO_4$ transport is at the level of the luminal $Na^+$-$PO_4$ cotransporter, $PO_4$ reabsorption by the kidney as a whole is a saturable process, characterized by a transport maximum (TmPi). However, the TmPi is not a fixed value and can be affected by hormones, dietary $PO_4$, and other factors, including age. Indeed, the TmPi in the neonate (corrected for body surface area, glomerular filtration rate (GFR), or kidney mass) is relatively greater compared with adults, and contributes to the elevated plasma $PO_4$ concentration. Thus, the high rate of renal $PO_4$ retention in the neonate is not a result of limited $PO_4$ excretion due to a low GFR, but rather the result of several different factors acting in concert specifically to elevate the tubular transport of $PO_4$ during development.

The principal hormonal regulator of $PO_4$ transport is PTH. Decreased plasma $Ca^{2+}$ concentrations stimulate PTH release, which acts to increase $Ca^{2+}$ and reduce $PO_4$ reabsorption by the kidney. Studies in both human infants and immature animals indicate that the response in newborns to the phosphaturic, but not the hypocalciuric, effects of PTH is reduced compared with adults. This occurs despite normal circulating concentrations of PTH postnatally and normal generation of the second messenger for PTH (cAMP). This aspect of reduced PTH responsiveness may account, in part, for the high renal retention of $PO_4$ in the young.

Another fundamental regulator of renal $PO_4$ transport is dietary $PO_4$. An increase in $PO_4$ intake in adults results in a rise in urinary $PO_4$ excretion because of a rapid decrease in TmPi. Although the neonate responds to an increase in dietary $PO_4$ with a reduction in TmPi, the change is much smaller. Ostensibly, this may serve to maintain $PO_4$ balance. However, because the TmPi remains high in the newborn fed high dietary $PO_4$, an excessive increase in dietary $PO_4$ could lead to hyperphosphatemia, resulting in decreased plasma $Ca^{2+}$ concentration and *secondary hyperparathyroidism*.

Conversely, dietary $PO_4$ deprivation increases renal $PO_4$ reabsorption, an effect that is relatively greater in the neonate compared with the adult. However, because of the very high requirements of the newborn for $PO_4$, a diet too low in $PO_4$ may lead to hypophosphatemia, $PO_4$ depletion, and reduced growth rate despite the complete tubular reabsorption of filtered $PO_4$.

Growth hormone is also an important factor regulating renal $PO_4$ reabsorption, particularly during the period of rapid growth. *Growth hormone deficiency* is associated with reduced growth rate, hypophosphatemia, and increased urinary $PO_4$ excretion, whereas the opposite has been reported with growth hormone hypersecretion. Recently, results from animal studies established an important link between the growth-promoting effects of growth hormone and renal $PO_4$ reabsorption. When the pulsatile release of growth hormone was specifically suppressed in weanling rats using a synthetic antagonist to growth hormone-releasing factor, the growth rate was attenuated and positive $PO_4$ balance was reduced due to a rapid decrease in the TmPi. Indeed, the TmPi was reduced to levels seen in adult rats. By contrast, no effect was seen on the tubular capacity to reabsorb $PO_4$ in adult rats. Furthermore, suppression of growth hormone release in weanling rats also restored a phosphaturic response to PTH similar to that seen in adults. Although the kidney contains growth hormone receptors, it is not clear whether the effects of growth hormone on $PO_4$ transport are direct, or occur indirectly through the action of insulin-like growth factor I (IGF-I), the purported mediator of the somatogenic effects of growth hormone. Indeed, IGF-I has been shown to directly stimulate $PO_4$ transport in tubules and cells. These findings suggest that the growth hormone/IGF-I system may play a critical role in enhancing renal $PO_4$ reabsorption during development, and in this way ensures that adequate amounts of $PO_4$ are provided to meet the demand for growth.

## SELECTED READING

Berndt TJ, Knox FG. Renal handling of phosphate. In: Massry SG, Glassock RJ, eds. *Textbook of nephrology*, 3rd edn, Vol 1, Chapter 22, Part 2. Baltimore: Williams & Wilkins, 1995: 389.

Caverzasio J, Bonjour JP. IGF-I, a key regulator of renal phosphate transport and 1,25-dihydroxyvitamin D3 production during growth. *News Physiol Sci*. 1991; 6: 206.

Friedman PA, Gesek, FA. Calcium transport in renal epithelial cells. *Am J Physiol* 1993; 264: F181.

Haramati A, Mulroney SE, Lumpkin MD. Regulation of renal phosphate reabsorption during development: implications from a new model of growth hormone deficiency. *Pediatr Nephrol* 1990; 4: 387.

Murer H. Cellular mechanisms in proximal tubular Pi-reabsorption: some answers and more questions. *J Am Soc Nephrol* 1992; 2: 1649.

Murer H, Werner A, Reshkin S, Wuarin F, Biber J. Cellular mechanisms in proximal tubular reabsorption of inorganic phosphate. *Am J Physiol* 1991; 260: C885.

Rouse D, Suki WN. Renal handling of calcium. In: Massry SG, Glassock RJ, eds. *Textbook of nephrology*, 3rd edn, Vol 1, Chapter 20, Part 2. Baltimore: Williams & Wilkins, 1995: 339.

Stewart CL, Devarajan P, Mulroney SE, Kaskel FJ, Haramati A. Transport of calcium and phosphorus. In: Polin RA, Fox WW, eds. *Fetal and neonatal physiology*, Vol II. Philadelphia: WB Saunders, 1992: 1223.

# 92

# Acid–Base Regulation

Pedro A. Jose and Gilbert M. Eisner

Selected reading 958

The kidneys maintain normal acid–base balance by reclaiming filtered bicarbonate and by excreting the salts of non-volatile acids produced each day by cellular metabolism. This is accomplished by the urinary secretion of $H^+$ produced by renal tubular cells. Qualitative and quantitative differences exist between the mature and developing organism. In particular, the rate of production of non-volatile acids by an infant [2 mEq/(kg · day)], as a result of a higher metabolic rate and protein intake, is twice that of the adult. Most nephron segments can reabsorb bicarbonate, but the majority (80 per cent or more) of filtered bicarbonate is reabsorbed in the proximal tubule. The thick ascending limb and distal convoluted tubule reabsorb 10 and 6 per cent, respectively. The cortical collecting system is capable of either net bicarbonate secretion or reabsorption (4 per cent).

The non-volatile acids produced by cellular metabolism are excreted by the kidney in the form of titratable acids and ammonium salts. The formation of titratable acid and ammonium ions ($NH_4^+$) results in the generation of new bicarbonate. As in the reclamation of filtered bicarbonate, the proximal tubule is also the major site of the formation of titratable acids and $NH_4^+$. Additional titratable acids are generated along the collecting ducts. After 3 days of an acid load, titratable acid production may increase two- to three-fold, while $NH_4^+$ production may increase six- to seven-fold. Titratable acid is determined by measuring the amount of hydroxyl ions (e.g. NaOH) required to titrate the urine back to the pH of blood. Filtered phosphate is the major component of titratable acids with some contribution from urate, creatinine, sulfate, and β-hydroxybutyrate.

The cellular mechanism involved in the secretion of $H^+$ is an essential step in the reabsorption of bicarbonate and formation of titratable acids. $H^+$ ions generated in the cell (resulting from the dissociation of $H_2CO_3$ into $H^+$ and $HCO_3^-$) are secreted at the luminal membrane by exchanging intracellular $H^+$ with luminal $Na^+$ and by electrogenic transport of $H^+$. The $Na^+$-$H^+$ exchanger (NHE-3) found in the apical membrane of the proximal tubule and thick ascending limb of Henle is responsible for most of the $H^+$ secretion in the proximal tubule (about 65 per cent). Electrogenic transport by $H^+$-ATPase accounts for the rest of $H^+$ secretion. $H^+$-ATPase is present throughout the nephron, but there is marked species variation. Two possible fates of $H^+$ ions secreted into the tubular lumen include: (1) reaction with filtered $HCO_3^-$ to form $H_2CO_3$, and (2) reaction with $HPO_4^{2-}$ to form $H_2PO_4^-$ (titratable acids). $H_2CO_3$ formed in the tubular lumen (from 1) is broken down to $H_2O$ and $CO_2$ by carbonic anhydrase (isoform 2) that is present in the brush border of proximal tubules. The luminal presence of this enzyme, by preventing too rapid a fall in intraluminal pH, allows relatively complete absorption of $HCO_3^-$ because proximal tubules cannot maintain a steep $H^+$ gradient. The tubular fluid pH at the late proximal convoluted tubule is 6.7. In more distal segments of the nephron, luminal $H_2CO_3$ slowly forms into $CO_2$ and $H_2O$ because the luminal membranes do not contain carbonic anhydrase. In the collecting ducts, where a steep $H^+$ gradient can be maintained, the pH of tubular fluid can decrease to as low as 4.5. In the proximal tubule, the $HCO_3^-$ remaining within the cell after the generation and secretion of $H^+$ is transported out of the cell at the basolateral membrane via a $Cl^-$-$HCO_3^-$ exchanger and a $Na^+$-$HCO_3^-$ cotransporter (Fig. 92.1).

The cortical collecting duct can reabsorb and secrete $HCO_3^-$ at its luminal membrane. $HCO_3^-$ reabsorption occurs as a result of $H^+$ secretion via the $H^+$-ATPase at the luminal membrane of the intercalated cell (type A). The intracellular $HCO_3^-$ exits at the basolateral membrane via the $Cl^-$-$HCO_3^-$ exchanger. When the $H^+$-ATPase is located at the basolateral side and the $Cl^-$-$HCO_3^-$ exchanger is located at the luminal side, the intercalated cell of the cortical collecting duct becomes a $HCO_3^-$ secreting cell (type B) (Fig. 92.2). The collecting ducts of the outer medulla also secrete $H^+$ via a $H^+$-ATPase mechanism.

The other mechanism by which the kidney excretes non-volatile acids depends on $NH_4^+$ production. This occurs in the proximal tubule by breakdown of glutamine. Two-thirds of glutamine comes from the plasma

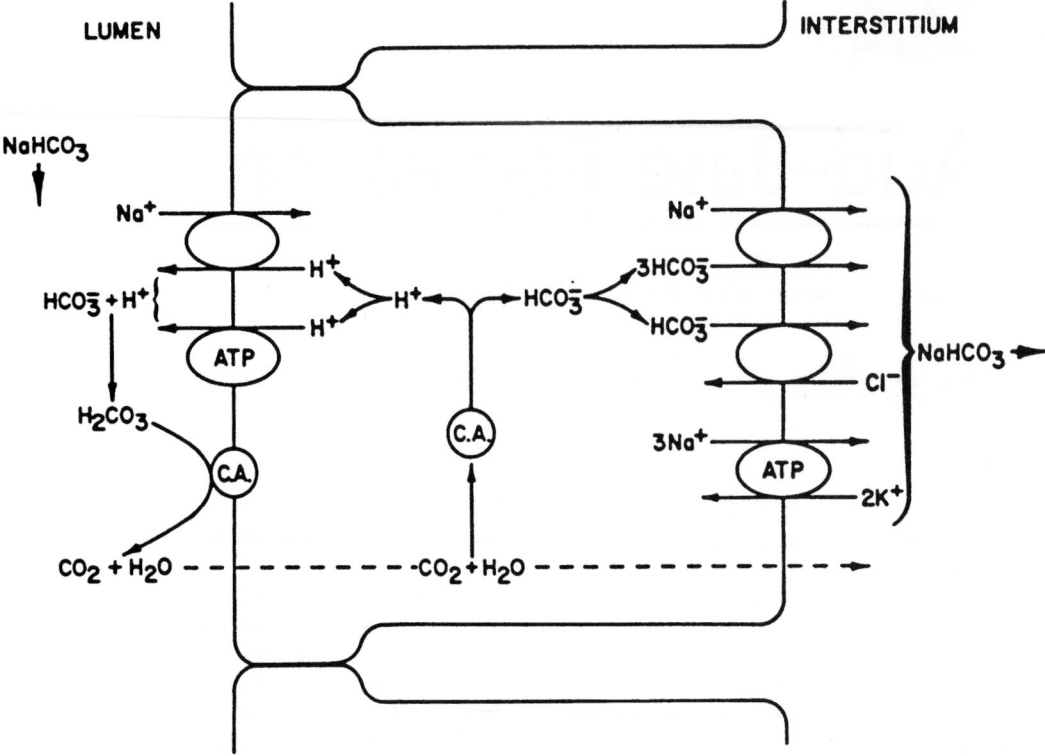

FIGURE 92.1 Cellular mechanisms for bicarbonate reabsorption by the proximal tubule and thick ascending limb of Henle. Carbonic anhydrase (C.A. type II) is responsible for the generation of $H^+$ ions inside the cell and the breakdown of $H_2CO_3$ at the luminal membrane. In the adult rat proximal tubule, secretion of $H^+$ ions in the luminal membrane occurs mainly via the $Na^+$–$H^+$ exchanger type III (65 per cent); the rest is accounted for by $H^+$-ATPase. The gradient favoring the entry of $Na^+$ into the cell in exchange for $H^+$ is generated by the sodium pump, $Na^+$-$K^+$-ATPase, located in the basolateral membrane. The transport of $HCO_3^-$ across the basolateral membrane into the interstitium is due mainly (90 per cent) to the action of a $Na^+$-$HCO_3^-$ cotransporter; the rest is due to the action of a $Cl^-$-$HCO_3^-$ exchanger. The $Na^+$-$H^+$ exchanger, type 1, expressed in basolateral membranes, is involved in the regulation of intracellular pH and volume and does not contribute to $HCO_3^-$ transport. Similar mechanisms exist in the thick ascending limb of Henle. (From Koeppen BM, Giebisch G. Segmental hydrogen ion transport. In: Seldin DW, Giebisch G, eds. *The regulation of acid–base balance*. New York: Raven Press, 1989: 139.)

and the rest from renal tubular metabolism. Glutamine is converted to glutamate and $NH_4^+$.

$$Glutamine + H_2O \rightarrow glutamate + NH_4^+$$

Glutamate thus formed is converted further to $\alpha$-keto-glutarate and another molecule of $NH_4^+$.

$$Glutamate + H_2O + NAD \rightarrow \alpha\text{-ketoglutarate} + NADH + NH_4^+$$

The metabolism of $\alpha$-ketoglutarate via the Krebs cycle results in the release of two molecules of $HCO_3^-$. The $NH_4^+$ formed is secreted into the proximal tubule and can be excreted into the urine. If $NH_4^+$ is not excreted in the urine, it is returned to the circulation where it is converted to urea in the liver, resulting in the generation of $H^+$ (*see also* Chapter 5).

$$2NH_4^+ + CO_2 \rightarrow 2H^+ + urea + H_2O$$

The $2H^+$ generated during urea formation in the liver would then neutralize the $2HCO_3^-$ generated by the proximal tubule during $NH_4^+$ formation. This results in zero net gain of $HCO_3^-$. As it turns out, under normal conditions, only 50 per cent of the $NH_4^+$ formed is secreted in the proximal tubule and 50 per cent is returned into the circulation. The $NH_4^+$ secreted into the proximal tubule is reabsorbed by the cells of the ascending loop of Henle, to a large extent by the $Na^+$-$K^+$ ($NH_4^+$)-$2Cl^-$ cotransporter and to a lesser extent by a $K^+$-$NH_4^+$ ($H^+$) cotransporter and by voltage-driven diffusion. The reabsorbed $NH_4^+$ exits at the basolateral membrane via several mechanisms [$Na^+$-$K^+$ ($NH_4^+$)-ATPase, barium, and furosemide-sensitive $K^+$ ($NH_4^+$)-$Cl^-$ cotransporter, NHE-1 exchanger, and $K^+$ ($NH_4^+$)-$HCO_3^-$ cotransporter]. In the medullary interstitium, the reabsorbed $NH_4^+$ splits into $NH_3$ and $H^+$. $NH_3$ can diffuse into the descending limb of Henle; $NH_4^+$ could also enter

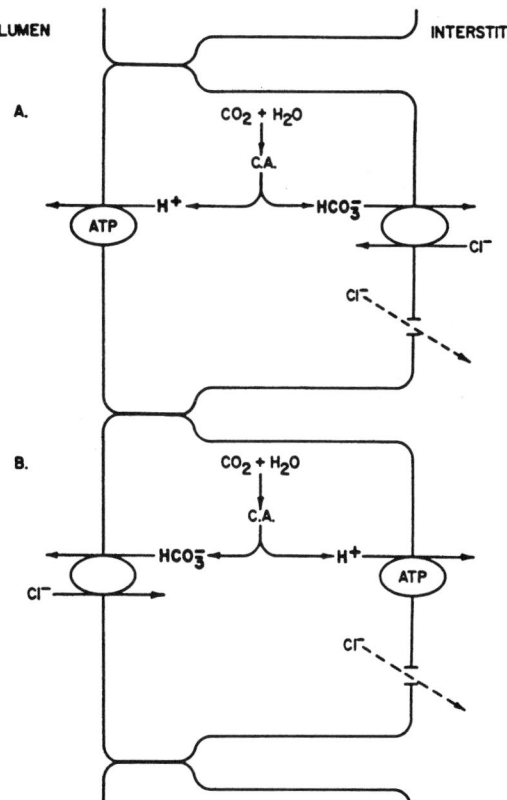

LUMEN INTERSTITIUM

A.

B.

FIGURE 92.2 Cellular mechanisms for bicarbonate reabsorption (A cell) and secretion (B cell) by the intercalated cells of the collecting duct. In the cortical collecting duct, the secretion of $H^+$ ions and reabsorption of $HCO_3^-$ ions occur in the A cells; the secretion of $HCO_3^-$ ions occurs in the B cells. Note that in the A cells, the $H^+$-ATPase is at the luminal membrane and the $Cl^-$–$HCO_3^-$ exchanger is at the basolateral membrane (interstitial side); the converse arrangement exists in the B cell. In the outer and inner medullary collecting duct, $HCO_3^-$ reabsorption occurs via the same mechanism as that in A cells; there is no $HCO_3^-$ secretion. (From Koeppen BM, Giebisch G. Segmental hydrogen ion transport. In: Seldin DW, Giebisch G, eds. *The regulation of acid–base balance*. New York: Raven Press, 1989: 139.)

at this site. This countercurrent multiplier mechanism contributes to the accumulation of $NH_4^+$ in the medulla. The high medullary concentration of $NH_3$ and luminal acidification at the collecting ducts create a favorable gradient for $NH_3$ diffusion, and therefore secretion of $NH_4^+$ into the medullary collecting duct. $NH_3$ cannot diffuse into the thin ascending limb of Henle because of its low permeability to $NH_3$.

Urine pH, under normal conditions with the usual diet (and after the first 2 weeks postnatally in term newborns), is usually acidic (pH 6.1). The minimum urinary pH is about 4.5 while the maximum urinary pH is about 8.5. The net amount of acid excretion (NAE) by the kidney is the sum of ammonium excretion and titratable acids minus urine bicarbonate.

$$NAE = NH_4^+ + \text{titratable acids} - HCO_3^-$$

Under these conditions, 50 per cent of NAE is contributed by $NH_4^+$ excretion while the other 50 per cent is contributed by titratable acids. Several factors affect urinary acid excretion in the normal state. These include distal $Na^+$ delivery, nature and quantity of anion delivered to the distal tubule, aldosterone, and ammoniagenesis. A reduction in distal $Na^+$ delivery decreases distal urinary acidification. The converse occurs; thus distal tubular acidification can be stimulated by natriuretic agents (e.g. furosemide). "Non-reabsorbable" anions delivered to the distal tubule increase $H^+$ secretion (e.g. sulfates, penicillins). Aldosterone modulates renal acid production by increasing $Na^+$ reabsorption and creating a positive transtubular potential gradient for $H^+$ secretion, by stimulating the $H^+$ pump, and by increasing ammoniagenesis. Several factors control $NH_4^+$ secretion into the tubular lumen. Factors that are inversely correlated with ammonium secretion include urine pH and $K^+$. Factors that are positively correlated with ammonium secretion include glomerular filtration rate, capillary blood flow, and tubular flow.

Acid–base balance in the fetus is mainly dependent on maternal control mechanisms. However, the fetal kidney, at least after the second half of pregnancy, is able to acidify the urine. Growth is associated with a positive $H^+$ balance. Moreover, the $H^+$ load (sum of intake and production) is 2 mmol/(kg·day) compared with 1 mmol/(kg·day) in adults. In healthy preterm infants, during the first weeks of postnatal life, the anion gap (serum $Na^+$ minus serum bicarbonate and $Cl^-$) ranges from 15–22 mmol/L, compared with values of 9–12 mmol/L in term newborns and adults. Serum bicarbonate concentrations in preterm infants may be as low as 14 mmol/L compared with 21–22 mmol/L in full-term newborns. Serum bicarbonate concentrations increase with age (22 mmol/L in infants, 24 mmol/L in children, 24–26 mmol/L in adults). The low serum bicarbonate concentration in the newborn is in part due to a lower threshold for bicarbonate. Because 80 per cent or more of the filtered bicarbonate is reabsorbed by the proximal tubule, immaturity of proximal tubular bicarbonate reabsorption is a significant factor.

The ability of the newborn to acidify the urine and excrete an acid load is limited compared with the adult. Rapid postnatal maturation is achieved so that by 2 weeks of age, urine pH can be as low as 4.5. The ability of the newborn to excrete an acute acid load also matures rapidly and is achieved by 1–2 months of age. This is mainly due to rapid maturation of titratable acid excretion. The ability of the newborn to excrete a chronic acid load matures more slowly. This may be due to a slower maturation of ammonia production where adult levels are not attained until 2 years of age. Several conditions can enhance renal tubular acidification mechanisms. Pretreatment of infants with phosphate, change of formula from breast milk to cows' milk, or increase in protein intake improve the ability of the newborn to excrete titratable acids and ammonia.

The driving force for $H^+$ secretion via the $Na^+$-$H^+$ exchanger is the low intracellular $Na^+$ concentration maintained by the basolateral $Na^+$-$K^+$-ATPase. In several animal species, $Na^+$-$K^+$-ATPase activity is lower in newborns compared with adults. In rabbits, both $Na^+$-$H^+$ exchanger and $Na^+$-$(HCO_3^-)_3$ cotransporter activities are lower in fetuses and newborns compared with adults. Thus, an immaturity of the transporters mediating $H^+$ transport may explain the decreased bicarbonate threshold in the newborn rabbit. The maturation of bicarbonate reabsorption in renal proximal tubules is mainly due to the increase in luminal $Na^+$-$H^+$ exchanger activity with contributions from luminal $H^+$-ATPase and basolateral $Na^+$-$HCO_3^-$ cotransporter activities. Glucocorticoids accelerate the maturation of neonatal bicarbonate reabsorption and renal proximal tubular $Na^+$-$H^+$ exchanger activity. The glucocorticoid-induced increase in proximal tubular $Na^+$-$H^+$ exchanger activity is specific to the type 3 isoform (NHE-3). However, glucocorticoids do not seem to increase the maturation of the overall $Na^+$ reabsorption. The role of neurohormonal factors in the maturation of proximal tubular $H^+$ transport remains to be determined. In the adult, angiotensin II and α-adrenergic receptors are associated with stimulation of $Na^+$-$H^+$ exchanger activity while dopamine and parathyroid hormone are inhibitory. Angiotensin II, the most potent of the hormonal factors, has been shown to increase $Na^+$-$H^+$ exchanger activity in the fetal kidneys as well; however, dopamine is slightly inhibitory of the renal proximal luminal $Na^+$-$H^+$ exchanger in the young. In the newborn, angiotensin II activity is increased, while the converse is true for dopamine.

Cortical collecting duct type A and type B intercalated cells also undergo postnatal proliferation and differentiation. The ability of the cortical collecting ducts to secrete bicarbonate increases with maturation, but the ability of the outer medullary collecting duct to reabsorb bicarbonate closely approximates the adult. The immature B ($HCO_3^-$ secreting) intercalated cell in the cortical collecting duct is able to secrete $HCO_3^-$ at one-third the rate observed in mature intercalated cells. This decreased ability of immature intercalated cells in cortical collecting ducts to secrete $HCO_3^-$ is associated with a decreased number of type B intercalated cells. In the outer medullary collecting duct, where the percentage of type B cells is low even in adults, the percentage of type A cells increases with maturation. In the inner medullary collecting ducts, the intercalated cells decrease with maturation. Basolateral $Cl^-$-$HCO_3^-$ exchanger expression in collecting ducts also increases with maturation. The expression of the two isoforms of carbonic anhydrase (II and IV) expressed in the kidney also changes with maturation, but their roles in the functional maturation of acid secretion remain to be defined. Whether the same situation applies to human newborns is yet to be determined.

In summary, urinary acidification is a highly regulated function of the kidney requiring a coordinated activity of nephron segments with specific capabilities. New knowledge of the roles of different transporters has provided important insights into the cellular mechanisms of renal $H^+$ transport. The concept that most $H^+$ secretion occurs in the proximal tubule remains true. New concepts are that titratable acid formation occurs mainly in the proximal tubule, and that generation of "new" bicarbonate due to ammoniagenesis occurs as a result of the formation of bicarbonate from α-ketoglutarate during the process of $NH_4^+$ production by renal tubules. Differences between the young and the adult in their ability to acidify the urine and excrete an acid load are due to the ontogeny of renal hemodynamics and transport proteins.

## SELECTED READING

Amlal H, Paillard M, Bichara M. $Cl^-$-dependent $NH_4^+$ transport mechanisms in medullary thick ascending limb cells. *Am J Physiol* 1994; **267**: C1607.

Baum M, Quigley R. Maturation of proximal tubular acidification. *Pediatr Nephrol* 1993; **7**: 785.

Flessner MF, Knepper MA. Ammonium transport in collecting ducts. *Miner Electrolyte Metab* 1990; **16**: 299.

Kurtz I, Dass PD, Cramer S. The importance of renal ammonia metabolism to the whole body acid–base balance: a reanalysis of the pathophysiology of renal tubular acidosis. *Miner Electrolyte Metab* 1990; **16**: 331.

Seldin DW, Giebisch G. *The regulation of acid–base balance.* New York: Raven Press, 1989.

Wrong O. Distal renal tubular acidosis: the value of urinary pH, $pCO_2$, and $NH_4^+$ measurements. *Pediatr Nephrol* 1991; **5**: 249.

# 93

# Regulation of Water Balance

Aníta Aperia

## TUBULAR WATER REABSORPTION, CONCENTRATION, AND DILUTION OF URINE

The bulk of filtered salt and water is reabsorbed in the proximal tubule. Approximately 20 per cent of the filtrate is delivered to the loop of Henle. This fluid is still isotonic because in the leaky proximal tubule the osmotic gradient created by the reabsorption of salt is almost immediately dissipated by water reabsorption.

In the distal part of the nephron, water and salt reabsorption are regulated by separate mechanisms. The thick ascending limb (TAL) of Henle is water impermeable and has a high capacity to transport $Na^+$ against a gradient. The $Na^+$ pump, $Na^+$-$K^+$-ATPase, is more abundant in the TAL than in most other cells. Active $Na^+$ reabsorption in TAL is generally considered to be the initial event in the creation of the hypertonic medullary interstitium that is a prerequisite for the process that leads to the concentration of urine. The hypertonicity of the renal medulla is potentiated by countercurrent flow in the vasa recta and the loops of Henle. It is also potentiated by recirculation of urea reabsorbed in the distal nephron. Arginine vasopressin (AVP), the antidiuretic hormone, acts by rendering the collecting duct cell water permeable (see also Chapters 40 and 41). In the presence of saturating concentrations of AVP, water will diffuse freely into the medullary interstitium, and the osmolality of the final urine will equal the osmolality of the inner medulla, which is 800–1200 mosmol/kg $H_2O$ in mature kidneys. In the absence of AVP, the urine will have approximately the same osmolality as the fluid in the distal tubule, i.e. approximately 60–80 mosmol/kg $H_2O$ in a healthy adult man.

The process that leads to concentration and dilution of urine will regulate not only water balance but also the tonicity of extracellular fluids. By concentrating the urine, water will be reabsorbed in excess of $Na^+$ and hypertonicity will be adjusted. Dilution of urine will adjust a state of hypotonicity.

## AVP: REGULATION OF RELEASE AND MECHANISM OF ACTION

An increase in blood osmolality excites osmoreceptors located in the hypothalamus. This leads to a chain of events that results in the release of AVP from the pituitary gland. There are at least two major types of AVP receptors involved in circulatory or fluid balance homeostasis (see also Chapters 40 and 41). $V_2$ receptors, present in epithelial cells such as the collecting duct cells, control water retention and $V_1$ receptors, present in vascular smooth muscle, regulate pressor responses. The $V_2$ receptors are coupled to a $G_s$-protein and stimulate adenylyl cyclase activity. The $V_1$ receptors stimulate phospholipase C activity. Activation of the $V_1$ receptors in the vessels causes vascular constriction. Activation of $V_1$ receptors plays an important role in the response to large blood losses. Activation of the $V_2$ receptors leads to incorporation of an intracellular pool of membrane fragments containing water channels. The effect of $V_2$ receptors on the collecting duct is counteracted by prostaglandins.

In individuals with healthy kidneys, there is a characteristic relationship between serum concentrations of AVP and urine osmolality. When serum concentrations exceed 2pg/mL, there is a sharp increase in the urine osmolality. Maximal osmolality is generally reached at serum concentrations of 8–10 pg/mL.

## DEVELOPMENTAL ASPECTS

Most mammalian neonates have a low concentrating capacity. The human newborn rarely excretes a concentrated urine. In contrast, the capacity to dilute the urine appears to be well developed, at least in the full-term infant. The capacity to concentrate urine increases almost linearly during the first year after birth. However, individual variations are large during this time.

Many factors contribute to the low concentrating capacity in the infant. The capacity to reabsorb $Na^+$ in the TAL is low due to a low content of $Na^+$-$K^+$-ATPase in the immature cells. The loop of Henle is relatively short, which will make the countercurrent system less efficient. Urea availability is generally limited. Finally, end-organ response to AVP is blunted, probably dependent on a deficient coupling between the AVP receptor and the adenylyl cyclase unit. The capacity to release AVP appears to be well developed during the late fetal period. Circulating levels of AVP are already high during the neonatal period. It has been suggested that in the neonatal period the main physiological role for AVP is to regulate regional vascular resistance.

## CLINICAL ASPECTS

The low concentrating capacity might serve a good purpose in the infant, where the water turnover needs to be very high. Low concentrating capacity, however, will render the infant much more sensitive to pathological fluid losses. Diarrheal disease therefore is always potentially dangerous in the infant. In the situation of dehydration, young infants are predisposed to develop hypertonic conditions because, due to the low concentrating capacity, salt can be retained more easily than fluid. The risk for hypertonic dehydration is higher in *diarrhea* of viral origin, where intestinal salt losses are relatively small. Preterm infants are also predisposed to develop hypertonic conditions because of the large transepithelial water losses.

Low urinary concentrating capacity can be due to lack of AVP (*central diabetes insipidus*) or to lack of responsiveness to AVP (renal diabetes insipidus). *Renal diabetes insipidus* can be due to either a genetic disorder of AVP receptors and/or signaling pathways coupled to the receptors or renal disease. A transient decrease in urinary concentrating capacity can occur in *pyelonephritis*.

## Tests of concentrating capacity

The capacity to concentrate urine can be determined with or without the administration of AVP. The osmolality of a urine sample obtained after 12 hours of food and fluid deprivation will test both central and renal mechanisms for urine concentration. The osmolality of a urine sample obtained 1–6 hours after the nasal administration of synthetic AVP will test the renal mechanism of urine concentration. Fluid intake should be avoided during this test. In children about 2 years of age, the osmolality should be above 800 mosmol/kg $H_2O$ using either test. *Caution:* in young children with diabetes insipidus, 12 hours of fluid deprivation might lead to shock. The administration of AVP, if there is a free fluid intake afterwards, might lead to a condition of hypotonic volume expansion with serum $Na^+$ falling to 120 mmol/L. Such a complication might result in convulsions.

## SELECTED READING

Aperia A, Celsi G. Ontogenic processes in nephron epithelia. Structure, enzymes, and function. In: Seldin DW, Giebisch G, eds. *The kidney: physiology and pathophysiology*, 2nd edn, Vol II. New York: Raven Press, 1992: 803.

Horster MF, Gilg A, Lory P. Determinants of axial osmotic gradients in the differentiating countercurrent system. *Am J Physiol* 1984; **246**: F124.

Polacek E, Vocel J, Neugebauerova L et al. The osmotic concentrating ability in healthy infants and children. *Arch Dis Child* 1965; **40**: 291. (Gives normal values for maximal urine osmolality at different ages.)

Seldin DW, Giebisch G, eds. *The kidney: physiology and pathophysiology*, 2nd edn, Vol II, Section 111: Water and electrolyte exchanges. New York: Raven Press, 1992: 1595.

# PART SIXTEEN

# Developmental Pharmacology

**Editor: Gideon Koren**

# 94

# Principles of Pharmacokinetics and Pharmacodynamics

Dennis Scolnik and Gideon Koren

In order to fully understand drug disposition in any given individual, a number of issues have to be addressed. First, the problem of compliance, i.e. whether the drug has been taken as prescribed, erratically, or not at all. Thereafter, knowledge of pharmacokinetics including drug absorption, distribution, metabolism, and elimination is necessary. Finally, the possibility of drug–drug interactions and of other factors, e.g. disease state influencing the actual mode of action of the drug at a molecular and receptor level (pharmacodynamics), must be considered. In the following sections we describe central pharmacokinetic and pharmacodynamic principles that are important for understanding drug effects during development.

## GENERAL PRINCIPLES

## Compliance

It is essential to quantify compliance in any assessment of drug efficacy; otherwise, a potentially efficacious drug will be said erroneously to lack any clinical effect. Four principal methods are used to assess compliance.

### Pill count

Although this method does not reveal when and how a drug was taken, and can easily be manipulated by the patient (or the patient's care givers), it has proven very useful when a "count" revealing low use concurs with lack of effect.

### Diary card

This method relies on patients' honesty, and it has been shown that many patients fill in details as they perceive the doctor would wish them to, thereby introducing a new source of bias.

### Patient interview

This is subject to serious bias from both inaccurate and selective recall of positive and negative events.

### MEMS

The "medication event monitoring system" consists of a computerized chip in the cap of the medication bottle that records the date and time every time the bottle is opened. This enables accurate correlation between adverse or favorable drug events and timing of doses.

## Absorption

After a drug has been administered, it must be absorbed in order to have any effect. The rate and extent of absorption obviously depend on the route of administration, whether it be gastrointestinal, intramuscular, percutaneous, intrathecal, or endotracheal.

The rate of absorption is especially pertinent when drug effect is proportional to peak concentrations obtained, as is thought to be the case with some antibiotics, or when adverse effects occur at high drug levels, such as with nifedipine. Rate of absorption is also important when the desired effect has to be achieved without delay, e.g. pain relief with acetaminophen or nitroglycerin.

Intravenous administration is considered to provide 100 per cent bioavailability of drug. Oral bioavailability is a measure of the extent of absorption and is exemplified by the following formula for oral drug administration (see below):

$$\text{Oral bioavailability} = \frac{\text{area under the curve from oral administration}}{\text{area under the curve from intravenous administration}}$$

The area under the curve refers to a graphical representation of drug concentration versus time. Many factors can affect oral bioavailability including vomiting, malabsorption, and changes in gastric pH. Low oral bioavailability can also be the result of the *first-pass effect*, even after complete absorption. This is a reflection of the amount of drug that is metabolized in the liver after absorption into the portal venous system and before reaching the systemic circulation. Saturation of intestinal absorption also has been demonstrated for some drugs and results in dose-dependent oral bioavailability.

# Distribution

After absorption a drug must be distributed to its site of action in order to exert an effect. The commonest measure of this is a drug's *volume of distribution* ($V_d$), the hypothetical blood volume that would be needed to account for the concentration of the drug in the blood assuming that the whole dose remained intravascular. It reflects how much of the drug remains in the blood after distribution is completed and is based on plasma concentration.

$$\text{Volume of distribution } (V_d) = \frac{\text{total amount of drug in body}}{\text{concentration of drug in plasma}}$$

Factors that influence drug distribution are as follows.

## Chemical characteristics

Lipid-soluble drugs cross membranes more easily than hydrophilic ones, and a drug's $pK_a$ (pH at which 50 per cent ionization occurs) often determines its movement as well. Some drugs have an affinity for certain tissues, e.g. aminoglycosides accumulate in renal tissue, possibly accounting for selective efficacy and toxicity.

## Method of administration

High peak serum concentrations can facilitate entry of a drug into a tissue that is otherwise relatively impermeable when only low serum concentrations are achieved.

## Protein and tissue binding

High levels of protein binding result in lower levels of free drug being available at the drug's site of action. Acidic drugs are usually bound to albumin and basic ones to $\alpha_1$-glycoproteins, lipoproteins, and $\gamma$-globulins. Additional drug therapy or derangements in blood chemistry, especially changes in pH, can lead to saturation of, and displacement from, binding sites.

## Perfusion

Poor perfusion of a tissue or organ decreases the amount of drug reaching its site of action.

# Metabolism and elimination

Most drugs are eliminated from the body via hepatic or renal routes. Hepatic metabolism usually serves to make more polar compounds, which can then be eliminated more efficiently through the bile or by the kidneys. Phase 1 (non-synthetic) hepatic reactions involve oxidation, reduction, or hydrolysis, while phase 2 (synthetic) reactions involve conjugation of new moieties to the drug molecule. In the kidney drugs can be filtered, with varying amounts of subsequent tubular reabsorption or secretion.

The *elimination constant* ($K_e$) is used to characterize drug elimination pattern and represents the fraction of drug eliminated per unit time. If a constant proportion of drug is eliminated per unit time, irrespective of drug levels, first-order kinetics are said to apply. Zero-order kinetics infer that the same amount of drug (not the same proportion) is eliminated per unit time. Half-life ($t_\frac{1}{2}$) is more useful than $K_e$ clinically. It is commonly used to tailor optimal dosing interval (see below):

$$\text{Dose interval} = 1.44 \times \text{half-life} \times \ln \frac{\text{maximum desired concentration}}{\text{minimum desired concentration}}$$

where ln is the natural logarithm. The half-life is also used to derive the *clearance*, which is the volume of blood totally cleared of a drug per unit time:

$$\text{Clearance} = 0.693 \times \frac{\text{volume of distribution}}{\text{half-life}}$$

Compartmental models are mathematical attempts to explain drug concentrations obtained after drug dosing. They reflect the balance between absorption, distribution, metabolism, and the redistribution that can occur when, for instance, a drug is released from tissue binding in response to falling plasma concentrations.

Mention will be made of one final formula that is frequently used. It describes the first-order kinetic behavior of drugs in mathematical terms:

$$\text{concentration at time } t' = \text{concentration at time } 0 \times (2.718)^{-Kt}$$

where $K$ is the rate constant and $t$ the time between samples $0$ and $t'$.

## DEVELOPMENTAL PERSPECTIVES

Children handle drugs differently compared with adults, as has been shown by the occurrence of the *gray baby syndrome* due to slow metabolism of chloramphenicol in young children, and *kernicterus* with sulfa therapy in jaundiced young infants. For some drugs, such as morphine, theophylline, and digoxin, the doses that are needed for clinical effect are highest between 6 and 12 months of age. For other drugs, such as sedatives, alcohol, and amphetamines, unusual effects are seen in children. Sedatives can cause hyperactivity, amphetamines are used to treat hyperactivity, and alcohol can cause fatal hypoglycemia even in low doses in children. For many drugs, such as psychotropics, sedatives, and analgesics, estimation of pharmacological response necessitates valid patient reporting, which is impossible to obtain from infants and young children. This reality has led to suboptimal pain therapy in young children who, on average, receive only a fraction of the adult dose per kilogram, despite apparently equivalent levels of pain. There is, moreover, a relative lack of knowledge about drug pharmacokinetics in children because such information is far more difficult to gather in children compared with adults due to ethical and technical considerations. The burgeoning of neonatal intensive care units has reversed this situation somewhat in the sphere of neonatology.

## Absorption

### Oral

Absorption of a drug after oral intake depends largely on gastric pH and emptying time.

### Gastric pH

At birth gastric pH is $\pm7.0$ due to the presence of amniotic fluid, but within a few hours acid secretion reduces it to 1.5–3.0. Milk then increases the pH to 7.0 for the next 24 hours, and there is a relative achlorhydria for the ensuing 10–15 days. The decrease in pH does not occur in the preterm infant. By age 3 years the child has achieved adult acid-producing capacity.

These changes contribute to the high levels that acid-labile drugs such as penicillin achieve in neonates, although decreased elimination could also play a part. Because acidic drugs such as nalidixic acid are better absorbed in the unionized form, the increased pH found in neonates increases the proportion of ionized drug and thereby decreases absorption.

### Gastric emptying

In preterm infants gastric emptying is slow and linear, whereas in later life there is an initial rapid phase followed by an exponentially slower phase. Gastric emptying remains relatively slow for the first 6 months after birth.

Although this slower gastric emptying might be thought to increase drug absorption, this is not the case for several drugs such as amoxycillin, chloramphenicol, cephalosporins, and rifampicin. However, in many cases absorption approaches, and even surpasses, adult absorption by the age of 3 months.

### Intramuscular

The bioavailability of a drug after intramuscular injection depends on the area that is infiltrated, the rate of penetration of the capillary membrane, and other pathological states affecting these parameters such as fever, hypovolemia, hypoperfusion, and hypoxemia. The rate of penetration of the capillary membrane is in turn dependent upon the ionization, lipid solubility, and osmolality of the drug; highly lipid-soluble drugs such as diazepam and chlordiazepoxide are less effectively and less rapidly absorbed, while water-soluble drugs such as phenobarbital are more readily absorbed. Neonates are much more prone to vasomotor instability and have decreased muscle mass and subcutaneous fat and increased body water, all leading to further variability in drug absorption after intramuscular injection.

The net effect of this is that some drugs, such as aminoglycosides and ampicillin, take the same time to peak after intramuscular injection in children as in adults, while others, such as benzylpenicillin, diazepam, and digoxin, undergo decreased or erratic absorption.

### Percutaneous

Percutaneous absorption is dependent upon the thickness of the stratum corneum of the epidermis, which is decreased in the neonate, and the degree of hydration, which is increased in the neonate. Thus the net effect is that neonates have increased percutaneous absorption, as has unfortunately been found with the cases of toxicity due to hexachlorophene, salicylic acid, and boric acid applied to the skin.

## Distribution

The amount of body water and its distribution as well as the degree of protein binding change throughout childhood, thereby influencing drug distribution. The proportion of blood reaching a given organ also varies with age. Thus increased cerebral perfusion may account for the increased toxicity seen in young children administered diazepam, clonazepam, phenobarbital, phenytoin, and theophylline.

## Protein binding

In the newborn there is relatively less albumin than in the adult, and much of it is fetal albumin, which has a decreased affinity for drugs. There are also decreased amounts of globulins and a relative acidemia and hypoxemia; in addition, maternal drugs as well as endogenous substances such as bilirubin and free fatty acids are found in increased amounts. Highly acidic drugs may displace bilirubin from plasma protein-binding sites, increasing the risk of *kernicterus*. Diminished protein binding persists until normal adult levels are reached by approximately 3 years of age for acidic drugs, and 7–12 years of age for basic ones. Although the increased free fraction of drugs could be expected to result in increased drug clearance, this is not the case as there is still a relative immaturity of the drug handling capacity of the nephron and hepatocyte in neonates.

## Body water

The water content of the newborn is up to 75 per cent, 40 per cent of which is extracellular. In the adult the figures are 40 and 20 per cent, respectively. Thus there is an increased volume of distribution of water-soluble drugs in neonates, resulting in lower peak drug concentrations, although the mean steady-state serum concentration is independent of the volume of distribution.

$$\text{Steady-state concentration} = \frac{\text{dose}}{\text{clearance}}$$

## Elimination

### Hepatic

Most hepatic metabolic functions are present at birth even in the preterm infant, but they are slower than in later life. The maturation rate of these functions varies for each enzyme complex, and some can be induced

prenatally and postnatally at a greater rate and to a larger extent than in adults. Since

$$\text{Drug half-life} = 0.693 \times \frac{\text{volume of distribution}}{\text{clearance}}$$

therapeutic and toxic concentrations can be achieved with lower doses, and longer dosing intervals are necessitated. The metabolism of low hepatic extraction drugs is reduced to a greater extent than that of high-extraction drugs. Hydroxylation and glucuronidation are the functions most modified after birth. Other factors that may lead to decreased drug metabolism in the newborn are maternal endogenous inhibitors, diminished liver blood flow, and relative hypoxemia. Adult doses of chloramphenicol, given to the neonate, accumulate due to decreased phase 2 hepatic elimination, and may lead to shock and death.

In the neonate the phase 1 functions of cytochrome $P_{450}$ and NADPH cytochrome $c$ reductase are approximately half of adult levels. Mildly depressed dealkylation and markedly depressed hydroxylation rates have been shown for many drugs. Esterase function reaches adult levels by 10–12 months of age. Phase 1 functions can increase 10–20-fold in 5 or 6 days in the neonate, and this possibility must be borne in mind when planning dosing schedules. The rates of phase 2 reactions generally reach adult levels by 18–24 months of age. The metabolic rate of hepatic microsomal drug metabolizing enzymes is markedly elevated for the first 2 years, after which it gradually decreases. At puberty there is a further sharp decrease to adult levels, presumably under hormonal control.

### Renal

Many drugs, such as penicillins, digoxin, and methotrexate, are eliminated unchanged by the kidneys. Some are only filtered, and others are reabsorbed and/or secreted by the tubules – functions that can sometimes be induced. Because even drugs that are hepatically metabolized are subsequently excreted in the kidneys, diminished renal function can lead to accumulation of drugs and/or their metabolites.

The preterm infant has fewer glomeruli than a baby born at term, and even in the term infant glomerular, and especially tubular, function is immature. In time there is lengthening and maturation of the tubule, increased renal blood flow, improvement in filtration coefficient, and use of more superficial nephrons, and adult functional levels are reached by 6–12 months. Clearance, corrected for body weight, of drugs such as digoxin and aminoglycosides may be up to 30 times slower in the preterm infant compared with adults. Although neonates may have higher serum concentrations of aminoglycosides, they experience less tubular reabsorption and accumulation secondary to relatively low glomerular filtration rate. Low urinary pH can lead to diminished reabsorption of weak bases and increased absorption of weakly acidic compounds. Lowered tubular secretion has been shown for penicillins and sulfonamides. The preterm infant, therefore, usually needs either decreased drug dosages or increased dosage intervals in many cases.

## Pharmacodynamic considerations

Maturation processes of target cells or receptors are evident for many drugs. As an example, immature animals need more digoxin than mature animals in order to obtain the desired clinical effect; similar experience has been accumulated with this drug in humans. This phenomenon can be partially explained by the higher density of the pharmacological receptors for digoxin in the neonate compared with the older individual. In the future researchers will have to be much more attuned to finding methods of measuring pharmacodynamic effect in the neonatal and pediatric age group.

## PATHOPHYSIOLOGY

Disease can alter drug disposition by affecting absorption, distribution, or metabolism and excretion.

## Absorption

Intestinal absorption of drugs can be affected by malabsorption syndromes, e.g. decreased rate and extent of absorption is found in celiac disease and cystic fibrosis. Peak and steady-state concentrations are thereby reduced, although in some cases increased mucous membrane permeability or luminal pH seem to account for increased peak concentrations. In *cystic fibrosis* and *protein-calorie malnutrition*, low pancreatic enzyme levels cause decreased bioavailability of drugs requiring hydrolysis for absorption. *Diarrhea* by itself decreases transit time, alters gut mucosa, and is associated with dehydration. Protein-calorie malnutrition and *Crohn disease* are associated with increased transit times. In Crohn disease there is also thickening of the bowel wall and decreased surface area for absorption if bowel resection has been performed. *Pyloric stenosis* is associated with secondary achlorhydria and delayed gastric emptying. Salicylate absorption has been shown to be diminished in the acute phase of *Kawasaki disease*, even though this is not the case with other febrile illnesses. Finally, drugs absorbed through formation of micelles could be affected by liver diseases, producing decreased levels of bile acids.

Extraintestinal diseases can also affect bowel absorption. For example, *cardiac failure* is thought to diminish absorption by inducing mucosal edema and because increased sympathetic tone diminishes splanchnic blood flow. Aberrations in thyroid function may affect transit time. Drug–drug interactions can occur; for example, antacids alter tetracycline solubility and may even chelate it.

## Distribution

An important determinant of drug distribution is the fraction of drug that is unbound in the serum. This in turn is proportional to plasma protein, especially albumin, concentrations. A greater unbound fraction, as may occur with true hypoproteinemia or dilutional hypoproteinemia, will allow more drug to distribute to peripheral compartments, increasing the drug's volume of distribution. More drug will then be available for clinical effect, metabolism, and excretion and this may require adjustments in dosing.

Many diseases lead to hypoproteinemia through decreased availability (*malabsorption syndromes*), decreased synthesis (*hepatic disease*), and increased losses (*nephrotic syndrome*) of proteins. Diseases associated with water retention, such as cardiac, renal, and hepatic failure, will also lead to low serum protein concentrations. Uremia and hyperbilirubinemia can cause displacement of drugs from protein-binding sites.

## Metabolism and elimination

Because the major sites for drug metabolism and elimination are the liver and the kidney, diseases affecting these organs will cause alterations in the pharmacokinetics of drugs. In the neonate the more common hepatic diseases encountered include *viral infections* such as herpes, echovirus, and adenovirus; bacterial sepsis; *inborn errors of metabolism*, such as galactosemia, hereditary fructose intolerance, $\alpha_1$-antitrypsin deficiency, and tyrosinemia; *congestive cardiac failure*; and fatty liver secondary to hyperalimentation. Later in life *viral hepatitides, graft-versus-host disease, cystic fibrosis*, and *intoxications* are common. Other conditions include protein-calorie malnutrition, cirrhosis and biliary tree obstruction, and poor hepatic blood flow secondary to cardiac failure.

The more completely a drug is excreted in the kidney, the more decreased renal function will diminish excretion and lead to drug retention. Lists are available of drugs whose doses need to be altered at different levels of renal impairment. Slowed renal excretion has been shown for penicillin and chloramphenicol in protein-calorie malnutrition, and in burn patients increased glomerular filtration rates and decreased half-life have been demonstrated for several aminoglycosides.

In cystic fibrosis lower serum concentrations, larger volumes of distribution, and more rapid total body clearance of many drugs have been demonstrated, e.g. aminoglycosides, co-trimoxazole, ceftazidime, cloxacillin and methicillin. Although the mechanisms for these changes are unclear, there is evidence for enhanced elimination of drugs at both hepatic and renal levels.

# 95

# Perinatal Toxicology

Doreen Matsui and Gideon Koren

Despite heightened awareness of the potential harmful effects to the fetus of *in utero* exposure to drugs and chemicals, their use during pregnancy remains common, and often unavoidable. According to various studies, 40–90 per cent of women consume one or more medications during pregnancy.

The prescribing of medication during pregnancy must include consideration of the alterations in pharmacokinetics and drug handling that arise as a result of maternal physiological changes. In general, during pregnancy the elimination rate of agents excreted by the kidney, e.g. digoxin, increases. Changes in hepatic elimination patterns are less consistent, although the possibility of increased hepatic clearance does exist with some drugs such as clindamycin. The volume of distribution may be altered by changes in various fluid and tissue compartments. In addition, the protein-binding of several anticonvulsant medications has been demonstrated to be decreased. Overall, the changes in drug disposition that occur during pregnancy tend to result in lower serum drug concentrations.

Placental transport is established at about the fifth week of fetal life with almost all drugs crossing to some extent.

Fetal and perinatal effects that are discussed include teratogenicity, direct drug toxicity or effect, and neonatal drug withdrawal.

## HUMAN TERATOGENS (*see* page 190)

The thalidomide tragedy of the late 1950s highlighted the possibility of drug-induced birth defects. However, overemphasis of the teratogenic potential of medications too often results in unnecessary anxiety due to unrealistic perceptions of the risk. Fortunately, only a few drugs have proved to be teratogenic in humans, and the vast majority probably do not pose a reproductive hazard when used in therapeutic amounts. An important issue to address when counseling women on teratogenic risks is the baseline risk of major malformations of around 3 per cent. Table 95.1 lists some of the drugs and chemicals that have proved to be teratogenic in humans.

Assessing the teratogenic potential of a drug in humans involves the analysis of case reports as well as retrospective and prospective studies. Often all available information has been gathered in animals. Animal data must be interpreted with caution as the drugs are often administered in doses and by routes that are not applicable to humans. Given the differences between various animal species it is not difficult to appreciate the reluctance to extrapolate such data to humans. However, almost all known human teratogens have been shown to cause similar effects in animals.

Time of exposure is an important factor to consider. Although it is commonly stated that the fetus is at greatest risk during the first trimester, some agents may have effects later in pregnancy, for example those that affect the developing brain. During the first 2 weeks of pregnancy, the "all-or-none" period, injuries to the embryo are likely to result in death of the conceptus or in repair and recovery. Vulnerability to teratogenic insult is greatest when the target organ is developing. For example, the neural tube closes during the fourth week of embryonic development; therefore,

TABLE 95.1 Known teratogens

| DRUG | TYPICAL MANIFESTATIONS |
|------|------------------------|
| Alcohol | Fetal alcohol syndrome (facial features and mental retardation) |
| Carbamazepine | Neural tube defects |
| Isotretinoin | Skeletal, ear, cardiovascular, and central nervous system malformations |
| Phenytoin | Fetal hydantoin syndrome (facial features, hypoplastic digits, and mental retardation) |
| Thalidomide | Limb anomalies |
| Valproic acid | Neural tube defects |
| Warfarin | Fetal warfarin syndrome (nasal hypoplasia and stippled epiphyses) |

if an agent is to be associated with the induction of a neural tube defect in the offspring, exposure must have occurred around that time. Thus if *in utero* exposure to valproic acid or carbamazepine, both of which have been associated with an increased risk of a neural tube defect, occurs during the first 4 weeks of pregnancy prenatal screening for this malformation may be indicated. Similarly it is important that adequate maternal folic acid intake, which has been demonstrated to have a protective effect against the occurrence of neural tube defects, be initiated early, preferably preconceptually.

The dose of the teratogenic agent may also play a key role. The risk of *fetal alcohol syndrome* has been proved only in chronic alcoholic women consuming at least 2 g/(kg · day) of alcohol (equivalent to six to seven alcoholic drinks per day). Occupational exposure to most organic solvents, provided appropriate precautions are taken, has not been shown to pose an increased fetal risk in humans; however, more extensive use, such as during substance abuse, has been shown to cause damage to the developing brain. A dose–effect relationship has also been suggested for vitamin A with doses greater than 10 000 IU considered not to be teratogenic.

Not all *in utero* exposures to teratogenic drugs result in malformations. Manifestation of the insult may depend on other factors such as genetic susceptibility. Variations in enzyme activity may be important when a toxic metabolite rather than the parent compound is the teratogenic agent. For example, it has recently been documented that fetuses suffering from *fetal hydantoin syndrome* are less likely to be able to detoxify a toxic intermediate of this antiepileptic drug. Consideration of the underlying maternal disorder is also required as many illnesses may adversely affect fetal well-being.

## DIRECT DRUG TOXICITY OR EFFECT

Most drugs cross the placenta and as a result may exert potential pharmacological and toxicological effects on the fetus. Only very large molecules such as heparin and insulin do not cross the placental barrier in appreciable amounts. Maternal use of tetracycline during pregnancy has been discouraged as this drug forms a complex with $Ca^{2+}$ orthophosphate and becomes incorporated into teeth undergoing calcification. Thus *in utero* exposure to tetracycline after 4–5 months' gestation may result in yellow-brown discoloration of teeth. Indomethacin, when administered to the mother to inhibit preterm labor, may have adverse secondary effects on the fetal circulation, such as ductus arteriosus constriction. With prolonged use during pregnancy, the probability exists of developing persistent pulmonary hypertension syndrome of the newborn. When maternal drug use occurs around the time of delivery, the newborn may experience prolonged effects due to slower neonatal drug elimination.

In most instances such effects can be explained by the known actions of the drug in older individuals.

The use of β-adrenergic antagonists (such as propranolol) late in pregnancy provides a typical illustration of this phenomenon. A proportion of neonates born in this situation will demonstrate transient symptoms and signs of β-adrenergic blockade (bradycardia, hypotension, and hypoglycemia). Examples of direct drug toxicity are listed in Table 95.2.

Recently, in addition to the study of the toxic effects noted shortly after birth, more attention is being paid to the potential long-term effects of *in utero* drug and chemical exposure on the offspring's subsequent development and behavior. For example, there is much interest in studies to determine the long-term sequelae of *in utero* cocaine exposure. Evidence exists suggesting that low-level lead exposure may result in significant long-term cognitive and neurobehavioral sequelae. Longitudinal epidemiological studies have found an association between prenatal or early infancy lead levels and later psychological scores even after adjustment for confounding variables.

Placental transfer of drugs to the fetus also has been exploited to benefit the fetus in the treatment of fetal medical conditions. For example, transplacental therapy of fetal supraventricular tachycardia with digoxin has become accepted management.

## DRUG WITHDRAWAL SYNDROMES

With chronic use of certain drugs during pregnancy, especially frequent and high-dose use late in gestation, dependence may develop in the fetus (as well as in the mother). After birth, when the supply of drug from the mother is no longer available, the neonate may manifest symptoms and signs of drug withdrawal.

The classic *neonatal withdrawal syndrome* is precipitated by opioids, the manifestations of which include irritability, tremors, hypertonicity, vomiting, high-pitched cry, respiratory distress, diarrhea, fever, and convulsions. Feeding difficulties and poor weight gain are not uncommon.

TABLE 95.2 Fetal toxicity of drugs

| DRUG | TOXIC EFFECT |
| --- | --- |
| Aspirin, indomethacin, ibuprofen | ? Premature closure or constriction of ductus arteriosus, abnormal hemostasis, ?IVH |
| β-Adrenergic blockers | β-Adrenergic blockade |
| Captopril, enalapril | Anuria/oliguria |
| Lithium | Hypotonia, cyanosis, bradycardia |
| Meperidine | Respiratory depression |
| Propylthiouracil | Hypothyroidism (goiter) |
| Streptomycin | Ototoxicity |
| Tetracycline | Yellow discoloration of teeth |

Not surprisingly, neonatal withdrawal has been described after maternal use of other classes of drugs including alcohol, barbiturates, and benzodiazepines. In some instances it is difficult to determine whether symptoms noted in the neonatal period are the result of drug intoxication or drug withdrawal. Such confusion exists with cocaine and tricyclic antidepressants, which exert toxic effects overlapping the withdrawal syndrome.

The clinical picture, including the time of onset and duration of symptoms, depends on the particular drug involved and the pattern of drug use during pregnancy (amount of dose, length of exposure, and time of last dose). For drugs with a relatively long elimination half-life (e.g. methadone) the withdrawal syndrome will become apparent much longer after that of drugs with a short half-life (e.g. morphine).

# 96

# Drug Transfer into Human Milk

Doreen Matsui and Gideon Koren

Breast-feeding is widely encouraged by pediatricians and other physicians due to many advantages to both the infant and mother. Despite the possibility of exposure of the infant to drugs and chemicals transferred via breast milk, a general recommendation to discontinue nursing while taking medications is not needed. Consideration of the determinants of drug transfer into milk and the clinical relevance of a specific drug's transfer will provide assistance in guiding the breast-feeding mother.

## MECHANISMS AND DETERMINANTS OF DRUG TRANSFER INTO MILK

To be present in human breast milk, drugs must reach the maternal circulation and then pass into breast milk. Thus, they must traverse a number of lipoprotein membranes, a process that occurs mainly by passive diffusion. Such transfer involves only the free fraction that is not bound to plasma proteins; therefore, drugs that are highly protein-bound are less likely to enter breast milk. High lipid solubility favors passage into breast milk. The $pK_a$ and degree of ionization of the drug in question are also important factors to consider. Weak bases, more likely to be non-ionized in the maternal circulation, tend to pass into breast milk to a greater extent. Once reaching the milk, a more acidic environment, the weak bases will be ionized. This "ion trapping" will create a gradient toward passage of the drug into breast milk. For most drugs, molecular weight is not an impediment to entrance into breast milk. As metabolites are generally more polar, they are less likely to be transferred into breast milk than their parent drug. Breast milk factors may also play a role. For example, composition of milk is not uniform (preterm vs term, foremilk vs hindmilk, etc.).

Estimation of the drug dose delivered via breast milk may be made using the following formula:

$$\text{Dose}\,(\text{mg}/[\text{kg} \cdot \text{day}]) = C_{ss} \times \text{M/P ratio} \times \text{milk volume}$$

where $C_{ss}$ is the maternal steady-state serum drug concentration, M/P ratio the milk/plasma ratio, and average milk volume = 150 mL/(kg of infant's body weight · day).

## CLINICAL RELEVANCE OF DRUG TRANSFER INTO MILK

Almost all maternally ingested drugs pass into the breast milk, usually in amounts less than 5 per cent of the maternal dose; however, this drug transfer in many cases is not clinically significant due to the small dose offered via this route to the suckling infant.

In addition to potential adverse effects to the nursing infant, maternal ingestion of medication may influence the process of lactation to decrease or increase milk yield. For example, bromocriptine, a dopamine agonist, may suppress lactation. On the other hand, metoclopramide may increase milk production.

Once the infant is fed the drug-containing breast milk, oral bioavailability, distribution, metabolism, and elimination of the drug by the infant must be considered. For example, reduced neonatal metabolism, due to decreased liver enzyme activity, and decreased neonatal renal excretion (lower glomerular filtration rate) may lead to accumulation of drug in the infant.

Drug effects in the breast-fed infant may be dose-related or idiosyncratic. Much of the information available to date has been gathered from single case reports. Studies are often conducted following a single dose, a somewhat unrealistic situation given that in practice most drugs are taken in repeated doses. Thus data gathered under such circumstances may not reflect the true picture.

Few drugs are absolutely contraindicated during breast-feeding (Table 96.1).

With most drugs a decision regarding breast-feeding must be reached based on a limited amount of information. Reluctance to encourage continuation of breast-feeding may arise if the inherent pharmacological action of the drug suggests that a toxic effect may occur (e.g. cytotoxic drugs) or if adverse effects have previously been noted in nursing infants. Experience with the direct use of the drug in infants for therapy may provide some reassurance.

TABLE 96.1 Drugs contraindicated during breast-feeding

Bromocriptine
Cocaine and other drugs of abuse
Cyclophosphamide
Cyclosporin
Doxorubicin
Ergotamine
Gold salts
Iodine-containing drugs
Lithium
Methotrexate
Phenobarbital
Radiopharmaceuticals

General recommendations include use of the lowest dose of drug necessary to achieve a therapeutic effect in the mother, nursing just before drug ingestion ("trough"), observation of the infant for unusual signs or symptoms suggestive of an adverse effect, and measurement of the breast milk and/or infant's serum drug concentration(s). Fortunately, in most situations, breast-feeding may continue without major consequences in the presence of maternally ingested drugs.

## SELECTED READING

American Academy of Pediatrics. The transfer of drugs and other chemicals into human milk. *Pediatrics* 1994; **93**: 137.

Bennett PN, ed. *Drugs and human lactation.* Amsterdam: Elsevier Science Publishers, 1988.

Briggs GG, Freeman RK, Yaffe SJ. *Drugs in pregnancy and lactation.* Baltimore: Williams & Wilkins, 1994.

Koren G, ed. *Maternal–fetal toxicology.* New York: Marcel Dekker, 1994.

Koren G, Ito S. Fetal drug therapy. *Clin Perinatol* 1994; **21**: 463.

Koren G, Prober CG, Gold R. *Antimicrobial therapy in infants and children.* New York: Marcel Dekker, 1988.

Schardein JL. *Chemically induced birth defects.* New York: Marcel Dekker, 1993.

Shepard TH. *Catalog of teratogenic agents.* Baltimore: The Johns Hopkins University Press, 1992.

# Index